FUNDAMENTALS *of* NURSING

ACTIVE LEARNING FOR COLLABORATIVE PRACTICE

FUNDAMENTALS *of* NURSING

ACTIVE LEARNING FOR COLLABORATIVE PRACTICE

BARBARA L. YOOST, MSN, RN, CNS, CNE, ANEF

Assistant Professor
Division of Nursing
Notre Dame College

LYNNE R. CRAWFORD, MSN, RN, MBA, CNE

Retired Faculty
College of Nursing
Kent State University

ELSEVIER

ELSEVIER

3251 Riverport Lane
St. Louis, Missouri 63043

FUNDAMENTALS OF NURSING: ACTIVE LEARNING FOR COLLABORATIVE PRACTICE ISBN: 978-0-323-29557-4

International Standard Book Number: 978-0-323-29557-4

Executive Content Strategist: Tamara Myers
Content Development Manager: Jean Sims Fornango
Senior Content Development Specialist: Laura Selkirk
Publishing Services Manager: Jeff Patterson
Senior Project Manager: Mary Stueck
Design Direction: Brian Salisbury

Printed in Canada

Last digit is the print number: 9 8 7 6 5 4

I dedicate this book to the love of my life, Charlie, who has supported my dreams throughout my adult life and nursing career, and graciously accepted my need to "vacation" with books and internet access for the last 6 years!
To our sons and "daughters," Tim, Jennie, Steve, and Mary, the greatest "kids" anyone could ever ask for, who shared their encouragement and professional expertise whenever needed.
To our five beautiful and handsome grandchildren, Vivian, Simon, Gwyneth, Thatcher, and Oscar, with whom we have been blessed since this project started.
To my closest and dearest nursing colleague, and friend of 34 years, Lynne, who graciously agreed to tackle this enormous undertaking in an effort to help twenty-first century nursing students more fully meet the challenges of contemporary health care.
And to my nursing colleagues at Notre Dame College, Kent State University, North Central State College, and Ohio Northern University for their tireless commitment to educating safe, ethical future nurses to care deeply about their patients and make a positive difference in the world.

Barbara L. Yoost

I dedicate this book to my loving and supportive husband, David. Thank you for your understanding during the years of writing and editing.
To our children and grandchildren, Deanna, Jake, Brian, Vicki, Jacob, and Alex. Your interest in the textbook encouraged me.
To my mother, Virginia. You inspired me by continuing to edit books at the age of 90, and helped me throughout this process with your knowledge of writing.
To my extended family, friends, and colleagues. You believed in me. I am thankful to have each of you in my life.

Lynne R. Crawford

CONTRIBUTORS

Loretta J. Aller, MSN, RN, CNS
Assistant Professor
College of Nursing
Kent State University
North Canton, Ohio

Carol A. Boswell, EdD, RN, CNE, ANEF
Co-Director, Center of Excellence in Evidence-Based Practice
Professor
School of Nursing
Texas Tech University Health Sciences Center
Odessa, Texas

Elizabeth Burkhart, PhD, RN, MPH
Associate Professor
Marcella Niehoff School of Nursing
Loyola University Chicago
Chicago, Illinois

Bridgett Carstens, MSN, RN
Medical Services Consultant
M Haynes
Hunt Valley, Maryland

Linda Crawford, MSN, RN
Nursing Instructor
Trident Technical College
Charleston, South Carolina

Barbara A. Cross, PhD, FNP-BC
Polytrauma Services Clinical Team
Chairperson
Department of Graduate Nursing
Hampton University
Hampton, Virginia

Leslee D'Amato-Kubiet, PhD, ARNP
Instructor and Lab Coordinator
Daytona Regional Campus Coordinator
College of Nursing
University of Central Florida
Daytona Beach, Florida

Bertha L. Davis, PhD, RN, ANEF, FAAN
Professor
School of Nursing
Hampton University
Hampton, Virginia

Cheryl DeGraw, MSN, RN, CNE
Nursing Instructor
Nursing Department
Florence-Darlington Technical College
Florence, South Carolina

Cheryl L. Delgado, PhD, APN-BC, CNL
Associate Professor
School of Nursing
Cleveland State University
Cleveland, Ohio

Larinda S. Dixon, MSN, EdD, RN
Professor
Nursing
College of DuPage
Glen Ellyn, Illinois

Cindy Ford, PhD, RN, CNE
Visiting Professor and Director Partnership Program
Department of Nursing
Lubbock Christian University
Lubbock, Texas

Elizabeth Hill, PhD, RN
Clinical Nursing Faculty
Towson University
Northwest Hospital Center
Hill Nurse Consulting
Towson, Maryland

Janice Hoffman, PhD, RN, ANEF
Assistant Dean for the Baccalaureate Program
Associate Professor, OSAH
School of Nursing
University of Maryland
Baltimore, Maryland

Jean Jones, MSN, RN, CNE
Associate Professor
North Central State College
Mansfield, Ohio

N. Kay Lenhart, MSN, RN
Director, Clinical Learning Resource Center
Drexel University
Philadelphia, Pennsylvania

Amy M. Kennedy, MSN, RN
Adjunct Faculty
ECPI University
Newport News, Virginia

Debra K. Mercer, MSN, RN
Assistant Professor
School of Nursing
Texas Tech University Health Sciences Center
Odessa, Texas

Timothy Meyers, MSN, RN
Lecturer
College of Nursing
Kent State University
Kent, Ohio

Maureen M. Mitchell, EdD, RN
Assistant Professor
Graduate Program Director
School of Nursing
Cleveland State University
Cleveland, Ohio

Susan Montenery, DNP, RN, CCRN
Interim Director
Chair
Department of Nursing
Ohio Northern University
Ada, Ohio

Diane Morey, PhD, MSN, RN, CNE
Assistant Director
Chair
Department of Nursing
College of the Canyons
Santa Clarita, California

Margaret Ross Kraft, PhD, RN
Assistant Professor
Marcella Niehoff School of Nursing
Loyola University Chicago
Chicago, Illinois

Pamela K. Rutar, EdD, MSN, RN, CNE
Assistant Professor
School of Nursing
Firelands Regional Medical Center
Sandusky, Ohio

Jane Greene Ryan, MSN, CNM
Assistant Clinical Professor
Division of Undergraduate Nursing
Bachelor of Science in Nursing Co-Op Department
College of Nursing and Health Professions
Drexel University
Philadelphia, Pennsylvania

Beverly Schaefer, EdD, RN
Assistant Professor
The Breen School of Nursing
Ursuline College
Pepper Pike, Ohio

Deanna Schaffer, MSN, RN, CNE, ACNS-BC
Assistant Clinical Professor
College of Nursing and Health Professions
Department Chair
Bachelor's of Science in Nursing Co-Op Nursing Program
Drexel University
Philadelphia, Pennsylvania

Debra Shelestak, PhD, RN
Assistant Professor
College of Nursing
Kent State University
North Canton, Ohio

Tracy Szirony, PhD, RN, CHPN, CNP
Associate Professor
School of Nursing
University of Toledo
Toledo, Ohio

Joan E. Thoman, PhD, RN, CNS, CDE
Associate Professor
Coordinator Community Health Nursing
School of Nursing
Cleveland State University
Cleveland, Ohio

Barbara V. Voshall, DNP, RN
Professor
Simulation Lab Co-Coordinator
School of Nursing
Graceland University
Independence, Missouri

Hilda M. Williamson, EdD, RN, FNP
Assistant Dean of Academic Affairs
Associate Professor
School of Nursing
Hampton University
Hampton, Virginia

Linda E. Wolf, PhD, RM, CNS
Associate Professor
School of Nursing
Cleveland State University
Cleveland, Ohio

Jean Yockey, MSN, FNP-BC, CNE
Associate Professor
Nursing, School of Health Sciences
University of South Dakota
Vermillion, South Dakota

Katherine M. Zimnicki, MSN, RN, APRN, BC, WOCN
Clinical Instructor
College of Nursing
Wayne State University
Detroit, Michigan

REVIEWERS

Faisal Aboul-Enein, PhD, RN
Nurse Practitioner
Associate Professor
Center for Health Care Thinking and Innovations, LLC.
Houston, Texas

Barbara S. Anderson, RN, MS, CNE
Professor
Nursing
Harper College
Palatine, Illinois

Marty Bachman, PhD, RN
Chair
Nursing Department
Front Range Community College
Larimer Campus
Fort Collins, Colorado

Debra W. Bensen, MSN,RN
Associate Professor
Nursing
University of Mary
Bismarck, North Dakota

Meg Blair, PhD, MSN, RN, CEN
Professor
Nursing
NE Methodist College
Omaha, Nebraska

Carolyn Boiman, PhD, RN
Instructor
Nursing
Cincinnati State Technical and Community College
Cincinnati, Ohio

Sharon Brubaker, MS, BSN, RN
Nursing Faculty
Nursing–RN
Northwest State Community College
Toledo, Ohio

Annette M. Burman, MSN, RN
Clinical Instructor
Nursing
C.S. Mott Community College
Flint, Michigan

Faith Caster, RN MSN
Instructor of Nursing
St. Louis Community College–Florissant Valley
St. Louis, Missouri

Barb Caton, MSN, RN, CNE
Assistant Professor
Nursing
Missouri State University–West Plains
West Plains, Missouri

Kimberly M. Clevenger, EdD, MSN, RN-BC
Associate Professor
Nursing
Bachelor's of Science in Nursing Program Coordinator
Morehead State University
Morehead, Kentucky

Barbara A. Coles, PhD(c), RN-BC
Academic Coach
Domiciliary Charge Nurse
James A Haley VAMC
Tampa, Florida

Dale A. Lange Crispell, RN
Associate Professor
Nursing
Rockland Community College
Suffern, New York

Marci L. Dial, DNP, ARNP, NP-C, MSN, BSN, RN-BC, LNC
Professor
Nursing
Valencia College
Orlando, Florida

Karen Eisenberg, MSN, RN, CNE
Lecturer
Clinical Instructor
Nursing
University of Nevada
Las Vegas, Nevada

Laura Fowler, MSN, RN
Assistant Professor
Luzerne County Community College, Geisinger Health System
Nanticoke, Pennsylvania

Karen Gonzol, MSN, RN
Assistant Professor
Nursing
Shenandoah University
Winchester, Virgnia

Wendy Greenspan, MSN, RN, CCRN, CNE
Assistant Professor
Nursing
Rockland Community College
Suffern, New York

Kelly Hemingway, RN, MSN
Instructor
Nursing
Delta College
University Center, Michigan

Pat Ketcham, MSN, RN
Director of Nursing Laboratories
School of Nursing
Oakland University
Rochester, Michigan

Vicky J. King, MS, RN, CNE
Nursing Instructor
Cochise College
Sierra Vista, Arizona

Linda S. Lewandowski MSN, RN
Division Chair
Full-time Faculty
Bay de Noc Community College
Escanaba, Michigan

Tiffany Losekamp-Roberts, MSN, RN
Assistant Professor
Clinical Nursing
University of Cincinnati
Cincinnati, Ohio

Sheri H. Mangueira, MSN, ARNP, APHN-BC, AGNPCP-BC
Adjunct Clinical Assistant Professor
Nursing
Unversity of Florida
Gainesville, Florida

Janice McKinney, MSN, RN
Assistant Professor
Nursing
Tarrant County College
Fort Worth, Texas

Lisa Miklush, PhD, RNC, CNS
Assistant Professor
Nursing
Gonzaga University
Spokane, Washington

Nancy Pea, MSN, RN
Instructor
Nursing
St. Louis Community College–Florissant Valley
St. Louis, Missouri

Kathleen Rockett, MSN, RN
Lecturer
Department of Nursing
Sonoma State University
Rohnert Park, California

Mindy Stayner, RN, MSN, PhD
Faculty
Nursing
Northwest State Community College
Archbold, Ohio;
Chamberlain College of Nursing
Addison, Illinois

Tetsuya Umebayashi, DNP, MSN, RN
Associate Professor
Nursing
Tarrant County College
Fort Worth, Texas

C.J. Voller, MSN, RN
Instructor
Nursing
Penn State–Mont Alto
Mont Alto, Pennsylvania

Cynthia Wachtel, MSN, RN, CDE
Instructor
Nursing
Siena Heights University
Adrian, Michigan

Jo Ellen Welborn, MSN, RN
Professor
Associate Degree in Nursing Program
Weatherford College
Weatherford, Texas

Georgia Wilson, MSN-ED, RN, CNN
Director of Nursing
Associate Dean of Health Science
Baker College of Flint
Flint, Michigan

Danielle Yocom, MSN, FNP-BC
Assistant Professor
Nursing
Massachusetts College of Pharmacy and Health Sciences University
Worcester, Massachusetts

Beth A. Zieman, MSN, RN
Professor
Nursing
Delta College
University Center, Michigan

Additional Reviewers

Janet H. Adams, MSN, RN, RT

Jane Anderson, RN

Amy Austin, MSN, RN

Kathy Batton, PhD, RN-BC

Ferrona Beason, PhD, ARNP

Kristin Benton, MSN, RN

Max Bishop, MSN, BSEd, RN

Diane Bridge, EdD, MSN, RN

Daryle Brown, EdD, RN

Stephen Campbell, RN, BSN, MSN, CCRN

Susan Carlson, MSN, RN, CS, NPP

Cheryl Cassis, MSN, RN

Barbara Celia, EdD, RN

Tobie Chapman, MAEd, BSN, RN

Esther Christian, MSN, RN

Angela Clem, PhD, RN

Margaret Clifton, MS, RN-BC

Charlotte K. Cooper, MSN, RN, CNS

Melody Corsom, MSN, RN

Karen Countryman, RN

Huberta Cozart, PhD, RN

Barbara Dagastine, MSN, RN

Catherine D'Amico, PhD, RN

Jennifer Delwiche, MSN, RN

Ann Denney, MSN, RN

Karla Dixon, BSN, RN

Lynda Dolphus, MSN, RN

Emily Droste-Bielak, PhD, RN

Peggy A. Ellis, PhD, RN

Sally Erdel, MS, RN, CNE ELNEC-Core

Marie Etienne, DNP, ARNP, PLNC

Mary Fabick, SN,MEd, RN-BC, CEN

Carol Fanutti, EdD, RN, CNE

Crystel Farina, MSN, RN, CNE

Cathy Green, RN, MSN, RN-CS

Annette Gunderman, DEd, MSN, RN

Claudia Haile, MSN, RN

Joan Hall, MS, RN

Nancy A. Hall, DNP, RN

Regina Hanchak, MSN, RN

Michelle Hawkins, MSN, RN

Kathleen Healy-Karabell, DNP, RN-CNS, CSN

Barbara Hebert, MN, RN

Anna Hefner, MSN, MAEd, CPNP, PhD

Beth Heydemann, RN, MSN, ANP-C

Jill Holmstrom, EdD, RN, CNE

Darcy Hostetter-Lewis, MSN, RN, PHN, PNE, CLE

Pam Hulstein, PhD, MSN, RN, CNM

Sherry James, MSN, RN

Shirley Jeandron, MBA, MSN, RN

Terri Jenkins, MSN, RN

Jane Kassens, MSN, CS, FNP

Cathleen Kunkler, MSN, RN, ONC, CNE

Donna Kubesh, PhD, RN

Carla Lee, PhD, ARNP-BC, FAAN, FIBA

Kimberly L. Leighton, PhD, RN

Greg Leonhard, MSN, RN, CNE

Doresea Lewis, DNP, GNP-BC

Valerie Love-Steward, BSN, RN

Lizy Mathew, EdD, RN, CCRN

Maryann McCarthy, EdD, RN, CNS, STAH, PHN

Emily McClung, MSN, RN

Janis McMillan, MSN, RN

Bernard McPherson, MSN, RN

Jody Mesches, MSN, RN

Candice Moore, MSN, BSN, AHN-BC, RN

Cindy Neff, RN, MSN

Eleanor Nixon, MSN, FNP-BC, RN

Noreen Nutting, MA, RN

Patricia Orender, BSN, RN

Tonya Passmonte, MSN, RN

Constance L. Peterson, PhD, RN

Patricia A. Plumer, MSN, RN

Teddie Potter, PhD, RN

Gina Purdue, DNP, RN

Amy Ragnone, MSN, MA, RN

Joscelyn Richey, MSN, ARNP, CDE

Margaret Richey, MSN, RN

Leland J. Rockstraw, PhD, RN

Slyvia Sheffler, PhD, RN

Kathleen Sheikh, MSN, CRNP, FNP-BC

Montray M. Smith, MSN, RN, LHRM, EMT-B

Dina Swearngin, MSN, RN

Mary L. Wallace, RN

Sara Washington, MSN, RN

Diane E. White, PhD, RN, CCRN

Joanne Yakumithis, MSN, RN

Mary Yost, PhD, MSN, RN

PREFACE

Fundamentals of Nursing offers a concise and contemporary approach to teaching nursing practice for today's students. It responds to the challenges faced in the nursing profession, including how to apply knowledge-based care and how to adapt to changes in innovations and technology. It guides student nurses through the professional and clinical concepts they will need to master in order to lead and educate in various settings, and to treat and maintain an individual's most healthy and safe state. Information is presented in a practical and easy to understand format that is desirable for achieving optimal patient care. It begins with a basic understanding of the nursing profession, and progresses students through the nursing process and into the safe and systematic methods of applying care. The nursing process is introduced in Chapters 5 to 9 and is then integrated and used throughout the text and clinical skills chapters.

Fundamentals of Nursing has three important criteria that will help students succeed as care providers in the twenty-first century.

RELEVANCY: CONCISE AND CONTEMPORARY APPROACH

The Yoost/Crawford team has introduced an approach to nursing practice that focuses on the essential "need to know" concepts. Nursing students have a lot of information they need to digest in a short amount time, and *Fundamentals of Nursing* presents that information in a clear and concise manner that prepares students to understand the role of the nurse, how to critically think and analyze, and how to confidently and accurately perform the nursing care skills and procedures that will make them successful. To reinforce this approach, every Learning Objective in *Fundamentals of Nursing* is directly tied to the content that elaborates that objective.

ORGANIZATION: BUILDING-BLOCK APPROACH TO TEACHING NURSING

Most nursing faculty agree that students get easily overwhelmed and confused trying to understand the art and science of nursing if the information is not presented in the appropriate way. And yet all other nursing books introduce difficult concepts early in their texts, thus bombarding students early in the course with an overload of concepts and terms. The Yoost/Crawford team believe that by slowing down the pace of the information and giving students time to practice and gain mastery, this building-block approach leads to greater student success.

Fundamentals of Nursing is organized in 6 units and 42 chapters. It is shorter than other nursing textbooks but still covers all essential fundamental concepts and skills—just in a clearer, more easy-to-understand manner. Students are not frustrated with repetitive discussions and unnecessary information.

TECHNOLOGY: POWERFUL TOOLS FOR TEACHING AND STUDY

Students have different learning styles and conflicting time commitments, so they want technology tools that help them study more efficiently and effectively. A rich amount of resources will help them maximize their study time and make their learning experience more enjoyable. *Fundamentals of Nursing* is accompanied by the interactive Conceptual Care Map creator, an online-only Case Study, a Fluid & Electrolytes tutorial, Body Spectrum (a program designed to help students understand or review anatomy and physiology), a Calculations tutorial, animations, skills videos clips, and other resources for the instructor and student.

PEDAGOGICAL FEATURES

A **Case Study** opens every chapter of *Fundamentals of Nursing*, and is designed to help students develop their analytical, critical thinking, and clinical reasoning skills. These case studies represent situations similar to those the nurse may encounter in daily practice. Students are encouraged to consider the case study as they read through the chapter, and to check their understanding by answering the **Critical Thinking Exercises**. These exercises appear throughout each chapter and tie directly to the case study scenario introduced at the beginning of the chapter. Students are required to use the case study content and what they have learned from the chapter materials to apply critical thinking and sound clinical judgment when answering the questions.

The **Conceptual Care Map** is a *unique*, interactive learning tool developed to assist students in their ability to make clinical judgments and synthesize knowledge about the whole patient. Although the first part employs some principles of a traditional concept map, the Conceptual Care Map requires the student to develop a plan of care after analyzing and clustering related patient assessment data. This tool assists students in recognizing the importance of each type of assessment data that provides the foundation for individualized, patient-centered care plan development.

BOXED FEATURES

- **Collaboration and Delegation** boxes stress the importance of effective and accurate communication among the health care team about a patient's condition and treatment, as well as the importance of assigning tasks appropriately.

- **Ethical, Legal, and Professional Practice** boxes address ethical and legal dilemmas commonly faced in nursing to prepare students to act in a professional and nonjudgmental manner while protecting patient rights.
- **Patient Education and Health Literacy** boxes stress the importance of patient education and how to deliver information in an understandable manner based on the patient's level of health literacy.
- **Health Assessment Question** boxes help students to learn how to properly ask and use assessment questions when interviewing patients.
- **Diversity Considerations** boxes prepare students to care for and communicate with patients of diverse ages, cultural, ethnic, and religious backgrounds, as well as various morphological characteristics.
- **Evidence-Based Practice and Informatics** boxes provide students with current research and resources that, combined with clinical expertise, will contribute to improved patient care outcomes.
- **Home Care Considerations** boxes highlight issues that pertain specifically to transitional nursing practice from the acute care setting to home.
- ***Safe Practice Alert!*** boxes underscore significant patient safety concerns and provide information to ensure the safety of both the patient and the nurse.
- ***QSEN Focus!*** boxes illustrate application of the six Quality and Safety Education for Nurses (QSEN) competencies for prelicensure nursing students: (1) patient-centered care, (2) teamwork and collaboration, (3) evidence-based practice, (4) quality improvement, (5) safety, and (6) informatics.

NURSING SKILLS

Skills are written in a clear and concise manner, with the nursing care actions and rationale presented in a straightforward, step-by-step format and supported by evidence-based practice notations, photographs, and illustrations.

Nursing Care Guidelines provide guidelines and resources to reduce risk and ensure safety for the patient and nurse.

END-OF-CHAPTER FEATURES

The **Summary of Learning Outcomes** reinforce key concepts integral to achieving a basic understanding of chapter content and applying theory to nursing practice.

Every chapter ends with **ten review questions**. An **additional five review questions** are available on the accompanying Evolve site. These questions help students review what they have learned and evaluate their understanding by providing complete answers and rationales.

ABOUT THE AUTHORS

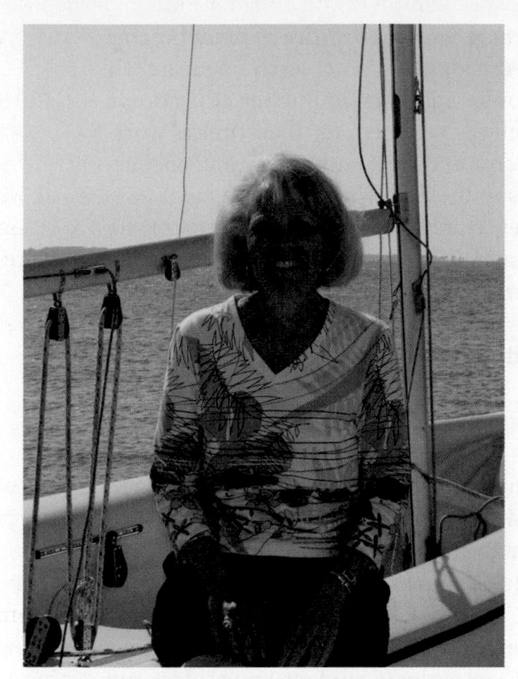

Barbara L. Yoost, MSN, RN, CNS, CNE, ANEF

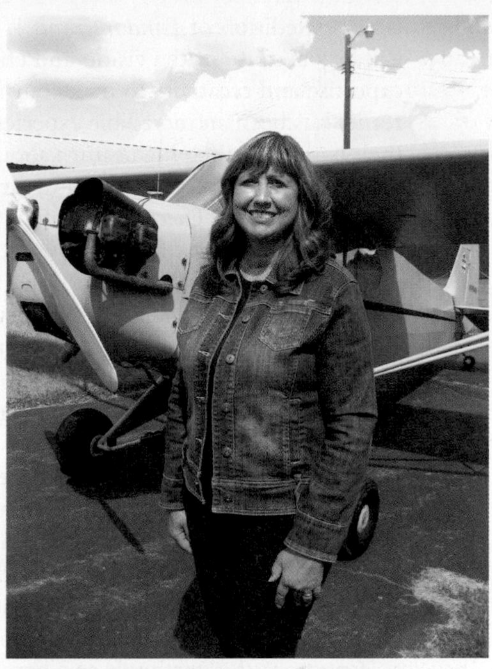

Lynne R. Crawford, MSN, RN, MBA, CNE

Barbara Yoost received her BSN from Kent State University and returned to complete her MSN with a concentration in Adult Medical Surgical Education. She is a Clinical Nurse Specialist, Certified Nurse Educator, and Fellow in the National League for Nurses Academy of Nursing Education. She practiced as in intensive care nurse while beginning her teaching career at the request of Kent State University's founding Dean Linnea Henderson. After practicing and teaching part time, Barbara taught full time at North Central State College in the ADN program; at Huron School of Nursing, part of the Cleveland Clinic Health System, in the Diploma program; and twice at her alma mater in the BSN program, giving her a unique perspective on the needs of prelicensure students in all types of programs. She is currently Assistant Professor of Nursing at Notre Dame College, where she teaches and coordinates the fundamentals, medical-surgical, international, and leadership nursing courses in their BSN program. For the past 30 years, Barbara's passion has been in the development and implementation of innovative teaching and active learning strategies. She is committed to engaging students in the educational process and providing faculty with practical methods to evaluate student outcomes. As a result of Barbara's early work with handheld technology and her innovative teaching style, she was invited to teach continuing nursing education courses in Turkey and the United Arab Emirates. Her commitment to servant leadership and service has resulted in her volunteering as a nurse at various senior high school youth camps, and developing and leading student study abroad immersion experiences in Geneva, Switzerland and San Juan LaLaguna, Guatemala. Barbara is a member of the American Nurses Association, National League for Nurses, Sigma Theta Tau International, and Phi Beta Delta, the Honors Society of International Scholars. An avid small boat sailor, Barbara and her husband, Charles, enjoy spending time near the water and with family.

Lynne Crawford graduated from Kent State University with her BSN. She began her nursing career working in pediatric neurology. She earned her MSN in Pediatric Nursing and Nursing Education from Frances Payne Bolton School of Nursing at Case Western Reserve University, and received the Cushing Robb Prize for academic achievement in the graduate program upon graduation. Her career in nursing education began at Kent State University College of Nursing, where she taught pediatric nursing. After receiving her MBA, she worked as an RN supervisor in long-term care facilities before coming back to Kent State University to teach fundamentals of nursing. Her passion for fundamentals grew as she witnessed the students' transformation during their fundamentals rotation. She is emerita faculty at Kent State University. Lynne has presented at national conferences in the areas of student-centered learning activities, handheld technology, and conceptual care mapping. She was a subject matter expert in the development of online simulations for nursing students. A charter member of the Delta Xi chapter of Sigma Theta Tau International, Lynne is also a member of the National League for Nursing and Beta Gamma Sigma Honor Society for Collegiate Schools of Business. Since 2010 she has been a Certified Nurse Educator, and in 2011 she was recognized as a Distinguished Alumna Honoree at KSU College of Nursing. Lynne and her husband, David, enjoy many hobbies including sailing on Lake Erie, flying in their single engine aircraft, motorcycling, and spending time with their family.

ACKNOWLEDGMENTS

This first edition of *Fundamentals of Nursing: Active Learning for Collaborative Practice* became a reality because of the vision and efforts of many talented people. To watch each one use their expertise and creativity to make our ideas for a contemporary approach to nursing education a reality has been an incredible experience. We want to thank each of them for their tireless work, their patience in helping us learn about the publishing process, and their enthusiasm and encouragement over many months and years, with special kudos to the following:

- Tamara Myers, Executive Content Strategist, whose energy, creative vision, and teamwork are unmatchable. The book, software, ancillary products, and online resources are a reality due to her hard work and leadership. It is difficult to imagine this project ever becoming a reality without the encouragement and support of Tamara.
- Michael Ledbetter, our former editor, who championed our efforts, a true professional in the publishing world and a cherished friend.
- Loren Wilson, Senior Vice President and General Manager, Content, who was the first person to welcome us to Elsevier.
- Laura Selkirk, Senior Content Developmental Specialist; Mary Stueck, Senior Project Manager; Jean Fornango, Content Development Manager; Tina Kaemmerer, Senior Content Development Specialist; and Savannah Davis, former Associate Content Development Specialist, for their exhaustive work in editing, finding photos, and turning manuscript into pages. We are honored to be working with the best team imaginable.
- Kathleen Schlesinger, our champion Marketing Manager, who helped us articulate the unique aspects of this textbook and how they support faculty to evaluate student knowledge, and students to provide safer, more informed patient care.
- Barnes-Jewish Hospital for allowing our film crew and the Mosby-Elsevier team to complete our photoshoot on site. They were wonderfully accommodating.
- All of our contributors and reviewers who shared their knowledge and time to write and thoughtfully consider the needs of fundamentals students, making sure the textbook presented the essentials in a user-friendly, accessible manner.
- Colleagues at Kent State University College of Nursing, especially Tim Meyers, who provided their support throughout our years of work and acknowledged our efforts by recognizing us as Distinguished Alumni even before the book was published!
- Former editors, Ken Kasee, Jonathan Joyce, and most significantly, Debbie Fitzgerald, who actually asked us to undertake this incredible project many years ago, and former developmental editors, Pat Gillivan, Jane Velker, and Kimberly Hooker.
- And last but not least, our current and former students, who have read and reviewed chapters, and utilized many of our innovative learning strategies during their nursing education. We are grateful for your feedback and enthusiasm. It is wonderful to see you progress in your nursing careers.

It is our hope that *Fundamentals of Nursing: Active Learning for Collaborative Practice* will help both students and faculty make a positive difference in the rapidly changing health care environment of the twenty-first century and beyond.

Barbara L. Yoost
Lynne R. Crawford

CONTENTS

UNIT III NURSING PRACTICE

UNIT IV NURSING ASSESSMENT

UNIT V NURSING PRINCIPLES

UNIT VI NURSING CARE

APPENDIXES

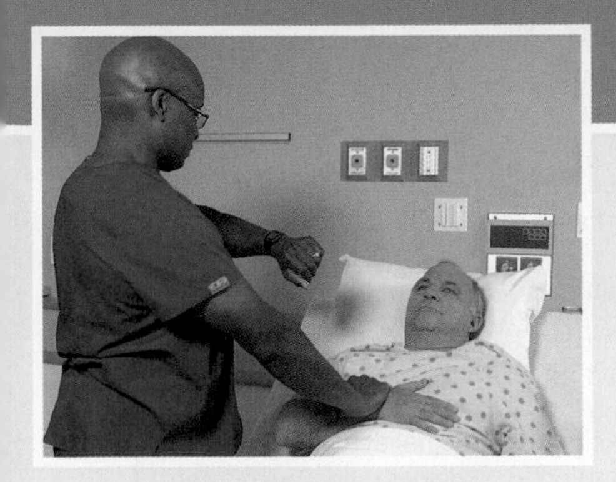

CHAPTER 1

Nursing, Theory, and Professional Practice

EVOLVE WEBSITE

http://evolve.elsevier.com/YoostCrawford/fundamentals/

- Additional Evolve-Only Review Questions With Answers
- Answers and Rationales for Text Review Questions
- Answers to Critical-Thinking Questions
- Case Study With Questions
- Glossary

LEARNING OUTCOMES

Comprehension of this chapter's content will provide students with the ability to:

LO 1.1 Define *nursing*.
LO 1.2 Differentiate among the functions and roles of nurses.
LO 1.3 Describe historical events in the evolution of nursing.
LO 1.4 Summarize nursing theories.
LO 1.5 Identify non-nursing theories that influence nursing practice.
LO 1.6 Articulate the criteria of a profession as applied to nursing.
LO 1.7 Discuss standards of practice and nurse practice acts.
LO 1.8 Describe the socialization and transformation process of a nurse.
LO 1.9 Explain the levels of educational preparation in nursing and differentiate among the nurse's roles depending upon education.
LO 1.10 List possible certifications in various arenas of nursing and professional organizations in nursing.
LO 1.11 Discuss the future directions in nursing.

KEY TERMS

advanced practice registered nurse (APRN), p. 15
collaboration, p. 4
conceptual framework or model, p. 6
cultural competence, p. 13
delegation, p. 5
discipline, p. 5
ethics, p. 12
evidence-based practice (EBP), p. 4
grand theory, p. 6
holistic, p. 3
licensure, p. 14
metaparadigm, p. 6
middle-range theory, p. 6
nurse practice acts, p. 13
nursing, p. 2
nursing process, p. 3
nursing theory, p. 6
philosophy, p. 6
profession, p. 3
socialization, p. 13
standards, p. 2

CASE STUDY

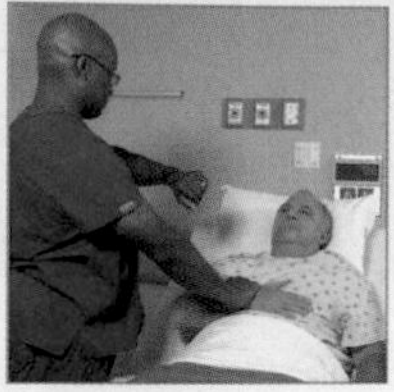

Chris, a registered nurse (RN), arrives for work on the day shift on an acute care medical unit and receives a patient assignment for the shift. The assignment includes care of five medical patients. After receiving the night shift report, the nurse makes rounds on the five patients, does a head-to-toe assessment of each, lists each patient's problems, sets patient goals, and plans their care for the day. During the shift Chris administers intravenous (IV) medications to all five patients; ensures that all oral medications are given by the licensed practical nurse (LPN); asks the unlicensed assistive personnel (UAP) to bathe two of the patients who need assistance; assists a patient with ambulation; provides education to a patient who will be discharged on a new medication; evaluates the plan of care for each patient, with updates as necessary; and notifies the primary care providers of critically abnormal blood work results for two patients.

One patient's friend comes to visit and stops Chris in the hallway to ask detailed questions about the patient's condition. Chris states that patient information is protected and cannot be shared without the consent of the patient.

At a recent continuing education conference, Chris learned that current evidence showed that aspirating the syringe after the needle is inserted into the muscle before administering deltoid intramuscular (IM) injections was no longer recommended. He remembers this new information while preparing to give a patient an IM immunization before discharge. Chris believes that self-care maintains wholeness, and meets patients' self-care needs by doing for, guiding, teaching, supporting, or providing the environment to promote self-care abilities.

Refer back to this case study to answer the critical-thinking questions throughout the chapter.

Registered nurses constitute the nation's largest health care profession. Nurses provide care to patients throughout the life span, from babies (and their parents) at the joyful occasion of birth to people who are at the end of life's journey. The privilege of caring for patients is the hallmark of this rewarding career. Those who follow this career path often are inspired by other nurses who have touched their lives, by stories they have read or heard about specific nurses, or by the concept of a helping profession that allows the nurse to make a difference in someone's daily life. The study of nursing requires a broad base of knowledge from the physical and behavioral sciences, humanities, nursing theories, and related non-nursing theories.

Within the field of nursing, various roles are performed in numerous arenas. Each of these roles is governed by nursing **standards** (minimum set of criteria) of practice to deliver quality care and by state nurse practice acts that provide legal criteria for adequate patient care. Nurses work in various areas within a hospital by focusing on a specific population, such as children or the elderly, or a specific department, such as critical care or surgery. They may concentrate on areas outside the hospital patient care environment, serving in positions such as nursing faculty member, school nurse, or legal nurse consultant, or be involved with computers in the field of nursing.

Nursing has continued to evolve throughout history to meet the needs of the patient and the changing health care environment. With a growing need for nurses, the future of nursing provides an incredible avenue for committed, caring practitioners to be involved in a profession which continues to progress to meet health care demands, utilizing innovative solutions related to the delivery of nursing care services. This complex profession that serves society by providing quality nursing care in a variety of settings is a career that combines the art of caring with scientific knowledge and skills.

DEFINITION OF NURSING LO 1.1

In 1860, Florence Nightingale (Figure 1-1) in her *Notes on Nursing* stated that nursing's role was "to put the patient in the best condition for nature to act upon him" (p. 133). As nursing has progressed to the 21st century, specific nursing definitions have been developed by professional organizations. The American Nurses Association (ANA) (2010) definition of nursing echoes the description first set forth by Nightingale but illustrates how nursing has evolved:

> **Nursing** is the protection, promotion, and optimization of health and abilities, prevention of illness and injury,

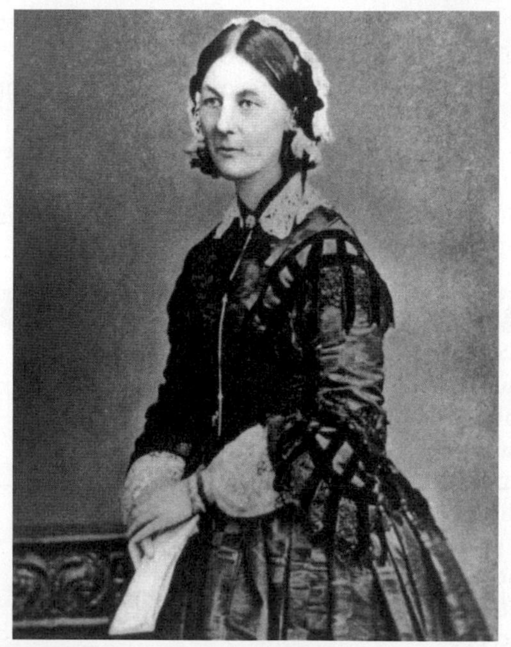

FIGURE 1-1 Florence Nightingale. (Courtesy Library of Congress, Washington, DC.)

alleviation of suffering through the diagnosis and treatment of human response, and advocacy in the care of individuals, families, communities, and populations (p. 1).

The International Council of Nurses (ICN) (2010) definition of nursing further illuminates the autonomous role of nurses and their part in not only patient care but also health policy:

> Nursing encompasses autonomous and collaborative care of individuals of all ages, families, groups and communities, sick or well and in all settings. Nursing includes the promotion of health, prevention of illness, and the care of ill, disabled and dying people. Advocacy, promotion of a safe environment, research, participation in shaping health policy and in patient and health systems management, and education are also key nursing roles.

Virginia Henderson (1966) is known for her specific definition of nursing:

> The unique function of the nurse is to assist the individual, sick or well, in the performance of those activities contributing to health or its recovery (or to peaceful death) that he would perform unaided if he had the necessary strength, will or knowledge. And to do this in such a way as to help him gain independence as rapidly as possible (p. 15).

As illustrated by these definitions, nursing is seen as a **holistic** (addressing physical, mental, emotional, spiritual, and social needs) profession that addresses the many dimensions necessary to fully care for a patient. A **profession** is an occupation that requires at a minimum specialized training and a specialized body of knowledge. The all-encompassing nature of the nursing profession sets it apart from the medical profession, which treats an illness with a specific medical diagnosis. Nurses build upon their broad education and understanding of illness to promote wellness and health maintenance. Nurses include the patient and family in their care while collaborating with all members of the health care team. Caring, which often is considered to be synonymous with nursing, is a fundamental value for nurses in both their personal and professional lives and a critical foundation of nursing practice.

PRIMARY ROLES AND FUNCTIONS OF THE NURSE LO 1.2

Nurses function in many roles each day to care for their patients. Nurses have various responsibilities within each role that relate to promotion of health, prevention of illness, and alleviation of suffering. Nurses assist patients with restoration of their health and help them to cope with illness, disability, and issues related to the end of their lives (ICN, 2012). The roles include care provider, educator, advocate, leader, change agent, manager, researcher, collaborator, and delegator.

CARE PROVIDER

"The nurse's primary professional responsibility is to people requiring nursing care" (ICN, 2012, p. 2). Through education, the nurse acquires critical-thinking skills to determine the necessary course of action, psychomotor skills to perform the necessary interventions, interpersonal skills to communicate effectively with the patient and family, and ethical and legal skills to function within the scope of practice and in accordance with the profession's code of ethics.

The scientific process that nurses use to care for their patients is a multistep approach called the **nursing process**. As a care provider, the nurse follows this process to assess patient data, prioritize nursing diagnoses, plan the care of the patient, implement the appropriate interventions, and evaluate care in an ongoing cycle. Chapter 5 provides a detailed description of the nursing process.

EDUCATOR

The nurse ensures that patients receive sufficient information on which to base consent for care and related treatment. The nurse assesses learning needs, plans to meet those needs through specific teaching strategies, and evaluates the effectiveness of patient teaching. Patients need to be informed about their medications, procedures, diagnostics, and health promotion measures. Education becomes a major focus of discharge planning so that patients will be prepared to handle their own needs at home. The nurse must understand literacy standards and regulatory guidelines related to patient rights, informed consent, educating patients, improving quality care, and meeting patient needs. The Joint Commission, an accrediting organization for health care facilities, publishes standards for patient and family education to improve health care outcomes. The Patient Education and Health Literacy box provides a definition of health literacy.

PATIENT EDUCATION AND HEALTH LITERACY

Definition of Health Literacy

- Health literacy is defined in *Healthy People 2020* as follows: "The degree to which individuals have the capacity to obtain, process, and understand basic health information and services needed to make appropriate health decisions" (U.S. Department of Health and Human Services, 2010).
- Low health literacy is associated with increased hospitalization, greater emergency care use, lower use of mammography and lower receipt of influenza vaccine (Agency for Healthcare Research and Quality, 2011).
- A goal of patient education by the nurse is to inform patients and deliver information that is understandable by examining their level of health literacy. The more understandable health information is for patients, the closer the care is coordinated with need.

ADVOCATE

As the patient's advocate, the nurse interprets information and provides the necessary education. The nurse then accepts and respects the patient's decisions even if they are different from the nurse's own beliefs. The nurse supports the patient's wishes and communicates them to other health care providers. It is up to the nurse to be an advocate for patients, especially in situations in which they cannot speak for themselves, such as during a severe illness or under general anesthesia.

LEADER

A leader provides direction and purpose to others, builds a sense of commitment toward common goals, communicates effectively, and assists with addressing challenges that arise in caring for patients in a health care setting. Other characteristics of a leader are integrity, creativity, interpersonal skills, and the ability to think critically and problem-solve. The nurse leader motivates others toward common goals. See Chapter 12 for more information about the nurse as a leader.

CHANGE AGENT

The nurse can be a change agent in a leadership role. This role requires knowledge of change theory, which encourages change and provides strategies for effecting change. In this role the nurse works with patients to address their health concerns and with staff members to address change in an organization or within a community. This role can be extended to bringing about change in the legislation on health policy issues.

MANAGER

A nurse manages all of the activities and treatments for patients. Promoting, restoring, and maintaining the patient's health requires coordinating all of the health care providers' services. This is accomplished efficiently and effectively within a reasonable time period for the welfare of the patient. In addition to managing a team of patients, the nurse may be the manager of a unit in a hospital. A nurse manager in a hospital oversees the staff on a patient care unit while managing the budget and resources required for necessary functions. See Chapter 12 for more information on nurses as managers.

RESEARCHER

Although not all nurses may have had research methodology in their coursework, nurses are often involved in research. Nurses concur research studies and apply research to practice. Nurses determine care concerns and ask questions about nursing practices. Nursing problems that are identified become the basis of research. By incorporating research into their practice, nurses are involved in evidence-based practice (EBP). The Evidence-Based Practice box defines EBP and the steps in the process. Larabee (2009) devised a model to guide nurses through a systemic process for change to evidence-based practice. Chapter 13 expands on these topics.

EVIDENCE-BASED PRACTICE

Definition of Evidence-Based Practice

- Evidence for nursing practice comes from nursing research. Potential problems are discovered during patient care, and nurse researchers gather and analyze data and report research findings in the literature.
- **Evidence-based practice (EBP)** is an integration of the best-available research evidence with clinical judgment about a specific patient situation.
- For EBP, the nurse assesses current and past research, clinical guidelines, and other resources to identify relevant literature.
- The application of EBP includes the following basic components:
  - Assessing the need for change and identifying a problem
  - Linking the problem with interventions and outcomes by formulating a well-built question to search the literature
  - Identifying articles and other evidence-based resources that answer the question
  - Critically appraising the evidence to assess its validity
  - Synthesizing the best evidence
  - Designing a change for practice
  - Implementing and evaluating the change by applying the synthesized evidence
  - Integrating and maintaining change while monitoring process and outcomes by reevaluating the application of evidence and assessing areas for improvement

From Larabee J: *Nurse to nurse: Evidence-based practice,* New York, 2009, McGraw-Hill.

COLLABORATOR

Collaboration is the process by which two or more people work together toward a common goal. In nursing, collaboration occurs when RNs, UAP, LPNs, primary care providers, social workers, clergy, and therapists all interact productively to provide high-quality patient care. The Collaboration box

COLLABORATION

Characteristics of Teamwork

- Clinical competence and accountability
- Common purpose
- Interpersonal competence and effective communication
- Trust and mutual respect
- Recognition and valuation of diverse complementary knowledge and skills
- Humor

describes the characteristics necessary for effective teamwork. All health care team members are responsible for patient care. The nurse plays an important role in the coordination of this care to make sure that all goals are met. The nurse is responsible for ensuring that all patient care orders are carried out and for communicating with the entire team.

DELEGATOR

In the process of collaboration, the nurse delegates certain activities to other health care personnel. **Delegation** is the process of entrusting or transferring the responsibility for certain tasks to other personnel, including UAP, licensed vocational nurses (LVNs), and LPNs. The RN needs to know the scope of practice or capabilities of each health care member. For example, UAP are capable of performing basic care that includes providing hygienic care, taking vital signs, helping the patient ambulate, and assisting with eating. The RN retains ultimate responsibility for patient care, which requires supervision of those to whom patient care is delegated. The *Five Rights of Delegation* as well as additional guidelines for consideration are discussed in Chapter 12.

All of these roles are interrelated as the nurse cares for patients on a daily basis (Figure 1-2). As a provider of care, the nurse assesses, leads, manages, and educates. The nurse is the patient advocate, researching appropriate care and collaborating with and delegating to other health care providers.

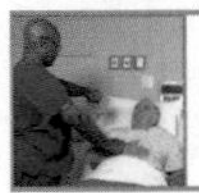

1. Which roles are exhibited by Chris, and when are they displayed?

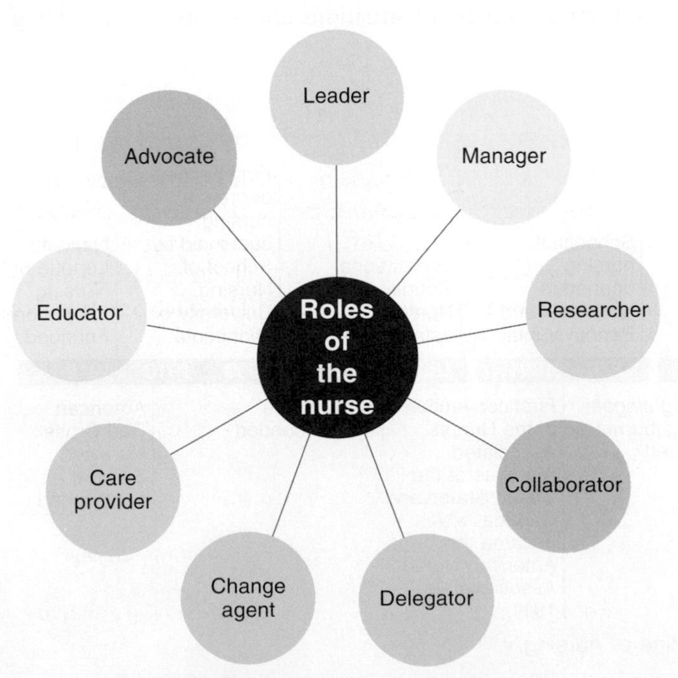

FIGURE 1-2 Roles of the nurse.

HISTORY OF NURSING — LO 1.3

Nursing had its beginnings in religious and military services in the Middle Ages, particularly during the Crusades. In 1860 Florence Nightingale's *Notes on Nursing* raised the profile of nursing with critical thinking and respect for patient needs and rights. Nightingale is considered the founder of modern nursing and is known for her care of the sick in the Crimean War. Her contributions influenced developments in the field of epidemiology by connecting poor sanitation with cholera and dysentery. Her role in nursing included establishing nursing as a respected profession for women that was distinct from the medical profession. She founded a nursing school and stressed the need for university-based and continuing education for nurses.

During the Civil War, two nurses emerged to further nursing. Dorothea Dix was the head of the U.S. Sanitary Commission, which was a forerunner of the Army Nurse Corps. Clara Barton (Figure 1-3) practiced nursing in the Civil War and established the American Red Cross. History continues to reveal other nurse leaders. Linda Richards was America's first trained nurse, graduating from Boston's Women's Hospital in 1873, and Lenah Higbee (Figure 1-4), superintendent of the U.S. Navy Nurse Corps, was awarded the Navy Cross in 1918.

After World War II, scientific and technologic advances brought changes to both principles and practices in health care delivery. This new approach required critical care specialty units and more experienced and skilled nurses. Health promotion became a greater focus, leading to a need for nurse practitioners. The timeline in Figure 1-5 provides a brief overview of modern nursing up to the present day.

NURSING THEORIES — LO 1.4

To enhance nursing as a profession, nursing works to establish itself as a scientific discipline. A **discipline** is a specific

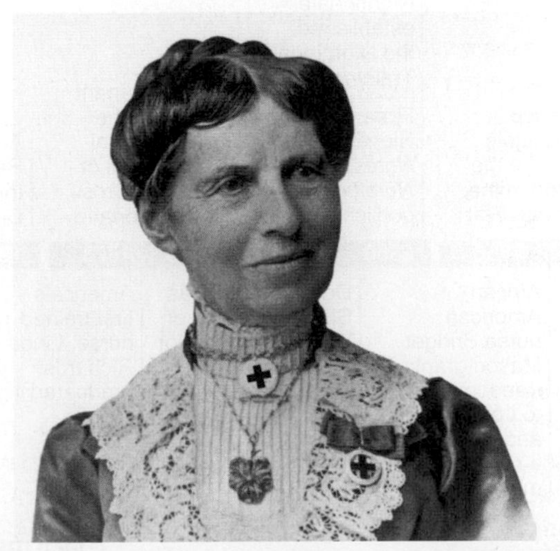

FIGURE 1-3 Clara Barton. (Courtesy National Park Service, U.S. Department of the Interior.)

field of study or branch of instruction or learning. Nursing leaders believe nursing needs a theoretical base that reflects its practice. With this belief, nursing theories have emerged from the time of Nightingale to the present to give substance to the body of knowledge of nursing.

DEFINITIONS

A **metaparadigm**, as the most abstract level of knowledge, is defined as a global set of concepts that identify and describe the central phenomena of the discipline and explain the relationship between those concepts (Fawcett and DeSanto-Madeya, 2013). For example, the metaparadigm for nursing focuses on the concepts of person, environment, health, and nursing. The next level of knowledge is a **philosophy**, which is a statement about the beliefs and values of nursing in relation to a specific phenomenon such as health. A philosophy provides guidance in practice.

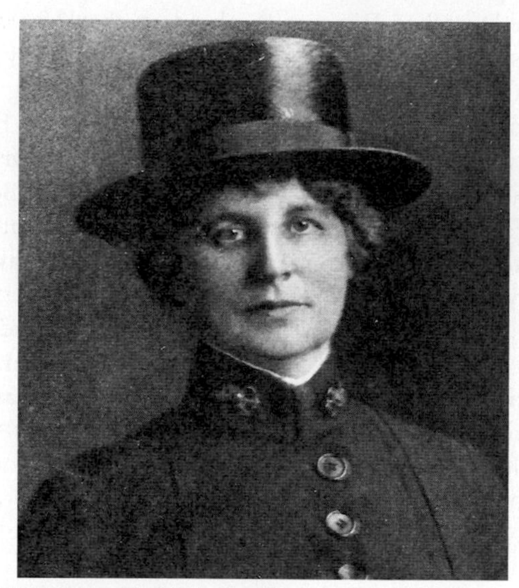

FIGURE 1-4 Lenah Higbee. (Courtesy U.S. Navy and the National Archives.)

The third level of knowledge is a nursing **conceptual framework**, or **model**, which is a collection of interrelated concepts that provides direction for nursing practice, research, and education. A conceptual model addresses the four concepts of the nursing metaparadigm: optimal functioning of the person, or patient, how people interact with the environment, illness and health promotion, and nursing's role (Alligood and Tomey, 2014). Each is defined and described by the theorist in the model. In nursing practice, nursing models approach the nursing process in a logical, systematic way. The model influences the data the nurse collects and the care of the patient. Conceptual models often are based on other non-nursing theories such as system or stress theory. The fourth level of nursing knowledge is a **nursing theory**, which represents a group of concepts that can be tested in practice and can be derived from a conceptual model.

Theories include both grand theories and middle-range theories, which are derived from conceptual models. A **grand theory** consists of a global conceptual framework that defines broad perspectives for nursing practice and provides ways of looking at nursing phenomena from a distinct nursing perspective. Although grand theories are derived from conceptual frameworks, they remain almost as broad as the framework itself. A grand theory defines key concepts and principles of the discipline in an abstract way (Alligood and Tomey, 2009).

A **middle-range theory** is moderately abstract and has a limited number of variables. Therefore middle-range theories are more concrete and narrowly focused on a specific condition or population than are grand theories (Fawcett and DeSanto-Madeya, 2013). They can be tested directly through application to practice situations and are useful in nursing

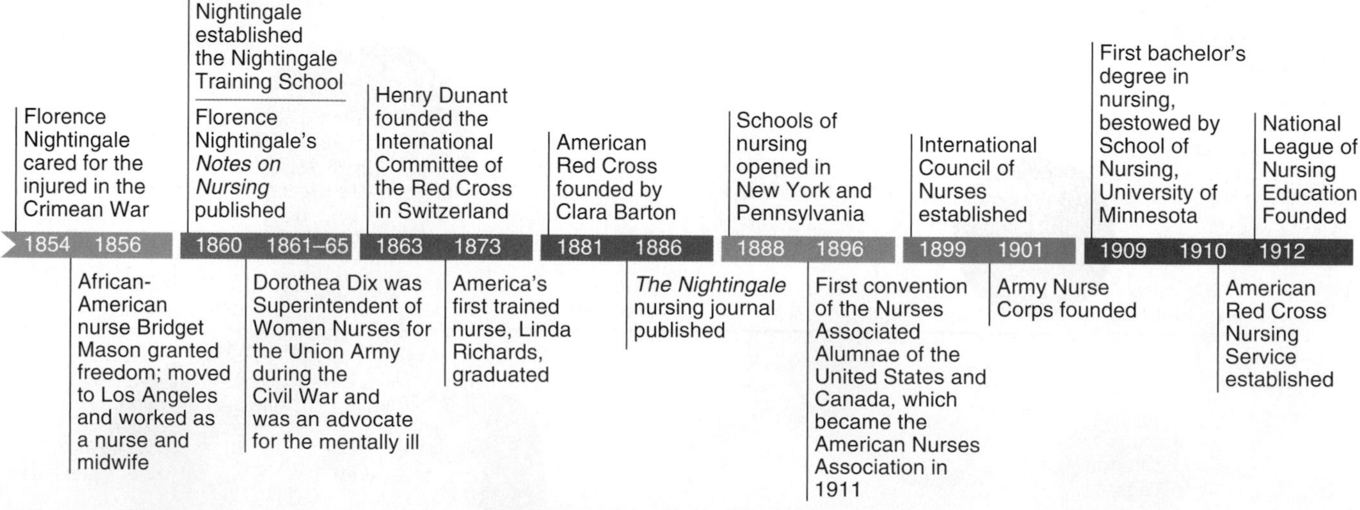

FIGURE 1-5 Timeline of nursing.

research and practice. These theories provide a map of how patients are assessed and how care is planned and delivered (McKenna and Slevin, 2008).

OVERVIEW OF KEY NURSING THEORIES

Florence Nightingale

Florence Nightingale's (1860) concept of the environment emphasized illness prevention, clean air, water, and housing. Her nursing theoretical work discussed environmental adaptation with appropriate noise levels, hygiene, light, comfort, socialization, hope, nutrition, and conservation of patient energy. This theory states that the imbalance between the patient and the environment decreases the capacity for health and does not allow for conservation of energy.

Hildegard Peplau

Hildegard Peplau (1952) focused on the roles played by the nurse and the interpersonal process between a nurse and a patient. The interpersonal process occurs in overlapping phases: (1) *orientation;* (2) *working,* consisting of two subphases—identification and exploitation; and (3) *resolution.* This theory has been used widely in psychiatric nursing and enhances the understanding of changing aspects regarding the goals and roles in the nurse-patient relationship.

Virginia Henderson

Virginia Henderson (1966) defined nursing as "assisting individuals to gain independence in relation to the performance of activities contributing to health or its recovery" (p. 15). Her 14 components were based on Maslow's hierarchy of human needs from the physiologic, psychological, sociocultural, spiritual, and developmental domains. She described the nurse's role as *substitutive* (doing for the person), *supplementary* (helping the person), or *complementary* (working with the person), with the ultimate goal of independence for the patient.

Martha Rogers

Martha Rogers (1970) developed the Science of Unitary Human Beings. She stated that human beings and their environments are interacting in continuous motion as infinite energy fields. The model includes four dimensions: energy fields, openness, patterns and organizations, and dimensionality. The dimensions are used in developing the three principles of *resonancy* (continuous change from lower to higher frequency), *helicy* (increasing diversity), and *integrality* (continuous process of the human and environmental fields). Well-being of the patient is illustrated by pattern and organization. Nurses assist the patient with repatterning to develop well-being. The resultant well-being of pattern and organization includes a symphonic interaction between the patient and the environment.

Sister Callista Roy

Sister Callista Roy's (1970) Adaptation Model is based on the human being as an adaptive open system. The person adapts by meeting physiological-physical needs, developing a positive self-concept–group identity, performing social role functions, and balancing dependence and independence. Stressors result in illness by disrupting the equilibrium. Nursing care is directed at altering stimuli that are stressors to the patient. The nurse helps patients strengthen their abilities to adapt to their illnesses or helps them to develop adaptive behaviors.

Dorothea Orem

Three interrelated theories of self-care, self-care deficit, and nursing systems constitute Dorothea Orem's (1971) Self-Care Deficit Theory of Nursing. A self-care deficit exists when

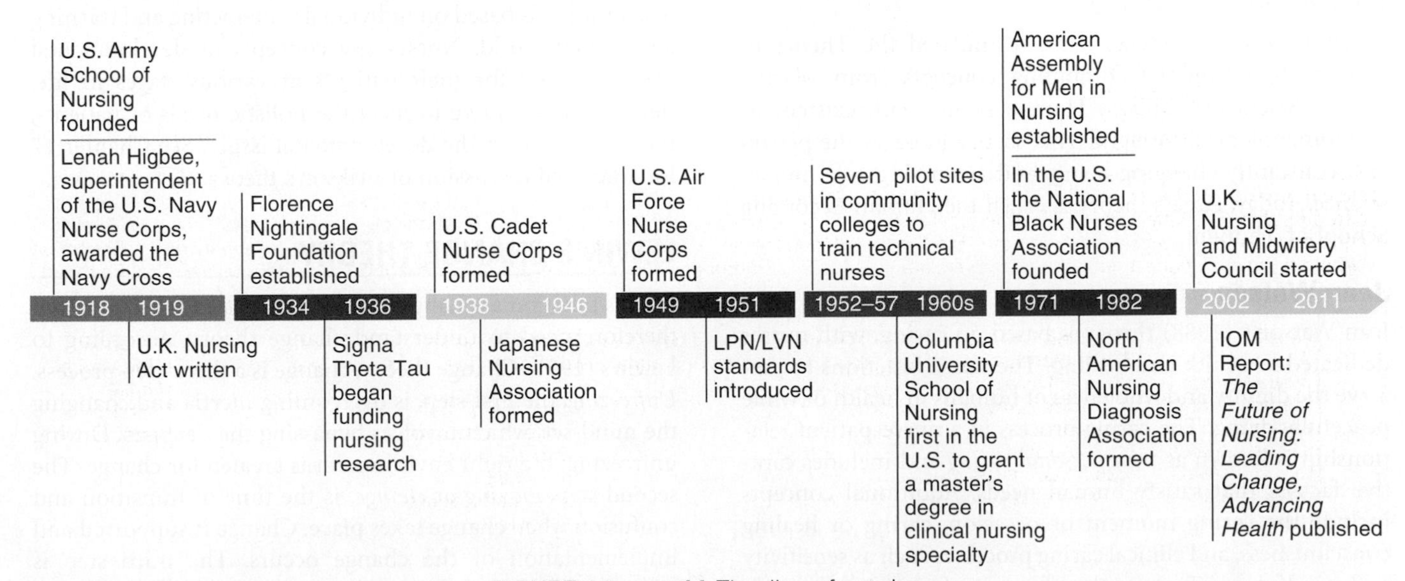

FIGURE 1-5, cont'd Timeline of nursing.

patients are unable to meet their self-care needs. Nursing systems care for patients who require assistance in one of three categories: (1) *wholly compensatory,* (2) *partly compensatory,* or (3) *supportive-educative.* The goal of nursing care is to help patients perform self-care by increasing their independence.

Imogene King

Imogene M. King (1971) developed a general systems framework that incorporates three levels of systems: (1) *individual or personal,* (2) *group or interpersonal,* and (3) *society or social.* The theory of goal attainment discusses the importance of interaction, perception, communication, transaction, self, role, stress, growth and development, time, and personal space. In this theory, the nurse and the patient work together to achieve the goals in the continuous adjustment to stressors.

Betty Neuman

Betty Neuman's (1972) Systems Model includes a holistic concept and an open-system approach. The model identifies energy resources that provide for basic survival, with lines of resistance that are activated when a stressor invades the system. The person has a normal response to stress, known as *normal lines of defense,* whereas a flexible line defends against unusual stress. Stressors may be intrapersonal, interpersonal, or extrapersonal. Three environments—*internal, external,* and *created*—are defined, and nursing actions involve three levels of prevention—primary, secondary, and tertiary (discussed in more detail in Chapter 16). The nurse's goal is to assist with attaining and maintaining maximum wellness, focusing on patients' responses to stressors, and strengthening their lines of defense. Two theories were produced from this model: optimal patient stability and prevention as intervention.

Rosemarie Rizzo Parse

In 1981 Rosemarie Rizzo Parse formulated the Theory of Human Becoming by combining concepts from Martha Rogers' Science of Unitary Human Beings with existential-phenomenological thought. This theory looks at the person as a constantly changing being, and at nursing as a human science. Today, Parse's theory is called the Human Becoming School of Thought.

Jean Watson

Jean Watson's (1988) theory is based on caring, with nurses dedicated to health and healing. The nurse functions to preserve the dignity and wholeness of humans in health or while peacefully dying. The caring process in a nurse-patient relationship is known as *transpersonal caring* and includes carative factors that satisfy human needs. Additional concepts include the caring moment or occasion, caring or healing consciousness, and clinical caring processes such as sensitivity and mindfulness. The practice of nursing focuses on the goals of growth, meaning, and self-healing. Table 1-1 compares the various nursing theories and models.

NON-NURSING THEORIES WITH SIGNIFICANT IMPACT ON NURSING LO 1.5

Nursing requires a strong scientific knowledge base in the natural, social, and behavioral sciences. Accordingly, nursing theories often are influenced by interdisciplinary theories. Nurses use these theories in their practice.

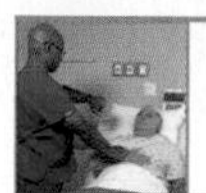

2. Which nursing theorist do Chris' beliefs parallel?

MASLOW'S HIERARCHY OF NEEDS

Maslow's hierarchy of needs specifies the psychological and physiologic factors that affect each person's physical and mental health (Figure 1-6). The nurse's understanding of these factors helps with formulating nursing diagnoses that address the patient's needs and values. Needs at the lower levels of the pyramid-shaped hierarchy must be met before needs at higher levels are addressed. At the base of the pyramid are physiologic needs, including oxygen, food, elimination, temperature control, sex, movement, rest, and comfort. These are followed by safety and security, love and belonging, self-esteem, and self-actualization. This hierarchy allows nurses to plan the care of patients by addressing their needs on the basis of priorities.

ERIKSON'S PSYCHOSOCIAL THEORY

Erikson's (1968) Psychosocial Theory of Development and Socialization is based on individuals' interacting and learning about their world. Nurses use concepts of developmental theory to care for their patients at various stages in life. Because nurses strive to meet the holistic needs of patients, they must address the developmental issues. See Chapter 17 for a detailed discussion of Erikson's theory.

LEWIN'S CHANGE THEORY

Nurses function as change agents in their leadership role and therefore need to understand change theory. According to Lewin's (1951) Change theory, change is a three-step process. *Unfreezing,* the first step, is overcoming inertia and changing the mind-set, which involves bypassing the defenses. During unfreezing, the right environment is created for change. The second step, *moving or change,* is the time of transition and confusion when change takes place. Change is supported and implementation of the change occurs. The third step is *refreezing,* during which the change is completed, reinforced

TABLE 1-1 **Nursing Model and Theory Comparison**

THEORIST AND THEORY OR CONCEPTUAL FRAMEWORK (YEAR)	GENERAL CONCEPT	METAPARADIGM			
		NURSING	PERSON	HEALTH	ENVIRONMENT
Nightingale Environmental Theory (1860)	Environment	Providing fresh air, warmth, quiet, cleanliness, and proper nutrition to facilitate reparative process.	Patient who is acted on by nurse and affected by environment has reparative powers.	Maintaining well-being by using a person's powers and control of environment.	Foundation of theory; included physical, psychological, and social.
Peplau Theory of Interpersonal Relations (1952)	Interpersonal	A therapeutic, interpersonal process that functions cooperatively with others to make health possible; involves problem solving.	An individual; a developing organism who tries to reduce anxiety caused by needs and lives in unstable equilibrium.	Implies forward movement of the personality toward creative, constructive, productive, personal, and community living.	Acknowledgment of the environment and influence of culture and other factors.
Henderson Humane and holistic care for patients (1966)	Helping the patient become as independent as possible	Temporarily assisting an individual who lacks the necessary will, strength, and knowledge to satisfy 1 or more of 14 basic needs.	The patient as a sum of parts with biopsychosocial needs, and the patient is neither client nor consumer.	Being as independent as possible with the 14 basic needs. Affected by age, culture, and physical, intellectual and emotional factors.	All external conditions and influences that affect life and development.
Rogers Science of Unitary Human Beings Model (1970)	Integrality, resonancy, and helicy; characterized by nonrepeating rhythmicities	Both an art and a humanistic science supported by an organized body of knowledge arrived at by scientific research and logical analysis.	A unitary human being is an "irreducible, indivisible, four-dimensional energy field."	Rogers defined health as an expression of the life process. Health and illness are part of the same continuum.	The environment is an "irreducible, four-dimensional energy field identified by pattern and integral with the human field."
Roy Adaptation Model (1970)	Adaptation	The science and practice that expands adaptive abilities and enhances person and environment transformation.	A biopsychosocial being with a unified system; an adaptive system in the four modes: physiologic-physical, self-concept–group identity, role function, and interdependence.	Equilibrium resulting from effective coping and a state of becoming integrated and whole that reflects person-environment mutuality.	Environment seen as all conditions that shape an individual's behavior.
Orem Self-Care Deficit Theory (1971)	Self-care maintains wholeness: theory of self-care, self-care deficit, and nursing systems	Meets self-care needs by acting or doing for, guiding, teaching, supporting, or providing the environment to promote patient's ability.	Patients require assistance either wholly or partially compensatory or supportive-educative.	Structurally and functionally whole or sound; self-care deficit occurs when the person cannot carry out self-care.	Components are internal and external; include environmental factors.

Continued

TABLE 1-1 Nursing Model and Theory Comparison—cont'd

THEORIST AND THEORY OR CONCEPTUAL FRAMEWORK (YEAR)	GENERAL CONCEPT	METAPARADIGM			
		NURSING	PERSON	HEALTH	ENVIRONMENT
King General systems framework (1971)	Importance of the interaction between nurses and patients	The nurse and patient mutually communicate, establish goals, and take action to attain goals.	Human beings bring a different set of values, ideas, attitudes, and perceptions to exchange.	Dynamic state in the life cycle; continuous adaptation to stress to achieve maximum potential for daily living.	Constant interaction with a variety of environmental factors.
Neuman Systems Model (1972)	Holistic concepts and open systems	Interventions are activated to strengthen lines of defense and resistance to stressors and maintain adaptation.	The person is a complete system: physiologic, psychological, sociocultural, developmental, and spiritual aspects.	Primarily concerned with effects of stress on health; wellness is equilibrium.	Balance between internal and external by adjusting to stress and defending against tension-producing stimuli.
Parse Human Becoming Theory (1981)	Man's reality is given meaning through lived experiences	A human science and art that uses an abstract body of knowledge to serve people.	Being who is more than the sum of the parts: reaching beyond the limits that a person sets and constantly transforms.	Open process of being and becoming; involves synthesis of values.	Energy is exchanged with the environment.
Watson Human Caring Theory (1988)	Humanitarian and science orientation to human caring processes	Human being to be valued, cared for, respected, nurtured, understood, and assisted.	Complete physical, mental, and social well-being and functioning.	Healing consciousness and self-healing.	Caring and society affect health.

and accepted. Change theory recognizes the dynamic nature of change and the need to constantly evaluate nursing practice. First, the nurse needs to recognize when change is needed. Next, the nurse analyzes the situation to determine what is maintaining the situation and what is working to change it. Then the nurse identifies methods to use in the change process and analyzes the influence of those involved in the change.

PAUL'S CRITICAL-THINKING THEORY

Critical thinking, according to Paul (1993), is an "intellectually disciplined process of actively and skillfully conceptualizing, applying, analyzing, synthesizing, and/or evaluating information gathered from, or generated by, observation, experience, reflection, reasoning, or communication, as a guide to belief and action" (p. 110). In applying Paul's definition, nurses analyze data, develop a patient care plan, implement a plan of action for the patient, and evaluate the plan of care. Certain intellectual values are recognized as pertinent to any subject matter, such as clarity, accuracy, precision, consistency, relevance, sound evidence, good reasons, depth, and fairness (Paul, 1993). Nursing expands upon this process of critical thinking and adapts it to the care of the patient.

Each of these critical-thinking skills is learned in the context of nursing and in the application to patient care. Chapter 4 explores more fully the concept of critical thinking in nursing.

ROSENSTOCK'S HEALTH BELIEF MODEL

Rosenstock (1974) developed the psychological Health Belief Model. Originally, the model was designed to predict responses of patients to treatment, but recently the model has been used to predict more general health behaviors. The model addresses possible reasons for why a patient may not

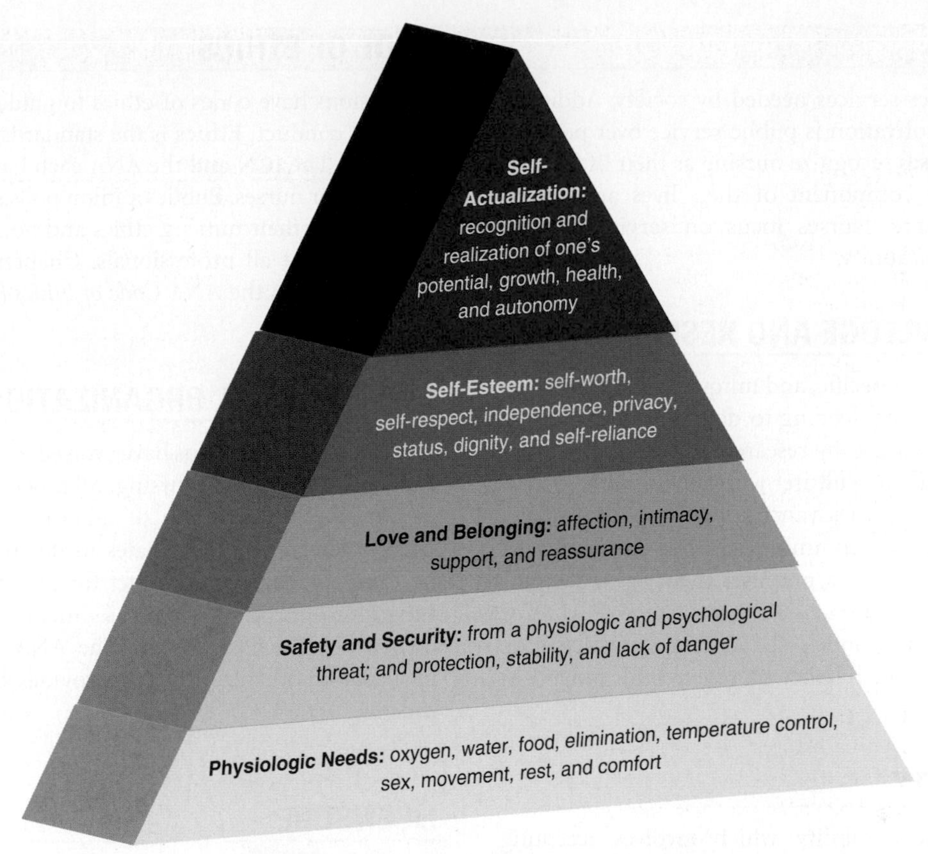

FIGURE 1-6 Maslow's hierarchy of needs.

comply with recommended health promotion behaviors. This model is especially useful to nurses as they educate patients. Rosenstock's Health Belief Model (Figure 1-7) is based on four core beliefs of people's perceptions by their own assessment:

- Perceived susceptibility of the risk of getting the condition
- Perceived severity of the seriousness of the condition and its potential consequences
- Perceived barriers of the influences that facilitate or discourage adoption of the promoted behavior
- Perceived benefits of the positive consequences of adopting the behavior

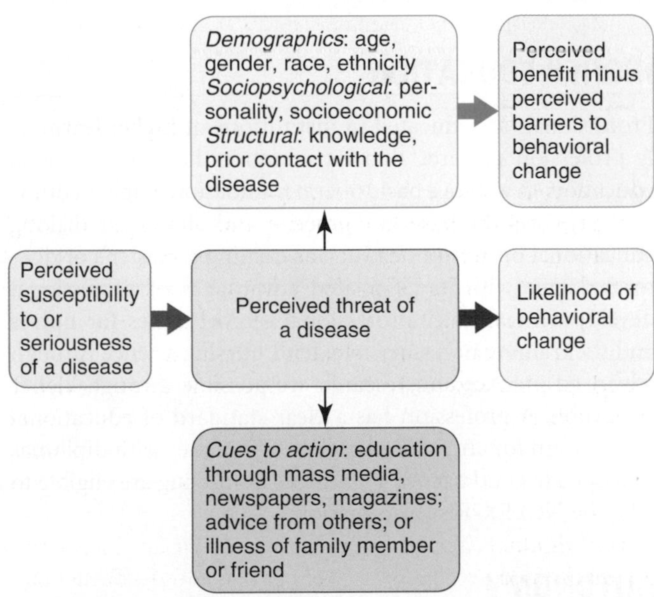

FIGURE 1-7 Rosenstock's Health Belief Model.

CRITERIA FOR A PROFESSION LO 1.6

As stated earlier, a profession is an occupation that requires at a minimum specialized training and a specialized body of knowledge. Nursing meets these requirements. Thus nursing is considered to be a profession. Specific criteria or characteristics are used to further define status as a profession. The sociologist Flexner (2001) first published a list of such criteria in 1915 that often is used as a benchmark for determining the status of an occupation as a profession.

ALTRUISM

A profession provides services needed by society. Additionally, practitioners' motivation is public service over personal gain (altruism). Nurses recognize nursing as their life's work, being an important component of their lives and clearly defining who they are. Nurses focus on service to their patients and the community.

BODY OF KNOWLEDGE AND RESEARCH

There is a well-defined, specific, and unique body of theoretical knowledge in nursing, leading to defined skills, abilities, and norms, that is enlarged by research. A profession is distinguished by a specific culture with norms and values common to its members. To advance knowledge in their field, professionals publish and communicate their knowledge. A profession develops, evaluates, and uses theory as a basis for practice. Nursing has been based on theory since the days of Nightingale. Numerous models for nursing practice have been developed. Nursing's reliance on research for practice is considered EBP.

ACCOUNTABILITY

Nursing requires accountability, which involves accepting responsibility for actions and omissions. Accountability has legal, ethical, and professional implications. It is essential for developing trusting relationships with patients and coworkers.

HIGHER EDUCATION

Professionals are educated in institutions of higher learning. A profession requires that its members have an extended education, as well as a basic liberal foundation. Higher education provides the basis for practice and allows for lifelong educational opportunities such as earning a master's or doctoral degree with its associated advantages of professional development. Greater professional opportunities for nurses and the training necessary to extend nursing science through advanced practice and research are possible through higher education. A profession has a clear standard of educational preparation for entry into practice. Graduates with diplomas or associate's and bachelor's degrees in nursing are eligible to take the NCLEX-RN examination.

AUTONOMY

Members of a profession have autonomy in decision making and practice and are self-regulating in that they develop their own policies in collaboration with one another. Nursing professionals make independent decisions within their scope of practice and are responsible for the results and consequences of those decisions.

CODE OF ETHICS

Professions have codes of ethics to guide decisions for practice and conduct. **Ethics** is the standards of right and wrong behavior. The ICN and the ANA each have developed a code of ethics for nurses. Public opinion polls show that nurses are admired for their nursing ethics and honesty by rating them the highest of all professionals. Chapter 11 provides more information on the *ANA Code of Ethics for Nurses.*

PROFESSIONAL ORGANIZATION

Numerous organizations have evolved to support and encourage high standards in nursing. Members participate in these organizations, which aim to support and advance nursing. Each organization participates in determining responsibilities and standards of conduct for individual members and the group and in regulating its members' adherence to its own professional standards. The ANA is an example of a professional organization that provides standards of nursing practice.

LICENSURE

A profession is committed to competence and has a legally recognized license. Members are accountable for continuing their education. An RN is committed to professional development and is required to continue to learn and maintain competency. All licensed nurses keep their knowledge base current by formal and informal continuing education and can demonstrate competency when required. Although there is more than one educational method of becoming a nurse, attainment of the legal right to practice as a RN in the United States is contingent on passing a standardized licensing examination.

DIVERSITY

"Inherent in nursing is respect for human rights, including cultural rights, the right to life and choice, to dignity and to be treated with respect. Nursing care is respectful of and unrestricted by considerations of age, colour, creed, culture, disability or illness, gender, sexual orientation, nationality, politics, race or social status" (ICN, 2012, p. 1). Diversity includes developmental aspects, morphologic aspects (body frame size/obesity), religion, and ethnicity. In providing care, the nurse promotes an environment in which the human rights, values, customs, and spiritual beliefs of the individual, family, and community are respected. To respect the diversity of patients, nurses practice culturally competent care as defined in the Diversity Considerations box. Chapter 21 discusses the topic of diversity in detail.

DIVERSITY CONSIDERATIONS

Culture

- *Cultural and linguistic competence* is a set of behaviors, attitudes, and policies that come together among health care professionals and allow for effective work in cross-cultural situations.
- *Culture* is the integrated patterns of human behavior that include the language, thoughts, communications, actions, customs, beliefs, values, and institutions of racial, ethnic, religious, or social groups.
- *Competence* implies having the ability to function effectively within the context of the cultural beliefs, behaviors, and needs presented by patients.
- **Cultural competence** is a method of bringing health care providers together to discuss health concerns whereby cultural differences enhance, rather than hinder, the conversation through a respectful atmosphere responsive to the health beliefs, practices, and cultural and linguistic needs of diverse patients.

PRACTICE GUIDELINES LO 1.7

The profession of nursing is guided by standards of practice and nurse practice acts. The Standards of Nursing Practice published by the ANA help to ensure quality care and serve as legal criteria for adequate patient care. ANA standards have two parts. The first part, the standards of practice, includes six responsibilities for the nursing process: assessment, diagnosis, outcomes identification, planning, implementation, and evaluation (ANA, 2010). Nurses providing direct patient care continuously follow these standards as they utilize the nursing process. Further discussion of the nursing process can be found in Chapter 5.

The second part of Standards of Nursing Practice focuses on professional performance, which includes ethics, education, evidence-based practice and research, quality of practice, communication, leadership, collaboration, professional practice evaluation, resource utilization, and environmental health (ANA, 2010). Nurses who attend continuing education conferences or further their education; use evidence to guide their nursing practice; or communicate and collaborate with patients and other professionals are practicing within the standards.

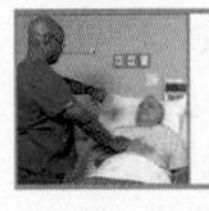

3. Which of the ANA Standards of Nursing Practice is Chris exhibiting during the shift?

Nurse practice acts provide the scope of practice defined by each state or jurisdiction and set forth the legal limits of nursing practice. These acts are laws that the nurse must be familiar with to function in practice. Nurse practice acts are worded in broad legal terms that need to be interpreted by nurses to be clearly understood within the context of their profession. A *scope of practice* defines the boundaries of the practice of nursing and clarifies how it may intersect with other professions or disciplines. In addition to adhering to nurse practice acts, nurses must function within the policies and procedures of the facility in which they are employed.

Guiding the nurse's professional practice are ethical behaviors. It is essential that nurses understand and incorporate basic concepts of ethics into their practice. The main concepts in nursing ethics are accountability, advocacy, autonomy (be independent and self-motivated), beneficence (act in the best interest of the patient), confidentiality, fidelity (keep promises), justice (relate to others with fairness and equality), nonmaleficence (do no harm), responsibility, and veracity (be truthful). As an example, the nurse holds in confidence personal information and uses judgment in sharing this information about a patient. Ethical guidelines direct the nurse's decision making in routine situations and in ethical dilemmas. *ANA's Principles for Social Networking and the Nurse* (ANA, 2011) outlines six principles that nurses must follow to protect patient privacy and maintain professional boundaries. The ANA *Code of Ethics for Nurses* is discussed in detail in Chapter 11.

SOCIALIZATION AND TRANSFORMATION INTO NURSING LO 1.8

Socialization to professional nursing is a process that involves learning the theory and skills necessary for the role of nurse. Internalizing this specific role allows the nurse to participate as a member of the profession. During this process of socialization to nursing, the student's knowledge base, attitudes, and values are affected regarding nursing practice. This process allows the person to grow both professionally and personally as the student internalizes a full understanding of the profession. This initial transformation continues after the student graduates and acquires experience while working and pursuing further education. Transformation to being a nurse requires students to become response-based practitioners with the abillity to recognize the complexity of a situation and prioritize concerns (Benner et al, 2010).

Benner (2001) used Dreyfus's (1980) model of skill acquisition in her description of novice to expert (Figure 1-8). Benner's model identifies five levels of proficiency: novice, advanced beginner, competent, proficient, and expert. The student nurse progresses from novice to advanced beginner during nursing school and attains the competent level after approximately 2 to 3 years of work experience after graduation.

The Essentials of Baccalaureate Education for Professional Nursing Practice are provided and updated by the American Association of Colleges of Nursing (AACN) (2008). The document offers a framework for the education of professional nurses with outcomes for students to meet. If students meet these outcomes, their socialization into the role of a

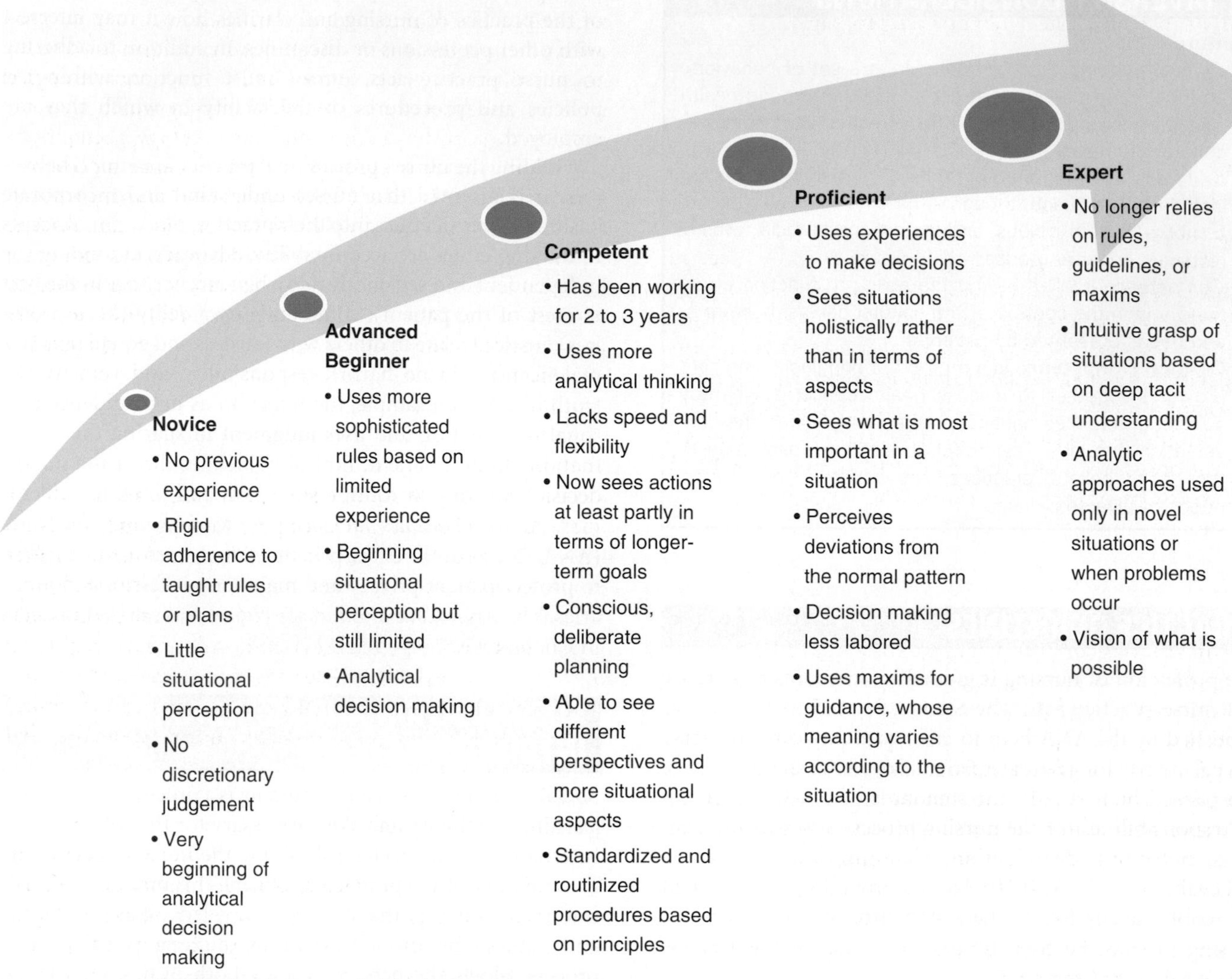

FIGURE 1-8 Benner's Novice to Expert Model. (From Benner P: *From novice to expert: excellence and power in clinical nursing practice,* Upper Saddle River, N.J., 2001, Prentice Hall.)

professional nurse will have begun. The first eight essentials describe the knowledge, skills, and attitudes required of the nursing student to meet the desired outcome. The ninth essential describes the practice of the nurse upon graduation from a baccalaureate program. In addition, other AACN documents outline competencies for nurses at the graduate education level.

The National League for Nursing (NLN) outlines and updates competencies for practical, associate, baccalaureate, and graduate nursing education programs. The titles of the competencies for each type of education program are "Human Flourishing," "Nursing Judgment," "Professional Identity," and "Spirit of Inquiry." The outcomes for each competency are progressively more complex at each educational level (NLN, 2010).

NURSING PRACTICE LICENSURE AND GRADUATE SPECIALTIES LO 1.9

Nursing provides various educational paths to practice. The two types of licensed nurses, the LVN/LPN and the RN, have different scopes of practice, but both must obtain a license to practice by passing a specific licensure examination. **Licensure** is the granting of a license that provides legal permission to practice. There are three accrediting bodies for schools and colleges of nursing: the AACN's Commission on Collegiate Nursing Education (CCNE), the Accrediting Commission for Education in Nursing (ACEN), and the recently formed NLN Commission for Nursing Education Accreditation (CNEA). The CCNE accredits baccalaureate and graduate nursing programs; the CNEA and the ACEN accredit a variety of different nursing programs including practical, diploma, associate, baccalaureate, and graduate programs.

LICENSED PRACTICAL NURSE OR LICENSED VOCATIONAL NURSE

LPNs, (or LVNs as they are called in California and Texas), are not RNs. They complete an educational program consisting of 12 to 18 months of training, and then they must pass the National Council Licensure Examination for Practical Nurses (NCLEX-PN) to practice as an LPN/LVN. They are under the supervision of an RN in most institutions and are able to collect data but cannot perform an assessment requiring decision making, cannot formulate a nursing diagnosis, and cannot initiate a care plan. They may update care plans and administer medications with the exception of certain IV medications. Later they may choose to complete an LPN/LVN-to-RN program to become an RN.

REGISTERED NURSE

To obtain the RN credential, a person must graduate from an accredited school of nursing and pass a state licensing examination called the National Council Licensure Examination for Registered Nurses (NCLEX-RN). The student may attend a 2- or 4-year degree program or a 3-year diploma program. Entry-level pay for graduates from all types of programs who have passed their NCLEX examinations is similar. In many facilities, nurses must have a bachelor's degree to advance into management or to hold specialized positions.

Associate Degree in Nursing

Associate Degree in Nursing (ADN) programs usually are conducted in a community college setting. Most programs require that students complete courses in psychology, human growth and development, biology, microbiology, and anatomy and physiology as a basis before they begin their nursing coursework. The nursing curriculum focuses on adult acute and chronic disease; maternal/child health; pediatrics; and psychiatric/mental health nursing. ADN RNs may return to school to earn a bachelor's degree or higher in an RN-to-BSN or RN-to-MSN program.

Diploma Programs

Generally associated with a hospital, the Diploma in Nursing program combines classroom and clinical instruction, usually over a period of 3 years. The number of such programs has decreased as nursing education has shifted to academic institutions.

Bachelor of Science in Nursing

The university-based Bachelor of Science in Nursing (BSN) degree provides the nursing theory, sciences, humanities, and behavioral science preparation necessary for professional nursing responsibilities and the knowledge base in research necessary for advanced education. Bachelor's degree programs include community health and management courses beyond those traditionally provided in an associate degree program. Nursing theory, bioethics, management, research and statistics, health assessment, pharmacology, pathophysiology, and electives in complex nursing processes are covered. The Institute of Medicine (IOM) report *The Future of Nursing: Leading Change, Advancing Health* recommends that 80% of nurses in the United States be at least baccalaureate-educated by 2020, while encouraging health care organizations to support nurses with associate degrees or diplomas to enter baccalaureate programs within 5 years of graduation (IOM, 2011).

MASTER OF SCIENCE IN NURSING

When obtaining a master's degree in nursing, called a Master of Science in Nursing (MSN) degree, the nurse may focus on a specific area of advanced practice. There are four specialties in which nurses provide direct patient care in advanced practice roles: certified nurse midwife (CNM), nurse practitioner (NP), clinical nurse specialist (CNS), and certified registered nurse anesthetist (CRNA). Four additional advanced practice roles that do not always involve direct patient care are clinical nurse leader (CNL), nurse educator, nurse researcher, and nurse administrator.

Advanced Practice Nurses

Advanced practice registered nurse (APRN) is a designation for an RN who has met advanced educational and clinical practice requirements at a minimum of a master's degree level and provides at least some level of direct care to patient populations. APRNs have acquired theoretical research–based and practical knowledge as part of the graduate education and are either certified or approved to practice in their expanded, specialized roles. Advanced practice nurses have a set of core competencies (Hamric, 2014):

- Direct clinical practice
- Collaboration
- Expert coaching and guidance
- Research
- Ethical decision making
- Consultation
- Leadership

CNMs provide well-gynecologic and low-risk obstetric care and attend births in hospitals, birth centers, and homes. NPs work in clinics, nursing homes, hospitals, or private offices and are qualified to provide a wide range of primary and preventive health care services, prescribe medication, and diagnose and treat illnesses and injuries. NPs may focus on a specific population, working in fields such as pediatrics or gerontology, or may have a more general family practice. NPs or physicians may be the patient's primary care provider.

CNSs work in hospitals, clinics, nursing homes, private offices, and community-based settings and manage a wide range of physical and mental health problems. They may work in consultation, research, or education. CRNAs, whose role is the oldest of the advanced nursing specialties, administer much of the anesthetics given to patients in the United States.

Other Advanced Roles

A new role is that of the CNL, who oversees the integration of care for a distinct group of patients and may actively provide direct patient care in complex situations utilizing evidence-based practice. This clinician functions as part of an interprofessional team and is not in an administration or management role. The CNL is a leader in the health care delivery system in all settings in which health care is delivered, not just the acute care setting. Implementation of this role varies across settings.

A master's degree can lead to one of the advanced practice roles that may not have a direct patient care component. The nurse educator option prepares nurses to practice as faculty in academic settings, such as colleges, universities, hospital-based schools of nursing, and technical schools, or as staff development educators in health care facilities. Nurse educators combine their clinical abilities with responsibilities related to designing curricula, teaching and guiding learners, evaluating learning and program outcomes, advising students, and engaging in scholarly work.

Two other options for nurses with master's degrees are researcher and administrator. Nurse researchers use statistical methodologies to discover or establish facts, principles, or relationships. They may be involved in clinical trials with patients or other clinical research regarding patient care. Nurse administrators coordinate the use of human, financial, and technological resources to provide patient care services. Positions include facilitator, manager, director, chief nurse executive, and vice president of nursing.

DOCTOR OF PHILOSOPHY AND DOCTOR OF NURSING PRACTICE

Doctoral nursing education can result in a doctor of philosophy (PhD) degree. This degree prepares nurses for leadership roles in research, teaching, and administration that are essential to advancing nursing as a profession. A newer practice-focused doctoral degree is the doctor of nursing practice (DNP), which concentrates on the clinical aspects of nursing. DNP specialties include the four advanced practice roles of NP, CNS, CNM, and CRNA. In addition, some DNPs focus on the CNL option.

CERTIFICATIONS AND PROFESSIONAL NURSING ORGANIZATIONS LO 1.10

Nurses may pursue certifications in specialty areas after they have practiced for several years. Nurses may choose membership in professional nursing organizations to network, remain current in their practice, and have access to current research.

CERTIFICATIONS

Nurses may become certified in a specialty. Each nursing certification has minimum work experience and education requirements. After meeting required criteria, nurses must pass an examination and maintain specific continuing education and work requirements. There are certifications for RNs as well as nurses with master's degrees and other advanced practice nurses.

The American Nurses Credentialing Center (ANCC) (2012) awards Magnet Recognition to hospitals that have shown excellence and innovation in nursing. Individual nurses in a variety of practice roles can seek certification through ANCC. For a complete list of specialties available, visit *www.nursecredentialing.org/certification.aspx#specialty*.

PROFESSIONAL ORGANIZATIONS

Belonging to a professional organization is an important aspect of one's profession. Nursing organizations enable the nurse to have access to current information and resources as well as a voice in the profession. Nursing organizations include the ANA, the NLN, the ICN, Sigma Theta Tau International Honor Society of Nursing, and the National Student Nurses Association (NSNA). Participating in NSNA while in nursing school is an important beginning to a nurse's professional career. There are also more than 80 specialty organizations, such as the American Association of Critical Care Nurses (AACN), the Emergency Nurses Association, the National Association of School Nurses (NASN), and the Oncology Nurses Society.

FUTURE DIRECTIONS LO 1.11

People worldwide are living longer and healthier lives (Figure 1-9). This increase in lifespan has led to a rapidly increasing population of those 65 years of age and older. Projections indicate that by 2030, this group will total 1 billion: One person of every eight in the world will be 65 or older (National Institute on Aging, 2011). The greatest increases are seen in developing countries. Life expectancy is increasing, placing a greater burden on health care systems worldwide.

Larger portions of the population are in retirement, with a consequent strain on both health and pension systems. As the Baby Boomers enter retirement, providing health care to this large portion of the population in the United States and other nations becomes a concern. This aging population will require more nurses to care for them. This need is one factor related to the current nursing shortage.

As the 21st century began, many organizations worked to make safety in health care a priority. The AACN's Quality and

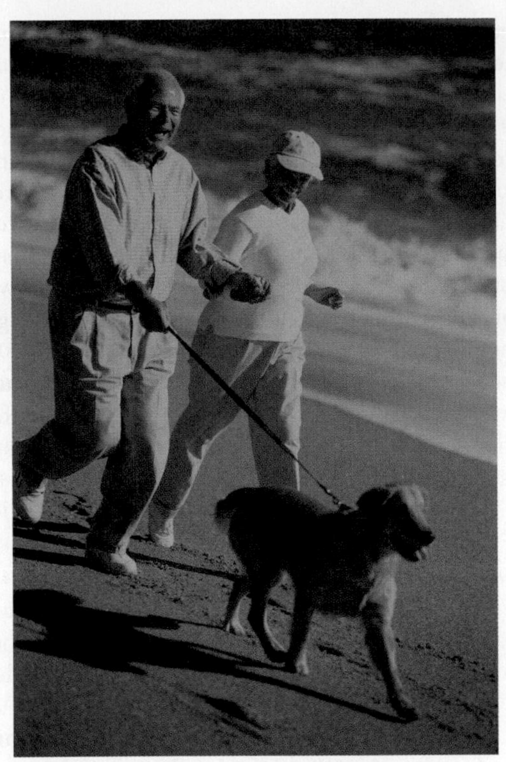

FIGURE 1-9 The growing population of older adults will require more nurses to care for them.

Safety Education for Nurses (QSEN) program, the IOM's report *The Future of Nursing: Leading Change, Advancing Health*, and The Joint Commission's National Patient Safety Goals will guide nurses into the future as safe and caring practitioners.

NURSING SHORTAGE

The World Health Organization's (WHO) report *A Global Survey Monitoring Progress in Nursing and Midwifery* (WHO, 2010) states that 70% of countries that participated in the survey were experiencing a nursing and midwifery shortage. The report called for improvements in training, recruitment, and retention of nurses.

Buerhaus and colleagues (Buerhaus, Staiger, and Auerbach, 2009) forecast that in the United States, the shortage of nurses could reach 500,000 by 2025. With the changing demographics of an increasing elderly population and the aging nursing workforce, the total number of new nurses needed continues to grow. In March 2008, the Council on Physician and Nurse Supply, an independent group of health care leaders based at the University of Pennsylvania, determined that 30,000 additional nurses should be graduated annually. To meet this need, more nursing faculty members are required. The lack of faculty is an impediment to increasing nursing school enrollment, and many faculty members are nearing retirement age.

With an insufficient number of nurses to care for patients, nurses face an increased level of stress, which can be expected to have an adverse impact on job satisfaction. This work situation can cause nurses to leave the profession, which further contributes to the nursing shortage and affects overall access to health care. Therefore nursing is a profession that will continue to be in demand.

QUALITY AND SAFETY EDUCATION FOR NURSES

The QSEN initiative, funded by the Robert Wood Johnson Foundation, adapted the IOM competencies for nursing. The IOM report *Health Professions Education: A Bridge to Quality* (IOM, 2003) outlined five core areas of proficiency for students and professionals: delivering patient-centered care, working as part of an interdisciplinary team, practicing evidence-based medicine, focusing on quality improvement, and using information technology. QSEN adds safety as a competency. The six QSEN competencies are patient-centered care, teamwork and collaboration, evidence-based practice, quality improvement, safety, and informatics. Knowledge, skills, and attitudes for each competency were developed for use in prelicensure nursing education (Cronenwett et al, 2007) and graduate education.

INSTITUTE OF MEDICINE REPORT

The Future of Nursing: Leading Change, Advancing Health (IOM, 2011) identified several goals for nursing in the United States:

- Nurses should practice to the full extent of their education and training.
- Nurses should achieve higher levels of education and training through an improved education system that promotes seamless academic progression.
- Nurses should be full partners with physicians and other health care professionals in redesigning health care in the United States.
- Effective workforce planning and policy making require better data collection and an improved information infrastructure.

The report outlined recommendations and specific actions to achieve these goals.

NATIONAL PATIENT SAFETY GOALS

The Joint Commission is the accrediting organization for health care facilities in the United States. In 2003 The Joint Commission established the first set of National Patient Safety Goals to improve patient safety for a variety of accredited health care facilities, including hospitals. The hospital goals for 2014 include the following broad categories:

- Identify patients correctly
- Improve staff communication

- Use medicines safely
- Use alarms safely
- Prevent infection
- Identify patient safety risks
- Prevent mistakes in surgery

Each category has specific elements of performance that are required for the health care worker to meet the goals (The Joint Commission, 2014). As new problems in patient care emerge, the safety goals are reassessed and revised.

INDEPENDENT NURSING PRACTICE

As previously mentioned, one characteristic of a profession is autonomy. Nurses have attained increased autonomy over time. Nursing has control over its education, practice, and legal recognition through licensure. State nurse practice acts regulate scope of practice, and state board examinations are required to practice. Nursing has a code of ethics that reflects current issues. This autonomy leads to functioning independently of any other profession or external entity. As employees of organizations, nurses do not always have full freedom in deciding on patient care within the defined scope of nursing practice. Striving toward this independence is a goal of nursing. Advanced practice nurses in some states work in collaboration with a physician, but NPs are increasing independence in their practice. The introduction of the DNP as the practice doctoral degree for advanced practice nurses is intended to place them on the same level as those with other professional degrees. Thus nursing continues to establish itself as a full-fledged profession.

SUMMARY OF LEARNING OUTCOMES

LO 1.1 *Define nursing:* Nursing is a holistic profession that addresses the many dimensions necessary to fully care for a patient.

LO 1.2 *Differentiate among the functions and roles of nurses:* Nurses provide care to patients while functioning in multiple roles as care provider, educator, advocate, leader, change agent, manager, researcher, collaborator, and delegator.

LO 1.3 *Describe historical events in the evolution of nursing:* Historically, the nursing profession has evolved from a religious and military background to meet the nursing needs of society.

LO 1.4 *Summarize nursing theories:* Nurses use nursing theories to guide their practice. Nursing theories began with Florence Nightingale's work in 1860 and continue to the present. Each theory discusses the four concepts of nursing, person, health, and environment.

LO 1.5 *Identify non-nursing theories that influence nursing practice:* Non-nursing theories that influence nursing practice include systems theory, developmental theory, change theory, theory of human needs, and leadership theories.

LO 1.6 *Articulate the criteria of a profession as applied to nursing:* Nursing is evaluated against the criteria of a profession, which include altruism, body of knowledge, accountability, higher education, autonomy, code of ethics, professional organization, and licensure.

LO 1.7 *Discuss standards of practice and nurse practice acts:* ANA standards of practice guide and direct the practice of nursing; state nurse practice acts define nurses' scope of practice.

LO 1.8 *Describe the socialization and transformation process of a nurse:* Socialization into the nursing profession follows a process from novice to advanced beginner during nursing school. The nurse reaches the competent level after several years of practice. Transformation takes place when the student gains the ability to perceive and prioritize the situational needs of complex care.

LO 1.9 *Explain the levels of educational preparation in nursing and differentiate among the nurse's roles depending on education:* Numerous levels of education (diploma, associate, baccalaureate, master's, and doctoral degrees) and career opportunities in nursing can be pursued.

LO 1.10 *List possible certifications in various arenas of nursing and professional organizations in nursing:* Many different certifications are available to nurses who meet specific requirements and pass qualifying examinations. Nursing organizations represent all nurses and nursing specialties.

LO 1.11 *Discuss the future directions in nursing:* Future directions in nursing include dealing with the nursing shortage, implementing new patient safety programs, and exploring the role of the independent nurse.

Responses to the critical-thinking questions are available at *http://evolve.elsevier.com/YoostCrawford/fundamentals/*.

REVIEW QUESTIONS

1. In comparing the American Nurses Association (ANA) and International Council of Nurses (ICN) definitions of nursing, what component does the ICN mention that is not included in ANA's definition and is indicative of a more global focus?
   a. Advocacy
   b. Health promotion
   c. Shaping health policy
   d. Prevention of illness
2. A profession has specific characteristics. In regard to how nursing meets these characteristics, which criteria are consistent and standardized processes? *(Select all that apply.)*
   a. Code of ethics
   b. Licensing
   c. Body of knowledge
   d. Educational preparation
   e. Altruism
3. Which specific aspect of a profession does the development of theories provide?
   a. Altruism
   b. Body of knowledge
   c. Autonomy
   d. Accountability
4. Health care workers are discussing a diverse group of patients respectfully and are being responsive to the health beliefs and practices of these patients. What important aspect of nursing professional practice are they exhibiting?
   a. Autonomy
   b. Accountability
   c. Cultural competence
   d. Leadership
5. A nurse makes a medication error, immediately assesses the patient, and reports the error to the nurse manager and the primary care provider. Which characteristic of a professional is the nurse demonstrating?
   a. Autonomy
   b. Collaboration
   c. Accountability
   d. Altruism
6. Which components are included in the American Nurses Association (ANA) standards? *(Select all that apply.)*
   a. Standards for professional performance
   b. A code of ethics
   c. Standards of care
   d. Legal scope of practice
   e. Licensure requirements
7. Which core competency of advanced practice nursing is the Master of Science in Nursing (MSN) nurse educator exhibiting when counseling a student in therapeutic communication techniques?
   a. Leadership
   b. Ethical decision making
   c. Direct clinical practice
   d. Expert coaching
8. Which statements describe a component discussed in nursing theories? *(Select all that apply.)*
   a. Optimal functioning of the patient
   b. Interaction with components of the environment
   c. Conceptual makeup of the hospital administration
   d. The illness and health concept
   e. Safety aspect of medication administration
9. Which factors are affecting the nursing shortage? *(Select all that apply.)*
   a. Aging faculty
   b. Increasing elderly population
   c. Job satisfaction due to adequate number of nurses
   d. Aging nursing workforce
   e. Greater autonomy for nurses
10. A nurse has performed a physical examination of the patient and reviewed the laboratory and diagnostic test results on the patient's chart. The nurse is performing which specific nursing function?
    a. Diagnosis
    b. Assessment
    c. Education
    d. Advocacy

Answers and rationales for the review questions are available at *http://evolve.elsevier.com/YoostCrawford/fundamentals/*.

REFERENCES

Agency for Healthcare Research and Quality: *Health literacy interventions and outcomes: An updated systematic review,* Evidence Report/Technology Assessment No. 199, Rockville, Md, 2011, Author.

Alligood M, Tomey A: *Nursing theorists and their work,* ed. 7, St. Louis, 2014, Mosby.

American Association of Colleges of Nursing: *The essentials of baccalaureate education for professional nursing practice,* Washington, D.C., 2008, Author.

American Nurses Association (ANA): *Nursing: Scope and standards of practice,* ed. 2, Silver Spring, Md, 2010, Author.

American Nurses Association (ANA): *ANA's principles for social networking and the nurse,* Silver Spring, Md., 2011, Author.
American Nurses Credentialing Center: ANCC certification center, 2012. Retrieved from *www.nursecredentialing.org/certification.aspx#specialty.*
Benner P: *From novice to expert: Excellence and power in clinical nursing practice,* Upper Saddle River, N.J., 2001, Prentice Hall.
Benner P, Sutphen M, Leonard V, Day L: *Educating nurses: A call for radical transformation,* San Francisco, 2010, Jossey-Bass.
Buerhaus P, Staiger D, Auerbach D: *The future of the nursing workforce in the United States: Data, trends, and implications,* Sudbury, Mass., 2009, Jones & Bartlett Publishers.
Cronenwett L, Sherwood G, Barnsteiner J, et al: Quality and safety education for nurses, *Nurs Outlook* 55(3):122-131, 2007.
Dreyfus HL, Dreyfus SE: *A five-stage model of the mental activities involved in directed skill acquisition,* Washington, D.C., 1980, Storming Media. Oxford, England, Basil Blackwell.
Erikson EH: *Identity: Youth and crisis,* New York, 1968, Norton.
Fawcett J, DeSanto-Madeya S: *Contemporary nursing knowledge: Analysis and evaluation of nursing models and theories,* ed. 3, Philadelphia, 2013, F.A. Davis.
Flexner A: Is social work a profession? *Res Soc Work Pract* 11(2):152-165, 2001.
Hamric AB: A definition of advanced practice nursing. In AB Hamric, JA Spross, CM Hanson (Eds): *Advanced practice nursing: An integrative approach* (pp. 75-94), St. Louis, 2014, Saunders.
Henderson V: *The nature of nursing: A definition and its implications for practice, research, and education,* New York, 1966, Macmillan.
International Council of Nurses: Definition of nursing, 2010. Retrieved from *www.icn.ch/about-icn/icn-definition-of-nursing.*
International Council of Nurses. *ICN code of ethics for nurses,* Geneva, Switzerland, 2012, Author.
The Joint Commission: 2014 national patient safety goals, 2014. Retrieved from *www.jointcommission.org/assets/1/6/HAP_NPSG_Chapter_2014.pdf.*
King IM: *Toward a theory of nursing,* New York, 1971, Wiley.
Larabee J: *Nurse to nurse evidence-based practice,* New York, 2009, McGraw-Hill.
Lewin K: *Field theory in social science,* New York, 1951, Harper & Row.
McKenna H, Slevin O: *Vital notes for nurses: Nursing models, theories and practice,* West Sussex, UK, 2008, Wiley-Blackwell.
National Institute on Aging: *Why population aging matters: A global perspective,* Washington, D.C., 2011, Author.
National League for Nursing (NLN): *Outcomes and competencies for graduates of practical/vocational, diploma, associate degree, baccalaureate, master's, practice doctorate, and research doctorate programs in nursing,* New York, 2010, Author.
Neuman B: *The Neuman Systems Model: Application to nursing education and practice,* New York, 1972, Appleton-Century-Crofts.
Nightingale F: *Notes on nursing: What it is and what it is not,* New York, 1860, D. Appleton & Co.
Orem DE: *Nursing: Concepts of practice,* ed. 3, New York, 1971, McGraw-Hill.
Parse RR: *Man-living-health: Theory of nursing,* New York, 1981, Wiley.
Paul R: *Critical thinking: How to prepare students for a rapidly changing world,* Rohnert Park, Calif., 1993, Center for Critical Thinking and Moral Critique.
Peplau HE: *Interpersonal relations in nursing,* New York, 1952, Putnam.
Rogers ME: *Theoretical basis of nursing,* Philadelphia, 1970, F.A. Davis.
Rosenstock I: Historical origin of the health belief model. *Health Educ Monogr* 2:334, 1974.
Roy C: Adaptation: A conceptual framework for nursing. *Nurs Outlook* 18:42-45, 1970.
U.S. Department of Health and Human Services: *Healthy People 2020: Understanding and improving health,* Washington, DC, 2010, U.S. Government Printing Office.
U.S. Institute of Medicine: *Health professions education: A bridge to quality,* Washington, D.C., 2003, National Academies Press.
U.S. Institute of Medicine: *The future of nursing: Leading change, advancing health,* Washington, D.C., 2011, National Academies Press.
Watson J: *Nursing: Human science, human care: A theory of nursing,* New York, 1988, National League for Nursing.
World Health Organization (WHO): A global survey monitoring progress in nursing and midwifery, 2010. Retrieved from *www.who.int/hrh/nursing_midwifery/en.*

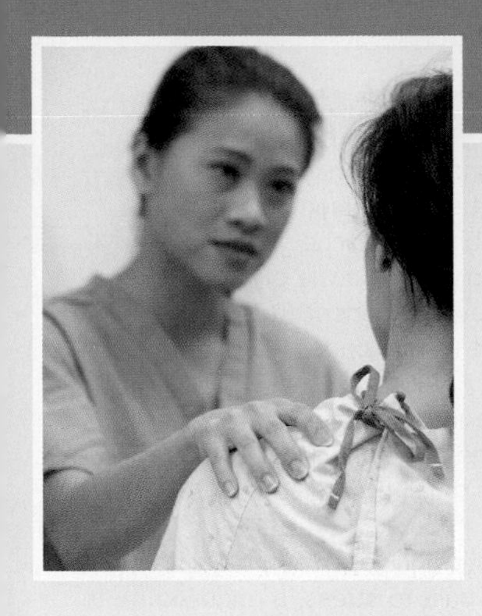

CHAPTER 2

Values, Beliefs, and Caring

EVOLVE WEBSITE

http://evolve.elsevier.com/YoostCrawford/fundamentals/

- Additional Evolve-Only Review Questions With Answers
- Answers and Rationales for Text Review Questions
- Answers to Critical-Thinking Questions
- Case Study With Questions
- Glossary

LEARNING OUTCOMES

Comprehension of this chapter's content will provide students with the ability to:

LO 2.1 Describe the differences between beliefs and values and how they develop.

LO 2.2 Explain the use of the values clarification process in dealing with a values conflict.

LO 2.3 Summarize how the beliefs of nurses and patients influence health care.

LO 2.4 Discuss the major concepts of four nursing theories of caring.

LO 2.5 Articulate ways in which nurses develop into caring professionals.

LO 2.6 Identify behaviors that demonstrate caring.

KEY TERMS

belief, p. 22
caring, p. 26
codependency, p. 29
first-order beliefs, p. 22
generalizations, p. 23
higher-order beliefs, p. 23
paradigms, p. 25
prejudice, p. 23
stereotype, p. 23
values, p. 22
values clarification, p. 24
values conflict, p. 24
values system, p. 23

CASE STUDY

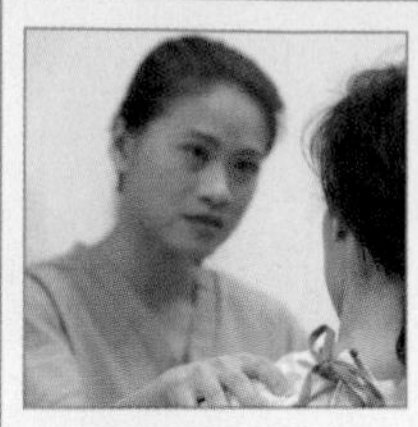

Hwa Yeon Lee calls herself "Clara" for the benefit of her American friends who cannot pronounce her Korean name. She is a 20-year-old college student who arrives in the emergency department accompanied by an older Korean man, who is a longtime friend of her family. Her major complaint is a throbbing headache, which she reports "has not let up for the past 3 days and nights." She rates the pain as an 8 or 9 on a scale of 0 to 10. Hwa expresses concern that "it might be something serious," because she has never experienced anything like this before. In fact, she states, "I can't remember ever having a headache that lasted longer than a half hour."

While awaiting diagnostic test results, Hwa tells the nurse that her parents still live in a small village in Korea and sacrificed a great deal to send her to the United States to attend college. She traveled to this country alone at the age of 16 and lived with her parents' friends until she graduated from high school. She now lives in a one-room apartment near the small private college that she attends.

When diagnostic test results show no abnormalities, the physician writes a prescription for a mild narcotic analgesic (pain medication) without asking Hwa what type of treatment she typically prefers for pain relief. He attributes the pain to stress, a migraine headache, or possibly hormones, because her menstrual period began the day before. When the nurse tries to administer the medication to Hwa, she respectfully refuses it, saying, "No, thank you." Hwa explains that she came to the emergency department only to find out if the cause was something serious, but now that she knows it is not, she prefers alternative therapy such as meditation or acupuncture for pain relief. After Hwa leaves, the nurse is bewildered and somewhat angry over her refusal to take the medication. The nurse turns to a colleague and asks, "Why did she come here if she didn't want our help?"

Refer back to this case study to answer the critical-thinking questions throughout the chapter.

Nurses are called on to provide care for patients with beliefs and values that may be vastly different from their own. In fact, the beliefs of many patients and their families may seem strange or, at times, perplexing to the nurse. In a multicultural practice environment, gaining an understanding of what beliefs and values are, how they develop, and in what ways they shape the behaviors of both patients and nurses will help nurses to assist patients toward better health outcomes (Pescosolido and Olafsdottir, 2010).

BELIEFS AND VALUES LO 2.1

Patients and their families look to nurses to support and guide them through some of the most difficult and vulnerable periods of their lives. They need to know that the nurse will be sensitive to their beliefs and values and will strive to understand how they want to be treated. It is important for nurses to have strong professional values to guide their practice that are consistent with society's expectations of a trusted professional. It is essential that nursing students develop and continue to adhere to critical professional nursing values throughout their careers (LeDuc and Kotzer, 2009). Understanding the importance and the relatedness of beliefs and values is a vital first step.

A **belief** is a mental representation of reality or a person's perceptions about what is right (correct), true, or real, or what the person expects to happen in a given situation (Miller, 2009). In a religious or spiritual sense, to have a belief means to place trust or have faith in a deity such as God or in something such as a religious ritual, tradition, or philosophy (Sartori, 2010). Three types of beliefs are recognized: *zero-order beliefs,* most of which are unconscious, such as object permanence; *first-order beliefs,* which are conscious, typically based on direct experiences; and *higher-order beliefs,* which are generalizations or ideas that are derived from first-order beliefs and reasoning (Bem, 2002).

Values are enduring ideas about what a person considers is the good, the best, and the "right" thing to do and their opposites—the bad, worst, and wrong things to do—and about what is desirable or has worth in life (Rassin, 2010). Values determine the importance and worth of an idea, a belief, an object, or a behavior. Personal values include the life principles that are most important to people and shape their thoughts, feelings, and, ultimately, actions. Values play a large part in how individuals view and evaluate themselves (self-concept) and others. Values strongly influence each person's selection of friends, professional decisions, organizational membership, and support of social causes (Carr and Mitchell, 2007; Rassin, 2010).

FIRST-ORDER BELIEFS

First-order beliefs serve as the foundation or the basis of an individual's belief system (Bem, 2002) (Table 2-1). People begin developing first-order beliefs about what is correct, real, and true in early childhood directly through experiences (e.g., most nurses are female) and indirectly from information shared by authority figures such as parents or teachers (e.g., anyone, regardless of gender, can become a nurse). People continue to develop first-order beliefs into adulthood through both direct experiences and the acquisition of knowledge from a vast number of sources with various degrees of expertise and levels of influence. People seldom question their first-order beliefs and rarely replace one, because to do so would require a great deal of rethinking about both that belief (which has been perceived as real or

TABLE 2-1 **Overview of Beliefs and Values Formation**

FIRST-ORDER BELIEFS	HIGHER-ORDER BELIEFS	VALUES
Purposes		
• Provide basic information about what is real or true • Indicate what a person expects on the basis of information shared or obtained from others • Are the foundation for the formation of all other beliefs	Categorize or bring order to a multitude of ideas	Establish the foundation of self-concept Indicate a person's judgments of ideas, objects, or behavior Provide a framework for decision making Guide life decisions on the basis of what a person views as most important
Derived From		

• Life experiences
• Respected authorities:
  • Parents or caregivers
  • Culture
  • Ethnicity
  • Education
  • Religion
  • Spirituality
	Assumptions based on first-order beliefs
	Inductive reasoning
	Deductive reasoning
		Personal experiences
		Family of origin
		Spirituality
		Religious beliefs
		Cultural/ethnic background
		Education
		Professional development

Examples		
• Most nurses are female. • Anyone, regardless of gender, can become a nurse.	*Generalization*: All nurses wear white uniforms. *Stereotype*: Nurses are more caring than other adults. *Prejudice*: Women are better nurses than men.	Professional nursing values include human dignity, the prevention of suffering, reliability, and faithful relationships between nurses and patients (Rassin, 2010). Others include trust, honesty, discretion, loyalty, integrity, caring, excellence, activism, professionalism, and justice (Grypma, 2009).

true) and similar or closely associated beliefs (Thompson, Teal, Rogers, et al, 2010). Nurses need to keep in mind that presenting information to patients that challenges their first-order beliefs may cause a great deal of emotional or cognitive upset (Rassin, 2010).

HIGHER-ORDER BELIEFS

Higher-order beliefs are ideas derived from a person's first-order beliefs, using either inductive or deductive reasoning (Bem, 2002). In the process of learning, people form **generalizations** (general statements or ideas about people or things) to relate new information to what is already known and to categorize the new information, making it easier to remember or understand. Generalizations may arise at an unconscious level. People may remain unaware of how they came to believe certain ideas in the first place, and even though generalizations are mental abstractions, they may be considered as real and true as first-order beliefs. One of the major problems with generalizations is that they are not true in all instances. When generalizations are treated as if they are always true, they are called *stereotypes.*

A **stereotype** is a conceptualized depiction of a person, a group, or an event that is thought to be typical of all others in that category (Acorn, 2006). One problem with stereotypes is that sometimes people use stereotypes to rationalize personal biases or prejudices. A **prejudice** is a preformed opinion, usually an unfavorable one, about an entire group of people that is based on insufficient knowledge, irrational feelings, or inaccurate stereotypes (Varkey, Chutka, and Lesnick, 2006). Most generalizations and even stereotypes seldom arise out of unkind or pathologic intent but are used by people to remember new information and to categorize their ideas and beliefs. Many stereotypes are of a harmless variety and are replaced as a person's knowledge or personal experiences broaden (Acorn, 2006).

VALUES SYSTEM

A **values system** is a set of somewhat consistent values and measures that are organized hierarchically into a belief system on a continuum of relative importance (Harris, 2010). Anthropologists and social scientists have noted that in every culture, a particular value system prevails and consists of culturally defined moral and ethical principles and rules that are learned in childhood. Each individual possesses a relatively small number of values and may share the same values with others, but to different degrees. A values system helps the person choose between alternatives, resolve values conflicts, and make decisions (Harris, 2010). Within every

DIVERSITY CONSIDERATIONS

Life Span

- Families and cultures have attitudes about what and how to eat that they transmit in the form of values.
- Parents and grandparents use many strategies to transmit their values about healthy eating to their children and grandchildren. Some of the strategies include limiting the purchase of unhealthy foods, involving children in shopping and meal preparation, and engaging children in ongoing conversations about healthful eating and the value of weight control (Kaplan, Kiernan, and James, 2006).

Culture, Ethnicity, and Religion

- In some cultures, parents may arrange marriages for their children. Because adolescents and young adults are exposed to differing values that allow for self-selection of a spouse, a values conflict may become increasingly evident (Seth, 2008).
- Pharmaceutical treatment may be rejected by individuals from some cultures based on traditional beliefs and values. Exploring the implementation of alternative or complementary therapies may help to meet patient needs while demonstrating respect.

Disability

- People with disabilities note that the real problem with being disabled often is not the physical or mental condition that places limits on what they can do but rather the situation of being excluded from society and not permitted to contribute that makes them feel devalued and isolated (Kurz, Saint-Louis, Burke, and Stineman, 2008).
- Nurses demonstrate respect for patients with disabilities by including them in their care as much as possible and seeking to understand what works best for each person, rather than generalizing treatment modalities (Figure 2-1).

Morphology

- Obesity is threatening to overtake malnutrition as the most serious global health problem in both developed and developing countries. The three major contributors to obesity are genetics, food marketing practices, and reduced physical activity. Food corporations have historically exerted a major impact on the values of young people through advertising focused on fast- and processed-food consumption (World Health Organization, 2013).
- Increasing the value that people place on exercise and the consumption of fresh fruits and vegetables is the focus of worldwide strategies to reduce the incidence of obesity.

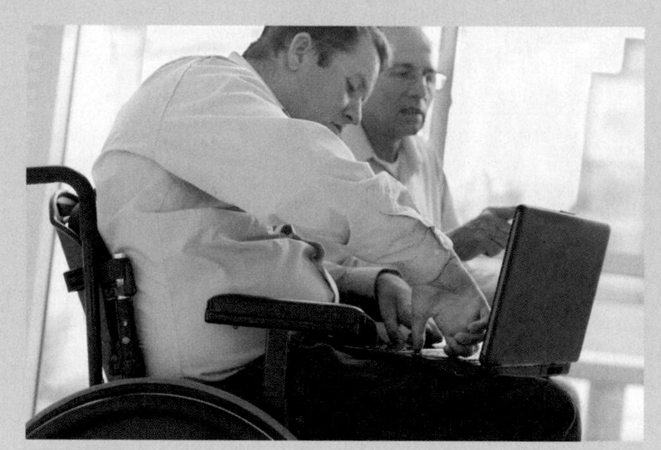

FIGURE 2-1 People with disabilities often can assist nurses in identifying care strategies that work best for them.

culture, however, values vary widely among subcultural groups and even between individuals on the basis of the person's gender, personal experiences, personality, education, and many other variables (Diversity Considerations box).

QSEN FOCUS

Collecting information on patient values during the interview and assessment process is essential to providing patient-centered care.

VALUES CONFLICT — LO 2.2

A **values conflict** occurs when a person's values are inconsistent with his or her behaviors or when the person's values are not consistent with the choices that are available (Edwards and Allen, 2008). Patients may experience a values conflict if evidence-based practice supports interventions that are inconsistent with their preferred, traditional treatment modalities. Providing care for a convicted murderer may elicit troubling feelings for a nurse, resulting in a values conflict between the nurse's commitment to care for all people and a personal repugnance for the act of murder. When people experience values conflicts or exhibit incongruent stated values and actions, values clarification may be helpful.

VALUES CLARIFICATION

Values clarification is a process used to help people reflect on, clarify, and prioritize personal values to increase self-awareness or to make decisions (Edwards and Allen, 2008). Nurses can use values clarification to help patients identify the nature of a conflict and reach a decision based on their values. Possibly the most helpful application of the values clarification process occurs when it is used by the nurse to assist a patient or family faced with making a health care decision or decisions concerning end-of-life care. Nurses may use the values clarification process to better identify their own personal values in challenging care situations.

While helping patients with values clarification and care decisions, nurses must be aware of the potential influence of their professional nursing role on patient decision making. Nurses should be careful to assist patients to clarify their own values in reaching informed decisions. This strategy will help to avoid the risk of unintended persuasion on the part of the nurse. Providing information to patients so that they can make informed decisions is a critical nursing role. Giving advice or telling patients what to do in difficult circumstances is both unethical and ill-advised (Patient Education and Health Literacy box). Figure 2-2 is an example of a values clarification tool that nurses can use with patients.

PATIENT EDUCATION AND HEALTH LITERACY

Teaching Pregnant Women Dealing With Substance Abuse or Addiction

Ackley and Ladwig (2014) note that the most effective approach for dealing with a values conflict in which substance abuse or an addiction is involved is to begin with an assessment interview, during which the nurse should:

- Listen for the subtle signs of denial, such as an unrealistic display of optimism or downplaying or minimizing the significance of the danger to the fetus.
- Avoid direct confrontation such as, "I hear you say you want a healthy baby, but I see that you are still smoking."
- Use a matter-of-fact approach to inform the patient of the reality of the consequences of the harmful behavior to the unborn child.
- Provide straightforward information about the effects of the substance abuse on the fetus to better equip the patient to understand the problem—an understanding that is integral to motivating change (Becker and Walton-Moss, 2001).

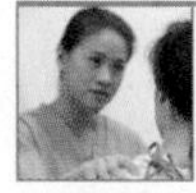

1. List five concerns related to beliefs and values that nurses should consider immediately when caring for a patient with a cultural background different from their own.

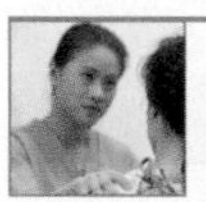

2. Identify two assessment questions regarding treatments that Hwa has used in the past to treat headaches that would have been helpful for the nurse to ask. What follow-up question should the nurse have asked after Hwa stated that she had never had a headache lasting longer than a half-hour?

BELIEFS, HEALTH, AND HEALTH CARE LO 2.3

Although personal beliefs are one of the most important factors in determining how a person responds to a health problem and its treatment, research shows that the beliefs of nurses and other health care workers are equally important factors in determining how patients are treated (Baumhover and Hughes, 2009; Heidal and Steinsbekk, 2009; Leiferman, Dauber, Heiseler, and Paulson, 2008). Patients listen to or do not listen to, trust or mistrust, and act upon or ignore information provided by members of the health care team on the basis of their previous experiences and, sometimes, stereotypes or prejudices.

This phenomenon is seen in research conducted to identify treatment disparities due to ethnic or racial differences. In a study of patients with sickle cell disease and the wait time they experienced in the emergency department, researchers found that African American race and a diagnosis of sickle cell disease contributed to longer wait times for care—between 25% and 50% longer than for patients without those characteristics (Haywood, Tanabe, Naik, et al, 2013). In another study of 34,203 patients hospitalized for hip fractures who were 65 years of age and older, on Medicare, and predominantly female, the Hispanic patients were almost three times more likely than the white patients, and the blacks were twice as likely as the whites, to be discharged to home self-care rather than to a rehabilitation facility. The researchers explained that the differences were due to the fact that the non-white families tended to have less favorable perceptions of rehabilitation facilities than the family members of white patients (Nguyen-Oghalai, Ottenbacher, and Kuo, 2009). The disturbing part of the findings is that those who went home to self-care seldom walked again.

Another example of how patients' beliefs may affect their health behaviors is found in a study that linked patients' feelings of hopelessness to poor participation in cardiac rehabilitation exercise (Dunn, Stommel, Corser, and Holmes-Rovner, 2009). When patients did not believe that rehabilitation would make a difference, they did not participate. Many studies have shown that a large number of health care disparities can be traced to the health beliefs of either patients or health care providers (Calloway, 2009; Leiferman et al, 2008; Pescosolido and Olafsdottir, 2010).

! SAFE PRACTICE ALERT

Nurses must collaborate effectively with patients to find treatment methods that are congruent with the patients' belief systems and that promote healthy outcomes. This approach requires excellent assessment skills and a willingness to listen carefully to determine how patients' personal beliefs impact their health beliefs.

Equally revealing are studies indicating the presence of a gap, in many cases, between what nurses believe to be true and real and what patients believe to be so (Dahlke, Fehr, Jung, and Hunter, 2009). This gap widens when nurses are formally educated in scientific causes of diseases and evidence-based practice. As nurses learn about their discipline, their **paradigm** (or worldview) gradually changes to one based on

Your values are your ideas about what is most important to you—what you want to live for and the values you want to live by. Values are the silent forces behind many of your actions and decisions. The goal of "values clarification" is to become fully conscious of their influence, and to explore and honestly acknowledge what you truly value. You can be more self-directed and effective when you know which values you choose to keep and live by as an adult, and which ones will get priority over others. Identify your values by designating them as a ***1*** (important), a ***2*** (somewhat important), or a ***3*** (not important), and then rank in order your top three ***1***s. When done, reflect on any lifestyle changes you might need to make so your lifestyle is more in line with what you value most.

_____ Achieving highly	_____ Being treated fairly	_____ Having prized possessions
_____ Avoiding boredom	_____ Being well-organized	_____ Having self-acceptance
_____ Being a creative person	_____ Being with people	_____ Having self-control
_____ Being a good parent (or child)	_____ Enjoying sensual pleasures	_____ Having someone's help
_____ Being a spiritual person	_____ Fighting injustice	_____ Having things in control
_____ Being admired	_____ Growing as a person	_____ Holding on to what you have
_____ Being appreciated	_____ Having a close family	_____ Learning and knowing a lot
_____ Being comfortable	_____ Having a purpose	_____ Living ethically
_____ Being competent	_____ Having a relationship with God	_____ Living life fully
_____ Being courageous	_____ Having a special partner	_____ Looking good
_____ Being emotionally stable	_____ Having an important position	_____ Loving someone
_____ Being free from pain	_____ Having companionship	_____ Making a contribution to the world
_____ Being healthy	_____ Having deep feelings	_____ Making a home
_____ Being independent	_____ Having enjoyable work	_____ Making money
_____ Being liked	_____ Having financial security	_____ Not being taken advantage of
_____ Being loved	_____ Having fun	_____ Preserving your roots
_____ Being married	_____ Having good friends	_____ Smelling the flowers
_____ Being physically fit	_____ Having it easy	_____ Striving for perfection
_____ Being popular	_____ Having peace and quiet	_____ Taking care of others
_____ Being productively busy	_____ Having people's approval	
_____ Being safe physically	_____ Having pride or dignity	

FIGURE 2-2 Values clarification tool. (Adapted from material at *www.smartrecovery.org.* Credited to Joyce Sichel, from Barnard ME, Wolf JL, eds: *The RET book for practitioners,* New York, 2000, Albert Ellis Institute.)

a body of knowledge that focuses on scientific principles and dismisses as superstition other explanations for the presence of disease or illness (Watson, 1988). This scientific or modern paradigm has been nursing's predominant paradigm since the early 1900s, when nurses began conducting research using the scientific method (Trafecanty, 2006). Patients, however, may hold a worldview very different from the scientific paradigm.

To determine a patient's values and beliefs, nurses must listen and ask relevant questions. Incorporating patient values and beliefs into a plan of care requires that patients and their families or primary caregivers be actively involved in establishing goals and outcome criteria. Patients should be included in determining what interventions will be implemented to assist them in achieving their goals. When patients speak a language different from that of the health care provider, use of a professional interpreter for over-the-phone or face-to-face interpretation can help to facilitate the inclusion of cultural beliefs and values in care planning (Collaboration and Delegation box).

NURSING THEORIES OF CARING LO 2.4

Caring, according to the American Nurses Association (ANA) Code of Ethics (2010), is having concern or regard for that which affects the welfare of another. As a profession, nursing can trace its earliest beginnings to the types of nurturing activities that demonstrate care, such as taking time to be with a suffering person, actively listening, advocating for the vulnerable, valuing and respecting all individuals, attempting to relieve pain, and making the healing process an act of the body, mind, and spirit.

The four nursing theories reviewed in this chapter have the concept of care as their primary focus and are used by

COLLABORATION AND DELEGATION

Guidelines for Working With an Interpreter

- It is always best to use an interpreter who has specialized training in health care terminology (Rosenberg, Seller, & Leanza, 2008) and, when possible, one whose age, gender, and background fit best with the patient or family (e.g., use of a female interpreter for female patients).
- Whether using over-the-phone or face-to-face translation, brief the interpreter before beginning by providing relevant information about the patient and the purpose of the conversation.
- If face-to-face translation is used, ask the interpreter to stand near the patient. Be sure to look at the patient and not at the interpreter when speaking.
- Ask the interpreter to speak to the patient in first person; for example, "Mrs. Carlos, you will need to travel by cart to the x-ray department early tomorrow morning," rather than "The nurse says. . . ."
- Use short sentences and stop often to allow time for the interpreter to translate (Rosenberg, et al, 2008).
- Tell the interpreter to ask for clarification if something that is said is not understandable.
- Ask the interpreter to translate everything the patient says and not to paraphrase or abbreviate anything.
- Follow up on every detail and seemingly unconnected issues or questions the patient raises. Sometimes the patient's questions uncover problems with the interpretation and lead to crucial diagnostic or assessment information (Galanti, 2008).

nurses around the world. These theories complement one another but approach the idea of caring and nursing from very different paradigms. A nurse's paradigm, or the way the nurse views the world, significantly affects how the nurse provides care. Understanding theories of caring can positively influence nursing practice. For example, a nurse who comprehends Watson's emphasis on holistic care will seek to include options of alternative or complementary therapies in patient care plans.

MADELINE LEININGER: CULTURAL CARE THEORY

Leininger's (1979) Cultural Care Theory is based on the belief that nursing is a transcultural care profession and that the concept of care is at its center. As a nurse and anthropologist, Leininger found that human caring was a universal phenomenon. *Nursing,* according to Leininger, is both an art and a science that provides culture-specific care to individual patients and groups to promote or maintain health behaviors or recovery from illness. Within the model, three nursing actions focus on finding ways to provide culturally congruent care. These three nursing actions include: (1) preserving or maintaining the patient's cultural health practices, (2) accommodating, adapting, or adjusting health care practices, and (3) repatterning or restructuring some cultural practices, as needed.

Leininger's (1979) model is based on a number of propositions and assumptions that relate closely to the earlier discussion of how a person's belief system influences that person's health beliefs. The focus of Leininger's theory is entirely on the patient's culture, almost to the exclusion of other factors such as the patient's educational experiences, peer social groups outside the traditional cultural setting, or even the influence of media, such as television, the Internet, and social networking.

JEAN WATSON: NURSING—HUMAN SCIENCE AND HUMAN CARE

Jean Watson's (1988) postmodern theory entails looking at patients holistically, which includes social, psychological, and spiritual aspects and may combine interventions that reflect both the science and art of nursing. Watson believes that health care needs to move from a total disease-cure focus based solely on scientific inquiry to a more holistic approach that incorporates values, beliefs, intentions, and the caring consciousness. Watson's theory is based on and is similar to an earlier nursing theory by Martha Rogers (1970) called the Science of Unitary Human Beings. However, Watson delves even deeper than Rogers into the mystical and paranormal realm. In Watson's view, *caring* is a metaphysical event with far-reaching effects on both humanity and the universe. Human bodies are manifestations of universal energy, and caring is transpersonal, transcending time, space, and the physical realm. The structure of Watson's theory originally was built on 10 carative (rather than curative) factors, which are now referred to as *caritas* processes (Box 2-1).

BOX 2-1 Watson's Caritas Processes

- Embrace altruistic values and practice loving kindness with self and others.
- Instill faith and hope and honor others.
- Be sensitive to self and others by nurturing individual beliefs and practices.
- Develop helping-trusting-caring relationships.
- Promote and accept positive and negative feelings while listening to another's story.
- Use creative, scientific problem solving for caring decision making.
- Share teaching and learning that addresses individual needs and comprehension styles.
- Create a healing environment for the physical and spiritual self that respects human dignity.
- Assist with basic physical, emotional, and spiritual human needs.
- Be open to mystery and allow miracles to enter.

From Watson J: *The philosophy and science of caring,* ed. rev, Boulder, Colo., 2008, University Press of Colorado.

TABLE 2-2 Swanson's Five Caring Processes With Subdimensions

KNOWING	BEING WITH	DOING FOR	ENABLING	MAINTAINING BELIEF
• Avoiding assumptions • Centering on the one cared for • Assessing thoroughly • Seeking cues • Engaging the self of both	• Being there • Conveying ability • Sharing feelings • Not burdening	• Comforting • Anticipating • Performing competently/skillfully • Protecting • Preserving dignity	• Informing/explaining • Supporting/allowing • Focusing • Generating alternatives/thinking it through • Validating/giving feedback	• Believing in/holding in esteem • Maintaining a hope-filled attitude • Offering realistic optimism • "Going the distance"

From Swanson K: Empirical development of a middle range theory of caring, *Nurs Res* 40(3):161–166, 1991.

JOYCE TRAVELBEE: HUMAN-TO-HUMAN RELATIONSHIP MODEL

Joyce Travelbee (1971), a psychiatric nurse practitioner, was inspired to develop the Human-to-Human Relationship Model after noting that nursing care being given to patients was so lacking in compassion that a humanistic revolution was needed. Travelbee predicted that if nurses did not become more caring, consumers would demand the services of a new and different kind of health provider to replace the nurse! The model describes steps toward "compassionate" and "empathetic" care. These steps are not included in other theories, making it as relevant today as it was when the theory was developed.

According to Travelbee (1971), the purpose of nursing is achieved through human-to-human relationships. The quantity and quality of nursing care delivered to an ill person are greatly influenced by the nurse's perception of the person and the relationship that is established. Travelbee points out that the human condition is shared by everyone. It is contradictory in its twofold nature. People will experience joy, contentment, happiness, and love at some point in life and also will at some time be confronted with illness and pain (mental, physical, or spiritual suffering) and eventually will encounter death.

Individual patients and families can be assisted to find meaning in the experience of illness and suffering. However, the spiritual and ethical values or the philosophical beliefs of the nurse about illness and suffering will determine the extent to which the nurse will be able to assist individuals and families to find meaning in these difficult experiences. The meaning can enable the individual to cope with the problems resulting from the experience.

KRISTEN SWANSON: MIDDLE RANGE THEORY OF CARING

In her Middle Range Theory of Caring, Kristen Swanson (1991) identifies five processes that characterize caring: knowing, being with, doing for, enabling, and maintaining belief. Swanson's theory is built on Watson's framework and resembles it, but Swanson brings caring theory into a more practical sphere by describing the five caring processes as well as practices for putting the processes into action (Table 2-2). Although Swanson defines *nursing* as informed caring for the well-being of others, the emphasis placed on the five caring processes is not unique to the nurse-patient relationship. The processes are present in any caring relationship, and they can and should be enacted throughout all levels of caring and in all healing organizations and by every health care worker (Koloroutis, 2004).

PROFESSIONAL CARING LO 2.5

There is widespread disagreement about whether it is possible to teach caring. The theories proposed by Leininger and Swanson seem to assume that all nurses care about and for patients. However, Travelbee and Watson, along with others, disagree and question whether it is possible to teach caring or whether all nurses know what caring is (Bartzak, 2010; Wolf, Zuzelo, Goldberg, and Crothers, 2006). Hudacek (2008) goes so far as to say that "no one can make another care; it has to be a free offering of oneself. No one can teach the true sentiment of caring; it is a gift, a talent" (p. 126).

DEVELOPING COMPASSION

In a study conducted by Lohri-Posey (2005) to evaluate how nursing students learned to be caring, the student subjects either emerged as "compassionate healers" or "they focused on tasks and the disease process" (p. 34). Those who were compassionate healers recognized the difference between themselves and their classmates and were able to articulate numerous instances in their short careers when the care they provided made a difference in patients' lives. Those students who were not compassionate healers were not even aware that a deeper practice level existed. Regarding timing of the emergence of this quality, those who were compassionate healers recognized in childhood a desire to become a nurse and were able to relate some incident in their lives, such as caring for an ill family member, during which they learned about the power of being compassionate toward others. Students who were compassionate healers were able to identify both positive and negative role models that inspired them to become even more compassionate. The surprising finding was that the negative role models inspired the students to not be like those people and motivated the students just as much as the positive role models. In her study, Lohri-Posey (2005) concluded that caring and compassion depended on personal qualities within the individual student, or on experiences that shaped the student's values, rather than on something that was taught in class.

Christiansen (2009) approached the topic of whether caring could be taught from a much more pragmatic perspective and reported quite different results. Instead of looking at caring as a personality trait that a nurse may or may not possess, Christiansen defined *caring* as the way nurses express themselves to patients or their family members in a sensitive and empathetic manner that communicates "authentic concern." Nursing students, in Christiansen's view, must take moral responsibility to develop and be able to display competency in caring skills just as they display other nursing skills. Developing the ability to demonstrate caring is an essential part of becoming a professional nurse. Not only can caring be taught, but according to Christiansen, it can be measured and evaluated by instructors in the clinical setting. The objective behaviors that constitute authentic concern typically are expressed by the nurse through eye contact, tone of voice and pace of speech, body language, and attention directed toward the patient.

It seems that for people who have not experienced caring as a product of their childhood and everyday life or as a part of their culture, values, and experiences, the concept may seem strange and foreign, making it difficult to act in caring ways. In their work with patients, however, as they witness the depth of suffering incurred with illness or injury, nurses may learn caring ways as part of their professional role (Ethical, Legal, and Professional Practice box).

ETHICAL, LEGAL, AND PROFESSIONAL PRACTICE

Ways in Which Values and Caring May Affect Professional Practice

- "Caring" was shown to be the common thread that linked critical care nurses with their patients and families in a high-tech nursing unit that could otherwise be a frightening and "alien environment" (McGrath, 2008).
- A student who sees a nurse turn his or her back on a weeping patient or learns about the use of touch by watching a "caring" nurse remembers and experiences a greater impact from both negative and positive examples than by hearing a lecture on "caring theories" in the classroom (Mackey, Goddard, and Warner, 2007).
- Cultural "desire" is the motivation of health care providers to "want to" engage in the process of cultural competence. Nurses must possess a genuine desire to care and motivation to work with culturally different patients (Campinha-Bacote, 1999).

CODEPENDENCY AND NURSING

Most people who choose nursing as a career do so out of a genuine desire to help others and because they find great satisfaction in the caring role. Sometimes, however, those who enter helping professions such as social work, nursing, or medicine have an intense need to be needed. The term that is commonly used to describe this type of behavior is *codependency*. **Codependency** is a dysfunctional relationship in which the person who wants to help acts in a manner that enables harmful behavior by another person. This unintended effect can be achieved through direct control over the dependent person, by making excuses for the dysfunctional behavior, or by protecting the person from negative consequences (Oakley, 2010).

Codependency may lead to controlling behaviors exhibited by nurses that prevent patients from healing and moving toward independence (Abernathy, 2006). Nurses who identify personal tendencies toward codependent behaviors should actively seek to overcome these controlling actions. To be truly effective in professional practice, nurses must recognize the role and responsibility of patients in attaining treatment goals and must demonstrate patient advocacy rather than codependency while providing compassionate care (Abernathy, 2006).

BEHAVIORS THAT DEMONSTRATE CARING IN NURSING LO 2.6

Many authors, theorists, and professional groups have identified qualities and behaviors that demonstrate caring in nursing practice. Several of the most important concepts include the nurse's presence, consistency and predictability, the use of touch, and the importance of listening in the nurse-patient relationship (Evidence-Based Practice box).

PRESENCE

Nurses are the only health care providers who are typically with patients 24 hours a day, 7 days a week. By simply being present in a patient's room, nurses have the potential to calm the fears of a patient and family and demonstrate caring. Research indicates that the interpersonal skills of nurses who demonstrate caring and compassion, such as being present with patients in times of crisis, often are the basis on which patients determine the competence of their nurses (Wysong and Driver, 2009).

Nurses often talk and write in their professional journals about what a great honor and privilege it is to be part of, or even to simply be present at, some of life's most important events, such as a birth or a death, in a pre-op room before surgery, or with patients and families as they go through a life-changing illness. Being present with patients and families at these critical times while applying the unique knowledge

EVIDENCE-BASED PRACTICE

Studies That Demonstrate Values and Caring in Nursing Practice

Patients in an acute care setting rated the quality of their health care experience on the basis of the nurses' caring behaviors.

- The most important caring behaviors, according to patients, included:
  - Respecting confidentially
  - Treating pain
  - Speaking in a soft and gentle voice
  - Being honest
  - Encouraging the patient to call if there was a problem
- The most important caring behaviors, according to the nurses, included:
  - Knowing how to give shots
  - Encouraging the patient to call if there was a problem
  - Giving information so that the patient could make decisions
  - Appreciating the patient as a human being and showing concern for the patient (Tanking, 2010)
- Nurses with a strong professional work ethic were consistently identified by patients as providing the highest-quality nursing care. The same nurses participated in nursing unit improvement projects and patient safety programs and provided patient-centered care, showed concern for patient safety, and incorporated evidence-based practices in their nursing care (Bartzak, 2010).
- Seven dimensions of caring that were identified as being universal by nurses from around the world include:
  - Caring
  - Compassion
  - Spirituality
  - Community outreach
  - Providing comfort
  - Crisis intervention
  - "Going the extra distance" (Hudacek, 2008)
- Nurses cannot pretend to care. Nurses' values are evident even to pediatric patients by what they do to genuinely care and by what they fail to do that shows lack of caring (Cantrell & Matula, 2009).
- Acts of caring, from a nursing perspective, are the result of the nurse's synthesis of scientific principles, artistry, and a deep sense of being present with patients (Cantrell, 2007).
- The professional values that have consistently been shown to be of highest value to nurses across the past two decades are:
  - Respect for human dignity
  - Prevention of suffering
  - Reliability
  - Maintaining a faithful relationship with patients (Rassin, 2010)

and skills of professional nursing practice demonstrates holistic care.

CONSISTENCY AND PREDICTABILITY

Patients who enter the health care system have two reasonable expectations. The first is not to be harmed, and the second is that the nurses providing care will be both competent and compassionate (Morath and Turnbull, 2005). In light of the number of injuries and incidents that take place in health care organizations each year, entering a hospital can be a frightening experience. Provision of care that is consistent and is delivered in a predictable way can make the experience less intimidating for the patient. The nurse provides predictable care by explaining what is going to take place beforehand or why things are happening, and by following through with the promised care in a timely fashion. Setting up a schedule with the patient and adhering to it can greatly reduce the anxiety the patient experiences and create a supportive environment that provides a sense of security. When nurses are consistent in providing competent care that is delivered on time and matches the patient's expectations, the patient is reassured that nursing care will be predictable and delivered as prescribed (Bartzak, 2010).

In an effort to ensure a more consistent approach to nursing care and to optimize patient outcomes, researchers have developed practice standards and clinical guidelines that are used by nurses in various health care settings to ensure that the quality of care delivered is based on best practices (Hill, Middleton, O'Brien, and Lalor, 2009). Providing treatment based on standardized best practices allows all patients, whether in small rural hospitals or in large teaching medical centers, to receive similar high-quality care.

TOUCH

Touch is the intentional physical contact between two or more people. It occurs so often in patient care situations that it has been deemed to be an essential and universal component of nursing care. Task-oriented touch and caring touch are common forms of physical contact used in nursing care. Both must be used carefully with patients to build trust and to provide appropriate professional care.

Task-Oriented Touch

Task-oriented touch includes performing nursing interventions such as giving a bath, changing dressings, suctioning an endotracheal tube, giving an injection, starting an IV line, or inserting an NG tube. Task-oriented touch should be done gently, skillfully, and in a way that conveys competence. Patients become alarmed when they detect that their nurse is unfamiliar with a procedure. It is best to seek assistance with any procedure or skill that the nurse cannot safely accomplish alone. Every task-oriented procedure should be explained to a patient, followed by feedback indicating patient understanding, before care is initiated.

Caring Touch

Caring touch is considered by most people to be a valuable means of nonverbal communication. In today's highly technical world of nursing, caring touch is an essential aspect of patient-centered care. Caring touch can be used to soothe, comfort, establish rapport, and create a bond between the nurse and the patient. Care may be conveyed by holding the hand of a patient during a painful or frightening procedure or when delivering bad news. This is an important way nurses let patients know that they are not alone and that another human being cares (Figure 2-3).

Even when the nurse's intentions are to provide comfort, however, touch can be perceived as being intrusive or, at times, hostile by some patients, such as those who are confused or suspicious, those who have been abused, or those who are aggressive or under the influence of drugs or alcohol. In the case of a patient who has been abused, it is especially important to ask permission before touching the patient. Nurses need to be culturally sensitive to how caring touch may be perceived by patients from a culture different from their own. Gender differences must be respected and may necessitate permission before initiation of care. Additional information on therapeutic touch as a nursing intervention is presented in Chapter 36 in the context of pain management.

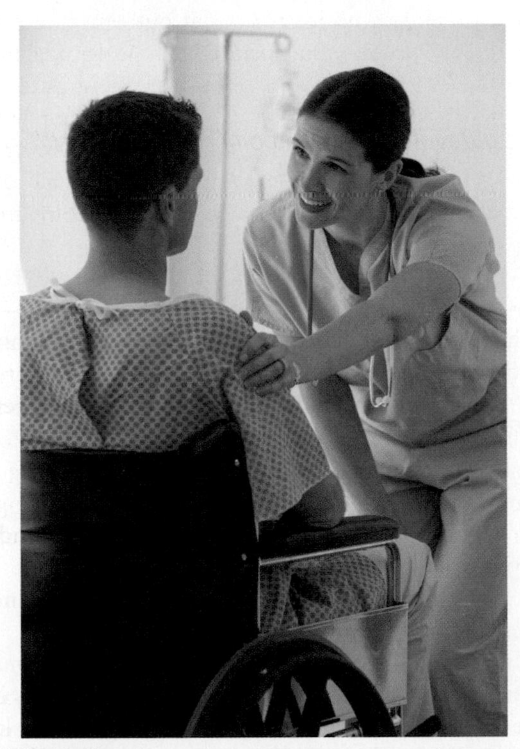

FIGURE 2-3 Touch can be used to communicate caring in difficult situations.

LISTENING

A vital aspect of providing effective and appropriate nursing care is being able to actively listen to a patient in a way that conveys understanding, sensitivity, and compassion. Caring involves interpersonal relationships and communication skills that require paying more attention to the details of communication than would be necessary in a social conversation. This type of listening is a highly developed skill that usually takes a great deal of time and many years of experience to acquire. It can be learned with practice and enhanced with sensitivity and attention to the feedback that is received during each interaction.

In a caring nurse-patient relationship, the nurse takes responsibility for establishing trust, making sure that the lines of communication are open and that the nurse accurately understands not only what the patient is saying but also that the nurse is clearly understood. Active listening means paying careful attention and using all of the senses to listen rather than just passively listening with the ears. It requires energy and concentration and involves hearing the entire message—what the patient means as well as what the patient says. This type of listening focuses solely on the patient and conveys respect and interest. For more information on active listening and other therapeutic communication techniques, refer to Chapter 3.

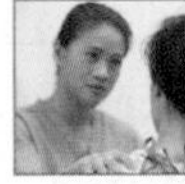

3. What actions by the nurse would have communicated caring and attention to Hwa's beliefs when she was first admitted to the emergency department? What action should the nurse have taken to exhibit concern when Hwa refused the prescribed medication?

Nurses must recognize the beliefs and values that are held by patients and families in order to provide culturally sensitive, relationship-based care. Incorporating patient concerns and outward displays of caring, such as touch and active listening, into patient treatment is essential to practicing evidence-based nursing. Nurses who have a commitment to respecting the ideas of others, lifelong learning, and caring are trusted by patients to provide safe, competent care.

SUMMARY OF LEARNING OUTCOMES

LO 2.1 *Describe the differences between beliefs and values and how they develop:* Beliefs are mental representations of reality, or what a person thinks is real or true; values are enduring beliefs that help the person decide what is right and wrong and determine what goals to strive for and what personal qualities to develop. Beliefs and values are developed through personal experiences, family influences, culture, ethnic background, spirituality, religion, and education.

LO 2.2 *Explain the use of the values clarification process in dealing with a values conflict:* The nurse needs to recognize when a values conflict exists and seek ways to identify the underlying factors causing the concern. A values clarification tool can be used to help patients examine past life experiences and consider where they spend their time, energy, and money to provide insight into what they truly value and believe. Values clarification can help nurses become more aware of their own personal values and beliefs that impact professional nursing practice.

LO 2.3 *Summarize how the beliefs of nurses and patients influence health care:* The beliefs of both nurses and patients influence how patients are treated, what patients listen to and act upon, and patient outcomes.

LO 2.4 *Discuss the major concepts of four nursing theories of caring:* Leininger's Cultural Care Theory states that culturally based nursing actions are intended to preserve, accommodate, or reconstruct the patient's meaningful health or life patterns. Watson's Human Science and Human Care Theory is a holistic model of care in which the nurse's focus is on 10 carative factors. According to Travelbee's Human-to-Human Relationship Model, the nurse assists the patient through five phases of a relationship and, if necessary, to find meaning in these experiences. Swanson's Middle Range Theory of Caring focuses on five processes of relationship-based caring for the nurse: maintaining belief, knowing, being with, doing for, and enabling the patient.

LO 2.5 *Articulate ways in which nurses develop into caring professionals:* Nurses develop caring skills through life experiences, observation of both positive and negative role models, and interaction with strong professional mentors.

LO 2.6 *Identify behaviors that demonstrate caring:* Nurses demonstrate caring through presence, consistency, predictability, touch, and listening.

Responses to the critical-thinking questions are available at *http://evolve.elsevier.com/YoostCrawford/fundamentals/*.

REVIEW QUESTIONS

1. A patient is struggling with the decision of whether to accept experimental treatment for cancer. The nurse begins to offer information to a patient and the patient says, "I've already heard all of that before and I don't agree with any of it." How should the nurse proceed?
   a. Ask why the patient is so defensive.
   b. Encourage the patient to discuss his beliefs.
   c. Question the patient's prejudicial attitude.
   d. Confront the patient about his values conflict.
2. Which nursing theory of care describes how the nurse's presence in the nurse-patient relationship transcends the physical and material world, facilitating development of a higher sense of self by the patient?
   a. Swanson's Middle Range Theory of Caring
   b. Madeline Leininger's Cultural Care Theory
   c. Watson's Theory of Human Science and Human Care
   d. Travelbee's Human-to-Human Relationship Model
3. Which statement best describes for new parents how and when children develop first-order beliefs?
   a. During infancy, and once developed, such beliefs seldom change
   b. From life experiences during the toddler and preschool years
   c. Throughout life from firsthand experiences and information provided by authority figures
   d. From teen and young-adult peer interaction and mentorship of professional role models
4. As the nurse is explaining preoperative instructions to a patient, the patient's older brother suddenly steps into the doorway and yells, "People who go under the knife always die. Don't do it! They're going to kill you." What type of higher-order belief is the patient's older brother displaying?
   a. Distress
   b. Stereotype
   c. Prejudice
   d. Denial

5. After admitting a homeless patient to the floor, the nurse tells a colleague that "homeless people are too dumb to understand instructions." What action should the colleague take first?
   a. Ignore the nurse's prejudicial comment without responding.
   b. Offer to trade assignments and care for the homeless patient.
   c. Ask the nurse about the patient's personal history assessment data.
   d. Challenge the nurse's thinking, pointing out the ability of all people.
6. The nurse in the emergency department is caring for an 8-year-old who has had a serious asthma attack. When the nurse attempts to explain the problem to the child's mother, she smells cigarette smoke on the mother's breath. The nurse asks the mother if she has been smoking and the mother responds, "Yes, and I know they've told me before I can't smoke around him." What should the nurse do next?
   a. Ask the patient's mother what she values most, her child or her habit.
   b. Ask the patient's mother to explain what she believes about smoking and asthma.
   c. Ask the patient's mother about her prejudicial feelings about continuing to smoke.
   d. Confront the patient's mother about the values conflict she's experiencing.
7. A nurse is working with a 35-year-old patient who needs to decide whether to donate a kidney to his brother who has been in renal failure for 5 years. The patient shares with the nurse that the decision is especially difficult because he would not be able to continue to work in his current profession and would be unable to support his three small children if he ever needed dialysis. Which interventions would be most appropriate for the nurse to implement in this situation? *(Select all that apply.)*
   a. Explain that it is unlikely that he will ever need dialysis even if he has only one kidney.
   b. Guide the patient through a values clarification process to help him make a decision based on his values.
   c. Provide factual information to the patient that may help him to make an informed decision.
   d. Ask for his permission to contact the kidney donation team to answer any questions he may have.
   e. Suggest that the patient seriously consider cancelling his plan to donate a kidney.
8. A 57-year-old male patient who was hospitalized with an admitting blood pressure of 240/120 asked the nurse if his family could bring in some meat and vegetable dishes from home. He explained that he cannot eat the foods on the hospital menu because it is summer and the hospital is offering only chicken and fish, which in his culture are "hot" foods that will interfere with his healing. Which response by the nurse would best demonstrate an application of Leininger's theory?
   a. Discourage the family from bringing in food, explaining that the idea of "hot" and "cold" foods is a superstition without scientific basis.
   b. Negotiate home-prepared food options with the patient and his family to ensure that treatment for the patient's blood pressure is supported.
   c. Explain that the patient will need to have home-prepared foods evaluated by the dietary staff to ensure that they are acceptable options.
   d. Tell the family to bring in any foods they want, to help preserve the patient's cultural practices and dietary preferences.
9. In Swanson's Middle Range Theory of Caring, the nurse demonstrates caring using several techniques. What action is included in the five caring processes?
   a. Call patients by their first name to demonstrate a caring attitude.
   b. Sit at the bedside for at least 5 minutes each hour.
   c. Use touch based on the nurse's judgment of what is appropriate.
   d. Ask the patient to identify the most important thing that the patient would like to accomplish during the nurse's shift.
10. A new nurse is about to insert a nasogastric tube for the first time but is not sure what equipment to gather or how to begin the procedure. The patient is an 80-year-old woman who is frightened and slightly confused. Which actions by the nurse would best demonstrate caring? *(Select all that apply.)*
    a. Offer the patient pain medication to help her calm down.
    b. Hold the patient's hand while inserting the nasogastric tube.
    c. Speak calmly while explaining the procedure to the patient beforehand.
    d. Ask another, more experienced nurse for assistance before initiating care.
    e. Obtain and insert the nasogastric tube as quickly as possible without explanation.

Answers and rationales for the review questions are available at *http://evolve.elsevier.com/YoostCrawford/fundamentals/*.

REFERENCES

Abernathy TM: Conflicting views about codependency. *J Gerontol Nurs* 32(11):7, 2006.

Ackley BJ, Ladwig GB: *Nursing diagnosis handbook: An evidence-based guide to planning care,* ed. 10, St. Louis, 2014, Mosby.

Acorn D: The role of self in social identity and the formation of stereotypes. Paper presented at the *American Sociological Association 2006 Annual Meeting, August 11-14.* Montreal, Canada, 2006.

American Nurses Association: *Code of ethics for nurses with interpretive statements,* Washington, D.C., 2010, Author.

Bartzak PJ: Professional work ethic strategies to motivate bedside nurse to deliver high quality patient care. *MEDSURG Nurs* 19(2):85-89, 2010.

Baumhover N, Hughes L: Spirituality and support for family presence during invasive procedures and resuscitation in adults, *Am J Crit Care* 18(4):357-366, 2009.

Becker KL, Walton-Moss B: Detecting and addressing alcohol abuse in women, *Nurse Pract* 26(10):13, 2001.

Bem D: Introduction to beliefs, attitudes and ideologies, 2002. Retrieved from *www.heart-intl.net/HEART/Stigma/Comp/Introductionbeliefsattitideologies.htm.*

Calloway SJ: The effect of culture on beliefs related to autonomy and informed consent, *J Cult Divers* 16(2):68-70, 2009.

Campinha-Bacote J: A model and instrument for addressing cultural competence in health care, *J Nurs Educ* 38(5):203-207, 1999.

Cantrell MA: The art of pediatric oncology nursing practice, *J Pediatr Oncol Nurs* 21(6):327-334, 2007.

Cantrell MA, Matula C: The meaning of comfort for pediatric patients with cancer, *Oncol Nurs Forum* 36(6):303-309, 2009.

Carr N, Mitchell J: The neglected role of religion and worldview in schooling for wisdom, character and virtue. In DN Aspin, JD Chapman (Eds): *Values education and lifelong learning: Principles, policies, programmes* (OhioLINK electronic book center; Lifelong Learning Book Series, Vol. 10), Dordrecht, Netherlands, 2007, Springer.

Christiansen B: Cultivating authentic concern: Exploring how Norwegian students learn this key nursing skill, *J Nurs Educ* 48(8):429-433, 2009.

Cronenwett L, Sherwood G, Barnsteiner J, et al: Quality and safety education for nurses, *Nurs Outlook* 55(3):122-131, 2007.

Dahlke S, Fehr C, Jung P, Hunter A: Attitudes toward aging: Implications for a caring profession, *J Nurs Educ* 48(7):374-380, 2009.

Dunn SL, Stommel M, Corser WD, Holmes-Rovner M: *Patient hopelessness is linked to poor participation in cardiac rehabilitation exercise. Research Activities* (DHHS Report No. 349). Washington, D.C., 2009, U.S. Government Printing Office.

Edwards A, Allen C: Values clarification used as intervention for urban, delinquent, pregnant adolescents and young mothers, *J Hum Behav Soc Environ* 18(1):1-14, 2008.

Galanti G: *Caring for patients from different cultures,* ed. 4, Philadelphia, 2008, University of Pennsylvania Press.

Grypma S: Nursing in need of transformation: What are we searching for? *J Christ Nurs* 26(3):166-173, 2009.

Harris S: *The moral landscape: How science can determine moral values,* New York, 2010, Free Press.

Haywood C, Tanabe P, Naik R, et al: The impact of race and disease on sickle cell patient wait times in the emergency department. *Am J Emerg Med,* 31(4):651-656, 2013.

Heidal F, Steinsbekk A: Norwegian healthcare professionals' perceptions of patient knowledge and involvement as basis for decision making in hematology, *Oncol Nurs Forum* 36(2):E93-E98, 2009.

Hill K, Middleton S, O'Brien E, Lalor E: Implementing clinical guidelines for acute stroke management: Do nurses have a lead role? *Aust J Adv Nurs* 26(3):53-58, 2009.

Hudacek SS: Dimensions of caring: A qualitative analysis of nurses' stories, *J Nurs Educ* 47(3):124-129, 2008.

Kaplan M, Kiernan NE, James L: Intergenerational family conversations and decision making about eating healthfully, *J Nutr Educ Behav* 18(5):298-306, 2006.

Koloroutis M (Ed): *Relationship-based care: A model for transforming practice,* Minneapolis, 2004, Creative Health Care Management.

Kurz AE, Saint-Louis N, Burke JP, Stineman MG: Exploring the personal reality of disability and recovery: A tool for empowering the rehabilitation process, *Qual Health Res* 18(1):90-105, 2008.

LeDuc K, Kotzer AM: A comparison of the professional nursing values of students, new graduates and seasoned professionals, *Nurs Educ Res* 30(5):279-284, 2009.

Leiferman JA, Dauber SE, Heiseler K, Paulson JF: Primary care physicians' beliefs and practices toward maternal depression, *J Womens Health (Larchmt)* 17(7):1143-1150, 2008.

Leininger MM: *Transcultural nursing,* New York,1979, MASSON International Nursing.

Lohri-Posey B: Becoming a compassionate healer, *J Christ Nurs* 22(4):34-37, 2005.

Mackey S, Goddard L, Warner P: Can you teach it? *Nurs Stand* 21(51):24-25, 2007.

McGrath M: The challenges of caring in a technological environment: Critical care nurse's experience, *J Clin Nurs* 17:1096-1104, 2008.

Miller SA: Children's understanding of second-order mental states, *Psychol Bull* 135(5):749-773, 2009.

Morath JM, Turnbull JE: *To do no harm: Ensuring patient safety in health care organizations,* San Francisco, 2005, Jossey-Bass.

Nguyen-Oghalai MD, Ottenbacher KJ, Kuo Y: *Blacks and Hispanics are less likely to receive outpatient rehabilitation after hip fractures, Research Activities* (DHHS Report No. 349), Washington, D.C., 2009, U.S. Government Printing Office.

Oakley B: Too kind? Maybe it's codependency, *Reflect Nurs Leadersh* 36(1):1527-1530, 2010.

Pescosolido BA, Olafsdottir S: The cultural turn in sociology: Can it help us resolve the age-old problem in understanding decision making for health care? *Sociol Forum* 25(4):655-676, 2010.

Rassin M: Values grading among nursing students: Differences between the ethnic groups, *Nurse Educ Today* 15(5):614-630, 2010.

Rogers ME: Roger's science of unitary human beings. In RR Parse (Ed): *Nursing science: Major paradigms, theories and critiques,* Philadelphia, 1970, Saunders.

Rosenberg E, Seller R, Leanza Y: Through the interpreter's eyes: Comparing roles of professional and family interpreters, *Patient Educ Couns* 70(1):87-93, 2008.

Sartori P: Spirituality 1: Should spiritual and religious beliefs be part of patient care? *Nurs Times* 106(28):14-17, 2010.

Seth R: *First comes marriage: Modern relationship advice from arranged marriages,* New York, 2008, Fireside.

Swanson K: Empirical development of a middle range theory of caring, *Nurs Res* 40(3):161-166, 1991.

Tanking J: Nurse caring behavior, *Kans Nurse 85*(4):3-5, 2010.

Thompson BM, Teal CR, Rogers JC, et al: Ideals, activities, dissonance, and processing: A conceptual model to guide educators' efforts to stimulate student reflection, *Acad Med* 85(5):902-908, 2010.

Trafecanty L: Biblical caring comes full circle: Identifying what constitutes caring in the 21st century remains imperative to defining nursing, *J Christ Nurs* 23(3):6-11, 2006.

Travelbee, J. (1971). *Interpersonal aspects of nursing,* ed. 2, Philadelphia, F.A. Davis.

Varkey P, Chutka DS, Lesnick TG: The aging game: Improving medical students' attitudes toward caring for the elderly, *J Am Med Dir Assoc* 7:224-229, 2006.

Watson J: *Nursing: Human science and human care. A theory of nursing,* New York, 1988, National League for Nursing.

Wolf SR, Zuzelo PR, Goldberg E, Crothers R: The caring behaviors inventory for elders: Development and psychometric characteristics, *Int J Hum Caring* 10(1):49-55, 2006.

World Health Organization (WHO): Obesity and overweight, 2013. Retrieved from *www.who.int/mediacentre/factsheets/fs311/en.*

Wysong P, Driver E: Patients' perceptions of nurses' skill, *Crit Care Nurse* 29(4):24-37, 2009.

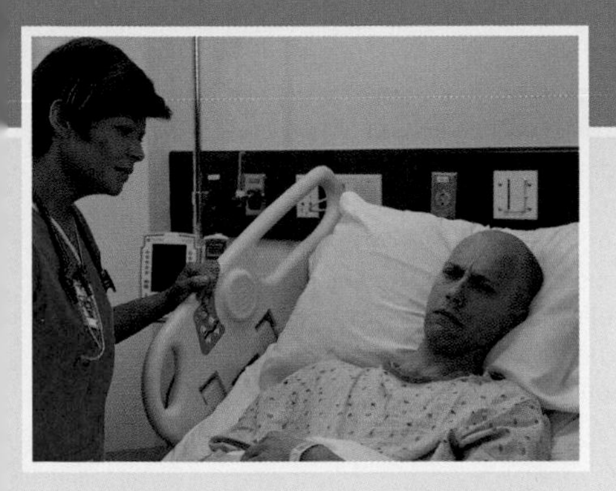

CHAPTER 3

Communication

EVOLVE WEBSITE

http://evolve.elsevier.com/YoostCrawford/fundamentals/

- Additional Evolve-Only Review Questions With Answers
- Answers and Rationales for Text Review Questions
- Answers to Critical-Thinking Questions
- Case Study With Questions
- Glossary

LEARNING OUTCOMES

Comprehension of this chapter's content will provide students with the ability to:

LO 3.1 Identify key components of the communication process.

LO 3.2 List examples of the verbal and nonverbal modes of communication.

LO 3.3 Recognize various types of communication.

LO 3.4 Describe how significant aspects of the nursing process are implemented in the nurse–patient helping relationship.

LO 3.5 Discuss factors affecting the timing of patient communication.

LO 3.6 Recognize the roles of respect, assertiveness, collaboration, delegation, and advocacy in professional nursing communication.

LO 3.7 Identify social, therapeutic, and nontherapeutic communication techniques.

LO 3.8 List defense mechanisms used by patients while they communicate.

LO 3.9 Illustrate methods of communicating in special situations.

KEY TERMS

assertiveness, p. 46
channel, p. 38
decode, p. 39
defense mechanisms, p. 49
encode, p. 39
feedback, p. 38
interpersonal communication, p. 42
intrapersonal communication, p. 42
meditation, p. 42
message, p. 38
negative self-talk, p. 42
nontherapeutic communication, p. 49
nonverbal communication, p. 39
positive self-talk, p. 42
prayer, p. 42
proxemics, p. 40
receiver, p. 38
referent, p. 38
role boundaries, p. 43
sender, p. 38
therapeutic communication, p. 46
verbal communication, p. 39

CASE STUDY

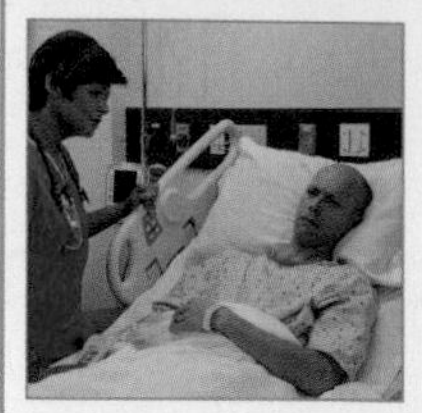

Mr. Beatrice, a married, 38-year-old father of two middle school–age children, was diagnosed with advanced melanoma. His doctor suggested an experimental treatment to stop further metastasis of the cancer. Mr. Beatrice was admitted within the past 24 hours to the oncology unit for treatment of anemia and fatigue. His medical history includes basal cell carcinoma diagnosed 10 years earlier and a concussion that occurred while in college. His surgical history includes repair of a fractured left tibia sustained while playing high school basketball.

Mr. Beatrice's vital signs are T 36.8°C (98.2°F), P 82 regular, R 18 and unlabored, BP 118/54, with a pulse oximetry reading of 99% on room air. He reports lower back and right hip pain at a level of 7/10 before administration of analgesics. He complains of feeling exhausted. His hemoglobin level is 8.2 g/dL. Mr. Beatrice appears tense and angry when the nurse goes into the room to see if he has ordered his lunch.

Refer back to this case study to answer the critical-thinking questions throughout the chapter.

Effective communication is an essential skill for the professional nurse. Critical nursing roles such as assessment and patient education require excellent and comprehensive communication to meet patients' needs. Patient advocacy, collaboration among health care team members, and safe patient care require the nurse to communicate in a way that clarifies a given situation. In more than 62% of sentinel health care events (i.e., unexpected death, injury, or serious risk of injury) that occurred between 2011 and June 2013, communication breakdown was identified as one of the top three causes (The Joint Commission, 2013).

To be viewed as competent, the nurse's communication skills must be professional and credible. Understanding the process of communication, the various modes in which individuals communicate, and the skills of therapeutic communication can greatly enhance the ability of a nurse to effectively care for patients and their families.

THE COMMUNICATION PROCESS LO 3.1

The dynamic process of communication occurs when six key elements interact (Figure 3-1). The elements of the communication process include a **referent** (event or thought initiating the communication), a **sender** (person who initiates and encodes the communication), a **receiver** (person who receives and decodes, or interprets, the communication), the **message** (information that is communicated), the **channel** (method of communication), and **feedback** (response of the receiver). For communication to be effective, the process must be interactive and ongoing. Realizing that a variety

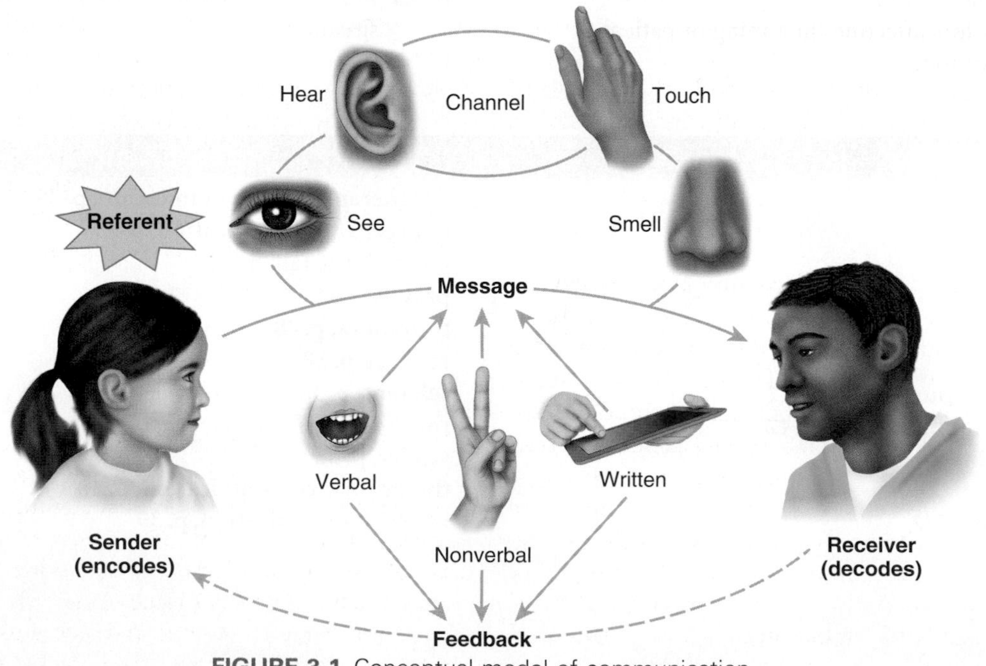

FIGURE 3-1 Conceptual model of communication.

of factors may initiate the communication process helps the nurse to critically analyze the purpose and meaning of interactions.

REFERENT

The referent, or initiating event or thought that leads one person to interact with another, may be anything, including a sensation. A patient may initiate a conversation due to feeling pain, having thoughts or concerns, recognizing a new lesion or symptom, hearing something unfamiliar or confusing, tasting a strange flavor, or smelling an unfamiliar scent. Each perceived event has the potential for initiating communication with others.

SENDER

Senders may be individuals or groups who have a message to share. Senders **encode** messages by translating their thoughts and feelings into communication with a receiver. The sender decides which mode of communication can most effectively convey the intended meaning of the message.

MESSAGE

A message is the content transmitted during communication. Messages are transmitted through all forms of communication, including spoken, written, and nonverbal modalities. Many factors influence whether a message is effectively communicated. The timing of conversations, educational levels of the people involved, modes of communication used, and physical and emotional factors may determine the outcome of interaction among individuals. For example, if a patient is experiencing significant pain, the nurse must address the patient's need for pain relief before attempting to obtain basic demographic data. The nurse must observe the patient's nonverbal messages to avoid missing essential elements of the communication.

CHANNEL

Messages are conveyed and received through a variety of channels. Any of the five senses may be used as channels, or methods, of communication. When a patient calls for help, the channel of communication is auditory. When a nurse observes a patient's gait for stability, communication is achieved through the visual channel. When a patient's wound smells noxious, the channel is olfactory. The accuracy of communication may be affected by the number of channels used to convey information. Typically, the more channels that are used to communicate, the more effectively the message is conveyed. This may not be the case, however, when the use of too many channels of communication overwhelms the receiver with information.

RECEIVER

There must be a receiver of information for the process of communication to take place. Receivers need to actively listen, observe, and engage in a conversation to **decode**, or sort out the meaning of, what is being communicated. Numerous factors may affect the ability of the receiver to accurately decode a message, including shared experiences with the sender, timing, educational background, cultural influences, and physical and emotional states. The message may be misinterpreted if clarity is not sought and achieved by the receiver.

FEEDBACK

To avoid misinterpretation of a message, it is essential that the receiver provide feedback to the sender regarding the conveyed meaning. By asking the receiver to restate the message, the sender is able to verify that the message was understood. This is especially important when a nurse and patient are communicating. If a nurse uses medical terminology that is not understood and a patient does not ask for clarification, effective communication cannot take place. Verification in the form of feedback is essential in nurse–patient interactions to ensure successful communication.

MODES OF COMMUNICATION LO 3.2

Although various methods can be used to convey information, there are only two basic forms of communication: verbal and nonverbal. **Verbal communication** may be spoken, written, or electronic. Most communication is nonverbal and provided in the form of body language such as gestures and eye contact. Nurses are bombarded with verbal and nonverbal communication throughout each workday. Understanding the significance of the two primary modes of communication and the various methods through which they take place is essential. Watching carefully for consistency or inconsistency between a patient's verbal and nonverbal communications allows the nurse to interpret and validate verbal statements.

NONVERBAL COMMUNICATION

Nonverbal communication is wordless transmission of information. According to seminal research by Mehrabian (1971), 93% of communication is nonverbal. Body language constitutes 55% of all nonverbal communication, and voice inflection accounts for 38%. Nonverbal communication is the more accurate mode of conveying information. Realizing the frequency and value of nonverbal communication helps the nurse to observe and assess patients more accurately. Nurses who perceive the potential effect of their own nonverbal behavior will communicate more professionally and consistently when interacting with others.

Body Language

Body language is conveyed in many ways. Posture, stance, gait, facial expressions, eye movements, touch, gestures, and symbolic expressions influencing personal appearance, such as jewelry and make-up, generally communicate a person's thoughts more accurately than simple verbal interactions. The nurse needs to observe the patient and family members for nonverbal cues while interviewing or completing assessments. Cultural and ethnic differences, mental health issues, and physical and emotional states affect the way people communicate.

Posture, Stance, and Gait

The way a person stands, sits, or ambulates can convey volumes to those observing. A relaxed body while sitting or standing indicates openness to what is being shared verbally in the conversation. If a patient sits with crossed legs or arms during an educational interaction with the nurse, the patient may be indicating a lack of openness to or acceptance of the information being shared. The manner in which patients and nurses ambulate communicates clearly without any words being spoken. A person's gait gives multiple cues to the nurse. If assistive devices are being used, the nurse knows that independent ambulation is at least temporarily impaired. A distinctive, intentional gait may communicate self-confidence, the need for immediate action, or a variety of potentially negative cues. A patient who is walking slowly with a bowed head may be feeling hopeless or exhausted or be in deep thought. Those observing a nurse running into a patient's room will certainly get the impression that there is an emergency. If a nurse walks quickly into a room and completes a task without making eye contact with the patient in the bed, the patient will have the impression that the nurse does not have time to address or does not care about the patient's needs and concerns.

Facial Expressions and Eye Movements

Grimacing or rolling the eyes communicates significant information. Some facial expressions may indicate fear or apprehension regarding impending diagnostic testing or surgery. The nurse must be especially perceptive when communicating with the patient and family members to observe the visual cues to their feelings. If there is incongruence between verbal communication and nonverbal facial expressions of patients or family members, the nurse must interview and assess the situation more carefully to identify and validate the most significant needs.

The facial expressions and eye movements of the nurse are of considerable concern. It is imperative to provide professional nursing care. Making inappropriate facial expressions may be offensive and hurtful to patients or their family members. The nurse must control his or her facial expressions to avoid communicating disdain or judgmental attitudes in challenging patient care situations. Maintaining a neutral facial expression establishes an environment of caring and openness in which the patient and family members can feel safe to share their innermost concerns.

Touch, Gestures, and Symbolic Expressions

Making physical contact in patient care situations can communicate caring or can be perceived as restrictive, depending on the type of touch used. Gently touching a blind patient's arm before providing care helps to alert the patient to the nurse's presence (Figure 3-2). Therapeutic touch, such as holding the patient's hand or touching the patient's shoulder, can provide comfort and may alleviate pain. This is especially true when a patient is undergoing a painful or stressful procedure. In most cases, it is important for the nurse to be aware of or verify a patient's openness to touch before implementing it as a nursing intervention.

Significant research has been conducted on human interaction. The anthropologist Edward Hall (1966) developed the theory of **proxemics** (i.e., study of the spatial requirements of humans and animals). He identified four specific distances in which people interact: intimate space (0 to 1.5 feet); personal space (1.5 to 4 feet); social space (4 to 12 feet); and public space (12 feet or more). Figure 3-3 illustrates these four basic distances. Nurses interact with patients within each of these distances, and they must become increasingly comfortable with and sensitive to interacting within the intimate-distance area while providing direct care. The Diversity Considerations box addresses cultural and other diversity factors that affect patients' comfort levels and tolerance with personal space and physical touch. Additional information on cultural differences related to communication and the use of

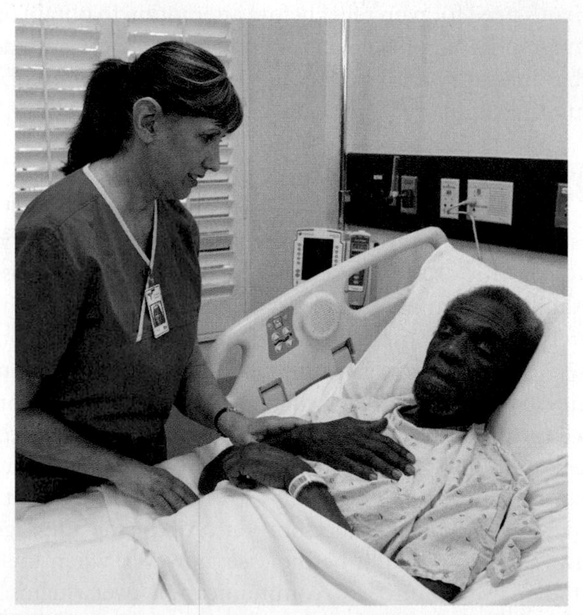

FIGURE 3-2 The nurse gently touches the arm of a blind patient to alert him to her presence.

interpreters while caring for patients whose native language is different from that of the nurse is provided in Chapter 21.

The use of gestures may be challenging to nurses practicing in a multicultural environment. Although they may enhance verbal communication, gestures may be viewed as inappropriate by patients of various cultures. Gestures may be most effective when used with people who have limited hearing. Establishing specific meanings for gestures before placing a patient on a ventilator or before a patient loses the ability to speak due to an advancing neurologic disease can facilitate communication when the patient is unable to speak.

Symbolic expression through the use of make-up, jewelry, or clothing may communicate self-esteem, economic resources, or mental health. Observing the appearance of a patient may provide the nurse with an indication of the patient's wellness or need for attention. Make-up and clothing may be used by a patient to hide inner feelings, or these symbols can indicate that the patient's condition is improving.

Nurses should be aware of their own use of symbolic expressions. Professionalism is best expressed without dramatic make-up and with minimal jewelry while performing patient care. Nurses who take pride in their professional appearance are more likely to be perceived by patients as competent and caring.

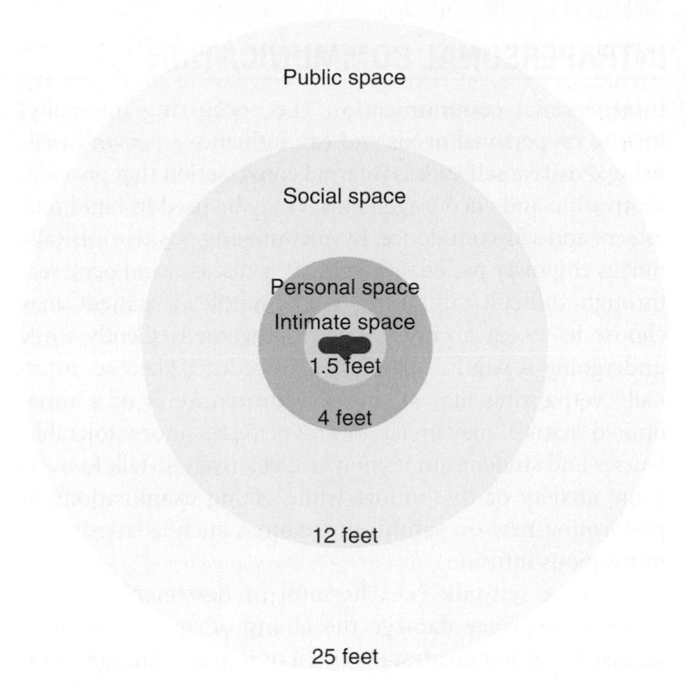

FIGURE 3-3 Hall's zones of interaction significantly affect communication in cross-cultural settings.

Voice Inflection

The second most significant form of nonverbal communication is voice inflection. Spoken words may be emphasized through tone, volume, and the rhythm or rate of speech. Nurses must actively listen to perceive the quality of speech used during interactions with others. Voice inflection provides insight into the significance of information being shared.

DIVERSITY CONSIDERATIONS

Life Span

- Children demonstrate a need for greater personal space as they age (Aiello and Aiello, 1974).
- Older adults of some cultures require personal care from younger, same-gender members of their family (Knott, 2002).

Gender

- Making direct eye contact immediately before touching a patient of the opposite sex may help to communicate caring and alleviate anxiety in the patient (Pullen, Barrett, Rowh, et al., 2009).
- In some cultures, nurses of the opposite sex may not be permitted to perform personal care or examine private areas of the patient's body (Pullen, 2007).

Culture and Ethnicity

- People born in more densely populated areas typically require less personal space for comfort.
- English-speaking people typically prefer at least 18 inches of distance between themselves and others when conversing. In contrast, Middle Eastern people may be comfortable standing very close while communicating (Purnell, 2013) (Figure 3-4).

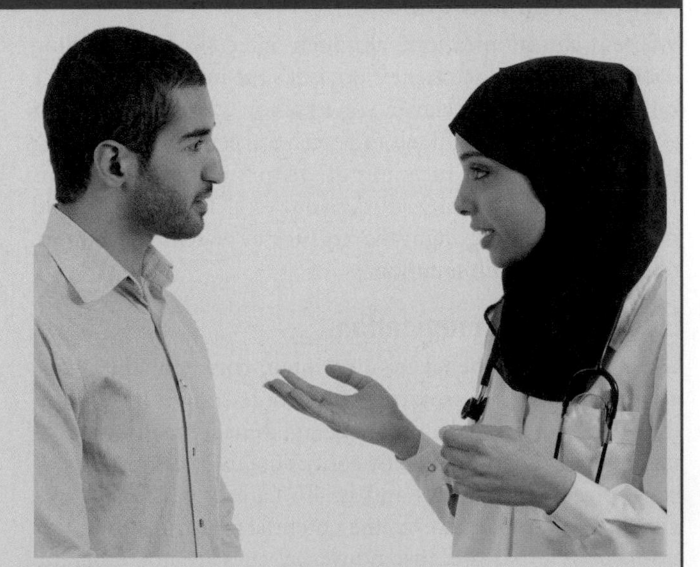

FIGURE 3-4 The nurse talks with a patient who requires little personal space.

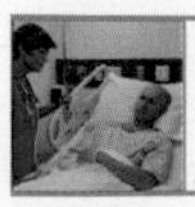

1. Describe nonverbal behaviors that may indicate tension and anger.

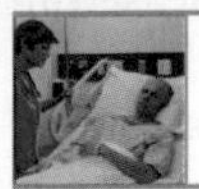

2. Identify at least two possible causes of Mr. Beatrice's nonverbal indications of tension and anger.

VERBAL COMMUNICATION

According to Mehrabian (1971), only 7% of communication about feelings and attitudes is verbal. This research finding underscores the critical need to integrate spoken, written, and electronic information with nonverbal cues garnered through observation and physical assessment.

Setting, Context, and Content

Spoken words may be communicated face to face, in a group setting, or through devices such as phones or intercoms. The setting of communication greatly influences what is or what can be shared. Depending on the confidentiality or privacy of the interaction, conversations may be overheard or taken out of context. Although it is important to get feedback when sharing patient information verbally to verify that the information is accurate, verbalizing potentially harmful or confidential information in a public setting may have legal ramifications for health care professionals. The context and content of verbal communication must be closely monitored by the nurse to avoid misinterpretation or errors in patient care.

Written Communication

Written communication, although effective in providing details and legal documentation, lacks the nuances that voice inflection and interactive conversation can provide. For example, it may be difficult to perceive urgency when reading progress notes. The meaning of written communication is often enhanced through discussion. Oral reports or grand rounds typically highlight the urgency of patient needs more than written documentation.

Electronic Communication

Special care must be taken to maintain confidentiality while communicating electronically. Electronic communication in the form of information referencing, e-mail, social networking, and blogging can quickly contribute to a person's knowledge, providing patients and health care professionals with vital information. However, the potential for miscommunication exists, in part because nonverbal cues are not apparent. When communicating verbally by electronic media, patients and nurses must take time to validate and verify shared information because misunderstandings can occur if feedback is inadequate. Chapter 10 provides additional information on the requirements of electronic documentation.

TYPES OF COMMUNICATION LO 3.3

Nurses engage in four basic types of professional communication: intrapersonal, interpersonal, small-group, and public communication. Each has a different focus and potential outcome.

INTRAPERSONAL COMMUNICATION

Intrapersonal communication (i.e., occurring internally) focuses on personal needs and can influence a person's well-being. **Positive self-talk** is internal conversation that provides motivation and encouragement; it may be used to build self-esteem and self-confidence. By encouraging positive self-talk, nurses empower patients to fight their diseases and persevere through difficult situations. For example, a patient may choose to repeat a phrase of encouragement silently while undergoing a painful diagnostic procedure; likewise, internally verbalizing that an invasive procedure is of a time-limited nature may make the experience more tolerable. Nurses and student nurses may use positive self-talk to overcome anxiety or discomfort while taking examinations or performing new or painful procedures, such as starting an intravenous infusion.

Negative self-talk (i.e., harmful or destructive internal conversation) may damage the ability of an individual to achieve his or her greatest potential or to overcome adversity. Negative self-talk may increase a patient's perception of pain, anxiety, or inability to meet the challenges of a poor prognosis.

Meditation (i.e., mindful reflection or contemplation) is another form of intrapersonal communication. Some people use it regularly as a means of self-encouragement and reassurance. Different from **prayer** (i.e., form of meditation traditionally directed to a deity), meditation is a continuous thought process that centers on one idea with the goal of achieving inner peace and relaxation.

INTERPERSONAL COMMUNICATION

Interpersonal communication takes place between two or more people. It may be formal or informal and conversational, and it may or may not have a stated goal or purpose. In the context of an interview, it may vary from the strictly formal to very casual. Health history interviews and patient–nurse interactions have a specific focus and intention and require confidentiality and setting of role boundaries. Effective interpersonal communication among health care

QSEN FOCUS!

Open communication among interdisciplinary teams of health care professionals creates a culture of safety, which is necessary to protect patients from harm and meet patient safety standards.

professionals is essential to ensure patient safety. Research indicates that 70% to 80% of medical errors involve issues of interpersonal communication (Agency for Healthcare Research and Quality, 2004).

Interprofessional Communication

Effective collaborative communication among various members of the interdisciplinary health care team is essential for patient safety. This is especially true when patient care is being transferred to new care providers. Data from The Joint Commission indicates that almost 70% of sentinel events were caused by communication breakdown, and 50% of those cases occurred during patient handoff (The Joint Commission, 2013). One method of interpersonal communication that has been adopted to increase interprofessional and hand-off communication is the SBAR model: situation, background, assessment, and recommendation (Ethical, Legal, and Professional Practice box).

ETHICAL, LEGAL, AND PROFESSIONAL PRACTICE

Hand-off Communication

SBAR (situation, background, assessment, and recommendation) is a widely accepted method of hand-off communication that involves interpersonal communication designed to enhance patient safety and outcomes.

- SBAR is used "to report to a health care provider a situation that requires immediate action, to define the elements of a hand off of a patient from one caregiver to another, such as during transfers from one unit to another or during shift report, and in quality improvement reports" (Iyer, 2007, p. 1).
- SBAR is often used by nursing as a hand-off tool and as a structured method for all communications between providers.
- SBAR communication requires the sharing of clear information focused on the four topical areas:
  - **S**ituation: What is happening right now?
  - **B**ackground: What led up to the current situation?
  - **A**ssessment: What is the identified problem, concern, or need?
  - **R**ecommendation: What actions or interventions should be initiated to alleviate the problem?
- Using SBAR format when documenting patient progress notes increases the clarity of shared information for legal purposes.

Chapter 10 provides additional information on SBAR methodology.

Ethical Implications

Information shared during informal and formal nurse–patient interaction is considered confidential. The nurse must maintain the patient's right to privacy to ensure that the Health Insurance Portability and Accountability Act (HIPAA) regulations are met. The American Nurses Association's *Principles for Social Networking and the Nurse* (2011) provides guidance to nurses on how to use social networking ethically while providing for the privacy and confidentiality required for professional nursing practice. Chapter 11 provides more information about ethical and legal interpersonal communication.

Professional **role boundaries** define the limits and responsibilities of individuals in a given setting. When undertaken by nurses, actions such as sharing personal phone numbers with patients, agreeing to meet patients outside the health care setting, and inappropriate touching violate these boundaries. Ethical or legal action may be taken against nurses who ignore professional role boundaries.

SMALL-GROUP COMMUNICATION

Communication in small groups focuses on meeting established goals or the needs of group participants. Focus groups, support groups, and task forces are examples of groups in which patients or nurses may be involved. Leaders of small groups may emerge from the group or be appointed before a first meeting. Nurses may be asked to lead small groups in their professional roles.

! SAFE PRACTICE ALERT

It is the nurse's responsibility to establish and maintain professional role boundaries when interacting with patients.

Small-Group Dynamics

When asked to lead small groups, nurses need to be aware of the phases of group development and group dynamics that may facilitate or hinder communication. In 1965, psychologist Bruce Tuckman identified four phases of group development: forming, storming, norming, and performing. He later added a fifth—adjourning—to denote the stage of closure in the small-group setting (Tuckman & Jensen, 1977). Aspects of these phases parallel those of the nurse–patient helping relationship. Although Tuckman's phases appear to be linear in nature, leaders should remember that group dynamics include individual personalities and that the arrival or departure of members may cause fluctuation among the various stages of group development.

During the forming phase, group members rely heavily on the leader to identify the mission and goals of the group. Ground rules are identified, and trust is established through the development of interpersonal relationships.

The storming phase of small-group development may involve some personality conflicts among the group participants. Group members with control issues may emerge. During the storming phase, the group leader needs to work with members to resolve conflicts and build cohesion. It is the group leader's responsibility to ensure that all members feel safe to share their thoughts and ideas freely without fear of ridicule.

Increased trust and openness emerge during the norming phase, resulting in productivity and meaningful sharing of information. During this phase, it is essential that the group leader encourage participation of all group members. The leader must redirect interaction if one member of the group tends to dominate the discussion. It is also important for group leaders to avoid sharing too many of their own thoughts or feelings. Sharing affirmations of what the group has accomplished and identifying future work constitute a vital role of an effective small-group leader.

Interdependence emerges during the performing phase of group development. During this phase, problem solving takes place within the group. Group members are typically highly committed during this time. Collaboration is effective in groups that perform at a high level.

The adjourning phase takes place as the small group disperses, having achieved the group's goals. By recognizing the various phases of group development and using strategies to encourage communication among all group members, nurses can be very effective small-group facilitators.

PUBLIC COMMUNICATION

Nurses communicate in a public forum through patient and community education on health care issues, including wellness. Public communication requires education, preparation, openness to diverse opinions, and communication skills that encourage acceptance and dialogue. Nurses may be asked to serve as professional experts on health care issues for the media. Training in public speaking may be beneficial for nurses who anticipate extensive public communication in their professional roles.

THE NURSE–PATIENT HELPING RELATIONSHIP LO 3.4

A helping relationship develops through ongoing, purposeful interaction between a nurse and a patient. Each helping relationship evolves as a result of systematic, intentional activities of the nurse. The focal point of the nurse–patient helping relationship is the patient and the patient's needs and concerns. Nurse–patient relationships focus on five areas: (1) building trust, (2) demonstrating empathy, (3) establishing boundaries, (4) recognizing and respecting cultural influences, and (5) developing a comprehensive plan of care.

PHASES OF THE HELPING RELATIONSHIP

The nurse–patient helping relationship consists of three phases: orientation or introductory phase, working phase, and termination (Table 3-1). Preinteraction activities, such as gathering assessment and diagnostic data, organizing the data, identifying areas of concern, and planning the interaction, prepare the nurse for the initial contact with the patient.

NURSING PROCESS IN THE HELPING RELATIONSHIP

The five steps of the nursing process are used in each phase of the helping relationship. During preinteraction and the orientation phase, the nurse gathers assessment data and formulates nursing diagnoses that are appropriate for the patient. Objective data are collected during preinteraction and the orientation phase, whereas subjective data are obtained almost exclusively while interacting with the patient during the orientation or introductory phase.

Nursing diagnoses for individual patients are identified during the orientation phase after assessment data are gathered and clustered. Nursing diagnoses commonly related to communication concerns include the following:

- *Impaired Verbal Communication*
- *Readiness for Enhanced Communication*
- *Powerlessness*
- *Risk for Powerlessness*
- *Social Isolation*
- *Situational Low Self-Esteem*

TABLE 3-1 Phases of the Nurse–Patient Helping Relationship

PHASE	FOCUS
Orientation or introductory	• Making introductions, establishing professional role boundaries (formally or informally) and expectations, and clarifying the role of the nurse • Observing, interviewing, and assessing the patient, followed by validation of perceptions • Identifying the needs and resources of the patient
Working	• Development of a contract or plan of care to achieve identified patient goals • Implementation of the care plan or contract • Collaborative work among the nurse, patient, and other health care providers, as needed • Enhancement of trust and rapport between the nurse and the patient • Reflection by the patient on emotional aspects of illness • Use of therapeutic communication by the nurse to keep interactions focused on the patient
Termination	• Alerting the patient to impending closure of the relationship • Evaluating the outcomes achieved during the interaction • Concluding the relationship and transitioning patient care to another caregiver, as needed

- *Anxiety*
- *Fear*

During the working phase of the helping relationship, goals or outcome statements and nursing interventions are developed in collaboration with patients and their families. It is important for the nurse to discuss assessment findings and concerns with the patient to establish realistic short-term and long-term goals. Communication with patients before initiating nursing interventions helps to alleviate anxiety and promotes goal attainment.

The evaluation step of the nursing process is completed during the termination phase of the helping relationship. During this phase, the nurse and patient determine the level of patient goal fulfillment and the possible need for further intervention. Outcomes of the nurse–patient helping relationship are greatly affected by the nurse's use of therapeutic communication and by the patient's receptivity.

FACTORS AFFECTING THE TIMING OF PATIENT COMMUNICATION LO 3.5

Many factors influence when communication with patients is best initiated, including the patient's pain or anxiety level and the physical location of the patient. Distractions in the patient's environment, including the presence of visitors, may also interfere with communication.

PAIN OR ANXIETY

Patients experiencing a moderate to high level of pain comprehend direct, empathetic communication most effectively. Short questions or specific instructions are the best methods for exchanging information with patients when they are suffering from acute or severe chronic pain. A similar approach is most effective with patients who are experiencing intense anxiety. If the nurse must provide an anxious patient with instructions for a diagnostic test or surgical procedure, short sentences that include only essential information should be used. Extensive patient education or preoperative teaching should be provided at an earlier or different time, when the patient is more relaxed or when the pain level is more tolerable.

LOCATION AND DISTRACTIONS

Several factors affect the location appropriate for communication with patients. Privacy and confidentiality are critical during the interviewing and assessment process. Patients should not be asked to share their health histories while visitors or non–health care providers are present. Simply pulling a cubicle curtain around a patient's bed does not prevent the transmission of sound beyond the curtain. If it is impossible to provide a private area in which to gather vital information, ask for the patient's permission to conduct the interview in the current setting before initiating the health history interview. Make every effort to talk with patients in an environment with as few interruptions and distractions as possible.

Effective communication can be challenging if the patient and nurse are distracted by technology and other people. Although technology, such as MP3 players, televisions, and cardiac monitors, may provide entertainment or valuable patient information, communication is enhanced when the people involved are totally attentive to the interaction. Ask the patient to turn off competing technology and to focus on the nurse–patient interaction as needed. Turn down the volume of audible monitor alerts during an extensive patient interaction. Remember to return the monitor alerts to their original levels before leaving the patient's bedside.

It is appropriate for the nurse to ask visitors to leave a patient's room for a few minutes to obtain critical, private information directly from the patient. The best source of information for an alert, oriented adult patient is the patient, not a spouse, another relative, or a visitor who happens to be present when the health history is taken. By focusing directly on the patient, the nurse communicates concern and is more attuned to subtle information communicated verbally and nonverbally.

With the patient's permission, relatives and friends may be considered secondary sources of subjective information. Data gathered from these persons may be helpful in validating or clarifying the information provided first by the patient. Relatives or friends of the patient may become sources of information after required permission has been secured, especially if the patient is disoriented, comatose, absent, or is a minor.

! SAFE PRACTICE ALERT

Make sure the patient is alert and oriented before conducting a health history or asking the patient to make significant health care decisions.

ESSENTIAL COMPONENTS OF PROFESSIONAL NURSING COMMUNICATION LO 3.6

Respect, assertiveness, collaboration, delegation, and advocacy are critical components of professional nursing communication that facilitate positive patient outcomes. Respecting patients and advocating on their behalf builds trust and conveys caring. Collaborating and delegating assertively with health care team members creates a positive work environment focused on patient needs.

RESPECT

Respect for patients and their families is conveyed by nurses verbally and nonverbally. Asking a patient's name preference during initial contact demonstrates respect and establishes the foundation for a trusting nurse–patient relationship.

Ensuring privacy, providing necessary health care information, and fostering autonomy in decision making are nursing actions that further strengthen the relationship. Controlling facial expressions and body language during challenging interactions with patients and health care team members is essential to consistently demonstrate respect.

ASSERTIVENESS

Assertiveness is the ability to express ideas and concerns clearly while respecting the thoughts of others. Assertive nurses communicate with patients, families, and other members of the health care team regularly and without hesitation. Assertive communication by nurses demonstrates confidence and elicits respect from patients and colleagues. Overly assertive nurses may be perceived as aggressive if they do not respect the rights and opinions of others. Nurses who communicate aggressively tend to receive negative or defensive responses from patients, family members, and health care team members.

COLLABORATION

Collaboration with other health care professionals is a key factor in communicating necessary health care information and providing comprehensive patient care. Most patients require the collaboration of many different health care professionals during hospitalization or outpatient treatment, and the nurse is often the coordinator of this team. Physicians, nurse practitioners, laboratory technicians, social workers, and respiratory, physical, occupational, and speech therapists, along with unlicensed assistive personnel, may share responsibility for patient care. The nurse must contact key health care professionals in an expedient manner and with respect and recognition of time and resource limitations. Ongoing communication with the patient about the status of the health care team collaboration is essential to allay unnecessary anxiety associated with not knowing what is happening.

QSEN FOCUS!

Requesting input from other members of the interdisciplinary health care team enhances a nurse's ability to meet the patient's needs. Each professional brings a different perspective and unique expertise that should be valued.

DELEGATION

Delegation is a multifaceted responsibility of the registered nurse. When communicating during delegation, nurses must show collegiality and respect for all members of the health care team. It is important to call other health care team members by their preferred names. Accuracy while communicating helps ensure positive patient outcomes. Receiving feedback from the person to whom care is delegated is required by law and provides an opportunity for clarity, which ensures greater accuracy. Chapter 11 provides further information on the legal requirements of delegation.

Communicating therapeutically with colleagues during the delegation process shows respect and recognizes the many stressors with which all members of the health care team cope while providing patient care. Offers of support and encouragement help convey empathy and promote teamwork. Chapter 12 focuses on the strengths of nursing leaders.

ADVOCACY

Patient advocacy is a hallmark of professional nursing. Advocacy involves defending the rights of others, especially those who are vulnerable or unable to make decisions independently. To be an effective advocate for patients, the nurse must be knowledgeable, organized, and able to communicate in a caring manner. Nurses who communicate therapeutically and assertively are better able to advocate for their patients.

SOCIAL, THERAPEUTIC, AND NONTHERAPEUTIC COMMUNICATION LO 3.7

Significant differences exist between social and **therapeutic communication** (i.e., beneficial, positive interaction). Nurses who understand this difference are effective in gathering information from patients and identifying their needs. Patients perceive nurses who develop strong therapeutic communication skills as caring, professional, and compassionate. Nurses who understand the impact of effective communication on patient care are less likely to engage in social conversation with patients and co-workers when it is not appropriate.

SOCIAL COMMUNICATION

Social communication most often occurs among individuals who know each other or who are getting to know each other informally. It typically involves mutual sharing of ideas, with a balanced focus on all parties engaged in the conversation. Friends may compare experiences, give advice, verbalize opinions, or make judgments on the behavior of others; anger and humor—appropriate or inappropriate—may be expressed. Most social conversations are multifaceted and change focus as topics of conversation evolve.

THERAPEUTIC COMMUNICATION

The primary focus of therapeutic communication between a patient and nurse is the patient. Nurses engaged in therapeutic conversations set their own opinions and judgments aside to listen more fully to their patients. Through various techniques, such as active listening, open posture, and reflection, nurses encourage patients to explore personal concerns (Figure 3-5). Patients often respond with open, honest sharing to nurses who are accepting of alternative ideas and empathetic to the circumstances of others. Nurses need to value the important role of therapeutic and open dialogue in the healing process.

The use of therapeutic communication techniques enhances nurse–patient relationships and helps to achieve positive outcomes. Consistent use demonstrates empathy and concern for patients. Various techniques greatly assist the nurse in gathering, verifying, and validating assessment data.

Table 3-2 provides examples and rationales for verbal therapeutic communication techniques that nurses should practice while providing care within all settings. Table 3-3 highlights examples and rationales for some essential nonverbal therapeutic techniques that nurses should implement when communicating with patients.

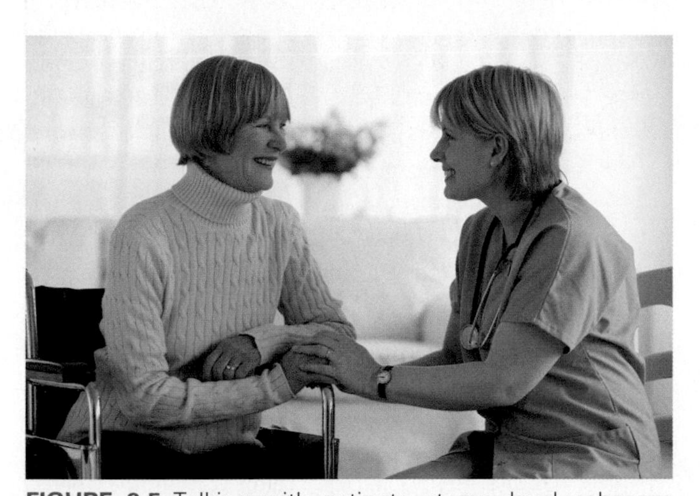

FIGURE 3-5 Talking with patients at eye level enhances communication.

A helpful reference for remembering the various aspects of active listening is the acronym SOLER (Egan, 2014). **S** encourages the listener to *sit* (if possible) facing the patient. **O** reminds the nurse to maintain an *open* stance or posture while listening. **L** suggests that the listener *lean* toward the speaker, positioning the body in an open stance. **E** refers to maintaining *eye* contact without staring. **R** reminds the nurse to *relax*. Demonstrating relaxation during a conversation encourages the person sharing to continue. It also conveys a sense of attention, interest, and comfort with the subject being shared.

Phrasing requests in a positive manner is a very effective communication technique that helps to promote patient cooperation and affirmation. Instead of saying, "Don't forget to use your incentive spirometer," reword the request with a positive focus by saying, "Remember to use your incentive spirometer every hour to help prevent pneumonia." Positive language tends to motivate individuals to comply with important activities. Practice on friends and family by rewording requests in a positive manner that supports cooperation.

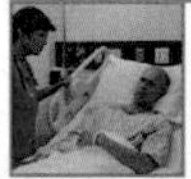

3. Write two opening statements or questions that may be used by the nurse to approach Mr. Beatrice and identify the underlying cause of his concern.

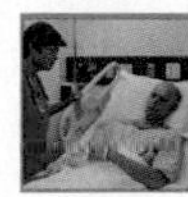

4. Name three therapeutic communication techniques that may be used by the nurse to encourage Mr. Beatrice to share his thoughts and concerns.

TABLE 3-2 Verbal Techniques for Initiating and Encouraging Communication

TECHNIQUE	EXAMPLES	RATIONALE
Offering self	"I'll sit with you for a while." "I'll stay with you until your family member arrives."	• Demonstrates compassion and concern for the patient • Establishes a caring relationship
Calling the patient by name	"Good morning, Mr. Trimble." "Hi, Ms. Martin. How are you feeling this evening?"	• Conveys that the nurse sees the patient as an individual • Shows respect and helps to establish a caring relationship
Sharing observations	"You look tense." "You seem frustrated." "You are smiling."	• Raises the patient's awareness of his or her nonverbal behavior • Allows the patient to validate the nurse's perceptions • Provides an opening for the patient to share possible joys or concerns
Giving information	"It is time for your bath." "My name is Pam, and I will be the RN taking care of you until 7 P.M." "Your surgery is scheduled for 10:30 A.M. tomorrow."	• Informs the patient of facts needed in a specific situation • Provides a means to build trust and develop a knowledge base on which patients can make decisions

Continued

TABLE 3-2 Verbal Techniques for Initiating and Encouraging Communication—cont'd

TECHNIQUE	EXAMPLES	RATIONALE
Using open-ended questions or comments	"What are some of your biggest concerns?" "Tell me more about your general health status." "Share some of the feelings you experienced after your heart attack."	• Gives the patient the opportunity to share freely on a subject • Avoids interjection of feelings or assumptions by the nurse • Provides for patient elaboration on important topics when the nurse wants to collect a breadth of information
Using focused questions or comments	"Point to exactly where your pain is radiating." "When did you start experiencing shortness of breath?" "How has your family responded to your being hospitalized?" "What is your greatest fear?" "Where were you when the symptoms started?" "Tell me where you live."	• Encourages the patient to share specific data necessary for completing a thorough assessment • Asks the patient to provide details regarding various concerns • Focuses on the immediate needs of the patient
Providing general leads	"And then?" "Go on." "Tell me more."	• Encourages the patient to keep talking • Demonstrates the nurse's interest in the patient's concerns
Conveying acceptance	"Yes." Nodding. "I follow what you are saying." "Uh huh."	• Acknowledges the importance of the patient's thoughts, feelings, and concerns
Using humor	"You are really walking well this morning. I'm going to have to run to catch up!"	• Provides encouragement • May lighten heavy moments of discussion • Used properly, allows a patient to focus on positive progress or better times and does not change the subject of a conversation
Verbalizing the implied	*Patient:* "I can't talk to anyone about this." *Nurse:* "Do you feel that others won't understand?"	• Encourages a patient to elaborate on a topic of concern • Provides an opportunity for the patient to articulate more clearly a complicated topic or feeling that could be easily misunderstood
Paraphrasing or restating communication content	*Patient:* "I couldn't sleep last night." *Nurse:* "You had trouble sleeping last night?"	• Encourages patients to describe situations more fully • Demonstrates that the nurse is listening
Reflecting feelings or emotions	"You were angry when your surgery was delayed?" "You seem excited about going home today."	• Focuses on the patient's identified feelings based on verbal or nonverbal cues
Seeking clarification	"I don't quite follow what you are saying." "What do you mean by your last statement?"	• Encourages the patient to expand on a topic that may be confusing or that seems contradictory
Summarizing	"There are three things you are upset about: your family being too busy, your diet, and being in the hospital too long."	• Reduces the interaction to three or four points identified by the nurse as being significant • Allows the patient to agree or add additional concerns
Validating	"Did I understand you correctly that...?"	• Allows clarification of ideas that the nurse may have interpreted differently than intended by the patient

TABLE 3-3 Nonverbal Techniques for Facilitating Communication

TECHNIQUE	EXAMPLES	RATIONALE
Active listening	• Maintaining intermittent eye contact • Matching eye levels • Attentive posturing • Facing the patient • Leaning toward the person who is speaking • Avoiding distracting body movement	• Conveys interest in the patient's needs, concerns, or problems • Provides the patient with undivided attention • Sends a clear message of concern and interest
Silence	• Being present with a person without verbal communication	• Provides the patient time to think or reflect • Communicates concern when there is really nothing adequate to say in difficult or challenging situations
Therapeutic touch	• Holding the hand of a patient • Providing a backrub • Touching a patient's arm lightly • Shaking hands with a patient in isolation	• Conveys empathy • Provides emotional support, encouragement, and personal attention • Relaxes the patient

NONTHERAPEUTIC COMMUNICATION

Nontherapeutic communication can be hurtful and potentially damaging to interaction. Changing the subject (e.g., in response to a patient who expresses a desire to talk about a concern that makes the nurse uncomfortable) or sharing personal opinions limits conversation between the nurse and the patient and discourages open conversation on sensitive topics. Many aspects of social conversation should be avoided when interacting with patients. Most are considered nontherapeutic and tend to shift the conversational focus away from the patient's concerns. Nurses engaging in nontherapeutic social conversation tend to be labeled by patients as uncaring and self-absorbed. Table 3-4 provides examples of nontherapeutic communication that should be avoided.

Avoiding nontherapeutic communication requires practice and experience. Intentionally incorporating as many therapeutic communication strategies as possible into conversations helps a nurse better meet patients' needs.

DEFENSE MECHANISMS LO 3.8

When individuals are under extreme stress or unable to comprehend and cope with the reality of a situation, they may use defense mechanisms to protect themselves and their psyches. **Defense mechanisms** are unconscious strategies that allow an individual to decrease or avoid unpleasant circumstances. Some defense mechanisms are protective when employed for short or long periods of time; others are consistently harmful. When used indefinitely, some defense mechanisms, such as denial, prevent an individual from effectively addressing critical issues. Others, such as compensation, may positively influence the productivity of an individual's life.

Patients faced with a situation perceived as hopeless may exhibit anger toward a nurse. When this happens, it is important for the nurse to recognize displacement and address the real concerns of the patient rather than taking the patient's expressions of anger personally. Table 3-5 defines common defense mechanisms that are important for the nurse to recognize when used by patients overwhelmed with the stress or realities of unpleasant situations in which they find themselves. Chapter 32 provides additional information on reactions to stress and defense mechanisms.

Nurses should document the use of defense mechanisms by patients. Use of unhealthy defense mechanisms over an extended period of time may require referral to a professional counselor.

! SAFE PRACTICE ALERT

Refer patients for professional counseling if they exhibit detrimental use of defense mechanisms while trying to cope with stressful situations.

SPECIAL COMMUNICATION CONSIDERATIONS LO 3.9

Many patients have sensory impairment, making nonverbal or verbal communication, or both, impossible. Communication with sensory-impaired patients requires patience, creativity, and adaptation to ensure that patient needs are met. The nurse's ability to modify the method of communication greatly impacts the quality of care delivered. Feelings of isolation, frustration, and depression by individuals with sensory impairment may be prevented if their caregivers use specific strategies to enhance communication. By assessing family dynamics and gathering community services information, nurses can better identify potential strengths and obstacles in patient support systems that affect effective communication.

TABLE 3-4 Nontherapeutic Communication

ACTION	EXAMPLES	RATIONALE
Asking "why" questions	"Why did you do that?" "Why are you feeling that way?" "Why do you continue to smoke when you know it is unhealthy?"	• Implies criticism • May make the patient defensive • Tends to limit conversation • Requires justification of actions • Focuses on a problem rather than a possible solution
Using closed-ended questions or comments	"Do you feel better today?" "Did you sleep well last night?" "Have you made a decision about radiation yet?" "Are you ready to take your bath?" "Will you let me give you your medicine now?"	• Results in short, one-word, yes or no responses • Limits elaboration or discussion of a topic • Allows patient to refuse important care • Differs from focused questions that direct an interview
Changing the subject	*Patient:* "I'm having a difficult time talking with my daughter." *Nurse:* "Do you have grandchildren?" *Patient:* "I just want to die." *Nurse:* "Did you sleep well last night?"	• Avoids exploration of the topic raised by the patient • Demonstrates the nurse's discomfort with the topic introduced by the patient
Giving false reassurance	"Everything will be okay." "Surgery is nothing to be concerned about." "Don't worry; everything will be fine."	• Discounts the patient's feelings • Cuts off conversation about legitimate concerns of the patient • Demonstrates a need by the nurse to "fix" something that the patient just wants to discuss
Giving advice	"If it were me, I would…" "You should really exercise more." "You should absolutely have chemotherapy to treat your breast cancer if you expect to live." "Of course you should tell your co-workers that you've been diagnosed with cancer."	• Discourages the patient from finding an appropriate solution to a personal problem • Tends to limit the patient's ability to explore alternative solutions to issues that need to be faced • Implies a lack of confidence in the patient to make a healthy decision • Removes the decision-making authority from the patient
Giving stereotypical or generalized responses	"It's for your own good." "Keep your chin up." "Don't cry over spilt milk." "You will be home before long."	• Discounts patient feelings or opinions • Limits further conversation on a topic • May be perceived as judgmental
Showing approval or disapproval	"That's good." "You have no reason to be crying."	• Limits reflection by patients • Stops further discussion on patient decisions or actions • Implies a need for patients to have the nurse's support and approval
Showing agreement or disagreement	"That's right." "I disagree with what you just said."	• Discontinues patient reflection on an introduced topic • Implies a lack of value for the thoughts, feelings, or concerns of patients
Engaging in excessive self-disclosure or comparing the experiences of others	"I had the same type of cancer 2 years ago." "I have several family members who drink too much, too." "I go to that restaurant every Friday for fish."	• Implies that experiences related to a disease process are similar for all patients • Takes the focus away from the patient • Limits further reflection or problem solving by the patient

TABLE 3-4 Nontherapeutic Communication—cont'd

ACTION	EXAMPLES	RATIONALE
Comparing patient experiences	"The lady in room 250 just had this surgery last week and did just fine." "My uncle had this type of inflammatory bowel disease and ended up having to have a colostomy."	• Removes the focus of conversation from the patient • Invalidates each individual patient experience as being unique and important • Breaches confidentiality
Using personal terms of endearment	"Honey." "Sweetie, it is time to take your medicine." "Sport, how about if you show me how well you can walk across the room?"	• Demonstrates disrespect for the individual • Diminishes the dignity of a unique patient • May indicate that the nurse did not take the time or care enough to learn or remember the patient's name
Being defensive	"The nurses here work very hard." "Your doctor is extremely busy." "This is the best hospital in the area." "You won't get any better care anywhere else."	• Moves the focus from the patient • Discounts the patient' feelings and thoughts on a subject • Limits further conversation on a topic of patient concern

TABLE 3-5 Defense Mechanisms

DEFENSE MECHANISM	DEFINITION
Compensation	Using personal strengths or abilities to overcome feelings of inadequacy
Denial	Refusing to admit the reality of a situation or feeling
Displacement	Transferring emotional energy away from an actual source of stress to an unrelated person or object
Introjection	Taking on certain characteristics of another individual's personality
Projection	Attributing undesirable feelings to another person
Rationalization	Denying true motives for an action by identifying a more socially acceptable explanation
Regression	Reverting to behaviors consistent with earlier stages of development
Repression	Storing painful or hostile feelings in the unconscious, causing them to be temporarily forgotten
Sublimation	Rechanneling unacceptable impulses into socially acceptable activities
Suppression	Choosing not to think consciously about unpleasant feelings

HEARING-IMPAIRED PATIENTS

Various approaches may be effective in providing patient care for those with impaired hearing. Patients who normally wear hearing aids should be encouraged to place them in their ears during morning care. Checking or replacing hearing aid batteries regularly helps to avoid most associated mechanical difficulties.

When communicating with a hearing-impaired patient, the nurse should make sure that the area is well lit with as little background noise as possible. Hearing aids amplify all sounds, making noisy environments confusing and frustrating. Raising the voice level slightly, speaking clearly, and making sure that the patient can see the nurse's face helps to facilitate communication. Adequate lighting enhances the patient's ability to see the speaker's mouth and face and interpret nonverbal communication. Stay within 3 to 6 feet of patients with hearing problems when conversing and avoid turning or walking away while talking. Consistent affirmative answers to the nurse's questions may be an indication that the patient is not hearing or understanding the information being shared. Care should be taken to verify that patients truly comprehend the content of verbal interaction. Extra patience may be required by the nurse to demonstrate caring while communicating with hearing-impaired patients.

Many of the strategies used when communicating with hearing-impaired patients are important when interacting with people who are deaf. Adequate lighting, avoiding over-enunciation, and speaking slowly while in direct proximity to deaf patients can help their ability to read lips and perceive the meaning of gestures and facial expressions. If deaf patients use sign language as their primary means of conversing, an interpreter should be contacted to help with communication of critical information (Collaboration and Delegation box). Gestures and the use of pictures can facilitate informal communication when an interpreter is unavailable.

Written communication is especially helpful when the nurse is providing detailed information to literate hearing-impaired or deaf patients and family members. A whiteboard and erasable marker or computer tablet kept at the bedside of a deaf patient may facilitate more effective communication. Institutional policies detailing the accommodations

COLLABORATION AND DELEGATION

Use of Interpreters

- Collaboration with the institutional department responsible for obtaining interpreters for deaf or limited English proficiency (LEP) patients should be initiated by the nurse as soon as the need is identified.
- Interpretation may be provided by a professional interpreter face-to-face with patients and families or by phone or video medical interpretation (VMI).
- Family members should not be used as interpreters of specific medical information to maintain the patient's right to privacy and to avoid possible misinterpretation of medical terminology.
- Access to interpretation or translation for deaf and LEP patients is required by Title VI of the Civil Rights Act of 1964, which mandates equal rights for people regardless of race, color, or national origin.

From U.S. Department of Health and Human Services: *Guidance to Federal Financial Assistance Recipients Regarding Title VI Prohibition against National Origin Discrimination Affecting Limited English Proficient Persons,* 2004. Retrieved from *http://onlineresources.wnylc.net/pb/orcdocs/LARC_Resources/LEPTopics/HC/hhsrevisedlepguidance.pdf.*

necessary to provide safe care to deaf patients should be followed.

VISUALLY IMPAIRED PATIENTS

An important factor to remember when caring for visually impaired or blind patients is that they are rarely hearing impaired. Typically, blind patients have heightened auditory and olfactory senses. Communication with blind patients can be characterized as anticipatory in nature, meaning that the nurse should alert visually impaired patients of potential hazards or object locations to provide necessary information and safe care. The position of numbers on an analogue clock is often used as a reference when communicating the location of food on the plate of a blind patient. For example, the nurse may inform the visually impaired patient that the meat entrée is in the 6 o'clock position and the coffee cup is at 2 o'clock on the tray. This system may be helpful in orienting blind patients to their hospital rooms. For example, from the vantage point of lying in bed, the bathroom may be at the 10 o'clock position and the phone at 5 o'clock on the bedside cabinet.

Large-print, Braille, audio, or e-books may be helpful in communicating effectively with visually impaired or blind patients. Many library materials and online resources are available to assist with patient education.

Gentle physical contact, such as a light touch on the arm, alerts the blind patient that someone is present. This is especially important if the patient has been sleeping, is in a noisy environment, or is hearing-impaired.

PHYSICALLY OR COGNITIVELY IMPAIRED PATIENTS

Communicating in ways that best meet the needs of physically or cognitively impaired individuals requires ongoing creativity and adaptation. Patients with severe respiratory difficulties requiring endotracheal intubation or a tracheostomy need special accommodations to communicate. Some of these patients may be able to use nonverbal cues such as head nodding or hand squeezing to communicate their needs. A whiteboard with erasable markers or a computer tablet can be particularly helpful. Patients with expressive aphasia may also benefit from these communication aids if their cognitive capacity and physical ability to write are intact. If a patient is weak, the caregiver should hold the board and help the patient write.

Communication with a semicomatose or postoperative patient still partially anesthetized may be realized through physical touch and hand squeezing and by observing for nonverbal signs. If the patient grimaces when touched or moved or responds when asked to squeeze the nurse's hand, communication is established. The nurse must talk to the patient before initiating care and throughout procedures, even if the patient is seemingly unaware of the surroundings. Individuals can hear even when they are physically unable to move or speak. This fact is important for nurses to remember when caring for patients who are temporarily noncommunicative or comatose.

Quadriplegic patients who have a tracheostomy or who are on a ventilator may use electronic devices and a variety of gestures or eye movements to communicate. Assistive devices that use eye movement technology help paralyzed patients who are mentally alert and have neuromuscular control of the head and neck to communicate. These devices include electronic transducers that connect remotely to computers. In addition to becoming familiar with assistive electronic equipment, nurses must pay close attention to the meaning of specific nods or shoulder shrugs to fully communicate with quadriplegic patients.

Patients diagnosed with intellectual disabilities or dementia require special attention by caregivers. Consulting with the family members of these patients often provides helpful hints and insights into what is most effective in gaining their cooperation with necessary nursing interventions. Avoiding confrontation is important. It is better to accept a demented patient's thought process than to argue or try to correct an erroneous line of thinking.

FAMILIES AND COMMUNITIES

Providing support for the families of hospitalized patients involves ongoing communication. Because the discipline of nursing addresses the effects of illness on patients rather than simply the illness itself, establishing and maintaining viable lines of communication among patients and their family members or friends is critical. Particularly helpful are therapeutic communication techniques, which may provide insight into the existence and strength of available support systems. Family dynamics are often revealed by listening and observing, providing a clearer picture of the impact of illness and the associated circumstances on patients and their families. Assessment data about patients' families and the communities in which they live are a significant resource for formulating patient-centered plans of care.

Nurses should become familiar with community services to provide for the ongoing needs of discharged patients and their families. Nurses should engage community leaders in dialogue related to health care access and home care services. By taking seriously their role as public communicators, nurses can influence the wellness and quality of life in the communities in which they work and live.

SUMMARY OF LEARNING OUTCOMES

LO 3.1 *Identify key components of the communication process:* A referent initiates communication between a sender and a receiver during which a message is sent through a channel and followed by feedback to ensure accuracy.

LO 3.2 *List examples of the verbal and nonverbal modes of communication:* The most common and accurate mode of communication is nonverbal, which uses various forms of body language and voice inflection. Verbal communication may be spoken, written, or electronic.

LO 3.3 *Recognize various types of communication:* Effective intrapersonal, interpersonal (including interprofessional), small-group, and public communication skills must be used by nurses to adequately meet the needs of patients, families, and the communities in which they practice.

LO 3.4 *Describe how significant aspects of the nursing process are implemented in the nurse–patient helping relationship:* The relationship focuses on addressing identified patient needs. The nurse must use all steps of the nursing process to build a trusting relationship focused on positive patient outcomes.

LO 3.5 *Discuss factors affecting the timing of patient communication:* Several factors influence the ability of patients to respond to nurse-initiated communication. They include pain level, anxiety, and environmental factors such as distractions or level of privacy.

LO 3.6 *Recognize the roles of respect, assertiveness, collaboration, delegation, and advocacy in professional nursing communication:* Nurses communicate professionally by showing respect, advocating for patients, and assertively conveying patient needs during collaboration and delegation.

LO 3.7 *Identify social, therapeutic, and nontherapeutic communication techniques:* Nurses must practice using a variety of therapeutic communication techniques to address the needs of patients. Nontherapeutic communication may be considered social in nature and shifts conversational focus away from the concerns of patients.

LO 3.8 *List defense mechanisms used by patients while communicating:* Individuals under extreme stress may use defense mechanisms to protect themselves and their psyches to better cope with the reality of life experiences.

LO 3.9 *Illustrate methods of communicating in special situations:* Nurses may use a variety of methods such as whiteboards, computer tablets, physical touch, and online resources to communicate effectively with sensory-impaired or nonverbal patients. Assessing family and community dynamics facilitates enhanced communication and patient safety.

Responses to the critical-thinking questions are available at *http://evolve.elsevier.com/YoostCrawford/fundamentals/.*

REVIEW QUESTIONS

1. A hospitalized patient experiences a sharp, stabbing pain while visiting with his spouse. Both the patient and his wife become very concerned, and the patient's call light is activated. What referent initiated communication between the patient and the nurse?
   a. Interaction between the patient and his wife
   b. Concern on the part of the patient's spouse
   c. Pain experienced by the patient
   d. Activation of the call light

2. Which factor influences whether a message is effectively communicated? *(Select all that apply.)*
   a. Timing of the conversation
   b. Educational level of participants
   c. Mode of communication used
   d. Physical environment of discussion
   e. Clothing that the nurse is wearing

3. When a patient is grimacing, what assessment statement or question would be most beneficial for identifying the underlying cause of the nonverbal communication?
   a. "Did you lose something?"
   b. "You appear to be having pain."
   c. "I will turn off the lights and let you rest."
   d. "May I get you something to relieve your tension?"
4. What action by the nurse would most ensure accurate interpretation of patient communication?
   a. Providing feedback regarding the conveyed message
   b. Writing down the patient's conversational highlights
   c. Assuming significant cultural differences exist
   d. Verifying the patient's emotional state
5. If a patient's verbal and nonverbal communication is inconsistent, which form of communication is most likely to convey the true feelings of the patient?
   a. Written notes
   b. Facial expressions
   c. Implied inferences
   d. Spoken words
6. What strategy would be most effective in communicating with a highly anxious adult immediately before surgery?
   a. Providing specific, concise information
   b. Detailing likely causes of their anxiety
   c. Focusing on postoperative details
   d. Using instructional multimedia DVDs
7. What action should the nurse take if an alert and oriented patient asks the nurse for personal contact information?
   a. Ask the patient why the personal information is needed.
   b. Report the interaction to the nursing supervisor immediately.
   c. State that it would not be appropriate to share that information.
   d. Change the subject, and hope that the patient does not ask again.
8. What would be the best therapeutic response to a patient who expresses indecision about recommended chemotherapy treatments?
   a. "Can you tell me why you are undecided?"
   b. "It's always a good idea to have chemotherapy."
   c. "What are you thinking about the treatments at this point?"
   d. "You should follow whatever your health care provider recommends."
9. Which statement is most accurate regarding symbolic expression?
   a. Skills confidence can be shared most effectively by nurses wearing distinctive clothing.
   b. Clothing choices by a hospitalized patient rarely reflect his or her economic resources.
   c. Make-up use by a patient is unnecessary for any reason during hospitalization.
   d. Nondramatic make-up use and minimal accessorizing by nurses demonstrates professionalism.
10. Which defense mechanism is being exhibited when a 27-year-old patient insists on having a parent present during routine care?
    a. Denial
    b. Regression
    c. Repression
    d. Displacement

Answers and rationales for the review questions are available at *http://evolve.elsevier.com/YoostCrawford/fundamentals/*.

REFERENCES

Agency for Healthcare Research and Quality: Interdisciplinary teamwork is a key to patient safety in the operating room, ICU and ER, January 2004. Retrieved from *http://archive.ahrq.gov/RESEARCH/jan04/0104RA25.htm*.

Aiello J, Aiello T: The development of personal space: Proxemic behavior of children 6 through 16. *Hum Ecol*, 2(3):177-189, 1974.

American Nurses Association: *ANA's principles for social networking and the nurse.* Silver Spring, Md., 2011, Author.

Cronenwett L, Sherwood G, Barnsteiner J, et al: Quality and safety education for nurses. *Nurs Outlook*, 55(3):122-131, 2007.

Egan G: *The skilled helper: A problem management and opportunity-development approach to helping*, ed. 10, Belmont, Calif., 2014, Wadsworth.

Hall E: *The hidden dimension*, Garden City, N.Y., 1966, Doubleday.

Iyer P: SBAR. *Med Legal News*, 31:1-2, 2007.

The Joint Commission: Sentinel event statistics, 2013. Retrieved from *www.jointcommission.org*.

Knott P: How does culture influence health care? *Physician Assistant*, 26(4):21-37, 2002.

Mehrabian A: *Silent messages: Implicit communication of emotions and attitudes*, Belmont, Calif., 1971, Wadsworth.

Pullen R, Barrett L, Rowh M, Wright K: Men, caring, & touch. *Nursing*, 39(Suppl):14-17, 2009.

Pullen R: Tips for communicating with patients of a different culture. *Nursing*, 37(10):48-49, 2007.

Purnell L: *Transcultural health care: A culturally competent approach*, ed. 4, Philadelphia, 2013, FA Davis.

Tuckman B, Jensen MA: Stages of small-group development revisited. *Group Organization Manage*, 2(4):419-427, 1977.

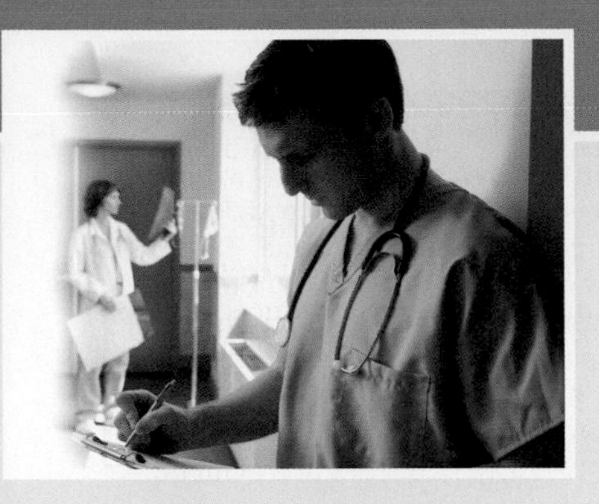

CHAPTER 4

Critical Thinking in Nursing

EVOLVE WEBSITE

http://evolve.elsevier.com/YoostCrawford/fundamentals/

- Additional Evolve-Only Review Questions With Answers
- Answers and Rationales for Text Review Questions
- Answers to Critical-Thinking Questions
- Case Study With Questions
- Glossary

LEARNING OUTCOMES

Comprehension of this chapter's content will provide students with the ability to:

LO 4.1 Identify the relationship between critical thinking and clinical reasoning.
LO 4.2 Summarize how theories of critical thinking apply to professional nursing practice.
LO 4.3 Describe the intellectual standards of critical thinking.
LO 4.4 Discuss critical-thinking components and attitudes.
LO 4.5 Apply principles of critical thinking in nursing practice.
LO 4.6 Explain errors to avoid in providing safe and competent patient care.
LO 4.7 Describe methods for improving critical thinking in nursing.

KEY TERMS

accuracy, p. 58
bias, p. 62
breadth, p. 58
clarity, p. 58
clinical reasoning, p. 56
critical thinking, p. 56
decision making, p. 56
deductive reasoning, p. 59
depth, p. 58
fairness, p. 58
inductive reasoning, p. 59
judgment, p. 56
logic, p. 58
precision, p. 58
problem solving, p. 56
reasoning, p. 56
relevance, p. 58
significance, p. 58
validation, p. 60

CASE STUDY

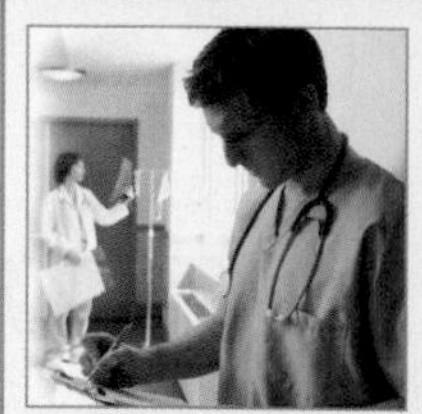

Sam is completing his first year as a nurse and works with a team of nurse practitioners and oncology surgeons in a private practice. He reviews each patient's chart at least 1 week before admission for surgery and develops a preliminary, individualized preoperative plan of care that best supports a positive patient outcome. The next chart Sam reads is that of Ms. Larchmere, who is a 24-year-old, intellectually disadvantaged woman from a local group home. She has been referred to the oncology practice for ovarian cancer surgery. A note on the chart states that Ms. Larchmere has a history of a congenital heart defect and seizures. She has limited verbal skills and physically lashes out or withdraws in unfamiliar situations.

Refer back to this case study to answer the critical-thinking questions throughout the chapter.

Survival and success in our complex society depends on critical thinking, which is an essential competency for registered nurses (Chaffee, 2012; Paul, 1993). The practice environment of nursing requires higher-order thinking so that the nurse can accurately assess and analyze clinical issues and make clinical judgments and decisions. As described by Paul (1988), **critical thinking** is a complex process that is "the art of thinking about your thinking while you're thinking so you make your thinking more clear, precise, accurate relevant, consistent and fair" (pp. 2-3). For the nurse, critical thinking provides a framework for reflection on judgments and actions that result in positive outcomes, increasing the accuracy of clinical decisions.

CRITICAL THINKING AND CLINICAL REASONING LO 4.1

Critical thinking has become a buzzword for all types of thinking, but it must be differentiated from casual or haphazard thinking, such as trial and error. Nurses make life-and-death decisions on the basis of critical thinking influenced by scientific research and best practices. "Critical thinking involves the application of knowledge and experience to identify patient problems and to direct clinical judgments and actions that result in positive patient outcomes" (Benner, Hughes, and Sutphen, 2008, p. 104). **Clinical reasoning** uses critical thinking, knowledge, and experience to develop solutions to problems and make decisions in a clinical setting (Carr, 2004). A nurse's clinical-reasoning skills develop over time with increased knowledge and expertise.

Many definitions for critical thinking can be found in social science, education, and health science literature. In nursing education and practice, the term *critical thinking* is often used synonymously with *problem solving, decision making, reasoning,* or *judgment.* Definitions of these related terms are given in Table 4-1. Although many of these terms are used interchangeably, for the purposes of this chapter, critical thinking is considered the foundation for the other processes.

In 1990, the American Philosophical Association published a Delphi report that focused on the conceptualization of critical thinking by a consensus of 46 experts, including theorists, educators, and specialists in critical-thinking assessment over a 22-month time frame. The report describes "the ideal critical thinker as habitually inquisitive, well-informed, trustful of reason, open-minded, flexible, fair-minded in evaluation, honest in facing personal biases, prudent in making judgments, willing to reconsider, clear about issues, orderly in complex matters, diligent in seeking relevant information, reasonable in the selection of criteria, focused in inquiry, and persistent in seeking results that are as precise as the subjects and the circumstances of inquiry require" (p. 3). Other themes from the Delphi report include honesty, trust, persistence, and precision. In the current health care delivery system, it is imperative that nurses maintain their professional practice and competency through seeking new knowledge, asking questions, making sound decisions, and remaining vigilant and open to changes and new developments.

THEORETICAL UNDERPINNINGS OF CRITICAL THINKING LO 4.2

The seminal works of Paul (1985, 1988, 1993; Paul and Elder, 2001, 2002), Ennis (1991, 2002), Schön (1983), and the later works of Alfaro-LeFevre (2012) have been used to understand critical thinking and its application to nursing practice,

TABLE 4-1 Processes That Depend on Critical Thinking

PROCESS	DEFINITION
Problem solving	Systematic, analytic approach to finding a solution to a problem
Decision making	Choosing a solution or answer from among different options; often considered a step in the problem-solving process
Reasoning	Logical thinking that links thoughts, ideas, and facts together in a meaningful way; used in scientific inquiry and problem solving
Judgment	The result or decision related to the processes of thinking and reasoning

education, and research. Critical thinking about any topic is a way to improve the quality of thought processes through analysis, assessment, and reconstruction. The interaction of these concepts is central to the development of critical thinking. Consistent theoretical underpinnings in these works include the following:

- *Reflection:* The results of deliberate thinking are used to guide further thinking. Benner (2001) and others assert that the ability to engage in reflection about and during practice and to make changes in practice based on the reflections is the hallmark of an experienced practitioner. Reflection is an effective tool that enables students and nurses to think about how best to improve their future caregiving in similar situations.
- *Evidence:* Identification and use of evidence is necessary to guide analysis of situations and decision making. Nursing practice must be based on evidence gained through research and review of findings.
- *Standards:* Critical thinking needs to be assessed and evaluated according to standards to ensure the quality of thinking. Nursing practice is based on standards established by the American Nurses Association in areas such as the nursing process, ethics, education, research, communication, leadership, and collaboration.
- *Attributes or traits:* Some personal characteristics are associated with critical thinking. Fairness, responsibility, and empathy are examples of traits that contribute to a nurse's ability to think critically while providing safe patient care.

The critical-thinking model of Alfaro-LeFevre (2012) has been specifically applied to nursing practice and includes four overlapping and integrated concepts: critical-thinking characteristics, theoretical and experiential knowledge, interpersonal skills, and technical competencies. To develop critical thinking, the nurse needs to develop a critical-thinking character, which includes maintaining high standards and developing critical-thinking qualities such as honesty, fair-mindedness, creativity, patience, persistence, and confidence.

The next step in the development of critical thinking includes taking responsibility for personal learning and seeking needed experiences that can provide the necessary knowledge on which to base the thinking. Fostering interpersonal skills, such as teamwork, conflict management, and advocacy, is important in the development of critical thinking. Self-evaluation and having thinking evaluated by others require the ability to accept and use constructive criticism.

The last step in Alfaro-LeFevre's critical-thinking model is technical competency. Until proficiency is achieved with technical skills, mental energy focused on psychomotor skills competes with other conceptual or knowledge gaps. This is often seen in clinical practice when a new skill or procedure is performed by the nurse. Being overly focused on the task may interfere with the nurse's ability to attend to the patient's questions and anxiety about the procedure.

INTELLECTUAL STANDARDS OF CRITICAL THINKING LO 4.3

According to Paul and Elder (2001), intellectual standards are foundational to thinking critically: "Critical thinkers routinely ask questions that apply intellectual standards to thinking. The ultimate goal is for these questions to become so spontaneous in thinking that they form a natural part of our inner voice, guiding us to better and better reasoning" (p. 84). The following intellectual standards are essential to critical thinking: clarity, accuracy, precision, relevance, depth, breadth, logic, significance, and fairness. Table 4-2 defines these intellectual standards and lists questions that facilitate the application of each standard. As with any skill, critical thinking can be enhanced through practice. The routine use of these questions should promote critical thought.

CRITICAL-THINKING COMPONENTS AND ATTITUDES LO 4.4

Critical thinking is not random or casual thinking. It is thinking characterized by accuracy, self-reflection, clarity, and soundness (Paul and Elder, 2001). Effective critical thinking depends on specific components such as a knowledge base, reasoning, inference, validation, and attitudes that promote learning.

KNOWLEDGE REVIEW

Because critical thinking is disciplined, this form of thinking is contextual and requires knowledge of the subject that is the focus of the thinking. It is not possible for a person to think critically about something if the person knows nothing about the subject matter.

Baseline Knowledge

In nursing, baseline knowledge includes content learned in prerequisite courses, such as human growth and development, nutrition, genetics, anatomy, physiology, biochemistry, and psychology; nursing-specific courses, such as fundamentals of nursing, pathophysiology, and pharmacology; and specialty information about specific patient populations, such as pediatrics, adult health, maternal-child, and critical care. These courses provide foundational knowledge that prepares the nurse to deal with practice and clinical issues.

Information Gathering

Data collection is an important concept for professional nursing practice and is integral to assessment, the first step in the nursing process. The focus of data collection often is based on knowledge gaps. The application of critical-thinking skills to information gathering assists the nurse in collecting relevant, precise, and accurate data. Because

TABLE 4-2 Intellectual Standards for Critical Thinking

DEFINITIONS	ASSESSMENT QUESTIONS
Clarity: being easily understood or precise in thought and style; considered a gateway standard because a statement cannot be evaluated for accuracy or precision if it is ambiguous	How can you elaborate on that point? How could you express that point differently? What is an illustration? What is an example? This is what I heard you say; am I correct about your meaning?
Accuracy: representing something in a true and correct way	Is that true? How can I determine whether this information is correct? How can this information be verified?
Precision: providing sufficient detail to understand exactly what was meant	What are additional details? Can you be more specific?
Relevance: focusing on facts and ideas directly related and pertinent to a topic	How is this related to the question? How does that relate to the issue? What is the relationship to other ideas?
Depth: getting beneath the surface of the topic or problem to identify and manage related complexities	How does this address the complexities of the issue? How does this take into account the problems associated with the question? What are the most significant factors in the problem?
Breadth: considering a topic, problem, or issue from every relevant viewpoint	Are there other points of view for consideration? How would this issue look from a different viewpoint? Is there another way to approach this problem?
Logic: using a mutually supportive and sensible combination of thoughts and facts to form a conclusion	Does this fit together logically? Does this make sense? How does the evidence lead to this solution or answer? How do the conclusions support the evidence?
Significance: concentrating on the most important information (e.g., concepts, facts) when considering an issue	What is the most significant information needed to address the issue? How is that fact important in this context? Which question or concept is most important to the issue?
Fairness: thinking or acting in accord with reason and without bias	How is the conclusion justified in relation to the evidence? Are the assumptions justified? Am I considering other points of view?

Adapted from Paul R, Elder L: *Critical thinking: Tools for taking charge of your learning and your life,* Upper Saddle River, N, 2001, Prentice-Hall.

clinical decisions are often based on such data collection, it is important that the nurse use critical-thinking skills during these assessments.

When a patient is initially interviewed and assessed, the nurse must complete a thorough analysis of the patient's physical, emotional, spiritual, and psychomotor status. Several tools are available to guide the nurse in conducting detailed, complete assessments, including Gordon's Functional Health Patterns. The nurse often works with unlicensed assistive personnel (UAP) to collect relevant data on height and weight, intake and output, and vital signs. Nurses collaborate with other health care professionals to coordinate care (Collaboration and Delegation box). Interdisciplinary clinical rounds, which include physicians, registered nurses, physical therapists, occupational therapists, and dietitians, are often undertaken to identify priorities of care, discuss overlapping areas of treatment, and ensure coordination of care.

COLLABORATION AND DELEGATION

Critical Thinking and Safe Patient Care

- Optimal patient management requires critical thinking and collaboration with all disciplines involved in the patient's care. Interdisciplinary clinical rounds are an effective approach to management of complex patient problems related to discharge planning, end-of-life decisions, and other ethical issues.
- Critical thinking is used by the registered nurse to guide decisions related to delegation of assignments and tasks. Before delegation of a task, the nurse must be knowledgeable about the role, scope of practice, and competency of the recipient of the delegated task.
- When developing preoperative plans of care, nurses use critical thinking, collaboration, and communication. Critical thinking helps the nurse to identify missing data. Collaboration and communication promote team-oriented decision making that supports positive patient outcomes (Mulcahy and Pierce, 2011).

Nurses must be equipped with a large knowledge base in addition to data collection and information-gathering skills to help them find answers when faced with new problems, questions, and situations. When the nurse is able to formulate a question when faced with a new problem or situation, possible solutions can be pursued.

REASONING

Paul and Elder (2006) explain that the terms *thinking* and *reasoning* are often used synonymously, although reasoning is more formal because it usually is aimed at finding answers, providing explanations, and forming conclusions. Wilkinson (2011) states, "Reasoning is logical thinking that links thoughts in meaningful ways. Reasoning is used in scientific inquiry, in examining controversial issues, and in problem solving (i.e., nursing process)" (p. 58). Nurses use clinical reasoning to monitor patients through ongoing assessment and evaluation and to guide decision making. Nurses use inductive reasoning and deductive reasoning in their practice.

Inductive Reasoning

Inductive reasoning uses specific facts or details to make conclusions and generalizations; it proceeds from specific to general. The nurse observes that a patient who recently had an indwelling urinary catheter removed complains of burning on urination and that the urine is cloudy and foul smelling. On the basis of this assessment, the nurse may reason that the patient has a urinary tract infection (UTI) because the findings are consistent with those seen in other patients with documented UTIs; this inductive argument is probably correct. The strength of inductive reasoning is closely related to the number of previous observations and the quality of the reasons (Wilkinson, 2011). However, because the conclusions are based on observations and assumptions, not valid proof, further actions may be required to substantiate the conclusion. In the example of the patient with burning on urination, a urine sample may be ordered for analysis to investigate the possibility of a UTI, a complication that can result from an indwelling urinary catheter.

Deductive Reasoning

Deductive reasoning involves generating facts or details from a major theory, generalization, or premise (i.e., from general to specific). In providing care for a patient with a suspected infection, the nurse observes for signs such as an elevated temperature and sources of infection to validate this deductive argument. These assessment findings may be consistent with an infection. However, as with inductive reasoning, other factors that may cause an elevated temperature need to be addressed to support this reasoning. For example, a patient who is dehydrated may also have an elevated temperature. It is generally accepted that if the premises or facts are true, the conclusions in deductive reasoning are also correct.

INFERENCES

Paul and Elder (2001) describe inferences as intellectual acts that involve a conclusion being made on the basis of something. The accuracy of an inference is directly related to the accuracy of what the inference is based on. Inferences are frequently based on assumptions, which are beliefs that are taken for granted and assumed to be true. Assumptions may be used to guide decision making even when they are based on something that was previously learned and not questioned.

It is important that nurses examine their assumptions and inferences about patients and their health care. When assessing an obese patient, the nurse may assume that the person eats too much and never exercises. On the basis of this assumption, the nurse may make the inference that the patient does not care about personal health. On further assessment, the nurse finds that the patient has severe hypothyroidism that is contributing greatly to the patient's obesity. This example reinforces the importance of the accuracy of assumptions and illustrates that inferences may be logical or illogical, accurate or inaccurate, justified or unjustified.

Intuition

Intuition is the feeling that you know something without specific evidence. Wilkinson (2011) describes intuition as a problem-solving approach that relies on an inner sense. Intuition is gaining favor as a valid characteristic of expert clinical judgment acquired through knowledge, practice, and experience. Alfaro-LeFevre (2012) explains that expert nurses use intuition to facilitate problem solving because their hunches (most likely intuition) are based on experiential knowledge. Less experienced nurses rely more on logic and a step-by-step approach when encountering the same issue (Figure 4-1). In either situation, intuition based on critical thinking requires analysis and evidence to support actions.

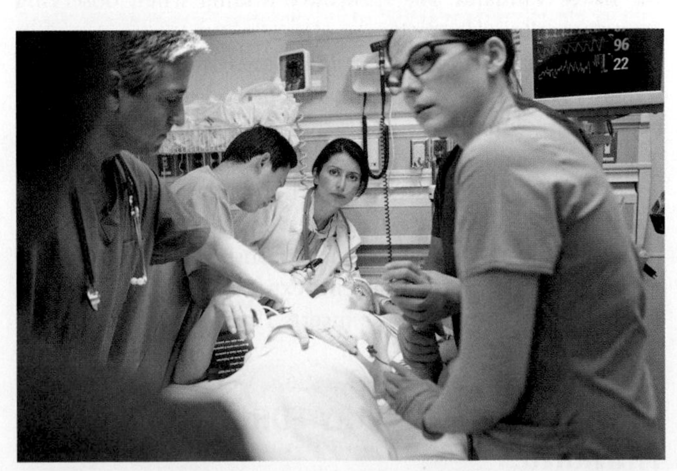

FIGURE 4-1 The intuition and knowledge of experienced nurses can help direct the practice of newer colleagues in emergency situations.

Interpretation

Examining how information is organized and given meaning guides the interpretation of the information. Interpretations must be differentiated from facts and evidence because they are based on personal conceptions, experiences, and perspective. Paul and Elder (2006) describe critical thinkers as being able to recognize their interpretations, differentiate the interpretations from the evidence, consider alternative interpretations, and reconsider their interpretations in light of new data.

Interpretation of data is an important aspect of professional nursing practice. Some data are objective (e.g., laboratory values, diagnostic examination results, clinical manifestations), and other data are subjective (e.g., facial expressions, mood, body language). However, in both situations, nurses are expected to interpret data and use it to guide their decisions and actions.

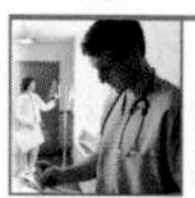

1. The critical-thinking skill of interpretation needs to be employed first to begin developing Ms. Larchmere's plan of care. Consider all that Sam knows about the patient, and identify a minimum of three people or resources Sam needs to consult to gather essential patient data. Provide a rationale for each of your answers.

VALIDATION

Along with the specific components of critical thinking—knowledge, reasoning, and inferences—validation of information is required before taking action. Alfaro-LeFevre (2012) defines **validation** as "the process of gathering information to determine whether the information or data collected are factual and true" (p. 292).

One aspect of validation is to find support for the findings or data. Subjective data are often validated with objective data; for instance, a patient complains of severe itching, and the nurse validates this subjective finding when observing scratch marks and a rash.

Validation is also pertinent to ensuring the competency of nurses in the clinical setting. When an experienced nurse begins employment at a new facility, competency assessments (i.e., validations) are frequently completed as part of the orientation process. For example, although a nurse might have been responsible for inserting intravenous (IV) catheters at a previous place of employment, demonstration of skill competency based on facility-specific expectations and standards is required before the nurse inserts IVs in patients at a new workplace.

ATTITUDES NECESSARY FOR CRITICAL THINKING

Critical-thinking attitudes promote learning, reasoning, and discipline. Particularly relevant to nursing, these attitudes foster critical thinking that focuses on clarity, precision, clarification, validation, and recognition of bias. Table 4-3 defines 11 intellectual traits identified by Paul (1993) as essential for competence in critical thinking.

TABLE 4-3 Essential Critical-Thinking Traits

INTELLECTUAL TRAIT	DEFINITION
Confidence	Feeling certain about one's ability to accomplish a goal
Thinking independently	Considering a wide range of ideas before coming to a conclusion
Fairness	Avoiding bias or prejudice and dealing with a situation in a just manner
Responsibility and accountability	Acting on sound knowledge and acknowledging actions as one's own
Risk taking	Being willing to try new ideas
Discipline	Following orderly thinking to do what is best
Perseverance	Staying determined to work until the goal is achieved
Creativity	Formulating new ideas and alternative approaches
Curiosity	Being motivated to achieve and asking why
Integrity	Being honest and willing to adhere to principles in the face of adversity
Humility	Admitting one's limitations

Adapted from Paul R: *Critical thinking: How to prepare students for a rapidly changing world,* Santa Rosa, Calif., 1993, Foundation for Critical Thinking.

THE ROLE OF CRITICAL THINKING IN NURSING PRACTICE LO 4.5

The rapid rate of change and increasing complexity of health care and information technology make critical thinking essential in nursing. No longer is rote memorization and recall of content sufficient for the complex decisions and judgment required in professional nursing practice. Because knowledge and technology continue to expand for nursing professionals, the content learned in nursing school is not sufficient to maintain competence in nursing practice.

Professional nursing requires a commitment to lifelong learning. Nurses must possess critical-thinking skills to maintain pace with ever-changing treatment modalities and technological advances. Outdated learning strategies that focus on remembering content must be replaced by a focus on understanding the rationales and outcomes. Nursing students and new graduates must be equipped to find answers to new situations (Ironside, 2004). It is an expectation of professional practice that nurses update and maintain their competency and knowledge base. Maintaining competency through professional development and reviewing research is facilitated by having critical-thinking abilities (Evidence-Based Practice box).

EVIDENCE-BASED PRACTICE

Point-of-Care Testing

During the past several years, recommendations have been made to base nursing care on the best and most reliable evidence, and patient-centered care has been emphasized.

- Point-of-care testing (POCT) evolved from these recommendations. The practice allows certain laboratory tests (e.g., urinalysis, urine specific gravity, fingerstick measurements) to be performed in patient care units.
- On the basis of differences found in practice and potential faulty results, the Institute of Medicine (Kohn, Corrigan, and Donaldson, 1999) recommended standards for POCT. These standards include routine assessment of the sampling practices, standardized evaluations of controls used in assessing the samples, and review of quality of testing procedures (The Joint Commission, 2012).
- The reliability of POCT is based on formal planning and systematic management to reduce errors and ensure the quality of patient testing.

Because nursing requires the application of knowledge to make clinical decisions and guide care, it involves active participation by the nurse. The application of knowledge requires development of a questioning attitude. This process is sometimes referred to as *thinking like a nurse.*

CRITICAL THINKING IN THE NURSING PROCESS

Nurses use critical-thinking skills to guide decision making and to solve problems. The scientific method, one approach to problem resolution, is systematic, logical, and based on data collection and hypothesis testing. The steps include (1) identification of the problem, (2) definition or clarification of the problem, (3) statement of the problem, (4) determination of criteria for evaluation, (5) data collection, (6) generation of solutions, and (7) hypothesis testing (Wilkinson, 2011). The scientific method is an established system of critical thinking that has been well studied.

Because nursing care is not always a problem, the scientific method is not always applicable to nursing practice. The nursing process, which consistently requires critical thinking, is based on assessment, diagnosis, planning, implementation, and evaluation, and it can be applied without a definitive problem. Lipe and Beasley (2004) apply essential critical-thinking skills to the nursing process in the following manner:

- *Interpretation:* Nurses use this skill to understand and explain the meaning of data. Drawing on knowledge of theory and application, the nurse uses interpretative skills to consider possible causes and implications of observed data, events, and actions. Using knowledge of the action of a medication, the nurse interprets the effects of the medication.
- *Analysis:* Investigating plans of action on the basis of examination of subjective and objective data is an example of nursing analysis. Considering the advantages, disadvantages, and consequences of all possibilities, the nurse determines appropriate explanations or actions. The nurse analyzes the clinical presentation of a patient in relation to admitting diagnoses and ordered treatments to ensure that they have an appropriate rationale.
- *Evaluation:* Information, including the reliability, credibility, and bias of the source, is assessed. Relevance, one of Paul's intellectual standards, is important in the evaluation of new information. Nurses also evaluate when determining whether the desired outcome for an intervention was achieved.
- *Inference:* According to Lipe and Beasley (2004), critical thinkers skilled in inference make accurate conclusions that are based on sound reasoning. Nurses gather relevant baseline data and compare them with other information, such as admitting diagnoses, medical history, and knowledge of disease processes, to make inferences.
- *Explanation:* The ability to explain conclusions is an important critical-thinking skill. Paul's intellectual standards of clarity, accuracy, and precision are important in this skill, as well as the ability to provide a sound rationale for thoughts and actions. In the acute care setting, the nurse should have sound rationales regarding which patient to assess first, which findings to report to the primary care provider (PCP), and what actions to delegate to UAP.
- *Self-regulation:* Similar to reflection, self-regulation requires monitoring of thinking, with specific emphasis on reflecting on the rationale for the conclusion drawn and action taken. The nurse ponders, "Did I collect all relevant data? Are my assumptions accurate?" As these statements demonstrate, the focus is on assessing personal thinking, decision making, and actions. With effective self-reflection, the nurse recognizes errors and makes changes to correct them.
- *Clinical decision making:* For nurses, the consistent use of the essential skills of critical thinking guides clinical decision making. Nurses make many decisions throughout a typical day, and data collection and interpretation guided by critical thinking are more likely to result in sound clinical decisions.

THINKING ERRORS TO AVOID LO 4.6

Critical thinking, reasoning, and decision making can be negatively influenced by errors in thinking. Factors that can influence thinking may be based on past experiences, cultural beliefs, emotions, states of mind, and other interpersonal and intrapersonal causes. Consider the following possible reasons for flawed thinking.

BIAS

Decisions may be unduly influenced by **bias**, which is an inclination or tendency to favoritism or partiality. Bias may be related to a preconceived notion or prejudice. For example, a nurse may consistently postpone care of elderly patients on the assumption that their care will take more time than caring for younger patients, without considering the actual acuity of the individual patients. It is important for nurses to examine personal biases because they can negatively impact care.

> **! SAFE PRACTICE ALERT**
>
> It is essential to thoroughly assess and validate the underlying reasons for patient concerns or problems. This can avoid unnecessary bias that may interfere with the nurse's ability to provide appropriate patient-centered care.

ILLOGICAL THINKING

Illogical thinking is characterized by a failure to follow rational, systematic processes when approaching an issue or problem. Often making hasty generalizations and assumptions that do not consider the evidence, the illogical thinker may jump to conclusions. Another trait associated with this type of thinking is an appeal to tradition (Lipe and Beasley, 2004): "We have always done it this way." When illogical thinking is used, creativity in thinking can be limited, and new ideas and approaches do not evolve. If nurses do not stay current, illogical thinking can occur, causing care to be compromised.

LACK OF INFORMATION

People cannot think critically about something without having knowledge about it. Knowledge deficit can cause errors in thinking. Nurses in practice must continue to build their knowledge base to provide safe and appropriate care. This is particularly relevant to the increased numbers of medications that nurses administer and the possible interactions with other medications and foods. The nurse can make a medication error if new or unfamiliar medications are not researched before administering them to patients.

> **! SAFE PRACTICE ALERT**
>
> It is the nurse's responsibility before administering medications to understand the reason that a medication is prescribed, the expected patient response, potential adverse reactions, and drug interactions. References are available for point-of-care, hand-held devices and in the health care facility electronic health record. If a new medication is not referenced in either of these places, requesting information from the pharmacist is recommended.

CLOSED-MINDEDNESS

Errors in thinking and decision making can result from intentionally overlooking alternatives suggested by others. When relevant information from patients or experts is ignored due to closed-mindedness, nursing care can be compromised. Closed-minded individuals often believe that their way is the best and preferred way. For example, a nurse may believe that it is best for all patients to be bathed in the morning and is resistant to the idea of patients bathing in the evening. However, there is a patient who prefers evening baths because he has a colostomy that he cares for in the evening and prefers to bathe after this is completed. The closed-minded nurse may ignore the individual needs and values of the patient.

> **QSEN FOCUS!**
>
> Open-mindedness is essential to ensure the development of therapeutic nurse–patient relationships and collaborative interdisciplinary practice that promotes patient safety and patient-centered care.

ERRONEOUS ASSUMPTIONS

Assumptions are beliefs that are taken for granted and assumed to be true. According to Paul and Elder (2001), assumptions can be unjustified or justified, depending on whether there are good reasons for them. Erroneous assumptions can lead to safety issues in the clinical setting. For example, the nurse observes that the breakfast tray of a diabetic patient has been removed from the patient's room and assumes that the patient ate. On the basis of this assumption, the ordered hypoglycemic agent to lower blood glucose levels is administered. However, the food might have been

> **QSEN FOCUS!**
>
> Asking questions for clarification before implementing patient care is essential to ensuring patient safety and providing patient-centered care. Actively listening to patients enhances a nurse's ability to communicate patient needs, values, and preferences to other members of the interdisciplinary health care team.

discarded by the patient or removed at the patient's request without having been eaten. In this scenario, the nurse should question the patient about food intake and check the amount of food left on the tray if possible before administering the medication.

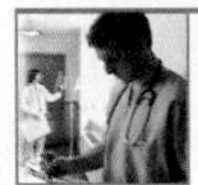

2. After consulting several resources and individuals, Sam decides that Ms. Larchmere can be assigned to a multibed preoperative area before surgery, even though it is often crowded and noisy. What critical-thinking skill should Sam employ regarding this decision? What change to the plan of care would you recommend and why?

METHODS FOR IMPROVING CRITICAL-THINKING SKILLS LO 4.7

Critical thinking is a skill that can be improved with practice. Reflection on one's thinking is an important exercise to facilitate critical-thinking skills. According to Wilkinson (2011), "Critical thinking requires reflection. Reflection means to ponder, contemplate, or deliberate on something. Reflective thinking integrates past experiences into the present and explores potential alternatives (Ethical, Legal, and Professional Practice box). In reflection, one considers an array of possibilities and reflects on the merits of each" (p. 40). Along with an attitude of reflection, the following strategies are intended to improve critical thinking.

ETHICAL, LEGAL, AND PROFESSIONAL PRACTICE

Caring and Competence

- Reflection and critical thinking are essential for providing competent and caring nursing care.
- Research indicates that caring encourages nurses to think critically while developing patient-centered plans of care (Zimmerman and Phillips, 2000).
- Combined competence and caring lead to more positive patient outcomes (Rhodes, Morris, and Lazenby, 2011).
- The thinking of student nurses is challenged through discussion of various views on and approaches to a subject, which enhances their ability to think critically and reflect and promotes transformative learning (Forbes and Hickey, 2009).
- Continuing education, certification, and The Joint Commission–required annual competency reviews are methods used to enhance critical thinking and ensure the competence of licensed nurses.

DISCUSSION WITH COLLEAGUES

Whether in an academic setting or in the clinical area, discussion of a problem, issue, or situation with colleagues may improve critical thinking. Through dialogue with others who have expertise or experience with the issue being faced, knowledge gaps can be filled, erroneous assumptions exposed, and unconscious biases addressed. Banning (2008) and Wendt, Kenny, and Marks (2007) describe "talk aloud" learning as a strategy to facilitate critical thinking. "Verbalizations (talk alouds) are a subset of the cognitive processes that generate action or behavior and can be used to address the cognitive processes encountered during problem solving" (Banning, 2008, pp. 10–11). Nurses can verify their assessments and diagnoses through discussion with colleagues to enhance clarity, precision, and accuracy.

AUDIBLE VERBALIZATION OF THOUGHTS

Nurses may use a type of "think aloud" as an inner dialogue to examine their thinking (Paul and Elder, 2001). In a process closely related to discussion with colleagues, the nurse verbally talks through data, assumptions, and plans for accuracy and relevance. This exercise incorporates elements of reflective thinking, which focuses on examining personal thinking. According to Banning (2008), the nurse who applies previously learned knowledge through verbalization may uncover knowledge gaps or areas of illogical thinking that can be addressed. The nurse who can recognize and verbalize what is unknown is better equipped to seek what is often a more creative answer or solution.

LITERATURE REVIEW

Because critical thinking cannot occur about subjects that are unknown, a review of literature may foster this type of thinking by addressing knowledge deficits. The process of literature review can be facilitated through the application of the intellectual standards described earlier. The more accurate, clear, and precise the reviewer can be in approaching the literature, the greater the likelihood that the information discovered addresses the original issue, question, or problem.

INTENTIONAL APPLICATION OF KNOWLEDGE

The application of knowledge through a case-based approach facilitates critical thinking (Hoffman, 2008). The case study is a type of problem-based learning strategy that focuses learning on solving real-world problems. Nursing practice is based on the application of knowledge to address patient problems.

Critical thinking can be improved by intentionally applying new concepts in the clinical setting. For example, when learning about acid-base and electrolyte balance, the student may review patients' laboratory values, analyze the results, and correlate the laboratory results with the patient's

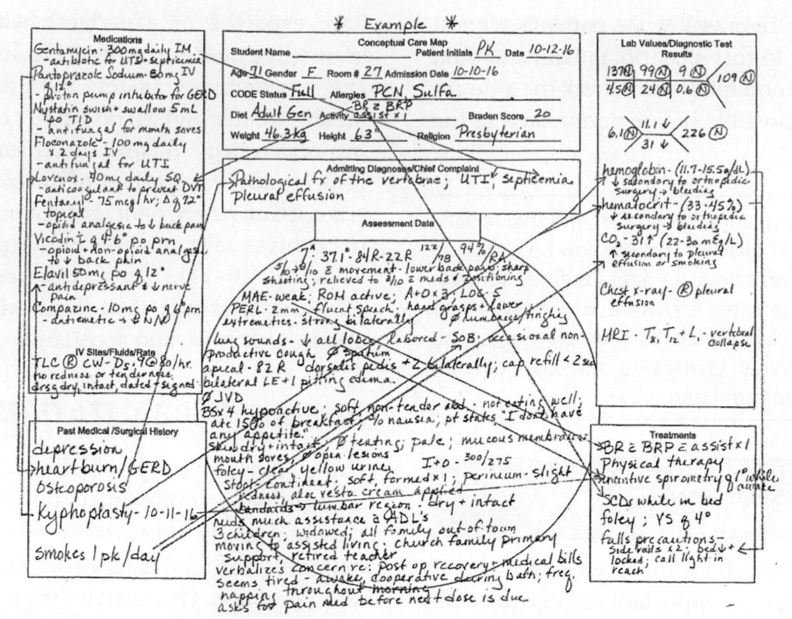

FIGURE 4-2 Use of the conceptual care map to organize and analyze information allows students to understand the relationship among patient data.

symptoms and diagnoses. This strategy encourages the learner to synthesize patient information and take more responsibility for learning (Thorpe and Loo, 2003).

CONCEPT MAPS

Concept mapping is a teaching-learning strategy that has been linked with improved critical-thinking skills in nurses (Vacek, 2009). St. Cyr and All (2009) describe the concept map as a way to organize and visualize data to identify relationships and solve problems. Concept maps can be used for note taking, mapping nursing care plans, and preparing for examinations. Through visual representations, the student can make correlations between related concepts (Alfaro-LeFevre, 2012). For example, when a student is studying or reviewing the pathophysiology and management of a patient with a brain tumor, the pathophysiology of the disease process can be the central theme. Main themes related to this disease process include representations of the clinical manifestations, treatment modalities, and nursing care. With a focus on correlating the main themes with the central theme, the pathophysiologic basis of the clinical manifestations is represented along with the rationales for the medical and nursing interventions.

Throughout this textbook, conceptual care maps are used to assist the student in organizing assessment data and applying critical-thinking skills to the development of nursing care plans. Conceptual care maps require students to organize, cluster, analyze, and synthesize data while identifying relationships among findings. This learning and organizational tool assists in the development of patient-centered goals, the recognition of evidence-based research interventions, and the evaluation of patient outcomes. The conceptual care map is a visual representation of a student's critical-thinking process and patient care plan (Figure 4-2).

SIMULATION

Facione and Facione (1996) describe critical thinking as a process of making judgments through interaction, reflection, and reasoning. Because this process develops over time and focuses on interactions in the discipline of nursing practice, it is important that learning environments be as realistic as possible. With the growing use of human patient simulators in nursing curricula, students are provided with realistic situations that foster increased confidence and competence. Simulated experiences enable the student to apply previously learned content in a safe and realistic environment that allows time for questioning, clarifying, and feedback. Students develop confidence in providing direct nursing care (Hilton and Pollard, 2005). According to Comer (2005), these opportunities for content application and skill practice are valuable in fostering the development of clinical judgment in students.

The learning effectiveness of simulated experiences largely depends on the feedback and debriefing that accompany the learning experiences (Murray, Grant, Howarth, et al, 2008; Rauen, 2004). Students need to critique their performance and to examine their understanding of the simulated learning experiences. If the simulation involved a patient experiencing respiratory distress from an exacerbation of asthma, in the debriefing, the student should be able to correlate the breath sounds with the pathophysiologic changes due to asthma and provide rationales for supplemental oxygen and any other nursing interventions played out in the scenario. These exercises require that students explore their thinking and reflect on the assumptions, inferences, and decisions made—all elements of critical thinking.

ROLE PLAYING

Many approaches to role playing can facilitate critical thinking. Simpson and Courtney (2008) describe a role-play strategy that involves assigning learners to different roles based on expected outcomes in a particular setting. Other learners and facilitators observe the role playing, and then all are involved in the debriefing or discussion of the scenario. As with simulation, this approach allows learners to interact in a safe, controlled environment. Simpson and Courtney integrated critical-thinking questions into the role playing, which allowed evaluation and validation of learning.

WRITTEN WORK

Strategies that focus on improving critical thinking through written work include reviewing and rewriting study or lecture notes, noting key facts while reading, identifying knowledge gaps while reading, and journaling. Alfaro-LeFevre (2012) explains that writing that is clear, organized, relevant, and focused requires the writer to apply critical-thinking principles.

Critical thinking is essential to safe, effective, professional nursing practice. It facilitates the collection of accurate patient data and the planning of patient-centered, evidence-based nursing care. Critical thinking is a skill that can be improved and facilitated through intentional and consistent application. Integrated into the nursing process, critical thinking is the method through which nurses think like a nurse.

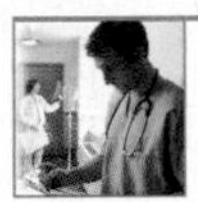

3. Sam is unfamiliar with all of the special needs of intellectually disadvantaged individuals. What critical-thinking methods should he undertake to improve his clinical decision-making skills and develop an individualized patient-centered plan of care for Ms. Larchmere?

SUMMARY OF LEARNING OUTCOMES

LO 4.1 *Identify the relationship between critical thinking and clinical reasoning:* Critical thinking is a required competency of professional nurses and is defined as a deliberate, reflective process that guides decision making and problem solving. Clinical reasoning requires critical thinking, knowledge, and expertise for decision making in clinical situations.

LO 4.2 *Summarize how theories of critical thinking apply to professional nursing practice:* The interaction of reflection, evidence, standards, and theoretical underpinnings fosters critical thinking. Critical thinking is used by nurses for decision making, clinical judgment, reasoning, problem solving, and organizing and prioritizing care.

LO 4.3 *Describe the intellectual standards of critical thinking:* Thinking critically requires competence in fundamental intellectual standards. These standards include clarity, accuracy, precision, relevance, depth, breadth, logic, significance, and fairness of the thinking process.

LO 4.4 *Discuss critical-thinking components and attitudes:* Effective critical thinking depends on specific components such as having an adequate knowledge base, reasoning, making inferences, and validating. Possessing the attributes of responsibility, accountability, creativity, perseverance, integrity, and humility assists nurses in the application of critical thinking to nursing practice.

LO 4.5 *Apply principles of critical thinking in nursing practice:* Critical thinking is essential at each step of the nursing process for clinical decision making. It is an expectation of professional practice that nurses update and maintain their competency and knowledge base. Maintaining competency through professional development and research reviews is facilitated by the nurse using critical-thinking skills. Decisions related to delegation, collaboration, and teamwork largely depend on the use of critical-thinking standards.

LO 4.6 *Explain errors to avoid in providing safe and competent patient care:* Patient safety is potentially threatened by errors in critical thinking that include bias, lack of knowledge, illogical thinking, closed-mindedness, and erroneous assumptions.

LO 4.7 *Describe methods for improving critical thinking in nursing:* Nurses can improve clinical decision making through discussions with colleagues, think aloud activities, literature review, intentional application of knowledge, concept mapping, simulation exercises, role playing, and written work.

Responses to the critical-thinking questions are available at *http://evolve.elsevier.com/YoostCrawford/fundamentals/*.

REVIEW QUESTIONS

1. The nurse receives a change of shift report on the five assigned patients and reviews prescriptions, treatments, and medications scheduled for the shift. Based on analysis of this information, the nurse chooses which patient to assess first. Which process of critical thinking best describes the nurse's action?
   a. Problem solving
   b. Decision making
   c. Judgment
   d. Reasoning
2. In approaching a new clinical situation, the nurse uses which question to facilitate precision in critical thinking?
   a. What do I know about this situation?
   b. What additional details do I need to gather?
   c. Does the clinical presentation correlate with the diagnosis?
   d. Are the treatments appropriate for the diagnosis?
3. Which question would be most appropriate for the nurse to ask while evaluating the relevance of patient data?
   a. Do these findings make sense?
   b. How can this information be verified?
   c. What are the most significant factors in the problem?
   d. What is the relation of this information to other data?
4. The nurse is assigned to develop a plan of care for a patient with a medical diagnosis that is unknown to the nurse. Guided by critical thinking, which action should the nurse take first?
   a. Ask the patient to describe the chief complaint.
   b. Request that another nurse be assigned to this patient.
   c. Review data about the medical diagnosis and routine management.
   d. Complete a physical assessment of the patient.
5. The nurse obtains a lower than normal (88% on room air) pulse oximetry reading on a patient. Which actions by the nurse result from accurately employing the critical-thinking skill of analysis in the nursing process? *(Select all that apply.)*
   a. Assessing the patient for symptoms of hypoxia
   b. Providing oxygen according to standing orders
   c. Elevating the head of the bed, if not contraindicated
   d. Allowing the patient to be alone to rest more comfortably
   e. Discussing adaptations needed for daily activities with the patient
6. Which of the following actions reflects inductive reasoning?
   a. Using subjective and objective data to confirm a diagnosis
   b. Assessing for specific clinical presentations based on a disease process
   c. Correlating elevated blood pressure with pathophysiology
   d. Validating an automatic blood pressure cuff reading with a manual measurement
7. The nurse is completing an assessment of a patient with sudden onset of abdominal pain. During the assessment, the nurse considers similar presentations and the underlying pathophysiology related to the patient's clinical manifestations. Which critical-thinking skill should the nurse use first to determine the cause of the patient's abdominal pain?
   a. Evaluation
   b. Interpretation
   c. Reflection
   d. Inference
8. The nurse can facilitate critical thinking through the use of which interpersonal skills? *(Select all that apply.)*
   a. Teamwork
   b. Intuition
   c. Judgment
   d. Conflict management
   e. Advocacy
   f. Reasoning
9. In providing care to a patient admitted to rule out human immunodeficiency virus (HIV) infection, wearing gloves during which activity may be an indication of bias?
   a. Collecting the patient's medical history
   b. Administering IV medications
   c. Performing oral care
   d. Completing a bed bath
10. During the assessment of a patient admitted for a total hip replacement, the nurse asks the patient to explain prior hospital experiences and, more specifically, any operative experiences. These questions reflect the nurse's use of which intellectual standard of critical thinking?
    a. Clarity
    b. Logic
    c. Precision
    d. Significance

Answers and rationales the review questions are available at *http://evolve.elsevier.com/YoostCrawford/fundamentals/*.

REFERENCES

Alfaro-LeFevre R: *Critical thinking, clinical reasoning, and clinical judgment: A practical approach*, ed. 5, St. Louis, 2012, Elsevier.

American Philosophical Association: Critical thinking: A statement of expert consensus for purposes of educational assessment and instruction. In *The Delphi report: Research findings and recommendations prepared for the Committee on Pre-College Philosophy*, ERIC document reproduction service no. ED315423, Millbrae, Calif., California Academic Press, 1990.

Banning M: The think aloud approach as an educational tool to develop and assess clinical reasoning in undergraduate students. *Nurse Educ Today*, 28:8-14, 2008.

Benner P: *From novice to expert: Excellence and power in clinical nursing practice*, Upper Saddle River, N.J., 2001, Prentice Hall.

Benner P, Hughes R, Sutphen M: *Patient safety and quality: An evidence-based handbook for nurses*, 2008. Retrieved from *www.ahrq.gov/qual/nurseshdbk/docs/BennerP_CRDA.pdf.*

Carr S: A framework for understanding clinical reasoning in community nursing. *J Clin Nurs*, 13(4):850-857, 2004.

Chaffee J: *Thinking critically*, ed. 10 Boston, 2012, Cengage Learning.

Comer SK: Patient care simulations: Role playing to enhance clinical reasoning. *Nurs Educ Perspect*, 26(6):357-361, 2005.

Cronenwett L, Sherwood G, Barnsteiner J, et al: Quality and safety education for nurses. *Nurs Outlook*, 55(3):122-131, 2007.

Ennis RH: Critical thinking: a streamlined conception. *Teach Philos*, 14(1):5-24, 1991.

Ennis RH: A super streamlined conception of critical thinking, 2002. Retrieved from *http://faculty.ed.uiuc.edu/rhennis.*

Facione NC, Facione PA: Assessment design issues for evaluating critical thinking in nursing. *Holist Nurs Pract*, 10(3):41-53, 1996.

Forbes M, Hickey M: Curriculum reform in baccalaureate nursing education: Review of the literature. *Int J Nurs Educ Scholarsh*, 6(1), 2009, doi: 10.2202/1548-923X.1797.

Hilton PA, Pollard CL: Enhancing the effectiveness of the teaching and learning of core clinical skills. *Nurse Educ Pract*, 5(5):289-295, 2005.

Hoffman JJ: Teaching strategies to facilitate nursing students' critical thinking. In M Oermann (Ed), *Annual review of nursing education*, New York, 2008, Springer.

Ironside PM: "Covering content" and teaching thinking: Deconstructing the additive curriculum. *J Nurs Educ*, 43(1):5-12, 2004.

Kohn LT, Corrigan JM, Donaldson MS (Eds): *To err is human: Building a safer health system*, Washington, D.C., 1999, National Academy Press.

Lipe SK, Beasley S: *Critical thinking in nursing: A cognitive skills workbook*, Philadelphia, 2004, Lippincott Williams & Wilkins.

Mulcahy M, Pierce M: Critical thinking, collaboration, and communication: The three "C's" of quality preoperative screening. *J Perianesth Nurs*, 26(6):388-394, 2011.

Murray C, Grant MJ, Howarth ML, Leigh J: The use of simulation as a teaching and learning approach to support practice learning. *Nurse Educ Pract*, 8(1):5-8, 2008.

Paul R: The critical thinking movement. *Natl Forum*, 65(1):32, 1985.

Paul R: *What, then, is critical thinking?* Paper presented at the Eighth Annual and Sixth International Conference on Critical Thinking and Educational Reform, Rohnert Park, Calif., 1988.

Paul R: *Critical thinking: How to prepare students for a rapidly changing world*, Santa Rosa, Calif., 1993, Foundation for Critical Thinking.

Paul R, Elder L: *Critical thinking: Tools for taking charge of your learning and your life*, Upper Saddle River, N.J., 2001, Prentice Hall.

Paul R, Elder L: *Critical thinking: Tools for taking charge of your professional and personal life*, Upper Saddle River, N.J., 2002, Prentice Hall.

Paul R, Elder L: *Critical thinking: Learn the tools the best thinkers use*, Upper Saddle River, N.J., 2006, Pearson-Prentice Hall.

Rauen CA: Cardiovascular surgery: Simulation as a teaching strategy for nursing education and orientation in cardiac surgery. *Critical Care Nurse*, 25(5):244-248, 2004.

Rhodes M, Morris A, Lazenby R: Nursing at its best: Competent and caring. *Online J Issues Nurs*, 16(2), 10, 2011. Retrieved from *www.nursingworld.org/MainMenuCategories/ANAMarketplace/ANAPeriodicals/OJIN/TableofContents/Vol-16-2011/No2-May-2011/Articles-Previous-Topics/Nursing-at-its-Best.html.*

Schön D: *The reflective practitioner: How professionals think in action*, New York, 1983, Basic Books.

Simpson E, Courtney M: Implementation and evaluation of critical thinking strategies to enhance critical thinking skills in Middle Eastern nurses. *Int J Nurs Pract*, 14(6):449-454, 2008.

St. Cyr S, All A: Concept mapping: A road to critical thinking. *J Nurses Staff Dev*, 25(2):70-74, 2009.

The Joint Commission: *2012 Comprehensive accreditation manual for laboratory and point-of-care testing (CAMLAB)*, Oakbrook Terrace, Ill., 2012, Joint Commission Resources.

Thorpe K, Loo R: Critical-thinking types among nursing and management undergraduate students. *Nurse Educ Today*, 23(8):566-574, 2003.

Vacek JE: Using a conceptual approach with concept mapping to promote critical thinking. *J Nurs Educ*, 48(1):45-48, 2009.

Wendt A, Kenny LE, Marks C: Assessing critical thinking using a talk-aloud protocol. *CLEAR Exam Rev*, 18(1):18-27, 2007.

Wilkinson JM: *Nursing process and critical thinking*, ed. 5, Upper Saddle River, N.J., 2011, Prentice Hall.

Zimmerman B, Phillips C: Affective learning: Stimulus to critical thinking and caring practice. *J Nurs Educ*, 39(9):422-423, 2000.

REFERENCES

[illegible] thinking, clinical reasoning, and [illegible] judgment [illegible]

American Philosophical Association: Critical thinking: a statement of expert consensus for purposes of educational assessment and instruction, The Delphi report: research findings and recommendations prepared for the Committee on Pre-College Philosophy, ERIC document reproduction services no. ED 315-423, Millbrae, Calif, 1990, California Academic Press.

Banning M: The think aloud approach as an educational tool to develop and assess clinical reasoning in undergraduate students, *Nurse Educ Today* 28:8-14, 2008.

Benner P: From novice to expert: Excellence and power in clinical nursing practice, [illegible], 2001, Prentice Hall.

Benner P, Hughes R, Sutphen M: [illegible] evidence-based handbook for nurses, 2008, accessed from [illegible].pdf.

Carr S: A framework for understanding clinical reasoning in community nursing, [illegible], 2004.

Chaffee J: Thinking critically, ed 10, Boston, 2012, Cengage Learning.

[illegible] role playing to enhance clinical [illegible], 2008.

[illegible], 2007.

[illegible] critical thinking [illegible].

[illegible] critical thinking, 2011. Retrieved from [illegible].

[illegible] for evaluating critical thinking in [illegible], 1996.

[illegible] in nursing: a systematic review of the literature, [illegible].

[illegible] the effectiveness of the teaching [illegible], 2009.

[illegible] teaching strategies [illegible] nursing students [illegible].

[illegible].

Kohn LT, Corrigan JM, Donaldson MS (eds): To err is human: building a safer health system, Washington, DC, 1999, National Academy Press.

Lipe SK, Beasley S: Critical thinking in nursing: a cognitive skills workbook, Philadelphia, 2004, Lippincott Williams & Wilkins.

[illegible] Critical thinking [illegible] collaboration and [illegible] quality [illegible] 26(?):388-391, 2011.

Marrow C, [illegible]: The [illegible] as a [illegible], 2008.

Paul R: The critical thinking movement, [illegible], 1985.

Paul R: Critical thinking: [illegible] rapidly changing world, [illegible], 1993, Foundation for Critical Thinking.

Paul R, Elder L: Critical thinking: tools for taking charge of your learning and your life, Upper Saddle River, NJ, 2001, Prentice Hall.

Paul R, Elder L: Critical thinking: tools for taking charge of your professional and personal life, Upper Saddle River, NJ, 2002, Prentice Hall.

Paul R, Elder L: Critical thinking: [illegible], Upper Saddle River, NJ, [illegible], Pearson Prentice Hall.

[illegible] students' critical thinking [illegible], 2007.

Rhodes MK, Morris AH, Lazenby RB: Nursing at its best: Competent and caring, *Online J Issues Nurs* 16(2):10, 2011. Retrieved from [illegible].

[illegible], 2011.

[illegible] critical thinking [illegible].

[illegible] in nursing [illegible], 2011.

[illegible] critical thinking among nursing and management undergraduate students, [illegible], 2012.

[illegible] approach with concept mapping [illegible], 2009.

[illegible] critical thinking [illegible].

Wilkinson JM: [illegible] critical thinking, ed 5, Upper Saddle River, NJ, 2011, Prentice Hall.

Zimmermann B, [illegible] critical thinking [illegible], 2008.

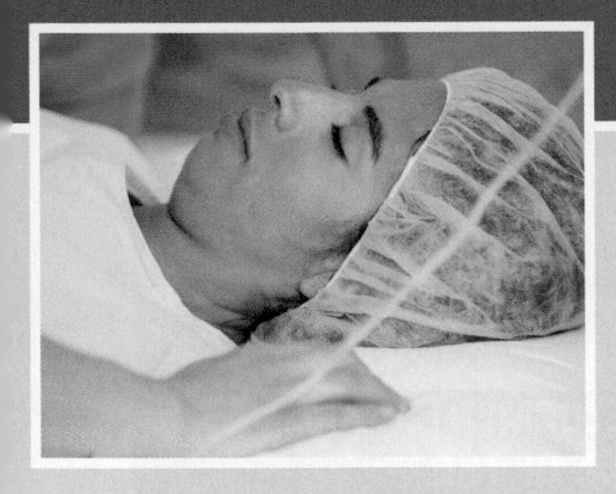

CHAPTER 5

Introduction to the Nursing Process

EVOLVE WEBSITE

http://evolve.elsevier.com/YoostCrawford/fundamentals/

- Online-Only Review Questions
- Answers to Review Questions
- Answers to Critical-Thinking Questions
- Case Study
- Glossary

LEARNING OUTCOMES

Comprehension of this chapter's content will provide students with the ability to:

LO 5.1 Define *nursing process.*
LO 5.2 Describe the historical development and significance of the nursing process.
LO 5.3 Articulate the characteristics of the nursing process.
LO 5.4 Describe the steps in the nursing process.
LO 5.5 Explain the significance of the cyclic and dynamic nature of the nursing process.

KEY TERMS

assessment, p. 74
evaluation, p. 79
implementation, p. 77
NANDA-I, p. 75
nursing diagnosis, p. 75
nursing process, p. 70
outcome identification, p. 77
planning, p. 76

CASE STUDY

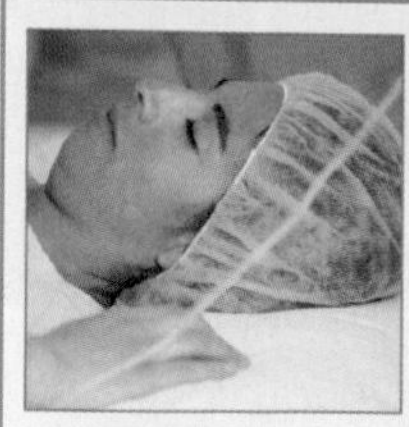

Mrs. Perez, a 48-year-old, Hispanic woman, is admitted to the nursing unit 2 hours after undergoing a right mastectomy (i.e., surgical removal of the breast). The floor nurse receives a report from the postanesthesia care unit (PACU) nurse that includes the patient's admitting diagnosis of breast cancer, latest vital signs, focused assessment, medication and intravenous (IV) orders, pain level and the time she was last medicated for pain, and the status of her surgical dressing. Initially, Mrs. Perez appears to be comfortable, dozing occasionally between short conversations with her husband, who is at her side. When Mrs. Perez fully awakens 3 hours after arriving on the nursing unit, she complains of sharp, constant pain on the right side of her chest. She rates her pain at 8 of 10 on the pain scale. She is grimacing and appears tense.

Refer back to this case study to answer the critical-thinking questions throughout the chapter.

Contemporary nursing practice is based on the **nursing process**, which is the systematic method of critical thinking used by professional nurses to develop individualized plans of care and provide care for patients. Similar to the scientific process, the nursing process is organized and methodical, with five primary steps: assessment, diagnosis, planning, implementation, and evaluation. Effective use of the nursing process depends on a nurse's knowledge, familiarity with standardized nursing diagnosis terminology, evidence-based practice, and ability to evaluate patient responses to interventions.

DEFINITION OF THE NURSING PROCESS LO 5.1

The nursing process is the foundation of professional nursing practice. It is the framework within which nurses provide care to patients in an organized and effective manner. Paul (1988) describes critical thinking as a complex process during which individuals think about their thinking to provide clarity and increase precision and relevance in a specific situation while attempting to be fair and consistent. Critical thinking using the nursing process allows nurses to collect essential patient data, articulate the specific needs of individual patients, and effectively communicate those needs, realistic goals, and customized interventions with members of the health care team. Chapter 4 provides additional information on its importance in nursing.

Thinking like a nurse is facilitated by nurses using the nursing process in the development of individualized patient plans of care. The Joint Commission requires a written plan of care that summarizes the treatment for every patient. Care plans can be handwritten or be part of the electronic medical record (EMR). Some standardized care plans may be available to nurses as basic templates for individual care plan development; however, all patients are required to have unique, patient-centered plans of care designed to meet their specific needs. Nursing care plans often incorporate aspects of multidisciplinary clinical pathways. Following the steps of the nursing process helps nurses to provide patient care that meets standards required by state boards of nursing and guided by the American Nurses Association's *Nursing: Scope and Standards of Practice* (2010).

HISTORICAL DEVELOPMENT AND SIGNIFICANCE OF THE NURSING PROCESS LO 5.2

The term *nursing process* was first used by Lydia Hall in 1955 (de la Cuesta, 1983). In the late 1950s and early 1960s, other nurses (Johnson, 1959; Orlando, 1961; Wiedenbach, 1963) began using the term to define the steps used for decision making while initiating and providing patient care. In 1973, the American Nurses Association (ANA) identified five specific steps of the nursing process in its *Standards of Clinical Practice* (1991). These five steps—assessment, diagnosis, planning, implementation, and evaluation—define how professional nursing practice is conducted. Outcome identification was added as an essential aspect of the nursing process by the ANA in 1991. Most nursing professionals and educators recognize outcome identification as part of the planning step of the traditional five-step nursing process.

Professional nursing practice in all types of settings is based on the nursing process. It is used to assess individuals, families, and communities; diagnose needs; plan attainable goals; identify outcome criteria; implement specific interventions; and evaluate degrees of goal attainment. Critical thinking, using the various steps of the nursing process, facilitates the development of safe, individualized, patient-centered care, which takes into consideration a patient's personal preferences, cultural traditions, values, and lifestyle. Professional nurses address the responses of people, families, and communities to health-related problems and promote healthy lifestyles through application of the nursing process.

CHARACTERISTICS OF THE NURSING PROCESS LO 5.3

The nursing process has several essential characteristics that must be recognized and understood by nurses to be effectively applied to the practice of nursing. The nursing process requires that nurses think critically. It is dynamic, organized, and collaborative, and it is universally adaptable to various types of health care settings.

ANALYTICAL

The nursing process requires nurses to think analytically using many aspects of critical thinking. Nurses must be able to assess patients accurately and then organize and analyze their findings to provide safe care. At each step of the process, nurses must address concerns:

- Is the data collection thorough and accurate?
- Are outcomes specific and realistic for the individual patient?
- Have all of the underlying factors contributing to the patient's response to illness been adequately addressed in the plan of care?
- Could any of the nursing interventions have a negative impact on the patient?
- Does each intervention provide for patient-centered care and the safety of the patient?
- Are there new data that necessitate modification of the existing plan of care?

The nursing process is dynamic and has overlapping steps (Figure 5-1). At any given time, nurses are required to think simultaneously about several steps of the nursing process to make sure all critical data are considered and to provide evidence-based, patient-specific care.

The nursing process is cyclic rather than linear. As an individual patient's condition changes, so does the way a professional nurse thinks about that patient's needs, forcing modification of earlier plans of care. At each step of the nursing process, nurses must consider the accuracy and effectiveness of their thought process. This form of reflective

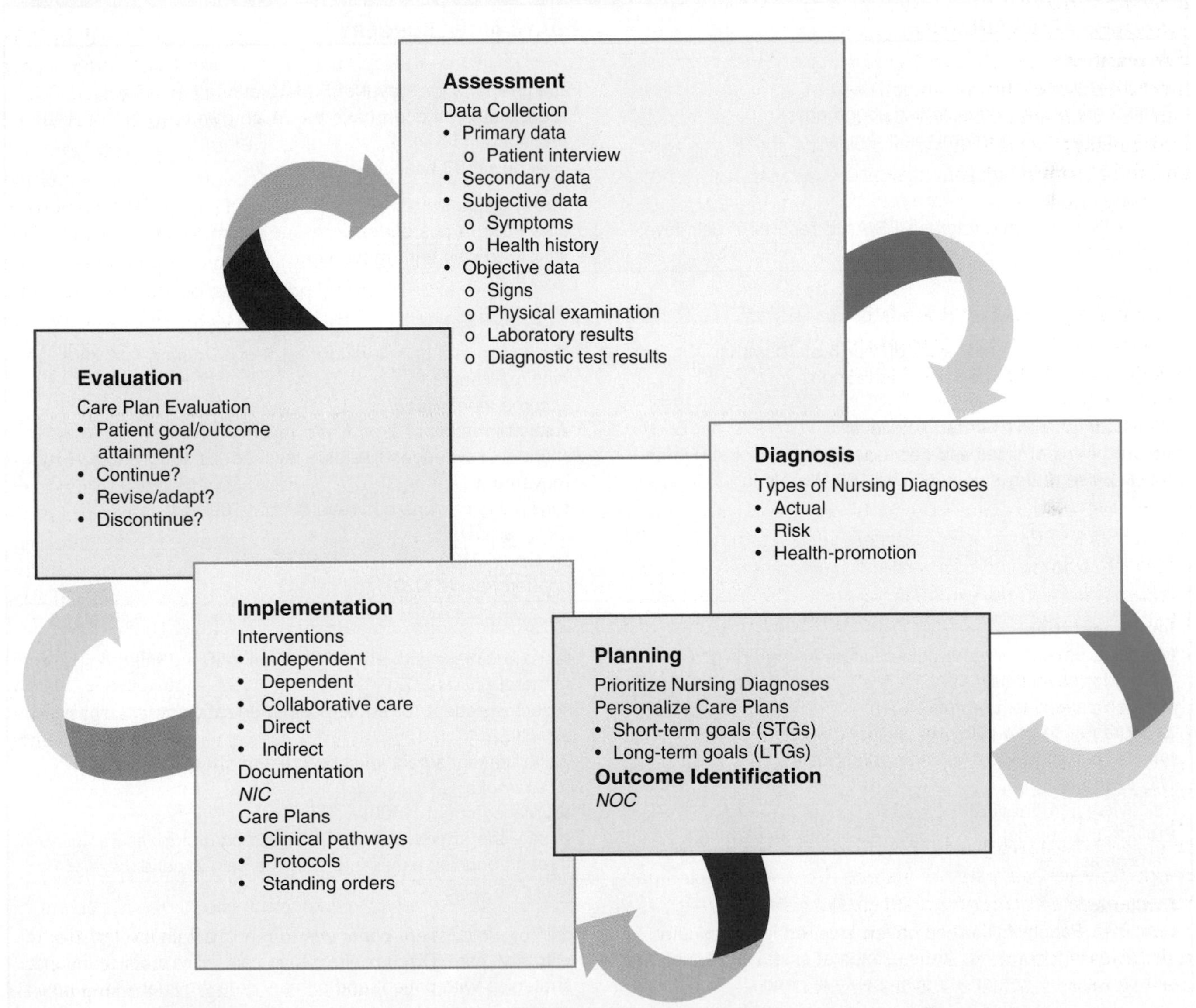

FIGURE 5-1 The dynamic nursing process includes five steps, with outcome identification as a subcategory of planning. *NIC*, Nursing Interventions Classification; *NOC*, Nursing Outcomes Classification.

thought is an essential aspect of critical thinking. The evolutionary nature of the nursing process allows nurses to adjust to changing patient needs. Plans of care must evolve as patients' needs change.

DYNAMIC

The nursing process is dynamic, changing over time in response to patients' individual needs. The dynamic, responsive nature of the nursing process allows it to be used effectively with patients in any setting and at every level of care, from the intensive care unit to outpatient wellness clinics. Keeping the five steps of the nursing process in mind, a nurse conducts ongoing assessment as a patient's condition changes and modifies the patient's plan of care on the basis of those findings.

Table 5-1 briefly describes the dynamic nature of the nursing process in caring for a patient recovering from surgery. Notice that the nursing diagnosis is *Acute Pain* in both situations; however, the plan of care is individualized for the patient on the basis of assessment findings, changing needs, setting, and timing of interaction. The dynamic nature of the nursing process makes this possible.

TABLE 5-1 Abbreviated Nursing Process for a Surgical Patient

2 HOURS AFTER SURGERY	3 DAYS AFTER SURGERY
Assessment Patient reports pain level of 8 of 10. Patient grimacing and clutching abdomen. Apical pulse: 104 beats/min and regular	Patient reports pain level of 5 of 10 during A.M. care. Patient states, "I don't have too much pain now except when I move around." Apical pulse: 68 beats/min and regular
Nursing diagnosis: *Acute Pain,* r/t tissue trauma AEB/AMB reports of pain level of 8 of 10	Nursing diagnosis: *Acute Pain,* r/t postoperative tissue inflammation AEB/AMB increased pain with movement
Planning *Short-term goal:* Patient verbalizes a pain level of 4 or 5 of 10 within ½ hour of receiving prescribed pain medication. *Outcome identification:* Verbal affirmation of 4 or 5 pain level Relaxed arms at sides and decreased guarding of abdomen Apical pulse rate between 60 and 100 beats/min *NOC example:* Pain Level (2102) Reported Pain (210201)	*Short-term goal:* Patient reports a pain level of 2 or 3 of 10 during A.M. care within 24 hours. *Outcome identification:* Verbal affirmation of 2 or 3 pain level Patient acknowledges tolerable level of discomfort with movement. Apical pulse remains between 60 and 100 beats/min *NOC example:* Pain Level (2102) Reported Pain (210201)
Implementation Medicate patient with morphine sulfate (4 mg IVP q 2 hr PRN) for severe pain. Position patient for comfort. Encourage use of a pillow for splinting areas of pain. Initiate relaxation techniques as appropriate. *NIC example:* Pain Management (1400) Provide the person optimal pain relief with prescribed analgesics.	Medicate patient with acetaminophen (650 mg PO q 4-6 hr) for moderate pain. Encourage patient to request pain medication before physical activity. Monitor patient's pain level before and after AM care. *NIC example:* Pain Management (1400) Evaluate the effectiveness of the pain control measures used through ongoing assessment of the pain experience.
Evaluation Goal met. Patient fell asleep on left side within 20 minutes of receiving morphine. Arms relaxed at sides. Continue plan of care during immediate postoperative period.	Goal not met. Patient continues to report a pain level of 5 or 6 with A.M. care. Discuss alternative pain relief medication and strategies with patient and primary care provider. Revise plan of care.

AEB/AMB, As evidenced by/as manifested by; *NIC,* Nursing Interventions Classification; *NOC,* Nursing Outcomes Classification; *r/t,* related to.

ORGANIZED

Following the steps of the nursing process ensures that patient care is well organized and thorough. The nursing process provides a standardized method of addressing patient needs that is understood by nurses worldwide. Due to its systematic nature, nurses use the nursing process as a framework for the development of individualized plans of care.

OUTCOME ORIENTED

The patient-centered nursing process is designed to achieve specific, well-defined outcomes. Patient care plans are developed to meet each patient's goals, not the goals of standardized patients or members of the health care team, including the nurse. Decisions regarding which nursing interventions and medical treatments to implement are made on the basis of safety and their effectiveness in meeting a patient's identified needs and desired outcomes. By referring to a patient's care plan developed within the nursing process context, nurses and other health care team members are able to treat a patient consistently and identify care that is effective while modifying efforts that are not helping the patient meet goals and achieve desired outcomes.

Care plans developed using the nursing process as a standardized framework hold nurses and other health care team members accountable for their actions. If the nurse's priority goals and the patient's goals are being met, the plan of care is effective. If not, the nurse needs to use critical-thinking skills, knowledge, and the nursing process to modify the plan to better address the patient's concerns.

QSEN FOCUS!

Nurses must identify the expectations of patients and their families to develop patient-centered plans of care. Acknowledging patient preferences empowers patients and their families to actively participate in the health care process.

COLLABORATIVE

Collaboration among several members of the health care team is often required to adequately address patient needs. In many cases, nurses incorporate orders from a primary care provider, nursing interventions, and input from others, such as physical therapists, social workers, or respiratory therapists, into a patient's plan of care to help alleviate patient problems and achieve established patient-centered goals and outcomes. For example, if a patient is experiencing shortness of breath, the nurse may place a nasal cannula for oxygen administration according to the physician's order, elevate the head of the patient's bed to reduce respiratory effort, and call the respiratory therapist to administer a breathing treatment to expand the patient's airways. Each of these interventions is part of the implementation step of the nursing process. In other cases, the nurse may incorporate actions by the patient or patient's family to address patient goals. This is especially true when the patient is not acutely ill or requires home care.

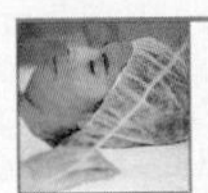

1. Identify two types of health care team members with whom the nurse would expect to collaborate while caring for Mrs. Perez.

ADAPTABLE

The nursing process is adaptable for developing plans of care for individuals who are hospitalized or are receiving care in an outpatient, long-term care, or home setting. It is an equally useful method for addressing the needs of a specific population.

Consider the problem of childhood obesity in a specific community. By using the nursing process, assessment data can be gathered regarding who is affected and what the underlying causes are. Analyzing these data allows nurse researchers to identify the problems and establish short- and long-term goals for improvement. After establishment of goals for alleviating childhood obesity in a community, area professionals from a variety of disciplines may collaborate on the implementation of programs designed to address the individualized needs of that specific population. After implementation of programs, evaluation is conducted to determine whether the goals were achieved.

The nursing process is adaptable in the community setting (Figure 5-2). At each step, revisions of the plan may need to take place, depending on a variety of concerns, including cost and availability of professionals to implement interventions. However, the universal nature of the nursing process enables this adaptability. Engaging the help of others in collaboration about how best to achieve patient or community goals can dramatically improve outcomes in all settings.

STEPS OF THE NURSING PROCESS LO 5.4

Each step of the nursing process—assessment, diagnosis, planning, implementation, and evaluation (ADPIE)—has a unique purpose.

1. During the assessment step, patient care data are gathered through observation, interviews, and physical assessment.
2. In the diagnosis step, patient data are analyzed, validated, and clustered to identify patient problems. Each problem is then stated in standardized language as a specific nursing diagnosis to provide greater clarity and universal understanding by all care providers.
3. During the planning step of the nursing process, the nurse prioritizes the nursing diagnoses and identifies short- and long-term goals that are realistic, measurable, and patient focused, with specific outcome identification for evaluation purposes.

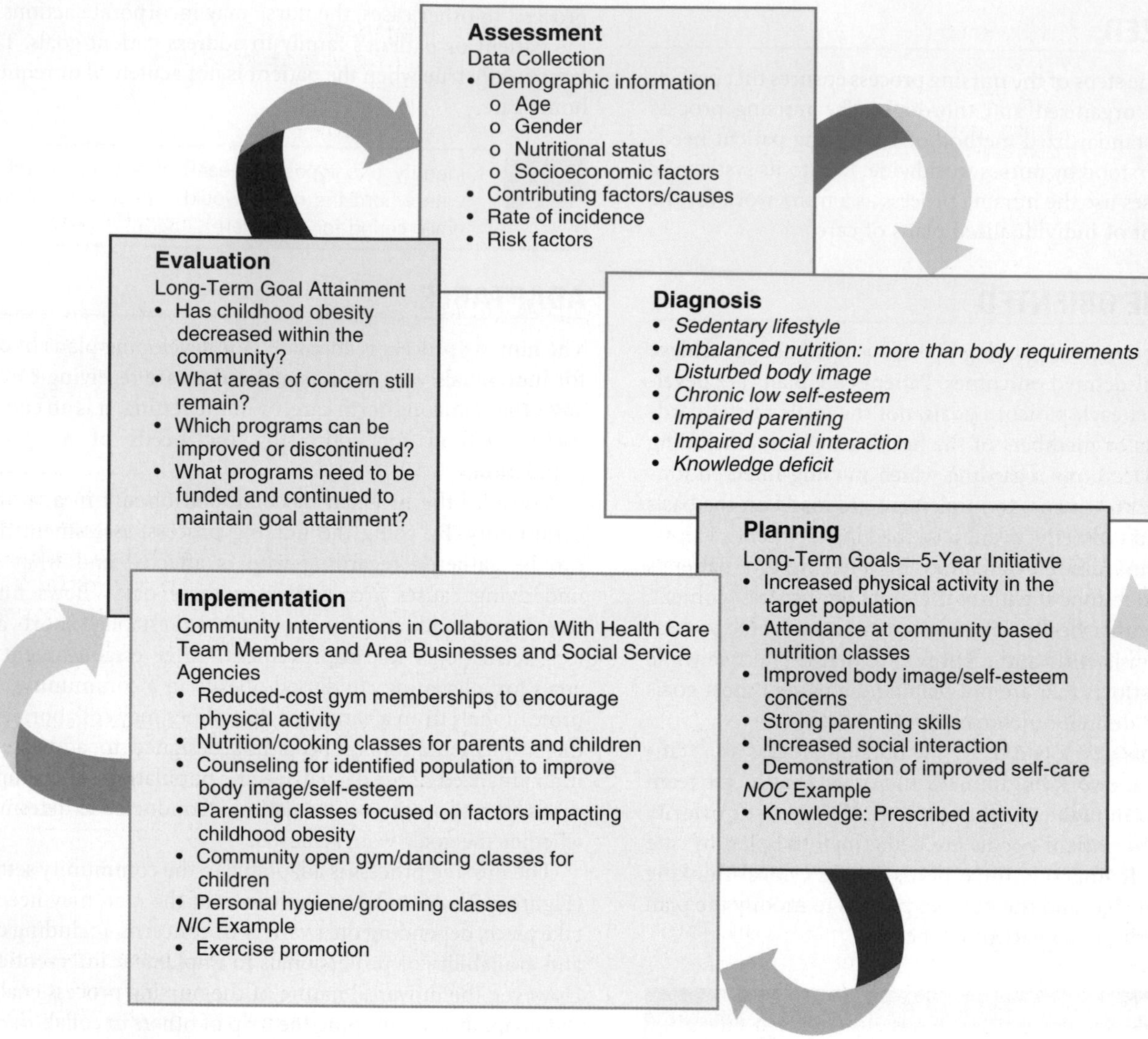

Assessment
Data Collection
- Demographic information
  - o Age
  - o Gender
  - o Nutritional status
  - o Socioeconomic factors
- Contributing factors/causes
- Rate of incidence
- Risk factors

Diagnosis
- *Sedentary lifestyle*
- *Imbalanced nutrition: more than body requirements*
- *Disturbed body image*
- *Chronic low self-esteem*
- *Impaired parenting*
- *Impaired social interaction*
- *Knowledge deficit*

Planning
Long-Term Goals—5-Year Initiative
- Increased physical activity in the target population
- Attendance at community based nutrition classes
- Improved body image/self-esteem concerns
- Strong parenting skills
- Increased social interaction
- Demonstration of improved self-care

NOC Example
- Knowledge: Prescribed activity

Implementation
Community Interventions in Collaboration With Health Care Team Members and Area Businesses and Social Service Agencies
- Reduced-cost gym memberships to encourage physical activity
- Nutrition/cooking classes for parents and children
- Counseling for identified population to improve body image/self-esteem
- Parenting classes focused on factors impacting childhood obesity
- Community open gym/dancing classes for children
- Personal hygiene/grooming classes

NIC Example
- Exercise promotion

Evaluation
Long-Term Goal Attainment
- Has childhood obesity decreased within the community?
- What areas of concern still remain?
- Which programs can be improved or discontinued?
- What programs need to be funded and continued to maintain goal attainment?

FIGURE 5-2 The nursing process can be adapted to the community setting to address childhood obesity. *NIC,* Nursing Interventions Classification; *NOC,* Nursing Outcomes Classification.

4. The implementation step includes initiating specific nursing interventions and treatments designed to help the patient achieve established goals or outcomes.
5. In the evaluation step, the nurse determines whether the patient's goals are met, examines the effectiveness of interventions, and decides whether the plan of care should be discontinued, continued, or revised.

Although each step of the nursing process has a clearly identified purpose, all of the steps are interdependent. Each requires information from the others for adequate development and revisions of an effective plan of care. The steps overlap and require thoughtful consideration by the nurse at each transition for the maintenance of accuracy and effectiveness.

ASSESSMENT

Assessment is the organized and ongoing appraisal of a patient's well-being (Figure 5-3). Assessment involves collecting data from a variety of sources that is needed to care for patients. Data collection begins at the first direct or indirect encounter with a patient. Specific data are collected during the patient interview, health history, and physical assessment. Nurses assess the state of a patient's physical, psychological, emotional, environmental, cultural, and spiritual health to gain a better understanding of his or her overall condition. This is known as a *holistic approach* to patient care.

Assessment data can be collected from a variety of sources, including patients, family members, friends, communities,

Assessment
Data Collection
- Primary data
  - o Patient interview
- Secondary data
- Subjective data
  - o Symptoms
  - o Health history
- Objective data
  - o Signs
  - o Physical examination
  - o Laboratory results
  - o Diagnostic test results

FIGURE 5-3 Assessment in the nursing process.

health care professionals, medical records, and laboratory and diagnostic test results. Data may be categorized as primary or secondary and as subjective or objective, depending on the source and form of the information. Primary data consist of information obtained directly from a patient. Secondary data are collected from family members, friends, other health care professionals, or written sources such as medical records and test results. Some nurses may subdivide secondary data to identify information as indirect if it is obtained from medical charts or a hand-off communication.

Subjective data (i.e., symptoms) are spoken. Patients' feelings about a situation or comments about how they are feeling are examples of subjective data. Data shared by a source verbally are considered subjective. Subjective data may be difficult to validate because they cannot be independently and objectively measured. Subjective data are most often gathered during a patient interview or health history. Use of an interpreter may be necessary when the patient or family members speak a language unfamiliar to the nurse. Subjective data are typically documented in the patient's medical record as direct quotations; for example, "I didn't get much sleep last night" or "I've had diabetes since I was 10 years old."

Data collected from medical records, laboratory, and diagnostic test results, or physical assessments are objective. Objective data (i.e., signs) consist of observable information that the nurse gathers on the basis of what can be seen, measured, or tested. Most objective data are collected by the nurse during physical assessment, which includes inspection, palpation, percussion, and auscultation, or during direct patient care.

Collecting an extensive health history and completing a thorough head-to-toe physical assessment are typically required when a patient is admitted to a hospital or seeking health care from a primary care provider for the first time. This information provides a baseline for future reference. Shorter, focused assessments are conducted by the nurse routinely throughout hospitalization or during repeated clinic visits to assess a patient's change of status. Collecting accurate information and documenting the findings in the patient's medical record are imperative for later comparison. The documentation process helps the nurse organize patient information so that it can be analyzed, validated, and clustered before the identification of accurate nursing diagnoses (see Chapters 6 and 20).

Diagnosis
Types of Nursing Diagnoses
- Actual
- Risk
- Health-promotion

FIGURE 5-4 Diagnosis in the nursing process.

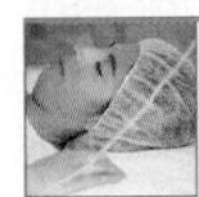

2. List five additional pieces of data that the nurse who admits Mrs. Perez to the nursing unit would want to know before initiating care. Next to each item, identify whether it is subjective or objective. Write examples of the five data that would be appropriate for a postoperative mastectomy patient.

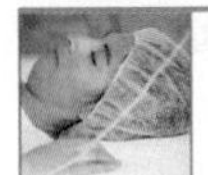

3. Write four questions that the nurse could ask to obtain primary data on Mrs. Perez. From what sources could the nurse obtain secondary data?

DIAGNOSIS

The second step of the nursing process is the nursing diagnosis (Figure 5-4). The **nursing diagnosis** identifies an actual or potential problem or response to a problem (NANDA-I, 2012). Accurate identification of nursing diagnoses for patients results from carefully analyzing, validating, and clustering related patient subjective (symptoms) and objective (signs) data. If data collection includes inaccurate or inadequate information or if data are not validated or clustered with related information, a patient may be misdiagnosed.

Diagnosis in the nursing process requires naming patient problems using nursing diagnostic labels. Nursing diagnoses are established and revised biannually by NANDA International, Inc. (**NANDA-I**), a professional nursing organization that provides standardized language to identify patient problems and plan customized care. Medical diagnoses are labels for diseases, whereas nursing diagnoses describe a response to an actual or potential problem or life process. NANDA-I (2012) identifies three types of nursing diagnoses (i.e., actual, risk, and health-promotion) that nurses should use when developing plans of patient care.

Actual nursing diagnoses are written with three parts, whereas risk nursing diagnoses and health-promotion nursing diagnoses contain only two parts. Three-part nursing diagnosis statements include (1) the patient's identified need or problem (i.e., NANDA-I nursing diagnostic label), (2) the etiology or underlying cause (i.e., related to [r/t]), and (3) signs and symptoms (i.e., as evidenced by [AEB] or as manifested by [AMB]). *Sleep Deprivation* related to frequent sleep interruption as evidenced by patient complaint of diarrhea 10 times throughout the night and feeling fatigued is an example of a three-part nursing diagnosis statement. Sometimes the acronym PES (problem, etiology, symptoms) is used to remind nursing students of how to structure an actual nursing diagnosis statement.

A two-part risk nursing diagnostic statement contains only (1) the patient's identified need or problem (i.e., NANDA-I nursing diagnostic label) and (2) factors indicating vulnerability (i.e., risk factors). This is an example of a two-part risk nursing diagnostic statement: *Risk for Injury* with the risk factor of impaired cognitive awareness. This risk nursing diagnosis might be appropriate for a patient coming out of anesthesia after surgery. In some cases, nurses may write a *risk for* nursing diagnosis using the words *related to* rather than *with the risk factors of.* Specific institutional guidelines should be followed.

A two-part health-promotion nursing diagnostic statement contains (1) the nursing diagnostic label and (2) defining characteristics. It always begins with the words *Readiness for Enhanced.* A health-promotion nursing diagnosis may state the following: *Readiness for Enhanced Self-Health Management* as evidenced by (as manifested by) expressed desire to manage illness more effectively.

Appendix B contains a complete list of accepted NANDA-I nursing diagnostic labels. Chapter 7 provides additional information on how to identify and formulate personalized nursing diagnoses for specific patients.

Through the use of well-defined nursing diagnoses, such as *Activity Intolerance* or *Risk for Spiritual Distress,* all nurses can clearly understand a patient's problems. Standardized lists of nursing diagnostic labels are available for quick reference in databases in electronic health records. It is the nurse's responsibility to accurately identify and use nursing diagnoses for every patient to develop patient-centered goals and realistic outcome criteria in individualized plans of care. Patients may have multiple problems, requiring a variety of nursing diagnoses. Regardless of how many nursing diagnoses a patient has, each must be considered in the planning process.

QSEN FOCUS!

Although NANDA-I no longer identifies specific collaborative nursing diagnostic labels, it is essential that nurses work with various members of the interdisciplinary health care team to plan holistic patient care. Respecting the unique skills and contributions of others on the health care team facilitates better communication and achievement of patient health goals.

Planning
Prioritize Nursing Diagnoses
Personalize Care Plans
- Short-term goals (STGs)
- Long-term goals (LTGs)

Outcome Identification
NOC

FIGURE 5-5 Planning in the nursing process. *NOC*, Nursing Outcomes Classification.

PLANNING

Planning is the third step of the nursing process (Figure 5-5). During **planning**, the nurse prioritizes a patient's various nursing diagnoses, establishes short- and long-term goals, chooses outcome indicators, and identifies interventions to address patient goals. Deciding the order in which nursing diagnoses are addressed depends on several factors, including the severity of symptoms and the patient's preference. Obviously, a patient's ability to breathe is of greater concern than the need to complete activities of daily living independently. After emergent needs are dealt with, less critical problems take priority. This aspect of the nursing process is another indication of its dynamic nature and interrelatedness.

Establishing short- and long-term goals to address nursing diagnoses involves discussion with the patient and often requires collaboration with family members and other members of the health care team (Collaboration and Delegation box). Coordinated, team-based patient care is called *collaborative care.* The patient's health care team members may include several nurses: the primary care provider; medical or surgical specialists; respiratory therapists; a dietician; a physical therapist; occupational, music, or art therapists; a spiritual adviser; and social workers. The patient's primary nurse is often the central figure in coordinating collaborative care.

COLLABORATION AND DELEGATION

Team-Based Patient Care
- Collaboration and delegation of care are integral to the implementation step of the nursing process. Nurses do not have the time or expertise to address all of the needs of patients.
- Effective collaboration with and delegation to various members of the health care team require the nurse to become familiar with the scope of practice and abilities of each member.
- After the nurse has established the scope of practice and abilities of the health care team members, their unique skills and abilities can be coordinated to benefit patient care and achieve positive patient outcomes.
- Planning comprehensive care that addresses the multiple needs of patients often facilitates shorter recovery or rehabilitation periods, leading to reduced length of hospitalization and greater patient satisfaction.

Short- and long-term goals are designed to meet the patient's immediate needs and future needs, which may extend over weeks or months. Some sources establish time parameters for short-term or long-term goals, but others do not. According to Carpenito-Moyet (2013), goals that are achievable within an immediate time frame of less than approximately 1 week are short-term goals, whereas goals that will take more time to achieve—weeks to months—are long-term goals. All short- and long-term goals must be (1) patient focused, (2) realistic, and (3) measurable. For example, a patient-focused, realistic, and measurable short-term goal may be written for a patient with the nursing diagnosis of *Activity Intolerance*: The patient walks to the bathroom without experiencing shortness of breath within 48 hours after surgery.

Goal setting creates a structure, or framework, within which nursing care takes place. Goals help to direct the patient's health care team and ensure that all members of the team work to achieve the same outcomes. Whenever possible, it is important to include patients in identifying their short- and long-term goals.

Outcome identification, added by the ANA in 1991 as a specific aspect of the nursing process, involves listing behaviors or observable items that indicate attainment of a goal. The Nursing Outcomes Classification (NOC) is one resource for outcome identification. Outcome classification for a patient with the nursing diagnosis of *Activity Intolerance* could be Endurance with an outcome indicator of uncompromised to severely compromised activity (Moorhead, Johnson, and Maas, 2013). Nursing interventions, including collaborative care interventions, are identified by the nurse during the planning stage to help patients meet goals, outcome classifications, and outcome indicators (i.e., criteria that can be observed or measured).

One method of determining interventions to meet patient outcome goals is use of Nursing Interventions Classification (NIC). NIC provides nurses with multidisciplinary interventions linked to specific NANDA-I–accepted nursing diagnoses and the NOC. For a patient with the nursing diagnosis of *Activity Intolerance,* the desired outcome of Endurance, and a goal of being able to walk to the bathroom without experiencing shortness of breath within 48 hours after surgery, the nurse may select interventions from NIC related to Exercise Therapy: Ambulation (Bulechek, Butcher H, Dochterman, et al, 2013). Using NIC as a reference, the nurse remains responsible for customizing and implementing appropriate interventions for each specific patient.

Developing a patient-centered plan to address identified short- and long-term goals requires that a nurse use critical thinking, creativity, expertise, and communication skills. The plan of care needs to be relevant to the patient's health status and goals, and the plan must be based on the latest evidence-based nursing practices. By identifying specific desired-outcome indicators for patient improvement, the nurse can more easily implement research-based nursing interventions to address the unique needs of a patient. Chapter 8 provides additional information on goal setting and outcome identification resources.

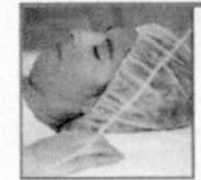

4. Write a patient-focused, measurable, and realistic short-term goal for Mrs. Perez, whose priority nursing diagnosis is *Acute Pain*.

IMPLEMENTATION

The **implementation** step of the nursing process focuses on initiation of appropriate interventions designed to meet the unique needs of each patient (Figure 5-6). Interventions may be independent, dependent, or collaborative nursing actions requiring direct or indirect nursing care. All should be derived from evidence-based practice standards that have evolved from research conducted to elicit the best patient outcomes possible.

QSEN FOCUS!

Nurses should read original research articles and systematic reviews of literature related to their specialties to stay current and implement new evidence into practice.

Clinical Pathways, Protocols, and Standing Orders

Clinical pathways, protocols, and standing orders often impact interventions carried out in the implementation phase of the nursing process. Clinical pathways, sometimes referred to as care pathways, care maps, or critical pathways, are multidisciplinary resources designed to guide patient care. Clinical pathways emerged in the 1980s in an effort to provide better-quality, standardized care for patients, and they were developed through evidence-based practice research

Implementation
Interventions
- Independent
- Dependent
- Collaborative

Care
- Direct
- Indirect

Documentation
NIC
Care Plans
- Clinical pathways
- Protocols
- Standing orders

FIGURE 5-6 Implementation in the nursing process. *NIC,* Nursing Interventions Classification.

(Kinsman, Rotter, James, et al, 2010). Nurses contribute to the formation of clinical pathways by using the nursing process to identify unique nursing interventions that assist patients in achieving desired outcomes. A clinical pathway for the care of a postmastectomy breast cancer patient is shown in Figure 5-7. Independent, dependent, direct, and indirect interventions are listed in the critical pathway.

Protocols are written plans that can be generalized to groups of patients with the same or similar clinical needs that do not require a physician's order. Health care agencies have established protocols outlining procedures for admitting patients or handling routine care situations. Because protocols are generalized to patient populations, they are often included in critical pathways.

Standing orders are written by physicians and list specific actions to be taken by a nurse or other health care provider when access to a physician is not possible or when care is common to a certain type of situation, such as what to do if a patient experiences chest pain or what actions to take after a colonoscopy. Standing orders are most commonly

Actual or Potential Problem	Activity/ Treatments	Postoperative Day 1 Outcome Date ______	Initials	Postoperative Day 2 Outcome Date______	Initials	Discharge Outcome Date ______	Initials
Comfort	Medications	IV fluids		IV fluid DC'd			
		Parenteral/oral analgesia		Oral analgesia		Oral analgesia provides pain relief	
		Antiemetic prn					
	Positioning	Assist with pillows for support Performs active ROM		Independent		Independent regular ambulation	
	Complementary therapy	*Circle type*: music, distraction, lighting, relaxation therapy, other		*Circle type*: music, distraction, lighting, relaxation therapy, other			
Mobility	Activity	Sits up in chair		Ambulates without assistance		Demonstrates physical therapy exercises	
		Ambulates q3hr with assistance		Physical therapy consult			
Respiratory	Respiratory therapy	Deep breathing and coughing		Deep breathing and coughing		Incentive spirometry and deep breathing, as needed	
		Incentive spirometry, as ordered		Incentive spirometry, as ordered			
Skin Integrity	Dressing	Assess dressing and drains		Remove incisional dressing; assess incision for redness		Oral temperature <102°F; incision without redness or pus	
		Empty and measure drain output		Maintain drain assessment		Understands drain care, as applicable	
		Bathes while keeping dressings and drains dry		Bathes, keeping drain sites dry		Maintains care around incision and drain sites	
Nutrition	Diet	DC IV fluids, as ordered		Tolerates regular diet without nausea		Tolerates regular diet	
		Clear liquids, advance as tolerated					
Self-Care	Activities of daily living	Completes self-care with minimal assistance		Performs drain care with minimal assistance		Completes self-care and drain care without assistance	
	Patient education	Discusses signs and symptoms (s/s) of infection and hematomas					
Psychosocial	Coping strategies	Spiritual, psychological, and/or social work consult, as needed		Visit from support group representatives		Verify follow-up appointments	
		Provide reconstructive surgery information, as requested		Provide breast prosthesis information, if requested			
Document initials when outcome is met. Record reason if not met in patient's electronic medical record or narrative note.							

FIGURE 5-7 Clinical pathway for treating a breast cancer patient after mastectomy. *DC,* Discontinue.

used in situations in which care is somewhat standardized, but the implementation of standing orders still requires extensive clinical judgment by the nurse. Community health nurses may practice with standing orders that identify how to treat emergency situations in a patient's home. However, all nurses must be able to recognize and act on changes in a patient's condition that are not covered by the standing orders.

! SAFE PRACTICE ALERT

Following protocols or implementing standing orders requires critical thinking and use of the nursing process to determine the applicability of interventions in specific patient care circumstances. Blindly following critical pathways, protocols, or standing orders is contraindicated in all nursing care situations.

All nursing interventions that are implemented for patients must be documented or charted. In some cases, this may involve checking off an intervention in the patient's EMR, or it may require completion of an additional form or area on the EMR designed to track the effectiveness of specific interventions. Many health care agencies have special requirements for documenting interventions such as the use of physical restraints or pain protocols. Proper documentation of interventions facilitates communication with all members of the health care team and provides an essential legal record (Ethical, Legal, and Professional Practice box). Accurate charting helps to alleviate omissions and repetition of care. Documentation also allows nurses to evaluate the effectiveness of nursing interventions in meeting patient goals and outcomes, which is the final step in the nursing process.

ETHICAL, LEGAL, AND PROFESSIONAL PRACTICE

Documentation

- All health care professionals are required to document patient interventions they implement in a traditional or an electronic medical record.
- Nurses must document the physical treatment and patient education that is provided.
- Follow-up evaluation of interventions must be documented to help the health care team determine the effectiveness of treatments, activities, and prescribed medications.
- Ethical and legal standards mandate that nurses chart or document only the interventions that they themselves implement.

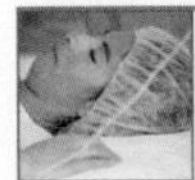

5. List three interventions that the nurse would want to implement to help Mrs. Perez achieve the identified short-term goal.

Evaluation

Care Plan Evaluation
- Patient goal/outcome attainment?
- Continue?
- Revise/adapt?
- Discontinue?

FIGURE 5-8 Evaluation in the nursing process.

EVALUATION

Evaluation focuses on the patient and the patient's response to nursing interventions and goal or outcome attainment (Figure 5-8). Evaluation is not a record of the care that was implemented. Evaluation must clearly identify the effectiveness of implemented interventions with the patient as its focus. During the evaluation step of the nursing process, nurses use critical thinking to determine whether a patient's short- and long-term goals were met and desired outcomes were achieved. Monitoring whether the patient's goals were attained is a collaborative process involving the patient.

Nurses need to ask some questions when evaluating the effectiveness of provided nursing interventions:
- Did the patient meet the goals and outcome criteria established during the planning phase?
- Since care began, have new assessment data been identified that should be taken into consideration?
- Does the care plan need to be modified in response to patient changes?
- Based on the patient's response to the implemented interventions, should the plan of care be continued, revised, or discontinued?

The answers to these and other questions determine how best to proceed with individualized patient care.

CYCLIC AND DYNAMIC NATURE OF THE NURSING PROCESS LO 5.5

The steps of the nursing process are cyclic and dynamic; one aspect of care leads into and informs the next. It is crucial that the professional nurse continuously reassess the patient, revise care as needed, and evaluate whether the patient's goals are being met. As the short-term goals are met, that section of the nursing plan can be eliminated or discontinued. Sometimes, nursing care needs to be modified to meet a patient's other needs that were not previously identified.

The ongoing process of evaluating and adjusting intervention strategies requires nursing care to be based on current evidence. This evaluation process is also based on the nurse's ability to critically think about what care was given and what care may be needed in the future. The nursing process is a professional nurse's best tool for application of the scientific method to patient care. It is the essential critical-thinking method used by nurses to provide safe, competent nursing care to patients, families, and communities.

SUMMARY OF LEARNING OUTCOMES

LO 5.1 *Define the nursing process*: The nursing process is the scientific method through which professional nurses systematically identify and address actual or potential patient problems. Critical thinking, using the nursing process, allows nurses to collect essential patient data, articulate the specific needs of individual patients, and effectively communicate those needs, establish realistic goals, and customize interventions with members of the health care team.

LO 5.2 *Describe the historical development and significance of the nursing process:* The five primary steps of the nursing process were clearly identified by the early 1960s and have remained virtually unchanged since then, with only the addition of a subcategory to planning, outcome identification, in the early 1990s. Professional nursing practice in all types of settings is based on the nursing process. It is used to assess individuals, families, and communities; diagnose needs; plan attainable goals; implement specific interventions; and evaluate degrees of goal attainment.

LO 5.3 *Articulate the characteristics of the nursing process:* The nursing process requires nurses to think critically. It is dynamic, organized, and collaborative, and it is universally adaptable to various types of health care settings.

LO 5.4 *Describe the steps in the nursing process:* During the assessment step of the nursing process, patient care data are gathered. In the diagnosis step, patient data are analyzed to identify patient problems and then are stated as specific nursing diagnoses. During the third step of the nursing process, planning, the nurse prioritizes the nursing diagnoses and identifies goals with specific outcome identification. The implementation step includes initiating specific nursing interventions designed to help achieve established goals. During the evaluation step, the nurse determines goal attainment, the effectiveness of interventions, and whether the plan of care should be discontinued, continued, or revised.

LO 5.5 *Explain the significance of the cyclic and dynamic nature of the nursing process:* Use of the nursing process requires the professional nurse to continuously reassess patients, revise care as needed, and evaluate whether goals are being met. As goals are met, portions of the nursing plan can be eliminated or discontinued. Nursing care sometimes needs to be modified to meet previously unidentified needs. The ongoing process of evaluating and adjusting intervention strategies requires nursing care that is based on current evidence-based practice.

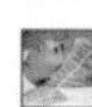
Responses to critical-thinking questions are available at *http://evolve.elsevier.com/YoostCrawford/fundamentals/.*

REVIEW QUESTIONS

1. What is the purpose of the nursing process?
   a. Providing patient-centered care
   b. Identifying members of the health care team
   c. Organizing the ways nurses think about patient care
   d. Facilitating communication among members of the health care team
2. A patient comes to the emergency department complaining of nausea and vomiting. What should the nurse ask the patient about first?
   a. Family history of diabetes
   b. Medications the patient is taking
   c. Operations the patient has had in the past
   d. Severity and duration of the nausea and vomiting
3. An alert, oriented patient is admitted to the hospital with chest pain. Who is the best source of primary data on this patient?
   a. Family member
   b. Physician
   c. Another nurse
   d. Patient
4. What is the primary purpose of the nursing diagnosis?
   a. Resolving patient confusion
   b. Communicating patient needs
   c. Meeting accreditation requirements
   d. Articulating the nursing scope of practice
5. On what premise is a nursing diagnosis identified for a patient?
   a. First impressions
   b. Nursing intuition
   c. Clustered data
   d. Medical diagnoses
6. Which statement is an appropriately written short-term goal?
   a. Patient will walk to the bathroom independently without falling within 2 days after surgery.
   b. Nurse will watch patient demonstrate proper insulin injection technique each morning.
   c. Patient's spouse will express satisfaction with patient's progress before discharge.
   d. Patient's incision will be well approximated each time it is assessed by the nurse.

7. What should be the primary focus for nursing interventions?
   a. Patient needs
   b. Nurse concerns
   c. Physician priorities
   d. Patient's family requests
8. Which nursing action is critical before delegating interventions to another member of the health care team?
   a. Locate all members of the health care team.
   b. Notify the physician of potential complications.
   c. Know the scope of practice for the other team member.
   d. Call a meeting of the health care team to determine the needs of the patient.
9. A patient reports feeling tired and complains of not sleeping at night. What action should the nurse perform first?
   a. Identify reasons the patient is unable to sleep.
   b. Request medication to help the patient sleep.
   c. Tell the patient that sleep will come with relaxation.
   d. Notify the physician that the patient is restless and anxious.
10. What action should the nurse take regarding a patient's plan of care if the patient appears to have met the short-term goal of urinating within 1 hour after surgery?
   a. Consult the surgeon to see if the clinical pathway is being followed.
   b. Discontinue the plan of care because the patient has met the established goal.
   c. Monitor patient urine output to evaluate the need for the current plan of care.
   d. Notify the patient that the goal has been attained and no further intervention is needed.

Answers and rationales for the review questions are available at *http://evolve.elsevier.com/YoostCrawford/fundamentals/*.

REFERENCES

American Nurses Association: *Standards of clinical nursing practice*. Washington, D.C., 1991, The Association.

American Nurses Association: *Nursing: Scope and standards of practice*, ed. 2, Silver Springs, Md., 2010, The Association.

Bulechek G, Butcher H, Dochterman J, Wagner C (Eds): *Nursing interventions classifications (NIC)*, ed. 6, St. Louis, 2013, Mosby Elsevier.

Carpenito-Moyet L: *Nursing diagnoses: Application to clinical practice*, ed. 14, Philadelphia, 2013, Lippincott.

Cronenwett L, Sherwood G, Barnsteiner J, et al: Quality and safety education for nurses. *Nurs Outlook*, 55(3):122-131, 2007.

de la Cuesta C: The nursing process: from development to implementation. *J Adv Nurs*, 8(5):365-371, 1983.

Johnson DE: A philosophy of nursing. *Nurs Outlook*, 7:198-200, 1959.

Kinsman L, Rotter T, James E, et al: What is a clinical pathway? Development of a definition to inform the debate, *BMC Med*, 8:31, 2010.

Moorhead S, Johnson M, Maas M, Swanson E (Eds): *Nursing outcomes classification (NOC)*, ed. 5, St. Louis, 2013, Mosby Elsevier.

NANDA International: *Nursing diagnoses: Definitions and classification, 2012–2014*. West Sussex, England, 2012, Wiley-Blackwell.

Orlando I: *The dynamic nurse-patient relationship*. New York, 1961, Putnam.

Paul R: *What, then, is critical thinking?* Paper presented at the Eighth Annual and Sixth International Conference on Critical Thinking and Educational Reform, Rohnert Park, Calif., 1988.

Wiedenbach E: The helping art of nursing. *Am J Nurs*, 63(11):54-57, 1963.

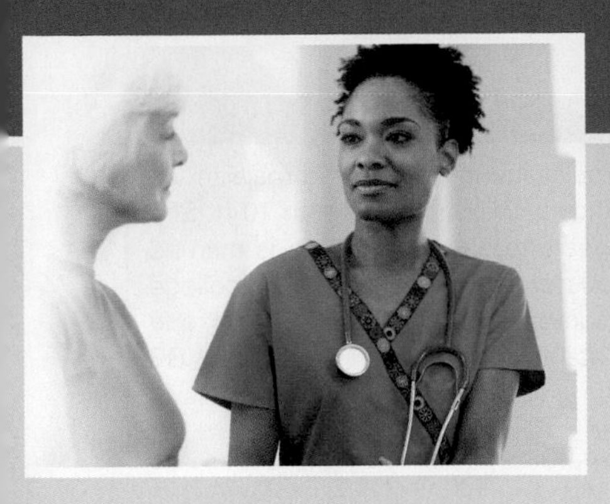

CHAPTER 6

Assessment

EVOLVE WEBSITE

http://evolve.elsevier.com/YoostCrawford/fundamentals/

- Additional Evolve-Only Review Questions With Answers
- Answers and Rationales for Text Review Questions
- Answers to Critical-Thinking Questions
- Case Study With Questions
- Glossary

LEARNING OUTCOMES

Comprehension of this chapter's content will provide students with the ability to:

LO 6.1 Identify methods used during the assessment phase of the nursing process.
LO 6.2 Describe techniques used during physical assessment.
LO 6.3 Differentiate among the three types of physical assessment.
LO 6.4 Categorize types of data collected during the assessment process.
LO 6.5 Use strategies to validate patient assessment data.
LO 6.6 Organize data according to established theoretical frameworks.

KEY TERMS

auscultation, p. 88
cue, p. 91
health history, p. 86
inferences, p. 91
inspection, p. 88
objective data, p. 91
palpation, p. 88
patient interview, p. 84
percussion, p. 88
primary data, p. 90
secondary data, p. 90
signs, p. 91
subjective data, p. 90
symptoms, p. 90

CASE STUDY

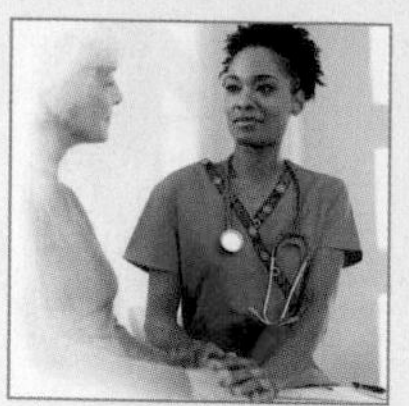

Ms. Kline, a 55-year-old white woman, arrived at an urgent care center complaining of generalized malaise, an overwhelming feeling of exhaustion that was not relieved with rest, and difficulty walking more than 10 ft. She has thinning scalp hair, scaly skin, and puffiness around her eyes. She appears to be anxious. She is married and responsible for raising three grandchildren (2, 4, and 8 years old). She is employed full time as a college professor, and is worried that she may have a serious condition that will compromise her ability to work and care for her grandchildren. She enjoys gardening and reading books. Her vital signs are T 36° C (36.8° F), BP 102/68, P 68 and regular, and R 12 and unlabored.

Refer back to this case study to answer the critical-thinking questions throughout the chapter.

Assessment is the first step in the nursing process (Figure 6-1). Assessment establishes the baseline on which each phase of the nursing process builds. As soon as the patient's records are accessed or a patient is first observed, the process of assessment begins. Valuable information about a patient is collected during the interview, health history, and physical examination. The assessment phase of the nursing process includes much more than collection of physical data. Physical, emotional, spiritual, socioeconomic, and cultural attributes unique to the individual are considered. After data are collected, they must be analyzed, validated, organized, and documented to provide the foundation for an individual patient-focused plan of care.

METHODS OF ASSESSMENT LO 6.1

Methods through which assessment is conducted include observation; the patient interview, including the completion of a health history and review of systems; and a physical examination. Assessment proceeds in a logical and organized fashion to various degrees of depth during each patient-nurse interaction.

OBSERVATION

A nurse can gather significant information about a patient's emotional condition and health status by observing the patient's affect, clothing, personal hygiene, and obvious physical conditions, such as a limp or an open wound. Using the senses of sight, hearing, and smell during the observation phase helps the nurse gather important patient information, which can guide later aspects of the assessment process.

Before initiating the patient interview, the nurse should review data collected previously by other health care professionals to avoid repetition. The nurse should be prepared with required forms and assessment tools to prevent disruption during the dialogue. All significant observations should be documented and verified for accuracy during the interview phase of assessment.

Assessment
Data Collection
- Primary data
  - o Patient interview
- Secondary data
- Subjective data
  - o Symptoms
  - o Health history
- Objective data
  - o Signs
  - o Physical examination
  - o Laboratory results
  - o Diagnostic test results

FIGURE 6-1 Assessment in the nursing process.

PATIENT INTERVIEW

The **patient interview** is a formal, structured discussion in which the nurse questions the patient to obtain demographic information, data about current health concerns, and medical and surgical histories. During the assessment phase of the nursing process, it is essential for the nurse to gather information regarding developmental, cultural, ethnic, and spiritual factors that may affect the patient. These factors can significantly influence patient outcomes and must be considered when developing a patient-centered plan of care.

Patients who feel accepted and relaxed in the health care environment are more likely to disclose vital information to the nurse during the interview and physical examination. The Diversity Considerations box lists some of the many factors that may affect patient cooperation and response to the assessment process.

The patient interview consists of three phases: orientation (introductory), working, and termination. Each phase contributes to the development of trust and engagement between the nurse and the patient.

Orientation Phase

During the orientation phase of the interview, the nurse should establish the name by which the patient prefers to be addressed. Some individuals prefer formal titles of respect (e.g., Dr., Mr., Ms., Professor) and the use of surnames, whereas others are comfortable with less formality. How a patient is addressed is the patient's choice.

The nurse should provide a personal introduction and state the purpose for the interview. This introductory phase is essential for establishing trust between the nurse and the

DIVERSITY CONSIDERATIONS

Life Span

- Establishing rapport is paramount to gaining the trust of the patient. The nurse should consider the patient's generational cohort, which may influence behavior and willingness to share personal information during the interview process.
  - Generational factors may influence behavior (Cannon and Boswell, 2012).
  - Veterans (born before 1945) respect authority; are detail oriented; communicate in a discrete, formal, respectful way; may be slow to warm up; value family and community; and accept physical touch as an effective form of therapeutic communication.
  - Baby Boomers (born 1946-1964) are optimistic; are relationship oriented; communicate by using open or direct speech, using body language, and answering questions thoroughly; expect detailed information; question everything; and value success.
  - Generation X members (born 1965-1976) are informal; are technology immigrants; multitask; communicate in a blunt or direct, factual, and informal style; may talk in short sound bites; share information frequently; and value time.
  - Millennials (born 1977-1997) are flexible; are technologically literate or are technology natives; multitask; communicate by using action verbs and humor; may be brief in the form of texting or email exchanges; like personal attention; and value individuality.
  - Children (born 1998-present) need to be included in discussions; are technology natives; have short attention spans; communicate in a short, focused way, primarily with parents or guardians; and value play.

Culture, Ethnicity, and Religion

- Cultural and ethnic norms affect the willingness of patients to speak openly about health concerns.
- Nurses should explain the need for information that may be considered intimate in nature.
- Privacy must be provided before interviewing patients regarding sensitive information such as the use of recreational drugs or sexual activity.
- Traditional treatment modalities common in a patient's culture or religion should be explored and documented during the interview process. It is important that this information be collected and recorded in a nonjudgmental manner.
- Electronic or live interpretation should be secured for patients who speak a language different from that of the health care providers.

Gender

- Personal space, communication patterns, and gender considerations unique to a patient's cultural background should be incorporated into the interview process in an effort to provide culturally competent care.
- Requests of patients for caregivers of the same gender should be honored whenever possible.

Morphology

- Physical assessment requires patient cooperation and positioning that may be difficult or impossible for individuals who are morbidly obese or physically disabled.
- Adjust the location in which the examination takes place on the basis of patient needs. For example, if a patient is unable to lie comfortably on a narrow examination table, arrange for a bed that can accommodate the patient.

Disability

- If a patient is paralyzed and unable to move independently from a wheelchair to a flat examination surface, seek help to safely transfer the patient so that a complete physical assessment can be done.
- Ask the trusted care providers of mentally challenged individuals to assist with the physical examination to ensure greater patient comfort and promote a feeling of safety and familiarity.
- Make any required adaptations during the physical assessment that are necessary to perform a thorough examination. The ability to provide safe patient care is challenged if the quality of the examination is compromised due to disability.

patient, which affects all future interactions. Demographic data should be collected by asking focused or closed-ended questions. More general information can be gathered by open-ended communication techniques. Identifying patient needs and determining the extent to which patients want to be involved in care planning are important aspects of the introductory phase.

The environment and timing of the interview are very important. Health Insurance Portability and Accountability Act (HIPAA) guidelines should be followed and privacy provided during patient interviews. The environment should be as private as possible. Privacy from other individuals and freedom from stressors that may affect the patient should be considered when determining when, where, and how to conduct the interview. The interview should be conducted in an area that is free from as many distractions as possible. Ensuring that the patient is comfortable and relaxed often takes prior thought and planning by the nurse. The patient should feel safe, because the questions raised may cause stress and anxiety.

When feasible, the nurse and the patient should be seated at eye level with each other (Figure 6-2). In this way, the interaction between the nurse and the patient is horizontal instead of vertical. Standing over someone implies control, power, and authority. The implication of power can result in less-than-optimal data collection and a potential conflict as the patient strives to regain control over the situation.

Nonverbal behaviors of the nurse can influence the information obtained from the patient. Negative nonverbal cues such as distracting gestures (e.g., tapping a pen, swinging a

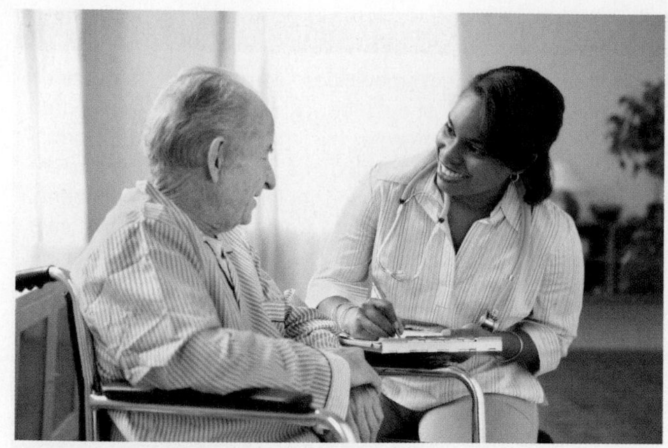

FIGURE 6-2 Sitting at eye level with a patient during the interview communicates caring and acceptance.

> **PATIENT EDUCATION AND HEALTH LITERACY**
>
> **The Role of Assessment in Patient Education**
> - The opportunity for teaching begins with a patient's entry into the health care environment, whether it is in an acute or community setting.
> - Prior to initiating patient education, the nurse needs to assess a patient's cognitive ability, reading level, and potential language barriers.
> - Assessment should include collecting information about what the patient already knows about her or his current condition and what additional knowledge is needed.
> - Assessment information about the patient's educational needs should be documented and should guide aspects of the patient's individualized plan of care.
> - Thorough assessment of the patient's knowledge should be used to determine the need for referrals and educational interventions.

foot, looking at a watch), inappropriate facial expressions, and lack of eye contact communicate disinterest. To establish a trusting relationship with the patient before the physical examination is conducted, the nurse should communicate professionally, sit close and lean in slightly toward the patient, listen attentively and demonstrate appropriate eye contact, smile, and use a moderate rate of speech and tone of voice.

Working Phase

During the working phase of the interview, the nurse must stay focused on the purpose of the interaction. The nurse needs to individualize the process on the basis of the health of the patient and concerns that emerge during the course of the interview. Active, engaged listening is imperative during this process. The nurse must stay alert to what the patient says and how information is presented. Sometimes, how the patient shares information is more important than what the patient says. The nurse should watch for emotional cues indicating fear or painful experiences and the appropriateness of verbal and nonverbal cues.

Educational needs are assessed during the patient interview (Patient Education and Health Literacy box). The nurse should document gaps in patient knowledge and areas in which clarification of disease processes or treatment would be beneficial. Knowing a patient's level of education and professional background is often helpful in designing appropriate patient teaching.

A variety of communication techniques can be incorporated into the interview process. Open-ended questions encourage narrative responses from patients. Closed-ended, focused, and direct questions elicit specific information, such as the exact location of a patient's pain. It is appropriate to use direct questions to gather data about a patient's health history or during the review of body systems, when a yes or no answer is adequate. Direct questions can be expanded on with open-ended questions if more extensive information is needed. Chapter 3 provides in-depth discussion on therapeutic communication techniques that are helpful during the patient interview.

During an admission interview, a thorough health history and review of systems should be conducted. If a patient being admitted to the hospital is too ill to interact for an extended period, the interview can be broken into smaller segments. Interviews with patients already hospitalized or established in the health care system are less extensive and more focused on newly identified patient concerns or problems.

Health History

An in-depth **health history** includes all pertinent information that can guide the development of a patient-centered plan of care. The health history includes demographic data, which is collected during the orientation phase of the interview; a patient's chief complaint or reason for seeking health care; history of current illness; allergies; medications; adverse reactions to medications; medical history; family and social history; and health promotion practices (Table 6-1). Because a patient's health history is continuously evolving, the data collection is ongoing, progressive, and methodical (Zastrow, 2009).

Thorough documentation of health history findings in the format prescribed by the health care facility contributes to better communication among health care team members and a more individualized plan of care. Ongoing efforts should be made to add missing data as they are obtained and to clarify any erroneous or confusing information.

Review of Systems

A review of systems, which is conducted by asking the patient questions pertaining to each body system, completes the health history. During the review of systems, the nurse collects subjective, patient-reported data. Questions asked during the review of systems usually are brief and inquire

TABLE 6-1 Framework for Collecting Health History Data

TYPE OF DATA	SPECIFIC INFORMATION
Demographic data	Name Address Telephone numbers Age Birth date Birthplace Gender Marital status Race Cultural background or ethnic origin Spiritual or religious preference Educational level Occupation
Chief complaint or current illness	Reason for seeking care Onset of symptoms
Allergies and sensitivities	Medication Food (e.g., peanuts, eggs) Environmental agents (e.g., latex, tape, detergents) Reaction to reported allergens (e.g., rash, breathing difficulty, nausea, vomiting) Contrast dye
Medications, vitamins, and herbal supplements	Prescription Over-the-counter medications and herbal remedies Dosage, frequency, and reason for use
Immunizations	Childhood and adult immunizations Date of last tuberculin skin test Date of last vaccines (e.g., flu, pneumonia, shingles)
Medical history	Childhood illnesses, accidents, and injuries Serious or chronic illnesses Hospitalizations, including obstetric history for female patients Date of occurrence and current treatment
Surgical history	Type of surgery Date Problems with anesthesia Any complications
Family history	Age and health status of living parents, grandparents, siblings, and children Age at death and cause of death of deceased immediate family members Genetic diseases or traits, familial diseases (e.g., cardiovascular disease, high blood pressure, stroke, blood disorders, cancer, diabetes, kidney disease, seizure disorders, drug or alcohol dependencies, mental illness)
Social history	Use of tobacco, alcohol, or recreational drugs Environmental exposures Animal exposures and pets Living arrangement Safety concerns (e.g., intimate-partner violence, emotional or physical abuse) Recent domestic or foreign travel
Cultural and spiritual or religious traditions	Primary language Dietary restrictions Religion Values and beliefs related to health care
Activities of daily living (ADLs)	Nutrition (e.g., meal preparation, shopping, typical 24-hour dietary intake); recent changes in appetite Caffeine intake Self-care activities (e.g., bathing, dressing, grooming, ambulation) Physical living environment (e.g., steps, access to toileting or sleeping areas, indoor plumbing, carpet or rugs) Use of prosthetics or mobility devices Leisure and exercise activities Sleep patterns (e.g., hours per night, naps, sleep aids)
Cognitive or emotional status	Cognitive functioning Personal strengths Self-esteem Support system (e.g., family, friend, support groups, professional counseling)

about the normal function of each area, such as "Are you experiencing any difficulty breathing?" or "Do you ever experience diarrhea or constipation?" Any deviation from normal triggers more directive questions and affects the physical assessment. Health assessment questions related to each body system can be found in Chapter 20.

After the collection of data, goals for care are established during the working phase in collaboration with the patient. Family members and other members of the health care team may be included in the goal-setting process. Information gathered during the interview and data gathered during the physical examination combine to form the foundation of a unique, patient-centered plan of care.

Termination Phase

As the end of the interview approaches, care is taken to review key findings and prepare the patient for the conclusion of the discussion. This can be done effectively by summarizing and validating the information covered with the patient. By reviewing the information with the patient, a consensus is established. As the interview concludes, the patient should be allowed an opportunity to interject additional pertinent information. The session is concluded with the nurse acknowledging the patient's participation and describing the next steps that the patient should expect.

PHYSICAL ASSESSMENT LO 6.2

On completion of the patient interview, health history, and review of systems, the nurse begins the physical assessment. During the physical assessment, the nurse collects objective data. If diagnostic tests, such as blood tests or x-rays, were ordered before the patient was seen, the results are reviewed by the nurse. Privacy for the patient is ensured, good lighting is established, and the equipment and instruments needed, such as a stethoscope, sphygmomanometer, and pulse oximeter, are gathered before the physical examination is started. A penlight, otoscope, and ophthalmoscope may be required, depending on the type of physical assessment being conducted. Hand hygiene is performed, and clean gloves are worn if contact with body fluids is anticipated. Vital signs are taken and recorded at the beginning of the physical examination.

The assessment techniques of inspection, palpation, percussion, and auscultation are performed one at a time in this order for each body system except during assessment of the abdomen. During abdominal assessment, auscultation precedes palpation and percussion. The altered sequence of abdominal assessment avoids stimulation of the bowel before auscultation of bowel sounds.

INSPECTION

Inspection involves the use of vision, hearing, and smell to closely scrutinize physical characteristics of a whole person and individual body systems. Distinguishing between normal and abnormal findings for patients of different age groups begins the moment the nurse first observes and meets the individual, and it continues throughout the examination. Symmetry should be assessed by comparing the right and left sides of the body. Because the human body is usually anatomically symmetric, observing for abnormalities on both sides is important for detecting anatomic deviations. After inspection, further examination is performed using palpation and percussion.

PALPATION

Palpation uses touch to assess body organs and skin texture, temperature, moisture, turgor, tenderness, and thickness. Palpation can determine organ location and size against the expected anatomic norm, any distention or masses, and vibration or pulsation associated with movement. Palpation is used to affirm details observed during inspection. Only light palpation should be applied to areas described by patients as sensitive or painful. Deep palpation is performed by physicians or advanced practice nurses to determine organ size and variation.

PERCUSSION

Percussion involves tapping the patient's skin with short, sharp strokes that cause a vibration to travel through the skin and to the upper layers of the underlying structures. Vibration is reflected by the tissues, and the character of the sound heard depends on the density of the structures that reflect the sound. Knowing how the various densities reflect or absorb sound helps to determine the approximate size, shape, and borders of organs, masses, and fluid. An abnormal sound implies that an organ or area is possibly compromised with another substance, such as air, blood, or other bodily fluids. Percussion is typically performed by an advanced practice nurse or physician.

AUSCULTATION

Auscultation is a technique of listening with the assistance of a stethoscope to sounds made by organs or systems such as the heart, blood vessels, lungs, and abdominal cavity. The characteristics of auscultated sounds depend on the body tissue or organ being assessed. Breath sounds, heart sounds, and bowel sounds are routinely assessed through auscultation. Practice is required to be able to differentiate normal from abnormal findings.

TYPES OF PHYSICAL ASSESSMENT LO 6.3

Three primary types of physical assessment are conducted by nurses in a variety of practice settings. Determining which is indicated depends on the situation and timing of the nurse-patient interaction. An initial comprehensive or complete physical examination should be performed by a nurse when a patient is admitted to the hospital. It can be followed by clinical or focused assessments at the beginning of each shift or more often, depending on the patient's condition and the health care facility's policies and guidelines. Emergency assessments, including triage, are conducted in emergent situations to quickly assess the extent of patient injuries and determine care priorities.

It is the responsibility of the professional nurse to determine if a patient's condition warrants more frequent or extensive assessment in any given situation. Although some aspects of assessment can be delegated to other members of the health care team or unlicensed assistive personnel, the nurse must know what can be legally and safely delegated and what requires the nurse's coordination of care and personal attention (Collaboration and Delegation box). A patient's plan of care is evaluated and modified on the basis of the assessment findings collected during every type of assessment.

COLLABORATION AND DELEGATION

The Registered Nurse's Critical Role in Assessment

- Initial and ongoing assessment of patients requiring critical care cannot be delegated to unlicensed assistive personnel (UAP).
- Initial patient assessment of unstable patients cannot be delegated to an Licensed Practical or Licensed Vocational Nurse (LPN/LVN). An LPN/LVN may contribute to the ongoing assessment of patients and document their observations and care.
- Routine assessment of vital signs of a patient in stable condition may be delegated to an LPN/LVN or qualified UAP.
- Nurses delegating assessment of vital signs must:
  - Determine the stability of the patient and complexity of the problem before delegation.
  - Verify that the UAP are trained and capable of accurately performing the skills.
  - Collaborate with the UAP to confirm completion of vital sign measurement and proper documentation.
- Specific patient assessment may require the assistance of other health team members, such as in these examples:
  - Determination of a patient's ability to swallow is commonly delegated to a speech therapist.
  - Establishing a patient's level of stability while using crutches is typically done by a physical therapist.

COMPREHENSIVE ASSESSMENT

A comprehensive or complete assessment includes a thorough interview, health history, review of systems, and extensive physical head-to-toe assessment, including evaluation of cranial nerves and sensory organs, such as with sight and hearing testing. A complete physical examination may be conducted on admission to a hospital, during an annual physical at the office of a physician or nurse practitioner, or on initial interaction with a specialist. Comprehensive assessments often include a variety of laboratory and diagnostic tests that are ordered by the primary care provider.

FOCUSED ASSESSMENT

A focused or clinical assessment is a brief individualized physical examination conducted at the beginning of an acute care–setting work shift to establish current patient status or during ongoing patient encounters in response to a specific patient concern. A focused assessment may be conducted when signs indicate a change in a patient's condition or the development of a new complication. This type of assessment is the most common type conducted by a nurse. Vital signs are assessed during each focused examination, which includes assessment of the pain level and pulse oximetry readings. The nurse examines the head, eyes, ears, nose, throat, neck, thorax (including lung and heart sounds), abdomen (including bowel sounds), and extremities.

During a focused examination, the edema, peripheral pulses, capillary refill, skin turgor, and muscle strength are routinely identified. Wounds, intravenous sites, supplemental oxygen levels and delivery systems, nasogastric tubes, cardiac monitoring, and urinary catheters are assessed and documented. While assessing extremities, the nurse evaluates edema, pulses, capillary refill, and strength. Intake and output levels are documented, as well as any unique concerns of the patient at the time of the assessment. After completion of the basic head-to-toe assessment, attention turns to any health concerns raised by the patient.

EMERGENCY ASSESSMENT

Emergency assessment is a physical examination done when time is a factor, treatment must begin immediately, or priorities for care need to be established in a few seconds or minutes. Patient treatment is based on a quick survey of accident or illness onset, followed by a narrowly focused physical examination of critical injuries or symptoms and signs.

Patient responsiveness is determined in an attempt to establish the potential extent of injury to vital organs. Attention is paid to the patient's airway, breathing, and circulation. Other concerns in the emergent setting are noticeable deformities such as compound fractures, contusions, abrasions, puncture wounds, burns, tenderness, lacerations, bleeding, and swelling. During an emergency, the nurse may never have time to do a complete assessment and may work to stabilize one body system at a time. In this event, the nurse must remember to continually reassess every 5 to 15 minutes, depending on the stability of the patient.

Triage, a form of emergency assessment, is the classification of patients according to treatment priority. Patients are categorized by the urgency of their condition. Most emergency departments use a three-tier or five-tier triage system;

TABLE 6-2 Five-Tier Triage System

TRIAGE TIER DESIGNATION	INDICATIONS FOR CARE
Level 1 Critical: life-threatening condition	Requires immediate and continuous care • Severe trauma • Cardiac arrest • Respiratory distress • Seizure • Shock
Level 2 Emergent: imminently life-threatening condition	Requires care within 30 min • Chest pain • Major fracture • Severe pain
Level 3 Urgent: potentially life-threatening condition	Requires care within 30-60 min • Minor fracture • Laceration • Dehydration
Level 4 Nonurgent: stable health condition	Requires care within 60-120 min • Sore throat • Abrasion
Level 5 Fast track: less urgent	Requires care when possible • Conditions with symptoms for a week or longer • Cold symptoms • Minor aches and pains

From O'Neill K, Molczan K: Pediatric triage: A 2-tier, 5-level system in the United States, *Pediatr Emerg Care* 19(4):285-290, 2003.

the trend is toward a five-tier system. The classifications in the three-tier system are emergent, urgent, and nonurgent. The five-tier system classifies patients by levels numbered 1 through 5 (Table 6-2). The triage nurse must remember that symptoms can change and ongoing reassessments are required.

Triage is usually conducted when a patient enters the emergency department. However, the increasing patient load at emergency departments has engendered a trend toward telephone triage, which can help a patient determine whether urgent care, along with a trip to the emergency department, is necessary or the patient can wait and make a physician or clinic appointment.

DATA COLLECTION LO 6.4

Throughout the assessment process, various types of data that contribute to the patient record are collected and documented. The combined data are grouped using an established organizing framework and serve as the foundation for a patient-centered plan of care.

Collecting data is a systematic process that must be ongoing throughout the nurse-patient interaction. A nurse must be able to assess a patient's response to treatment, evaluate changes in the patient's evolving health status, and make clinical decisions based on those changes. The nurse must realize that the assessment process is cyclic and should be fluid and dynamic (Broom, 2007). The two forms of data, subjective and objective, that are elicited during the nurse-patient interaction and physical assessment are categorized as primary and secondary.

PRIMARY AND SECONDARY DATA

Primary data come directly from the patient. Patients are the best source of information about their conditions, feelings, and what they have done to address their concerns before seeking professional health care. In some cases, it is best to collect data from the patient before seeking information from secondary sources.

! SAFE PRACTICE ALERT

Remember that patients are most familiar with their bodies and feelings. Nurses must actively listen to patients to better understand their concerns and care preferences. Involving patients in their care enhances patient satisfaction and outcomes.

If an adult patient is cognitively impaired or unconscious or if the patient is an infant or young child, subjective data about how the patient has been acting or feeling needs to be obtained from the patient's family or guardian. Information shared by family members, friends, or other members of the health care team is **secondary data**. Likewise, data obtained from reviewing a patient's chart, medical records, results of laboratory and diagnostic tests, and literature reviews are secondary. Verification of primary and secondary data is vitally important to avoid a plan of care based on inaccurate information. Primary caregivers and family members can be extremely helpful in providing valuable assessment data on patients with disabilities.

SUBJECTIVE DATA

Subjective data are spoken information or **symptoms** that cannot be authenticated. Subjective data usually are gathered during the interview process if patients are well enough to describe their symptoms. Alert and oriented adult patients are the source of primary, subjective data. Family members, friends, and other members of the health care team can contribute valid secondary, subjective data.

Subjective data should be documented as direct quotations (within quotation marks). Statements may include descriptions of feeling dizzy or ill, emotions, concerns, and other types of knowledge that cannot be quantified objectively. For example, if a patient is experiencing chest pain and says, "It feels like an elephant is standing on my chest," the nurse should include the patient's statement in his or her medical record.

OBJECTIVE DATA

Objective data, also referred to as **signs**, can be measured or observed. The nurse's senses of sight, hearing, touch, and smell are used to collect objective data. Objective assessment data are acquired through observation, physical examination, and analysis of laboratory and diagnostic test results. Examples of objective data are blood pressure readings, pulse measurement, and hemoglobin levels—any information that can be compared with established norms.

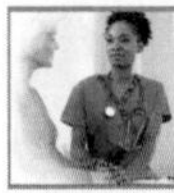

1. Identify data that the nurse collected by looking at Ms. Kline.

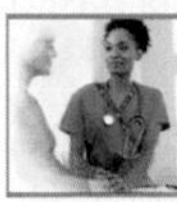

2. Classify each piece of Ms. Kline's data in the case study as subjective or objective.

VALIDATING DATA LO 6.5

Sometimes during assessment of a patient, the nurse observes nonverbal cues that imply possible physical or emotional concerns (Figure 6-3). A **cue** is a hint or an indication of a potential disease process or disorder. For instance, if a patient winces, it may indicate pain, or if a patient resists being touched, the patient may be a victim of physical abuse. Crying, a disheveled appearance, and lack of eye contact may be cues of depression. However, conclusions about the underlying cause of the patient's actions cannot be assumed. All cues need to be interpreted and validated to verify the data's accuracy.

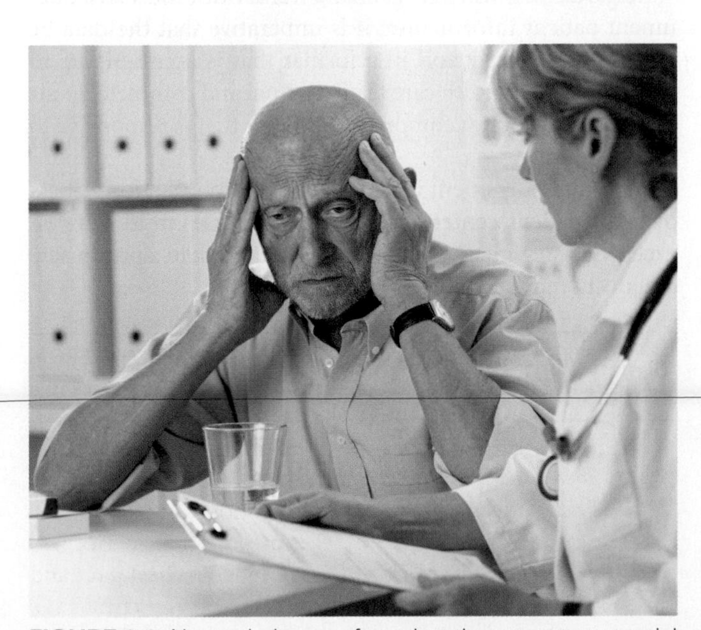

FIGURE 6-3 Nonverbal cues often alert the nurse to potential physical or emotional concerns of the patient.

Validating data is making sure that the data are accurate. As patient information is collected, consistency between subjective and objective data must be confirmed. Confirming the validity of collected data often requires verbally checking with the patient to see whether assumptions or conclusions at which the nurse arrived are correct. Sometimes, the nurse can use laboratory and diagnostic test results to validate the subjective data. For example, objective data can validate patient subjective data when the patient's hemoglobin level is low, indicating anemia, and the patient complains feeling fatigued and dizzy. In the day-to-day process of caring for the patient and family, pertinent information becomes available to corroborate initial assessment data. Although data validation should be done on a continual basis, care should be taken to avoid repetition.

DATA INTERPRETATION

Careful observation and attention to detail help the nurse to notice subtle cues and recognize how best to validate and interpret patient data. While interpreting data, the nurse must be careful to avoid inaccurate **inferences** (i.e., conclusions) based on the nurse's personal preferences, past experiences, generalizations, or outdated and inaccurate health care information. Interpreting data and making inferences that determine patient care must involve ongoing interaction with patients and others, which includes sensitivity to the patient's expectations, cultural and ethnic traditions, and values.

QSEN FOCUS!

Patient-centered care requires the nurse to understand patient and family preferences and values. The nurse must recognize patients' expectations for care and provide care with respect for the diversity of human experience.

Accurate interpretation of patient data requires that the nurse have a wide breadth of knowledge, including disease processes, vital sign parameters, and normal values and outcomes for laboratory and diagnostic tests. The nurse must know typical signs and symptoms of disease processes and which laboratory and diagnostic test results should be monitored on the basis of a patient's condition and medical diagnosis.

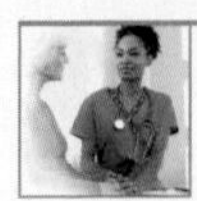

3. Write a minimum of five follow-up questions that the nurse should ask Ms. Kline to obtain additional assessment data.

Review of current references and evidence-based practice research is essential for implementing safe patient care (Evidence-Based Practice and Informatics box). Care must be taken to ensure that materials accessed online are accurate and scholarly. Information from reliable sources is valuable for determining appropriate interventions that should be included in a patient's plan of care.

EVIDENCE-BASED PRACTICE AND INFORMATICS

Electronic Resources for Evidence-Based Nursing Practice

Many reliable mobile resources, websites, and research databases that are available to nurses provide information that can guide patient care:

- Reference software is available for every type of mobile device, making assessment, diagnostic, and medication information accessible at the point of care.
- Information from online websites—including the Centers for Disease Control and Prevention (CDC), the National Institutes of Health (NIH), and Agency for Healthcare Research and Quality (AHRQ)—contain evidence-based practice research and can be used to help interpret assessment information.
- Research databases such as Joanna Briggs, the Cumulative Index of Nursing and Allied Health Literature (CINAHL), and the Cochrane Review provide nurses with current evidence-based practice research and applications.

DATA ORGANIZATION LO 6.6

After the patient's data are collected, validated, and interpreted, the nurse organizes the information in a framework (format) that facilitates access by all members of the health care team. In some cases, health care facilities have their own organizing formats, but most use formats based on one of the three traditional organizing frameworks.

BODY SYSTEMS MODEL

The body systems model organizes data on the basis of each system of the body: integumentary, respiratory, cardiovascular, nervous, reproductive, musculoskeletal, gastrointestinal, genitourinary, and immune systems. It follows a sequence similar to the medical model for physical examination. The body systems model for data organization tends to focus on the physical aspects of a patient's condition rather than a more holistic view.

HEAD-TO-TOE MODEL

Organizing assessment data in a head-to-toe (cephalic-caudal) pattern ensures that all areas of concern are addressed. The nurse documents information regarding the patient's general health status first, including data related to psychosocial concerns, emotional status, cultural and ethnic influences, and living conditions. Vital sign assessment data are then recorded, followed by objective and subjective patient information. Physical assessment data are documented, starting with the head and ending with findings related to the lower extremities.

GORDON'S FUNCTIONAL HEALTH PATTERNS

A third method of organizing health assessment data is based on areas of function. Marjory Gordon (2010) developed functional health patterns to help nurses focus on patient strengths and related but sometimes overlooked data relationships. For instance, one of the functional health patterns is activity and exercise. In this health pattern, the patient data related to cardiac, respiratory, and musculoskeletal function are recorded because the ability of a patient to initiate and continue activity depends on the condition of the heart, lungs, and muscles and bones.

Table 6-3 illustrates each functional health pattern with an example of patient assessment data that would be recorded in it. This method of organizing patient data is a more holistic approach than the others. Its comprehensive structure is beneficial when organizing vast amounts of patient information and when clustering related patient data before formulating nursing diagnoses, patient goals, and treatment outcomes.

Regardless of which organizing framework is used to document patient information, it is imperative that the data be recorded accurately and in a format that is accessible to all members of the health care team. Factual and complete documentation facilitates comprehensive care that is responsive to patient needs.

Accurate assessment is essential to the overall effectiveness of every patient-centered plan of care. Nurses must develop excellent assessment skills to accurately aid in appropriate diagnosis and treatment of their patients.

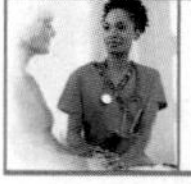

4. Organize the assessment findings from Ms. Kline in functional health patterns.

TABLE 6-3 Functional Health Patterns

FUNCTIONAL HEALTH PATTERN	FOCUS	FUNCTIONAL HEALTH PATTERN	FOCUS
Health perception and health management	Patient's perceived level of health Social habits Living conditions Health and safety concerns	Sleep and rest	Sleep patterns Rest and relaxation activities Fatigue levels
Nutrition and metabolism	Food consumption Fluid intake and balance Tissue integrity	Self-perception and self-concept	Identity Body image Self-worth Self-esteem
Elimination	Excretory concerns • Bowel • Urinary	Roles and relationships	Role satisfaction Role strain Relationship function or dysfunction
Activity and exercise	Activities of daily living Exercise and leisure Cardiac status Respiratory status Musculoskeletal status	Sexuality and reproduction	Sexuality patterns Satisfaction with intimacy
		Coping and stress tolerance	Coping abilities, stress tolerance Support system evaluation
Cognition and perception	Sensory intactness Cognitive ability Level of consciousness Neurologic function	Values and beliefs	Values Spiritual beliefs Cultural patterns Influences on decision making

From Gordon M: *Manual of nursing diagnosis,* ed. 12, Sudbury, Mass., 2011, Jones & Bartlett.

SUMMARY OF LEARNING OUTCOMES

LO 6.1 *Identify methods used during the assessment phase of the nursing process:* Assessment requires observation; a patient interview, including collection of demographic data; a health history; a review of systems; and a physical examination.

LO 6.2 *Describe techniques used during physical assessment:* The assessment techniques of inspection, palpation, percussion, and auscultation are performed one at a time in this order for each body system except during assessment of the abdomen. During abdominal assessment, auscultation precedes palpation and percussion.

LO 6.3 *Differentiate among the three types of physical assessment:* A complete physical examination is typically performed on admission to the hospital, at an initial visit to a specialist, or during an annual physical. Focused assessments are most often done at the beginning of each shift but can be done more often, depending on the patient's condition, evolving complications, and health care facility policies and guidelines. Emergency assessments, including triage, are conducted in emergent situations to quickly assess the extent of patient injuries and determine care priorities.

LO 6.4 *Categorize the types of data collected during the assessment process:* Primary data are obtained directly from a patient, whereas secondary data consist of information collected from family members, other members of the health care team, and medical records. Subjective data are symptoms or spoken information. Objective data are signs or information that is observed.

LO 6.5 *Use strategies to validate patient assessment data:* Sometimes, the nurse can use laboratory and diagnostic test results to validate subjective data. In some cases, cues validate symptoms reported by patients. In other cases, confirming the validity of collected data requires verbally checking with the patient to see whether the nurse's assumptions or conclusions are correct.

LO 6.6 *Organize data according to established theoretical frameworks:* Three commonly used methods of organizing patient data are by body system, in head-to-toe format, and by functional health patterns. The first two methods focus on the medical model and illness, whereas the functional health pattern approach is more holistic.

Responses to the critical-thinking questions are available at ***http://evolve.elsevier.com/YoostCrawford/fundamentals/.***

REVIEW QUESTIONS

1. Which action by a patient marks the beginning of the physical assessment process?
   a. Redressing after a physical examination
   b. Breathing normally during auscultation
   c. Greeting the nurse in the examination room
   d. Sharing work environment information
2. Which factors should be taken into consideration by the nurse before and during a patient interview? *(Select all that apply.)*
   a. Distance between the chairs in which the nurse and patient are sitting
   b. Traditional treatments typically used by the patient to treat disease
   c. Gender preference for primary care providers
   d. Physical condition of the patient
   e. Music preference of the patient
3. Which action by the nurse is most appropriate during the orientation phase of the patient interview?
   a. Always position patients in a comfortable reclined position to ensure their comfort during questioning
   b. Ask which name a patient prefers to be called during care to show respect and build trust
   c. Quickly conduct a review of systems to determine the need for a complete or focused assessment
   d. Begin with questions about intimacy and sexuality to address sensitive issues first
4. Which activity by the nurse best demonstrates part of the working phase of a patient interview?
   a. Summarizing previously discussed key topics
   b. Including selected family members in care planning
   c. Transferring care responsibilities to the home health nurse
   d. Verifying the name by which a patient prefers to be addressed
5. Which entry in a patient's electronic health record best indicates the need for a nurse to gather secondary rather than primary subjective data?
   a. Complaining of chest pain
   b. Apical pulse 110
   c. Comatose
   d. Difficulty swallowing
6. Which line of questioning by the nurse best represents an appropriate approach to the review of systems aspect of the assessment process?
   a. "What do you do for a living? Can you describe your work environment?"
   b. "Is there a family history of heart disease, cancer, high blood pressure, or stroke?"
   c. "When was your last annual physical? What immunizations did you receive at that time?"
   d. "Do you have any chest tightness, shortness of breath, or difficulty breathing while exercising?"
7. Which cue by a patient can be validated by laboratory and diagnostic test results?
   a. Deeply sighing with fatigue
   b. Bilateral crackles in the lungs
   c. Oxygen saturation of 98% on room air
   d. 2+ pitting edema of the ankles and feet
8. A patient discusses his job stress and family relationships with the nurse during his health history interview. In which organizational framework is this type of data likely to be recorded most extensively?
   a. Body systems model
   b. Physical assessment model
   c. Head-to-toe assessment model
   d. Functional health patterns model
9. When initiating a physical examination, which action should the nurse take first?
   a. Review of the patient's prior medical records
   b. Gather admission health history forms
   c. Assess the patient's vital signs
   d. Perform light and deep palpation for fluid
10. If the nurse discovers that a patient's right elbow is swollen and painful during a physical examination, which action should the nurse take next?
    a. Apply ice to decrease swelling and reduce pain
    b. Percuss the area to determine the presence of fluid
    c. Perform passive range of motion to promote flexibility
    d. Inspect the patient's left elbow to compare its appearance

Answers and rationales for the review questions are available at *http://evolve.elsevier.com/YoostCrawford/fundamentals/*.

REFERENCES

Broom M: Exploring the assessment process. *Paediatr Nurs*, 19(4):22-25, 2007.

Cannon S, Boswell C: *Evidence-based teaching in nursing: A foundation for educators*, Sudbury, Mass., 2012, Jones & Bartlett.

Cronenwett L, Sherwood G, Barnsteiner J, et al: Quality and safety education for nurses. *Nurs Outlook*, 55(3):122-131, 2007.

Gordon M: *Manual of nursing diagnosis*, ed. 12, Sudbury, Mass, 2010, Jones & Bartlett.

Zastrow SL: Perioperative nursing assessments made simple. *OR Nurse*, 3(4):16-17, 2009.

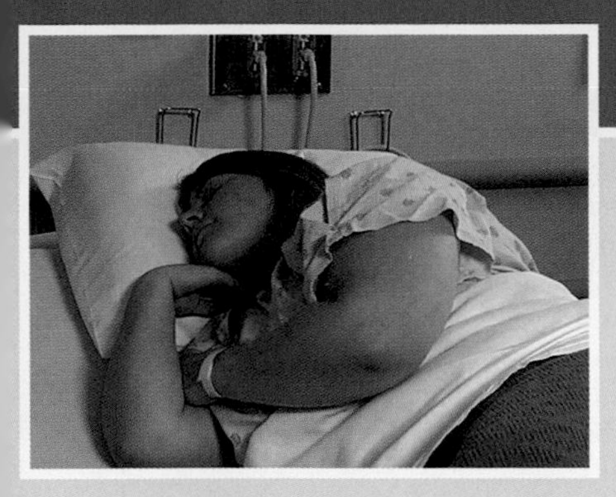

CHAPTER 7

Nursing Diagnosis

EVOLVE WEBSITE

http://evolve.elsevier.com/YoostCrawford/fundamentals/

- Additional Evolve-Only Review Questions With Answers
- Answers and Rationales for Text Review Questions
- Answers to Critical-Thinking Questions
- Case Study With Questions
- Glossary

LEARNING OUTCOMES

Comprehension of this chapter's content will provide students with the ability to:

LO 7.1 Explain basic nursing diagnosis methodology.
LO 7.2 Describe the historical development of NANDA-I and the nursing taxonomy.
LO 7.3 Differentiate among the three types of nursing diagnostic statements.
LO 7.4 Outline nursing diagnoses with appropriate components.
LO 7.5 Implement the steps for accurately identifying nursing diagnoses.
LO 7.6 Discuss how to avoid common problems associated with the diagnostic process.
LO 7.7 Articulate the contribution of nursing diagnosis to the individualized care of patients.

KEY TERMS

actual nursing diagnoses, p. 96
clustering, p. 100
defining characteristics, p. 99
diagnosis label, p. 98
health-promotion nursing diagnoses, p. 96
nursing diagnosis, p. 96
related factors, p. 99
risk factors, p. 99
risk nursing diagnoses, p. 96
taxonomy, p. 96

CASE STUDY

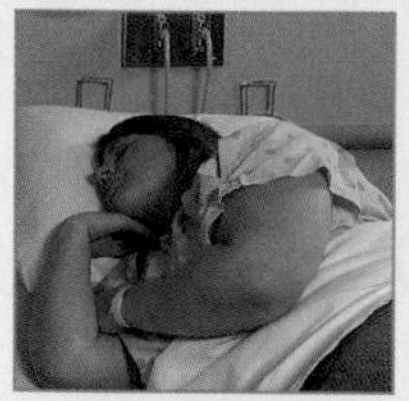

Ms. Hayes is a 34-year-old woman admitted to the emergency room yesterday complaining of nausea, vomiting, and right upper quadrant pain. An upper right quadrant sonogram revealed several large stones in the gallbladder and possibly smaller stones in the common bile duct, requiring an open cholecystectomy.

On the first postoperative day, Ms. Hayes's vital signs are BP 170/98, P 92 and regular, R 28 and unlabored, and T 38.1° C (100.6° F). She reports a pain level of 7 of 10, and her pulse oximetry reading is 92% on room air. Her incision is 5 inches long, running parallel to the right upper quadrant ribs; it is secured with retention sutures. Because of her obesity, the incision is taut in certain sections. There is no swelling and only slight redness along the incision. The sterile gauze dressing has a minimal amount of dried blood. She has an intravenous line of 5% dextrose running at 125 mL/hr.

Ms. Hayes has been medicated for pain three times during the 12-hour night shift and is currently requesting more pain medicine. Crackles are audible during lung auscultation. She does not want to turn, cough, and breathe deeply because "it hurts." She has gotten up once to urinate 750 mL of concentrated urine and has not had a bowel movement. She denies having nausea and vomiting. She is asking when she can eat but remains on a clear liquid diet. She states that she is not comfortable in her bed. She appears anxious, expresses concern about her job, and wants to know when she can leave.

Refer back to this case study to answer the critical-thinking questions throughout the chapter.

Nursing diagnosis is the second step of the nursing process. Formulation of nursing diagnoses follows patient data collection and involves the analysis and clustering of related assessment information. The use of nursing diagnosis labels facilitates clear communication of patient needs and promotes professional accountability and autonomy by defining and describing the independent area of nursing practice (ANA, 2010). Nursing diagnostic statements clearly communicate to legislators, consumers, and insurance providers the unique care nurses deliver and the specific nature of the health conditions they treat (Ethical, Legal, and Professional Practice box). Use of a unified language classification system, or **taxonomy**, is an effective vehicle for communication among nurses and other health care professionals. Nursing diagnostic labels are identified from the NANDA International, Inc. (NANDA-I) list of approved nursing diagnostic statements.

ETHICAL, LEGAL, AND PROFESSIONAL PRACTICE

Responsibilities of the Professional Nurse

Accurate identification of nursing diagnoses for patients is critical to professional nursing practice, as delineated in the American Nurses Association's *Nursing: Scope and Standards of Practice* (2010). Professional nurses are required to:

- Make accurate, applicable nursing diagnoses to guide quality, individualized nursing care of patients.
- Consider ethical and legal consequences for failure to identify areas of concern requiring treatment.
- Understand the implications of delayed recovery, further negative health issues, and if it occurs, the death of the patient.
- Realize the ultimate risk for litigation involving the nurse in the event of lack of or poor performance of identification of nursing diagnostic statements.
- Formulate individualized nursing diagnostic statements at all levels of professional practice, and assign medical diagnoses within the scope of the nurse practice acts governing advanced practice nursing.

QSEN FOCUS!

The use of standardized nursing diagnosis language to communicate patient data enhances the accurate transfer of information among nurses, which is essential for patient safety. Because a nursing diagnosis consolidates a great volume of information in a concise statement, it provides an effective shorthand means of communicating the patient's status.

NURSING DIAGNOSIS METHODOLOGY LO 7.1

Nursing diagnosis, the identification of actual or potential health problems or life processes and responses to a problem (NANDA-I, 2012), follows assessment in the nursing process. In this step, the nurse makes clinical judgments about a patient's experiences and responses to problems or life events identified during the data collection process. Identification of correct nursing diagnoses depends on accurate collection, validation, analysis, and clustering of patient data (Evidence-Based Practice box).

Careful consideration of the patient's subjective (symptoms) and objective (signs) data yields one of three types of nursing diagnoses from which an individualized plan of care is created (Figure 7-1). **Actual nursing diagnoses** identify existing problems or concerns of a patient. **Risk nursing diagnoses** apply when there is an increased potential or vulnerability for a patient to develop a problem or complication. **Health-promotion nursing diagnoses** are used in situations in which patients express interest in improving their health status through a positive change in behavior. Although most nursing diagnoses are used for individual patients, nursing

Diagnosis
Types of Nursing Diagnoses
- Actual
- Risk
- Health-promotion

FIGURE 7-1 Diagnosis in the nursing process.

EVIDENCE-BASED PRACTICE

Applying the Nursing Process to Practice

- Professional nursing practice demands that nurses continually develop their knowledge and critical-thinking skills to apply them to patient care using the nursing process. Use of the nursing process maintains focus on the patient; the patient's needs, potential concerns, and/or response to situations.
- Proper identification and articulation of nursing diagnoses guide the dynamic nursing process.
- Changes in patient status and life experiences require the addition, modification, and discontinuation of nursing diagnoses on the basis of nursing judgment and evidence-based research findings.
- Evidence-based practice enhances a nurse's ability to use the nursing process for clinical judgment and inquiry during patient care.
- Clinical research, documenting the study findings of nurses who practice using the nursing process, is required to support the addition of new nursing diagnoses to the NANDA-I taxonomy.

diagnosis taxonomy can be applied to families, groups of individuals, and communities.

DIFFERENTIATING BETWEEN MEDICAL AND NURSING DIAGNOSES

Whereas medical diagnoses identify and label medical (physical and psychological) illnesses, nursing diagnoses are much broader in focus. Nursing diagnoses consider a patient's response to medical diagnoses and life situations in addition to making clinical judgments based on a patient's actual medical diagnoses and conditions. Risk nursing diagnoses guide the initiation of treatments to avoid potential problems. Health-promotion nursing diagnoses identify opportunities for patient improvement. Nursing diagnoses take into consideration a patient's attitudes, strengths, and resources—not just the medical problems identified—which are critical for planning holistic, individualized care.

NANDA INTERNATIONAL LO 7.2

Before the 1970s, there was no uniform, systematic method used by nurses to identify patients' health concerns. Assessments were completed and data collected, leading to identification of patient problems without a standardized method of communicating the findings. Nursing care was primarily guided by physicians' orders and directed at treating the signs and symptoms specific to medical diagnoses.

EVOLUTION

The first unofficial nursing diagnosis conference, with 100 nurses in attendance, was held in 1973 to develop a nursing taxonomy (Gebbie, 1976). The nurses continued to meet every 2 years until 1982, when the group officially became the North American Nursing Diagnosis Association, or NANDA (Kim, McFarland, and McLane, 1984). NANDA pioneered work in nursing language and classification with its identification of nursing diagnoses.

The organization is composed of nurses from all areas of nursing, including practice, research, education, administration, and specialty areas of practice. In 2002, it became NANDA International (NANDA-I) to acknowledge the increased interest in nursing taxonomy worldwide (NANDA-I, 2011). The initial goals were to generate, name, and implement nursing diagnostic categories. These goals exist today in addition to the goals of revising the taxonomy, promoting research to validate diagnostic labels, and encouraging nurses to use the taxonomy in practice.

CYCLE OF REVISION

The NANDA-I taxonomy is dynamic. Every 2 years, NANDA-I members meet to focus on revision of the taxonomy and evaluation of nursing research conducted to validate current and evolving nursing diagnoses. Nursing diagnoses are developed through comprehensive research and data collection to support the eventual confirmation of actual nursing diagnostic statements. Diagnoses are evaluated according to how well they are developed and supported by research. The complete NANDA-I taxonomy, including new nursing diagnoses, is published biannually in *Nursing Diagnoses: Definitions and Classification* (see Appendix B).

TYPES OF NURSING DIAGNOSTIC STATEMENTS LO 7.3

The three types of nursing diagnostic statements are actual, risk, and health promotion. Determining which type is needed for each patient can be challenging. Figure 7-2 is an algorithm to help nurses with the decision-making process. Nurses may identify one or more of each type of nursing diagnosis for a patient, depending on the patient's current health status or situation. It is important that all applicable nursing diagnoses are recognized to guide patient care. Determining the priority in which to address each nursing diagnosis takes place during the planning phase of the nursing process.

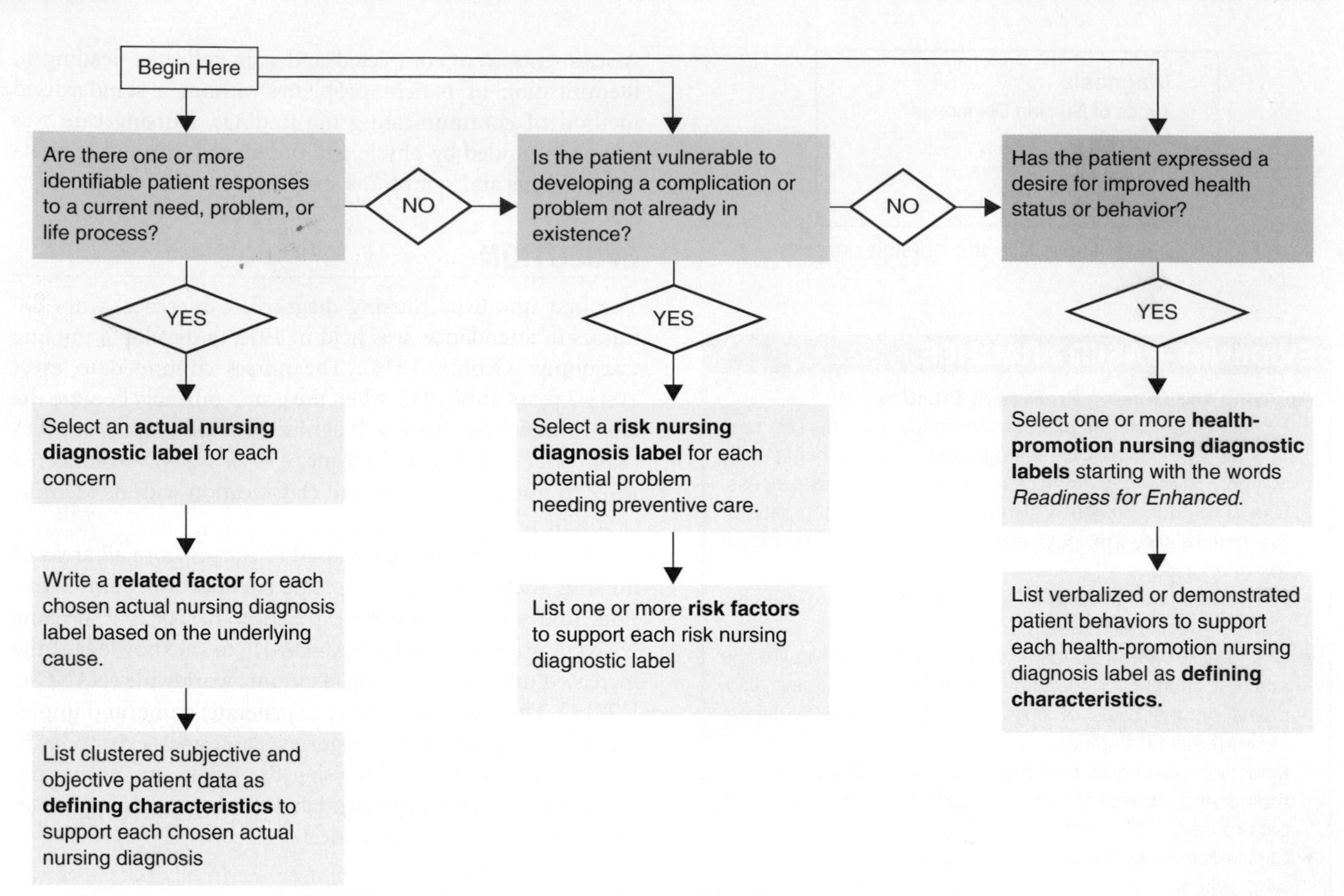

FIGURE 7-2 Algorithm for writing the three types of nursing diagnoses.

Actual nursing diagnoses describe the response of a patient to a current need, problem, or life process (NANDA-I, 2012). Risk nursing diagnoses are used to identify specific potential problems of individuals vulnerable to developing complications due to their current disease state or life experience. Health-promotion nursing diagnoses are clinical judgments based on the expressed desire of patients, families, or groups for change (NANDA-I, 2012). The clustered supporting data (i.e., defining characteristics) should reflect a readiness to address positive lifestyle changes and increase healthy behaviors.

After nursing diagnoses have been established and goals and interventions are planned, patient care is provided, often in collaboration with a variety of health care professionals or agencies (Collaboration and Delegation box). Patient education needs to be included as a part of patient care in most cases. Each of the three types of nursing diagnoses requires the nurse's clinical judgment, which is based on patient assessment data, knowledge, and nursing experience.

COMPONENTS OF NURSING DIAGNOSES LO 7.4

Each type of nursing diagnostic statement contains sections or parts. Actual nursing diagnostic statements are written with three parts: a diagnosis label, related factors, and defining characteristics. Risk nursing diagnoses have two segments: a diagnosis label and risk factors. Depending on the institutional guidelines, nurses may include related factors rather than risk factors when writing risk nursing diagnoses. Health-promotion nursing diagnoses are written with only two sections: the diagnosis label and defining characteristics.

DIAGNOSIS LABEL

The **diagnosis label** is a concise term or phrase that represents a pattern of related, clustered data (NANDA-I, 2012). It is taken from the official NANDA-I list. The diagnosis label is the first section of every nursing diagnosis. It describes the diagnostic focus and requires nursing judgment before its assignment to a patient. Impaired Gas Exchange is a diagnosis label that is defined as "excess or deficient in oxygenation and/or carbon dioxide elimination at the alveolar-capillary membrane" (NANDA-I, 2012). This example demonstrates that the nurse must be familiar with the patient's impaired respiratory status and its underlying cause before determining that Impaired Gas Exchange is an appropriate nursing diagnosis label. To accurately identify diagnosis labels for a patient, the nurse must (1) know the definition of a diagnostic label, (2) cluster and analyze related assessment findings, and (3) make a clinical judgment based on the patient's

COLLABORATION AND DELEGATION

Engaging Others in Patient Care

The provision of excellent care to patients requires a team approach to achieve success. The nurse plays an important role, but many other individuals and disciplines are involved in the provision of excellent care:

- Social workers
- Pharmacists
- Dietitians
- Occupational and physical therapists
- Chaplains
- Physicians
- Unlicensed assistive personnel
- Environmental services
- Maintenance department staff

The successful implementation of a plan of care requires the nurse to delegate at certain times and collaborate at other times:

- Nurses are well trained in providing patient education, but the primary care nurse may delegate patient teaching regarding glucometer use to test blood sugar levels for a newly diagnosed diabetic patient to the clinical nurse specialist whose practice focus is diabetic teaching.
- Collaboration may occur among the chaplain, physician, and nurse to meet the various spiritual needs of a patient.
- The rooms must be clean and the equipment working correctly for patients to recover well. The environmental and maintenance staffs are crucial for excellence in patient care.
- Even though collaboration and delegation may occur, the nurse is ultimately responsible for the continued assessment of patient needs and progress. Detection of additional problems or lack of progress with the patient should prompt the nurse to reconsider the nursing process steps.

condition. All risk nursing diagnoses begin with the words *Risk for*. All health-promotion nursing diagnosis labels begin with the words *Readiness for Enhanced* (NANDA-I, 2012).

RELATED FACTORS AND RISK FACTORS

According to the NANDA-I guidelines, the second part of the nursing diagnosis consists of related factors (for actual nursing diagnoses) and risk factors (for risk nursing diagnoses). **Related factors** are the underlying cause or etiology of a patient's problem. **Risk factors** are environmental, physical, psychological, or situational concerns that increase a patient's vulnerability to a potential problem or concern. Depending on the institutional guidelines, nurses may include related factors rather than risk factors when writing risk nursing diagnoses.

DEFINING CHARACTERISTICS

Defining characteristics are traditionally written as the third section of an actual nursing diagnostic statement. Only in the case of a health-promotion nursing diagnosis are defining characteristics the second, rather than the third, component of the nursing diagnostic statement. **Defining characteristics** are cues or clusters of related assessment data that are signs, symptoms, or indications of an actual or health-promotion nursing diagnosis. Examples of each type of nursing diagnostic statement are presented in Box 7-1.

BOX 7-1 Actual, Risk, and Health-Promotion Nursing Diagnoses

Actual Nursing Diagnosis Statements

Acute Pain (r/t) physical injury as evidenced by/as manifested by (AEB/AMB) (1) complaint of pain at a level 8 on a scale of 0 to 10, (2) fracture of the right femur, and (3) inability to move without grimacing and yelling.

Ineffective Airway Clearance r/t retained secretions AEB/AMB (1) dyspnea, (2) rhonchi in the left lung fields, (3) thick, copious secretions, and (4) unproductive cough.

Self-Care Deficit r/t inability to feed self AEB/AMB (1) right-sided paralysis, (2) weakness, and (3) limited left-arm movement.

Risk Nursing Diagnosis Statements

Risk for Infection with the risk factor of a suppressed inflammatory response indicated by leukopenia.

Risk for Self-Mutilation with the risk factors of low self-esteem and history of harming self.

Risk for Falls with the risk factors of advanced age, dizziness, low blood pressure, and anemia.

Health-Promotion Nursing Diagnosis Statements

Readiness for Enhanced Immunization Status AEB/AMB expressed desire to identify providers of pneumonia vaccine.

Readiness for Enhanced Family Processes AEB/AMB verbalized willingness to attend family counseling.

Readiness for Enhanced Nutrition AEB/AMB recognition of healthy food choices and the need to eat a daily minimum of six servings of fruits and vegetables.

r/t, Related to.

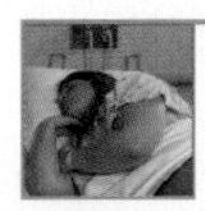

1. Identify three pieces of assessment data (i.e., defining characteristics) that the nurse could use to support the actual nursing diagnosis of *Acute Pain* for Ms. Hayes.

STEPS FOR IDENTIFICATION OF ACCURATE NURSING DIAGNOSES LO 7.5

Accurate identification of nursing diagnoses requires analysis of assessment data and clustering of related cues and information. All patient information should be considered as potentially contributing to the identification of diagnostic labels. This information includes subjective and objective data collected through physical assessment of the patient, interview of the patient and family members, and laboratory and diagnostic test results, including x-rays, physicians' orders, and documentation from health care providers. Verifying specific nursing diagnoses for a particular patient or situation follows accurate analysis and clustering of data.

DATA CLUSTERING

After collecting and reviewing all of the assessment data, the nurse looks for patterns and related data to support specific nursing diagnoses. This process is referred to as *clustering data.* Clustering involves organizing patient assessment data into groupings with similar underlying causes. The nurse looks for cues among the data that support the diagnosis of a problem. For example, objective and subjective data related to mobility can be clustered. Data related to nutritional status, such as weight, height, and dietary intake, can be clustered.

One patient may have several problems simultaneously, requiring the nurse to understand the potential relatedness of signs and symptoms from various body systems. The nurse combines an understanding of pathophysiology, normal structure and function, disease processes, and symptomatology to accurately cluster data. For example, a patient with congestive heart failure may have the following seemingly diverse but related assessment findings:

Subjective data:

- Patient reports weight gain of 10 lb in 48 hours.
- Patient complains of "shortness of breath."
- Patient complains of "feeling tired all the time."

Objective data:

- Bilateral basilar crackles in the lungs on auscultation
- Bilateral 2+ pitting edema of the ankles and feet

Although these individual assessment findings may seem unrelated at first glance, they are all signs and symptoms of heart failure that should be clustered to support the nursing diagnosis of *Excess Fluid Volume.* In other circumstances, clustered data relate to only one body system in support of a nursing diagnosis. The following data would be clustered to support the nursing diagnosis of *Impaired Gas Exchange:*

Subjective data:

- Patient states, "I am having difficulty breathing."
- Patient complains of "getting winded" with activity.

Objective data:

- Dyspnea on exertion
- Pulse oximetry reading of 88% on room air

The nurse finds that some data or cues may support more than one type of nursing diagnosis. For example, difficulty with mobility or ambulation observed by the nurse and verbalized by the patient can be a defining characteristic for an actual nursing diagnosis stated as *Impaired Physical Mobility* related to limited range of movement as evidenced by slow, unsteady gait and patient states, "I am having a very difficult time walking."

The patient's difficulty with mobility may also make the patient vulnerable to developing constipation or decreased peripheral blood circulation. In this case, the patient's plan of care may include the risk nursing diagnoses of *Risk for Constipation* with the risk factors of decreased peristalsis and limited ambulation and *Risk for Ineffective Peripheral Tissue Perfusion* with the risk factors of limited mobility, increased potential for deep vein thrombosis, and patient states, "I am having a very difficult time walking."

Analysis of patient assessment data may yield several clusters of related data or cues. It is common to apply several nursing diagnostic statements to one patient. This is especially true for acutely ill patients with multiple problems related to complex physical or psychological needs. For example, one patient may have nursing diagnoses such as *Acute Pain, Risk for Falls, Powerlessness,* and *Disturbed Sleep Pattern.*

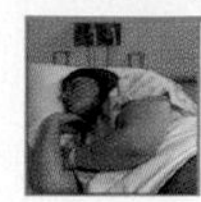

2. List a minimum of three actual nursing diagnostic labels (not including *Acute Pain*) applicable to Ms. Hayes' current condition.

DIAGNOSTIC VALIDITY

Before assigning diagnostic labels, the nurse consults the official NANDA-I list to ensure accurate use of the nursing diagnostic label. The nurse writes nursing diagnostic statements as needed to address the highest-priority needs of the patient. These diagnostic statements are uniquely based on the assessment data of each patient (Diversity Considerations box). Accurate nursing diagnoses are foundational to the development of an effective, personalized plan of care.

AVOIDING PROBLEMS IN THE DIAGNOSTIC PROCESS LO 7.6

A variety of errors in identification, statement structure, and statement content may occur when formulating nursing diagnoses. These include clustering unrelated data, accepting erroneous data, using medical diagnoses as related factors in the nursing diagnostic statement, missing the true underlying etiology of a problem, and identifying multiple nursing diagnosis labels in one nursing diagnostic statement.

DATA CLUSTERING

Clustering unrelated data most often occurs when the nurse has not completed a thorough review of the patient's assessment information or is missing important data. For example, at first glance, a patient's inability to urinate and minimal oral fluid intake may seem related. However, after further review of the data the nurse should realize that they are not related; the patient has an intravenous infusion running at 150 mL/hr that provides adequate hydration, as well as the patient's postoperative status after abdominal surgery. In this case, the patient's inability to urinate most likely results from having had abdominal surgery and may be expected, depending on when the operation was performed. Clustering unrelated data can be avoided with more information.

DIVERSITY CONSIDERATIONS

Life Span

- Assessment that is specific for each individual, regardless of age, is important to establish accurate, applicable nursing diagnoses.
- Making assumptions based solely on a patient's chronologic age without thorough assessment may lead to impersonal, generalized diagnostic statements that do not reflect a patient's true condition or circumstances.

Culture, Ethnicity, and Religion

- Although some medical diagnoses are more common for specific ethnic groups, how patients respond to illnesses varies dramatically, requiring individualized identification of nursing diagnoses.
- Consider the impact of cultural food practices and their influence on patient health when identifying nursing diagnoses.
- Some care plan interventions may conflict with patients' religious practices. A thorough assessment of each individual is crucial for accuracy in nursing diagnostic statements and subsequent interventions.

Disability

- The incidence of chronic diseases and conditions, especially high blood pressure, diabetes, and cancer, varies widely by race and ethnicity. The primary focus of nursing diagnosis in the acute care setting is current illness or exacerbation of chronic illness rather than long-term, permanent disabilities.
- When patients with disabilities are being treated for acute or chronic illness, the nurse needs to understand their capabilities and limitations. This enables the nurse to identify appropriate nursing diagnostic statements that address current patient needs and provide individualized, patient-centered care.

Morphology

- There has been an increase in the number of morbidly obese patients admitted to hospital care and subsequently to home health care services. Nursing diagnostic statements for these patients should include a focus on long-term needs to support their personal goals and improve their health status.

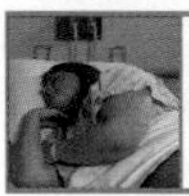

3. Write two risk nursing diagnoses for Ms. Hayes.

ACCURATE DATA COLLECTION

Errors in data collection (e.g., omitting key information) or an incomplete understanding or knowledge of assessment techniques or a patient's condition may lead to the inclusion of erroneous data in a nursing diagnostic statement. It is the nurse's responsibility to collect accurate, extensive assessment data and analyze them on the basis of accurate scientific knowledge. Poor assessment skills or misinterpretation of assessment findings may lead to improper treatment and poor-quality patient care. It is the nurse's responsibility to stay current in nursing research to provide the best care possible.

SAFE PRACTICE ALERT

Research is being conducted on a continuous basis in the discipline of nursing. Evidence-based nursing practice should always be the realm within which the nurse practices. To ensure safe nursing practice founded on empirical research results, the professional nurse must commit to reading about, discussing, and disseminating the most current and best practices for nursing care.

Inaccurate documentation of data may lead to errors in diagnosis. Accurate documentation is essential to ensure patient safety and to facilitate communication among health care professionals. For example, misinterpretation of a critical laboratory value or recording the absence of dependent edema although it exists prevents the accurate diagnosis of patient needs and may endanger a patient's life.

QSEN FOCUS!

Effectively collecting and documenting patient data contribute to evidence-based practice research and support the accurate diagnosis of patient problems and implementation of best nursing practice.

FORMULATING RELATED FACTORS

The underlying etiology, or cause of a patient's concern or situation, rather than a medical diagnosis, should be used as a related factor when writing a nursing diagnosis. By doing so, the nurse articulates an understanding of the pathophysiology or situation with which the patient is faced. For instance, for a patient who has the medical diagnosis of pneumonia and has an oxygen saturation of 88% on room air, the first two sections of a proper nursing diagnostic statement may be *Impaired Gas Exchange* related to poor alveolar perfusion. The medical diagnosis of pneumonia can be clustered with the other data as defining characteristics. Some additional assessment findings that may be listed as defining characteristics are restlessness, change in mental status, and dyspnea.

IDENTIFYING THE CORRECT CAUSE

The related factor in an actual nursing diagnosis needs to address the underlying etiology of the patient's problem expressed by the nursing diagnostic label rather than listing data that are defining characteristics. This can be achieved by thinking of the related factor as a broad statement of causality rather than specific data or cues that support the diagnosis.

The related factor in an actual nursing diagnosis needs to be significantly comprehensive in nature to direct the focus of future nursing interventions. For instance, this is a properly stated nursing diagnosis: Impaired Swallowing related to neuromuscular impairment as evidenced by aspiration with liquids noted during swallowing study, observed choking when trying to take liquids, and patient verbalization, "I can't swallow without choking!" Remember that the *related to* section needs to identify the underlying cause of the nursing diagnosis, which is supported by the data listed as defining characteristics.

FOCUSING ON ONE PROBLEM AT A TIME

When writing nursing diagnoses, the nurse should avoid inclusion of more than one label in the statement. Regardless of the type of nursing diagnosis being written, only one label should be used in each statement. For example, a preoperative patient who is anxious about surgery and has diarrhea due to the surgical preparation should have these two problems addressed in separate nursing diagnoses. The nurse would not start off by stating "Anxiety and Diarrhea related to … ." To address the separate concerns of this patient accurately, the nurse would write two nursing diagnostic statements. One would begin "Anxiety related to"; the other would begin "Diarrhea related to." Both are approved nursing diagnoses in the NANDA-I taxonomy. Including more than one nursing diagnosis label in a diagnostic statement causes confusion and may prevent the identification and treatment of critical patient concerns due to lack of organization and focus.

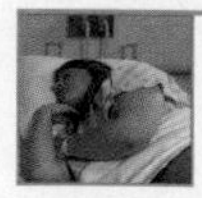

4. On discharge, Ms. Hayes expresses a desire to improve her health status. Identify two health-promotion nursing diagnosis labels that may apply to her situation, and give a rationale for each.

APPLICATION TO PATIENT CARE LO 7.7

By identifying and writing clear nursing diagnostic statements, the nurse enables accurate development of individualized patient plans of care. The nursing diagnosis step of the nursing process leads the nurse to the planning phase, which begins with prioritizing the identified nursing diagnoses. Nursing diagnoses and patient outcomes, which are established during the planning step, help the nurse to determine appropriate interventions for patient care. Chapters 8 and 9 provide more information on nursing interventions and individualized plans of care based on nursing diagnostic statements and identified patient outcomes.

Ultimately, nurses are accountable for formulating accurate nursing diagnoses and intervening appropriately. By collecting accurate and complete assessment data and articulating concise nursing diagnoses for each patient, the professional nurse has a significant impact on patient care outcomes, the quality of patient care, and patient satisfaction.

SUMMARY OF LEARNING OUTCOMES

LO 7.1 *Explain basic nursing diagnosis methodology:* Nursing diagnosis is the second step of the nursing process. When deciding on an accurate nursing diagnosis for a patient, the nurse makes clinical judgments about a patient's experiences and responses to identified problems or life events expressed during the data collection process.

LO 7.2 *Describe the historical development of NANDA-I and the nursing taxonomy:* In 1973, the first conference of nurses met to develop a nursing taxonomy. The group continued to meet every 2 years and officially became the North American Nursing Diagnosis Association in 1982. In 2002, the group became NANDA International to acknowledge worldwide interest in nursing taxonomy. It continues with the original goals of generating, naming, and implementing nursing diagnostic categories, as well as revising the taxonomy, promoting research, and encouraging nurses to use the taxonomy in practice.

LO 7.3 *Differentiate among the three types of nursing diagnostic statements:* Actual nursing diagnoses describe the response of a patient to a current need, problem, or life process. Risk nursing diagnoses identify specific potential problems in individuals vulnerable to developing complications due to their current disease state or life experience. Health-promotion nursing diagnoses are clinical judgments based on the expressed desire of patients, families, or groups for change (NANDA-I, 2012).

LO 7.4 *Outline nursing diagnoses with appropriate components:* Actual nursing diagnostic statements are written with three parts: a diagnosis label, related factors, and defining characteristics. Risk nursing diagnoses have two segments: a diagnosis label and risk factors. Health-promotion nursing diagnoses are also written with only two sections: a diagnosis label and defining characteristics.

LO 7.5 *Implement the steps for accurately identifying nursing diagnoses:* Accurate identification of nursing diagnoses for patients is achieved through careful analysis and clustering of patient data, followed by verification of the specific nursing diagnoses for use with each individual patient.

LO 7.6 *Discuss how to avoid common problems associated with the diagnostic process:* To write concise, properly developed nursing diagnoses, the nurse must avoid clustering unrelated data, accepting erroneous data, using medical diagnoses as related factors in the nursing diagnostic statement, missing the true underlying etiology of a problem, and identifying multiple nursing diagnoses labels in one nursing diagnostic statement.

LO 7.7 *Articulate the contribution of nursing diagnoses to the individualized care of patients:* As the second step of the nursing process, the nursing diagnosis provides a framework on which nurses provide care to patients in an organized and effective manner. An accurate nursing diagnosis promotes positive patient outcomes, quality patient care, and patient satisfaction.

Responses to the critical-thinking questions are available at ***http://evolve.elsevier.com/YoostCrawford/fundamentals/.***

REVIEW QUESTIONS

1. What is the most important reason for nurses to use a standardized taxonomy such as NANDA-I?
   a. Insurance documentation
   b. Professional autonomy
   c. Role delineation
   d. Patient safety
2. Which of the following nursing diagnoses is appropriately written? *(Select all that apply.)*
   a. *Risk for Infection* related to elevated temperature and white blood count
   b. *Readiness for Enhanced Relationship* as evidenced by mutual respect verbalized by spouses and expressed desire for improved communication
   c. *Noncompliance* related to an inability to access care as evidenced by failure to keep appointments, homebound status
   d. *Risk for Bleeding* with the risk factor of prolonged clotting time
   e. *Chronic Pain* related to osteoarthritis as manifested by verbalized postoperative discomfort.
3. Which phrase best represents a related factor in an actual nursing diagnosis?
   a. Unsteady gait requiring the assistance of two people
   b. Redness and swelling around the incision site
   c. Ineffective adaptation to recent loss
   d. Patient complaint of restlessness
4. Which action does the nurse need to take before determining the types of nursing diagnoses that are applicable to a patient? *(Select all that apply.)*
   a. Thoroughly review the patient's medical history
   b. Analyze the nursing assessment data to determine whether information is complete
   c. Outline an individualized plan of care to address each concern
   d. Consider potential complications to which the patient is susceptible
   e. Evaluate how the patient has responded to treatment
5. What is the primary difference between a risk nursing diagnosis and an actual nursing diagnosis?
   a. Defining characteristics are not part of a risk diagnosis.
   b. There is no cause and effect relationship established.
   c. Defining characteristics are subjective in a risk diagnosis.
   d. There are no nursing interventions prescribed in a risk diagnosis.
6. What is the most important action for a nurse to take in order to have a new nursing diagnosis considered for inclusion in the NANDA-I taxonomy?
   a. Share concerns with the nurse manager on the nursing unit.
   b. Offer alternative care for a patient and family members.
   c. Discuss how to address patient needs with physicians.
   d. Provide evidence-based research to support nursing care.
7. What is the most significant problem that may result from improperly written nursing diagnostic statements?
   a. Lack of direction for formulating patient plans of care
   b. Omission of physician or primary care provider orders
   c. Combining of two unrelated patient concerns
   d. Increased team collaboration needs
8. Which statement best describes the relationship of medical diagnoses and nursing diagnoses?
   a. Medical diagnoses are imbedded in nursing diagnoses.
   b. Nursing diagnoses are derived from medical diagnoses.
   c. Medical diagnoses are not relevant to nursing diagnoses.
   d. Medical diagnoses may be interrelated to nursing diagnoses.

9. A patient has just experienced a cardiac arrest on the unit. The nurse has implemented the acute care plan for management of code situations. What is the next step the nurse should take?

a. Resume all interventions for previously identified nursing diagnoses.
b. Perform the steps of the nursing process related to the patient's current condition.
c. Seek physician input related to updating the nursing diagnostic statements.
d. Evaluate the success of the acute care plan for management of the cardiac arrest.

10. What signs and symptoms would the nurse appropriately cluster for a patient with extreme anxiety? *(Select all that apply.)*

a. Denies any difficulty falling asleep
b. Elevated pulse rate auscultated at 140 BPM
c. Continuous foot tapping throughout intake interview
d. Demonstrates how to give insulin self-injection without hesitation
e. Patient states, "I feel nervous all the time, especially when I am alone."

Answers and rationales for the review questions are available at ***http://evolve.elsevier.com/YoostCrawford/fundamentals/.***

REFERENCES

American Nurses Association (ANA): *Nursing: Scope and standards of practice*, ed. 2, Silver Springs, Md., 2010, The Association.

Cronenwett L, Sherwood G, Barnsteiner J, et al: Quality and safety education for nurses. *Nurs Outlook*, 55(3):122-131, 2007.

Gebbie K: Development of taxonomy of nursing diagnosis. In J Walter (Ed), *Dynamics of problem-oriented approaches: Patient care and documentation*, Philadelphia, 1976, Lippincott.

Kim M, McFarland G, McLane A: *Proceedings of the Fifth National Conference of the North American Nursing Diagnosis Association*, St. Louis, 1984, Mosby.

NANDA International: *NANDA-I history, 2011*. Retrieved from *www.nanda.org/AboutUs/History.aspx*.

NANDA International: *Nursing diagnoses: Definitions & classification, 2012–2014*. West Sussex, England, 2012, Wiley-Blackwell.

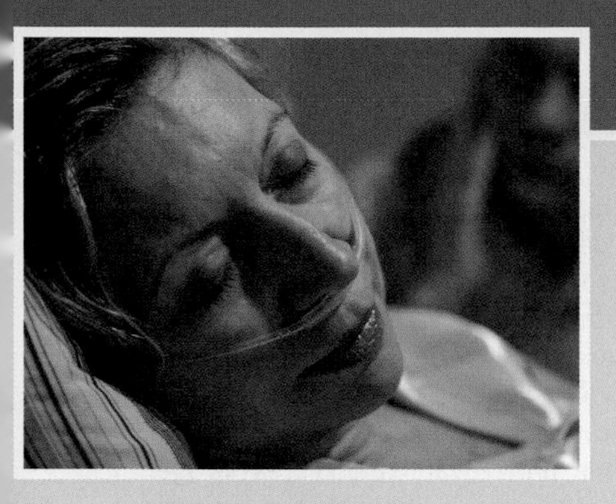

CHAPTER 8

Planning

EVOLVE WEBSITE

http://evolve.elsevier.com/YoostCrawford/fundamentals/

- Additional Evolve-Only Review Questions With Answers
- Answers and Rationales for Text Review Questions
- Answers to Critical-Thinking Questions
- Case Study With Questions
- Glossary

LEARNING OUTCOMES

Comprehension of this chapter's content will provide students with the ability to:

LO 8.1 Articulate nursing actions that take place during the planning process.

LO 8.2 Describe various measures used in prioritizing patient care.

LO 8.3 Illustrate an understanding of goal development.

LO 8.4 Describe the relationship between outcome identification and goal attainment.

LO 8.5 Identify formats in which patient-centered plans of care can be developed.

LO 8.6 Distinguish among the types of interventions.

LO 8.7 Discuss the importance of planning throughout patient care.

KEY TERMS

long-term goals, p. 109
***Nursing Interventions Classification,* p. 112**
***Nursing Outcomes Classification,* p. 110**
outcome indicators, p. 110
short-term goals, p. 109

CASE STUDY

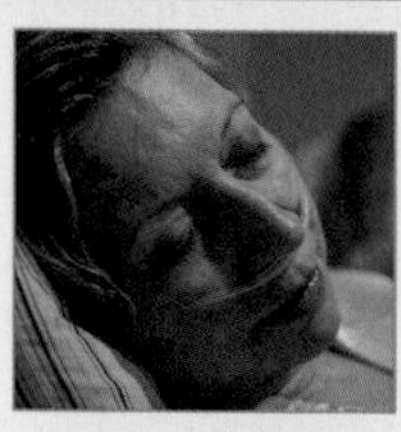

Mrs. Rizzi is a 64-year-old woman who was diagnosed 1 year earlier with end-stage renal disease. On Monday, she is admitted to the hospital with a 15-lb weight gain over the past 4 days, blood pressure of 210/120, pulse of 104 and regular, and respirations at 32 with shortness of breath and crackles heard bilaterally on auscultation. Her pulse oximetry reading is 92% on 2 L of oxygen. She states, "I am so short of breath!" Her ankles are swollen with 3+ pitting edema, and she verbalizes that she is tired. Mrs. Rizzi typically has hemodialysis treatments through an arteriovenous (AV) graft three times each week on Tuesday, Thursday, and Saturday. She reports that she had transportation problems on Saturday and has not had dialysis since last Thursday. Her AV graft, located on the right forearm, is functional, with a strong thrill and bruit without redness, swelling, or drainage. Her laboratory work reveals elevated potassium, low calcium, low hematocrit and hemoglobin, low serum albumin, and elevated blood urea nitrogen (BUN) and creatinine levels. Mrs. Rizzi is placed on telemetry to monitor her cardiac function until her fluid volume overload and hyperkalemia are resolved.

Treatment includes vital signs taken every 4 hours, fluid restriction to 1000 mL/day, intake and output measurements, daily weight measurement, complete blood count (CBC) and chemistry evaluations every morning, urinalysis when urine is available, hemodialysis initially and daily for 2 days, monitoring with a telemetry unit, a bone density x-ray, a chest x-ray, and an electrocardiogram. The patient was maintained on a 1500-calorie renal diet and bed rest with bathroom privileges.

The nurse on the previous shift admitted Mrs. Rizzi and identified the following nursing diagnoses:

- *Excess Fluid Volume* related to (r/t) compromised renal function as evidenced by/as manifested by (AEB/AMB) a 15-lb weight gain, compromised lung function, crackles, swollen ankles, and elevated blood pressure and heart rate.
- *Ineffective Breathing Pattern* r/t increased fluid in lungs AEB/AMB increased respiratory rate, crackles on auscultation, and shortness of breath observed and stated by the patient.
- *Risk for Injury* with the risk factor of hypocalcemia; possible phosphorous retention, bone reabsorption of calcium, increased parathyroid hormone level, and inadequate calcium absorption.
- *Risk for Infection* with the risk factors of hemodialysis access and AV graft cannulation.
- *Ineffective Self-Health Management* r/t limited transportation options AEB/AMB stated inability to get to dialysis appointment on Saturday, fluid retention due to missing dialysis, and electrolyte imbalance.

Refer back to this case study to answer the critical-thinking questions throughout the chapter.

Planning is the third step of the nursing process. During the planning phase, the professional nurse prioritizes the patient's nursing diagnoses, determines short- and long-term goals, identifies outcome indicators, and lists nursing interventions for patient-centered care. Each of these actions requires careful consideration of assessment data and a thorough understanding of the relationship among nursing diagnoses, goals, and evidence-based interventions.

THE PLANNING PROCESS LO 8.1

Critical decisions regarding the patient are made during the planning step of the nursing process (Figure 8-1). To begin planning, the nurse prioritizes each nursing diagnosis that is identified and establishes goals in collaboration with the patient. The nurse identifies the most urgent goals to be addressed, considers the patient's capabilities, and then selects interventions to include in the patient's individualized plan of care. The order in which nursing diagnoses are addressed depends on factors such as the severity of symptoms and the patient's preference. For example, a patient's ability to breathe is of greater concern than the ability to complete activities of daily living independently. After emergent needs are met, less critical needs are addressed. The nurse's ability to prioritize patient needs expressed through nursing diagnosis statements is essential for establishing realistic outcome criteria and interventions to help meet them. Goals are set for short- and long-term attainment.

Planning
Prioritize nursing diagnoses
Personalize care plans
- Short-term goals (STGs)
- Long-term goals (LTGs)

Outcome Identification
NOC
NIC

FIGURE 8-1 Planning in the nursing process. *NOC*, Nursing Outcomes Classification; *NIC*, Nursing Interventions Classification.

Patients should be included in the planning process. Involving patients in planning their care helps them to (1) be aware of identified needs, (2) accept realistic and measurable goals, and (3) embrace interventions to best achieve the mutually agreed-on goals. Inclusion of patients in the planning process tends to improve goal attainment and patient cooperation with interventions. By accepting guidance and input from patients during the planning process, the nurse provides them with a greater sense of empowerment and control. A large portion of the success in or progress toward achieving the goals remains within the patient's power!

Depending on the patient's condition or circumstances, it may be advantageous to include members of the patient's support system (i.e., family, friends, and caregivers) in the planning phase. Including patients and their families enhances their understanding of identified needs and increases their sense of ownership in working toward the established goals. The professional nurse is instrumental in communicating and teaching the steps necessary for patient improvement. It is imperative for the patient to understand the plan of care and be an active participant in the nursing interventions.

PRIORITIZING CARE — LO 8.2

Setting priorities among identified nursing diagnoses is the first step in the planning process. The nurse is responsible for monitoring patient responses, making decisions culminating in a plan of care, and implementing interventions, including interdisciplinary collaboration and referral, as needed (Ethical, Legal, and Professional Practice box). The nurse is significantly accountable for achieving the desired outcomes. Providing safe and effective care to all patients is a national priority. Nurses are constantly challenged by increasing patient comorbidities and greater complexity of patient needs.

ETHICAL, LEGAL, AND PROFESSIONAL PRACTICE

Standards of Care Guide Practice

- Professional nurses have more accountability now than at any other time in the history of nursing.
- Standards of care are met through the prudent performance of the nursing process.
- The planning step is critical for guiding patient care to acceptable patient outcomes.
- Standards of care are determined by governmental and nongovernmental committees and may be defined as local standards or national standards (Cartwright-Vanzant, 2011).
- The planning step provides concrete evidence to support the accuracy and pertinence of the patient care plan.
- Conscientious practice of the nursing process in development of the patient care plan ensures that professional standards of care are being met.

MASLOW'S HIERARCHY OF NEEDS

Use of Maslow's (1987) hierarchy of needs helps to organize the most urgent to less urgent needs. This framework organizes patient data according to basic human needs common to all individuals. Maslow's theory suggests that basic needs, such as physiologic needs, must be met before higher needs, such as self-esteem (Table 8-1). Applying this theory to the prioritization of nursing diagnoses means that a patient's nursing diagnosis of *Nausea* is of more immediate concern than the patient's *Impaired Social Interaction.* Even in this case, the needs of the patient may be related. A patient experiencing nausea (because of chemotherapy treatment or as a reaction to medication) may increase interactions with others after the nausea is relieved. This example underscores the interrelatedness of patient responses to illness and life situations.

TABLE 8-1 Maslow's Hierarchy of Needs Applied to Patient Data

LEVEL OF NEEDS	EXAMPLES OF DATA
Physiologic: basic survival needs	Airway patency, breathing, circulation, oxygen level, nutrition, fluid intake, body temperature regulation, warmth, elimination, shelter, sexuality, infection, pain level
Safety and security: need to be safe and comfortable	Physical safety (falls and drug side effects), psychological security (knowledge of routines and procedures, bedtime rituals, fear of isolation and dependence needs)
Love and belonging: need for love and affection	Compassion of care provider, information from family and significant others, strength of support system
Self-esteem: need to feel good about oneself	Changes in body image (injury, surgery, puberty), changes in self-concept (ability to perform usual role functions), pride in abilities
Self-actualization: need to fulfill maximum potential; need for growth and change	Goal attainment, autonomy, motivation, problem-solving abilities, ability to provide and accept help, feeling of accomplishment, desired roles

Adapted from Maslow AH: *Motivation and personality,* ed. 3, New York, 1987, Harper & Row.

LIFE-THREATENING CONCERNS VERSUS ROUTINE CARE

It is essential that the nurse identify life-threatening concerns and patient situations that need to be addressed most quickly. The ABCs of life support, in the health care setting (airway, breathing, and circulation) are a valuable tool for directing the nurse's thought process. Depending on the severity of a problem, the steps of the nursing process may be performed in a matter of seconds. For instance, if a patient is in respiratory arrest, the most critical goal is for the patient to begin breathing.

In critical situations, the steps of the nursing process are performed through instant clinical reasoning by the nurse and do not involve patient input. The necessity for this type of rapid clinical judgment requires the nurse to have the ability to recognize the existence of crises, have extensive knowledge of current best practice, and have excellent professional skills. Optimal patient safety requires nurses to acquire and continually improve their assessment and critical-thinking skills (Jacobson, Soto, Hsu, et al, 2010). After a patient is stabilized, the nurse continues assessment to evaluate the patient's updated status, determine possible causes of complications, and identify less urgent goals and interventions for care.

QSEN FOCUS!

Nursing care should consistently acknowledge the worth of the individual, recognizing that each person views life and makes treatment choices on the basis of unique life experiences.

Some situations fall between life-threatening and routine, and the patient's needs require a proportional response. For example, a patient's need for medication to relieve pain rated 3/10 is not as urgent as a patient's need for relief of pain rated 10/10. Likewise, a pain level of 10 that does not appear to impact the patient's ability to breathe is severe, but it is not as life-threatening as an ABC problem. The patient's feelings about which concerns are most important influence the ranking of nursing diagnoses in addition to clinical judgment. For situations in which no life-threatening concern exists, goal setting for a patient-centered plan of care must take patient preferences into consideration.

CONFLICTING PRIORITIES

Occasionally, the nurse and patient have conflicting priorities. The nurse and patient may have different beliefs and values regarding health practices. On the basis of prior experiences, each may reach conclusions before fully understanding the other's perspective. Patients may have difficulty accepting and making necessary lifestyle changes. Finding time to exercise when a patient typically works 12 hours each day or giving up traditional cultural foods due to medication interactions can be challenging. Identifying realistic goals that are acceptable to patients and include adherence to sound health care regimens requires time and cooperation by everyone involved in the goal-setting process. Nurse-patient collaboration in the goal-setting process can help to alleviate the incidence of conflicting priorities.

Planning that includes patient teaching to support goal attainment and explain the importance and implementation of interventions is a core nursing responsibility. If patients do not understand what has been taught, the potential for goal achievement is diminished. The nurse must account for individual differences in goal planning to facilitate effective teaching and positive patient outcomes (Diversity Considerations box).

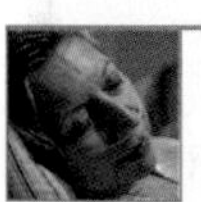

1. Prioritize the nursing diagnoses identified for Mrs. Rizzi from most important to address first to the least urgent.

DIVERSITY CONSIDERATIONS

Life Span

- Fifty-nine percent of the elderly have limited health literacy (Kutner, Jin, and Jin, 2006).
- Older adults have particular problems with medical issues when they must assimilate new information or make complex decisions about treatments.
- The ability of a patient to grasp the importance of goals is directly related to the patient's comprehension of the purpose for recommended treatments and interventions. Patient education by nurses facilitates greater understanding of all aspects of the planning process.

Gender

- Patients of both genders, including those who are well educated and highly literate but have limited health care experience, may struggle with the complexity of health care terminology and procedures (Cornett, 2009; National Research Council, 2004).
- Time taken to educate all patients during the goal-setting process is valuable for achieving positive outcomes.

Culture, Ethnicity, and Religion

- High numbers of minority populations (particularly black and Hispanic) and immigrants are unable to understand health teaching (Kutner, Jin, and Jin, 2006; Rudd, 2007; Singleton, 2009).
- Interpretation should be made available to all patients whose primary language is different from that of the care provider.
- Nurses need to pay particular attention to cultural norms, religious traditions, and convictions while formulating patient care goals for individuals of many ethnic backgrounds.

Disability

- Before implementing teaching strategies to support goal attainment, the nurse must explore a patient's disabilities and the effects they may have on achieving specific goals. Successful accommodation of a patient's disabilities should yield attainable goals that lead to positive outcomes.

Morphology

- For the morbidly obese patient, success in addressing healthy interventions and moving toward a healthier body mass index can depend on the success of realistic goal setting and patient teaching. These patients require keen assessment by the nurse and accommodation considerations for success in goal achievement.

GOAL DEVELOPMENT LO 8.3

Goals are broad statements of purpose that describe the aim of nursing care. Goals represent short- or long-term objectives that are determined during the planning step. Some sources establish time parameters for short- and long-term goals, whereas others do not. According to Carpenito-Moyet (2013), goals that are achievable in less than a week are **short-term goals**, and goals that take weeks or months to achieve are **long-term goals**. A short-term goal for a morbidly obese patient might be "Patient will lose 1 lb during 1 week's hospitalization." A long-term goal for this patient might be "Patient will lose 50 lb in 1 year."

Useful and effective goals have certain characteristics. They are mutually acceptable to the nurse, patient, and family. They are appropriate in terms of nursing and medical diagnoses and therapy. The goals are realistic in terms of the patient's capabilities, time, energy, and resources, and they are specific enough to be understood clearly by the patient and other nurses. They can be measured to facilitate evaluation (Osborn, Watson, and Wraa, 2010).

The nurse creates goals with the patient and possibly with the family by discussing the patient's current condition, the condition the patient wants to progress to, and the actions the patient and nurse undertake to accomplish the goal. The nurse's input into this process is critical to developing reasonable goals and interventions. Without the nurse's guidance during this step, the goals and interventions may be too weak to promote the patient's success or too aggressive for the patient to achieve. The nurse works with the patient to develop a plan of care that is reasonable, is appropriately challenging, and promotes patient success for goal attainment.

GOAL CHARACTERISTICS

Goals are statements designed in collaboration with patients to provide guidance and ultimately a measure of progress when addressing nursing diagnoses (i.e., patient problems). The goals should be realistic, patient centered, and measurable.

Realistic Goals

Realistic goals consider the patient's physical, mental, and spiritual condition in relation to the ability to attain goals. The nurse must consider the effects of conditions, such as severe pain related to recent surgery or clinical depression or hopelessness, on the ability of the patient to reach goals in a timely manner. Other barriers to goal attainment may be related to economic issues or available resources. Some goals may be too ambitious to attain and need to be reevaluated and revised.

Patient-Centered Goals

Patient-centered goals are written specifically for the patient. The goal should specify the activity the patient is to exhibit or demonstrate to indicate goal attainment. The activity may be the patient ambulating, eating, turning, coughing and deep breathing, or any number of other activities. These goals are written to reflect patient, not nursing, activities.

BOX 8-1 Measurable Verbs for Writing Goals and Outcomes

Administer	Inject
Ambulate	List
Articulate	Perform
Attend	Report
Call	Schedule
Cough	Select
Create	Share
Decide	Sit
Demonstrate	Stand
Describe	State
Design	Touch
Discuss	Verbalize
Exercise	Walk
Express	Watch
Identify	Weigh

Measurable Goals

Measurable goals are specific, with numeric parameters or other concrete methods of judging whether the goal was met. When writing a goal statement with a patient, the nurse needs to clearly identify how achievement of the goal will be evaluated. When terms such as *acceptable* or *normal* are used in a goal statement, goal attainment is difficult to judge because they are not measurable terms, unless they refer to laboratory values or diagnostic test findings. For example, although there is a normal range for blood pressure, the goal "The patient's morning blood pressure will be between 120 and 140 mm Hg systolic and 70 and 90 mm Hg diastolic" is preferable to "Blood pressure will be within the normal range." Physiologic norms vary somewhat from person to person and sometimes depend on age and ability. The use of measurable verbs when writing goals and outcomes is essential for establishing criteria with which attainment can be evaluated (Box 8-1).

Time-Limited Goals

In most cases, goal statements need to include a time for evaluation. The time depends on the intervention and the patient's condition. Some goals may need to be evaluated daily or weekly, and others may be evaluated monthly. The health care setting affects the time of evaluation. If the goal is set during hospitalization, the goal may need to be evaluated within days, whereas a goal set for home care may be evaluated weekly or monthly. At the time of evaluation, the goal is assessed for goal attainment, and new goals are set or a new evaluation date for the same goal may be chosen if the goal is still applicable for the patient care plan.

OUTCOME IDENTIFICATION AND GOAL ATTAINMENT LO 8.4

Outcome identification, which was added by the American Nurses Association (ANA) in 1991 as a specific aspect of the

TABLE 8-2 Goal Statement and Nursing Outcome Classification and Indicator

NANDA-I NURSING DIAGNOSIS LABEL WITH NURSING DIAGNOSIS STATEMENT	MEASURABLE GOAL	NURSING OUTCOME CLASSIFICATION (NOC) AND INDICATOR
Hyperthermia related to (r/t) illness as evidenced by/as manifested by (AEB/AMB) temperature elevation of 102.4° F and skin warm to touch	Patient's temperature will return to between 98.2° and 98.6° F within 48 hr.	*Vital signs* (0802) Body temperature (080201)

From Bulechek G, Butcher H, Dochterman J, et al (Eds): *Nursing interventions classification (NIC),* ed. 6, St. Louis, 2013, Mosby; Moorhead S, Johnson M, Maas M, et al (Eds): *Nursing outcomes classification (NOC),* ed. 5, St. Louis, 2013, Mosby; NANDA International: *Nursing diagnoses: Definitions and classification, 2012–2014,* West Sussex, England, 2012, Wiley-Blackwell. Reprinted with permission from NANDA International, Inc.

nursing process, involves listing observable behaviors or items that indicate attainment of a goal. Just as universal nursing taxonomy has been created for nursing diagnosis statements (i.e., NANDA-I), there is a taxonomy for nursing outcomes: ***Nursing Outcomes Classification*** **(NOC)**. It is a standardized vocabulary used for describing patient outcomes. In this system, an outcome is "an individual, family, or community state, behavior, or perception that is measured along a continuum in response to nursing interventions" (Moorhead, Johnson, Maas, et al, 2013). **Outcome indicators** are criteria by which goal attainment is observed or measured.

Moorhead and colleagues (2013) believe that for the nursing profession to become a full participant in clinical evaluation research, policy development, and interdisciplinary work, patient outcomes influenced by nursing care must be identified and measured. Nurses play a critical role in achievement of positive outcomes and in outcome identification. An example of a measurable goal statement and a NOC and indicator is provided in Table 8-2.

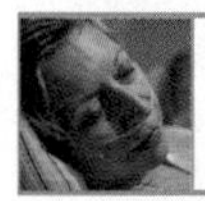

2. Write one short-term goal or desired outcome for each of Mrs. Rizzi's identified nursing diagnoses.

CARE PLAN DEVELOPMENT LO 8.5

There are multiple formats in which to develop individualized care plans for patients, families, and communities. Each health care agency has its own form, including electronic formats, to facilitate the documentation of patient goals and individualized patient-centered plans of care. All formats contain areas in which the nurse identifies key assessment data, nursing diagnostic statements, goals, interventions for care, and evaluation of outcomes. In many agencies and specialty units, standardized care plans that must be individualized for each patient are available to guide nurses in the planning process. These types of plans, including clinical pathways, are addressed in Chapter 9.

In formulating patient care plans, students can use the conceptual care map (CCM). This tool facilitates the organization of assessment data, nursing orders, and physician orders (i.e., treatments); analysis of medication orders and laboratory and diagnostic testing results; and development of a plan of care based on the patient's total picture. Figure 8-2 shows a partially completed CCM. It is a combination of a concept map and a care plan. This format for care plan development enhances the nursing student's ability to accurately collect, analyze, and synthesize patient data for identifying appropriate nursing diagnoses, goals, and interventions. It can be used to organize patient data and develop a plan of care. The patient data in the assessment area of the CCM can be organized in a variety of ways, including by a head-to-toe approach, body systems, or Gordon's functional health patterns.

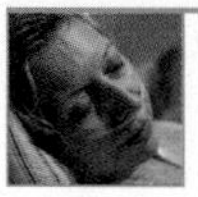

The conceptual care map provided in Figure 8-2 is partially completed to indicate how to use the map as a learning tool. Using it as an example, complete Nursing Diagnoses 2 and 3.

TYPES OF INTERVENTIONS LO 8.6

During the planning phase of the nursing process, the nurse works with the patient, family, and other caregivers to design activities that can assist the patient in improving health and attaining goals. These activities are called *interventions.* The three types of interventions—independent, dependent, and collaborative—take into consideration five key elements:

- Patient assessment findings indicating signs and symptoms that have resulted from or occurred in response to an illness or life experience
- The underlying etiology or related factor identified in each nursing diagnosis
- Realistic patient outcomes in light of the patient's health status and resources for improvement
- Evidence-based interventions aligned with patient acceptance and practicality
- Expertise of the nurses and other health care professionals and agencies involved in the patient's care

The nurse is primarily responsible for making decisions about which interventions are best suited to meet a patient's individual needs. There is no substitute for an extensive understanding of the nursing process, excellent skill set,

Medications

Furosemide: 80 mg PO BID x 2 days for diuresis

Conceptual Care Map

Student name__________ Patient Mrs. R Date ___

Age 64 Gender F Room # ___ Admission date ____

CODE Status Full Allergies NKDA Braden score _______

Diet 1500 cal renal Activity Bedrest c/BRP

Weight ______ Height ______ Religion __________

Admitting Diagnoses/Chief Complaint

15-lb weight gain

Lab Values/Diagnostic Test Results

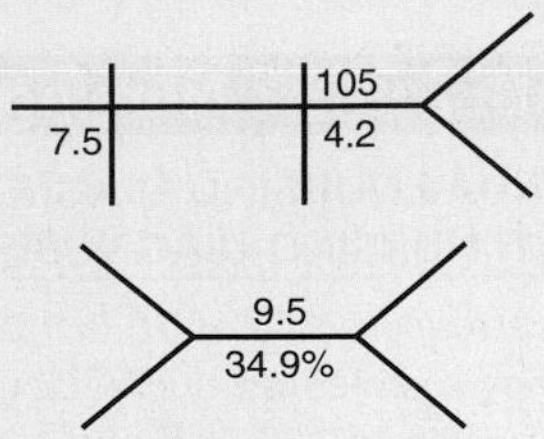

7.5 | 105 | 4.2

9.5 | 34.9%

Potassium: 7.5
Norm: 3.5-5.0 mEq
Blood urea nitrogen (BUN): 105
Norm: 5-20 mg/dL
Creatinine: 4.2
Norm: 0.5-1.3mg/dL
Hemoglobin: 9.5
Norm: Women: 12-16 g/dL
Hematocrit: 34.9%
Norm: Women: 38%-47%
Serum albumin: 2.7
Norm: 3.5-5.5 mg/dL
Calcium: 7.1
Norm: 8.2-10.2 mg/dL
Chest x-ray: results pending

IV Sites/Fluids/Rate

IV heplock: L forearm; no redness or swelling at site; transparent dressing dry and intact; initialed
A-V fistula: R forearm; patent with excellent bruit and thrill; no redness, swelling, or drainage at site

Assessment Data

P: 104 regular, R: 32 labored, B/P: 210/120,
O_2 saturation: 92% on 2 liters (L) of oxygen
15-lb weight gain in past 4 days
Patient states, "I am so short of breath!"
Bilateral crackles audible in all lung fields
3+ pitting edema of both ankles
Patient states that she is tired
Patient missed most recent scheduled hemodialysis treatment due to transportation issues

Past Medical/Surgical History

Hypertension
End-stage renal disease

Treatments

Telemetry
VS q 4 hr
CBC and chemistry q AM
I&O
Hemodialysis now and daily × 2 days
Daily weight
1000 mL/day fluid restriction
Bone density x-ray
Routine urinalysis

Primary Nursing Diagnosis

Excess Fluid Volume related to compromised renal function

Supporting Data

15 lb weight gain. Compromised lung function; bilateral crackles.
3+ pitting edema of both ankles.
Elevated BP and HR.

STG/NOC

Bilateral crackles will no longer be present following hemodialysis treatment.
NOC: Fluid volume severity (0603)
Crackles (060310)

Interventions/NIC With Rationale

1. Weigh daily to measure fluid removal.
2. Limit fluid intake throughout 24-hr periods to reduce patient thirst while restricting fluid overload due to inability to excrete urine.
3. Assess lung sounds, dyspnea, and possible ECG changes to monitor presence of repiratory and systemic venous overload.
4. Monitor pulse and blood pressure to assess level of fluid overload.

NIC: Hemodialysis therapy (2100)
Initiate hemodialysis according to protocol.

Rationale Citation/EBP

Yoost BL, Crawford LR: *Fundamentals of nursing: Active learning for collaborative practice*, St. Louis, 2016, Mosby.

Evaluation

Patient continues to experience some shortness of breath. Minimal crackles audible in bases of both lungs, immediately following hemodialysis. Goal unmet. Continue plan of care.

Nursing Diagnosis 2

Supporting Data

STG/NOC

Interventions/NIC With Rationale

Rationale Citation/EBP

Evaluation

Nursing Diagnosis 3

Supporting Data

STG/NOC

Interventions/NIC With Rationale

Rationale Citation/EBP

Evaluation

FIGURE 8-2 Partially completed conceptual care map based on Mrs. Rizzi, the case study patient in this chapter. *EBP*, Evidence-based practice; *IV*, intravenous; *Lab*, laboratory; *NIC*, Nursing Interventions Classification; *NOC*, Nursing Outcomes Classification; *STGs*, short-term goals.

TABLE 8-3 Nursing Intervention Classification and Associated Activities

NANDA-I NURSING DIAGNOSIS LABEL WITH NURSING DIAGNOSIS STATEMENT	NURSING INTERVENTION CLASSIFICATION (NIC)	ASSOCIATED ACTIVITIES
Hyperthermia related to (r/t) illness as evidenced by/as manifested by (AEB/AMB) temperature elevation of 102.4° F and skin warm to touch	*Temperature regulation* (3900)	1. Monitor temperature at least q 2 hr, as appropriate. 2. Monitor skin color and temperature. 3. Administer antipyretic medication, as appropriate.

From Bulechek G, Butcher H, Dochterman J, et al (eds): *Nursing interventions classification (NIC)*, ed. 6, St. Louis, 2013, Mosby; Moorhead S, Johnson M, Maas M, et al (eds): *Nursing outcomes classification (NOC)*, ed. 5, St. Louis, 2013, Mosby; NANDA International: *Nursing diagnoses: Definitions and classification, 2012–2014*, West Sussex, England, 2012, Wiley-Blackwell. Reprinted with permission from NANDA International, Inc.

knowledge of best nursing practices, and compassion for a patient's situation. Professional nursing practice guides each aspect of decision making in the planning process (Evidence-Based Practice box).

EVIDENCE-BASED PRACTICE

Encouraging Nurses to Integrate Evidence-Based Practice Into Patient Care Requires Innovation

Nurses are accountable for the quality and systematic improvement of nursing practice (ANA, 2010).

- Research has found that lack of knowledge, time, and resources limits nurses from providing evidence-based care.
- Nurses often choose interventions on the basis of tradition rather than research findings.
- Plans of care tend to focus on the primary care provider's orders rather than independent nursing interventions.
- Frequently, communication between nurses at a change of shift neglects to include plan-of-care information.
- Integrating modifiable, evidence-based plans of care into the electronic health record helps to guide practice and focus on nurse-driven outcomes.

From Bennett T, Fowler K, Harne-Britner S: Promoting evidence-based practice at the point of care, *Clin Nurse Specialist* 23(2): 106, 2009.

INDEPENDENT NURSING INTERVENTIONS

The ability of nurses to enact independent interventions has expanded in recent years, allowing nurses to initiate care that they recognize as essential in meeting patient needs or preventing complications. Ordering heel protectors for patients susceptible to skin breakdown and initiating preventive measures (e.g., activity regimens, consultations with social workers, preadmission teaching) are often independent, nurse-initiated interventions.

One method of determining interventions to meet patient outcome goals is to use the ***Nursing Interventions Classification (NIC)***, a comprehensive, research-based, standardized collection of interventions and associated activities. NIC provides nurses with multidisciplinary interventions linked to each NANDA-I nursing diagnosis and a corresponding NOC. It is useful for clinical documentation, communication of care across settings, integration of data across systems and situations, effectiveness research, productivity measurement, competency evaluation, reimbursement, and curricular design. Each NIC includes associated activities that nurses do on behalf of patients, independent and collaborative interventions, and direct and indirect care (University of Iowa, 2011). An example of a NIC with associated activities is provided in Table 8-3.

DEPENDENT NURSING INTERVENTIONS

Some interventions originate from health care provider orders. The nurse incorporates these orders into the patient's overall care plan by associating each with the appropriate nursing diagnosis. Dependent nursing interventions include orders for oxygen administration, dietary requirements, medications, and diagnostic tests. Dependent interventions complement independent nursing interventions to more fully address patient needs. As the role of the advanced practice nurse expands, nurse practitioners are becoming increasingly responsible for what were traditionally considered only physician-initiated interventions. The associated activities shown in Table 8-4 are both independent and dependent nursing interventions. Monitoring the patient's temperature and skin color are independent nursing interventions, whereas administering antipyretics is a dependent action.

COLLABORATIVE INTERVENTIONS

Collaborative interventions require cooperation among health care professionals and unlicensed assistive personnel (UAP). Collaborative interventions include activities such as physical therapy, home health care, personal care, spiritual counseling, medication reconciliation, and palliative or hospice care (Collaboration and Delegation box). These types of interventions require consultation with other health care professionals or referrals to specialists or agencies for assistance.

TABLE 8-4 Care Plan With Independent and Dependent Nursing Interventions

NANDA-I NURSING DIAGNOSIS LABEL WITH NURSING DIAGNOSIS STATEMENT	MEASURABLE GOAL	NURSING OUTCOME CLASSIFICATION (NOC) AND INDICATOR	NURSING INTERVENTION CLASSIFICATION (NIC)	ASSOCIATED ACTIVITIES
Hyperthermia r/t illness AEB/AMB temperature elevation of 102.4° F and skin warm to touch	Patient's temperature will return to between 98.2° and 98.6° F within 48 hr.	*Vital signs* (0802) Body temperature (080201)	*Temperature regulation* (3900)	1. Monitor temperature at least q 2 hr, as appropriate. 2. Monitor skin color and temperature. 3. Administer antipyretic medication, as appropriate.

From Bulechek G, Butcher H, Dochterman J, et al (eds): *Nursing interventions classification (NIC)*, ed. 6, St. Louis, 2013, Mosby; Moorhead S, Johnson M, Maas M, et al (eds): *Nursing outcomes classification (NOC)*, ed. 5, St. Louis, 2013, Mosby; NANDA International: *Nursing diagnoses: Definitions and classification, 2012–2014*, West Sussex, England, 2012, Wiley-Blackwell. Reprinted with permission from NANDA International, Inc.

COLLABORATION AND DELEGATION

Medication Safety

- One of the greatest concerns during transitional care from hospital to home is medication reconciliation.
- Accurate communication among members of the interdisciplinary health care team is essential to ensure that patients receive medications that are ordered and avoid adverse drug events due to omission or overdose.
- To provide for the safety of patients, nurses must collaborate with pharmacists, primary care providers, and caregivers in the home.
- Implementation of interventions to ensure patient medication safety during transition includes access to electronic patient information by all interdisciplinary health care team members.
- Nurses should employ interventions designed to reduce adverse drug events, treatment duplication, and hospital readmissions and to improve patient compliance with the prescribed medication regimen.

From Setter S, Corbett C, Neumiller J: Transitional care: Exploring the home healthcare nurse's role in medication management, *Home Healthc Nurse* 30(1): 19-26, 2012.

Collaborative interventions may involve the expertise of a few or many members of the health care team. In the case of home or hospice care, the nurse is most often the care planner and coordinator of care among many health care team members before, during, and after acute care. Care planning cannot be delegated to UAP.

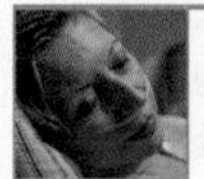

3. Considering each identified short-term goal or desired outcome, identify at least one intervention per goal or outcome that should be included in Mrs. Rizzi's care plan.

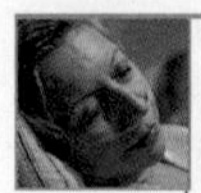

4. Provide a list of interdisciplinary team members that Mrs. Rizzi's physician or nurse may need to consult with during her hospitalization.

PLANNING THROUGHOUT PATIENT CARE LO 8.7

Planning patient care is an ongoing process that takes place at a variety of times and in many settings. Care planning begins when a patient and nurse first interact, and it continues until the patient no longer requires care. The process of planning is similar in all circumstances, even if the setting or timing varies. Seamless communication throughout a patient's care ensures continuity of treatment and improved patient outcomes.

Preadmission teaching is a significant role for the outpatient surgery or office nurse who contacts patients before testing or surgery to educate them on preadmission procedures and facilitate their cooperation (Patient Education and Health Literacy box). Through early intervention, patients learn what will happen, and they are better prepared for health care experiences. This increased understanding aids patients as they approach diagnostic testing or surgery. Research studies indicate improved outcomes, including reduced perioperative complications, increased postoperative pain control, and decreased anxiety in patients experiencing nurse-initiated preoperative teaching and counseling through early intervention (Kearney, Jennrich, Lyons, et al, 2011; Zhang, Jiang, Yin, et al, 2012).

Acute care, community, and home care nurses continually review patient data to determine the need for revised goal setting and care plans. Discharge planning plays an important role in the success of a patient's transition to the home setting after hospitalization (Home Care Considerations box). Because most patients are in the hospital for only a short time, nurses must begin discharge planning on admission and continue until a patient is dismissed. Research shows that comprehensive discharge planning reduces complications and readmissions (Dedhia, Kravet, Bulger, et al, 2009). Home care planning adapts to the situation as the patient's condition improves or deteriorates due to advancing disease.

PATIENT EDUCATION AND HEALTH LITERACY

The Impact of Health Literacy

- There is a strong, independent association between health literacy and health outcomes.
- These outcomes include emergency department use, hospitalization, self-reported physical health, and mortality.
- According to the National Assessment of Adult Literacy, only 12% of Americans have proficient health literacy skills (Kutner, Jin, and Jin, 2006). Most adults may have difficulty completing routine health tasks such as understanding a drug label or vaccination table.
- Patients with lower health literacy levels experience higher rates of hospitalization and emergency room use. The estimated annual health care costs resulting from low levels of health literacy range from $106 to $238 billion (Vernon, Trujillo, Rosenbaum, et al, 2007).
- The health care environment is rapidly changing and becoming increasingly complex for patients to navigate. Nurses must recognize when patients are struggling to understand health-related instructions, identify a patient's usual means of compensating for health literacy limitations, and intervene appropriately.
- It is imperative that nurses and all health care workers intervene appropriately and ensure patients' understanding of their health conditions and required self-care behaviors (Sand-Jecklin, Murray, Summers, et al, 2010).

HOME CARE CONSIDERATIONS

Discharge Planning

- Early, structured discharge planning ensures a smoother transition of patients from hospital to home.
- Discharge documentation should include medical information, patient goals, and interventions developed to accelerate recovery and provide needed care.
- Research has demonstrated that inadequate discharge planning may lead to an increase in patients returning to the hospital, more frequent emergency room encounters, and adverse events.
- A structured, collaborative approach that focuses specifically on the needs of at-risk patients has proved beneficial.
- Various resources for improving the discharge planning process have been developed by nurses. Use of these planning and documentation tools has improved patient outcomes and satisfaction associated with hospital-to-home transition (Dedhia, Kravet, Bulger, et al, 2009).

The significance of developing organized plans of care for patients cannot be stressed enough. The nurse must take seriously the responsibility of prioritizing patient needs, developing mutually agreed-on goals, determining outcome criteria, and identifying interventions that can help patients to achieve positive outcomes. After these actions are completed in the planning phase of the nursing process, it is time for implementation of the patient's plan of care.

SUMMARY OF LEARNING OUTCOMES

LO 8.1 *Articulate nursing actions that take place during the planning process:* During planning, the professional nurse prioritizes the patient's nursing diagnoses, determines short- and long-term goals, identifies outcome indicators, and lists nursing interventions for patient-centered care.

LO 8.2 *Describe various measures used in prioritizing patient care:* Maslow's hierarchy of needs and the ABCs of life support in the health care setting are helpful resources in prioritizing care. Collaboration with patients while developing goals can decrease the incidence of conflicting priorities.

LO 8.3 *Illustrate an understanding of goal development:* Goals need to be patient centered, realistic, and measurable. Using measurable verbs and time limits when writing goals assists the nurse in evaluation of patient goal attainment.

LO 8.4 *Describe the relationship between outcome identification and goal attainment:* Outcome identification, added by ANA in 1991 as a specific aspect of the nursing process, involves listing observable behaviors or items that indicate attainment of a goal.

LO 8.5 *Identify formats in which patient-centered plans of care can be developed:* Each health care facility or agency has its own electronic health record or form on which patient care plans are formulated and documented. In some agencies and specialty units, standardized care plans, which must be individualized for each patient, are available to guide nurses in the planning process. The conceptual care map (CCM) is a format for nursing students to use when developing patient care plans. It helps students to accurately collect, analyze, and synthesize patient data that are used to identify appropriate nursing diagnoses, goals, and interventions.

LO 8.6 *Distinguish among the types of interventions:* Independent interventions are nurse initiated, and dependent nursing interventions require an order from a patient's health care provider. Collaborative interventions require cooperation among a few or many members of the interdisciplinary health care team.

LO 8.7 *Discuss the importance of planning throughout patient care:* Care planning begins when a patient and nurse first interact and continues until the patient no longer requires care. It takes place at a variety of times and places. It can include preadmission, acute care, home care, and discharge planning. Seamless communication throughout a patient's care ensures continuity of treatment and improved patient outcomes.

Responses to the critical-thinking questions are available at *http://evolve.elsevier.com/YoostCrawford/fundamentals/.*

REVIEW QUESTIONS

1. Which action would the nurse undertake first when beginning to formulate a patient's plan of care?
   a. List possible treatment options.
   b. Identify realistic outcome indicators.
   c. Consult with health care team members.
   d. Rank patient concerns from assessment data.
2. Which resource is most helpful when prioritizing identified nursing diagnoses?
   a. *Nursing Interventions Classification (NIC)*
   b. Gordon's functional health patterns
   c. Maslow's hierarchy of needs
   d. *Nursing Outcomes Classification (NOC)*
3. If a patient is exhibiting signs and symptoms of each of the following nursing diagnoses, which should the nurse address first while planning care?
   a. *Fatigue*
   b. *Acute Pain*
   c. *Knowledge Deficit*
   d. *Body Image Disturbance*
4. Which statement illustrates a characteristic of goals within the care planning process?
   a. Goals are vague objectives communicating expectations for improvement.
   b. Short-term goals need not be measurable, unlike long-term goals.
   c. Goal attainment can be measured by identifying nursing interventions.
   d. Long-term goals are helpful in judging a patient's progress.
5. Which nursing goal is written correctly for a patient with the nursing diagnosis of *Risk for Infection* after abdominal surgery?
   a. Nurse will encourage use of sterile technique during each dressing change.
   b. Patient's white blood count will remain within normal range throughout hospitalization.
   c. Patient's visitors will be instructed in proper handwashing before direct interaction with patient.
   d. Patient will understand the importance of cleaning around the incision with a clean cloth during bathing.
6. If the nurse chooses the *Nursing Outcome Classification (NOC)* Appetite (1014) for a chemotherapy patient, which outcome indicators would be acceptable for evaluation of goal attainment? *(Select all that apply.)*
   a. Expressed desire to eat
   b. Report that food smells good
   c. Use of relaxation techniques before meals
   d. Preparation of home-cooked meals for self and family
   e. Uses nutritional information on labels to guide selections
7. Which action by the nurse would be most important in developing a patient-centered plan of care for an alert, oriented adult?
   a. Providing a written copy of care options to the patient and family
   b. Collaborating with the patient's social worker to determine resources
   c. Listening to the patient's concerns and beliefs about proposed treatment
   d. Engaging the patient's family, friends, or care providers in conversation
8. Which interventions can the nurse initiate independently while providing patient care? *(Select all that apply.)*
   a. Ordering a blood transfusion
   b. Auscultating lung sounds
   c. Monitoring skin integrity
   d. Applying heel protectors
   e. Adjusting antibiotic dosages
9. The nurse notices that a patient is becoming short of breath and anxious. Which of the following interventions is a dependent nursing action, requiring the order of a primary care provider?
   a. Elevating the head of the patient's bed
   b. Administering oxygen by nasal cannula
   c. Assessing the patient's oxygen saturation
   d. Evaluating the patient's peripheral circulation
10. Which situation indicates the greatest need for collaborative interventions provided by several health care team members?
    a. Hospice referral
    b. Physical assessment
    c. Activities of daily living
    d. Health history interview

Answers and rationales for the review questions are available at *http://evolve.elsevier.com/YoostCrawford/fundamentals/.*

REFERENCES

American Nurses Association (ANA): *Nursing: Scope and standards of practice*, ed. 2, Silver Spring, Md., 2010, *www.Nursebooks.org*.

Carpenito-Moyet LJ: *Nursing diagnosis: Application to clinical practice*, ed. 14, Philadelphia, 2013, Lippincott.

Cartwright-Vanzant R: Standards of care. *J Legal Nurse Consult*, 22(1):14-18, 2011.

Cornett S. Assessing and addressing health literacy. *Online J Issues Nurs*, 14(3):12, 2009.

Cronenwett L, Sherwood G, Barnsteiner J, et al: Quality and safety education for nurses. *Nurs Outlook*, 55(3):122-131, 2007.

Dedhia P, Kravet S, Bulger J, et al: A quality improvement intervention to facilitate the transition of older adults from three hospitals back to their homes. *J Am Geriatr Soc*, 57(9):1540-1546, 2009.

Jacobson H, Soto M, Hsu C, et al: Self-assessed emergency readiness and training needs of nurses in rural Texas. *Public Health Nurse*, 27(1):41-48, 2010.

Kearney M, Jennrich M, Lyons S, et al: Effects of preoperative education on patient outcomes after joint replacement surgery. *Orthop Nurs*, 30(6):391-396, 2011.

Kutner ME, Jin Y, Jin CP: *The health literacy of America's adults: Results from the 2003 National Assessment of Adult Literacy*, NCES no. 2006-483, Washington, D.C., 2006, U.S. Department of Education, National Center for Educational Statistics.

Maslow AH: *Motivation and personality*, ed. 3, New York, 1987, Harper & Row.

Moorhead S, Johnson M, Maas M, Swanson E: *Nursing outcomes classification (NOC)*, ed. 5, St. Louis, 2013, Mosby.

NANDA International: *Nursing diagnoses: Definitions and classification, 2012–2014*, West Sussex, England, 2012, Wiley-Blackwell.

National Research Council: *Health Literacy: A prescription to end confusion*, Washington, D.C., 2004, The National Academies Press.

Osborn K, Watson A, Wraa C: *Medical surgical nursing: Preparation for practice*, Vol. 1, Upper Saddle River, N.J., 2010, Pearson Health Science.

Rudd RE: Health literacy skills of U.S. adults. *Am J Health Behav*, 3(suppl 1):S8-S18, 2007.

Sand-Jecklin K, Murray B, Summers B, Watson J: Educating nursing students about health literacy: From the classroom to patient bedside. *Online J Issues Nurs*, 15(3):1, 2010.

Singleton K: Understanding cultural and linguistic barriers to health literacy. *Online J Issues Nurs*, 14(3):10, 2009.

University of Iowa College of Nursing: CNC—Overview: Nursing interventions classification (NIC), 2011. Retrieved from *www.nursing.uiowa.edu/cncce/nursing-outcomes-classification-overview*.

Vernon J, Trujillo A, Rosenbaum S, Debuono B: Low health literacy: Implications for national health policy, 2007. Retrieved from *http://hsrc.himmelfarb.gwu.edu/sphhs_policy_facpubs/172/*.

Zhang C, Jiang Y, Yin Q, et al: Impact of nurse-initiated preoperative education on postoperative anxiety symptoms and complications after coronary artery bypass grafting. *J Cardiovasc Nurs*, 27(1):84-88, 2012.

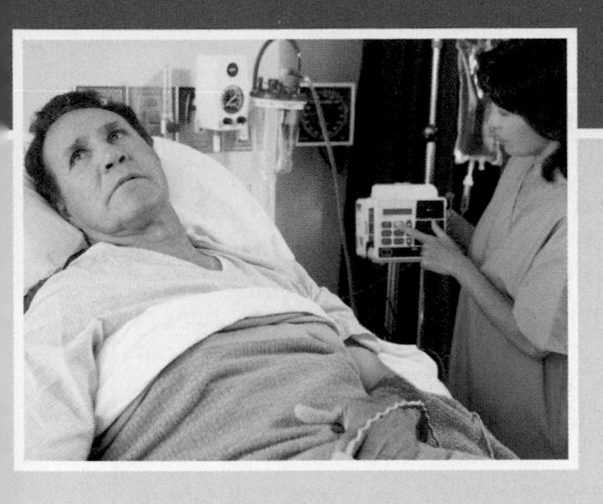

CHAPTER 9

Implementation and Evaluation

EVOLVE WEBSITE

http://evolve.elsevier.com/YoostCrawford/fundamentals/

- Additional Evolve-Only Review Questions With Answers
- Answers and Rationales for Text Review Questions
- Answers to Critical-Thinking Questions
- Case Study With Questions
- Glossary

LEARNING OUTCOMES

Comprehension of this chapter's content will provide students with the ability to:

LO 9.1 Explain the significance of implementation and evaluation in the nursing process.

LO 9.2 Describe different types of direct-care interventions.

LO 9.3 Differentiate among various forms of indirect-care interventions.

LO 9.4 Identify examples of independent nursing interventions.

LO 9.5 Recognize dependent nursing interventions.

LO 9.6 Identify the significance of documentation in the implementation step.

LO 9.7 Apply evaluation principles used in the nursing process.

LO 9.8 Describe the relationship between care plan modification and quality improvement.

KEY TERMS

dependent nursing interventions, p. 122
direct care, p. 118
evaluation, p. 123
implementation, p. 118
independent nursing interventions, p. 122
indirect care, p. 120

CASE STUDY

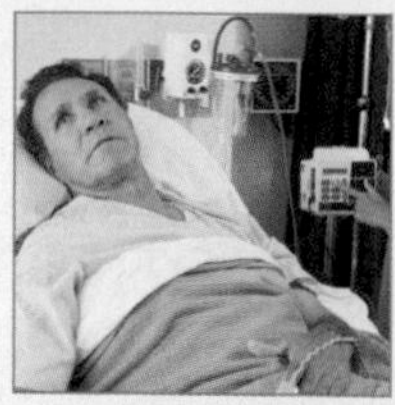

Mr. Khalek is a 57-year-old man with a 20-year history of smoking who came to the emergency department complaining of shortness of breath and anxiety. He is allergic to penicillin and has a medical history of hypertension and a high cholesterol level. His vital signs are T 101.6°F (38°C), P 96 and regular, R 24, BP 132/74, O_2 saturation 89% on room air, and pain level of 3/10. Mr. Khalek's respiratory assessment reveals slightly labored respirations with diminished breath sounds in both upper lobes and rhonchi in the left base, orthopnea, pain in his chest, and a productive cough of thick, yellow sputum. He states that he has been unable to shower without becoming dizzy and sleeps only about 4 hours each night in a recliner. Mr. Khalek expresses concern that he has not been able to go to work for a week and may lose his job. After being diagnosed with pneumonia, Mr. Khalek is transferred to a telemetry unit.

Treatment included vital signs taken every 4 hours, intake and output measurements, oxygen at 2 to 4 L per nasal cannula to maintain O_2 saturation above 92%, intravenous (IV) administration of 0.9 NaCl at 75 mL/hr, and incentive spirometry every hour while awake. The patient was maintained on a 4-g sodium, low-fat, low-cholesterol, no-caffeine diet and on bed rest with bathroom privileges. Medication orders included the following:

- Ciprofloxacin (Cipro): 400 mg IV q 12 hr
- Methylprednisolone (Solu-Medrol): 40 mg IVP q 8 hr
- Albuterol (Ventolin) breathing treatments: q 4 hr and PRN for shortness of breath
- Lorazepam (Ativan): 1 mg PO q 8 hr and PRN for anxiety

Refer back to this case study to answer the critical-thinking questions throughout the chapter.

After the first three phases of the nursing process (i.e., assessment, diagnosis, and planning) are completed, the nurse proceeds to implementation and evaluation. In these steps, the plan of care is carried out, and patient outcomes are evaluated. On the basis of evaluation findings, the nurse revises, continues, or discontinues the plan of care.

IMPLEMENTATION OF NURSING CARE LO 9.1

Nurses and other members of the interdisciplinary health care team provide care through interventions designed to promote, maintain, or restore a patient's health during the implementation phase of the nursing process. Interventions may be direct or indirect activities, and they may be independent or dependent nursing actions. Each intervention is included in the patient-centered plan of care to support patient goals identified during the planning process. **Implementation** consists of performing a task (e.g., giving a backrub, repositioning the patient, assessing vital signs, calling pastoral care) and documentation of each intervention (Figure 9-1).

Implementation

Interventions
- Independent
- Dependent
- Collaborative

Care
- Direct
- Indirect

Documentation

NIC

Care plans
- Clinical pathways
- Protocols
- Standing orders

FIGURE 9-1 Implementation in the nursing process.

DIRECT CARE LO 9.2

Direct care refers to interventions that are carried out by having personal contact with patients. For example, direct-care interventions include cleaning an incision, administering an injection, ambulating with a patient, and completing patient teaching at the bedside. Some direct-care interventions must be carried out by the registered nurse (RN), but others may be delegated to another care provider, such as unlicensed assistive personnel (UAP), with proper training and supervision by the nurse.

! SAFE PRACTICE ALERT

Before implementing all interventions, the nurse must check the patient's identity using a minimum of two methods. Asking a patient to state his or her name and birth date while cross-checking what the patient says with the patient's armband information are the two most common ways to verify patient identity. This critical safety step prevents interventions from being performed on the wrong person.

REASSESSMENT

One form of direct care that is ongoing throughout all stages of the nursing process is reassessment. After the nurse completes a patient's initial assessment and develops a plan of care, continual reassessment of the patient detects noticeable changes in the patient's condition, requiring adjustments to interventions outlined in the plan of care. For example, a patient may initially be unresponsive and unable to breathe independently, requiring the aid of a ventilator. As the patient's condition improves and he or she is able to breathe without the ventilator, this intervention can be deleted from the plan of care, and oxygen administered by nasal cannula may take its place. The need for continual patient reassessment underscores the dynamic nature of the nursing process and is crucial to providing essential care.

ACTIVITIES OF DAILY LIVING

Activities of daily living (ADLs) include tasks that are undertaken on a regular basis: eating, dressing, bathing, toileting, and ambulation. Because patients perform ADLs at different levels, it is important for the nurse to assess where deficits exist and to determine whether patients require short- or long-term interventions to address their needs. For example, patients who have limited mobility after knee surgery need short-term interventions for ambulation assistance. Patients who have debilitating strokes (i.e., cerebrovascular accidents [CVAs]) or amputations require long-term interventions, which may or may not change as the severity of disability changes or the duration since the initiating event lengthens.

PHYSICAL CARE

Many interventions focus on physical care that is performed when treating patients. These interventions may include invasive procedures, such as starting an intravenous line or inserting a catheter, or they may be noninvasive, such as administering oral medications and repositioning. The nurse must perform the procedures competently and safely, taking into consideration any special needs of the patient (Diversity Considerations box). Some procedures may be unfamiliar to the nurse, and some techniques vary among health care facilities. The state boards of nursing provide some procedural guidance; however, each institution adheres to internal policies and procedures. Nurses must take responsibility for learning and adapting procedures to ensure proper technique and practice within regulatory guidelines.

Skills manuals and software are excellent references for nurses seeking information on approved nursing care procedures. Point-of-care references in the form of hand-held technology provide bedside nurses with evidence-based interventions to implement during patient care. In 2000, the Institute of Medicine (IOM) endorsed point-of-care reference use by all health care professionals in its landmark report, *To Err Is Human: Building a Safer Health System* (Kohn, Corrigan, and Donaldson, 2000).

DIVERSITY CONSIDERATIONS

Life Span

- Interventions must always be age- or developmental-level appropriate.
- Older individuals with cognitive deficits may require care that would typically be provided only for children or adults with physical disabilities.
- Encouraging patients of all ages to actively participate in their care provides them with a sense of control, even in the most serious circumstances.

Gender

- Identify gender roles that may affect care delivery.
- Some patients may prefer care from nurses of the same gender. This preference may stem from generational norms, personal comfort, or cultural considerations.

Culture, Ethnicity, and Religion

- Culture plays an important role in communicating with patients. Professional interpretation services should be implemented when detailed care information needs to be shared.
- It is important to know whether eye contact or physical contact should be avoided.
- Proper explanation of all procedures is essential for individuals of all cultures.
- Asking patients to share their understanding of a procedure that has just been explained is a valuable way to verify that communication has been successful.
- Some interventions may be declined because of religious affiliation (e.g., blood transfusion for a Jehovah's Witness, pork-based insulin for a Muslim patient).

Disability

- Interventions must be individualized for each patient and adapted for any limitations (e.g., amputation, learning disability, blindness, deafness).

Morphology

- The nurse must ensure safe practice in relation to patient body size and should seek additional support or equipment when necessary (e.g., mechanical lift equipment, sliding boards).
- Some institutions have units that are dedicated to the care of morbidly obese patients.

INFORMAL COUNSELING

In some cases, nurses provide support and intervene with patients through informal counseling. Counseling is the process through which individuals use professional guidance to address personal conflicts or emotional problems. Nurses counsel patients by providing a "listening ear" or stimulating a patient's thought process or decision-making process. Informal counseling may occur when the patient is faced with a new diagnosis (e.g., breast cancer), a chronic condition (e.g., diabetes), a loss (e.g., death of a parent), or acute illness (e.g., pneumonia). Informal counseling encourages patients to express their concerns and emotions and to ask questions.

The nurse uses counseling techniques to identify the need for indirect interventions (e.g., consultations for other services) that should be implemented. When the need for in-depth or formal counseling is perceived, the nurse can recommend that a patient be referred for psychotherapy, which is outside the scope of practice of a nurse without advance practice training.

TEACHING

Teaching is an essential professional nursing intervention. Each interaction with a patient is an opportunity to teach. While administering medications at the bedside, the nurse assesses the patient's knowledge of the prescribed medications and provides supplemental information, reinforcement, and clarification as needed. During ambulation, a nurse may teach a patient about safe ambulation or the correct way to use a walker. At other times, teaching is more formalized, such as discharge teaching after open heart surgery.

Each teaching method and patient interaction involving teaching requires the nurse to individualize the teaching plan for the patient. The nurse must keep in mind the best way that the patient learns, the patient's educational and knowledge level, cultural considerations, and potential communication barriers. Readiness to learn is also an important consideration. For example, when a patient returns from surgery, it is essential that some information be reviewed (e.g., how to use the patient-controlled analgesia pump and incentive spirometer), but completing all discharge teaching at this time would not be effective. Choosing opportunities in which the environment and the patient's condition are most conducive to learning is recommended.

Another teaching plan consideration is whether to involve family and care providers in the teaching process. Spouses, children, and friends often are involved in the care of a patient after discharge. With the patient's permission, the nurse should share instructions with the people who may assist with care. Nurses empower patients and their support systems through effective teaching. When nurses provide patients and their families with opportunities to ask questions and comprehend health care information, they become an integral part of the health care process.

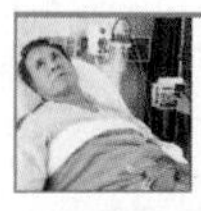

1. What health-promotion teaching interventions would be most appropriate for Mr. Khalek before he leaves the hospital?

INDIRECT CARE LO 9.3

Indirect care includes nursing interventions that are performed to benefit patients but do not involve face-to-face contact with patients. Examples of indirect care include giving change-of-shift report, communicating and collaborating with members of the interdisciplinary health care team, and ensuring availability of needed equipment. These activities assist in providing comprehensive care to patients, although their impact may not be obvious to or known by patients.

COMMUNICATION AND COLLABORATION

Effective communication and collaboration regarding patient care are essential for patient safety and positive patient outcomes. Change-of shift-reports, ongoing communication with primary care providers (PCPs) and specialists, and accurate documentation of assessment findings provide continuity of care. The use of electronic health records (EHRs) allows patients' records to be accessed in an efficient manner and by multiple organizations, increasing communication while decreasing the time necessary to transfer information. Their use connects pieces of the patient care puzzle and reduces the potential for transcription errors. Patient status reports may lead to the addition of physician orders, such as consultations with specialists or services (e.g., physical therapy, social services, mental health services) that can be added to the plan of care and substantially benefit the patient. Effective communication and collaboration between the nurse and all members of the health care team, including patients, is essential for providing patient-centered, comprehensive care.

REFERRALS

Referrals in health care involve sending a patient to another member of the interdisciplinary health care team or agency for a consultation or other services. In some cases, a PCP may refer a patient to a medical or surgical specialist for further assessment, testing, or treatment. Referral information provided by a specialist can provide the nurse and PCP with ideas for a more structured plan of care to address specific patient concerns.

Referrals for specialized services can support and protect patients. Nurses are often instrumental in initiating these types of referrals. For instance, if a patient is experiencing extreme anxiety during chemotherapy treatments, the nurse may set up a referral with the music therapist to assist the patient with relaxation. Nurses initiate referrals for specific dietary requests and adaptive care devices, such as bedside commodes or specialized beds, depending on the patient's unique circumstances. In collaboration with social services, a nurse may refer discharged patients to community agencies that provide in-home assistive services. Some referrals may require the order of a physician or an advanced practice nurse.

RESEARCH

Implementation of evidence-based care is not unique to nursing; it involves interventions provided by all members of the interdisciplinary health care team. The best methods for treating patients with a variety of signs and symptoms are researched by nurses with input from the research findings of other disciplines. Nursing care continues to evolve as nursing research provides new knowledge and recognizes best practices to improve patient care and outcomes. Evidence-based practice guidelines and updated information must be included in plans of care. To implement research-based interventions, nurses must read recent literature and remain current in practice. Accurate communication of care plans among health care team members and the use of informatics to locate relevant research and treatment options support the implementation of best practices (Evidence-Based Practice and Informatics box).

EVIDENCE-BASED PRACTICE AND INFORMATICS

The Role and Impact of Technology on Patient Care

Electronic resources have enhanced the ability of nurses to communicate patient needs and explore new treatment modalities available for patient care:

- Electronic health records (EHRs) often include care plan formats that enhance nurses' ability to formulate individualized plans of care and facilitate coordination of care. Documentation of evaluative criteria and data in a patient's EHR allows nurses and other health care providers to collaborate electronically while responding to changes in the patient's health status.
- Hand-held technology users have significantly better awareness and broader use of research, resulting in improved quality of care (Doran, Straus, Haynes, et al, 2009).
- Hand-held technology assists in the transformation of assessment data, interventions, and outcome documentation to evidence-based decision making (Hardwick, Pulido, and Adelson, 2007).

ADVOCACY

Nurses advocate by supporting and working on behalf of patients or people for whom they have concern. Advocacy can be easy or challenging, depending on the situation. Nurses advocate for patients by coordinating care and supporting the changes necessary to improve conditions and outcomes. Excellent negotiation techniques are required for nurses who advocate on behalf of patients' rights with insurance companies or legislative leaders. As resources for patient care become increasingly limited, nurse advocacy is critical for ensuring patient access to needed services.

DELEGATION

Delegation is the transfer of responsibility for performing a task to another person while the nurse who delegated the task still remains accountable (ANA, 2010). Delegation is an indirect intervention based on assessment findings and established care priorities. Nurses must be familiar with the nurse practice act in their practice jurisdiction to ensure legal delegation. The nursing process cannot be delegated. In most jurisdictions, licensed practical nurses (LPNs) function in a dependent role and may not delegate (Kelly and Marthaler, 2011). The RN is most responsible for incorporating delegation into practice.

Delegation principles focus on the appropriate intervention being performed under the correct circumstances, by the correct personnel, and with the correct direction and supervision (Collaboration and Delegation box). In the United States, the National Council of State Boards of Nursing (1997) developed the Delegation Decision-Making Tree, adapted from an original Ohio Board of Nursing tool, to assist RNs in the application of delegation to practice. It is available at *www.ncsbn.org/delegationtree.pdf.*

COLLABORATION AND DELEGATION

The Five Rights of Delegation

Collaboration among health care team members sometimes results in the nurse delegating some aspects of patient care to unlicensed assistive personnel. The National Council of State Boards of Nursing has provided the Five Rights of Delegation to support safe delegation of patient care:

- *Right task:* Is this a task that can and should be delegated?
- *Right circumstance:* Is this appropriate at this time with what is going on?
- *Right person:* Does this person have the skills, scope of practice, understanding, and expertise to perform this task?
- *Right direction or communication:* Has proper information about what tasks need to be completed been shared so that what needs to be done is clear?
- *Right supervision or evaluation:* Has the nurse followed up to ensure that care was adequate to meet the needs of the patient?

Adapted from National Council of State Boards of Nursing: *The five rights of delegation,* 1997. Retrieved *from www.ncsbn.org/fiverights.pdf.*

PREVENTION-ORIENTED INTERVENTIONS

Some interventions prevent illness or complications and promote healthy activities or lifestyles (Patient Education and Health Literacy box). Interventions such as patient education and immunization programs are prevention oriented. These interventions influence patient outcomes and may be as important as intervening in crisis situations. Cleansing an incision is a nursing intervention that can help prevent infection. Educating a patient about risk-factor modification for cardiovascular disease may prevent a future myocardial infarction. Placing infants on their backs to sleep may reduce the risk of sudden infant death syndrome (American Academy of Pediatrics Task Force, 2000). Being current in evidence-based practice enhances a nurse's ability to include preventive interventions in patient plans of care.

PATIENT EDUCATION AND HEALTH LITERACY

The Patient's Role in Care Provider Hand Hygiene

- Research has indicated that educating patients regarding their role in monitoring handwashing by health care workers can increase compliance and reduce hospital-acquired infections.
- Written material in the form of a brochure is most often used to instruct patients on when and how to ask staff members to wash their hands.
- Patients should be instructed to ask their care providers to wash their hands if they have not observed them doing so.
- Although patients are less likely to ask physicians to wash their hands than to ask nurses, the intervention of having patients ask staff to wash their hands has increased hand-washing practices in study sites by approximately 50%.

Adapted from McGuckin M, Waterman R, Porten L, et al: Patient education model for increasing handwashing compliance, *Am J Infect Control,* 27(4): 309-314, 1999; McGuckin M, Waterman R, Storr IJ, et al: Evaluation of a patient-empowering hand hygiene programme in the UK, *J Hosp Infect,* 48(3): 222-227, 2001.

INDEPENDENT NURSING INTERVENTIONS LO 9.4

Independent nursing interventions are tasks within the nursing scope of practice that the nurse may undertake without a physician or PCP order. Determining what nursing interventions to include in a patient's plan of care and prioritizing that care are independent nursing interventions based on nursing knowledge. Repositioning a patient in bed, performing oral hygiene, and providing emotional support through active listening are examples of other independent nursing interventions.

The extent to which nurses can implement independent nursing interventions is often determined by the area in which care is taking place. For instance, community nurses or those working in international field hospitals may have the authority to initiate interventions traditionally reserved for other health care professionals in a formal inpatient setting. Safe nursing practice requires nurses to know (1) how to perform interventions before their independent implementation and (2) whether the initiation of independently chosen interventions is permitted in their practice setting.

DEPENDENT NURSING INTERVENTIONS LO 9.5

Dependent nursing interventions are tasks the nurse undertakes that are within the nursing scope of practice but require the order of a primary care provider to be implemented. They require nurses to pay strict attention to the details of what is ordered and to recognize when implementing a dependent nursing intervention is appropriate or should be withheld. Administering patient medications or administering oxygen to a patient are examples of common dependent nursing interventions that require clinical judgment before implementation. These interventions are based on a collaborative effort of the nurse and the PCP to provide care to patients.

BOX 9-1 Standing Orders for Patients With Chest Pain

Standing orders for patients experiencing chest pain include independent and dependent nursing interventions:

- Assess vital signs.
- Obtain an electrocardiogram (ECG).
- Initiate or maintain telemetry.
- Initiate oxygen therapy beginning at 2 L per nasal cannula; monitor pulse oximetry levels.
- Administer sublingual nitroglycerin (0.4 mg SL); repeat up to three times, as needed.
- Initiate intravenous access if not already available.
- Notify laboratory to assess cardiac enzymes.
- Notify physician for further orders.

STANDING ORDERS

Some physician orders are received through a preapproved standardized order set known as *standing orders.* For example, when patients return to their rooms after cardiac catheterization, standing orders may indicate that the patients are to remain on bed rest for a specified period of time. To follow the standing orders, the nurse maintains patients on bed rest for the indicated amount of time. When the specified time period ends and a patient's condition remains unstable, the nurse contacts the physician for further orders rather than continuing to follow the standing orders. Regardless of the existence of standing orders, it is the nurse's responsibility to continually reassess individual patients and not blindly follow orders. Box 9-1 provides an example of standing orders for patients with chest pain.

MEDICATION ADMINISTRATION

Medication administration is within the scope of nursing practice and is performed as a dependent nursing intervention. Nurses must complete three checks and follow the six rights of medication administration to safely carry out this type of dependent action. Nurses check the primary care provider's orders, the patient's allergies, and the expiration date of the medication to be administered, and then address the six rights. They include administering the right medication and dosage, by the correct route, to the right patient, at the right time, and documenting correctly (see Chapter 35). All forms of prescription medication (i.e., oral, topical, and parenteral) require an order before administration, as does providing oxygen to a patient.

MEDICAL TREATMENTS

Medical treatments are dependent nursing interventions. Examples of medical treatments requiring a physician order include urinary catheterization, 24-hour urine collection, dressing changes, incision irrigation, intubation, and placement of a nasogastric tube. The nurse collects data and gathers supplies and necessary information to carry out these interventions. Nurses must use sound clinical judgment to perform interventions and should seek clarification as needed. For example, if a patient has been ordered to ambulate four times daily, but a recent ultrasound confirms the presence of a deep vein thrombosis in the patient's left leg, the nurse would contact the physician about the ultrasound results to obtain updated orders before ambulating the patient.

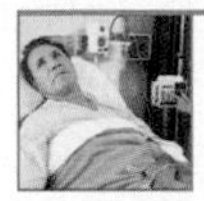

2. The admitting nurse identified five initial nursing diagnosis labels for Mr. Khalek: *Impaired Gas Exchange, Fatigue, Ineffective Airway Clearance, Risk for Falls,* and *Anxiety.* List a minimum of two nursing interventions to implement for each of these nursing diagnoses.

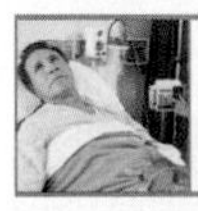

3. Highlight all of the independent nursing actions listed as interventions for Mr. Khalek's care.

DOCUMENTATION OF INTERVENTIONS LO 9.6

All interventions that are performed by nurses or other health care personnel need to be documented. A common adage states, "If it's not documented, it's not done." Nurses must document to accurately convey information to other care providers. If a nurse does not document that a medication was administered, for example, the patient may receive an additional dose. If completion of patient orders is not documented—such as if laboratory results were not reported and the patient needs to have another blood draw—the patient may be adversely affected medically and financially (e.g., a repeated blood draw is painful and costly).

Documentation most often is charted in the patient's EHR and standardized flow sheets according to agency policy. Patient health records are legal documents. Within the Health Insurance Portability and Accountability Act (HIPAA) guidelines, patient documentation is provided to insurance companies and others for billing and reimbursement. All documentation entries should be completed in a timely, accurate, and professional manner. More information on documentation is provided in Chapter 10.

EVALUATION OF THE NURSING CARE PLAN LO 9.7

Evaluation is the final step in the nursing process (Figure 9-2). **Evaluation** focuses on the patient and the patient's response to nursing interventions and outcome attainment. Evaluation is not a record of care that was implemented. Patient outcomes serve as the criteria against which the success of a nursing intervention is judged (Bulechek, Butcher, Dochterman, et al., 2013). Information on the effectiveness of nursing interventions is a by-product of the evaluation process. During the evaluation phase, nurses use critical thinking to determine whether a patient's short- and long-term goals were met and whether desired outcomes were achieved. Monitoring whether the patient's goals were attained is collaborative, involving the patient in the decision-making process.

Evaluation

Care plan evaluation
- Patient goal/outcome attainment?
- Continue?
- Revise/adapt?
- Discontinue?

FIGURE 9-2 Evaluation in the nursing process.

GOAL ATTAINMENT IN THE PLAN OF CARE

The evaluation process begins with determining whether patient goals have been met. Although interventions may or may not be performed, evaluation examines the extent to which interventions affected patient outcomes. Did the patient achieve the goal that was set?

Each nursing care plan is tailored to meet the specific needs of a patient. Ideally, when patient outcomes are evaluated, they will be positive, indicating improved patient status. Unfortunately, this is not always the case. For instance, a patient may have a nursing diagnosis of *Acute Pain* after a motor vehicle accident. The goal is for the patient to report a pain level of less than 6 of 10 during the nurse's shift. Nursing interventions include assessing pain, administering analgesic medication, repositioning the patient, distracting the patient, providing a quiet environment, and giving the patient an opportunity to share concerns. The patient consistently rates his pain level at 8 of 10 for the entire shift. In this case, evaluation reveals that the patient's goal was unmet and that revision of the patient-centered care plan is required to more effectively address his needs.

CONTINUATION, ADAPTATION, OR REVISION OF THE PLAN OF CARE

When a patient goal is unmet or only partially met, the plan of care may need to be revised or adapted to support goal attainment. Patients may develop complications (e.g., deep vein thrombosis) that limit the ability to ambulate four times each day, making a goal of increased ambulation unattainable. When complications arise or patient goals are only partially met, the nurse revises the plan of care in response to the evaluation findings. It is common for plans of care to change to meet evolving needs. Reassessment occurs with each patient-nurse interaction. As changes in a patient's condition occur, the plan of care should be revised.

Evaluation of a patient goal or outcome may be positive when the patient's goal is met and the problem resolved. When this happens, the nurse needs to determine whether the patient's plan of care should be continued to support sustained or greater improvement or should be discontinued. Decisions such as this are made by the nurse on the basis of patient preference and the nurse's clinical judgment.

DISCONTINUING THE PLAN OF CARE

Goal attainment is one reason that plans of care are discontinued. Another is changing circumstances. If the goal was for the patient to demonstrate proper injection of enoxaparin (Lovenox) before discharge and the patient did so safely and accurately for three consecutive injections, the outcome has been met, and this aspect of the plan of care can be discontinued.

However, if a goal was for a patient to ambulate three times daily without assistance, but the patient became unresponsive due to a cerebrovascular accident (CVA), the ambulation goal is no longer realistic or appropriate, and this aspect of the plan of care needs to be discontinued. Table 9-1 illustrates goal and evaluation statements in the context of the nursing process. Table 9-2 shows examples of how to formulate evaluation statements in various situations.

REFLECTION ON UNMET GOALS

If patient goals are not achieved, the nurse reflects on questions such as these: What barriers did the patient have in meeting these goals? Were the goals realistic? What happened that was not anticipated? What can be done differently? These questions assist the nurse in revising the plan of care.

Reassessment should occur every time the nurse interacts with a patient or reviews updated diagnostic laboratory or test results. The nurse must continually monitor for changes in a patient's condition that affect the plan of care. Higher-priority goals sometimes emerge through the reflection process.

TABLE 9-1 Goal and Evaluation Statements

NANDA-I NURSING DIAGNOSIS LABEL WITH NURSING DIAGNOSIS STATEMENT	NURSING OUTCOME CLASSIFICATION (NOC) AND INDICATOR	NURSING INTERVENTION CLASSIFICATION (NIC) AND ASSOCIATED ACTIVITIES
Impaired Physical Mobility r/t recent surgical intervention AEB/AMB limited range of motion, pain with movement, and difficulty moving	*Ambulation* (0200) Walks moderate distance (020011)	*Activity therapy* (4310) 1. Determine patient's commitment to increasing range of activity. 2. Assist with choosing activities consistent with physical capabilities.
Goal: Patient will increase walking to a minimum of 100 yards four times per day before discharge.		
Evaluation statement: Goal met. Patient ambulating 200 yards four or five times each day. Continue plan of care until discharge.		

From Bulechek G, Butcher H, Dochterman J, et al (eds): *Nursing interventions classification (NIC),* ed. 6, St. Louis, 2013, Mosby; Moorhead S, Johnson M, Maas M, et al (eds): *Nursing outcomes classification (NOC),* ed. 5, St. Louis, 2013, Mosby; NANDA International: *Nursing diagnoses: Definitions and classification, 2012–2014,* West Sussex, England, 2012, Wiley-Blackwell. Reprinted with permission from NANDA International, Inc.

NANDA-I, North American Nursing Diagnosis Association International; *NIC,* Nursing Interventions Classification; *NOC,* Nursing Outcomes Classification.

TABLE 9-2 Types of Evaluation Statements

Goal: Patient will ask for assistance by using the call light and waiting for help before toileting every time ambulation to the bathroom is required.	
Evaluation statement *when goal is met*	Goal met. Patient consistently requests assistance before toileting. Continue plan of care to ensure patient safety, or discontinue plan of care because patient no longer requires assistance for safe use of the toilet.
Evaluation statement *when goal is partially met*	Goal partially met. Patient forgetting to ask for assistance with toileting during the day. Revise plan of care to include use of bed alarm.
Evaluation statement *when goal is unmet*	Goal is unmet. Discontinue plan of care. Patient is no longer able to call for assistance due to diminished level of consciousness.

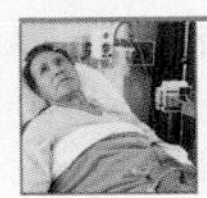

4. A goal for Mr. Khalek was "Patient's oxygen saturation will remain above 96% on 2 L of O_2 per nasal cannula throughout the first 24 hours of hospitalization." When evaluating whether or not the goal was met, the nurse notices that since he was admitted 25 hours earlier, the only time his oxygen saturation fell to 93% on 2 L of O_2 was right after dinner, and then it returned to 95% within 30 minutes. Write an evaluative statement for this goal to be documented in Mr. Khalek's patient-centered plan of care.

CARE PLAN MODIFICATION AND QUALITY IMPROVEMENT LO 9.8

Care plans should be updated regularly after patient evaluations. The nursing process is ongoing in an attempt to meet patient needs. The nursing process is not linear in nature but is dynamic and cyclic, constantly adapting to a patient's health status. Care plan modifications may be necessitated due to deterioration or improvement of a patient's condition.

The Joint Commission requires patient care plans to be evaluated on a continual basis. In many agencies, nurses are required to evaluate patient outcomes at least once during every shift. Making modifications to plans of care as a patient's status changes is a necessary component of providing safe patient care.

As a patient-centered plan of care changes, new goals are developed. After new goals are formulated, additional interventions are developed and implemented to assist the patient in achieving them. The patient care plan remains the cornerstone of nursing care. Evaluation is the means by which nurses determine a care plan's effectiveness in meeting the patient's needs. Thorough evaluation of patient outcomes contributes to quality improvement (QI) research and initiatives that affect future patient care implementation.

QUALITY IMPROVEMENT

Quality improvement (QI) is a formal way to look at patient and treatment outcomes and to determine what can be done differently to affect a situation in a positive way. During the evaluation phase of the nursing process, nurses consider the effectiveness of interventions to meet goals and improve patient outcomes. QI processes benefit patients and ultimately affect patient care. If certain patient outcomes are consistently improved by the implementation of specific nursing interventions, procedures can be changed on the basis of the QI research. This performance-based approach seeks excellence in patient care and contributes to evidence-based practice. Chapter 12 provides more information on quality improvement.

Although implementation and evaluation are considered the last two steps of the nursing process, they are as integral to helping patients achieve positive outcomes, as are the other steps. Providing individualized, patient-centered care and evaluating whether that care has helped to achieve positive patient outcomes are essential to safe, professional nursing practice.

SUMMARY OF LEARNING OUTCOMES

LO 9.1 *Explain the significance of implementation and evaluation in the nursing process:* Nurses and other members of the interdisciplinary health care team provide care through interventions designed to promote, maintain, or restore a patient's health during the implementation phase of the nursing process. Implementation consists of performing a task and documenting each intervention. Evaluation focuses on the patient and the patient's response to nursing interventions and outcome attainment. Evaluation data are used by the nurse to adapt a plan of care on the basis of the patient's changing health status.

LO 9.2 *Describe different types of direct-care interventions:* Direct care refers to interventions that are carried out by having personal contact with patients. Direct nursing interventions include reassessing patients, assisting with ADLs, giving physical care, counseling, and teaching.

LO 9.3 *Differentiate among various forms of indirect-care interventions:* Indirect care includes nursing interventions performed to benefit patients without face-to-face contact. Indirect nursing interventions include communicating and collaborating with other health care team members, making referrals, doing research, advocating, delegating, and engaging in preventive actions such as patient education and health promotion.

LO 9.4 *Identify examples of independent nursing interventions:* Independent nursing interventions are tasks within the nursing scope of practice that the nurse may undertake without a physician or PCP order. The extent to which nurses can implement independent nursing interventions is often determined by the area in which care is taking place.

LO 9.5 *Recognize dependent nursing interventions:* Dependent nursing interventions are tasks the nurse undertakes that are within the nursing scope of practice but require the order of a physician or PCP to implement. They require nurses to pay strict attention to the details of what was ordered and to recognize when implementing a dependent nursing intervention is appropriate or should be withheld in consultation with the PCP.

LO 9.6 *Identify the significance of documentation in the implementation step:* Nurses must document effectively to convey information accurately to other care providers. Within the HIPAA guidelines, patient documentation is provided to insurance companies and others for billing and reimbursement.

LO 9.7 *Apply evaluation principles used in the nursing process:* Evaluation focuses on the patient and the patient's response to nursing interventions and outcome attainment. Evaluation is not a record of the care that was implemented. Information on the effectiveness of nursing interventions is a by-product of the evaluation process. During the evaluation phase, nurses use critical thinking to determine whether a patient's short- and long-term goals were met and the desired outcomes were achieved.

LO 9.8 *Describe the relationship between care plan modification and quality improvement:* Care plan modification is based on the effectiveness of interventions to meet and improve desired patient outcomes. QI processes benefit patients and ultimately affect patient care. If certain patient outcomes are consistently improved by the implementation of specific nursing interventions, procedures can be changed on the basis of the QI research.

Responses to the critical-thinking questions are available at *http://evolve.elsevier.com/YoostCrawford/fundamentals/*.

REVIEW QUESTIONS

1. What should the nurse consider before implementation of all nursing interventions? *(Select all that apply.)*
   a. Potential communication barriers
   b. Diverse cultural practices
   c. Scope of nursing practice
   d. Functional status of the patient
   e. Time of most recent shift change
2. Which intervention would be most important for the nurse to include in the care plan if the patient is unable to complete activities of daily living without becoming fatigued?
   a. Instruct the patient to shower and shave simultaneously.
   b. Discourage the patient from bathing while hospitalized.
   c. Encourage the patient to rest between bathing activities.
   d. Ask the patient's spouse to assist with all bathing.
3. Which nursing intervention is most important to complete before giving medication to a patient?
   a. Provide water to aid in the patient's ability to swallow the medication.
   b. Double-check the patient's allergies before giving the drug.
   c. Ask the patient to verify having taken the medication before.
   d. Place the patient in a side-lying position to prevent aspiration.
4. Which direct-care intervention would be most effective in helping a patient cope emotionally with a new diagnosis of cancer?
   a. Reassessing for changes in the patient's physical condition
   b. Teaching the patient various methods of stress reduction
   c. Referring the patient for music and massage therapy
   d. Encouraging the patient to explore options for care
5. What should be taken into consideration by the nurse when deciding on interventions to include in a patient's plan of care? *(Select all that apply.)*
   a. Patient's treatment preferences
   b. Cultural and ethnic influences
   c. Professional level of expertise
   d. Current evidence-based research
   e. Convenience to the nursing staff
6. Which task may the registered nurse safely delegate to unlicensed assistive personnel without prior intervention?
   a. Ambulating a patient with ataxia and new right-sided paresthesia
   b. Feeding a patient with cerebral palsy who recently aspirated
   c. Transporting a patient to the hospital entrance for discharge
   d. Administering prescribed programmed medications

7. Which actions are a part of the evaluation step in the nursing process? *(Select all that apply.)*
   a. Recognizing the need for modifications to the care plan
   b. Documenting performed nursing interventions
   c. Determining whether the nursing interventions were completed
   d. Reviewing whether a patient met the short-term goal
   e. Identifying realistic outcomes with patient input
8. Which action by the day-shift nurse provides objective data that enables the night-shift nurse to complete an evaluation of a patient's short-term goals?
   a. Encouraging the patient to share observations from the day
   b. Leaving a message with the charge nurse before the shift change
   c. Documenting patient assessment findings in the patient's chart
   d. Checking with the pharmacist regarding possible drug interactions
9. Which notation is most appropriate for the nurse to include in a patient's chart regarding evaluation of the goal, "Patient will ambulate three times daily in the hallway before discharge without shortness of breath (SOB)"?
   a. Goal not met; patient states he is tired.
   b. Goal not met; patient ambulated three times in room.
   c. Goal met; patient ambulated three times in the hallway.
   d. Goal met; patient ambulated three times in the hallway without SOB.
10. What is the primary purpose of quality improvement?
   a. Recognizing the need to discipline employees violating policies
   b. Preventing patient injury that may contribute to the death of others
   c. Increasing institutional profits to support further scientific research
   d. Enhancing current practice to improve patient outcomes and care

Answers and rationales for the review questions are available at *http://evolve.elsevier.com/YoostCrawford/fundamentals/*.

REFERENCES

American Academy of Pediatrics Task Force on Infant Sleep Position and Sudden Infant Death Syndrome: Changing concepts of sudden infant death syndrome: Implication for infant sleeping environment and sleep position. *Pediatrics,* 105(3), 650-656, 2000.

American Nurses Association (ANA): *Nursing: Scope and standards of practice,* ed. 2, Silver Spring, Md., 2010, *www.Nursebooks.org*.

Bulechek G, Butcher H, Dochterman J, Wagner C (Eds): *Nursing interventions classifications (NIC),* ed. 6, St. Louis, 2013, Mosby Elsevier.

Doran D, Straus S, Haynes B, et al: Improving workplace learning at the point of care through information technology. *Comput Inform Nurs,* 27(5), 332-333, 2009.

Hardwick M, Pulido P, Adelson W: The use of handheld technology in nursing research and practice. *Orthop Nurs,* 26(4), 251-255, 2007.

Kelly P, Marthaler MT: *Nursing delegation, setting priorities, and making patient care assignments,* ed. 2, Clifton Park, N.Y., 2011, Delmar Cengage Learning.

Kohn L, Corrigan J, Donaldson M (Eds): *To err is human: Building a safer health system,* Washington, D.C., 2000, National Academies Press.

National Council of State Boards of Nursing: *Delegation decision-making tree,* 1997. Retrieved from *https://www.ncsbn.org/delegationtree.pdf*.

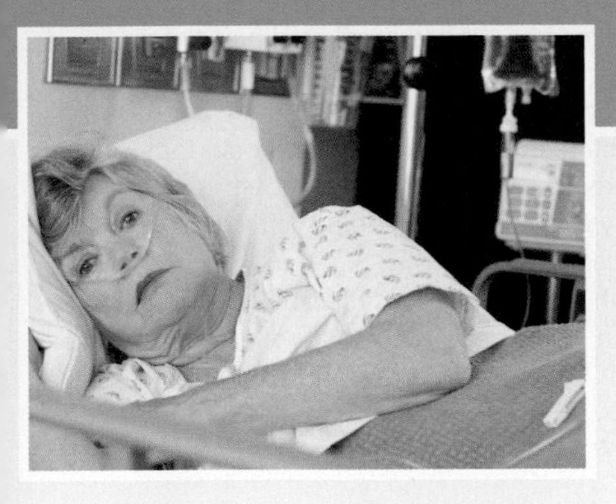

CHAPTER 10

Documentation, Electronic Health Records, and Reporting

EVOLVE WEBSITE

http://evolve.elsevier.com/YoostCrawford/fundamentals/

- Additional Evolve-Only Review Questions with Answers
- Answers and Rationales for Text Review Questions
- Answers to Critical-Thinking Questions
- Case Study with Questions
- Glossary

LEARNING OUTCOMES

Comprehension of this chapter's content will provide students with the ability to:

LO 10.1 Identify the standards for effective documentation by nurses.

LO 10.2 Discuss the functions of the medical record, including the electronic health record.

LO 10.3 List the important attributes of nursing documentation in the medical record.

LO 10.4 Define *privacy* and *confidentiality* as they relate to information in a medical record.

LO 10.5 Describe standardized formats for use in hand-off reports and change-of-shift reports.

LO 10.6 Explain the process of accepting verbal and telephone orders.

LO 10.7 Discuss the proper use of incident reports.

KEY TERMS

ANTICipate model, p. 138
APIE note, p. 134
bar-coded medication administration, p. 134
charting by exception, p. 134
computerized provider order entry, p. 131
confidentiality, p. 135
DAR note, p. 134
electronic health record, p. 131
electronic medical record, p. 131
hand-off, p. 136
Health Insurance Portability and Accountability Act, p. 136
medication administration record, p. 134
PIE note, p. 134
privacy, p. 136
problem-oriented medical record, p. 133
SBAR, p. 137
sentinel event, p. 137
SOAP note, p. 134
SOAPIE note, p. 134
SOAPIER note, p. 134

CASE STUDY

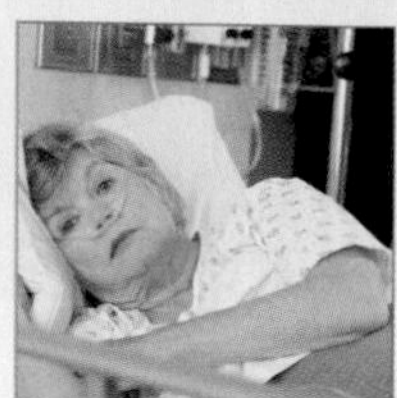

Mrs. Schmidt is a 73-year-old, widowed female admitted to the hospital after a right hip fracture sustained when she tripped off a curb and fell. She had open reduction and internal fixation of her hip 24 hours earlier. Her medical history indicates that she is in good health with no other medical diagnoses. She is employed part time at her community library. She is allergic to penicillin.

Mrs. Schmidt's vital signs are T 36.6° C (97.9° F), P 80 and regular, R 18 and unlabored with SpO2 of 97% on 2L O2 via nasal cannula, and BP 140/80. She rates her pain at 7 of 10 and states that she has "sharp pain that shoots from my hip to mid-calf when I move." She ambulated to the bathroom twice with assistance but grimaced while walking. She transferred from bed to chair with assistance to eat lunch. The physical therapist worked with her on ambulation during the afternoon. She indicates that she is anxious to get moving so that she can go home.

Her incision is well approximated, without swelling or excessive redness, and there is no drainage on the dressing. She received oral Vicodin at 8 A.M., 12 noon, and 4 P.M. 45 minutes after being medicated she reported pain of 3 of 10. The nurse responsible for her care on the 12-hour day shift needs to document care according to facility policy, which mandates the SOAPIE format.

Refer back to this case study to answer the critical-thinking questions throughout the chapter.

Health care documentation is any written or electronically generated information about a patient that describes the patient, the patient's health, and the care and services provided, including the dates of care. These records may be paper or electronic documents, such as electronic medical records, faxes, e-mails, audiotapes, videotapes, and images. The primary purpose of health care documentation and record-keeping systems is facilitation of information flow that supports the continuity, quality, and safety of care. The goal in documenting care is to describe the facts clearly and concisely to improve intradisciplinary and interdisciplinary communication.

Nurses are largely responsible for coordinating the patient's care, implementing the plan for nursing care, and documenting the patient's care and progress toward goals. As a result, nurses spend considerable time doing information work (i.e., accessing, generating, and sharing information), to ensure that appropriate, accurate information is available to all members of the care team (Agency for Healthcare Research and Quality [AHRQ], 2008).

DOCUMENTATION STANDARDS AND PRINCIPLES LO 10.1

Standards for documentation are established by each health care organization's policies and procedures. They should be in agreement with The Joint Commission's standards and elements of performance, including having a medical record for each patient that is accessed only by authorized personnel. General principles of medical record documentation from the Centers for Medicare and Medicaid Services (2010) include the need for completeness and legibility; the reasons for each patient encounter, including assessments and diagnosis; and the plan of care, the patient's progress, and any changes in diagnosis and treatment.

The American Nurses Association (ANA, 2010) has identified principles of nursing documentation related to the characteristics of documentation, education and training, policies and procedures, protection systems, entries, and standardized terminologies. The ANA's model for high-quality nursing documentation reflects the nursing process and includes accessibility, accuracy, relevance, auditability, thoughtfulness, timeliness, and retrievability.

Accurate documentation is necessary for hospitals to be reimbursed according to diagnostic-related groups (DRGs). DRGs are a system used to classify hospital admissions. Each DRG is reimbursed at a specific rate, and payment is often based on the documentation supporting the hospital stay.

THE MEDICAL RECORD LO 10.2

The medical record is a document with comprehensive information about a patient's health care encounter, as well as demographic, administrative, and clinical data. The record serves as the major communication tool between staff members and as a single data access point for everyone involved in the patient's care. It is a legal document that must meet guidelines for completeness, accuracy, timeliness, accessibility, and authenticity.

The medical record promotes continuity of care and ensures that patients receive appropriate health care services. The record can be used to assess quality-of-care measures, determine the medical necessity of health care services, support reimbursement claims, and protect health care providers, patients, and others in legal matters. It is a clinical data archive. The medical record serves as a tool for biomedical research and provider education, collection of statistical data for government and other agencies, maintenance of compliance with external regulatory bodies, and establishment of policies and regulations for standards of care (Ethical, Legal, and Professional Practice box).

WRITTEN MEDICAL RECORDS

The use of paper medical records requires no special technical training. Information entry on paper is often in narrative form. The paper-based medical record has served clinical practice for many years, but the formal structure of the

ETHICAL, LEGAL, AND PROFESSIONAL PRACTICE

The Medical Record

- The medical record is the legal documentation of care provided to a patient.
- In the event of litigation, the medical record is often the only available evidence of the event in question.
- Medical record documentation should be based on fact, not opinions.
- Every note in a medical record must include a date, time, and signature with credentials.
- Ethical practice dictates that nurses document only interventions that are performed.
- Medical record entries cannot be altered or obliterated.

information within the record has changed significantly over time, moving from an unstructured or semistructured chronologic record of events to a problem- or task-oriented structure.

Paper records have several potential problems. It may be difficult to locate a particular chart because it is being used by someone else, it is in a different department, or it is misfiled. The paper chart is available to only one person at a time. Paper is fragile, susceptible to damage, and can degrade over time. Handwriting may be illegible. Storage and control of paper records can be a major problem.

Entries into paper medical records are traditionally made with black ink to enable copying or scanning, unless a facility requires or allows a different color. The date, time, and signature, with credentials of the person writing the entry, are included in the entry. No blank spaces are left between entries because they could allow someone to add a note out of sequence.

! SAFE PRACTICE ALERT

Paper records must be available only to people with an appropriate need for access. When not in use, paper charts must be secured in a location accessible to staff members but not accessible to patients, families, and visitors.

ELECTRONIC HEALTH RECORDS

The term *electronic medical record* is often used interchangeably with *electronic health record* or *computerized patient record*. The **electronic medical record** (EMR) is a record of one episode of care, such as an inpatient stay or an outpatient appointment. The **electronic health record** (EHR) is a longitudinal record of health that includes the information from inpatient and outpatient episodes of health care from one or more care settings (Collaboration and Delegation box). In the American Recovery and Reinvestment Act of 2009, the government mandates the use of a certified EHR for each person in the United States by 2014 (U.S. House of Representatives, 2009).

COLLABORATION AND DELEGATION

Use of the Electronic Health Record

- The electronic health record (EHR) includes documentation over time from inpatient and outpatient sources.
- Physicians, nurse practitioners, nurses, medical assistants, physician assistants, unlicensed assistive personnel (UAP), social workers, and therapists may contribute to the EHR. Check the facility policy for documentation guidelines.
- Laboratory data and other test results are available in inpatient and outpatient settings so that care decisions can be made.
- In some circumstances, care such as taking vital signs, assisting with activities of daily living, and documenting their outcomes can be delegated to UAP.
- Registered nurses are responsible for reviewing documentation by UAP for all patients under their care.

Although the EHR varies among health facilities, the major components are health information, diagnostic test results, an order-entry system, and decision support. Health information comprises patient data such as demographics, assessment findings, flow sheets that include point-of-care results, diagnoses, nursing treatments, and a medication profile listing historical and currently active medication orders. The nursing process is integrated in the EHR through documentation related to each of the five steps (i.e., assessment, diagnosis, planning, implementation, and evaluation). Diagnostic findings include current and historical results from procedures, laboratory tests, and x-rays.

Computerized provider order entry (CPOE) allows clinicians to enter orders in a computer that are sent directly to the appropriate department. Decision support in the electronic record may include medication interaction screening and reminders for preventive health actions such as vaccinations. More sophisticated decision support systems assist the diagnostic process and include recommendations for treatment. The electronic record provides connectivity to enhance communication between all members of the health care team, who can access and update the record simultaneously. The EHR supports administrative processes with more efficient and timely data abstraction for scheduling, billing, and claims management.

Adoption of an EHR system produces major cost savings through gains in productivity and error reduction, which ultimately improves patient health status (Hillestad, Bigelow, Bower, et al, 2005). The most common benefits of electronic records are increased delivery of guideline-based care, better monitoring, and reduced medication errors (Chaudhry, Wang, Wu, et al, 2006). Use of EHRs can reduce storage space, allow simultaneous access by multiple users, facilitate easy duplication for sharing or backup, and increase portability in environments using wireless systems and hand-held devices. Although data are often entered by keyboard, they can also be entered by means of dictated voice recordings, light pens, or handwriting and pattern recognition systems. Computer programs can convert these types of data entry to text.

Electronic Health Record Documentation

As more health care facilities implement EHRs and EMRs, the quality of nursing documentation improves, enhancing patient safety and communication with other providers. However, implementation of electronic records does involve a learning curve as staff become accustomed to the new system. Consideration must be given to how the new system fits into the existing workflow. The nurse must have a basic level of computer competency in addition to an understanding of documentation principles. Disadvantages of use of computers for documentation include computer and software failure and problems if there is a power outage. Therefore any facility using an EHR system must have computer support and maintenance available at all times, and have a back up plan in place in the event of a power outage.

> **QSEN FOCUS!**
>
> Effective use of technology and standardized best practice facilitated by the EHR enable the nurse to provide safer patient care.

Access to an EHR is controlled through assignment of individual passwords and verification codes that identify people who have the right to enter the record. Passwords should never be shared with anyone. Health care information systems have the ability to track who uses the system and which records are accessed. These organizational tools contribute to the protection of personal health information.

Computer Availability

The move to electronic documentation requires computers to be readily available to health care staff. Originally, computers were located in the nurses' stations for use by all. Many facilities now support point-of-care documentation, with computers in each patient's room and mobile devices such as computer tablets (Figure 10-1) or workstations on wheels (WOWs) that can be rolled to a patient's bedside (see Chapter 15). The ability to document at the point of care supports the goals of timeliness and accuracy of documentation.

> **! SAFE PRACTICE ALERT**
>
> When reviewing patient information, ensure that computer screens are not visible to others in the area. Always log off when finished documenting in an EHR.

NURSING DOCUMENTATION LO 10.3

The delivery of safe, evidence-based, high-quality nursing practice requires nursing documentation to be "clear, accurate, and accessible" (ANA, 2010). Nursing documentation is

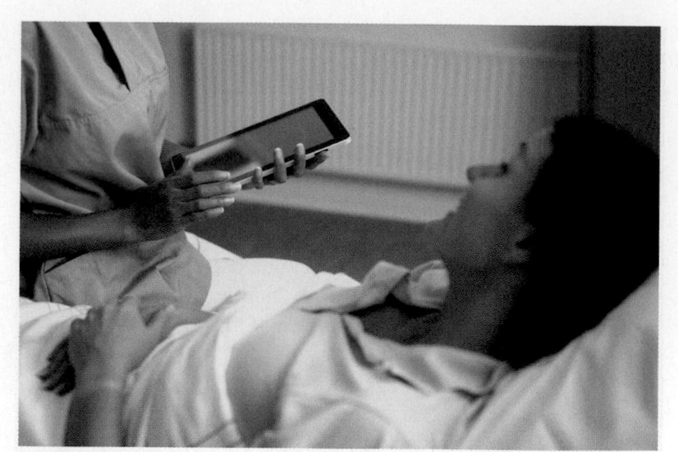

FIGURE 10-1 A nurse documents on a tablet at a patient's bedside.

an important part of effective communication among nurses and with other health care providers. Nursing documentation is part of a permanent medical record. It is a record of the nursing care that identifies the nurses providing care and the contribution of that care to patient outcomes. Documentation is a way of demonstrating that professional and legal standards of care are met. In some instances, the nursing documentation is directly related to reimbursement (Hentschke, 2009).

Documentation guidelines require accessible, accurate, timely nursing documentation that is clear, concise, complete, and objective (ANA, 2010). Documentation should be factual and nonjudgmental, with proper spelling and grammar. Events should be reported in the order they happened, and documentation should occur as soon as possible after assessment, interventions, condition changes, or evaluation. Each entry includes the date, time, and signature with credentials of the person documenting. Double documentation of data should be avoided because legal issues can arise due to conflicting data.

The documentation format used should reflect the care needs of patients and the practice setting. Specific documentation formats, including narrative, charting by exception, and flow charts, are discussed later in this chapter. Nursing documentation should clearly describe the patient's health status and include a care plan that reflects the needs and goals of the patient, the nursing interventions, and the impact of the interventions on the patient outcomes. Interactions with physicians and other health care providers are included (ANA, 2010).

CRITICAL ASPECTS OF DOCUMENTATION

Some health care facilities combine different methods of charting to improve the effectiveness of documentation. Nursing documentation is guided by the five steps of the nursing process: assessment, diagnosis, planning, implementation, and evaluation. Expected nursing documentation

TABLE 10-1 Do-Not-Use Abbreviations

DO NOT USE	POTENTIAL PROBLEM	USE INSTEAD
U, u (unit)	Mistaken for the number 0 or 4 or for cc	Write *unit*
IU (international unit)	Mistaken for IV (intravenous) or the number 10	Write *international unit*
QD, Q.D., qd, q.d. (daily) QOD, Q.O.D., qod, q.o.d (every other day)	Mistaken for each other Period after *Q* mistaken for *I*, and the *O* mistaken for *I*	Write *daily* Write *every other day*
MS, MSO_4, and $MgSO_4$	Confused with one another Can mean morphine sulfate or magnesium sulfate	Write *morphine sulfate* Write *magnesium sulfate*
Trailing zero (X.0 mg) Lack of leading zero (.X mg)	Decimal point is confusing	Write as *X mg* Write as *0.X mg*

From The Joint Commission: Facts about the official "Do Not Use" list of abbreviations, *Patient Safety Fact Sheets,* 2014b. Retrieved from *www.jointcommission.org/facts_about_the_official_/.*

includes a nursing assessment, the care plan, interventions, the patient's outcomes or response to care, and assessment of the patient's ability to manage after discharge. Care plans provide treatment guidelines for individual patients and are part of the permanent health record. The care plan should clearly identify patient preferences, with goals mutually developed by the patient and nurse.

The use of standardized nursing language has many advantages for direct patient care. Standardized nursing terminologies such as the NANDA International, Inc. (NANDA-I) nursing diagnoses, *Nursing Interventions Classification (NIC),* and *Nursing Outcomes Classification (NOC)* may be used in the documentation process. Use of standardized language provides consistency, improves communication among nurses and with other health care providers, increases the visibility of nursing interventions, improves patient care, enhances data collection to evaluate nursing care outcomes, and supports adherence to care standards (Rutherford, 2008). Chapters 5 and 15 provide more information on these topics.

Do-Not-Use Abbreviations

Nurses must be aware of the danger of using abbreviations that may be misunderstood and compromise patient safety. The Joint Commission (2014b) has compiled a list of do-not-use abbreviations, acronyms, and symbols to avoid the possibility of errors that may be life-threatening (Table 10-1). The Joint Commission supplies a toolkit to help facilities reach compliance in this area, and it recommends that each facility implement a "spell it out" campaign rather than using risky abbreviations.

! SAFE PRACTICE ALERT

Document using only accepted abbreviations and acronyms to facilitate effective communication among care providers that supports safe patient care.

DOCUMENTATION FORMATS

Nurses use a variety of documentation formats, usually based on facility policy. Source-oriented charting gives each profession a separate section of the record in which to do narrative charting. The **problem-oriented medical record** (POMR) integrates charting from the entire care team in the same section of the record. The POMR format provides a framework for documentation. The nurse's notes may be in a narrative format or in a problem-oriented structure such as the PIE, APIE, SOAP, SOAPIE, SOAPIER, DAR, or CBE format. The elements in each of these types of charting are listed in Table 10-2.

Narrative Charting

Narrative charting is chronologic, with a baseline recorded on a shift-by-shift basis. Data are recorded in the progress notes, often without an organizing framework. Narrative charting may stand alone, or it may be complemented by other tools, such as flow charts, flow sheets, and checklists. This charting format may be time-consuming and contain lengthy notes that may not add to the care process.

TABLE 10-2 Charting Formats

FORMAT	ELEMENTS
PIE	Problem, intervention, evaluation
APIE	Assessment, problem, intervention, evaluation
SOAP	Subjective data, objective data, assessment, plan
SOAPIE	Subjective data, objective data, assessment, plan, intervention, evaluation
SOAPIER	Subjective data, objective data, assessment, plan, intervention, evaluation, revisions to plan
DAR	Data, action, response
CBE	Charting by exception

Formatted Charting

Problem-oriented documentation can be completed in a variety of formats and follows a selected structure.

PIE Notes

A **PIE note** is used to document problem *(P)*, intervention *(I)*, and evaluation *(E)*. For example, a PIE note may read as follows:

P: Acute pain rated by postsurgical patient as 8 of 10.
I: Morphine sulfate (5 mg IV) given at 0930 per order for pain relief.
E: Patient reported a 3 of 10 pain level 20 minutes after an analgesic was administered.

APIE Notes

An **APIE note** adds assessment *(A)*, combining subjective and objective data in the PIE format. For example, an APIE note may read as follows:

A: Patient holding hand over surgical site and grimacing while reporting pain at a level of 8 of 10 on the pain scale.

SOAP Notes

A **SOAP note** is used to chart the subjective data *(S)*, objective data *(O)*, assessment *(A)*, and plan *(P)*. The format is sometimes expanded to a **SOAPIE note**, which includes the actual interventions *(I)* and an evaluation *(E)* of intervention outcomes. Another form of the SOAP note is the **SOAPIER note**, which adds revision *(R)* of the plan of care as necessary to meet the follow-up needs of the patient. Documentation is usually organized in the following way:

S: What do the patient and others tell you?
O: What are the results of the physical examination, relevant vital signs, or other tests?
A: What is the patient's current status?
P: What interventions are necessary?
I: What treatments did the nurse provide?
E: What are the patient outcomes after each intervention?
R: Does the plan stay the same? What changes are needed to the care plan?

DAR Notes

A **DAR note** is used to chart the data *(D)* collected about the patient problems, the action *(A)* initiated, and the patient's response *(R)* to the actions. A DAR note may read as follows:

D: Patient grimacing. Holding hand at surgical site. Pulse 98. States pain at a level of 8 of 10.
A: Given pain medication and repositioned for comfort.
R: 20 minutes after medication is given, Patient states relief with a pain level at 2 of 10.

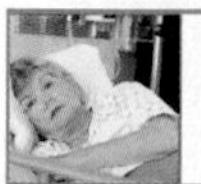

1. Develop a SOAPIE note for Mrs. Schmidt.

Charting by Exception

Charting by exception (CBE) is documentation that records only abnormal or significant data. It reduces charting time by assuming certain norms. For this type of charting, each facility must define what is normal. Any assessment finding outside normal is charted as an exception.

Case Management Documentation

The case management process of documentation is focused on providing and documenting high-quality, cost-effective delivery of patient care. This documentation uses standards of care to monitor patient outcomes on a regular basis, often using a predetermined care path format. The goal of case management is to achieve realistic and desired patient and family outcomes within appropriate lengths of stay and with appropriate use of resources. Clinical pathways based on nursing assessments provide standardized, evidence-based patient care that leads to achievement of outcomes. These ideas are discussed in greater detail in Chapter 5.

Flow Sheets

Flow sheets and checklists may be used to document routine care and observations that are recorded on a regular basis, such as vital signs, medications, and intake and output measurements (Figure 10-2). Data collected on flow sheets may be converted to a graph, which pictorially reflects patient data. Flow sheets and checklists are part of the permanent medical record.

A **medication administration record** (MAR) is a list of ordered medications, along with dosages and times of administration, on which the nurse initials medications given or not given. A paper MAR usually includes a signature section in which the nurse is identified by linking the initials used with a full signature. The EHR includes an electronic medication administration record (eMAR).

! SAFE PRACTICE ALERT

Medications administered must be documented immediately to avoid confusion about what has been given and the possibility of double dosing.

Bar-Coded Medication Administration

Many facilities using electronic records have incorporated **bar-coded medication administration** (BCMA) into the process of medication administration. Using a portable scanner, the nurse scans the patient's wristband and the medication to be given. In some facilities, the nurse's bar-coded identification is also scanned. If the eMAR and the scanned medication do not agree, the nurse receives an alert about a potential problem. The use of BCMA and eMAR allows the nurse to obtain a report of medications given, held, or due. Chapter 35 provides more information on medication administration.

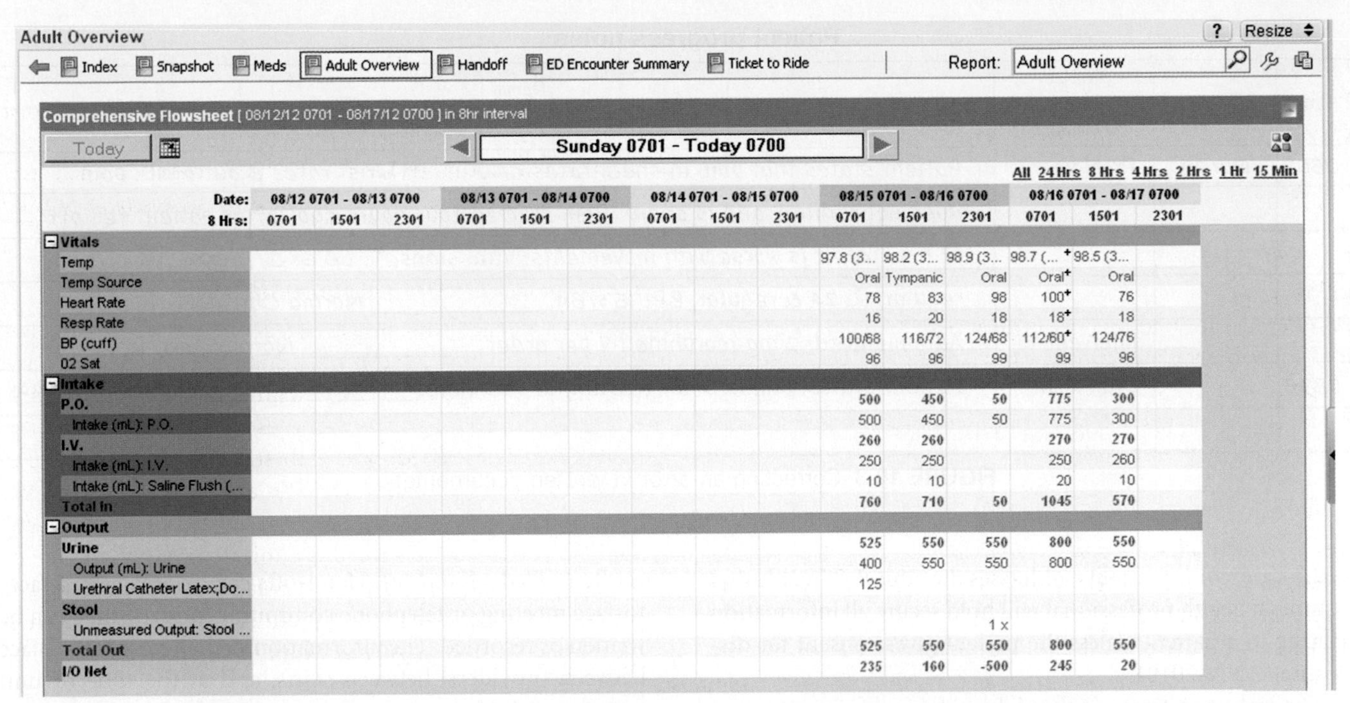

Date:	08/12 0701 - 08/13 0700			08/13 0701 - 08/14 0700			08/14 0701 - 08/15 0700			08/15 0701 - 08/16 0700			08/16 0701 - 08/17 0700		
8 Hrs:	0701	1501	2301	0701	1501	2301	0701	1501	2301	0701	1501	2301	0701	1501	2301
Vitals															
Temp										97.8 (3...	98.2 (3...	98.9 (3...	98.7 (... +	98.5 (3...	
Temp Source										Oral	Tympanic	Oral	Oral+	Oral	
Heart Rate										78	83	98	100+	76	
Resp Rate										16	20	18	18+	18	
BP (cuff)										100/68	116/72	124/68	112/60+	124/76	
02 Sat										96	96	99	99	96	
Intake															
P.O.										500	450	50	775	300	
Intake (mL): P.O.										500	450	50	775	300	
I.V.										260	260		270	270	
Intake (mL): I.V.										250	250		250	260	
Intake (mL): Saline Flush (...										10	10		20	10	
Total In										760	710	50	1045	570	
Output															
Urine										525	550	550	800	550	
Output (mL): Urine										400	550	550	800	550	
Urethral Catheter Latex;Do...										125					
Stool															
Unmeasured Output: Stool ...												1 x			
Total Out										525	550	550	800	550	
I/O Net										235	160	-500	245	20	

FIGURE 10-2 Flow sheet. (Courtesy Epic Systems, Corporation Verona, Wis., 2012.)

Kardex

Originally, the Kardex was a nonpermanent filing system for nursing records, orders, and patient information that was held centrally on the unit. The Kardex contained patient orders and demographic information. Although computerization of records may mean that the Kardex system is no longer active, the term *kardex* continues to be used generically for certain patient information held at the nurses' station.

Admission and Discharge Summaries

An admission summary includes the patient's history, a medication reconciliation, and an initial assessment that addresses the patient's problems, including identification of needs pertinent to discharge planning and formulation of a plan of care based on those needs. The discharge summary addresses the patient's hospital course and plans for follow-up, and it documents the patient's status at discharge. It includes information on medication and treatment, discharge placement, patient education, follow-up appointments, and referrals.

LEGAL ISSUES OF DOCUMENTATION

Nurses' notes are legal documents. The medical record is seen as the most reliable source of information in any legal action related to care. When legal counsel is sought because of a negative outcome of care, the first action taken by an attorney is to acquire a copy of the medical record. Documentation that meets specific guidelines can prevent a case from going to court or can provide protection if a case does go to trial.

Every entry into the medical record should include a date, time, and signature. Notes should never be altered or obliterated. Documentation mistakes must be acknowledged. If an error is made in paper documentation, a line is drawn through the error and the word *error* is placed above or after the entry, along with the nurse's initials (Figure 10-3) and followed by the correct entry. If an error is made in electronic documentation, it can be corrected on the screen view but the error and correction process remains in the permanent electronic record. Log-on access to the electronic record identifies the person making the change. Any correction in documentation that indicates a significant change in patient status should include notification of the primary care provider.

Charting should be completed as soon as possible after care is given. Timeliness of documentation depends on the patient's condition. When the patient's acuity and complexity of care are high, documentation occurs more frequently. Waiting until the end of a shift to chart creates the potential for documentation errors that may result in missing information regarding nursing assessments and patient outcomes.

The principles of documentation remain the same regardless of whether it is completed on paper or in an EHR. However, electronic recording, transmitting, and receiving of patient information poses significant challenges for nurses in regard to confidentiality and security of patient information.

CONFIDENTIALITY AND PRIVACY LO 10.4

The **confidentiality** of patient information must be safeguarded and the information shared only with individuals who have a need and a right to know. Nurses have a professional and legal obligation to protect patient information. In

Patient progress notes

Time	Discipline	Problem intervention evaluation	Remar
			4/22/2014
0800	Nursing	Problem	Patient states that pain ~~in sheet rates 4/10~~ (error nc) in left wrist rates 8 out of 10. pain
			does not radiate, and is sharp. Pain started four hours ago' after patient fell off
			of his bike. It is worse with movements. Vital signs: T: 36.6°C, P : 92 and
			regular, R: 24 & regular, BP: 153/84. ______ Norma Carr, RN
		Intervention	Administered 2 mg morphine I V per order. ______ Norma Carr, RN
0830		Evaluation	Patient states pain is 3/10. Resting at this time. ______ Norma Carr, RN

FIGURE 10-3 Correcting an error in written documentation.

health care, confidentiality addresses the ethical principle that assumes a health professional will hold secure all information relating to a patient unless the patient gives consent for disclosure (ANA, 2010).

The right to **privacy** is the right to be free from intrusion or disturbance in a person's private life (ANA, 2010). In the context of recorded information, it refers to the expectation of controlling or, in some cases, the legal right of a person to control access to personal information.

The **Health Insurance Portability and Accountability Act** (HIPAA), originally passed in 1996, created standards for the protection of personal health information, whether conveyed orally or recorded in any form or medium. The act clearly mandates that protected health information may be used only for treatment, payment, or health care operations. Nurses share the responsibility for preventing a breach of this information. Chapter 11 provides more information on HIPAA.

HIPAA privacy standards should be applied during phone, fax, e-mail, or Internet transmission of protected patient information. Patient information should be shared and the EHR accessed only in private work areas. EHR access is password protected. Nursing care guideline 11-A of the HIPAA principles lists procedural and documentation concerns associated with HIPAA.

Patients' rights include obtaining, viewing, or updating a copy of their own medical records. Methods for implementation vary by facility and type of medical record. The American Recovery and Reinvestment Act (ARRA) of 2009 updated some aspects of HIPAA. It requires requested EHRs to be transmitted to the patient within 30 days, at a cost not to exceed the expenses incurred (Center for Democracy and Technology, 2009).

HAND-OFF REPORTS LO 10.5

The real-time process of passing patient-specific information from one caregiver to another or among interdisciplinary team members to ensure continuity of care and patient safety is often called a ***hand-off***. Hand-offs can be oral, as in a face-to-face meeting or telephone communication, or they can be written or recorded. The information exchange can take place between providers, between shifts, and at the time of unit transfer or discharge referral.

Transitioning patients from one type of care to another (e.g., acute care to long-term care, inpatient to outpatient care) involves risks due to a lack of uniformity in the hand-off process and inadequate training on how to communicate during the transfer of care. Staff may not fully realize the importance of the specific patient information needed in the care transition process (Boutwell and Frankel, 2009). When complete and accurate information is not shared during a hand-off report, patients may not get needed care, proper medications, or recommended therapies.

The process of making a change-of-shift report serves several functions. Hand-offs provide accurate and timely information about the care, treatment, and services rendered to a patient, addressing the patient's current condition and anticipated changes. Information in a hand-off includes the transfer of authority and responsibility for the patient's care (AHRQ, 2008). Patient information that supports care delivery and clinical decision making must be shared to facilitate continuity of care. The hand-off process can be an opportunity for collaborative problem solving. Improvement in the hand-off process can increase patient safety and promote positive patient outcomes. During an average hospital stay of approximately 4 days, as many as 24 hand-offs can occur for just one patient because shifts change every 8 to 12 hours and many individuals are responsible for care. An ineffective hand-off may lead to wrong treatments, wrong medications, or other life-threatening events, increasing the length of stay and causing patient injury or death.

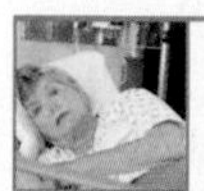

2. What information is important to share with the nurse who will be responsible for Mrs. Schmidt's care on the next shift?

Unfortunately, wide variations exist in the quality and quantity of information shared in the shift report. The Joint Commission (2010) data analysis indicated that communication problems were the primary cause of 65% of sentinel events between 1995 and 2004. A **sentinel event** is an unexpected occurrence involving death or serious physical or psychological injury or the risk of injury (The Joint Commission, 2014c). These events are called *sentinel* because they signal the need for an immediate investigation and response. In 2005, 70% of sentinel events were caused by communication breakdowns, and 50% of those occurred during patient hand-off. To improve the effectiveness of communication among caregivers, The Joint Commission (20014a) introduced a national patient safety goal in 2006, which became a standard in 2009, requiring implementation of a standardized approach to hand-off communications (Evidence-Based Practice box).

Boutwell and Frankel (2009) believe that patient hand-offs can be improved and suggest using a face-to-face discussion rather than electronic or written communication. Implementing a standardized process for hand-offs is the best way to avoid errors. In many sites, the move to standardized shift reports consists of bedside reports that include incoming staff, outgoing staff, and the patient (Figure 10-4). Successfully implemented, bedside reporting is seen as "providing a real-time exchange of information that increases patient safety, improves quality of care, increases accountability, and strengthens teamwork" (Federwisch, 2007). Interdisciplinary patient care conferences and rounds are a major source of communication between health care professionals and patients (Patient Education and Health Literacy box).

EVIDENCE-BASED PRACTICE

Hand-off Reports

One multihospital system piloted a new intershift hand-off process on a unit in seven hospitals to test improvements in patient and nurse satisfaction. The goal of the pilot program was to use evidence-based practice to implement a new hand-off process to improve patient safety and satisfaction and promote patient-centered care.

Pilot Hand-off Program

- The hospital system implemented an evidence-based hand-off process.
- A standardized tool was used for nurses to exchange information in the hand-off report to ensure that pertinent information was passed on to the next shift.
- Patients and their families were invited in writing to participate in the intershift hand-off, which occurred at the bedside.
- Patients and their families were at the center of the hand-off, and nurses deliberately sought input from them.

Results of the Program

- Nurses had increased knowledge about patient priorities.
- New nursing graduates reported feeling empowered.
- Nurses were able to jointly teach at the bedside and collaboratively assess patients.
- Nurses perceived that appropriate information was being exchanged and that relationships between shifts improved.
- Patient satisfaction scores improved significantly in all three categories measured:
  - Nurses kept patients informed
  - Friendliness and courtesy of the staff
  - Likelihood to recommend the hospital

From Thomas L, Donohue-Porter P: Blending evidence and innovation: Improving intershift handoffs in a multihospital setting, *J Nurs Care Quality* 27(2): 116-124, 2012.

PATIENT EDUCATION AND HEALTH LITERACY

"Patient Participation in Handoff Reports"

Handoff reports are enhanced with patient participation. Nurses should:

- Teach patients to actively participate with staff during the bedside rounds.
- Ask patients to validate the information shared during the rounding process.
- Encourage patients to ask questions during the rounding process.

Current hand-off mechanisms vary from hospital to hospital and even from unit to unit. A communication format specifically suggested for use in nurse-physician interactions is **SBAR** (i.e., situation, background, assessment, and recommendation), a situation-briefing tool used by the U.S. Navy (Table 10-3). SBAR was adapted for health care at Kaiser Permanente of Colorado and has become widely used in the United States and in the British National Health Service. SBAR is used "to report to a health care provider a situation that requires immediate action; to define the elements of a hand-off of a patient from one caregiver to another, such as during transfers from one unit to another or during shift report; and in quality improvement reports" (Iver, 2007,

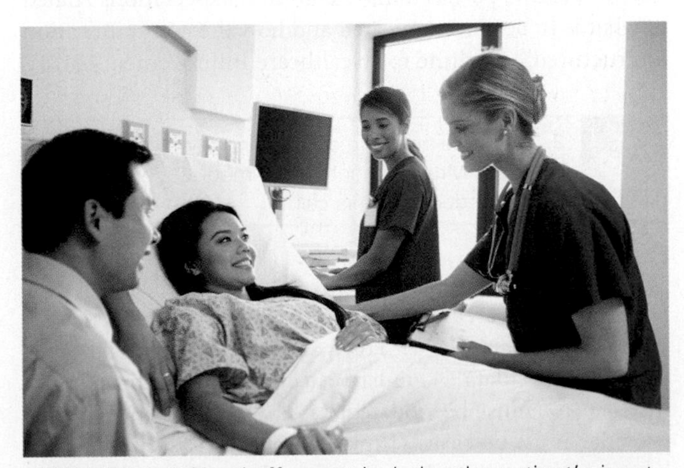

FIGURE 10-4 Hand-off report includes the patient's input.

TABLE 10-3 SBAR Communication Tool

ELEMENT	DESCRIPTION
Situation	What is happening at the current time?
Background	What are the circumstances leading up to this situation?
Assessment	What does the nurse think the problem is?
Recommendation	What should we do to correct the problem?

SBAR, Situation, background, assessment, and recommendation. From Institute for Healthcare Improvement: *SBAR Toolkit*, 2014.Retrieved from *www.ihi.org/knowledge/pages/tools/sbartoolkit.aspx*.

TABLE 10-4 ANTICipate Model

ELEMENTS	DESCRIPTION
Administrative data	Name, record number, location
New clinical information to be updated	Real-time information
Tasks to be performed	Must be clearly explained
Illness severity	Must be communicated
Contingency	Plans for change in clinical status

From Agency for Healthcare Research and Quality: *PSNet Patient Safety Primer*, 2012. Retrieved from *www.psnet.ahrq.gov/primer.aspx?primerID=9*.

p. 1). SBAR is often used by nursing as a hand-off tool and as a structured method for all communications between providers.

The SBAR model, not unlike the nursing process, begins with the active situation, the related background, the assessment of the problem, and a recommendation for a solution. "SBAR offers a simple way to help standardize communication and allows parties to have common expectations related to what is to be communicated and how the communication is structured" (Institute for Healthcare Improvement, 2014).

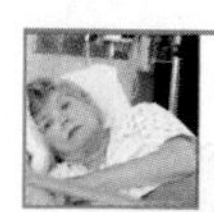

3. The nurse needs to call the primary care provider to renew Mrs. Schmidt's pain medication. Develop a SBAR report for this call.

Another hand-off mechanism, endorsed by the Agency for Healthcare Research and Quality (AHRQ), is the **ANTICipate model** (Table 10-4). For a safe and effective hand-off, administrative data *(A)* must be accurate; new clinical information *(N)* must be updated; tasks *(T)* performed by the provider must be clearly explained; illness *(I)* severity must be communicated; and contingency plans *(C)* for changes in clinical status must be outlined to assist cross-coverage of the patient overnight (AHRQ, 2012). Research is being conducted to identify the most effective methods for patient hand-offs.

Use of EHRs supports development of a standardized and integrated shift report to facilitate better communication of significant information. When documentation is completed electronically at the point of care, the potential for errors and omitted information is decreased. A hand-off report can be printed that is specifically designed to address all pertinent information for a patient assignment. Strople and Ottani (2006) found that using electronic systems in this process ensured a more effective and efficient shift report centered on patients' needs. Even with computerized systems, nurses should continue to ask questions and seek additional information for handoff reports.

QSEN FOCUS!

Teamwork and collaboration are demonstrated when the nurse appreciates the risks associated with hand-offs among providers and across transitions of care and follows communication practices that minimize those risks.

Patient safety issues are heightened when information is transferred during intrahospital transport. Some facilities have developed a structured "ticket-to-ride" communication tool that includes important information to ensure adequate care during transport and at the destination hospital. This process decreases the risk of adverse events while increasing patient satisfaction (Pesanka, Greenhouse, Rack, et al, 2009).

VERBAL AND TELEPHONE ORDERS LO 10.6

With the advent of EMRs, CPOEs, and widespread access to information technology, many facilities limit verbal or telephone orders to emergency situations. The primary care provider can access the EMR from a smartphone, hand-held device, or personal computer and enter or send orders directly to the appropriate department. This removes the nurse or unit secretary from the ordering process and decreases the possibility of error.

If a verbal or phone order is necessary in an emergency, the order must be taken by a registered nurse (RN) who repeats the order verbatim to confirm accuracy and then enters the order into the paper or electronic system, documenting it as a verbal or phone order and including the date, time, physician's name, and RN's signature. Most facility policies require the physician to cosign a verbal or telephone order within a defined time period.

INCIDENT REPORTS LO 10.7

When an unusual and unexpected event involving a patient, visitor, or staff member occurs, an incident report is completed. An incident may be the occurrence of a fall, a medication error, or an equipment malfunction. The purpose of this report is to document the details of the incident immediately to ensure accuracy. Incident reports are objective, nonjudgmental, factual reports of the occurrence and its consequences. The incident report is not part of a medical record but is considered a risk management or quality-improvement document. The fact that an incident report was completed is not recorded in the patient's medical record; however, the details of a patient incident are documented.

> **! SAFE PRACTICE ALERT**
>
> Incident reports, which are used in the risk management process, must include only facts, not suppositions or opinions.

SUMMARY OF LEARNING OUTCOMES

LO 10.1 *Identify the standards for effective documentation by nurses:* Standards for documentation should be in agreement with The Joint Commission's standards, the general principles of medical record documentation from the Centers for Medicare and Medicaid Services, and the ANA principles.

LO 10.2 *Discuss the functions of the medical record, including the electronic health record:* The medical record may be written or electronic. It is an accurate, comprehensive record of a patient's health care encounter and a major communication tool between health care providers.

LO 10.3 *List the important attributes of nursing documentation in the medical record:* Nursing documentation demonstrates nursing contributions to patient care and must be accurate, timely, comprehensive, and relevant.

LO 10.4 *Define* privacy *and* confidentiality *as they relate to information in a medical record:* Nurses must maintain the confidentiality and privacy of patients' personal health information.

LO 10.5 *Describe standardized formats for use in hand-off reports and change-of-shift reports:* Nurses must be able to determine the critical information necessary to ensure patient safety when communicating with other nurses and other health care professionals. Use of standardized formats for hand-offs and shift reports helps to ensure the accurate exchange of pertinent information.

LO 10.6 *Explain the process of accepting verbal and telephone orders:* Only RNs can accept a verbal or telephone order, and they must immediately enter the order into the paper or electronic record.

LO 10.7 *Discuss the proper use of incident reports:* Incident reports are factual accounts of an incident involving a patient, visitor, or staff member that are not part of the medical record.

Responses to the critical-thinking questions are available at *http://evolve.elsevier.com/YoostCrawford/fundamentals/*.

REVIEW QUESTIONS

1. The hospital has just implemented the use of electronic health records (EHRs). While learning to use this new system, the nurse realizes that EHRs may do which of the following?
   a. Limit access to the patient record to one person at a time
   b. Improve access to client information at the point of care
   c. Negate the use of nursing documentation
   d. Increase the potential for medication errors

2. Which statement best contributes to the nurse's documentation of assessment of patient status in the patient's medical chart?
   a. "Patient had a good day with minimal complaints. Patient was pleasant and cooperative during morning care."
   b. "Patient complained that the nurse didn't come quickly enough when she pressed the call button."
   c. "Patient complained of pain 7 of 10 at 7:45 A.M. Received pain medication at 8 A.M., reporting pain 3 of 10 at 8:30 A.M."
   d. "Patient was grumpy today, even after administration of pain medication, a back massage, and a nap."

3. A patient requests a copy of his medical record. What is the correct response by the nurse?
   a. Inform him that his record is the property of the facility and cannot be accessed by anyone but staff.
   b. Tell him that the Code for Nurses does not allow you to give him access to his records.
   c. Acknowledge that he has the right to have a copy his records, and make arrangements per facility policy.
   d. Refer his request to the hospital administrator since all such requests need to go through proper channels.
4. A patient's sister comes to visit and asks to read the patient's chart. What is the best response by the nurse?
   a. Settle her in a chair at the nurses' station and give her the chart.
   b. Respond that the contents of a patient's chart are private and confidential.
   c. Tell her she can read the chart only if the patient sits with her.
   d. Distract the sister by changing the subject and then walking away.
5. Which are reasons that accurate documentation in the medical record is important? *(Select all that apply.)*
   a. Reimbursement for care
   b. Evidence of care provided
   c. Communication between health care providers
   d. Nonlegal documentation of a nurse's actions
   e. Promotion of continuity of care
6. Which note is an example of the *S* in SBAR?
   a. Patient resting; 1 hour after receiving narcotic analgesic pain was rated 3 of 10
   b. Patient was admitted on evening shift with a fractured right femur after a fall at home.
   c. Patient's pain was rated 8 of 10 before administration of narcotic pain medication.
   d. Assess pain ever 2 hours, continue pain medication as prescribed, and provide backrub.
7. Which attributes are important in nursing documentation? *(Select all that apply.)*
   a. Inconsequentiality
   b. Timeliness
   c. Relevancy
   d. Accuracy
   e. Factual basis
8. When should administered medications be documented?
   a. At the end of a shift when all meds have been given
   b. As given to avoid the possibility of double dosing
   c. After every meal to document at least three times daily
   d. In pencil to allow for changes to be made
9. What is an advantage of the use of paper medical records?
   a. Charts with paper records are always available to all health care team members.
   b. Paper records do not need much storage space in the health care facility.
   c. Recording on paper does not require any special computer knowledge.
   d. Writing implements are always available on nursing units and patient rooms.
10. What is a purpose of a hand-off report?
    a. Ensures continuity of care and patient safety
    b. Keeps the doctor informed
    c. Completed when a patient is discharged to his home
    d. Determines patient assignments

ⓔ Answers and rationales for the review questions are available at *http://evolve.elsevier.com/YoostCrawford/fundamentals/*.

REFERENCES

Agency for Healthcare Research and Quality (AHRQ): *Patient safety and quality: An evidence-based handbook for nurses,* Rockville, Md., 2008, Author.

Agency for Healthcare Research and Quality (AHRQ): PSNet patient safety primer, 2012. Retrieved from *www.psnet.ahrq.gov/primer.aspx?primerID=9.*

American Nurses Association (ANA): *Principles for documentation,* ed. 2, Silver Spring, Md., 2010, Author.

Boutwell A, Frankel R: Patient handoffs can always be improved. *Healthc Risk Manage,* 28(9), 105-107, 2009.

Center for Democracy and Technology: Summary of health privacy provisions in the 2009 economic stimulus legislation. Retrieved from *www.cdt.org/files/healthprivacy/20090324_ARRAPrivacy.pdf.*

Centers for Medicare and Medicaid Services: *Evaluation and management services guide,* Washington, D.C., 2010, U. S. Department of Health and Human Services.

Chaudhry B, Wang J, Wu S, et al.: Systemic review: Impact of health information technology on quality, efficiency and costs of medical care. *Ann Intern Med,* 144(10):E12-E22, 2006.

Cronenwett L, Sherwood G, Barnsteiner J, et al: Quality and safety education for nurses. *Nurs Outlook,* 55(3):122-131, 2007.

Federwisch A: Passing the Baton: Bedside shift report ensures quality handoff. *NurseWeek Calif* 20(21):14, 2007.

Hentschke P: 24-hour rehabilitation nursing: The proof is in the documentation. *Rehabil Nurs,* 34:128-132, 2009.

Hillestad R, Bigelow J, Bower A, et al: Can electronic medical records systems transform health care? Potential health benefits, savings, and costs. *Health Affairs,* 24(5):1103-1117, 2005.

Institute for Healthcare Improvement. SBAR toolkit, 2014. Retrieved from *www.ihi.org/knowledge/pages/tools/sbartoolkit.aspx.*

Iver P: SBAR. *Med Legal News,* 31:1, 2007.

The Joint Commission: National patient safety goals, 2014a. Retrieved from *http://www.jointcommission.org/assets/1/6/HAP_NPSG_Chapter_2014.pdf.*

The Joint Commission: Sentinel event statistics, 2010. Retrieved from *www.jointcommission.org/search/default.aspx?Keywords=Sentinel+event+statistics&f=sitename&sitename=Joint+Commission.*

The Joint Commission: Facts about the official "Do Not Use" list of abbreviations, 2014b. Patient safety fact sheets. Retrieved from *http://www.jointcommission.org/facts_about_the_official_/.*

The Joint Commission: Sentinel event definition, 2014c. Retrieved from *www.jointcommission.org/sentinel_event.aspx.*

Pesanka DA, Greenhouse PK, Rack LL, et al: Ticket to ride: Reducing handoff risk during hospital patient transport. *J Nurs Care Qual,* 24:109-115, 2009.

Rutherford M: Standardized nursing language: What does it mean for nursing practice? *Online J Issues Nurs,* 13(1), 2008.

Strople B, Ottani P: Can technology improve intershift report? What the research reveals. *J Prof Nurs,* 22(3):197-203, 2006.

U.S. House of Representatives: *H.R. 629 (Report No. 111-7, Part I).* Washington, D.C., 2009, U.S. Government Printing Office. Retrieved from *www.gpo.gov/fdsys/pkg/BILLS-111hr629rh/pdf/BILLS-111hr629rh.pdf.*

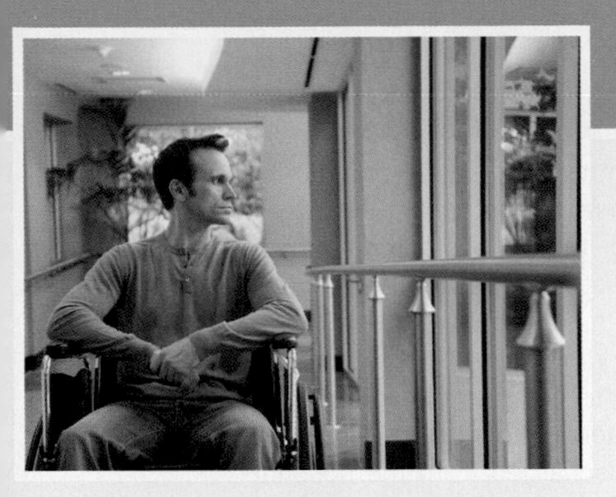

CHAPTER 11

Ethical and Legal Considerations

EVOLVE WEBSITE

http://evolve.elsevier.com/YoostCrawford/fundamentals/

- Additional Evolve-Only Review Questions With Answers
- Answers and Rationales for Text Review Questions
- Answers to Critical-Thinking Questions
- Case Study With Questions
- Glossary

LEARNING OUTCOMES

Comprehension of this chapter's content will provide students with the ability to:

LO 11.1 Identify key ethical theories that affect nursing practice.

LO 11.2 Apply ethical concepts to professional nursing practice.

LO 11.3 Describe how the American Nurses Association (ANA) Code of Ethics for Nurses applies to nursing education and practice.

LO 11.4 Recognize the role of ethics in genetic, biomedical, and end-of-life health care decision making.

LO 11.5 Discuss the legal implications of nursing practice.

LO 11.6 Differentiate among constitutional, statutory, regulatory, and case laws as they relate to professional nursing practice.

LO 11.7 Identify various types of statutory law, including intentional and unintentional torts, and their potential effect on nurses providing patient care.

LO 11.8 Explain liability issues such as professional boundaries, delegation, and documentation that are pertinent to nursing practice.

LO 11.9 Summarize the legal issues that guide patient care.

LO 11.10 Describe the effect of federal and state laws on nursing practice.

KEY TERMS

accountability, p. 145
advance directives, p. 156
advocacy, p. 145
assault, p. 152
assisted suicide, p. 160
autonomy, p. 145
battery, p. 152
beneficence, p. 145
bioethics, p. 148
case law, p. 151
civil law, p. 151
civility, p. 148
code of ethics, p. 147
confidentiality, p. 145
constitutional law, p. 150
criminal law, p. 151
defamation of character, p. 152
deontology, p. 144
do-not-resuscitate (DNR) order, p. 157
durable power of attorney, p. 156
ethics, p. 144
euthanasia, p. 146
false imprisonment, p. 152
felony, p. 151
fidelity, p. 146
futile care, p. 149
health care proxy, p. 156
informed consent, p. 155
intentional torts, p. 151
invasion of privacy, p. 152
justice, p. 146
libel, p. 152
living will, p. 156
malpractice, p. 153
misdemeanor, p. 151
negligence, p. 152
nonmaleficence, p. 146
nurse practice act, p. 151
regulatory law, p. 151
responsibility, p. 146
slander, p. 152
standards of care, p. 157
statutory law, p. 151
torts, p. 151
unintentional torts, p. 152
utilitarianism, p. 144
veracity, p. 146

CASE STUDY

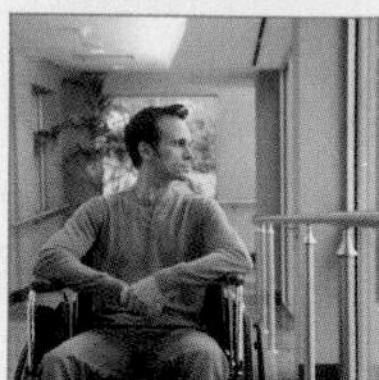

Mr. Finch is a single, 27-year-old, paraplegic veteran. He was injured 8 months earlier while riding in a jeep that hit a roadside bomb. On returning home from his military service, he began rehabilitation and has been learning to adapt to life confined to a wheelchair. Mr. Finch uses a straight catheter to empty his urinary bladder three or four times each day. He was admitted to the hospital yesterday for treatment of a persistent urinary tract infection. When asked, Mr. Finch states that he "prefers to be called Tom." He answers questions abruptly with one-word responses and expresses a lack of trust in his physicians and nurses.

Tom has a high school sweetheart to whom he is engaged, and she visits him each evening after work. During the day, Tom makes an occasional sexually suggestive remark to his 24-year-old, female registered nurse. Tom asks the nurse for her personal contact information and permission to call her for help with his care after he is discharged from the hospital.

Refer back to this case study to answer the critical-thinking questions throughout the chapter.

High ethical and legal standards must be maintained within professional nursing practice to ensure safe and comprehensive patient care. It is the responsibility of every nurse to be familiar with the rights of patients and with the ethical and legal requirements of professional nursing. To provide safe and compassionate patient care, nurses must base their decisions and actions on the ethical and legal standards of care, current clinical facility policies, and evidence-based practice guidelines.

Nurses are consistently considered to be honest and ethical professionals by most respondents in an annual Gallup poll (Gallup, 2014). This designation carries with it significant responsibility. Nurses are required to advocate for patients and their families and build trusting relationships. Professional nurses are encouraged to model healthy lifestyle choices and work for equal health care access for all individuals in their communities. By focusing on the needs of others and maintaining a commitment to excellence, nurses maintain high ethical and legal standards of care.

ETHICS AND ETHICAL THEORIES LO 11.1

The study of **ethics** considers the standards of moral conduct in a society. Personal ethics are influenced by values, societal norms, and practices (Burkhardt and Nathaniel, 2014). Family, friends, beliefs, education, culture, and socioeconomic status influence the development of ethical behavior. Behaviors that are judged as ethical or unethical, right or wrong, reflect a person's character.

ETHICAL THEORIES

Decision making in health care is influenced by theories that view ethical behavior from a variety of philosophical perspectives. Personal ethical dilemmas arise when values conflict and individuals are required to make choices among equally undesirable alternatives. For instance, when a middle-aged patient who does not believe in organ transplantation is diagnosed with chronic renal failure, the patient may need to (1) decide to begin hemodialysis treatments three times per week indefinitely, which will significantly limit the patient's ability to work full time and travel, (2) accept impending death without treatment, or (3) undergo kidney transplantation. None of these three options is without significant consequences, and at least one of them is in direct opposition to the patient's values. A nurse's ability to empathize with patients and families who are faced with challenging health care decisions is enhanced by the nurse's knowledge of ethical theories and their potential impact on behavior.

Deontology

Deontology is an ethical theory that stresses the rightness or wrongness of individual behaviors, duties, and obligations without concern for the consequences of specific actions (Aiken, 2015). Immanuel Kant, an 18th-century German philosopher, developed many aspects of deontologic theory. With its focus on duty, deontology is the foundation of most professional codes of ethics, including the Code of Ethics for Nurses (Burkhardt and Nathaniel, 2014). Meeting the needs of patients while maintaining their right to privacy, confidentiality, autonomy, and dignity is consistent with the tenets of deontology.

Kant believed that the ethical rules of deontology were consistent and could be understood by all rational individuals (Burkhardt and Nathaniel, 2014). However, Kant's assertion that moral rules were applicable to all people, all of the time, and in every situation is particularly challenging in a modern, multicultural society. His rigid, universal conceptualization of deontologic theory is difficult to apply in complex situations. For instance, when a patient is sedated and decisions need to be made regarding care, should the nurse act on what the nurse knows to be the desire of the patient, or is the nurse obligated to listen to a spouse whose wishes conflict with those of the patient?

Utilitarianism

Compared with deontology, utilitarianism is on the opposite end of the ethical theory continuum. **Utilitarianism** maintains that behaviors are determined to be right or wrong solely on the basis of their consequences (Aiken, 2015). The father of modern utilitarianism is Jeremy Bentham, a political philosopher of the late 18th century. Bentham's work was further developed by John Stuart Mill, a 19th-century British moral philosopher who posited the principle of *greatest happiness.* The utilitarian concept of greatest happiness maintains that the right action is one that brings the greatest happiness to the most people (Mill, 1910). "The end justifies the means" is a phrase that expresses the essence of pure utilitarianism. Unlike the rigidity of deontology, utilitarianism views actions as neither right nor wrong without knowing how they benefit the greater good or society. Advocates of utilitarian thought tend to be highly concerned with social justice while exhibiting resistance to rules and regulations (Aiken, 2015).

Decision making in health care based on pure utilitarianism becomes challenging when the individual rights of patients are inconsistent with the needs of society. For example, a cancer patient may be asked to participate in the trial of a new chemotherapy regimen. Although society may benefit from information gained during the drug trial, the patient undergoing treatment may react violently to the medication and become more ill. In this case, which action is best? Should the nurse support the patient's participation in the drug trial so that many people may benefit from the findings of the study, or should the nurse support the patient's right to refuse treatment because it may cause him additional suffering?

Although many additional ethical theories exist, most are variations of deontology or utilitarian thought. Although theoretical approaches to ethical dilemmas vary widely, the essential ethical concepts on which each theory is based are fundamentally the same.

ESSENTIAL CONCEPTS OF ETHICS IN NURSING LO 11.2

Nursing practice requires ethical decision making on a consistent basis. Nurses make judgments about patients' rights and benefits in many situations. Becoming familiar with essential ethical concepts can help nurses understand how values and morals impact patient care.

AUTONOMY

A patient who makes independent health care decisions is demonstrating autonomy. **Autonomy**, or self-determination, is the freedom to make decisions supported by knowledge and self-confidence. Nurses promote autonomy when they include patients in the process of developing care plans with realistic goals and interventions.

Nurses demonstrate personal autonomy in many different situations. When nurses stand up for their beliefs in critical situations or pursue continuing education without being required to do so, they are acting autonomously. Autonomy is a defining characteristic of a well-adjusted, independent adult.

ACCOUNTABILITY

Accountability is the willingness to accept responsibility for one's actions. Accountability is required to provide safe patient care and address potential problems. Accountability is a personal attribute that does not require the encouragement of others to be expressed. A nurse who is accountable readily admits to actions without having to be questioned by others.

An important aspect of accountability is tested when a nurse inadvertently makes a mistake. A nurse who is being accountable reports the error and takes responsibility to ensure patient safety, regardless of the personal consequences. Nurses who exhibit accountability are honest, accept the consequences of their actions, and initiate best nursing practices based on current evidence-based research.

ADVOCACY

Supporting or promoting the interests of others or of a cause greater than ourselves defines **advocacy**. Patient advocacy is an essential aspect of nursing. A nurse is ethically required to advocate for the rights of all patients, including those who are unable to express themselves and those with whom the nurse disagrees philosophically. Advocacy is an important aspect of collaboration and coordination of patient care. Frequently, nurses must contact various referral agencies and network with several health care professionals to meet patient needs. The process of advocacy requires nurses to focus on patients' needs and benefits.

BENEFICENCE

In its simplest form, **beneficence** can be defined as doing good. Nurses demonstrate beneficence by acting on behalf of others and placing a priority on the needs of others rather than on personal thoughts and feelings. Nursing practice is motivated by the concept of beneficence. Nurses are socialized to focus on patient needs and concerns, even if they differ significantly from those of the nurse. One of the most challenging situations in which beneficence must take precedence over a nurse's personal feelings occurs when a nurse is assigned to care for an incarcerated murderer or rapist. The ethical concept of beneficence necessitates providing care for the prisoner without reproach. Nurses are required by beneficence to provide compassionate care for all people in all circumstances.

CONFIDENTIALITY

Confidentiality is the ethical concept that limits sharing private patient information. Maintaining the confidentiality of patient information means that its disclosure is limited to authorized individuals and agencies. Confidentiality is the cornerstone of a nurse-patient relationship in which trusting, unguarded communication takes place.

All health care professionals are required by law to maintain the confidentiality of patient information. This protects patients from being ridiculed or judged inappropriately on the basis of personal information. Confidentiality also protects patients from being denied jobs or benefits because of their health care history.

Due to the critical nature of confidentiality and patient care, this concept is discussed throughout the textbook in relation to various aspects of patient care. The Health Insurance Portability and Accountability Act (HIPAA) is explored in detail later in this chapter.

FIDELITY

Keeping promises or agreements made with others constitutes **fidelity**. In nursing, fidelity is essential for building trusting relationships with patients and their families. Fidelity in relationships with colleagues is necessary to ensure comprehensive care. When a nurse acknowledges a patient's request for pain medication, assesses the patient's pain level and quality, and returns within a few minutes with the analgesic medication, the nurse is demonstrating the ethical concept of fidelity. Following through on promises is a critical factor in establishing strong professional relationships with patients and their families.

JUSTICE

To do **justice** is to act fairly and equitably. Although justice may seem easy to achieve, the concept is often challenging to apply in health care. Human, material, and financial resources are limited. Many patients may deserve the attention of a nurse simultaneously, which requires the nurse to prioritize. While a nurse is caring for one patient, others may feel that their needs are being ignored.

Justice mandates that all people be treated impartially. Fairness implies that all individuals should have ready access to health care regardless of their ability to pay. However, how are the costs of health care to be covered? Is it fair for some to bear the burden of care for all?

Organ donation is another challenging issue in health care justice. Many potential recipients are in need of transplants, but a limited number of organs are available for transplantation. How can fair decisions be made regarding who will receive the limited number of donor organs? As with many ethical concepts, justice is important but difficult to apply universally.

NONMALEFICENCE

First, do no harm is the colloquial definition of **nonmaleficence**. Unlike beneficence, which requires actively doing good, nonmaleficence requires only the avoidance of harm. It is a fundamental ethical mandate for all health care professionals. The phrase *do no harm* appears in the original Hippocratic oath describing the ethical practice of medicine. Nonmaleficence requires nurses to provide compassionate care for all patients, especially those who are undergoing painful medical interventions developed to cure debilitating diseases. Nurses are often required to weigh the benefits of medical treatments with their risks and potential harm to patients.

The ethical concept of nonmaleficence is challenged most when health care professionals are involved in end-of-life decisions. Some health care professionals may contend that **euthanasia** (act of painlessly ending the life of another) is murder. Others believe that patients should have the autonomy to make their own decisions regarding end-of-life care, including the option of a painless death facilitated by a health care professional. This issue has ethical and legal implications for nursing practice. Does hospice care, which is endorsed by nurses as an appropriate and holistic approach to end-of-life care, border on euthanasia because it includes withholding extreme medical treatment? Alternatively, is hospice the most compassionate method of caring for individuals whose death, rather than life, would be extended if extreme medical interventions were implemented? Chapter 42 provides additional information on hospice care.

RESPONSIBILITY

Responsibility is the concept of being dependable and reliable. A nurse who is responsible adheres to professional standards of care, complies with institutional policies, meets requirements of continuing education, and follows the orders of physicians and nurse practitioners. The nature of responsibility depends on the specific role in which an individual is functioning. For example, the responsibilities of nurses caring for older adults are very different from those practicing in the delivery room. Each nurse has specific responsibilities to fulfill to adequately meet the requirements of individual patient care.

VERACITY

Truthfulness defines the ethical concept of **veracity**. Honesty promotes unrestricted communication among individuals, demonstrates respect for others, and builds trust. Veracity is considered a virtue by deontologic and utilitarian philosophers. Challenges to this ethical ideal arise when nurses are faced with situations in which individuals perceive the truth as potentially harmful. For example, some family members of a seriously ill patient may prefer that the patient not be told about a poor prognosis. Keeping secrets from patients is in direct conflict with the ethical concepts of autonomy and veracity. Withholding information violates a patient's rights, and it may permanently damage the nurse-patient relationship if the patient discovers the truth. Opposing the wishes of well-intentioned family members can be extremely difficult. However, as with all ethical decisions, nurses must carefully weigh the potential benefits and risks of their actions.

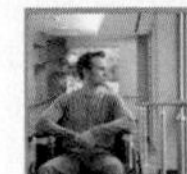

1. Name four ethical concepts that, when implemented by the RN, will help Mr. Finch establish trust in his health care providers.

CODES OF ETHICS LO 11.3

A **code of ethics** is a formalized statement that defines the values, morals, and standards guiding practice in a specific discipline or profession. These principles should be reflected in the actions of professionals in a particular group. Codes of ethics delineate group expectations and identify specific behaviors that are required by members. Ethical codes promote behavior that is of a higher standard than is required by law.

HISTORY

The foundation of ethical codes of professional conduct for nurses is the original Nightingale Pledge, which was written in 1893 by Lystra Gretter, a nurse educator, to be recited by nursing graduates at their commencement. The Nightingale Pledge was an adaptation of the Hippocratic oath for physicians.

The first official Nursing Code of Ethics was adopted in 1950 by the American Nurses Association (ANA). It evolved from earlier documents, formulated as early as 1896, by American and Canadian nurses who were members of precursor organizations to the ANA (Fowler, 2010). Periodic revisions are made to the Nursing Code of Ethics in response to societal changes and evolution of the professional role of nurses.

CODE OF ETHICS FOR NURSES

The current nursing code, the Code of Ethics for Nurses with Interpretive Statements, was published in 2015. It includes a glossary of terms and links to support documents that provide a foundation for the Code. The Code of Ethics for Nurses is "a succinct statement of the ethical values, obligations, duties, and professional ideals of nurses individually and collectively," the profession's "nonnegotiable ethical standard," and "an expression of nursing's own understanding of its commitment to society" (ANA, 2015, p. viii). The nursing code identifies nine basic provisions under which nursing practice is to take place. In the complete Code of Ethics for Nurses, specific professional expectations such as respect for others, advocacy, and a commitment to the rights of patients, families, and groups are described under each of the basic provisions.

Provision 1.5 states, "Respect for persons extends to all individuals with whom the nurse interacts. Nurses maintain professional, respectful, and caring relationships with colleagues, and are committed to fair treatment, transparency, integrity-preserving compromise, and the best resolution of conflicts" (ANA, 2015, p. 4). The provision continues by saying, "This standard of conduct includes an affirmative duty to act to prevent harm. Disregard for the effects of one's actions on others, bullying, harassment, intimidation, manipulation, threats, or violence are always morally unacceptable behaviors" (p. 4). It is expected that nurses (including student nurses) will not engage in behaviors that show "disregard for the effect of one's actions on others." This is a powerful mandate for all nurses to communicate and act professionally to prevent inflicting physical or emotional pain on others while pursuing nursing education and engaging in nursing practice.

Responsibility of Nurse Educators

The responsibilities of nursing faculty are addressed specifically in the Code of Ethics for Nurses. Nurse educators are required to advise and supervise their students. Faculty members are expected to collaborate with students to identify individual learning needs in the clinical setting and facilitate the educational process. According to the Code of Ethics for Nurses, faculty members share responsibility and accountability for the patient care provided by their students (Figure 11-1).

Nurse educators are required to instill in students the values and professional standards of nursing. Faculty members are expected to enhance student commitment to all ethical concepts and to socialize nursing students in the fundamental requirements of the profession. Expecting nursing students to meet professional standards while pursuing their education is a primary responsibility of nursing faculty.

Provision 3.3 of the Code of Ethics for Nurses states that, "... professional nursing is a process of education

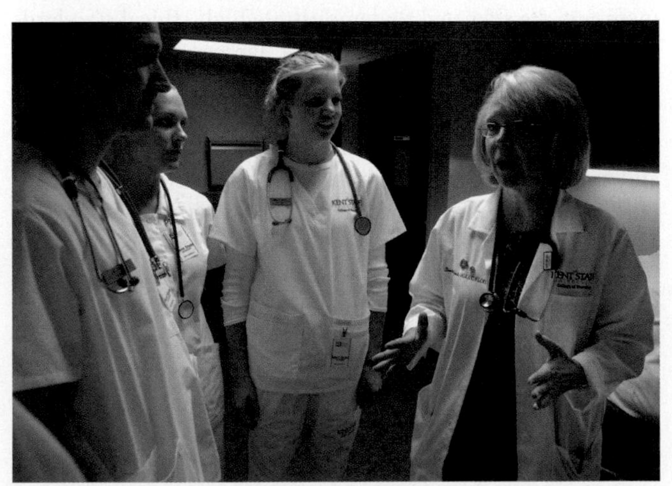

FIGURE 11-1 Nursing faculty members advise and support student learning in the clinical setting. (From Bob Christy, Kent State University, Kent, Ohio.)

and formation . . . that involves the ongoing acquisition and development of the knowledge, skills, dispositions, practice experiences, commitment, relational maturity, and personal integrity essential for professional practice. Nurse educators, whether in academics or direct care settings, must ensure that basic competence and commitment to professional standards exist prior to entry into practice" (ANA, 2015, p. 11).

Responsibility of Student Nurses

Student nurses are held to the same ethical standards as professional nurses. This requires that students pursuing nursing education behave responsibly and respectfully toward all people, be accountable for their actions, develop professionally, and strive to learn all that is necessary to safely care for patients and their families. In 2001, the National Student Nurses Association adopted the Code of Academic and Clinical Conduct, in which students agree to "promote the highest level of moral and ethical principles" and "promote an environment that respects human rights, values, and choice of cultural and spiritual beliefs."

Nursing is a difficult discipline requiring that students be committed to excellence, compassion, and integrity. Preparing to be responsible for the lives of others requires nursing students to be disciplined in their studies and practice communication and clinical skills with which students in other academic majors are not concerned. Students can successfully meet the professional standards expected by the Code of Ethics for Nurses by attending class, laboratories, and clinical experiences regularly; studying and practicing skills; and actively seeking to apply concepts to patient care.

PROFESSIONAL ETHICAL STANDARDS IN THE ACADEMIC SETTING

Adhering to the ethical principles of nursing is a lifestyle commitment that may require significant or minimal personal behavior modification. Student nurses and faculty members are expected to demonstrate high ethical standards at all times—in the classroom, the laboratory, and clinical areas and during all electronic and interpersonal communication. If a peer is acting inappropriately, it is every student's responsibility to call the behavior to that student's attention and solicit the help of a faculty member if the student does not respond to peer intervention. Any form of cheating cannot be tolerated, because a student who engages in cheating may be unable to acquire the knowledge necessary to safely care for patients and their families. Faculty should be addressed with respect consistently, and students should expect to be treated with dignity and respect while being held to a high level of accountability by nurse educators.

Civility (acting politely) is essential in all interactions among faculty and nursing students. Respectful interaction between students and faculty members establishes professional communication patterns and affects the way in which students interact with patients. Nurse educators and students report instances of incivility in the education setting. Faculty members report student behaviors such as tardiness, inattentiveness (e.g., texting during class), disrespectful remarks, and more aggressive offenses. Students report being belittled or treated with disrespect by clinical staff, instructors, or classmates (Luparell, 2013). The Evidence-Based Practice and Informatics box describes the effects of incivility on nurse educators and students and lists methods for coping with uncivil situations. If nurses are to maintain high standards of ethical practice, adherence to those standards must begin in the academic setting and be applied in all professional, personal, and clinical encounters.

EVIDENCE-BASED PRACTICE AND INFORMATICS

Incivility in Nursing Education

Nurse educators and students who have been the victims of incivility report experiencing the following:

- Loss of sleep
- Increased stress and depression
- Feelings of powerlessness
- Decreased confidence

Strategies for use by nurse educators and students to cope with incivility in the academic setting include the following:

- Treat others respectfully on a consistent basis by avoiding nonverbal indications of frustration, refraining from talking about people who are not present, and using the terms *please* and *thank you* when making requests.
- Avoid escalating the problem. Talk with the perpetrator privately as quickly as possible after an act of incivility to gain a better understanding of the situation.
- Intervene professionally using appropriate conflict management strategies.

Adapted from Luparell S: Incivility in nursing education: Let's put an end to it, 2008. Retrieved from *www.nsna.org/Portals/0/Skins/NSNA/pdf/Imprint_AprMay08_Feat_Incivility.pdf.*

BIOETHICS CHALLENGES IN HEALTH CARE LO 11.4

Bioethics is the study of ethical and philosophical issues in biology and medicine. Bioethical dilemmas arise on a consistent basis in health care, and nurses are faced with such decisions throughout their practice. Patients often seek information regarding bioethical concerns from nurses. Changing mores within society and cultural differences among people require nurses and other health care professionals to consider alternatives that were previously unknown. Advances in scientific research, innovative treatments, and advanced technology have increased the bioethical issues in our society.

GENETIC TESTING

The ability to test individuals for potentially debilitating or fatal genetic diseases has increased significantly in the past decade. Genetic testing can assist in determining the likelihood of disorders such as cystic fibrosis, Huntington disease, and breast cancer. On the basis of the outcome of genetic testing, individuals may decide to abort an abnormally developing fetus, choose not to have children to avoid passing on a serious genetic disorder, or have preventive surgery such as a prophylactic mastectomy to prevent breast cancer. None of these decisions is easily made. All have an ethical component and require the support of a professional counselor, loved ones, and friends to decide what is best in each unique circumstance.

The results of genetic testing may indicate the existence or future development of a severely debilitating or fatal disorder, or genetic testing may identify only the potential for development of a serious disease. Both circumstances make decisions based solely on genetic test results difficult. How does a person decide whether to have a bilateral prophylactic mastectomy on the basis of genetic testing when medical research does not clearly identify best practice? As is evident, such types of decisions require time and counseling from professionals and health care team members who are familiar with possible options for care.

CLONING AND EMBRYONIC STEM CELL RESEARCH

Cloning of organs and embryonic stem cell research are extremely controversial ethical issues faced by nurses practicing in various specialty areas. The ability to grow cloned organs and tissues that can be transplanted into humans in acute need of surgery is a major scientific accomplishment. Embryonic stem cell research has the potential to save lives through the development of effective treatment or cures for disorders such as severe spinal cord injury, Alzheimer disease, cystic fibrosis, and multiple sclerosis. However, ethical dilemmas exist worldwide among health care professionals, scientists, theologians, politicians, and others about what types of cells can be cloned or used for research, for what purposes, and by whom.

There are no clear solutions to these dilemmas. Responsible individuals who have studied all aspects of these issues differ greatly on how research should proceed. While research endeavors in cloning and embryonic stem cells offer great potential for reducing human suffering, ethical dilemmas and research requirements in these areas continue to evolve. Studying research issues in depth and completing values clarification (see Chapter 2) can help nurses to identify their feelings about controversial ethical topics.

END-OF-LIFE CARE

One of the greatest challenges in nursing is helping patients and families cope with end-of-life decisions that focus on quality-of-life issues. Due to cultural, spiritual, educational, and philosophical differences among people, these decisions are often emotionally charged and rarely based solely on intellectual knowledge. Two major roles of a nurse caring for a dying patient are (1) providing accurate information regarding the disease process and treatment options and (2) offering support for the patient and family without interjecting personal opinions. An essential ethical concept is autonomy, which underscores the importance of allowing patients to make their own health care decisions.

Ethical dilemmas in end-of-life care exist regarding the establishment of do-not-resuscitate (DNR) orders, adherence to living will and organ donation requests, removal of extraordinary measures already initiated, and continuance of **futile care** (i.e., care that is useless and prolongs the time until death rather than restoring life). End-of-life institutional policies and DNR order requirements guide individual nursing practice in these ethically challenging situations. Chapter 42 provides further discussion of issues related to the dying patient.

RESOURCE ALLOCATION AND ACCESS

The allocation of human and material resources and provision of access to those resources are major concerns for nurses. These bioethical challenges are evident when staffing levels for safe patient care are sought, when few organs are available for transplantation but many patients are awaiting life-saving transplants, and when lack of transportation or financial limitations prevents individuals from obtaining adequate health care.

Studies published in the *New England Journal of Medicine* and *Journal of the American Medical Association (JAMA)* indicate that increased staffing of registered nurses correlates with better patient care outcomes and fewer preventable postoperative patient deaths (Aiken, Clarke, Cheung, et al, 2003; Needleman, Buerhaus, Mattke, et al, 2002). The ANA supports the Registered Nurse Safe Staffing Act, which attempts to address the issues of patient safety and responsible, professional nursing practice. The economic limitations of hospitals and other health care facilities make providing safe staffing levels a challenge for nurse managers and hospital administrators. The need to decide between two equally undesirable situations underscores the ethical nature of adequate staffing.

Organ transplantation and the extensive number of decisions surrounding it raise endless ethical questions. If a patient who is a strong organ transplant candidate decides that the postoperative care is too extensive, is the patient allowed to die without undergoing the recommended transplantation? Who should undergo organ transplantation and based on what priorities? Should a person who has a history of alcoholism receive a liver transplant? Are there enough donor livers available for transplantation in a person who has been previously diagnosed with pancreatic cancer? Does a child with Down syndrome deserve to receive a much-needed heart transplant? Allocation of organs and decisions on when and how donor organs are to be assigned involve endless ethical decision making of multidisciplinary teams of health care professionals, including bioethicists.

Whether all clinical facilities should have expensive diagnostic equipment and where such resources should be located are ethical dilemmas. Should state-of-the-art diagnostic equipment be available only to patients who can pay for its use? With limited numbers of nurses and other health care professionals available to provide care, how many should be assigned to clinics for the uninsured? There are no easy answers to these concerns. Although some nurses might argue that no preference should be given to patients with greater financial resources, who will pay for new technologies and research if the patients with the greatest philanthropic potential are denied care while the uninsured receive extensive services? These types of ethical dilemmas and financial challenges have motivated great change in the health care system in recent years, requiring nurses to provide more care with fewer material resources.

ETHICAL DECISION MAKERS

All nurses are faced with ethical decisions each day in practice, and some choose to obtain further education and experience in the field of bioethics and participate on institutional ethics committees along with physicians, ethicists, attorneys, and academicians (Figure 11-2). Ethics committees are required by The Joint Commission (TJC), formerly the Joint Commission on the Accreditation of Healthcare Organizations (JCAHO), to respond to ethical challenges related to patient care requiring consultation. The work of the ethics committees in health care institutions helps to prevent unnecessary legal intervention in patient care matters. The Ethical, Legal, and Professional Practice box identifies the roles of ethics committees in clarifying health care dilemmas. If acceptable resolutions are not achieved through consultation with the ethics committee, patients, families, and health care providers, the legal system may become involved.

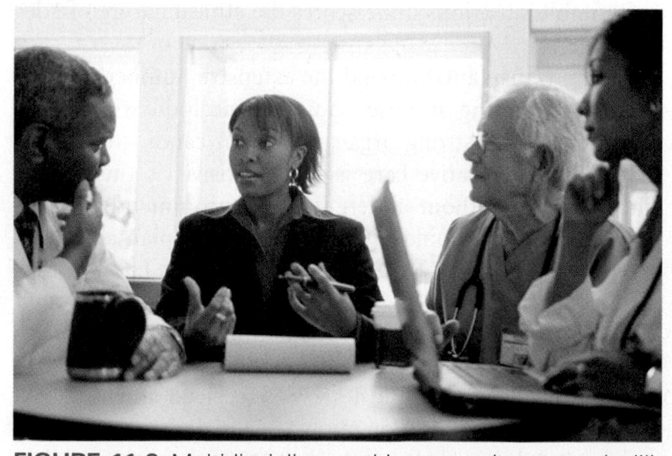

FIGURE 11-2 Multidisciplinary ethics committees work diligently to resolve bioethics dilemmas.

ETHICAL, LEGAL, AND PROFESSIONAL PRACTICE

The Role of Ethics Committees

The role of ethics committees in health care facilities is essential for providing equitable and legal patient care. Ethics committees

- Provide educational resources on ethical issues to committee members and institutional staff.
- Establish policies that govern health care decision making.
- Review cases in which clarity is needed.
- Identify sets of values relevant to cases requiring consultation.
- Determine any values conflicts that may exist.
- Interview key individuals impacting the case being reviewed.
- Provide unbiased input that is not possible from a patient, family members, or close caregivers.
- Clarify potential legal implications of the medical or nursing interventions.

LEGAL IMPLICATIONS IN NURSING PRACTICE LO 11.5

Laws delineate acceptable nursing practice, provide a basis on which many health care decisions are determined, and protect nurses from liability in cases in which safe practice is maintained. Each state has a nurse practice act that establishes the standards of care required for legal nursing practice. Licensure, laws, rules, and regulations governing nursing practice are enforced to protect the public from harm. Errors in health care occur too frequently. In many cases, the nurse is the last line of defense to prevent an error in medication administration or other types of patient care. Keeping current with changing laws related to nursing practice and technology can ensure safety for nurses and their patients.

SOURCES OF LAW IMPACTING PROFESSIONAL NURSING LO 11.6

There are four major sources of law: constitutional, statutory, regulatory, and case law (Judson and Harrison, 2012). Aspects of each type of law help to govern the practice of nursing.

CONSTITUTIONAL LAW

Constitutional law is derived from a formal, written constitution that defines the powers of government and the responsibilities of its elected or appointed officials. Constitutional law in the United States is based on the U.S. Constitution. Each state has a constitution that must be consistent with the U.S. Constitution. In the United States, constitutional law impacts nursing indirectly because the legislative bodies that enact statutory law are established and governed by the Constitution. The Bill of Rights and other amendments to the U.S. Constitution further identify the rights of individuals, such as freedom of speech and religion, that affect the ethical practice of nursing.

STATUTORY LAW

Statutory law is created by legislative bodies such as the U.S. Congress and state legislatures. Statutory laws are often referred to as *statutes.* State statutes should be consistent with all federal laws. Statutes governing health care, such as provisions for care of the uninsured and the actions that constitute child abuse, originally became law after they were introduced and passed as bills in a legislative body. Legislators introduce bills in Congress or state legislatures in response to the rapidly changing health care environment, nursing and medical research, and constituents' concerns.

Each state's legislature passes laws referred to collectively as a **nurse practice act** (NPA). The NPA defines the scope of nursing practice in the state. Matters pertaining to licensure, accreditation of schools and colleges of nursing, and professional roles are outlined in a state's NPA. It is the responsibility of all nurses to become familiar with the nurse practice act in the state of their residence and to adhere to the laws that govern practice.

REGULATORY LAW

State legislatures give authority to administrative bodies, such as state boards of nursing, to establish **regulatory law**, which outlines how the requirements of statutory law will be met. Nursing rules and regulations are categorized as regulatory law. Rules and regulations, written by members of boards of nursing, articulate how nurses practice within the laws of the state nurse practice act. The rules and regulations set the standards for safe practice.

Because of the evolving nature of medical and nursing knowledge, emerging technologies, and economic factors that impact health care, nurses must actively seek to keep current to avoid practicing illegally. Some of the nursing rules and regulations identify who is permitted to administer medications in various institutions, the procedure for reporting unsafe or unethical nursing practice, and the number of continuing education hours required for licensure.

> **! SAFE PRACTICE ALERT**
>
> Rules and regulations governing nursing practice are reviewed and revised on a regular basis. To stay current, nurses must read updates from their boards of nursing and seek continuing education in the legal aspects of nursing practice.

CASE LAW

Judicial decisions from individual court cases determine **case law**. Case law was historically referred to as *common law* because it originally was determined by customs or social mores that were common at the time. The decisions of cases used to be shared only orally by judges with one another (Judson and Harrison, 2012). In contemporary society, case law is established by judicial decisions based on the outcome of specific court cases. These court decisions are documented and published. They set legal precedents on which similar cases are decided in the future. The rights of patients to informed consent were established through case law.

TYPES OF STATUTORY LAW — LO 11.7

Statutory laws may be criminal or civil in nature. **Criminal law** is the body of state and federal laws written to prevent harm to the country, state, and individual citizens. Criminal laws define the nature of specific crimes and the required punishment. Federal criminal law violations include treason and kidnapping or serious offenses that occur across state borders. State criminal laws address crimes such as murder, rape, theft, and practicing nursing without a license (Judson and Harrison, 2012).

Depending on the nature of the committed crime, it may be designated as a misdemeanor or a felony. A **misdemeanor** is a crime of lesser consequence that is punishable by a fine or incarceration in a local or county jail for up to 1 year. A **felony** is a more serious crime that results in the perpetrator's being imprisoned in a state or federal facility for more than 1 year. Practicing nursing without a license, child abuse, and illegal drug dealing are examples of felonies. Felonies are classified by levels of seriousness. Class A felonies may result in punishment by death or life imprisonment.

Civil law governs unjust acts against individuals, rather than federal or state crimes. In civil law, court judgments require the payment of restitution in the form of services or money to the victim or family members. Lawsuits are filed under civil law for offenses such as defamation of character, slander, libel, invasion of privacy, negligence, or malpractice. Civil law includes a category of law known as **torts**, which are wrongs committed against another person that do not involve a contract. Torts against another person may cause injury, damage property, or infringe on an individual's personal rights. Torts can be classified as intentional or unintentional.

INTENTIONAL TORTS

Intentional torts are wrongs committed by individuals who deliberately seek to injure or hurt another person. It is imperative that nurses be familiar with intentional tort law to avoid acting irresponsibly while providing nursing care. Intentional torts may be committed by nurses and other individuals, including students, if they act in an unprofessional manner. Nurses should be particularly aware of intentional torts such as assault, battery, defamation of character, false imprisonment, and invasion of privacy.

Assault

Assault is a threat of bodily harm or violence caused by a demonstration of force by the perpetrator. A feeling of imminent harm or feeling of immediate danger must exist for assault to be claimed.

Battery

Actual physical harm caused to another person is **battery**. The threat to hurt someone is carried out. Battery may involve angry, forceful touching of people, their clothes, or anything attached to them (Guido, 2013). Performing a surgical procedure without informed consent is an example of battery. Actions much more subtle, such as inserting an intravenous catheter or urinary catheter against the will of a patient, also may be classified as battery.

> **! SAFE PRACTICE ALERT**
>
> Inform patients of procedures before initiating care. If there is any doubt about a patient's comprehension of a procedure, asking the patient to explain what is to be done will alert the nurse to any areas of ambiguity that need clarification and ensure patient understanding.

Defamation of Character

Defamation of character occurs when a public statement is made that is false and injurious to another person. Written forms of defamation of character are considered **libel**. Broadcasting or reading statements aloud that have the potential to hurt the reputation of another person is considered libel.

Oral defamation of character is **slander**. Slander is spoken information that is untrue, causing prejudice against someone or jeopardizing that person's reputation. For instance, if a nursing student says that a classmate cheated on an examination despite this being untrue, the student has committed slander. A nurse who falsely judges a patient as uncooperative or drug seeking and shares that information during a shift report may be charged with slander if the patient perceives that the nurse's accusations negatively influenced the patient's care.

> **! SAFE PRACTICE ALERT**
>
> Nurses must be careful when discussing information about patients and colleagues. As professionals, nurses are required to share only accurate information in writing and conversation. Nurses should avoid making judgmental statements while documenting or orally communicating information.

False Imprisonment

Unauthorized restraint or detention of a person is considered **false imprisonment**. Preventing patients from leaving a health care facility at their request may be considered false imprisonment (Judson and Harrison, 2012). To prevent health care providers and institutions from being held liable if a patient chooses to leave a facility when physicians and nurses think that it is in the patient's best interest to remain hospitalized, the patient is asked to sign an *against medical advice* (AMA) form. A signed AMA form documents that the patient has chosen to leave the facility when leaving could jeopardize the patient's condition.

Depending on the situation, physically restraining a patient may be considered false imprisonment and battery. Health care institutions are required to have procedures in place to document and allow temporary restraint of individuals who are mentally unstable or disoriented or who suffer from a contagious disease. Sometimes, the legal system must become involved to deem a patient incompetent, allowing the appointment of a temporary guardian.

Invasion of Privacy

Public disclosure of private information, use of a person's name or likeness without permission, intrusion into a person's place of solitude, and meddling into another's personal affairs are examples of **invasion of privacy**. Accessing the medical record of a patient for whom a nurse does not have the responsibility of providing care is an example of invasion of privacy. Other examples include making confidential information about anyone public without permission and asking patients specific information regarding their wills or personal affairs that do not directly affect nursing care.

> **! SAFE PRACTICE ALERT**
>
> Even sharing with others that a friend or colleague is hospitalized is an invasion of privacy if authorization to share that information publicly has not been secured. Asking a patient, "Is it all right if I share with others that you are hospitalized?" is an appropriate way to ask permission.

UNINTENTIONAL TORTS

Unintentional torts are omissions or acts by individuals that cause unintended harm. The unintentional torts of negligence and malpractice are charged when individuals, health care providers, or institutions fail to act responsibly, causing injury to others.

Negligence

Creating a risk of harm to others by failing to do something that a reasonable person would ordinarily do or doing something that a reasonable person would ordinarily not do constitutes **negligence**. For instance, if water is spilled on a hospital corridor floor, a reasonable person would recognize it as a potential fall hazard, seek to alert others to its presence, and have it cleaned up as quickly as possible. Nurses are held to the same standards as the public to avoid charges of simple negligence. Nurses, physicians, and other health care providers also are held to a higher standard due to the professional nature of their education and work.

Malpractice

Malpractice is negligence committed by a person functioning in a professional role. Malpractice may occur when a professional such as a nurse acts unethically, demonstrates deficient skills, or fails to meet standards of care required for safe practice. Examples of these types of malpractice include engaging in sexual activity with a patient; calculating medication dosages inaccurately, resulting in a patient's drug overdose; and administering penicillin to a patient with a documented penicillin allergy, resulting in the patient's death from a severe allergic (anaphylactic) reaction. Even if a physician or nurse practitioner inadvertently orders a medication to which the patient is allergic, it is the nurse's responsibility to check the patient's allergies before administering all medications to meet standards of care for safe practice. To avoid a charge of malpractice, a nurse must provide care commensurate with care provided by other nurses with similar levels of education and experience (Burkhardt and Nathaniel, 2014).

Judson and Harrison (2012) stress the four *D*s of negligence, which are four components that must exist to prove professional negligence or malpractice:

- *Duty:* It must be proved that the nurse or other health care provider owed a duty of care to the accusing patient.
- *Dereliction:* There must be evidence that the nurse's actions did not meet the standard of care required or that care was totally omitted.
- *Damages:* Actual injury to the accusing patient must be evident.
- *Direct cause:* A causal relationship must be established between harm to the accusing patient and the actions or omitted acts of the nurse.

Burden of proof (i.e., responsibility for establishing that the four Ds of negligence exist) lies with accusing patients and their attorneys. All health care professionals, including nurses, must remember that the intent to harm someone is not a requirement for malpractice. Good intentions are not a defense against malpractice.

Actions especially helpful in avoiding charges of malpractice include maintaining (1) current professional practice knowledge, (2) competent practice skills, and (3) professional relationships with patients and their families. Additional measures for practicing within the law are listed in Box 11-1.

All nurses should purchase professional malpractice insurance to provide legal support in the event that legal action is brought against them for any type of professional misconduct. Nursing students and faculty may be covered by the school's malpractice insurance during clinical experiences. However, practice outside an assigned clinical experience is typically not covered by an educational or health care institution's insurance policy, and every nurse and nursing student should obtain an individual malpractice insurance policy.

BOX 11-1 Guidelines for Professional Nursing Practice Within Legal Boundaries

In addition to maintaining current professional practice knowledge, competent practice skills, and professional relationships with patients and their families, nurses should follow guidelines to practice legally and avoid charges of malpractice:

- Maintain confidentiality.
- Follow legal and ethical guidelines when sharing information.
- Document promptly and accurately.
- Adhere to established institutional policies governing safety and procedures.
- Comply with legal requirements for handling and disposing of controlled substances.
- Meet licensure and continuing education requirements.
- Practice responsibly within the scope of personal capabilities, professional experience, and education.

PROFESSIONAL LIABILITY ISSUES LO 11.8

Three professional liability issues are of particular concern for nurses: (1) professional practice conduct, (2) adherence to the Principles for Delegation established by the ANA and legally binding within each state's nurse practice act, and (3) accurate and timely documentation.

PROFESSIONAL PRACTICE CONDUCT

Building and maintaining trusting relationships with patients and colleagues requires professional communication and competent practice. Focusing on the needs of patients and their families helps nurses to avoid crossing professional boundaries that breach patients' rights. Nurses are in a position of power due to their professional role and access to private patient information. In all patient care situations, it is imperative that nurses recognize their authority and take intentional steps to avoid misconduct.

High degrees of patient vulnerability and prolonged patient contact are two situations in which violations of professional boundaries tend to occur (Ohio Board of Nursing, 2009). The National Council of State Boards of Nursing (n.d.) recognizes specific nurse behaviors that indicate a potential for professional boundary violations, including the following:

- Engaging in excessive self-disclosure of personal information to a patient
- Keeping secrets with a patient; limiting others from conversation and patient information
- Spending excessive amounts of time with one patient
- Acting as if a patient is a family member or close personal friend
- Failing to protect the patient from inappropriate sexual involvement with the nurse

BOX 11-2 Boundary Issues That Violate Ethical and Legal Standards in Nursing

- Stealing a patient's property
- Personally gaining at a patient's expense
- Intervening in a patient's personal relationships
- Making seductive or sexually disparaging statements
- Engaging in sexual conduct with a patient or patient's family member

Examples of professional boundary violations are listed in Box 11-2.

Social Networking

Use of the Internet and social networking sites to exchange knowledge and share information has increased exponentially in recent years. Nursing students and nurses must understand their professional obligations associated with sharing online information. The ANA's *Principles for Social Networking and the Nurse* (2011) and the National Student Nurses' Association's *Recommendations for: Social media usage and maintaining privacy, confidentiality and professionalism (n.d.)* provide guidelines for online nursing practice and assist nurses and nursing students in understanding the limitations and consequences associated with violating online boundary issues.

In addition to professional boundary violations, nursing practice misconduct may include illegally obtaining patient medication (including narcotics), engaging in drug abuse, or practicing incompetently. All of these are serious offenses punishable by law.

Nurses must be alert to the potential for violating professional conduct standards in all patient care situations and act intentionally to avoid breaking the law or the Code of Ethics for Nursing. Nurses who engage in professional misconduct are subject to legal and disciplinary action in their state or jurisdiction. In addition to being charged with a misdemeanor or felony, depending on the seriousness of the action, nurses may have their nursing licenses permanently or temporarily taken away or restricted to allow only specific employment.

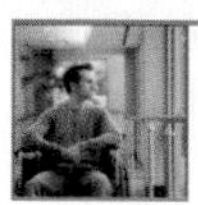

2. Identify a charge that could be made against the registered nurse if she engages in a social relationship with Mr. Finch that violates nursing standards of care.

ADHERENCE TO PRINCIPLES OF DELEGATION

Appropriate delegation by registered nurses seeks to ensure patient safety and meet nursing standards of care. The ANA (2013a) Principles for Delegation clearly delineate the basic nursing responsibilities related to delegation. The document is supplemental to each state's nurse practice act. Additional information on delegation is found in Chapter 12. All nurses must become familiar with and adhere to their specific state or jurisdictional requirements for delegation to prevent patient injury and legal action.

ACCURATE AND TIMELY DOCUMENTATION

Nurses are required to document patient information in written or electronic format. This documentation becomes the legal record of care provided by the nurse. Falsification of patient records is unethical and illegal.

Documentation must be accurate to provide a realistic view of a patient's condition. Serious documentation errors include (1) omitting documentation from patient records, (2) recording assessment findings obtained by another nurse or unlicensed assistive personnel (UAP), and (3) recording care not yet provided. Nurses sometimes document that a patient has received medication before its administration. This is a serious violation of the law and becomes a medication error of omission if the nurse is distracted before administering the patient's medication.

A second major legal concern related to documentation is the issue of timeliness. For patient care to proceed smoothly, nurses must record assessment findings and concerns as soon after their discovery as possible. Documentation of assessment data in a timely manner allows other health care professionals to accurately address a patient's concerns or change in status. For instance, if a nurse finds patient A's blood pressure and apical pulse elevated during the morning assessment but fails to document those findings before proceeding to another patient's room, the physician responsible for patient A's care may make rounds while the nurse is in the other patient's room and fail to realize patient A's change in condition. Nurses must always record patient findings as quickly and as accurately as possible to ensure safety and provide appropriate care. The use of an incident report for documenting unusual patient circumstances is discussed in Chapter 10, which also provides extensive guidelines that must be followed to meet the legal and ethical requirements for documentation.

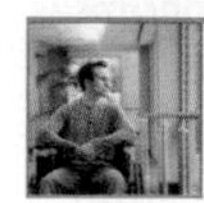

3. Write four interventions that the registered nurse should initiate to avoid crossing professional boundaries with Mr. Finch.

LEGAL ISSUES GUIDING PATIENT CARE LO 11.9

Some issues affect nursing practice regardless of the setting in which care is provided. To ensure safe and legal patient care, nurses need to be aware of their responsibilities in regard to informed consent, patients' rights, organ donation, advance directives, and DNR orders.

INFORMED CONSENT

Giving permission or consent for treatment is implied when a patient makes an appointment to see a physician or nurse practitioner. General consent forms giving permission for treatment in a hospital are signed by a patient before being admitted. Patients undergoing surgery and invasive diagnostic procedures are required to provide informed consent.

Informed consent is permission granted by a patient after discussing each of the following topics with the physician, surgeon, or advanced practice nurse who will perform the surgery or procedure: (1) exact details of the treatment, (2) necessity of the treatment, (3) all known benefits and risks involved, (4) available alternatives, and (5) risks of treatment refusal. Legal regulations mandating the content of an informed consent document and the procedure for obtaining informed consent are typically outlined in a state's medical practice act (Judson and Harrison, 2012). Ultimately, it is the responsibility of the physician (or advanced practice nurse in some states) who is performing the surgery or procedure to explain the content of the informed consent form and acquire the patient's signature. Nurses are usually asked to witness the patient's signing of the form. By witnessing a patient's signing of an informed consent, the nurse verifies that the patient is mentally competent and that the signature is that of the patient.

Informed consent for minors, except in the case of emancipated or married minors, must be obtained from their parents or legal guardians. Patients who are mentally incompetent or are under the influence of alcohol or drugs are not legally permitted to give informed consent due to their inability to comprehend the required information. Informed consent for these patients must be obtained from a legal guardian, power of attorney, or health care proxy. Securing informed consent from competent adults who have already received preoperative medications that may impair their ability to comprehend and make sound decisions is not permissible.

Acting as a patient advocate, the nurse is responsible for ensuring that the patient has received adequate information regarding the proposed procedure, understands the content of the informed consent form, and was not coerced into giving informed consent. Discussing the surgery or procedure with a patient and allowing the patient to ask questions and receive answers to any questions is an excellent method of ensuring that a patient's autonomy in decision making has been respected. Although physicians and nurses are allowed to make recommendations to patients regarding the necessity of treatment, coercing or forcing a patient to sign an informed consent form is not permitted (Burkhardt and Nathaniel, 2014).

QSEN FOCUS!

Intervening on behalf of a patient who needs additional information before giving informed consent is one method of providing safe, patient-centered care. Helping patients to locate high-quality electronic sources for health care information increases their health literacy and their ability to make informed health care decisions.

When obtaining informed consent, nurses must be concerned with the legal implications of a patient's ability to read the informed consent document and the patient's cultural beliefs regarding decision making. If a patient is illiterate or requires an interpreter, the method of obtaining informed consent must be adapted appropriately. Use of a professional interpreter rather than a family member is essential to provide detailed medical information accurately.

A patient whose culture prefers to allow other family members to make final health care decisions is inconsistent with nursing's ethical belief in autonomy. However, in this situation, the method of obtaining informed consent may need to be adapted to meet the patient's beliefs within the scope of the law. The solution may be as simple as providing information regarding the surgery or procedure to the patient and family members involved in the decision-making process and then verifying that adequate opportunity for asking questions and receiving clarification has been given.

PATIENT'S BILL OF RIGHTS

In 1992, the American Hospital Association (AHA) adopted the Patient's Bill of Rights to inform consumers of health care about specific privileges of which they should be aware. The original list of 12 rights has been revised and formatted as a brochure entitled *The Patient Care Partnership: Understanding Expectations, Rights and Responsibilities* (AHA, 2003). The brochure informs patients that they should expect (1) excellent care, (2) a safe environment, (3) participation in planning their care, (4) privacy, (5) help with discharge arrangements, and (6) assistance with fulfilling financial responsibilities.

QSEN FOCUS!

To provide patient-centered care, nurses need to discuss with patients the level to which they want to be involved in planning their care. Factors such as culture, age, level of education, cognitive ability, physical health, and energy affect a patient's ability and desire to actively participate in the process.

ORGAN DONATION

Organ donation is encouraged to address the tremendous need of individuals who are suffering from life-threatening illnesses and could benefit from organ transplantation. According to the United Network for Organ Sharing (UNOS), over 123,000 people in the United States were waiting for organ transplants in September, 2014. Only 11,845 organ transplantations of all types took place in the first 8 months of 2014. Organs for those procedures were received from 9565 deceased donors and 2280 living donors (UNOS, 2014). These statistics underscore the critical need for organ donation. The UNOS establishes the policies and procedures for obtaining and allocating donated organs to waiting recipients. The National Organ Transplant Act of 1984 made the sale or purchase of organs illegal in the United States.

In 1968, the Uniform Anatomical Gift Act was approved to allow people over the age of 18 to donate their bodies or body parts after death for transplantation, deposit in tissue banks, or research. Consent for organ donation must be given in writing. In many states, licensed drivers are permitted to sign organ donation forms on the back of their licenses. Adults who do not have a driver's license can obtain a separate organ donation card to carry in their wallets. However, having a signed form indicating the desire to be an organ donor is not enough in most states. Individuals must make their desire to donate organs known to family members before their death to ensure that their wishes are fulfilled. In some states, regardless of the existence of signed organ donation forms, final permission for organ and tissue donation must be received from family members of the deceased.

All nurses need to be aware of institutional policies and procedures for organ donation. Often, hospitals contact designated personnel who are specially trained in talking with family members about organ donation. These organ procurement professionals help in relaying vital information and facilitating the process of donation.

ADVANCE DIRECTIVES

In 1990, the federal government passed the Patient Self-Determination Act, which requires health care providers to supply all patients with written information regarding their rights to make medical decisions and implement advance directives (Judson and Harrison, 2012). **Advance directives** consist of three documents: (1) living will, (2) durable power of attorney, and (3) health care proxy, commonly referred to as a *durable power of attorney for health care.* It is the responsibility of nurses and other health care providers to document the existence of advance directives in patient's medical records. If a patient has signed and notarized advance directives, a copy of each document should be placed in the patient's medical record on admission to a health care facility.

Living Will

A **living will** specifies the treatment a person wants to receive when he or she is unconscious or no longer capable of making decisions independently. Specifications in a living will may address end-of-life care and the circumstances under which treatment should be withheld or stopped. A living will may indicate when a person wants to have extraordinary measures, such as cardiopulmonary resuscitation (CPR) or ventilator treatment, terminated. Preferences regarding organ donation, performance of an autopsy, and a designated spokesperson also may be specified in a living will.

All states recognize the legitimacy of living wills, although individuals need to communicate their wishes with family members and provide copies of their living wills to health care providers and family members as documentation of their preferences. The existence of a signed living will alleviates confusion and may help to avoid legal disputes regarding the care of loved ones.

Durable Power of Attorney

A **durable power of attorney** is a legal document that allows a designated person to make legal decisions on behalf of an individual unable or not permitted to make legal decisions independently. It sets limits on the powers of the person designated as having power of attorney and is not limited to matters related to medical care. Spouses, domestic partners, and attorneys are the most common people to be granted power of attorney.

Health Care Proxy

The specific durable power of attorney for medical care is called a **health care proxy**. This document specifies the person who can make health care decisions for an individual who is unable to comprehend information or communicate his or her wishes for any reason. The health care proxy limits the scope of power of the designated person or people to medical care and treatment decisions. One or more alternates should be named in the health care proxy document in case the primary designate is unavailable in an emergency. For U.S. residents, the Patient Education and Health Literacy box provides information on the process of completing advance directives and how to obtain advance directive forms.

PATIENT EDUCATION AND HEALTH LITERACY

Advance Directives

Completing advance directive forms is a process that involves personal reflection, information gathering, discussion with loved ones, decision making, and documentation of individual choices. State agencies and all health care facilities can provide copies of blank advance directive forms on request. The online U.S. Living Will Registry at *http://liv-will1.uslivingwillregistry.com/forms.html* provides information for individuals, family members, heath care professionals, and institutions. Resources on this site include the following:

- Personal-choice options and benefits of advance directives
- Definitions of terms used on all advance directive documents
- Organ donation information and registration
- Printable living will and heath care proxy forms for each of the 50 states

Signed and notarized advance directive documents allow an individual's health care choices to be followed when resuscitation or other extraordinary measures are being considered.

DO-NOT-RESUSCITATE ORDERS

Patients who are faced with life-threatening illness or their designated family members acting as health care proxies may choose to refuse or limit treatment. This designation is documented as a **do-not-resuscitate (DNR) order**. Sometimes, DNR orders are referred to as *no codes,* indicating that no extraordinary measures are to be taken to prolong a patient's life in the case of a natural death. DNR orders are written documents that indicate the extent of resuscitation efforts preferred by a patient or legally designated family members in the case of cardiac or respiratory arrest.

Each state has laws and every health care institution has policies that must be followed to designate a patient as DNR. In most cases, the written DNR order must be renewed on a regular basis, similar to that of an order for antibiotic therapy or narcotic medication administration. Some states have different levels of designations for DNR orders, such as DNR-CC (i.e., do not resuscitate, comfort care), that identify specific protocols for administering medications and providing treatment in addition to instructions on CPR or endotracheal intubation. Nurses should become familiar with their state's statutes and health care institution's policies to ensure compliance with DNR orders.

LAWS IMPACTING PROFESSIONAL PRACTICE LO 11.10

Many laws guide the practice of nursing throughout the world. The discussion of laws in this chapter is limited to those pertaining specifically to the practice of nursing in the United States. These laws impact professional practice within and outside hospitals, extended care facilities, mental health institutions, public health clinics, private practice offices, and many other institutions.

LICENSURE

Licensure and certification of nurses seek to ensure professional competence. The laws of each state require graduates of accredited nursing schools and colleges pass the National Council Licensure Examination (NCLEX) before beginning professional practice (see Chapter 1). Most states recognize only their own licenses. However, beginning in 2000, the Nurse Licensure Compact (NLC), which is a multistate licensure model, was initiated to allow nurses licensed in one state to practice physically and electronically in other states in the consortium. As of September 2014, 24 states participate in the NLC. Nurses must legally reside in a state participating in the NLC to obtain privileges to practice outside the state in which they hold a nursing license *(https://www.ncsbn.org/nlc.htm)*. The NLC is an especially significant legal initiative in light of technologic advancements that allow electronic transfer of medical information and consultation among medical and nursing professionals across state lines and around the world.

Although not required by law, specialty certification seeks to ensure safe, competent nursing practice. Certification is available to nurses in a wide variety of specialties, including critical care, gastroenterology, oncology, pediatrics, and education. Becoming certified in a nursing specialty requires years of practice, a recognized level of expertise, and a commitment to excellence in addition to the time and financial resources needed to prepare for and successfully complete the certification examination. Nurses who are certified in their areas of practice display a high level of clinical competence and a commitment to comprehensive, safe patient care *(www.nursingcertification.org)*. An Institute of Medicine (2011) report, *The Future of Nursing: Leading Change, Advancing Health,* recommends that 80% of nurses in the United States be baccalaureate educated by 2020 and that health care organizations encourage nurses with associate degrees or diplomas to enter baccalaureate programs within 5 years of graduation. These recommendations complement the Advanced Practice Registered Nurse regulatory model for licensure, accreditation, certification, and education (LACE) (National Council of State Boards of Nursing, 2008). The LACE model addresses the need for all nurses to be licensed, graduate from accredited nursing programs, achieve certification in their chosen specialty, and seek graduate education. Chapter 1 provides additional information on specialty certification.

STANDARDS OF CARE

Standards of care are the minimum requirements for providing safe nursing care. Federal and state laws, rules and regulations, accreditation standards, and institutional policies and procedures are used to formulate nursing standards of care. Institutional policies and procedures must be consistent with state laws, rules, and regulations, which must comply with federal law.

The ANA identifies standards for safe practice and regularly releases policy statements and current practice information to guide and update the standards of care for nurses. Each state's board of nursing establishes accreditation standards for schools and colleges of nursing that must be met. These accreditation standards help to ensure that graduates of nursing programs meet standards-of-care requirements in their nursing practice. Academic accreditation standards established by the Commission for Nursing Education Accreditation (C-NEA), the Accrediting Commission for Education in Nursing (ACEN), and the Commission on Collegiate Nursing Education (CCNE) and the accreditation standards for health care institutions required by The Joint Commission contribute to a large body of safe-practice requirements.

By adhering to standards of care, nurses can avoid accusations of unsafe, negligent care and malpractice. Standards of care are used as the benchmark against which a nurse's actions are evaluated. These standards are fairly universal for all nurses practicing in similar specialties. For instance, the standards of care for intensive care unit (ICU) nurses practicing in Kentucky are consistent with the expected standards of care for ICU nurses in California. The same is true for advanced practice nurses, including certified registered nurse anesthetists, certified nurse midwives, clinical nurse specialists, and certified nurse practitioners. The conduct of advanced practice nurses is required to meet the standards of care in their specialty areas. General nursing standards of care are defined for each specialty. Pursuing continuing education, reading professional journals, and actively participating in professional organizations such as the ANA, the National League for Nursing (NLN), and state or specialty nursing associations are the best ways for practicing nurses to remain current on standards of care.

HEALTH INSURANCE PORTABILITY AND ACCOUNTABILITY ACT

The Health Insurance Portability and Accountability Act (HIPAA) was enacted in 1996 to protect the privacy of health care information. HIPAA contains four sets of standards, each with rules that must be implemented by all health care facilities (Judson and Harrison, 2012). The accessibility aspect of HIPAA allows sharing of protected health information (PHI) with those who need it to properly care for individuals seeking treatment, and limits access by individuals and agencies that may use the information prejudicially or for monetary gain. PHI includes physical or mental health data, health care treatment locations and occurrences, and payment information related to all health care treatment (U.S. Department of Health and Human Services, 2013). The HIPAA portability section prevents individuals who have had health care coverage through an employer for a minimum of 12 months from losing their coverage during a job change, even in the case of preexisting health conditions.

Privacy and confidentiality are the two expectations of HIPAA most relevant to nursing practice. By requiring predisclosure authorization, the HIPAA Privacy Rule enables an individual to control the sharing of personal information (Harman, 2006). The Privacy Rule limits disclosure of patient health care information to the patient and only those people and health care agencies to which the patient has granted specific permission. Confidential treatment of patient records involves limiting access to documentation of interactions between patients and health care providers.

Electronic transmission of health care information heightened the necessity for HIPAA. Nurses should pay particular attention to the rules of privacy and confidentiality while engaging in phone, fax, e-mail, or Internet transmission of protected patient information. The information should never be shared in public areas, and all electronic health record software should be closed by the nurse after documentation to ensure patient privacy and prevent a breach of confidentiality. In some health care institutions, a patient is asked to identify a code word that the patient's family member or friend must share with the nurse before receiving any information on the patient's condition from the nurse. Nurses must refrain from sharing patient information with unauthorized individuals. Many web resources are available that provide helpful information on HIPAA privacy and confidentiality issues for health care professionals. The Nursing Care Guideline box lists procedural and documentation concerns associated with HIPAA.

American Recovery and Reinvestment Act of 2009

The American Recovery and Reinvestment Act (ARRA) of 2009 refined some aspects of HIPAA and improved standards governing the privacy and security of health information. This act prevents the sale of protected health information without a patient's knowledge of payment and authorization, except in the case of public health records, research, and rare, specified business transactions. It also requires patients to receive requested copies of their electronic health records within 30 days and at a minimal cost (Center for Democracy and Technology, 2009).

GOOD SAMARITAN ACTS

All 50 states have enacted Good Samaritan laws offering protection for physicians and other health care professionals who provide emergency care at the scene of a disaster, emergency, or accident (Figure 11-3). Good Samaritan laws protect health care professionals from charges of negligence in providing emergency care if (1) the care is within the professional's scope of knowledge and standards of care and (2) no fee is received or charged for services.

In some states, the Good Samaritan law includes a *duty-to-assist clause,* which requires health care professionals to provide care at the scene of an emergency. In Minnesota, failure to provide emergency care may result in being charged

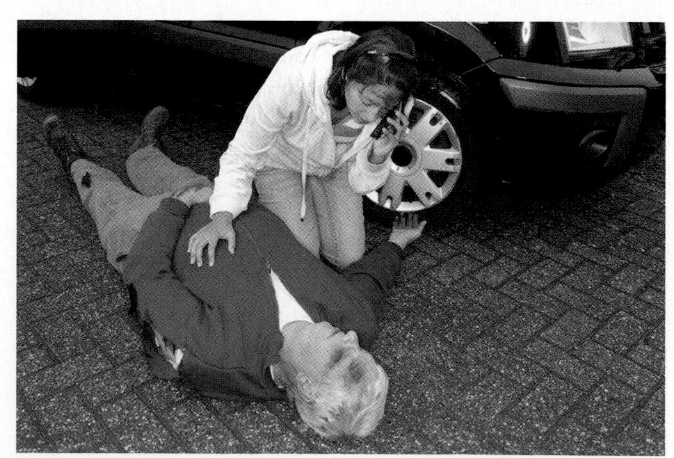

FIGURE 11-3 Good Samaritan laws protect nurses who provide assistance to accident victims while maintaining standards of care.

NURSING CARE GUIDELINE

Background

- The Health Insurance Portability and Accountability Act (HIPAA) of 1996 was established to protect patients' privacy and personal information. It encompasses accessibility, privacy, security, and confidentiality.
- The act makes provisions for verbal, written, and electronic information.
- Health care providers of all disciplines and at all levels must remain current on the principles of this act through continuing education at their facility or an accredited educational institution.
- Civil and criminal penalties are set forth in the act for violation of any provision of the act.

Procedural Concerns

- Patients must be offered or have access to a notice of their rights under this act.
- Patient names cannot be posted or released.
- Discussion of patient information cannot be held in public-access areas, and discussions in nursing areas must be held using soft voices.
- Using a camera and/or recorder or not concealing patient information while preparing school assignments is considered a violation of the act, resulting in penalties.
- Paper or electronic charts cannot be visible or left in an open, public-access area.
- Fax transmissions
  - Include a cover sheet with the word *Confidential* (set in a highly visible way) and instructions for destroying or returning the information if it is inadvertently delivered to a wrong number.
  - Call ahead, and ensure that the facility is ready to receive the transmission and that the fax machine is in a confidential area.
  - Require the facility to confirm receipt of the transmission.
- Electronic medical records (EMRs) must be password protected, with access given only to those who need it to provide care or those whom the patient has authorized.
- Personnel must log off computers when finished working with patient records. Computers must have the protection of an automatic log off after a certain period of inactivity.
- Passwords can never be shared.
- Patient information should never be e-mailed or faxed unless special arrangements have been made for receiving the data.
- Firewalls and other Internet technology (IT) protections should be installed to prevent unwarranted intrusions and identity theft.

Documentation Concerns

- Patients' rights include
  - Obtaining, viewing, and/or updating a copy of their own medical records.
  - Obtaining information regarding HIPAA and how the facility will use personal information that is collected and requesting variants on those uses.
  - Choosing how to receive information and education about their health.
- Signatures and consents are usually obtained for accessing personal health information.
- Paper documentation should not be thrown in the trash; it must be shredded. This includes scrap paper and report memorandums.
- The Joint Commission requires individual facilities to have written policies and procedures in place for the protection of personal health information that is conveyed by verbal, electronic, or printed means.

with a petty misdemeanor (Minnesota Office of the Revisor of Statutes, 2013). Vermont statutes allow a fine of up to $100 if the duty to assist is violated (Vermont Good Samaritan Act, 1967).

Good Samaritan laws may require health care professionals to ask for and receive permission for treatment before initiating care. If a patient is intentionally injured or gross negligence occurs during emergency care, Good Samaritan laws do not protect nurses or other health care professionals from legal consequences.

SAFE PRACTICE ALERT

Before leaving the scene of an accident in which a nurse has provided emergency treatment, the nurse should transfer the care of injured individuals to equally competent professionals. They may be paramedics or emergency department personnel.

UNIFORM DETERMINATION OF DEATH

Advancements in life support technology caused the original case law definition of death—absence of spontaneous respiratory and cardiac functions—to become limited in scope (National Conference of Commissioners on Uniform State Laws, 1980). The Uniform Determination of Death Act of 1981 identified a comprehensive and medically sound basis for declaring a person dead. As a result, most states have enacted laws establishing two criteria for death: (1) all spontaneous respiratory and circulatory function stops or (2) all brain function, including that of the brainstem, ends. If brain death has been established, organ procurement for donation may take place.

ASSISTED SUICIDE AND EUTHANASIA

Assisted suicide and euthanasia are related but different actions. Both involve facilitating the death of another person

(Marker and Hamlon, 2013). **Assisted suicide** occurs when a person causes his or her own death with the assistance of medication or an intravenous injection supplied by a physician or other health care provider. Euthanasia occurs when a person who willingly requests to die is injected with a lethal drug dosage by another individual. Both actions typically occur when the person requesting assistance to die is suffering unbearably; experiencing excruciating, chronic pain; or facing certain death as a result of a terminal illness.

As of late 2013, assisted suicide is legal in Oregon, Washington, and Montana, and euthanasia is permitted in the Netherlands, Belgium, and Luxembourg. Physician-prescribed suicide is considered a legal medical treatment in Vermont (Marker and Hamlon, 2013). Nurses must be familiar with state laws regarding these issues. The participation of nurses in assisted suicide is opposed by the ANA (2013b) on the basis of the Code of Ethics for Nurses. Nurses are encouraged to provide comprehensive end-of-life patient care that alleviates pain and minimizes suffering.

NATURAL DEATH ACTS

Laws known as *natural death acts* exist in some jurisdictions that permit competent patients to make health care decisions that may result in their deaths. This includes nursing actions such as discharging patients who are likely to die without acute care and withholding or withdrawing life-sustaining treatments under the direction of a physician when requested by a competent patient. The acts prevent civil liability, criminal liability, and professional sanctions against health care providers who explain the medical risks associated with the decisions before their initiation.

AMERICANS WITH DISABILITIES ACT

The Americans With Disabilities Act (ADA), adopted in 1990 and amended in 2008, provides protection against discrimination for individuals who have a physical or mental impairment that interferes with one or several life activities, have a history of impairment, or are perceived as having a disability. Impairment of life activities is identified by the ADA (2008) as difficulty performing the activities of daily living (ADLs): "seeing, hearing, eating, sleeping, walking, standing, lifting, bending, speaking, breathing, learning, reading, concentrating, thinking, communicating, and working" [Section 12102, (2) (A)].

The ADA delineates requirements for reasonable physical accommodation and services that allow individuals with disabilities to be employed and live reasonably unobstructed lives. This includes readers for the blind and sign language interpreters for those who are deaf. The ADA law mandates accessibility requirements for public and private institutions.

Employment concerns for individuals with communicable diseases, such as human immunodeficiency virus (HIV) infection, are addressed in the ADA. Heath care workers infected with HIV and infected patients are not to be discriminated against under this law. ADA rules specify that alternative gender preference such as homosexuality or bisexuality is not considered a disability nor is the illegal use of drugs. Students who are immigrants to the United States need to be aware that having English as a second language is not a disability requiring accommodation. The Diversity Considerations box highlights some accommodations that can be made for individuals with documented disabilities. Most include collaboration with other professionals and referrals to community agencies.

DIVERSITY CONSIDERATIONS

Disability

- Assistive devices, including individually sized walkers and wheelchairs, are available to assist children, youths, and adults with ambulation.
- Voice-activated computer programs may be provided for quadriplegic individuals of all ages who are unable to use a keyboard.
- Eyeglasses, special contacts, and hearing aids can be fitted for toddlers, children, and adults in need of sensory assistance.
- Instruction for teachers and support staff in monitoring the status of children or adults with mental retardation or severe physical conditions can be facilitated by the school nurse to avoid preventable medical emergencies.

Culture, Ethnicity, and Religion

- Foreign-language interpreters are accessible by phone or video link or in person to assist a patient in understanding medical care.
- Religious beliefs, education, culture, and socioeconomic status influence health care decisions.

Morphology

- Special lifts, beds, and wheelchairs are available for use with morbidly obese patients to provide for their safety and the safety of care providers.

PHYSICAL RESTRAINTS

Under the law, nurses are responsible for providing safe patient care, which includes preventing patient injury from physical restraint and unrestrained, accidental falls. Historically, physical restraints were used as a primary nursing intervention to prevent patients from injuring themselves or others and to avoid the removal of medical equipment such as endotracheal tubes or intravenous lines. Federal and state laws and guidelines from The Joint Commission have mandated that physical restraints be used only in the event that alternative, less restrictive interventions to prevent patient injury have been unsuccessful and a written order for restraints is in place. The written order must include dates, indicating the start and stop times for use of physical restraints, and it must be updated frequently according to institutional policies. In an effort to prevent injury from restraints, accredited health care facilities have flow sheets on which nurses routinely document the use of physical restraints and the patient's mental and circulatory status. Using physical restraints without proper orders and documented indications of need may result in charges of abuse.

Innovative equipment such as rapid-lift beds that lower to ground level and rise to waist height in a few seconds is being used to reduce falls from bed in extended care facilities. The employment of sitters to be present with patients when health care providers are out of a patient's room is another creative solution commonly used in hospitals to avoid the use of restraints while providing for patient safety.

ADDITIONAL ACTS INTRODUCED IN CONGRESS

The Registered Nurse Safe Staffing Act and the Nurse and Health Care Worker Protection Act have been introduced in the U.S. Congress for several years in an effort to increase patient safety and prevent the loss of registered nurses from the workforce because of physical injury. One landmark research study published in *JAMA* found that an increase of one patient in the average nurse's assigned workload contributes to a 7% increase in the rate of patient deaths within 30 days of admission and a 7% increase in "failure to rescue" from a life-threatening emergency (Aiken, Clarke, Sloane, et al, 2002). The same study addressed the effect of high patient-nurse ratios on nurse burnout and employment dissatisfaction.

The primary research supporting the Nurse and Health Care Worker Protection Act was conducted by the ANA in collaboration with the U.S. Department of Veteran Affairs. Chapter 28 provides additional information on the Safe Patient Handling and Movement research and initiative. Both of the bills and the research supporting their enactment underscore the importance of nurses' being involved politically to inform and educate their local, state, and national legislators on issues related to public safety and nursing.

ULTIMATE RESPONSIBILITY OF PROFESSIONAL NURSES

It is ultimately the responsibility of all professional nurses to practice ethically and within the laws of the state and nation in which they reside. Ignorance of the rules and regulations governing nursing practice is not a defense against malpractice or employment dismissal.

To prevent breaches of ethical behavior, nurses must reflect on their personal values, become familiar with the Code of Ethics for Nurses, and implement strategies to protect all patients in their care. To avoid unsafe patient care, nurses must maintain their licensure and competency through continuing education and provide care consistent with their level of expertise and the standards of care for their specialty. Individual nurses must accept the responsibility to act ethically and legally in all situations.

SUMMARY OF LEARNING OUTCOMES

LO 11.1 *Identify key ethical theories that affect nursing practice:* Deontology and utilitarianism are the two fundamental ethical theories on which other ethical theories and codes of ethics are based.

LO 11.2 *Apply ethical concepts to professional nursing practice:* Nurses are expected to demonstrate accountability, advocacy, autonomy, beneficence, confidentiality, veracity, and other ethical concepts in their professional practice.

LO 11.3 *Describe how the American Nurses Association (ANA) Code of Ethics for Nurses applies to nursing education and practice:* The ANA Code of Ethics for Nurses articulates ethical standards with which all nurses, including nursing students, are expected to comply.

LO 11.4 *Recognize the role of ethics in genetic, biomedical, and end-of-life health care decision making:* Decisions regarding genetic testing, biomedical issues such as cloning and stem cell research, and end-of-life care involve intellectual knowledge and ethical evaluation. Specially trained members of ethics committees can help to guide institutional policies and procedures that affect nursing practice in ethically challenging situations.

LO 11.5 *Discuss the legal implications of nursing practice:* Each state has a nurse practice act that establishes the standards of care required for legal nursing practice. Licensure, laws, rules, and regulations governing nursing practice are enforced to protect the public from harm.

LO 11.6 *Differentiate among constitutional, statutory, regulatory, and case laws as they relate to professional nursing practice:* Laws are established through various means to address criminal and civil violations that may occur during the practice of nursing.

LO 11.7 *Identify various types of statutory law, including intentional and unintentional torts, and their potential effect on nurses providing patient care:* Intentional torts such as assault, battery, defamation of character, false imprisonment, and invasion of privacy may be committed by nurses who are unfamiliar with the law and their facility's policies and procedures intended to ensure safe patient care. Nurses may be charged with malpractice (i.e., professional negligence), an unintentional tort, if their actions do not meet professional standards of care.

LO 11.8 *Explain liability issues such as professional boundaries, delegation, and documentation that are pertinent to nursing practice:* Practicing nursing in a manner consistent with ethical and legal standards requires that nurses set professional practice boundaries, follow the Principles for Delegation, and document care expediently and accurately.

LO 11.9 *Summarize legal issues that guide patient care:* Informed consent, patient rights, organ donation, advance directives, and DNR orders guide members of the interdisciplinary health care team to care for patients in a manner consistent with their requests.

LO 11.10 *Describe the effect of federal and state laws on nursing practice:* The American Disabilities Act and the Uniform Determination of Death Act are examples of federal laws that were enacted to guide professional practice. Good Samaritan laws and laws governing assisted suicide and organ donation are specific to states. Nurses are responsible for becoming familiar with the laws of their state of residence and practicing within those laws.

Responses to the critical-thinking questions are available at ***http://evolve.elsevier.com/YoostCrawford/fundamentals/.***

REVIEW QUESTIONS

1. On which ethical theory do nurses implement their care when they act on the basis of the needs of one specific patient rather than the potential consequences to other patients?
   a. Deontology
   b. Autonomy
   c. Utilitarianism
   d. Nonmaleficence
2. Which nursing intervention is the best example of patient advocacy?
   a. Collecting blood samples according to the physician's order each morning
   b. Assessing the vital signs of a patient who is receiving a blood transfusion
   c. Seeking an additional analgesic medication order for a patient who is experiencing severe pain
   d. Accompanying an ambulating patient who is walking for the first time after undergoing surgery
3. What action should nurses who demonstrate accountability take if they forget to administer a patient's medication at the ordered time?
   a. Document the medication as refused by the patient.
   b. Administer the medication as soon as the error is discovered.
   c. Record the medication as given after making sure the patient is okay.
   d. Follow the administration and documentation procedures for medication errors.
4. Nursing students are held to which standard by the Code of Ethics for Nurses? *(Select all that apply.)*
   a. Clinical skills performance equal to that of an experienced nurse
   b. Demonstration of respect for all individuals with whom the student interacts
   c. Avoidance of behavior that shows disregard for the effect of those actions on others
   d. Accepting responsibility for resolving conflicts in a professional manner
   e. Incorporating families in patient care regardless of patient preference
5. If a student nurse overhears a peer speaking disrespectfully about a patient, nurse, faculty member, or classmate, what is the most ethical first action for the student nurse to take?
   a. Discuss the peer's actions during group clinical conference.
   b. Ignore the initial occurrence and observe if it happens again.
   c. Report the actions of the classmate to the clinical instructor.
   d. Speak to the peer privately to prevent further occurrences.
6. What nursing intervention is best when a patient is struggling with the decision to abort an abnormally developing fetus discovered during genetic testing in the first trimester of pregnancy?
   a. Recommend additional testing.
   b. Refer the patient to an abortion clinic.
   c. Listen to the patient's concerns.
   d. Discuss regional adoption agencies.
7. Making prejudicial, untrue statements about another person during a conversation may expose a nurse to being charged with what offense?
   a. Libel
   b. Assault
   c. Slander
   d. Malpractice

8. What consequences may a nurse experience if the nurse is convicted of a crime? *(Select all that apply.)*
   a. Loss of nursing licensure
   b. Employment affirmation
   c. Monetary penalty
   d. Imprisonment
   e. Promotion
9. What is the best way for a nurse to avoid crossing professional practice boundaries with patients?
   a. Spend extensive time with a patient without visitors.
   b. Focus on the needs of patients and their families.
   c. Intervene in problematic patient relationships.
   d. Discuss personal information excessively.
10. What action should a nurse take if a patient who needs to sign an informed consent form for nonemergency surgery appears to be under the influence of drugs or alcohol?
   a. Contact the physician to see what should be done.
   b. Ask the patient's spouse to sign the form.
   c. Request permission to bypass the need for a signed consent form.
   d. Wait to have the informed consent form signed when the patient is alert and oriented.

Answers and rationales for the review questions are available at *http://evolve.elsevier.com/YoostCrawford/fundamentals/.*

REFERENCES

Aiken T: *Legal and ethical issues in health occupations,* ed. 3 St. Louis, 2015, Saunders.

Aiken L, Clarke S, Cheung R, et al: Educational levels of hospital nurses and surgical patient mortality. *JAMA,* 290(12), 1617-1623, 2003.

Aiken L, Clarke S, Sloane D, et al: Hospital nurse staffing and patient mortality, nurse burnout, and job dissatisfaction. *JAMA,* 288(16), 1987-1993, 2002.

American Hospital Association (AHA): The patient care partnership: Understanding expectations, rights and responsibilities, 2003. Retrieved from *www.aha.org/content/00-10/pcp_english_030730.pdf.*

American Nurses Association (ANA): *Code of ethics for nurses with interpretive statements,* Washington, D.C., 2015, Author. Also available at *Nursebooks.org.*

American Nurses Association (ANA): *ANA's Principles for social networking and the nurse: Guidance for registered nurses,* Silver Spring, Md., 2011, Author.

American Nurses Association (ANA): Principles for delegation by registered nurses to unlicensed assistive personnel (UAP), 2013a. Retrieved from *www.nursingworld.org/MainMenuCategories/ThePracticeofProfessionalNursing/NursingStandards/ANAPrinciples/PrinciplesofDelegation.pdf.aspx.* [only available to members]

American Nurses Association (ANA): Euthanasia, assisted suicide, and aid in dying, 2013b. Retrieved from *www.nursingworld.org/euthanasiaanddying.*

Americans with Disabilities Act (ADA) of 1990, as Amended, 2008. Retrieved from *www.ada.gov/pubs/adastatute08markscrdr.htm#12113d.*

Burkhardt M, Nathaniel A: *Ethics and issues in contemporary nursing,* ed. 4, Stanford, Conn., 2014, Cengage.

Center for Democracy and Technology: Summary of health privacy provisions in the 2009 economic stimulus legislation, 2009. Retrieved from *https://cdt.org/insight/summary-of-health-privacy-provisions-in-the-2009-economic-stimulus-legislation/.*

Cronenwett L, Sherwood G, Barnsteiner J, et al: Quality and safety education for nurses. *Nurs Outlook,* 55(3):122-131, 2007.

Fowler M: *Guide to the code of ethics for nurses: Interpretation and application.* Silver Spring, Md., 2010, American Nurses Association.

Gallup: Honesty/ethics in professions, 2014. Retrieved from *www.gallup.com/poll/1654/honesty-ethics-professions.aspx.*

Guido G: *Legal issues in nursing,* ed. 6, Upper Saddle River, N.J., 2013, Pearson.

Harman L: *Ethical challenges in the management of health information,* ed. 2, Boston, 2006, Jones & Bartlett.

Institute of Medicine: *The future of nursing: Leading change, advancing health,* Washington, D.C., 2011, National Academies Press.

Judson K, Harrison C: *Law & ethics for the health professions,* ed. 6, New York, 2012, McGraw-Hill.

Luparell S: Incivility in nursing education: Let's put an end to it, 2008. Retrieved from *www.nsna.org/Portals/0/Skins/NSNA/pdf/Imprint_AprMay08_Feat_Incivility.pdf.*

Luparell S:. Dealing with challenging student situations, 2013. Retrieved from *www.aacn.nche.edu/membership/members-only/presentations/2013/13facdev/Luparell.pdf.*

Marker R, Hamlon K: Euthanasia and assisted suicide: Frequently asked questions, 2013. Retrieved from *www.patientsrightscouncil.org/site/frequently-asked-questions/.*

Mill JS: *Utilitarianism,* London, 1910, Dent & Sons.

Minnesota Office of the Revisor of Statutes: Good Samaritan Law, 604A.01, Minnesota Statutes, 2013. Retrieved from *https://www.revisor.mn.gov/statutes/?id=604a.01.*

National Conference of Commissioners on Uniform State Laws: Uniform Determination of Death Act, 1980. Retrieved from *http://pntb.org/wordpress/wp-content/uploads/Uniform-Determination-of-Death-1980_5c.pdf.*

National Council of State Boards of Nursing: Consensus model for APRN regulation: Licensure, accreditation, certification, & education, July 7, 2008. Retrieved from *www.aacn.nche.edu/education-resources/APRNReport.pdf.*

National Council of State Boards of Nursing: Professional boundaries: A nurse's guide to the importance of appropriate professional boundaries, n.d. Retrieved from *www.ncsbn.org/ProfessionalBoundariesbrochure.pdf.*

National Student Nurses Association: Code of academic and clinical conduct, 2001. Retrieved from *www.nsna.org/Portals/0/Skins/NSNA/pdf/Pieces_Appendix_B.pdf.*

National Student Nurses Association: Recommendations for social media usage and maintaining privacy, confidentiality and professionalism, n.d. Retrieved from *www.nsna.org/Portals/0/Skins/NSNA/pdf/NSNA_Social_Media_Recommendations.pdf.*

Needleman J, Buerhaus P, Mattke S, et al: Nurse-staffing levels and the quality of care in hospitals. *N Engl J Med,* 346(22), 1715-1722, 2002.

Ohio Board of Nursing: Professional boundaries violations: Case studies. *Momentum,* 25, 7-9, 2009.

United Network for Organ Sharing (UNOS): U.S. transplantation data, 2014. Retrieved from *optn.transplant.hrsa.gov/data/default.asp.*

U.S. Department of Health and Human Services: Health information privacy, 2013. Retrieved from *www.hhs.gov/ocr/privacy/hipaa/understanding/summary/index.html.*

Vermont Statutes: Good Samaritan Act, 1967. Retrieved from *http://vem.vermont.gov/sites/vem/files/H%20VT%20Good%20Samaritan%20Law12.doc.*

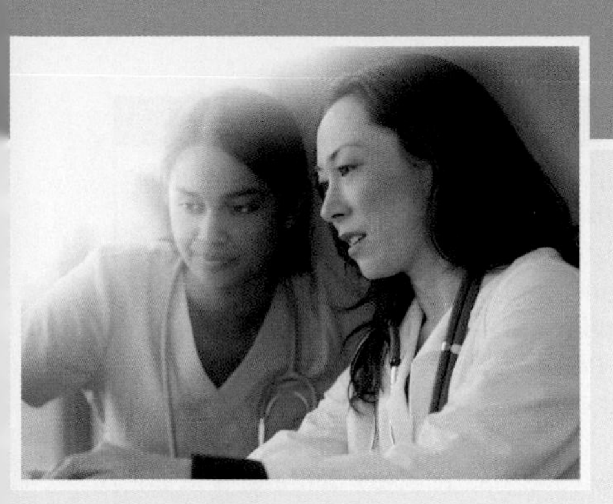

CHAPTER 12

Leadership and Management

EVOLVE WEBSITE

http://evolve.elsevier.com/YoostCrawford/fundamentals/

- Additional Evolve-Only Review Questions With Answers
- Answers and Rationales for Text Review Questions
- Answers to Critical-Thinking Questions
- Case Study With Questions
- Glossary

LEARNING OUTCOMES

Comprehension of this chapter's content will provide students with the ability to:

LO 12.1 Compare leadership and management.
LO 12.2 Describe the styles of leadership, including the qualities of effective leaders.
LO 12.3 Discuss various management theories, including qualities of effective managers.
LO 12.4 Characterize nursing leadership roles in health care.
LO 12.5 Explain the underlying principles of delegation in health care.

KEY TERMS

accountability, p. 166
advocate, p. 171
autocratic leader, p. 167
behavioral theories, p. 167
bureaucratic leader, p. 168
creativity, p. 168
dedication, p. 168
delegation, p. 172
democratic leader, p. 167
formal leadership, p. 168
humility, p. 168
informal leadership, p. 168
integrity, p. 168
laissez-faire leader, p. 168
leadership, p. 166
magnanimity, p. 168
management, p. 166
openness, p. 168
situational theories, p. 167
supervision, p. 173
trait theories, p. 167
transactional leaders, p. 167
transformational leaders, p. 167

CASE STUDY

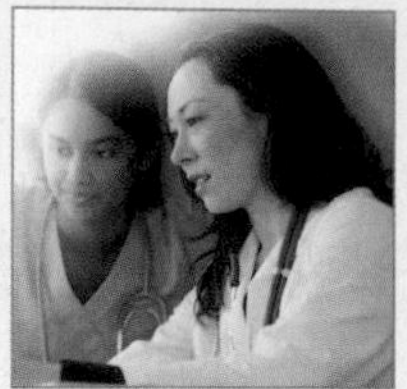

The registered nurse (RN) is assigned to care for six patients. Working with the nurse is a licensed practical nurse (LPN) and unlicensed assistive personnel (UAP). The nurse reviews the list of patients:

- Mr. Solomon is a 76-year-old male with chronic obstructive pulmonary disease (COPD) and Alzheimer dementia who was admitted with increasing shortness of breath. He has been living at home with his wife but recently has been having increasing episodes of confusion and disorientation to self, place, and time. He is unable to communicate his level of pain or discomfort. His vital signs at 0400 were T 37.2° C (99° F), P 102 and regular, R 24 and labored, BP 134/86, with a pulse oximetry reading of 88% on 2 L of oxygen by nasal cannula.
- Mrs. Jarvis is a 45-year-old female on postoperative day 1 after an abdominal hysterectomy. She has a Foley catheter and an intravenous (IV) line. Overnight, she received morphine twice for pain rated as 8 of 10. She has the original abdominal dressing in place. She was afebrile overnight, and other vital signs were within normal limits.
- Mrs. Kimball is a 92-year-old female with urosepsis who was admitted from home 3 days earlier. She is on IV antibiotics every 8 hours. She is awaiting placement at a local nursing home. She rates her pain at 0 of 10 consistently and is alert and oriented. She needs assistance with ambulation and meal setup. She was afebrile overnight, and vital signs were stable.
- Mr. Lowe is a 29-year-old male admitted 2 days earlier after a motorcycle accident. He was wearing a helmet. His cervical spine x-rays were normal. He is alert and oriented. He had an open fracture of the radius, which was surgically set. An external fixator is in place. He is ambulatory but requires assistance of one person when moving from the bed to a standing position. He has a saline lock in place and receives IV antibiotics twice each day. At 0600, he received oral medication one time for pain rated 6 of 10. His vital signs overnight were reported as afebrile and stable.
- Mr. Fox is an 88-year-old, nonambulatory male admitted from a nursing home 2 days earlier and diagnosed with stage IV lung cancer. His code status is a do-not-resuscitate (DNR) order. He is on oxygen and is having Cheyne-Stokes respirations. He responds only to painful stimuli. The local hospice organization is working with the family.
- Ms. Tomcik is a 22-year-old female admitted from a group home yesterday with pneumonia. She has a history of Down syndrome but has no history of major medical problems. She is receiving respiratory treatments q 4 hr and IV fluids and IV antibiotics q 4 hr. She is not complaining of pain, but she needs to be encouraged to use her incentive spirometer often. She has an order for ambulation twice each shift. Night shift reports vitals at 0400 as T 38.3° C (101° F), P 72 and regular, R 22 and labored, with a pulse oximetry reading of 98% on room air.

Refer back to this case study to answer the critical-thinking questions throughout the chapter.

New nurses may not consider themselves to be leaders or managers as they enter the realm of nursing care. However, all RNs use leadership and management skills in their daily work. They manage, plan, and coordinate care for their patients. Many nurses are responsible for directing the work of others in providing patient care. It is important that the beginning nurse have an understanding of the processes involved in leading and managing others.

DEFINITIONS OF LEADERSHIP AND MANAGEMENT LO 12.1

The terms *leadership* and *management* are often used interchangeably. Although these concepts are related, they are different in definition and in practice. Leadership behaviors and management skills complement each other. However, a manager may not possess leadership traits, and a leader may lack management skills.

Leadership is the ability to influence, guide, or direct others. Leadership focuses on relationships, using interpersonal skills to persuade others to work toward a common goal. Leaders may or may not have the authority that comes with a formal position in an organization; their power lies in their ability to form relationships and alliances with those around them. The leader is able to develop followers by sharing a common vision and values. Traditionally, leaders are visionaries who set the overall direction for a group or organization.

Management is the process of coordinating others and directing them toward a common goal. Management is focused on the task at hand. A manager holds a formal position of authority in an organization; that position includes **accountability** and responsibility for accomplishing the tasks within the work environment. Managers demonstrate accountability when they are answerable for their own actions and the actions of those under their direction.

LEADERSHIP LO 12.2

Leaders have the ability to influence and motivate others while maintaining relationships to accomplish a goal. There are many different ideas and theories about why some people are better leaders than others.

LEADERSHIP THEORY OVERVIEW

Researchers have conducted many studies to determine which traits are associated with good leadership and what styles of leadership are most effective. Despite the research, no one leadership style has proved to be best because different situations require different styles of leadership.

Trait Theories

Early theories about leadership focused on the traits of leaders. **Trait theories** assumed that leaders were born with the personality traits necessary for leadership, which few people were thought to possess. Bass (1990) classified these traits in three categories: intelligence, personality, and abilities. Specific qualities of good leaders include good interpersonal skills, self-confidence, and a willingness to take risks. One problem with the early research on leadership was that it focused on males, and feminine characteristics were not included in the lists of traits. However, this early research laid the groundwork for further studies of leadership behaviors.

Behavioral Theories

Behavioral theories assume that leaders learn certain behaviors. These theories focus on what leaders do, rather than on what characteristics they innately possess. Characteristics that were consistent in leaders included task-oriented behavior and consideration for others. Various models were developed on the basis of behavioral research.

Situational Theories

The next wave of leadership theories appeared in the 1970s and 1980s. Situational theorists proposed that behavioral theories did not account for the effect of the environment, or situation, in which the leadership behaviors occurred. Evidence suggests that although no one leadership style is best, leaders who focus on the person and the task are most effective (Taylor, 1994).

Situational theories suggest that leaders change their approach depending on the situation. The situation includes a number of factors, such as characteristics of the group, the type of business, and the economic climate (Whitehead, Weiss, and Tappen, 2010).

Contemporary Theories

The latter part of the past century saw increasing numbers of women in management and leadership positions. Researchers began to study and identify the different leadership styles of women and their influence on organizations. From this research, a variety of new theories developed.

In the late 1970s, Burns (1978) identified transactional leaders and transformational leaders. **Transactional leaders** use reward and punishment to gain the cooperation of followers. One advantage of transactional leadership is that employees know exactly what is expected. The employees realize that if they do what is expected or more, there will be a reward, usually a salary increase or bonus. If the employees fail, some sort of negative consequence is anticipated, ranging from being reprimanded to losing a position. This type of leadership focuses on getting the job done or making change happen. The nurse who is a transactional leader rewards other health care team members who provide safe and effective care and uses reprimands for those who do not meet performance goals for safe patient care.

Transformational leaders employ methods that inspire people to follow their lead. Transformational leaders work toward transforming an organization with the help of others. These individuals think that the interaction between leaders and followers can raise both to higher levels of morality and motivation (Burns, 1978).

Transformational leadership is sometimes confused with charismatic leadership. Charismatic leaders use charm and emotion to form allegiances with others. Although this is not necessarily a negative trait, charismatic leaders can be motivated by many things, including personal gain. Although transformational leaders share some characteristics with charismatic leaders, the main difference is that the aim of a transformational leader is to enact change in an organization. The nurse who is a transformational leader inspires other members of the health care team to achieve goals for the sake of excellent patient care by exhibiting safe and effective care measures. This nurse may use stories of satisfied patients and families to motivate staff.

STYLES OF LEADERSHIP

In the late 1930s, Kurt Lewin (1951) conducted studies of teenage boys to identify patterns of leadership behaviors. He identified three basic styles of leadership: autocratic, democratic, and laissez-faire. In addition to these three types, bureaucratic leadership has been identified.

Autocratic Leadership

The authoritarian or **autocratic leader** exercises strong control over subordinates. This type of leader assumes that employees are motivated by external forces, such as the need for approval by the supervisor and the need to avoid punishment. Information flows in a top-down style and is primarily directive in nature. The leader demands respect and obedience from employees. If necessary, the autocratic leader uses coercion to ensure accomplishment of the goal.

Although this is a strict form of leadership, it is useful in crisis situations. A nurse may act as an autocratic leader when taking charge after a patient is found unresponsive. In this situation, it is helpful to have a leader who takes control and directs other members of the health care team.

Democratic Leadership

The participative or **democratic leader** believes that employees are motivated by internal means and want to participate in decision making. The primary function of the leader in this situation is to foster communication and develop relationships with followers. Leaders of this type view themselves as equal to their followers even if they hold formal positions of authority. Followers usually are satisfied with this type of leadership and feel that their ideas are valued. However, decision making can be a lengthy process. This type of leadership is not appropriate in a crisis environment, in which decisions must be made rapidly and without debate.

Nurses who are in charge during a shift may have patient assignments and work with other health care team members to provide care. These nurses may see themselves as equals with other team members and may consult with other nurses, exhibiting a democratic form of leadership. This style of leadership can be utilized in unit council meetings where nurses collaborate together to identify solutions to common problems.

Laissez-Faire Leadership

Like the democratic leader, the permissive or **laissez-faire leader** thinks that employees are motivated by their own desire to do well. The laissez-faire leader provides little or no direction to followers, who develop their own goals and make their own decisions. Few policies and procedures are in place. Although this type of leadership benefits followers by allowing them autonomy over their own work, it usually does not succeed in highly structured organizations such as hospitals. It is most useful in situations in which employees are highly educated, trustworthy, motivated, and experienced. A nurse in a leadership position who uses the laissez-faire style of leadership assigns patient care and expects all team members to set goals for the day and manage their time to complete the assignment. Successful implementation of this leadership style in nursing requires a highly efficient and reliable staff, such as seen in some specialized operating room nursing teams with a history of working together on a set type of cases.

Bureaucratic Leadership

Like the autocratic leader, the **bureaucratic leader** assumes that employees are motivated by external forces. This type of leader relies on policies and procedures to direct goals and work processes. The nurse using bureaucratic leadership tends to relate impersonally to staff and exercises power on the basis of established rules.

QUALITIES OF EFFECTIVE LEADERS

Bennis (2003) identified six qualities of effective leaders. They are integrity, dedication, magnanimity, humility, openness, and creativity.

Integrity is the quality of having clear ethical principles and aligning one's actions with the stated values. This is extremely important for health care professionals. Nurses are expected to follow personal and professional ethics, as outlined in the American Nurses Association (ANA) Code of Ethics for Nurses (2010b). To maintain the trust necessary for the provision of safe and effective care, nurses must do everything possible to protect shared information and maintain the dignity of every person.

Dedication is the ability to spend the time necessary to accomplish a task. Effective leaders persist in working toward accomplishment of a goal even when doing so is difficult. They encourage others to continue working toward the goal. Nurses persevere through difficult situations to provide care that helps patients reach their goals.

Magnanimity means giving credit where credit is due. Good leaders reflect the work and success of accomplishing a goal by crediting those who helped reach it. Magnanimous leaders accept personal responsibility for failure to accomplish objectives. The nurse leader who is magnanimous gives credit to other health care team members who were instrumental in reaching goals.

Humility is the ability to recognize that no one is superior to another. Effective leaders recognize their own worth while respecting the worth of those around them. The nurse in a leadership position who is humble recognizes the valuable contributions made by others and thus helps foster community.

Openness refers to the leader's ability to listen to other points of view without prejudging or discouraging them. An effective leader considers others' opinions with an open mind because a wider variety of solutions to problems is offered. Openness by the nurse leader encourages creative solutions by providing an environment in which people feel comfortable "thinking outside the box." A nurse leader who demonstrates openness maintains approachability for others when questions arise.

Creativity is the ability to think differently. A creative leader examines all possible solutions to a problem even if at first glance they appear to be unrealistic or outside the norm. This ability allows the nurse leader to inspire followers to consider broader visions and goals.

FORMAL AND INFORMAL LEADERSHIP

Leadership may emerge in many circumstances. **Formal leadership** is practiced in an organization as part of an official position, which may or may not be a management position. For example, a nurse can exercise formal leadership in the role of nurse director or supervisor. However, other nurses in the same organization can exercise formal leadership but not have a management role. Examples are nurse practitioners and clinical nurse specialists.

Informal leadership emerges outside the structure of a formal position. For example, staff nurses on a unit demonstrate informal leadership when they take responsibility for coordinating the staff schedule or act as part of the unit governance committee. Informal leadership is exhibited by individuals with strong interpersonal skills who can build relationships to help guide others.

MANAGEMENT LO 12.3

The function of a manager is to accomplish the organization's goals by coordinating and directing the work of others. Successful managers rely on a variety of abilities, including strong communication, organizational proficiency, and critical-thinking skills.

MANAGEMENT THEORY OVERVIEW

Over the years, research has been conducted on the functions of management, management styles and behaviors, and the qualities of effective managers. The resulting theories provide a framework for nurses and nurse managers in understanding how effective managers operate in the health care organization to ensure high-quality patient care.

Fayol's Functions of Management

In the early part of the 20th century, Henri Fayol described the functions of management. They are still applicable today and include planning, organizing, directing, and controlling (Fairholm and Fairholm, 2010).

Planning

The planning function of a manager is comparable to the assessment, diagnosis, and planning portions of the nursing process. It includes four stages:

1. Setting goals
2. Assessing the current situation and future trends
3. Setting the plan
4. Converting the plan into an action statement

The nurse assesses the patient during the planning function of management. The patient's medical diagnosis and prognosis are considered. The nurse works with the family to decide on the best course of action in light of the information gathered, and a plan is formulated, which includes the list of nursing interventions necessary to accomplish the goals (Figure 12-1).

Organizing

The second function of management is organizing. After the plan has been developed, the manager coordinates the work to be done while avoiding duplication of effort. In a hospital setting, the RN organizes the care to be delivered to the patient. The RN delegates care to other health care team members, including LPNs and UAP, matching the team members' skills to the patient's needs to ensure care in the most expedient and cost-effective manner.

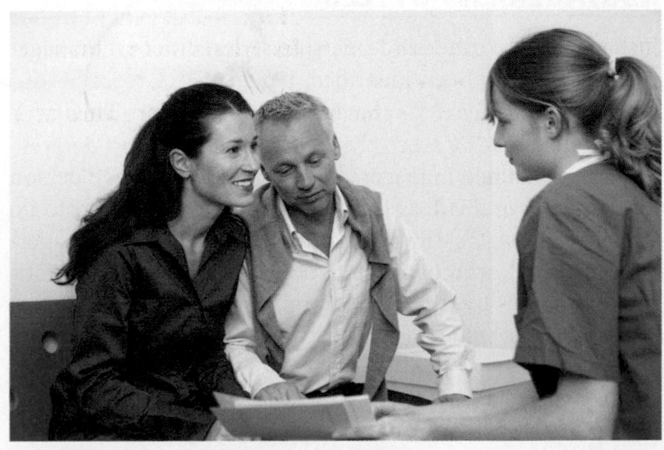

FIGURE 12-1 The nurse works with the patient and family members to establish a plan of care.

Directing

Directing is the management function that ensures the work of the organization is done. Clear direction is essential for smooth operation of any nursing unit. Examples can be seen on nursing units as the charge nurse or unit manager coordinates admissions, discharges, and patient assignments while the RN often directs the work of LPNs and UAP in the course of patient care. Skills required for efficient and clear direction include good communication, organization, and delegation. The ability to motivate others toward a common goal is helpful, because the nurse must work with other, more autonomous professional personnel in patient care situations and in hospital committee work.

Controlling

The act of controlling involves comparing expected results of the planned work with the actual results. In the nursing process, evaluation is comparable to controlling. Evaluation is the process by which outcomes are compared with goals. In the situation of patient care, the patient's progress is measured on the basis of goals set forth in the nursing care plan. The nurse manager participates in organization-wide monitoring of quality of care through the hospital's quality management processes. These processes help to determine care standards and monitor the quality of care delivered.

Mintzberg's Behavioral Model

In 1973 Mintzberg described management in terms of behaviors. Underlying his descriptions were two assumptions: much of a manager's time is spent in human relations, and managers are more reactive than proactive. These assumptions provided the basis for three categories of behaviors: interpersonal roles, informational roles, and decisional roles. Mintzberg described three interpersonal roles: figurehead, leader, and liaison. The three informational roles he described are monitor, disseminator, and spokesperson. The third category of Mintzberg's behavioral roles is composed of the four decisional roles: entrepreneur, disturbance handler, resource allocator, and negotiator.

Mintzberg's Contemporary Model

Mintzberg (1994) later proposed another model of management. The two Mintzberg models are related, but the later version takes into consideration the experience, knowledge, and values of the manager. It describes managerial work as occurring at three different levels, rather than by role. The three levels are information, people, and action.

Information Level

The manager brings to the role a collection of experiences, knowledge, values, and competencies. The manager then develops a framework for what the job is supposed to be and includes the purpose of the job, the work to be done, and the way it should be performed. The information level of work includes communicating and controlling. At this level, the manager gives and receives information and then uses that information to manage the work of others. The nurse manager accomplishes this through staff meetings, message boards, and one-on-one interactions with staff.

People Level

The second level of Mintzberg's contemporary model involves people. At this level, the manager focuses on leading and linking people. Leading entails motivating and encouraging others to take action. Linking occurs when the manager networks with individuals outside the work unit to communicate needs and to develop liaisons. Nurse managers motivate the staff to provide high-quality patient care, and they network through multidisciplinary meetings in the hospital and in the community.

Action Level

At the action level, the focus is doing. At this third level, the manager directs the work of others and works with other departments to gain the resources necessary to achieve the work unit's objective. A nurse manager is working at the action level when contacting the central supply department to get additional dressing supplies when the unit runs short.

QUALITIES OF EFFECTIVE MANAGERS

Many articles describe the qualities of a good leader. The lists of qualities necessary to be an effective manager can be confusing and are as varied as the number of articles dealing with the topic. Hiscock and Shuldham (2008) describe the personal qualities necessary for effective leadership and management in nursing, including self-belief, self-awareness, self-management, personal integrity, and a drive for improvement. Hiscock and Shuldham state that it is important for nurse leaders to be focused on the patients rather than themselves to deliver good patient-focused care. Nurses must desire to improve the status quo to provide higher levels of quality in the care delivered. These qualities are also discussed in other works concerning effective managers (Forsyth, 2004).

SKILLS OF EFFECTIVE MANAGERS

A *skill* is a developed aptitude. Skills are the tools by which a manager carries out the work. The American Organization of Nurse Executives (AONE, 2005) has outlined the competencies necessary for nurse leaders and managers:

- Communication and relationship building
- Knowledge of the health care environment
- Leadership
- Professionalism
- Business skills

Communication is the foundation of nursing practice. Communication skills are essential for the work of the nurse manager and every nurse. By developing excellent communication skills, the nurse can obtain information, relay a plan, delegate, and evaluate a plan of care. The nurse develops relationships—with patients, families, co-workers, and other health care professionals and managers—that are necessary for functioning in the work environment.

An effective nurse manager must have knowledge of the health care environment. This environment includes trends in the local market area and state and national trends. The nurse manager must be aware of regulations and patient care standards so that clinical policies and procedures implemented at the unit level are in compliance with regulatory body expectations.

Leadership is often mentioned as a quality, but it is also a skill. Leadership as a skill is the application of personal traits to promote change. It is the willingness to take action and motivate others with words and by example.

Professionalism refers to the ability to hold others and oneself accountable for actions and outcomes. The professional nurse is aware of and holds high standards of ethics. Advocacy for the patient is part of this skill. The nurse manager is responsible for ensuring that the patient is the center of all decisions in the health care organization.

An effective manager must have business skills and a business sense. Part of quality care is ensuring that the care the patient receives is cost-effective. The nurse manager must understand concepts of budgeting, staffing, marketing, and information management. An understanding of human resource management is equally important. The skillful nurse manager understands the way these elements interact and their influence in achieving expected outcomes in an economically responsible manner.

MANAGEMENT STYLES

Just as there are different leadership styles, different management styles have been identified. Douglas McGregor (1960) identified managers as having Theory X or Theory Y characteristics.

Theory X–style managers believe that the average person dislikes work and will avoid it if given the opportunity to do so. These managers think subordinates must be closely supervised, directed, and coerced into doing their work. They motivate employees by threatening punishment. They think that most workers value job security and have little ambition beyond it.

Theory Y–style managers think that if employees are satisfied in their work, they will view it as being as acceptable as play. These managers believe that satisfied workers are capable of self-direction, self-control, and initiative. They think that given the proper conditions, employees will accept and seek out responsibility on the job.

NURSING LEADERSHIP ROLES LO 12.4

A nurse does not have to be a manager to be a leader. Even at the bedside, nurses use leadership skills, although possibly in different ways than a nurse manager.

PATIENT CARE PROVIDER

The nurse must be able to plan, organize, deliver, and evaluate nursing care for patients. Depending on the mode of nursing care delivery, the patient care nurse may delegate care to licensed and unlicensed personnel. Communication skills are essential to effectively convey information about patients to colleagues in other disciplines, such as medicine. An example of a nurse in this role is an RN on a hospital unit who assesses, plans, and provides care for a group of patients. The RN also delegates certain aspects of care to other members of the health care team.

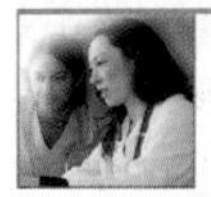

1. Which patients in the case study should the RN consider as priorities in terms of assessment and care? What are the reasons?

PATIENT ADVOCATE

An **advocate** is someone who supports and promotes the interests of others. The RN acts as a patient advocate during the course of treatment (ANA, 2010b). The nurse's unique knowledge and relationship with the patient imparts the responsibility for speaking on the patient's behalf (Patient Education and Health Literacy box). Nurse advocacy roles are discussed in Chapter 1.

PATIENT EDUCATION AND HEALTH LITERACY

Patient Advocate

- Educating patients about their conditions and about the purposes and expected outcomes of the planned treatment empowers them to act as their own advocates and can improve their cooperation with the treatment plan.
- After patients have information about their conditions, they can seek further information on their own and discuss treatment options with their health care provider.
- Discussing topics such as the purposes and side effects of medication can give patients the awareness they need to monitor their response to treatment, including untoward effects, which can then be reported in a timely manner.

CASE MANAGER

Although many health care organizations have case managers to aid in moving the patient through the health care system, the bedside nurse also acts as a case manager. One important way a nurse can do this is by beginning discharge planning on admission. The data gathered from the patient and family during the admission assessment contain important information about the patient's prehospitalization condition, functional ability, and knowledge of disease. During the admission process, areas of difficulty or lack of function are identified, and planning for discharge is placed into an electronic care plan.

QSEN FOCUS!

The nurse exhibits teamwork and collaboration when recognizing the contributions of other team members in helping the patient achieve health goals and when assuming the role of a team member or leader, depending on the situation.

CLINICAL NURSE LEADER

The clinical nurse leader (CNL) has a master's degree and certification from the American Association of Colleges of Nursing (AACN) Commission on Nurse Certification. In this newer nursing role, the CNL oversees patient care or provides direct patient care using evidence-based practice, evaluates patient outcomes, and updates care plans. The CNL's role may vary in different care settings (AACN, 2014).

FINANCIAL RESOURCE MANAGER

The nurse is in a unique position to help manage financial resources. Wise use of supplies is one way the nurse can contain costs and manage charges for the patient. For example, a nurse who is going to perform a dressing change on a patient in the hospital should gather and take into the patient's room only the supplies needed for that procedure. After supplies have been taken into a patient room, they cannot be returned to the clean utility room and would be wasted if not used. The nurse has a responsibility to the patient to consider the cost of prescribed therapies. To do this responsibly, nurses must have an understanding of Medicare, Medicaid, and insurance provisions.

COLLABORATIVE TEAM MEMBER

Coordination of patient care makes the nurse an integral part of the health care team. The nurse works as a collaborative team member with physicians and allied health colleagues for the benefit of the patient. In recognition of the importance of the need for collaboration among nursing and other health care disciplines, the American Nurses Credentialing Center (ANCC, 2014) included interdisciplinary relationships as one of the "forces of magnetism" (Ethical, Legal, and Professional Practice box) that determine certification in the Magnet Recognition Program.

ETHICAL, LEGAL, AND PROFESSIONAL PRACTICE

Magnet Recognition Program

The Magnet Recognition Program developed by the American Nurses Credentialing Center (ANCC, 2014) recognizes health care organizations for exemplary practice in the areas of patient care, nursing excellence, and innovation in nursing practice. Health care organizations can apply to become Magnet certified. The forces of magnetism that determine certification are as follows:

- Quality of nursing leadership
- Organizational structure
- Management style
- Personnel policies and programs
- Professional models of care
- Quality of care
- Quality improvement
- Consultation and resources
- Autonomy
- Community and the health care organization
- Nurses as teachers
- Image of nursing
- Interdisciplinary relationships
- Professional development

Magnet recognition is beneficial to the health care organization, because it recognizes a professional environment that supports development of the nursing staff. The evaluation for Magnet status is based on quality indicators and standards found in the ANA (2010a) publication *Nursing Administration: Scope and Standards of Practice*.

The quality indicators and standards put forth in the Magnet Recognition Program are designed to create a professionally satisfying environment for nurses. By enacting nurse-friendly policies and programs, Magnet hospitals are able to recruit and retain nurses at higher rates than non-Magnet organizations. Other professions also benefit from the professional values and collaboration in Magnet-status organizations. Some hospitals have found it easier to recruit and retain other in-demand professionals, such as pharmacists, because of the increased job satisfaction that comes from true interprofessional collaboration (Brahm, Kelly-Rehm, and Farmer, 2009). Patients also benefit, because Magnet organizations with more stable staffing patterns are better able to consistently provide safe, competent patient care.

DELEGATION

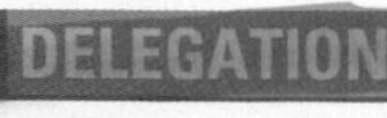

LO 12.5

For patient care to be completed in a safe and timely manner, it is sometimes necessary for the nurse to delegate tasks to other health care providers. The National Council of State Boards of Nursing (NCSBN) offers support in this process. In their joint statement (ANA and NCSBN, 2005), the ANA describes **delegation** as the transfer of responsibility, and the NCSBN calls it a transfer of authority. This transfer gives a competent individual the authority to perform a selected nursing task in a selected situation. The nurse retains accountability for the delegation. When a nurse assigns the hygienic care of a group of patients to the UAP, the nurse is ultimately responsible for making sure the care is completed. Any significant findings during the care such as alterations in skin integrity, shortness of breath, or changes in a patient's condition should be reported to the nurse. The nurse is then responsible for assessing the alterations and addressing them in the plan of care.

QSEN FOCUS!

Through quality improvement, the nurse appreciates the value of what each team member can do to improve patient care.

PRINCIPLES OF DELEGATION

First Principle of Delegation

Nurses must have knowledge of the nurse practice act in the state where they are licensed. Each state's nurse practice act defines the RN scope of practice and discusses appropriate delegation. A second resource in delegation is the employing organization's policy and procedure manual. Employers must have job descriptions for each job class that outline the responsibilities and limitations of each position. The NCSBN website and journal articles are other resources for understanding delegation.

In considering the delegation of nursing tasks, the nurse must ask the following questions:

- Is this task within the RN scope of practice, knowledge, and skill?
- Is this task within the scope and abilities of the person to whom it is being delegated?
- Is this task something that can be delegated?
- Are there adequate resources available to the delegatee to complete the task?
- Does the patient's condition require ongoing or frequent assessment or intervention?
- What are the potential risks to patient safety related to this task?
- Does this task entail assessment, evaluation, or nursing judgment?

Second Principle of Delegation

The RN cannot delegate assessment, planning, evaluation, or accountability for the assigned task. This means that even though the task has been assigned, the RN is still responsible for following up with the delegatee to ensure that the task has been completed. If the delegatee does not carry out the task in a satisfactory manner, the RN is responsible for seeing that it is completed.

! SAFE PRACTICE ALERT

The RN is responsible for assessment of patients even if certain tasks are delegated to others.

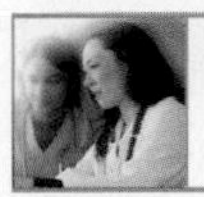

2. Which tasks cannot be delegated to the UAP? Why?

Third Principle of Delegation

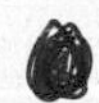

The person to whom the assignment was delegated cannot delegate that assignment to someone else. If the person cannot carry out the assignment, the individual needs to notify the delegating RN so that the task may be reassigned or completed by the RN (Ethical, Legal, and Professional Practice box).

ETHICAL, LEGAL, AND PROFESSIONAL PRACTICE

Delegation

Before delegation, the nurse should do the following:

- Identify
  - The task to be performed.
  - The specific time frame for the task to be completed.
- Assess
  - The patient.
  - The type of nursing care needed.
  - The complexity and frequency of needed care.
  - Patient stability.
  - Assessments of other providers.
- Determine that all of the following apply:
  - The task requires no nursing judgment.
  - The outcomes are reasonably predictable.
  - There is no need to alter the procedure for completing the task.
  - The task does not require complex observations or critical decisions.
  - Repeated nursing assessments are not required.
  - The consequences of delegating the task are not a risk to the patient.

From Ohio Board of Nursing: *Standards and practice relative to registered nurse or licensed practical nurse,* Ohio Revised Code 4723-4-01, 2011.

! SAFE PRACTICE ALERT

Remember to follow up with the UAP to ensure that the delegated task has been completed and properly documented.

FIVE RIGHTS OF SAFE DELEGATION

The Joint Statement on Delegation by the ANA and NCSBN (2005) identifies Five Rights of Delegation. Applying these rights while working with licensed and unlicensed personnel takes some practice. The new nurse may want to enlist the support of more experienced co-workers when first using these rights of delegation (Collaboration and Delegation box).

COLLABORATION AND DELEGATION

Five Rights of Delegation

1. *Right task:* one that is delegable for a specific patient
2. *Right circumstances:* appropriate patient setting, available resources, and other relevant factors considered
3. *Right person:* the right person delegating the right task to the right person to be performed on the right patient
4. *Right direction or communication:* clear, concise description of the task, including its objective, limits, and expectations
5. *Right supervision:* appropriate monitoring, evaluation, intervention, and feedback

Right Task

Wise use of the skills and knowledge available through support staff frees the RN to perform the aspects of care that only a nurse can do. The RN must remember to delegate tasks that do not require nursing judgment. Only tasks that are routine and do not require variation from a standardized procedure should be delegated.

Right Person

The definition of delegation states that a task must be assigned to a competent person in a selected situation. Most states have a certification process for UAP. LPNs or licensed vocational nurses (LVNs) are licensed. Work settings have job descriptions and approved skills or competency lists as part of the hiring and orientation process. In working with a group of people, the nurse becomes knowledgeable about individual skills, strengths, and weaknesses.

Right Circumstance

Delegation depends on the patient care situation. The nurse evaluates a situation and determines whether it is appropriate for delegation. Depending on the unit type and patient acuity, the nurse may elect to negotiate a modified assignment or a different staffing combination.

Right Communication

The first component of supervision is communication. The ANA and NCSBN (2005) state that communication regarding delegation should be clear, concise, correct, and complete. The information that needs to be communicated includes the specific data to be collected, along with methods for reporting; the activities to be carried out, along with patient-specific instructions and limitations; and the expected outcomes, possible complications, and specific timelines for reporting the information. Cultural differences should be considered when communicating tasks (Diversity Considerations box).

Right Supervision

Supervision means monitoring an activity being carried out by someone else and making sure that it is performed

DIVERSITY CONSIDERATIONS

Culture, Ethnicity, and Religion

Consider these transcultural phenomena when delegating tasks. Be sure to address any racial or gender prejudices among the staff. Avoid always delegating tasks to the new person; use the expertise of experienced staff. Be sure not to overextend by delegating exclusively to one person or group of people, even if doing so is viewed as conferring higher status.

Cultural phenomena should be considered when delegating to a diverse staff:

- Culture in the form of ethnic values or religious beliefs affects verbal and nonverbal communication. Factors such as eye contact, posture, and use of assertive or passive terms must be considered in communicating with a diverse staff.
- Of the four zones of interpersonal space (intimate, personal, social, and public), some cultures prefer a closer interpersonal space while others prefer more distance.
- For most cultural groups, the family is the most important social organization, and family responsibilities may be placed above all else, including work.
- Cultural groups may be past, present, or future oriented. Past- and present-oriented cultural groups tend not to focus on long-range goals.
- Individuals and cultural groups with an internal locus of control need to feel in control of their environment and focus on planning. Those with an external locus of control think that fate or chance plays a role in life events and focus more on the obstacles they face.

Gender

- Be aware of gender differences in communication. Males and females transmit and interpret messages differently.

Disability and Morphology

- Disease, health, body habitus, and wellness all play a role in alertness and stamina.

From Poole VL, Davidhizar RE, Giger JN: Delegating to a transcultural team. *Nurs Manag*, 26(8), 33-34, 1995.

correctly. Supervision and accountability go hand in hand. Supervision does not mean that the nurse has to directly observe the delegatee carry out the assigned task. However, the nurse does conduct periodic follow-up inquiries with the individual to ascertain that the task is being completed, that clarification of instructions is provided, and that the assignment is adjusted if necessary.

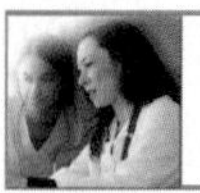

3. What tasks are appropriate to delegate to the UAP at the start of the shift? Why?

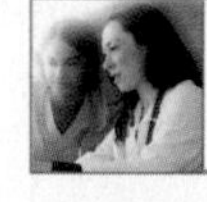

4. What tasks are appropriate to delegate to the LPN or LVN? Why?

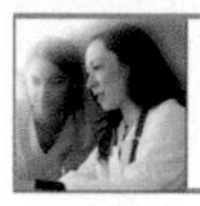

5. What information should the nurse include for the UAP when delegating the tasks?

SUMMARY OF LEARNING OUTCOMES

LO 12.1 *Compare leadership and management:* Leadership and management are related but different concepts. Leadership is the ability to influence others. Management is the ability to motivate people to accomplish a goal.

LO 12.2 *Describe the styles of leadership, including the qualities of effective leaders:* There are different styles of leadership based on leadership theories. No one style fits every situation. The six qualities of an effective leader are integrity, dedication, magnanimity, humility, openness, and creativity.

LO 12.3 *Discuss various management theories, including qualities of effective managers:* Management theories provide a framework for nurse managers in understanding how to effectively operate within the health care organization to ensure high-quality patient care. Successful managers possess qualities of self-belief, self-awareness, self-management, personal integrity, and a drive for improvement. Leadership, professionalism, and communication skills are also desirable. Nurse managers must be able to influence change, communicate clearly, solve problems, and be effective organizers.

LO 12.4 *Characterize nursing leadership roles in health care:* Nurses act as leaders in various roles. All nurses have a responsibility to provide safe patient care, to act as patient advocates, be fiscally responsible in care, and collaborate with other team members to provide high-quality, cost-effective care.

LO 12.5 *Explain the underlying principles of delegation in health care:* Appropriate delegation is the responsibility of the RN. The Five Rights of Delegation are right task, right person, right circumstance, right communication, and right supervision. The nurse cannot delegate assessment, planning, evaluation, or accountability for the assigned task.

Responses to the critical-thinking questions are available at ***http://evolve.elsevier.com/YoostCrawford/fundamentals/.***

REVIEW QUESTIONS

1. Processes used in management parallel the nursing process. Which sentence describes a nurse using a management principle paralleled with the nursing process?
   - **a.** Planning is demonstrated when the nurse motivates others.
   - **b.** Directing is demonstrated when the nurse plans care for the patient.
   - **c.** Organizing is demonstrated when the nurse coordinates care for patients.
   - **d.** Controlling is demonstrated when the nurse tells other staff members what to do.
2. Which statement most closely reflects the differences between nurse leaders and managers?
   - **a.** Nurse leaders are always in formal positions of authority.
   - **b.** Nurse managers use transactional principles to accomplish goals.
   - **c.** Nurse leaders rely primarily on interpersonal skills to accomplish goals.
   - **d.** Nurse managers rely on supervisors for accountability and responsibility.
3. The nurse manager is monitoring overtime for the unit. She closely monitors staff hours and does not allow staff to come in for extra hours if they are over their allotted time per week. This is an example of which of Mintzberg's decisional roles of the manager?
   - **a.** Entrepreneur
   - **b.** Disturbance handler
   - **c.** Negotiator
   - **d.** Resource handler
4. A nurse manager is trying to improve patient satisfaction ratings for her area of responsibility. The manager meets with the staff and forms an ad hoc committee to address the issues around the problem. This is an example of what style of leadership?
   - **a.** Bureaucratic
   - **b.** Democratic
   - **c.** Laissez-faire
   - **d.** Autocratic
5. A nurse is volunteering in the community to educate parents to increase the number of children in the school district who are immunized. The nurse oversees the activities of a group of volunteers. Which role best describes the nurse's activity in this situation?
   - **a.** Management
   - **b.** Leadership
   - **c.** Volunteerism
   - **d.** Activism
6. Which statement is an example of the use of situational leadership?
   - **a.** The emergency room manager takes a vote on holiday coverage and then responds to a Code Blue by directing orders at the nursing staff.
   - **b.** The manager in surgery uses the vacation policy to grant time off and then performs a surgical count in an operating room using a checklist.
   - **c.** A vice president of nursing allows the department directors to make a decision about a hospital policy on holiday time and then sides with a nurse who does not want to work the required time.
   - **d.** The CEO of the hospital instructs the nursing senate to develop a dress code and then changes the dress code after determining he does not like it.
7. Effective nurse managers focus on which area?
   - **a.** Cost-effective operation of the unit
   - **b.** Motivation of staff
   - **c.** Accomplishing organizational goals
   - **d.** The patients and their needs
8. A nurse states she believes in the dignity of each patient. At break, she is overheard talking about a patient in a persistent vegetative state as a "lump." This represents an inconsistency in which quality of an effective leader?
   - **a.** Dedication
   - **b.** Magnanimity
   - **c.** Integrity
   - **d.** Humility
9. A nurse delegates a bed bath to unlicensed assistive personnel (UAP). After lunch, the patient complains that he has not yet been cleaned up. He is very upset and angry. What should the nurse's next action be?
   - **a.** Assist the patient in getting cleaned up.
   - **b.** Write up the UAP for not carrying out the assignment.
   - **c.** Report the UAP to the unit manager.
   - **d.** Go find the UAP, and tell her to complete the bath immediately.
10. The registered nurse on an inpatient medical unit delegates vital signs and morning care to the UAP for five stable patients. The nurse asks the UAP to document the vital signs and report any abnormal results immediately. Which rights of delegation is the nurse demonstrating? *(Select all that apply.)*
    - **a.** Right person
    - **b.** Right circumstance
    - **c.** Right time
    - **d.** Right supervision
    - **e.** Right patient

Answers and rationales for the review questions are available at *http://evolve.elsevier.com/YoostCrawford/fundamentals/*.

REFERENCES

American Association of Colleges of Nursing (AACN): What is CNL certification?, 2014. Retrieved from *www.aacn.nche.edu/cnl/cnc/what-is-cnl-certification.*

American Nurses Association (ANA): *Nursing administration: Scope and standards of practice*, Silver Springs, Md., 2010a, Author.

American Nurses Association (ANA): *Guide to the Code of ethics for nurses: Interpretation and application.* Silver Springs, Md., 2010b, Author.

American Nurses Association (ANA), National Council of State Boards of Nursing (NCSBN): Joint statement on delegation, 2005. Retrieved from *https://www.ncsbn.org/Delegation_joint_statement_NCSBN-ANA.pdf.*

American Nurses Credentialing Center (ANCC): Magnet Recognition Program overview, 2014. Retrieved from *www.nursecredentialing.org/Magnet/ProgramOverview.*

American Organization of Nurse Executives (AONE): AONE nurse executive competencies. *Nurse Leader* 3(1), 15-22, 2005. Retrieved from *www.nurseleader.com/article/S1541-4612(05)00007-8/fulltext.*

Bass B: *Bass & Stodgill's handbook of leadership: Theory, research, and managerial applications*, ed. 3, New York, 1990, Free Press.

Bennis W: *On becoming a leader: The leadership classic,* Reading, Mass, 2003, Perseus.

Brahm N, Kelly-Rehm M, Farmer K: Collaboration: What can health-care organizations learn about pharmacist retention from Magnet status hospitals? *Res Soc Admin Pharm*, 5(4), 382-389, 2009.

Burns JM: *Leadership,* New York, 1978, Harper Torchbooks.

Cronenwett L, Sherwood G, Barnsteiner J, et al.: Quality and safety education for nurses. *Nurs Outlook*, 55(3):122-131, 2007.

Fairholm G, Fairholm M: *Understanding leadership perspectives: Theoretical and practical approaches*, New York, 2010, Springer.

Forsyth R: M-A-N-A-G-E-M-E-N-T defined subordinates' expectations. *FBI Law Enforce Bull*, 73(3):23-27, 2004.

Hiscock M, Shuldham C: Patient centered leadership in practice. *J Nurs Manage*, 16:900-904, 2008.

Lewin K: *The field theory in social science*, New York, 1951, Harper & Row.

McGregor DM: *The human side of enterprise*, New York, 1960, McGraw-Hill, pp. 37-57.

Mintzberg H: *The nature of managerial work*, New York, 1973, Harper & Row.

Mintzberg H: Managing as blended care. *Nurs Admin*, 24, 29-36, 1994.

Ohio Board of Nursing: Standards and practice relative to registered nurse or licensed practical nurse, Ohio Revised Code 4723-4-01, 2011.

Poole VL, Davidhizar RE, Giger JN: Delegating to a transcultural team. *Nurs Manage*, 26(8):33-34, 1995.

Taylor P: Leadership in education. *Emerg Librarian*, 21(3), 1994.

Weiss SA, Tappen RM: *Essentials of nursing leadership and management*, ed. 6, Philadelphia, 2015, FA Davis.

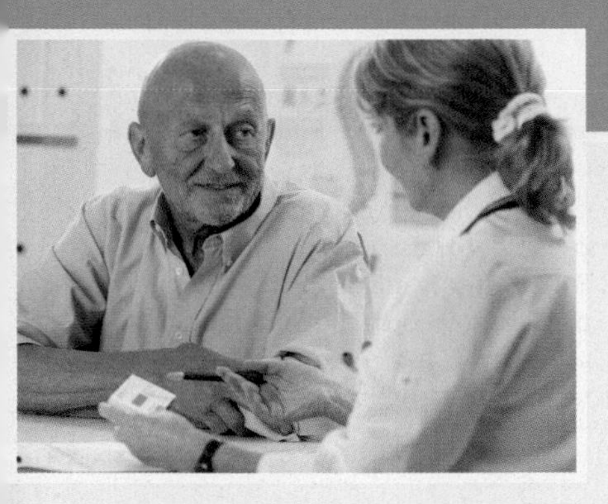

CHAPTER 13

Evidence-Based Practice and Nursing Research

EVOLVE WEBSITE

http://evolve.elsevier.com/YoostCrawford/fundamentals/

- Additional Evolve-Only Review Questions With Answers
- Answers and Rationales for Text Review Questions
- Answers to Critical-Thinking Questions
- Case Study With Questions
- Glossary

LEARNING OUTCOMES

Comprehension of this chapter's content will provide students with the ability to:

LO 13.1 Define various types of nursing research.
LO 13.2 Compare quantitative and qualitative research methods.
LO 13.3 Explain the steps involved in the research process.
LO 13.4 Explain research and its relationship to evidence-based practice.
LO 13.5 Discuss the steps required in conducting evidence-based research.
LO 13.6 Identify considerations for implementing research in nursing practice.
LO 13.7 Explain the relationship of hospital Magnet status with nursing research and practice.

KEY TERMS

anonymity, p. 181
applied research, p. 178
basic research, p. 178
clinical research, p. 178
confidentiality, p. 181
control group, p. 180
correlational research, p. 179
critical appraisal, p. 185
data, p. 179
data analysis, p. 182
deductive reasoning, p. 179
dependent variable, p. 180
descriptive research, p. 179
dissemination, p. 182
ethnography, p. 179
evidence-based practice, p. 178
experimental research, p. 179
grounded theory research, p. 179
historical research, p. 179
human subject, p. 180
hypothesis, p. 180
independent variable, p. 180
inductive reasoning, p. 179
informed consent, p. 181
institutional review board, p. 180
instruments, p. 180
literature review, p. 179
meta-analysis, p. 180
phenomenological research, p. 179
phenomenon, p. 179
PICO, p. 184
research use, p. 183
sample, p. 180
stakeholder, p. 183
systematic review, p. 179
qualitative research, p. 179
quantitative research, p. 179
quasi-experimental research, p. 179
validity, p. 185
variable, p. 179

CASE STUDY

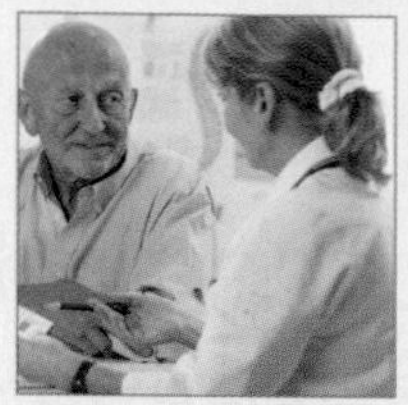

Mr. Tregalin is a 60-year-old male with a 30-year history of smoking. He asks the nurse at his annual physical about quitting smoking. He wants to know the best method for him to use that will provide long-term abstinence. He inquires about oral medications that he has heard about and nicotine replacement therapy such as nicotine patches, lozenges, or gum. He cannot remember the name of the medication that he saw advertised on TV and in magazines. The nurse uses research and evidence-based practice principles to develop a patient-centered plan of care for Mr. Tregalin.

Refer back to this case study to answer the critical-thinking questions throughout the chapter.

Evidence for the practice of nursing is derived from research in nursing, medicine, health care, and disciplines outside of health care. **Evidence-based practice** (EBP) is the integration of best research evidence with (1) clinical expertise, (2) patient values and needs, and (3) the delivery of quality, cost-effective health care. The ultimate goal is to promote positive outcomes for the patient. Nurses often identify potential research problems while caring for patients, such as how best to treat pressure ulcers. Some nurses are involved in collecting data for research, whereas others analyze and disseminate findings that affect practice. All nurses need to be familiar with how to review research findings to guide their EBP. Each research study helps to expand the nursing knowledge base, and this further defines nursing as a discipline and profession.

DEFINITION OF NURSING RESEARCH LO 13.1

RESEARCH

Research is a "systematic inquiry that uses disciplined methods to answer questions or solve problems" (Polit and Beck, 2013, p. 4). Research is also defined as "a diligent, systemic inquiry or study that validates and refines existing knowledge and develops new knowledge" (Burns and Grove, 2011, p. 3). Federal regulations define research as "systematic investigation, including research development, testing, and evaluation, designed to develop or contribute to generalizable knowledge" (Office of Human Research Protection, 2008, para. 2). These general descriptions provide a basis for understanding research conducted in nursing.

NURSING RESEARCH

Nursing research "provides the scientific basis for the practice of the profession" (American Association of Colleges of Nursing, 2012). A more specific definition is that "nursing research is a formal, systematic, and rigorous process of inquiry used to generate and test theories about the health related experiences of human beings within their environments and about the actions and processes that nurses use in practice" (Fawcett and Garity, 2009, p. 5).

Research conducted to generate theories is **basic research**. These theories help to provide explanations for phenomena. Testing theories in different situations with different populations is **applied research**. **Clinical research** is conducted to test theories about the effectiveness of interventions. Each type of research contributes to the theoretical base for the practice of nursing.

AMERICAN NURSES ASSOCIATION RESEARCH STANDARDS

The American Nurses Association (ANA) standards of professional performance require nurses to use research findings in practice. Two criteria are measured. The first criterion is that nurses need to use the best available evidence, which includes research findings, to guide their practice decisions (ANA, 2010). The second criterion is that nurses participate in research activities that are appropriate for their position and level of education. Activities may include identifying problems in the clinical setting that may be researched; participating in data collection; participating as a member of a research committee or a research program; sharing research findings the nurse has found with others; conducting research; critiquing research that may be used in practice; using research findings to develop policies, procedures, and standards for patient care at health care facilities; and incorporating research as part of ongoing learning as a nurse. Nurses may participate in one or more of these activities during their careers. The ANA (2012) Research Toolkit was developed to help nurses to provide evidence-based care that improves patient outcomes. In 1981, the ANA Commission on Nursing Research published guidelines for the investigative function of nurses according to their level of education.

In 1985, the ANA created the National Center for Nursing Research. This organization evolved into the National Institute of Nursing Research (NINR) in 1993, affording it equal status with other National Institutes of Health. "The mission of NINR is to promote and improve the health of individuals, families, communities, and populations. NINR supports and conducts clinical and basic research and research training on health and illness across the lifespan" (NINR, 2011).

METHODS OF RESEARCH LO 13.2

Three methods of research are used in studies: quantitative, qualitative, and combined qualitative and quantitative. Each method is used to gather data. **Data** are facts collected and analyzed by the researcher from the participants in a study. Data are expressed as numbers or in words, and the form of data expression determines which method of research is used.

QUANTITATIVE RESEARCH

Quantitative research usually produces data in the form of numbers. Quantitative research is based on a postpositivist philosophy, which assumes that reality is objective, fixed, stable, observable, measurable, and value free (Sale, Lohfeld, and Brazil, 2002). Positivism assumes that the approach is deductive in nature (Newman, 2000), and it seeks to gain knowledge through scientific and experimental research (Erzberger and Kelle, 2003). **Deductive reasoning** formulates a specific conclusion from a large amount of data. Clinical trials of medications that are used to treat certain diseases, such as high blood pressure, employ quantitative research methodology. A nurse may be involved in quantitative research while investigating, for example, the effectiveness of a specific intervention for the prevention of skin breakdown.

There are several types of quantitative research, including descriptive, correlational, and experimental research. **Descriptive research** identifies data and characteristics about the population or phenomenon. A **phenomenon** is a fact, event, or circumstance that can be observed or experienced. Descriptive research can provide a starting point for future research or generate a hypothesis or theory through observation or documentation of a particular situation.

Correlational research is used to explore a relationship between two variables. A **variable** is a concept or item that has values that can change and that can be measured, manipulated, or controlled in the study. Correlational research examines the relationship between two items such as weight and age. In correlational research, there is no control over the variables. Research may be done by looking retrospectively at a phenomenon and at the variables that can affect its occurrence. Originally, retrospective lung cancer research looked at patients who had or did not have cancer and at possible correlations with specific behaviors such as smoking.

Experimental research explores the causal relationships between variables. Experimental research examines whether or not one variable has a cause-and-effect relationship with another, such as a blood pressure medication having an effect on decreasing blood pressure. Experimental research examines a cause, whereas correlational research determines only whether or not the two variables are related to each other. Correlation cannot prove causation.

Quasi-experimental research examines a causal relationship between variables, but it may not meet the strict guidelines of experimental research. Some research of the effects of nursing interventions on patient outcomes may fall into this category. Outcome research includes studies of patient and family responses to interventions or patient satisfaction related to care in the hospital.

QUALITATIVE RESEARCH

Qualitative research is based on a constructivist philosophy, which assumes that reality is composed of multiple socially constructed realities of each person or group (Sale, Lohfeld, and Brazil, 2002) and is therefore value laden, focusing on personal beliefs, thoughts, and feelings. Constructivism assumes an approach that is inductive (Newman, 2000). **Inductive reasoning** generalizes from specific facts. Qualitative research usually results in data expressed in words, often in the form of a narrative.

There are several types of qualitative research, including phenomenology, grounded theory, ethnography, and historical. **Phenomenological research** explores the reactions of a specific group of people who experienced a similar event in their lives.

Grounded theory research derives theories from the data collected in studies. The grounded theory method has been used to study postpartum depression, communication processes, and the way people with human immunodeficiency virus (HIV) infection manage their illness.

Ethnography focuses on the sociology of meaning through close field observation of a sociocultural phenomenon. The term *ethnography* is sometimes applied to the field notes or case studies produced from ethnographic research. **Historical research** studies historical documents to determine an accurate picture of a past event or time period.

COMPONENTS OF RESEARCH LO 13.3

The research process involves many different components. The literature review is conducted after a research problem is identified. Ethical procedures must be addressed before the study begins. Data are then collected and analyzed before discussion of the research results.

LITERATURE REVIEW

After a research problem is identified, the purpose of the study is defined. This purpose states why the problem is important. A review is conducted to determine what is already known on the topic and identify any gaps in the literature. A **literature review** is a critical analysis of current information on the subject that will be studied in the research. The literature is searched for relevant articles on the topic, and the resulting information is then analyzed. A literature review typically appears near the beginning of published research articles.

Literature reviews include scholarly analyses of research. An integrative literature review synthesizes research findings and formulates ideas about future research. A **systematic review** of the literature provides a comprehensive, unbiased analysis through the use of a strict scientific design to select and assess each of the studies. A **meta-analysis** merges statistical results from related studies to discover similarities and differences in their findings.

The literature review process includes an overview of the subject, which involves dividing the literature into categories of articles that support a particular position and those that do not. The review should explain how each of the articles is similar to or different from the other articles. Conclusions are drawn about their contributions on the basis of the persuasiveness of the research findings. When reading each article, the researcher needs to determine the type of evidence that is provided: history, statistics, recent findings, or narrative or case study. The analysis includes the objectivity of the author, the credibility of the findings, and the overall value of the study. The purpose of the review is to describe the relationship of each article to the others, interpret the findings, and identify any gaps in the literature, which may provide a need for further research. The literature review provides a rationale for conducting the research proposed for the study.

DATA COLLECTION

After the literature review is conducted, hypotheses or research questions are formulated. A **hypothesis** is a statement about two or more variables and their relationship to each other. The design of the research is then selected to provide a plan for how to collect and analyze the data; the design includes the population to be studied and the specific sample for the study. The **sample** consists of the individuals in the population from whom the data will be collected.

Data can be collected by many different methods. **Instruments** are data collection tools. An example of an instrument is a questionnaire, which may be created in a Likert scale format, showing the degree of satisfaction with each item, or as open-ended questions. Degree of agreement can be shown with 5 being the most satisfied and 1 being the least satisfied. Figure 13-1 is an example of a Likert scale. Interviews and focus groups are other means of obtaining data that may have structured questions or a more unstructured format. The data can also include diagnostic information concerning patients, such as laboratory values or information such as age, gender, ethnicity, vital signs, height, and weight.

DEPENDENT AND INDEPENDENT VARIABLES

In experimental research, the independent variable is referred to as an *experimental variable* or *treatment variable.* An **independent variable** is a concept or idea whose value determines the value of other (dependent) variables. In research, the independent variable comprises the experimental treatment or intervention, and it is manipulated by the researcher to yield various outcomes. The **dependent variable** is the outcome that is affected by manipulation of the independent variable. For example, in researching the effectiveness of an antihypertensive medication, the medication is the independent variable and the person's blood pressure is the dependent variable.

In a controlled study, some of the participants are assigned to the treatment group, and others are assigned to the control group by a random process. The **control group** does not receive the treatment. In the clinical trial of a medication, the control group receives a placebo. The purpose of a control group is to prevent bias and ensure that the outcome results from the treatment rather than some other factor.

Institutional Review Board

An **institutional review board** (IRB) is a review committee established to help protect the rights and welfare of human research subjects. Regulations require IRB review and approval for research involving human subjects if it is funded or regulated by the federal government. Most research institutions, professional organizations, and scholarly journals apply the same requirements to all human research. The IRB must approve the research and procedure for data collection from human subjects.

A **human subject** is defined as "a living individual about whom an investigator conducting research obtains (1) data through intervention or interaction with the individual or (2) identifiable private information" (Office of Human Research Protection, 2008, para. 3). *Interventions* may include procedures such as gathering diagnostic information or manipulating the subject's environment. *Interaction* refers to any communication or contact during the research. *Private information* includes anything not expected to be made public, such as a medical record.

The IRB addresses three ethical principles that are inherent in research. The beneficence principle reminds researchers to minimize harms and maximize benefits. The principle of justice requires researchers to treat people fairly and design research to select subjects equitably and avoid exploitation of vulnerable populations. Autonomy includes the ability to understand and process information (i.e., mental capacity) and the ability to volunteer (i.e., freedom from the control or influence of others). Elements of autonomy and justice are related to issues concerning vulnerable populations and need

I was satisfied with the care I received during my stay in the hospital.

Strongly Agree	Agree	Neither	Disagree	Strongly Disagree
5	4	3	2	1

FIGURE 13-1 Likert scale.

DIVERSITY CONSIDERATIONS

Research participation by all human subjects is voluntary. However, nurses need to be sensitive to unique circumstances that may affect the willingness or ability of persons to engage in research. Individuals may choose not to participate because of cultural or religious reasons. When providing information to participants, the researcher must assess their level of understanding and ensure that the information is provided at the appropriate level.

Situations of Vulnerability

- When participants have limitations in volunteerism or capacity, they are vulnerable.
- Vulnerable subjects are more likely to have their rights abused through:
  - Physical control, as occurred during the Holocaust in the Nazi concentration camps, where research was conducted on the prisoners.
  - Coercion, which exists when subjects are told to participate and have reason to fear they will be harmed or threatened if they refuse.
  - Undue influence of someone in authority.
  - Manipulation of the information provided, such as by lying, withholding information, or exaggerating.

Vulnerable Subjects

- Children
- Embryos or fetuses
- Mentally disabled subjects
- Subjects experiencing an emergency situations (e.g., being in an ambulance on the way to the hospital may cause a person to make a hasty decision about participating in research)
- Subjects in hierarchical social structures (e.g., hospitalized patients, nursing home residents, students, prisoners, military personnel), who may feel pressured to volunteer
- Educationally disadvantaged subjects, who may be illiterate or unable to comprehend the materials provided
- Economically disadvantaged subjects, who may be influenced by monetary compensation
- Members of marginalized social groups, who may not have access to the legal system
- Individuals with a fatal or incurable illness, who may accept high risks in the hope of a cure even if there is no direct benefit

to be considered when conducting research (Diversity Considerations box). Vulnerable subjects are those with diminished autonomy. Additional information on these ethical concepts is provided in Chapter 11.

Respect for persons requires researchers to treat individuals as autonomous human beings, allowing them to choose for themselves. Rules derived from respect for persons include the requirement to obtain informed consent and the requirement to respect the privacy of research subjects. **Informed consent** begins when the subjects are recruited and continues throughout the research process (Ethical, Legal, and Professional Practice box).

ETHICAL, LEGAL, AND PROFESSIONAL PRACTICE

Patient Rights Regarding Informed Consent

- Research participants require an explanation of the study in which they are subjects. Any information provided needs to be in a language that is understandable to them.
- Procedures and the purpose of the study need to be explained.
- The manner in which subject anonymity and confidentiality will be protected needs to be explained.
- Any potential harm, including physical or mental discomfort, and possible benefits from participation should be explained.
- Questions should be answered so that participants fully understand the research and their part in the process.
- All subjects need to be given time to decide about participation.
- Study participants are voluntary, may withdraw at any time, or may choose not to complete tasks.

Confidentiality and Anonymity

The way in which data will be used and made available to others is part of the agreement researchers make with study participants, and it is described in the informed consent. There are procedural design guidelines for anonymity and confidentiality. **Confidentiality** is the assurance that information can be viewed only by those requiring access. **Anonymity** means that a person's identity or personal information is not known. When collected, this type of data must be kept anonymous. If identifiers are used, they should be identification codes that are kept secure and destroyed on completion of the study. When data are to be reported, the researcher must determine whether to use names or pseudonyms. Participants' permission is needed if the data include quotations or can reveal the subject's identity.

The ultimate goal is to protect the identity of those participating, especially if there is any information that they would not want revealed about themselves. The data must be protected in some way. If the data are on a computer, password-protected access is required. Regulations under the Health Insurance Portability and Accountability Act (HIPAA) and its Privacy Rule, which outlines handling of protected health information, must be followed during research and addressed in the IRB application.

Any videos, photos, or audiotapes require releases if they are to be shown in the dissemination of research findings. The participants have the right to review these tapes before allowing them to be used for research. If subjects are involved in a group, they should be reminded that exchange of information in the group and the identities of participants must remain confidential.

DATA ANALYSIS

Data analysis techniques are procedures used to summarize words or numbers and create a meaningful result for interpretation. Quantitative analysis involves statistical analysis. Many types of statistical analyses may be performed on the data, and the appropriate technique needs to be applied. Qualitative analysis involves content analysis. This process requires coding of themes and analysis of the narrative content. The qualitative data may contain quotations and require their interpretation. Quotations from study participants support the evidence that is provided by the study.

DISSEMINATION OF OUTCOMES

The next stage of the research process is dissemination of the findings. **Dissemination** is communication and distribution of the information. Dissemination may occur by publication in a journal or through a poster, an oral presentation, or a workshop at a conference. Researchers also may discuss study findings with their colleagues in less formal settings. If study participants want the research progress and findings reported to them, the material should be provided in understandable terms.

Nursing research with practical implications may need to be reported to agencies and health care providers to initiate necessary changes. If the research has a large-scale impact, study results should be disseminated to the community, those who funded the research, and policy makers. Research reports can be published by a university on a website or in printed newsletters to provide more public dissemination. A dissemination plan should be devised at the beginning of the research.

APPLICATION TO PRACTICE

When most nursing research is conducted, the goal is to apply the findings to practice. Patient education regarding the latest findings is one method of application (Patient Education and Health Literacy box).

PATIENT EDUCATION AND HEALTH LITERACY

Research Findings

- Patients require research results to be translated into understandable language that is practical for them.
- Brochures and fact sheets that provide brief but pertinent information about different topics have the greatest impact on patients.
- Short videos can relay information about health practices to patients.
- Websites provided by the health care facility or by state or federal health care agencies can be a source of accurate information.
- Public service announcements, such as antismoking campaigns based on research, are a means of educating the community.

One obstacle to applying research to practice is the difficulty in bedside access to information by nurses. Nurses often lack the time to participate in research-related activities. Not all nurses have the educational preparation for research (Yoder, Kirkley, McFall, et al, 2014). However, even a novice nurse can identify problems related to improving patient care. By reading research articles, the nurse may notice discrepancies in what is recommended in current practice and what is found in the literature. Research about nursing practice, nursing administration, and nursing education has an impact on patient care.

Nurses often feel that their bedside nursing care is removed from the research process. However, nurses participate every day in the care of patients, which is based on the nursing process. The nursing process is based on the scientific method used in research. Nurses should use research to improve the quality of patient care and should understand the research base before initiating nursing interventions. To further apply research to practice, nurses need to implement EBP. Nurses are patient advocates who should consistently provide the best possible care for patients. Patient safety and quality improvement must be the focus of nursing practice. Nurses are accountable for their practice and must prevent errors by using the best evidence. Society expects high-quality health care, and nurses are in the forefront of providing that care.

EVIDENCE-BASED PRACTICE LO 13.4

Evidence-based practice (EBP) is integration of the best available research evidence and the nurse's clinical expertise to make patient care decisions. EBP allows a nurse to address questions and problems by reviewing the research, clinical guidelines, and other resources to determine practice. EBP results in better patient outcomes, keeps nursing practice current, and increases the nurse's confidence in professional decision making.

The Centers for Disease Control and Prevention published the *Guideline for Hand Hygiene in Health-Care Settings,* which provides a review of data regarding handwashing in health care environments and makes recommendations for improving hand hygiene practices and reducing pathogenic transmissions. Clinical practice guidelines such as this are the result of an emphasis on EBP.

HISTORICAL CONTEXT

Evidence-based practice plays a significant role in nursing, medicine, and other health care disciplines by improving clinical decision making, which results in better-quality patient care. Nurses provide holistic care when determining the best treatment for patients. In addition to the best evidence, clinical decision making includes factors such as acceptability to the patient and cost-effectiveness.

Nightingale

Florence Nightingale, in her *Notes on Nursing* in 1859, outlined basic principles of nursing science. Nightingale's method of nursing included rigorous monitoring of the effectiveness of interventions and treatments. This provided the initial basis for EBP. Her work was based on trial and error, careful observation, discussion with patients, and clinical experience (McDonald, 2001). She used statistical data to improve sanitation, health, nursing education, and health administration. Nightingale applied a statistical approach to the study of public health and mortality data and used a pie chart to display research findings. However, nursing did not publish its first EBP journal, *Evidence-Based Nursing,* until 1998 (Melnyk, Fineout-Overholt, Stone, et al, 2000).

Cochrane

During the 1970s, physicians began the EBP movement. This occurred after Archie Cochrane, a British epidemiologist, criticized health professionals' lack of evaluation of their treatment methods. Cochrane's *Effectiveness and Efficiency: Random Reflections on Health Services* is credited with being the impetus for evidence-based medicine. *JAMA* published an article in 1992 that focused on evidence-based medicine in physician education. Named for Cochrane, the Cochrane Library is a collection of research databases for health care. This collection includes the Cochrane Reviews, which are systematic reviews and meta-analyses that interpret the results of medical research.

RESEARCH USE VERSUS EVIDENCE-BASED PRACTICE

Research use is a subset of EBP. **Research use** is the application of research findings to clinical practice (Polit and Beck, 2013). As research is conducted, evidence accumulates over time on a topic. Eventually, the evidence becomes accepted into practice. Often, there is a considerable gap in the amount of time between conducting the research and its acceptance. Research use is the direct application of findings from a single study to patient care (e.g., tracheal suctioning techniques).

In contrast, EBP integrates theoretical background, clinical judgment, and patient preferences. This is accomplished while the findings are being critically appraised, a process that requires knowledge of research to evaluate scientific evidence. EBP then applies cost-effective and clinically effective evidence to nursing practice (Polit and Beck, 2013). EBP includes research use with a complex skill set and larger knowledge base to provide the nurse with enough information to make decisions about the research evidence. EBP involves comparing interventions and determining the best evidence derived from a review of the literature. EBP includes (1) the best possible evidence, (2) clinical expertise, (3) patient values and needs, and (4) cost-effectiveness.

> **QSEN FOCUS!**
>
> To adequately integrate EBP into patient care, nurses must critique research to differentiate between opinion and evidence and must regularly read current professional journals.

BARRIERS TO EVIDENCE-BASED PRACTICE

Some barriers are common to research use and EBP, including the difficulty of communicating how to conduct EBP and the individual nurse's skills in determining the quality of research available for review. Another limitation is the reluctance of organizations to fund research and subsequently make potentially costly practice changes based on the best evidence.

The proliferation of research available to health care providers has led to an increase in the quality and quantity of evidence on diagnostic tests, treatments, and models of health care delivery. Due to the copious amount of literature on a specific topic, it is difficult to analyze the literature in an efficient and effective manner. Health care literature with clinically applicable findings is published at a rate that is impossible for individual health care professionals to keep up with. Alper and colleagues (2004) estimated that a physician would need to read 17 articles per day, 7 days per week, 20 hours per day (Alper, Hand, Elliott, et al, 2004).

There are delays of approximately 17 years for implementation of clinical research into practice (Balas, 2001). For example, the research on sudden infant death syndrome conducted in the 1970s that led to the recommendation of placing infants on their backs was not relayed to parents until the early 1990s (Gilbert, Salanti, Harden, et al, 2005). Such situations have led to a need for better EBP resources and an improved process for conducting evidence-based research and disseminating the results.

CONDUCTING EVIDENCE-BASED RESEARCH LO 13.5

A specific process is required for evidence-based research (EBR). It begins with assessment and has six phases. The steps for conducting EBR parallel Larrabee's (2009) model for EBP change (Figure 13-2).

ASSESSING THE PROBLEM

The first phase of evidence-based research consists of assessing the need for change in practice by identifying a problem. For a practicing nurse, problems present themselves in the context of caring for patients. This may occur while the nurse is determining the best intervention for a reoccurring problem or addressing a problem specific to a group of patients. The nurse collects data about the current practice to determine what is being done in response to the identified problem. Major stakeholders such as staff nurses, patients, or administrators are involved in this process. A **stakeholder** is someone

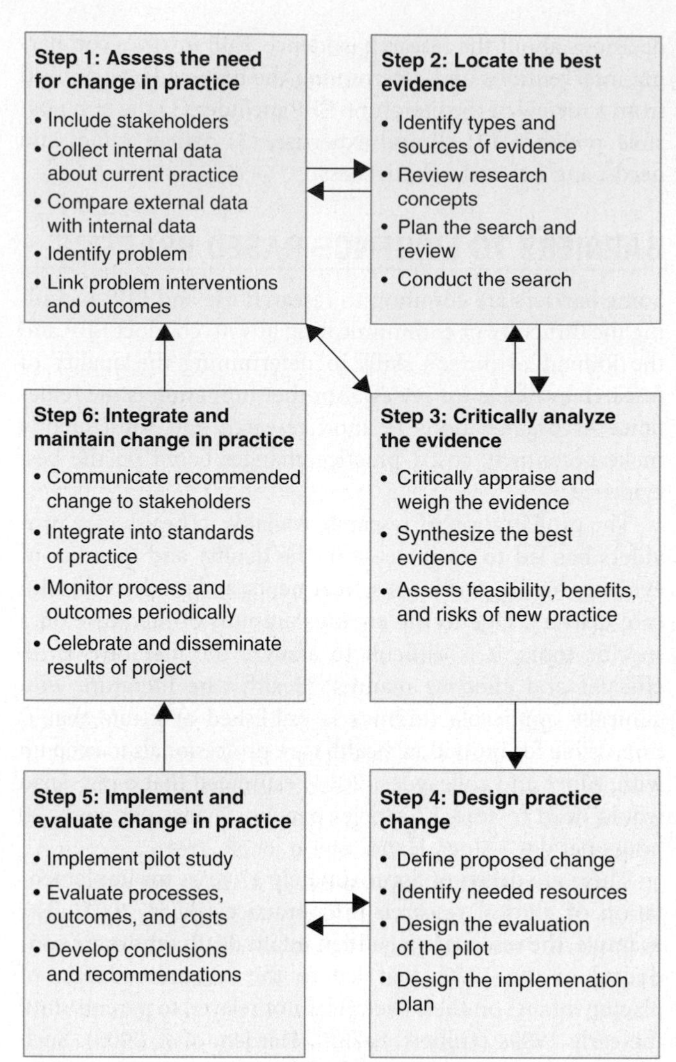

Step 1: Assess the need for change in practice
• Include stakeholders
• Collect internal data about current practice
• Compare external data with internal data
• Identify problem
• Link problem interventions and outcomes
Step 2: Locate the best evidence
• Identify types and sources of evidence
• Review research concepts
• Plan the search and review
• Conduct the search
Step 6: Integrate and maintain change in practice
• Communicate recommended change to stakeholders
• Integrate into standards of practice
• Monitor process and outcomes periodically
• Celebrate and disseminate results of project
Step 3: Critically analyze the evidence
• Critically appraise and weigh the evidence
• Synthesize the best evidence
• Assess feasibility, benefits, and risks of new practice
Step 5: Implement and evaluate change in practice
• Implement pilot study
• Evaluate processes, outcomes, and costs
• Develop conclusions and recommendations
Step 4: Design practice change
• Define proposed change
• Identify needed resources
• Design the evaluation of the pilot
• Design the implemenation plan

FIGURE 13-2 Larrabee's model for evidence-based practice change. (From Rosswurm MA, Larrabee JH: Clinical scholarship: A model for change to evidence-based practice, *Image J Nurs Sch* 31(4):317-322, 1999.)

who is an integral part of the process and may be the end user of the process or anyone who may be affected by the process.

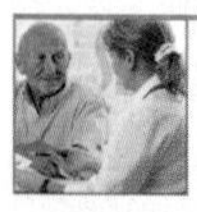

1. If the nurse is not familiar with the medication Mr. Tregalin is referring to, how will the background information be obtained? What resources are available for this type of information?

DEVELOPING A QUESTION

The second phase of evidence-based research consists of formulating a specific research question so that the nurse can effectively search the literature databases. To generate a specific question, a nurse needs to link the problem, interventions, and outcomes. One method of formulating a research question is identified by the acronym **PICO** (i.e., patient, population, or problem; intervention; comparison intervention; and outcomes) (Stone, 2002) (Box 13-1).

BOX 13-1 Constructing a Good Research Question

The acronym PICO assists in remembering the steps of research question formulation. The following approach may be used to construct a good research question:

- *P (patient, population, problem):* Describe the subject of the problem. The nurse determines how best to describe the group of patients participating in the research.
- *I (intervention):* Define which intervention is being considered for the specific patient or population.
- *C (comparison intervention):* Describe a second intervention to compare with the first if appropriate. An example is comparison of traditional x-rays with magnetic resonance imaging (MRI).
- *O (outcome):* Define the type of outcome to assess. An outcome may be the change in a physical sign, the result of a diagnostic test, a patient response to a treatment or intervention, or the cost-effectiveness of a treatment.

A clinical question that can be researched includes specific components:

- The patient's disorder or disease
- The intervention or finding that is being reviewed
- A comparison intervention (if applicable, not always used)
- The outcome

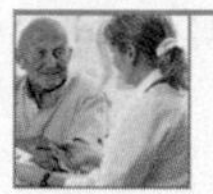

2. After determining which medication Mr. Tregalin is referring to, write a clinical question using PICO model as a guide.

SEARCHING FOR AND EVALUATING EVIDENCE

The third phase of evidence-based research involves searching the database for relevant evidence. This phase also includes evaluating and critically appraising the information that has been identified.

Searching

Searching the database for the evidence begins the third phase. The nurse may need to consult three categories of information resources, which are reviewed in sequential order depending on need and applicability. The categories are general information (background) resources, filtered resources, and unfiltered resources.

Nurses may encounter conditions outside their specialty area and need an overview. Background resources provide detailed information. If the nurse is looking for a presentation of information or types of therapies, the best source is a background resource. Background resources include UpToDate, STAT!Ref, and MD Consult, which are web-based databases. Another source of background information is a current nursing textbook.

When trying to determine the best treatment or course of action and incorporate the most reliable evidence into the decision, the nurse can use a filtered resource such as the Cochrane Reviews or the Joanna Briggs Institute Library of Systematic Reviews. Filtered resources provide the best available evidence. In filtered resources, clinical and subject experts have asked a question and then synthesized evidence to establish conclusions based on the research. This pre-evaluation process is already completed for nurses and allows the resources to be used while caring for patients. The conclusions from filtered resources still need to be evaluated by clinicians in terms of a specific patient. Filtered resources produce systematic reviews of the literature.

Systematic reviews such as those of the Cochrane Collaboration are a mechanism of assisting health care providers in EBP. These reviews are typically conducted by an expert or group of experts in a particular field. The purpose of critiquing a series of studies is to provide health care professionals with recommendations to guide their practice. Some of the groups that systematically review scientific evidence are described in the Evidence-Based Practice and Informatics box.

EVIDENCE-BASED PRACTICE AND INFORMATICS

Research Resources

Systematic Reviews

- *Cochrane Collaboration:* This international collaboration facilitates the creation, maintenance, and dissemination of systematic reviews that are published as *Cochrane Reviews* in the Cochrane Library. These reviews usually are medically oriented, and they are considered the gold standard of reviews.
- *Database of Abstracts of Reviews of Effects (DARE):* This database contains systematic reviews produced and maintained by the National Health System's Centre for Reviews and Dissemination in the United Kingdom.

Clinical Practice Guidelines

- *Agency for Healthcare Research and Quality (AHRQ):* In the United States, AHRQ launched its initiative to promote evidence-based practice in everyday care through establishment of Evidence-based Practice Centers (EPCs). The EPCs develop evidence reports and technology assessments on topics relevant to clinical, social science or behavioral, economic, and other health care organization and delivery issues by reviewing all relevant scientific literature on clinical, behavioral, organizational, and financing topics. These scientific syntheses may include meta-analyses and cost analyses.
- *National Guideline Clearinghouse (NGC):* This is a public resource for evidence-based clinical practice guidelines and measurement tools. The NGC is sponsored by the AHRQ.

If a resource is not found in a filtered resource that addresses the question, an unfiltered resource may be used. Unfiltered resources include MEDLINE/PubMed, PsychINFO, and the Cumulative Index to Nursing and Allied Health Literature (CINAHL). The nurse can also check journals for original research studies. The nurse may consult an unfiltered resource to determine whether any new studies have been conducted since the systematic review in the filtered resource was written.

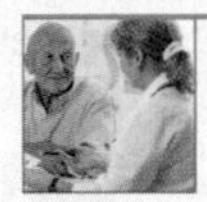

3. On the basis of the clinical question developed for Mr. Tregalin, determine the best clinical resources that address the question, and provide the necessary information to guide the patient care decision.

Critically Appraising Information

After identifying an article or systematic review resource that seems appropriate to the question, the nurse must critically appraise the information. Nurses should not accept research without carefully reviewing the study. **Critical appraisal** is a balanced evaluation of the strengths, benefits, weaknesses, and flaws of the research. Critical appraisal requires a systematic assessment of the evidence to assess validity, results, and relevance before using the research in a clinical situation (MacDermid, Walton, and Law, 2009). This process requires the use of critical-thinking skills. Articles in peer-reviewed journals provide a measure of quality control, but even they may vary in their quality (Benos, Basharia, Chaves, et al, 2007).

If the study is from a primary source that provides original data on a topic with no commentary, the nurse needs to check its validity. Interpreting the data depends on skill and experience, and the nurse may also consult with a peer. To determine validity, the nurse must address a number of issues in the appraisal. **Validity** generally refers to the strength or the degree to which a concept, conclusion, or measurement is justifiable and corresponds accurately to the truth. Understanding the components of a research article can help to find the information needed to critique it (Figure 13-3).

Internal Validity

To determine a study's validity, the nurse must first address the internal validity of the research and examine whether the results of the study are reasonable on the basis of how the study was conducted. The study should address a clearly focused issue. The literature review must be appropriate to the topic. The participants should have been randomly assigned to the experimental and accepted treatment groups, with each group treated equally apart from the experimental treatment itself. By having a control group and random assignment in experimental research, the study has more validity.

All ethical issues related to the research should be addressed. All participants should be accounted for at the end

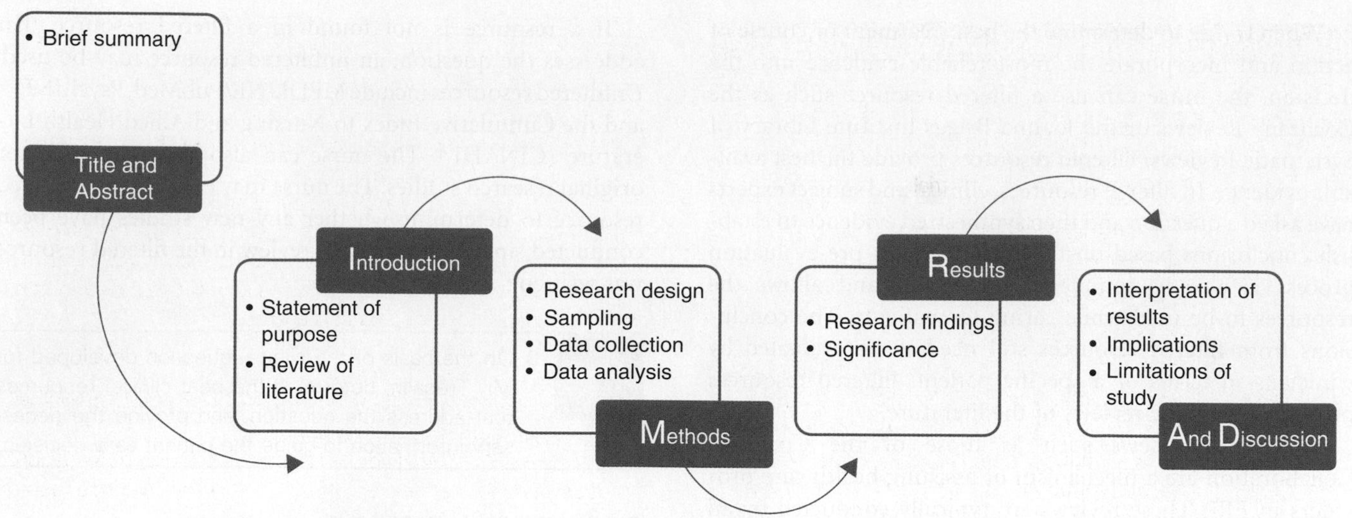

FIGURE 13-3 Components of a research article: introduction, methods, results, and discussion (IMRAD). (From Huth E: Structured abstracts for papers reporting clinical trials, *Ann Intern Med* 106(4):626-627, 1987.)

of the study. Measures should be objective and without bias. The subjects and clinicians should be blinded, remaining unaware of which treatment was being received by whom until the end of the study. In all studies, the data collection methods need to be clearly defined, and the analytic methods must be appropriate.

Result Analysis

The nurse must analyze the results of the study. The findings need to be reported in terms of significance. The size and precision of the treatment effect needs to be assessed to determine the significance of the results.

External Validity

External validity and relevance are determined last. External validity is a measure of whether a study can be applied to any other setting. When studies have large numbers of participants, it is easier to generalize the results. Quantitative studies often have large numbers of subjects, whereas qualitative studies frequently have smaller numbers of participants, which does not allow for generalization. A determination needs to be made on whether the outcomes of the study can be applied to a current clinical nursing situation. The treatment needs to be feasible in the current setting. The benefit of the intervention must be weighed against any harm to the individual patient.

Critical appraisal tools have been developed that can assist with this process (MacDermid, Walton, and Law, 2009). For example, a form with check boxes can list individual points to be addressed during the study. In determining questions, some forms give information regarding the sections where the information can be found in the articles about the study. Various critical appraisal tools are available *(www.gla.ac.uk/media/media_64037_en.pdf)*.

If a systematic review is being critically appraised, different criteria are needed to determine whether the results of the review are valid. The review should include appropriate studies and not eliminate any that are pertinent. The quality and results of the studies included in the review should be similar. The review requires a clear presentation of the results of each study and the value of its evidence. Various levels of evidence should be considered. The systematic review or meta-analysis of randomized, controlled trials (RCTs) or evidence-based clinical practice guidelines based on systematic reviews of RCTs are the highest level of evidence. Levels of evidence are listed in descending order in Table 13-1. Each level of evidence provides a different level of assurance about the validity of the information provided.

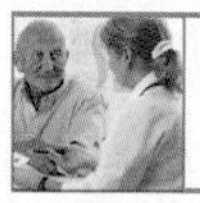

4. What questions should the nurse ask to critically appraise the identified clinical resources?

SYNTHESIZING THE EVIDENCE AND DEVELOPING A PLAN

The fourth phase in the EBR process requires the nurse to design a practice change based on the evidence found in the literature. The plan needs to include how the findings will be conveyed to the nurses who will use the new information. Workshops and in-service or focused training may be necessary if the plan involves a comprehensive change in care or it affects the entire health care agency or community. A bulletin can be provided that lists several safe practice concerns with rationales in the form of a safe practice alert.

IMPLEMENTING THE PLAN

The fifth phase in the EBP process requires implementation of the change by applying the evidence. At this point, nurses begin to use the new information in their practice. In the

TABLE 13-1 Classification of Evidence

EVIDENCE LEVEL	DESCRIPTION
Ia	Evidence obtained from meta-analysis of randomized, controlled trials
Ib	Evidence obtained from at least one randomized, controlled trial
IIa	Evidence obtained from at least one well-designed, controlled study without randomization
IIb	Evidence obtained from at least one other type of well-designed, quasi-experimental study (situation in which implementation of an intervention is outside the control of the investigators but an opportunity exists to evaluate its effect)
III	Evidence obtained from well-designed, nonexperimental, descriptive studies, such as comparative studies, correlation studies, and case studies
IV	Evidence obtained from expert committee reports or opinions and/or clinical experiences of respected authorities

From LoBiondo-Wood G, Haber J: *Nursing research: Methods and critical appraisal for evidence-based practice*, ed. 7, St. Louis, 2010, Mosby.

process of implementing EBP, the nurse develops a clinical question, seeks answers to verify and support a clinical decision, and ultimately applies the findings to patients.

MAINTAINING THE CHANGE AND REEVALUATING

After the change has been integrated and maintained in practice, the final phase in the EBR process consists of evaluating the effectiveness of the decision in terms of the patient's response. The nurse determines whether the diagnosis and treatment were successful, whether there has been any new information in the literature since implementation, and how the clinical decision can be improved or updated. All of these evaluations prompt the nurse to keep up to date with the current literature. Box 13-2 provides an example of evidence-based research.

IMPLEMENTING RESEARCH IN NURSING PRACTICE LO 13.6

EBP has a role to play in improving the care of patients. Nurses should be able to recognize the different types of evidence levels to identify best practices. Any single means to establishing care, even if it is an accepted method, may not meet the complex needs of individual patients. For EBP to be safe and effective, nurses must be able to evaluate the strength and relevance of research findings. Nurses need to understand that there are different types of evidence that should be used to respond appropriately to individual patient preferences (Nolan and Bradley, 2008). Nurses must use critical thinking to implement different care practices that are consistent with patients' values. Collaboration with others

BOX 13-2 Evidence-Based Research Example

Phase 1: Assess the Problem

The nurses questioned the effectiveness of the nasogastric tube (NGT) placement verification procedure in their facility and wanted to determine the best practice. Most nurses in the facility were checking placement by aspiration of contents, but other nurses said that a chest x-ray was the preferred method. The pediatric nurses were interested in the best practice for neonates and children.

Phase 2: Develop a Question

The PICO components of the question for this problem were:

- *Patient:* Pediatric and neonates
- *Intervention:* Verification of NGT by radiologic confirmation
- *Comparison:* Verification of NGT by another method (aspiration or auscultation)
- *Outcome:* Confirmation of NGT placement

Phase 3: Search for Evidence and Evaluate

The nurses initially reviewed articles about pediatric and adult NGT insertion and verification. They then focused on the articles for pediatrics and critically appraised the evidence. A review of the literature on NGT verification revealed a clinical practice guideline for pediatric patients published through the National Guideline Clearinghouse and AHRQ in 2009. These recommendations were derived from the research.

- Multiple, nonradiologic verification methods are strongly recommended to confirm placement of an NGT in neonatal, pediatric, and adolescent patients.
- Radiologic verification is strongly recommended when results for nonradiologic methods conflict and for high-risk patients:
  - Patients in pediatric and cardiac intensive care units
  - Patients with an altered level of consciousness
  - Patients with swallowing problems*

Phases 4 Through 6: Develop the Plan, Implement the Plan, and Reevaluate

From review of the evidence, a plan was developed to design a practice change in the pediatric unit. Staff nurses were educated on the new policy for NGT verification. The nurses implemented the change and planned an evaluation of the change.

AHRQ, Agency for Healthcare Research and Quality; *NGT,* nasogastric tube; *PICO,* patient (population or problem), intervention, comparison intervention, and outcome.
*NGT guidelines are available at *www.guideline.gov/content.aspx?id=35117&search=nasogastric+tubes.*

COLLABORATION AND DELEGATION

Research Participation and Implementation

Interpret and use research in clinical decision making:

- Incorporate evidence-based practice (EBP) into individual practice, and assist colleagues to incorporate research findings into their individual practices.
- Collaborate with colleagues to use research when caring for the same patient on various shifts and days.

Implement EBP beyond personal practice, such as on the nursing unit, at an informational program, for an entire department, or at the organizational level:

- Collaborate with colleagues to use research on the nursing unit to influence the clinical microsystem (i.e., small, functional unit where care is provided).
- Educate unlicensed assistive personnel before delegating care on the importance of EBP for positive patient outcomes.
- Collaborate with administrators to use research to influence the larger practice environment.

Participate in collaborative research:

- Function as a participant or co-researcher in a collaborative, knowledge-generating research project.

provides a mechanism for implementing best practices for patient care (Collaboration and Delegation box).

MAGNET HOSPITAL STATUS AND THE ROLE OF NURSING RESEARCH IN PRACTICE LO 13.7

Magnet status is recognition given by the American Nurses' Credentialing Center (ANCC), an affiliate of the ANA. To receive this recognition, hospitals must satisfy a set of criteria designed to measure the strength and quality of nursing. A Magnet hospital is characterized by excellent patient outcomes due to nursing, a high level of nursing job satisfaction with a low nurse turnover rate, and appropriate resolution of any grievances (Box 13-3). The Magnet Recognition Program supports an evidence-based environment, which includes the nurses' autonomy to improve quality of care by using evidence (Reigle, Stevens, Belcher, et al, 2008). Research and EBP must therefore become a part of the nurses' care of the patients.

BOX 13-3 Qualities of a Magnet Hospital

Magnet hospitals have the following qualities:

- Nurses are involved in data collection and decision making in the process of delivering patient care.
- The relationship between nursing leaders and staff nurses indicates appreciation and respect and rewards them for advancing nursing practice.
- The administration involves staff nurses in research-based practice through ongoing open communication and collaboration between nurses and other members of the health care team.
- The hospital has an appropriate mix of personnel that allows for the best patient outcomes.

RESEARCH AND BEST PRACTICES

With the increasing emphasis on EBP, nurses must understand research and its application to patient care. A criticism of EBP is that it will become a standard formula. However, a key element of EBP is including the patient in the process to individualize care. There must always be personalization of the evidence to specific patient circumstances. High-quality nursing care is the priority of EBP. Nursing practice must be based on research evidence rather than tradition. As they begin their practice, new nurses should actively seek opportunities to become involved in EBP immediately, because doing so enables EBP to further evolve and can increase its acceptance in the nursing community.

SUMMARY OF LEARNING OUTCOMES

LO 13.1 *Define various types of nursing research:* Basic research generates theories, applied research tests the application of research in different situations and populations, and clinical research is used when testing theories about the effectiveness of interventions.

LO 13.2 *Compare quantitative and qualitative research methods:* Quantitative research designs are descriptive, correlational, experimental, and quasi-experimental. Qualitative research designs include phenomenological, grounded theory, ethnographic, and historical.

LO 13.3 *Explain the steps involved in the research process:* Research includes a literature review, data collection, data analysis, dissemination of outcomes, and application to practice. Before conducting research, permission must be sought from an IRB, whose responsibilities include protecting the rights and welfare of the participants.

LO 13.4 *Explain research and its relationship to evidence-based practice:* EBP is integration of the best available research evidence and the nurse's clinical expertise to make patient care decisions. EBP allows a nurse to address questions and problems by reviewing the research, clinical guidelines, and other resources to determine practice. EBP results in better patient outcomes, keeps nursing practice current, and increases the nurse's confidence in professional decision making.

LO 13.5 *Discuss the steps required in conducting evidence-based research:* Evidenced-based nursing research consists of assessing a need for change; developing a question that links the problem, interventions, and outcomes; searching for and synthesizing the best evidence; designing a plan for change; implementing the change; and integrating, maintaining, and evaluating the change.

LO 13.6 *Identify considerations for implementing research in nursing practice:* Nurses should be able to recognize the different types of evidence levels to identify best practices. Nurses must understand that any single means to establishing care, even if it is an accepted method, may not meet the complex needs of individual patients or be consistent with patients' preferences or values. Collaboration among health care professionals can help with individualizing patient care while incorporating research into practice.

LO 13.7 *Explain the relationship of hospital Magnet status to nursing research and practice:* The Magnet Recognition Program for hospitals supports an evidence-based environment, which includes the nurses' autonomy to improve quality of care by using evidence.

Responses to the critical-thinking questions are available at *http://evolve.elsevier.com/YoostCrawford/fundamentals/.*

REVIEW QUESTIONS

1. A nursing student is taking care of a patient with possible appendicitis and is curious about the best method of diagnosing this disorder. What does the nursing student have to consider in formulating a question using the PICO format (patient, population, or problem; intervention; comparison intervention; outcomes) to determine evidence-based practice?
   a. Problem: appendicitis; interventions: ultrasound versus computed tomography (CT) scan; outcome: diagnosis of appendicitis
   b. Problem: pain; interventions: meperidine versus morphine; outcome: pain free
   c. Problem: fever; interventions: cooling measures versus antipyretics; outcome: normal temperature
   d. Problem: appendicitis; interventions: complete blood count versus chemistry panel tests; outcome: painless
2. The nurse decides to access a systematic review database to determine evidence-based practice related to the patient's treatment plan for a diagnosis of otitis media (i.e., ear infection). What database can provide that type of resource?
   a. Cumulative Index of Nursing and Allied Health Literature (CINAHL)
   b. Cochrane
   c. PubMed
   d. MD Consult
3. The nurse researcher provides participants with informed consent so that what ethical principle is upheld?
   a. Respect for persons
   b. Beneficence
   c. Justice
   d. Ethics
4. The nurse thinks the results of a recent literature search and analysis about hand washing should be implemented in the entire hospital system. With whom would the nurse be required to collaborate?
   a. Colleagues caring for patients in her unit
   b. Colleagues in the community
   c. Administrators at the hospital
   d. Others in her department
5. Knowledge gained from research in the 1970s about placing infants on their backs to prevent sudden infant death syndrome was not recommended to parents until the 1990s. This is an example of what barrier to evidence-based practice?
   a. Proliferation of research
   b. Implementation delay
   c. Information needs not being met
   d. Lack of readily available resources
6. A patient is on the way to the hospital in an ambulance and is asked to participate in a research protocol for a new treatment for myocardial infarction. What is this an example of? *(Select all that apply.)*
   a. Standard practice
   b. An ethical dilemma
   c. A violation of informed consent
   d. A patient who is in a vulnerable population category
   e. Compliance with important ethical issues of justice and autonomy
7. Patients are participating in a study to identify genetic disorders. What are potential concerns? *(Select all that apply.)*
   a. Violation of confidentiality if a disorder is revealed
   b. Possible adverse consequences related to employment
   c. Possible adverse consequences related to reputation
   d. Possible adverse consequences to insurability
   e. Inability to prevent the progression of genetic disorders

8. Which entities or documents specifically address the role of the nurse in research? *(Select all that apply.)*
   a. American Nurses Association standards of practice
   b. Institutional review board
   c. Hospital Magnet status
   d. The Joint Commission
   e. MD Consult
9. Which factors contribute to the nurse having difficulty keeping up with the latest patient care information? *(Select all that apply.)*
   a. Implementation delays
   b. Proliferation of research
   c. Volume of health care literature
   d. Hours spent in direct patient care
   e. The need to read three articles every day
10. After reading various research articles and reviews on a subject, the nurse designs a practice change based on the literature. What stage of evidence-based practice is this?
   a. Maintaining the change
   b. Implementing the change
   c. Evaluating and critically appraising
   d. Synthesizing the evidence and developing a plan

Answers and rationales for the review questions are available at *http://evolve.elsevier.com/YoostCrawford/fundamentals/.*

REFERENCES

Alper BS, Hand JA, Elliott SG, et al: How much effort is needed to keep up with the literature relevant for primary care? *J Med Libr Association*, 4, 430-437, 2004.

American Association of Colleges of Nursing: Nursing research, 2012. Retrieved from *www.aacn.nche.edu/publications/position/nursing-research.*

American Nurses Association (ANA): Research toolkit, 2012. Retrieved from *www.nursingworld.org/Research-Toolkit.*

American Nurses Association (ANA): *Nursing: Scope and standards of practice*, ed. 2, Silver Springs, Md., 2010, Author. Also available at *Nursebooks.org*.

Balas E: Information systems can prevent errors and improve quality. *J Am Med Inform Assoc*, 8(4):398-399, 2001.

Benos DJ , Basharia E, Chaves J, et al: The ups and downs of peer review. *Adv Physiol Educ*, 31:145-152, 2007.

Burns N, Grove S: *Understanding nursing research: Building evidence based practice*, ed. 5, St. Louis, 2011, Saunders.

Cronenwett L, Sherwood G, Barnsteiner J, et al: Quality and safety education for nurses. *Nurs Outlook*, 55(3):122-131, 2007.

Erzberger C, Kelle U: Making inferences in mixed methods: The rules of integration. In A Tashakkori, C Teddlie (Eds), *Handbook of mixed methods in social & behavioral research*, Thousand Oaks, Calif., 2003, Sage, pp 457-488.

Fawcett J, Garity J: *Evaluating research for evidenced-based nursing practice*, Philadelphia, 2009, FA Davis.

Gilbert R, Salanti G, Harden M, See S: Infant sleeping position and the sudden infant death syndrome: Systematic review of observational studies and historical review of recommendations from 1940 to 2002. *Int J Epidemiol*, 34(4):874-887, 2005.

Larrabee J: *Nurse to nurse evidence-based practice: A step-by-step handbook*, New York, 2009, McGraw-Hill.

MacDermid J, Walton D, Law M: Critical appraisal of research evidence for its validity and usefulness. *Hand Clinics*, 25(1): 29-42, 2009.

McDonald L: Florence Nightingale and the early origins of evidence-based nursing. *Evid Based Nurs*, 4(3):68-69, 2001.

Melnyk BM, Fineout-Overholt E, Stone P, Ackerman M: Evidence-based practice: The past, the present, and recommendations for the millennium. *Pediatric Nurs*, 26(1):77-80, 2000.

National Institute of Nursing Research (NINR): *NINR strategic plan*, Washington, D.C., 2011, National Institutes of Health.

Newman I: *A conceptualization of mixed methods: A need for inductive/deductive approach to conducting research.* Paper presented at the annual meeting of the American Educational Research Association, 2000, New Orleans, La. (ERIC document reproduction service no. ED443849).

Nolan P, Bradley E: Evidence-based practice: Implications and concerns. *J Nurs Manag*, 16(4):388-393, 2008.

Office of Human Research Protection: *Guidance on research involving coded private information or biological specimens*, Washington, D.C., 2008, U.S. Department of Health and Human Services.

Polit D, Beck C: *Essentials of nursing research: Methods, appraisal, and utilization*, ed. 8, Philadelphia, 2013, Lippincott.

Reigle B, Stevens K, Belcher J, et al: Evidence-based practice and the road to Magnet status. *J Nurs Admin*, 38(2):97-102, 2008.

Sale JE, Lohfeld LH, Brazil K: Revisiting the quantitative-qualitative debate: Implications for mixed-methods research. *Qual Quant*, 36(1):43-53, 2002.

Stone PW: Popping the PICO question for research and evidence-based practice. *Appl Nurs Res*, 15(3):197-198, 2002.

Yoder L, Kirkley D, McFall D, et al: Original research: Staff nurses' use of research to facilitate evidence-based practice, *Amer J Nurs*, 114(9):26-37, 2014.

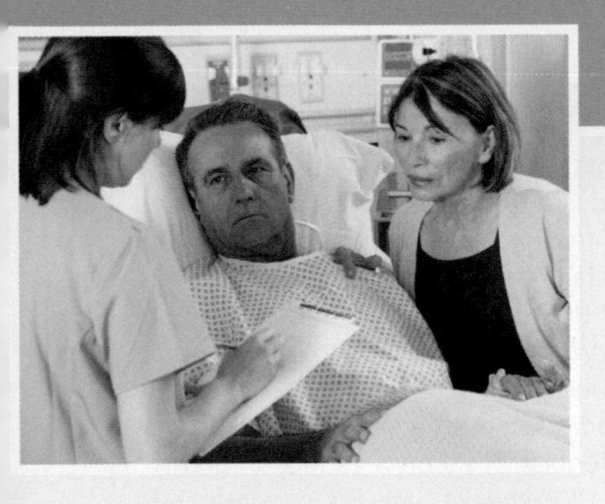

CHAPTER 14

Health Literacy and Patient Education

EVOLVE WEBSITE

http://evolve.elsevier.com/YoostCrawford/fundamentals/

- Additional Evolve-Only Review Questions With Answers
- Answers and Rationales for Text Review Questions
- Answers to Critical-Thinking Questions
- Case Study With Questions
- Glossary

LEARNING OUTCOMES

Comprehension of this chapter's content will provide students with the ability to:

LO 14.1 Define *health literacy.*
LO 14.2 Explain the role of health literacy in nursing and patient education.
LO 14.3 Identify the types of patient education and the settings in which patient education occurs.
LO 14.4 Differentiate among the three domains of learning.
LO 14.5 Explain how learning styles affect patient teaching.
LO 14.6 Describe factors affecting health literacy and patient education.
LO 14.7 Carry out an assessment of the patient's health literacy and education needs.
LO 14.8 Choose nursing diagnoses appropriate for use with patient education.
LO 14.9 Determine goals and outcome criteria for patient education.
LO 14.10 Implement teaching plans and evaluate their effectiveness.

KEY TERMS

affective domain, p. 195
cognitive domain, p. 195
health literacy, p. 192
learning, p. 194
multimodal learner, p. 195
psychomotor domain, p. 195
teaching, p. 194

CASE STUDY

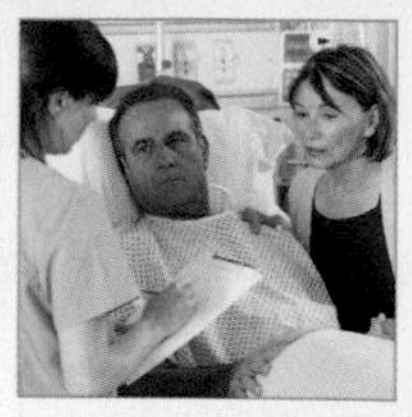

Mr. Lubic, a 53-year-old male patient with a 1-week history of night sweats, shortness of breath, and cough, was seen in the office of the primary care provider (PCP). A chest x-ray and laboratory tests were ordered, and he was diagnosed with bilateral pneumonia and pleural effusions, with a white blood cell (WBC) count of 27,000/mm^3. The PCP advises Mr. Lubic that he needs to be admitted to the hospital for treatment. Mr. Lubic tells the PCP that he does not have insurance and states, "I can't be admitted." The PCP agrees to send him home with prescriptions for an antibiotic, a steroid, and an inhaler. The nurse gives him written instructions to call the office immediately if he feels worse or does not begin to feel better within 48 hours.

Three days later, Mr. Lubic is brought to the emergency room by ambulance and is intubated, placed on a ventilator, and transferred to the intensive care unit (ICU). Mr. Lubic's vital signs are T 38° C (100.4° F), P 92 and regular, R 20 on a ventilator, and BP 153/84. He expressed chest pain as 6 of 10 before being placed on the ventilator. When the PCP speaks with the patient's wife the next day in the waiting room, he asks if her husband seemed to get any better after he started the prescribed medicines. Mrs. Lubic appears confused, and after a few more minutes of conversation, she pulls "the receipt for his office visit" from her purse. However, the papers are not a receipt but the written prescriptions and instructions provided during the visit. The PCP then learns that neither Mr. nor Mrs. Lubic is able to read.

Refer back to this case study to answer the critical-thinking questions throughout the chapter.

Not all patients in need of health care information can easily grasp the concepts provided during patient teaching. Nurses have a responsibility to present health-related information to patients and their families and to do everything possible to ensure their ability to comprehend and integrate the information. To teach effectively, nurses must recognize that patients of all ages come from diverse cultural, educational, and socioeconomic backgrounds. Each has a different ability to comprehend health care information. The unique ability of a patient to understand and integrate health-related knowledge is known as **health literacy**.

Health literacy "is about consumers being able to understand the medical information their caregivers give them or they find through the Internet and being able to use that information to make good decisions about their own course of care" (Schardt, 2011). The most recent comprehensive data exploring health literacy in the United States are from a research project called Assessing the Nation's Health Literacy: Key Concepts and Findings of the National Assessment of Adult Literacy (NAAL), which was conducted in 2003 (White, 2008). The NAAL was the first assessment of the nation's progress in adult literacy since the National Center for Education (NCES) adult literacy assessment performed a decade earlier, the 1992 National Adult Literacy Survey (NALS) (White, 2008).

Results of the NAAL research indicate that among American adults, 30 million (14%) had below basic health literacy in English and 47 million (22%) had basic health literacy. This means that 77 million (36%) American adults possessed very rudimentary literacy skills that allowed them to read only short, simple printed and written materials (White, 2008).

HEALTH LITERACY LO 14.1

Nurses have been providing educational information to patients since the late 1800s, but health literacy is a recent concept. Florence Nightingale's efforts incorporated the importance of patient education into the nursing profession. Chapter 1 provides additional information on Nightingale.

Although discussion of Nightingale's work often focuses on her efforts to distinguish nursing as a profession and address the impact of sanitation on health, she advocated exploring all aspects of the patient. She thought that patients needed care that is "delicate and decent" and that demonstrates "the power of giving real interests to the patient" (Quixley, 1974). Exploring patients' interests and abilities was an early acknowledgment that nurses must be aware of patients' ability to comprehend the health care information provided.

The realization that consumers need to be able to understand the medical information delivered by health care providers has gained recognition at many governmental levels. The *Healthy People 2020* publication describes a national movement that addresses the priorities of prevention and public health in the United States. Health literacy with its impact on this initiative is being recognized and has become a key component of the project (Riegelman and Garr, 2011).

As the health care community explores the concept of health literacy, many organizations recognize that before improvements can be made, operational definitions are needed. According to the American Medical Association (AMA, n.d.), health literacy is "the ability to obtain, process, and understand basic information and services needed to make appropriate health decisions and follow instructions for treatment." A similar and perhaps more global definition of health literacy is "the degree to which individuals have the capacity to obtain, process, and understand basic health information needed to make appropriate health decisions and services needed to prevent or treat illness" (Health Resources and Services Administration, n.d.).

In exploring communication patterns and techniques between health care providers and patients with low health literacy, Schwartzberg and colleagues (2007) defined health literacy as "an individual's ability to read and understand health information and use it to make appropriate health decisions. Low health literacy refers to the condition in which individuals are unable to comprehend health-related information or instructions and may fail to make appropriate decisions regarding their care" (p. 96). The results obtained in their study further explain that while low literacy and low health literacy are related terms, they are not interchangeable. Low health literacy is content-specific, meaning that the individual may not have difficulty reading and writing outside the health care arena. These patients may struggle to comprehend the complicated, unfamiliar terms and ideas found in health-related materials or instructions (Schwartzberg, Cowett, VanGeest, et al., 2007).

Interest in effective patient education is not a phenomenon unique to the United States. The Institute of Medicine Roundtable on Health Literacy held a workshop in 2012 focused on international health literacy. The workshop combined the strengths of the United States' research, Europe's multilingual and multinational experience, and developing countries' community-based programs (Institute of Medicine, 2013). The American Medical Association definition of health literacy is used in this chapter, but nurses should recognize that there are other definitions of the term.

ROLE OF HEALTH LITERACY IN NURSING AND PATIENT EDUCATION LO 14.2

Understanding that effective patient education is key to health promotion and wellness, nurses must be aware of the concept of health literacy and determine how it affects the care of every patient. "Patient education is a primary responsibility of nurses" (Scheckel, Emery, and Nosek, 2010). Often, health care professionals assume that the explanations and instructions given to patients and families are readily understood. In reality, research has shown that these instructions are frequently misunderstood, sometimes resulting in serious errors (Cornett, 2009).

As part of the health care team, nurses have direct contact with patients and their families throughout the life span. Teaching that is not effective can have negative implications, as Squellati (2010) describes:

> Health literacy is a significant concern for Americans. Understanding health information is vital in addressing issues of access, quality, and affordability. If nurses are not able to teach patients effectively about their conditions and treatments, outcomes will be adversely affected. Providing information in ways that are appropriate for the patient's health literacy level is a step toward decreasing health disparities and increasing patient compliance.

Preventing disease, promoting health, providing treatment instructions, clarifying information, and teaching patients to cope with limitations are all components of patient education. In exploring disease prevention, consider the complexity

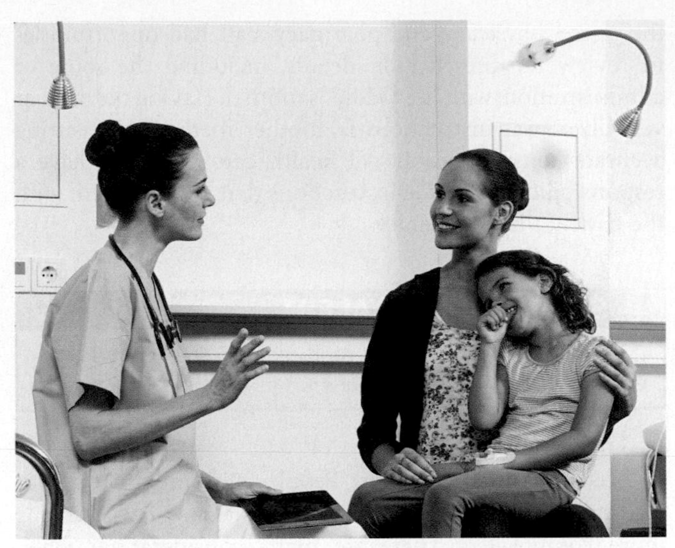

FIGURE 14-1 Nurses teach parents about immunizations.

of immunization information given to parents regarding their newborn infant. The volume of materials, including the rationale for giving vaccines and the potential side effects and risks, can be overwhelming even for parents with no literacy challenges (Figure 14-1). Imagine the difficulty parents may have if they are unable to read or write or unable to understand the language or reading level in which the instructions are given.

Health promotion activities such as smoking cessation and weight management and management of conditions such as diabetes, chronic renal failure, and heart failure are examples of areas affected by a gap between health care teaching and the patient's health literacy. Treatment instructions are another area in which nurses teach patients about some component of their health. Examples include preoperative instructions, those before a procedure, and those given on discharge from the hospital, urgent care, or emergency room. Misunderstanding instructions in any of these settings can be detrimental to the patient.

An example of a gap between the health care information provided and the health literacy of the caregiver is seen in this scenario:

> A toddler was diagnosed with an inner-ear infection and prescribed an antibiotic. Her mother understands that her daughter should take the prescribed medication twice each day. After carefully studying the label on the bottle and deciding that it does not tell how to take the medicine, she fills a teaspoon and pours the antibiotic into her daughter's painful ear (Parker, Ratzan, and Lurie, 2003).

Although the child's mother was able to read, she did not understand that the medication was to be taken orally. If the health care provider caring for this patient had written out the words *by mouth* rather than using the medical abbreviation *PO*, the situation could have been avoided. Most likely, the nurse, physician, and pharmacy staff had opportunities to review the prescription details, including the route of administration, with the toddler's mother. Having the mother verbally repeat instructions is another method of ensuring accurate comprehension. All health care providers have a responsibility to provide instructions that are consistent with the patient's health literacy.

SAFE PRACTICE ALERT

Do not use abbreviations or medical terminology when providing patients with instructions.

According to the Healthy People 2020 initiative, health information and the associated access issues have become more complicated. There are many considerations when determining whether an individual has proficient health literacy. The patient should be able to exhibit certain competencies:

- Read and identify credible health information
- Understand numbers in the context of the patient's health care
- Make appointments
- Fill out forms
- Gather health records and ask appropriate questions of physicians
- Advocate for appropriate care
- Navigate complex insurance programs, Medicare or Medicaid, and other financial assistance programs
- Use technology to access information and services (USDHHS, 2010a)

TYPES OF PATIENT EDUCATION LO 14.3

Patient education occurs in a wide variety of settings, which can be categorized as formal and informal. Formal patient education is delivered throughout the community in the form of media, in a variety of educational and group settings, or in a planned, goal-directed, one-on-one session with a patient in the acute care setting. Formal education usually has goals set by the educator or, in the case of patient education, the nurse.

Informal education is usually learner or patient directed. This type of education may occur when a patient asks a question about a medication, treatment, or procedure. The health care information is considered informal because it is situation and patient specific. Some patient education sessions have formal and informal elements, because the nurse and patient may set goals together before the nurse formulates and implements the plan of care, and the patient is free to ask questions that may direct the session.

Patients are inundated with information from the Internet, television, radio, newspapers, and community programs. Nurses can help patients recognize reliable sources and accurate information.

QSEN FOCUS!

Nurses are responsible for evaluating sources of health care information and using high-quality electronic sources for patient education.

Many health care consumers begin receiving information as children through their primary education. Handwashing, proper dental care, and nutrition are examples of early instructions. The dangers and risks associated with smoking, drug or alcohol abuse, and drunk driving are taught throughout their secondary education. College students are provided with education intended to promote health and well-being. Health care education continues in adulthood in the form of medication commercials, nutritional food labels, and information obtained from Internet sites.

Teaching is imparting knowledge or giving instruction, whereas **learning** is acquiring knowledge or skills through instruction or experience. Teaching may be delivered in acute care, long-term care, and outpatient settings. Examples are instructions given regarding a new prescription at a doctor's appointment, information about the need for dietary supplements in a long-term care setting, or postoperative or discharge instructions for the patient in a hospital or other acute care facility. An example of patient education provided for

PATIENT EDUCATION AND HEALTH LITERACY

Sick-Day Guidelines for People With Diabetes

In one part of diabetic teaching, the nurse instructs the patient about what to do if flulike illness occurs:

- Continue taking diabetes pills or insulin.
- Test blood glucose levels every 4 hours, and keep track of the results.
- Drink extra (calorie-free) liquids, and try to eat normally. If unable to eat normally, eat an equivalent amount of carbohydrates.
- Track weight daily. Losing weight without trying may be a sign of high blood glucose levels or be from other causes. Further evaluation is needed.
- Check temperature every morning and evening. A fever may be a sign of infection.
- Call the health care provider or go to an emergency room if you:
  - Are too sick to eat normally or are unable to keep down food for more than 6 hours.
  - Are having severe diarrhea.
  - Lose 5 pounds or more.
  - Have a temperature higher than 38.3° C (101° F).
  - Have blood glucose levels lower than 60 mg/dL or that remain higher than 300 mg/dL.
  - Are having trouble breathing.
  - Feel sleepy or cannot think clearly.

Adapted from Centers for Disease Control and Prevention: Sick day guidelines for people with diabetes, 2012. Retrieved from *www.cdc.gov/diabetes/news/docs/flu_protect.htm#sickday*.

diabetics is outlined in the Patient Education and Health Literacy box.

Consideration must be given to the patient's background, readiness to learn, and current condition before education can occur. A patient's ability to read, write, and comprehend health care materials enhances health literacy.

DOMAINS OF LEARNING LO 14.4

To provide effective patient teaching, the nurse must be aware of the three domains, or types, of learning: cognitive, psychomotor, and affective (Bloom, 1956). Effective patient teaching requires knowledge about how the individual learns. **Cognitive domain** learning comprises knowledge and material that is remembered. Memorization and recall of information is needed for the learner to remember, understand, apply, analyze, evaluate, and create the new material.

Learners in the cognitive domain integrate new knowledge through first learning and then recalling the information. They then categorize and evaluate, making comparisons with previous knowledge that result in conclusions related to the new content (Bloom, 1956). Some examples of teaching methods in the cognitive domain include reading-level-appropriate written literature, demonstration, and use of examples. A patient who remembers the information taught during an education session, applies that information during a return demonstration, and is able to ask questions to further enhance knowledge gained is functioning in the cognitive domain.

The **psychomotor domain** incorporates physical movement and the use of motor skills in learning. Teaching the newly diagnosed diabetic how to check blood sugar is an example of a psychomotor skill. Having the patient observe the nurse demonstrating the skill and then demonstrate it and receive feedback is an effective method of teaching learners in the psychomotor domain. When the patient has successfully demonstrated how to perform the task, psychomotor learning has occurred.

Bloom's (1956) third style of learning is the affective domain. **Affective domain** learning recognizes the emotional component of integrating new knowledge. Successful education in this domain takes into account the patient's feelings, values, motivations, and attitudes. Exploring these patient-specific attributes enhances the value of the learned information. A patient who readily receives the information taught, responds to the nurse with active participation, and values the importance of the teaching session is operating in the affective domain.

LEARNING STYLES LO 14.5

Understanding how individuals learn is important for nurses when considering the written or verbal information they are teaching. Although research has shown that most adults read at an eighth-grade level, 20% of the U.S. population reads at or below a fifth-grade level. Nurses can supplement materials that are written at a high reading level with photos, drawings, and explanations of terms that are difficult to understand.

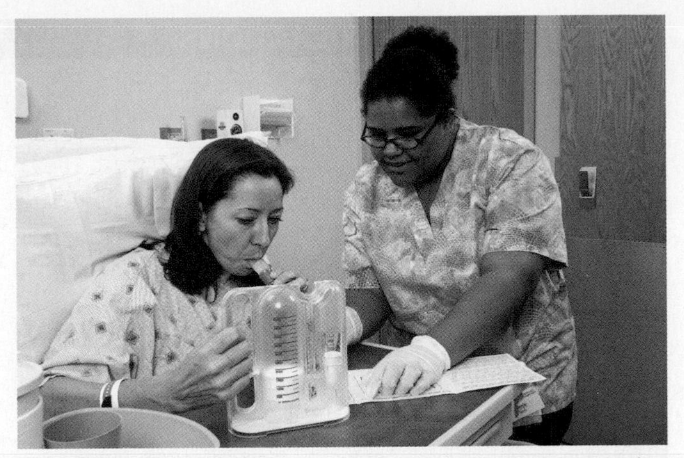

FIGURE 14-2 A nurse uses a variety of teaching strategies to show a patient how to use an incentive spirometer.

In addition to being aware of learning domains and the materials used to teach patients, nurses must give consideration to the learning styles, strengths, and abilities of the individual. Tools have been developed to help health care workers evaluate the health literacy of their patients. One such tool is the VARK (*v*erbal, *a*ural, *r*ead/write, *k*inesthetic) assessment of learning styles of people who are having difficulty learning (Fleming, 2010). The VARK areas are evaluated to educate individuals on the basis of their learning preferences.

The VARK developers have written other assessment aids that are available online. Some are designed to assess learning styles on the basis of language, age, and purpose of the evaluation. Some versions are directed at business, and others are specific to education and may provide valuable learner-specific information to assist the provider of health care information and the patient (Fleming, 2010).

Individuals typically learn through more than one method. For example, a patient's VARK assessment may indicate learning through VAR or ARK. When the use of more than one style facilitates learning, the individual is considered a **multimodal learner**, meaning that the person does best when more than one teaching strategy is used or that the person is able to adapt to a variety of teaching strategies (Figure 14-2) on the basis of what is being presented (Fleming, 2010). Understanding how patients learn best makes collaborative learning plans most effective. It is good practice to provide multiple means of learning, because most individuals learn through more than one style and repetition enhances learning.

FACTORS AFFECTING HEALTH LITERACY AND PATIENT TEACHING LO 14.6

Many factors affect patients' health literacy. The educational level of the learner and the instructional materials was

DIVERSITY CONSIDERATIONS

Life Span

- Patient education provided for children should be age-specific.
  - Use pictures and simple words for young children.
  - Use clear, simple explanations for school-age children.
- Before health care teaching sessions for adults, assess reading level, learning styles, and readiness to learn.

Culture and Religion

- Patient education may not be understood because of language, beliefs, and values.
- For patients who do not speak or understand the language of the nurse:
  - Use a professional nonfamily member as an interpreter. Family members should not be used as interpreters of specific medical information to maintain the patient's right to privacy and to avoid possible misinterpretation of medical terminology.
  - Use photos, drawings, or video to enhance understanding.
- Different cultural and religious practices, beliefs, and values may interfere with certain medical treatments:
  - Nurses who are culturally sensitive tailor education to align with cultural beliefs.
  - A patient whose cultural beliefs and values are considered is more likely to demonstrate compliance.

Disability

- Patients with physical impairments may not be able to perform skills requiring psychomotor learning.
  - Provide visual and auditory materials as needed.
  - A caregiver or significant other may need to be involved in the patient education session.
- Patients with learning disabilities or cognitive alterations need individualized instruction geared to their special needs.
- Patients with vision loss may not be able to read regular printed material. Use other methods:
  - Verbal instructions
  - Demonstration
  - Large-print material
  - Braille or audio materials
- Patients with hearing loss may not be able to hear and understand verbal instructions. Use other methods:
  - Printed material
  - Demonstration
  - Recorded materials amplified through headsets
  - Interpretation:
    - Interpretation for the hearing impaired may be provided by a professional interpreter face-to-face with patients and families or by phone or video medical interpretation (VMI).
    - Access to interpretation or translation for deaf and limited English proficiency (LEP) patients is required by Title VI of the Civil Rights Act of 1964, which mandates equal rights for people regardless of race, color, or national origin.
  - Simulations, photos, drawings, or video to enhance understanding.

discussed previously. Factors such as age, culture, language, environment, nature of the content, and current situation, including level of pain, timing of instruction, and economic resources, also must be considered. The Diversity Considerations box addresses some diversity issues that should be considered in planning patient education. Adjustments to factors that are within the nurse's control, such as timing of instruction, are often necessary to achieve the maximum benefit of the nurse-patient interaction.

AGE AND DEVELOPMENTAL STAGE

The patient's age directly affects the instructional methods and materials used. Effective patient education involving a child requires the presence of a parent or caregiver, who is likely the target of teaching. Children should not be excluded from the learning session unless exclusion is deemed appropriate by the parent or caregiver; a presentation using an age-appropriate strategy may complement the instructions reviewed with the adult. The stages of development (see Chapter 17) should be explored as the foundation for the choice of educational materials. Learning theories as they relate to developmental stages are also discussed in Chapter 17.

Adult learners tend to be self-motivated and able to participate in planning their health education. During a visit to an outpatient facility or inpatient hospital, an adult learner may learn independently, may have learning facilitated by the nurse, or may need a spouse or significant other for support, depending on the diagnosis and current condition of the patient. The pace of adult education sessions depends on the patient, the situation, and the difficulty of the content.

Teaching should be tailored to elderly patients. Reports indicate that two thirds of U.S. adults 66 years old and older have inadequate or marginal literacy skills, and 81% of patients 60 years old and older at a public hospital could not read or understand basic materials such as prescription labels (National Network of Libraries of Medicine, 2013). Although each patient must be assessed individually, cognitive and sensory alterations often occur with aging, and the teaching materials should be adjusted accordingly.

ROLE

Exploration of the patient's roles is an important task that must be done before development of a patient education plan. For example, a 32-year-old, single mother of five young children who has just undergone a hysterectomy may require a different perspective in her discharge instructions than that in the instructions of a 67-year-old female living with her husband who recently retired after 35 years as a family practice physician. The first patient may have less support and less flexibility regarding rest, lifting limitations, and cost of prescriptions than the second. It is important not to stereotype and assign roles but rather to develop a plan in collaboration with the individual. The patient's support system should be taken into consideration when the nurse plans patient education.

ENVIRONMENT

The location of patient education influences the outcome. The setting should be quiet, and the session should have minimal interruptions. Providing privacy is difficult in settings such as emergency rooms, outpatient surgery centers, and semiprivate inpatient rooms, but the nurse should make every effort to ensure confidentiality. Environmental considerations such as good lighting and the availability of resources should be explored to enhance the outcome of patient education.

TIMING

The nurse should examine the patient's situation and comfort level before beginning teaching. For example, a postoperative patient who is rating pain at 7 of 10 will be much more receptive to learning after being medicated for pain. A patient who just received a diagnosis of metastatic cancer will learn and assimilate more information later in the day or perhaps the next day. Asking whether a patient would like a family member or caregiver to sit in on the session may affect the timing. The nurse should end the session if the patient shows signs of fatigue. Prioritizing the key points of patient education ensures that the most important aspects are taught at the beginning of a session.

ECONOMIC RESOURCES

Learning objectives should be determined collaboratively between the nurse and the patient to ensure that the patient's economic resources are congruent with the plan. For example, a patient with limited health care insurance and no prescription plan may not be able to obtain necessary medications or dressing supplies after discharge from the hospital. If a need for support services is identified, the nurse should contact the social services department, discharge planning personnel, or community agencies about assistance for the patient and family.

EVIDENCE-BASED PRACTICE

Nurses play a key role in providing patients with accurate, unbiased, scientifically sound information. Individuals may not be able to judge the validity of advertisements or medical treatment claims they see in the media. Evidence-based practice is used in patient education to "help consumers think more critically about the evidence used to substantiate medical claims" (Schardt, 2011).

Although evidence-based practice is important, it is sometimes insufficient when making patient care decisions. Attention to the patient's values and informed preferences is necessary when planning treatments that are required by expertise and practical wisdom. Patients may choose to have, or not to have, a recommended treatment (Montori, Britto, and Murad, 2013). Health literacy is woven into treatment plans because nurses must ensure that patients comprehend health care information before determining their preferences in making decisions. Patients trust nurses to share with them valid and legitimate information and resources (Evidence-Based Practice and Informatics box).

EVIDENCE-BASED PRACTICE AND INFORMATICS

Patient Involvement in Education

- Many patient safety advocates—including The Joint Commission in *National Patient Safety Goals* (2014) and Cronenwett and colleagues in *Quality and Safety Education for Nurses* (2007)—encourage the active involvement of patients and their families in patient-centered care.
- To promote involvement, nurses must ensure that patients understand the information relevant to their care.
- Nurses need to provide patients with easy-to-understand information and speak in a clear, distinct voice, using short sentences and understandable terminology.
- Multiple teaching methods should be used to meet the needs of all types of learners.
- Patient education sessions should be reassessed after two to three key points to ensure that the patient is still engaged in learning and ready to assimilate more information.
- Information taught at previous sessions can be reviewed before proceeding with new key points.

QSEN FOCUS!

Nurses read original research and clinical practice guidelines to prepare patient education. By using evidence-based practice, nurses provide patients with the most up-to-date information available.

When exploring the concepts of health literacy and patient education, nurses must recognize the need to work collaboratively with health care professionals in other disciplines, such as physicians, social workers, dieticians, and occupational, speech, and physical therapists. "There is a need for a framework that connects … the health professions" in the development of patient education (Riegelman and Garr, 2011).

Engaging in multidisciplinary discussions and planning with the patient facilitate the most effective results.

ASSESSMENT LO 14.7

Assessment of health literacy occurs with each patient encounter. Nurses observe patient behavior during interactions to determine if further assessment is needed. Certain patient behaviors may indicate inadequate health literacy which have the potential to affect patient education. These behaviors are exhibited in the following examples:

- Information on forms is incomplete or inaccurate.
- Patient wants to take written documents home to discuss with family or asks health care provider to read information aloud, stating, "I left my glasses at home."
- Patient misses appointments or comes to appointments at an unscheduled time.
- Patient misses appointments or doesn't follow through with laboratory tests, imaging tests, or referrals to specialists.
- Patient is noncompliant with medication and treatment regimens.
- Patient claims to be taking medication or following a treatment regimen, but laboratory or imaging tests do not show expected results.

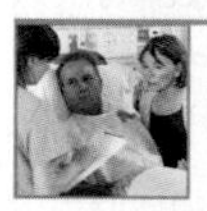

1. What cues could have helped the primary care provider (PCP) and nurse realize that Mr. Lubic and his wife were unable to read?

Knowledge or discovery of literacy limits in the assessment stage can aid the nurse in developing the education plan and decrease the potential for life-threatening outcomes. The Health Assessment Questions box provides examples of questions to ask the patient. Limited literacy skills may result from a lack of educational opportunity (high school level or less education), learning disabilities, or cognitive declines in older adults. Patients' reading abilities may be below standard. Reading abilities are typically three to five grade levels below the last year of school completed. People with a high school diploma typically read at a seventh- or eighth-grade reading level (National Network of Libraries of Medicine, 2013).

HEALTH ASSESSMENT QUESTIONS

Patient Education Focus

- Who will be taking care of you? Who do we need to educate?
- What do you already know about your diagnosis or care of this condition?
- What is your preferred language?
- Do you have access to the Internet?
- What is the highest grade level that you completed in school?
- Can you read the local newspaper? Do you like to read books? Magazines?
- What do you hope to learn from our teaching sessions?
- What information do you feel is most important?
- Have you ever had instruction on this subject? (If so, ask for details.)
- How do you learn best? (If needed, give examples such as "by watching and doing" and "by reading.")
- Do you have any difficulty with hearing or vision?
- Are you having pain or discomfort?

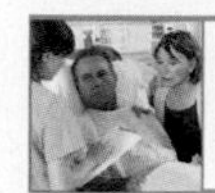

2. What could the office nurse have done differently during the initial visit with Mr. Lubic?

The patient's ability to learn or perform health-related care is essential. Low health literacy (i.e., basic or below basic) and cognitive impairments such as memory issues, impaired vision or hearing, or poor hand-eye coordination are factors to be considered in the development of the teaching plan. Special attention should be given to determining patients' learning styles; asking how they learned best or easily retained information in the past elicits valuable information. Determining the patient's physical, emotional, and cognitive readiness to learn is an essential component of the preeducation assessment.

Educational assessment includes designating the learner: patient, family, significant other, or caregiver. Infants, children, and individuals with developmental disabilities need to have an adult as the primary learner. Terminally ill patients and some elderly patients may view themselves as dependent on their caregivers, and they may not want to be involved in learning or may want to have their caregivers present during educational sessions.

In ensuring a comprehensive assessment of patient education and health literacy, the nurse should discuss the motivation and willingness of patients or caregivers to learn and review their previous experiences with health care learning. Helping the patient to identify priorities in learning can determine how to proceed with development of the teaching plan. Adults must place value on the need for or purpose of learning (Gulanick and Myers, 2014).

NURSING DIAGNOSIS LO 14.8

On completion of assessment, a nursing diagnosis relevant to the educational needs of the patient or caregiver can be determined. Diagnoses specifically related to patient education include *Deficient Knowledge, Readiness for Enhanced Knowledge,* and *Noncompliance.*

Individualized nursing diagnostic statements written for patients depend on the related factors and defining characteristics. Examples of nursing diagnostic statements are:

- *Deficient Knowledge* (i.e., self-administration of insulin) related to (r/t) new-onset hyperglycemia as evidenced by patient's verbalized fear of needles and blood sugar levels ranging from 210 to 305 mg/dL.

- *Readiness for Enhanced Knowledge* (i.e., diabetes management) with defining characteristics of patient found in bed reading diabetes information or literature left on the bedside table yesterday by the nurse and patient asking questions about management of the blood glucose level.
- *Noncompliance* related to (r/t) barrier to comprehension (i.e., anxiety) as evidenced by trembling hands, getting up from chair every 3 to 5 minutes, and verbalizing, "I'm just so nervous!"

PLANNING LO 14.9

After working with the patient or caregiver to determine the appropriate nursing diagnosis, the next step is developing the patient education plan (Table 14-1). Considering the patient's support system is an integral part of this step, because it may be necessary or helpful to have someone monitor progress. Collaboration with the patient, caregiver, and health care professionals in other disciplines enhances the potential for a positive outcome (Collaboration and Delegation box). The patient and caregiver, to the extent agreed to by the patient, should be directly involved in determining the goals of teaching. Determining the outcome statements early in this process directs the remainder of the plan.

COLLABORATION AND DELEGATION

Multidisciplinary Patient Education

- Assessment and development of a patient teaching plan may not be delegated to unlicensed assistive personnel (UAP).
- Collaboration with the patient, caregiver, and physician is imperative in creating and implementing an effective teaching plan.
- Social workers or discharge planners are able to assist with socioeconomic issues. (For example, the patient may not have insurance coverage for the supplies or medications needed; social workers or discharge planners are familiar with community resources, fee waivers, and other sources of assistance.) These individuals also coordinate and facilitate referrals to home care or other settings that are most appropriate for the patient's situation and educational needs.
- Physical, occupational, and speech therapists can collaborate with nurses to enhance a comprehensive teaching plan.

QSEN FOCUS!

Patient education is coordinated by the nurse but involves other members of the health care team. Teamwork and collaboration are demonstrated when the nurse recognizes and integrates the contributions of the primary care provider, therapists, dietitians, and social workers and respects the unique attributes that each brings in helping the patient achieve health education goals.

As health care educators, nurses should allow patients to identify what is most important to them. If a newly diagnosed diabetic patient is interested in learning techniques of care that will allow discharge to home rather than to an extended care facility, the patient is more likely to be receptive to learning about self-monitoring blood sugar levels. After the learning goals related to the issues the patient feels are a priority have been met, the patient may then be able to focus on health promotion and avoiding complications (Home Care Considerations box).

HOME CARE CONSIDERATIONS

Patient Education in the Home

- The nurse is a guest in the patient's home when providing care or teaching in this setting (Figure 14-3).
- Visits by nurses and other staff in the home setting are less frequent than those in other settings.
- Insurance coverage available for staff visits, supplies, and equipment must be considered when developing the teaching plan in the home.
- To promote continuity, documentation of the teaching plan and progress toward goals must be readily available to all staff visiting the home care patient.

TABLE 14-1 Care Planning

NANDA-I NURSING DIAGNOSIS LABEL WITH NURSING DIAGNOSIS STATEMENT	NURSING OUTCOME CLASSIFICATION (NOC)	NURSING INTERVENTION CLASSIFICATION (NIC)
Deficient Knowledge (self-administration of insulin), related to new-onset hyperglycemia as evidenced by patient's verbalized fear of needles and blood sugars ranging from 210 to 305 mg/dL	*Knowledge: Diabetes management* (1820) Proper technique to draw up and administer insulin (182027)	*Medication administration: subcutaneous* (4130) Determine the patient's knowledge of medication and understanding of method of administration

From Bulechek G, Butcher H, Dochterman J, et al (Eds): *Nursing interventions classification (NIC),* ed. 6, St. Louis, 2013, Mosby; Moorhead S, Johnson M, Maas M, et al (Eds): *Nursing outcomes classification (NOC),* ed. 5, St. Louis, 2013, Mosby; NANDA International: *Nursing diagnoses: Definitions and classification, 2012–2014,* West Sussex, England, 2012, Wiley-Blackwell. Reprinted with permission from NANDA International, Inc.

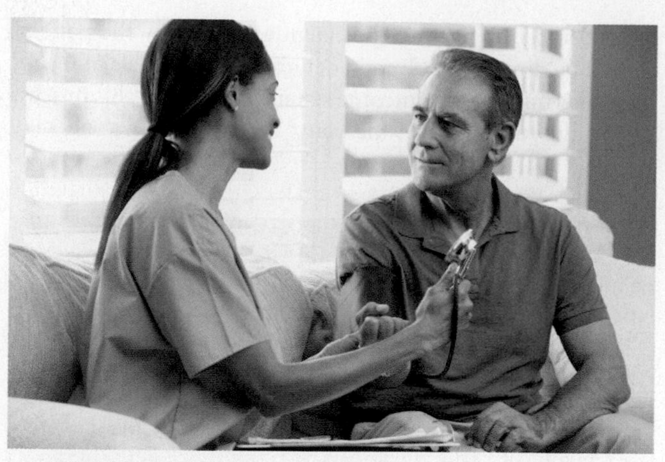

FIGURE 14-3 A nurse teaches a patient how to check pulse and blood pressure before taking medication.

The following are examples of goals or outcome statements:

- Patient will demonstrate the correct technique for administering insulin within 48 hours.
- Patient will verbalize the need to learn diabetes-related information within 24 hours.
- Patient will verbalize a decrease in anxiety at the next outpatient visit.

Before developing the interventions to be used in the patient education plan, the nurse should again consider the health literacy of the patient or caregiver. Strategies of assessment were discussed earlier in this chapter, but it is important to understand that patients with low health literacy may have difficulty with the following:

- Locating providers and services
- Filling out complex health forms
- Sharing their medical history with providers
- Seeking preventive health care
- Knowing the connection between risky behaviors and health
- Managing chronic health conditions
- Understanding directions on medicine (Health Resources and Services Administration, n.d.)

◆ IMPLEMENTATION AND EVALUATION LO 14.10

In all patient education situations, a return demonstration by the patient (i.e., repeating what has been taught), helps the nurse to assess the level of learning that has taken place. Healthy People 2020 reiterates the three As of health information identified in the National Action Plan to Improve Health Literacy, which states that health information must be accurate, accessible, and actionable (USDHHS, 2010b).

Keeping these concepts in mind when implementing the teaching plan can guide the information, the approach, and the evaluation of progress. Accessibility needs to encompass getting the learning content to the learner and planning for the use of alternative methods of instruction for individuals with sensory limitations (e.g., use of Braille boards or magnified fonts for those with visual difficulties and amplified media with headphones for those with auditory issues). The Diversity Considerations box earlier in the chapter provides guidelines for patients with specific needs.

Nurses often advocate for patients when other members of the health care team have provided information that needs clarification. Making sure that patients understand instructions and terminology and seeking clarification from other providers when needed are part of the nurse's role as patient educator.

ENVIRONMENT

To facilitate learning, care should be taken to ensure physical comfort for the learner, whether in a group or individual session. In setting the stage for effective learning, it is important, for example, to schedule teaching sessions when pain medication has been administered but the patient is not too cognitively affected by the pharmacologic side effects of the medication. Attempting to minimize interruption in a quiet atmosphere of respect and trust is also important. Nurses may have different values or priorities from those of patients, and they must take care to provide a nonjudgmental environment.

PACE

Teaching sessions should focus on one idea at a time and should be kept short. Patients are likely to experience a sense of accomplishment when they are focusing on and mastering one task at a time. Because learners who are ill may be facing fatigue or decreased stamina and attention, lengthy sessions are less beneficial.

DATA INTEGRATION

Patient education plans require steps to assist the learners with integrating the newly acquired information into their lives. When presenting health care materials, the nurse should use basic terminology that is easily understood by the learner and is consistent with the individual's health literacy level. Instructions should be presented in a clear, concise way at a learner-appropriate level. Information should be presented by starting with familiar concepts and progressing to the less familiar, complex, or abstract ideas.

A variety of teaching methods can be combined to match content with learning style. Examples include verbal instruction, media such as computer-assisted programs and digital media, demonstration and return demonstration, and written instructions. Providing patients with material written in their native language at the end of the session gives them the opportunity to review what they have learned, allowing effective integration of the information.

REPETITION AND DEMONSTRATION

Newly presented information or techniques should be reviewed at the end of the session, with adequate time allowed for questions and demonstration. Having the patient practice a task is extremely beneficial because it enables the nurse to provide immediate feedback, correct errors, and ensure that the patient comprehended the material as it was intended. In some instances, the patient may observe by computer or other format a skill being performed in a simulation scenario until the patient is able to perform the skill. These sessions give the nurse ample opportunity to provide praise and positive feedback to the learner. In all patient education situations, return demonstration by the patient helps the nurse to assess the level of learning that has taken place.

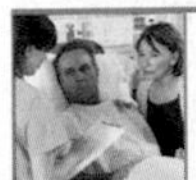

3. What alternative methods could the nurse and other members of the health care team have used to convey the essential information to the Lubics without relying on written patient discharge instructions?

EVALUATION

Ongoing evaluation of patient education occurs by each member of the health care team who provides teaching according to the patient's teaching plan. Having the learner repeat what has been learned can help the nurse evaluate the teaching plan and adjust the plan for future patient education sessions. Future sessions should review what was learned previously and continue to add to what has been taught. Health care team members can view documentation on the electronic health record (EHR) before beginning an education session to determine the patient's progress in meeting educational goals.

DOCUMENTATION

Teaching sessions—including topics and skills reviewed, methods and materials used, and patient progress—must be documented (Figure 14-4). EHRs document the progress of patient teaching with detailed descriptions of the goals, what was taught, how it was taught, and the patient's reaction to the teaching. In many settings, the learner may be instructed

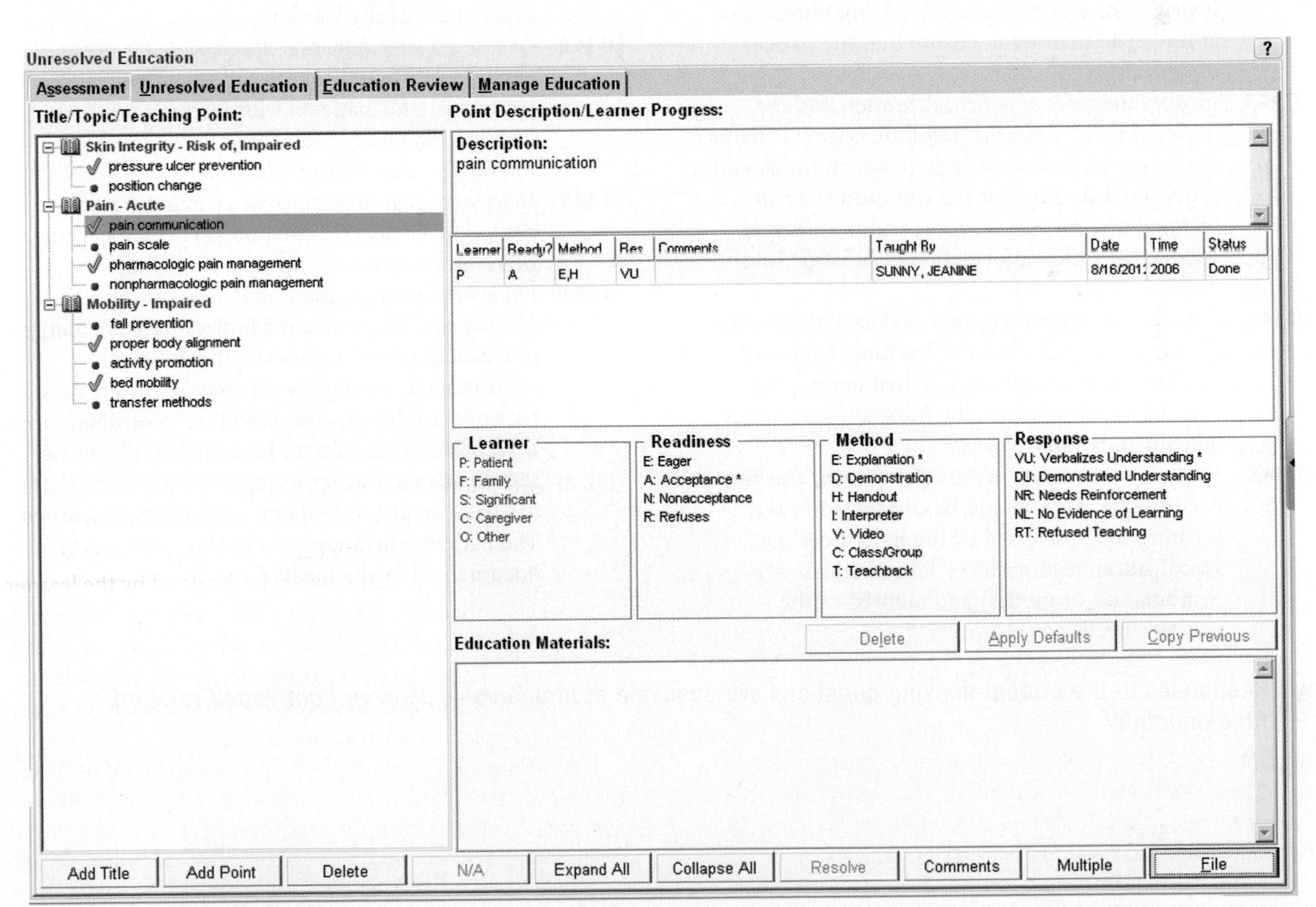

FIGURE 14-4 An electronic teaching plan shows documentation of unresolved education, learners and their response to the teaching, methods used, and completed instruction. (Courtesy Epic Systems Corporation, Verona, Wis, 2012.)

by different individuals in a discipline (e.g., nurses on different shifts) or by multidisciplinary teams. All members of the teaching team need accurate, up-to-date information regarding the patient's progress toward achieving patient education goals.

Some agencies have multiple-copy forms that are signed by the nurse and patient to indicate the teaching that has taken place. It is important for the nurse to document what was taught, to whom, by which method, and how the patient responded. Paper or electronic copies of any information necessary for use at home should be made available to the patient.

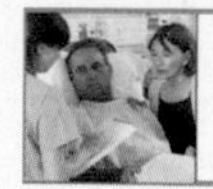

4. Describe what to include in the care plan that would better meet the needs of teaching Mr. Lubic.

SUMMARY OF LEARNING OUTCOMES

LO 14.1 *Define health literacy:* Health literacy refers to a patient's ability to seek and understand information related to health care, disease prevention, and treatment of illness. Patients are unique in their ability to comprehend health care information. Health literacy directly affects the patient's ability to comprehend and integrate knowledge.

LO 14.2 *Explain the role of health literacy in nursing and patient education:* Knowledge of a patient's health literacy level assists nurses in communicating instructions and educational information in an appropriate manner to ensure that the patient understands.

LO 14.3 *Identify the types of patient education and the settings in which patient education occurs:* Patients are taught in formal settings, in which information is delivered throughout the community or in planned one-on-one sessions, and in informal settings, in which information is situation and patient specific.

LO 14.4 *Differentiate among the three domains of learning:* There are three domains of learning: cognitive, psychomotor, and affective. When developing effective teaching plans, the nurse must consider *how* the individual learns.

LO 14.5 *Explain how learning styles affect patient teaching:* Patient education should be conducted in the learning style preferred by the individual (i.e., verbal, aural, read/write, or kinesthetic or a combination of modes) and tailored to the patient's needs.

LO 14.6 *Describe factors affecting health literacy and patient education:* Health literacy and patient education are affected by numerous factors, including cultural background, socioeconomic level, age or developmental stage, role, environment, and timing.

LO 14.7 *Carry out an assessment of the patient's health literacy and education needs:* An assessment must be done before developing a patient teaching plan and should take into consideration the learner and the learning level, educational needs, and previous experiences of the learner.

LO 14.8 *Choose nursing diagnoses appropriate for use with patient education:* Examples of nursing diagnoses appropriate for patients with learning needs are *Deficient Knowledge, Readiness for Enhanced Knowledge,* and *Noncompliance.*

LO 14.9 *Determine goals and outcome criteria for patient education:* Goals are based on particular learning needs and established nursing diagnoses.

LO 14.10 *Implement teaching plans and evaluate their effectiveness:* The nurse maximizes implementation of teaching plans by choosing the best environment, pacing the sessions according to the patient's condition, and providing information that is accurate, accessible, and actionable. The nurse should ask the learner to repeat or perform what has been taught to evaluate what has been learned. The patient education session should be documented in the medical record.

Responses to the critical-thinking questions are available at *http://evolve.elsevier.com/YoostCrawford/fundamentals/*.

REVIEW QUESTIONS

1. The nurse is caring for a 6-year-old patient in the emergency department who just had a full left leg cast placed for a fracture. As the nurse is reviewing the discharge instructions with the patient's mother, she states, "You don't have to go over those—I'll read them at home." What should the nurse do?
   a. Contact the physician immediately.
   b. Consider the possibility of health literacy limitations and assess further.
   c. Stop the teaching, because the mother obviously has taken care of casts before.
   d. Explain to the mother that reading the instructions with her is required.
2. A 58-year-old male is admitted for a small-bowel obstruction late Saturday night. The nurse obtains admitting orders, which include the need to place a nasogastric (NG) tube to low intermittent suction. During the assessment, the nurse determines that the patient does not speak English. What should the nurse do before placing the tube?
   a. Assess the presence of any family members who may speak English and the patient's native language.
   b. Take two additional staff members into the room when placing the tube so the patient can be restrained if needed.
   c. Request an interpreter by leaving a voicemail on his or her office extension.
   d. Do not place the NG tube because the physician would not want to frighten the patient.
3. Which nursing diagnoses are used in developing a patient teaching plan? *(Select all that apply.)*
   a. *Noncompliance*
   b. *Readiness for Enhanced Knowledge*
   c. *Ineffective Coping*
   d. *Health-Seeking Behaviors*
   e. *Anxiety*
4. Which nursing diagnosis is appropriate if a patient expresses an interest in learning?
   a. *Readiness for Enhanced Knowledge*
   b. *Knowledge Deficit*
   c. *Information Processing*
   d. *Health-Seeking Behaviors*
5. A 61-year-old male is undergoing an emergency cardiac catheterization when the nurse gives his wife a packet of registration paperwork and asks her to complete the forms. Which observed actions may indicate a health literacy issue? *(Select all that apply.)*
   a. Putting on glasses before beginning the paperwork
   b. Asking someone in the waiting area to read the forms to her "because I need to get new glasses—these just don't work"
   c. Waiting until her daughter arrives to begin the paperwork so that her daughter can complete the forms
   d. Setting the clipboard aside and staring tearfully out the window
   e. Returning the forms only partially filled out, with missing or inaccurate information
6. A weight-loss program that combines nutrition instruction with exercise is an example of teaching based on which domain of learning?
   a. Psychomotor
   b. Affective
   c. Psychosocial
   d. Cognitive
7. The nurse is providing home care to a 62-year-old female who was recently diagnosed with insulin-dependent diabetes mellitus. What is the most important reason for the nurse to document the teaching session?
   a. The patient's insurance company requires documentation.
   b. The nurse's employer requires documentation of home care sessions.
   c. Other members of the health care team need to know the patient's progress.
   d. Insulin is a potentially dangerous medication and needs to be documented.
8. Written instructions showing pictures of the steps necessary to test a blood sugar, along with demonstration and a return demonstration of the steps, would most benefit which learners?
   a. Affective
   b. VARK
   c. Psychomotor
   d. Cognitive

9. The nurse is providing care to an 88-year-old male patient who just returned from the recovery room after a right hip replacement. The nurse plans to teach the patient prevention techniques for deep vein thrombosis. What is the best time to provide teaching?
   a. Do it right before the patient's next intravenous pain medication.
   b. Wait until tomorrow morning because he is in too much pain today.
   c. Leave written materials on his over-the-bed tray that he can read at his convenience.
   d. Wait until 10 to 15 minutes after his next intravenous pain medication.

10. Which is true about patient teaching sessions?
    a. Present all of the information so the patient can learn all that is needed.
    b. Present the patient with one idea at a time.
    c. Ensure the presence of a family member at each session.
    d. End with a written quiz to ensure understanding of the information.

Answers and rationales for the review questions are available at *http://evolve.elsevier.com/YoostCrawford/fundamentals/*.

REFERENCES

American Medical Association (AMA): Health literacy program, n.d. Retrieved from *www.ama-assn.org/ama/pub/about-ama/ama-foundation/our-programs/public-health/health-literacy-program.page.*

Bloom BS: *Taxonomy of educational objectives, Handbook I*, New York, 1956, David McKay.

Cornett S: Assessing and addressing health literacy. *Online J Issues Nurs*, 14(3):1-18, 2009.

Cronenwett L, Sherwood G, Barnsteiner J, et al: Quality and safety education for nurses. *Nurs Outlook*, 55(3):122-131, 2007.

Fleming N: VARK: A guide to learning styles, 2010. Retrieved from *www.vark-learn.com/english/index.asp.*

Gulanick M, Myers J: *Nursing care plans: Diagnoses, interventions and outcomes*, ed. 8, St. Louis, 2014, Mosby.

Health Resources and Services Administration: About health literacy, n.d. Retrieved from *www.hrsa.gov/healthliteracy.*

Institute of Medicine: Health literacy: Improving health, health systems, and health policy around the world, 2013. Retrieved from *www.iom.edu/Reports/2013/Health-Literacy-Improving-Health-Health-Systems-and-Health-Policy-Around-the-World.aspx.*

The Joint Commission: National patient safety goals, 2014. Retrieved from *www.jointcommission.org/assets/1/6/HAP_NPSG_Chapter_2014.pdf.*

Montori VM, Britto JP, Murad M: The optimal practice of evidence-based medicine: Incorporating patient preferences in practice guidelines. *JAMA* 310(23):2503-2504, 2013.

National Network of Libraries of Medicine: Health literacy, 2013. Retrieved from *http://nnlm.gov/outreach/consumer/hlthlit.html#A2.*

Quixley J: Introduction. In *Notes on nursing: What it is and what it is not*, Glasgow, Scotland, 1974, Blackie & Son (originally published 1859).

Parker RM, Ratzan SC, Lurie N: Health literacy: A policy challenge for advancing high-quality health care. *Health Affairs* 22(4):147, 2003.

Riegelman R, Garr D: Healthy People 2020 and education for health: What are the objectives? *Am J Prev Med*, 40(2):203-206, 2011.

Schardt C: Health information literacy meets evidence-based practice. *J Med Libr Assoc*, 99(1):1-2, 2011.

Scheckel M, Emery N, Nosek C: Addressing health literacy: The experiences of undergraduate nursing students. *J Clin Nurs*, 19:794-802, 2010.

Schwartzberg J, Cowett A, VanGeest J, Wolf M: Communication techniques for patients with low health literacy: A survey of physicians, nurses and pharmacists. *Am J Behav Health*, 31(1):S96-S104, 2007.

Squellati R: Health literacy: Understanding basic health information. *Creat Nurs*, 16(3):110-114, 2010.

U.S. Department of Health and Human Services (USDHHS): *Healthy People 2020: Understanding and improving health*, Washington, D.C., 2010a, U.S. Government Printing Office.

U.S. Department of Health and Human Services (USDHHS): *National action plan to improve health literacy*, Washington, D.C., 2010b, U.S. Government Printing Office.

White S: *Assessing the nation's health literacy: Key concepts and findings of the National Assessment of Adult Literacy*, Chicago, 2008, American Medical Association Foundation.

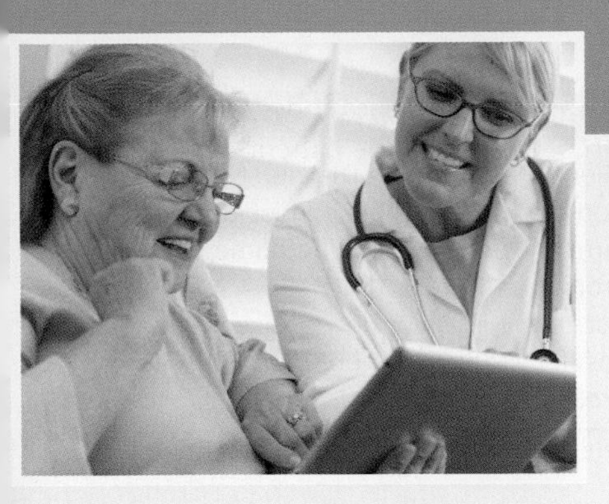

CHAPTER 15

Nursing Informatics

EVOLVE WEBSITE

http://evolve.elsevier.com/YoostCrawford/fundamentals/

- Additional Evolve-Only Review Questions With Answers
- Answers and Rationales for Text Review Questions
- Answers to Critical-Thinking Questions
- Case Study With Questions
- Glossary

LEARNING OUTCOMES

Comprehension of this chapter's content will provide students with the ability to:

LO 15.1 Define *nursing informatics.*
LO 15.2 Discuss the uses of technology in health care.
LO 15.3 Summarize the benefits of informatics.
LO 15.4 Compare competency levels of nursing informatics.
LO 15.5 Explain the importance of using standardized terminologies in electronic health records.
LO 15.6 Implement the use of information technology in obtaining health information for consumers and in educating nurses.
LO 15.7 Summarize potential ethical issues related to the use of health care information technology.
LO 15.8 Outline future directions of informatics in nursing.

KEY TERMS

bar-code medication administration, p. 208
blog, p. 209
computer literacy, p. 211
computerized provider order entry, p. 208
decision support systems, p. 208
electronic health record, p. 209
electronic medical record, p. 209
informatics, p. 206
information literacy, p. 211
International Classification for Nursing Practice, p. 213
Internet, p. 209
listserv, p. 209
nursing informatics, p. 206
Nursing Minimum Data Set, p. 212
social media, p. 209
standardized nursing terminology, p. 212
telehealth or telemedicine, p. 207

CASE STUDY

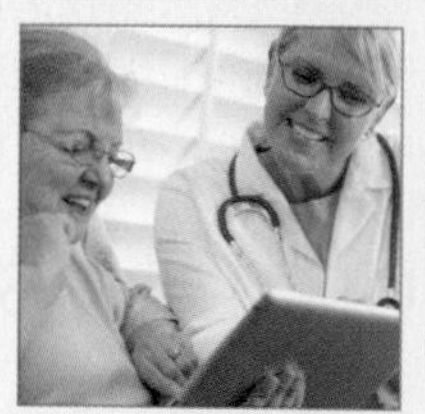

The nurse is caring for Mrs. Henkle, a patient with diabetes on an inpatient medical unit. The nurse enters Mrs. Henkle's admission history and nursing assessment into the bedside computer, checks the admission laboratory test results, and reads the patient's current orders entered by the primary care provider. The nurse plans Mrs. Henkle's care for the day on the basis of the information in the electronic health record.

Mrs. Henkle tells the nurse that a friend mentioned a great new product that will allow her to discontinue insulin. The patient looked it up on the Internet and wants to stop taking insulin and try the new product.

Refer back to this case study to answer the critical-thinking questions throughout the chapter.

There is growing recognition of the importance of informatics in health care. Nursing represents a large percentage of the workforce in U.S. health care, and it is a profession that is critical to successful widespread adoption of health care information technology (IT). If nursing can advocate, adopt, and integrate IT initiatives in practice, the positive impact will be felt beyond the practice of nursing. As the U.S. health care system considers reform, it is important that nurses are able to use the information and communication technologies that address issues of quality, cost-effectiveness, and outcomes of care.

DEFINITION OF INFORMATICS LO 15.1

Informatics is a broad academic field encompassing artificial intelligence, cognitive science, computer science, information science, and social science. *Medical informatics* refers to informatics related to health care and describes a distinct specialty in the discipline of medicine. It deals with the resources, devices, and methods required for the acquisition, storage, retrieval, and use of information in health and biomedicine. In addition to computers, informatics tools in health care include clinical guidelines, formal medical terminologies, and information and communication systems.

Nursing informatics is a specialty area of informatics that addresses the use of health information systems to support nursing practice. The American Nurses Association (ANA, 2008) states that the specialty of nursing informatics integrates nursing computer and information science for the management and communication of data, information, knowledge, and wisdom.

DATA COLLECTION

As a nurse assesses a patient, data are collected and organized as a source of information. The computerization of nursing practice data enables capture, storage, retrieval, organization, processing, and analysis of information. The information can be used to make a diagnosis, plan for care, provide nursing decision support, enhance documentation, and identify nursing care trends and costs. Systems that support data collection at the point of care can directly enhance patient care by decreasing the time spent on documentation, reducing the potential for errors, and supporting improved assessment and data communication. Computers, tablets, or pocket devices used at the bedside for documentation are examples of point-of-care technology. Patient data collected by a nurse and recorded electronically are immediately available to all members of the health care team.

! SAFE PRACTICE ALERT

Nurses must ensure the accuracy of recorded data. Documentation should occur on a timely basis. Bedside and mobile computers enable real time charting.

DATA, INFORMATION, KNOWLEDGE, AND WISDOM

Data are facts, observations, and measurements that can be used as a basis for reasoning, discussion, or calculation, but until they are organized and processed, data are meaningless. *Information* is organized and processed data that can be communicated and are meaningful and useful to the recipient. *Knowledge* is organized and processed information that can be applied to problem solving and decision making. The transformation of patient data to clinical information becomes nursing knowledge. *Wisdom* addresses the use of knowledge and experience to manage and solve problems. Wisdom is the appropriate application of knowledge. At the wisdom level, a nurse uses critical thinking to interpret and evaluate nursing knowledge. At each level of processing, some type of knowledge is produced. Figure 15-1 shows this progression.

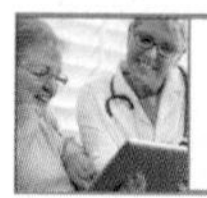

1. How is the nurse caring for Mrs. Henkle using nursing informatics?

TECHNOLOGY IN THE INFORMATION AGE LO 15.2

Nurses working surrounded by computers and mobile IT must develop skills in the use of all available technology. At the same time, it is important to recognize that the rapid advancement of IT means that the technology in use today may be entirely different tomorrow. Some facilities have computer access at every bedside, and others have mobile computers, sometimes called *workstations on wheels* (WOWs), that can be taken to each bedside (Figure 15-2). Cell phones

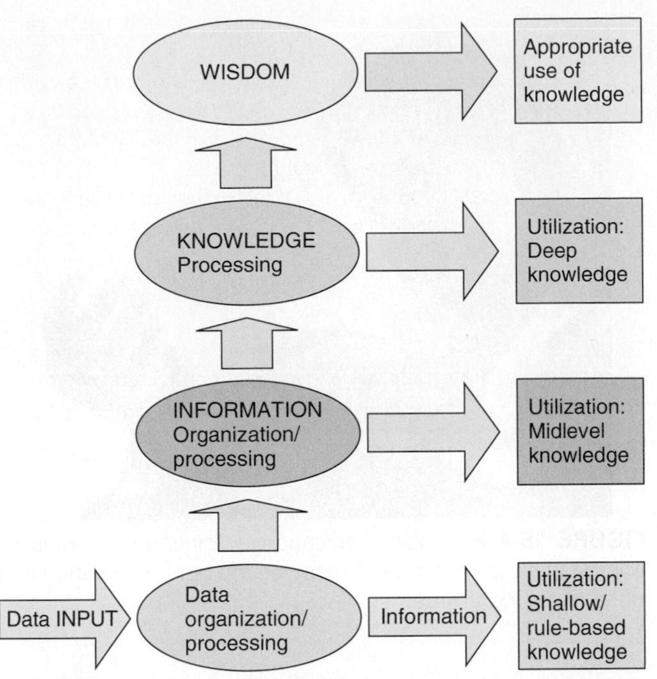

FIGURE 15-1 Data are the foundation of information, knowledge, and wisdom. (Courtesy Margaret Ross Kraft, Maywood, Ill.)

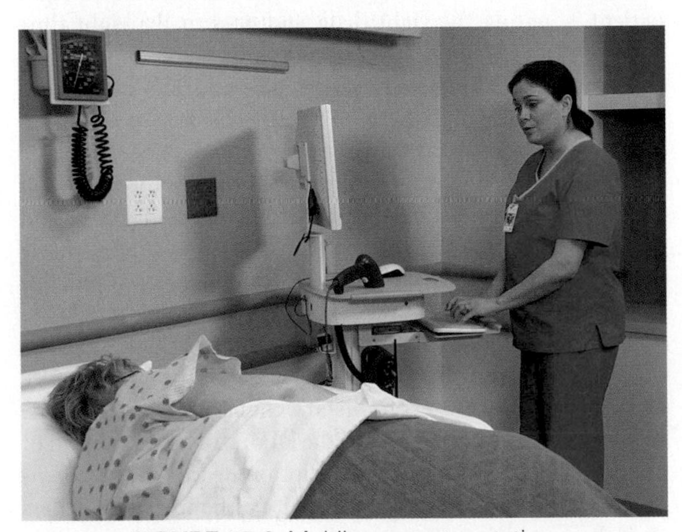

FIGURE 15-2 Mobile computer station.

have cameras, global positioning systems, and Internet connections. Pagers, iPods, fax machines, tablet computers, and personal digital assistants (PDAs) are being used in health care for communication, reference, and documentation. Nurses using technology as part of patient care need to work within facility policy and HIPAA guidelines as outlines in Chapter 11.

Many mobile devices include handwriting recognition software, some support voice recognition, and some have an internal cell phone and modem to link with other computers or networks. The technology supports bedside charting and remote charting. Nurses may use a portable device such as a smartphone or tablet computer to access reference materials, including medical information and vast amounts of drug information. Some facilities issue these devices to staff (Evidence-Based Practice and Informatics box).

EVIDENCE-BASED PRACTICE AND INFORMATICS

Use of Mobile Technology

- The 2010 Institute of Medicine report, *The Future of Nursing: Leading Change, Advancing Health,* emphasizes that nurses use technology resources that "require skills in analysis and synthesis to improve the quality and effectiveness of care" (IOM, 2010).
- The most obvious advantage of mobile technology is prevention of medication errors. As the final providers in the administration process, nurses are in a position to prevent a medication error. Mobile technology provides nursing students and nurses with instant access to safe dose, compatibility, and pharmacokinetic information that is essential for safe medication administration (Yoost, 2011).
- Among hand-held technology users, there is a significant improvement in research awareness and valuing, quality of care, job satisfaction, and reduction in barriers to research use (Doran, Straus, Haynes, et al, 2009).
- Hand-held technology assists in the transformation of assessment data, interventions, and outcome documentation into evidence-based decision making in nursing (Hardwick, Pulido, and Adelson, 2007).

Robots in operating rooms facilitate less invasive surgical procedures. Robots in pharmacies support safer medication selection. Information systems have moved from strict alphanumeric data to multimedia information that can include graphics and sound. X-rays are in digital form. **Telehealth** or **telemedicine** is the use of the Internet to link medical experts with other clinicians, allowing remote consultations with clear video images and high-fidelity links. Telehealth nursing is the transmission by a nurse of electronic data, images, or audio from a patient's bedside or home to other health providers for the purpose of providing care and improving outcomes. Patients may have telehealth hardware in their homes to provide in-home monitoring and direct reporting to their health care providers (Figure 15-3). The use of telemonitoring offers the opportunity to reduce the cost of health care while improving outcomes and patient satisfaction.

BENEFITS OF INFORMATICS LO 15.3

In health care, treatment decisions are based on information derived from data. If data are faulty or incomplete, the quality of the derived information may be poor, and decisions may be inappropriate and possibly harmful. Health care depends on information. Nursing is an information-intensive profession, and nurses must be able to work in data-rich

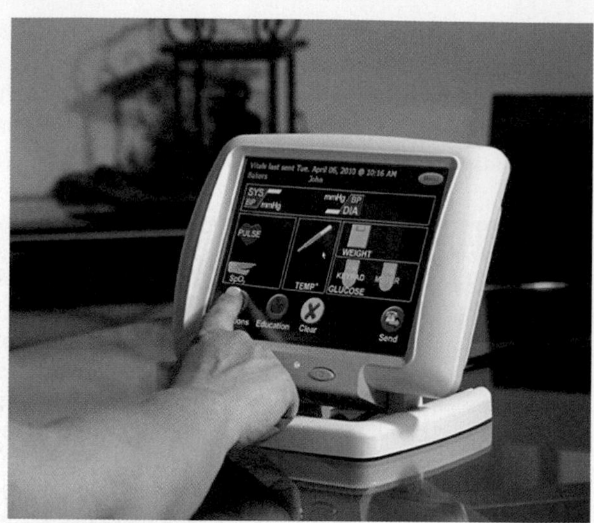

FIGURE 15-3 Telehealth can be used for in-home monitoring of patients.

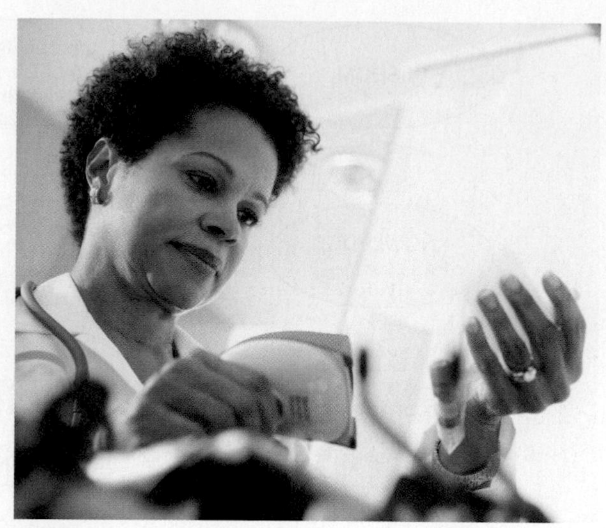

FIGURE 15-4 Bar-code medication administration helps to ensure that the right patient receives the right medication and dose at the right time.

environments. The actions nurses take depend on the information and knowledge available. The ability to quickly review laboratory results or review a complete medication profile can help the nurse to choose appropriate interventions. Long before the development of computers and their widespread use in health care, Florence Nightingale became the first nurse informaticist. She thought that accurate data must be used for nursing decisions (Saba and McCormick, 2011). She used data and statistics to address the health care issues encountered in the Crimean War.

Use of health care IT has improved organization, communication, and decision making; reduced duplicate orders, charting time, and paperwork; made medication administration safer; and enhanced information access and administrative functions. Current initiatives in health care IT are focused on admission systems that capture demographic patient data and bed availability; the electronic health record, which moves the traditional paper patient chart online; computerized provider order entry; bar-code medication administration; and e-prescribing, telehealth, personal health records, and radiofrequency identification (RFID).

! SAFE PRACTICE ALERT

Technology at the point of care can provide the right data on the right patient at the right time.

PATIENT SAFETY

IT can be used to increase patient safety. Errors are analyzed to develop strategies for prevention. Diagnostic test results are available sooner to support treatment decisions and avoid redundancy in orders. When technology such as a **bar-code medication administration** (BCMA) system is used as part of the process of medication administration, fewer errors are made. After signing into the system or scanning his or her identification (ID) badge, the nurse electronically scans the bar codes of the patient ID, the medication administration record (MAR), and the drug to ensure that the right patient is getting the right drug and dose at the right time (Figure 15-4). An alert signals a potential error, and it is the nurse's responsibility to verify all information before administration.

Computerized **decision support systems** (DSSs) include safe practice alerts and reminders that improve the quality of care. Some DSSs assist in determining a correct diagnosis and choosing an appropriate medication. Access to needed information at the point of care supports evidence-based practice initiatives.

Computerized provider order entry (CPOE) allows orders to be directly communicated to the appropriate department—diet orders to dietary, medication orders to the pharmacy, laboratory orders to the laboratory. Elimination of an intermediary for order transcription decreases the potential for errors related to the ambiguity of handwritten orders and allows quicker responses by appropriate departments. Legibility and availability of computerized documentation improve provider communication. The Agency for Healthcare Research and Quality (AHRQ) recommends CPOE as one of the safe practices for better health care. CPOE systems ensure legible orders and have the potential to reduce ordering and transcribing errors. Disadvantages of CPOE include workflow issues, provider resistance to new technology, and overdependence on technology (AHRQ, 2012).

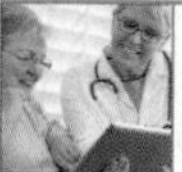

2. How can the nurse share the conversation that occurred with Mrs. Henkle about the new diabetic treatment with the primary care provider?

! SAFE PRACTICE ALERT

Medication administration requires the nurse to perform three checks—patient allergies, the order, and drug expiration—and then check the Six Rights: Right patient, Right medication, Right dose, Right time, Right route, and Right documentation.

Computerized clinical decision support systems (CDSSs) are usually paired with CPOE. When used with a CPOE system, the CDSS suggests dosages, frequencies, and routes of administration for drugs; cross-checks for drug allergies and drug-drug interactions; and may suggest laboratory tests, depending on the drugs ordered (AHRQ, 2012).

RECORD MANAGEMENT

Implementation of computerized or electronic medical records makes patient records readily available through remote access to multiple providers at the same time. This availability of patient information supports efficient delivery of effective care. The **electronic medical record** (EMR), which is the documentation of a single episode of care (i.e., outpatient visit or inpatient stay), becomes a part of the **electronic health record** (EHR), which is a longitudinal record of care. EHRs are becoming widely used for individual health care encounters and for maintaining patients' health records over long periods. As EHRs become fully implemented, they include provider order entries, progress notes for all disciplines, computerized medication profiles, access to diagnostic test results on a timely basis, DSSs, and online clinical reminders and alerts. Because nurses have access to drug formularies and the National Library of Medicine, the latest literature on a specific medical problem is readily available.

As care records are aggregated in a data storage system, the patient data can be searched for cases, trends, and outcomes that can be analyzed to determine the best evidence for practice. The ability to quickly review a patient's longitudinal data at the point of care supports the improved management of each patient. Being able to see blood pressure documented over time enables the nurse to assess the effect of an ordered medication. The longitudinal data allow the nurse to see trends in responses to specific interventions and patterns of vital signs and laboratory results. Chapter 10 provides a complete discussion of the EHR.

Another advantage of the EHR is that work lists are created on the basis of the information in the database. Nursing measures can be organized according to the time they are due or the type of task (Figure 15-5). Use of work lists helps to ensure that important patient care and medication administration are carried out at the appropriate times.

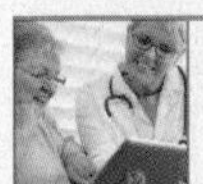

3. What can the nurse do with the information found in Mrs. Henkle's EHR?

RESEARCH ACCESS

The goal of research is knowledge. The computerization and storage of health care data provide a source of information that contributes to the knowledge base of nursing and that of other health care professions. Computer applications are available for quantitative and qualitative research designs. Data management programs can analyze data to identify trends and patterns, allowing meaningful organization of information. Comparisons of nursing care data at the nurse-patient level can initiate comparisons across patient populations, and findings can support evidence-based nursing, evidence-based staffing, and specific billing for nursing services (Welton and Sermeus, 2010). Analysis and comparison of electronically captured health data identifies evidence to support nursing practice. For example, analysis of nursing interventions necessary for care delivery on a particular unit can produce a staffing pattern based on the needs of patients.

NETWORKING

The growth of IT has created many new avenues for connecting with friends, family, and other professionals. The shared global computing network of the **Internet** provides connections with many kinds of resources that can be useful in the delivery of nursing care. Electronic access to libraries is available. E-mail has become a common means of communication. A **listserv** is a computer program that automatically sends messages to multiple e-mail addresses on a mailing list. Listservs can be used in health care to connect groups of patients with common problems or to send updated information to large groups.

Social media include online technologies such as Facebook, Twitter, and LinkedIn that allow people to communicate easily via the Internet to share information and resources. These technologies enable a potentially massive community of participants to collaborate, providing a mechanism for tapping into collective power in ways previously unachievable. Nurses should always follow confidentiality and HIPAA guidelines as outlined in Chapter 11 when using social media. A **blog** is a social medium that is usually maintained by an individual and has regular entries of commentary, descriptions of events, or other material such as graphics or videos. Most blogs are interactive, allowing visitors to leave comments and message each other. Many blogs focus on health care issues.

NURSING INFORMATICS SKILLS AND ROLES LO 15.4

Descriptions of nursing informatics competencies often focus on levels that include beginner, experienced, specialist, and innovator (Staggers, Gassert, and Curren, 2001). All levels identify specific knowledge and skills involved in using IT to enter, retrieve, and manipulate data to produce

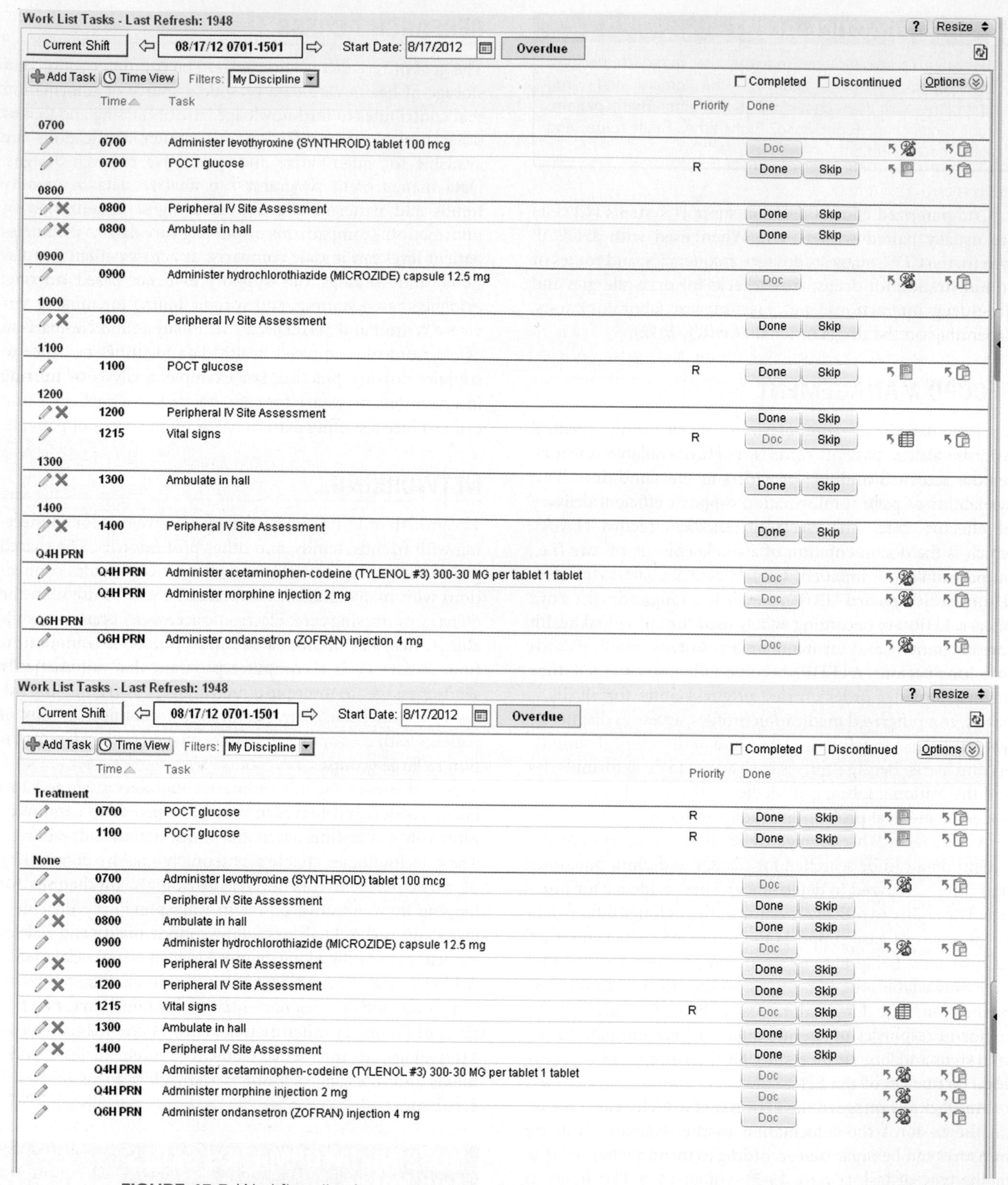

FIGURE 15-5 Workflow list from a patient's electronic health record. (Courtesy Epic Systems Corporation, Verona, Wisc., 2012.)

information for nursing practice and contribute to nursing knowledge. Beginner skills include computer, information, and web literacy; fundamental skills in information management and computer technology; and the ability to identify and collect relevant data. The nurse at the beginning level may have keyboarding skills, can document in the EHR, and look up medications and other health information on reputable Internet reference sites.

The nurse at the experienced level of informatics competencies is able to see data relationships and make judgments based on trends and patterns in data, is skilled in information management and the use of computer technology, and is able to suggest areas for IT system improvement. Examples of experienced competencies include relating data posted by others to the nursing assessment, basing the nursing process and clinical decisions on the data, and devising better ways of using data from the EHR.

The nurse at the specialist level of competency focuses on information needs for the practice of nursing; integrates and applies information science, computer science, and nursing science; and applies skills in critical thinking, data management, processing, and system development. At the specialist level of competency, the nurse may conduct research based on information trends or patient data, devise applications for computer technology in nursing, or develop new software to enhance nursing care. Nursing informatics innovators conduct research and generate theory. They develop solutions and understand the interdependence of systems, disciplines, and outcomes.

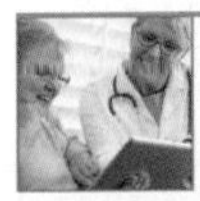

4. At what level of informatics competency is the nurse functioning? Give examples of the level from the case study.

QSEN FOCUS!

Nurses need to be proficient in navigating the EHR—documenting and planning patient care in an EHR—and diligent in seeking lifelong learning of information technology skills.

One classification system for nursing informatics competencies uses technical, utility, and leadership categories. Technical competencies pertain to the use of computers and other technological equipment and the use of a variety of software programs for word processing, spreadsheet and database development, presentation, referencing, and e-mail. Utility competencies address critical thinking and evidence-based practice applications. Nurses who have a utility competency recognize the relevance of nursing data for improving practice and can access multiple information sources for gathering evidence for clinical decision making.

Leadership competencies address the ethical and management issues related to using IT in nursing practice, education, research, and administration. Specific leadership competencies include the application of accountability, maintenance of privacy and confidentiality, and quality assurance (Herbert, 2008). Using informatics is a core competency required of all health care professions, but many nurses lack the skills they need as professionals to integrate IT seamlessly into their practice.

Nursing informatics specialists are experts who assume a variety of roles, including training others and supervising the use of information systems, designing systems particularly for use by nurses, and using data for establishing best-practice guidelines. Goals are to improve patient care and safety and establish best-care practices. After meeting the educational and experience requirements, the nurse can receive certification in nursing informatics from the Health Care Information and Management Systems Society (HIMSS) and through the American Nurses Credentialing Center (ANCC).

QSEN FOCUS!

Nurses must be involved in the design, selection, implementation, and evaluation of information technologies to support patient care.

Basic competencies include computer and information literacy. **Computer literacy** is knowledge of computers and the ability to use them efficiently. Computers are everywhere, and their applications continue to grow at an astounding rate. As health care becomes increasingly dependent on technology, the value of a nurse may be partly measured in terms of technological competency. A computer-literate nurse is able to easily learn and use new computer programs with minimal assistance. **Information literacy** is the ability to recognize when information is needed and to locate, evaluate, and effectively use the needed information (American Library Association, 2000). As the amount of available information increases exponentially, individuals must acquire the skills to select, evaluate, and use needed information.

The Technology Informatics Guiding Education Reform (TIGER) initiative (2014) identified a set of skills needed by all nurses practicing in the 21st century. The TIGER Vision Pillars include management and leadership, education, communication and collaboration, informatics design, and IT policy and culture. This skill set includes informatics competencies that range from basic computer skills to advanced-level IT and literacy competencies and expertise. TIGER's vision for the future of nursing addresses informatics and emerging technologies to provide safer, patient-centered care by using evidence and technology in practice, education, and research.

As nurses progress through levels of competency in the use of IT, many informatics roles are possible. Software capability expands as rapidly as IT hardware, and nurses are very involved in information system implementation. They may function as database managers and data analysts. Nurses are involved in the design and development of systems that offer the ability to document each element of the nursing process—assessment, diagnosis, planning, implementation, and evaluation—in an electronic format. Nurses are often responsible for informatics and health IT education.

STANDARDIZED TERMINOLOGIES LO 15.5

A **standardized nursing terminology** is a structured vocabulary that provides a common means of communication among nurses. A standardized language ensures that when a nurse talks about a specific patient problem, another nurse fully understands the problem. An example is the choice between *pressure ulcer, decubitus ulcer,* and *bedsore*. Do all nurses in all settings have a shared understanding of these labels for a patient problem?

Implementation of electronic records increases the necessity for standardized terminologies for documentation, because computers cannot make the association between different expressions meaning the same thing. The use of standardized terminologies promotes consistent documentation and allows the description and comparison of nursing care across a variety of settings, facilitating measurement of the impact of nursing interventions on patient outcomes (Lunney, Delaney, Duffy, et al, 2005).

The **Nursing Minimum Data Set** (NMDS) represents the first attempt to standardize the collection of essential nursing data. These core data, used on a regular basis by most nurses in the delivery of care across settings, provide accurate descriptions of the nursing diagnoses, nursing care, outcomes of care, and nursing resources used. Collected on an ongoing basis, the NMDS enables nurses to compare data across populations, settings, geographic areas, and time (Werley and Lang, 1988).

Implementation of a standardized nursing terminology has made a significant impact on patient outcomes. Smith and Smith (2007) showed that nurse-driven care supported by a standardized nursing terminology decreased the number of average ventilation days for all ventilator-associated pneumonia patients from 14 to 10 days. The ANA recognizes specific standardized nursing terminologies (Table 15-1) and multidisciplinary terminologies (Table 15-2) that support

TABLE 15-1 Nursing Terminologies Recognized by the American Nurses Association

TERMINOLOGY	CONTENT
NMDS: Nursing Minimum Data Set	Clinical data elements for use in all nursing settings
NMMDS: Nursing Management Minimum Data Set	Nursing administrative data elements for use in all nursing settings
CCC: Clinical Care Classification	Diagnoses, interventions, and outcomes
ICNP: International Classification of Nursing Practice	Diagnoses, interventions, and outcomes
NANDA-I: NANDA International	Nursing diagnoses
NIC: Nursing Interventions Classification	Nursing interventions
NOC: Nursing Outcomes Classification	Outcomes related to nursing care
Omaha System	Diagnoses, interventions, and outcomes for home care, public health, and community
PNDS: Perioperative Nursing Data Set	Diagnoses, interventions, and outcomes for use in the perioperative area

TABLE 15-2 Multidisciplinary Terminologies Recognized by the American Nurses Association

CODE NAME	CODE CONTENTS
ABC: Alternative Billing Codes	More than 4500 descriptions of integrative health care services, remedies, and supplies; ABC fills the gaps of traditional medical code sets
LOINC: Logical Observation Identifiers Names and Codes	A universal code system for identifying laboratory and clinical observations
SNOMED CT: Systematic Nomenclature of Medicine Clinical Terms	A coding system, controlled vocabulary, classification system, and thesaurus; designed to capture information about a patient's history, illnesses, treatment, and outcomes

nursing practice. The use of a standardized nursing terminology provides visibility to the nursing profession and documents the value of professional nursing. A patient's EHR is based on information in the NMDS. The nursing diagnoses, interventions, and outcomes use standardized nursing terminology. Each nurse reading and documenting in the EHR understands the diagnosis and can provide the interventions and measure the outcomes. Use of multidisciplinary terminologies aids health care team members in understanding each other when communicating about a patient.

The **International Classification for Nursing Practice** (ICNP), developed under the auspices of the International Council of Nurses (ICN), provides a standard that facilitates the description and comparison of nursing practice locally, regionally, nationally, and internationally. The ICNP articulates the contributions of nursing to health and health care, enhances communications, and improves the quality and continuity of health care on a global basis. The World Health Organization Family of International Classifications (WHO-FIC) accepted ICNP as a related terminology in 2008.

INFORMATION AND EDUCATION LO 15.6

The age of information has expanded the need for health literature. As nurses promote consumer responsibility for health, the Internet is increasingly used to search for information about a specific disease or medical problem. A survey (Fox and Duggan, 2013) found that 72% of Internet users searched for health information online. Of the health seekers, 77% initiated their most recent online health inquiry at a search engine, and 13% began at a health-related website. Positive and negative search results were reported. Unfortunately, only about 20% of health seekers research online reviews and the rankings of health care service providers and treatments.

As patient advocates, nurses must be prepared to teach consumers how to evaluate the online sources of information and the information provided as they promote health literacy (Patient Education and Health Literacy box). *Health literacy* "is about consumers being able to understand the medical information their caregivers give them or they find through the Internet and being able to use that information to make good decisions about their own course of care" (Schardt, 2011). Table 15-3 offers a guide to website evaluation.

PATIENT EDUCATION AND HEALTH LITERACY

Health Information Online

- Ask patients where and how they get health-related information.
- Explore with patients their use of computers and how they decide whether information obtained from the Internet is reliable, accurate, and current.
- Teach patients how to evaluate a health-related website.

TABLE 15-3 Website Evaluation Criteria

CRITERION	EVALUATION QUESTIONS
Authority	Who is the sponsor or publisher? Is this a personal page? Where does it come from? Is the author or organization listed? What are the author's credentials?
Purpose	Does the site inform? Explain? Share? Disclose? Sell? What is the intended audience?
Coverage	Are citations correct? Is there a balance of text and images?
Currency	When was the site created? How often is it updated?
Objectivity	What are the goals and objectives of the site? Is there evidence of bias? Is bias explicit or hidden?
Accuracy	Are there footnotes or links to information sources?
Verification	Can the information be found in other sources?

STANDARDS FOR INTERNET HEALTH SITES

Ethical standards and guidelines for Internet health sites are being developed and promoted by several organizations. The Health on the Net Foundation (HON) is an international initiative created in 1995 that focuses on the promotion and use of reliable online health information (HON, 2013). The Internet Healthcare Coalition, founded in 1997, was created to promote quality health resources online and to ensure that consumers and professionals are able to find reliable, high-quality information online. This organization consults with various government agencies, including the World Health Organization, the U.S. Food and Drug Administration, and the U.S. Federal Trade Commission, on efforts to promote credible online health care information and combat online health fraud (Mack, 2000).

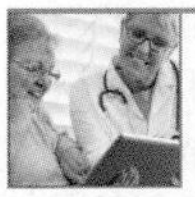

5. How should the nurse respond to Mrs. Henkle's statement about the new product? What strategy should the nurse use to educate her on how to evaluate a health care–related website?

NURSING INFORMATICS AND NURSING EDUCATION

As nurse educators work with students who have been raised in a "wired" world with widespread information access, IT has become integrated into the curriculum and become part of the educational delivery system. Distance learning opportunities are widely available for formal degree programs and continuing education. Virtual realities and simulations allow the learner to participate in immersion scenarios that help in the development of critical-thinking and decision-making skills. Online discussion boards, classrooms, and support groups, as well as social media sites, are used for educational activities. An important part of the TIGER vision is the reform of nursing education to provide the 21st-century nurse with informatics skills that enable the use of IT to provide the most knowledgeable and safe care possible.

ETHICAL, LEGAL, AND PROFESSIONAL PRACTICE CONCERNS LO 15.7

Key areas of possible ethical conflict related to IT in health care include the creation and retention of documentation, ownership of software, ownership and integrity of data, preservation of privacy and confidentiality, and prevention of computer fraud and misuse. Patients' rights must be protected. It is important that nurses know about applicable laws and regulations, policies, procedures, the ethical codes of their employers, and the ethical codes of their professional organizations.

Data security and confidentiality of patient information are major issues. Access to electronic records requires a user to have system access and verification codes as a measure of security and protection of the patient's privacy. The codes leave an electronic trail of authorized users that can be audited. The Health Insurance Portability and Accountability Act (HIPAA) of 1996 sets the standards on how security and confidentiality of health care information must be maintained. The act also sets the penalties for any breach in security of health care data. HIPAA is discussed in detail in Chapter 11.

! SAFE PRACTICE ALERT

Sign-on and password codes for access to an electronic health record system must never be shared with anyone.

COMPUTER ETHICS

The Computer Ethics Institute (CEI) was founded in 1985 to serve as a forum and resource for identifying, assessing, and responding to ethical issues associated with the advancement of information technologies and to facilitate the recognition of ethics in the development and use of computer technologies. CEI developed the Ten Commandments of Computer Ethics (Ethical, Legal, and Professional Practice box).

eHEALTH CODE OF ETHICS

The goal of the eHealth Code of Ethics, developed by Health Informatics Europe (2005), is "to ensure that people worldwide can confidently and with full understanding of known risks realize the potential of the Internet in managing their own health and the health of those in their care." The principles that provide the framework for this ethical code are candor, honesty, quality, informed consent, privacy, professionalism in online health care, responsible partnering, and accountability.

ETHICAL, LEGAL, AND PROFESSIONAL PRACTICE

Ten Commandments of Computer Ethics

1. Thou shalt not use a computer to harm other people.
2. Thou shalt not interfere with other people's computer work.
3. Thou shalt not snoop around other people's computer files.
4. Thou shalt not use a computer to steal.
5. Thou shalt not use a computer to bear false witness.
6. Thou shalt not copy or use proprietary software for which you have not paid.
7. Thou shalt not use other people's computer resources without authorization or proper compensation.
8. Thou shalt not appropriate other people's intellectual output.
9. Thou shalt think about the social consequences of the program you are writing or the system you are designing.
10. Thou shalt always use a computer in ways that ensure consideration and respect for your fellow humans.

From Computer Ethics Institute: Ten commandments of computer ethics, 1999. Retrieved from *http://cpsr.org/issues/ethics/cei/*.

THE FUTURE OF NURSING INFORMATICS LO 15.8

The nursing profession is critical to successful adoption of IT in health care. The focus of nursing informatics is not on direct patient care but on how the process of patient care can be improved and patient safety ensured. Nurses need a working knowledge of how IT can support and improve clinical processes (Sensmeier, 2009). There are challenges to advancements in IT, such as increased amount of time spent documenting, cost of equipment, protection of patient privacy, use of different EHRs in different facilities, and resistance by health care providers to new technology. However, the advantages of IT, particularly the EHR, outweigh the challenges. Nurses competent in informatics can help to overcome some of the obstacles and advocate for the use of technology in patient care.

As nursing information systems are further refined to completely encompass the work of nurses, the ability to determine the evidence of best practice will be enhanced. Practice models and care delivery systems will integrate more IT. The technology in use today will not be the technology of tomorrow. Nurses can expect a wide range of mobile technology tools that permit greater access to information, data processing, and decision support. While adopting new technology that enhances patient care and safety, it is the nurse's responsibility to continue to provide compassionate care.

National strategies for information and communication technologies extend IT investment beyond the hospital setting and physician practices to the home and community. The spread of IT supports consumer empowerment and self-management of wellness and disease. Consumers can electronically access their own health information, communicate with their health care providers, and seek needed education about health care (Weaver, Delaney, Weber, et al, 2010). Nursing must transform itself as a profession to make full use of the capabilities that information and communication technologies provide.

SUMMARY OF LEARNING OUTCOMES

LO 15.1 *Define nursing informatics:* Nursing informatics is a specialty area of informatics that addresses support of nursing practice in health information systems.

LO 15.2 *Discuss the uses of technology in health care:* Mobile workstations, bedside computers and tablets, cell phones, pagers, iPods, fax machines, and personal digital assistants are used in health care for communication, reference, and documentation. Robots are used in operating rooms and pharmacies, x-rays are in digital form, and telehealth or telemedicine is used to link medical experts with other clinicians and to provide in-home monitoring of patients.

LO 15.3 *Summarize the benefits of informatics:* The benefits include improved organization, communication, and information access; safer medication administration; reduction of duplicate orders and paperwork; better decision making; reduced charting time; and improved administrative functions.

LO 15.4 *Compare competency levels of nursing informatics:* Levels of competency in nursing informatics are beginning, experienced, specialists, and innovator, and they determine specific roles for nursing. The nurse's role in the use of informatics intensifies as the competency level increases.

LO 15.5 *Explain the importance of using standardized terminologies in electronic health records:* The use of standardized nursing terminologies supports the capture of important data and nursing information.

LO 15.6 *Implement the use of information technology in obtaining health information for consumers and in educating nurses:* As the Internet becomes a widely used source of health information, nurses need to know how to evaluate websites and direct consumers to sites that are reliable.

LO 15.7 *Summarize potential ethical issues related to the use of health care information technology:* Nurses must be aware of potential legal and ethical issues related to computer applications in health care, such as patients' rights and protection of patients' information.

LO 15.8 *Outline future directions of informatics in nursing:* Advancements in nursing informatics will enable nurses to improve patient care and safety, gather evidence of best practice, use point-of-care documentation and references, and advocate for consumer access to health care information.

Responses to the critical-thinking questions are available at *http://evolve.elsevier.com/YoostCrawford/fundamentals/.*

REVIEW QUESTIONS

1. Which descriptions are advantages of health care information technology (IT)? *(Select all that apply.)*
   - **a.** Increases health care delivery costs
   - **b.** Improves communication among providers
   - **c.** Improves administration functions
   - **d.** Increases time necessary to document care
   - **e.** Decreases the safety of providing care
2. Which description is an example of data?
   - **a.** A printout of a patient's history and physical examination
   - **b.** A patient's blood pressure and pulse rate
   - **c.** The nurse's knowledge of a disease
   - **d.** A nurse's interpretation of a change in the patient's condition
3. Which items are supported by point-of-care use of information technology? *(Select all that apply.)*
   - **a.** More accurate documentation
   - **b.** Direct access to diagnostic results
   - **c.** Confidentiality
   - **d.** Direct access to records by patients
   - **e.** Access to medication profiles
4. The hospital has implemented a new electronic medication administration record (MAR). What is true about the use of this new tool?
   - **a.** Verifies medication dosages
   - **b.** Reduces medication administration errors
   - **c.** Eliminates the need to count narcotics
   - **d.** Requires a hard copy of the MAR to be printed

5. A famous rock star has just been admitted to Unit 12A after an automobile accident. A nurse on Unit 12B who is a fan of the musician uses the electronic health record (EHR) to find out how the patient is doing. Which is true regarding the use of a patient's EHR?
   a. Only staff caring for the patient should access this record.
   b. Permission from a supervisor is needed to read this record.
   c. The patient's record can be discussed with the nurse's co-worker.
   d. The nurse can call a friend who works at the local newspaper.
6. Which activity by a unit nurse demonstrates information literacy?
   a. Researching a patient's diagnosis online
   b. Entering patient data into the electronic health record (EHR)
   c. Organizing patient data to study trends
   d. Learning a new electronic health record system
7. The nurse is assigned to administer medications to a patient on a unit that has just implemented bar-code medication administration (BCMA). Which step is proper for the nurse to follow?
   a. Open the medication packages at the nurses' station.
   b. Ask the patient to verify his or her address.
   c. Scan the nurse's ID, the patient's ID, and the code on the medication package.
   d. Ask the patient to name two patient identifiers.
8. Which statement is correct concerning the implementation of computerized provider order entry (CPOE)?
   a. The unit secretary transcribes the physician's orders into the computer.
   b. The nurse must ensure that orders go to the appropriate departments.
   c. Physician orders go directly to the appropriate department.
   d. Handwriting legibility is a major problem.
9. Which behaviors are expected of the nurse at the experienced informatics competency level? *(Select all that apply.)*
   a. Collect accurate assessment data.
   b. Conduct informatics research.
   c. Group assessment data.
   d. Document data appropriately on the electronic health record (EHR).
   e. Integrate information science, computer science, and nursing science.
10. Which description is true about the Nursing Minimum Data Set (NMDS)?
   a. An admission assessment tool
   b. A discharge summary
   c. The core nursing data for collection across all sites
   d. An organization of nursing diagnoses

Answers and rationales for the review questions are available at *http://evolve.elsevier.com/YoostCrawford/fundamentals/*.

REFERENCES

Agency for Healthcare Research and Quality (AHRQ): Patient safety primers: Computerized provider order entry, 2012. Retrieved from *http://psnet.ahrq.gov/primer.aspx?primerID=6*.

American Library Association: Information literacy competency standards for higher education, 2000. Retrieved from *www.ala.org/acrl/standards/informationliteracycompetency*.

American Nurses Association (ANA): *Scope and standards of nursing informatics practice*, Washington, D.C., 2008, Author.

Cronenwett L, Sherwood G, Barnsteiner J, et al: Quality and safety education for nurses. *Nurs Outlook*, 55(3):122-131, 2007.

Doran DM, Straus S, Haynes B, et al: Improving workplace learning at the point of care through information technology. *Comput Inform Nurs* 27(5):332-333, 2009.

Fox S, Duggan M: Health online 2013: Information triage. Retrieved from *www.pewinternet.org/Reports/2013/Health-online/Part-One/Section-2.aspx*.

Hardwick M, Pulido P, Adelson W: The use of handheld technology in nursing research and practice. *Orthop Nurs*, 26(4):251-255, 2007.

Health Informatics Europe: eHealth code of ethics, 2005. Retrieved from *www.ihealthcoalition.org/ehealth-code-of-ethics/*.

Health on the Net Foundation (HON): HONcode, 2013. Retrieved from *www.hon.ch*.

Herbert M: A national education strategy to develop nursing informatics competences. *Electr Healthc*, 7(1), 2008.

Institute of Medicine (IOM): The future of nursing: Leading change, advancing health, 2010. Retrieved from *www.iom.edu/Reports/2010/The-Future-of-Nursing-Leading-Change-Advancing-Health.aspx*.

Lunney M, Delaney C, Duffy M, et al: Advocating for standardized nursing languages in electronic health records. *J Nurs Admin*, 35(1):1-3, 2005.

Mack J: The Internet Healthcare Coalition. *J Med Internet Res*, 2(1), 2000.

Saba V, McCormick K (Eds): *Essentials of nursing informatics*, ed. 5, New York, 2011, McGraw-Hill.

Schardt C: Health information literacy meets evidence-based practice. *J Med Libr Assoc*, 99(1):1-2, 2011.

Sensmeier J: Don't overlook the role of nurses in the digital revolution, 2009. Retrieved from *www.govhealthit.com/news/dont-overlook-role-nurses-digital-revolution*.

Smith V, Smith K: Supporting evidence-based practice through the use of standardized nursing language [HIMSS webinar], 2007. Retrieved from *www.himss.org/ResourceLibrary/ResourceDetail.aspx?ItemNumber=8445.*

Staggers N, Gassert C, Curran C: A Delphi study to determine competencies for nurses at four levels of practice. *Nurs Res* 51(6):383-390, 2001.

TIGER Initiative: TIGER: Advancing the integration of health informatics to transform practice, education and consumer engagement, 2014. Retrieved from *http://thetigerinitiative.org/default.aspx.*

Weaver C, Delaney C, Weber P, Carr R: Nursing and nursing informatics: Current context to preferred future. In C Weaver, C Delaney, P Weber, R Carr (Eds): *Nursing and informatics for the 21st century*, ed. 2, Chicago, 2010, Health Information Management Systems Society, pp. 575-593.

Welton J, Sermeus W: Use of data to make nursing visible: Business and efficiency of healthcare system and clinical outcomes. In C Weaver, C Delaney, P Weber, R Carr (Eds): *Nursing and informatics for the 21st century*, ed. 2, Chicago, 2010, Health Information Management Systems Society, pp. 179-192).

Werley H, Lang N (Eds): *Identification of the nursing minimum data set*, New York, 1988, Springer.

Yoost B: Mobile technology & nursing education, practice: Instant, current information can be available to any student or nurse, 2011. Retrieved from *http://nursing.advanceweb.com/Columns/Nursing-Informatics/Mobile-Technology-Nursing-Education-Practice.aspx.*

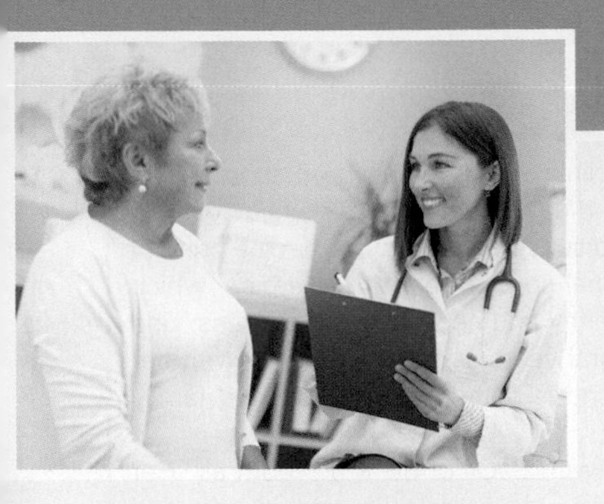

CHAPTER 16

Health and Wellness

EVOLVE WEBSITE

http://evolve.elsevier.com/YoostCrawford/fundamentals/

- Additional Evolve-Only Review Questions with Answers
- Answers and Rationales for Text Review Questions
- Answers to Critical-Thinking Questions
- Case Study with Questions
- Glossary

LEARNING OUTCOMES

Comprehension of this chapter's content will provide students with the ability to:

LO 16.1 Define the concept of *health* in an individual and a corporate context.

LO 16.2 Compare the theoretical models of health and wellness that provide the basis for nursing practice.

LO 16.3 Discuss health promotion and its relationship to wellness.

LO 16.4 Explain the three levels of preventive care and the nursing interventions associated with each.

LO 16.5 Summarize key aspects of each type of illness and the stages of illness behavior.

LO 16.6 Identify factors influencing health and their impact on illness.

KEY TERMS

acute illness, p. 226
Behavioral Risk Factor Surveillance System, p. 229
chronic illness, p. 226
exacerbation, p. 226
genetic vulnerability, p. 228
health, p. 220
Health Belief Model, p. 221
health promotion, p. 222
Health Promotion Model, p. 222
health protection, p. 222
***Healthy People 2020,* p. 224**
holistic health models, p. 222
humanistic, p. 221
illness, p. 226
Maslow's hierarchy of needs, p. 221
opportunistic infections, p. 227
preventive action, p. 221
primary prevention, p. 225
remission, p. 226
risk factor reduction, p. 224
secondary prevention, p. 225
self-actualization, p. 221
self-concept, p. 230
self-efficacy, p. 221
social determinants of health, p. 227
Stages of Illness Model, p. 227
tertiary prevention, p. 225
wellness, p. 224

CASE STUDY

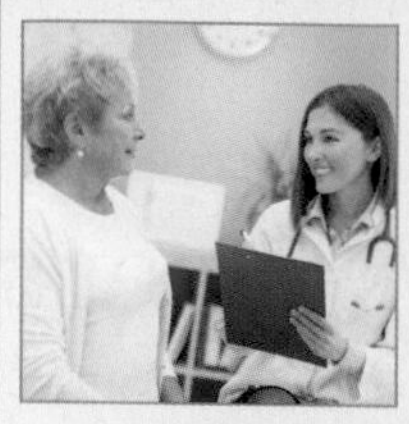

Mrs. Wolford is a 46-year-old female being evaluated at her local walk-in clinic for dyspnea on exertion (DOE). She has noticed a gradual increase in shortness of breath (SOB), fatigue, and daytime sleepiness since "gaining a few pounds" several years ago. She has no known history of illness or disease and does not have a primary care provider. Mrs. Wolford claims she is rarely ill, except for the occasional cold or seasonal allergies, which she treats using over-the-counter remedies. Mrs. Wolford is otherwise healthy and appears in no distress. She is currently unemployed, having left her former position as a teacher several years ago to stay home with her only child, who has required around-the-clock care since birth. Her husband is self-employed, and the family currently carries minimal health insurance except for their child, who is a Medicaid recipient.

Vital signs are T 37.5° C (99.5° F), P 92 and regular, R 22 and unlabored at rest, BP 170/94, with SaO_2 of 96% on room air. Her height is 5 feet 5 inches, and she weighs 200 pounds. She complains of occasional headaches, which are relieved with rest and ibuprofen. Mrs. Wolford states she has smoked one pack per day of low-tar cigarettes since the age of 17 and has two or three mixed alcoholic drinks per week, drinking almost exclusively on the weekends. She denies the use of recreational drugs but states her husband "smokes weed." She does not exercise and has a sedentary lifestyle except when assisting her child with activities of daily living. Her diet is mostly fried foods, diet soft drinks, and very few vegetables or fruits. Mrs. Wolford states she has been "eating more since quitting her job several years back" and has "a sweet tooth for candy and cakes."

Refer back to this case study to answer the critical-thinking questions throughout the chapter.

At the turn of the nineteenth century, good health and overall wellness were defined as the absence of disease; health and wellness were not viewed as multidimensional concepts. During the latter half of the twentieth century, with the discovery of antiinfective drugs and the rapid growth of the biomedical industry, disease was no longer the primary focus for defining a person's health status.

In the twenty-first century, the concept of health has evolved into a multifaceted model focused on the need to maintain individual health and prevent chronic disease. Current news headlines bombard the general public with topics ranging from the rise in childhood obesity to the increase of smoking among adolescents to the comparable rates in men and women of chronic conditions such as cardiovascular disease, chronic obstructive pulmonary disease (COPD), and stroke. Because noncommunicable diseases claim the lives of three of five people worldwide, the United Nations General Assembly convened a high-level meeting in September 2011 to launch a global campaign for their prevention and control (UN, 2011).

There has never been a more important time to focus on health and wellness in our society. The professional nurse is poised to navigate the challenges of promoting health and wellness among patients by helping them achieve and maintain the highest level of physiologic functioning and mental well-being possible. Likewise, nurses who understand how individuals react to a real or perceived illness in themselves or their loved ones have the advantage of an experiential and scientifically based education to assist in achieving the optimal level of functioning.

THE CONCEPT OF HEALTH LO 16.1

Capturing the total meaning of health and wellness for all people in a universal context is a challenging task. However, the World Health Organization (WHO, 1948) offers a definition for **health**: "a state of complete physical, mental, and social well-being and not merely the absence of disease or infirmity" (p. 100). The word *health* has several meanings. Individuals define health in terms of their own values, experiences, and ways of living. Organizations and businesses define health in the context of their goals and objectives. Familiar uses of the term *health* in the names of government organizations and businesses include World Health Organization (WHO), Occupational Safety and Health Administration (OSHA), National Institutes of Health (NIH), and health maintenance organization (HMO). *Health* is understood in the context of the name of the organization, but the value each organization, industry, or government office assigns to the meaning of the word varies.

Nurses must balance the requirements of the health care industry in which they are employed with the needs of the individuals for whom they care. Sometimes, this can be extremely challenging. Nurses are responsible for helping patients reach their optimal levels of physiologic and mental health, but they also must provide health care in a system that requires cost containment and fiscal responsibility. This can place nurses at ethical odds as they seek to meet the perceived health care needs of individuals and remain sensitive to the fiscal limits of their employers. Addressing the fiscal challenges of health care in the twenty-first century while adequately meeting the needs of patients requires creativity and the ability to help individuals identify and achieve their wellness goals.

HEALTH MODELS LO 16.2

Health models describe the relationship between health and wellness. These models provide a foundation for defining optimal physiologic and mental status. Patients' beliefs, values, and attitudes about health and wellness are based on a complex series of experiences that can have positive and negative effects on their health status. Several health models have been developed to guide practice using the nursing process.

BASIC HUMAN NEEDS MODEL

Maslow's hierarchy of needs describes the relationships between the basic requirements for survival and the desires that drive personal growth and development. The model is most often presented as a pyramid consisting of five levels (see Chapter 1, Figure 1-6). The lowest level is related to physiologic needs, and the uppermost level is associated with self-actualization needs, specifically those related to purpose and identity. According to this model, deficiency needs must be met first. This means that until basic physiologic requirements are achieved, attaining the higher levels of the pyramid will not be a priority. **Self-actualization** is considered the highest level of optimal functioning and involves the integration of cognitive ability, compassion, acceptance of self, and autonomy. In later years, Maslow described a level above self-actualization called *self-transcendence.* He refers to self-transcendence as a peak experience, in which analysis of reality or thought changes a person's view of the world and his or her position in the greater structure of life.

In nursing, the hierarchy of needs model implies that basic physiologic needs are more immediate and therefore of greater importance in terms of survival than higher-level needs. Maslow's hierarchy of needs model supplies a **humanistic** approach (i.e., promotion of human welfare) to health and wellness. Nurses apply this model when developing interventions focused on preventive care and patient education. A humanistic approach to health care focuses on strengths of individuals rather than weaknesses or illness (i.e., physiologic disease or mental disorder) (Maslow, 1954).

Nurses should also consider that applying a fixed hierarchical order is not always the most accurate method for predicting patient behavior or actions concerning optimal health. Areas of need categorized above basic physiologic function, such as self-esteem and love, often override essential physiologic needs when a patient is confronted with certain circumstances. For example, nurses encounter a variety of approaches to death and dying when patients are faced with end-of-life issues. Nutrition and fluid needs may not be as much of a priority to the dying as the need for dignity, spiritual guidance, or comfort from loved ones. Nurses regularly witness emotional and self-esteem issues that outweigh physiologic needs. Patients with life-threatening conditions related to anorexia nervosa frequently refuse medical therapies due to issues of self-esteem or lack thereof, which nurses find particularly challenging. A nurse should never assume that one patient's needs are the same as those of another patient with a similar health condition or that a patient's choices follow a hierarchal model of care. Nursing care aimed at the individual's specific level of need during the current health care encounter is the most effective method for prioritizing patient care using Maslow's hierarchy of needs model.

HEALTH BELIEF MODEL

The **Health Belief Model** (HBM) was developed by psychologists Hochbaum, Rosenstock, and Kegels (Rosenstock, 1974). It explores how patients' attitudes and beliefs predict health behavior.

The model has been adapted and reorganized since its original inception. The latest addition to the construct, self-efficacy, was added in 1988. **Self-efficacy** is defined as the belief in one's ability to perform a task (Bandura, 1992). When applied to the nursing process, the HBM is used as a measure for determining the patient's readiness and motivation to act.

There are three primary components to the model that seek to predict how likely individuals are to change their health care behaviors. The first is an individual's perception of susceptibility to illness; for example, a patient with a family history of colon cancer may have several first-degree relatives who have been diagnosed and treated for the disease. The second component is the individual's perception about the seriousness of the illness. If the person does not perceive the need for periodic colonoscopy screenings or does not attempt to lose weight despite warnings that obese people have a higher incidence of colon cancer, the threat of the disease appears to be minimized. The third component is the probability that the individual will act to prevent avoidable health risks. **Preventive action** involves lifestyle change and information gathering about a health topic that leads to a change in behavior.

In the three primary components of the HBM, six main constructs influence an individual's decision to take action about disease prevention, screening, and controlling illness. The model suggests that individuals are motivated to take action if they have certain beliefs or experiences such as the following:

- They are susceptible to the condition (i.e., perceived susceptibility).
- The condition has serious consequences (i.e., perceived severity).
- Taking action would reduce the susceptibility or severity of the condition (i.e., perceived benefit).
- The costs of taking action (i.e., perceived barriers) are outweighed by the benefits.
- They are exposed to factors that prompt action, such as media campaigns, postcard reminders, and advice from others (i.e., cues to action).
- They have confidence in their ability to perform an action (i.e., perceived self-efficacy).

Together, the six constructs of the HBM provide a useful framework for implementing the nursing process (Table 16-1). Nurses can use measures in the model to assess

TABLE 16-1 Health Belief Model

CONCEPT	DEFINITION	CHANGE STRATEGIES
Perceived susceptibility	Beliefs about the chances of getting a condition or disease	Define the populations at risk. Tailor risk information to the individual's characteristics or behaviors. Help the individual develop an accurate perception of his or her own risk.
Perceived severity	Beliefs about the seriousness of a condition and its consequences	Specify the consequences of a condition, and recommend action or intervention.
Perceived benefits	Beliefs about the effectiveness of taking action to reduce risk or seriousness	Explain how, where, and when to take action and describe likely positive results.
Perceived barriers	Beliefs about the material and psychological costs of taking action	Offer reassurance, incentives, and assistance; correct misinformation or allegations.
Cues to action	Factors that activate readiness to change	Provide how-to information, promote awareness, and employ reminder systems.
Self-efficacy	Confidence in one's ability to take action	Provide training and guidance in performing action. Use progressive goal setting. Give verbal reinforcement. Demonstrate desired behaviors.

Adapted from National Cancer Institute: *Theory at a glance: A guide for health promotion practice,* ed. 2, Washington, D.C., 2005, U.S. Department of Health and Human Services, National Institutes of Health.

the value of short- and long-term behavioral change strategies designed for optimizing patients' health and wellness status.

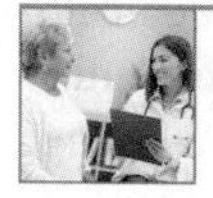

1. Which two of the three primary components of the Health Belief Model did Mrs. Wolford exhibit by coming to the walk-in clinic for evaluation of her dyspnea on exertion?

HEALTH PROMOTION MODEL

The **Health Promotion Model** (HPM) developed by Pender and colleagues (Pender, Murdaugh, and Parsons, 2011) defines health as a positive, dynamic state of well-being rather than the absence of disease in the physiologic state. The model relies on the premise that a multidimensional interaction exists between an individual and the environment, and health promotion consists of behaviors directed at improving the individual's level of well-being.

The model focuses on three areas: (1) individual characteristics and experiences, (2) behavior-specific knowledge and affect, and (3) behavioral outcomes. The concepts that define the model are health promotion and health protection. **Health promotion** is behavior motivated by the desire to increase well-being and optimize health status. **Health protection** includes intentional behaviors aimed at circumventing illness, detecting it early, and maintaining the best possible level of mental and physiologic function within the boundaries of illness (Pender, Murdaugh, and Parsons, 2011). The variables in the HPM promote desired health outcomes as determined by an individual's motivation to achieve a better quality of life and improve functional capacity. Patients may seek nursing care for illness or preventive health maintenance. Through use of the nursing process, nurses can educate patients about acute, chronic, and preventive health care interventions (Figure 16-1) (Pender, Murdaugh, and Parsons, 2011).

HOLISTIC HEALTH MODELS

Holistic health models in nursing care are based on the philosophy that a synergistic relationship exists between the body and the environment. Holistic care is an approach to applying healing therapies. Holistic models focus on the interrelatedness of body and mind. Incorporating features of spirituality, emotional security, and environment into natural, holistic care supports the premise that the body knows how to heal itself if given the proper support. When applied to the nursing process, holistic health models strive to include the patient as an active participant in the healing process rather than a passive receiver of therapeutic interventions.

Nurses participate in holistic care through the use of natural healing remedies and complementary interventions. These include the use of art and guided imagery, therapeutic touch, music therapy, relaxation techniques, and reminiscence. Eastern holistic therapists have been using techniques such as acupuncture, yoga, and tai chi for thousands of years as methods of healing and, more recently, in conjunction with modern allopathic medical therapies.

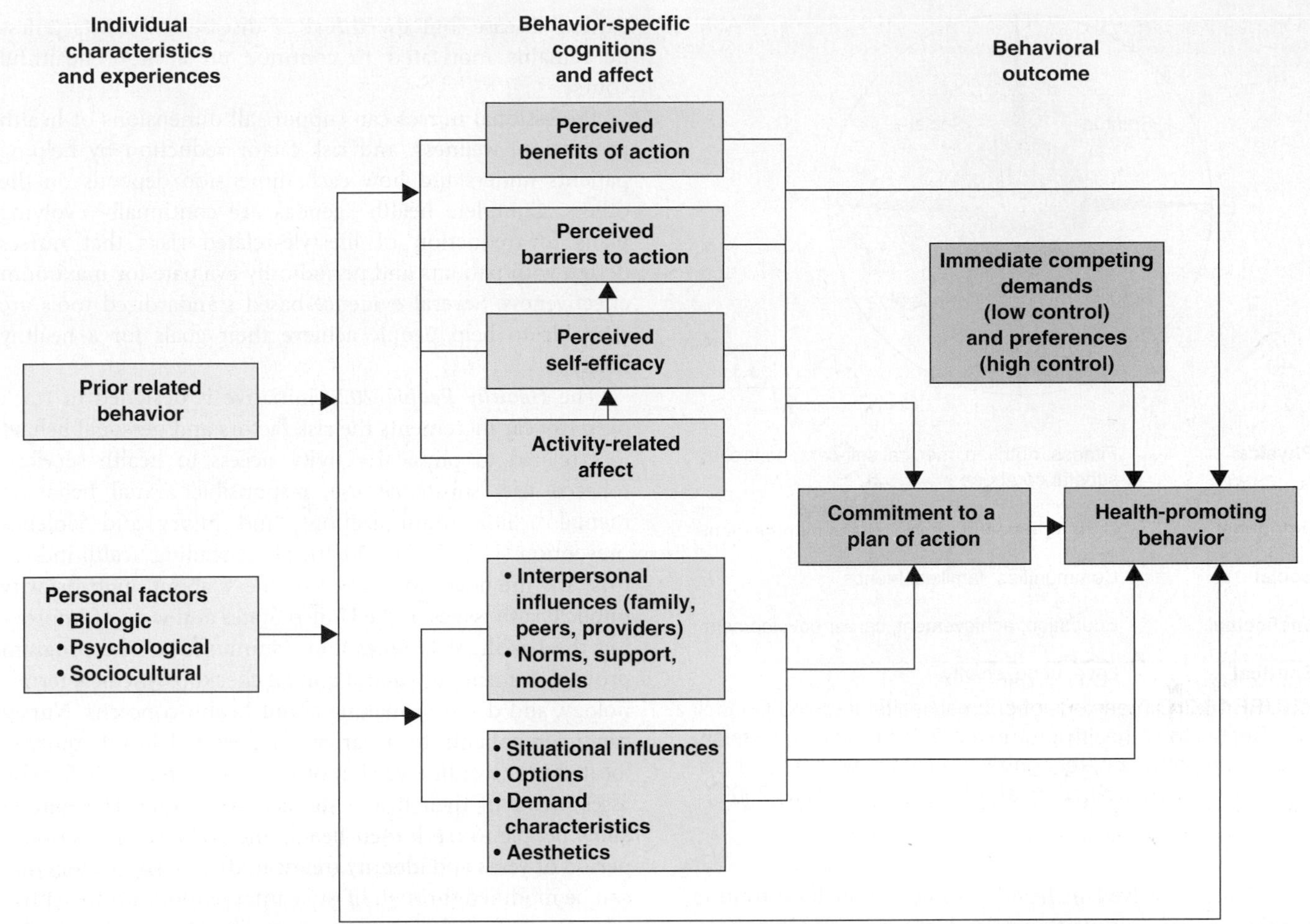

FIGURE 16-1 The Pender Health Promotion Model. (From Pender NJ, Murdaugh CL, Parsons MA: *Health promotion in nursing practice*, ed. 6, Upper Saddle River, N.J., 2011, Prentice Hall.)

The holistic model provides nurses with strategies to help patients learn how to manage illness and optimal health. Guided imagery and therapeutic communication are used for patients undergoing chemotherapy and radiation therapy to help relieve pain and to discuss fear related to cancer outcomes. Relaxation and breathing techniques are used for patients in wound care settings to focus attention away from painful dressing changes and wound debridement while supporting the need to improve oxygenation to sensitive tissues (Van Kuiken, 2004).

Holistic nursing practice has rapidly expanded to meet the growing consumer demand for alternative and complementary interventions. Consumers of health services have become more familiar with alternative care through the Internet, and they have sought alternatives because of increasing health care costs and expectations of management of their own care. Holistic nursing interventions are more readily recognized and accepted by patients because mind-body-spirit therapies are emerging as proven, feasible options in contemporary medical treatment.

HEALTH PROMOTION AND WELLNESS LO 16.3

Health promotion and wellness are increasingly emphasized in health care visits and outcome planning for chronic disease. Rising health care costs have increased government and consumer demands to decrease the incidence of disease and minimize risk factors that predispose to illness. Concepts of health promotion, wellness, and risk reduction influence individual motivation for setting and achieving health goals.

HEALTH PROMOTION

Health promotion has been defined as "the art and science of helping people discover the synergies between their core passions and optimal health and become motivated to strive for optimal health" (O'Donnell, 2009, p. 5). Optimal health implies a balance of physical, emotional, social, spiritual, and intellectual well-being (Figure 16-2).

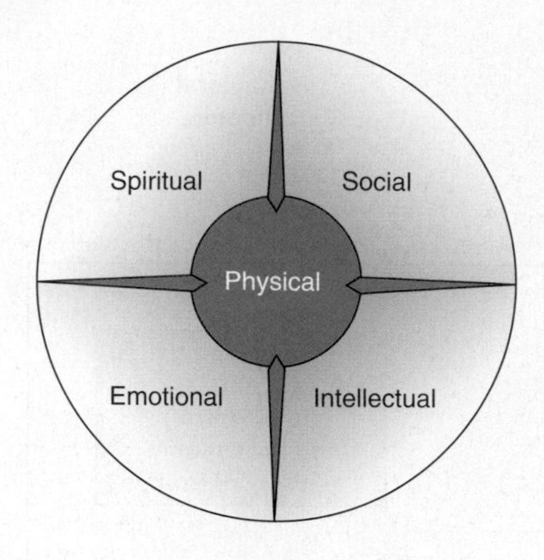

Physical	Fitness, nutrition, medical self-care, control of substance abuse
Emotional	Care for emotional crisis, stress management
Social	Communities, families, friends
Intellectual	Education, achievement, career development
Spiritual	Love, hope, charity

FIGURE 16-2 Dimensions of optimal health. (From O'Donnell MP: Definition of health promotion 2.0: Embracing passion, enhancing motivation, recognizing dynamic balance, and creating opportunities, *Am J Health Promotion* 24(1):iv, 2009.)

Activities involved in health promotion include routine exercise, meeting nutritional and vitamin requirements, maintaining a body mass index within range for weight and height, good sleep habits, and stress reduction. Health promotion activities are effective when the individual is consistently motivated and committed to lifestyle changes that support positive health behaviors.

WELLNESS

Wellness is a process of self-care achieved by making choices leading to a healthy life. Wellness knowledge empowers a person to become more aware of bodily needs and how to meet those needs. Individuals seeking wellness need to take environmental, occupational, intellectual, spiritual, emotional, physical, and social lifestyle choices into consideration.

Risk factor reduction is step-by-step improvement of individual health factors. These combined improvements lower the likelihood of developing a disease. For example, an overweight, sedentary middle-aged smoker with a family history of cardiac disease has noticed a steady rise in resting blood pressure over a 3- to 4-year period. The patient is concerned about his slightly elevated blood pressure and begins walking 20 to 30 minutes in the evenings with his wife and reduces his pack-a-day cigarette habit to 10 cigarettes per day. He has taken the first steps in reducing risk factors for cardiac disease, but the threat of disease still exists unless he remains motivated to continue on a more healthful course.

Professional nurses can support all dimensions of health promotion, wellness, and risk factor reduction by helping patients understand how each dimension depends on the others. Complete health agendas are continually evolving plans for reduction of lifestyle-related risks that nurses design with patients and periodically evaluate for maximum effectiveness. Several evidence-based standardized tools are available to help people achieve their goals for a healthy lifestyle.

The ***Healthy People 2020*** initiative is designed to track over 10-year increments the risk factors and personal behaviors related to physical activity, access to health services, tobacco use, substance use, responsible sexual behavior, mental health, immunizations, and injury and violence prevention (U.S. DHHS, 2010). These leading health indicators are intended to raise awareness about high-priority public health issues in the United States and ways of improving the health of families and communities. The program provides information about annual checkups, medical terminology, and decision making about health concerns. Nurses can refer patients to a variety of personal health quizzes, located in the online version of *Healthy People 2020,* for risk assessments of their health status and lifestyle. The quizzes allow people to track their health and wellness status over a period of years and identify trends in disease risk factors that can be modified through lifestyle interventions or preventive measures before the disease occurs. The *Healthy People 2020* initiative helps nurses provide educational materials for individuals, families, and communities, enabling them to lead healthier lifestyles and to make permanent changes in wellness habits.

Additional methods nurses can use to identify specific demographic areas for health and wellness promotion activities are found in the U.S. health agency links for state departments of public health. International information is available from the United Nations WHO website. Links of interest to nurses include hospital mortality rates, disease prevalence, epidemiology statistics, and behavioral risk factor analysis (Patient Education and Health Literacy box). Nursing goals for all individuals and their families seeking preventive care are improvement of quality of life through positive lifestyle choices and taking responsibility for health and wellness.

LEVELS OF PREVENTION LO 16.4

Illness and disease prevention involves activities and interventions that delay or prevent clinical manifestations, complications, and death. Leavell and Clark (1965) identified health-related measures as primary, secondary, and tertiary levels of preventive care from a public health perspective. Signs or symptoms to be prevented depend on the stage of health or disease of individuals receiving preventive care.

PATIENT EDUCATION AND HEALTH LITERACY

Web Links to Health Promotion and Statistics Data

Cardiac Health
- *www.heart.org/HEARTORG*
- *www.nlm.nih.gov/medlineplus/heartdiseases.html*

Neurologic Care
- *www.nlm.nih.gov/medlineplus/neurologicdiseases.html*
- *www.ninds.nih.gov*
- *www.nlm.nih.gov/medlineplus/stroke.html*

Pulmonary Health
- *www.nhlbi.nih.gov/health/public/lung/index.htmwww.lungusa.org*

Cancer Prevention
- *www.cancer.org*
- *www.cancer.gov*
- *www.cancer.gov/cancertopics*

General Topics for Health and Wellness
- *www.nhlbi.nih.gov*
- *www.nih.gov*
- *http://nihseniorhealth.gov*
- *www.who.int/topics/en*

PRIMARY PREVENTION

Primary prevention is instituted before disease becomes established by removing the causes or increasing resistance. The goal of intervention during this phase is to modify risk factors to avoid the onset of disease and prevent pathologic processes from occurring (Leavell and Clark, 1965). Health promotion and specific protection strategies are appropriate methods of primary prevention nurses can use for patients. Many health-promoting activities are nonmedical, such as lifestyle changes, nutrition improvement, and environmental alterations. They contribute to the prevention of many diseases and enhance patients' overall vigor and health.

Specific protection strategies are undertaken when health promotion efforts are unsuccessful or inappropriate. The objective is to address a specific disease or potential injury. Examples include the use of seatbelts and airbags in automobiles, helmet use when riding bicycles or motorcycles, and the occupational use of mechanical devices when lifting heavy objects. Immunizations against specific diseases, such as human papillomavirus infection or pneumonia, are also types of primary prevention.

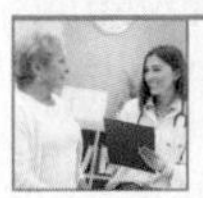

2. List three or four risk factors identified in Mrs. Wolford's health history and physical assessment that the nurse should address during this or subsequent clinic visits. Place an asterisk next to preventable lifestyle-related risk factors that Mrs. Wolford can change with mutually agreed-on interventions.

SECONDARY PREVENTION

Secondary prevention is undertaken in cases of latent (hidden) disease. Although the patient may be asymptomatic, the disease process can be detected by medical tests. Secondary prevention may be directed at individuals who are at risk for complications. The goal for health intervention during this phase is early detection and diagnosis of health problems before patients exhibit symptoms of disease (Leavell and Clark, 1965).

Screening tests may be used to assess for latent disease in vulnerable populations. Although screening examinations do not prevent disease or the cause of disease, they may influence progression to the symptomatic phase. Examples of screening tests used as secondary prevention strategies include the purified protein derivative (PPD) skin test for tuberculosis, fecal occult blood test for colorectal cancer, and mammograms for breast cancer. Nursing care implemented as secondary prevention occurs wherever nurses interact with patients, including in acute care or home care settings and during community health care functions. While implementing secondary prevention measures, nurses can provide preventive health education, which is considered a primary prevention effort.

TERTIARY PREVENTION

Tertiary prevention, also known as the treatment or rehabilitation stage of preventive care, is implemented when a condition or illness is permanent and irreversible. The aim of care is to reduce the number and impact of complications and disabilities resulting from a disease or medical condition. Interventions are intended to reduce suffering caused by poor health and assist the patients in adjusting to incurable conditions.

QSEN FOCUS!

Patient-centered care plans for addressing tertiary prevention should be developed in collaboration with patients, families, and other health care providers to ensure sensitivity to patient needs and to coordinate care.

Nursing care is focused on rehabilitation efforts in the tertiary stage of prevention. Outcomes are evaluated on the basis of patient responses. The goal is to help patients attain the highest level of physical and mental health achievable within the parameters of impairment caused by disease or disability. The professional nurse assumes a leadership role in coordinating all members of the patient's health care team with collaborative efforts to maximize health outcomes (Collaboration and Delegation box). Collaborative efforts are a necessary function of tertiary prevention because the patient often has health needs encompassing numerous health

COLLABORATION AND DELEGATION

Collaboration in Preventive Care

- Prevention is not solely the responsibility of the nurse; it involves active participation by the individual and the combined services of practitioners in a spectrum of health care disciplines as varied as nutrition, physical therapy, exercise physiology, and pharmacy.
- Collaborative health care partnerships are designed to deliver well-balanced care to the patient as a whole, rather than rendering fragmented care involving a single element of a disease process.
- Collaborative preventive care can be mandated in the form of health care legislation, with rates for reimbursement of practitioners determined by the individual provider's ability to collaborate and develop innovative methods for delivering high-quality, cost-effective health care services.
- The role of the professional nurse is to collaborate and communicate health education to the patient and family, care provider, or surrogate. Patient education responsibilities are not delegated to assistive personnel or other members of the health care team and are considered a cornerstone of nursing care.
- More information about collaborative efforts in preventive health care services that are patient centered and value driven is available at *www.icsi.org.*

disciplines that might not have been involved in the initial stage of illness.

ILLNESS LO 16.5

Illness is a state of health characterized by decreased or impaired abilities to engage in physical or mental functioning that was previously experienced (Segen, 2006). People respond to illness in a variety of subjective and objective ways. Response to illness is determined by an individual's emotional and cognitive development and by the physiologic response to stress experienced by the body. For example, pneumonia is an infectious disease that is highly curable when treated promptly and with patient compliance throughout therapy. One person with pneumonia identifies alterations in health status by the symptoms of illness associated with decreased function (e.g., fever, malaise, cough), seeks treatment, and has a positive physiologic response, maintaining usual daily activities. Another person may ignore or disregard physiologic alterations in health, with the possible result of increasing the duration of the illness, the length of treatment, and the severity of impairment. Perception of illness and the experience of illness go beyond the physical dimension, and the nurse must recognize that a patient's illness is not necessarily synonymous with disease status.

Illness can be categorized as acute or chronic depending on the clinical course and prognosis of disease. Both acute and chronic illnesses can be lethal or cause permanent disability in the host organism.

ACUTE ILLNESS

Acute illness is typically characterized by an abrupt onset and short duration (<6 months). Clinical manifestations of acute illness appear quickly. They may be severe or lethal, or they may soon resolve because they respond to treatment or are self-limiting. The physiologic and psychological consequences of an acute illness can affect a patient's immediate functional ability. Residual effects of acute illness may last beyond the course of the disease itself.

CHRONIC ILLNESS

Chronic illness is of greater concern than communicable diseases in many areas of the world, including some developing countries. This focus on chronic illness results from factors such as people living longer; improved health care and medications; high-fat, high-sugar diets and sedentary lifestyles that contribute to obesity; and substance abuse, including tobacco, alcohol, and illegal drugs.

Chronic illness is characterized by a loss or abnormality of body function that lasts longer than 6 months and requires ongoing long-term care. Chronic health conditions may be controlled with lifestyle management or drug therapy, but they are considered to be irreversible. The ability to carry out activities of daily living varies from person to person, depending on progression of the disease process. Chronic illness may be characterized by periods of wellness (**remission**) and **exacerbation** (worsening) of clinical manifestations, which can be life-threatening. Individuals learn to adjust their lifestyles accordingly. The drug regimen, laboratory tests, health care provider visits, and changes in nutritional intake often interfere with the lifestyle the chronically ill individual led before disease onset.

Nurses play a pivotal role in providing care, support, and education for people with chronic illness. Many individuals living with the burden of chronic disease initially find the daily disease management overwhelming. Nurses can help patients establish a daily routine of care by educating them about how to manage their care and the symptoms associated with the condition, including emergency or life-threatening situations. Emphasis is on improving quality of life through preventive behaviors. The attitude of being a victim, suffering with, or being afflicted by a chronic illness is viewed by nurses as a counterproductive behavior that needs positive intervention. Nurses can assist patients with strategies that help them cope with their chronic conditions and associated feelings of anger, frustration, and depression. Encouragement and positive support from a professional nurse can help individuals gain control over the alternating periods of health and illness and improve their quality of life.

ILLNESS BEHAVIORS

Social and environmental factors are important components of health and illness. Recognition that the health of an individual is more than just a biologic process related to physiologic function has increased awareness about the sociologic dimension of health that influences illness behaviors.

Several stages of illness behavior have been identified by medical sociologists to describe how people monitor their physical well-being, label and interpret their symptoms, take curative actions, and enter the health care system (Mechanic, 1995). People react to illness in a variety of ways based on history, family upbringing, personal values, community constraints, and cultural norms (Mechanic, 1995).

For the purpose of providing nursing care, Suchman's **Stages of Illness Model** (1965) best describes illness behavior and how individuals arrive at the coping mechanisms necessary for the management of disease conditions. According to the model, the process of being ill is composed of five components—or stages—of the illness experience. Each stage is characterized by certain decisions, behaviors, and end points comparable to parts of the nursing process.

During stage I (Symptom experience) of Suchman's model, a clinical manifestation of disease is experienced, and the person acknowledges that something is wrong and seeks a cure. The outcome of stage I is that the person accepts the reality of symptoms and decides to take action in seeking care.

During stage II (Assumption of the sick role), the person decides that the illness is genuine and that care is necessary. This stage gives an individual permission to act sick and to be excused temporarily from typical social and personal obligations. The results of this stage are either acceptance of the sick role or rejection of its necessity.

In stage III (Medical care contact), professional advice from health care providers is sought by the individual. A professional health care provider identifies and validates the illness and legitimizes the sick role. During this stage, the condition still may be denied, or the patient may seek additional medical care or may accept the adverse condition, the medical diagnostic authority, and the plan for treatment.

During stage IV (Dependent patient role), the person, who is designated as a patient, usually undergoes treatment. During this stage, patients often feel dependent on others and may experience ambivalent or fearful thoughts that cause them to reject treatment, the advice of health care providers, and the illness. More often, care is accepted and administered to an ambivalent patient. In this stage, the sick individual has a significant need to be educated and provided with emotional support.

During stage V (Perceived recovery), the patient abandons the sick role and resumes usual tasks and roles to the greatest degree possible. Some people do not willingly give up the sick role; they begin to view themselves as chronically ill, or they malinger in the health care setting, acting sick for secondary gain. Patients with permanent disabilities may require therapy to assist them in making adjustments necessary for performing activities of daily living (ADLs) (Suchman, 1965).

FACTORS INFLUENCING HEALTH AND THE IMPACT OF ILLNESS LO 16.6

Identifying variables that affect health and wellness is a key component in guiding health promotion activities and preventive behaviors. The variables are often referred to as **social determinants of health**, and they are affected by resource distribution throughout the world. The value a patient assigns to a real or perceived health risk can influence health beliefs, behaviors, and practices that will ultimately determine a positive or negative health outcome. Understanding the effects of these factors affords the nurse an opportunity to initiate the steps of the nursing process to plan and implement individualized care.

AGE

The chronologic age of an individual is a strong indicator of susceptibility to disease or disabling conditions. Assessment of the patient begins with risk factors that take into account the person's age and the associated level of immune system function. The very young, especially neonates and infants born prematurely, are more susceptible to infections because of the immaturity of their immune systems. Likewise, older adults have decreased immune system function as a result of the aging process. Older patients are at risk for **opportunistic infections** caused by harmless organisms that become pathogenic and illness from the spread of community-acquired disease. Complications from comorbidities of chronic disease may also increase in the aged population.

Nurses need to educate the parents of newborns, infants, children, and adolescents about the importance of regular, age-appropriate checkups and screening examinations. Young adults, adults, and older adults should be instructed to undergo age-appropriate screening examinations, schedule regular health care provider visits, and receive recommended immunizations to promote wellness and prevent illness (Diversity Considerations box). A schedule of immunizations *(www.cdc.gov/vaccines/schedules/index.html)* has been provided by the Centers for Disease Control (CDC), and the U.S. Department of Health and Human Services (DHHS) provides links to health screening and disease prevention sites (*www.hhs.gov/diseases/index.shtml#screenings*). Nurses should encourage adults of all ages to act as role models for good health and to promote wellness behaviors. Access to peer-reviewed research on age-related preventive services and best-practice guidelines can be found at *http://healthyamericans.org*.

GENDER

Gender-related risk factors for disease are assessed according to the characteristics of each disease. Nurses in primary and acute care settings are often the first health care providers to approach individuals about gender-specific health and wellness issues. Preventive screening examinations take into

DIVERSITY CONSIDERATIONS

Life Span

- Parents need to have scientific, evidence-based information about immunizations and their consequences before choosing to accept or reject immunizations for their children. The parent's ability to make an informed decision is the primary goal for nurses educating people about childhood immunizations.
- The cost of drug therapy is often a serious financial concern and stressor for older adults on fixed incomes who are living with chronic disease.

Gender

- Although the risk for breast cancer in men is low compared with the risk for women, all men past puberty should be taught and encouraged to perform breast self-examinations for cancer. This is particularly important if there is a family history of malignancies.
- Genital human papillomavirus (HPV) testing is recommended for all women who are sexually active. Although there are no definitive tests for the 40 strains of HPV that cause infection in humans, tests for HPV strains that cause cervical cancer are available and are performed at the same time as the Pap test (CDC, 2012).

Disability

- Children born with genetic or chromosomal disorders, such as cystic fibrosis, Down syndrome (also called trisomy 21), and sickle cell disease, are at increased risk for opportunistic infections and communicable diseases because of the comorbidities associated with the underlying conditions (Baum, Nash, Foster, et al, 2008).
- Health and wellness guidelines are being expanded to accommodate children and older adults with special needs because they are outliving previous life expectancies as a result of tailored drug therapies and biotechnology advances.

Morphology

- Screening for metabolic syndrome, a precursor of chronic disease, and preventive interventions are aimed at young and middle-aged adults. Components of metabolic syndrome include overweight and obesity (i.e., waist circumference >102 cm [40 inches] in men and >88 cm [35 inches] in women), serum triglyceride levels greater than 150 mg/dL, serum concentration of high-density lipids less than 40 mg/dL in men and less than 50 mg/dL in women, hypertension (i.e., blood pressure >130/85 mm Hg), and insulin resistance (i.e., fasting blood glucose >100 mg/dL) (Ervin, 2009).

account reproductive anatomy and follow the current CDC guidelines for age and sexual maturity. For example, a priority assessment task for nurses in a variety of care settings is to ask female and male patients about breast self-examination. An adolescent male should be assessed for testicular self-examination habits, and older males should have an annual prostate examination. Menstrual history should be obtained from female patients, and an annual Papanicolaou (Pap) test is recommended (Box 16-1). Pregnancy and childbirth issues, such as gestational diabetes, gestational hypertension, or rectoceles and cystoceles, should be evaluated by the nurse as potential alterations in health status that may need continued monitoring.

BOX 16-1 Age-Related Guidelines for Pap Smears

- All women should begin cervical cancer screening at the age of 21 years. Women between the ages of 21 and 29 years should have a Pap test every 3 years.
- Women between the ages of 30 and 65 years should have a Pap test plus a HPV test (i.e., co-testing) every 5 years.
- Women 65 years of age or older who have had normal results for previous Pap tests should no longer be screened.
- Women who have had a total hysterectomy (i.e., removal of the uterus and cervix) should not be tested, unless the surgery was done as a treatment for cervical cancer or precancer.

Adapted from American Cancer Society: American Cancer Society guidelines for the early detection of cancer, 2012. Retrieved from *www.cancer.org/healthy/findcancerearly/cancerscreeningguidelines/american-cancer-society-guidelines-for-the-early-detection-of-cancer.*

Nurses are knowledgeable resources with whom people can discuss sensitive issues and questions about gender-specific illness and health-promotion activities. Nurses must display sensitivity and comfort in dealing with these issues, which may be awkward or difficult for people to discuss with friends, family, or other members of the health care team.

GENETICS AND INHERITED TRAITS

Preventive health care based on principles of human genetics is the next frontier for patient care. The **genetic vulnerability**, or risk of disease expression based on genotype, is involuntarily passed from biologic parents to their offspring. Societal attitudes about testing and management of high-risk populations depend on the potential for expression of genetic disorders possibly triggered by environmental factors. Controlling factors that place stress on physiologic function can reduce pathologic genetic expression and susceptibility to disease. For example, a person with a family history of hyperlipidemia and atherosclerosis is at risk for developing cardiovascular disease later in life. Lifestyle-modifying factors, such as weight reduction, daily exercise, and balanced nutritional intake, can help reduce the likelihood that the genetic risk factor for heart disease will be expressed. Diabetes, cancer, mental illness, and renal disease also have genetic components and are amenable to interventions that reduce risk.

LIFESTYLE

Health and wellness risk factors are inherent in the choice to engage in and continue particular behaviors. Habitual lifestyle behaviors can produce health benefits or intensify the effects of pathologic risk factors.

Information on lifestyle behaviors that lead to disease is available at research-sponsored websites that have peer-reviewed material and expert analyses. Website content should be easy to read and understandable for the general population. Most sites that discuss the latest information about health risks, lifestyle behaviors, and outcomes have separate information specifically for health care providers (Evidence-Based Practice and Informatics box). Examples of risky lifestyle behaviors that can lead to poor outcomes include excessive alcohol intake, which can cause liver damage and gastrointestinal distress, and poor dietary choices and lack of exercise, which can lead to overweight or obesity in adults and children.

EVIDENCE-BASED PRACTICE AND INFORMATICS

Research Opportunities and Resources Related to Health and Wellness

- Health and wellness topics for each body system offer a broad range of research opportunities.
- Research that evaluates positive and negative lifestyle-behavior outcomes is constantly evolving as discoveries are made about the physiologic changes bodies experience with disease and illness.
- Nurses are at the forefront of medical breakthroughs and are expected to be knowledgeable about the latest technology and pharmaceutical interventions.
- Up-to-date information about government-sponsored best-practice guidelines regarding nutrition, physical activity, and healthy living is available at *www.health.gov/default.asp*.
- For older adults, best-practice guidelines for health and wellness can be found at *www.aarp.org/health*.

The CDC weekly morbidity and mortality report follows trends in modifiable risk factors in the United States by age, socioeconomic status, and other demographic indicators. Behavioral risk factors such as smoking, poor diet, physical inactivity, and excessive drinking are linked to the leading causes of death in the U.S. population. The **Behavioral Risk Factor Surveillance System** (BRFSS) is an ongoing, state-based, random-digit-dialed telephone survey of the noninstitutionalized U.S. population older than 18 years of age. The BRFSS collects data on health risk behaviors and preventive health services related to the leading causes of death. The results from the BRFFS and other surveys about lifestyle-related risk factors are available online from the National Center for Health Statistics (NCHS) at *www.cdc.gov/nchs*.

The NCHS (2013) provides the latest data about modifiable risk factors that correlate with disease and illness. These data are available for most areas of the United States and emphasize the need for health promotion and preventive care initiatives tailored to individual, community, and statewide levels of the health care system. The economic impact of modifiable lifestyle-related risk factors that contribute to chronic disease is a serious concern to all communities due to the drain on health care and financial resources needed to accommodate an ailing population. Nurses are often asked to participate in education efforts to promote health and wellness and reduce disease risk factors as part of their communities' public health agendas.

Nutrition and dietary intake have a direct link to modifiable lifestyle-related risk factors that predispose an individual to obesity, hyperlipidemia, and atherosclerosis. Nurses can assist people with weight loss and maintenance techniques by educating them about the food choices and portion sizes suggested by the CDC's My Plate Food Guide for daily caloric requirements. Chapter 30 provides additional information on these requirements.

Exercise is essential for the prevention of illness and promotion of wellness. Physical exercise is any bodily activity or movement that enhances or maintains physical fitness levels and overall health. Exercise strengthens muscles, improves cardiovascular performance, enhances athletic skills and endurance, and reduces or maintains weight, and it is performed for enjoyment (Powers and Howley, 2012). Regular physical exercise boosts the immune system, builds and maintains healthy bone density, increases joint mobility, and helps to prevent cardiovascular disease, type 2 diabetes, and obesity. Exercise also improves mental health and helps to prevent depression through the release of endorphins and other neurotransmitters that are responsible for exercise-induced euphoria (Powers and Howley, 2012).

There are definitive recommendations for the amount of physical activity adults, children, and the elderly population should include in their weekly routines. Nurses should advise healthy adults to engage in moderate-intensity physical activity for at least 30 minutes 5 or more days per week. As an alternative, adults can participate in vigorous-intensity physical activity for at least 20 minutes 3 or more days per week. Children and adolescents should participate in at least 60 minutes of moderate-intensity physical activity most days of the week. For older adults, the recommendations are 30 minutes of moderate-intensity aerobic activity 3 to 5 days per week, daily stretching, and participation in strength-building activities two or three times per week (Powers and Howley, 2012).

Nurses should warn patients that severe physical pain, shortness of breath, blurred vision, changes in mental status, or any type of symptomatic response to exercise indicates they should immediately stop the exercise and seek help.

ENVIRONMENT

Where individuals live determines their access to food, water, shelter, and clean air. Indoor and outdoor environmental factors influence 85 of the 102 categories of disease and injury listed in *The World Health Report* (WHO, 2012) and determine the disease-producing organisms and substances to which an individual is exposed.

Indoor environments may harbor toxic household cleaning agents, chemicals (e.g., radon, carbon monoxide, unused drugs), tobacco smoke, and energy sources (e.g., microwave ovens). Exposure to mold, household pests (e.g., dust mites, spiders), inside cooking fumes, and unsanitary living conditions in an enclosed space increases the likelihood of respiratory illness and skin disorders.

Outdoor environments affect individual health in the areas of sanitation and waste disposal, water quality, air quality, and safety. Children living in areas where there are safety issues related to gang activity, sexual predators, or heavy traffic are less likely to engage in outdoor play activities. Their limited access to safe outdoor play space increases their risk for sedentary behaviors, excessive calorie intake, and obesity.

Nursing assessment is critical in identifying and minimizing modifiable environmental risks that can affect the health status of community members. Nurses familiar with community resources can dramatically impact the health of individuals by making necessary referrals and exploring creative options with community members to minimize negative health factors. The role of the nurse in addressing environmental concerns is often as a change agent and advocate for people with limited financial and educational resources.

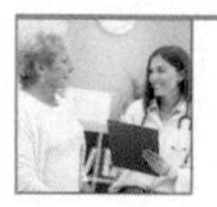

3. List nursing interventions to address each of Mrs. Wolford's preventable lifestyle-related risk factors that the nurse can discuss with Mrs. Wolford before including them in an individualized plan of care.

ATTITUDES AND EMOTIONS

Individuals respond differently to illness or the threat of illness. Their attitudes, behaviors, and emotional reactions depend on the severity of the illness and its perceived impact on their health. An individual's unique illness behaviors are influenced by self-concept, opinions of peers and family, and cultural customs.

A short-term, self-limited illness that is not life-threatening does not evoke emotions or actions that cause fundamental changes in daily lifestyle. More often, illnesses such as the flu, ear infections, and sore throats are viewed as minor irritations or inconveniences. They usually require a short-term adjustment in daily routines, and treatment of symptoms is the priority so that the individual can continue with normal activities. The emotional and behavioral changes associated with non–life-threatening illness are usually minimal, and the individual quickly returns to the previous baseline level of emotional functioning.

Chronic, debilitating disease and severe illness can produce a broad range of emotional or behavioral responses in patients and their families. Patients commonly react to the diagnosis of a disease or disorder with a poor prognosis with shock and feelings of numbness or bewilderment. Shock may soon be replaced by anger, denial, anxiety, and withdrawal from others. Emotional responses may be heightened in people who previously had controlled reactions to stressful situations.

After assessment and diagnosis of emotional distress, nurses can plan interventions in collaboration with patients and their families to help identify coping mechanisms and support systems that are appropriate to each situation. Identification and mobilization of patients' support networks help the patients and their families deal with the crisis of severe illness. Interventions that promote stress reduction and encourage positive behaviors are essential to healing. To promote positive patient outcomes, nurses must use their therapeutic communication skills when patients express concerns and wish to discuss their treatment options.

SELF-CONCEPT

Self-concept refers to the way in which individuals perceive unchanging aspects of themselves, such as social character, cognitive abilities, physical appearance, and body image. It is a mental image of self in relation to others and the surroundings. If the image is positive, the person will develop strengths, compensate for weaknesses, and experience life in a healthy way. If the image is negative (e.g., frail), the person will find life's challenges devastating and sometimes insurmountable. The impact of illness on the self-concept of a patient and the patient's family members depends on how secure the parties' relationships are with one another.

Changed behaviors that may reflect altered self-concept when a person is faced with a severe or terminal illness range from minimally noticeable to extreme. Extreme shifts in behaviors occur when the individual engages in an activity that was uncharacteristic before the illness, for example, a patient diagnosed with terminal cancer who takes up skydiving despite a long-held fear of heights. Family, friends, and peers may be confused by the deviation from characteristic behaviors, including unmet social obligations, interpersonal tension, and increased interpersonal conflict.

Nurses coordinating care for patients with end-stage disease must learn to recognize subtle and blatant changes in self-concept. The nurse can assist patients and their families in developing effective coping strategies to adapt to differences resulting from alterations in health status.

DEVELOPMENTAL LEVEL

Intellect and behavior can be attributed to genetic traits and environmental stimuli. An individual's developmental level, as characterized by mastery of expected milestones and interactions with surroundings, reflects more than chronologic age and physical size. The developmental level depends on a person's ability to reason and learn from life experiences in predictable stages at age-appropriate intervals. When planning care, the nurse must create strategies and integrate activities that conform to the patient's cognitive level of development to achieve a specific outcome.

For many years, sociologists focused primarily on the rapid physical and cognitive growth of children and adolescents during development. Recent research has focused on adult developmental changes because people are living longer and are exposed to illnesses and age-related changes that few individuals in previous centuries lived long enough to experience.

The concept of illness is different at each level of development. Fear and anxiety are common and appropriate traits for children and adults. The impact of disease may be beyond the ability of a child or developmentally-delayed adult to comprehend. Painful procedures and fear of the unknown are often part of treatment. Patients may associate the white coat of a health care provider with pain, anxiety, or unwanted physical touch. An adult may experience fear or anxiety related to illness, but unlike the child, the adult usually can control the associated emotions through reason and fully participate in care. Knowledge of the individual's developmental level helps the nurse to plan care according to the patient's expectations and ability to participate.

INFLUENCE OF PEERS AND FAMILY

The value that friends and family place on health status can positively or negatively influence the health of an individual. Typically, the developmental level of the patient determines whether peers or family members have more influence. Children and adults tend to be affected more by family members, whereas adolescents may be influenced more by their friends.

Regardless of the age of the patient, family is the principal collective framework for health promotion and disease prevention. Families weigh health choices and care decisions in each situation of illness according to beliefs, values, and their way of life. Family members typically use health care resources in similar ways, and health practices follow the norms established by parental influence over minors. In some cases, parental figures can send mixed messages about health issues. Consider the parent who drives home intoxicated after telling the children not to drink and drive or the parents who accept the use of recreational drugs in their home because they would rather have their children use drugs where they can monitor them.

BOX 16-2 Child and Adolescent Reactions to Trauma and Loss

- *Preschoolers:* Thumb sucking, clinging to parents, bedwetting, sleep disturbances, fear of the dark, loss of appetite, regression in behavior, and withdrawal from friends and routines.
- *Elementary school children:* Poor concentration, irritability, aggressiveness, clinging to parents, nightmares, school avoidance, and withdrawal from friends and activities.
- *Adolescents:* Agitation, sleeping and eating disturbances, increased conflicts, physical complaints, delinquent behavior, and poor concentration.

From the National Association of School Psychologists: Helping children deal with tragic events in unsettling times: Tips for parents and teachers, 2003. Retrieved from *www.nasponline.org/resources/crisis_safety/helpingchildrencope.aspx*.

Peers and generational norms influence the health behaviors and risk-taking attitudes of adolescent patients. Encouraging open communication and nonjudgmental attitudes among parents or trusted adult authority figures regarding the adolescent patient's health issues is a high-priority educational opportunity for nurses. Peer influence affects adolescent risk behaviors but tends to have less impact on health care matters.

Nurses should stress the importance of parental or adult supervision of adolescent health care. Nurses need to openly discuss family lifestyle and preventive health issues with each family member. Supporting families and assisting parents with coping techniques when dealing with devastating illness or tragedy is a vital aspect of nursing care. It is accomplished by being a good listener and observer and being attentive to emotional cues (Box 16-2). Teaching families to adhere to good health and wellness habits helps members to feel positive and productive.

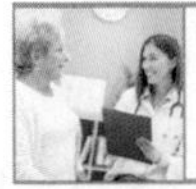

4. Identify at least three family factors that place Mrs. Wolford at risk for additional concerns.

TRADITIONS, BELIEFS, AND VALUES

Cultural traditions, spiritual beliefs, and the value an individual places on ethnic heritage greatly influence illness behaviors and therapeutic practices. Some people have ethnic practices or religious beliefs that nurses must consider before treatment or diagnostic procedures are performed. For instance, a patient may observe a day of fasting for religious reasons despite the detrimental effects the lack of nutrients has on the disease process.

Religious and cultural practices sometimes interfere with medical treatment to the point that life and death issues become secondary to beliefs. Patients make health care decisions based on cultural background and religious beliefs, and it is the patient's right to accept or refuse medical therapies. To improve compliance with prescribed treatments, nurses can incorporate patients' religious and cultural views into the plans of care.

HEALTH CARE ACCESS AND AVAILABILITY

Gaining access to any type of health care can be an intimidating task for healthy and sick individuals. Socioeconomic factors can compound the need for care if it is not affordable. For individuals or families deciding whether to seek treatment, the cost may be a less significant issue than the availability of health care. People living in isolated or less densely populated areas may have little or no access to health care providers or facilities within a reasonable distance. The circumstances affecting access to care may confound nurses' attempts to assist patients to comply with drug therapy, diagnostic test schedules, and follow-up appointments.

The economic stability of individuals or families can determine whether they are willing to seek preventive care or screening examinations. Even if screening is free or low cost, the patient or family members may decline because of the potential for testing positive for a disease. Treatment of a disorder often requires time spent away from work, lost wages, and expensive drug therapies and diagnostic tests. The financial impact can be devastating to families or individuals who have a limited or fixed income and fear that employment stability may be compromised.

Diminished availability of care has a major impact on the health and wellness of the people residing in rural areas and less densely populated regions. The length of time it takes to travel to the nearest health care provider or facility can inhibit patients from seeking care for illness or initiating preventive measures. For example, treatment can be delayed for so long that a minor, non–life-threatening, treatable infection becomes a severe, life-threatening, systemic infection requiring hospitalization and intravenous drug therapy.

Patients who must drive long distances to seek medical care and treatment often bring the entire family for evaluation. During visits, it is not uncommon for the health care provider to address multiple problems with different degrees of severity that have been "saved up" for the long trip. This puts the nurse in an advantageous position to assess the needs of the patient and the family in one visit. The nurse can perform detailed examinations and engage many family members in long-term strategies to address issues of health and wellness.

Urban settings often have more highly specialized health care systems but may lack the availability of primary and preventive care venues. Challenges to meeting personal health needs in urban communities center on poor air quality, crowded living and working conditions, and decreased access to exercise and recreational activities because of availability and safety issues. In these instances, nurses are instrumental in identifying barriers to health maintenance habits and routines. Finding opportunities to maximize health access for patients living in urban areas can include adding an air-purifying system to an existing air-conditioning unit; reinforcing the necessity and technique of good hand hygiene, especially during seasonal outbreaks of illness; and encouraging exercise routines that accommodate the buddy system or group activities during daytime hours.

The Institute of Medicine report, *The Future of Nursing: Leading Change, Advancing Health* (2011), calls for nurses to be full partners in transforming health care in the United States. Nurses have the responsibility and the expertise to help educate, enable, and encourage people of all ages to adopt healthier lifestyles and to become proactive about health care practices that can prevent or minimize illness and disease. Day to day, nurses continue the commitment of contributing to the wellness of patients, families, and communities by supporting initiatives, programs, and projects that promote a culture of health and self-care, which improves patients' quality of life.

SUMMARY OF LEARNING OUTCOMES

LO 16.1 *Define the concept of health in an individual and a corporate context:* Individuals define health in terms of their values, experiences, and ways of living. Organizations and businesses define health in the context of their goals and objectives.

LO 16.2 *Compare the theoretical models of health and wellness that provide the basis for nursing practice:* The Basic Human Needs Model, Health Belief Model, Health Promotion Model, and holistic health models provide a foundation for defining optimal physiologic and mental status while approaching health care delivery from different viewpoints.

LO 16.3 *Discuss health promotion and its relationship to wellness:* The concepts of health promotion, wellness, and risk reduction are interconnected with a person's motivation and goals for achieving a predetermined level of health.

LO 16.4 *Explain the three levels of preventive care and the nursing interventions associated with each:* Health promotion and specific protection strategies are two examples of appropriate ways in which nurses can work with their patients in primary prevention. The goal for health intervention during secondary prevention is early detection and diagnosis of health problems before patients exhibit symptoms of disease. Nursing care is focused on rehabilitation efforts in the tertiary stage of prevention.

LO 16.5 *Summarize key aspects of each type of illness and the stages of illness behavior:* Acute illness is typically characterized by an abrupt onset and short duration (<6 months), with clinical manifestations that appear quickly, may be severe, and resolve within a short period because they respond to treatment or are self-limited. Chronic illness is any condition in which a loss or abnormality of body function occurs that lasts longer than 6 months and requires ongoing, long-term care. Chronic health conditions may be controlled with lifestyle management or drug therapy, but they are considered to be irreversible. Stages of illness may progress from the acceptance of being ill to the resumption of previously assumed roles and activities.

LO 16.6 *Identify factors influencing health and their impact on illness:* Many factors influence health and illness, including social determinants of health such as age; gender; availability of and access to health care; cultural, spiritual, and ethnic considerations; attitudes; monetary resources; environmental factors; genetics; lifestyle choices; self-concept; and health policies.

Responses to the critical-thinking questions are available at *http://evolve.elsevier.com/YoostCrawford/fundamentals/.*

REVIEW QUESTIONS

1. Which of the listed basic needs identified by Maslow must be addressed first when providing nursing care?
   a. Self-esteem
   b. Love and belonging
   c. Self-actualization
   d. Nutrition and elimination
2. Which activity best illustrates use of the Health Promotion Model (HPM) by the nurse to increase the level of well-being for a patient immediately after surgery?
   a. Holding a pillow across his chest when coughing and deep breathing
   b. Encouraging the patient to eat his entire evening meal
   c. Changing his surgical dressing daily as ordered by the physician
   d. Asking his family to step out of the room during dressing changes
3. A nurse providing preventive care to an overweight patient with a family history of diabetes should engage in which priority care-planning activity for this patient?
   a. Calculating the patient's body mass index (BMI) and recommending a daily exercise routine
   b. Instructing the patient to perform blood glucose monitoring once daily
   c. Giving the patient a month's supply of insulin needles and syringes
   d. Participating in diabetes education classes offered at a local health facility
4. A normally active, older patient has been frequently evaluated for minor problems at the clinic since the death of her husband 3 months earlier. During one of her visits she states that she has no energy to get through the day and no desire to keep up with her Tuesday night bridge club. Which type of holistic health model intervention should the nurse use to help the patient cope with the loss of her husband?
   a. Encouraging use as needed of a drug for anxiety ordered by her provider
   b. Teaching the value of music therapy to address anxiety about her loss
   c. Explaining that she will be over the loss of her husband in a few months
   d. Encouraging a gradual reentry into social interaction and activities with friends
5. An 8-year-old girl is newly diagnosed with type 1 diabetes. The nurse may expect fear and crying when teaching the child how to self-administer insulin injections because of which influencing factor?
   a. Self-concept
   b. Self-esteem
   c. Developmental level
   d. Hierarchy of needs
6. Three weeks after delivery, a patient started a diet of 800 calories per day and began jogging 2 miles twice per day. The nurse recognizes the patient's behavior may be influenced by which motivating factor?
   a. Body image
   b. Family roles
   c. Illness behavior
   d. Chronic illness
7. A 65-year-old male patient has been a one-pack-a-day smoker for 40 years. He was recently diagnosed with early stage chronic obstructive pulmonary disease (COPD) and would like to attend a smoking cessation class. The nurse recognizes smoking cessation as which level of prevention for this patient?
   a. Primary prevention
   b. Secondary prevention
   c. Statutory prevention
   d. Tertiary prevention

8. A patient diagnosed with an aggressive cancer is estimated to have 6 months to live. Two months later, the patient's wife calls the nurse's office because she is upset that her husband has taken up motorcycle racing and has already been injured twice. The nurse knows that the patient is experiencing a behavioral change in which factor because of the prognosis of his illness?
   a. Spirituality
   b. Physical attributes
   c. Self-concept
   d. Personal affect
9. The nurse enters a patient's room to deliver a dinner tray and notices that the patient has not been out of bed since the previous day. The patient states that his condition has made him bedridden, although the nurse knows that he is capable of independent ambulation. Which type of reaction is the patient exhibiting?
   a. Ambivalence to symptoms
   b. Illness behavior
   c. Diminished functional ability
   d. Overreaction to illness
10. A patient is seeking information about leading indicators that show the importance of health promotion and illness prevention in the United States. To which government-sponsored program would the nurse refer the patient for the best source of information?
   a. American Cancer Society website
   b. *Healthy People 2020* website
   c. Centers for Disease Control and Prevention (CDC) morbidity and mortality reports
   d. American Association of Hospitals home page

Answers and rationales for the review questions are available at *http://evolve.elsevier.com/YoostCrawford/fundamentals/.*

REFERENCES

Bandura A: Exercise of personal agency through the self-efficacy mechanism. In R Schwarzer (Ed), *Self-efficacy: Thought control of action*, Washington, D.C., 1992, Hemisphere, pp. 3-38.

Baum RA, Nash PL, Foster JE, et al: Primary care of children and adolescents with Down syndrome: An update. *Curr Probl Pediatr Adolesc Health Care*, 38(8):241-261, 2008.

Centers for Disease Control and Prevention (CDC): *Human papillomavirus*, 2012. Retrieved from *www.cdc.gov/hpv/WhatIsHPV.html.*

Cronenwett L, Sherwood G, Barnsteiner J, et al: Quality and safety education for nurses. *Nurs Outlook*, 55(3):122-131, 2007.

Ervin RB: Prevalence of metabolic syndrome among adults 20 years of age and over, by sex, age, race and ethnicity, and body mass index: United States, 2003–2006. *Natl Health Stat Rep*, 13, 1-8, 2009.

Institute of Medicine: *The future of nursing: Leading change, advancing health*, Washington, D.C., 2011, National Academies Press.

Leavell HR, Clark EG: *Preventive medicine for the doctor in his community*, ed. 3, New York, 1965, McGraw-Hill.

Maslow AH: *Motivation and personality*, New York, 1954, Harper & Row.

Mechanic D: Sociologic dimensions of illness behavior. *Soc Sci Med*, 41(9):1995-1207, 1995.

National Center for Health Statistics (NCHS): *Health risk factors*, 2013. Retrieved from *www.cdc.gov/nchs/hus/healthrisk.htm.*

O'Donnell MPL: Definition of health promotion. *Am J Health Promot*, 23(5i), 2009.

Pender NJ, Murdaugh CL, Parsons MA: *Health promotion in nursing practice*, ed. 6, Upper Saddle River, N.J., 2011, Prentice Hall.

Powers S, Howley ET: *Exercise physiology: Theory and application to fitness and performance*, ed. 8, New York, 2012, McGraw-Hill.

Rosenstock IM: Historical origins of the Health Belief Model. In MH Becker (Ed), *The Health Belief Model and personal health behavior*, Thorofare, N.J., 1974, Charles B. Slack, pp. 1-8.

Segen J: *McGraw-Hill concise dictionary of modern medicine*, New York, 2006, McGraw-Hill.

Suchman EA: Stages of illness and medical care. *J Health Hum Behav*, 6:114-128, 1965.

United Nations (UN): Leaders gather at UN headquarters for a high-level meeting on non-communicable diseases (NCDs), 2011. Retrieved from *www.un.org/en/ga/ncdmeeting2011.*

U.S. Department of Health and Human Services (DHHS): *Healthy People 2020: Healthy people in healthy communities*, Washington, D.C., 2010, U.S. Government Printing Office.

Van Kuiken D: A meta-analysis of the effect of guided imagery practice on outcomes. *J Holist Nurs*, 22:164-179, 2004.

World Health Organization (WHO): Preamble to the constitution of the World Health Organization, 1948. Retrieved from *http://apps.who.int/gb/bd/PDF/bd47/EN/constitution-en.pdf.*

World Health Organization (WHO): 10 Facts on preventing disease through healthy environments, 2012. Retrieved from *www.who.int/features/factfiles/environmental_health/environmental_health_facts/en/index7.html.*

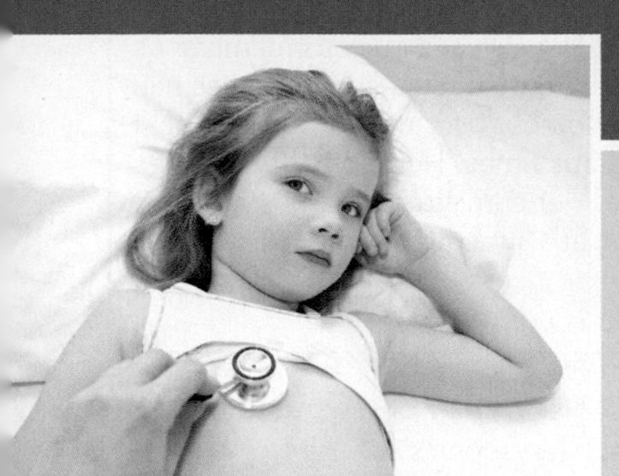

CHAPTER 17

Human Development: Conception Through Adolescence

EVOLVE WEBSITE

http://evolve.elsevier.com/YoostCrawford/fundamentals/

- Additional Evolve-Only Review Questions With Answers
- Answers and Rationales for Text Review Questions
- Answers to Critical-Thinking Questions
- Case Study With Questions
- Conceptual Care Map Creator
- Glossary

LEARNING OUTCOMES

Comprehension of this chapter's content will provide students with the ability to:

LO 17.1 Describe major theories of human development.
LO 17.2 Explain human development from conception to birth.
LO 17.3 Identify the primary developmental tasks of the newborn.
LO 17.4 Outline infant developmental milestones.
LO 17.5 Describe the physical, psychosocial, and cognitive development of the toddler.
LO 17.6 Summarize growth and development during the preschool years.
LO 17.7 Discuss development that occurs during the school-age years.
LO 17.8 Articulate physical, psychosocial, and cognitive adolescent development.

KEY TERMS

accommodation, p. 239
adaptation, p. 239
assimilation, p. 239
centration, p. 240
conception, p. 242
conservation, p. 240
continuous theories, p. 236
development, p. 236
discontinuous theories, p. 236
ego, p. 236
egocentric, p. 240
embryo, p. 242
equilibration, p. 239
fetus, p. 242
growth, p. 236
id, p. 236
nature versus nurture, p. 236
negative reinforcement, p. 242
object permanence, p. 239
operant conditioning, p. 242
positive reinforcement, p. 242
puberty, p. 251
reversibility, p. 240
seriation, p. 240
superego, p. 236
zygote, p. 242

CASE STUDY

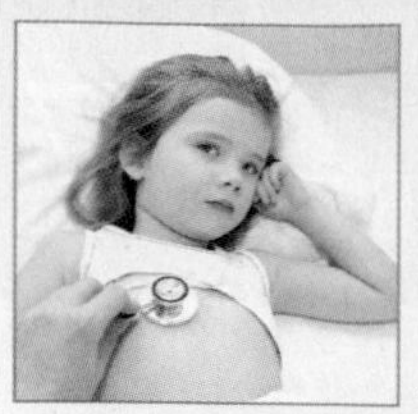

Four-year-old Eva is admitted to the pediatric unit for dehydration related to diarrhea from gastroenteritis. Vital signs are T 39.6° C (103.3° F), P 137 and regular, R 28 and unlabored, BP 80/45, and weighs 34 pounds. She had been taking sips of electrolyte solution orally at home but is now lethargic. Her skin and mucous membranes are dry. Her mother is with her, and her father is at home with her siblings. Her mother states that Eva has had multiple episodes of diarrhea at home today, but she is unsure about urine output. Her mother explains that Eva is toilet-trained but the diarrhea has caused her to be incontinent numerous times. Her mother also states that Eva sleeps in a youth bed at home. Eva's immunizations are up to date. Her admission history is negative for any major illnesses, and she has met all of her developmental milestones, including walking at 13 months, being toilet-trained at 2 years 3 months, and speaking in full sentences. She attends preschool two times per week.

Refer back to this case study to answer the critical-thinking questions throughout the chapter.

The terms *growth* and *development* are closely related but differ as follows: **Growth** is the process by which an increase in size occurs, measured in humans as height and weight. Growth proceeds in an orderly, predictable pattern, from head to tail (cephalocaudal) and in a proximal to distal (near to far) direction. **Development**, on the other hand, is the increasing maturation of physical ability, thought processes, and behaviors over time. The focus of this chapter is development from conception through the teen years.

THEORIES OF HUMAN DEVELOPMENT LO 17.1

Over the years, many theories have been written about how children develop. From these theories emerged a major debate regarding whether development is predetermined at birth (nature) or whether the child's environment (nurture) controls how development progresses (**nature versus nurture**). At present, many developmental experts agree on a middle-of-the road approach to this debate, believing that a combination of environment and heredity affects the developmental process.

Schools of thought also debate whether development is continuous or discontinuous. **Continuous theories** of development subscribe to the belief that development occurs in a smooth and gradual process from infancy to adulthood. **Discontinuous theories** describe development as progressing through a series of distinct and predictable stages triggered by inborn factors. As in the nature-versus-nurture debate, most modern theorists acknowledge that both inborn and external factors influence development.

PSYCHOSOCIAL THEORIES

Certain events in the lives of humans, such as the decision to marry, occur when a person has reached the psychological and social maturity to make such a decision. This maturity is achieved in part as an internal process of maturation and in part is influenced by social and cultural norms. Psychosocial theorists who have attempted to explain this process are Sigmund Freud, Erik Erikson, and Robert Havighurst.

Freud's Theory

Freud (1923/1974) viewed the mind as mostly unconscious. He compared the mind to an iceberg, with the majority of it below the surface in the unconscious, rather than conscious, realm. He believed that there were three basic components to the personality: the id, ego, and superego. The **id** is the part of personality consisting of instincts. The id operates on a totally unconscious level and is not centered in reality. The id functions by seeking out pleasure and avoiding pain. According to Freud, very young children start out functioning at the id level. However, as children mature, the ego part of the personality is formed. As children experience the demands of real life, they learn that they must make decisions on the basis of rational rules and not just for pleasure. The **ego** is the part of the mind that functions in reality. It allows people to seek out pleasure within the norms of society. The ego is partially conscious. However, the id and the ego do not consider right or wrong. The **superego** is the structure that houses the "moral" branch of personality. It often is referred to as the *conscience.* The superego is partially conscious. In considering a moral dilemma, the superego is the structure that makes us think about whether an action is right or wrong.

In addition to theorizing on the structures of personality, Freud conceptualized five stages of psychosexual development in childhood. The ability of the child to progress successfully through these stages determines whether the person will be a well-adjusted adult. These stages are the oral stage, the anal stage, the phallic stage, the latency stage, and the genital stage (Table 17-1).

Oral Stage

The oral stage is the period of life from birth to 18 months. During this stage, the child gains pleasure primarily from the mouth area. Chewing, sucking, and biting are all activities believed to reduce tension during this phase.

Anal Stage

The anal stage is the time between 18 months and 3 years of age. The primary source of pleasure and tension release at this phase is the anus and eliminative functions associated with

TABLE 17-1 Freud's Stages of Psychosexual Development

AGE RANGE	STAGE	BEHAVIORS	CONFLICT
Birth to 18 mo	Oral	Mouthing, chewing, sucking, biting	Weaning
18 mo to 3 yr	Anal	Bowel elimination	Toilet training
3 to 6 yr	Phallic	Genital stimulation	Triggering of Oedipus/Electra complex
6 yr to puberty	Latency	Sexual urges sublimated into other social activities; friends of the same sex	Avoiding stress of conflicts
Puberty and beyond	Genital	Sexual reawakening, sexual gratification	Revisiting previous unresolved conflicts with parents

it. It is during this stage that many children learn bowel and bladder control.

Phallic Stage

Freud believed that the phallic stage extends between the ages of 3 and 6 years. Pleasure at this stage centers on the child's discovery that self-stimulation is enjoyable. Freud viewed the phallic stage as an important stage in personal development because this stage triggers the Oedipus complex. The Oedipus complex is the strong attachment the young male child develops to the parent of the opposite sex. The Electra complex is the same feeling in the female child. Freud believed that the child wants to replace the same-sex parent so as to gain the exclusive attention and affection of the opposite-sex parent. He theorized that later during the phallic stage, the child begins to fear punishment by the same-sex parent for this feeling. The child then begins to identify with the same-sex parent, to reduce this conflict.

Latency Stage

According to Freudian theory, between the age of 6 years and the onset of puberty, the child experiences the latency stage, during which all interest in sexuality is repressed. The child puts energy into emotionally safe activities, thereby avoiding the stress of the conflicts experienced in the phallic stage.

Genital Stage

The genital stage extends from puberty onward, and it is the fifth and final stage in Freud's theory of development. During this stage, sexual feelings are reawakened. Previous conflicts with parents that were unresolved from earlier stages of development reemerge. When these conflicts are resolved, the individual becomes able to develop mature adult relationships.

Erikson's Theory

Erik Erikson (1963) was trained by Freud as a psychoanalyst. He developed a theory of psychosocial development adapted from Freud's theory. Erikson believed that as people grow, they face a series of psychosocial crises that shape their personality. This series of psychosocial crises is divided into eight stages: trust versus mistrust, autonomy versus shame and doubt, initiative versus guilt, industry versus inferiority, identity versus role confusion, intimacy versus isolation, generativity versus stagnation, and integrity versus despair (Table 17-2). Nurses, particularly in psychiatrics, utilize these stages to assess whether an individual is in the appropriate state for their age, or whether progression has been delayed based on social behaviors observed.

Trust versus Mistrust

The first of Erikson's stages is trust versus mistrust, which extends from birth to the age of 18 months. During this phase, the consistent caregiver plays an important role in meeting the affection and food needs of the child. If the caregiver is inconsistent or unable to meet these needs, the child becomes frustrated and develops a sense of mistrust in those around him or her. Children who do not have a consistent caregiver during this phase may have difficulty with emotional attachments at later stages in life.

Autonomy versus Shame and Doubt

The second stage extends between the ages of 18 months and 3 years. In autonomy versus shame and doubt, the child has begun to walk and to speak in basic terms. Children in this stage strive to do things for themselves. The conflict lies in children's dual desires to hold on and to let go. The parents' role at this stage is best served by providing flexible but firm guidance, thereby allowing autonomy while providing safety and security. The child is given choices within reasonable boundaries. With parents who are overly controlling and restrictive, children may develop a sense of shame and doubt in their own abilities.

Initiative versus Guilt

Between the ages of 3 and 6 years, the child is in the stage of initiative versus guilt according to Erikson. In this stage, children's maturing physical and verbal abilities encourage them to expand their world. Families can best encourage this sense of initiative by allowing children to run, jump, play, and throw. Children at this time are exploring what kind of people they may become. Parents who limit their children's attempts at initiative cultivate a sense of guilt in children during this stage that may persist into later life as well.

TABLE 17-2 Erikson's Developmental Stages

AGE RANGE	STAGE OF PSYCHOSOCIAL CRISIS	BEHAVIOR	RESOLUTION OF CRISIS
Birth to 18 mo	Trust versus mistrust	Caregiver must meet all needs of the child.	Develop a sense of trust in others by having needs met.
18 mo to 3 yr	Autonomy versus shame and doubt	Child strives to make decisions for himself or herself.	Achieve a balance between holding on and letting go.
3 to 6 yr	Initiative versus guilt	Child explores his or her world and abilities (running, jumping, throwing).	Initiate activities without fear of reprimand from caregivers.
6 to 12 yr	Industry versus inferiority	Child refines skills acquired previously and develops a peer social network that exerts great influence on him or her.	Develop a sense of self-worth based on accomplishments while avoiding feelings of failure.
12 to 18 yr	Identity versus role confusion	Adolescent explores and integrates multiple roles: student, athlete, child, adult. Emotional fluctuation and stress are common as the adolescent struggles to sort out his or her identity.	Emerge from the stage with a strong sense of individuality.
18 to 35 yr	Intimacy versus isolation	Person searches for a partner who supports and complements him or her. Starting a family is common.	Seek fulfilling love and family relationships.
35 to 55 yr	Generativity versus stagnation	Person seeks involvement in creative and meaningful work and transmits culture and values to younger generations.	Develop a sense of self-worth as children leave the home.
55 yr and beyond	Integrity versus despair	Person reviews life events and accepts the finality of death.	Achieve a sense of fulfillment over life's accomplishments.

Industry versus Inferiority

Industry versus inferiority is the stage that encompasses the ages of 6 to 12 years. When children enter school, their social realm expands. Peers and teachers take on more importance, while parental influence decreases. Children in this stage take great pride in accomplishments. Failure, whether incurred in a real sense or through an inability to meet one's own expectations, can lead to a sense of inadequacy or inferiority. It is the responsibility of parents and other adult role models to help children understand what constitutes success and failure.

Identity versus Role Confusion

Erikson's fifth stage of development is identity versus role confusion, which coincides with adolescence. During this stage, the teen attempts to determine a sense of who he or she is. This stage is experienced as a time of great change. Not only is the body undergoing major physical changes, but pressures are emerging for the young person to make decisions about future education and career choices. Teens typically experiment with different sexual, occupational, and educational roles while they try to develop a sense of identity as they approach adulthood. When adolescents fail to figure out their sexual, occupational, or educational path, conflict results.

Intimacy versus Isolation

On entering the phase of intimacy versus isolation, the young adult has achieved a sense of identity and has set a path for where he or she is going. The main task of this phase is to develop an intimate and trusting relationship with another person. The ideal relationship should complement the individuality of each partner without stifling growth. People who fail at developing such a relationship may retreat into isolation.

Generativity versus Stagnation

Generativity versus stagnation is the stage of middle adulthood. Generativity can be accomplished by successfully rearing one's own children or by engaging in other activities that promote creativity and productivity. If the person fails to grow during this phase, the result may be stagnation with self-absorption (egocentric behavior) and self-indulgence.

Integrity versus Despair

Erikson's eighth and final stage, integrity versus despair, begins with late adulthood, when the person looks back over his or her lifetime and resolves any final identity crisis. Accomplishments must be reconciled with failures and limitations for the person to develop a sense of integrity. The finality of death must be accepted. A person who fails to do so risks developing a sense of despair and regret over the way his or her life has turned out.

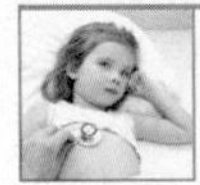

1. According to Erikson, what is Eva's stage of development? How might hospitalization affect her in this stage? What can be done to encourage continued development?

Havighurst's Theory

Robert Havighurst (1972) is credited with identifying the concept of developmental tasks. Havighurst's theory defines a developmental task as one that arises during certain periods in life. Successful achievement of the task allows the person to move on toward new experiences and challenges. Failure to accomplish such tasks can lead to feelings of inadequacy and failure in achieving future developmental tasks. The three sources from which developmental tasks arise are physical changes, personal sources, and societal pressures. Havighurst identifies six major age periods, each with its own developmental tasks (Table 17-3). See Chapter 18 for detailed information on adult development.

TABLE 17-3 Havighurst's Stages of Development

STAGE	TASKS
Infancy and early childhood	Taking food, learning to talk, and learning sex differences and sexual modesty
6 to 12 yr	Learning to get along with age-mates, developing a sense of conscience and morality, and achieving personal independence
12 to 18 yr	Preparing for marriage/relationship and a career, acquiring a set of values, and achieving socially responsible behavior
Early adulthood (19 to 29 yr)	Selecting a partner, starting a family, managing a home, establishing a career, and assuming civic responsibilities
Middle adulthood (30 to 60 yr)	Fulfilling civic and social responsibilities, maintaining a standard of living, assisting children into adulthood, adjusting to aging parents, adjusting to physiologic changes
Late adulthood (61 yr and beyond)	Adjusting to physiologic changes and health status changes associated with aging, adjusting to retirement and altered income, establishing living arrangements, and fulfilling civic and social responsibilities

COGNITIVE DEVELOPMENT THEORY

Cognitive development theory addresses how the process of thought develops in humans. Mental activities addressed in these theories include thinking, remembering, and developing language. The primary theorist in cognitive development is Jean Piaget.

Piaget's Theory

Jean Piaget (1969) was educated as a biologist but later became interested in psychology. His background in biology influenced his views on the process of cognitive development. He theorized that children progress through four stages (described next). He also believed that young children develop patterns of behavior called *schemes* (adaptation, assimilation, accommodation, and equilibrium), which older children and adults use to deal with objects in the environment. **Adaptation** is the process of adjusting behavior in response to stimuli within the environment. The person adapts by using assimilation and accommodation. With **assimilation**, the child attempts to use a new object in the same way as that applied with more familiar objects. A young child encountering a tomato for the first time, for example, displays assimilative behavior in grasping it, saying "ball," and then squeezing it—the child perceives a familiar toy and a tomato as identical in terms of size and shape. **Accommodation** occurs when the child discovers that the tomato cannot be played with in the same way as a more familiar toy ball. The child finds that the tomato bursts when squeezed; the child accommodates this discovery by changing the pattern of behavior on subsequent encounters with new, similar objects.

Equilibration is the process by which a balance between present understanding and new experiences is restored. Piaget believed that this process is critical to cognitive development. When equilibration is upset, the child has the opportunity to learn and grow. From the disequilibrium, new ways of thinking and dealing with the environment develop, preparing the child to progress to the next stage of development.

Sensorimotor Stage

As noted, Piaget described four distinct stages of development (Table 17-4). The first of these is the sensorimotor stage, extending from birth to 2 years of age. Children in this stage explore their environment by using their senses and developing motor skills. Initially, infants interact with the environment primarily through reflexes. For example, if a parent puts an object into the infant's hand, the infant will reflexively grasp it. As the child grows, however, learning occurs, and reflexes are controlled to produce desirable effects. Gradually, trial-and-error behaviors are replaced by planned behaviors. The child becomes capable of simple problem solving.

Children at this stage develop an understanding of the concept of **object permanence**. Early on, children do not understand that something still exists when it is out of sight.

TABLE 17-4 Piaget's Stages of Development

AGE RANGE	STAGE	BEHAVIORS
Birth to 2 yr	Sensorimotor	The child explores the environment by using the senses.
2 to 7 yr	Preoperational	The child begins to use images and symbols to represent the world; is still unable to repeat mentally what he or she can do physically.
7 to 11 yr	Concrete operational	Logical reasoning gradually replaces intuitive thought.
11 yr and beyond	Formal operational	The person refines his or her ability to think logically; is capable of abstract thought.

For example, if a parent covers a toy with a blanket, the child does not understand that the toy is still there. By the age of 2 years, the child understands that the toy still exists even when it is out of sight. Attainment of this ability is key to development toward more advanced thinking skills.

Preoperational Stage

The preoperational stage encompasses the preschool and early school-age years, between the ages of 2 and 7 years. During this stage, children acquire the use of symbols to represent objects. This ability allows language skills to grow rapidly. However, other thinking skills are not yet developed. Children at this age still lack an understanding of the concept of conservation. **Conservation** is the ability to recognize that objects remain the same even if they change in appearance. The child can focus on only one aspect of a dilemma. For example, if the preoperational child is confronted with two 6-ounce glasses of water, one tall and narrow and one short and wide, the child typically will insist that the taller glass contains more water. The child focuses only on the height of the glass as an indication of volume. Likewise, the child may think a cookie broken into two pieces is more than the same cookie in one piece. By focusing on only one aspect of an object, the child is exhibiting **centration** in his or her thought process.

Preschoolers demonstrate irreversibility in their thinking patterns. **Reversibility** is an important development in thinking patterns that enables older children and adults to change direction in their thinking to return to the starting point. If the preschooler had the ability of reverse thinking, he or she would understand that 6 ounces of milk initially poured into a tall narrow glass can then be poured into the short glass—mentally reversing the pouring process and accepting the implication that the volumes in the glasses are the same.

The preoperational stage is characterized by **egocentric** thinking. Children in this stage believe that everyone else sees the world exactly as they see it. They tend to interpret situations and events in terms of their own perceptions. For example, when these children are asked to describe a toy, they typically define the toy in terms of how they use it. When asked to describe a ball, the preoperational child may say, "I throw it."

Concrete Operational Stage

The concrete operational stage extends between the ages of 7 and 11 years—that of the school-age child. At this stage, the child develops the ability to think logically and has acquired an understanding of conservation. The child's thinking is still grounded in familiar situations and concrete objects, however, and is not yet capable of abstraction.

One important skill that develops at this age is **seriation**, the ability to arrange things in a logical order. To do this, the child must be able to sort and classify objects using some criterion or characteristic. School-age children enjoy sorting and classifying objects and often have collections of a variety of items. Children in this age-group are moving from egocentric to decentered or objective thought, which allows them to view things from another's perspective.

Formal Operational Stage

Around the time of the onset of puberty, the child's thought patterns begin to take on adult characteristics. The child develops the ability to think abstractly and to problem-solve in a more systematic fashion than that seen in a child in the concrete operational stage. Adolescents in formal operations can reason about hypothetical situations and are not restricted to situations in which they have experience. This ability to think abstractly and to form and test hypotheses in a systematic fashion continues into adulthood, although it is thought that some people may never fully function in this stage.

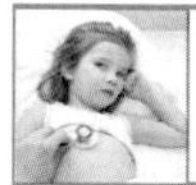

2. According to Piaget, what is Eva's cognitive stage? What does this mean for Eva?

MORAL DEVELOPMENT THEORY

Moral development refers to how children develop a sense of right and wrong. As children develop, they internalize values and cultural norms that provide a framework for decisions later in life. Lawrence Kohlberg developed his theory of moral development on the basis of the cognitive theory of Jean Piaget and others.

Kohlberg's Theory

Kohlberg (1987) theorized that people progress through three levels of moral reasoning as they develop (Table 17-5). Each

TABLE 17-5 Kohlberg's Stages of Moral Development

LEVEL	STAGE	BEHAVIORS
Preconventional level	Stage 1	*Obedience and punishment orientation:* Rules are imposed by others, and punishment is to be avoided.
	Stage 2	*Individualism and exchange:* Judgments are guided by values of exchange, with the person's own wants and needs taking priority.
Conventional level	Stage 3	*Good/bad orientation:* The person is motivated by wanting to meet expectations of parents and other close family members; in return, the person receives love, respect, and admiration.
	Stage 4	*Law and order orientation* (doing what is right, respecting authority, maintaining the social order): The focus is on meeting the needs of society and doing one's duty in order to maintain social order. Many adults do not progress beyond this stage.
Postconventional morality	Stage 5	*Social contract and individual rights:* The person recognizes the need for order in society but is able to examine rules and respect the differing views of others.
	Stage 6	*Universal principles:* The person is able to ponder and identify universal principles of justice that are applicable to all. Most people do not consistently achieve this level of moral reasoning.

TABLE 17-6 Westerhoff's Theory of Faith Development

STAGE	AGE	BEHAVIOR
Experienced faith	Preschool and early childhood	The child explores, tests, observes, and copies adults. Children learn faith by what they see and experience from those around them.
Affiliative faith	Childhood and early adolescent years	The child acts with others in a community of faith, participating in community activities offered in youth groups, choirs, and service organizations.
Searching faith	Early adulthood	The person goes through three characteristic steps: doubt/critical judgment, experimentation, and commitment. These steps are needed to move from an understanding of community faith to ownership of faith.
Owned faith	Adulthood	The person attains full ownership of faith. Such people want to share their experience with others and are willing to stand up for their beliefs.

level is divided into sublevels, called *stages.* According to Kohlberg, reasoning is the important part of the process, not the end decision. Kohlberg believed that the person cannot comprehend or function at higher levels until he or she works through the lower levels.

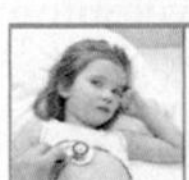

3. How might Eva view why her illness happened to her from a moral standpoint?

FAITH DEVELOPMENT THEORY

Whereas moral development involves *how* the person makes moral decisions, faith development is the *way* in which a person develops spiritually. Kohlberg and others did not focus on the development of religious beliefs. However, theorists such as Westerhoff did address the process of a person's committing to a set of religious beliefs.

Westerhoff's Theory

John Westerhoff described a process of faith development. Faith, according to Westerhoff (2012), is a way of behaving that comprises knowing, being, and willing. He described four distinctive styles of faith through which a person may progress, given proper interactions and experiences: experienced faith, affiliative faith, searching faith, and owned faith (Table 17-6).

BEHAVIORIST THEORY

Behaviorist theory focuses on measuring observable behaviors that occur in response to stimuli. It is concerned not with how or why knowledge is obtained but with producing behaviors. Behaviorist theory focuses on the influences of the external environment on the person's behavior.

Skinner's Theory

B. F. Skinner (1953) believed that personality developed not as a result of inherited traits but as a result of the influences of the external environment. He believed that operant conditioning influences the development of behavior. **Operant conditioning** is a form of learning based on reinforcement or punishment. **Positive reinforcement** occurs when a behavior is met with a positive consequence. **Negative reinforcement** occurs when a behavior is strengthened by removal of an unpleasant stimulus. Both types increase the chance that the behavior will be repeated.

SOCIAL LEARNING THEORY

Social learning theory holds that people learn from observations, interactions, and imitation of others. It bridges concepts between behaviorist and cognitive theories.

Bandura's Theory

Albert Bandura (1977) believed that people learn from one another through their interactions, observations, and imitation of others. He theorized that there is a continuous interaction of cognitive, environmental, and behavioral influences. Bandura believed that four conditions are necessary for effective modeling of behaviors:

- *Attention:* Certain variables affect how much attention is given to a behavior. Some of these variables are the complexity of the situation and the personal characteristics of the observer of the situation.
- *Retention:* The ability to store the information that was given attention for later recall. Examples of tools used to aid retention are mental coding and symbolic images.
- *Reproduction:* The ability to reproduce the behavior at a later time.
- *Motivation:* The reason for imitating the behavior. Tradition, imagined incentives, reinforcement, and punishment are motivators.

Bandura believed that the interaction of the environment and the person is what shapes behaviors. He termed this concept *reciprocal determinism.*

DEVELOPMENT FROM CONCEPTION TO BIRTH LO 17.2

The process of physiologic development begins at conception and is ongoing, continuing up to death. It is predictable, proceeding in both cephalocaudal and proximal to distal directions. At times, growth occurs rapidly; at other times, it is slowed. Regardless of its speed, change in the human organism is occurring continuously.

Conception occurs with fertilization and implantation. The process of a sperm and an ovum uniting is called *fertilization.* The fertilized ovum is called a **zygote**, which begins as a single cell. Fertilization triggers a process of cell division.

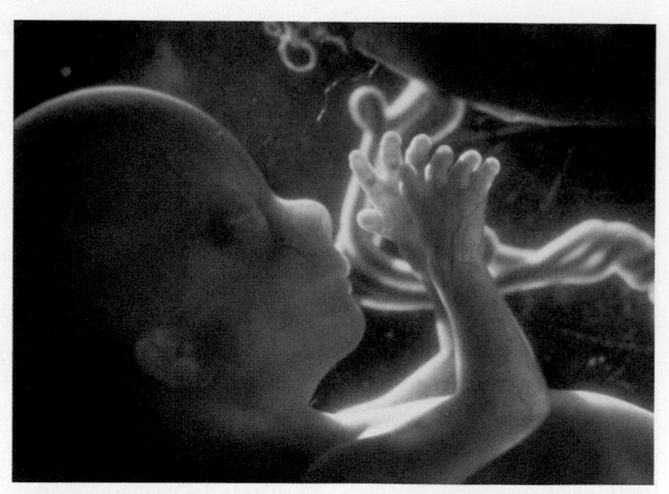

FIGURE 17-1 A fetus at 16 weeks of development.

During the first 2 weeks, the developing zygote travels through a fallopian tube and into the uterus, where *implantation* into the uterine wall occurs. The period before implantation is the germinal period.

After 3 weeks, the zygote is known as an **embryo**. During this phase, the rate of cell differentiation increases and organs begin to form. By week 3, the neural tube that eventually becomes the spinal cord forms. The eyes appear at around 21 days, and by the 24th day, the cells of the heart begin to differentiate and soon will be beating rhythmically. By 8 weeks, an embryo weighs close to 1/30 of an ounce and is approximately an inch long. Most of this rapid development occurs before many women realize that they are pregnant.

Two months after conception, an embryo is now called a **fetus**. The fetal period lasts until delivery of the infant. During this time, the fetus continues to grow and organs continue to mature (Figure 17-1). Weight increases to between 4 and 7 ounces and length to approximately 6 inches by 4 months. By completion of the pregnancy between 37 and 41 weeks of gestation, the fetus has gained considerably more weight, and organs have matured enough to function outside the womb.

The developing fetus is susceptible to a variety of substances from the outside environment called *teratogens,* or agents which can disrupt development. Teratogens include certain medications, illegal drugs, alcohol, radiation, and infectious agents. A pregnant woman's choices, health, and prenatal care have well-recognized impact on the developing fetus. Nurses should ask pregnant women about medications, drug use, alcohol use, tobacco use, and safe sex practices (Health Assessment Questions: Prenatal box). They also should ask pregnant women about the home and work environments, to screen for possible teratogens in these areas. Prenatal screening is discussed in the Ethical, Legal, and Professional Practice: Prenatal Screening box, and diversity considerations related to pregnancy are listed in the Diversity Considerations box. Members of the health care team collaborate when caring for the expectant mother (Collaboration and Delegation: Prenatal Care box).

HEALTH ASSESSMENT QUESTIONS

Prenatal

Present Health

- What is your age?
- How many pregnancies have you had?
- What is your ethnic background?
- Do you drink alcohol? If so, how many drinks do you have per week?
- Do you smoke tobacco? If so, how many packs per day?
- Do you use any over-the-counter medications or herbal supplements? If so, what are they, and how much do you take?
- Do you use any illegal or street drugs?
- Where do you work? Are you exposed to any chemicals or radiation at home or at work?
- Do you have a cat? Who in the family is responsible for changing the litter box?
- What have you eaten in the past 24 hours? Is this a typical day's intake for you?
- Do you consume products with caffeine, such as coffee, cola, or chocolate?

Health History

- Have you ever had any infectious diseases such as rubella?
- Do you have any health problems like diabetes or epilepsy?
- Are you taking any medications? If so, what are they and how often do you take each one?

Family History

- Are any of the following diseases present in your family: diabetes, heart disease, hypertension, stroke, respiratory problems, kidney problems, thyroid problems, bleeding disorders, epilepsy, or other disorders?
- Has anyone in your family had a child with a birth defect?

COLLABORATION AND DELEGATION

Prenatal Care

Collaboration with other health care professionals may be necessary to offer the best care possible to the expectant mother.

- Referral to a dietitian is indicated when the pregnant woman is malnourished or suffering from hyperemesis. These disorders can adversely affect the developing fetus.
- Having a significant other or family member present at prenatal visits provides support for the expectant mother.
- Health care providers work closely together to provide referrals and support for smoking cessation and alcohol avoidance programs during pregnancy, to avoid risks to the fetus that are associated with the use of tobacco or alcohol.
- Women who are older than 35 years of age, are pregnant with multiple babies, or have other medical conditions should be followed closely by their medical provider and may be referred to an obstetrician who specializes in high-risk pregnancies.

ETHICAL, LEGAL, AND PROFESSIONAL PRACTICE

Prenatal Screening

- Fetal chromosome screening is recommended for all women, regardless of age, by the American College of Obstetricians and Gynecologists (ACOG).
- First-trimester screening includes a blood test to check for possible neural tube defects and for trisomy 21 (Down syndrome).
- An ultrasound examination is performed to check for fluid collection at the back of the fetus's neck. This nuchal translucency measurement may indicate the presence of chromosomal abnormalities, congenital heart defects, abdominal wall defects, diaphragmatic hernias, and other defects.
- More invasive procedures such as chorionic villus sampling and amniocentesis, along with genetic counseling, may be considered if the screening tests indicate a high risk for defects.
- ACOG recommends second-trimester *quad screening,* a four-part test that detects neural tube defects, trisomy 18, and trisomy 21 with a high degree of accuracy. The timing of this test in the second trimester is important because the levels of the substances measured change during pregnancy. The combination of first- and second-trimester results increases the chances of detecting Down syndrome to 90% to 95%.
- Other testing includes complete blood count, blood type and Rh, rubella titer, TB skin testing (before 20 weeks of gestation), urinalysis, urine culture, renal function testing, and PAP test. Testing for sexually transmitted infections such as those due to HIV, *Neisseria gonorrhoeae,* and HPV are completed at the first prenatal visit.
- A 1-hour glucose tolerance test is performed between 24 and 28 weeks of gestation to screen for gestational diabetes. If the result is elevated, a 3-hour glucose tolerance test is ordered.
- At 35 to 37 weeks of gestation, a vaginal smear is obtained to check for group B streptococci.

Adapted from American College of Obstetricians and Gynecologists: ACOG's screening guidelines on chromosomal abnormalities, 2007. Retrieved from *www.acog.org/About_ACOG/News_Room/News_Releases/2007/ACOGs_Screening_Guidelines_on_Chromosomal_Abnormalities*; Driggers R, Seibert D: Prenatal screening: New guidelines, new challenges. *J Nurse Pract, 4*:351-356, 2008.

DEVELOPMENT DURING THE NEWBORN PERIOD LO 17.3

The newborn, or neonatal, period is from birth to 28 days of life (Figure 17-2). The primary developmental task of the newborn is to adapt to the external environment. A full-term infant is born between 37 and 41 weeks of gestation. Some health concerns for newborns are infections, oxygenation, feeding difficulties, and safety issues. An infant is considered

DIVERSITY CONSIDERATIONS

Life Span

- Pregnant women older than 35 years of age are at increased risk for having a child with Down syndrome. Women older than 35 have the option of screening tests that are offered to all pregnant women, or they can elect to have more invasive tests performed.

Culture, Ethnicity, and Religion

- Women of Eastern European and Ashkenazi Jewish descent are at increased risk for having children affected by Tay-Sachs disease. This is a fatal genetic lipid disorder. A simple blood test can identify carriers of the disease.
- Women of African, Southeast Asian, and Mediterranean descent are at increased risk for having children with red blood cell disorders, called *hemoglobinopathies,* such as sickle-cell disease and should have screening tests during pregnancy.
- Cultural diversity may encompass maternal diet, infant care beliefs, and cultural birth practices. It is important for the nurse to provide patient teaching that is culturally sensitive. The nurse helps parents plan ways to ensure a healthy pregnancy while honoring the family's cultural and religious beliefs.
- In discussions about prenatal screening, it is important to respect the patient's personal religious and cultural beliefs about the process. For example, some religions prohibit abortion for any reason.

preterm if born earlier than 37 full weeks of gestation. Term births are further divided into subcategories of early term, term, and late term, given findings that demonstrate differences between a 37-week and a 41-week infant (London et al, 2014). Preterm infants are at increased risk for developmental delays and health problems, depending on gestational age at birth and birth weight as well as other physical and socioeconomic factors. Sample health assessment questions for a newborn's office visit are listed in the Health Assessment Questions: Newborn box.

SAFE PRACTICE ALERT

Always use good handwashing technique when caring for newborns. Check facility protocols for additional requirements when entering and exiting newborn care areas.

Patient teaching during newborn visits is focused on helping parents with feeding, elimination, and sleep concerns. The nurse is a primary resource person for new parents, and a supportive atmosphere is important during this time.

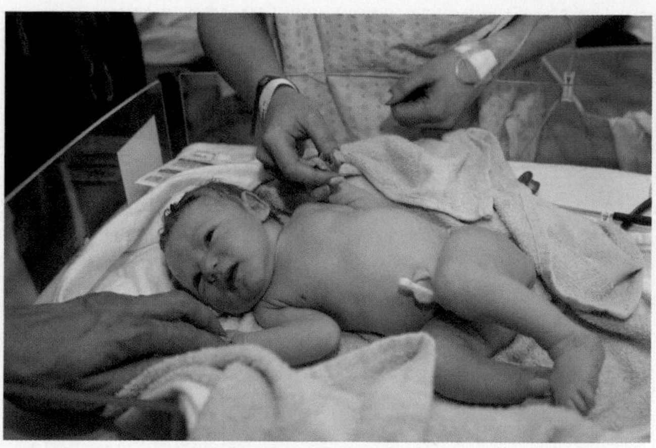

FIGURE 17-2 A full-term infant.

HEALTH ASSESSMENT QUESTIONS

Newborn

When examining a newborn, it is important to ask the mother about her pregnancy.

- Were there any problems experienced during the pregnancy?
- Was the baby born early or on time?
- What was the method of delivery? If the baby was delivered by cesarean section, do you know the reason?
- Were any medications, drugs, alcohol, or tobacco products used during pregnancy?
- Is your baby breast- or bottle-fed? If bottle-fed, what type of formula? Do you have to wake the baby to eat or does the baby awake on his own to eat? How long does it take the baby to eat?
- Can you tell me about the baby's eating patterns? bowel patterns?
- How about the baby's sleeping patterns?
- Does the baby seem to look at you?
- Does the baby startle when a loud sound occurs?
- Are you getting enough rest?
- Is the baby floppy (flaccid) when awake or is the baby wiggly?

INFANT DEVELOPMENT LO 17.4

From 28 days after birth until 1 year of age, the child is considered an infant. Physical development progresses in a rapid, yet sequential, pattern. Physical growth progresses in cephalocaudal and proximodistal directions. At birth, the infant is dependent on the caregiver for everything from feeding to positioning. By 1 month of age, babies can lift the head when placed in a prone position. At approximately 4 months of age, babies can lift the head and chest. As neural connections increase and mature, so do the child's physical abilities. Some reflexes evident in the infant will persist into adulthood. These include blinking, coughing, and yawning. However, other reflexes will disappear. In some cases, these reflexes must diminish so that intentional skills can develop.

TABLE 17-7 Developmental Milestones by Age

3 MONTHS	7 MONTHS	12 MONTHS
Raises head and chest when prone	Rolls from front to back and from back to front	Gets to sitting position without assistance
Brings hands to mouth	Sits with support and then without it	Crawls forward on belly, using arms and legs to push
Follows a moving object with eyes	Transfers object from one hand to another	Assumes hands-and-knees position
Smiles at the sound of caregiver's voice	Responds to own name	Uses pincer grasp
Smiles socially	Uses voice to express pleasure	Says "da-da" and "ma-ma"
Babbles	Finds partially hidden objects	Tries to imitate words

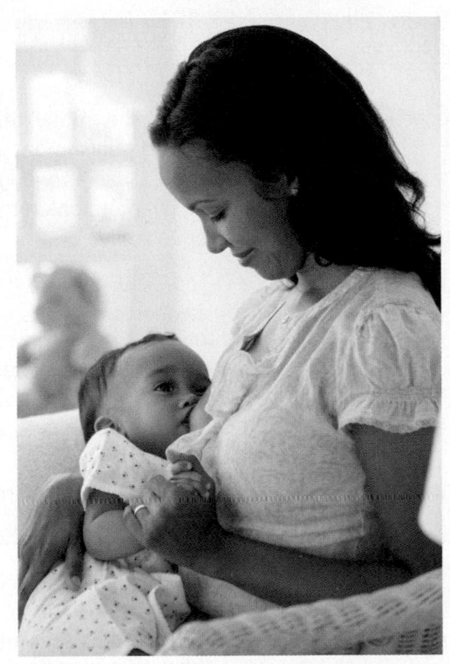

FIGURE 17-3 Breast milk is the ideal nutrition during the first 6 months of life.

Important developmental milestones to watch for in infants, as recommended by the American Academy of Pediatrics (2007a), include those presented in Table 17-7. At well-child visits, the nurse performs screening tests, such as the Denver Developmental Screening Test, to make sure that each child is meeting developmental milestones.

Ideally, infants need only their mother's breast milk for nutrition for the first 6 months of life (Figure 17-3). Iron supplementation is recommended between the ages of 4 and 6 months. Additionally, infants being exclusively breast-fed may require vitamin D supplements in the first 2 months of life. Babies who are formula-fed should receive an iron-fortified infant formula. Whole milk should not be introduced until after the child is 1 year of age. Gradual introduction of solid foods usually begins somewhere between 4 and 6 months of life. Bland foods such as rice cereal are introduced first with the addition of complex, richer foods one at a time in order to monitor for possible allergies.

In addition to meeting basic biologic needs, a stimulating environment is necessary for the infant to develop properly. Toys and mobiles with high-contrast color patterns are a good choice. Soft music, rattles, and chimes provide auditory stimulation. Fabrics of various textures and textured toys offer tactile stimulation (Patient Education and Health Literacy: Infant Safety box). Use of swings and push/pull toys as the child grows older encourages mobility.

PATIENT EDUCATION AND HEALTH LITERACY

Infant Safety

The nurse provides education for parents at each well child visit, which may include:

- Caregivers should keep infant cribs clear of overstuffed pillows, blankets, and stuffed animals. Such objects present a suffocation hazard, especially to small infants.
- Caregivers should never leave small objects within the reach of an infant because of the risk of choking.
- Infants should never be put to sleep in the prone position because of this position's link with sudden infant death syndrome (SIDS).
- Parents should use good handwashing technique to prevent infections, especially before infant feedings and after diaper changes. Visitors should wash their hands when they come to an infant's home.

! SAFE PRACTICE ALERT

To prevent burns, microwaving breast milk or infant formula is not recommended. To warm milk or formula, place the container in a lukewarm or warm water bath for several minutes. Test the temperature by squirting a couple drops on the inner portion of caregiver's wrist before offering to infant. Never add water into a bottle to cool it down as this upsets the precisely formulated concentration considered safe for the infant.

TABLE 17-8 Age and Developmental Stages Across Theories

AGE GROUP	ERIKSON (PSYCHOSOCIAL)	PIAGET (COGNITIVE)	KOHLBERG (LEARNING)
Infant	*Trust versus mistrust* Dependent on others to meet needs	*Sensorimotor: primary circular reactions* Actions reflexive in nature	*Preconventional* No sense of "good" or "bad" behavior Later, motivation is to avoid punishment
Toddler	*Autonomy versus shame* Beginning to assert authority over own actions	*Sensorimotor: tertiary circular reactions* Realizes own actions cause reactions in others	*Preconventional* Behavior based on rules imposed by others; main motivation is to avoid punishment
Preschool child	*Initiative versus guilt* Focus is on energetic learning	*Preoperational* Preconceptual (2-4 yr): egocentric thought processes, magical thinking Intuitive thought (4-7 yr): beginning sense of others' perspectives	*Preconventional* Motivation for behavior is to avoid punishment; rules imposed by others. Does not understand reasons for the rules
School-age child	*Industry versus inferiority* Eager to develop skills; motivated to complete tasks	*Concrete operations* Able to use thought processes to experience events Less egocentric; able to see others' viewpoints Concept of conservation is mastered Able to classify objects	*Conventional* Early school age: motivated by reward and punishment After age 7 yr: able to judge actions by intentions rather than consequences
Adolescent	*Identity versus confusion* Focuses on who the adolescent is and who he or she wants to become	*Formal operations* Capable of abstract thought Can manipulate more than two categories of data at the same time Can think about the way others think	*Conventional to postconventional* Able to make decisions based on own set of internal moral values Questions the status quo and established rules

The hospitalized infant is at risk for developing mistrust (Table 17-8). If parents are unable to stay and provide care for the infant in the hospital, the nurse must ensure that infant needs such as feeding, bathing, and changing are met. Additionally, it is important to ensure that the environment is both safe and stimulating for the infant. The use of developmentally appropriate toys, such as mobiles, encourages continued progress toward developmental milestones.

In assessing an infant's development, the nurse is not always able to observe behaviors. The nurse evaluates progress by asking the parent or caregiver questions about developmental behaviors (Health Assessment Questions: Infant box).

Some health concerns during infancy are sudden infant death syndrome (SIDS), colic, and abuse. SIDS is diagnosed when a baby dies while sleeping and no known cause can be found. Placing babies on their backs to sleep is believed to reduce the occurrence of SIDS, as does putting babies to sleep in their own cribs. Placing babies in the parents' bed is dangerous, because suffocation can occur from clothing or bedding, or as a consequence of inadvertent pressure from a sleeping parent. Babies become colicky when they have intestinal spasms, causing pain and making the infant very fussy. The cause is not known, but some babies respond well to a change in formula and others to a calmer environment. Shaken-baby syndrome is a form of abuse that occurs in infants. This syndrome occurs when a frustrated or angry caregiver shakes the baby, causing trauma to the brain from the force of its hitting against the skull. Nurses should be aware of cues from parents, such as exhaustion, frustration, and anger that might lead to abuse of the infant. Helping parents with coping skills and education about the risk of injury to infants are important components of the nurse's role.

! SAFE PRACTICE ALERT

SIDS is a health risk during infancy. The best way to reduce the risk of SIDS is to instruct parents to always put babies to sleep on their backs (National Institutes of Health, 2014).

HEALTH ASSESSMENT QUESTIONS

Infant

1 to 3 Months

- Does your baby smile at you?
- Does your baby follow objects like a rattle with her eyes?
- Does your baby turn her head from side to side when she hears a noise?
- Does your baby seem to try to talk to you when you talk to her?
- Does your baby hold an object if you put it in her hand?
- Do you ever see your baby looking at her own hand?
- Does your baby ever squeal when she is excited?

4 to 6 Months

- Does your baby roll from back to side?
- Can your baby sit if propped?
- Does your baby play with his hands, clothing, and blankets?
- Does your baby try to reach for objects held in from of him?
- Does your baby put toys in his mouth?
- Does your baby laugh out loud?
- Does your baby hold his own bottle?
- Does your baby imitate sounds?
- Does your baby say "da-da" or "ma-ma"?
- Does your baby look for toys that are dropped?

7 to 9 Months

- Can your baby sit up either supported or unsupported?
- Does your baby pass toys from one hand to another?
- Can your baby focus on an object for longer periods of time than in previous months?
- Does your baby get upset when you leave the room?
- Is your baby crawling or trying to stand?
- Does your baby resist diaper changes or washing her face?

10 to 12 Months

- Can your child move from lying face down to sitting unassisted?
- Is your child trying to walk? If so, with or without support?
- What words does your child say?
- Does your child search for objects you hide?
- Does your child play games like peek-a-boo?

PHYSICAL, PSYCHOSOCIAL, AND COGNITIVE DEVELOPMENT OF THE TODDLER LO 17.5

The toddler stage begins around 1 year of age and ends around 3 years. Physical growth slows after the infant stage, but the child continues to develop rapidly in many ways. Visual acuity improves, and binocular vision is developed. Most body systems are matured. Heart and respiratory rates slow. The gastrointestinal system has matured, and the toddler can tolerate a variety of foods. By 12 to 13 months of age, children usually begin to ambulate, using a wide stance to support themselves and falling easily at first. This skill is gradually refined between the ages 2 and 3 years. By age 2, toddlers are able to walk up and down stairs; by age 2½, they are able to jump on two feet (Figure 17-4). Fine motor development is evident in increased skills. At 1 year of age, children can grasp small objects. By the time they are 15 months old, children can drop small objects into a bottle. They enjoy throwing objects down to watch others retrieve them. By 18 months of age, children can throw a ball overhand while maintaining balance (American Academy of Pediatrics, 2007a). Some sample questions to ask at the well-child visit for a toddler are listed in the Health Assessment Questions: Toddler box.

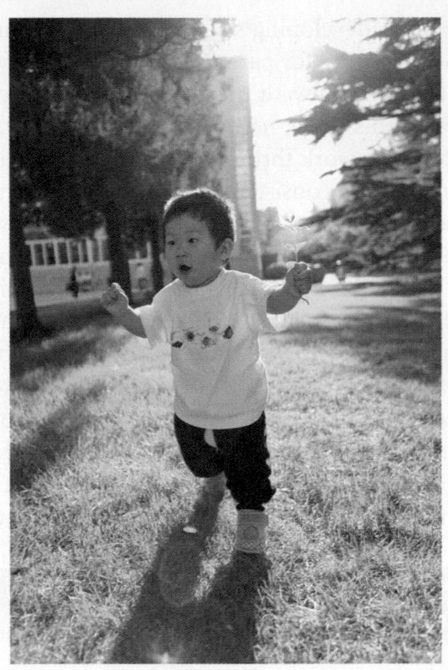

FIGURE 17-4 The toddler progresses from standing to walking to climbing stairs.

HEALTH ASSESSMENT QUESTIONS

Toddler

- At what age did your toddler start walking?
- Is your toddler sleeping through the night?
- What kinds of foods does your toddler eat?
- Is your toddler saying words?
- Does your toddler interact with you and others?

Nutrition often is a concern for the toddler's parents. Growth rate slows during this time, so the child's need for calories and other nutrients also decreases. Toddlers often become picky eaters. It is important that mealtimes be enjoyable, without pressure to "clean your plate." The general guide to a serving size is 1 tablespoon of solid food per year of age. Toddlers often require planned snacks in addition to regular meals. Planned snacks that offer a variety of nutritious foods are a good way to avoid empty calories.

The toddler's developing sense of autonomy can be frustrating and confusing for parents. Often, toddlers will say *no* even when they really want to say *yes*. Two behaviors typical of toddlers in this stage, *negativism* and *ritualism*, are ways that help toddlers work through this conflict. It is important for toddler to have a consistent bedtime ritual, such as a calm environment, a darkened room, and reading books, to aid in readiness for sleep. Frustration often is exhibited in the form of temper tantrums. Parents must be supported in dealing with these often exasperating behaviors. Ritualism aids the child in maintaining security and sameness, which provides a sense of comfort. This security enables the toddler to explore the environment with the comfort of knowing that familiar people, places, and routines exist. The Patient Education and Health Literacy: Car Safety box offers suggestions for teaching parents how to keep young children safe in a car.

PATIENT EDUCATION AND HEALTH LITERACY

Car Safety

- Advise parents to insist on car seat use for all trips. The National Highway Traffic Safety Administration (NHTSA) recommends that children from birth to 3 years old travel in the back seat in a rear-facing car seat until they reach the car seat manufacturer's height or weight limit for the seat. Once children reach the limit, a forward-facing car seat with a harness is used in the backseat (NHTSA, 2011).
- Instruct parents to follow the instructions provided by the car seat manufacturer and their vehicle manufacturer for car seat installation.
- Recommend that parents have their car seat installation checked by a certified inspector. The geographically closest inspector can be located at *www.nhtsa.gov*.

! SAFE PRACTICE ALERT

Avoid feeding toddlers foods that present choking hazards, such as hot dogs, hard candy, and fruit with pits.

Toddlers are beginning to understand that objects exist even when they do not see them. Parents must be constantly on the lookout for potential household dangers that can attract the curious toddler. It is helpful that toddlers are motivated to avoid punishment at this stage (see Table 17-8). To keep them safe, the parent should provide simple rules with just punishments for offenses, and consistently follow the same rules. A simple explanation of what the child did wrong and, usually, a time-out are good ways to set limits with the toddler.

QSEN FOCUS!

Vigilance and monitoring by the nurse, family members, and other members of the health care team are valued in providing safe caring for toddlers.

Toddlers in the hospital often find the experience upsetting, in part because it disrupts the comfort of their routine and separates them from their caregivers. The nurse may find it helpful to ask the parents about rituals and routines at home and try to incorporate them into the care of the child. The nurse can expect some regression to earlier behaviors in a child who is hospitalized. Often, toddlers will react with temper tantrums to even minor procedures or routine hygienic care. If possible, having the parents nearby to provide comfort and care is preferred.

! SAFE PRACTICE ALERT

Toddlers are mobile. Ensure that hospital crib side rails are up and locked into position and overhead rails are down and locked into position before leaving the bedside.

GROWTH AND DEVELOPMENT DURING THE PRESCHOOL YEARS LO 17.6

Biologic growth slows for the preschool child. The average weight gain is approximately 5 pounds per year, and the average increase in height is 2½ to 3 inches per year. Physical appearance changes from that of the toddler to the more streamlined appearance of the child. As gross and fine motor skills develop, the child becomes more graceful and agile than a toddler. By 3 years, the child not only can walk but also run, jump, and climb. Three-year-olds enjoy activities like riding a tricycle and throwing a ball. By 4 to 5 years, the child can skip, hop on one foot, and turn somersaults. Fine motor skill development is exhibited by increased interest and ability in drawing and printing letters. The child is able to dress without assistance. Sample health assessment questions for parents or caregivers of preschoolers are shown in the Health Assessment Questions: Preschooler box.

HEALTH ASSESSMENT QUESTIONS

Preschooler

- Has your child had frequent infections or colds?
- Is your preschooler toilet-trained?
- What types of activities does your preschooler enjoy? Can your preschooler ride a tricycle? skip? hop on one foot?
- Does your preschooler play with other children?
- What is your child's typical diet during the day?
- Does your child talk in sentences?
- Can your child write his or her own name?
- Does your preschooler play make-believe?

Nutrition requirements for the preschooler stay more or less the same as those for toddlers, although calorie and fluid requirements increase slightly. After 24 months of age, low-fat milk can replace whole milk. Whole fruits and vegetables are preferred to fruit and vegetable juices. Nonnutritive fruit drinks and soda should be avoided, because they add empty calories and contribute to tooth decay. A variety of fruits and vegetables should be offered.

The preschool years are a period of active learning. Play is the primary method through which learning occurs. Preschoolers are physically active. They often are seen running, jumping, and rolling around (Evidence-Based Practice and Informatics box). They have vivid imaginations. It is not uncommon for some preschool children to have imaginary friends. These imaginary friends serve many purposes: They are there when the child is lonely, they can accomplish what the child is still working on, and they can experience situations that the child does not want to remember, such as breaking Mom's cell phone. Preschoolers like to imagine themselves in roles they see in their parents and other adults. It is common for preschoolers to pretend to be parents, nurses, firefighters, carpenters, or police personnel, or to assume other adult roles they have seen modeled (Figure 17-5).

EVIDENCE-BASED PRACTICE AND INFORMATICS

Minimizing Aggressive Behavior in Children

Aggression is behavior that hurts a person or property. Preschoolers often exhibit aggressive behavior. Ways to avoid or minimize aggressive behavior include:

- Limit exposure to media (television, video games) to 1 to 2 hours of quality programming per day.
- Discourage television viewing for children younger than 2 years of age. Instead, focus on activities that promote brain development, such as talking, playing, singing, and reading together.
- Remove televisions, Internet connections, and video games from children's bedrooms.
- Monitor television programs that children are watching.
- View television programs with children to monitor content. Discuss controversial or violent content with children, and explore other methods of problem solving as alternatives to the violent solutions shown on programs.
- Encourage alternative activities to television, such as athletics, hobbies, and creative play.

From American Academy of Pediatrics: Policy statement on media violence. *Pediatrics 124*(5), 2009. Retrieved from *http://aappolicy.aappublications.org/cgi/content/full/pediatrics;124/5/1495.*

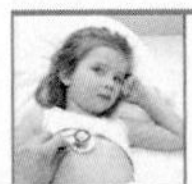

4. The nurse receives a new order to start an IV line for Eva. What reaction might the nurse expect from Eva when the IV line is started? What might cause this reaction? How can the nurse help to alleviate Eva's concerns about the procedure?

Preschoolers are very egocentric in their thought processes. Objects are defined in terms of how the child uses them. If asked to define a crayon, the child will say, "I color with it." Another characteristic of preschool thought is *magical thinking.* Because of their egocentric thought processes, preschoolers believe that they can cause events by simply wishing them to happen. Often, hospitalized preschoolers will blame their illness on something they perceive they did wrong (see Table 17-8). The nurse must take this into consideration when caring for a preschool child. Even if the hospitalization is a result of injuries the child sustained as a result of not following rules, such as the rule of wearing a bicycle helmet, the nurse should avoid blaming the child or telling the child that this is punishment for breaking the rules.

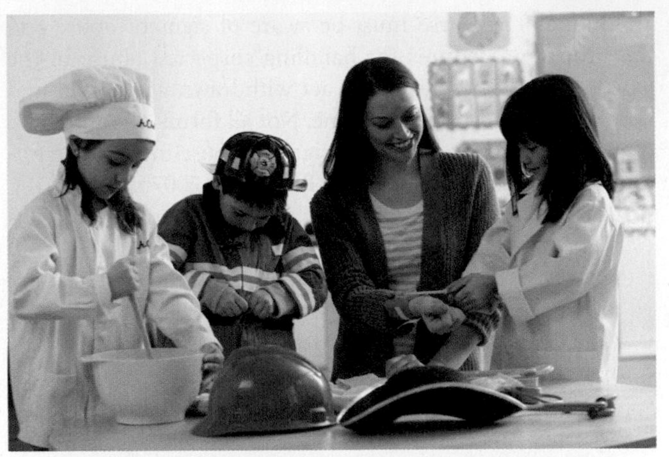

FIGURE 17-5 Preschoolers have vivid imaginations.

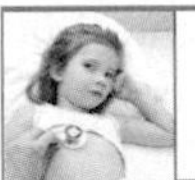

5. What approach can the nurse use in explaining the illness to Eva?

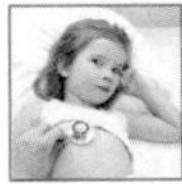

The conceptual care map for Eva can be found at *http://evolve.elsevier.com/YoostCrawford/fundamentals/.* It is partially completed to indicate how to use the map as a learning tool. Complete the nursing diagnoses using the example conceptual care maps shown in Chapters 8 and 25-33.

QSEN FOCUS!

The nurse should remove barriers to the presence of families and value an active partnership with parents and other caregivers in planning, implementing, and evaluating care for children.

The nurse may notice a child who demonstrates inappropriate behavior, such as trying to touch another child in a sensitive area. This would alert the nurse that this child may either be experiencing or observing such behaviors in the home. These observations warrant further investigation since the child may be a victim of abuse.

Child maltreatment is a term used to describe intentional physical abuse or neglect, emotional abuse or neglect, and sexual abuse of children. It is a significant problem in childhood. The nurse must be aware of signs of abuse and the proper procedures for handling suspected abuse in the work setting. The child may act withdrawn and afraid and may express fear of going home. Not all forms of abuse have obvious signs. Some warning signs of abuse include the following (American Academy of Pediatrics, 2007b):

- Physical evidence of abuse or neglect, including previous injuries
- A vague explanation of how an injury occurred, or failure to offer any explanation at all
- An explanation that is inconsistent with the pattern, age, or severity of the injuries
- Markedly different stories from different witnesses about how an injury occurred

! SAFE PRACTICE ALERT

The presence of viral infection and the use of aspirin in children are linked to Reye syndrome, a potentially fatal toxic encephalopathy. Avoid use of aspirin and non–aspirin-containing salicylates during febrile illnesses in children.

DEVELOPMENT DURING THE SCHOOL-AGE YEARS LO 17.7

Between the ages of 6 and 12 years, the child is said to be in middle childhood, or the school-age years. The pace of physical growth is slower than in preceding years, with the child growing an average of 2 inches per year and gaining approximately 4 to 6 pounds per year. The child's physical appearance becomes slimmer and even more graceful, and the child is more adept than in the preschool years. Fat diminishes further, and the skeleton lengthens along with an increase in muscle tissue. Boys and girls of this age have similar physical growth characteristics during the early years of the school-age period.

The body systems of the school-age child are more mature than they were in the preschool years. They are better able to fight infection, although early in this period children often have an increased rate of illness because of more exposure to other children. They are able to maintain a more stable blood glucose pattern. Caloric needs decrease, and an increase in stomach capacity enables children to eat less frequently. In most cases, full bowel and bladder control have been achieved, although young school-age children occasionally have toileting accidents as they adjust to the more controlled school environment. The skeletal system continues to develop, with bones lengthening and ossifying. Some sample health assessment questions for parents of school-age children are presented in the Health Assessment Questions: School-age Child box.

Safety is a concern for the active school-age child. As children play outdoors, they are at risk for accidents while riding bicycles and skateboards. Bicycle safety is discussed in the Patient Education and Health Literacy box. Children who are sedentary are at risk for developing childhood obesity and its

HEALTH ASSESSMENT QUESTIONS

School-age Child

- Does your child get along with classmates?
- What are your child's favorite activities?
- Can your child ride a two-wheeled bike? play ball?
- Does your child eat a well-balanced diet?
- Is your child sick frequently?
- Does your child have any problems seeing the blackboard at school or seeing words in a book?

PATIENT EDUCATION AND HEALTH LITERACY

Bicycle Safety

Teach parents and children about bicycle safety. Include the following information:

- All bicyclists must wear a properly fitting helmet that meets Consumer Product Safety Commission (CPSC) standards (Figure 17-6).
- Young children riding as passengers must wear a properly fitted helmet. They must ride in a bicycle-mounted seat or in a bicycle-towed child trailer. Children should never ride on the handlebars or cross bar.
- Helmets that are involved in a crash or are damaged must be replaced immediately. All helmets should be replaced every 5 years, or sooner if the child outgrows the helmet.
- Parents and children should be knowledgeable about bicycle safety rules and traffic laws.

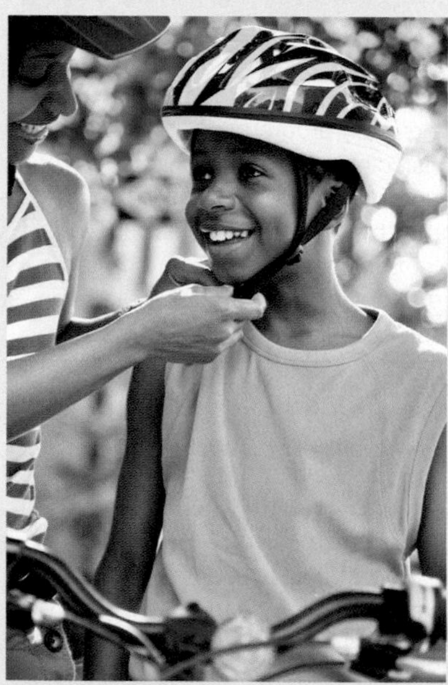

FIGURE 17-6 Wearing a properly fitting helmet is important for bicycle safety.

Adapted from American Academy of Pediatrics: Committee on injury and poison prevention: Bicycle helmets. *Pediatrics, 108*(4), 2013. Retrieved from *www.healthychildren.org/English/safety-prevention/at-play/Pages/Bicycle-Helmets-What-Every-Parent-Should-Know.aspx.*

side effects. This risk is higher in children who watch too much television or play video games instead of engaging in activities that involve movement.

A growing concern that emerges in the school-age years and continues into adolescence is bullying. Bullying can be in the form of verbal taunts, physical abuse, or cyberbullying through e-mail and social media. Parents need to be vigilant in monitoring their children's activities and computer use and be aware when their child exhibits a change in behavior that may indicate feelings of sadness or depression. Bullying can lead to mental health problems including depression, low self-esteem, and suicide in both children and young adults. Emotional support from the nurse along with education about setting safe limits on social media, being able to access their child's accounts for monitoring, and maintaining communication help promote the school-age child's well-being and safety.

The school-age child may continue to have strong food preferences. Children at this age, however, are more open to exploring a variety of foods. It is important that they be offered nutritious choices for meals and snacks, to avoid consumption of empty-calorie snack foods and high-fat fast foods. Parents should encourage children to make good choices by using the U.S. Department of Agriculture (USDA) MyPlate guidelines in planning meals and snacks (USDA, 2014). These dietary guidelines are discussed in detail in Chapter 30. Good oral hygiene and food choices can help prevent tooth decay.

! SAFE PRACTICE ALERT

Children's bones are susceptible to injury or deformity from prolonged or excessive pressure and the pull of strong muscle groups. Talk to parents about limiting the weight of book bags and the possibility of accessing ebooks available from some schools. Backpacks distribute the weight more evenly, reducing strain on growing bones and joints. Specific limits have been set for safe backpack weights and vary by the size of the child.

Toward the end of the school-age period, the child enters preadolescence. During this time, discrepancies in growth patterns and maturation appear between boys and girls. Girls often are taller and heavier than boys.

School-age children delight in developing new skills (see Table 17-8). They gain confidence and a sense of satisfaction from peer interactions and from activities that they can carry through to completion. They enjoy competition and working together to accomplish goals. They become capable of making judgments based on reasoning, rather than on just what they see. Around the ages of 5 to 7 years, children grasp the concept of conservation. This knowledge is transferred to mathematical equations, and children become able to reverse the arrangement to solve problems.

School-age children develop the ability to classify objects. They often enjoy sorting and grouping objects by different characteristics. For example, many children keep collections of items such as rocks, stamps, and stickers.

School-age children in hospitals present some challenges for nurses. Fears are common at this stage, particularly fear of being hurt or of experiencing unknown procedures. Simple explanations before procedures are helpful in alleviating some of these fears. Additionally, separation from peers can be stressful. Encouraging visits, cards, phone conversations, and supervised email and social media activities with friends and family can reduce anxiety and feelings of isolation. Preventive health is important during this time, as immunizations are brought up to date before starting school.

PHYSICAL, PSYCHOSOCIAL, AND COGNITIVE DEVELOPMENT IN ADOLESCENTS LO 17.8

Adolescence is a time of great change, both physically and socially. This period of development is referred to as **puberty**. Hormonal changes that occur with the onset of puberty trigger the process of physical and sexual maturity.

In females, changes include the following:

- Breast enlargement
- Increasing height and weight
- Growth of pubic and axillary hair
- Menarche (onset of menstruation)

In males, changes include the following:

- Enlargement of testicles
- Growth of pubic, axillary, facial, and body hair
- Rapid increase in height
- Changes in larynx, causing lowering of the voice
- Nocturnal emissions

In both males and females, the final 20% to 25% of height generally is achieved during a 24- to 36-month period known as the *adolescent growth spurt*. In females, this usually begins between the ages of 9 and 14 years and ends 1 to 2 years after onset of menstruation. It occurs somewhat later in males, with the onset between the ages of 10 and 16 years and the end between the ages of 18 and 20 years.

Body systems mature, with increased size of the heart and lungs. As the heart and lungs grow to adult size, blood volume and blood components expand with them. The adolescent is better able to meet the physiologic demands of exercise. Subsequently, development of muscle mass and definition is apparent, particularly in males. Health assessment questions should be directed to the adolescent, rather than to parents. Some sample questions are listed in the Health Assessment Questions: Adolescent box.

Nutritional needs increase during adolescence owing to increased rates of growth in height, weight, and muscle mass and with sexual maturation. Caloric and protein needs increase to one of the highest levels during the life span. These increased needs, combined with often hectic schedules, may lead to excessive consumption of high-fat and high-calorie

HEALTH ASSESSMENT QUESTIONS

Adolescent

- What are your favorite activities?
- What do you eat on a normal day?
- Tell me about school.
- Do you have friends?
- Do you get along with your parents? siblings?
- Do you have a boyfriend or girlfriend?
- Are you having sex? If so, what type? How many partners?
- Have you ever used drugs? tobacco products?
- Do you drink alcohol?
- Do you ever feel sad?

snack foods. It is important to be sure that teens avoid skipping meals and have healthy, filling snacks such as fruits and vegetables available. Overeating, fad dieting, and nutritional misinformation are common in this age group. Healthy dietary habits should be discussed with adolescents and periodically reinforced during office visits, at school, and at home. Emphasis should be placed on good nutritional choices and physical activity as means of maintaining a healthy weight. Bulimia and anorexia are psychological problems that develop during adolescence leading to nutrient deficiencies and underweight. Some children may develop obesity due to sedentary lifestyle, overeating of high-fat, high-calorie foods, or psychosocial factors. Obesity can cause problems such as early puberty and premature closure of growth plates. For further discussion of these disorders see Chapter 30.

! SAFE PRACTICE ALERT

Nonthreatening, nonjudgmental approaches work best when nurses are interviewing adolescents about their health practices.

Adolescence is a time of great physical and emotional upheaval. The need for privacy at this stage is very strong. Often, this need is triggered as teens struggle to accept the body image changes associated with adolescence. Adolescents often isolate themselves from the rest of the household in an attempt to exercise their independence and separate from their parents (see Table 17-8). At the same time, peer-group influence peaks (Figure 17-7). Parents are often concerned about maintaining open communication with their teens. Although it may not seem so to them, parents still exert influence in the teen's life. Parents should be guided in exercising appropriate authority in the teen's decisions while encouraging increasing autonomy for the adolescent.

Teens are able to make decisions based on the context of the situation, with consideration of all possible outcomes. However, this does not mean teens will always make good decisions. Teens commonly are exposed to drugs, tobacco, alcohol, and situational influences on sexual behavior. Nurses are in a position to educate teens about the risks of drugs, tobacco, and alcohol use and the consequences of unprotected sex.

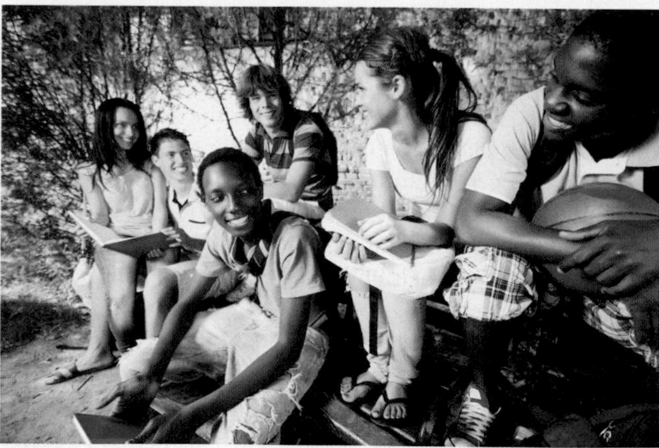

FIGURE 17-7 The adolescent relies on peers for friendship and support.

! SAFE PRACTICE ALERT

Ensure confidentiality and privacy when interviewing adolescents. Conduct the interview without the presence of parents.

Because of the concurrent increase in physical size and ability, teens often develop a false sense of security and invincibility. Injuries, including those from sports accidents, are prominent in this age group. The Centers for Disease Control and Prevention (CDC) (Eaton, Kann, Kinchen, et al, 2012), through its Youth Risk Behavior Surveillance project, monitors health risk behaviors. Behaviors that contribute to the leading causes of death and disability among youths and adults include the following:

- Behaviors that contribute to unintentional injuries and violence
- Sexual behaviors that contribute to unintended pregnancy and sexually transmitted diseases, including HIV
- Alcohol and other drug use
- Tobacco use
- Unhealthy dietary behaviors
- Inadequate physical activity

In the United States, 72% of all deaths among youths and young adults aged 10 to 24 years result from four causes: motor vehicle crashes, other unintentional injuries, homicide, and suicide (CDC, 2012). Teens are experimenting, often with risky behavior. Some may have the feeling that they have to try drugs or sex just to "fit in." Others may feel as if they will never fit in at all. Suicide or suicide attempts may be the result of feelings of inadequacy, depression over bullying or breaking up with a boyfriend or girlfriend, or mental illness. Suicide is also more common in this age group because their impulse control has not fully developed, thus they may act on an impulse without considering the consequences. Early identification of mood pattern changes is important in this age group. Nurses working with the adolescent population should be attuned to signs of depression and suicide. Accidents, particularly those involving motor vehicles, constitute the single most important cause of death in this age group (Patient Education and Health Literacy: Safety Education for Teens box).

Most adolescents who are hospitalized can understand a lot of what is happening to them. Nurses should explain reasons for procedures and treatments in terms that adolescents can understand and should encourage them to ask questions. Both teens and their parents need to be included in the plan of care. Socialization is very important to adolescents, and they should be encouraged to keep in touch with their peers through phone calls, texting, social media, e-mail, or visits.

PATIENT EDUCATION AND HEALTH LITERACY

Safety Education for Teens

Teach teens to do the following:

- Use seat belts at all times.
- Use protective gear such as helmets and long pants when riding all-terrain vehicles (ATVs) and motorcycles.
- Participate in an approved driver education program.
- Avoid texting and other distractions while driving.

SUMMARY OF LEARNING OUTCOMES

LO 17.1 *Describe major theories of human development:* Many theories have evolved to describe human growth and development in cognitive, psychosocial, sexual, behavioral, and spiritual dimensions. Most of these theories outline developmental tasks and/or stages through which the person progresses toward higher levels of functioning.

LO 17.2 *Explain human development from conception to birth:* Conception occurs with fertilization and implantation. The zygote is known as an embryo after 3 weeks and then as a fetus after 8 weeks. Rapid development and cell differentiation occur during the early weeks of pregnancy. The fetus continues to grow and develop until delivery. The developing fetus is susceptible to a variety of teratogens, including certain medications, illegal drugs, alcohol, radiation, and infectious agents.

LO 17.3 *Identify the primary developmental tasks of the newborn:* The primary developmental tasks in the newborn period (birth to 1 month) involve adaptation to life outside the uterus and include learning to eat, developing sleep-wake patterns, and laying the groundwork for trust by having needs consistently met by the caregivers.

LO 17.4 *Outline infant developmental milestones:* The infant period (1 month to 1 year) is marked by rapid growth. Primary developmental tasks include developing trust, adapting to the environment, and beginning refinement of fine and gross motor skills.

LO 17.5 *Describe the physical, psychosocial, and cognitive development of the toddler:* The toddler attains control of bowel and bladder function, increases mobility, refines development of fine and gross motor skills, and expands language acquisition. Safety concerns in the toddler period include protection from injury as the child gains increased mobility in the environment.

LO 17.6 *Summarize growth and development during the preschool years:* Preschoolers develop a sense of initiative as they continue to refine gross and fine motor skills. Safety concerns in this period include protection from injury as preschoolers become more active.

LO 17.7 *Discuss development that occurs during the school-age years:* The school-age child grows in stature and weight and becomes capable of logical thought. Peer relationships exert a greater influence on the school-age child than on children in previous stages. Health and safety concerns in the school-age years include prevention of injury, particularly from play equipment such as bicycles.

LO 17.8 *Articulate physical, psychosocial, and cognitive adolescent development:* Adolescents go through many physical changes. Peers become very important, and adolescents often try to isolate themselves from their parents. Teens make decisions based on the context of the situation and can understand much of what is happening when hospitalized. Safety concerns during the adolescent years include protection from injury. Health concerns include the promotion of a healthy diet and safe sexual practices and the support of mental health as the teen struggles with multiple physiologic and psychological changes.

Responses to the critical-thinking questions are available at *http://evolve.elsevier.com/YoostCrawford/fundamentals/*.

REVIEW QUESTIONS

1. Which action by a 3-month-old infant would the nurse interpret as an example of Piaget's stage of primary circular reaction?
   a. Deliberately placing the thumb into the mouth
   b. Accidentally kicking a ball
   c. Searching for an object under a blanket
   d. Shaking a rattle
2. The mother of a 5-month-old infant is concerned because her child is not yet sitting on his own. What is the nurse's best response to her concerns?
   a. Informing the mother that this is not normal and recommending further evaluation
   b. Telling the mother that this is normal development for a 5-month-old
   c. Encouraging the mother to do sit-ups with the child to encourage muscle development
   d. Asking the mother if the child had any trauma at birth
3. A 1-year-old child grabs an Easter egg and attempts to throw it across the room. The nurse knows that the child is exhibiting which scheme according to Piaget?
   a. Adaptation
   b. Assimilation
   c. Accommodation
   d. Equilibration
4. A preschooler's mother is concerned because her child behaves in a mean fashion toward her younger brother. The mother states, "She acts like she has no sympathy for him!" What is the nurse's best response?
   a. "She is very young to exhibit sibling rivalry."
   b. "What does her brother do to her to make her act this way?"
   c. "Do you fight at home? She is probably imitating you."
   d. "Preschoolers are not capable of putting themselves in another's place."
5. A 2-year-old child insists on having a drink of water, having a story read to him, and says "Good night, sleep tight" at bedtime every night. The nurse knows the child is exhibiting which type of behavior?
   a. Controlling
   b. Ritualism
   c. Obsession
   d. Compulsion
6. How is the toddler's need for autonomy best met?
   a. The parents' consistently meeting the child's needs
   b. Allowing the child limited choices
   c. Encouraging imaginative play
   d. Promoting experimentation to determine cause and effect
7. The nurse is performing a health assessment on a 15-year-old female patient. Which is the best way to obtain accurate information regarding her sexual activity?
   a. Ask the mother about the girl's sexual activity.
   b. Privately ask the girl about her sexual activity.
   c. Warn the girl about the dangers of sexual activity.
   d. Ask the girl if she wants birth control.
8. When an injury to a child is suspicious for abuse, which findings are important to document? *(Select all that apply.)*
   a. Size and location of bruising
   b. Distinguishing characteristics of injuries
   c. Height and weight of the child
   d. Time of last meal
   e. General state of health of the child
9. What is the best activity for a hospitalized school-age child to encourage continued appropriate development?
   a. Watching favorite television shows for 2 hours per day
   b. Keeping a journal of feelings while in the hospital
   c. Working on a paint-by-number project that can be completed in an afternoon
   d. Playing a favorite video game each afternoon
10. A teenage girl faces a long hospitalization after surgery. How can the girl's continued development be fostered?
   a. Encourage her to write her feelings in a journal.
   b. Divert her attention by playing video games.
   c. Encourage her to work on craft projects.
   d. Make sure her parents are constantly by her side.

Answers and rationales for the review questions are available at *http://evolve.elsevier.com/YoostCrawford/fundamentals/*.

REFERENCES

American Academy of Pediatrics: Developmental stages. *Children's health topics*, 2007a Retrieved from *www.aap.org/healthtopics/stages.cfm.*

American Academy of Pediatrics: Evaluation of suspected child abuse. *Pediatrics*, 119(6), 2007b. Retrieved from *http://aappolicy.aappublications.org/cgi/content/full/pediatrics;119/6/1232.*

Bandura A: *Social learning theory*, New York, 1977, General Learning Press.

Centers for Disease Control and Prevention (CDC). Youth risk behavior surveillance—United States, 2011. *MMWR, Surveillance Summaries, 61*(4). Atlanta, 2012, Author.

Cronenwett L, Sherwood G, Barnsteiner J, et al: Quality and safety education for nurses. *Nurs Outlook*, 55(3):122-131, 2007.

Eaton DK, Kann L, Kinchen S, et al: Youth risk behavior surveillance—United States, 2011. *MMWR Surveill Summ*, 61(4):1-162, 2012.

Erikson EH: *Childhood and society*, ed. 2, New York, 1963, Norton.

Freud S: *The ego and the id*, London, England, 1974, Hogarth (original work published 1923).

Havighurst R: *Developmental tasks and education*, New York, 1972, Random House.

Kohlberg L: *Child psychology and childhood education: A cognitive-developmental view*, New York, 1987, Longman.

London ML, Ladewig PW, Davidson MC, et al: *Maternal and child nursing care*, ed. 4, Upper Saddle River, NJ, 2014, Pearson Prentice Hall.

National Highway Traffic Safety Administration: *Car seat recommendations for children. 4 Steps flyer.* Washington, D.C., 2011, Author.

National Institutes of Health: *Sudden infant death syndrome.* National Institute of Child Health and Human Development, 2014. Retrieved from *www.nlm.nih.gov/medlineplus/suddeninfantdeathsyndrome.html.*

Piaget J: *The theory of stages in cognitive development*, New York, 1969, McGraw-Hill.

Skinner BF: *Science and human behavior*, New York, 1953/1969, Free Press.

U.S. Department of Agriculture: Dietary guidelines for Americans, 2014. Retrieved from *www.choosemyplate.gov/food-groups.*

Westerhoff J: *Will our children have faith?* rev ed. 3, New York, 2012, Morehouse.

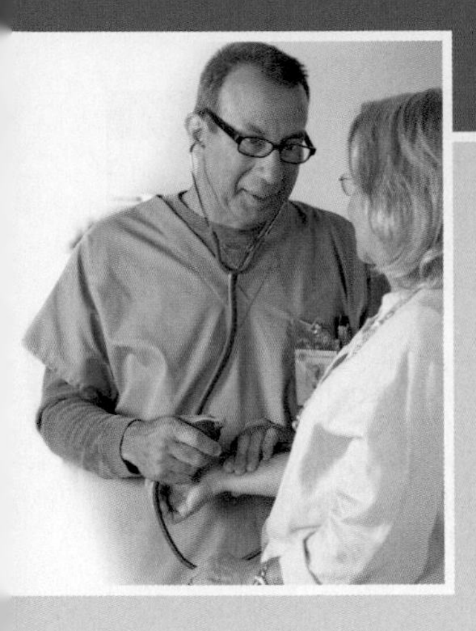

CHAPTER 18

Human Development: Young Adult Through Older Adult

EVOLVE WEBSITE

http://evolve.elsevier.com/YoostCrawford/fundamentals/

- Additional Evolve-Only Review Questions With Answers
- Answers and Rationales for Text Review Questions
- Answers to Critical-Thinking Exercises
- Case Study With Questions
- Conceptual Care Map Creator
- Glossary

LEARNING OUTCOMES

Comprehension of this chapter content will provide students with the ability to:

LO 18.1 Discuss theories on aging and adult development.
LO 18.2 Describe changes that occur as the body ages.
LO 18.3 Identify physiologic, cognitive, emotional, and social changes that affect the young adult.
LO 18.4 Articulate health risks and concerns for the young adult.
LO 18.5 Summarize the physiologic, cognitive, emotional, and social changes that occur in the middle adult age group.
LO 18.6 Explain health risks and concerns for the middle adult.
LO 18.7 Recognize the physiologic, cognitive, emotional, and social changes that affect the older adult.
LO 18.8 Outline health risks and concerns for the older adult.

KEY TERMS

adaptive cognition, p. 263
angina pectoris, p. 272
angioplasty, p. 272
arrhythmia, p. 272
atherosclerosis, p. 272
Cross-Linking Theory of Aging, p. 259
crystallized intelligence, p. 270
dualistic thinking, p. 262
emerging adulthood, p. 262
fluid intelligence, p. 270
free radicals, p. 259
generativity, p. 270
life expectancy, p. 258
myocardial infarction (MI), p. 272
postformal thought, p. 262
relativist thinking, p. 262
sandwich generation, p. 274
sarcopenia, p. 270
senescence, p. 258
skipped generation, p. 273
stagnation, p. 271
Wear-and-Tear Theory of Aging, p. 258

CASE STUDY

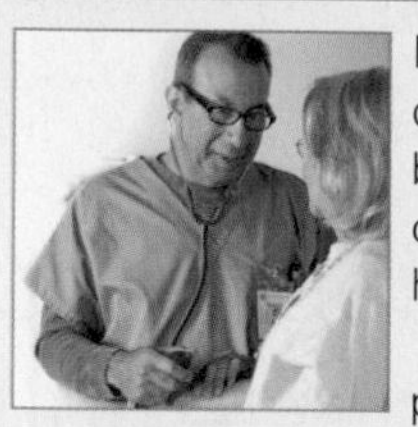

Ms. Dubois is a 58-year-old woman who has spent the past 2 years caring for her 82-year-old mother who had dementia. Ms. Dubois, who is divorced, had a managerial position in a corporate office with a good salary and benefits. She tried to continue working while caring for her mother, but eventually resigned her position and cared for her mother full time until her mother's death 3 months ago. While caring for her mother, she used her personal savings and borrowed from her retirement savings.

After her mother died, Ms. Dubois was unable to get another job at the same managerial level as that of her previous position. She took a job that pays an hourly wage with minimal health insurance benefits and a retirement plan to which employees can contribute.

Ms. Dubois came to her primary care provider's office complaining of a throbbing headache, swelling in her feet, and dizziness. She stated that she feels restless. Multiple BP readings taken by the nurse were above 160/100. Vital signs were T 36.6° C (97.9° F), P 96 and regular, R 22 and unlabored, pulse oximetry 97% on room air, height 160 cm (5 ft 3 in.) and weight 66.2 kg (198 lb), and head pain level 6 on a scale of 0 to 10. She had pitting edema of her ankles and feet. Ms. Dubois was diagnosed with hypertension, uncontrolled.

Patient teaching and outpatient plan are as follows:

- Low-sodium, low-calorie diet
- Referral to social service/grief counseling
- Exercise program
- Stress management/relaxation program
- Patient education: hypertension

Laboratory/diagnostic test orders are as follows:

- Laboratory studies pending: CBC, BUN, serum electrolytes, creatinine, fasting lipid panel, and urinalysis
- Chest x-ray
- 12-lead ECG

Medication orders are as follows:

- Hydrochlorothiazide 25 mg PO once daily
- Metoprolol 50 mg PO twice a day
- Tylenol 500 mg two tablets q 6 hr PRN

Refer back to this case study to answer the critical-thinking questions throughout the chapter.

Adulthood is divided into three age groups: young adulthood, middle adulthood, and older adulthood. Young adulthood spans the ages of 18 to 34 years; middle adulthood includes people 35 to 65 years of age; and older adulthood includes those 66 years of age and beyond. At each stage, the person is tasked with achieving specific developmental milestones. Various researchers have developed theories and specified tasks that can be identified as evidence of transition through these life stages.

THEORIES ON AGING AND ADULT DEVELOPMENT LO 18.1

Biologic aging, or **senescence**, is defined as a normal physiologic process that occurs at the cellular and molecular levels and is universal and irreversible (McCance and Heuther, 2014). This process is the genetically influenced decline in the functioning of organs and systems that is universal in all living creatures. It can occur asynchronously, with some organ systems aging faster than others. Individual differences are great owing to genetics, lifestyle, stress, and culture. **Life expectancy** is the average number of years of life remaining at a given age. Life expectancy varies by gender, culture, and socioeconomic status and from country to country.

Loss of hormones, as the endocrine system gradually fails, contributes to aging. Menopause affects many body functions. A drop in growth hormone leads to loss of muscle and bone mass, additional fat, thinning of the skin, and a decline in cardiovascular function. Diet and physical exercise can slow some of these effects. Hormone therapy can reduce the loss of growth hormone, but side effects include risk of cancer. Declines in immune system function lead to susceptibility to infections, risk of cancer, and changes in blood vessel walls.

WEAR-AND-TEAR THEORY

The **Wear-and-Tear Theory of Aging** proposed that the body wears out from hard use. This theory was first introduced in 1882 by Dr. August Weismann, a German biologist. He believed that the body and its cells are damaged by overuse and abuse. The organs and organ systems are worn down by the adverse effects of toxins in the diet and in the environment; excessive consumption of fat, sugar, caffeine, alcohol, and nicotine; the ultraviolet rays of the sun; and the many other physical and emotional stresses to which the body is subjected. Wear and tear is not confined to organs; it also takes place on the cellular level (Moody, 2010). Biologic changes occur at both the DNA/cellular level and the organ system level.

AGING AT THE LEVEL OF DNA AND BODY CELLS

Cells vary in shape, size, and function; however, they all endure the aging process. According to McCance and Heuther (2014), it is difficult to determine the physiologic changes from the pathologic changes of aging. Areas of primary focus in the biology of aging include endocrine regulation through endocrine signaling pathways, nuclear architecture, genomic instability, decline in cell renewal by adult stem cells, and accumulation of cellular damage related to cancer and aging (McCance and Heuther, 2014). Cellular changes related to aging include atrophy, cell loss, and decreased cellular function. Loss of cellular function leads to hypertrophy and to hyperplasia of the remaining cells. DNA and RNA in aged cells are susceptible to injurious stimuli, increasing the cells' demise. Research suggests that in the aged cell the processes of DNA repair, which usually occur over time, are decreased, leading to the cells' being susceptible to mutations and neoplasia (McCance and Heuther, 2014). Theories that emphasize the cumulative effects of random events suggest that DNA is gradually damaged owing to changes in the DNA caused by internal or external forces. This leads to mutations that accumulate, and thus cell repair becomes less efficient or cancerous cells develop.

Free radicals are one cause of cellular abnormalities. They are naturally occurring, highly reactive chemicals that form in the presence of oxygen. These by-products of molecular oxygen chemical reactions can cause harmful alterations in cellular function similar to those seen in aging. Free radicals are related to many disorders of aging, including cancer, cataracts, heart disease, and arthritis. Antioxidants, vitamins C and E, and beta carotene can limit this damage.

CROSS-LINKING THEORY OF AGING

The **Cross-Linking Theory of Aging** also is referred to as the *Glycosylation Theory of Aging.* The Cross-Linking Theory of Aging suggests that, over time, protein fibers that make up the body's connective tissue form bonds, or links, with one another. When these normally separate fibers cross-link, tissue becomes less elastic, leading to negative outcomes such as loss of flexibility, clouding of the lens of the eye, clogged arteries, and damaged kidneys (Bjorksten, 1968). The longer a person lives, the greater the possibility that cross-linking will occur, causing certain disorders.

GOULD'S THEORY ON ADULT DEVELOPMENT

In his book *Transformations,* Roger Gould (1979) describes adulthood as a stage of life during which people dismantle protective devices that gave them an illusion of safety as children. Gould postulates that this is a process of freeing oneself from childhood restraints and beginning the establishment of personal identity. According to Gould, this transformation occurs in a series of stages divided into the following age groups:

- Ages 18 to 22 years: leaving the parents' world
- Ages 22 to 28 years: getting into the adult world
- Ages 28 to 34 years: questioning and reexamination
- Ages 34 to 43 years: midlife decade
- Ages 43 to 50 years: reconciliation and mellowing
- Ages 50 to 60 years: stability and acceptance

Gould (1979) also identifies the following four false assumptions that adults need to resolve during their lifetimes:

1. "I'll always live with my parents and be their child."
2. "I'll always be there to help when my parents can't do things on their own."
3. "Life is simple, and I can control it."
4. "Death and evil are not real."

Gould's theory assumes that people are redefining their identities as they take on adult roles and the related task of adulthood.

PHYSICAL CHANGES DUE TO AGING LO 18.2

As aging occurs, the body goes through physical changes that are universal and irreversible. The changes that occur during young adulthood often go unnoticed. Many age-related functions peak before age 30 and gradually decline thereafter. Certain physical changes that may lead to illness and disease begin to take shape during young adulthood if prevention and wellness are not a specific focus of self-care. Disorders, rather than normal aging, appear to be the primary cause of functional loss during old age. In many cases, declines that occur with aging may be due, at least in part, to environmental factors, lifestyle behaviors, and diet. Table 18-1 highlights some of the normative changes seen with aging.

YOUNG ADULTHOOD: AGES 18 TO 34 LO 18.3

Compared to past generations, individuals transitioning into young adulthood today have more options to consider as they branch out from the protective shelter of their parents' homes. Some of the issues they face are decisions about college, vocational choices, gender identity and sexual preference, and gender stereotypes (e.g., men who choose nontraditional careers). In 2009, young adults accounted for 35.4% of the labor force in the United States (U.S. Census Bureau, 2011). Between 2006 and 2009 the annual average health care expenditure among young adults was $2400, which was spent on health care insurance, medical services, drugs, and medical supplies (U.S. Census Bureau, 2011).

TABLE 18-1 Physical Changes Associated With Normal Aging

BODY SYSTEM	PHYSICAL CHANGES
Bones and joints	Bones become less dense so are weaker and more likely to break. In women, loss of bone density speeds up after menopause because less estrogen is produced.
Muscles and body fat	Loss of muscle mass begins around age 30 and continues throughout life. Muscles are used less and begin to shrink, and the levels of growth hormone and testosterone, which stimulate muscle development, decrease.
Eyes	The lens of the eye stiffens, making focusing on close objects harder. The lens becomes denser, making seeing in dim light more difficult. The pupil reacts more slowly to changes in light. The lens yellows, changing the way colors are perceived. The number of nerve cells decreases, impairing depth perception. The eyes produce less fluid, making them feel dry.
Ears	Changes in hearing are due to noise exposure and to aging. Exposure to loud noise over time damages the ear's structures involved in the ability to hear. Some changes in hearing occur as people age, regardless of their exposure to loud noise. As people age, hearing high-pitched sounds becomes more difficult. This change is considered age-associated hearing loss (presbycusis).
Mouth and nose	As people age, taste buds on the tongue decrease in number and sensitivity. This change affects tasting sweet and salt more than bitter and sour. The ability to smell diminishes because the lining of the nose becomes thinner and drier and the nerve endings in the nose deteriorate.
Skin	The skin becomes thinner, less elastic, drier, and finely wrinkled. However, exposure to sunlight contributes to wrinkling and to making the skin rough and blotchy. The fat layer under the skin thins. This layer acts as a protective cushion for the skin, and helps conserve body heat.
Brain and nervous system	The number of nerve cells in the brain decreases with aging. However, the brain can partly compensate for this loss in several ways: • As cells are lost, new connections are made between the remaining nerve cells. • New nerve cells may form in some areas of the brain, even during old age. • The brain has more neural pathways than it needs to do most activities—a characteristic called *redundancy*. Nerve cells may lose some of their receptors for messages. Blood flow to the brain decreases.
Heart and blood vessels	The heart and blood vessels become stiffer. The heart fills with blood more slowly. The stiffer arteries are less able to expand when blood is pumped through them. Thus blood pressure increases.
Muscles of breathing and the lungs	The muscles used in breathing weaken. The number of air sacs (alveoli) and capillaries in the lungs decreases. Thus slightly less oxygen is absorbed from air that is breathed in. The lungs become less elastic.
Digestive system	The digestive system is less affected by aging than most parts of the body. The muscles of the esophagus contract less forcefully, but movement of food through the esophagus normally is not affected. Food is emptied from the stomach more slowly, and the stomach cannot hold as much food because it is less elastic. In the large intestine, materials move through a little more slowly. The liver becomes smaller because the number of cells decreases and less blood flows through it. Liver enzymes that help the body process drugs and other substances work less efficiently.
Kidneys and urinary tract	The kidneys become smaller because the number of cells decreases. Less blood flows through them, and by the age of approximately 30 years, they begin to filter blood less efficiently. They may excrete too much water and too little salt as aging occurs, making dehydration more likely.
Reproductive organs	*Women:* The effects of aging on sex hormone levels are more obvious in women than in men. In women, most of these effects are related to menopause, when the levels of female hormones (particularly estrogen) decrease, menstrual periods end permanently, and pregnancy is no longer possible. The decrease in female hormone levels causes the ovaries and uterus to shrink. The tissues of the vagina become thinner, drier, and less elastic (a condition called *atrophic vaginitis*). *Men:* In men, changes in sex hormone levels are less sudden. Levels of the male hormone testosterone decrease, resulting in fewer sperm and a decreased sex drive (libido), but the decrease is gradual. Although blood flow to the penis tends to decrease, many men can have erections and orgasms throughout life. However, erections may not last as long, may be slightly less rigid, or may require more stimulation to maintain. Erectile dysfunction (impotence) becomes more common as men age.

TABLE 18-1 Physical Changes Associated With Normal Aging—cont'd

BODY SYSTEM	PHYSICAL CHANGES
Endocrine system	The levels and activity of some hormones, produced by endocrine glands, decrease. Growth hormone levels decrease, leading to decreased muscle mass. Aldosterone levels decrease, making dehydration more likely. Insulin is less effective, and less insulin may be produced. The changes in insulin mean that the sugar level increases more after a large meal and takes longer to return to normal. For most people, the changes in the endocrine system have no noticeable effect on overall health. But in some, the changes may increase the risk of health problems. For example, the changes in insulin increase the risk of type 2 diabetes.
Immune system	The cells of the immune system act more slowly. These cells identify and destroy foreign substances such as bacteria, other infecting microbes, and probably cancer cells. This immune slowdown may partly explain several findings associated with aging: • Cancer is more common among older people. • Vaccines tend to be less protective in older people. • Infections, such as pneumonia and influenza, are more common among older people and result in death more often. • Allergy symptoms may become less severe.

Adapted from Porter RS, Kaplan JL (Eds): Changes in the body, *Merck Manual Online*, 2013. Retrieved from *www.merckmanuals.com/professional/index.html*.

AGE GROUP CHARACTERISTICS

The transition phase from adolescence to young adulthood, for people 18 to 34, is marked by many changes physically, psychologically, and socially. Approximately 27% of the population is between the ages of 18 and 34 years. A career, marriage, and economic independence are the signal for many that they have reached adulthood. Taking on career, household, and financial responsibilities brings a set of stressors for young adults, who often are inexperienced in dealing with these new issues. This experience is influenced by cultural and societal values, beliefs, and expectations, which make the journey an individual experience that cannot be ascribed to everyone in this age group. Little is normative, or socially expected, during this time, so routes to adult roles and responsibilities are highly diverse (Coté, 2006).

Significant cultural, economic, and demographic changes have occurred in the span of a few generations, and these changes are challenging youths' psychological and social development. Some are adapting well and choosing educational or vocational paths. Others struggle with this transition period in which definitive decisions about work, school, and life may be constrained by lack of education, early parenthood, and low-paying jobs or unemployment (Berlin, Furstenberg, and Waters, 2010; Schulenberg, Bryant, and O'Malley, 2004). This transition phase may be marked by periods of experimentation with drugs, multiple casual or intimate relationships, and reckless behaviors that can and may have untoward consequences (Berk, 2011). Young adults may find themselves needing assistance from family, friends, their community, and society to successfully complete this phase of life. Some U.S. Census Bureau statistics for this age group are cited in the Diversity Considerations box.

DIVERSITY CONSIDERATIONS

The following are statistics collected by the U.S. Census Bureau in 2011 for marriage and educational diversity in the young adult age group:

Life Span

- Among people aged 25 to 34 years, 88.4% held a high school diploma or higher.
- Among high school graduates, 70% enrolled in college the year after graduating, compared with 60% in 1990 and 52% in 1970.
- Advanced degrees were attained by 8.9% of people aged 25 to 34.

Gender

- Age 20 to 24: 10.8% of males were married, compared with 19.2% of females.
- Age 25 to 29: 34.7% of males were married, compared with 47.6% of females.
- Age 30 to 34: 57.1% of males were married, compared with 63.8% of females.

From the U.S. Census Bureau, *Statistical abstract of the United States: 2012*, ed. 131, Washington, D.C., 2011, Author. Retrieved from *www.census.gov/compendia/statab*.

EMERGING ADULTHOOD

In generations past, the transition to adulthood occurred rapidly. Enrollment in higher education and marriage were goals set in late adolescence, and high school graduation marked the beginning of the pathway to those goals. As recently as the late 1970s and early 1980s, the typical 21- to 22-year-old was engaged to be married or already married, caring for a newborn child or expecting one soon, about to graduate from college or done with education, or settled into a long-term job or full-time motherhood. Young adults grew up quickly and made serious, enduring choices about their lives at a relatively early age.

Today there is a much slower transition to adulthood, marked by indecision and lack of commitment to one fixed goal in life. This prolonged transition phase is now being called **emerging adulthood**. The life of a typical 21-year-old is quite different from that of his or her counterpart 40 or 50 years ago. Marriage is at least 5 to 10 years in the future. Some individuals begin parenting during this transition phase, but the commitment to marriage may be on hold until a later time. Education is often extended; the average undergraduate enrollment period is now 5 to 6 years in length, and the pursuit of graduate and/or professional school often follows. Changing jobs occurs frequently, as emerging adults look for work that pays well and is personally fulfilling.

According to Arnett (2006), the explorations of emerging adults and their shifting choices in love and work make emerging adulthood an exceptionally full and intense period of life but an unstable one. From the late teens to the late 20s, a prolonged exploration of the possibilities available in love and work precedes commitment to enduring choices. To be a young-adult American today is to experience excitement and uncertainty, wide-open possibility and confusion, and new freedoms and fears (Arnett, 2006).

PHYSICAL DEVELOPMENT IN YOUNG ADULTHOOD

The young-adult stage is full of major changes in both physical and cognitive attributes. The body has finished fully developing, and the thinking process is carried out in a more complex manner. It is during this developmental stage that young adults can contemplate the views of another and put themselves in the other's place to gain a better understanding, thus achieving mature empathy.

During the young adult phase of life, individuals reach their peak growth physically. Young adults are at top physical condition between their late teens and early 30s, after which they may start to slow down physically and mentally (Figure 18-1).

This is an opportune time to do a complete assessment of the individual's lifestyle, emphasizing wellness, health-promotion activities, and disease prevention for those individuals who see a health care provider on a regular basis. Areas that are assessed include family history, mental health, environmental and work-related exposures to hazardous materials, military service, and travel abroad, as these activities can expose individuals to health hazards. Assessment of lifestyle includes such sensitive issues as sexual orientation, safe-sex practices, sexually transmitted diseases (STDs), pregnancy prevention, domestic and intimate partner violence, and substance use and abuse.

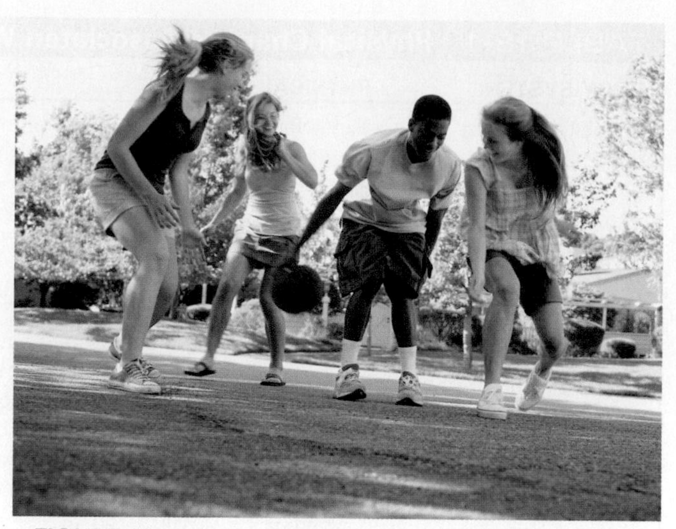

FIGURE 18-1 Young adults engaged in physical activity.

CHANGES IN COGNITIVE DEVELOPMENT

Cognitive abilities are strong during young adulthood. Also typical is an increase in rational-thinking, motor, conceptual, and problem-solving skills as a result of formal education, occupational training, and overall life experiences.

According to Piaget (1969), by this stage the person no longer requires concrete objects to make rational judgments. The young adult is capable of deductive and hypothetical reasoning and has an ability for abstract thinking very similar to that of the more mature adult. For more information on Piaget's theory, see Chapter 17.

Postformal thought is cognitive development past Piaget's formal operational stage. William Perry, a professor of education at Harvard University, studied college students to understand development during the college years. Perry (1981) found that students gradually changed their thinking in the face of reality and adult responsibility. He found that young adults engage in **dualistic thinking**, or dividing information, values, and authority into right and wrong, good and bad, "we" and "they." Truth is compared against abstract standards, and authority figures are respected simply because of their authority base.

In Perry's scheme, students have a nine-stage progression from dualistic to **relativist thinking**. Learners move from viewing truth in absolute terms of right and wrong (obtained from "good" or "bad" authorities) to recognizing multiple, conflicting versions of "truth" representing legitimate alternatives. The intent of the original research was to describe students' experience during the college years (Perry, 1981). Relativistic thinking occurs as students age and become aware of the diversity of opinions on any topic. Knowledge is seen as being embedded in a framework of thought. Truth is seen as being relative, based on context, rather than absolute. Thinking becomes more flexible, tolerant, and realistic. This transition in thinking may be unique to people pursuing extended education, with the diversity of opinions that they encounter in that environment. The underlying theme is **adaptive cognition**, in which thought is more responsive to context and less constrained by the need to find only one answer to a question (Berk, 2011).

Young adults are faced with many difficult decisions that involve relationship issues, home life, and work or occupation. An understanding of theories of cognitive development and learning regarding young adults allows the nurse to individualize patient education on the basis of knowledge of young-adult cognitive functioning.

PRIMARY DEVELOPMENTAL TASKS

Many theories offer help in understanding human development and the tasks associated with stages of development. According to the life span perspective, no age period is superior to another in terms of impact on the life course. The psychoanalytic perspective hypothesizes that individuals progress through a series of stages in which they confront conflicts between biologic and social expectations. The resolution of these conflicts determines the individual's ability to thrive. Conversely, those individuals who experience a life trauma during a developmental stage may have greater difficulty overcoming the conflicts specific to that stage even as the individual may have success achieving resolution in future stages.

According to Sigmund Freud (1923/1974), an individual's basic personality is developed during the preschool years as relations between the id, ego, and superego are established. Freud's theory has been criticized for its overemphasis on sexual feelings in child development. It should be noted that Freud's patients were not children but adults, who were asked to recall events that may have occurred very early in life. Adults are in what Freud called the *genital stage,* which occurs from puberty onward. Sexual feelings are reawakened. When conflicts from previous stages reemerge and are resolved, the individual is able to develop a mature adult relationship. See Chapter 17 for more information on Freud's theory.

According to Erikson, the initial stage of being an adult is intimacy versus isolation. Work is done on establishing intimate relationships with others. Young adults try to find satisfying relationships, primarily through marriage and friends, and many start a family. In today's society, family life may begin much later, with many individuals not having children until their late 30s. If people are able to negotiate this stage successfully, intimacy is experienced on a deeper level. For some, because of earlier disappointments in life, this intimacy is not achieved, resulting in isolation or limited interpersonal relationships (Erikson, 1963). Erikson explained that culture and life situations impact development. See Chapter 17 for more information on Erikson's theory.

For the young adult, Havighurst (1953) identifies the following developmental tasks:

- Achieving new and more mature relations with age-mates of both sexes
- Achieving a masculine or feminine social role
- Accepting one's physique and using the body effectively
- Achieving emotional independence of parents and other adults
- Preparing for marriage and family life
- Acquiring a set of values and an ethical system as a guide to behavior
- Desiring and achieving socially responsible behavior
- Selecting an occupation

See Chapter 17 for more information on Havighurst's theory in the context of development in childhood and adolescence.

PSYCHOSOCIAL CHANGES IN YOUNG ADULTHOOD

Young adulthood is a time of dramatic change in personal relationships. Young adults seek emotional and physical intimacy in relationships with peers and romantic partners. Self-disclosure and a sense of belonging are important aspects of intimacy. Intimate relationships are associated with physical and mental health. Although the Internet, social media, and smartphone use offer expanded opportunities for communication, lack of personal contact may lead to a weakening of intimacy and a decline in psychological well-being. Most young adults have friends but have increasingly limited time to spend with them. Women's friendships usually are more intimate than men's. Attitudes toward premarital sex have been greatly liberalized, but men and women are less promiscuous than is sometimes believed.

LIFESTYLES

Many nontraditional family options are seen in the United States as people postpone marriage or chose to cohabit. The traditional family design still exists but has gone through some transformations over the years. Reasons for evolution of nontraditional lifestyles vary in accordance with environment, life situation, socioeconomic level, and relevant legislation. Many young adults have postponed marriage until educational goals are met or career objectives accomplished. Being single can afford opportunities to travel for work and pleasure.

During these changing times, young adults face many stressors that may have an adverse impact on their lives. Attention is focused on the attainment of higher education and jobs that pay well in an attempt to improve lifestyle. With today's economic downtrends, increases in unemployment, and corporate downsizing, many college graduates are forced to accept employment in positions that are less fulfilling and for pay that will meet only basic needs. These factors and others require that family and friends provide financial and social support to sustain young adults.

HEALTH RISKS AND CONCERNS DURING YOUNG ADULTHOOD LO 18.4

The challenge for nurses in planning and delivering care is to adequately account for how factors such as age, gender, race, culture, lifestyle, and religious practices influence young adults' lives. Thus strategies must be in place to address these influences as part of the provision of health care for young adults. The focus of nurses providing care for young adults should be on identifying factors that lead to unhealthy lifestyles and increase the risks of illness and injury.

HEALTH RISKS DURING YOUNG ADULTHOOD

As parental and other adult oversight decreases, young people assume increasing responsibility for their own decisions. These decisions include those that will directly affect their current and future health status—such as alcohol, cigarette, and illicit drug use; sexual activity; childbearing; exercise; and eating habits—as well as decisions that will indirectly affect their future health (National Center for Health Statistics, 2013).

Cigarette Smoking and Alcohol Use

By age 19 young adults can legally purchase tobacco in all 50 states, and by age 21 they can legally purchase alcohol. Among young adults, approximately 20% are cigarette smokers (Centers for Disease Control and Prevention [CDC], 2012a). E-cigarettes are growing in popularity and the health effects are not yet known.

Alcohol use contributes to increased mortality from unintentional injuries, including motor vehicle accidents while people are driving under the influence. Drinking in excess and binge drinking can cause immediate danger and long-term effects. For example, alcohol consumption accounts for 50% of all cases of pancreatitis. Holiday syndrome is another acute condition related to alcohol consumption; this syndrome occurs generally after individuals engage in binge drinking over a period of time. Withdrawal of alcohol can result in atrial and ventricular arrhythmias of the heart. Acute skeletal myopathy can occur after an individual consumes large amounts of alcohol. Chronic alcohol consumption can result in esophageal varices, erosive gastritis, cirrhosis of the liver, and hepatitis.

Illicit Drug Use

Use of illicit drugs—such as marijuana, heroin, cocaine (including crack cocaine), methamphetamine, hallucinogens, and other illegal drugs used recreationally—and nonmedical use of prescription drugs—such as pain relievers, stimulants, and depressants—is associated with serious health and social consequences. These include injury, illness, disability, and death, as well as crime, domestic violence, and lost school or workplace productivity (U.S. Department of Health and Human Services, 2010). Table 18-2 lists commonly abused drugs and the side effects of overuse and abuse of these drugs. Nurses need to ask young adults about illicit drug use and know the signs and symptoms of overuse and abuse of the most commonly used drugs.

Other drugs abused by young adults include anabolic steroids, which can have serious side effects, and inhalants such as glues and gases, which can cause neurologic impairment and death. Education about the harmful aspects of drug, alcohol, and tobacco use should be provided at every health care visit.

In 2012, the rate of current illicit drug use in 18- to 25-year-olds was 21.3%. Levels in the 18-to-25 age group were higher than those among teenagers younger than 18 years or people 30 years of age and older (Substance Abuse and Mental Health Services Administration, 2013). Marijuana and hashish were the most commonly reported illicit drugs. Almost one third of 18- to 20-year-olds reported marijuana use in the past year and nearly one fifth in the past month.

Prescription drugs used for nonmedical purposes were the next most commonly reported illicit drugs; this category included pain relievers, tranquilizers, stimulants, and sedatives but not over-the-counter (OTC) drugs. Of young adults 18 to 29 years of age, 11% to 17% reported using prescription drugs for nonmedical reasons in the past year (Substance Abuse and Mental Health Services Administration, 2013).

! SAFE PRACTICE ALERT

Always ask patients about their use of alcohol, nicotine products, and recreational drugs such as marijuana, cocaine, crack, and heroin. Use of these substances has increased among young adults, thereby increasing the risk of associated diseases.

Intimate Partner Violence and Sexual Violence

Intimate partner and domestic violence, dating violence, and sexual violence are pervasive problems in the United States and other countries. Abuse can result in death or injuries, or in mistrust or a shattered sense of well-being that is a barrier to moving forward in life for some victims. Sexual violence may result in unwanted pregnancy. The United States has made progress in the last few decades in addressing this type of violence, resulting in a decline in its occurrence, but more work needs to be done to implement strategies to end it. Younger generations should be taught that exposure to violence in movies or video games and on television may influence behaviors negatively in the future. Health care providers need training to assess patients for signs of abuse. Workplace prevention and victim support programs are needed, with the goal of making services available to all. On average, more than three women are murdered each day by their husbands or

TABLE 18-2 Commonly Abused Drugs

SUBSTANCE CATEGORY WITH DRUG NAMES	SOME COMMERCIAL AND STREET NAMES	DEA SCHEDULE AND HOW DRUG IS USED	INTOXICATION EFFECTS AND POTENTIAL HEALTH PROBLEMS
Cannabinoids • Marijuana • Hashish	*Marijuana:* blunt, dope, grass, herb, joints, Mary Jane, pot, reefer, weed, boom, chronic, gangster, hemp *Hashish:* hash, hash oil	Schedule I Swallowed, smoked	Increased heart rate, anxiety; panic attacks; euphoria, slowed thinking and reaction time, confusion, impaired balance and coordination; impaired memory and learning; cough, frequent respiratory infections; tolerance, addiction
Opioids and morphine derivatives • Codeine • Fentanyl • Heroin • Morphine • Oxycodone • Hydrocodone	*Codeine:* Captain Cody, schoolboy; *with glutethimide:* doors and fours, loads, pancakes and syrup *Fentanyl (Actiq, Duragesic, Sublimaze):* Apache, China girl, China white, dance fever, friend, goodfella, jackpot, murder 8, TNT, Tango and Cash *Heroin:* brown sugar, dope, H, horse, junk, skag, skunk, smack, white horse *Morphine sulfate (Roxanol, Duramorph):* M, Miss Emma, monkey, white stuff *Oxycodone (Oxycontin):* Oxy, O.C., killer *Hydrocodone-acetaminophen (Vicodin):* vike, Watson-387	Schedules II, III, IV, V Injected, swallowed	Respiratory depression and arrest; euphoria, drowsiness, confusion, sedation, unconsciousness, coma, death; nausea, constipation; tolerance, addiction
Stimulants • Amphetamine • Cocaine • DOM (dimethoxy-methylamphetamine) MDMA (methylenedioxy-methamphetamine) • Methylphenidate • Nicotine	*Amphetamine (Dexedrine), amphetamine-dextroamphetamine (Biphetamine)* *Adderall:* bennies, black beauties, crosses, hearts, LA turnaround, speed, truck drivers, uppers *Cocaine hydrochloride:* blow, bump, C, candy, Charlie, coke, crack, flake, rock, snow, toot *MDMA:* Adam, clarity, ecstasy, Eve, lover's speed, peace *DOM:* STP, X, XTC *Methylphenidate (Ritalin):* JIF, MPH, R-ball, Skippy, the smart drug, vitamin R *Nicotine:* cigarettes, cigars, smokeless tobacco, snuff, spit tobacco, chew	Schedule II Injected, swallowed, smoked, snorted, chewed	Rapid or irregular heart beat, increased blood pressure, heart failure, cardiovascular disease, stroke; increased metabolism; feelings of exhilaration, energy, increased mental alertness, nervousness, insomnia, tremor, loss of coordination; impulsive behavior, aggressiveness, psychosis, panic attacks, mild hallucinogenic effects, headaches; reduced appetite, weight loss; adverse pregnancy outcomes; chronic lung disease, seizures, cancer; tolerance, addiction
Hallucinogens • LSD (lysergic acid diethylamide) • Mescaline • Psilocybin	*LSD:* acid, blotter, boomers, cubes, microdot, yellow sunshines *Mescaline:* buttons, cactus, mesc, peyote *Psilocybin:* magic mushroom, purple passion, shrooms	Schedule I Swallowed, absorbed through oral tissues	Altered states of perception and feeling, nausea, persisting perception disorder (flashbacks) *Also for LSD and mescaline:* increased body temperature, heart rate, blood pressure; loss of appetite, sleeplessness, numbness, weakness, tremors, persistent mental disorders

Continued

TABLE 18-2 Commonly Abused Drugs—cont'd

SUBSTANCE CATEGORY WITH DRUG NAMES	SOME COMMERCIAL AND STREET NAMES	DEA SCHEDULE AND HOW DRUG IS USED	INTOXICATION EFFECTS AND POTENTIAL HEALTH PROBLEMS
Sedatives (depressants, hypnotics, tranquilizers) • Barbiturates • Benzodiazepines (other than flunitrazepam) • Flunitrazepam GBH (gamma-hydroxybutyrate)	*Barbiturates (Amytal, Nembutal, Seconal, phenobarbital):* barbs, reds, red birds, phennies, tooies, yellows, yellow jackets *Benzodiazepines (Ativan, Halcion, Librium, Valium, Xanax):* candy, downers, sleeping pills, trank *Flunitrazepam (Rohypnol):* forget-me pill, Mexican Valium, R2, Roche, roofies, roofinol, rope, rophies *GBH:* G, Georgia home boy, grievous bodily harm, liquid ecstasy	Schedules II, III, IV, V Injected, swallowed	Slowed pulse and breathing, lowered blood pressure; reduced anxiety, feeling of well-being, lowered inhibitions; poor concentration/fatigue, confusion; impaired coordination, memory, judgment; addiction

DEA, Drug Enforcement Agency.
From National Institute on Drug Abuse: Commonly abused drugs, 2011. Retrieved from *www.drugabuse.gov.*

boyfriends in the United States (Catalano, 2007). In 2010, 1181 women were murdered by their intimate partners. According to data collected by the CDC, women experience 2 million injuries from intimate partner violence each year. Nearly 3 in 10 women in the United States report experiencing violence by a current or former spouse or boyfriend at some point in their lives (CDC, 2012b).

Consequences of Domestic Violence

In the United States the cost of intimate partner rape, physical assault, and stalking was estimated to be $8.3 billion in 2003 for direct medical and mental health care services and lost productivity from paid work and household chores (CDC, 2012b). Both physical health and mental health are affected by intimate partner violence that results in injury, disability, flashbacks, panic attacks, and low self-esteem. The stress can lead to depression and harmful health behaviors such as smoking, drinking, using drugs, and having risky sex as a way of coping with the trauma (CDC, 2012b). Current technologies, such as smartphones, social media, texting, and webcams have increased the methods employed by people to stalk, monitor, and harass victims.

Nurses have a responsibility to ask patients whether they are being abused. Knowing how to ask requires training on addressing such a sensitive issue without offending the patient. Phrasing the question correctly during a patient encounter can mean the difference between life and death (Health Assessment Questions box). Many screening tools are available that allow the patient to self-report abuse. It may not be practical to screen all patients, but some screening tools make this simple to do and can be incorporated into the health assessment forms used by most health care organizations. Most health care organizations have counselors and nurses trained to handle cases of abuse, so the novice nurse should seek help when needed (Collaboration and Delegation box). See Chapter 24 for more information on handling cases of sexual abuse.

HEALTH ASSESSMENT QUESTIONS

Intimate Partner Violence

- Are you in a relationship with a person who physically hurts or threatens you?
- Has your partner or ex-partner ever hit you or physically hurt you? Has he or she ever threatened to hurt you or someone close to you?
- Do you feel controlled or isolated by your partner?
- Do you ever feel afraid of your partner? Do you feel you are in danger? Is it safe for you to return home?
- Has your partner ever forced you to have sex when you did not want to? Has your partner ever refused to practice safe sex?

COLLABORATION AND DELEGATION

Domestic Violence

- Nurses and other health care providers are uniquely positioned to address issues related to domestic and intimate partner violence.
- Health care providers in every discipline should collaborate to remove barriers to identifying and treating victims of domestic violence.
- All health care providers should:
  - Ask about abuse.
  - Identify barriers for detection of abuse.
  - Facilitate screening.
  - Provide training on signs and symptoms and detection of abuse.
  - Provide services.
  - Empower patients.

! SAFE PRACTICE ALERT

Nurses should include screening for domestic violence as part of the assessment of all patients, female and male, knowing that abuse occurs in both homosexual and heterosexual relationships.

Accidents and Violence

According to the National Adolescent Health Information Center (NAHIC), motor vehicle accidents accounted for 31% of deaths among adolescents and young adults in 2003, followed by homicides at 14.8%, suicides at 11.2%, and other unintentional injuries at 13.7% (NAHIC, 2006) (Diversity Considerations box). Excessive drinking is the leading risk factor for injury in the United States, and the third leading cause of preventable death (CDC, 2010b). Texting, eating, or being otherwise distracted while driving contribute to motor vehicle accidents.

DIVERSITY CONSIDERATIONS

Life Span and Gender

Accidents and Fatal and Nonfatal Injuries

- Young males have a higher homicide mortality rate than females.
- Nonfatal violent crimes are more common than homicide.
- The homicide rate in 15- to -19-year-old males is much higher among African Americans compared with other ethnic groups:
  African American (38.47/100,000)
  Hispanics (13.99/100,000), whites (2.61/100,000)
  American Indians and Alaska Natives (8.21/100,000)
  Asian and Pacific Islanders (3.19/100,000).
- The leading causes of nonfatal, unintentional injuries among 18- to 34-year-olds of all races and both sexes were unintentional falls, unintentionally being struck by or against an object, and being an occupant in a motor vehicle.

From National Adolescent Health Information Center: Demographics: Young Adults Fact Sheet, 2008. Retrieved from *http://nahic.ucsf.edu.*

HEALTH CONCERNS DURING YOUNG ADULTHOOD

Physical changes occur gradually and often go unnoticed during early adulthood. Now that health issues such as diabetes, hypertension, obesity, alcohol abuse, drug abuse, and smoking are prevalent among young adults, health insurance is a key factor in these adults' access to medical services. In the United States, adults aged 20 to 29 years are more likely than adults aged 30 and older to lack health insurance (National Center for Health Statistics, 2011). With the Affordable Care Act, more young adults will have at least minimal health insurance.

Health Screenings and Health Promotion

Early detection of illness and disease can best be accomplished when young adults participate in periodic health screenings. For young women these screenings include annual Pap smears for those who are sexually active and regular breast self-examination (BSE). Pap smears are the most accurate method of detecting cervical cancer in women. When young women become sexually active, the risk of exposure to the HPV increases, thus increasing the risk for cervical cancer. BSE is a great tool for detection of breast lumps and/or abnormalities. Testicular self-examination can alert young men to changes in their testicles and should serve as a stimulus to seek medical advice if an abnormality is found. Screenings for changes in the skin are advised, as many young adults spend a lot of time exposed to ultraviolet rays whether at work or at play. Nurses can serve as a catalyst to move young adults to action when it comes to health promotion activities. Nurses provide education on health-promotion activities, as well as performing screenings at health fairs, in schools, and at employment sites.

Diet and Physical Activity

Young adults are often fixated on their bodies and on the idea of being appealing to the opposite sex. They are constantly bombarded by images of beautiful people in movies, on television, and in magazines. Advertisements for diets, makeup, and skin creams are prevalent. The desire to be thin and beautiful has led many young men and women to be anorexic or bulimic, two conditions that have led to death for some young adults. Most young adults want to be healthy but can be confused about what being healthy truly means. An abundance of food is available in the United States. However, healthy eating and maintaining a proper diet can be a challenge for some. Many young adults have grown up in the age of the microwave, where cooking fresh food and sitting down to eat has been replaced by microwaving frozen foods and eating on the run. Fast-food restaurants have added to this trend by offering quick food that is high in saturated fats, which is filling but does not contain recommended nutrients. Nurses should emphasize proper nutrition and exercise to promote good health among young adults.

Nurses are equipped to teach the importance of good nutrition and the consequences of not having a proper diet. Patients in lower socioeconomic situations may feel that they cannot adhere to proper nutrition because of cost. Nurses can use the U.S. Department of Agriculture (USDA) MyPlate guidelines to teach patients about food substitutions that are nutrient-rich and economical.

Young adults often are very active, and many pursue exercise as a part of their daily routines. Others have not made physical activity a priority, and nurses should try to impress on them the benefits of exercise. Exercise helps decrease the risk of heart disease, obesity, diabetes, and cancer. It strengthens the heart, reduces anxiety, improves mood, and enhances overall subjective sense of well-being. Nurses can teach

PATIENT EDUCATION AND HEALTH LITERACY

Exercise

- Teach patients that most adults need at least 30 minutes of moderate physical activity such as brisk walking or bicycling at least 5 days per week.
- Encourage patients to find an exercise that they enjoy and to start slowly if they haven't been exercising regularly. Walking with a friend or joining a class may help to keep motivated.
- Advise patients that adding stretching and weight training to their routine will improve strength and fitness.

From National Library of Medicine: Exercise and physical fitness, MedlinePlus, 2011. Retrieved from *www.nlm.nih.gov/medlineplus/exerciseandphysicalfitness.html.*

patients the current recommendations for exercise (Patient Education and Health Literacy box).

Mental Health

Mental, emotional, and behavioral (MEB) disorders—which include depression, conduct disorders, bipolar disorder, schizophrenia, and substance abuse—are seen in a large number of young adults. Posttraumatic stress disorder and depression are being diagnosed frequently among young men and women returning from combat. High rates of suicide are seen in these young adults. Studies indicate that MEB disorders constitute a major health threat and are commonplace today among young people. Almost one in five young people will have one or more MEB disorders at any given time. Among adults, half of all MEB disorders were first diagnosed by age 14 and three fourths by age 24 (O'Connell, Boat, and Warner, 2009).

Many disorders have lifelong effects that include high psychosocial and economic costs, not only for the young people but also for their families, schools, and communities. The financial costs in terms of treatment services and lost productivity are estimated at $247 billion annually (O'Connell, Boat, and Warner, 2009). Beyond the financial costs, MEB disorders interfere with the young person's ability to accomplish age and culturally appropriate developmental tasks, such as establishing healthy interpersonal relationships, succeeding in school, and making their way in the workforce. The Health Assessment Questions box lists questions the nurse should ask to assess the mental health status of young adults.

Screening should be a part of nurses' assessment of young adults, with referral for mental health services when indicated. A quick assessment for depression and anxiety can be performed in approximately 5 to 10 minutes.

HEALTH ASSESSMENT QUESTIONS

Mental Health Conditions

Anxiety Disorders

- How often have you been feeling anxious, on edge, or nervous?
- How often have you been unable to stop or control worrying?
- Do you feel that you worry too much about different things?
- Do you have trouble relaxing?
- Are you able to fall asleep within 15 to 30 minutes of going to bed?
- How often are you restless or do you have problems sitting still?
- Do you easily become annoyed or irritable?
- How often do you feel afraid that something bad will happen?
- Do your thoughts seem like they are racing?

Depression

- Have you recently lost pleasure or interest in things that previously brought you pleasure?
- Have you been having feelings of helplessness, hopelessness, or sadness?
- Are you having trouble falling asleep or staying asleep?
- Do you feel tired often?
- Has your appetite increased or decreased recently?
- Have you been feeling bad about yourself or feeling like a failure recently?
- Have you had thoughts of harming yourself or someone else?

Adapted from Spitzer RL, Williams JB, Kroenke K, et al: GAD-7 and PHQ-SADS. Retrieved from *www.phqscreeners.com.*

Sexual Behavior and Sexually Transmitted Diseases

Some young adults engage in risky sexual behaviors that can result in negative health outcomes. These behaviors, while signaling a certain freedom from commitment, can increase the risk of sexually transmitted diseases (STDs) in both males and females. The most common sexually transmitted diseases include gonorrhea, chlamydial infection, herpes simplex, human immunodeficiency virus (HIV) infection, syphilis, and human papillomavirus (HPV) infection (Evidence-Based Practice and Informatics box). According to the CDC (2012c), in the United States, chlamydial genital infection is the most frequently reported infectious disease, and the prevalence is highest among people 20 to 24 years of age. For more information about signs and symptoms of STDs and their prevention, see Chapter 24.

Because of the temporary nature of many relationships among young adults, nurses should encourage all sexually active adults to get screened for STDs. Nurses have the knowledge and skills necessary to teach patients safe sex practices and signs and symptoms that need to be reported and investigated (Patient Education and Health Literacy box). Assure patients that their health information is confidential and that no disclosure will be made except if required by law.

EVIDENCE-BASED PRACTICE AND INFORMATICS

HPV, Genital Warts, and Oral Cancer

- At least 50% of sexually active people will have genital human PPV infection at some time in their lives.
- HPV is passed on through genital contact via vaginal or anal sex. There is no cure for HPV infection.
- Many strains of the HPV virus have been recognized. Some are considered low-risk strains, and some are considered high-risk.
- Low-risk HPV infections can cause genital warts.
- High-risk HPV infections can cause lesions that sometimes develop into cancer over time.
- Females and males can get vaccinated to protect against the types of HPV that most commonly cause health problems. The vaccine is most effective when people receive it before they have sexual contact with their first partners.
- HPV may contribute to the development of 20% to 30% of oral cancers.

From Centers for Disease Control and Prevention: Genital HPV infection fact sheet, 2012. Retrieved from *www.cdc.gov*; American Cancer Society: Oral cancer, 2013. Retrieved from *www.cancer.org*.

PATIENT EDUCATION AND HEALTH LITERACY

Sexually Transmitted Disease

- Teach patients the signs and symptoms of common sexually transmitted diseases.
- Ask patients to verbalize an understanding of the importance of practicing safe sex.
- Teach patients that latex condoms, when used consistently and correctly, are highly effective in preventing the sexual transmission of HIV, the virus that causes AIDS, and reducing the risk of other STDs, including diseases transmitted by genital secretions and, to a lesser degree, genital ulcer diseases.
- Demonstrate proper condom application to both males and females, with a return demonstration to assess knowledge.

MIDDLE ADULTHOOD: AGES 35 TO 65 LO 18.5

Middle adulthood is a time of adjustment for many adults. This transitional stage of life is marked by physical changes and adaptation to challenges such as making career changes, children's leaving home for college or returning home after college, and caring for aging parents. These changes produce increased stress, which manifests itself in different ways. In 2009, middle adults accounted for 60.3% of the U.S. labor force (U.S. Census Bureau, 2011). Middle adults' annual average health care expenditure between 2006 and 2009 was $9254, which was spent on health care insurance, medical services, drugs, and medical supplies (U.S. Census Bureau, 2011). Each person's transition is an individual process, and no two people experience middle adulthood in exactly the same way. Some diversity considerations for middle adults are listed in the Diversity Considerations box.

DIVERSITY CONSIDERATIONS

Life Span and Gender

Marital Status

- Ages 35 to 39: 67.3% of males were married, compared with 69.4% of females.
- Ages 40 to 44: 68.0% of males were married compared with 70. 1% of females.
- Ages 45 to 54: 69.7% of males were married compared with 68.3% of females.
- Ages 55 to 64: 73.9% of males were married compared with 66.9% of females.

Educational Attainment

- A high school diploma was *not* attained by 11.7% of adults ages 35 to 44, 10.4% of adults 45 to 54, and 10.4% of adults 55 to 64.
- A bachelor's degree or higher was attained by 33.1% of people ages 35 to 44, compared with 29.4% of people 45 to 54 and 31.7% of people 55 to 64.

From U.S. Census Bureau: Statistical abstract of the United States: 2012, ed. 131, Washington, D.C., Author, 2011. Retrieved from *http://www.census.gov/compendia/statab.*

AGE GROUP CHARACTERISTICS

Middle adulthood has its own developmental changes and issues not common to young adulthood. Middle adulthood is difficult to define, however, because people in this life stage exhibit wide variation in attitudes and behaviors. For some, certain personal choices have led to a very fulfilling life, whereas for others, such choices have led to significant changes and stresses in their lives. Children may leave home during this time, and retirement often looms. Attitudes about life determine the extent to which people act young or old during this period. Recent advances in medicine and technology offer the opportunity to live a better-quality life, with a slower transition to old age. Some predictable physical declines occur at this stage of life. It was long thought that some cognitive decline was associated with the normal aging process. This belief has since been disputed: One study by Wilson, Aggarwal, Barnes, Mendes de Leon, Hebert, and Evans (2010) contradicts the idea of inevitable mental deterioration and asserts that forgetfulness and memory lapses are early changes that may signal dementia later in life.

PHYSICAL CHANGES IN MIDDLE ADULTHOOD

Physical changes are evident as wrinkles begin to appear on the face, hair thins, and the waist thickens in most middle-aged adults. Muscle tissue (muscle mass) and muscle strength tend to decrease beginning in the thirties. This process is called **sarcopenia**, which means loss of flesh. Other physical changes with aging are listed in Table 18-1 earlier in this chapter.

CHANGES IN COGNITIVE DEVELOPMENT

Crystallized intelligence refers to skills that depend on accumulated knowledge, experience, good judgment, and mastery of social conventions. These skills are acquired because they are valued in our culture. Crystallized intelligence is evaluated through vocabulary tests, general information tests, verbal analogies, and logical-reasoning tests. This type of intelligence increases through middle adulthood, as adults add to their knowledge and skills at work and in leisure activities and practice the skills daily (Berk, 2011).

Fluid intelligence represents basic information-processing skills, that is, the ability to detect relationships among stimuli, the speed with which information is analyzed, and the capacity of working memory (Berk, 2011). This type of intelligence supports reasoning, abstraction, and problem solving and is more inherited than culturally trained. Fluid-intelligence skills are evaluated through number-series tests, spatial visualization, picture sequencing, and symbol search (Berk, 2011). This type of intelligence peaks in adolescence and progressively declines beginning around age 30 (Horn and Cattell, 1967).

Changes in mental abilities seem to be related to a general slowing of the central nervous system (CNS). The neural processing speed decreases. Well-practiced skills aren't noticeably affected, and adults find ways to compensate. Generalities do not explain individual and group differences. Some people lose cognitive function as a consequence of illness or adverse environments. Others remain creatively intellectual into very old age. Those who keep their intellect active usually are busy using their skills in work, leisure pursuits, travel, reading, cultural and arts endeavors, or civic commitments. People who have flexible personalities, have a lasting marriage to an intellectually challenging partner, are healthy, and live at a higher socioeconomic level will maintain their intellect longer (Berk, 2011). Some diversity considerations are listed in the Diversity Considerations box.

DIVERSITY CONSIDERATIONS

Life Span

- Numeric ability has declined, especially in younger middle adults, because of the reliance on calculators today.
- People who maintain higher levels of perceptual speed tend to have advantages in other mental abilities as well (Belsky, 2009).

Gender

- In early adulthood, women outperform men on verbal tasks and perceptual speed. Men excel at spatial skills. Losses over time are similar for both men and women.
- Aging women of the Baby Boomer generation perform better than aging women from earlier groups. This reflects the Baby Boomers' greater opportunities for education, technology, stimulation from work, and health care.

Ethnicity

- Ethnicity is not associated with rates of decline in cognition (Massel and Peek, 2009).
- Education and physical activity may be mediators of differences in cognitive test scores among white, African American, and Hispanic middle-aged adults (Massel, Raji, and Peek, 2010).

PRIMARY DEVELOPMENTAL TASKS IN MIDDLE ADULTHOOD

Middle adulthood is the time when many people reevaluate their lives, look for meaning in their existence, refine and strengthen their identities, and reach out to younger generations. For some middle-aged adults, this is a time for making adjustments in their daily lives, their outlook on life, and their goals. For others, it can be a time of crisis that can greatly affect their outlook on life and their future path in life (Berk, 2011).

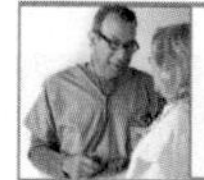

1. Which developmental issues is Ms. Dubois dealing with?

Erikson's Theory: Generativity versus Stagnation

Generativity means reaching out to others in ways that guide and give to the next generation. In midlife this activity extends beyond the nuclear family to social groups and communities (Figure 18-2). Personal life goals are now viewed in context with the welfare of the greater society. Generativity includes anything a person can develop and produce that can improve society and continue after the person's death. It is expressed through activities such as mentoring in the workplace or with youth groups, volunteering at shelters and organizations, being involved in community issues of importance to the individual, and engaging in creative endeavors in fields such

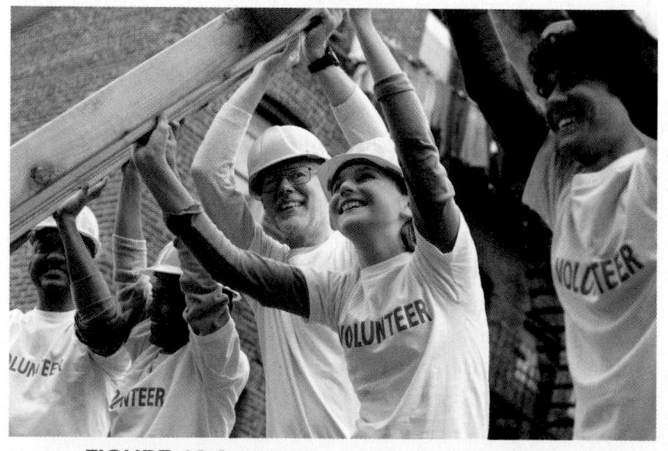

FIGURE 18-2 Volunteering in the community.

as art, music, and dance. People want to be needed and to feel that they have had a lasting effect on the world.

The alternative to generativity is **stagnation**—becoming self-centered and narcissistic. In stagnation, people place their own comfort and security above challenges that include other people. They have a detachment even from their own children, with a self-centered focus on what they can get from others, not what they can give. They lose interest in being productive at work or developing talents.

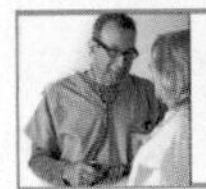

2. Discuss Ms. Dubois's status in regard to Erikson's stages.

Generative people are well adjusted, low in anxiety and depression, and high in self-acceptance and life satisfaction. They are more open to others' differences and points of view, have leadership qualities, care about the welfare of others, and care about more than financial gain in their work. Parenthood seems to enhance generativity in men more than in women. Women may have many ways to awaken to the needs of others, whereas men may need to feel the nurturance of a child to develop that outward concern. African Americans score higher in generativity in connection to religious groups, social support, and a view of themselves as models of wisdom for children (Belsky, 2009).

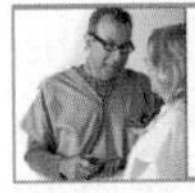

3. How can the nurse help Ms. Dubois to achieve generativity?

Levinson's Seasons of Life

In Levinson's (1996) Seasons of Life Theory, middle adulthood begins with a transition (at ages 40 to 45 years), followed by entry into a life structure (45 to 50). This structure is reevaluated (50 to 55) and ends in a culminating life structure (55 to 60). Midlife transition occurs around age 40, when people evaluate their success in meeting adult goals. In response to this self-evaluation, some people make big changes in their lives, such as career changes, divorces, remarriages, and expressions of creativity, whereas others make smaller changes but remain in their marriages and maintain their current careers. The self often becomes the middle adult's focus as the person is less distracted by other people and things. Levinson's theory identifies the following four developmental tasks of middle adulthood:

1. *Young-old:* Seeking new ways of being young and old and finding positive meaning in changes
2. *Destruction-creation:* Reevaluating past hurtful acts and attempting to be kinder, more creative, and other-focused
3. *Masculinity-femininity:* Integrating masculine and feminine aspects of the personality
4. *Engagement-separateness:* Finding a balance between engagement with the outside world and interior needs

Havighurst's Developmental Tasks for Middle Adulthood

In Havighurst's theory of development, middle adulthood tasks are age-dependent, and all serve pragmatic functions dependent on age. According to Havighurst (1953), "The developmental tasks of middle years arise from changes within the organism, from environmental pressures, and above all from demands or obligations laid upon the individual by his own values and aspirations" (p. 268). Primary developmental tasks as hypothesized by Havighurst (1953, pp. 268-276) are as follows:

- Achieving adult civic and social responsibility
- Establishing and maintaining an economic standard of living
- Assisting teenage children to become responsible and happy adults
- Developing adult leisure activities
- Relating oneself to one's spouse as a person
- Accepting and adjusting to the physiologic changes in middle age
- Adjusting to aging parents

HEALTH RISKS AND CONCERNS DURING MIDDLE ADULTHOOD LO 18.6

People in middle adulthood continue to have some of the health risks discussed in young adulthood. During middle adulthood, deaths due to complications from disease outnumber deaths due to accidents.

HEALTH RISKS DURING MIDDLE ADULTHOOD

Some leading causes of death in middle age are cancer and cardiovascular disease. The leading causes of nonfatal injury in middle adulthood are unintentional falls, unintentional overexertion, being struck by or against an object, and being an occupant in a motor vehicle accident (CDC, 2010a). Health promotion factors suggested by Berk (2011) are listed in the Patient Education and Health Literacy box.

PATIENT EDUCATION AND HEALTH LITERACY

Factors That Promote Well-Being in Midlife

- Good health and exercise
- Sense of control and life investment
- Positive social relationships
- A good marriage
- Mastery of multiple roles

From Berk LE: *Exploring lifespan development*, ed. 2, Boston, Mass., 2011, Pearson.

Cancer

Cancer is the second leading cause of death in the U.S. The death rates for all cancers has been declining in the past 15 years due to earlier detection and advance of treatment. Lung cancer is the leading cause of cancer deaths in women and men in the United States. Cigarette smoking is the primary cause of lung cancer. Death rates from lung cancer began to decline in 1991 for men and 2003 for women. Over the past decade, the number of lung cancer deaths is still declining, although lung cancer remains the top cause of cancer deaths.(American Cancer Society, 2014). Patient teaching tips from the Mayo Clinic are listed in the Patient Education and Health Literacy box.

PATIENT EDUCATION AND HEALTH LITERACY

Reducing Cancer Risk

To reduce the incidence of cancer and cancer deaths, teach patients to:

- Know the symptoms of cancer.
- Perform self-examinations.
- Get regular check-ups, screenings, and immunizations.
- Avoid tobacco, sun exposure, pollutants, and x-ray exposure.
- Eat a healthful diet and maintain an appropriate weight.
- Drink alcohol only in moderation.
- Exercise daily.

From Mayo Clinic: *Cancer:* Prevention, 2012. Retrieved from *http://www.mayoclinic.com/health/cancer/DS01076/DSECTION=prevention.*

Cardiovascular Disease

Cardiovascular disorders affect 28% of middle-aged Americans, many of whom die from complications and effects of cardiovascular disorders. These disorders include high blood pressure, high blood cholesterol, and **atherosclerosis**, or buildup of plaque in coronary arteries around the heart. **Myocardial infarction (MI)**, blockage of blood flow to the heart, is the most extreme symptom and is largely due to a blood clot in a coronary artery. Lack of oxygen and blood flow to the heart muscle produces excruciating pain. Approximately 50% of the victims of MIs die before getting to the hospital; of those who survive, 5% to 10% die within the first year after the MI, and approximately 50% of the survivors are rehospitalized within the first year (Zafari et al, 2012). **Arrhythmia** is an irregular heartbeat that can prevent the heart from pumping enough blood. **Angina pectoris** is the crushing chest pain that is the first indication of an oxygen-deprived heart. Heart disease is treated with bypass surgery, medicines, pacemakers, and **angioplasty**—balloon surgery that flattens fatty deposits to open blood flow in blocked arteries. Diet and exercise are essential in the prevention of cardiovascular disease. Nearly three quarters of all strokes occur in people aged 65 years or older. The chances of having a stroke double each decade after the age of 55. Strokes can—and do—occur at *any* age. Nearly 25% of strokes occur in people younger than 65 years of age. Stroke death rates are higher for African Americans than for whites, even at younger ages (CDC, 2010b). Preventive measures suggested by the American Heart Association (AHA) are listed in the Patient Education and Health Literacy box.

PATIENT EDUCATION AND HEALTH LITERACY

Reducing the Risk of Cardiovascular Disease

To reduce the risk of myocardial infarction, teach patients to:

- Eat a healthy diet and exercise regularly.
- Quit smoking.
- Reduce intake of foods that are high in cholesterol.
- Identify and treat high blood pressure.
- Maintain ideal weight.
- Take a low-dose aspirin under physician direction.

From American Heart Association: Lifestyle changes, 2012. Retrieved from *www.heart.org/HEARTORG/Conditions/HeartAttack/PreventionTreatmentofHeartAttack/Lifestyle-Changes_UCM_3039.*

HEALTH CONCERNS DURING MIDDLE ADULTHOOD

Health assessments conducted in people in middle adulthood should address the physiologic and psychological problems that can be experienced during this period in life, such as heart disease, diabetes, obesity, hypertension, arthritis, chronic obstructive pulmonary disease (COPD), migraines, anxiety, and depression (Health Assessment Questions box). Information obtained should be used to guide the care and education of patients.

Health Screening and Health Promotion

Health promotion activities for middle adulthood should address adequate rest, leisurely activities, regular exercise, good nutrition, satisfactory sexual function, and reduction and cessation of tobacco and alcohol use. Adults should be encouraged to have regular health screenings, such as blood pressure checks, colonoscopies, prostate examinations for men, and mammograms and Pap smears for women. Domestic violence should be assessed in both men and women, as discussed in the young adulthood section of this chapter.

Relationships at Midlife

Nine of ten middle-aged adults live in families, most of them with a spouse (U.S. Census Bureau, 2011). This period of the family life cycle is called the "launching children and moving on" stage. In the past it was known as the "empty nest" period, but it is no longer seen in such a negative light (Berk, 2011). This period may last as long as 20 years before retirement. It relates to establishing different relationships with children and finding new relationships with in-laws and grandchildren. In addition, midlife adults must cope with elderly parents and their needs.

HEALTH ASSESSMENT QUESTIONS

Middle Adulthood

General Information

- Have you experienced any recent weight loss or gain?
- Have you experienced any fatigue lately?
- Do you have trouble falling asleep or staying asleep?
- Do you smoke? How many packs per day?
- Do you exercise regularly?
- Do you drink alcohol? How many drinks per week?
- Do you use any recreational drugs or substances?

Cardiovascular System

- Have you had chest pains?
- Do you have any rapid heartbeats?
- Do you become short of breath with exertion?

Respiratory System

- Have you been experiencing any shortness of breath?
- Do you snore loudly?
- Do you experience coughing or wheezing?

Gastrointestinal/Genitourinary System

- Do you have heartburn or indigestion?
- Have you had a change in your bowel habits?
- Have you noticed any bloody or black, tarry stools?
- Do you have pain with urination?
- Do you have to get up during the night to use the bathroom?
- Do you have concerns about your sexual function?

Integumentary System

- Have you noticed any changes to moles or any new moles?
- Do you have any rashes or itching or changes to your skin?

Endocrine System

- Have you experienced any recent heat or cold intolerance?
- Have you experienced any excessive sweating?

Neurologic System

- Have you experienced any of the following recently?
  - Headaches
  - Dizziness
  - Fainting
  - Falls
  - Memory problems

Women Only

- Are you experiencing hot flashes or night sweats?
- Are you having irregular menstrual periods?
- When was your last mammogram?
- Does your spouse or partner hit, slap, or punch you?
- Are you afraid to return home?
- Are there firearms or guns in your home?

Marriage and Divorce

Households at the midlife stage tend to be better positioned economically and financially than they were previously. However, recent changes in economic stability in the United States have affected the middle-aged adult as well as other age groups. Adults between 45 and 54 years of age in the United States have the highest average annual income (U.S. Census Bureau, 2011), which in the past allowed for expansion of opportunities to learn or travel. Recently, many middle-aged adults have found that more savings are needed for retirement than was the case in the past. In addition, this period often is when marriages that have experienced some turmoil will end and former partners venture out for a new start. Most divorces occur in the first 5 to 10 years of marriage, but 10% occur after 20 years or more (Berk, 2011). At midlife, divorce seems to be more manageable emotionally. People who are better educated and employed are more likely to divorce because they can better support themselves. STDs are a concern in this age group when high-risk behavior is present, such as having an affair or dating and engaging in sexual activity with multiple partners after a divorce.

Grandparents Rearing Grandchildren

In the United States, approximately 4% to 5% of the child population live with grandparents and apart from parents, who are called the **skipped generation**. This arrangement may occur as a consequence of parental substance abuse, emotional illness, or physical illness. Sometimes a child welfare agency is involved and tries to place an at-risk child with a grandparent rather than in foster care. This arrangement may be difficult for the grandparent to maintain financially. Custodial grandparents often face high levels of stress and frustration and a decline in health as they attempt to provide stability for their grandchildren. In the children themselves, the disruption of normal family relations can lead to learning disabilities, depression, and even antisocial behavior. The grandparents often report being tired and emotionally drained, even depressed. They become important to the grandchildren, however, and these children often describe close relationships with their caregiving grandparents (Berk, 2011).

Middle-Aged Adults and Their Aging Parents

According to a University of Michigan (2011) study on health and retirement, almost 10 million adults over the age of 50 care for their aging parents. The study gives an updated look at adults who work and care for their parents and at the impact of caregiving on their earnings and lifetime wealth. The results found that the proportion of adults providing personal care and/or financial assistance to a parent has more than tripled since the mid-1990s. Currently, 25% of adults—primarily Baby Boomers—provide care to a parent. Working and nonworking adults are almost equally likely to provide care to parents in need. Adults ages 50 and older who work

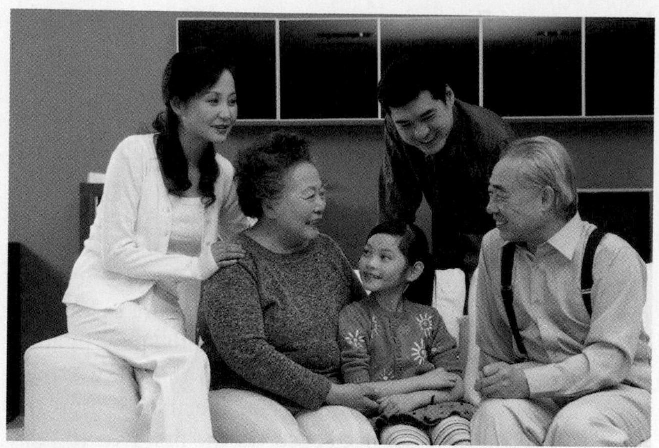

FIGURE 18-3 Many middle adults care for their children and for their aging parents as well.

and provide care to a parent are more likely to have fair or poor health than those who do not provide such care.

The term **sandwich generation** refers to middle-aged adults who are the caretakers of multiple generations of their families. More middle-aged adults are now caring for their children or grandchildren, and for their aging parents, who may no longer be able to care for themselves. Many Baby Boomers provide financial support to adult children and financial assistance to a parent. This multiple-generation caretaker role generates many stressors that can lead to a breakdown in the caretaker's health and functioning. It also can lead to role overload, or conflicting demands of worker, spouse, parent, and child roles (Cohn, 2008) (Figure 18-3).

The role of caring for a parent often has been compared with that of taking care of children, but the two are not the same. In caring for a child, the expectation is that the child will grow up and eventually leave home to prosper. In caring for an elderly parent, there is little hope that the parent will return to independence as the slow decline of aging takes place. Watching this process and feeling helpless to slow or stop it can lead to depression, exhaustion, and illness in the middle-aged caregiver (Evidence-Based Practice and Informatics box and Patient Education and Health Literacy box). Respite care is available for some at a cost, but not all families can afford this. In some cases, nursing home placement must be explored; however, it too can pose a financial burden on the middle-aged caregiver and family.

EVIDENCE-BASED PRACTICE AND INFORMATICS

Chronic Stress Can Shorten Caregivers' Lives

- The chronic stress incurred by spouses and children caring for a patient with Alzheimer's disease may shorten their lives by as much as 4 to 8 years, according to a study by Glaser and Kiecolt-Glaser (2007).
- This study showed that chronic caregiver stress affects the body at both the genetic and molecular levels.

PATIENT EDUCATION AND HEALTH LITERACY

Tips for Dealing With Caregiver Stress

Advise caregivers to:

- Accept help from others.
- Join a support group or attend caregiver classes offered by organizations such as the American Red Cross or the Alzheimer's Association local chapter.
- Use community resources such as respite care services or adult day care.
- Commit to keeping healthy.
- Avoid feeling guilty.
- Communicate with lawmakers and officials for information on policies that relieve financial burdens (Mayo Clinic, 2012).

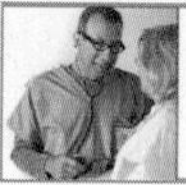

4. What issues may have to be addressed by the nurse before Ms. Dubois can lead a fulfilling life?

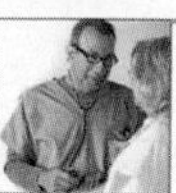

The conceptual care map for Ms. Dubois can be found at *http://evolve.elsevier.com/YoostCrawford/fundamentals/*. It is partially completed to indicate how to use the map as a learning tool. Complete the nursing diagnoses using the example conceptual care maps shown in Chapters 8 and 25-33.

OLDER ADULTHOOD: AGE 65 AND OLDER — LO 18.7

The American population is growing older. Society has defined the older adult as anyone older than 65 years of age. In some literature and textbooks, this age group is further divided into the *young-old* (up to 74 years old), *middle-old* (75 to 84 years), and *old-old* (85 years and older). According to the U.S. Census Bureau (2011), the average annual expenditure on health care between 2006 and 2008 was $4779 for adults 65 to 74 years of age and $4413 for those 75 years and older.

AGE GROUP CHARACTERISTICS

There are 41 million older Americans, with the number estimated to more than double to approximately 92 million by 2060. It is predicted that by 2040 people aged 65 and older will constitute 21% of the population (as compared with 13.3% in 2011), with those 85 and older increasing from 5.7 million to 14.1 million. Older women outnumber older men in a ratio of 3 to 2. The proportion of older people is higher among whites than in other populations, although the number of older adults in racial and ethnic minority populations is projected to increase from 21% in 2011 to 28% by 2030 (Administration on Aging, 2012). The older population in the United States is becoming increasingly more racially and ethnically diverse as the overall minority population grows and experiences increased longevity. As a result, it is critical that nurses understand that each person is unique, whether along the dimensions of race, ethnicity, gender, sexual orientation, socioeconomic status, age, physical abilities, religious beliefs, political beliefs or other ideologies. The increase in diversity can be expected to have an impact on almost every facet of nursing care for older adults because cultural background affects communication, values, health beliefs and health related-behaviors, and other aspects of functioning (Miller, 2012).

Dr. Robert Butler (1969) coined the term *ageism* and defined it as "the prejudices and stereotypes that are applied to older people on the basis of their age." According to Miller, ageism is an outcome of urbanization and industrialization resulting from the emphasis on the negative and debilitative aspects of old age, and is based on perceptions that older people are unproductive.

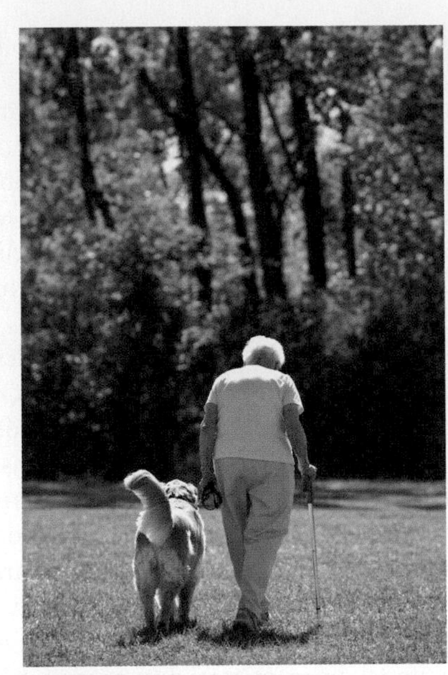

FIGURE 18-4 Older adult's posture.

PHYSICAL CHANGES DURING OLDER ADULTHOOD

Physical alterations seen in older adults include some of the changes listed in Table 18-1. Age-specific differences in physical appearance and mobility involve changes in the skin, hair, facial structure, and body build. The physical capabilities of older adults are not the same as they were in earlier stages of life, although many older adults remain agile and physically fit in later life. There are obvious signs of aging: Hair becomes gray, and facial skin and other parts of the body become wrinkled because of loss of skin elasticity and collagen content (Feldman, 2014). Height declines as the spine collapses with bone loss and decreased muscle tone. Reactions slow, and the senses become less acute. Cataracts and glaucoma may affect the eyes, and hearing loss is common. Mobility declines as muscle strength declines by 30% to 50% after age 70. Stretching exercises can reduce this decline (Figure 18-4).

The changes of aging that affect the internal functioning of the organ systems are occurring simultaneously with the alterations that can be seen. The brain decreases in size but retains its structure and function in the absence of disease. The heart pumps less blood through the body. The respiratory system is less efficient. The digestive system produces smaller amounts of digestive juices, which affects the movement of food through the intestines and therefore increases the likelihood of constipation.

Taste and smell decrease in acuity over time, causing food to be less appetizing. This has an unfortunate side effect for older adults, who tend to eat less, because it can lead to undernutrition.

COGNITIVE CHANGES DURING OLDER ADULTHOOD

During the normal aging process, mental health and cognition remain relatively stable. Severe changes in behavior and sudden loss of cognitive function usually are symptoms of a physical or mental illness, such as Alzheimer's disease or serious depression. In 2014, the number of adults with Alzheimer's disease was 5.2 million, or one in eight people (13%). Of people aged 85 and older, 38% have Alzheimer's disease (Alzheimer's Association, 2014). Alzheimer's disease is the most common form of dementia (a group of disorders occurring almost entirely in the older adult population), in which structural and chemical brain deterioration is associated with gradual loss of many aspects of thought and behavior (Berk, 2011). Among the earliest warning symptoms are severe memory problems such as forgetting names, appointments, and travel routes to familiar places in the community. Depression can often appear in the earlier stages of Alzheimer's disease. The life expectancy of a person with Alzheimer's disease can range from 1 year to as long as 15 years. At this time, a cure for this disease is lacking; however, several categories of drugs have been found to slow its progression. Researchers are testing drugs and nondrug approaches to treatment of this condition.

Depression is one of the psychiatric illnesses appearing most frequently in the older adult population. The prevalence of serious depression at any given time among adults aged 65 and older in community settings ranges from 1% to 5%; among medical outpatients, 5% to 10%; among medical inpatients, 10% to 12%; and among residents of long-term care facilities, 14% to 42% (Fiske, Wetherell, and Gatz, 2009). Depression is still underdiagnosed, because patients and health care providers believe that isolation, sleep problems, and diminished appetite are part of the normal aging process. People with severe depression typically report increased numbers of days in bed, increased pain, and decreased physical activities compared with older adults without depression.

Arthritis, diabetes, and hypertension are risk factors for depression (Fiske, Wetherell, and Gatz, 2009).

Delirium is not a disease but a syndrome with multiple causes that result in a similar constellation of symptoms. *Delirium* is defined as a transient, usually reversible cause of cerebral dysfunction, and it manifests clinically with a wide range of neuropsychiatric abnormalities. The clinical hallmarks are decreased attention span and a waxing-waning type of confusion.

Delirium often is called *acute confusion,* which is a syndrome characterized by confusion, memory loss, disorientation, disorganized thinking, fatigue, sleep disturbance, fearfulness, excessive energy, altered perceptions including hallucinations and delusions, and personality changes. Delirium is a serious, preventable, and treatable disorder. Some factors that increase the risk for onset of delirium are advanced age, pain, polypharmacy, hospitalization, surgery, and physiologic and pathologic conditions (Miller, 2012). An attempt should be made to differentiate acute confusion (delirium) from chronic confusion (dementia), which has a gradual onset and is not irreversible, as with Alzheimer's disease.

Nursing interventions are based on history—what previously has been effective in patients with cognitive changes. Drug therapies have been effective in slowing Alzheimer's disease and managing serious depression. Important strategies for nurses caring for patients in this age group are to maximize safety by modifying the environment to compensate for cognitive losses, to plan and maintain a consistent routine, and to teach caregivers how to identify burnout from the daily care of older adults with cognitive changes.

! SAFE PRACTICE ALERT

Stimulating leisure activity helps to facilitate cognitive functioning. Keeping the mind and body active is essential for older adults.

PRIMARY DEVELOPMENTAL TASKS

According to Erikson (1963), the developmental task of older adults is ego integrity versus despair. Older adults who attain ego integrity view life as wholeness, receiving satisfaction from past accomplishments and accepting death as a completion of life. By contrast, older adults with despair often believe they made poor choices during the life journey and wish they could live their lives over again. Older adults have accumulated a lifetime of self-knowledge that leads to more secure and complex conceptions of themselves than at earlier ages (Berk, 2011). Some of the challenges of the older adult years center on retirement and maintaining independence and self-esteem.

According to Havighurst (1953), people who are 60 years of age and older must adjust to decreasing physical strength and health, retirement and reduced income, death of a spouse, and the processes of establishing an explicit affiliation with their age group, adopting and adapting to social roles in a flexible way, and establishing satisfactory physical living arrangements. A complete discussion of developmental tasks by age can be found in Chapter 17.

PSYCHOSOCIAL CHANGES IN THE OLDER ADULT

A majority of the people in the United States older than 65 years of age are unemployed, according to statistics from the Federal Interagency Forum on Aging-Related Statistics (FIFAS) (2012). Those who are still able to work have a better income and sense of worth and are able to continue long-established routines. The retirement age established to receive federal benefits through the Social Security system has no relationship to the abilities of the worker. Some older adults need to work for economic reasons because actual retirement would mean loss of essential income. In general, however, nonworking retired people are no longer governed by an alarm clock, and they have time to pursue projects, hobbies, or recreational activities that were deferred earlier in life.

The financial needs of older adults vary considerably (FIFAS, 2008). Problems with income often are related to low retirement benefits, lack of pension plans, and increased life span with prolonged duration of retirement years (Johnson, Soto, and Zedlewski, 2008). Meeting food and medical costs can be a financial strain. Adequate financial resources, however, allow the older adult to remain independent. Older adults of minority groups have greater financial problems than white older adults, and older women of all ages usually have lower incomes than older men (FIFAS, 2008).

QSEN FOCUS!

The nurse engages older adult patients in an active partnership that promotes health, safety, well-being, and self-care management and appreciates shared decision making with empowered patients and families.

Living Arrangements

Living arrangements are influenced by a variety of factors, including marital status, financial well-being, the value placed on living independently or with family members, the availability of social services and social support, health status, family size and structure, and cultural traditions. As people are living longer, more living choices are becoming available. During late adulthood, many people relocate when their house or apartment becomes too large, expensive, or burdensome to maintain, or when decreased mobility requires different living arrangements (Administration on Aging, 2012). Chronic health problems may require an environment that is adapted to meet the older adult's physical limitations, such as a larger bathroom to accommodate a wheelchair or a home with living space on one level. Making the decision to relocate is stressful even if it is voluntary, because the older adult often has to leave the neighborhood, friends, and home that have been a part of his or her life for many decades.

With increasing age, living arrangements may need to change to adapt to changing life circumstances. Many different types of living arrangements are available, and the selection should be based on the older adult's requirements. The Diversity Considerations box lists some of these options.

DIVERSITY CONSIDERATIONS

Life Span

Living Arrangements for Older Adults

- Assisted living is an option for older adults who need assistance with activities of ADLs. Assisted-living facilities provide older adults with the freedom to live in a semi-independent manner, with help with those tasks that they can no longer perform themselves on a daily basis, such as cooking, cleaning, and doing laundry.
- Adult day care is a solution for older adults who are incapable of caring for themselves and whose caregivers are not able to look after them during work hours.
- Adult foster care and group homes are suitable for older adults who can care for themselves but require some form of supervision for safety purposes.
- Long-term care facilities or nursing homes provide care for older adults who can no longer care for themselves, often because of mobility or memory impairment. These facilities can also provide short-term rehabilitation services for older adults until they are able to return to their independent living situation.
- Palliative care and hospice care are available for patients suffering from chronic illnesses. Hospice care differs slightly from palliative care in that the aim is to provide the patient with the best quality of life by relieving pain and other symptoms during the final days of life. In palliative care, the aim is symptom control in people with chronic illnesses, and the care is not related to life expectancy of the affected person.
- Retirement homes and communities are multiunit housing facilities that accommodate older adults with many different levels of care needs. Offering a wide range of living services, amenities, and activities, retirement homes give older adults a sense of daily enjoyment and personal belonging. A retirement community is a private, planned community for retirees or older adults. Such communities consist of a group of houses in a particular geographic area that share common amenities and features.
- Home care has become a preferred solution for many older adults who want to live in the comfort of their own homes but need some assistance with day-to-day responsibilities. Some of the types of care available are nursing care, housekeeping, and therapy.

Most older adults thrive on independence even if they are slow in performing activities of daily living (ADLs). Most prefer to live in an independent living environment as long as they can. Older adults appreciate the same respect for and acceptance of their abilities as expected for people of other age groups. Therefore nurses need to acknowledge the older adult's ability to think, reason, and make decisions.

! SAFE PRACTICE ALERT

Patients returning home from a hospital stay may require the assistance of a home care nurse until they are able to manage their own care. This potential need should be evaluated and be part of the nursing care plan before discharge.

Sexuality in Older Adulthood

Nurses may find it embarrassing or uncomfortable to discuss sexuality with older patients. Often, nurses working with older-adult patients are much younger than their patients; therefore, nurses must have strong communication skills, scientific knowledge, and self-awareness when working with this population. Older adults, whether healthy or frail, need to express sexual feelings, which include passion, affection, and admiration. Sexuality is a basic human need that has psychological, social, moral, and biologic components.

Sexuality in the older adult shifts from procreation to companionship, intimate communication, and a pleasure-seeking physical relationship. Sexual activity depends on the state of the person's sex drive and the presence of illness or chronic conditions that affect activity and mobility, as well as on individual interpersonal circumstances, opportunities, and moral and religious beliefs. Pain, fatigue, joint stiffness, other musculoskeletal limitations, heart disease, cerebrovascular accident (stroke), chronic obstructive pulmonary disease, diabetes, cancer, and other conditions and diseases may interfere with sexual activity but need not curtail enjoyment of sexual intercourse. Nurses must have the requisite knowledge to assist the older adult in making the appropriate behavioral and practice changes to accommodate the health care condition.

! SAFE PRACTICE ALERT

Many older adults remain sexually active until late in life; nurses should include education and counseling on safe sex practices for the older adult.

Cultural Differences in Aging

Older adults fare best when they retain social status and opportunities for community participation. When older adults are excluded from social roles, their sense of well-being is reduced. Instead of fostering the integration and enhancement of wisdom that can be learned from the older adults, such exclusion can cause resentment between the generations. Ethnic and socioeconomic status variations in health tend to diminish with age. Still, compared with majority whites, minority older adults 65 to 80 years of age tend to have more health problems, and more of these adults exist at or below poverty (U.S. Census Bureau, 2011).

HEALTH RISKS AND CONCERNS IN OLDER ADULTHOOD LO 18.8

Disease is not a normal outcome of aging, but chronic health problems and disabilities increase as age increases. Nurses need to recognize that assessing and promoting functional abilities in ADLs is vital for people 65 years of age and older, who have another 10 or more years to enjoy life. Emerging issues in the health care of older adults include the following:

- Coordinating care
- Helping older adults manage their own care
- Establishing quality measures
- Identifying minimum levels of training for people who care for older adults
- Researching and analyzing appropriate training to equip providers with the tools they need to meet the needs of older adults (U.S. Department of Health and Human Services, 2010)

HEALTH RISKS DURING OLDER ADULTHOOD

Older adults are major users of health care services from acute care, rehabilitation, and long-term care facilities and from the community (Stanley, Blair, and Beare, 2005). The overall goal in the facilities providing care is improving the patient's health to encourage independent functioning in an environment of safety.

Many of the illnesses and diseases that are seen in older adults are not peculiar to this population; people of other age groups also suffer from cancer and heart disease. However, the probability that an older adult will become ill increases with age.

Common causes of death in the older adult are heart disease, cancer, cerebrovascular accident (stroke), lower respiratory disease, pneumonia, influenza, and complications from diabetes mellitus (FIFAS, 2008). Because aging is associated with a weakening of the body's immune system, older adults are more susceptible to infectious diseases (Feldman, 2014). Common chronic illnesses associated with significant impairment of function in older adulthood are osteoporosis, osteoarthritis, rheumatoid arthritis, chronic obstructive pulmonary disease, hearing and visual alterations, and cognitive dysfunctions such as dementia. In addition, acute illnesses such as pneumonia, fractures, and trauma from falls and motor vehicle accidents may create chronic health problems (CDC, 2011).

Cardiovascular Disease

Stroke is the leading cause of long-term disability among adults in the United States. Strokes are cerebrovascular accidents that affect the cerebral circulation through blockage with occlusive thrombi and emboli in the subarachnoid and intracerebral spaces. Risk factors for stroke include diabetes, obesity, hypertension, hyperlipidemia, and some cardiac disorders such as atrial fibrillation, myocardial infarction, and valvular disease. Many older adults do not know the signs and symptoms of stroke; thus, when they seek medical attention, permanent damage may already have occurred.

! SAFE PRACTICE ALERT

Many patients in older adulthood who have had a stroke are maintained on anticoagulant medications. It is essential that caregivers and other family members be taught how to administer these medications and be instructed about signs to look for indicating bleeding or hemorrhage.

Hypertension is a major risk factor for experiencing other cardiac-related illnesses. An estimated 43 million Americans have hypertension. *Hypertension* refers to elevated blood pressure readings, either diastolic or systolic, or both, over a period of time. Systolic hypertension is common in older adults. The underlying causes of hypertension are not known in most cases. In a small percentage of affected people, specific causes can be identified; these include (1) genetic differences in renal absorption of sodium, (2) dysfunction of the renin-angiotensin-aldosterone system, (3) insulin resistance, and (4) autonomic nervous system dysfunction.

Untreated hypertension results in several physical changes in the body. Hypertension accelerates the rate of atherosclerosis formation in the arteries. Arteries become stiff as elastin is lost and collagen increases. Stroke rates are increased in hypertensive patients. Assessment of the patient with hypertension includes taking accurate blood pressure readings and looking for evidence of target organ damage by means of urine analysis for the presence of protein. Regular ophthalmologic examinations are encouraged for hypertensive patients.

! SAFE PRACTICE ALERT

The changes caused by aging to the baroreceptors makes it vital for nurses to check postural blood pressures in the older adult to prevent postural hypotension and falls.

Cancer

Older adults are less likely than younger adults to be screened for cancer, so cancers in older adults often go undiagnosed or are discovered in later stages of the disease. Common cancers in older adults include lung, skin, breast, colon, ovarian, and brain cancers. In some older adults, the disease may lead to cognitive compromise; decision making about care may then become the responsibility of a family member or other caregiver (Miller, 2012). Decisions about treatment can be complicated by comorbid conditions. Although the numbers of cancers found among older adults are higher than the numbers in other age groups, research, education, and public health policies regarding cancer among older adults are scarce.

Respiratory Diseases

The exchange of oxygen and carbon dioxide is the primary function of the respiratory system. Age-related changes occur over time that can affect the maximal inspiratory and expiratory force. For example, kyphosis (increased curvature of the spine), poor posture, a shortened thorax, chest wall stiffness, and an increase in the anteroposterior diameter of the chest wall result in diminished respiratory efficiency. Tobacco use (smoking) is a major factor in development of lung disease and impaired respiratory function. Chronic exposure to tobacco smoke has been confirmed to be harmful not only to the smoker but to everyone who is exposed to secondhand smoke. Secondhand smoke is known as *environmental tobacco smoke* (ETS) or *passive smoke.* The effects of chronic exposure to air pollution and environmental toxins such as housecleaning products can cause complications in patients with chronic respiratory conditions.

COPD is a prevalent respiratory condition that may necessitate hospitalization of the older adult. Age and smoking are the two major risk factors for COPD, which is a group of diseases, including emphysema, chronic bronchitis, and a subset of asthma characterized by chronic airflow obstruction (Miller, 2012). The most common signs and symptoms are cough, dyspnea, wheezing, and increased sputum production. The condition is progressive, meaning that it will become more disabling as the person ages. In the interview with the older adult or caregiver, the nurse identifies risk factors that may affect the patient's respiratory system. Identifying potential and actual risk factors is an opportunity to address health promotion behavioral changes such as cessation of smoking. Some assessment questions regarding COPD that the nurse may ask are shown in the Health Assessment Questions box.

HEALTH ASSESSMENT QUESTIONS

COPD

- Have you had any respiratory problems in the past such as asthma, pneumonia, or frequent respiratory infections?
- Have you ever had tuberculosis?
- Do you smoke?
- Do you experience shortness of breath with walking or lying down?
- Have you ever lived or worked in an area with heavy pollution from traffic, factories, or mining?

! SAFE PRACTICE ALERT

Check the patient's electronic health record for immunization dates for pneumonia and influenza vaccines.

Musculoskeletal Disorders

Normal changes of aging often bring about complaints of musculoskeletal pain and various joint limitations. These chronic conditions can limit mobility and impair the ability to perform self-care activities such as bathing, dressing, and cooking; these changes may result in loss of independence. Osteoporosis and osteomalacia are metabolic bone diseases. Osteoarthritis, rheumatoid arthritis, and gout are joint diseases.

Nursing assessment of an older adult with any musculoskeletal conditions must include assessing the patient's functional ability to perform self-care activities—the skills of dressing, toileting, bathing, eating, and ambulating. An inability to perform any of these skills will affect the patient's independence. The nurse should assess the patient's ability to prepare a meal and safely use medications, monitor the patient's pain level, and check for risk factors that may impair musculoskeletal function, including the following:

- *Nutritional status:* Daily proteins and vitamin D maintain optimal skeletal function.
- *Activity:* Exercise helps to prevent age-induced declines in mobility.
- *Lifestyle factors:* Smoking, daily high intake of caffeine, inadequate calcium intake, sodium, and phosphorus can negatively affect calcium balance and increase the risk factors for osteoporosis (Miller, 2012).

! SAFE PRACTICE ALERT

Falls are a common problem in later adulthood. The combination of decreased visual acuity, loss of muscle strength, and slowed reaction time contributes to the increased risk of falls.

Diabetes Mellitus

Diabetes mellitus (DM) is a highly prevalent disease that increases in incidence among people older than 65 years of age, particularly in racial and ethnic minorities (Tabloski, 2014). DM is a complex disorder of hyperglycemia that results from defects in insulin secretion, insulin action, or both, which lead to abnormalities in carbohydrate, protein, and fat metabolism (American Diabetes Association, 2006). Two major types of DM affect the older adult: type 1 DM and type 2 DM. Type 1 DM, formerly called *juvenile-onset* or *insulin-dependent diabetes,* is the result of pancreatic islet cell destruction and a total deficit of circulating insulin. Type 2 DM, formerly called *non–insulin-dependent* or *adult-onset diabetes,* results from insulin resistance with a defect in compensatory insulin secretion.

The clinical signs and symptoms of DM in older adults include dehydration, confusion, delirium, decreased visual acuity, fatigue, nausea, recurrent infections, delayed wound healing, and paresthesia (Touhy and Jett, 2012). Complications that can develop due to poor glycemic control include the following (Tabloski, 2014):

- Eye disease, which can lead to partial loss of vision or even blindness
- Kidney failure
- Heart disease

- Nerve damage, which can cause pain or a loss of feeling in the hands, feet, legs, or other parts of the body (peripheral neuropathies)
- Stroke
- Peripheral vascular disease
- Poor wound healing due to impaired immune response and to poor tissue perfusion (Tabloski, 2014)

When assessing an older adult with newly diagnosed diabetes, the nurse focuses on acute and chronic complications and provides education about the factors that increase risk, such as smoking, lack of exercise, and elevated blood pressure and blood sugars. Treating adult-onset diabetes requires lifestyle changes including monitoring dietary intake, exercising regularly, and losing weight. Adherence to these practices will promote glucose absorption, decrease abdominal fat, and lessen disease symptoms.

! SAFE PRACTICE ALERT

Examine the diabetic patient's feet at every clinical encounter.

HEALTH CONCERNS DURING OLDER ADULTHOOD

People in the United States are living longer than ever before. Many older adults live active and healthy lives, but as aging occurs, bodies and minds change. According to the National Institute on Aging (2010), to stay healthy, adults should eat a balanced diet, keep active both mentally and physically, refrain from smoking, practice safety habits, and get regular health care check-ups. Screening tests needed depend on the person's age, gender, family history, and risk factors for certain diseases. For example, being overweight may increase the risk of developing diabetes and exacerbate many other comorbid conditions.

Health Screening and Health Promotion

Screening should be a primary focus of health promotion because of the potential for early detection of cancers such as breast and colorectal cancer. Nurses should focus patient education on cancer prevention; vaccinations that protect against influenza and pneumococcal disease; screenings for the early detection of diabetes, lipid disorders, osteoporosis, and hypertension; fall risk assessment; elder abuse; and smoking cessation counseling (Miller, 2012). The nurse must remember to be sensitive to cultural, language, and other differences among older adults when providing health-promotion information.

Changing Roles and Relationships

According to statistics from the Administration on Aging (2012), the older-adult population, 65 years and older, numbered 41 million in 2011, which represented 13.3% of the U.S. population. The older adult population will continue to grow significantly. In 2011, a small number (1.5 million), or 3.6%, of older adults lived in institutional settings such as nursing homes (Ethical, Legal, and Professional Practice box). In 2009, 2.7% lived in senior housing with at least one supportive service available to them.

ETHICAL, LEGAL, AND PROFESSIONAL PRACTICE

Ethical and Legal Issues in Nursing Homes

- The Nursing Home Residents' Bill of Rights is a federal law requiring all long-term care facilities to have a procedure in place whereby patients are informed of their rights, participate in their own care, have the right to complain, make independent choices, and have the right to privacy and confidentiality.
- Autonomy, individual rights, and quality of life for residents of long-term care settings create ethical issues because it is not easy to balance individual patients' needs with those of the institution.

Miller CA: *Nursing for wellness in older adults,* ed. 6, Philadelphia, 2012, Lippincott, Williams & Wilkins.

The median income of older adults in 2011 was $27,707 for males and $15,362 for females. Households headed by a person aged 65 or older in 2009 reported median income of $48,538. Almost all noninstitutionalized older adults were covered by Medicare in 2011; some had private health insurance, military-based insurance, or Medicaid (Administration on Aging, 2012).

Limitations in activities because of chronic conditions increase with age. In 2011, among Medicare beneficiaries, 92% of those institutionalized had difficulties with one or more ADLs, in contrast with 28% of those who were community residents (Administration on Aging, 2012). Many community-resident older adults with chronic disabilities receive either informal care from family or friends or formal care from services (Collaboration and Delegation box). Nurses compromise their care of older adults when they fail to recognize the unique manifestations of aging and disease

COLLABORATION AND DELEGATION

Home Care of Older Adults

Collaboration among health care agencies and providers is needed to provide care to older adults in the home.

- Home health care should be considered for older adults being discharged from the hospital.
- Services include skilled nursing care; physical, occupational, and speech-language therapies; medical social services; and home health aide care.
- Home health agencies conduct assessment in the patient's environment and determine the patient's ability to perform ADLs independently.
- Patient and family education is provided so that proper care continues even when the agency is not present.

(Miller, 2012). Nurses must include assessment for abuse in older adults, especially those who are experiencing cognitive changes and those who rely on others for their care.

> **QSEN FOCUS!**
>
> Integrating the contribution of others who help patients achieve health goals and valuing the expertise of health team members demonstrate teamwork and collaboration.

Assistive Technology

Technologically, the world is advancing, and many more devices are being developed that permit people with disabilities to improve function. Such devices include computers and phones that can be dialed by voice command or can print out the spoken words of the caller, allowing blind or deaf people to remain independent. A computer chip can be placed on medicine bottles to remind older adults to take medicines on schedule. Architects are building "smart homes" with features that promote safety and mobility.

SUMMARY OF LEARNING OUTCOMES

LO 18.1 *Discuss theories on aging and adult development:* Senescence is the biologic process of aging influenced by genetic factors. Theories on aging include the Wear-and-Tear Theory, aging at the cellular level, and the Cross-Linking Theory. Developmental theories include Gould's Theory on Adult Development and the life stages theories of Havighurst, Erikson, and Piaget.

LO 18.2 *Describe changes that occur as the body ages:* Physical changes occur within all body systems as aging progresses and can affect mobility, cognition, and independence.

LO 18.3 *Identify physiologic, cognitive, emotional, and social changes that affect the young adult:* The transitions that occur during young adulthood are influenced by cultural beliefs, societal values, and individual beliefs and expectations. Emerging adulthood is signified by a prolonged transition to adulthood as people pursue education and employment. The young adult is at a peak of cognitive and physical development.

LO 18.4 *Articulate health risks and concerns for the young adult:* Many young adults tend to ignore health issues and adopt a "wait and see" attitude. Health risk behaviors associated with young adulthood include increased alcohol use, illicit drug use, and frequent STDs. Domestic violence is seen throughout adulthood but frequently begins in young adulthood.

LO 18.5 *Summarize the physiologic, cognitive, emotional, and social changes that occur in the middle adult age group:* Middle adulthood may be difficult to define as attitudes about life often determine the extent to which individuals feel and act young or old. During middle adulthood, men and women begin to experience changes that, if unacknowledged, can lead to illness and disability.

LO 18.6 *Explain health risks and concerns for the middle adult:* Cancer and cardiovascular disease are leading causes of death in middle adults. Disease prevention is an important aspect of patient education for this age group. Many middle adults are caring for children, grandchildren, and/or parents, adding unique stressors to life as they juggle career and family responsibilities.

LO 18.7 *Recognize the physiologic, cognitive, emotional, and social changes that affect the older adult:* Older adults are living longer, and many remain independent until death. Others experience cognitive and physical changes that require care in the home or in a health care facility.

LO 18.8 *Outline health risks and concerns for the older adult:* Many older adults are affected by aging in the form of chronic diseases that alter their independence. Musculoskeletal problems, respiratory disorders, cardiovascular diseases, cancers, and diabetes are increasingly common in this age group.

Responses to the critical-thinking questions are available at *http://evolve.elsevier.com/YoostCrawford/fundamentals/*.

REVIEW QUESTIONS

1. From the nurse's knowledge about the emerging adult according to Arnett's theory, which behavior by a 21-year-old hospitalized male patient is most appropriate for his age group?
   a. Talking about college courses that he is taking while working part-time at a restaurant
   b. Requesting that his mom be present when his IV line is started
   c. Stating that he cares for his disabled father and his 2-year-old daughter
   d. Becoming upset that he is not giving back to his community
2. The nurse knows that which patient is an example of the Wear-and-Tear Theory of Aging?
   a. A patient who is dying of cancer at age 35
   b. A 55-year-old who runs half-marathons
   c. A patient with depression and suicidal thoughts who is 65
   d. An 88-year-old with heart failure, kidney failure, and osteoarthritis
3. The nurse is caring for a group of older adults. Which patients in this group are exhibiting normal signs of aging? *(Select all that apply.)*
   a. The patient with knee pain and wrinkles around the eyes
   b. The patient who needs reading glasses and states that the food tastes bland
   c. The patient who is confused and does not know the current year
   d. The patient who states that constipation is an increasing problem
   e. The patient who is showing signs of depression and hopelessness
4. Which behavior by the young adult patient indicates an understanding of patient education aimed at reducing the health risks for that age group?
   a. Smoking only one pack of cigarettes per day
   b. Limiting alcohol use to an occasional drink
   c. Using drugs found in a roommate's drawer for anxiety
   d. Having a relationship with a partner who was threatening in the past
5. While assessing a patient for domestic violence, the nurse knows that which statement is true regarding domestic violence?
   a. It is a health risk factor only during young adulthood.
   b. It occurs across socioeconomic levels and cultural boundaries.
   c. Young women aged 20 to 24 have the lowest incidence of rape and sexual assaults.
   d. Women are the only victims of domestic violence whom nurses should be concerned about.
6. Which steps can nurses and health care providers take to remove barriers to identifying and treating victims of domestic violence? *(Select all that apply.)*
   a. Call the police.
   b. Ask about abuse.
   c. Ask for proof of domestic violence.
   d. Screen for domestic violence with all patients.
   e. Disregard reported abuse in spouses.
7. Which group is referred to as the "sandwich generation"?
   a. Older adults who are caretakers for their elderly parents
   b. Younger adults who are reexamining their life choices
   c. Middle adults who are caretakers for multiple generations of their family
   d. Younger adults who are changing employment constantly
8. Which term indicates a mental health disorder that is frequently seen in older adults?
   a. Schizophrenia
   b. Bipolar disorder
   c. Depression
   d. Posttraumatic stress disorder
9. For which person seen at a physician's office appointment would patient and family education be most critical?
   a. A 24-year-old male patient with a cold virus and on no medications
   b. A 45-year-old male patient on metformin for type 2 diabetes for the past 3 years
   c. A 75-year-old female patient just prescribed the anticoagulant warfarin
   d. A 40-year-old male asthmatic patient diagnosed 10 years ago and on albuterol
10. Which factors are likely to influence the transition from adolescence to adulthood? *(Select all that apply.)*
    a. Cultural beliefs
    b. Societal values
    c. Personal beliefs and expectations
    d. Governmental rules
    e. Societal expectations

Answers and rationales for the review questions are available at *http://evolve.elsevier.com/YoostCrawford/fundamentals/*.

REFERENCES

Administration on Aging: *A profile of older Americans: 2012*, Washington, D.C., 2012, U.S. Department of Health and Human Services.

Alzheimer's Association: Alzheimer's Disease Facts and Figures. *Alzheimer's & Dementia*, 10(2), 2014.

American Cancer Society: Cancer facts & figures 2014, Atlanta, 2014, Author. Retrieved from *www.cancer.org*.

American Diabetes Association: Diagnosis and classification of diabetes mellitus. *Diabetes Care*, 29(S1):S43-S48, 2006.

Arnett JJ: The psychology of emerging adulthood: What is known, and what remains to be known? In JJ Arnett, JL Tanner (Eds): *Emerging adults in America: Coming of age in the 21st century* (pp. 303-330). Washington, D.C., 2006, American Psychological Association.

Belsky J: *Experiencing the lifespan*, ed. 2, New York, 2009, Worth.

Berk LE: *Exploring lifespan development*, ed. 2, Boston, 2011, Pearson.

Berlin G, Furstenberg F, & Waters M: Transition to adulthood: Introducing the issues. *Fut Child*, 20(1), 2010, Spring.

Bjorksten J: Crosslinkage theory of aging. *J Am Geriatr Soc* 16:408-427, 1968.

Butler RN: Ageism: Another form of bigotry. *Gerontologist*, 9:243-246, 1969.

Catalano S: *Intimate partner violence in the United States*. Office of Justice Programs, U.S. Department of Justice, 2007. Retrieved from *www.ojp.usdoj.gov*.

Centers for Disease Control and Prevention: Leading causes of non-fatal violence-related injury in the United States in 2009, 2010a. Retrieved from *www.cdc.gov/injury*.

Centers for Disease Control and Prevention: Summary of health statistics for US adults. National health interview survey, 2009, 2010b. Retrieved from *www.cdc.gov/nchs/data/series/sr_10/sr10_249.pdf*.

Centers for Disease Control and Prevention: Healthy aging: Helping people to live long and productive lives and enjoy a good quality of life, 2011. Retrieved from *www.cdc.gov/chronicdisease/resources/publications/aag/aging.htm*.

Centers for Disease Control and Prevention: Adult cigarette smoking in the United States: Current estimate, 2012a. Retrieved from *www.cdc.gov/tobacco/data_statistics/fact_sheets/adult_data/cig_smoking/index.htm*.

Centers for Disease Control and Prevention: Understanding intimate partner violence fact sheet, 2012b. Retrieved from *www.cdc.gov*.

Centers for Disease Control and Prevention: 2011 Sexually transmitted diseases surveillance, 2012c. Retrieved from *www.cdc.gov/std/stats11/chlamydia.htm*.

Cohn D: Baby boomers: The gloomiest generation. *Pew Social and Demographic Trends Project*, 2008. Retrieved from *http://pewresearch.org/pubs/880/baby-boomers-the-gloomiest-generation*.

Coté J: Emerging adulthood as an institutional moratorium. In JJ Arnett, JT Tanner (Eds): *Emerging adults in America: Coming of age in the 21st century* (pp. 85-126), Washington, D.C., 2006, American Psychological Association.

Cronenwett L, Sherwood G, Barnsteiner J, et al: Quality and safety education for nurses. *Nurs Outlook*, 55(3):122-131, 2007.

Erikson EH: *Childhood and society*, ed. 2, New York, 1963, Norton.

Federal Interagency Forum on Aging-Related Statistics: *Older Americans 2012: Key indicators of well-being*, Washington, D.C., 2012, U.S. Government Printing Office.

Feldman RS: *Development across the life span*, ed. 7, Upper Saddle River, N.J., 2014, Prentice Hall.

Fiske A, Wetherell JL, Gatz M: Depression in older adults. *Annu Rev Clin Psychol* 5:363-389, 2009.

Freud S: *The ego and the id*, London, England, 1974, Hogarth (original work published 1923).

Glaser R, Kiecolt-Glaser J: Chronic stress can steal years from caregivers' lifetimes. *OSU Res*, 2007. Retrieved from *http://researchnews.osu.edu/archive/telomeres.htm*.

Gould R: *Transformations: Growth and change in adulthood*. New York, 1979, Simon & Schuster.

Havighurst RJ: *Human development and education*. New York, 1953, McKay.

Horn J, Cattell R: Age differences in fluid and crystallized intelligence. *Acta Psychol* 26:107-129, 1967.

Johnson RW, Soto M, Zedlewski SR: How is the economic turmoil affecting older Americans? *Urban Institute Fact Sheet on Retirement Policy*, 2008. Retrieved from *www.urban.org/retirement_policy*.

Levinson DJ (with Levinson JD): *Seasons of a woman's life*, New York, 1996, Knopf.

Massel M, Peek M: Ethnic differences in cognitive function over time. *Ann Epidemiol*, 19(11):778-783, 2009.

Massel M, Raji M, Peek M: Education and physical activity mediate the relationship between ethnicity and cognitive function in late middle-aged adults. *Ethn Health*, 15(3): 283-302, 2010.

Mayo Clinic: Caregiver stress: Tips for taking care of yourself, 2012. Retrieved from *www.mayoclinic.com/health/caregiver-stress/MY01231*.

McCance K, Heuther S: *Pathophysiology: The biological basis for disease in adults and children*, ed. 7, St. Louis, 2014, Mosby.

Miller CA: *Nursing for wellness in older adults*, ed. 6, Philadelphia, 2012, Lippincott, Williams & Wilkins.

Moody H: *Aging: Concepts and controversies*, Thousand Oaks, Calif., 2010, Pine Forge Press/Sage.

National Adolescent Health Information Center: 2006 fact sheet on mortality: Adolescents and young adults, 2006. Retrieved from *http://nahic.ucsf.edu*.

National Adolescent Health Information Center: Demographics: Young adults fact sheet, 2008. Retrieved from *http://nahic.ucsf.edu*.

National Center for Health Statistics: *Health, United States, 2013*, Hyattsville, Md., 2009, Author.

National Center for Health Statistics: *Young adults seeking medical care: Do race and ethnicity matter?* NCHS Data Brief No. 55, Hyattsville, Md., 2011, Author.

National Institute on Aging: Healthy aging: Lessons from the Baltimore longitudinal study of aging, 2010. Retrieved from *www.nia.nih.gov*.

O'Connell M, Boat T, Warner K: *Preventing mental, emotional, and behavioral disorders among young people: Progress and possibilities*, Washington, D.C., 2009, Institute of Medicine, National Research Council.

Perry WG: Cognitive and ethical growth: The making of meaning. In AW Chickering et al (Eds), *The modern American college* (pp. 76-116), San Francisco, 1981, Jossey-Bass.

Piaget J: *The theory of stages in cognitive development*, New York, 1969, McGraw-Hill.

Schulenberg JE, Bryant AL, O'Malley PM: Taking hold of some kind of life: How developmental tasks relate to trajectories of well-being during the transition to adulthood. *Dev Psychopathol*, 16:1119-1140, 2004.

Stanley M, Blair KA, Beare PG: *Gerontological nursing: Promoting successful aging with older adults*, ed. 3, Philadelphia, 2005, F.A. Davis.

Substance Abuse and Mental Health Services Administration: *Results from the 2012 national survey on drug use & health: Summary of national findings*, Rockville, Md., 2013, Department of Health and Human Services. Retrieved from *www.samhsa.gov/data/NSDUH.aspx.*

Tabloski PA: *Gerontological nursing: The essential guide to clinical practice*, ed. 3, Upper Saddle River, N.J., 2014, Pearson Prentice-Hall.

Touhy TA, Jett K: *Ebersole and Hess' toward healthy aging: Human needs and nursing response*, ed. 8, St. Louis, 2012, Mosby.

University of Michigan: *Health and retirement study*, Ann Arbor, Mich., 2011, Author.

U.S. Census Bureau: *Statistical abstract of the United States: 2012*, ed. 131, Washington, D.C., 2011, Author. Retrieved from *www.census.gov/compendia/statab.*

U.S. Department of Health and Human Services: *Healthy people 2020*, Washington, D.C., 2010, U.S. Government Printing Office. Retrieved from *http://healthypeople.gov/2020.*

Wilson RS, Aggarwal NT, Barnes LL, et al: Cognitive decline in incident Alzheimer disease in a community population. *Neurology*, 75:1070-1078, 2010.

Zafari AM, Afonso LC, Aggarwal K, et al: Myocardial infarction. *Medscape Reference*, 2012. Retrieved from *http://emedicine.medscape.com/article/155919-overview#a0104.*

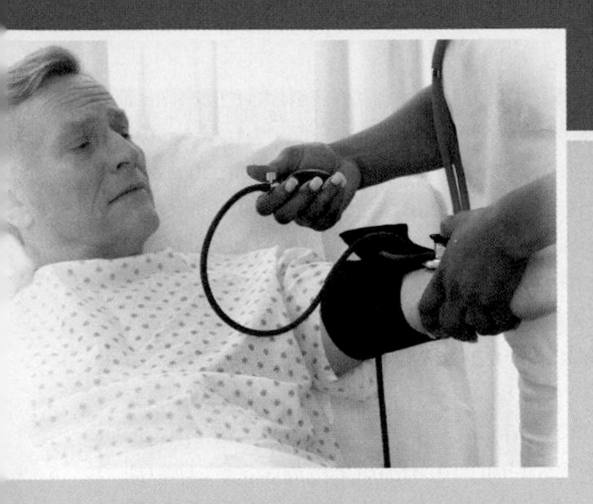

CHAPTER 19

Vital Signs

EVOLVE WEBSITE

http://evolve.elsevier.com/YoostCrawford/fundamentals/

- Additional Evolve-Only Review Questions with Answers
- Answers and Rationales for Text Review Questions
- Answers to Critical-Thinking Exercises
- Case Study with Questions
- Video Clips
- Conceptual Care Map Creator
- Body Spectrum
- Animations
- Skills Checklist
- Glossary

LEARNING OUTCOMES

Comprehension of this chapter's content will provide students with the ability to:

LO 19.1 Explain the purpose of assessing vital signs.
LO 19.2 Describe techniques for obtaining accurate temperature measurement.
LO 19.3 Identify common assessment sites and techniques for assessing pulse.
LO 19.4 Discuss assessment of respirations and blood oxygenation.
LO 19.5 Summarize correct methods for measuring blood pressure.
LO 19.6 Perform pain assessment in diverse populations.

KEY TERMS

afebrile, p. 289
apical pulse, p. 294
apnea, p. 298
arrhythmia, p. 296
auscultation, p. 295
auscultatory gap, p. 304
blood pressure, p. 286
bradycardia, p. 296
bradypnea, p. 298
core temperature, p. 289
cyanosis, p. 299
diastolic pressure, p. 300
dyspnea, p. 298
dysrhythmia, p. 296
eupnea, p. 298
febrile, p. 290
fever, p. 290
frostbite, p. 290
heat exhaustion, p. 290
heatstroke, p. 290
hypercapnia, p. 297
hypertension, p. 287
hyperthermia, p. 290
hyperventilation, p. 298
hypotension, p. 290
hypothermia, p. 290
hypoventilation, p. 298
hypoxemia, p. 297
Korotkoff sounds, p. 304
orthopnea, p. 298
orthostatic hypotension, p. 301
oxygen saturation, p. 298
pain, p. 286
palpation, p. 305
peripheral pulse, p. 294
pulse, p. 286
pulse deficit, p. 296
pulse oximetry, p. 286
radial pulse, p. 296
respiration, p. 286
systolic pressure, p. 300
tachycardia, p. 296
tachypnea, p. 298
temperature, p. 286
vital signs, p. 286

CASE STUDY

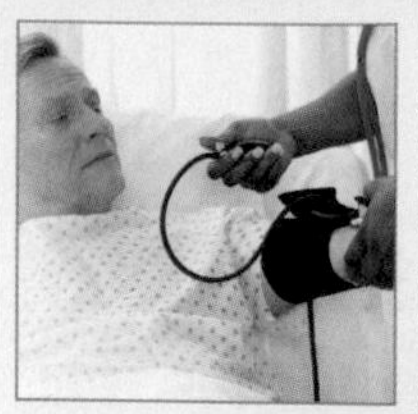

Mr. Donley, a 79-year-old male, was just admitted from the emergency department with complaints of shortness of breath, dizziness, green-tinged sputum, and pain with deep inspiration. He started sleeping with two pillows 2 nights ago to ease his breathing. Chest x-ray shows pneumonia and exacerbation of heart failure. The arterial blood gas report is pending. Serum K (potassium) is 3.0 mEq/L, and the white blood cell (WBC) count is 19,000/mm^3. A urinalysis (UA) is ordered, but Mr. Donley has not voided yet. His medical history includes hypertension, high cholesterol, and previous episodes of heart failure. He smoked one pack per day of cigarettes for 30 years but quit 20 years ago.

Mr. Donley's admission vital signs (VS) are T 38.89°C (102°F), P 104 regular, R 32 and shallow and labored, BP 160/94, pulse oximetry (SpO_2) of 89% on room air (RA), and chest pain 5 of 10 with deep breathing. During assessment, the nurse notes a "barrel chest," bilateral crackles, diminished lung sounds in the left lower lobe, pedal pulses that are not palpable but can be heard on Doppler examination, and 3+ pedal edema. The patient experiences dyspnea on exertion and when lying flat and exhibits use of accessory muscles to breathe. A 15-pound weight gain is noted over that measured at the outpatient clinic where Mr. Donley visited 1 week ago. His Braden score is 17, and his Morse Fall score is 48.

Treatment orders are as follows:

- VS q 4 hr with pulse oximetry
- Fluid restriction of 1200 mL/24 hr
- No-added-salt diet
- Up with assistance; fall precautions
- Intake and output
- Administer supplemental O_2 up to 4 L to keep SpO_2 ≥92%
- Incentive spirometer (IS) and coughing and deep breathing (CDB) q 2 hr

Medication orders are as follows:

- Digoxin 0.125 mg PO q day
- Furosemide 40 mg IV q day
- KCl 40 mEq PO q day
- Levofloxin 750 mg IV q 24 hr × 5 days

Refer back to this case study to answer the critical-thinking questions throughout the chapter.

Vital signs are a basic but very important component of physiologic assessment of the patient. They are used to monitor the functioning of body systems. Assessment of vital signs allows the nurse to detect changes in the health status of the patient, identify early warning signs of life-threatening health conditions, and evaluate the effectiveness of interventions.

Vital signs consist of body temperature (T), pulse (P), respirations (R), and blood pressure (BP). **Temperature** refers to the measurable heat of the human body. **Pulse** is the detectable rhythmic expansion of an artery that occurs with the pumping action of the beating heart; thus, the pulse rate is measured as number of heartbeats per minute (bpm), with pulse strength and pattern often specified as well. **Respiration** is the act of breathing, so respirations are assessed for frequency, or breaths per minute (BPM); abnormal quality and pattern of breathing also should be noted. **Blood pressure** is the measurable pressure of blood within the systemic arteries.

Since 2001, The Joint Commission has required that every patient be assessed and treated for **pain** (refer to Chapter 36). Accordingly, pain often is referred to as the *fifth vital sign.*

Results of **pulse oximetry**, which measures the amount of oxygen available to tissues, typically are included with reported vital signs. The pulse oximeter reading is the saturation of peripheral oxygen (SpO_2).

VITAL SIGN MEASUREMENT LO 19.1

Baseline values, or initial vital signs, are used to identify changes in patient status; a series of vital sign measurements establishes patient trends. The task of obtaining vital signs is relatively easy to learn, but interpreting the meaning of the values and incorporating the results into the management of patient care require knowledge, problem solving, and clinical judgment. Although determination of vital signs is one of the most frequently performed nursing tasks, it is also important to assess the patient's clinical status (see Chapter 20).

The frequency of assessing vital signs is determined individually for each patient and is dependent on patient status. Patients may have vital signs checked every time they visit an outpatient clinic or once a week in some psychiatric settings or long-term care settings. Health care providers may order specific parameters for vital signs. Most inpatient facilities have a policy specifying the minimum frequency at which vital signs are obtained. Vital sign assessments typically are done every 4 or 8 hours for stable patients, every 15 to 60 minutes for postprocedure or postsurgical patients, and every

BOX 19-1 Situations That Require Vital Sign Assessment

- On admission to a health care agency, to establish baselines
- As part of a physical assessment
- During an inpatient stay, as routine monitoring
- With any change in health status, especially complaints of chest pain and shortness of breath or feeling hot, faint, or dizzy
- Before and after surgery or invasive procedures to establish baselines and monitor effects
- Before and after administration of medications that impact cardiac, respiratory, or thermal regulation systems
- Before and after interventions such as ambulation
- In ongoing care, to detect improvement in patient condition
- Before discharge or transfer from a unit, to validate patient readiness

5 minutes or continuously for critical or unstable patients. Technology-based devices provide continuous monitoring of vital signs in critical care and surgical settings. The nurse providing care uses clinical judgment to determine the need to assess vital signs more frequently on the basis of the patient's condition. Situations in which vital signs are assessed are listed in Box 19-1. Vital signs may be affected by many factors. Asking specific assessment questions (Health Assessment Questions box) related to vital signs helps the nurse interpret the measurement findings.

Vital signs are interpreted on the basis of current health status and previously established (baseline) normal values for the patient. Normal values vary with patient age, and normal ranges for each vital sign component have been established for various age groups (Table 19-1).

To interpret vital signs, the nurse begins by comparing the patient's measurements with expected normal values (see Table 19-1) and with that patient's baseline values, recognizing that it is always appropriate to recheck vital signs to verify any changes that occur. The nurse compares the most recent measurements with previous readings. Values may have increased or decreased from previous readings; such variations may indicate an improving or worsening condition or even a sudden change in status requiring emergency interventions. It is part of nursing judgment to determine that vital signs need to be assessed, sometimes as often as every 5 minutes, to monitor changes in the patient's condition. Understanding the patient's medical history and diagnosis is part of the nurse's interpretation of vital sign findings. For example, a patient with **hypertension** may have a blood pressure reading higher than normal. Blood pressure also may be increased in the patient experiencing pain, and pain medications may slow the respiratory and cardiovascular system, lowering the blood pressure, heart rate, and respiratory rate.

Many medical factors influence vital signs, such as infection and renal, respiratory, and cardiovascular disease. Other

HEALTH ASSESSMENT QUESTIONS

Focus on Temperature

- Have you had anything to eat or drink or chewed gum in the last 15 minutes?
- Have you been exercising in the last 30 minutes?
- Have you been sleeping?
- Do you smoke? When was your last cigarette?
- Have you been feeling hot, sweaty, or cold?

Focus on Pulse

- Have you been exercising within the last 30 minutes?
- Are you feeling short of breath? tired?
- Are you having chest pain? feeling of racing pulse?
- Do you have swelling in your hands or feet?
- What medications are you taking?
- Do you smoke?
- Do you have a history of heart disease?

Focus on Respiratory Rate

- Are you feeling short of breath?
- Have you been exercising recently?
- Do you have a history of respiratory illness or diabetes?
- Have you had pain medication recently?
- Are you having pain?
- Are you a smoker?

Focus on Blood Pressure

- Have you recently been engaged in activity, exercise, or eating?
- What medications are you taking?
- Do you have a family history of hypertension?
- Do you exercise regularly?
- What do you eat in a typical day?
- How would you rate your pain level? stress level?
- What surgeries have you had?

Focus on Pain

Special care should be taken in assessing pain. Completing a thorough pain assessment requires that nurses ask patients about several critical areas of concern: pain location, onset, quality, intensity, and pattern; precipitating and alleviating factors; and associated symptoms. The acronym *SOCRATES* is used by many health care professionals to track each area of pain assessment *(www.valuemd.com/clinical.php)*. The letters in SOCRATES stand for:

- ***S**ite:* Where is the pain located?
- ***O**nset:* When did the pain start? Was it gradual or sudden?
- ***C**haracter:* What is the quality of the pain? Is it stabbing, burning, or aching in nature?
- ***R**adiation:* Does the pain radiate anywhere?
- ***A**ssociations:* What signs and symptoms are associated with the pain?
- ***T**ime course:* Is there any pattern to the pain?
- ***E**xacerbating/relieving factors:* Does anything make the pain worse or help it?
- ***S**everity:* On a scale of 0 to 10, what is its intensity?

TABLE 19-1 Vital Sign Ranges Across the Life Span

AGE GROUP	TEMPERATURE	PULSE (bpm)	RESPIRATIONS (bpm)	SpO_2	BLOOD PRESSURE (mm Hg)	
					SYSTOLIC	DIASTOLIC
Newborn	35.5°-37.5° C (96°-99.5° F)	80-160	30-80	>95%	60-90	20-60
1 yr old	37.4°-37.6° C (99.4°-99.7° F)	80-140	24-40	>95%	74-100	50-70
6 yr old	36.6°-37° C (98°-98.6° F)	75-110	15-25	>95%	84-120	54-80
15 yr old	36.1°-37.2° C (97°-99° F)	50-90	15-20	>95%	94-120	62-80
Adult	35.5°-37.5° C (95.9°-99.5° F)	60-100	12-20	>95%	90-120	60-80
Older adult	35°-37.2° C (95°-99° F)	60-100	15-20	>95%	90-120	60-80

factors that affect vital signs include, but are not limited to, the physical environment, emotional state of the patient, medications, food and fluid intake, and activity level and tolerance. The nurse takes these factors into account when interpreting vital sign results for each patient.

Accuracy of vital sign values obtained depends on the precision of measurement. Careless measurement can result in inappropriate or missed interventions and care decisions. Expertise in the skill of vital sign determination is a critical nursing function, although this task may be delegated (Collaboration and Delegation box). It is important to provide patient education for people who need to monitor vital signs in the home setting to manage their own or a family member's health. For example, patients receiving chemotherapy may need to have their temperature taken as ongoing monitoring for infection. Patients with hypertension may need to routinely check their blood pressure.

COLLABORATION AND DELEGATION

Vital Signs

- The task of taking vital signs may be delegated to unlicensed assistive personnel (UAP), but before delegating this task, the nurse assesses patients to determine that they are medically stable.
- UAP may measure, record, and report vital signs for the stable patient, but interpretation of vital signs remains the responsibility of the licensed or registered nurse. Interpreting vital signs is done in relation to other assessment findings.
- The nurse ensures that the UAP knows the proper technique for taking vital signs and knows what values need to be reported immediately for each patient.
- It is the nurse's responsibility to ensure the accuracy of vital sign data and to report abnormal values in conjunction with additional physical symptoms.
- The nurse should double-check vital signs to verify abnormal values.

Both normal and abnormal vital sign results are appropriately documented and communicated to all members of the health care team. Values are recorded on the specified form or the electronic medical record used by the facility. With such documentation, multiple sets of vital signs typically are easily visible at a time, thereby showing trends for the patient.

QSEN FOCUS!

Nurses use informatics when identifying essential information such as vital signs that must be available in a common database to support patient care. Nurses must be able to navigate the electronic health record to view baseline patient data, and they must understand the technology that supports clinical decision making.

SAFE PRACTICE ALERT

Sudden alterations in vital signs or values outside the normal range are indicators of a priority situation for the nurse. Further assessments and emergency measures should be initiated as indicated by the patient's status. The health care provider is notified of alterations in vital signs.

TEMPERATURE LO 19.2

Healthy people are able to maintain body temperature within the normal range even when exposed to temperature extremes for short periods. A person's ability to manage body temperature depends on certain behavioral abilities and thought processes, such as adequate mobility to leave an area of extreme heat or cold, the capacity to sense temperature discomfort, and the physical ability to add or remove clothing. For example, infants can sense discomfort but are unable to change their circumstances to adjust their temperatures. They cannot adjust the amount of clothing they wear or leave an environment that is too hot or too cold. Older adults may need assistance in adjusting to temperature changes because of cognitive impairment or physical issues, or both. Illness or an altered level of consciousness puts the affected person at risk for inability to maintain proper thermal control.

TABLE 19-2 Average Normal Adult Temperature Ranges at Different Body Sites

ORAL	AXILLARY	RECTAL	TYMPANIC	TEMPORAL
36.0°-37.6° C (96.8°-99.68° F)	35.5°-37.0° C (95.9°-98.6° F)	34.4°-37.8° C (93.92°-100.04° F)	35.6°-37.4° C (96.08°-99.32° F)	36.1°-37.3° C (96.98°-99.14° F)

From Davie A, Amoore J: Best practice in the measurement of body temperature, *Nurs Stand* 24(42):42-49, 2010.

NORMAL PARAMETERS OF BODY TEMPERATURE

Temperature is measured in degrees, represented by the symbol °. The core body temperature remains relatively constant within the range of 36.5° to 37.5° C (97.6° to 99.6° F); the average oral temperature is 37° C (98.6° F). A person who maintains this normal body temperature is considered to be **afebrile**. Body tissue and cells function best within this range. Axillary temperatures may be approximately 1° less than oral readings, which in turn are approximately 1° less than rectal temperatures. Normal tympanic temperatures fall between normal oral and rectal temperatures. Table 19-2 compares average normal adult temperatures at different body sites.

PHYSIOLOGY OF HEAT PRODUCTION AND LOSS

Humans are warm-blooded, which means that they maintain a consistent internal temperature independent of the outside environment. Body temperature reflects the difference between the amount of heat produced by body processes and the amount of heat lost to the external environment. Heat is generated by metabolic processes in core tissues of the body and is transferred by circulating blood to the skin, where it is dissipated into the environment.

Thermoregulation comprises the physiologic and behavioral mechanisms that regulate the balance between heat production and heat loss. Regulation by neurologic mechanisms maintains this relationship of heat production and loss.

The hypothalamus in the brain acts as the body's thermostat. Even minor changes in body temperature are transmitted by thermal receptors located throughout the body to the hypothalamus by way of the spinal cord. The anterior hypothalamus controls heat loss through the mechanisms of diaphoresis (sweating) and vasodilation of blood vessels, which enable heat loss. The posterior hypothalamus conserves heat through mechanisms such as vasoconstriction to reduce heat loss and shivering. Disease or trauma to the hypothalamus or spinal cord can therefore cause alterations in temperature control.

Heat Production

Heat produced in the body is a by-product of metabolism, the chemical process that is responsible for generating energy for cellular functions. Food is the primary fuel source for metabolism. The amount of heat produced is related to the rate of metabolism. Exercise, increased release of epinephrine and norepinephrine, and increased production of thyroid hormones all can increase heat production.

Heat Loss

Heat production and loss occur simultaneously. The skin regulates temperature through insulation of the body with subcutaneous tissue and fat, and in conjunction with the circulatory system, it is the primary source of heat loss. Circulating blood brings heat to the skin surface, where connections between the arterioles and venules below the skin's surface open (vasodilate) to allow heat to dissipate or close (vasoconstrict) to retain heat. The sympathetic nervous system controls the opening and closing of these connections in response to changes in the **core temperature** (temperature of deep tissues) or environmental temperature (Porth, 2011). Because skin is exposed to the environment, there is constant heat loss through radiation, conduction, convection, and evaporation:

- *Radiation:* Radiation is the transfer of heat as waves or particles of energy. No actual contact occurs between the object transmitting the heat and the object absorbing it. For example, peripheral vasodilation increases blood flow to the skin, thereby increasing radiant heat loss. Vasoconstriction minimizes heat loss from the skin. If the environmental temperature is higher than the skin temperature, the body also will absorb heat by radiation.
- *Conduction:* Conduction is the transfer of and reaction to heat through direct contact. Heat from the body is lost when it comes in contact with a cooler object, such as an ice pack or cool cloth.
- *Convection:* Convection is the transfer of heat by movement or circulation of warm matter such as air or water.
- *Evaporation:* Evaporation is the process by which a liquid is changed to a vapor through heat. Diaphoresis increases during exercise, emotional or mental stress, and fever. The process of evaporation lowers body temperature.

FACTORS AFFECTING BODY TEMPERATURE

Many factors can alter the relationship between heat production and heat loss. Part of the nursing assessment is evaluating factors that are affecting the temperature of a patient. Typical factors that affect patient temperature include age (very young and very old), recent exercise, hormone fluctuations, circadian rhythms, stress, and environment (Box 19-2).

BOX 19-2 Factors Affecting Body Temperature

- *Age:* Newborns have unstable body temperatures because of immature regulatory mechanisms. Even a mild rise in temperature is significant in infants younger than 3 months of age. It is common for the baseline temperature to drop as the person ages. Infants and elderly people are more susceptible to environmental temperature extremes.
- *Exercise:* Body temperature increases with exercise as carbohydrates and fats are metabolized to provide energy.
- *Hormone fluctuations:* Women typically have a higher temperature during ovulation. Thyroxine, epinephrine, and norepinephrine increase heat production and therefore can increase temperature.
- *Circadian rhythms:* The temperature of most people is lowest around 3 A.M. and highest around 6 P.M.
- *Stress:* The levels of epinephrine and norepinephrine can increase during emotional or physical stress.
- *Environment:* Extended exposure to extreme heat or extreme cold can affect core body temperature. Heat and cold application used as treatment for pain, injuries, or swelling can affect body temperature.
- *Smoking:* Smoking causes vasoconstriction, which can cause a drop in the temperature of the skin and mucous membranes.

EVIDENCE-BASED PRACTICE AND INFORMATICS

Preventing Hypothermia in Older Adults

Advise patients to:

- Dress in layers, even while at home. Long underwear may be worn under clothing, along with socks and slippers.
- Use a blanket or throw to keep legs and shoulders warm.
- When outside in cold weather, wear a scarf and gloves. A hat is especially important to maintain body heat.
- Keep extremities covered to prevent heat loss.
- Keep the thermostat at a minimum of 68° F.

Assistance with heating costs may be available through utility companies, local nonprofit organizations such as the United Way, or the Low Income Home Energy Assistance Program (LIHEAP). Refer patients for assistance if they are unable to pay heating costs.

From National Institute on Aging: Hypothermia: staying safe in cold weather, *NIH News*, Jan 14, 2010. Retrieved from *www.nih.gov/news/health/jan2010/nia-14.htm.*

Clothing allows the wearer to lose heat when it is hot or retain heat when it is cold. When a person is exposed to extreme cold without adequate protective clothing, heat loss can lead to **hypothermia** (low body temperature). Likewise, exposure to extreme heat for a prolonged time can lead to **hyperthermia** (high body temperature). Either of these extremes can cause serious illness or even death. The thermoregulation systems of the very young and the very old are not as efficient as in people of other age groups, placing them at higher risk for hypothermia and hyperthermia.

Signs of hypothermia include decreased body temperature and respirations, pale and cool skin, **hypotension** (decreased blood pressure), decreased muscle coordination and urinary output, disorientation, and drowsiness progressing to coma. The Evidence-Based Practice and Informatics box identifies measures recommended for elderly people to prevent hyperthermia. **Frostbite** occurs from exposure to subnormal temperatures. Ice crystals form inside the cells, which may cause permanent circulatory and tissue damage. Common sites for frostbite are earlobes, the tip of the nose, fingers, and toes. The skin becomes white and firm, with a loss of sensation. Interventions for frostbite include gradual warming, pain management, and protection of the injured area.

Fever (pyrexia) is a rise in body temperature above normal, caused by trauma or illness. A person with a fever is described as **febrile**. Fever may be associated with an infection, tissue injury, cancer, trauma, or surgery. Patients with a fever can experience loss of appetite (anorexia), headache, malaise, hot and dry skin, flushing, thirst, shivering, and a general feeling of not being well. Signs of fever include dehydration, decreased urinary output, and rapid heart rate. Older people may demonstrate only a slight rise in temperature despite an illness process such as pneumonia.

Heatstroke occurs when prolonged exposure to the sun or high environmental temperatures overwhelms the body's heat loss mechanisms. This health emergency carries a high mortality rate. Risk factors include very young or very old age, cardiovascular disease, diabetes, and alcoholism, along with exercise or work out of doors in predisposing conditions. Signs and symptoms include confusion, delirium, excessive thirst, nausea, muscle cramps, and high temperature and heart rate. Hot, dry skin and absence of sweating are other features of heat stroke. **Heat exhaustion** occurs when extreme or prolonged environmental heat exposure leads to profuse sweating with consequent excessive water and electrolyte loss. Clinical manifestations are those of fluid volume deficit (see Chapter 39 for a discussion of this metabolic disturbance).

ASSESSMENT OF TEMPERATURE

Body temperature is measured in degrees on either the Fahrenheit or the Celsius scale. The reliability of temperature values depends on selecting the most appropriate site, using the correct equipment, and using the correct procedure to obtain the measurement. The five sites commonly used to measure temperature are the mouth, ear, rectum, forehead (where the temporal artery is close to the skin), and axilla. Depending on patient status, any of these sites may be appropriate if the proper technique is used. Site selection is affected by patient age, state of consciousness, amount of pain the patient is suffering, and treatment the patient is undergoing, such as oxygen supplementation. Normal temperature varies

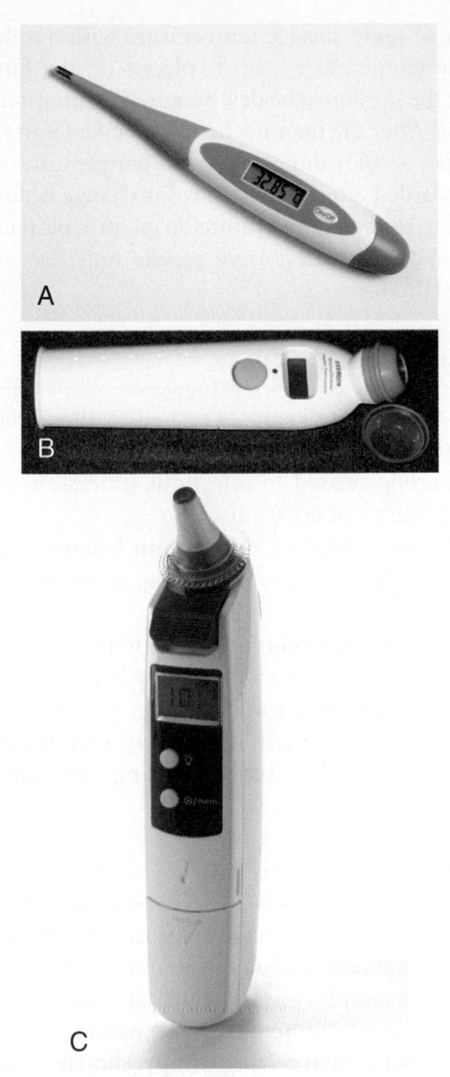

FIGURE 19-1 Types of thermometers: **A,** electronic; **B,** temporal artery; **C,** tympanic.

among sites (see Table 19-2). Core temperatures can be measured with specialized equipment through the esophagus or pulmonary artery sites. The measuring device used is dependent on the site (Figure 19-1). Skill 19-1 describes the procedures for measuring body temperature at different sites with different types of thermometers.

Oral Temperature

The most common site for measuring temperature is under the tongue. The patient must be able to close the mouth around the thermometer. Advantages of this site are that it is readily accessible and comfortable for the patient. Eating, drinking, smoking, and the use of oxygen by cannula or mask can affect measurements obtained at the oral site. It is not a preferred site for infants and young children, unconscious patients, post–oral surgery patients, or people with seizure disorders.

Rectal Temperature

Rectal temperature readings are considered to be very accurate. The rectum, however, is not a site preferred by patients. The rectal route is contraindicated in newborns, in patients who are neutropenic (manifested as a low white blood cell count), and in patients with spinal cord injury. It should not be used for patients with diarrhea or rectal disease, post–rectal surgery patients, or quadriplegic patients.

! SAFE PRACTICE ALERT

Taking rectal temperatures can cause rectal perforation in young infants, and the site should be used only when no other feasible option is available. If a rectal temperature must be taken, a well-lubricated thermometer, inserted no more than the length of the thermometer's bulb, should be used.

! SAFE PRACTICE ALERT

Taking the patient's temperature using the rectal route can cause bleeding in people with hemorrhoids.

Ear (Tympanic) Temperature

The tympanic membrane temperature is a core temperature. The thermometer does not touch the tympanic membrane. This site is easily accessed for both adults and children. Use of the tympanic route is appropriate for patients who are confused or those who are unconscious. Readings are not significantly affected by otitis media (infection of the middle ear). Spread of infection from patient to patient is less of a concern with use of the tympanic site than with the oral and rectal sites. False-low readings from the tympanic site reflect poor technique, leading to an inaccurate temperature measurement at the site (Mackechnie and Simpson, 2006). An accurate tympanic reading is obtained by grasping the pinna and gently pulling up and back for the adult, or down and back for a child younger than 3 years of age; placing the covered probe snugly in the ear canal; and angling it toward the jaw line before activating the sensor.

The tympanic thermometer is battery-powered. The sensor probe, covered with a disposable cover, is placed in the ear canal, and the degree of infrared heat radiation is read from the tympanic membrane (eardrum). It is important to train users in proper technique to obtain accurate readings. Readings are obtained in approximately 2 seconds, making use of this site appropriate in young children older than 2 months of age and in emergency settings in which assessments need to be completed quickly. It is not appropriate for patients with ear drainage or eardrum scarring.

Forehead (Temporal Artery) Temperature

Technology now allows measuring temperature from the temporal artery, and results may closely reflect the body's core temperature (Davie and Amoore, 2010). This measurement is well tolerated by infants and young children. It is not affected by mild perspiration when performed correctly.

The temporal artery thermometer is a small handheld unit that is scanned across the forehead to measure heat emitted from the temporal artery. This thermometer actually measures ambient air temperature and corrects the temperature reading for radiant heat loss. A covering on the head can affect the accuracy of the reading.

Axillary Temperature

The axillary site may be used when the oral and rectal sites are contraindicated or inaccessible. It is the site frequently used for healthy newborns. The thermometer is placed in the center of the patient's axilla until the reading is obtained. The end of the sensor must remain in contact with the skin. The axillary route is acceptable for infants, children, and patients who cannot tolerate measurement by other routes.

Electronic Thermometers

Electronic and digital thermometers are commonly used in health care facilities to measure oral, rectal, or axillary temperature in less than 1 minute. The thermometer is battery-powered, with a temperature-sensitive probe attached to the unit. A disposable probe cover is used for infection control. Readings are given on a digital screen within several seconds. The same probe can be used for oral and axillary measurements. A separate probe, color-coded red, is used for rectal measurements. Inexpensive disposable digital thermometers often are used for patients in isolation.

Disposable Thermometers and Temperature-Sensitive Strips

Disposable paper thermometers are single-use or reusable strips of paper with liquid crystal dots or bars and a temperature sensor at one end that changes color to reflect body temperature. To obtain the temperature, the nurse reads the highest reading among the dots that have changed color. These strips are an excellent choice when asepsis must be maintained for infection control. The strips can be used for oral (1-minute reading) or axillary (3-minute reading) sites. Temperature-sensitive strips may be used to obtain a general indication of body surface temperature within a designated range. The temperature strip is placed on the forehead or abdomen; the skin must be dry, because perspiration can alter the reading. After the manufacturer's specified wait time (e.g., 15 seconds), a color appears on the temperature strip. The strip is discarded after the initial color change is noted. With use of color-change temperature strips in children younger than 2 years of age, abnormal results must be verified by another method.

NURSING DIAGNOSIS

Examples of nursing diagnoses related to altered body temperature are:

- *Hyperthermia* related to infectious process, as evidenced by temperature of 40° C (104° F)
- *Hypothermia* related to exposure to below-freezing temperature without adequate clothing, as evidenced by temperature of 93.6° F
- *Ineffective Thermoregulation* related to premature infant of 32 weeks' gestation, as evidenced by inability to maintain temperature within normal range
- *Risk for Imbalanced Body Temperature* with the risk factor of trauma to the brain causing damage to the hypothalamus

PLANNING

The planning stage of the nursing process involves prioritizing nursing diagnoses, evaluating resources, and setting goals (Table 19-3). Examples of goal statements are:

- Patient will exhibit temperature within normal range within 1 hour of receiving antipyretic (fever reducing) medication.
- Patient will maintain temperature within normal range within 1 hour of placement on an aquathermia pad and initiation of warmed intravenous fluids.
- Patient will maintain temperature within expected parameters before discharge from the newborn intensive care unit.
- Patient's temperature will measure within normal range throughout recovery from head injury.

TABLE 19-3 Care Planning

NANDA-I NURSING DIAGNOSIS LABEL WITH NURSING DIAGNOSIS STATEMENT	NURSING OUTCOME CLASSIFICATION (NOC)	NURSING INTERVENTION CLASSIFICATION (NIC)
Hyperthermia related to infectious process, as evidenced by temperature of 40° C (104° F)	*Thermoregulation* (0800) Reported thermal comfort (080015)	*Fever treatment* (3740) Administer medications to treat the cause of fever, as appropriate.

From Bulechek G, Butcher H, Dochterman J, et al (Eds): *Nursing interventions classification (NIC),* ed. 6, St. Louis, 2013, Mosby; Moorhead S, Johnson M, Maas M, et al (Eds): *Nursing outcomes classification (NOC),* ed. 5, St. Louis, 2013, Mosby; NANDA International: *Nursing diagnoses: Definitions and classification, 2012–2014,* West Sussex, England, 2012, Wiley-Blackwell. Reprinted with permission from NANDA International, Inc.

For vital signs, planning focuses on selection of the best site and method for measuring each vital-sign component. Gathering the correct equipment before approaching the patient is important; equipment for measuring temperature includes electronic or digital thermometers, tympanic membrane thermometers, temporal artery (forehead) thermometers, and disposable paper thermometers. Glass mercury thermometers are no longer manufactured or sold and should not be used because of the risk of exposure to mercury (Home Care Considerations box).

HOME CARE CONSIDERATIONS

Proper Disposal of Mercury

Although use of glass mercury thermometers in health care settings is obsolete, many such thermometers are still used in the home. Mercury exposure can cause respiratory and gastrointestinal irritation and renal damage. Prolonged exposure can cause neurologic impairment.

Patients should be encouraged to properly dispose of glass thermometers and purchase a safer type. Teach patients what to do if a glass thermometer breaks:

- Do not touch spilled mercury droplets. If skin contact occurs, immediately flush the area with water for 15 minutes.
- Have everyone leave the area and close the door to the contaminated room. Do not allow children to help clean up the area.
- Using gloves, remove any items contaminated with mercury and place them in a zip-top bag.
- Wipe up mercury beads with a wet paper towel and place it in a zip-top bag.
- Shaving cream on a small paint brush or duct tape may be applied to small beads to facilitate pickup; place the item in a zip-top bag.
- Consult the local health department or fire department for disposal instructions.
- After the spill is cleaned, keep the area well ventilated for at least 24 hours.

From Environmental Protection Agency: What to do if a mercury thermometer breaks, 2010. Retrieved from *www.epa.gov/mercury/spills/#thermometer*.

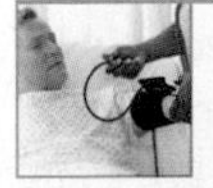

The conceptual care map for Mr. Donley can be found at *http://evolve.elsevier.com/YoostCrawford/fundamentals/*. It is partially completed to indicate how to use the map as a learning tool. Complete the nursing diagnoses using the example conceptual care maps shown in Chapters 8 and 25 to 33.

IMPLEMENTATION AND EVALUATION

Information from the patient history and assessment are used to formulate an individualized treatment plan. Nursing interventions are chosen on the basis of nursing diagnoses for each patient and are based on the patient's thermoregulation problem. Interventions for an increased or decreased temperature must be evaluated for appropriateness for the specific patient.

When treatment is indicated for an increased temperature, nonsteroidal drugs with antipyretic effect, such as aspirin and acetaminophen, may be ordered to lower the set-point of the hypothalamus. Cool sponge baths, cooling blankets, and cool packs are used to reduce fever, but they can increase energy expenditure by stimulating shivering. Aspirin should not be given to children younger than 2 years of age without medical supervision, nor should it be given to children or teenagers with a viral illness because of the associated risk of Reye's syndrome (a serious illness affecting the liver and brain). If the fever is a result of bacterial infection, an antibiotic is administered as prescribed. Blood cultures may be ordered to identify causative organisms. Oxygen may be necessary to meet increased metabolic needs. Other interventions include monitoring the patient's temperature frequently, monitoring other vital signs, monitoring intake and output, increasing the intake of fluids as appropriate, and maintaining oral hygiene. Removal of extra blankets can help dissipate excessive heat. Because diaphoresis occurs with fever, a change of clothing and bedding often is needed. Nursing activities to restore normal body temperature include:

- Identify the underlying cause of the fever in order to plan and provide effective treatment or obtain ordered culture specimens.
- Assess the patient frequently for changes.
- Monitor body temperature and other vital signs by appropriate route every 2 hours or more frequently, as indicated by patient status, to measure treatment response, because the increased metabolic rate that accompanies fever increases pulse and respirations.
- Provide oral and/or intravenous fluids to replace fluid loss from increased respirations and diaphoresis.
- Provide prescribed interventions such as antibiotics to treat the underlying cause of the fever. Note that blood and other culture specimens may need to be obtained before antibiotics are started.
- Implement nonpharmacologic measures to reduce the fever without causing shivering, as shivering produces additional body heat.
- Keep clothing and bedding dry to reduce shivering.
- Encourage physical rest to reduce metabolic demands and oxygen use.
- Provide nutritional support to meet increased metabolic demands.

Hypothermia requires measures to raise body temperature. Gradual warming through external wraps, a head covering to prevent heat loss, and warm intravenous fluids are means of warming the body. Patients who are alert can drink hot liquids such as soup. Alcohol and caffeine beverages should be avoided. Some facilities have blanket warmers.

Survival of extreme cold situations, such as nearly drowning in cold water or being buried in snow, has occurred in some instances due to the cold body's decreased metabolic demands for oxygen.

QSEN FOCUS

Through patient-centered care, the nurse provides physical comfort and emotional support while treating symptoms of altered body temperature.

! SAFE PRACTICE ALERT

Fires may result from attempting to warm blankets in a microwave oven or other nonapproved warming devices.

When evaluating a temperature reading, the nurse must compare the temperature measurement obtained against any baseline data, previous readings, and the normal range for the patient. The nurse interprets the findings by considering the patient's diagnosis, time of day, and other factors such as medications administered. The nurse performs any needed follow-up activities, such as medication administration, changes in the environment, increased fluid intake, or notification of the primary care provider (PCP) for additional orders. Nursing interventions are evaluated by comparing patient responses with the expected outcomes. If the nursing interventions are effective, the patient's temperature will return to normal range and other vital signs will stabilize.

PULSE LO 19.3

The pulse is the palpable, bounding blood flow created by the contraction of the left ventricle of the heart. It can be assessed at various points on the body. The pulse is an indicator of circulatory status. Electrical impulses originating in the sinoatrial (SA) node of the heart stimulate cardiac muscle contraction, which sends a pulse wave. The number of pulsing sensations occurring in 1 minute is the pulse rate. Mechanical, neural, and chemical factors regulate the strength of ventricular contraction and the subsequent cardiac output. As the heart rate increases, less time is available for the heart to fill. An abnormally slow, rapid, or irregular pulse reflects an alteration in cardiac output, which may result in an inability to meet the physiologic demands of the body. The **apical pulse** is a central pulse that can be auscultated over the apex of the heart at the point of maximal impulse (PMI). **Peripheral pulses** are those that can be palpated over arteries located away from the heart—at the wrist or foot, for example. Normal pulse rates are listed in Table 19-1.

FACTORS AFFECTING PULSE RATE

As noted earlier, pulse rate is expressed in bpm. The pulse rate is variable and is dependent on physiologic and emotional factors. The nurse should consider several patient-specific factors when assessing the pulse, including age, gender, exercise, presence of fever, medications, fluid volume status, stress, and underlying disease processes (Box 19-3).

BOX 19-3 Factors Affecting Pulse Rate

- *Age:* As age increases from infancy to adulthood, the pulse rate decreases.
- *Gender:* After puberty, the average-male pulse is lower than that of the average female.
- *Fever:* Pulse increases with fever due to the increased metabolic rate and peripheral vasodilation that occurs.
- *Medications:* Various medications may either increase or decrease the pulse rate.
- *Hypovolemia:* Loss of blood normally increases the pulse rate from sympathetic nervous system stimulation.
- *Hypoxia and hypoxemia:* When oxygen levels decrease, cardiac output increases to attempt to compensate, resulting in an increased pulse rate.
- *Stress:* Sympathetic nervous system stimulation from stress (e.g., fear, anxiety, and the perception of pain) increases the heart rate.
- *Pathology:* Heart conditions or illnesses that impair oxygenation can alter the pulse rate as cardiac output attempts to compensate for low oxygen levels. Head injuries can cause a drop in pulse to compensate for increased intracranial pressure.
- *Electrolyte balance:* Changes in potassium and calcium affect pulse rate and rhythm.

SITES FOR ASSESSING PULSE

Peripheral pulses are assessed where arteries lie over bony prominences. A pulse may be measured in several sites that are easily accessible (Box 19-4). These sites include the temporal artery of the head; the carotid artery in the neck; the brachial and radial arteries in the arms; and the femoral, popliteal, dorsalis pedis, and posterior tibial arteries in the legs and feet. The most definitive site used for pulse assessment is over the apex of the heart, where the apical pulse can be auscultated.

The most common site for assessing the quality, rate, and rhythm of the pulse is the radial artery. In an emergency or during cardiopulmonary resuscitation, the carotid or femoral pulse may be used to assess the pulse rate and adequacy of cardiac compressions. The brachial pulse is used in children during emergencies. The dorsalis pedis and posterior tibial artery pulses are used to evaluate the effectiveness of the peripheral vascular system but not to assess heart rate or rhythm.

! SAFE PRACTICE ALERT

Never palpate both carotid arteries at the same time. Doing so could limit blood flow to the brain, causing the patient to experience syncope (fainting).

BOX 19-4 Pulse Sites

1. *Temporal:* Where the temporal artery passes over the temporal bone of the head, above and lateral to the eye; used when the radial pulse is not accessible
2. *Carotid:* At the side of the neck where the carotid artery runs between the trachea and the sternocleidomastoid muscle; used in cases of cardiac arrest and for determining circulation to the brain
3. *Apical* or *PMI:* Apical, at the apex of the heart, and PMI, at the fifth intercostal space, midclavicular line; used for infants and children up to 3 years of age, placed in the supine position, to determine discrepancies with radial pulse, and used in adults in conjunction with some diseases and medications and during a head-to-toe assessment
4. *Brachial:* At the inner aspect of the arm; used to assess pulse in pediatric emergencies and to measure blood pressure
5. *Radial**:* On the thumb side of the inner aspect of the wrist where the radial artery runs along the radial bone
6. *Femoral:* Where the femoral artery passes alongside the inguinal ligament; used in cases of cardiac arrest and for assessing circulation to the leg
7. *Popliteal:* Behind the knee where the popliteal artery passes; used to determine circulation to the lower leg
8. *Posterior tibial:* Medial surface of the ankle; used to determine circulation to the foot
9. *Pedal (dorsalis pedis):* Where the dorsalis pedis artery passes across the top of the foot; used to determine circulation to the foot

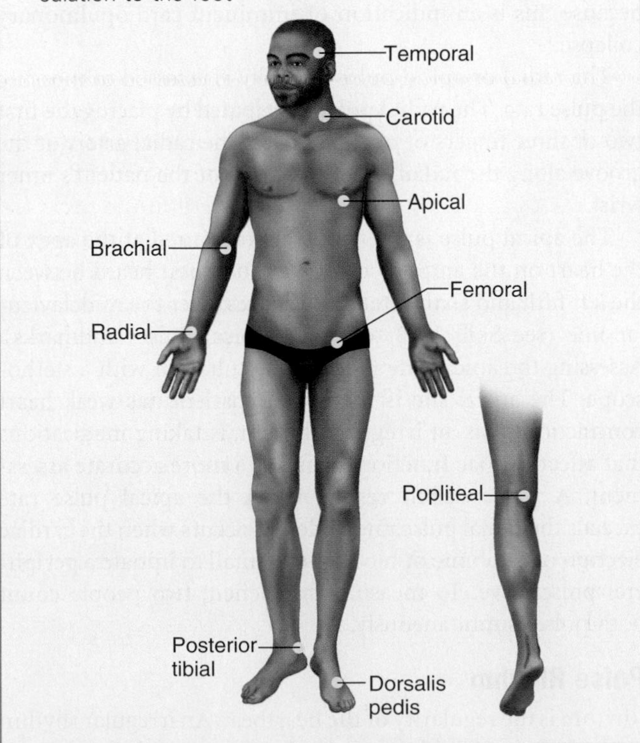

*The radial pulse typically is readily accessible. In elderly people, however, palpating the radial pulse may pose a challenge if tremors are present. Peripheral pulses also may be decreased in general as a consequence of cardiovascular changes with aging.

ASSESSMENT OF PULSE

Assessing the pulse includes measuring the rate, rhythm, and volume and comparing the findings on both sides of the body. The pulse is assessed by palpation (feeling with the middle three fingertips), **auscultation** (listening with a stethoscope) (Evidence-Based Practice and Informatics box), or electronic monitoring through specifically placed sensors. Too much pressure of the fingertips can obliterate the pulse, and pressure that is too light may not capture the pulsations. A Doppler ultrasound unit is used to assess pulses that are otherwise difficult to detect, especially pedal pulses (Nursing Care Guideline box). Skill 19-2 reviews the steps for measuring a pulse.

EVIDENCE-BASED PRACTICE AND INFORMATICS

Using a Stethoscope

A stethoscope is a medical device that is critical in listening to internal sounds of the body. It commonly is used to listen to lung and heart sounds. It also is used to listen to intestinal activity and blood flow in arteries and veins. In combination with a sphygmomanometer, it is used for measurements of blood pressure. It is important that a stethoscope be used and cared for correctly.

- The earpieces should fit snugly and point toward the nose. This position follows the path of the ear canal. The chin is dropped toward the chest to determine the position where the earpieces fit the ears the best and room sounds are blocked out.
- If the stethoscope has a dual head, with a diaphragm and bell end piece, and if this end piece rotates, it must be rotated to be open to the head in use. The bell is designed to hear low-pitched tones; the diaphragm is designed to hear higher-pitched sounds.
- The end piece is placed against the patient's skin with light pressure.
- The stethoscope should not be worn against the skin. Tubing made of polyvinyl chloride (PVC) will harden over time from skin oils.
- The stethoscope must be kept away from extreme heat or cold.
- Infection control issues include the following:
  - The end piece must be cleaned with an antimicrobial wipe before using it on a patient to prevent infection.
  - The stethoscope must not be sterilized with steam heat.
  - The earpieces should be cleaned routinely, as well as whenever shared with anyone else, to prevent infection. Earpieces may be removed for thorough cleaning.
  - The stethoscope should not be submerged in water; the tubing may be gently wiped with an antimicrobial wipe if needed.
  - To prevent the spread of infection, decorative coverings should not be placed over the stethoscope tubing.

From 3M: Use of your stethoscope, 2014. Retrieved from *http://solutions.3m.com/wps/portal/3M/en_US/Littmann/stethoscope/products/stethoscope*.

NURSING CARE GUIDELINE

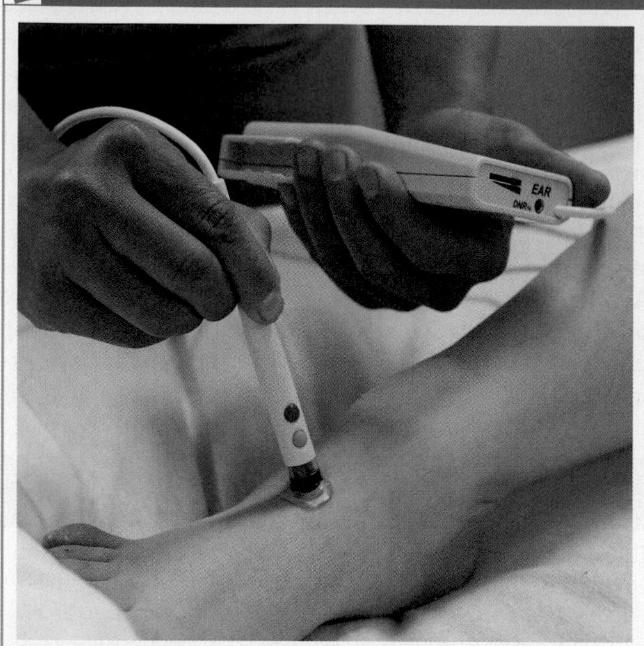

Using a Doppler Ultrasound Unit to Obtain a Pulse

Background

- A Doppler ultrasound unit may be used to assess peripheral circulation when a pulse cannot be palpated.
- Each pulse wave makes a sound that the Doppler ultrasound unit amplifies.
- Pulses may be difficult to palpate for many reasons, including poor circulation, edema, obesity, and other obstructive issues.

Procedural Concerns

- Apply a small amount of special gel to the skin or the tip of the ultrasound probe. The gel helps to further transmit and amplify the sound waves.
- Turn on the machine, and adjust the volume control.
- Hold the tip of the ultrasound unit (also called the *transducer*) at a 45- to 90-degree angle against the skin and directed toward the site of the pulse.
- Slide the transducer until the pulse (similar to a "whoosh" sound) can be heard. The pressure used to hold the unit against the skin may need to be varied to obtain the strongest signal.
- Ensure presence of a consistent sound at the point where the pulse wave is heard before documenting that a pulse was obtained via Doppler technique.
- The transducer should be cleaned with a water-based solution.

Documentation Concerns

- Note the rate and rhythm of the pulse.
- Note the location of the pulse and use of the ultrasound unit for the assessment.

! SAFE PRACTICE ALERT

If the peripheral pulse is irregular, count an apical pulse for 1 full minute to ensure accurate measurement.

! SAFE PRACTICE ALERT

In infants and children younger than 2 years of age, the pulse rate is obtained by auscultating the apical pulse.

Pulse Rate

Pulse rate is an indirect measurement of cardiac output obtained by counting pulse waves over a pulse point. An excessively fast heart rate (>100 bpm in the adult) is termed **tachycardia**. A slow heart rate (<60 bpm in the adult) is called **bradycardia**. Tachycardia decreases cardiac filling time, leading to a decreased cardiac output. Factors that lead to tachycardia include a drop in blood pressure; an elevated temperature; conditions such as anemia, which result in poor oxygenation; exercise; prolonged application of heat; pain; strong emotions, such as fear or anxiety; and some medications, including bronchodilators.

Bradycardia can occur in athletes, during sleep, in a state of hypothermia, in association with medications such as beta blockers, during tracheal suctioning, in association with increased intracranial pressure, and in myocardial infarction. Bradycardia accompanied by difficulty breathing and decreased blood pressure should be reported immediately, because this is an indication of imminent cardiopulmonary collapse.

The radial or apical pulse typically is assessed to measure the pulse rate. The **radial pulse** is palpated by placing the first two or three fingers of one hand over the radial artery at the groove along the radial, or thumb, side of the patient's inner wrist.

The apical pulse is the heart rate measured at the apex of the heart on the anterior chest wall. It is best heard between the left fifth and sixth intercostal spaces, over the midclavicular line (see Skill 19-2 to review apical pulse landmarks). Assessing the apical rate requires auscultation with a stethoscope. The apical site is used if the patient has weak heart contractions, has an irregular rhythm, is taking medications that affect cardiac function, or needs a more accurate assessment. A **pulse deficit** results when the apical pulse rate exceeds the radial pulse rate. A deficit occurs when the cardiac ejection of a volume of blood is too small to initiate a peripheral pulse wave. To measure this deficit, two people count both pulses simultaneously.

Pulse Rhythm

Rhythm is the regularity of the heartbeat. An irregular rhythm in the pulse, caused by an early, late, or missed heartbeat, is referred to as a **dysrhythmia** or an **arrhythmia**. When an irregular rhythm is detected, the apical pulse is assessed. An electrocardiogram (ECG) is necessary to define the specific dysrhythmia.

TABLE 19-4 Pulse-Volume Scale

SCALE	DESCRIPTION OF PULSE
0	Absent pulse
1+	Weak and thready pulse, difficult to palpate
2+	Normal pulse, able to palpate with normal pressure
3+	Bounding pulse, may be able to see pulsation

Pulse Volume

The pulse volume, also called *amplitude,* is the strength of the pulse with each beat. It is described as normal (full and easily palpable), weak (thready and rapid), or strong (bounding). A normal pulse can be felt with moderate pressure of the fingers and obliterated with greater pressure. A forceful volume that is obliterated only with difficulty is a bounding pulse, which may be caused by vasodilation and overhydration. A pulse readily obliterated is described as weak or thready. Causes include vasoconstriction, stiff vessel walls from disease, and shock.

A standard pulse-volume scale is used to document findings, with descriptions recorded using a range of 0 to 3+ (Table 19-4).

NURSING DIAGNOSIS

- *Ineffective Peripheral Tissue Perfusion* related to decreased peripheral circulation, as evidenced by pedal edema and need to use Doppler ultrasound to detect pedal pulses
- *Activity Intolerance* related to immobility, as evidenced by shortness of breath with ambulation and increased pulse with activity
- *Decreased Cardiac Output* related to altered contractility of the heart, as evidenced by shortness of breath, peripheral edema, and tachycardia
- *Deficient Fluid Volume* related to fluid volume loss, as evidenced by increased temperature, decreased blood pressure, thirst, and change in mental status

PLANNING

Goals for the patient experiencing abnormal pulse rate could include:

- Patient will exhibit increased perfusion as indicated by less than 1+ edema in lower extremities within 48 hours of beginning medication interventions.
- Patient will exhibit respirations, pulse, and blood pressure within patient's usual range during activity before discharge.
- Patient will demonstrate decreased episodes of shortness of breath, edema, and tachycardia after initiation of treatment plan.
- Patient will maintain adequate fluid volume as evidenced by stable vital signs, adequate urinary output, and moist mucous membranes within 12 hours.

IMPLEMENTATION AND EVALUATION

Hand hygiene is performed before caring for a patient. After selection of the appropriate site and method, the pulse rate is measured. An irregular pulse of new onset should be reported to the PCP. Interventions for an increased pulse rate include identification and treatment of the cause. Fluid replacement is used for tachycardia caused by hypovolemia. Measures to decrease anxiety are implemented for tachycardia related to emotional stress. By contrast, fluid removal by use of diuretic medications would be an appropriate intervention for tachycardia from fluid overload. Oxygenation status often is closely linked to pulse rates and should be stabilized for the patient who experiences deviations in pulse rate. Evaluation is accomplished by comparing the pulse rate with baseline data or to the normal range for the age of the patient. The pulse rate and volume are related to other vital signs, assessment data, and health status.

RESPIRATIONS LO 19.4

As noted, respiration is the act of breathing. Breathing (pulmonary ventilation) is the movement of air into and out of the lungs: Inspiration (inhalation) is the act of breathing in, and expiration (exhalation) is the act of breathing out. To survive, cells of the body must receive enough oxygen to meet metabolic requirements and release carbon dioxide. The purpose of respiration is to allow the exchange of oxygen and carbon dioxide among the alveoli, circulating blood, and tissue cells. Several physiologic events work together to meet the gas exchange needs of the body. Nurses assess for signs of changes in gas exchange. The process that is measured as a vital sign is pulmonary ventilation, or respirations. A normal respiratory rate is 12 to 20 BPM for an adult (see Table 19-1).

PHYSIOLOGY AND REGULATION OF BREATHING AND VENTILATION

Respiratory centers in the medulla and pons are stimulated by impulses from chemoreceptors located throughout the body. Chemoreceptors located in the aortic arch and carotid arteries are especially sensitive to low oxygen levels in the blood (**hypoxemia**). Receptors in the medulla are especially sensitive to high levels of carbon dioxide (**hypercapnia**) and changes in pH. Additional stretch receptors in the lungs and receptors in muscles and joints provide input to the medulla and pons. Respiratory rate and depth change on the basis of input from these receptors, but the strongest respiratory stimulant is an increase in carbon dioxide, which causes an increase in respiratory rate and depth. The cerebral cortex of the brain allows voluntary control of breathing, for example, when singing.

BOX 19-5 Factors Affecting Respiratory Rate and Depth

- *Age:* Respiratory rate decreases with age through late adolescence, when it stabilizes.
- *Exercise:* Respiratory rate and depth increase with exercise.
- *Illness processes:* Cardiovascular disease and hematologic disorders such as anemia cause an increased respiratory rate. Sickle cell disease reduces the ability of hemoglobin to carry oxygen, resulting in increased respiratory rate and depth. Respiratory diseases can be manifested by difficulty breathing, use of accessory muscles, increased rate, and shallower depth. Smoking alters airways, resulting in an increased rate.
- *Acid-base balance:* Acidosis results in increased rate and depth of respirations in an attempt to rid the body of excess carbon dioxide. Alkalosis results in decreased respiratory rate as the body tries to retain carbon dioxide.
- *Medications:* Some medications, such as narcotics and general anesthesia, slow respirations. Alternatively, drugs such as amphetamines and cocaine increase respirations. Bronchodilators slow the respiratory rate by dilating the airways.
- *Pain:* Acute pain increases respiratory rate while decreasing respiratory depth.
- *Emotions:* Fear or anxiety can cause increased respiratory rate and decreased depth.

FACTORS AFFECTING RESPIRATION

Inspiration and expiration should be smooth and without conscious effort. Environmental or physiologic factors may cause increases or decreases in respiratory rate or depth. Factors that affect respiratory rate and depth include age, exercise, respiratory and cardiovascular disease, alterations in fluid and electrolyte balance acid-base disturbances, medications, pain, and emotions (Box 19-5).

ASSESSMENT OF RESPIRATIONS

Assessment of respirations always includes measurement of the breathing rate, depth, and rhythm, and it routinely includes measurement of levels of **oxygen saturation** (amount of oxygen in the arterial blood) by pulse oximetry. Before assessing respirations, the nurse needs to be aware of the patient's normal respiratory pattern, how the patient's health status affects respirations, any medications that may affect respirations, and the impact of cardiovascular system factors on the respiratory system.

Respiratory Status

The assessment of respirations begins with observing the chest and abdominal movements for effort and symmetry (Skill 19-3). The rate is assessed by counting the number of breaths taken per minute. One inspiration and expiration cycle is counted as one breath.

On inspiration, the rib cage raises and the diaphragm lowers, allowing air to fill the lungs. The muscles relax in expiration, causing the rib cage to lower and the diaphragm to rise, forcing the air out of the lungs. A complete respiratory assessment, including abnormal respiratory sounds, is described in Chapter 20.

Respiratory Rate

Normal respiration with a normal rate and depth for the patient's age is termed **eupnea**. **Tachypnea** is an increase in respiratory rate to more than 24 BPM in the adult. Any condition that causes an increased need for oxygen or an increased metabolic rate (e.g., high altitude or fever) or an increase in carbon dioxide levels (e.g., chronic lung disease) will cause tachypnea. **Bradypnea** is a decrease in respiratory rate to less than 10 BPM in the adult. Bradypnea can be caused by medications, especially opioids, metabolic disorders, or brain injury.

Depth of Respirations

The depth of respirations normally varies from shallow to deep. Periodic sighs are deep inhalations that fill the lungs with more air than during normal inspiration. **Hypoventilation** is characterized by shallow respirations; it is associated with drug overdose and obesity, as well as COPD and cervical spine injury. **Hyperventilation** is exhibited by deep, rapid respirations; it is often caused by stress or anxiety. Different respiratory patterns have characteristic rates, rhythms, and depths (Table 19-5).

Quality of Respirations

Apnea is an absence of breathing; brain damage occurs after 4 to 6 minutes of apnea. **Dyspnea** is difficult, labored breathing, usually with a rapid, shallow pattern, that may be painful. Anxiety usually is present as well. Accessory muscles in the chest and neck are used in dyspneic breathing. Many patients experiencing dyspnea find it easier to breath in an upright position, in which gravity lowers the organs of the abdomen away from the diaphragm, giving the diaphragm room to expand downward as the lungs expand with inspiration.

TABLE 19-5 Respiratory Patterns

PATTERN	DESCRIPTION	ASSOCIATED FACTOR(S)
Eupnea	Quiet, regular breathing; 12-20 BPM	Normal pattern
Tachypnea	Breathing rate increased (>24 BPM), with quick, shallow breaths	Fever, exercise, anxiety, respiratory disorders
Bradypnea	Breathing rate abnormally slow (<10 BPM)	Depression of respiratory center by increased intracranial pressure, brain damage, or medications
Hyperventilation	Overexpansion of the lungs, characterized by rapid and deep breaths	Extreme exercise, fear, anxiety, diabetic ketoacidosis, aspirin overdose
Hypoventilation	Underexpansion of the lungs, characterized by shallow, slow respirations	Drug overdose, head injury
Cheyne-Stokes respirations	Rhythmic respirations, going from very deep to very shallow or apneic periods	Heart failure, renal failure, drug overdose, increased intracranial pressure, impending death
Kussmaul's breathing	Respirations abnormally deep, regular, and increased in rate	Diabetic ketoacidosis
Apnea	Absence of breathing for several seconds	Respiratory distress, obstructive sleep apnea
Biot's breathing	Respirations abnormally shallow for two or three breaths, followed by irregular period of apnea	Meningitis, severe brain injury

Difficulty breathing experienced in positions other than sitting or standing is termed **orthopnea**.

! SAFE PRACTICE ALERT

Patients with dyspnea experience more distress when lying flat. Placing the patient in a semi-Fowler or Fowler position facilitates a better respiratory pattern. Maximal lung expansion can be achieved by having the patient assume a sitting position, leaning forward over a raised bedside table with arms resting on the table, in what is called a *tripod position*.

OXYGEN SATURATION

Measurement of respiratory rate is not a measurement of how much oxygen actually enters the bloodstream. The SpO_2, which reflects the percentage of hemoglobin that combines with oxygen, normally is 95% to 100%. Factors that affect the SpO_2 include lung disease, decreased circulation, and hypotension. **Cyanosis**, bluish discoloration of the skin and mucous membranes, results from decreased oxygen levels in arterial blood. The level of consciousness is affected by changes in oxygen levels. Patients displaying signs of reduced oxygen require additional assessment of mental status, activity tolerance, and measurement of oxygen saturation.

Measurement of oxygen saturation is performed noninvasively and painlessly by means of pulse oximetry. A pulse oximeter is a small device that is clipped to a fingertip, a toe, the nose, or an earlobe. The most desirable site is the fingertip; alternate sites are used only when use of the fingertip is not appropriate. The device has an electronic display for oxygen saturation and pulse rate. Infrared light from one side of the sensor is read by a photo detector on the other side, which measures the amount of light absorbed by oxygenated and deoxygenated hemoglobin. Cold or injury to extremities, peripheral edema, and jaundice interfere with obtaining an accurate value. Movement at the site of sensor attachment, shivering, and some types of nail polish also affect the accuracy of the reading.

Skill 19-4 explains how to measure oxygen saturation. The role of oxygen saturation readings in identifying changes in patient status is critical. It is important to maintain vigilance in monitoring the patient's clinical condition, especially when abnormalities in vital signs or changes in vital sign measurements are present; any significant change must be reported promptly.

ARTERIAL BLOOD GASES

Measurement of arterial blood gases (ABGs) is a way of assessing the respiratory component of acid-base balance and the adequacy of oxygenation. ABG values include the carbon dioxide level and pH, and they are used to determine the need for and response to treatment. (Refer to Chapter 39 for a detailed discussion of ABG results.) Arterial blood is used for assessment because values for venous blood gases are highly variable, depending on the metabolic demands of the tissues that empty into the vein where the sample is drawn. ABG studies are used to establish baseline values, identify respiratory disorders, and evaluate the effectiveness of interventions. ABG samples also are drawn to monitor patients who are critically ill.

! SAFE PRACTICE ALERT

Signs of respiratory distress include the use of accessory muscles of the chest and neck and/or an exaggerated effort to breathe. Children and infants may exhibit nasal flaring or sternal retractions if they are having trouble breathing.

NURSING DIAGNOSIS

Respiratory assessment data are a defining characteristic of many nursing diagnoses, including:

- *Ineffective Breathing Pattern* related to increased intracranial pressure from traumatic head injury as evidenced by hypoventilation
- *Impaired Gas Exchange* related to alveolar changes as evidenced by oxygen saturation of 89% on room air
- *Activity Intolerance* related to decreased oxygenation levels as evidenced by dyspnea on exertion
- *Ineffective Airway Clearance* related to thick secretions as evidenced by inability to clear sputum with cough

PLANNING

Goals related to respiratory rate assessment focus on ensuring adequate level of oxygen to meet the physiologic needs of the body. Examples are:

- Patient will exhibit regular breathing pattern with assistance from ventilator while in the ICU.
- Patient will be free of signs of hypoxia with ABGs within the patient's normal range within 8 hours of admission.
- Patient will demonstrate ability to complete activities of daily living with no increase in dyspnea before discharge.
- Patient will be able to cough up secretions within 24 hours of beginning respiratory treatments.

IMPLEMENTATION AND EVALUATION

Changes in respiratory rate and rhythm are a sign of many physiologic and emotional disorders. Interventions for the underlying disorder should improve an altered respiratory pattern, and they include positioning, supplemental oxygen, suctioning, and medications such as bronchodilators.

A watch with a sweep second hand is needed to count respirations for 1 minute. To ensure an accurate measurement, respirations are counted when the patient is unaware of the procedure to prevent voluntary control of breathing by the patient. If respirations are shallow and slow, a stethoscope may be needed to auscultate breath sounds. Respirations can be palpated by placing a hand on the lower chest or abdomen and counting the breaths felt. An apnea monitor is used to monitor chest movement with leads that are placed on the chest and set off an alarm according to preset parameters. Apnea monitors are used for ill or preterm infants, as well as adults who may have periods of apnea, especially during sleep. Apnea monitors may be used in the home or during hospital admissions.

Evaluation of respiration must be done in conjunction with the other vital signs obtained and the medical status of the patient. A respiratory rate significantly above or below normal, any notable changes in pattern, and inadequate oxygenation must be reported to the PCP. Appropriate follow-up to prescribed interventions, such as evaluating the response to oxygen therapy, medications, and positioning, is essential.

BLOOD PRESSURE LO 19.5

Blood pressure can adapt to various stimuli and still remain within a normal range. Knowing the baseline, or usual, blood pressure of an individual is important to be able to interpret a single measurement in a potential illness process. An increase or decrease of 20 to 30 mm Hg in a person's blood pressure is considered a significant change. Sustained change in blood pressure is considered abnormal.

PHYSIOLOGY OF BLOOD PRESSURE

Blood pressure is the force of the blood against arterial walls. The left ventricle pushes blood through the aortic valve and into the aorta. The pressure rises as the ventricle contracts, and it falls as the heart relaxes, creating a pressure wave through the arterial system. The peak of the pressure wave is **systolic pressure**. The lowest pressure on arterial walls, which occurs when the heart rests, is **diastolic pressure**. Blood pressure is measured in millimeters of mercury (mm Hg) and is recorded as a fraction: The numerator, or top number, is the systolic pressure and the denominator, or bottom number, is the diastolic pressure. Pulse pressure is the difference between the diastolic and systolic pressures. For example, for a patient with a normal blood pressure of 120/80 mm Hg, 120 is the systolic pressure, 80 is the diastolic pressure, and the pulse pressure is 40 mm Hg.

The body regulates blood pressure by several mechanisms to maintain tissue perfusion. Arteries, arterioles, capillaries, venules, and veins form a continuous loop for circulation. Arterioles regulate the distribution of blood to the organs, tissues, and cells. To respond to the body's needs at any given moment, the arterioles are normally partially contracted, creating peripheral resistance. This resistance is a major factor affecting blood pressure. Arteries have elastic tissue that allows stretching and distention, or compliance. The arteries stretch with the systolic pressure and relax with diastolic pressure, although a certain amount of pressure is always present in the arteries. This constant pressure maintains a continuous flow into capillaries rather than intermittent bursts of circulation. The arteries provide compliance, while the arterioles supply resistance. With the normal aging process, arterioles become less elastic, and this can contribute to increased pressure within the cardiovascular system.

The autonomic nervous system (ANS) manages mechanisms to maintain short-term regulation of blood pressure. The ANS responds to circulatory system signals as well as to triggers such as pain and cold. Additionally, the renin-angiotensin-aldosterone system controls vasoconstriction and water retention that affects circulatory fluid volume. Antidiuretic hormone (ADH) is released in response to decreased blood pressure, decreased blood volume, or increased blood osmolarity. Water is retained when ADH is released, and this increases blood pressure. The cardiac output is the amount of blood pumped per minute. An increase in cardiac output results in increased blood pressure; a decrease in cardiac output leads to a decrease in blood pressure.

Hypotension

Hypotension is systolic blood pressure of less than 90 mm Hg (or 20 to 30 mm Hg below the patient's normal blood pressure) or diastolic blood pressure of 60 mm Hg or less. Hypotension is caused by a disruption in cardiovascular dynamics, such as decreased blood volume (hemorrhage), decreased cardiac output (heart attack or heart failure), or decreased peripheral vascular resistance (shock). An initial compensatory response to decreased blood pressure is an increase in pulse. If the falling blood pressure is not treated, the body's compensatory mechanisms will fail and the patient will manifest signs of shock: clammy skin, thready pulse, decreased urinary output, and confusion from decreased cerebral blood flow. Note that a consistently low blood pressure can be normal in highly trained athletes.

Orthostatic hypotension is a sudden drop of 20 mm Hg in systolic pressure and 10 mm Hg in diastolic pressure when the patient moves from a lying to sitting to standing position. The low pressure occurs from peripheral vasodilation with no rise in cardiac output for compensation. It occurs with aging and is a common side effect of several medications. Other risk factors for orthostatic hypotension include prolonged immobility, dehydration, and blood loss.

Hypertension

Hypertension, or elevated blood pressure, is the leading cause of cardiovascular disorders and the most important risk factor for stroke. It is the leading cause of death in the United States (National Heart, Lung, and Blood Institute, 2011). The animation "Hypertension" shows the changes that occur in patients with high blood pressure.  Hypertension occurs when there is dysfunction of the neurohormonal system. When angiotensin and aldosterone are overstimulated, blood pressure increases, and the result may be permanent thickening of the blood vessels, leading to increased peripheral resistance. This resistance affects the brain, heart, and kidneys. Systolic blood pressure of 120 to 139 mm Hg or diastolic pressure of 80 to 89 mm Hg is classified as prehypertension. Pressures above these values are classified as either stage 1 or stage 2 hypertension (Table 19-6). Primary (essential) hypertension occurs when there is no known cause for the high blood pressure. Secondary hypertension is caused by a known illness process, such as renal failure. Risk factors for hypertension include a family history of the disorder, sedentary lifestyle, obesity, and ongoing stress, as well as smoking, alcohol use, and a high-salt, high-fat-calorie diet (see Table 19-6). Important factors in self-management for patients with prehypertension or hypertension are outlined in the Home Care Considerations box.

HOME CARE CONSIDERATIONS

Hypertension

Patients with risk factors for hypertension, or those who are prehypertensive, should be educated about the need to adopt health-promoting lifestyle changes. According to the National Heart, Lung, and Blood Institute (2011), the lifestyle changes that have been shown to lower blood pressure are:

- Maintain normal body weight.
- Adopt the Dietary Approaches to Stop Hypertension (DASH) eating plan, which includes reduced fat intake and increased intake of fruits and vegetables.
- Reduce dietary sodium intake to 2.4 g daily.
- Engage in regular aerobic physical activity at least 30 minutes a day, on most days of the week.
- Limit alcohol consumption: for men, two drinks a day; for women, one drink a day.

FACTORS AFFECTING BLOOD PRESSURE

Many factors affect blood pressure. Activities throughout the day, emotions, fluid balance, exercise, and medications can alter blood pressure (Box 19-6). It is important to maintain vigilance in monitoring vital signs in patients receiving narcotic pain medication. If any abnormalities in vital signs develop, they must be reported promptly.

TABLE 19-6 Categories for Blood Pressure Levels in Adults*

CATEGORY	SYSTOLIC (mm Hg)		DIASTOLIC (mm Hg)
Hypotension	Less than 90	*or*	Less than 60
Normal	Less than 120	*and*	Less than 80
Prehypertension	120-139	*or*	80-89
High blood pressure			
Stage 1 hypertension	140-159	*or*	90-99
Stage 2 hypertension	Greater than 160	*or*	Greater than 100

From National Heart, Lung, and Blood Institute: The seventh report of the Joint National Committee on prevention, detection, evaluation, and treatment of high blood pressure—complete report (JNC7), 2004. Retrieved from *www.nhlbi.nih.gov*.
*People 18 years of age and older who are not on medications for high blood pressure or other conditions that affect blood pressure.

BOX 19-6 Factors Affecting Blood Pressure

- *Age:* With age, elasticity in arteries decreases; this increases peripheral resistance, leading to higher blood pressure.
- *Gender:* Blood pressure usually is lower in women than in men until menopause.
- *Race:* Hypertension is more prevalent in African American men and women.
- *Medications:* Oral contraceptives cause an increase in blood pressure in some women.
- *Weight:* Blood pressure usually is higher in people who are obese.
- *Circadian rhythm:* Blood pressure usually is lower in the morning and slightly higher by late afternoon.
- *Head injury:* Increased intracranial pressure from head injury causes increased blood pressure.
- *Increased blood volume:* Increased fluid in the cardiovascular system increases blood pressure.
- *Food intake:* Blood pressure increases after eating.
- *Emotions:* Anger, fear, and excitement cause blood pressure to rise until the emotion passes.
- *Pain:* Pain increases blood pressure.

ASSESSMENT OF BLOOD PRESSURE

Blood pressure is measured during physical examination, at initial admission, and with routine vital signs, as well as whenever the patient status changes (Diversity Considerations box). Blood pressure assessment requires excellent technique, correctly calibrated equipment, and proper interpretation of the sounds obtained. Blood pressure can be measured manually, through the use of a stethoscope and sphygmomanometer, or electronically, through intermittent or continuous monitoring (Skill 19-5) or through placement of an arterial catheter. If the patient has severe hypotension or shock, a Doppler ultrasound may need to be used in place of a stethoscope to amplify the diminished sounds.

Blood pressure measurements should be taken after the patient rests for at least 5 minutes and has not smoked or ingested caffeine for at least 30 minutes before the measurement. Because of the variations that occur during a typical day, readings on two or more occasions should be averaged before diagnosing high blood pressure. Hypotension accompanied by tachycardia, pallor, increased sweating, and confusion should be reported to the PCP immediately. These signs can indicate the critical loss of cardiovascular function, such as an impending acute myocardial infarction (heart attack).

DIVERSITY CONSIDERATIONS

Life Span

- *Children:* All children aged 3 years and older need to have blood pressure assessed at least annually. Readings are difficult to obtain and may be inaccurate in a child who is upset or restless. A child can be prepared for the measurement by describing the procedure in terms of "a tight squeeze on your arm." A pediatric stethoscope bell is helpful in hearing the Korotkoff sounds in a child.
- *Elderly people:* The skin of elderly patients may be fragile. Therefore, the cuff pressure should not be left on any longer than necessary. The timing of antihypertensive medications affects blood pressure readings. Antihypertensive medications that cause vasodilation increase the risk of orthostatic hypotension. If the patient has contractures of the arm, the blood pressure may be taken by the palpation method or from the popliteal artery.

Gender

- After puberty, females usually have lower blood pressure than males of the same age. Although this difference is not fully understood, female hormones may affect renal sodium handling and/or vascular resistance. After menopause, females generally have higher blood pressure than they did before (Oparil and Miller, 2005).

Culture, Ethnicity, and Religion

- African Americans older than 35 years of age tend to have higher blood pressure than European Americans of the same age (Ong, Cheung, Man, et al., 2007).

Morphology

- Obesity in children and adults is linked to a higher incidence of hypertension (Bhan, Yan, Leiter, et al, 2010).

Sites for Assessing Blood Pressure

Blood pressure can be measured in the upper or lower extremity. It is usually assessed manually, or indirectly. The most common site for indirect blood pressure measurement is the upper arm at the brachial artery. A brachial artery reading should not be taken on a patient's arm if an arteriovenous fistula or shunt is present; when the arm, shoulder, or hand is diseased; if a cast or bulky dressing is in place; or when intravenous fluids are being infused. Blood pressure should not be taken on the side of the body where axillary nodes were dissected or a mastectomy was performed. The pressure exerted on the site when taking a reading in such patients can increase the risk of lymphedema. Clinical judgment is an important aspect of determining the appropriate site, with the appropriate equipment, for obtaining blood pressure.

In some cases, blood pressure is assessed by palpating the radial artery at the wrist or the posterior tibial or dorsalis pedis artery of the lower leg. Palpation requires only a sphygmomanometer. The nurse places two or three fingers over the artery pulse point, and the cuff is inflated 30 mm Hg above the point where the pulsation in the artery is no longer felt. As the air in the bladder is released, the nurse feels for the return of the pulse. As an example, if the palpated value was felt at 70 mm Hg, the blood pressure typically would be recorded as "70 palpable," with the understanding that it is a measurement of palpated systolic pressure.

If the brachial artery is not accessible, the popliteal artery behind the knee can be used for blood pressure measurement. Injuries such as trauma or burns or the presence of a cast, intravenous line, or arteriovenous shunt may mean that the blood pressure must be obtained on a lower extremity. The popliteal artery, found behind the knee in the popliteal space, is the site used for auscultation. The cuff is sized specifically to fit around the thigh, and the cuff is positioned 2.5 cm (1 inch) above the popliteal artery, with the cuff bladder over the posterior aspect of the thigh. The technique is the same as that used for the brachial artery. Systolic blood pressure in the leg is approximately 20 mm Hg higher than it is in the brachial artery; diastolic pressure usually is the same in the leg as in the brachial artery. It is necessary to document the site if one other than the brachial artery is used to take a blood pressure reading.

Orthostatic hypotension is measured by taking the blood pressure reading and pulse while the patient is in the lying position, sitting position, and standing position (Nursing Care Guideline box). A drop in blood pressure of 20 mm Hg systolic or 10 mm Hg diastolic, or an increase in heart rate of 20 bpm, is indicative of orthostatic hypotension.

Blood Pressure Devices

Many styles of electronic, or automatic, blood pressure measurement devices are available (Figure 19-2). Electronic blood pressure devices use an electronic sensor to detect vibrations caused by blood moving through the artery. It is appropriate to measure blood pressure electronically in the critically ill, potentially unstable patient or during or after invasive procedures.

Low blood pressure may not be read as accurately with an electronic blood pressure device. If the accuracy of the blood pressure reading is questionable, manual measurement is used to ensure accuracy. It is inappropriate to use an electronic blood pressure device in patients with an irregular heart rate, shivering, seizure activity, or blood pressure less than 90 mm Hg systolic, because the device will not be able to accurately sense the blood pressure.

Arterial Lines

An arterial line is an indwelling catheter inserted into an artery by a physician or an advanced practice nurse to monitor blood pressure. This invasive procedure is used for patients with unstable blood pressure necessitating frequent monitoring. It may be used for patients who are dangerously hypotensive or hypertensive or who are receiving blood pressure medications requiring titration, or regulating, and monitoring. Special training is required for the use, care, and monitoring of an arterial line.

NURSING CARE GUIDELINE

Assessing Orthostatic Hypotension

Background

- Orthostatic hypotension, also known as *postural hypotension,* is a condition in which there is an abrupt decline in blood pressure when a person moves from a supine to a sitting or standing position. An accompanying increase in heart rate is typical. An accurate assessment of orthostatic hypotension requires identifying a blood pressure decline of 20 mm Hg in the systolic pressure or 10 mm Hg in the diastolic pressure, or an increase in heart rate of 20 bpm, within 1 to 3 minutes of postural change.
- Orthostatic hypotension can be indicative of dehydration (leading to low blood volume) or anemia, or it may occur in conjunction with prolonged immobilization.
- Orthostatic hypotension is most commonly due to a problem with the autonomic nervous system and/or a delay of the circulatory response to adjust to rapid movement.
- Symptoms may include dizziness, fainting, changes in mental status, and anxiety. Nausea, rapid onset of pallor, and fast, shallow breathing also are common during an episode of orthostatic hypotension.
- Because the condition has several different causes that vary from person to person, no single treatment for orthostatic hypotension can be recommended. However, its prevalence increases with age.

Delegation

- Assessment cannot be delegated to a UAP, but UAP may assist in obtaining the measurements and in positioning the patient for safety.

Procedural Concerns

- It is best to evaluate the patient in the morning rather than during the afternoon and/or after meals.
- Have the patient remain in a supine position for 5 to 10 minutes before the procedure.
- Three blood pressure and heart rate measurements are taken 1 to 3 minutes apart while the patient is in three different positions:
  - Supine
  - Sitting
  - Standing
- The blood pressure and heart rate measurements must be taken as soon as the position change occurs.
- Assess the patient throughout the procedure for signs and symptoms of syncope: dizziness, weakness, pale skin, diaphoresis, light-headedness, blurry vision, nausea, headache, and similar complaints.
- To ensure patient safety, stay with the patient throughout the procedure.

Documentation Concerns

- Vital signs are documented in conjunction with the position and time.
- Any signs, symptoms, or other complaints during the procedure should be documented.

Evidence-Based Practice

- An official diagnosis of orthostatic hypotension requires a 20 mm Hg drop in systolic blood pressure or a 10 mm Hg drop in diastolic blood pressure, with or without symptoms, within 3 minutes of the positional change. There usually is a corresponding increase in heart rate, although certain medications may prevent the heart rate from increasing (Mayo Clinic, 2014).

! SAFE PRACTICE ALERT

An arterial line is *never* used for infusion of intravenous medications or fluids. These solutions are irritating to the vessel and may impair tissue perfusion beyond the catheter.

Korotkoff Sounds

The sounds for which the nurse listens when assessing blood pressure are called **Korotkoff sounds**. In some adults these sounds are distinct, and in other adults only the beginning and ending sounds are heard. Table 19-7 summarizes the features of Korotkoff sounds by specific phases.

An **auscultatory gap** may occur in the latter part of phase I and during phase II. The auscultatory gap is the absence of Korotkoff sounds noted in some patients after the initial systolic pressure; the gap may cover a range as wide as 40 mm Hg. Failure to recognize an auscultatory gap may lead to major errors in measuring blood pressure.

TABLE 19-7 Korotkoff Sounds

PHASE	DESCRIPTION
Korotkoff I	The initial presentation of faint but clearly audible tapping sounds, which gradually increase in intensity to a thud or loud tap; the first sound is recorded as the systolic pressure
Korotkoff II	Muffled, swishing sounds
Korotkoff III	Crisp, loud sounds as the blood flows through an opening artery
Korotkoff IV	A distinct, abrupt muffling sound
Korotkoff V	The last sound heard before silence—this is the diastolic measurement

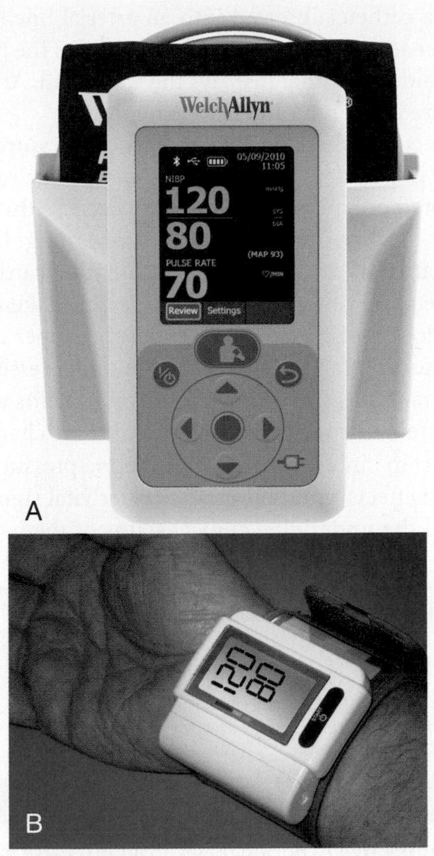

FIGURE 19-2 Electronic blood pressure device. (**A,** From Welch Allyn, Inc., New York, N.Y.)

Normally, blood pressure is recorded as a two-number fraction. The first sound heard during measurement, the onset of phase I, represents the systolic pressure and is recorded as the top number on the blood pressure fraction. The second number, the bottom of the fraction indicates the level at which the sounds stop. For example, if the blood pressure is recorded as 122/78, the number 122 represents the systolic pressure, and the number 78 represents the diastolic pressure. The American Heart Association recommends that when an abrupt change followed by the cessation of sounds occurs, all three numbers be recorded, such as 122/86/78. The middle number would be the Korotkoff phase IV sound. On some occasions, sounds may be heard all the way to zero on the blood pressure cuff. This measurement would be recorded as 122/78/0. Each facility will have a procedure on how to record blood pressure; this procedure should be followed for consistency in measurements.

> **! SAFE PRACTICE ALERT**
>
> When using a continuous blood pressure device, be sure to set high and low alarm limits for systolic and diastolic pressures. Do not turn off alarms. Check the position of the cuff frequently, and remove the cuff regularly to assess skin integrity.

NURSING DIAGNOSIS

Sample nursing diagnoses for altered blood pressure are:

- *Risk for Falls* with risk factor of orthostatic hypotension and dizziness when standing; blood pressure 136/70 lying and 96/60 standing
- *Decreased Cardiac Output* related to altered stroke volume as evidenced by estimated blood loss of 500 mL during surgery and irregular heart rate
- *Excess Fluid Volume* related to renal compromise as evidenced by increased blood pressure, dyspnea, and orthopnea

PLANNING

Patient goals related to blood pressure focus on maintaining blood pressure throughout the body to maintain functioning of all organs. Examples of goals or outcome statements are:

- Patient will be free from injury throughout hospitalization and in the home environment.
- Patient's blood pressure and peripheral pulses will be within defined parameters for patient within 24 hours postsurgery.
- Patient will have vital signs within patient's expected norm within 48 hours of admission.

IMPLEMENTATION AND EVALUATION

Different devices are available to measure blood pressure. The most common equipment used by the nurse is a stethoscope and sphygmomanometer (blood pressure cuff). Blood pressure can be measured with a Doppler stethoscope, estimated by **palpation** (assessment by feeling with the hand or fingers), or measured by an electronic, or automated, cuff. Equipment needs to be monitored to ensure that it is in proper working order, with recalibration or repair as needed.

A stethoscope is used to hear the sounds created by blood flowing through the artery. The stethoscope used should be properly fit to the person using it and should be used accurately. A sphygmomanometer consists of a cuff and the manometer. The cuff consists of a flat, rubber bladder covered with stiff cloth. Two tubes are attached to the bladder within the cuff. One is connected to the manometer, and the other is attached to the bulb used to inflate the bladder. The bladder is inflated until the blood flow through the artery is obstructed. A valve on the bulb allows the bladder in the cuff to be deflated, releasing the pressure and allowing blood to flow through the artery again, which creates the first sound, or systolic pressure reading. Electronic blood pressure devices sense vibrations within the artery wall and display the pressure readings in digital numbers. Electronic sphygmomanometers frequently are used by patients who self-measure their blood pressure.

Cuff sizes range from neonate to adult thigh sizes (Figure 19-3). The width of the cuff should be approximately 40% of

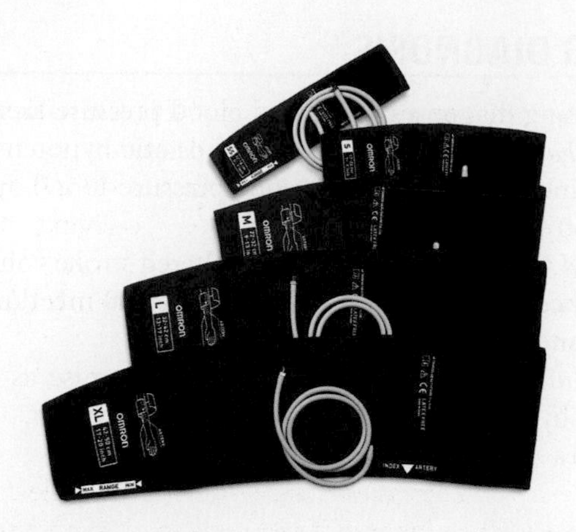

FIGURE 19-3 Blood pressure cuffs come in different sizes.

TABLE 19-8 Factors That Contribute to Blood Pressure Assessment Errors

ERROR	CONTRIBUTING FACTORS
Inaccurate reading	Defective equipment Equipment not calibrated Improper use of equipment Patient not positioned correctly
Falsely low reading	Hearing deficit in assessing person Arm positioned above heart level Extraneous noise in surrounding environment Use of a cuff that is too wide Ear tips of stethoscope placed incorrectly Breaks or kinks in cuff tubing Cuff deflated too rapidly Stethoscope bell not placed directly over artery Failure to follow all steps in recommended blood pressure procedure
Falsely high reading	Assessing blood pressure too soon after patient smoking or exercise Use of a cuff that is too narrow Releasing the pressure valve too slowly Reinflating the bladder before it has completely deflated

the circumference of the extremity being used, and the bladder of the cuff should be approximately 60% to 80% of the circumference of the extremity being used. If the cuff is too narrow, the reading can be erroneously high. (A common source of this error is use of a normal-size cuff on an overweight person.) Conversely, if the cuff is too wide, the reading can be erroneously low. Table 19-8 presents a review of factors that contribute to blood pressure assessment errors. It is possible to measure blood pressure directly in the artery by means of a catheter inserted into an arterial line. The tip of the catheter senses the pressure and transmits the readings to an electronic device that displays the waveform. Arterial lines typically are used in an intensive care unit.

Many factors cause an inaccurate blood pressure measurement. It is important that the nurse not take the routine task of blood pressure measurement lightly because this measurement can give critical information regarding the overall cardiac status of the patient. Because the cardiovascular system affects all other body systems, care is taken to obtain accurate blood pressure readings by using proper equipment and technique. Many factors affect blood pressure values. It is important to compare current measurements with previous measurements to identify any significant changes. Considerations in interpretation of blood pressure include medication effects, correlation with other vital sign measurements, and the underlying clinical status of the patient.

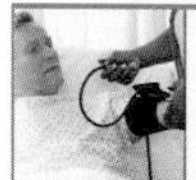

1. The nurse administers the IV dose of a diuretic, furosemide, to reduce fluid volume overload. Which assessments will assist the nurse in evaluating whether the medication was effective?

PAIN LO 19.6

Pain is a subjective experience, and the intensity and quality of pain are whatever the patient says they are. Pain can be caused by disease processes, medical or surgical procedures, trauma, immobility, wounds, and routine nursing care such as repositioning, changing a dressing, or starting an intravenous line. Pain is a means of monitoring a patient's illness and health progress. Management of pain is discussed in Chapter 36.

Pain may be acute (it resolves when the underlying injury heals) or chronic (it lasts longer than the healing period). The perception of pain can be intensified by the emotional state of the patient. Poor assessment of pain is the primary barrier to effective pain management (American Pain Society, 2005). In 2001, The Joint Commission issued guidelines requiring that pain assessment be conducted when other vital signs are measured.

ASSESSMENT OF PAIN

Because pain is a subjective experience, the level of pain will vary from person to person. It is important to believe the patient's subjective report of pain. Many patients exhibit objective signs of pain, such as grimacing or refusing to move or take breaths. Physiologic signs of pain, such as increases in the vital signs of respiratory rate or depth, pulse rate, and blood pressure, are less sensitive indicators of pain (American Pain Society, 2005).

Although pain is subjective, varying from one patient to another and from one day to the next, health care providers attempt to measure pain as objectively as possible. Various tools and scales have been developed to assess pain. Pain usually is determined by asking the patient to describe the pain and rate the pain level on a scale. In adult patients, this pain rating often is a numeric measurement between 0 and 10, with 0 meaning "no pain" and a score of 10 indicating "the worst pain imaginable" (see Figure 36-4).

Because children may be unable to grasp the concept of numbers and how they relate to pain, a pediatric pain scale is utilized for them. This scale consists of expressions on pictured faces. Six faces are normally displayed in front of the child, with the first face depicting a happy expression and the sixth face showing a grimace (see Figure 36-4). A scale using faces may be used with patients who have cognitive impairment. Specific questions regarding the patient's pain help determine what interventions should be implemented. Be sure to allow patients enough time to respond to the questions.

Alternate tools are used when assessing pain in circumstances in which the patient is not able to report the pain level, such as a pediatric, cognitively impaired, or unconscious patient. The American Society for Pain Management in Nursing (2006) has published a position statement with clinical practice recommendations for nonverbal patients. The focus is on elderly people with advanced dementia, infants and preverbal toddlers, and intubated or unconscious patients. Such a patient's pain measurements are determined by closely monitoring the patient's other vital signs (heart rate, respiration, pulse, and temperature) as well as behaviors such as the patient's level of agitation, irritation, and restlessness. See Chapter 36 for a thorough discussion of pain assessment in diverse populations using pain scale tools.

> **! SAFE PRACTICE ALERT**
>
> Ongoing nursing assessment for pain should include the intensity, quality, duration, and location of any pain. Assumptions about pain location may delay treatment for new symptoms and problems.

NURSING DIAGNOSIS

- *Acute Pain* related to abdominal surgery as evidenced by a pain rating of 10, reluctance or refusal to reposition, and request for medication
- *Chronic Pain* related to chronic inflammatory process as evidenced by inability to perform ADLs or work at place of employment

PLANNING

Patient goals related to pain focus on enabling the patient to complete needed or desired tasks. Examples are:

- Patient will report pain level of less than 3 on a 0-to-10 pain scale within 45 minutes of receiving pain medication.
- Patient will initiate modifications of lifestyle to meet ADLs within the next 3 months.

IMPLEMENTATION AND EVALUATION

Assistive devices such as glasses, large-print pain scale tools, pictures, and hearing aids are offered to patients to help them use pain assessment scales. Physiologic and objective signs are assessed in conjunction with subjective reports of pain. A pain assessment scale that is appropriate for the individual patient is chosen. Assessment for alternative pain management methods the patient may prefer, especially for chronic pain, also is done.

Various nursing measures may be implemented to address the patient's pain. Positioning with proper support of extremities and back massage can relax muscles and increase comfort. Encouraging the patient to use complementary interventions such as music and imagery, as appropriate, is helpful. Ongoing assessment of pain enables timely treatment before pain levels increase. Prescribed medications can be very effective in managing pain but must include patient monitoring for adverse effects.

Selection of an appropriate pain assessment scale is important. When used consistently, the selected tool becomes an important communication pathway between the patient and caregivers in identifying needs and measuring the outcome of pain relief interventions. Evaluation of pain focuses on the patient's report of pain relief and effectiveness of treatment. Pain management is an important component of a patient's care. Interventions should be adapted and changed as needed for patient comfort.

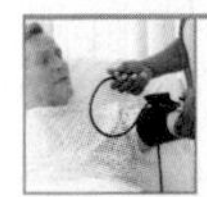

2. The nurse evaluates the patient's vital signs. What data would account for the observed deviations from normal values?

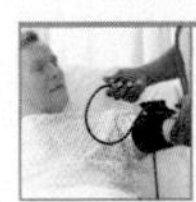

3. The patient requests pain medication for the chest pain related to the pneumonia. What assessment data does the nurse consider before administering pain medication in this patient? How might administration of pain medication change the patient's vital signs?

SKILL 19-1 Measuring Body Temperature

PURPOSE

- Determine the patient's baseline temperature. Body temperature may be measured in degrees Fahrenheit or Celsius.
- Identify whether the body temperature is within normal range.
- Monitor the patient for fever or an inability to maintain normal body temperature.
- Monitor the patient for change in physical condition.
- Monitor temperature changes for response to medications.

RESOURCES: ALL METHODS

- Thermometer
- Vital-sign flow sheet and pen or an electronic health record (EHR)

COLLABORATION AND DELEGATION

- Measuring a temperature may be delegated to UAP after the initial assessment of the patient.
- Assistive personnel should report the following to the nurse:
  - Deviations from baseline temperature
  - Complaints related to temperature regulation
  - Sores, wounds, irritations, and/or lesions in the area where the temperature is being measured
  - Any difficulties performing the procedure
- UAP should be instructed in:
  - Appropriate placement of the thermometer/probe
  - Appropriate use of equipment (verifying accurate results)
  - Appropriate documentation

EVIDENCE-BASED PRACTICE

- Bradypnea may cause high temperature readings. Hot and cold beverage intake influences oral temperature assessment. Both situations require an average of 15 minutes for a return to baseline measurements (Quatrara, Coffman, Jenkins, et al., 2007).
- Baseline oral temperature does not deviate between older and younger cohorts, but room temperature affects elderly adults' oral temperature readings more than it does those of younger people (Lu and Dai, 2009).
- All noninvasive temperature measurement methods have been shown to be just as accurate as the rectal temperature method (core temperature) provided the nurse or caregiver is utilizing the equipment properly and has been well-trained on the procedure, including the anatomy and physiology involved (Giantin, Toffanello, Enzi, et al., 2008; Langham, Maheshwari, Contrera, et al., 2009; Smitz, Van de Winckel, and Smitz, 2009; Spitzer, 2008).

SPECIAL CIRCUMSTANCES: ALL METHODS

1. **Assess:** Has the patient undergone exercise or physical therapy within the last 30 minutes?
   Intervention: Physical exercise increases body temperature; have the patient rest for 30 minutes before assessing temperature.
2. **Assess:** Does the temperature deviate from the normal range in either direction?
   Intervention: Validate equipment accuracy and proper use.
   - Assess the room temperature.
   - Assess the patient for clinical manifestations of hyperthermia or hypothermia.
   - Retake the patient's temperature using different equipment or a different method (if needed).
   - Check the PCP orders and care plan for further interventions.

RESOURCES AND SPECIAL CIRCUMSTANCES: SPECIFIC METHODS

Oral Method

Resources

- Electronic or digital thermometer
- Disposable probe covers or plastic thermometer sheaths

Special Circumstances

1. **Assess:** Has the patient consumed cold or hot food or beverages, chewed gum, or smoked within the past 15 minutes?
   Intervention: Wait 15 minutes from the last oral intake to assess oral temperature, or use a different method.
2. **Assess:** What is the patient's level of consciousness? Is the patient awake, alert, and oriented?
   Intervention: Select an alternative method to measure temperature, if necessary.
3. **Assess:** Are there any mouth lesions or sores?
   Intervention: Select an alternative method to measure temperature, if necessary.

Temporal Artery Method

Resources

- Temporal artery thermometer
- Alcohol wipes

Special Circumstances

1. **Assess:** Does the patient exhibit extreme perspiration?
   Intervention: Use a different method. Extreme perspiration interferes with the accuracy of the temperature reading.

2. **Assess:** Is the patient lying on his or her side?
   Intervention: Use the side of the patient's face that is not on the pillow. The side of the face that is on the pillow has an artificially high temperature.
3. **Assess:** Do you suspect an inaccurate or unreliable result?
   Intervention: Wait 30 seconds before repeating the temperature measurement. It takes at least 30 seconds for the skin temperature to normalize.

Axillary Method

Resources

- Electronic or digital thermometer
- Disposable probe covers or plastic thermometer sheaths

Special Circumstances

1. **Assess:** Has the skin recently been washed?
   Intervention: Wait 15 minutes after bathing before assessing axillary temperature to allow time for the skin temperature to normalize, or use a different method.
2. **Assess:** Is the axilla moist or diaphoretic?
   Intervention: Use the other arm; use a different method; or dry the axillary region with a towel, using a patting motion because perspiration causes inaccurate results.
3. **Assess:** Are lesions, wounds, skin irritations, or sores present?
   Intervention: Use the other axilla or use a different method because skin problems may raise temperature.

Rectal Method

Resources

- Electronic or digital thermometer
- Disposable probe covers or plastic thermometer sheaths
- Lubricant (water-soluble)
- Toilet paper or cloth
- Paper towel or tissue (for rectal temperature)
- Waterproof pad

Special Circumstances

1. **Assess:** What is the reason for using this method?
   Intervention: If a less invasive method can be used, use it. Patient comfort is important, and other methods have been shown to be as accurate as the rectal method.
2. **Assess:** Is there a patient history of rectal surgery or bleeding?
   Intervention: Rectal method is contraindicated. Use a different method to avoid risk of injury.
3. **Assess:** Is the patient on an anticoagulant or having diarrhea?
   Intervention: Use a different method to avoid the risk of bleeding or stimulating a bowel movement.
4. **Assess:** Are lesions, wounds, hemorrhoids, or other sores present?
   Intervention: Use a different method to avoid risk of injury.

Special Circumstances Arising During Procedure

1. **Assess:** Is there difficulty in inserting the temperature probe?
   Intervention: Remove the probe; assess the site; use a different method; and document the methods and findings.
2. **Assess:** Does the patient faint or become lightheaded or dizzy?
   Intervention: Remove the probe; assess blood pressure and heart rate; obtain assistance if needed; notify the PCP; use a different method; document; and notate "no rectal temps" because of the risk of vasovagal response.

Tympanic Method

Resources

- Tympanic thermometer
- Disposable probe covers
- Alcohol wipes

Special Circumstances

1. **Assess:** Is there a history of recent or current ear surgery or infection?
   Intervention: Use the other ear or a different method to avoid risk of injury.
2. **Assess:** Are there hearing aids or personal stereo or other listening device(s) in the ear(s)?
   Intervention: Use the other ear if one device is present; if two devices are present, remove one and wait 5 minutes before taking the temperature. These devices have retained heat inside the ear canal, artificially making the temperature higher; it takes at least 3 minutes for the ear canal to normalize its temperature.
3. **Assess:** Is the patient lying on his or her side?
   Intervention: Use the ear that has not been resting on the pillow. The ear on the pillow has an artificially high temperature.
4. **Assess:** Is cerumen present in the ear?
   Intervention: Use the other ear if only one ear is affected, or use a different method if both are affected; document excessive cerumen accumulation. Cerumen obstructs the probe's interaction with the tympanic membrane, so the result is inaccurate.
5. **Assess:** Do you suspect an inaccurate or unreliable result?
   Intervention: Wait 5 minutes before repeating the measurement. Taking a temperature with a tympanic probe causes the ear canal to cool because the probe is at room temperature, which is cooler than ear temperature. It takes at least 3 minutes for the ear canal temperature to normalize.

PREPROCEDURE

I. Check PCP orders and the patient care plan.
Knowledge of patient-specific orders is critical for safe patient care.

II. Gather supplies and equipment.
Preparing for the patient encounter saves time and promotes patient trust.

III. Perform hand hygiene.
Frequent hand hygiene prevents the spread of microorganisms.

IV. Maintain standard precautions.
Use of the correct personal protective equipment (PPE) is required whenever contact with bodily fluids is possible, to reduce the transfer of pathogens.

V. Introduce yourself.
Initial communication establishes the role of the nurse and begins a professional relationship.

VI. Provide for patient privacy.
It is important to maintain patient dignity.

VII. Identify the patient, using two identifiers.
Identifying a patient involves scanning barcodes or comparing the patient's stated name and birthdate to information on the patient's wristband or health record. The correct person must receive the correct treatment.

VIII. Explain the procedure to the patient.
The nurse has a responsibility to inform a patient before initiating care. Information may ease patient anxiety and facilitate cooperation.

PROCEDURE

Oral Temperature

Follow preprocedure steps I through VIII.

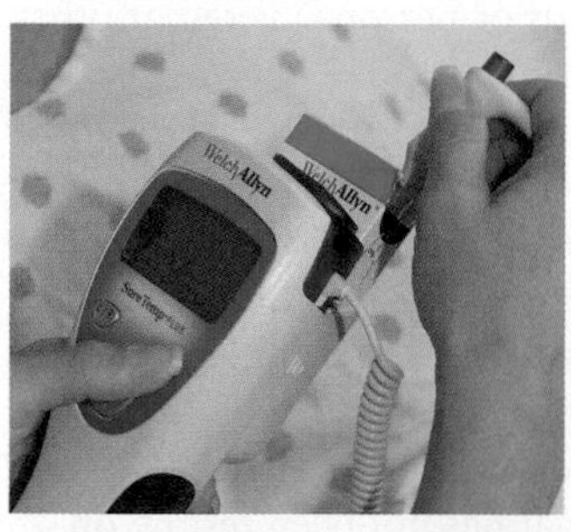

STEP 3

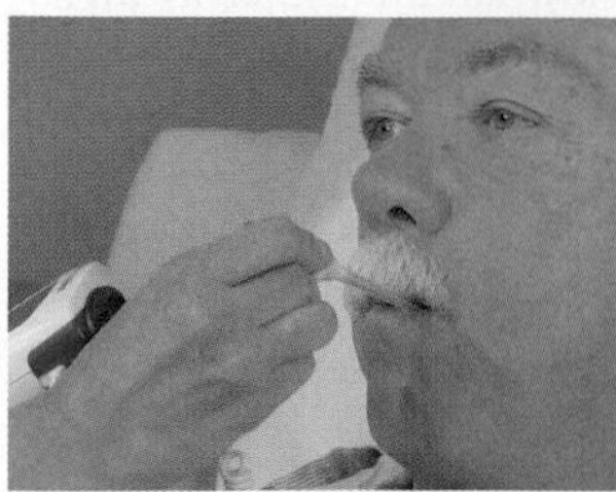

STEP 4

1. Obtain electronic thermometer with blue probe.
   Blue is standard for oral use.
2. Remove temperature probe; machine will beep, and digital display will appear.
   Indicates the machine is charged, accurate, and ready for use.
3. Place probe in disposable cover; cover will click into place.
   Secures the fit so that the cover will not fall off. The cover reduces transmission of microorganisms.
4. Insert probe tip into posterior sublingual pocket of mouth, holding it along slightly off the center of the jaw; patient's lips must be closed around probe.
   Provides the best location to achieve the most accurate temperature in the mouth. Holding along the side of the probe prevents accidentally pushing the button that ejects the probe cover.
5. Hold probe in place until reading is completed; machine will beep to indicate measurement is completed.
   Keeps the probe tip in place for accuracy.
6. Remove probe from patient.
7. Note temperature reading on display.
   Needed for documentation.
8. Discard probe cover; push ejection button at the end of the probe to release cover into trash can.
   Prevents the spread of microorganisms.

Follow postprocedure steps I through VI.

Rectal Temperature

Follow preprocedure steps I through VIII.

1. Obtain electronic thermometer with red probe.
   ***R**ed probe = **R**ectal. Red probe is standard for rectal use; use of a dedicated probe prevents the spread of microorganisms.*

2. Raise bed to comfortable working height, and flatten bed as tolerated by patient.
   Prevents provider discomfort and possible injury; the flat bed provides for patient comfort.
3. Position patient in Sims position, with upper leg flexed and lower leg straight.
   Promotes comfort; allows visualization of the buttocks.

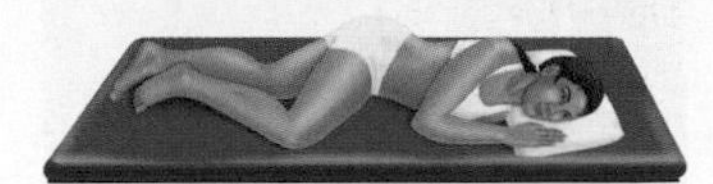
STEP 3

4. Apply clean gloves. Cover patient, except for buttocks.
   Gloves are standard precautions when there is possible exposure to blood and body fluids. Provides warmth, comfort, and privacy.
5. Remove temperature probe; machine will beep, and digital display will appear.
   Indicates the machine is charged, accurate, and ready for use.
6. Place probe in disposable cover; cover will click into place.
   Secures the fit so that the cover will not fall off. The cover reduces transmission of microorganisms.
7. Apply water-soluble lubricant to 1 to 1½ inches of the probe tip; can be done three different ways:
   Lubricant allows the probe to be inserted into the rectum without injury.
   a. *Packets:* Dip probe in packet.
      Use with single-use packets to prevent the spread of microorganisms; packets are an appropriate size to cover the tip.
   b. *Direct application:* Squeeze directly onto probe; cover all around tip; do *not* touch tube tip to probe tip.
      Use with single-use packets or multiuse tubes to prevent the spread of microorganisms.
   c. *Indirect application:* Squeeze onto paper towel or tissue; dip probe to cover tip; do *not* touch tube tip to paper towel or tissue.
      Use with single-use packets or multiuse tubes to prevent the spread of microorganisms.

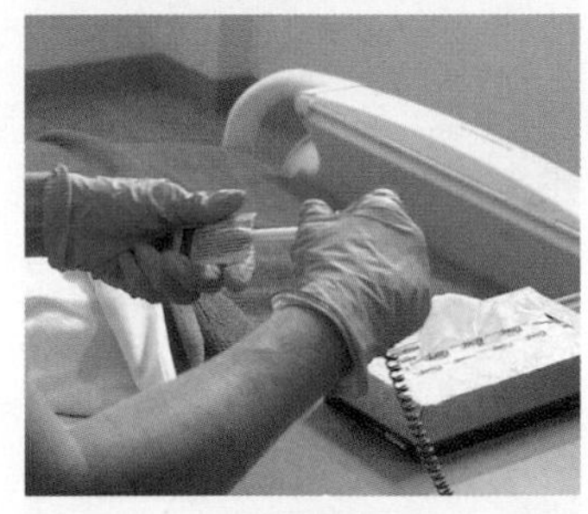
STEP 7

8. Separate buttocks with one hand.
   Visualize anus.
9. Ask patient to breathe slowly and relax.
   Relaxes muscles; allows for easier insertion.
10. Insert probe tip 1 to 1½ inches, pointing toward the umbilicus.
    Location for obtaining the most accurate temperature; blood vessels are against the rectal wall.

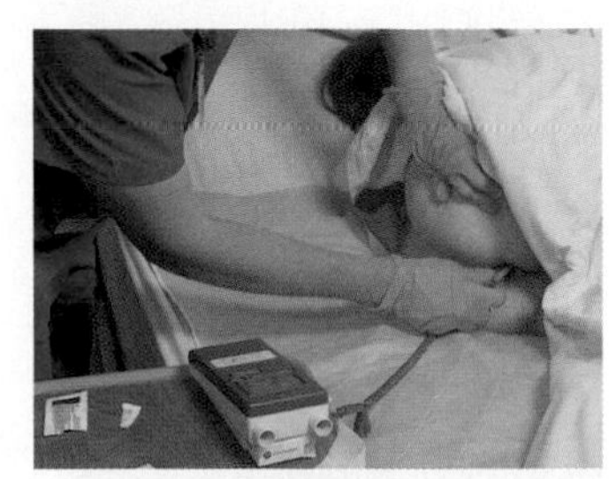
STEP 10

11. Hold probe in place until reading is completed; machine will beep to indicate measurement is completed.
    Keeps the probe tip in place for accuracy.
12. Remove probe from patient.
13. Note temperature reading on display.
    Needed for documentation.
14. Discard probe cover; push end of probe to release cover into trash can.
    Prevents the spread of microorganisms.
15. Clean probe tip with alcohol wipe before returning probe to case.
    Prevents the spread of microorganisms.
16. Clean patient; reposition.
    Removes extra lubricant and possible feces; provides comfort.

Follow postprocedure steps I through VI.

Axillary Temperature

Follow preprocedure steps I through VIII.

1. Obtain electronic thermometer with blue probe.
   Blue is standard for oral use and is also used for axillary temperatures.
2. Remove temperature probe; machine will beep, and digital display will appear.
   Indicates the machine is charged, accurate, and ready for use.
3. Place probe in disposable cover; cover will click into place.
   Secures the fit so that the cover will not fall off. The cover reduces transmission of microorganisms.

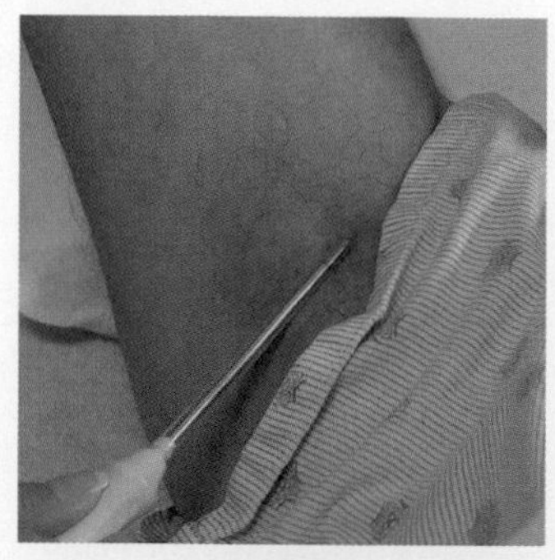

STEP 4

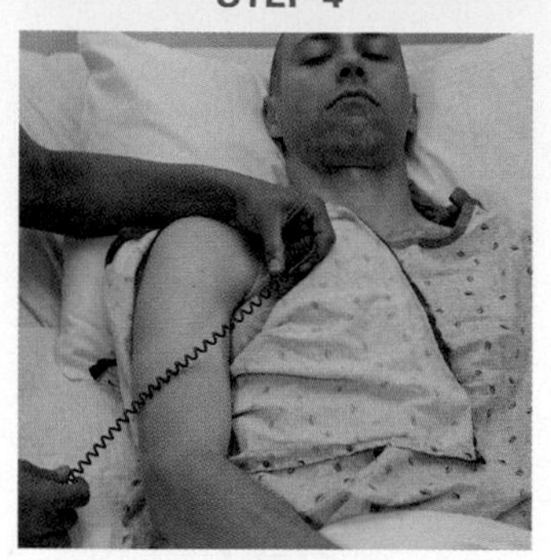

STEP 5

4. Remove clothing from axillary area; place probe tip in middle of the axilla.
   Location for obtaining the most accurate temperature; blood vessels are closest to the skin.
5. Arm should be held down, close to the body or across chest.
   Keeps the probe tip in place for accuracy.
6. Hold probe in place until reading is completed; machine will beep to indicate measurement is completed.
   Keeps the probe tip in place for accuracy.
7. Remove probe from axilla.
8. Note temperature reading on display.
   Needed for documentation.
9. Discard probe cover; push end of probe to release cover into trash can.
   Prevents the spread of microorganisms.

Follow postprocedure steps I through VI.

Tympanic Temperature

Follow preprocedure steps I through VIII.

1. Obtain tympanic thermometer unit; remove thermometer portion from base.
   The special unit is needed for measuring temperature in the ears.
2. Inspect lens; if dirty, clean with alcohol wipe and allow to air-dry for 5 minutes.
   Interference from dirt on the lens can cause an inaccurate reading; using a cloth to dry off the alcohol may smudge the lens.
3. Insert probe tip into disposable probe tip cover until it clicks into place.
   The cover reduces transmission of microorganisms; maintains accuracy of temperature reading by keeping the lens clean.
   a. Some units beep, and digital display appears; proceed to step 4.
      Indicates the machine is on and ready.
   b. Some units have manual on/off: Push the on/off button; wait for beep to sound and for digital display to appear; proceed to step 4.
      Indicates the machine is on and ready.
4. Remove hearing aids if present, and make sure ear canal is clean. Insert probe tip snugly into ear: Are you right-handed? Measure temperature in right ear. Are you left-handed? Measure temperature in left ear.
   Ear canal must be accessible. This angle of approach (less acute) provides a snug fit, ensuring accuracy.

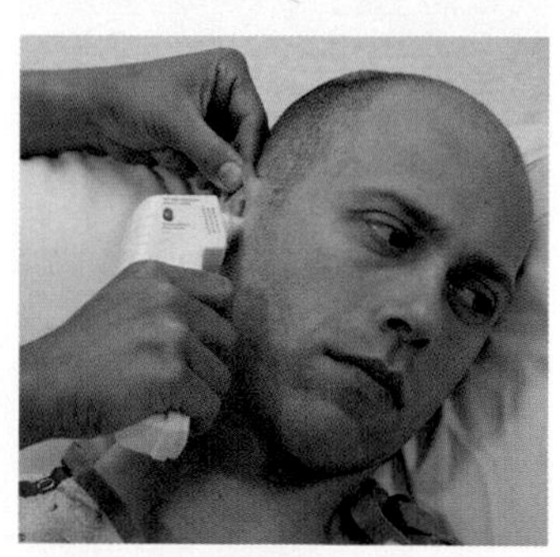

STEP 5

5. Pull top of ear up and back for adults and children older than 3 years of age, down and back for children younger than 3; rotate thermometer in line with jaw.
   Lines up the tympanic membrane with the lens to get an accurate reading.
6. Push "Start" or "Activate" button
   Tells the machine that probe is in place.
7. Support probe until reading is complete; machine will beep.
   Keeps the probe tip in place for accuracy.
8. Remove probe from patient.
9. Note temperature reading on display.
   Needed for documentation.
10. Discard probe cover; push end of probe to release cover into trash can.
    Prevents the spread of microorganisms.

Follow postprocedure steps I through VI.

Temporal Artery Temperature

Follow preprocedure steps I through VIII.

1. Obtain temporal thermometer unit; remove protective cap from lens.
   The special unit is needed for measuring temperature on the forehead near the temporal artery.
2. Inspect lens; if it is dirty, clean with alcohol wipe and allow to air-dry for 5 minutes.
   Interference from dirt on the lens can cause an inaccurate reading; using a cloth to dry off the alcohol may smudge the lens.
3. Place probe on center of the patient's clean, dry forehead; push "Scan" button; keep button pressed throughout steps 4 and 5.
   The temporal artery is located midline center of the forehead, 1 mm beneath the skin; keeping the button depressed signals the device that a temperature measurement is occurring. Moisture affects temperature measurement when using this device.
4. Slide probe straight across forehead to hairline near the temple (see step 3 above).
   Ensures accurate reading; takes an average of 1000 readings while scanning the forehead.
5. Lift probe; if perspiration is present, touch probe behind earlobe on skin over mastoid process.
   Ensures an accurate reading; averages skin, temporal artery, and room temperatures.
6. Release "Scan" button.
   Signals to the device that temperature measurement is completed.
7. Remove probe from patient.
8. Note temperature reading on display.
   Needed for documentation.
9. Clean lens with alcohol wipe; allow to air-dry for 5 minutes.
   Prevents spread of microorganisms. Interference from dirt on the lens can cause an inaccurate reading; using a cloth to dry off the alcohol may smudge the lens.
10. Replace cap on lens.
    Keeps the lens protected; maintains equipment for optimal use and accuracy.

Follow postprocedure steps I through VI.

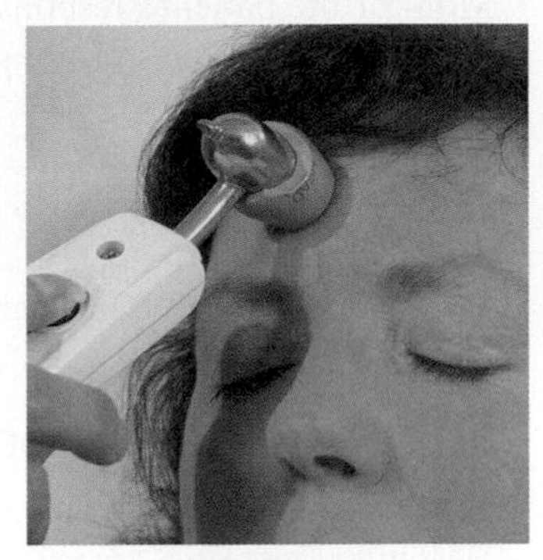

STEP 3

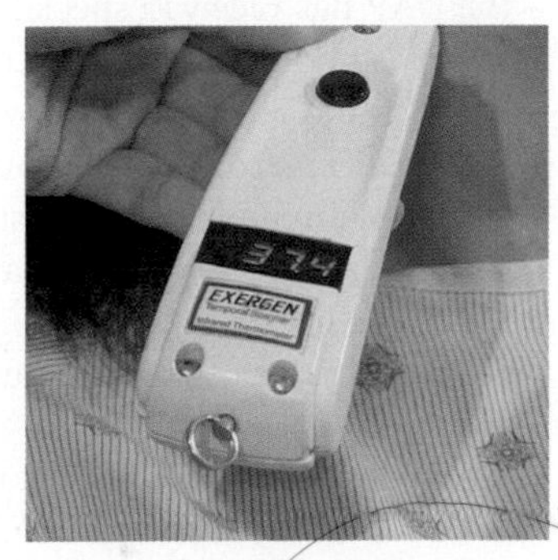

STEP 8

POSTPROCEDURE

I. Return the bed to its lowest position, raise the top side rails, and verify that the call light is within reach for the patient.
   Precautions are taken to maintain patient safety. Top side rails aid in positioning and turning. Raising four side rails is considered a restraint.

II. Assess for additional patient needs and state the time of your expected return.
   Meeting patient needs and offering self promote patient satisfaction and build trust.

III. Properly dispose of PPE.
   Gloves, gowns, and masks must be appropriately discarded to prevent the spread of microorganisms.

IV. Clean equipment if it was in contact with the patient; see specific manufacturer instructions.
   Disinfection eliminates most microorganisms from inanimate objects.

V. Perform hand hygiene.
   Frequent hand hygiene prevents the spread of infection.

VI. Document the date, time, assessment, procedure, and patient's response to the procedure.
   Accurate documentation is essential to communicate patient care and to provide legal evidence of care.

SKILL 19-2 Assessing Pulses

PURPOSE

- Determine the baseline heart rate and rhythm.
- Monitor the heart rate and rhythm.
- Assess blood flow from the heart to the body.
- Monitor the patient for changes in physical condition.
- Monitor the patient's response to medications.
- Monitor the patient's response to therapy.

RESOURCES

- Clock or watch that has a second (or "sweep") hand or a digital display
- Vital signs flow sheet and pen or electronic health record
- Stethoscope

COLLABORATION AND DELEGATION

- Assessing a radial or peripheral pulse may be delegated to UAP after the initial assessment of the patient.
- Assessing an apical pulse usually is not delegated unless the UAP has received special training. Check with the facility's guidelines and procedures.
- UAP should report the following to the nurse:
  - Deviations from normal pulse range
  - Complaints related to chest pain or discomfort
  - Irregular pulse, including a weak or thready pulse
  - Pulse less than 60 bpm or greater than 100 bpm
  - Difficulties in obtaining pulse (strength and/or quality)
  - Any changes in pulse rate, rhythm, or strength
- UAP should be instructed in:
  - The appropriate technique and method required for obtaining a pulse
  - Appropriate use of equipment (verification of accurate results, Doppler, stethoscope, electronic vital sign machines)
  - Appropriate documentation

SPECIAL CIRCUMSTANCES

1. **Assess:** Has the patient participated in exercise or physical therapy within 10 minutes?
   Intervention: Physical exercise increases the heart rate; have the patient rest 10 minutes before assessing pulse.
2. **Assess:** Is the patient upset or anxious because of stress or pain?
   Intervention: Stress raises the heart rate; therapeutic communication may calm the patient before assessing pulse.
3. **Assess:** What is the patient's history for medications? pacemakers? cardiac disease? cardiac clinical manifestations?
   Intervention: Know the baseline pulse measurement; measure the pulse for 1 minute; notify the PCP of any change and document the findings.
4. **Assess:** What should you do if you are unable to find the point of maximal impulse (PMI) when measuring apical pulse?
   Intervention: Turn the patient slightly to the left side. (Heart disease may obscure the PMI when the patient is in a supine or sitting position; using the left-side position moves the apex of the heart closer to the chest wall and may assist in locating the PMI.)
5. **Assess:** Is the pulse irregular, with strength and/or quality differences? Has there been a new onset of clinical manifestations?
   Intervention: Assessment should not be delegated if the pulse is irregular, with strength and or quality differences. Perform apical and radial pulse measurements:
   - Measure both radial and apical pulses simultaneously to determine any further assessment needs. Auscultate the apical pulse at the PMI, and palpate the radial pulse. If a pulse deficit (apical pulse exceeds the radial pulse) is present, two nurses should assess the patient's pulse at the same time, with one nurse counting the radial pulse and one counting the apical.
   - Document the apical and radial (AR) pulse rates and rhythm and any pulse deficit.
6. **Assess:** Is the patient's pulse outside the normal range?
   Intervention: If the pulse deviates from the normal range of 60 to 100 bpm for adults:
   - Retake the patient's pulse, using a different site.
   - Check the documentation for the previous site assessment.
   - Check the documentation for rhythm comma and strength or quality notations.
   - Assess the patient for clinical manifestations of an abnormal pulse.

   If the patient has a fever, give antipyretics, as ordered; fever raises the pulse rate.
   - Check the PCP orders and care plan for further interventions.

PREPROCEDURE

I. Check PCP orders and the patient care plan.
Knowledge of patient-specific orders is critical for safe patient care.

II. Gather supplies and equipment.
Preparing for the patient encounter saves time and promotes patient trust.

III. Perform hand hygiene.
Frequent hand hygiene prevents the spread of microorganisms.

IV. Maintain standard precautions.
Use of the correct personal protective equipment (PPE) is required whenever contact with bodily fluids is possible, to reduce the transfer of pathogens.

V. Introduce yourself.
Initial communication establishes the role of the nurse and begins a professional relationship.

VI. Provide for patient privacy.
It is important to maintain patient dignity.

VII. Identify the patient, using two identifiers.
Identifying a patient involves scanning barcodes or comparing the patient's stated name and birthdate to information on the patient's wristband or health record. The correct person must receive the correct treatment.

VIII. Explain the procedure to the patient.
The nurse has a responsibility to inform a patient before initiating care. Information may ease patient anxiety and facilitate cooperation.

PROCEDURE

Radial Pulse

Follow preprocedure steps I through VIII.

1. Patient may be sitting or supine. Support the patient's arm. Find pulse with your index and middle fingertips by gently placing fingertips over the area next to the radius and applying just enough pressure to palpate pulse.
Fingertips are sensitive to pulsation; feeling with both fingers ensures not feeling other vibrations. The thumb cannot be used because it has its own pulse, which would interefere with an accurate reading. Too much pressure might occlude the pulse and make measurement difficult or inaccurate. Radial pulse used to count heart rate and assess blood flow to the hand.

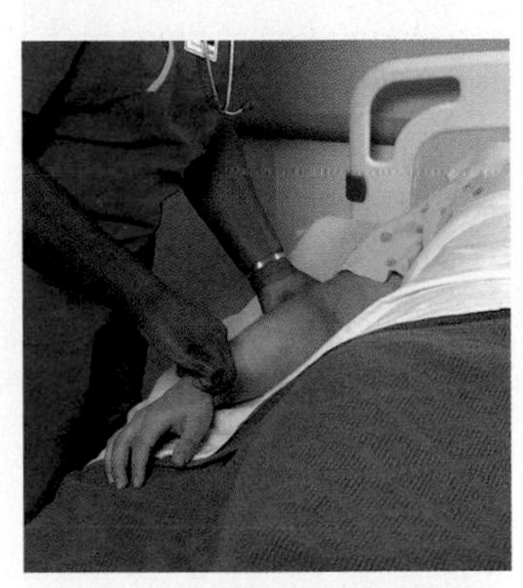

STEP 1

2. Instruct patient to remain still and not to talk.
Ensures an accurate reading.
3. Count beats for 30 seconds; if beat is irregular or rate or rhythm changes during that time, count for 1 minute.
Ensures precise reading if pulse is irregular.
4. Calculate rate: If pulse is regular, count beats for 30 seconds and multiply by 2 to calculate bpm; if pulse is irregular, count beats for 60 seconds and record findings as bpm. (Some facilities allow pulse to be counted for 15 seconds and multiplied by 4 in patients who have a regular rhythm.)
Pulse typically is recorded as bpm.
5. Note pulse rhythm (regular versus irregular) and strength (quality).
Data for documentation.
6. *For other sites:* Follow steps 1 to 5 above. Note the guidelines for the different pulse areas described next.
Other sites usually are not used to assess the pulse rate. Most sites are used to assess strength and rhythm only.
   a. *Temporal:* Both sides of the head may be assessed simultaneously.
   Temporal sites may be compared for strength.

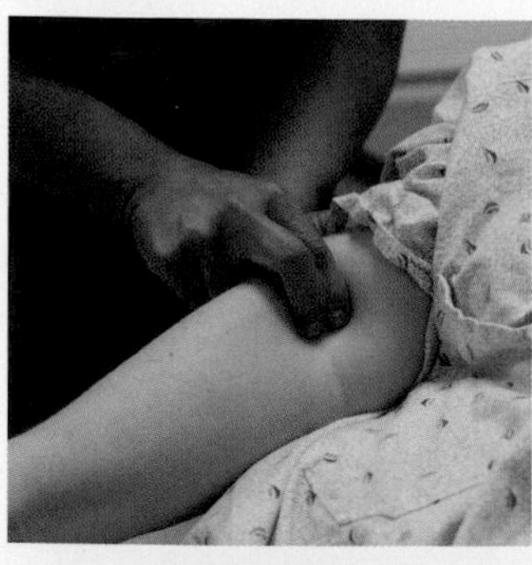

STEP 6C

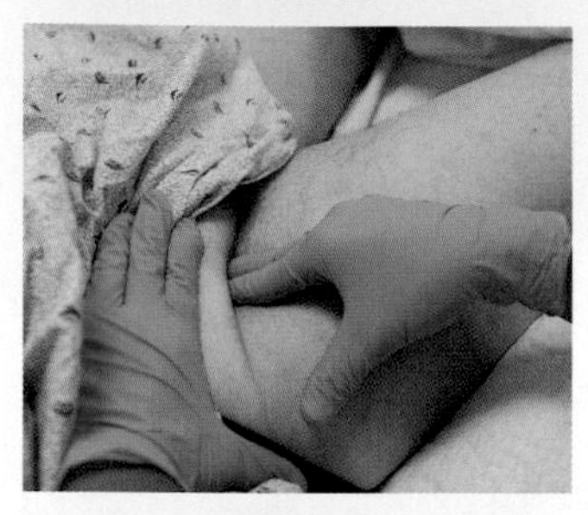

STEP 6D

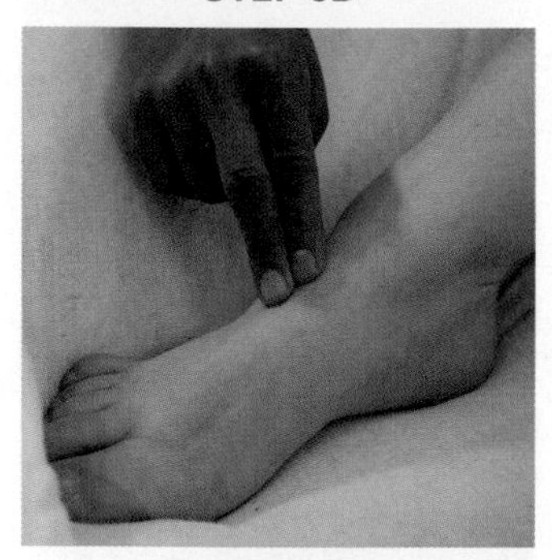

STEP 6F

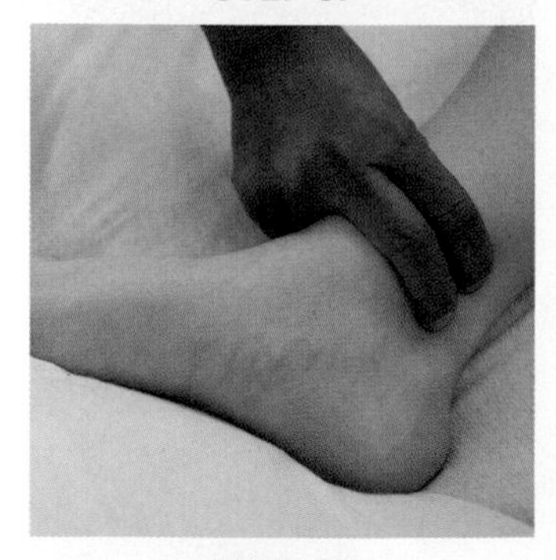

STEP 6G

b. *Carotid:* The pulse must be assessed on one side of the neck at a time.
Compares strength and/or quality of carotid pulses. This site often is used in children. Bilateral palpation of carotid pulses could block blood flow to the brain, causing the patient to experience syncope. The carotid is a main vessel often used in emergencies when the pulse is not obtainable from other sites.

c. *Brachial:* The arm is held straight out and supported.
This arm position prevents muscle contraction. The site is used to assess blood flow to the lower arm and most often to measure blood pressures. It is easily palpated in infants and young children but can be difficult to palpate in adults because of their heavier muscle mass.

d. *Femoral:* Assessment involves deeper palpation in groin area.
Large, deep main vessel in thigh. This site often is used in emergencies when pulse at other sites is not palpable. It is used to assess blood flow to the legs.

e. *Popliteal:* Knee flexed slightly; leg muscles relaxed.
Used to assess blood flow to the lower leg.

f. *Dorsalis pedis (pedal):* If this pulse is not palpable, use of a portable Doppler ultrasound machine may be required.
The pulse often is difficult to find. This site is used to assess blood flow to the foot.

g. *Posterior tibial:* may feel both extremities simultaneously.
Compares strength of the pulse between both extremities. This site is used to assess blood flow to foot.

Follow postprocedure steps I through VI.

Apical Pulse

Follow preprocedure steps I through VIII.

1. Locate PMI.
   a. Place hand at angle of Louis (sternal notch near neck where second rib attaches).
   Easy anatomic landmark for use in locating the correct site to find the PMI.
   b. Starting with left second intercostal space, count down to the left fifth intercostal space.
   The angle of Louis intersects at the second intercostal space; the PMI usually is felt at the left fifth intercostal space.
   c. Follow the left fifth intercostal space laterally to midclavicular line; stop halfway between shoulder and angle of Louis.
   The PMI usually is located near this point, called the left midclavicular line.
   d. Palpate pulsations near this point with fingertips; this is the PMI.
   The PMI is where the apex of the heart is located (usually within 1 to 2 inches of this area); the apex is closest to the skin, and it is easy to feel heart pulsations in this area.
   e. Turn patient slightly onto left side if difficulty is encountered palpating pulse.
   This brings the heart closer to the chest wall, enabling palpation of the pulse.
2. Place a clean, warm stethoscope on PMI to count apical pulse for 1 minute.
Because the PMI is at the apex and closest to the skin, it is easiest to hear heart sounds in this area.
3. Listen to heartbeat; "lub-dub" is one beat.
Normally, one heartbeat has two sounds: S_1 and S_2; listening before counting ensures accuracy.
4. Instruct patient to remain still and not to talk.
Ensures an accurate reading.
5. Count beats for 30 seconds; if beat is irregular, rate or rhythm changes during that time or the patient is on cardiovascular drugs, count for 1 full minute.
Ensures precise reading if pulse is irregular.

6. Calculate rate: If pulse is regular, count beats for 30 seconds and multiply by 2 to calculate bpm; if pulse is irregular, count beats for 60 seconds and record findings as bpm. (Some facilities allow pulse to be counted for 15 seconds and multiplied by 4 in patients who have a regular rhythm.)
   Pulse is typically recorded as bpm.
7. Note pulse rhythm (regular vs. irregular) and strength (quality).
   Data for documentation.

Follow postprocedure steps I through VI.

POSTPROCEDURE

I. Return the bed to its lowest position, raise the top side rails, and verify that the call light is within reach for the patient.
   Precautions are taken to maintain patient safety. Top side rails aid in positioning and turning. Raising four side rails is considered a restraint.

II. Assess for additional patient needs and state the time of your expected return.
   Meeting patient needs and offering self promote patient satisfaction and build trust.

III. Properly dispose of PPE.
   Gloves, gowns, and masks must be appropriately discarded to prevent the spread of microorganisms.

IV. Clean equipment if it was in contact with the patient; see specific manufacturer instructions.
   Disinfection eliminates most microorganisms from inanimate objects.

V. Perform hand hygiene.
   Frequent hand hygiene prevents the spread of infection.

VI. Document the date, time, assessment, procedure, and patient's response to the procedure.
   Accurate documentation is essential to communicate patient care and to provide legal evidence of care.

SKILL 19-3 Assessing Respirations

PURPOSE

- Determine the rate, rhythm, quality, and depth of respiration.
- Monitor the patient's respirations and respiratory changes.
- Monitor for change in the patient's physical condition.
- Monitor the patient's response to medications.
- Monitor the patient's response to therapy.

RESOURCES

- Clock or watch with a second hand or digital display.
- Vital sign flow sheet and pen or an electronic health record.

COLLABORATION AND DELEGATION

- Assessing a respiratory rate may be delegated to UAP after the initial assessment of the patient.
- UAP should report any of the following findings to the nurse:
  - Difficulty breathing or any change in respiratory rate, rhythm, or depth (report immediately)
  - Patient's complaints related to breathing difficulty or chest discomfort
  - Irregular respiratory rhythm
  - Rates less than 12 or greater than 20 BPM
  - Any difficulties in obtaining respiratory rates
- UAP should be instructed in:
  - Appropriate technique
  - Appropriate documentation

SPECIAL CIRCUMSTANCES

1. **Assess:** Has the patient undergone exercise or physical therapy within the past 5 minutes?
   Intervention: Physical exercise increases respiratory rate; have the patient rest 5 minutes before measuring respirations.
2. **Assess:** Is the patient experiencing pain?
   Intervention: Pain changes breathing characteristics; administer pain medication if prescribed, and reassess respirations after an appropriate time interval.
3. **Assess:** Is the patient upset, anxious, or emotional?
   Intervention: Emotional stress increases respiratory rate; therapeutic communication or medication may calm the patient before assessing a respiratory rate.
4. **Assess:** Does the patient's respiratory rate deviate from the normal breathing pattern?
   Intervention:
   - Respirations vary with age; know the normal range parameters expected for the patient.
   - Assess the environment for factors such as increased temperature and altitude. These conditions can increase respirations.
   - Assess the patient for clinical manifestations.
   - Reposition the patient, and reassess the respiratory rate.
   - Check the chart for respiratory side effects from any administered medications, and monitor the patient.
   - Reassess respiratory rate if needed.
   - Check the PCP orders and care plan for further interventions.
5. **Assess:** Is the patient experiencing changes in respiratory rhythm?
   Intervention: Assess the respiratory rhythm. Variations or change in respiratory rhythm (e.g., Cheyne-Stokes respirations, Kussmaul's breathing) may indicate a change in the patient's condition.

PREPROCEDURE

I. Check PCP orders and the patient care plan.
Knowledge of patient-specific orders is critical for safe patient care.

II. Gather supplies and equipment.
Preparing for the patient encounter saves time and promotes patient trust.

III. Perform hand hygiene.
Frequent hand hygiene prevents the spread of microorganisms.

IV. Maintain standard precautions.
Use of the correct personal protective equipment (PPE) is required whenever contact with bodily fluids is possible, to reduce the transfer of pathogens.

V. Introduce yourself.
Initial communication establishes the role of the nurse and begins a professional relationship.

VI. Provide for patient privacy.
It is important to maintain patient dignity.

VII. Identify the patient, using two identifiers.
Identifying a patient involves scanning barcodes or comparing the patient's stated name and birthdate to information on the patient's wristband or health record. The correct person must receive the correct treatment.

VIII. Explain the procedure to the patient.
The nurse has a responsibility to inform a patient before initiating care. Information may ease patient anxiety and facilitate cooperation.

PROCEDURE

Follow preprocedure steps I through VIII.
It is recommended that this procedure be performed while measuring the pulse.

1. Keep hand or stethoscope placed as if taking pulse; see Skill 19-2 (under "Radial Pulse" or "Apical Pulse").
   Observation or auscultation of respiratory rate occurs after taking the pulse, either by radial or apical site.
2. *Radial pulse method:* Observe rise and fall of chest.
   Apical pulse method: Observe rise and fall of chest; feel rise and fall of chest by placing hand over chest wall, or auscultate respiratory rate with stethoscope on chest.
   Patients may alter respiration rate when aware that rates are being measured.
3. Count breaths for 1 full minute; rise and fall of chest = 1 breath. Or, if respirations are regular, count for 30 seconds and multiply by 2 to get BPM or respiratory rate.
   Ensures accuracy.
4. Note rate, rhythm, and depth of respirations.
   Data for documentation.

Follow postprocedure steps I through VI.

POSTPROCEDURE

I. Return the bed to its lowest position, raise the top side rails, and verify that the call light is within reach for the patient.
Precautions are taken to maintain patient safety. Top side rails aid in positioning and turning. Raising four side rails is considered a restraint.

II. Assess for additional patient needs and state the time of your expected return.
Meeting patient needs and offering self promote patient satisfaction and build trust.

III. Properly dispose of PPE.
Gloves, gowns, and masks must be appropriately discarded to prevent the spread of microorganisms.

IV. Clean equipment if it was in contact with the patient; see specific manufacturer instructions.
Disinfection eliminates most microorganisms from inanimate objects.

V. Perform hand hygiene.
Frequent hand hygiene prevents the spread of infection.

VI. Document the date, time, assessment, procedure, and patient's response to the procedure.
Accurate documentation is essential to communicate patient care and to provide legal evidence of care.

SKILL 19-4 Assessing Pulse Oximetry

PURPOSE

- Determine the patient's baseline SpO_2 (saturation of peripheral oxygen).
- Monitor any underlying respiratory disease.
- Monitor the patient's recovery from anesthesia.
- Assess the patient for any change in physical condition.
- Assess complaints of respiratory difficulty.
- Monitor patient response to medications.
- Monitor patient response to oxygen therapy.

RESOURCES

- Pulse oximeter with probe attachment
- Alcohol wipes
- Nail polish remover
- Vital sign flow sheet and pen or an electronic health record

COLLABORATION AND DELEGATION

- Assessing SpO_2 may be delegated to UAP after initial assessment of the patient.
- UAP should report any of the following to the nurse:
  - Readings less than 92% or other designated saturation, as determined by the nurse or PCP
  - Complaints related to breathing difficulty or chest discomfort
  - Situations in which the patient is not using oxygen or it is not at the appropriate level according to the PCP orders
  - Any difficulties in procedure
- UAP should be instructed in:
  - Appropriate placement of oximeter probe (finger, toe, bridge of nose, or earlobe)
  - Appropriate equipment use (verifying accurate results)
  - Patient oxygen use and frequency of monitoring
  - Appropriate documentation

SPECIAL CIRCUMSTANCES

1. **Assess:** Has the patient undergone exercise or physical therapy within the past 5 minutes?
   Intervention: Have the patient rest 5 minutes before measuring SpO_2; if the PCP order is for exercise oximetry, see the respiratory therapist for assistance.
2. **Assess:** Is the patient wearing fingernail polish or artificial nails?
   Intervention: Remove polish or artificial nails before measuring SpO_2, or use an alternative location to take the measurement if permitted by equipment and facility policy.
3. **Assess:** Are there any sores, wounds, or irritations at the site?
   Intervention: Use a different site, and document the location and reason for using it.
4. **Assess:** Does the patient have hand or arm tremors?
   Intervention: Use the patient's other arm or a different site (toe, earlobe, bridge of nose).
5. **Assess:** Does the patient have carbon monoxide poisoning?
   Intervention: Obtain an order for arterial blood gas instead, because the SpO_2 is falsely elevated.
6. **Assess:** Does the SpO_2 differ from the baseline measurement?
   Intervention:
   - Assess the patient for clinical manifestations of hypoxemia resulting in hypoxia, such as cyanosis or pallor, dyspnea, restlessness, decreased level of consciousness, increased pulse and blood pressure, or use of accessory muscles for breathing.
   - Reposition the patient and reassess SpO_2.
   - Check the oxygen therapy equipment/flow rate, orders, and weaning status.
   - Check the PCP orders and care plan for further interventions.
7. **Assess:** Is there impaired circulation to the extremity on which the oximeter probe is applied?
   Intervention: Impaired circulation might result in a false SpO_2; apply the probe to a different site.

PREPROCEDURE

I. Check PCP orders and the patient care plan.
Knowledge of patient-specific orders is critical for safe patient care.
II. Gather supplies and equipment.
Preparing for the patient encounter saves time and promotes patient trust.
III. Perform hand hygiene.
Frequent hand hygiene prevents the spread of microorganisms.
IV. Maintain standard precautions.
Use of the correct personal protective equipment (PPE) is required whenever contact with bodily fluids is possible, to reduce the transfer of pathogens.
V. Introduce yourself.
Initial communication establishes the role of the nurse and begins a professional relationship.
VI. Provide for patient privacy.
It is important to maintain patient dignity.
VII. Identify the patient, using two identifiers.
Identifying a patient involves scanning barcodes or comparing the patient's stated name and birthdate to information on the patient's wristband or health record. The correct person must receive the correct treatment.
VIII. Explain the procedure to the patient.
The nurse has a responsibility to inform a patient before initiating care. Information may ease patient anxiety and facilitate cooperation.

PROCEDURE

Follow preprocedure steps I through VIII.
1. Obtain pulse oximeter and appropriate probe.
2. Place probe on appropriate site; instruct patient to breathe normally and not to move body part where oximeter is attached.
A finger is the most common site; the oximeter will give an inaccurate reading with movement.
3. Turn on oximeter.
Sends signal to oximeter that probe is in place and ready for reading.
4. Observe oximeter reading when pulse waveform is present and beats are constant; compare oximeter pulse reading with patient's radial pulse.
Ensures accuracy of the SpO_2 reading. Most oximeters display the pulse, which can then be compared with the pulse measurement taken by the nurse.

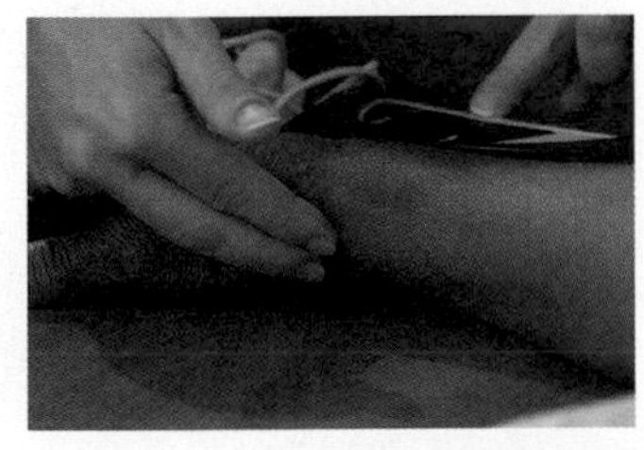
STEP 4

5. *Reading:* Depending on model of oximeter, device may emit audible beep when a single reading is complete (when SpO_2 reaches a constant value) or, if continuous monitoring is necessary (e.g., with critical care), may beep with each heartbeat to indicate that device is detecting pulse.
Knowledge of how the equipment works ensures an accurate reading.
6. Note SpO_2 reading on display, and note whether patient is on supplemental oxygen.
Data for documentation.
7. Remove probe from patient (if not performing continuous monitoring).
8. Clean probe and wire with alcohol wipe.
Prevents the spread of microorganisms.

Follow postprocedure steps I through VI.

POST-PROCEDURE

I. Return the bed to its lowest position, raise the top side rails, and verify that the call light is within reach for the patient.
Precautions are taken to maintain patient safety. Top side rails aid in positioning and turning. Raising four side rails is considered a restraint.

II. Assess for additional patient needs and state the time of your expected return.
Meeting patient needs and offering self promote patient satisfaction and build trust.

III. Properly dispose of PPE.
Gloves, gowns, and masks must be appropriately discarded to prevent the spread of microorganisms.

IV. Clean equipment if it was in contact with the patient; see specific manufacturer instructions.
Disinfection eliminates most microorganisms from inanimate objects.

V. Perform hand hygiene.
Frequent hand hygiene prevents the spread of infection.

VI. Document the date, time, assessment, procedure, and patient's response to the procedure.
Accurate documentation is essential to communicate patient care and to provide legal evidence of care.

SKILL 19-5 Measuring Blood Pressure: Manual and Electronic

PURPOSE

- Determine the baseline blood pressure.
- Monitor blood pressure.
- Assess the heart's pumping ability and the patency of blood vessels.
- Monitor for changes in physical condition.
- Monitor the patient's response to medications.
- Monitor the patient's response to therapy.

RESOURCES

- Sphygmomanometer with bladder and cuff
- Stethoscope with a bell and diaphragm
- Electronic blood pressure or vital sign machine with bladder and cuff
- Vital sign flow sheet and pen or an electronic health record

COLLABORATION AND DELEGATION

- Electronic measurement of blood pressure may be delegated to UAP after initial assessment of the patient.
- Manual measurement of blood pressure may be delegated if the UAP has received special training. Check the facility's guidelines and procedures.
- UAP should report any of the following findings to the nurse:
  - Deviations from normal range of blood pressure
  - Complaints related to chest pain or discomfort
  - Systolic blood pressure greater than 140 or less than 90 or diastolic blood pressure greater than 100 or less than 70
  - Difficulties in obtaining blood pressure
- UAP should be instructed in:
  - The appropriate technique and method required for the patient
  - Appropriate equipment use (verifying accurate results with stethoscope, sphygmomanometer, electronic vital sign devices, appropriate cuff size, and site choice)
  - Sites and conditions that are contraindicated—intravenous lines, arteriovenous (AV) fistulas or shunts, amputations, breast surgery, and casts or bandages
  - Appropriate documentation

EVIDENCE-BASED PRACTICE

- Blood pressure does not always rise in response to emotion. The patient's culture may affect whether blood pressure is elevated or lowered from normal range in response to emotion (Butler, Lee, and Gross, 2009).
- Automated blood pressure measurements are not always accurate, especially in hypertensive patients and the elderly population (Heinemann, Sellick, Rickard, et al., 2008).
- The two-step method, palpating a systolic pressure, is the most accurate technique, especially in hypertensive and geriatric populations in whom the auscultatory gap may be widened considerably. When the two-step method is not employed, manual blood pressures are frequently inaccurate (Cork, 2007; Curran, 2009).

SPECIAL CIRCUMSTANCES

1. **Assess:** Has the patient undergone exercise or physical therapy within the past 15 minutes?
   Intervention: Physical exercise raises blood pressure; have the patient rest 15 minutes before assessing blood pressure.
2. **Assess:** Is the patient upset, anxious, or emotional?
   Intervention: Emotional stress raises blood pressure; therapeutic communication may calm the patient before assessing blood pressure.
3. **Assess:** What is the patient's medication, pacemaker, and cardiac history?
   Intervention: Compare current findings to the baseline; review the chart and history; determine possible effects of medications on blood pressure; notify the PCP of any change; and document all findings.
4. **Assess:** Is the patient complaining of cardiac clinical manifestations?
   Intervention: Compare the current findings to the baseline; compare other assessments with the baseline; review the patient's chart and history; obtain assistance if needed; notify the PCP of any changes; and document all findings and actions.
5. **Assess:** What is the patient's arm size?
   Intervention: Obtain the correct cuff size for the patient. A cuff size that is too small could result in a false-high reading, while a cuff size that is too large could result in a false-low reading.
6. **Assess:** Has the patient had any caffeine or tobacco intake within the past 30 minutes?
   Intervention: Caffeine intake or smoking can raise blood pressure. If possible, wait 30 minutes from intake; if waiting is not possible, document the intake.
7. **Assess:** Does the patient have special circumstances that prevent taking blood pressure in one or both arms?
   Intervention: If the patient has an IV or has had a mastectomy, use the opposite arm. If both arms are affected, blood pressure can be taken on the lower extremity.
8. **Assess:** Does the blood pressure deviate from the normal range?
   Intervention:
   - Check the documentation for previous site assessment and method.

- Check the documentation for trends and the most recent medications.
- Assess the following factors, because they may influence blood pressure: pain, time of day, patient position, emotional stress, environmental temperature, patient's temperature, and lab values.
- Assess the patient for clinical manifestations of hypertension and hypotension.
- Reassess blood pressure using a different site or method.
- Check the PCP orders and care plan for further interventions.

PREPROCEDURE

I. Check PCP orders and the patient care plan.
Knowledge of patient-specific orders is critical for safe patient care.

II. Gather supplies and equipment.
Preparing for the patient encounter saves time and promotes patient trust.

III. Perform hand hygiene.
Frequent hand hygiene prevents the spread of microorganisms.

IV. Maintain standard precautions.
Use of the correct personal protective equipment (PPE) is required whenever contact with bodily fluids is possible, to reduce the transfer of pathogens.

V. Introduce yourself.
Initial communication establishes the role of the nurse and begins a professional relationship.

VI. Provide for patient privacy.
It is important to maintain patient dignity.

VII. Identify the patient, using two identifiers.
Identifying a patient involves scanning barcodes or comparing the patient's stated name and birthdate to information on the patient's wristband or health record. The correct person must receive the correct treatment.

VIII. Explain the procedure to the patient.
The nurse has a responsibility to inform a patient before initiating care. Information may ease patient anxiety and facilitate cooperation.

PROCEDURE

Two-Step Manual Method: Upper Extremity

Follow preprocedure steps I through VIII.

1. Obtain blood pressure cuff (correct size for patient) and stethoscope.
Ensures accuracy: cuff too small = false high; cuff too large = false low. The bladder of the blood pressure cuff should be approximately 60% to 80% of the circumference of the extremity being used, and the width of the cuff should be approximately 40% of the circumference of the extremity.
2. Remove clothing and bedding from upper arm. Patient is in sitting or supine position with arm at level of heart, supported by mattress or table; feet on floor or supported by mattress; legs uncrossed.
Placing the cuff directly on the arm ensures accuracy; supporting the arm keeps the patient from flexing muscles; and having the arm at the level of the heart and feet uncrossed ensures accuracy.
3. Palpate brachial and radial pulses (see Skill 19-2: Assessing Pulses).
Provides a baseline; checks for adequate circulation in the arm; and locates placement for the stethoscope.

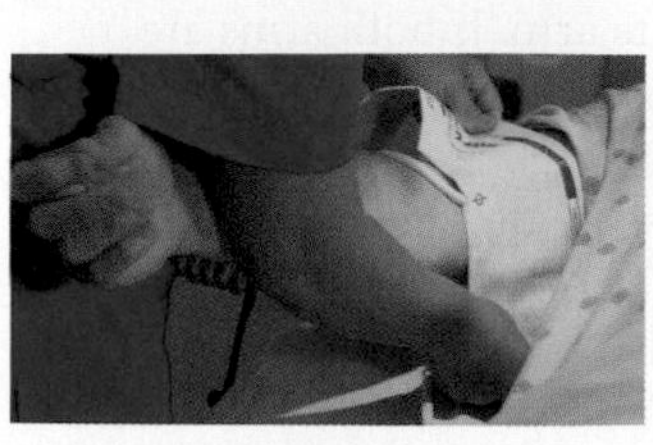
STEP 4

4. Position appropriately sized cuff 1 inch above antecubital fossa, with arrow pointing to brachial artery. Position of manometer gauge is vertical and at eye level.
Positioning the cuff with the bladder centered on the brachial artery ensures accuracy.
5. Palpate brachial pulse; instruct patient to remain still and not to talk; close valve on pump by turning implement clockwise.
Prepares for reading and ensures accuracy.

6. Inflate cuff to 30 mm Hg above point at which brachial pulse disappears; note that point.
   Starting point for determining how much to inflate the cuff. Overinflation may be painful for the patient and damage small blood vessels.
7. Deflate cuff slowly; note point at which pulse reappears; then fully deflate cuff quickly.
   Approximates systolic blood pressure.
8. Wait 2 minutes before taking additional measurement.
   Allows blood pressure to return to baseline as the blood refills the veins; ensures accuracy.
9. Place clean stethoscope diaphragm over brachial pulse, and insert ear attachments, positioning them slightly forward.
   Sound is heard more clearly when earpieces are positioned to follow the direction of the ear canal.

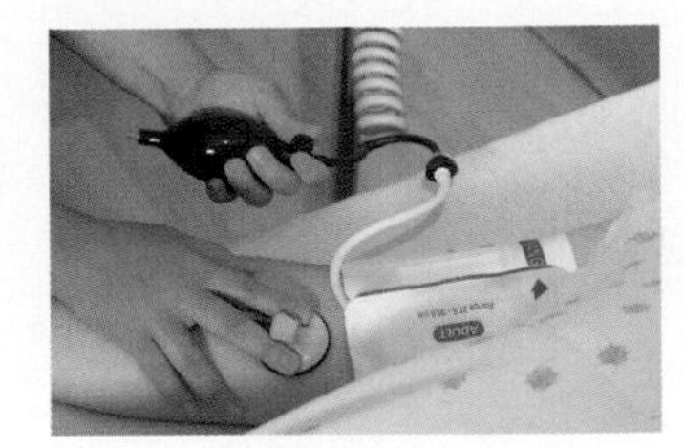

STEP 9

10. Inflate cuff to 30 mm Hg above point noted in step 6.
    Ensures that the cuff is inflated above the level of the systolic blood pressure.
11. Deflate cuff slowly (2 mm Hg/second): Note reading at first sound (when heartbeat first becomes audible); note reading at last sound (when individual heartbeats are no longer audible).
    Deflating quickly results in inaccurate measurement. First sound = systolic blood pressure; last sound = diastolic blood pressure.
12. Deflate cuff quickly and completely; remove equipment from patient.
    Keeps the equipment calibrated to ensure accuracy; keeps the patient comfortable; and prevents wounds and skin irritation.
13. Clean equipment as needed.
    Prevents the spread of microorganisms.

Follow postprocedure steps I through VI.

Two-Step Manual Method: Lower Extremity

Follow preprocedure steps I through VIII.

1. Obtain blood pressure cuff (correct size for patient) and stethoscope.
   Ensures accuracy: cuff too small = false high; cuff too large = false low. The bladder of the blood pressure cuff should be approximately 60% to 80% of the circumference of the extremity being used, and the width of the cuff should be approximately 40% of the circumference of the extremity.
2. Remove clothing and bedding from lower extremity. Patient is the supine, side-lying or prone position with legs uncrossed.
   Placing the cuff directly on the leg ensures accuracy; supporting the leg with the mattress keeps the patient from flexing muscles.
3. With patient in the supine, side-lying or prone position, check popliteal and pedal pulses (see Skill 19-2).
   Provides a baseline; checks for adequate circulation in the leg; locates placement for the stethoscope.
4. Position appropriately sized cuff 1 inch above knee, with arrow pointing to popliteal artery; make sure gauge is in direct line of vision.
   Positioning the cuff with the bladder centered on the popliteal artery ensures accuracy.

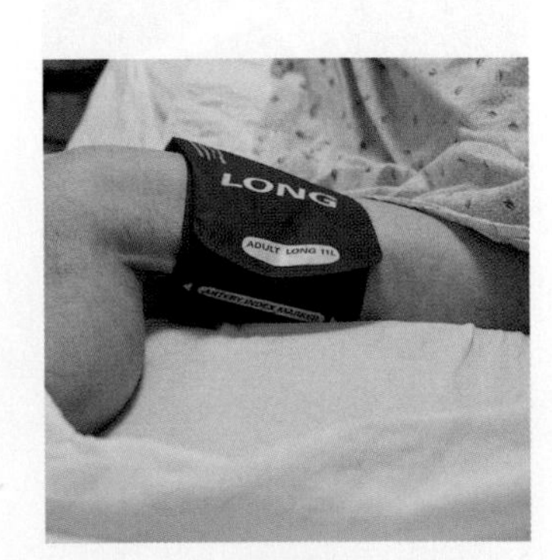

STEP 4

5. Palpate popliteal pulse; instruct patient to remain still and not to talk; close valve on pump by turning implement clockwise. Make sure that gauge is in direct line of vision.
   Prepares for reading and ensures accuracy.
6. Inflate cuff to 30 mm Hg above point at which popliteal pulse disappears; note that point.
   Starting point for determining how much to inflate the cuff. Overinflation may be painful for the patient and damage small blood vessels.
7. Deflate cuff slowly; note point at which pulse reappears; then fully deflate cuff quickly.
   Approximates systolic blood pressure.

8. Wait 2 minutes before taking additional measurement.
   Allows blood pressure to return to baseline as the blood refills the veins; ensures accuracy.
9. Place stethoscope diaphragm over popliteal artery.
   Stethoscope diaphragm is meant for lower sound frequency.
10. Inflate cuff to 30 mm Hg above point noted in step 6.
    Ensures that the cuff is inflated above the level of the systolic blood pressure.
11. Deflate cuff slowly (2 mm Hg/second): Note reading at first sound (when heartbeat first becomes audible); note reading at last sound (when individual heartbeats are no longer audible).
    Deflating quickly results in inaccurate measurement. First sound = systolic blood pressure; last sound = diastolic blood pressure.
12. Deflate cuff quickly and completely; remove equipment from patient.
    Keeps the equipment calibrated to ensure accuracy; keeps the patient comfortable; and prevents wounds and skin irritation.
13. Clean equipment as needed.
    Prevents the spread of microorganisms.

Follow postprocedure steps I through VI.

Electronic Method

Follow preprocedure steps I through VIII.

1. Obtain electronic blood pressure machine with appropriate cuff size for patient.
   Ensures accuracy: cuff too small = false high; cuff too large = false low. The bladder of the blood pressure cuff should be approximately 60% to 80% of the circumference of the upper arm.
2. Remove clothing and bedding from upper arm. Patient is in sitting or supine position with arm at level of heart, supported by mattress or table; feet on floor or supported by mattress; legs uncrossed.
   Placing the cuff directly on the arm ensures accuracy; supporting the arm keeps the patient from flexing muscles; and having the arm at the level of the heart and feet uncrossed ensures accuracy.
3. Palpate brachial and radial pulses (see Skill 19-2: Assessing Pulses).
   Provides a baseline; checks for adequate circulation in the arm; and locates placement for the stethoscope.
4. Position cuff snugly.
   Ensures accuracy.
5. Instruct patient to remain still and not to talk.
   Prepares for reading and ensures accuracy.
6. Push on/off button: Machine will beep; digital display will appear.
   Indicates machine is charged and ready for use.

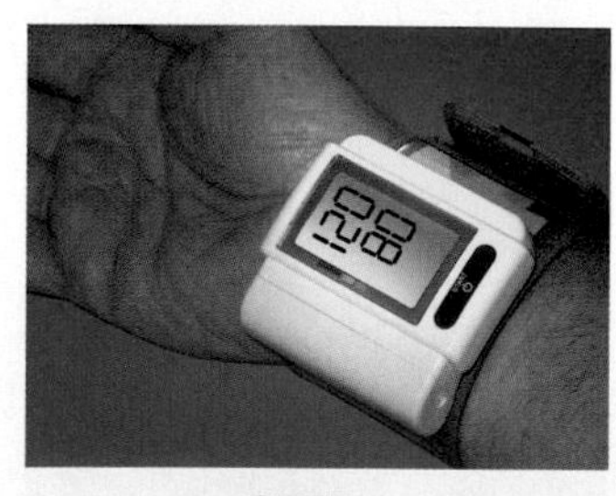

STEP 6

7. Push Start button: Cuff will inflate and deflate; display will appear.
   Machine detects pulses in conjunction with cuff pressure.
8. Note readings or obtain readings from the memory of the unit.
   Data needed for documentation; most machines have a built-in memory.
9. Remove equipment from patient.
   Keeps patient comfortable; prevents wounds and skin irritation.
10. Clean equipment as needed; plug unit into electrical outlet.
    Prevents the spread of microorganisms. Most units require recharging after use.

Follow postprocedure steps I through VI.

POSTPROCEDURE

I. Return the bed to its lowest position, raise the top side rails, and verify that the call light is within reach for the patient.
   Precautions are taken to maintain patient safety. Top side rails aid in positioning and turning. Raising four side rails is considered a restraint.

II. Assess for additional patient needs and state the time of your expected return.
Meeting patient needs and offering self promote patient satisfaction and build trust.

III. Properly dispose of PPE.
Gloves, gowns, and masks must be appropriately discarded to prevent the spread of microorganisms.

IV. Clean equipment if it was in contact with the patient; see specific manufacturer instructions.
Disinfection eliminates most microorganisms from inanimate objects.

V. Perform hand hygiene.
Frequent hand hygiene prevents the spread of infection.

VI. Document the date, time, assessment, procedure, and patient's response to the procedure.
Accurate documentation is essential to communicate patient care and to provide legal evidence of care.

SUMMARY OF LEARNING OUTCOMES

LO 19.1 *Explain the purpose of assessing vital signs:* Vital signs include temperature, pulse, respirations with oxygen saturation, and blood pressure, as well as pain assessment. The measurement of vital signs gives critical information about a patient's psychological and physiologic status. Nursing judgment determines how frequently vital signs are assessed.

LO 19.2 *Describe techniques for obtaining accurate temperature measurement:* Body temperature can be measured orally, tympanically, rectally, and temporally, as well as by axillary methods and internally through an arterial probe. The most appropriate route is dependent on patient status and age.

LO 19.3 *Identify common assessment sites and techniques for assessing pulse:* The radial pulse is the most common site to measure pulse rate. There are eight other sites that can be used to assess the character and strength of the pulse. The apical pulse is measured in specific cases such as when the rate is irregular, the patient is taking certain medications, or the radial pulse is not palpable.

LO 19.4 *Discuss assessment of respirations and blood oxygenation:* Normal respirations are quiet, effortless, and automatic. Assessment of respirations includes observing the patient's breathing and assessing the effectiveness of ventilation, perfusion, and diffusion. Pulse oximetry measures the percentage of hemoglobin saturated with oxygen that is available for use by body tissues.

LO 19.5 *Summarize correct methods for measuring blood pressure:* Blood pressure reflects cardiac output, peripheral vascular resistance, and blood volume and viscosity. It measures the highest pressure (systolic) and lowest resting pressure (diastolic) of the blood in the vessels. A blood pressure cuff that is too small or too large or is applied improperly will cause errors in the reading.

LO 19.6 *Perform pain assessment in diverse populations:* Pain perception is influenced by age, past experiences, culture, and values. Pain is assessed in conjunction with other vital signs with appropriate assessment tools.

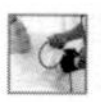

Responses to the critical-thinking questions are available at *http://evolve.elsevier.com/YoostCrawford/fundamentals/*.

REVIEW QUESTIONS

1. The nurse is measuring blood pressures as part of a community health fair. Which blood pressure reading would cause the nurse to refer the patient for follow-up regarding potential hypertension?
   a. 118/78
   b. 126/84
   c. 136/90
   d. 144/94
2. The nurse is admitting a stable patient for a minor outpatient procedure. What site would the nurse most commonly use to assess pulse rate?
   a. Radial site
   b. Apical site
   c. Brachial site
   d. Carotid site
3. The unlicensed assistive personnel reports vital signs for a patient to the nurse: temperature 99.2° F oral, pulse 88 bpm and regular, respirations 18 BPM and regular, blood pressure 178/112, oxygen saturation 96%, and pain score of 3 of 10 for headache. Which vital sign should the nurse be most concerned about?
   a. Temperature
   b. Pulse
   c. Respirations
   d. Blood pressure
4. From the nurse's understanding, which statements regarding temperature and heat production in the body are accurate? *(Select all that apply.)*
   a. Heat generates energy for cellular functions.
   b. Hormones such as thyroid decrease metabolism and heat production.
   c. Exercise decreases heat production through muscular activity.
   d. Body temperature is 1° to 2° higher in the morning than in late afternoon.
   e. Expected temperature readings vary by the route selected for measurement.
   f. Women tend to have more fluctuations in temperature than do men.
5. The nurse is performing an initial assessment of a patient with a severe infection at hospital admission. Vital signs for the patient indicate hypotension and tachycardia. Which data pair would support this evaluation?
   a. Pulse 88, blood pressure 140/88
   b. Pulse 96, blood pressure 120/76
   c. Pulse 100, blood pressure 118/80
   d. Pulse 114, blood pressure 98/60

6. The nurse places a patient with a high fever on a cooling blanket. How is heat loss achieved with this treatment?
   a. Radiation
   b. Convection
   c. Conduction
   d. Evaporation
7. Which clinical patient scenario is associated with the most critical need for the nurse to obtain vital signs?
   a. Ambulating for the first time after surgery
   b. Complaining of pressure in the chest
   c. Completes ambulating 100 feet after a stroke
   d. Complaining of a hunger while NPO (nothing by mouth)
8. The nurse understands that which statement is correct regarding respiratory rates?
   a. Infants have a lower respiratory rate than adults.
   b. Healthy adults breathe between 12 and 20 times a minute.
   c. A compensatory response to a fever is to breathe at a slower rate.
   d. An increase in intracranial pressure results in an increased rate.
9. The nurse is caring for a patient who has a blood pressure of 184/110. An hour after administering an antihypertensive medication, the nurse returns to rechecks the blood pressure, only to find the patient in the chair pale, sweaty, and feeling faint. Which is the expected explanation for the nurse's observations?
   a. The blood pressure is 184/110; the medication has not had an effect.
   b. The blood pressure is 118/76; the sudden drop has caused the signs.
   c. The blood pressure is 174/96; the medication has made the patient sick.
   d. The blood pressure is 130/82; the symptoms are from another cause.
10. It is 6 A.M. and the UAP reports to the nurse that the patient has a temperature of 96.7° F tympanic. Which factor explains this reading?
   a. The patient's room is cold.
   b. The patient was drinking cold water.
   c. The patient is exhibiting a normal circadian rhythm.
   d. The patient just completed a warm shower.

Answers and rationales for the review questions are available at *http://evolve.elsevier.com/YoostCrawford/fundamentals/.*

REFERENCES

American Pain Society: *Guidelines for the management of cancer pain in adults and children*, Glenview, Ill., 2005, Author.

American Society for Pain Management in Nursing: Pain assessment in the nonverbal patient: Position statement with clinical practice recommendations. *Pain Manag Nurs* 17(2):44-52, 2006.

Bhan V, Yan R, Leiter L, et al: Relation between obesity and the attainment of optimal blood pressure and lipid targets in high vascular risk outpatients. *Am J Cardiol* 106(9):1270-1276, 2010.

Butler EA, Lee TL, Gross JJ: Does expressing your emotions raise or lower your blood pressure? The answer depends on cultural context. *J Cross- Cult Psychol* 40(3):510-517, 2009.

Clinical mnemonics, 2014. Retrieved from *www.valuemd.com/clinical.php.*

Cork A: Theory and practice of manual blood pressure measurement. *Nurs Stand* 22(14-16):47-50, 2007.

Cronenwett L, Sherwood G, Barnsteiner J, et al: Quality and safety education for nurses. *Nurs Outlook* 55(3):122-131, 2007.

Curran R: The vital signs: Part 1. Blood pressure. *EMS Acad Clin Track* 38(3):62-66, 2009.

Davie A, Amoore J: Best practice in the measurement of body temperature. *Nurs Stand* 24(42):42-49, 2010.

Giantin V, Toffanello ED, Enzi G, et al: Reliability of body temperature measurements in hospitalized older patients. *J Clin Nurs* 17:1518-1525, 2008.

Heinemann M, Sellick K, Rickard C, et al: Automated versus manual blood pressure measurement: A randomized crossover trial. *Int J Nurs Pract* 14:296-302, 2008.

Langham GE, Maheshwari A, Contrera K, et al: Noninvasive temperature monitoring in postanesthesia care units. *Anesthesiology* 111(1):90-96, 2009.

Lu SH, Dai YT: Normal body temperature and the effects of age, sex, ambient temperature and body mass index on normal oral temperature: A prospective, comparative study. *Int J Nurs Stud* 46:661-668, 2009.

MacKechnie C, Simpson R: Traceable calibration for blood pressure and temperature monitoring. *Nurs Stand* 21(11): 42-47, 2006.

Mayo Clinic: Orthostatic hypotension (postural hypotension), 2014. Retrieved from *www.mayoclinic.com.*

National Heart, Lung, and Blood Institute: Eighth report of the Joint National Committee on prevention, detection, evaluation, and treatment of high blood pressure—complete report (JNC8), 2011. Retrieved from *www.nhlbi.nih.gov/.*

Ong KL, Cheung BM, Man YB, et al: Prevalence, awareness, treatment, and control of hypertension among United States adults 1999–2004. *Hypertension* 49:69-75, 2007.

Oparil S; Miller AP: Gender and blood pressure. *J Clin Hypertens* 7(5):300-309, 2005.

Porth CM: *Essentials of pathophysiology,* ed. 3, Philadelphia, 2011, Lippincott Williams & Wilkins.

Quatrara B, Coffman J, Jenkins T, et al: The effect of respiratory rate and ingestion of hot and cold beverages on the accuracy of oral temperatures measured by electronic thermometers. *MEDSURG Nurs* 16(2):100, 105-108, 2007.

Smitz S, Van de Winckel A, Smitz MF: Reliability of infrared ear thermometry in the prediction of rectal temperature in older inpatients. *J Clin Nurs* 18:451-456, 2009.

Spitzer OP: Comparing tympanic temperatures in both ears to oral temperature in the critically ill adult. *Dimens Crit Care Nurs* 27(1):24-29, 2008.

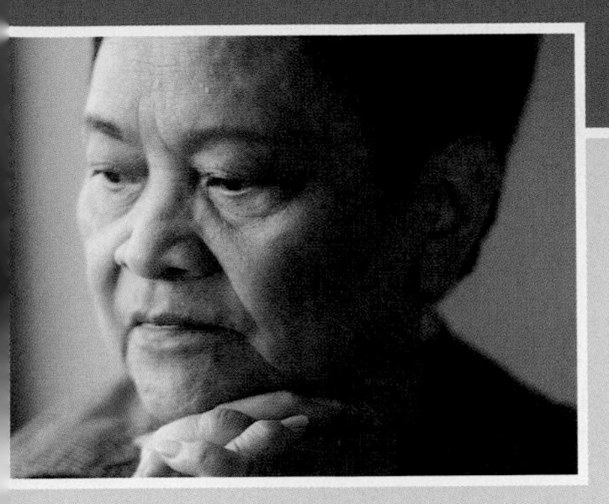

CHAPTER 20

Health History and Physical Assessment

EVOLVE WEBSITE

http://evolve.elsevier.com/YoostCrawford/fundamentals/

- Additional Evolve-Only Review Questions With Answers
- Answers and Rationales for Text Review Questions
- Answers to Critical-Thinking Questions
- Case Study With Questions
- Body Spectrum
- Glossary

LEARNING OUTCOMES

Comprehension of this chapter's content will provide students with the ability to:

LO 20.1 Apply strategies used to conduct a patient interview, health history, and review of systems.

LO 20.2 Discuss the environmental and patient care activities that should be completed before and during history taking and physical examination.

LO 20.3 Use the four physical assessment techniques when examining each body system.

LO 20.4 Discuss factors for consideration during the general survey.

LO 20.5 Demonstrate a focused and head-to-toe physical assessment, noting opportunities for patient education.

LO 20.6 Describe the activities and specific documentation that are required at the completion of the physical assessment.

KEY TERMS

accommodation, p. 354
adventitious breath sounds, p. 368
albinism, p. 343
alopecia, p. 349
atelectasis, p. 368
auscultation, p. 338
borborygmi, p. 384
bruit, p. 364
capillary refill, p. 350
cardiac murmurs, p. 371
cataracts, p. 354
cerumen, p. 357
cheilitis, p. 362
chief complaint, p. 335
clinical manifestations, p. 335
clonus, p. 376
comorbid, p. 335
consistency, p. 337
crepitation (crepitus), p. 337
cyanosis, p. 343
diplopia, p. 353
dysrhythmia, p. 371
ecchymosis, p. 348
edema, p. 348
epistaxis, p. 361
erythema, p. 343
excoriation, p. 361
focused assessment, p. 335
guarding, p. 337
hirsutism, p. 349
hydrocephalus, p. 352
hypertonicity, p. 376
hypotonicity, p. 376
inspection, p. 337
jaundice, p. 343
kyphosis, p. 376
lordosis, p. 376
nystagmus, p. 355
pallor, p. 343
palpation, p. 337
paresthesia, p. 375
percussion, p. 337
peristalsis, p. 384
petechiae, p. 344
phlebitis, p. 375
physical assessment, p. 333
pruritus, p. 349
ptosis, p. 353
pulse deficit, p. 371
purpura, p. 343
purulent, p. 357
rebound tenderness, p. 337
scoliosis, p. 376
smegma, p. 389
stenosis, p. 384
strabismus, p. 353
striae, p. 384
tactile fremitus, p. 367
thrill, p. 372
tinnitus, p. 359
tortuosity, p. 372
turgor, p. 337
vertigo, p. 359
vitiligo, p. 343

CASE STUDY

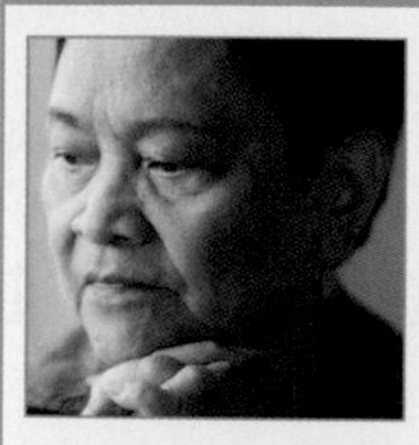

Mrs. Thatcher, an 85-year-old recent widow, comes to the health clinic for her annual physical examination. She reports feeling more tired than usual and has noticed that her feet are swelling. Mrs. Thatcher states that sometimes she feels short of breath after climbing the steps to her bedroom on the second floor. Her intake vital signs are T 36.78° C (98.2° F), P 100 and slightly irregular, R 24 and shallow, and BP 116/68. The nurse is acquainted with Mrs. Thatcher and notices that she is walking more slowly than usual to the examination room.

Refer back to this case study to answer the critical-thinking questions throughout the chapter.

Physical assessment is an integral part of the first step in the nursing process, which begins with comprehensive data collection followed by systematic physical examination. Collecting a patient's health history is achieved through two methods: conducting a patient interview to gather subjective data or symptoms and reviewing past medical records for significant medical and surgical history, which is objective data. (Refer to Chapter 6 for additional information on subjective and objective data.) The physical assessment that follows is a head-to-toe examination of each body system during which the nurse gathers more objective data, or signs. The patient's health status and the extent of physical impairment, as well as the location and timing of the patient's interaction with the nurse, influence the accuracy and intensity of physical assessment. It is the RN's responsibility to gather either comprehensive or focused assessment data during each patient encounter. Assessment findings are used to formulate individualized plans of care.

PATIENT INTERVIEW LO 20.1

Obtaining a health history begins with a patient interview. The patient's first impression of the health care system during the interview often sets the tone for subsequent interactions with members of the health care team (Evidence-Based Practice and Informatics box). The interview has three phases: orientation (or introductory), working, and termination. During the interview process patients express their emotional and physical concerns. Some of the factors that affect the patient interview include privacy, interruptions, the environment, and communication techniques. A sense of privacy may be achieved by using a private room or curtain partitions as well as by minimizing interruptions during the interview. The environment should be comfortable and conducive to a professional interaction. A comfortable room temperature, sufficient lighting, reduction of extraneous sound, and removal of distracting objects contribute to patient comfort. The patient and the nurse conducting the interview should be comfortably seated at eye level, without barriers.

Nurses need to be attentive throughout the interview process. Maintaining a relaxed and open posture, leaning slightly toward the patient, and showing interest with occasional gestures all communicate concern. Negative nonverbal cues such as distracting gestures (e.g., tapping a pen, swinging a foot, looking at a watch), inappropriate facial expressions, or lack of eye contact communicate disinterest.

EVIDENCE-BASED PRACTICE AND INFORMATICS

Nursing Behaviors During the Interview

Research has identified several nursing behaviors that contribute to patient satisfaction and safety and should be implemented during the interview process:

- Summarizing and repeating information
- Explaining medical terminology
- Providing a room with adequate privacy
- Involving family and friends as requested by the patient

From Uphoff E, Wennekes L, Punt CJ, et al: Development of generic quality indicators for patient-centered cancer care by using a RAND Modified Delphi Method, *Cancer Nurs* 35(1):29-37, 2012.

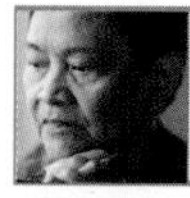

1. What action is required by the nurse before initiating Mrs. Thatcher's patient interview?

Different forms of communication can be used to obtain patient information. Open-ended questions encourage narrative responses from patients. Closed-ended, focused, or direct questions elicit specific information such as a patient's address or birth date. It is appropriate to use direct questions to gather information about a patient's past health history or during the review of body systems when a yes or no answer is adequate. Direct questions can be expanded on with open-ended questions if more extensive information is needed. Refer to Chapter 3 for an in-depth discussion on therapeutic communication techniques that are helpful during the patient interview.

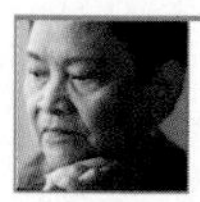

2. Identify four activities by the nurse that might communicate disinterest or the need to hurry through Mrs. Thatcher's examination.

HEALTH HISTORY

A patient's health history is collected through the interview process. The health history consists primarily of subjective data obtained from verbal interaction with the patient or

BOX 20-1 Framework for Collecting Health History Data

- *Demographic data:* Name, address, telephone numbers, stated age, birth date, birthplace, gender, marital status, race, cultural background or ethnic origin, spiritual or religious preference, educational level, occupation
- *Chief complaint or present illness:* Reason for seeking care, onset of symptoms
- *Allergies and sensitivities:* Medication, food (e.g., peanuts, eggs), environmental agents (e.g., latex, tape, detergents), reaction to reported allergens (e.g., rash, breathing difficulty, nausea and vomiting)
- *Medications, vitamins, and herbal supplements:* Prescriptions; over-the-counter medications and herbal remedies; dosage, frequency, and reason for use, including as-needed (PRN) medications
- *Immunizations:* Childhood and adult immunizations, date of last tuberculin skin test, date of last vaccines (e.g., flu, pneumonia, shingles)
- *Medical history:* Childhood illnesses, accidents, and injuries; serious or chronic illnesses; hospitalizations, including obstetric history for female patients; dates of occurrence; present treatments
- *Surgical history:* Type of surgery, date, any complications
- *Family history:* Age and health status of parents, grandparents, siblings, and children; age and cause of death of immediate family members; genetic diseases or traits, familial diseases (e.g., cardiovascular disease, high blood pressure, stroke, blood disorders, cancer, diabetes, kidney disease, seizure disorders, drug or alcohol dependencies, mental illness)
- *Social history:* Caffeine intake; use of tobacco, alcohol, or recreational drugs; environmental exposures; animal exposures and pets; living arrangement; safety concerns (e.g., intimate partner violence, emotional or physical abuse, recent domestic or foreign travel)
- *Cultural and spiritual or religious traditions:* Primary language, dietary restrictions, values and beliefs related to health care
- *Activities of daily living (ADLs):* Nutrition (e.g., meal preparation, shopping, typical 24-hour dietary intake), any recent changes in appetite, self-care activities (e.g., bathing, dressing, grooming, ambulation), use of prosthetics or mobility devices, leisure and exercise activities, sleep patterns (e.g., hours per night, naps, sleep aids)
- *Cognitive and emotional status:* Cognitive functioning (long-term and short-term memory), personal strengths, self-esteem, support system (e.g., family, friends, support groups, professional counseling)

family and objective data gathered through observation and review of past medical records. A significant amount of demographic data can be obtained from the electronic health record (EHR) before meeting the patient. The health history is organized to make essential patient data available for reference by all members of the health care team. During the last phase of the health history, the nurse conducts a review of systems before initiating a thorough physical assessment. There are several ways to organize health history and physical assessment data: by body systems, from head to toe, or by Gordon's Functional Health Patterns (Gordon, 2011). Refer to Chapter 6 for more information on data organization during assessment. Using a structured order for collecting data during the interview process facilitates completion of a thorough patient health history. Box 20-1 provides a framework for collecting health history data.

REVIEW OF SYSTEMS

Completion of a patient's health history through the interview process continues with a review of systems. The review of systems begins by having patients describe their general health status. The nurse then asks about current conditions or concerns related to each body system. Questions that can be asked to obtain a patient's general health information at the beginning of the review of systems are listed in the Health Assessment Questions box. Questions for each body system can be found in a box at the beginning of each physical examination section in this chapter.

HEALTH ASSESSMENT QUESTIONS

General Health Information

- How are you feeling?
- Do you have any general concerns about your health?
- Are you in pain? If so, where is the pain located? On a scale of 0 to 10 with 10 being the most severe pain, how do you rate your pain? What type of pain is it? How long have you had the pain? Does it radiate anywhere? Does anything relieve the pain or make it worse?
- How is your energy level? Are you fatigued with normal daily activities?
- Are you experiencing any significant life stresses at the present time?

PREPARATION FOR PHYSICAL ASSESSMENT LO 20.2

Before initiating a **physical assessment** (physical examination, or physical exam), the nurse needs to organize the environment and gather necessary equipment to enhance patient cooperation and attention throughout the examination. Too many interruptions or disorganization during the physical examination can lead to the collection of erroneous information, resulting in incomplete or insufficient data.

PHYSICAL ENVIRONMENT

Physical examination requires privacy, whether the exam is conducted in the patient's home setting, a hospital room, or a clinic. In the home, a physical exam is often performed in the patient's bedroom, while in clinics or hospitals, a ward or private room may serve as the assessment environment. Any room or setting needs to have adequate lighting for clear assessment of patient anatomy and physiologic features. The room should have a space where the patient can safely stand, sit, and lie down. Controlling room temperature, eliminating drafts, and providing warm blankets or towels help to ensure patient warmth and comfort.

Examination tables should be cleaned between patients with a bactericidal cleanser, and exam table paper or barrier surface material should be replaced. Since exam tables often are firm and unsupportive to back muscles and spinal curvature when the patient lies supine, the head of the table should be raised to a 30-degree angle and a small pillow offered for placement beneath the patient's head. If the patient is being examined in bed, the bed should be raised to allow the nurse easier access to the patient during the examination.

EQUIPMENT

The equipment used during the physical examination should be readily available and arranged in the order in which it will be used by the nurse. Medical asepsis is used in preparation of the equipment, and all devices are checked for proper function before the start of the exam. Hand hygiene is performed by the nurse before setup and as needed during the examination. Soiled equipment is discarded in the appropriate receptacle (if one-time-use or disposable devices) or placed in a designated container for recycling or decontamination according to facility policy.

Equipment should be warmed to a comfortable temperature for the patient. The head of the stethoscope may be rubbed between the palms of the hands before applying it to the patient's skin. See Box 20-2 for equipment used during the physical examination.

BOX 20-2 Equipment Used for Physical Examination

- Patient gown
- Scale
- Height assessment tool
- Sphygmomanometer with cuff
- Stethoscope with bell and diaphragm
- Thermometer
- Wristwatch
- Pulse oximeter
- Disposable pads and/or examination table paper
- Bath blanket or sheet
- Gloves
- Cotton applicators and/or cotton balls
- Eye chart
- Flashlight or penlight
- Otoscope and ophthalmoscope
- Tuning fork
- Tongue depressor
- Reflex hammer
- Tape measure or ruler
- Specimen containers, as needed

PATIENT PREPARATION

The patient's physical and emotional comfort and safety are top priorities for ensuring optimal cooperation and accuracy during the examination. The patient's identity should be verified. Patients should be given the opportunity to empty their bladder and bowels before the start of the examination. This facilitates a more thorough and comfortable abdominal exam for patients. If needed, proper collection of urine or fecal material is explained at this time, as well as disposal of any contaminated specimens. All specimen containers should be handled with gloves, wiped clean of debris, and properly labeled following collection and before sending the specimen to the laboratory.

Preparation of the patient for physical examination requires that the patient be properly dressed and covered to ensure privacy. Hospitalized patients can be dressed in gowns and covered with a sheet or bath blanket. In an outpatient setting, such as a clinic or health care provider's office, the patient will need to undress and wear a paper or light-cloth gown. If the examination involves only specific body systems, the patient may not have to undress entirely but may be asked to expose certain areas. In any case, allowing for privacy and an ample amount of time for undressing is necessary to reduce the embarrassment that can occur from walking into a room while the patient is in the process of disrobing. After donning appropriate attire, the patient may sit or lie on the examination surface with a cover or blanket draped discreetly over the lower torso or lap.

In addition to providing for physical needs, nurses must be sensitive to the emotional needs of patients. This may include the need for others to be present during a physical exam. It is entirely appropriate for a patient to request the presence of a third person (or chaperone) during a physical assessment. Former abuse or cultural norms, as well as the level of comfort felt by patients, are all factors that influence the desire for a support person to be present. Evaluation of the mental stability of patients, their potential for falling, and the use of protective equipment such as side rails can help to ensure the safety of patients throughout the physical examination process.

PRIVACY AND CONFIDENTIALITY

Patients' emotional and physical responses often depend on their level of comfort or anxiety about the physical assessment. Ideally, an examination room is soundproof or separated from other patients and staff in the vicinity. The patient should be reassured that confidentiality will be maintained throughout the examination and that data collected during the interview will be released only to providers or caregivers directly involved with the patient's care.

QSEN FOCUS!

Nurses must protect the confidentiality of protected information in EHRs.

Patients may ask to review their charts. When this happens, a written request from the patient may be required by the health care institution before a personal chart review. Patients are better able to understand their health records if a nurse or a primary care provider knowledgeable in health care documentation is present during the review to decipher medical terminology used to document health visits or conditions. The patient's written permission, with a witness's signature, is required for the release of the patient's health records to a third party, such as an insurance company or employer, unless the release is associated with a worker compensation claim. See the Ethical, Legal, and Professional Practice box for specific guidelines on sharing patient medical information.

ETHICAL, LEGAL, AND PROFESSIONAL PRACTICE

Nurses who are conducting patient physicals need to be aware of the following guidelines for sharing medical information:

- Patients are permitted to review their personal medical records.
  - This is one of many reasons that documentation should always be factual and nonjudgmental in nature.
  - Patients' review of their records should take place in the presence of the primary care provider to ensure accurate interpretation of the documentation.
- Family members may review the patient's medical records only with the written consent of the patient.
- Primary care providers are permitted to share patient medical information with specialists to whom the patient is referred without additional consent.
- Health care facilities require that patients sign a release form when requesting copies of their medical records or diagnostic test records.
- Nurses must respect the right of patients to know with whom their medical information can be legally shared.

From U.S. Department of Health and Human Services. Retrieved from *www.hhs.gov/ocr/privacy/hipaa/understanding/consumers/index.html*.

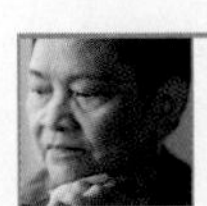

3. List three or more physical considerations that the nurse should address before having Mrs. Thatcher enter the exam room.

POSITIONING THE PATIENT

The ability to assume the positions required for physical assessment depends on the patient's level of mobility, physical strength, and **comorbid** conditions (i.e., two or more medical conditions existing simultaneously). Age and level of cognitive ability can be an issue when the patient is expected to follow directions for position changes. For example, a child often requires an adult's assistance when changing clothes. An older patient with arthritis or limited joint mobility also may need help and extra time for clothing and position changes. Small children, infants, and older patients should never be left unattended in an examination room or on an examination table. Likewise, confused, uncooperative, combative patients or those who are physically or chemically restrained should never be left unsupervised during examination because of the potential for falls or injury from medical equipment.

To limit the patient's time and energy spent in changing positions, a sequential organization of steps for the examination is helpful. All techniques requiring a sitting position are done at the same time, followed by techniques requiring a supine position, until the physical examination is complete. At times, it may be necessary to have the patient return to a position that was previously examined to verify a result. In such instances, explain to the patient the reason for verifying that portion of the exam and assist the patient to the position needed. Table 20-1 illustrates specific positions used during physical examination. Attention to draping provides for exposing only the area being examined.

INTEGRATION OF ASSESSMENT SKILLS WITH NURSING ACTIVITIES

A complete physical examination requires systematic assessment of each body system. However, the patient's **chief complaint** (presenting problem) or **clinical manifestations** (signs and symptoms) or the timing of the exam may require a **focused assessment**, in which only specific, relevant areas are examined. A patient with an acute problem, such as a cut or wound, who is otherwise healthy may not require a full physical examination; assessment of only the affected area may be appropriate. Typically, when a patient is admitted to the hospital or enters the health care system for the first time, a complete physical examination is performed. Nurses assess patients already hospitalized at least once per shift.

A patient undergoing an annual physical for preventive care is evaluated on the basis of the patient's age or health risk. General health promotion information, such as nutritional recommendations, optimal weight maintenance, and abstinence from at-risk behaviors such as smoking and excessive alcohol use, should be shared during all patient visits, even when a complete physical examination is not indicated. Nurses who routinely conduct annual physical exams should

TABLE 20-1 Physical Examination Positions

POSITION	USES AND POTENTIAL CONCERNS
Supine position	To examine the head and neck, anterior thorax and lungs, breasts, axillae, heart, abdomen, extremities, and pulses Relaxed position; easy access to critical anatomy Patient may become short of breath; this position is difficult for a patient who has back pain or kyphosis of the spine
Dorsal recumbent position	To examine the head and neck, anterior thorax and lungs, breasts, axillae, heart, and abdomen Promotes relaxation of abdominal muscles and removes pressure from the lower spine Patients with weak lower extremities and knees will find this position challenging
Fowler position	To examine the head and neck, anterior thorax and lungs, breasts, axillae, heart, abdomen, lower extremities, and pulses Comfortable position for patients who are short of breath; most relaxing position Difficult to assess the abdomen owing to shortened space
Lithotomy position	To examine the female genitalia Provides maximal exposure of genitalia and facilitates the progress of speculum examination Uncomfortable and embarrassing position; minimize patient's time in lithotomy position
Prone position	To examine the back, spine, posterior aspect of the head, neck, thorax, buttocks, and lower extremities Promotes airflow and facilitates assessment of skin and lungs Uncomfortable for large-breasted women; excessive pressure on neck and spine
Sims position	To examine the rectal and perineal areas Left side-lying flexion of the right hip and knee improves exposure of rectal anatomy Not tolerated well by patients with shortness of breath or other breathing difficulty
Knee-chest position	Provides maximal exposure of rectal area Uncomfortable; many patients will not be able to assume this position owing to physical limitations

be knowledgeable about current seasonal and scheduled immunizations and preventive health screening information based on government research guidelines that help to define standards of care.

Nursing skills for physical assessment require a well-organized approach so that important details are not overlooked. A head-to-toe technique is systematic and includes all body systems, allowing the nurse and the patient to anticipate the next system to be examined. A systematic examination method allows continuity between providers that, in turn, helps to ensure consistency in examination outcomes.

ASSESSMENT TECHNIQUES LO 20.3

The four assessment techniques used to complete a comprehensive physical examination are inspection, palpation, percussion, and auscultation. Hand hygiene is a standard precaution before, during, and after performing a physical examination. Clean gloves should be readily available for use by the nurse at various stages of the assessment. Appropriate personal protective equipment (PPE) should be worn as needed. See Chapter 26 for detailed instructions on donning gowns, masks, and sterile gloves.

INSPECTION

Inspection involves the use of vision and smell to closely scrutinize physical characteristics of a whole person and individual body systems. Distinguishing between normal and abnormal findings for patients of different age groups begins the moment the nurse first observes and meets the individual and continues throughout the examination.

Begin an assessment by observing a patient's ability to ambulate. Then conduct the examination of individual body systems, using each person as his or her own control. Symmetry should be assessed by comparing the right and left sides of the body. The human body is usually anatomically symmetric, so observing for abnormalities on either side is vitally important to noting anatomic deviations.

The quality of the inspection phase of physical examination depends on several variables, including (1) the nurse's ability to identify normal variations among patients, (2) good lighting, with adequate exposure of anatomic surfaces, and (3) the time allotted for attention to detail. After inspection, further examination is performed using palpation. In many instances, palpation is done at the same time as inspection or shortly afterward.

PALPATION

Palpation uses touch to assess body organs and skin texture, temperature, moisture, **turgor** (tension due to fluid content), tenderness, and thickness. **Consistency** measures organ location and size against the expected anatomic norm, any distention or masses, and vibration or pulsation associated with movement. Palpation can be used to affirm details observed during inspection. Rigidity, **crepitation (crepitus)** (crackling or rubbing), and the presence of lumps can be detected through palpation. Ask the patient to describe areas that are sensitive or painful, and note any nonverbal signs of distress or discomfort the patient may express, such as **guarding** (positioning to prevent movement of a painful body part) or **rebound tenderness** (discomfort experienced after stimulation is discontinued). During palpation, the patient should be relaxed and comfortable. Muscle tension during palpation may be misinterpreted by the nurse. Palpation is performed immediately after inspection, except during assessment of the gastrointestinal system. Palpation and percussion of the abdomen are delayed until after inspection and auscultation to prevent false assessment findings secondary to stimulation of the bowel.

Various parts of the hand are best suited for assessing different anatomic areas. The fingertips are used for fine tactile discrimination of texture, vibration, or pulsations. The palmar surface of the fingers and finger pads, the most sensitive parts of the hand, are used to determine the position, size, consistency, and shape of an organ or mass and its surrounding structures. The back, or dorsal, surface of the hand is best for determining temperature because the skin is thinner than that on the palms.

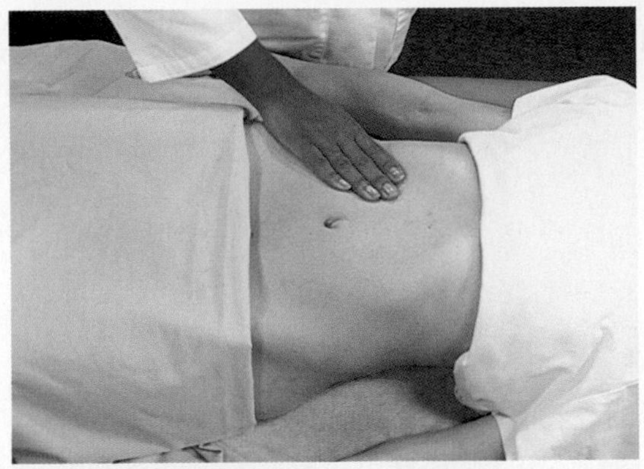

FIGURE 20-1 Light palpation. (From Ball JW, Dains JE, Flynn JA, et al: *Seidel's guide to physical examination*, ed. 8, St. Louis, 2015, Mosby.)

Palpation should be completed in a relaxed, gentle, and systematic way, with tender areas palpated last. The nurse should have warm hands and short fingernails; hands can be warmed by rubbing them together or holding them under warm water. Begin with light palpation, depressing the area approximately 1 cm (½ inch). Intermittent pressure is applied for brief intervals during light palpation, using the fingertips of three to four fingers held together (Figure 20-1).

After light palpation, deep palpation is used to examine organ structures. Deep palpation typically is performed by an advanced practice nurse or a physician. The area being examined is depressed approximately 4 cm (2 inches), using one hand to identify organ location and consistency. Caution is exercised to avoid injury to the patient during deep palpation. When using two hands, or bimanual deep palpation, the nurse places one hand lightly over the area to be examined, and the top hand is used to apply pressure to the hand closest to the skin (Figure 20-2).

When performing palpation, the nurse must consider the body area being palpated, the reason for palpation, and the patient's condition. For example, palpation should not be performed on an enlarged thyroid gland or neck mass. In this instance, palpation or rubbing the area may release excessive thyroid hormone or cause pain. Palpation over major arteries or vascular structures is contraindicated as it may obstruct blood flow, causing damage or dysfunction to the area and surrounding tissues.

PERCUSSION

Percussion is an advanced practice examination technique used to assess body tissues and structures. **Percussion** involves tapping the patient's skin with short, sharp strokes that cause a vibration to travel through the skin and to the upper layers of the underlying structures (Figure 20-3). Vibration is reflected by the tissues, and the character of the sound heard

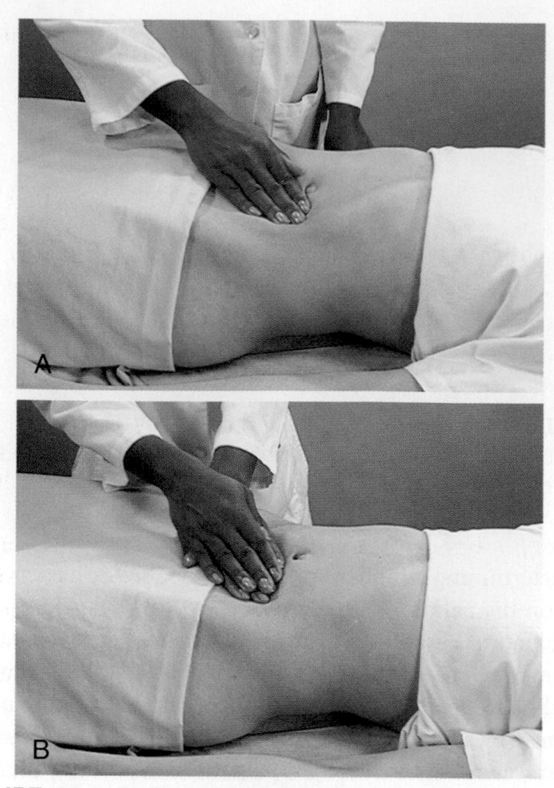

FIGURE 20-2 **A,** Deep palpation. **B,** Deep bimanual palpation. (From Ball JW, Dains JE, Flynn JA, et al: *Seidel's guide to physical examination*, ed. 8, St. Louis, 2015, Mosby.)

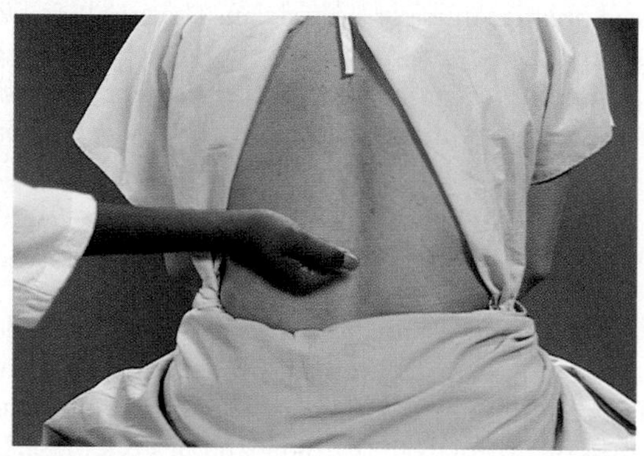

FIGURE 20-3 Percussion can help to identify the outline of organs and the possible presence of masses. (From Ball JW, Dains JE, Flynn JA, et al: *Seidel's guide to physical examination*, ed. 8, St. Louis, 2015, Mosby.)

depends on the density of the structures that reflect the sound. Knowing how the various densities reflect or absorb sound helps the advanced practice nurse to locate or approximate the size, shape, and borders of organs, masses, and fluid. An abnormal sound implies that an organ or area is possibly compromised with another substance, such as air, blood, or other bodily fluids. Percussion requires dexterity and practice for useful data to be obtained.

AUSCULTATION

Auscultation is the technique of listening to sounds made by body organs or systems such as the heart, blood vessels, lungs, and abdominal cavity, with and without the assistance of a stethoscope. Some sounds, such as stridor, wheezing, or congestion, may be heard by the naked ear. The characteristics of auscultated sounds are dependent on the body tissue or organ being assessed. Sounds are typically documented according to their duration, frequency, intensity, and quality. A stethoscope is required to hear more distant sounds.

It is important for the nurse to be able to recognize normal body sounds. This knowledge will contribute to the nurse's ability to identify abnormalities as well as areas within the body that typically remain silent. To auscultate correctly, the nurse needs intact hearing, an adequate stethoscope, and an understanding of how to use a stethoscope.

A stethoscope typically has two different heads, a diaphragm and a bell. The diaphragm is flat and is used to hear high-pitched sounds, such as breath sounds, bowel sounds, and normal heart sounds. The bell is a concave, cuplike shape used for assessing soft, low-pitched sounds, such as extra or distant heart sounds and murmurs. Both are held directly on the patient's skin to ensure contact and prevent auditory interference. Before contact with the patient's skin, the stethoscope head can be warmed by rubbing it between the nurse's hands. Practicing auscultation with a stethoscope will help establish good technique, to avoid auditory interference from inadvertent movement of the tubing or rubbing of the diaphragm or bell head against the body's surface, clothing, or other fabric.

During auscultation, difficulty hearing sounds may be due to extraneous noise in the room or poor skin contact with the head of the stethoscope. The nurse may need to ask patients or visitors to refrain from talking and may need to turn down audio on televisions or radios during auscultation. Special amplified stethoscopes are available for purchase by nurses with hearing limitations.

Auscultation normally is the last step in physical assessment for all body systems except the abdomen. When examining the abdomen, the nurse performs auscultation before palpation to prevent stimulation of bowel sounds that may cause hyperactivity, leading to false assessment findings. Stethoscopes should be cleaned between patients to help prevent the spread of nosocomial infections.

GENERAL SURVEY LO 20.4

The general survey is the visual assessment and evaluation of the whole patient. It covers the patient's primary reason for seeking care and current health status, as well as any obvious deviations from normal. The general survey expands on findings recorded in the patient's health history and includes initial observations. The nurse begins a general survey by noting the patient's overall appearance and behavior and then observes hygiene, body image, affect and mood, gait, speech, and developmental status. The general survey compares patients with typical characteristics associated with accepted cultural, societal, and behavioral norms. Observing significant cultural norms is critical to providing culturally competent care during physical assessment. See the Diversity Considerations box for special considerations related to the examination process.

AGE

Patients should appear to be their stated age. If they do not, because of premature aging, sun exposure, or tobacco use, the phrase "appears older/younger than stated age" may be used in documentation. Chronologic age determines which screening exams and general health maintenance activities are recommended for patients to prevent illness and promote healthy lifestyle choices.

RACE

Physical features, such as skin color or pigmentation, hair texture, and stature, related to genetic background are noted. Certain conditions are more prevalent among people of specific races, such as hypertension in people of African and Mediterranean descent and skin cancer in people of Northern European backgrounds.

SEX AND GENDER ORIENTATION

The patient's sex is noted as well as gender orientation, when relevant. Some conditions are specific to or more prevalent in one sex. Certain conditions specific to the anatomy and physiology of the female and male genitalia are explored through physical examination, discussed later in the chapter.

CLOTHING

Many factors affect how a patient dresses. Personal preferences are based on culture, lifestyle, and socioeconomic level, as well as age and activity level. Note whether the patient's clothing is appropriate to the climate and current weather conditions, looks clean, and fits the body. Infants and older adults often wear several layers of clothing to preserve body temperature and may have clothing with Velcro or large-button closures due to issues with dexterity. If a patient appears unkempt or inappropriately dressed for the season or circumstance (e.g., wearing undergarments on top of outerwear), this should be documented. It may be a manifestation of an underlying medical condition such as cognitive impairment or dementia or a psychiatric–mental health disorder.

DIVERSITY CONSIDERATIONS

Life Span

- A parent or guardian should be present during the assessment of an infant, child, or adolescent minor. The adult should be able to verify subjective data shared by the school-age child or adolescent. If abuse is suspected, ask the adult to step out of the room before an in-depth interview or further investigation.
- Assistance is required to safely assess an infant or small child. This is also true for individuals with special physical or psychological needs and for elderly patients who have limited dexterity and mobility.

Gender

- Honor a patient's request to have a nurse or care provider of a certain gender. Even though many elderly women have male physicians, they may prefer to have a female nurse, which they view as traditional.
- Ask patients if they would prefer to have an additional person in the room during the physical examination. If so, invite a professional colleague to stay in the examination room for support. Be sure to provide for the patient's privacy regardless of who is present during the examination.

Culture

- Provide interpretation for patients whose native language is different from that of the health care environment.
- A person's economic and educational levels can impact the person's appearance and ability to interact within the health care system. Be sure to assess these factors and avoid judgmental attitudes or actions when interacting with all patients.
- If unfamiliar with the customs of a patient's cultural background, ask about personal patient preferences that would allay the patient's fears and enhance the examination experience.

Morphology

- Patients who are morbidly obese need to be assessed by using special equipment, including large blood pressure cuffs and adapted scales to ensure accuracy. Make sure the appropriate equipment is assembled before initiating the physical examination, to limit potential embarrassment to the patient.
- During the annual physical, provide a referral to local programs, if available, that focus on exercise, nutrition, and emotional support for obese children and their families.
- Refer patients who exhibit signs of anorexia nervosa or bulimia to programs and health care providers specializing in treatment of these conditions. Early nutritional and emotional intervention is critical to behavior modification.

HYGIENE AND GROOMING

Note whether patients appear clean and appropriately groomed for their age, occupation, socioeconomic level, or activity immediately before seeking care. Note the appearance of nails, skin, and hair. If the patient is a female, note whether her makeup is appropriate for her age and culture. Notice the condition of facial hair on male patients. Unpleasant body odors are evaluated to determine whether they are caused by physical activity or exercise, poor hygiene, or specific disease states. Be sensitive to religious or cultural beliefs about bathing that may have an impact on the perceived hygienic condition.

AFFECT AND MOOD

A patient's affect can be observed or assessed through various displays of emotion. The nurse should note whether a patient's verbal and nonverbal communication is congruent. Observations should include whether the patient's mood is appropriate to the situation, with specific attention to the patient's facial expressions during data collection.

In most situations, the patient's level of distress or comfort is obvious in the form of clinical manifestations or behavior. For example, symptoms of pain or discomfort can be indicated through facial grimacing, splinting the painful area, or displaying a flat affect, as in some cases of emotional pain. Cultural norms related to the appropriate expression of emotion must be taken into account. In some cultures, extremely dramatic behavior is accepted as normal, and free verbalization or display of emotion is expected, whereas in others, stoic behavior in times of pain or crisis is promoted. Detection of symptoms that cause a change in mental status or are potentially life-threatening is a high priority in the examination.

SAFETY

Issues of patient safety fall into three general categories: (1) use of assistive devices or equipment, such as walkers, scooters, hearing aids, or eyeglasses; (2) environmental safety; and (3) personal safety and security. The nurse should observe and ask patients about the use of assistive devices. If patients use any assistive equipment, such as walkers or canes, they should be able to demonstrate the proper technique for use of the devices. Lack of attention to maintaining assistive equipment in working order, such as not replacing batteries for hearing aids or improperly fitting prostheses, may be a sign of busyness, neglect, economic hardship, or mental health alterations, which require follow-up evaluation by the nurse.

Some environmental concerns about which patients should be asked are living conditions, air quality at home and work, the presence of stairs or rugs, and means of transportation. These are especially important issues for the chronically ill, infants, children, and elderly people. Overcrowded living conditions predispose people to communicable diseases, and smoke from air pollution or cigarettes and cigars increases the affected person's susceptibility to an asthma attack and diseases such as lung cancer. Presence of rugs and stairs, especially in the home, can affect the ability to ambulate safely and are of particular concern when patients are prone to dizziness or are unable to walk without using assistive devices or dragging their feet. Depending on the patient's age and physical condition, driving safety should be evaluated. The use of public transportation or assistance from a family member or friend for transportation to reach appointments should be noted to facilitate planning clinic visits accordingly. To address personal safety, the nurse is required to ask patients directly if they feel safe in their living environment. Questions related to personal safety are asked when the patient and nurse are in a totally private setting to promote honesty and protection from potentially abusive family or friends. Observe for signs of withdrawal or hesitation when patients are answering. The prevalence of domestic violence and emotional abuse makes it imperative that nurse-patient interactions include concern for this critical aspect of patient safety.

Providing for patient safety in each category may require that the nurse complete an extensive community assessment, which is discussed in Chapter 23. All nurses who discharge patients for home care should become familiar with community resources available to patients and their families. See the Home Care Considerations box for aspects of a community that affect the ability of patients of all ages to live in their own homes while undergoing medical treatment and nursing care.

HOME CARE CONSIDERATIONS

Community Resources

Government and Community Resources

- Transportation
- Schools and tutoring services
- Library resources
- Fire and safety resources
- Economic resources
- Recreation

Social Service Agencies

- Meal preparation and delivery
- Utility assistance
- Day care facilities for all age groups
- Cleaning and home maintenance assistance

Public and Home Health Services

- Immunizations
- Environmental surveillance
- Medical equipment
- Medication delivery

ALCOHOL, TOBACCO, OR RECREATIONAL DRUG USE

Ask patients about their level of alcohol, tobacco, and recreational drug use. Inquire in a nonjudgmental manner so that the impact of these substances on the patient's health and lifestyle can be accurately determined. Knowing a patient's level of alcohol, tobacco, or drug use will assist in planning health promotion activities and avoid unanticipated complications with anesthesia if the patient is scheduled for surgery.

SPEECH

Speech patterns typically are assessed by their rate, clarity, tone, and volume. Normal speech is understandable, neither rapid nor too slow and loud enough to be heard without excessive volume. Difficulty with articulation may indicate neurologic impairment. The pace of conversation should be moderate, with a steady stream of talking that is fluent. Word choice should be effortless and appropriate to a person's age and educational level, with older children and adults speaking in complete sentences, including occasional pauses for thought. Note when a patient is multilingual. Remember that speech patterns of foreign patients may vary.

Listen for patients who are speaking too rapidly or slowly. Patients whose lips are moving without speech, talking to themselves, or whispering to real or imagined people or objects may be demonstrating signs of emotional or mental disturbances. Speech impediments can be warning signals of impaired emotions or neurologic damage.

GAIT

Observe patients when they are walking into the exam room or at the bedside (if they are ambulatory). Erect body posture with a straight spine, freely swinging arms, and slightly rounded shoulders is normal. If the patient is slumped over, limping, or holding a certain part of the body, this should be noted. Ambulation should be smooth, purposeful, and well balanced. Observe the patient for asymmetric steps or hesitant forward motion of one or both feet with movements that are coordinated or uncoordinated. Note tremors, shuffling, limping, and cogwheel movement of the limbs or gait as abnormal findings.

VITAL SIGN ASSESSMENT

Vital sign assessment is conducted at the beginning of the physical examination. The findings serve as a baseline for future assessments to determine the patient's status. Vital sign measurements include temperature, pulse, respirations, blood pressure, and pain level. Refer to Chapter 19 for in-depth information on determination of vital signs.

HEIGHT AND WEIGHT

Assessment of height and weight is helpful in screening for overall changes in health status. A person's weight will vary daily and throughout each day, depending on food intake and fluid retention or loss. Weight gain or loss can be intentional or unintentional. Height is most often affected by normal growth, aging, or degenerative diseases such as osteoporosis. A patient's baseline height and weight are used to determine medication dosages and to properly size antiembolitic stockings, splints, and other assistive devices such as crutches.

Height and weight are measured throughout the person's life span. Head circumference is measured for infants and children up to age 3. The findings are compared with standardized clinical growth charts to determine the percentile into which the child falls relative to physical development. The clinical growth charts are available at *www.cdc.gov/growthcharts/clinical_charts.htm.*

To accurately evaluate trends in weight, it is important to weigh patients at the same time of day, on the same calibrated scale, and in clothes similar or identical to the ones worn when the previous weight was taken. Accuracy of weight can be the deciding factor in many instances of care, including changes in treatment decisions or admission to an acute care facility. Standing scales, bed scales, platform scales, and chair scales are available for weight measurement in most clinic or hospital settings. Scales should be properly calibrated to zero with sheets or other objects, such as diapers, that will be weighed with the patient. Attention to patient transfers is critical to prevent falls or injury to the provider or patient. More than one care provider should be used in any instance of uncertainty about a safe transfer of the patient to the measurement device.

Measure height vertically by using the post attached to a standing scale or horizontally with a measuring tape for infants, children, or adults lying in a supine position. A complete listing of healthy height and weight assessments for adults, children, and infants can be found at the CDC website, *www.cdc.gov/healthyweight/assessing/index.html.*

PHYSICAL EXAMINATION LO 20.5

Examination of each body system should progress in an organized fashion. Typically, this is achieved by starting with skin assessment and proceeding head to toe. Clinical judgment is used by the nurse to determine how extensive a physical exam needs to be on the basis of the patient's condition, timing, and the location of the interaction.

SKIN, HAIR, AND NAILS

The integumentary system is made up of the skin, hair, scalp, and nails. As the largest organ of the body, the skin helps to regulate body temperature, sense stimuli, and protect underlying structures. Figure 20-4 illustrates the three skin layers,

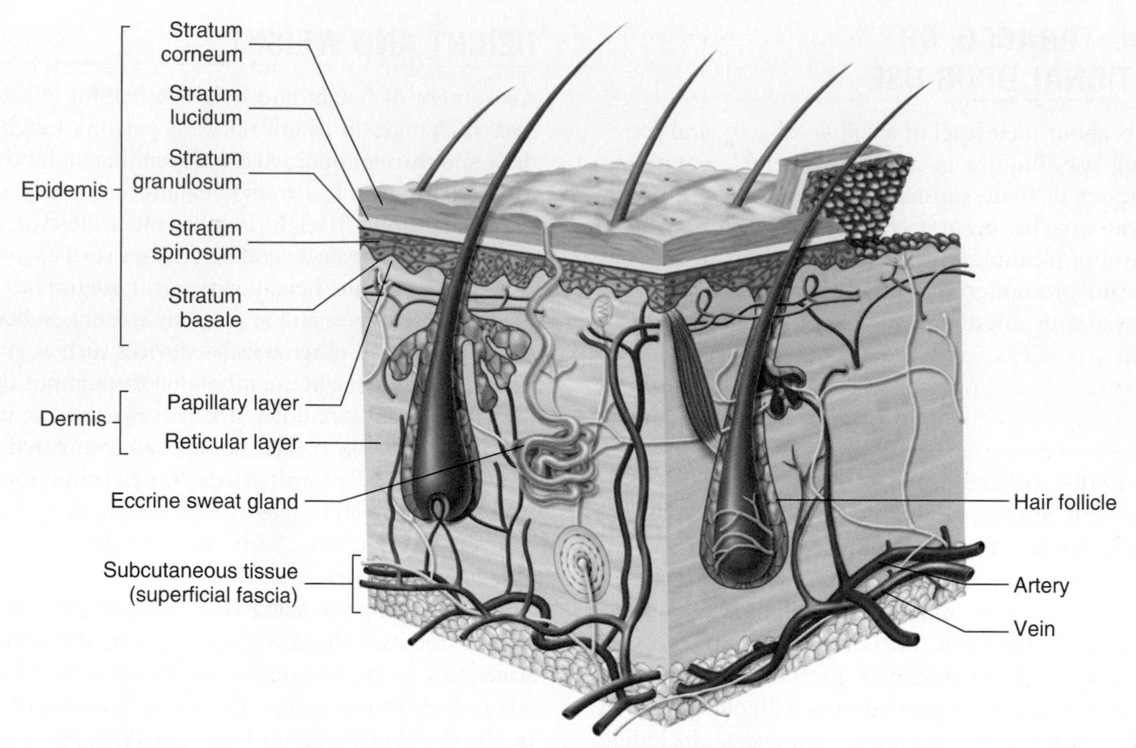

FIGURE 20-4 Cross section of skin layers. (From Ball JW, Danis JE, Flynn JA, et al: *Seidel's guide to physical examination,* ed. 8, St. Louis, 2015, Mosby.)

nerve endings, and blood supply. The condition of the skin is a reflection of overall well-being. Nutritional, metabolic, and hydration status are evident during skin assessment, as is a person's oxygenation and circulatory condition. Skin appearance may also indicate a person's emotional state, reaction to medications, and daily work or leisure activities.

Examination of various parts of the integumentary system begins with inspection of the entire skin surface. The Health Assessment Questions box provides skin assessment questions to assist with completing a thorough nursing history. Collection of subjective data can take place both before and during visual inspection. The technique of palpation is performed after inspection, with special care taken in patients who bruise easily, have open skin lesions, or have painful skin surfaces.

Natural light is best for assessing skin color in all patients and is especially preferred for inspecting dark skin. An overly warm room can lead to superficial dilation of the skin, causing increased redness and sweating, whereas an overly cool room can induce vasoconstriction, causing the patient to appear pale or cyanotic. Clean, disposable gloves should be worn for palpation to inspect skin folds or for protection if the patient

HEALTH ASSESSMENT QUESTIONS

Skin, Hair, and Nails

- Have you observed any noticeable changes in the consistency, color, or texture of your skin, hair, or nails recently? Is your skin normally dry, oily, or a combination of both?
- Has anyone in your family ever had skin cancer? Do you have any birthmarks, moles, or tattoos? Have any of them changed in color, size, or shape?
- List any allergic skin reactions you have ever had to food, drugs, plants, or other daily encountered substances.
- Do you have any problems with perspiration, malodorous skin in the absence of perspiration, or itching?
- How much sun or tanning-bed exposure do you have in the average week? What type of sun protection do you use, and how often?
- In your daily activities or occupation, is your skin exposed to chemicals, excessive temperatures, petroleum, bleach, or caustic cleaning products?
- Describe your normal hair texture. How often do you wash your hair? What types of grooming products do you typically use, and how often? Do you ever use chemicals on your hair?
- Have you noticed any generalized hair loss, bald spots, or loss of hair in a specific location? Have you noticed any lumps or painful areas around hair follicles?
- Have you experienced recent changes in your diet or appetite?
- Have you recently undergone chemotherapy or radiation treatment? Are you on any new medications that may cause hair loss or growth?
- Do you have a familial history of male pattern baldness? If so, at what age did it begin?
- Describe any changes you have had in the appearance or condition of your nails.
- Do any skin, hair, or nail problems limit your normal activities?

has any open wounds or unusual skin lesions. Visualizing the entire skin surface and palpating skin folds or lesions ensures a thorough skin assessment.

Skin Inspection

The major portion of the skin assessment can be conducted while the patient is sitting on an examination table or bed. To properly inspect the skin of the buttocks and dorsal aspects of the legs or lower torso, the nurse can ask the patient to stand or can position the patient on the side or abdomen. During skin assessment, privacy is maintained by exposing only the body part being examined. If abnormalities are noticed during inspection, the involved areas should be palpated. A mental note should be made of the distribution and symmetry of hair, skin coloring, markings, and lesions. Observations of each part of the body are precisely documented, including pressure areas, skin breakdown, skin odors, unusual position of leg folds, condition of axillae skin and the area under the breasts, and any lesions or incision sites. For patients at risk for development of pressure ulcers, the Braden scale is used by nurses and other health care professionals to reliably score the potential for this complication. Refer to Chapter 29 for the complete Braden scale.

Skin Color Alterations

The amount of pigment in skin determines its color intensity and hue. Small amounts of melanin are common in whiter skin, whereas larger amounts of melanin result in darker or olive-hued skin tones. Carotene is responsible for yellow-tinted skin tones. Exposed skin on the hands, neck, face, and lower legs usually has darker pigmentation than areas less exposed to the sun and elements, such as skin on the abdomen and genitalia. Normal skin pigmentation varies in tone, depending on the location of the skin and on age, culture, and ethnicity.

Each person's skin color has fairly uniform characteristics of tone and shading. Normal skin color variations include ivory or light pink, ruddy to light tan, light to dark black, and bronze or olive tone. In older patients, skin color tends to be uneven owing to varying pigmentation or more pronounced birthmarks.

Abnormalities in skin color are most easily identified in areas where **pallor** (lack of color, paleness) can be most readily observed, such as the oral mucosa, nail beds, palms of the hands, and conjunctiva of the eye. It is more difficult to detect skin color changes and rashes in patients with dark or olive-toned skin. Skin located in skin folds and creases is darker than skin at other areas of the body in people with darker skin tones. Several common skin alterations should be looked for during inspection.

Absence of Pigment

Albinism is a congenital loss of pigmentation characterized by a generalized lack of melanin pigment in the eyes, skin, and hair or, in rare instances, in the eyes alone. It is a hereditary trait that causes the affected person to have pale skin, pinkish eyes, and almost white hair from birth.

Cyanosis

Cyanosis is a blue discoloration of the skin, nail beds, or mucous membranes that results from vasoconstriction or deoxygenated hemoglobin in blood vessels near the skin's surface. Central cyanosis is often due to cardiac or respiratory conditions that lead to poor blood oxygenation. Peripheral cyanosis, causing blue discoloration in the fingers or extremities, is most often due to local vasoconstriction or inadequate peripheral circulation. All factors contributing to central cyanosis also can lead to peripheral symptoms; however, peripheral cyanosis is most often observed in the absence of heart or lung conditions, such as exposure to cold for an extended period of time.

Erythema and Purpura

Erythema is redness of the skin caused by congestion or dilation of the superficial blood vessels in the skin, signaling circulatory changes to an area. It can occur with any skin injury, sunburn, infection, fever, or inflammation and disappears when pressure is applied. A temperature elevation may accompany erythema if the redness is associated with dilation of blood vessels in the deeper layers of the skin. Erythema is not easily detected in dark-skinned people but may be present in an area of the skin that is edematous (swollen) or warmer than the surrounding skin. **Purpura** (bleeding underneath the skin) and red pigmentation that does not blanch with pressure are nonspecific signs. Purpura may indicate vascular, coagulation, or platelet disorders.

Jaundice

Jaundice is a yellow hue to the skin, mucous membranes, or eyes seen in both light- and dark-skinned people. The yellow pigment results from excess bilirubin, a by-product of red blood cell destruction, or liver failure. The best site for evaluation of the patient for jaundice is the sclera or, in darker-skinned people, the hard palate.

Pallor

Pallor, a pale or lightened skin tone, usually is uniformly disseminated throughout the skin surface. Pallor can be caused by illness, emotional shock or stress, decreased exposure to sunlight, or anemia or may be a genetic trait. It is most evident on the face, nail beds, lips, and palms. Pallor can develop suddenly or gradually, depending on the cause. Localized pallor usually is not clinically significant unless it is accompanied by general pallor that is not typical of the patient's normal skin tone. It should be noted as unique from conditions such as vitiligo.

Vitiligo

Vitiligo is a loss of skin pigment. It is thought to result from an autoimmune response. Patches of depigmented skin most often are noted on the hands, face, and genital areas. Although vitiligo may occur in people of all skin types, it is most noticeable in dark-skinned people.

Skin Lesions

Benign, age-related skin conditions include age spots, skin tags, cherry angiomas (ruby red, often slightly raised papules), keratosis (thickened patches of skin), warts, and freckles. Inspection and palpation evaluates for lesions or disruptions in continuity of the skin. Skin lesions appear in a variety of shapes, sizes, and colors. When a lesion is identified, it is inspected for size, shape, color, location, and distribution. Measure skin lesions with a clear, flexible ruler, documenting the breadth, circumference, and height, as appropriate. Measure a lesion's depth if it extends below the skin's surface. Any type of exudate associated with a lesion is documented in terms of color, approximate amount of drainage, consistency, and odor. Pressure ulcers that develop as a consequence of poor circulation, inactivity, infection, or traumatic injury require extensive assessment and treatment, which is discussed in Chapter 29, in the context of wound care.

Skin lesions are classified as primary lesions (arising from normal skin) or secondary lesions (resulting from changes in primary lesions due to scratching, trauma, infection, or the healing process). Primary skin lesions include **petechiae** (tiny, dark red spots that indicate hemorrhage under the skin), warts, psoriasis, poison ivy, or insect bites. Examples of secondary lesions are pressure ulcers, scars, and wound dehiscence. Table 20-2 presents a review of skin lesions, with illustrations, as they appear both above and below the skin's surface.

Skin Malignancies

Inspection of the skin is a key component for early detection of abnormalities and malignancy of the integumentary system. When detected and treated early, many skin cancers are highly curable. Research indicates that indoor tanning increases a person's risk for the most deadly form of skin cancer, melanoma, by 75% (American Academy of Dermatology, 2014). Nurses are responsible for screening exams and preventive education that helps protect patients from risk factors associated with skin cancer. Encourage patients to inspect their own skin regularly for lesions that are growing, changing shape, bleeding, or itching (American Academy of Dermatology, 2014). Types of skin cancer with perceptible changes on inspection during screening include basal cell carcinoma, squamous cell carcinoma, and melanoma (Table 20-3). The American Cancer Society and American Academy of Dermatology have established a mnemonic, ABCDE, to aid in screening for melanoma, which is presented in Table 20-4.

> **! SAFE PRACTICE ALERT**
>
> Early detection of melanoma is essential to prevent or limit metastasis to other areas of the body. Once a melanoma lesion elevates or ulcerates below the skin, metastasis is more likely to have begun.

Palpation

Palpation is performed to assess the patient's skin for texture, warmth, turgor, edema, and moisture. Palpation can be used to corroborate suspicious results noted during inspection. Gloves are worn during palpation when potentially infectious or contagious exudate may be present on the skin that that may not be visible during inspection. Palpation helps to identify the characteristics of lesions with consideration to the contour (flat, raised, or sunken), stability, and consistency (soft or firm). Use gentle pressure to palpate both over and around the lesion. Gently assess areas of tenderness, noting the extent of any discomfort.

Texture

Skin texture is palpated using two or three fingertips. Patient skin can be described as soft, supple or firm, smooth or rough, and thin or thick. Skin typically is thicker on the palms of the hands and the soles of the feet. Age and environmental exposure are contributing factors to skin consistency. In older patients, skin becomes thinner, wrinkled, and more prone to variations in temperature because of reduced collagen, muscle tone, subcutaneous fat, and sweat glands. People repeatedly exposed to extreme environmental elements such as the sun or extreme cold tend to have thicker, more leathery, wrinkled skin with numerous freckles or moles. Skin texture may be altered because of underlying disease or illness.

Temperature

Skin temperature is dependent on the amount of blood circulating through the dermis. Temperature is assessed by palpating the skin with the back of the hand, and it is compared symmetrically on each body area. Skin temperature should be uniform throughout the body, with minor variations from one area to another. Environment often determines the temperature and appearance of the skin. In warmer environments, blood vessels close to the skin dilate, producing a flushed or reddened appearance, whereas in cooler environments, constricted blood vessels shunt blood away from the skin surface, causing it to be pale and cool to touch. Detailed assessment is always performed on patients at risk for impaired circulation. Areas of redness often are warmer owing to increased blood flow. Palpation is especially critical to determine the level of circulation distal to injuries or immobilized areas.

Turgor

Turgor describes the skin's elasticity or ability to resist deformity after being displaced. Skin turgor is assessed by grasping a fold of skin (½ to 1 inch in thickness) on the back of the forearm or over the sternum along the second or third

TABLE 20-2 Primary Skin Lesions

DESCRIPTION	EXAMPLES	SKIN CUTAWAY	ACTUAL CASE
Macule/Patch Flat, not detectable with palpation Changes in color Size <1 cm >1-cm macule: called a *patch*	Port wine stain Flat moles	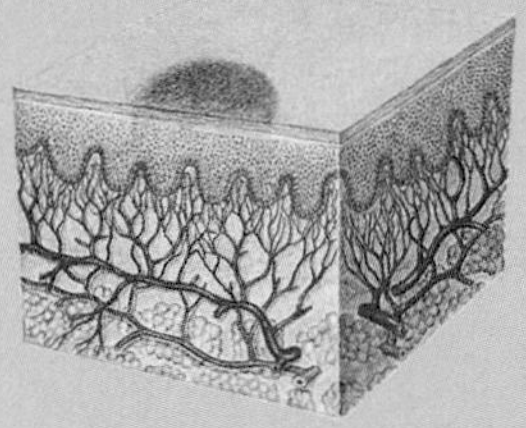	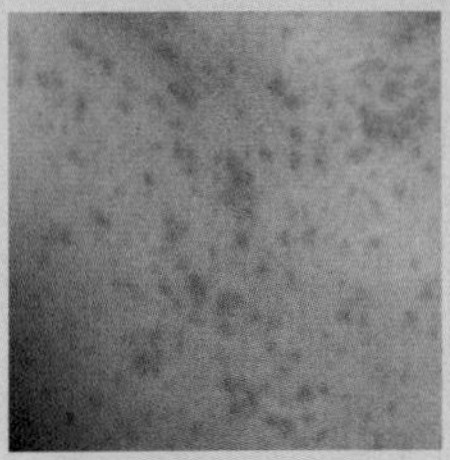 (Habif, 2004)
Papule/Plaque Solid, raised lesion with distinct borders Variety of shapes: domed, flat-topped, umbilicated Often associated with secondary features: crusts or scales Size <0.5 cm >0.5-cm papule: referred to as a *plaque*	Wart Psoriasis Actinic keratosis	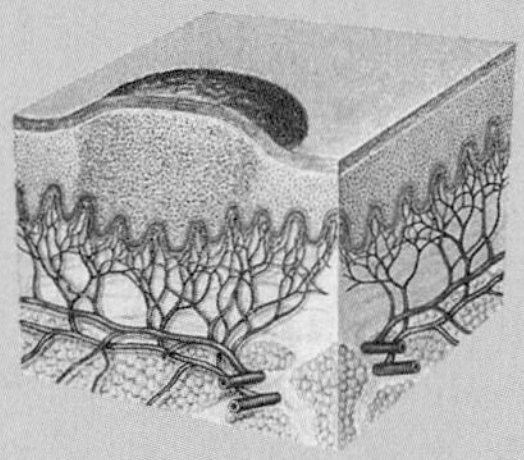	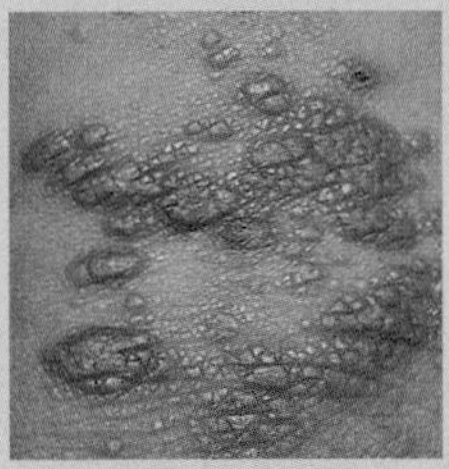 (Weston and Lane, 2007)
Nodule Raised solid mass with defined borders Extends into the dermis or beyond Deeper and more solid than a papule Size 0.5-2 cm	Lipomas Squamous cell cancers	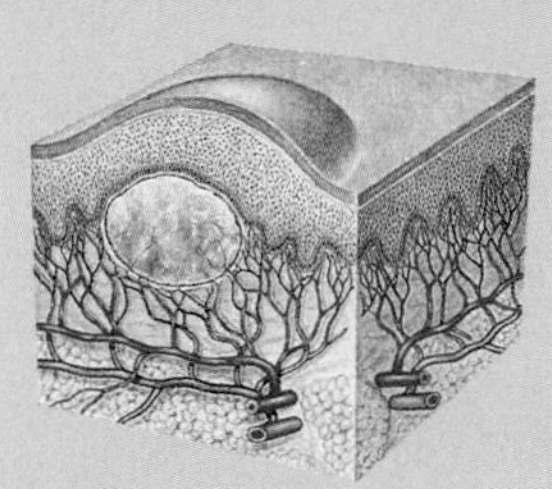	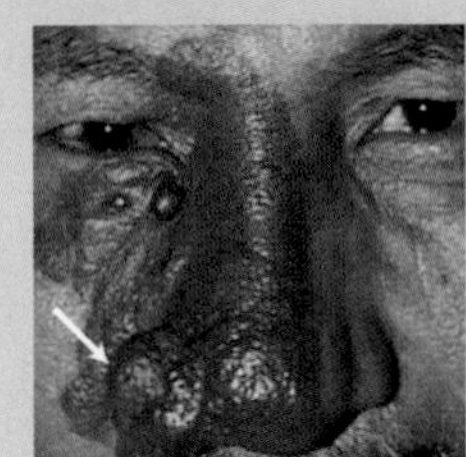 (Goldman and Fitzpatrick, 1994)
Tumor Solid mass that extends through subcutaneous tissue May have undefined borders Not always cancerous; may be larger lipomas Nodules that typically are >1-2 cm	Larger lipomas Cancerous lesions	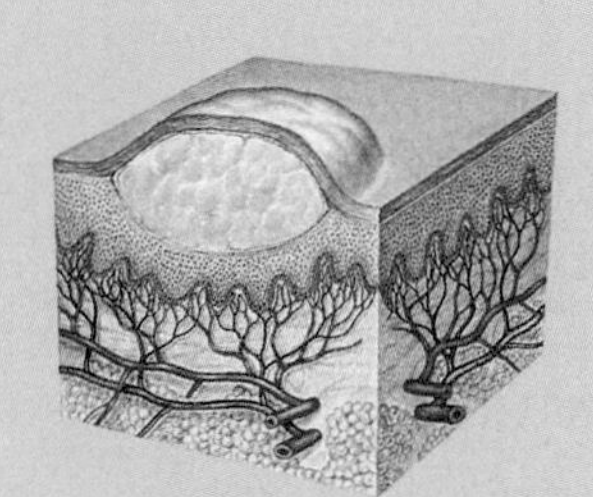	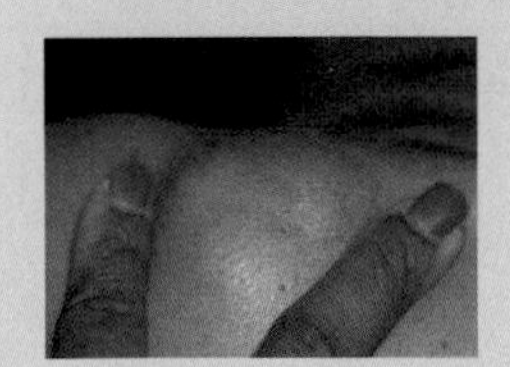 (Lemmis and Lemmi, 2000)
Vesicle/Bulla Circumscribed, raised lesions Filled with serous (clear) fluid Size <0.5 cm Vesicles >0.5 cm: referred to as *bullae*	Chickenpox (varicella) Poison ivy Second-degree burn blisters	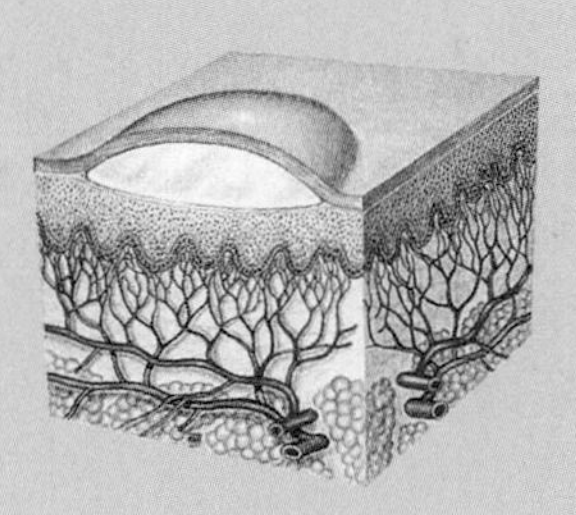	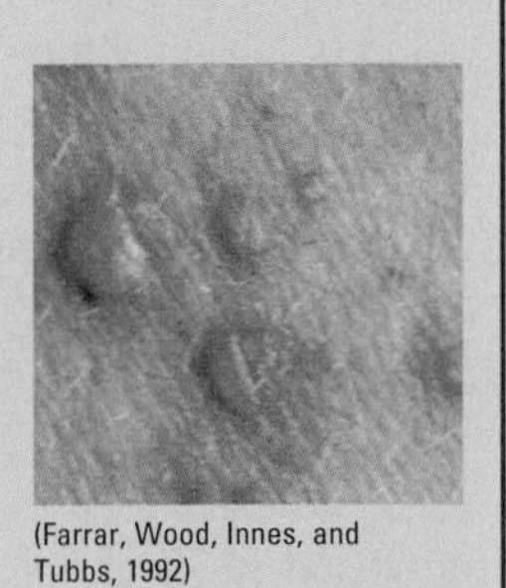 (Farrar, Wood, Innes, and Tubbs, 1992)

Continued

TABLE 20-2 Primary Skin Lesions—cont'd

DESCRIPTION	EXAMPLES	SKIN CUTAWAY	ACTUAL CASE
Pustule Similar to vesicle Circumcised, elevated lesion containing pus instead of clear fluid Most commonly infected	Impetigo Acne		(Weston, Lane, and Morelli, 1996)
Wheal Irregularly shaped area of edema Caused by serous fluid in the dermis Varies in color and size	Hives (urticaria) Insect bites		(Farrar, Wood, Innes, and Tubbs, 1992)
Burrow Linear or circular in appearance Caused by infestation and tunneling of parasitic organisms	Scabies mites Ringworms		(Marks and Miller, 2014)
Cyst Encapsulated fluid-filled or semisolid mass Extends into the dermis or subcutaneous tissue	Sebaceous cyst		(Weston and Lane, 2007)

(From Habif TP: *Clinical dermatology,* ed. 4, St. Louis, 2004, Mosby; Weston WL, Lane AT: *Color textbook of pediatric dermatology,* ed. 4, St. Louis, 2007, Mosby; Goldman MP, Fitzpatrick RE: *Cutaneous laser surgery,* St. Louis, 1994, Mosby; Lemmi FO, Lemmi CAE: *Physical assessment findings CD-ROM,* Philadelphia, 2000, Saunders; Farrar WE, Wood MJ, Innes JA, Tubbs H, et al: *Infectious diseases,* ed. 2, London, 1992, Gower; Weston WL, Lane AT, Morelli JG: *Color textbook of pediatric dermatology,* ed. 2, St. Louis, 1996, Mosby; Marks JG, Miller JJ: *Lookingbill and Marks' principles of dermatology,* ed. 5, St. Louis, 2014, Saunders.)

intercostal space and gently pinching the fingertips together and then releasing (Figure 20-5). Skin that is well hydrated and free of underlying disease lifts easily and returns without delay to its original position. Avoid assessing turgor over areas that are wrinkled or scarred, because they are consistently loose or indurated.

When skin turgor is poor, the skin will stay pinched or will return to its original state more slowly. Decreased skin turgor is a sign of moderate to severe dehydration. If skin turgor remains poor or compromised, the patient is susceptible to skin breakdown or invasion by opportunistic organisms, against which healthy skin acts as a barrier.

TABLE 20-3 Types of Skin Cancer

DESCRIPTION	RISK FACTORS	SYMPTOMS	PHOTO
Basal Cell Carcinoma (BCC)			
Most common skin cancer worldwide Slow growing Usually does not metastasize May cause destruction and disfigurement of surrounding tissues	Sun exposure Fair complexion Familial history of skin cancer Weakened immune system History of radiation therapy Increased age	Bump or scaly growth Does not heal within 2 wk Begins to itch or bleed May begin at size of 0.5-1 cm and grow Slightly raised or flat	(Kumar, Abbas, and Aster, 2015)
Squamous Cell Carcinoma (SCC)			
Second most common form of skin cancer Grows more rapidly than BCC May metastasize if left untreated	Chronic sun exposure Additional risk factors same as those for BCC	Red, crusted or nonhealing nodule or ulcer	(Kumar, Abbas, and Aster, 2015)
Melanoma			
Least common skin cancer Accounts for 75% of skin cancer deaths* Elevation indicates a more advanced stage	Sun exposure Fair complexion, freckling, light hair Multiple moles Male gender Familiar or personal history of melanoma Immune suppression†	Brown, flat, lesion with irregular borders Variegated pigmentation with poorly defined margins May begin as only 0.5-1.0 cm in diameter Changing size and shape of an existing mole Possible tenderness, bleeding or itching	(Kumar, Abbas, and Aster, 2015)

*From National Cancer Institute: SEER stat fact sheets: Melanoma of the skin, 2014. Retrieved from *http://seer.cancer.gov/statfacts/html/melan.html.*

†From American Cancer Society: Melanoma skin cancer, 2014. Retrieved from *www.cancer.org/cancer/skincancer-melanoma/detailedguide/melanoma-skin-cancer-risk-factors.*

(All figures in table from Kumar V, Abbas AK, Aster JC: *Robbins and Cotran pathologic basis of disease*, ed. 9, Philadelphia, 2015, Saunders.)

TABLE 20-4 Screening for Melanoma: ABCDE

A = ASYMMETRY	B = BORDER	C = COLOR	D = DIAMETER	E = EVOLVING
One half of lesion does not match the other half	Irregular, uneven, or notched borders	Variable in color Ranges from tan, brown, or black to white, red, or blue	Typically exceeds size of pencil eraser: >6 mm	Looks different from other moles Changes in size, shape, or color

From American Academy of Dermatology: Melanoma: Signs and symptoms, 2014. Retrieved from *www.aad.org/dermatology-a-to-z/diseases-and-treatments/m—p/melanoma/signs-symptoms.*

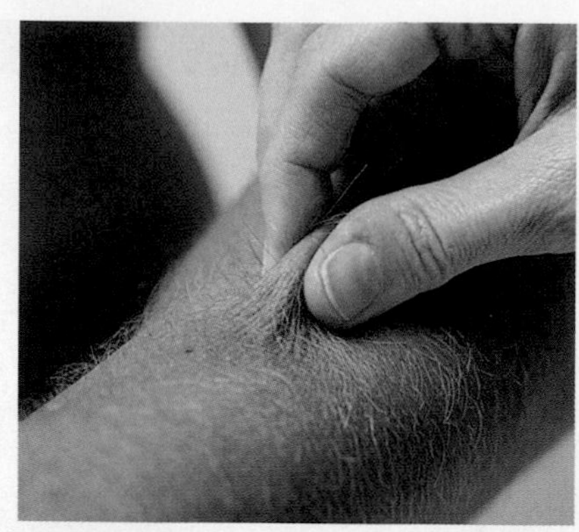

FIGURE 20-5 Skin turgor assessment of the forearm. (From Ball JW, Dains JE, Flynn JA, et al: *Seidel's guide to physical examination*, ed. 8, St. Louis, 2015, Mosby.)

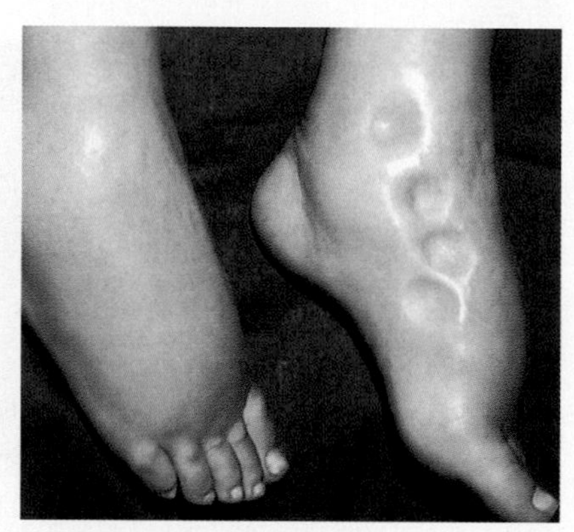

FIGURE 20-6 Pitting edema. (From Patton KT, Thibodeau GA: *Anatomy and physiology*, ed. 7, St. Louis, 2010, Mosby.)

Edema

Edema (swelling) is caused when there is a buildup of fluid in underlying tissues. Common causes of edema are localized trauma to an area and impairment of venous return. Edema secondary to poor venous return usually is most prominent in the lower extremities or dependent areas of the body (e.g., the feet, ankles, and lower legs).

Edematous skin usually appears stretched and glossy, depending on the amount of fluid in the underlying tissues and the elasticity of the skin. In older patients, edematous skin can have more subtle changes, often appearing boggy as a result of decreased underlying muscle tone and loss of skin elasticity. Edematous areas should be palpated to determine pain, mobility, and consistency of the underlying tissue involvement.

If the palpation causes an indentation that persists for some time after the release of the pressure, the edema is referred to as *pitting edema* (Figure 20-6). The degree of pitting edema is assessed by pressing the edematous area with the thumb or forefinger for 1 to 2 seconds and then releasing. Pitting edema is documented according to the depth of indentation (Box 20-3). Caution should be exercised when assessing pitting edema in patients with underlying conditions associated with venous or arterial insufficiency. Even slight pressure that causes indentation in edematous skin can produce tissue trauma, leading to ecchymosis (bruising), ulceration, or permanent damage requiring skin grafting.

BOX 20-3 Documentation of Pitting Edema

1+	Slight pitting, 2 mm
2+	Deeper pit, 4 mm
3+	Deep pit, 6 mm; dependent extremity enlarged
4+	Very deep pit, 8 mm; dependent extremity extremely distorted

Hair and Scalp Inspection and Palpation

Normal hair structure consists of keratinized cells. Hair is found over most parts of the body except lips, palms of the hand, soles of the feet, nipples, labia minora, and the penis. Two general types of hair cover body surfaces: vellus and terminal. *Vellus* hair is short, fine, and pale and covers most of the body's surfaces. *Terminal* hair (e.g., on the scalp and in the axillae) is coarse and darker, more visible, and longer than vellus hair. Puberty initiates the development of terminal hair in both sexes in the perineum, axillae, and legs. Pigment production determines the color and type of hair of an individual. A lack of pigment or inclusion of air spaces within the hair follicle produces gray or white hair color variations. Hair serves as a protective covering for the body (e.g., scalp) and filters airborne debris and dust to prevent it from entering body orifices, such as the ears, nose, and eyes.

Inspection begins with noting the condition and distribution of body hair and continues through all phases of the physical assessment. Ask the patient to remove any hair pins, clips, or wigs. Explain that assessment of the hair and scalp requires separating layers of the hair to detect irregularities beginning at the hair shaft. Obtain subjective data by asking questions similar to those found in the Health Assessment Questions box. Inspect the patient's hair color, quantity, distribution, thickness, and texture, as well as moisture surrounding areas of body hair. When inspecting scalp hair color, remember that variations range from pale blonde or flaxen to black to silver or gray. Understand that color variations can be chemically altered due to the patient's use of rinses or dyes. Patients of African American and African heritage often have coarse or wiry hair texture that requires less frequent washing to maintain a healthy sheen.

Recognize that normal hair growth and distribution vary with age and gender. In older adults, scalp hair often becomes light gray, yellow, or white, and terminal hair in the pubic areas, scalp, and axillae becomes thinner and more sparse. Older men usually experience decrease in density of facial hair, whereas older women tend to develop hair on the upper lip and chin with a decrease in estrogen levels. Dry, brittle hair may occur with overuse of chemical products for coloring and/or straightening, and such changes are commonly seen with aging. Note whether younger patients have

HEALTH ASSESSMENT QUESTIONS

Head, Ears, Eyes, Nose, and Throat (HEENT)

Head and Neck

- Do you have a history of any head injuries (e.g., concussion), subdural hematoma, or recent lumbar punctures? Have you ever experienced dizziness or had a tumor or seizure disorder? Have you lost consciousness for any period of time or become confused and/or dazed for an unknown reason? Do you have a history of high or low thyroid hormone levels?
- Do you have a history of headaches? If so, what are the typical onset, duration, and resolution of the headaches? Have you ever been diagnosed with migraines?
- Is there a risk of head injury in your employment? Do you wear a hard hat? Do you wear head protection when participating in sports? Do you wear a motorcycle or bicycle helmet?

Eyes

- Have you noticed any change in your vision? Have you experienced halos around lights, floaters, light sensitivity, or double vision (diplopia)?
- Do you have a history of glaucoma or cataracts? Have you ever had eye surgery?
- Do you wear contact lenses or glasses?
- Do you have any superficial or deep pain in or around the eye? Have you noticed any burning, itching, or discharge?
- When was your last eye examination?

Nose

- Do you have a history of allergies, sinus infections, or trauma to the nose? Do you experience nasal discharge? If so, describe its character, including color, odor, amount, and duration.
- Do you experience sinus pain or tenderness, postnasal drip, daytime cough, headache, or face pain?
- Do you snore? If so, when is it most common for you to snore? Does it wake you or your partner? Do you feel tired after sleeping all night? Do you need frequent naps?
- Do you have a history of nosebleeds? If so, describe the frequency, amount of bleeding, and treatment.

Ears

- Do you have a history of dizziness or vertigo, earache, or hearing loss?
- Do you ever experience ringing in the ears?
- Do you wear hearing aids or use another type of hearing assistive device? Do you wear ear protection for your work?
- When was your last hearing test?

Mouth and Throat

- Is there a personal or family history of mouth or throat cancer?
- Do you experience frequent bleeding of the gums, tooth pain, tonsillitis, cold sores, dry mouth, or cracked lips?
- Do you have any difficulty swallowing or do you feel as though something is caught in your throat?
- When was your last dental examination?

experienced hair growth associated with puberty in the pubic and axillary areas, as well as coarsening of facial hair in adolescent boys. Both genders experience an increase in coarse hair growth, evenly distributed, on the lower extremities during changes associated with puberty. Cultural norms, religion, or style trends usually dictate whether body hair, including scalp hair, is groomed in a particular method.

Changes in hair growth or loss can have either positive or negative effects on the patient's sense of well-being or body image. Patients with hormone disorders often report and exhibit unusual patterns of hair growth and distribution. **Hirsutism** is a condition affecting both men and women in which hair growth on the upper lip, chin, and cheeks becomes excessive and vellus body hair becomes thicker and coarser. This condition is common in patients with hormone imbalances. Permanent or temporary hair loss (**alopecia**) and extreme thinning of hair, in which the scalp is clearly visible, often are related to genetic predisposition, endocrine disorders, severe febrile illness, chemotherapy, or scalp disease. In patients with thyroid disease and diabetes, hair becomes sparser, brittle, and fine, because of decreased blood flow to underlying capillary beds supplying the skin. Dull, dry, stringy-looking hair is characteristic of poor grooming practices and nutritional deficits, such as in anorexia nervosa, alcoholism, or malabsorption syndromes. Venous or atrial insufficiency can be the cause of hair loss or lack of growth in areas where circulation is compromised, usually involving the lower extremities.

Parasites can be found in scalp and pubic hair follicles. Observe for the presence of head lice, bedbugs, cockroaches, or other parasitic insects. Lice infestations usually produce severe **pruritus** (itching) from bites that also are visually detectable. When bites become infected from the host's scratching the affected area, or as a consequence of the body's immune response, pustular eruptions can be observed close to the hair roots where skin surfaces come in contact with each other, such as in the axillae and the groin.

Palpate the patient's scalp and hair while wearing gloves for protection from any hidden lesions, parasites, or hygiene concerns. Scalp palpation should evaluate for lesions or bumps by separating strands of hair in a systematic method until every portion of the scalp is evaluated. The scalp normally is smooth, even-toned, and supple, with hair follicles evenly dispersed. If scalp lesions or bumps are found, ask the patient about any recent trauma to the area. Describe characteristics associated with abnormalities (e.g., pain, size, drainage), and note whether the patient has been scratching the area or using home remedies on the site for relief. Moles and birthmarks on the scalp are common and can bleed if combed or brushed too hard. Dry patches of scalp can be

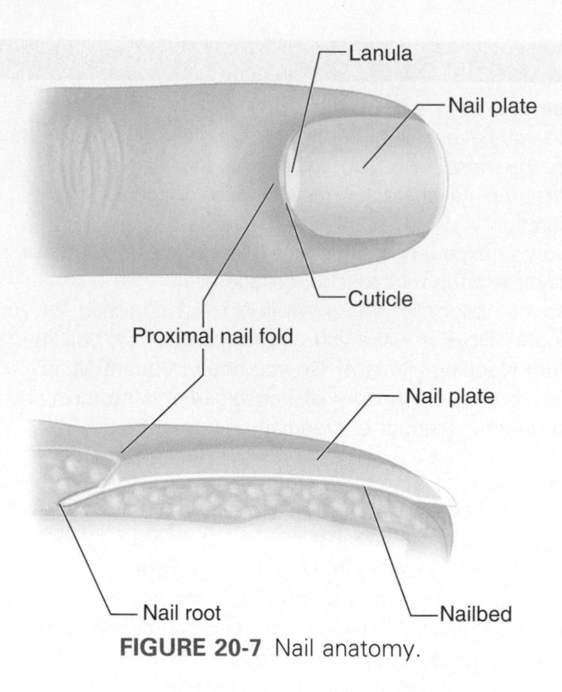

FIGURE 20-7 Nail anatomy.

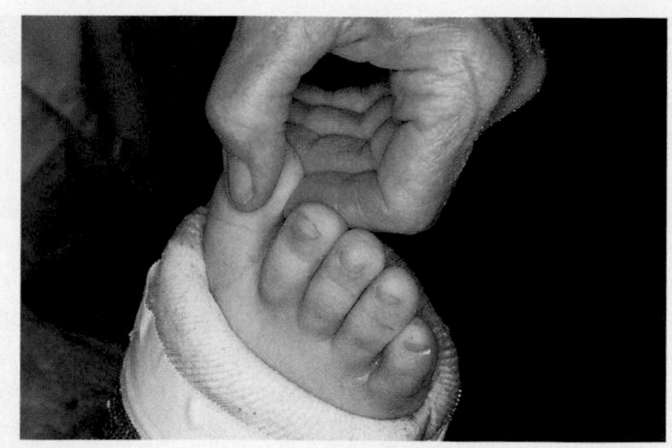
FIGURE 20-8 Assessment of capillary refill. (From Perry AG, Potter PA, Elkin MK: *Nursing interventions and clinical skills,* ed. 5, St. Louis, 2012, Mosby.)

found in patients with decreased sebum production in skin covering the scalp. More commonly, overuse of products that wash away the skin's natural oils and lubricants leads to dandruff or to aggravation of underlying skin conditions, causing flakiness, dryness, and pruritus of the scalp.

Nail Inspection and Palpation

Nails are hard, keratinized plates of epidermal cells that originate and grow from a root beneath a skin crease called the *cuticle* or *eponychium.* The crescent-shaped, whitish area located at the base of the nail, where it meets the cuticle, is called the *lunula.* The most visible portion of the nail is the nail plate, a transparent layer of epithelial cells that extends over the entire nailbed (Figure 20-7). The underlying nailbed normally is light pink to reddish brown–tinged. Nailbed color results from the supply of superficial capillary blood vessels found in the skin beneath the nail and is dependent on the patient's race or genetic makeup. The nails' primary function is to protect the distal ends of the fingers and toes.

The nails often are reflective of the patient's general level of health, nutritional status, and hygiene habits. The nailbed should be inspected for grooming and cleanliness, color, markings, and shape. The length of the nail is taken into consideration; however, nail length can vary greatly from person to person on the basis of personal preference and is not always indicative of poor grooming or health problems.

Observe the angle between the nail plate and nail and the condition of the lateral and proximal nail folds. The nail folds and the cuticles should be smooth, with intact skin that is without redness or inflammation. The patient's occupation, grooming habits, or culture can influence the nail appearance and texture. For example, people who are employed as mechanics or construction workers tend to have damaged, dirty, or brittle nails. Such changes occur despite adequate nail care and frequent handwashing performed by the patient. All components of the nail and nailbed should be clean and intact; otherwise, the patient is at greater risk for infection or permanent damage to the nail and its underlying structures.

Nails normally develop at a steady rate and can grow slightly faster on one side of the body than the other. The thickness of nails changes with aging, usually becoming harder and thicker, with nail growth occurring more slowly than in younger patients. As a patient ages, nails appear more opaque, yellow, and striated, rather than transparent, smooth, and pinkish. Such changes often are due to decreased calcium and mineral intake, poor circulation, or the progression of generalized disease processes.

On inspection, the nailbed is normally at a 160-degree angle between the nail and the nail plate. Nails should be hard and relatively immobile. A larger angle and decreased firmness of the nailbed can indicate chronic circulation or oxygenation concerns (Table 20-5). For example, clubbing of the nails typically is a result of chronic peripheral oxygen deprivation, as seen in cardiac or pulmonary disease.

Palpate nails to assess for texture and consistency, noting if the nail plate is firmly attached to the nailbed. To test for **capillary refill** (an indication of peripheral blood flow), use the thumb to gently depress the patient's nail tip for approximately 1 second and release (Figure 20-8). As pressure is applied, the nailbed will blanch or appear white. The pink tone should return immediately when the pressure on the nail is released. Capillary refill is measured in seconds, and blanching that occurs with pressure should reverse, with return of the nailbed to normal color in less than 2 to 3 seconds; this response is referred to as *brisk.* Capillary refill lasting longer than 2 to 3 seconds (slow or sluggish capillary refill) usually is a sign of respiratory or cardiac disease associated with hypoxia, anemia, or conditions linked to circulatory insufficiency.

Calluses and corns are areas of thickened skin that may occur in areas of pressure, typically on the fingers or toes as a result of continuous rubbing, tight footwear, or gait abnormalities. For example, professional guitarists often develop calluses on their strumming fingers. A callus is generally a more diffuse thickening of the skin. Corns are more focused

TABLE 20-5 Nail Shape and Curvature Abnormalities

ABNORMALITY	CAUSE(S)
Splinter hemorrhage: Red or purple-brown streak in nailbed	Minor trauma, trichinosis, subacute bacterial endocarditis
Paronychia: Inflammation of the skin at the base of the nail	Local infection • Acute: *Staphylococcus aureus,* herpes simplex virus • Chronic: *Candida albicans, Pseudomonas* spp
Clubbing: Enlargement of the fingertips, softening of the nailbed, and flattening of the nail; angle between the nail plate and the nail often greater than 180 degrees Clubbing—early: almost 180° Clubbing—middle: 180° Clubbing—severe: >180°	Chronic hypoxia from heart and/or pulmonary disease
Beau's lines: Transverse ridging in nails due to a temporary halt in nail growth	Nail injury, systemic injury, eczema, psoriasis, paronychia
Koilonychia: Concave curves of the nail, with thinning of the nail plate; also called "spoon nail"	Iron deficiency anemia, repeated chemical trauma, syphilis
Muehrcke's lines: Double band of white lines (leukonychia)	Renal disease

areas that appear as horny, thickened, or cone-shaped masses, typically found over bony prominences on the feet.

Serious complications can occur in people with poor circulation and peripheral neuropathy. Document any abnormalities such as thickening or ulceration of the nails and skin surfaces of the hands or feet.

! SAFE PRACTICE ALERT

Toenails should be cut straight across and filed with an emery board or nail file. Remind diabetic patients to seek professional help immediately if they notice an ingrown toenail developing. Failure to act quickly may result in a serious infection that can be difficult to treat and can spread systemically.

HEAD, EARS, EYES, NOSE, AND THROAT

Examination of the head and neck requires general assessment of the head as well as external and limited internal assessment of the eyes, ears, nose, mouth, throat, and neck. The Health Assessment Questions: Head, Ears, Eyes, Nose and Throat box can provide a foundation for collecting health history information related to each of these areas. Advanced practice nurses and physicians conduct extensive internal examination of these organs. Assessment of the carotid arteries, jugular veins, lymph nodes, thyroid gland, and trachea are included during this part of the physical exam. Assessment techniques for the head and neck frequently incorporate inspection and palpation simultaneously, followed by systematic auscultation of individual anatomic landmarks.

Head Inspection and Palpation

Begin examination of the head and neck by inspecting the patient's head position. The patient's head should be held upright, in a midline to trunk position, and remain motionless during inspection. Tremors or other neurologic disorders may be present if jerking movements are noted.

Inspect the skull contour for size, shape, and symmetry. Make note of any abnormal lesions, incisions, masses, or nodules that are distinct in appearance, texture, or contour from the skin nearby. Gently palpate the skull in a circular pattern, progressing systematically from front to back. The adult skull should feel smooth and seamless, with the bones indistinguishable from one another. Overall, the scalp should move freely over the skull without tenderness, swelling, or depressions. Enlargement of the skull due to **hydrocephalus** (accumulation of cerebrospinal fluid in the ventricles of the brain) in children most often is a congenital condition, whereas in adults it may occur as a result of tumor growth. In adults with disorders of the adrenal glands that cause excessive growth hormone secretion, enlarged jaws and facial bones may result in acromegaly in both male and female patients.

The size, shape, and contour of the head and eye and ear location should be mostly symmetric. Inspection of the eyes, eyebrows, and mouth should yield consistency and overall uniformity in the shape and contour of the features during rest, movement, and expression. If facial asymmetry is present, note whether all features on one side or portion of the face are affected and whether there are any accompanying abnormalities, such as edema, swelling, pallor, or pigmentation. Suspect facial nerve paralysis when an entire side or hemisphere of the face is involved. Facial nerve weakness is seen primarily in cases in which the lower half of the face is symptomatic. When only the mouth is involved, consider peripheral trigeminal nerve damage as the causative factor. Spasmodic muscular contraction or tics noted in the face, head, or neck of the patient are often associated with varying amounts of pressure on facial nerves and/or with psychogenic or degenerative changes to underlying facial structures. Examples are nerve damage caused by cosmetic procedures, traumatic injury from airbag deployment, and varicella-zoster virus infection.

Eye Inspection and Palpation

Eye examination includes assessment of normal eye structures (Figure 20-9), extraocular movements, and visual acuity. The nurse should determine the patient's level of eye function in relation to deficits or alterations that impact ambulation, self-care, and completion of activities of daily living.

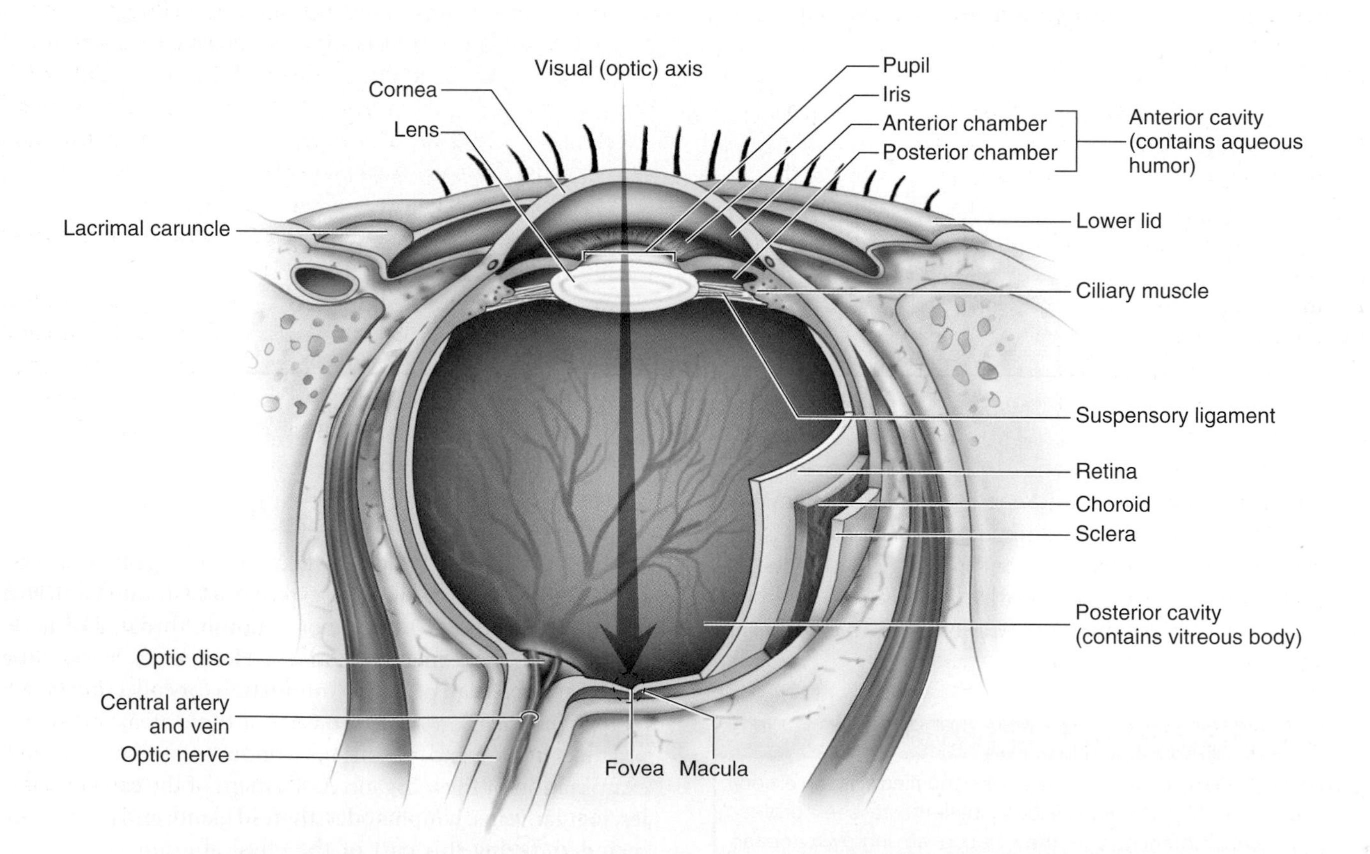

FIGURE 20-9 Normal eye anatomy. (From Thibodeau GA, Patton KT: *The human body in health and disease,* ed. 4, St. Louis, 2005, Mosby.)

Alignment

Normally, both eyes move together, receiving the same image on corresponding areas of both retinas simultaneously. The brain fuses these images into a single three-dimensional image. **Strabismus** (crossed eyes) is a disorder in which one or both eyes deviate out of alignment owing to muscle weakness or paralysis, most often outwardly (divergent strabismus) or toward the nose (convergent strabismus). In this case, the brain receives two different images, and either it suppresses one or the condition results in the person's seeing double (**diplopia**). Depending on the underlying cause, by maneuvers to weaken or strengthen the appropriate muscles to center the eyes, the affected person may be able to correct strabismus. For example, if an eye turns upward, the muscle at the bottom of the eye could be strengthened to correct the misalignment.

Positioning

The eyes are positioned on each side of the nasal bone, approximately 1 to 2 inches apart from one inner canthus to the other, and are housed in the anterior portion of the skull. On inspection, they appear equally situated below the forehead and eyebrows and above the nose and mouth, just above or at the midline of the patient's ears. Abnormal eye protrusion can be due to tumors or inflammation of the orbit. "Bulging" eyes often indicate hyperthyroidism or severe increased intraocular pressure from trauma or glaucoma.

Eyebrows and Eyelids

The eyebrows and eyelids should be inspected for position, color, alignment, and movement. Eyebrows normally grow symmetrically and extend to the temporal canthus of the eye. Excessive coarseness, flakiness, or brittleness of hair and failure to extend beyond the temporal canthus can be due to conditions such as hypothyroidism or adrenal disease. Thinned or lightened eyebrows can result from grooming techniques such as plucking, coloring, or waxing or can be caused by normal aging. Ask patients to raise and lower the eyebrows. Observe for symmetry in movement. Difficulty performing this task can indicate a facial nerve palsy or facial cranial nerve VII dysfunction.

When the eye is open, the superior (upper) eyelid should cover a portion of the iris but not the pupil itself. Observe the patient's ability to completely open and close the eyelid and to blink. The lids normally close symmetrically. Under normal circumstances, people blink both eyes simultaneously and involuntarily up to 25 to 30 times a minute. The blink reflex serves to lubricate the cornea and surrounding tissues. Fasciculation (twitching) or tremors noted with the eyelids closed tightly can be a sign of hyperthyroidism.

Note whether the superior eyelid covers more of one iris than the other or whether it extends over the pupil. When abnormal drooping of the eyelid occurs, the condition is known as **ptosis**. It can indicate a congenital or acquired weakness of the levator muscle or can result from paralysis affecting all or portions of the oculomotor cranial nerve III. Ptosis more often is seen in older adults, in whom age-related loss of elasticity, muscle weakness, and excessive skin can interfere with eyelid opening or movement. The nurse should note whether the lids are turned inward, a condition known as *entropion,* or whether the lids are turned away from the eye, a condition called *ectropion.* Entropion causes the lashes to turn inward, which may cause corneal and conjunctival irritation that increases the risk of secondary eye infection. Ectropion may result in excessive tearing or watery-appearing eyes, because the tear-collecting structure cannot collect the secretions of the lacrimal gland, causing them to spill over onto the face.

A hordeolum, or stye, may result from the blockage or infection of a sebaceous gland at the base of an eyelash, causing an erythematous or yellow lump on the upper or lower eyelid. Styes are painful but typically do not cause any lasting damage.

Inspect the orbital area for edema, puffiness, or sagging tissue below the orbit. Although these signs may also be congruent with the normal aging process, periorbital edema is never a normal finding. It can indicate the presence of thyroid hypoactivity, allergies, renal disease, or infection. Slightly raised, flat, irregularly shaped, yellow-tinted lesions on the periorbital tissues are called *xanthelasma* and are suggestive of an abnormality of lipid metabolism. These elevated plaques of cholesterol most commonly are deposited on the nasal portion of either the upper or lower lid. Edema of the eyelid can prevent the lids from closing entirely. Conditions such as facial nerve paralysis, unconsciousness, or drug use can prevent the lids from closing entirely, which can expose the cornea to drying that leads to risk for infection. Note how often the lids close and whether closing is symmetric, infrequent, rapid, or uniocular (one-eyed).

Palpate the eyelids for nodules, and then gently palpate the eye itself with the eyelids closed. Determine whether it feels hard or if gentle pressure causes discomfort. Extreme firmness and rigidity of the eyeball on palpation can be a sign of glaucoma, hyperthyroidism, or retroorbital tumor. The lids should feel smooth and typically are the same color as that of facial skin.

Conjunctiva and Sclera

The conjunctiva covers the visible surface of the sclera and extends to the external border of the cornea. The conjunctiva normally is free of redness or exudate. The presence of erythema, exudate, or discoloration can indicate an allergic response or infective conjunctivitis. Conjunctivitis ("pinkeye") is a highly contagious infection that is spread through contact with the crusty drainage that collects on the eyelid margins. It is characterized by intense itching and redness of the sclera.

The sclera is examined to check its color and to ensure that it is intact, without lesions. In white patients, the appearance of the sclera is a pearly white color. In dark-skinned patients, the sclera is light yellow to pale gray. In the presence of certain conditions, such as liver disease, the sclera becomes pigmented or discolored, turning yellow (jaundice) or copper-colored. A sunken appearance of the orbit or sclera can indicate dehydration, retinal damage, or trauma.

> **! SAFE PRACTICE ALERT**
>
> Hand hygiene should be performed before and after examination of the eye. Wear gloves in the presence of any exudate or irritation. Examine the healthy eye first. Take special precautions to avoid transferring organisms found in one eye to the other eye.

Clarity of the Lens and Cornea

The cornea is the transparent front layer of the eye that covers the iris, pupil, and anterior chamber. Together with the l ens, the cornea refracts light and accounts for approximately two thirds of the eye's total optical power. The refractive power of the lens is roughly one third of the eye's total power. Examine the cornea for clarity by asking the patient to focus on a point straight ahead while shining a light at an angle that covers the entire corneal surface. The corneal surface should appear transparent, glossy, and even. Because the cornea is avascular, blood vessels should not be present. Any irregularities or blood present on the corneal surface can indicate a corneal abrasion or tear, leaving the area susceptible to infection or pain with movement. Corneal sensitivity is tested by touching a wisp of cotton to the outer edge of the cornea. The expected response is a blink, demonstrating that the sensory fibers of cranial nerve V and the motor nerve of cranial nerve VII (facial nerve) are intact.

The lens is examined by shining a light indirectly toward the cornea. It may appear gray or yellow; however, clarity is better assessed during examination of the lens with the ophthalmoscope. **Cataracts** cause the lens of the eye to become cloudy and impair vision. They grow slowly over time and often are left untreated until they become opaque or dense, significantly compromising the patient's ability to see clearly and adversely affecting quality of life.

Lacrimal Glands

The lacrimal glands are responsible for tear production and assist in lubrication of the outer surface of the eye. They are located in the upper, anterolateral aspect of the bony orbit of each eye and normally are not palpable. Inspect the area of the lacrimal gland, and palpate the upper and lower rim of the eye orbit, working from the inner canthus outward. If the lateral aspect of the upper lid feels full or elicits a pain response, gently evert the lid and examine the area around the lacrimal gland. Lacrimal ducts may be blocked, with obstruction of the flow of tears, causing redness or swelling of the eyelids and conjunctiva.

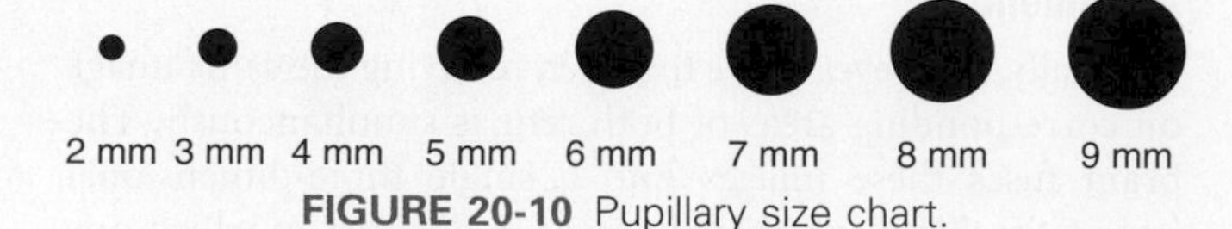

FIGURE 20-10 Pupillary size chart.

Iris and Pupil

The anterior surface of the iris reveals the color of a person's eyes. The iris of both eyes should be clearly visible and the same color. The iris has a deeply pigmented posterior surface and prohibits the entrance of light, except through the pupil.

Pupils are examined for size, shape, symmetry, reaction to light, and accommodation. The pupils should be round, black, and equal in size; normally 3 to 7 mm in diameter. Estimate individual pupil size while referring to a standardized chart (Figure 20-10), and then compare the pupils for equality and size variation.

Cloudy pupils indicate the presence of cataracts. Verify whether a patient has had surgery to reduce intraocular pressure (as in glaucoma) if a V-shaped portion of the pupil is missing. Pupillary constriction to less than 2 mm (pinpoint pupils) and failure to dilate generally are caused by ingestion of opioids such as morphine or medications that control glaucoma. Pupillary dilation of more than 6 mm and failure of the pupils to constrict with light stimulation may result from trauma, neurologic dysfunction, glaucoma, or ophthalmic drugs introduced into the eye for examination or surgery. In situations in which extreme trauma or permanent neurologic damage has taken place, pupils that do not respond to light and remain dilated over time may be documented as fixed and dilated.

Pupillary Reflexes and Accommodation

Pupillary reflexes are evaluated in a darkened environment using a penlight. To check for light reflexes, approach the patient's eyes from one side while asking the patient to focus straight ahead into the distance (Figure 20-11). Ask the patient to avoid looking directly into the light. The pupil closer to the light should constrict immediately in response to exposure to the indirect light, followed by constriction of the opposite pupil (consensual constriction) more distant from the light. Repeat the procedure on the opposite eye.

Testing pupillary reflexes for **accommodation** evaluates the ability of the eyes to focus on near objects. Assessment of accommodation is necessary only if pupillary reflexes are sluggish, absent, or abnormal in any way (Jun, 2014). Accommodation is facilitated by movement of ciliary muscles and increased curvature of the lens, neither of which is visible. It is assessed by observing whether the pupils converge and constrict when focused on an object at close range. Have the patient focus on a distant object, and then on a pen or unlit penlight held just a few inches in front of the patient's nose. Slowly move the pen or penlight closer to the patient's nose, observing for bilateral convergence and constriction of the pupils. Documentation of a normal pupillary reflex

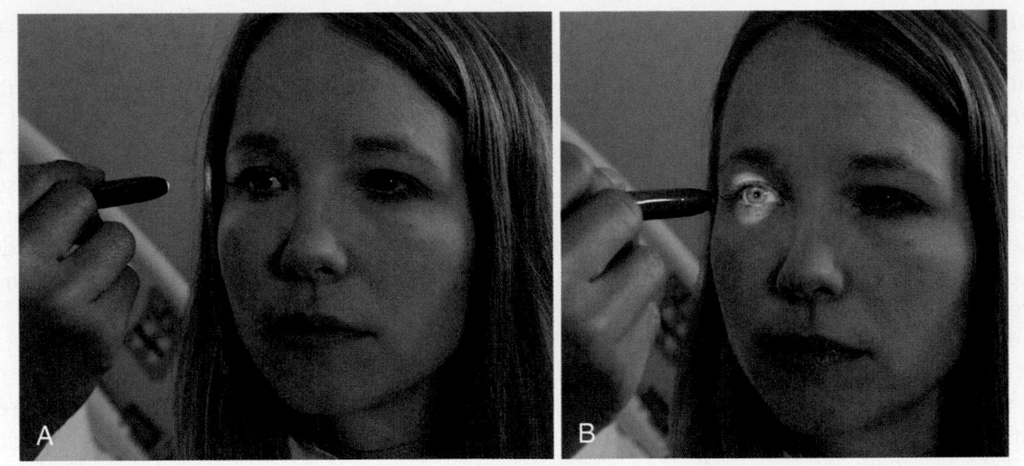

FIGURE 20-11 Assessing pupillary light reflex. **A,** Begin by approaching one eye with a penlight from the side. **B,** Observe the closest pupil for immediate constriction followed by consensual constriction of the opposite pupil.

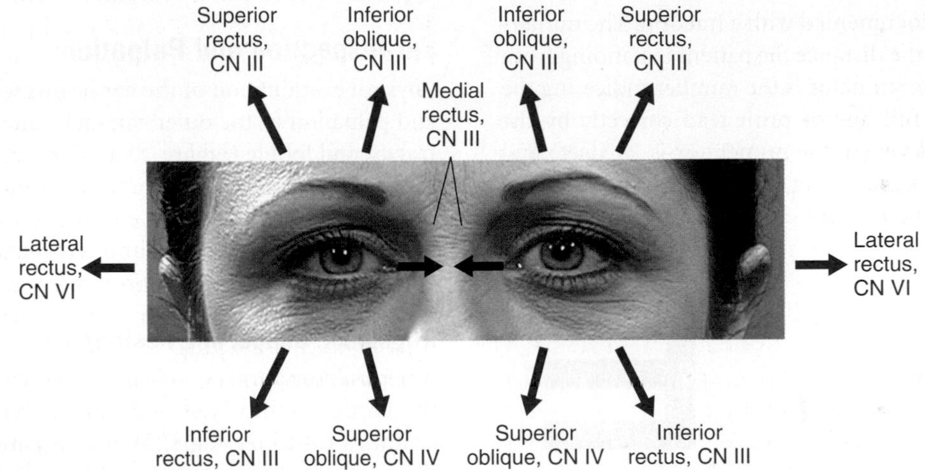

FIGURE 20-12 Examining the six fields of vision. (From Ball JW, Dains JE, Flynn JA, et al: *Seidel's guide to physical examination*, ed. 8, St. Louis, 2015, Mosby.)

examination is recorded as PERRLA (pupils equal, round, reactive to light and accommodation).

Extraocular Movement

Movement of the eyes in all directions is controlled by the combined function of three cranial nerves (III, oculomotor; IV, trochlear; and VI, abducens) and six extraocular muscles. A critical aspect of assessing extraocular movement is examination of the six fields of vision. This exam is completed by having the patient and the nurse seated or standing approximately 2 feet away from each other at eye level. Ask the patient to follow a finger (or pen) with just the eyes, as it proceeds through the six fields of gaze (Figure 20-12). Move the finger (or pen) in a smooth, gliding motion to the right, the left, and diagonally within each of the patient's fields of vision, approximately 6 to 12 inches from the patient's eyes. Then ask the patient to move the eyes to the extreme lateral position (toward the ears), both left and right. As the patient looks in each direction, note the presence of normal parallel and equal eye movement and lid position or any signs of abnormal movement.

Nystagmus is rapid, shaking, involuntary movement of the eyes. It is especially noticeable when the patient is asked to look to the side and quickly return the gaze to the front. Depending on the cause, movements can be in both eyes or in just one eye. Prolonged nystagmus (lasting longer than 1 to 2 seconds) can be due to inner ear disorders, multiple sclerosis, narcotic use, or brain injury (secondary to motor vehicle accidents, strokes, or tumors).

Visual Acuity

Assessment of visual acuity examines the patient's ability to see at a distance and at close range. It evaluates cranial nerve II (optic nerve) patency and central vision. To assess near vision, ask the patient to read printed material at a comfortable distance (approximately 35 cm, or 14 inches) from the eyes in adequate lighting. If the patient normally wears glasses, the patient should wear them during this part of the assessment. Be sure to take language and reading ability into consideration before initiating this test. If the patient has difficulty reading, move on to other aspects of the examination.

A Snellen chart comprises increasingly smaller lines of letters and is used to test distant or far vision. The Snellen chart should be placed on a wall or door at eye level. Patients stand 20 feet from the chart and cover one eye at a time, reading each line of letters until they can no longer identify them. An E chart can be used to test visual acuity with patients who are unable to read or are unfamiliar with the English alphabet. Patients are asked to point in the direction of the open end of the E (Figure 20-13). Vision usually is tested first without glasses or corrective lenses.

Each line of the Snellen or E chart is followed by a fraction indicating 20 over the distance at which a person with normal vision would be able to see the line without assistance. Results of acuity testing are documented with a fraction: The numerator is 20 (indicating the distance the patient is standing from the chart) and the denominator is the number indicating the distance for the last full line of print read correctly by the patient. With normal vision, the numerator is 20 (feet) and the denominator also is 20 (feet), and the person is documented as having 20/20 vision. If the denominator in the fraction is greater than 20, the patient's visual acuity for distance is reduced, and the myopia (ability to see close objects clearly but not distant objects) worsens as the denominator increases. Thus vision measured as 20/200 means that the patient can read at 20 feet what the average person can read at 200 feet. Various conditions that affect visual acuity, along with associated risk factors, prevention strategies, and treatments, are listed in the Patient Education and Health Literacy box. Vision not improved with correction to better than 20/200 is considered legal blindness.

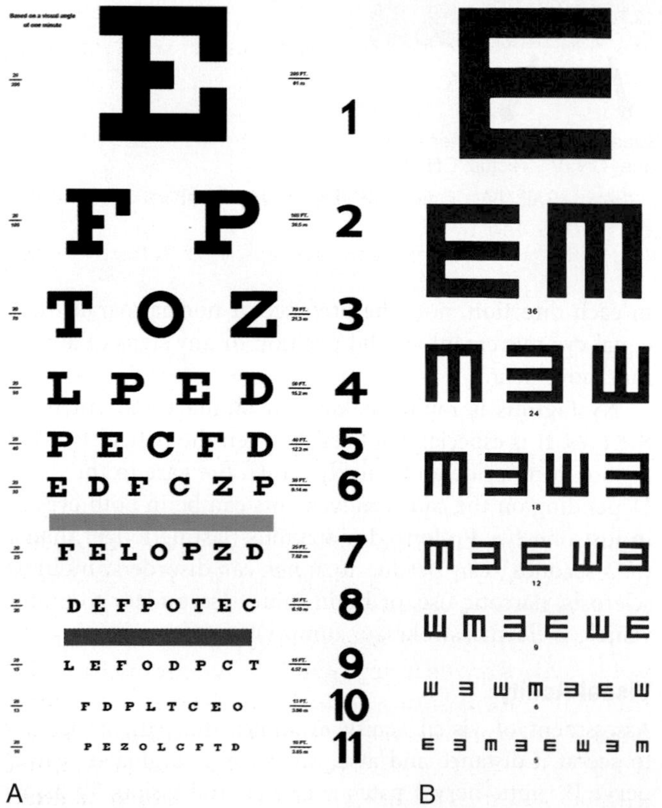

A B

FIGURE 20-13 Visual acuity assessment tools. **A,** Snellen chart. **B,** E chart.

Use of the Ophthalmoscope

Examination of the internal structures of the eye is performed by an advanced practice nurse using an ophthalmoscope. The appearance of the optic disc and retinal vasculature is the main focus of examination during ophthalmoscopy. Abnormalities in the appearance of the internal ocular structures may indicate eye disease or a chronic condition such as hypertension, diabetes, or brain injury.

Ear Inspection and Palpation

Physical examination of the ear begins with direct inspection and palpation of the outer ear, including the auricle (pinna), tragus, and lobule (Figure 20-14). Inspection of the auditory canal and tympanic membrane (eardrum) is then completed using an otoscope. Assessment of the middle and inner ear by testing hearing acuity, sound conduction, and equilibrium is the final step in examination of the auditory system.

Alignment, Shape, and Positioning

A person's ear auricles typically are equal in size, aligned with the corner of the eyes, and almost vertical in orientation (within a 10-degree angle). While the patient is seated, inspect the size and shape of the auricle, tragus, and lobule. Note symmetry, color, earlobe attachment, and positioning in relation to facial features. Misaligned or low-positioned ears can be a feature of genetic disorders associated with genitourinary tract malformations or of chromosomal anomalies such as Down syndrome. Auricles should have the same color as that of the facial skin and be free of lesions. Erythema may be due to elevated temperature or inflammation; pallor can indicate decreased circulation, frostbite, skin disease, or hypoxia.

Auricles should be smooth and curved and should shape the upper ear. Earlobes may be "soldered" (tightly attached with no visible lobe), attached, or free. People of Asian ancestry are more likely to have soldered or attached lobes than are those of African or European descent. Darwin's tubercle, a thickening on the upper ridge of the outer auricle but sometimes present on the front of the upper auricle, is a normal variation in appearance.

Palpate the auricles and mastoid area for tenderness, nodules, or swelling. The auricles should be firm and pliant, without masses. Gentle pushing or palpation during any portion of the external ear examination should not cause

PATIENT EDUCATION AND HEALTH LITERACY

Conditions Affecting Visual Acuity

Cataracts

- Opacity or clouding of the eye lens
- Risk factors include:
  - Increasing age, female gender
  - Prolonged sun exposure
  - Cigarette smoking, alcohol or steroid use
  - Diet low in antioxidants
- Prevention strategies include:
  - Wearing sunglasses and hats when outside
  - Quitting smoking and limiting alcohol consumption
  - Increasing intake of vitamins E and B
- Treatment is:
  - Surgery to replace the cloudy lens with a clear, artificial lens implant

Glaucoma

- Optic neuropathy, usually associated with increased intraocular pressure
- Risk factors include:
  - Increased age, African or Hispanic ancestry
  - Migraines, diabetes, low blood pressure
  - Increased intraocular pressure
  - Family history
  - Eye injury
- Prevention strategies include:
  - Having regular eye examinations by an ophthalmologist
  - Wearing protective eyewear at work, during construction projects, or while participating in sports to prevent injury
  - Limiting caffeine intake, increasing water consumption
  - Engaging in regular physical exercise
- Treatments are:
  - Medicated eyedrops to lower intraocular pressure
  - Laser or open-eye surgery

Macular Degeneration

- Deterioration of the macula, the area on the retina that is responsible for central vision, allowing for clear vision of fine details
- Risk factors include:
  - Family history, white ancestry
  - Overactive immune system causing inflammation
  - Smoking, hypertension, hypercholesterolemia
- Prevention strategies include:
  - Wearing sunglasses when outside
  - Taking dietary supplements including vitamins E, C, B_6, and B_{12} as well as beta carotene, zinc oxide, and copper
  - Eating a healthy, well-balanced diet
- Treatments are:
  - Medication injection treatments
  - Thermal laser therapy
  - Photodynamic therapy

Myopia

- Nearsightedness, caused by a refractive error focusing objects on the front of the retina
- Associated with increased risk for detached retina, glaucoma, and cataracts
- Risk factors include:
  - Familial history
- Treatment is:
  - Eyeglasses, contact lenses, or Lasik surgery

Hyperopia

- Farsightedness, caused by a refractive error focusing objects behind the retina
- Risk factors include:
  - Familial history
- Treatment is:
  - Eyeglasses, contact lenses, or Lasik surgery

Presbyopia

- Age-related loss of near vision due to increased lens rigidity
- Risk factors include:
  - Age older than 40 years
- Treatments are:
  - Reading glasses, bifocal or progressive eyeglasses or contacts
  - Conductive keratoplasty (CK), Lasik or refractive lens exchange surgery

From American Academy of Ophthalmology: Diseases and conditions, 2012. Retrieved from *www.geteyesmart.org/eyesmart/diseases/index.cfm.*

pain. If the auricle or tragus is painful, otitis externa may be present; pain behind the ear can indicate otitis media. Mastoiditis is suspected if there is tenderness or swelling over the mastoid process. There should be no discharge from the external ear.

Cerumen and Discharge

Inspect the external ear canal for discharge or drainage. If any is present, note the color and presence of odor. Discharge that is **purulent** (containing pus) or is accompanied by an odor can indicate infection or foreign body penetration of the middle ear. Severe head trauma or brain injury can produce bloody or serous discharge, suggestive of a skull fracture or cerebrospinal fluid leakage.

A small amount of earwax (**cerumen**), which may be yellow to dark brown in appearance, is the only discharge that should be present during inspection of the external auditory canal. Cerumen assists the ear with removal of particles and debris that may cause damage to the inner ear or tympanic membrane. Excess cerumen, when visible, should be gently cleaned away from the outer ear canal, before the otoscopic examination.

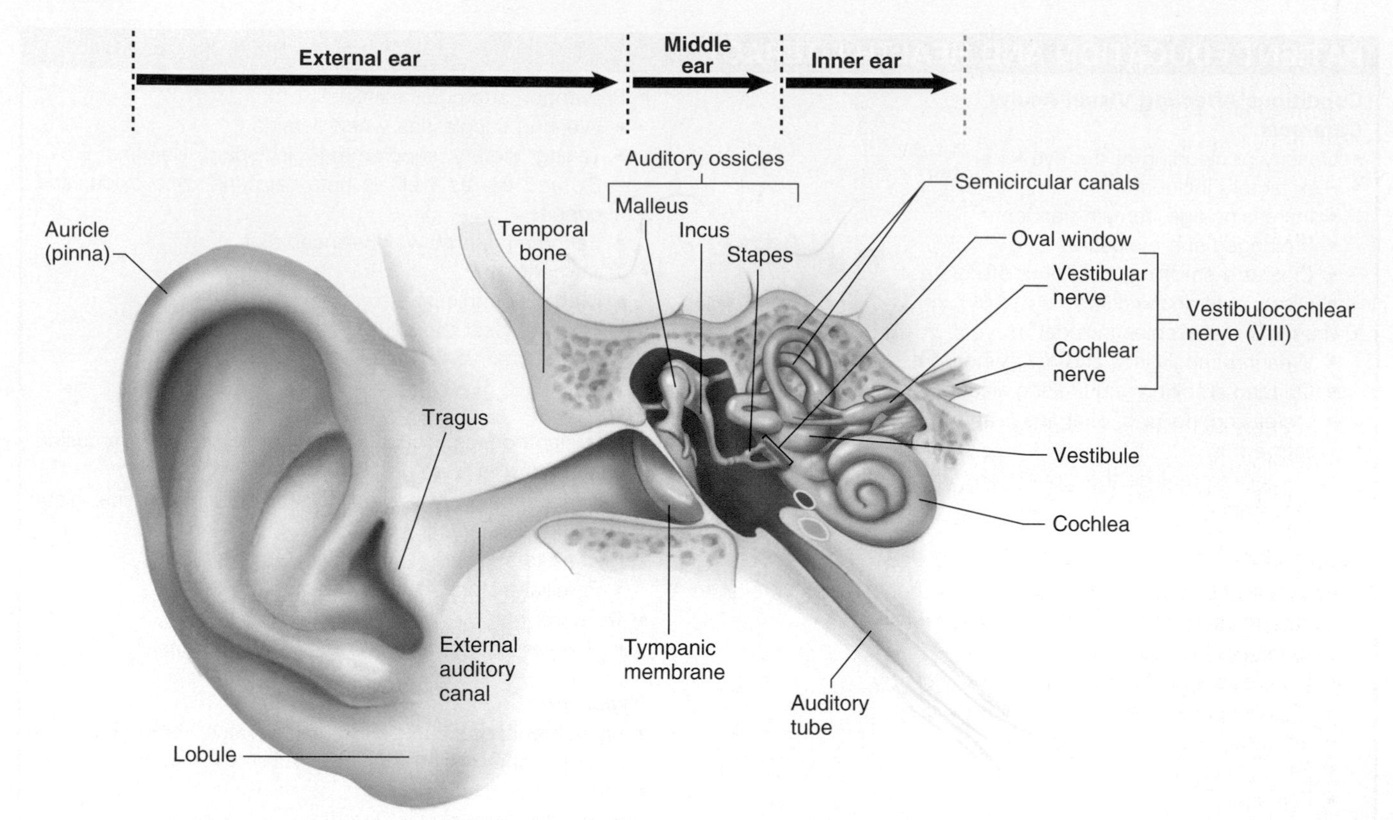

FIGURE 20-14 Normal ear anatomy. (From Thibodeau GA, Patton KT: *The human body in health and disease,* ed. 4, St. Louis, 2005, Mosby.)

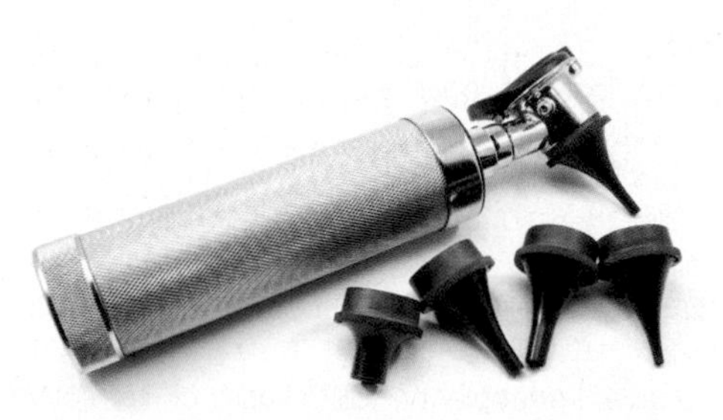

FIGURE 20-15 An otoscope is used to examine the ear canal and tympanic membrane.

Otoscopic Examination

Although complete otoscopic examinations typically are conducted by advanced practice nurses, it is helpful for all nurses to be familiar with ear examination procedures because they often are involved in checking the ears for cerumen and in hearing aid care. An otoscope is used to inspect the auditory canal and tympanic membrane. The otoscope is an ophthalmoscope handle with a magnified lens and cone-shaped viewer, called a *speculum,* which fits into the ear canal (Figure 20-15). Disposable plastic speculum covers are available in a variety of sizes for one-time use. To properly visualize structures, the nurse should select the largest speculum size that fits comfortably into the patient's ear (usually 5 mm for an adult).

The ear canal is straightened by gently pulling the auricle of the ear up and back in adults and down and back in small children. Insert the speculum no more than 1 to 1.5 cm (½ inch) into the ear canal, being careful not to touch the canal wall, because touching it will cause pain.

Do not advance the speculum past the inner third of the auditory canal or as far as the tympanic membrane. Advancing it that far may cause severe pain or damage the auditory canal. Inspect the ear canal, looking for discharge, redness, foreign bodies, or swelling. The ear canal normally appears uniformly pink, with tiny hairs located in the outer third of the canal. A small amount of dry or moist cerumen may be present. During the examination, it is appropriate to ask patients what techniques they use to clean the ear canal and surrounding structures. If piercings are present, inquire about cleaning techniques, infections, or previous allergic reactions.

! SAFE PRACTICE ALERT

Patients with excessive cerumen production should be instructed to clean the outer-ear canals by using a warm, damp cloth or by gently flushing the ear canals with warm water from an ear syringe to promote motility and softening of the cerumen, allowing it to move outward. A softening agent may be needed in some cases. Impacted cerumen in the external auditory canals can contribute to conductive hearing loss.

Light from the otoscope allows the nurse to visualize landmarks characteristic to the tympanic membrane. The normal tympanic membrane is slightly concave and has a translucent, pearly-gray, shiny appearance. The surface should be smooth. Look for retraction, perforation, or a bulging tympanic membrane. Red, bulging eardrums indicate acute otitis media, while visible white spots most often are due to scarring secondary to infection. Eardrum retraction results from an obstructed eustachian tube. Any deviation from normal requires follow-up treatment to prevent hearing loss.

Hearing Evaluation

Assessment of auditory function begins when a patient responds to the nurse's questions and instructions. Hearing loss becomes apparent when a patient fails to respond to conversation or verbal cues. Speech without inflection or appropriate volume may indicate a hearing deficit. All patients should be asked if they experience **tinnitus** (ringing, buzzing, or roaring in the ears), which may contribute to hearing loss, indicate overuse of salicylates, or be symptomatic of diseases that cause **vertigo** (disequilibrium, spinning sensation) such as Ménière's disease. Hearing loss may result from trauma, aging, heredity, disease, medication, and prolonged exposure to high-decibel sound.

The three primary types of hearing loss are sensorineural, conductive, and mixed. *Sensorineural* hearing loss is due to inner-ear damage that prevents sound from being converted to nerve impulses. Possible causes include prolonged exposure to loud sounds and ototoxic medications, such as aminoglycosides, loop diuretics, and antineoplastic agents. Presbycusis is a form of gradual sensorineural hearing loss common in older people that is due to degeneration of the cochlea or vestibulocochlear nerve.

Conductive hearing loss occurs when something interferes with the transmission of sound via vibration to the inner ear. Fluid in the middle ear and cerumen accumulation are the most common causes of vibration interruption. Atrophy of the tympanic membrane or otosclerosis results in conductive hearing loss in older adults. *Mixed* hearing loss results from middle-ear and nerve damage.

Patency of the eighth cranial (acoustic or vestibulocochlear) nerve is assessed in evaluating a patient's hearing acuity. Although the nurse can conduct a primitive evaluation of a patient's ability to hear by whispering and asking the patient to repeat what is heard, the only precise method of determining the quality and limits of a person's hearing is audiometry. Audiometry is conducted by a professional audiologist in a controlled, soundproof environment with equipment that transmits various sound frequencies through headphones.

Weber Test

The Weber test can be conducted if a patient complains of hearing loss in one ear. Through use of a tuning fork, the advanced practice nurse can determine whether the patient is experiencing conductive or sensorineural hearing loss. If the patient reports "hearing" sound from the tuning fork in the poor ear, lateralization of sound to the poor ear has occurred, and conductive hearing loss is indicated. If the patient reports lateralization of sound to the good ear, sensorineural hearing loss is the most likely cause.

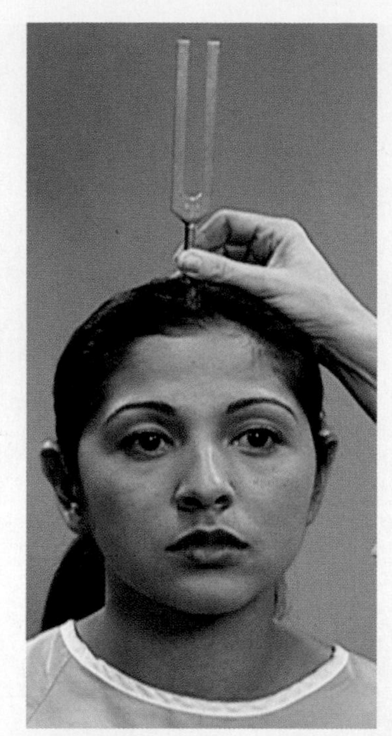

FIGURE 20-16 The Weber test evaluates lateralization of sound via bone conduction. (From Ball JW, Dains JE, Flynn JA, et al: *Seidel's guide to physical examination*, ed. 8, St. Louis, 2015, Mosby.)

To conduct the Weber test, strike the tuning fork softly with the back of the hand and place the base of the vibrating tuning fork against the center of the patient's head or forehead (Figure 20-16). Placement on the midline is critical. Ask the patient if the sound is heard better in one ear or the other or heard the same in both. Vibration detected equally in both ears indicates no hearing loss.

Rinne Test

The Rinne test compares bone and air conduction. It is carried out by gently placing the base of a vibrating tuning fork against the mastoid process behind the ear. The nurse asks the patient to indicate when sound is no longer audible. After the patient has indicated that sound is no longer audible, the tines of the tuning fork are placed in front of the external auditory canal and the patient is again asked to indicate when sound is no longer heard (Figure 20-17). The length of time sound was heard by bone conduction (BC) versus air conduction (AC) is determined. Air-conducted sound should be heard twice as long as bone-conducted sound. Patients with conductive hearing loss will hear bone conduction sound for

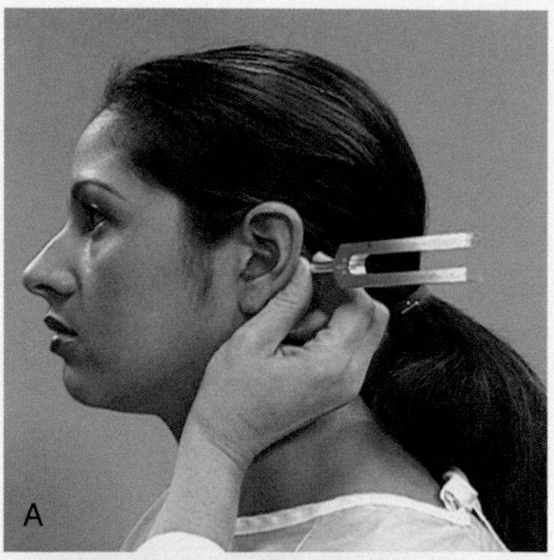

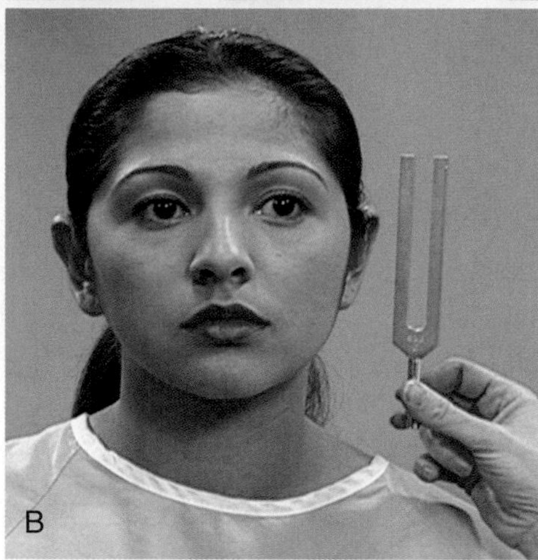

FIGURE 20-17 The Rinne test assesses the patient's ability to hear sound via bone versus air conduction. **A,** Place the tuning fork on the mastoid bone for bone conduction. **B,** To test for air conduction, hold the tuning fork 1 to 2 cm (½ to 1 inch) from the ear with the tines facing forward. (From Ball JW, Dains JE, Flynn JA, et al: *Seidel's guide to physical examination*, ed. 8, St. Louis, 2015, Mosby.)

longer than, or as long as, air conduction sound (BC ≥ AC). If the patient has sensorineural hearing loss, air conduction sound is heard for only slightly longer than bone conduction sound (AC > BC), if sound is heard at all.

Equilibrium

An important function of the inner ear is to aid the person's ability to maintain balance by sensing head movements and position. Patients with inner-ear disorders often experience a loss of equilibrium and vertigo.

Romberg Test

The Romberg test is conducted to assess the patient's equilibrium (Figure 20-18). Patients are asked to stand with their feet together and arms at their sides, first with their eyes open and then with their eyes closed. Patients should be able to maintain balance for at least 20 seconds without moving their feet or starting to fall. Inability to stay balanced with eyes closed may indicate some type of vestibular disease.

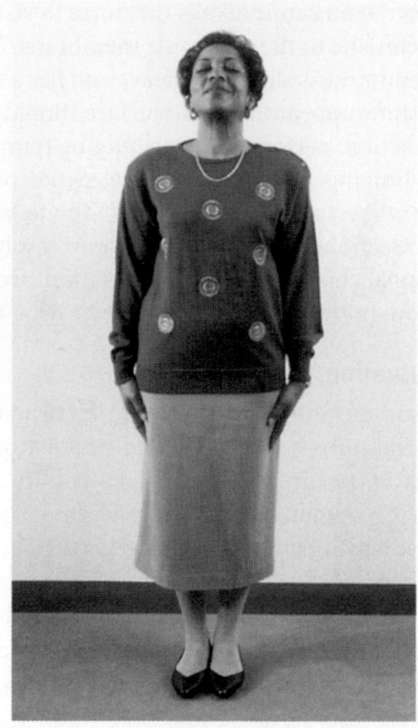

FIGURE 20-18 Romberg test. (From Monahan FD, Sands, JK, Neighbors M, et al: *Phipps' medical-surgical nursing*, ed. 8, St. Louis, 2007, Mosby.)

> **! SAFE PRACTICE ALERT**
>
> Nurses should instruct the patient to open the eyes during the Romberg test if he or she feels about to fall. The nurse also should "spot" the patient (encircling the patient with the nurse's arms, without touching the patient) while conducting the test. This will avoid patient injury from falling.

Nose and Sinus Inspection and Palpation

The nose and sinuses are inspected and palpated with the patient seated. Inspection involves the use of a penlight for examination of each naris and surrounding structures. Assessment of the deeper nares using a nasal speculum or otoscope is conducted by an advanced practice nurse. However, knowledge pertaining to results of speculum examination of the nose is useful for providing nursing care in a patient with nasal or sinus conditions. Each of the sinus cavities is palpated to assess for tenderness or swelling.

Nose

Inspect the nose for color, shape, symmetry, swelling, and tenderness. The nares should be without drainage, and the patient should be free of nasal flaring or narrowing. The skin on and around the nose should be smooth, even, and consistent with the color of facial skin tones.

The central column (septum) of the nose should be straight and midline. A nose that appears crooked may have a deviated septum caused by a traumatic injury or congenital condition. The nares (nostrils) usually are semioval or oval in shape and are symmetrically positioned on each side of the nasal column. The overall shape of the nose extending to the tip varies, depending on the patient's genetic makeup, history of fractures, and clinical manifestations of disease (e.g., skin cancer, alcoholism).

Inspect the mucosa of the patient's nares. Normal mucosa is pink and moist, without lesions or tears. Nasal mucosa may appear swollen or bluish gray in patients with allergies. The mucosa becomes red and swollen in upper respiratory infections. Watch for polyps, which appear as small, round, firm masses. Polyps typically are seen in patients with chronic allergies. Observe for inflammation, ulceration, or a perforated septum, which may be secondary to trauma, chronic infection, or cocaine use. Treatment with nasogastric tubes or nasal cannulas may cause skin breakdown and drying of the nasal mucosa. Frequent assessment of the skin and nares will prevent redness or skin **excoriation** (abrasion due to rubbing or scratching).

Air should pass freely through the nose when the patient breathes. Ask the patient to breathe through one nostril at a time, while the opposite nostril is pressed closed with a fingertip. Inability to sniff through each nostril independently may be due to congestion, swelling, or obstruction by a foreign object. Flaring of the nostrils during breathing may indicate difficulty with inhalation of air.

If nasal discharge is present, note the character, amount, and color of the discharge and whether it is unilateral or bilateral. Drainage may range from excessive watery discharge to thick yellowish-green, purulent mucous to blood. Watery discharge accompanied by sneezing and nasal congestion often indicates an allergy or a response to environmental irritants. A clear, watery discharge occurring after head trauma can be cerebrospinal fluid leakage from a skull fracture. Mucous or purulent discharge is typical of rhinitis, abscess, and upper respiratory tract infection. Bloody nasal discharge often results from **epistaxis** (nosebleed) or trauma, but it can be caused by conditions such as high blood pressure or diabetes.

Palpate the ridge and soft tissues of the nose by placing one finger on each side of the nasal arch and gently pressing the fingers from the nasal bridge to the tip of the nose. Note any displacement of bone or cartilage, tenderness, masses, or lumps. The nasal structures should feel firm yet slightly flexible and should return to their previous shape after palpation. A depression of the nasal bridge can result from a fracture. Palpation should not elicit nasal discharge or irritation.

Sinuses

Inspect the maxillary sinus areas below the eyes for swelling and discoloration, which may be associated with a history of sinusitis, allergies, or recent viral illness. Next, palpate the frontal sinuses by using the thumbs to press up on the eyebrows without pushing on the eyes. Move down to both sides of the nose, and press gently with thumbs up to palpate the maxillary sinuses. Figure 20-19 illustrates palpation of the frontal and maxillary sinuses. No tenderness or swelling should be elicited when light pressure from palpation is applied to soft tissue over sinus areas. Further assessment for tenderness, using percussion, and transillumination of the sinuses, using a light source, is best performed by nurses with advanced clinical experience.

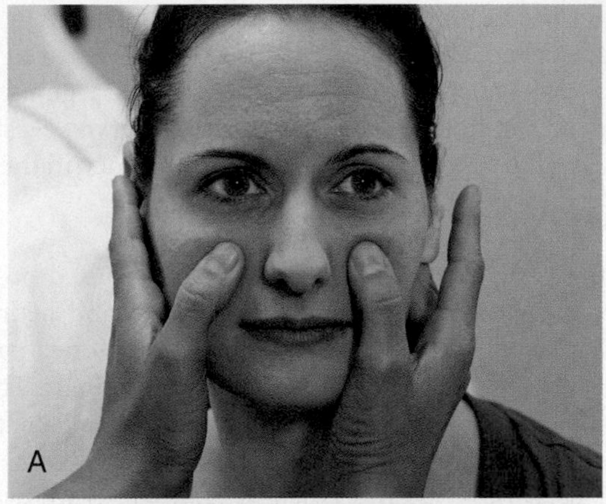

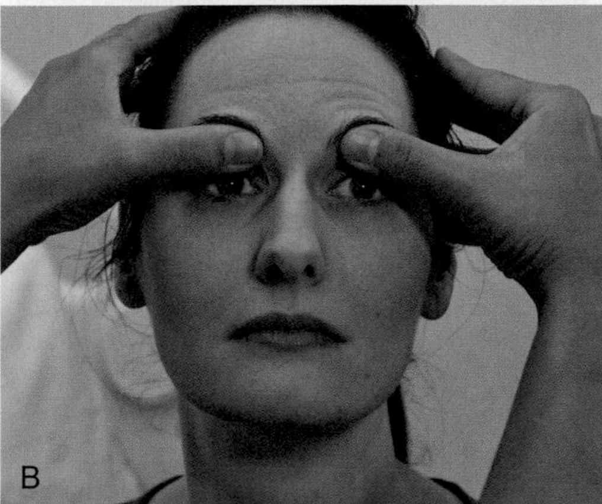

FIGURE 20-19 Palpating the frontal and maxillary sinus cavities. **A,** Maxillary. **B,** Frontal.

Mouth, Throat, and Neck Inspection and Palpation

Assessment of the mouth, throat, and neck provides the nurse with the opportunity to evaluate many aspects of the patient's health status, including:

- Oral hygiene
- Condition of the teeth and gums
- Hydration status
- Airway patency
- Ability to meet nutrition needs
- Patency of cerebral blood flow

The patient may be seated or lying down, with the head of the table or bed elevated approximately 45 degrees during this aspect of the examination. Clean gloves, a penlight, a single 2 × 2 gauze pad, and a tongue depressor are needed to assess the oral cavity, including the lips, buccal mucosa, gums, teeth, tongue, palate, floor of the mouth, and pharynx. A stethoscope is required to assess carotid artery patency in the neck.

Mouth

With the patient's mouth in a closed and relaxed position, inspect the lips for color, patency, scarring, and hydration. Lip color varies, ranging from pink in light-skinned patients to bluish or freckled in darker-skinned individuals. The lips normally are moist, smooth, and symmetric. Palpate the surface of the lips and the skin around them. All surfaces should be without lesions (such as cold sores) or swelling. Patients who had cleft lip repair during childhood may have residual scarring. Note the presence of any piercings or lip enhancement.

Changes in the color or texture of the lips can be influenced by various conditions. Edema most often is the result of an allergic reaction. Pallor is seen if a patient is anemic or in shock, whereas a vibrant red color is typical in cases of ketoacidosis or carbon monoxide poisoning. Acute or chronic respiratory and cardiovascular disorders cause circumoral cyanosis (a bluish-purple hue of the lips and surrounding skin), often extending to the facial tissue around the mouth. Dry, cracked lips (**cheilitis**) often indicate dehydration from limited oral intake or exposure to excessive heat (hyperthermia) or cold. Some nutritional deficiencies may result from poor dental hygiene or jaw dysfunction.

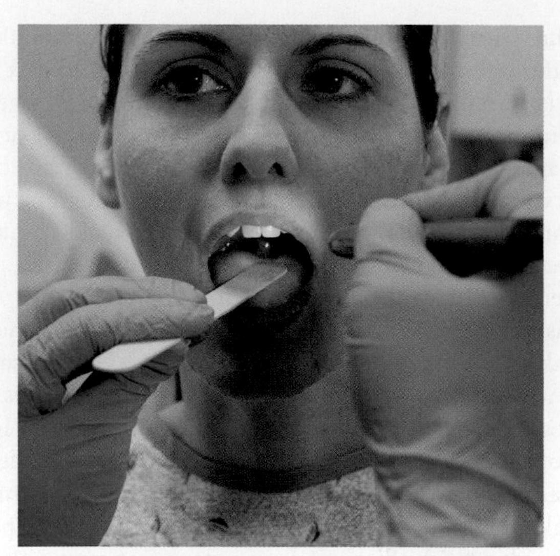

FIGURE 20-20 Oral cavity assessment.

> **! SAFE PRACTICE ALERT**
>
> A variety of patients with artificial heart valves, congenital heart conditions, and artificial joint replacements should be referred to their dentists for prophylactic antibiotics before dental care to prevent infective endocarditis or infection at the joint replacement site. Guidelines developed in cooperation among the American Dental Association (2014), the American Heart Association, and the Academy of Orthopedic Surgeons are available at *www.ada.org/2157.aspx*.

Dental Assessment

Inspection of the teeth determines the quality of dental hygiene and the ability of the patient to chew food for nutritional intake. Inspection begins with asking the patient to smile broadly, observing the teeth for occlusion and alignment. Generally, the upper incisors slightly override the lower incisors, and the upper molars are directly over the lower molars, without spaces or gaps. To test cranial nerve VII (facial nerve) function, ask the patient to demonstrate clenching the teeth and then smiling. The ability to perform this maneuver indicates normal facial nerve functioning.

Next, inspect the teeth for color, irregular shape, and cavities (caries). Loose and missing teeth should be noted, as well as rotted, blackened, or severely decayed teeth. The teeth generally appear ivory or white and are smooth and glossy. A tongue depressor can be used to retract the lips, cheeks, and tongue when viewing the upper and lower molars. The risk for systemic, bacterial infection is greater in teeth with compromised surfaces or cracks that extend below the gum line.

Oral Mucosa, Gums, Tongue, Uvula, Tonsils, and Palate

Using a tongue blade and penlight, inspect the buccal mucosa, teeth, gums, tongue, uvula, tonsils, and palate for color, texture, lesions, ulcers, bleeding, and patency (Figure 20-20). Move the light source systematically throughout the mouth to illuminate and view both the anterior and posterior oral cavities. The mucous membranes should be pale pink to pinkish red in appearance, with a moist, smooth, uninterrupted surface.

Gently insert a clean tongue blade into the patient's mouth, and depress the anterior half of the tongue 2 to 3 cm. This maneuver causes the soft palate to rise, offering better visualization of the oropharynx. Be careful not to insert the tongue depressor onto the posterior aspect of the tongue or near the uvula, because this may stimulate the gag reflex. View the condition of the hard palate, which forms the anterior roof of the mouth, and the soft palate, which forms the posterior roof of the mouth. Observe for any clefts (splits or elongated openings) or signs of palate repair. A yellow or whitish coating over the lining of the pharynx suggests postnasal drip or sinus inflammation. Ask the patient to vocalize the "ah" sound when the tongue is depressed. The soft palate should move symmetrically, with the uvula slightly retracting but remaining centered in the oral cavity. This movement verifies proper function of the glossopharyngeal and vagus nerves (cranial nerves IX and X). If the soft palate does not rise bilaterally with vocalization, the vagus nerve may be damaged, causing the uvula to move to the unaffected side.

Observe the uvula and tonsils for enlargement, edema, and discoloration. Tonsils reach their largest size at puberty and gradually atrophy with aging. Enlarged or inflamed tonsils (tonsillitis) may necessitate surgical removal (tonsillectomy) to prevent chronic infections, airway obstruction, or sleep apnea. White patches or pustules on the tonsils or pharynx typically indicate a bacterial infection requiring antibiotic treatment. Infection within the pharynx may cause palpable enlargement of exterior lymph nodes.

Gently retract the patient's lower lip away from the teeth to inspect the gum line and gums. Gum color should be consistent with the buccal mucosa and covered with a light sheen of saliva, causing the gums to appear shiny. Normal gum tissue appears slightly ridged, with a distinct, firm margin bordering each tooth. Repeat the process for the gum line of the upper jaw. Small, yellow-white, raised areas that appear on the buccal mucosa are an expected variant known as Fordyce spots, which are ectopic sebaceous glands. Discoloration due to jaundice, anemia, or cardiopulmonary conditions is readily observed in the oral mucosa.

Note any abnormalities of the tongue, including unusual size, deep fissures, or lesions, by asking the patient to stick out the tongue. Observe for alignment and tremors that may indicate hypoglossal (cranial nerve XII) damage. A small tongue suggests malnutrition, and an enlarged tongue implies hypothyroidism or Down syndrome. Color deviations suggest various vitamin or nutritional deficiencies. Deep fissures may be due to dehydration.

Before palpating the oral cavity, describe the procedure to the patient to ensure cooperation with manual examination of the mouth. While wearing gloves, insert the index finger into the patient's mouth and carefully palpate the gums and oral mucosa for any lesions, masses, pain, or thickening. No tenderness, bleeding, or swelling should be present.

Using the 2 × 2 gauze pad, gently grasp the tongue and visualize the bottom of the mouth to check for possible lesions or abnormalities. Enlargement or thickening of the gums is expected during pregnancy and at puberty. Leukoplakia (precancerous white spots or patches) may be present owing to chronic irritation or smoking. Oral thrush (candidiasis) is a fungal infection that manifests as a white film over red tissue that bleeds easily. Thrush develops in a variety of patients, including those with a weakened immune system secondary to chemotherapy or steroid therapy. Gingivitis or periodontal disease often is associated with swollen gums that bleed easily and pitted crevices between the teeth and the gum margins. Debris or plaque buildup along the tooth margins significantly contributes to oral mucosa infection, gum disease, and tooth decay. Patients with any of these conditions should be referred for further evaluation by a specialist.

Jaw

Two bones, the maxilla (upper) and the mandible (lower), hold the teeth and form the jaw. The mandible meets the temporal bone at the temporomandibular joint (TMJ). Jaw examination includes inspection for redness or swelling and palpation for edema or warmth. Facing the patient, look for facial asymmetry, indicating swelling or malocclusions. Ask the patient about recent trauma, surgery, or dental procedures. Consider that jaw pain may accompany symptoms of life-threatening disorders such as an impending myocardial infarction. While the patient opens and closes the mouth, listen for any clicking, and note any reported pain. Refer the patient to a specialist for further evaluation for possible temporomandibular joint disorder (TMD).

Lymph Nodes

The lymph system produces lymphocytes and antibodies that serve as a defense against infection and abnormal cells. Several lymph nodes are located in the head and neck (Figure 20-21). The superficial lymph nodes in the neck, which are not palpable under normal circumstances, are readily accessible for examination. An entire group (or chain) of lymph nodes becomes enlarged when it receives drainage from a specific area of infection or disease. For this reason, an understanding of drainage patterns of the lymph system is necessary for the nurse to focus the assessment on the corresponding affected area of the body.

To begin examination of the lymph nodes of the neck, ask the patient to raise the chin and slightly tilt the head to one side and then the other. Inspect the neck for bilateral symmetry and abnormalities by comparing the superficial skin features. Ask the patient to face directly forward with the chin slightly elevated. Using the pads of the middle two or three fingers of both hands, gently palpate the lymph nodes on each side of the patient's neck simultaneously, comparing one side with the other. Begin palpation at the top of a lymph group, rotating the fingers in a circular motion down the sides of the neck.

Note the size, shape, location, and consistency of any palpable nodes. Consider the warmth of the skin over the area, and note whether palpable nodes are mobile or stationary

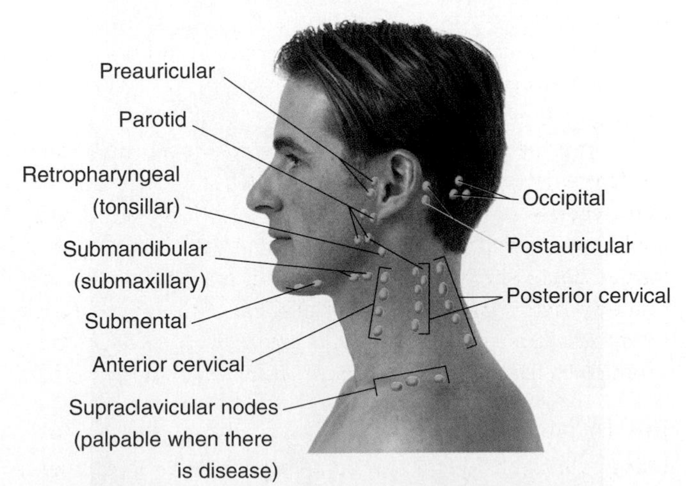

FIGURE 20-21 Lymph nodes of the head and neck. (From Ball JW, Dains, JE, Flynn JA, et al: *Seidel's guide to physical examination,* ed. 8, St. Louis, 2015, Mosby.)

compared with the surrounding structures. Any tenderness with palpation or movement of the neck should also be documented. Small, soft, nontender nodes are typically benign discoveries during routine examination. Abnormal results consist of lymph nodes that are hard, fixed (immobile), or enlarged and usually are associated with pain and/or inflammation. Enlarged lymph nodes are common in patients with immunocompromised and autoimmune conditions, such as HIV infection, allergies, malignancy, or systemic lupus erythematosus (SLE).

Neck

Assessment of the neck includes inspection, palpation, and auscultation. Neck muscles are examined for flexibility, strength, and discomfort. Patients should be able to move the head up and down and from side to side without limitation or pain. Strength and full range of motion of the neck is assessed during the musculoskeletal part of the physical examination.

Jugular Veins

The jugular veins are observed for distention and blood flow. Increased blood volume or conditions interfering with the flow of blood into the right side of the heart can increase jugular vein distention (JVD). Observe the jugular veins while the patient is seated, with the head of the table or bed elevated approximately 45 degrees (Figure 20-22). Document the findings of jugular vein assessment by noting whether JVD is present or absent.

Carotid Arteries

The carotid arteries, which provide blood supply to the head, are assessed for patency of blood flow. The nurse inspects the carotid arteries to see whether bounding pulses are visible. One at a time, palpate each carotid artery. It is vital to palpate only one carotid artery at a time, to avoid limiting blood flow to the brain and causing the patient to experience syncope and pass out. After completion of palpation, each carotid artery is auscultated (Figure 20-23) for the presence of a **bruit** (abnormal "swooshing" sound). Bruits are audible during auscultation when blood flow is partially or significantly obstructed.

Thyroid Gland and Trachea

The last two areas of the neck to examine are the thyroid gland and the trachea. Inspect the thyroid gland for position and enlargement. The thyroid gland is the largest endocrine gland in the body. It produces thyroid hormones necessary to increase the metabolic rate of cells in the body. The thyroid gland should appear midline in the neck (Figure 20-24, *A*) and move up and down without discomfort when the patient swallows. Any thyroid enlargement (Figure 20-24, *B*) should be noted for further palpation by an advanced practice nurse or physician.

The trachea consists of cartilage rings and is positioned anterior to the esophagus and midline in the neck directly above the sternal notch. It provides a passage for air from the lungs to the upper respiratory system. It should be palpated by feeling for the cartilage rings at the sternal notch. Tumors, thyroid gland enlargement, or conditions such as pneumothorax may cause the trachea to be deviated to one side.

Any abnormalities, limitations to movement, or emergent conditions found in the neck region should be promptly identified and addressed to prevent permanent disability or loss of function.

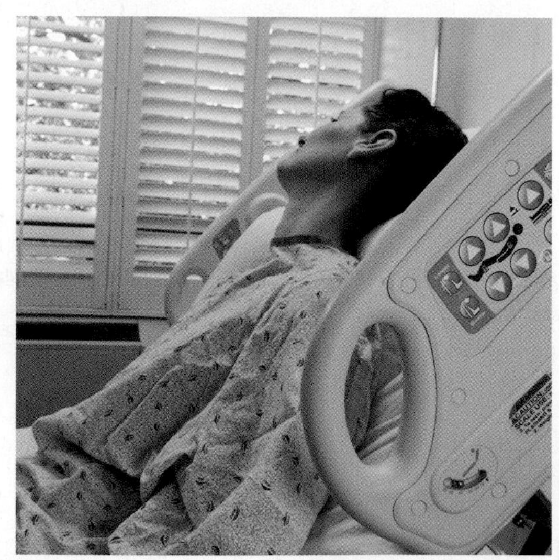

FIGURE 20-22 Position for assessment of jugular vein distention.

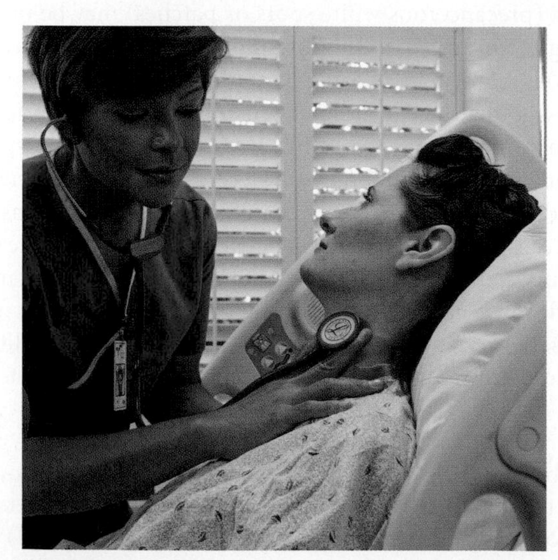

FIGURE 20-23 Auscultation of the carotid artery.

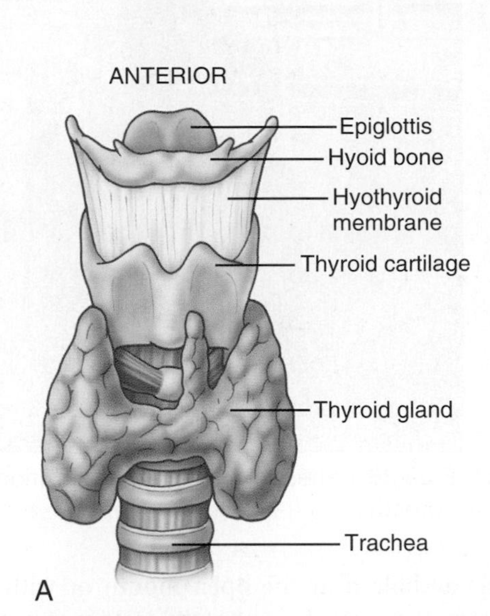

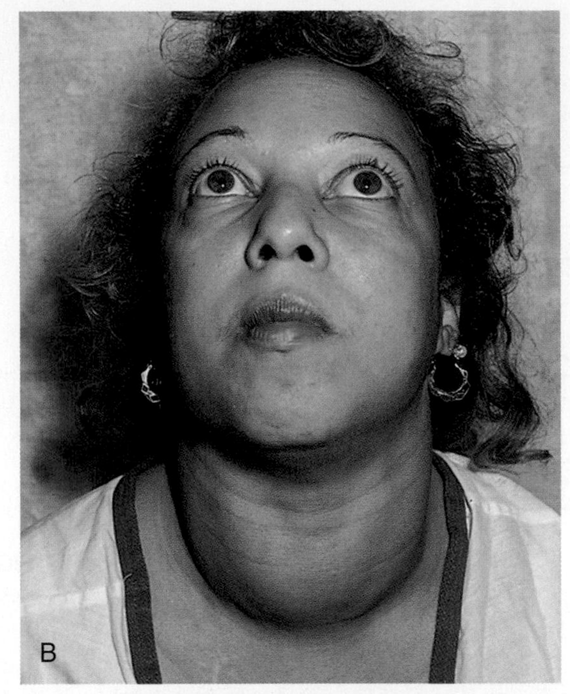

FIGURE 20-24 Thyroid gland. **A,** Location. **B,** Enlargement. (**A,** from Rothrock JC: *Alexander's care of the patient in surgery,* ed. 15, St. Louis, 2015, Mosby. **B,** from Swartz MH: *Textbook of physical diagnosis,* ed. 7, St. Louis, 2015, Saunders.)

RESPIRATORY ASSESSMENT

Assessment of respiratory status begins with questioning the patient about risks for pulmonary complications by using the health assessment questions in the Health Assessment Questions box. Data gathered on all body systems are synthesized to determine the extent and effect of lung alterations within the body, because oxygenation affects all tissues and organs.

> **! SAFE PRACTICE ALERT**
>
> If at any time a patient appears to be in significant respiratory distress or complains of severe chest pain or shortness of breath, help should be sought immediately.

The nurse performs the assessment with knowledge of the structure and function of the respiratory system. Figure 20-25 illustrates the organs of respiration.

Inspection of the Chest and Breathing

Inspection of the chest requires access to the patient's thoracic area. Patients are asked to disrobe to the waist. A gown is offered to preserve privacy. Sitting is the best position for assessment of the posterior and lateral chest. For examination of the anterior chest, the patient can sit or lie down.

Shape and Configuration

Inspect the anterior and posterior thorax for symmetry and shape. Observe chest hair for color, thickness, and even

> **HEALTH ASSESSMENT QUESTIONS**
>
> **Respiratory System**
>
> - How far can you walk on level ground?
> - How many stairs are you able to climb without becoming short of breath?
> - Do you have a cough? If so, when did it start?
> - Do you cough up mucus or blood?
> - Can you lie flat when sleeping?
> - Do you snore?
> - Do you use oxygen or breathing machines at home?
> - Do you ever experience shortness of breath either at rest or with exercise?
> - Do you have any pain with breathing?
> - Is the pain associated with coughing, shortness of breath, trauma, nasal congestion, or sore throat?
> - Does chest pain cause splinting, shallow breathing, or uneven chest expansion, or does it radiate to the back, neck, or arms?
> - What relieves the chest pain associated with respiration?
> - Do you have any recent history of trauma or infection?
> - Do you have a history of chronic conditions that affect respiration, including allergies, emphysema, chronic obstructive pulmonary disease, tuberculosis, cystic fibrosis, or asthma?
> - Do you have a history of tumors or lung cancer?
> - Do you use tobacco or marijuana? If so, how many years and packs per day?
> - Have you been exposed to dust, fumes, or smoke in the environment at work or home?
> - Have you traveled out of the country recently?

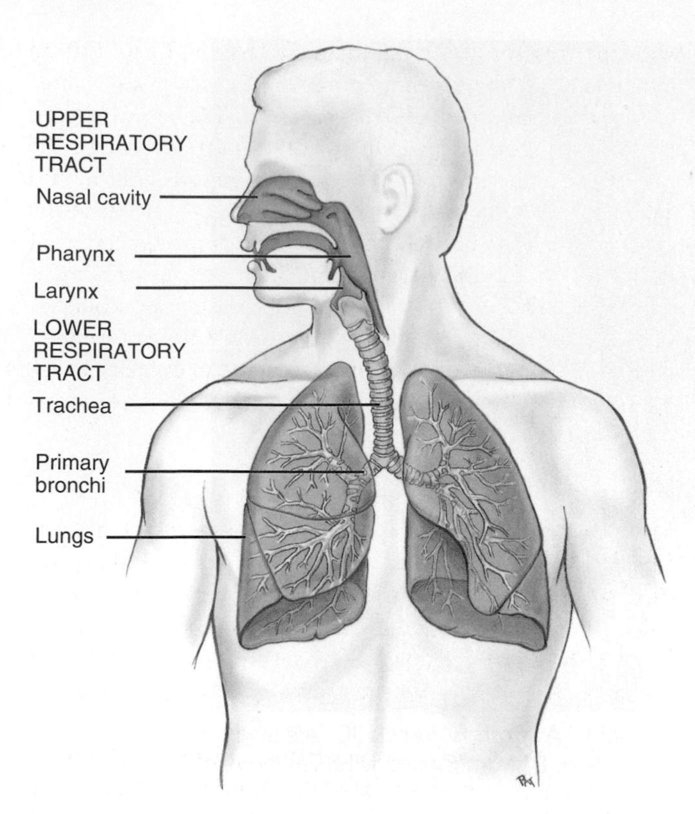

FIGURE 20-25 Respiratory system. (From Applegate E: *The anatomy and physiology learning system,* ed. 3, St. Louis, 2007, Saunders.)

distribution across the chest and upper abdomen. Nipples should be centered on either side of the sternum. Observe the spine, which normally is midline and straight. Ribs should slope downward, with symmetric intercostal spaces. The scapulae lie flat on either side of the spine. The normal anteroposterior (AP) diameter of the chest is less than the transverse (across-the-chest) diameter, with normal ratios of 1:2 to 5:7. Note any lesions, scarring, or grossly asymmetric features.

Accessory muscles of breathing—the sternocleidomastoid, intercostal, trapezius, and abdominal muscles—require little effort or movement with normal, passive respiration. In situations in which effort is needed to breathe, such as with exercise or pulmonary disease, the accessory muscles respond to the increased demand by contracting and relaxing to provide respiratory support. In such situations, retraction of the intercostal muscles can be seen during inspiration.

Breathing Patterns

Observation of the patient's breathing pattern is done during inspection of the anterior chest while the patient breathes passively. Normal breathing patterns are relaxed, automatic, and effortless. Respiratory rates in adults usually are between 12 and 20 bpm. The chest expands symmetrically, with regular and even inspiratory and expiratory effort. Normal breathing is quiet and produces no noise. Respirations are

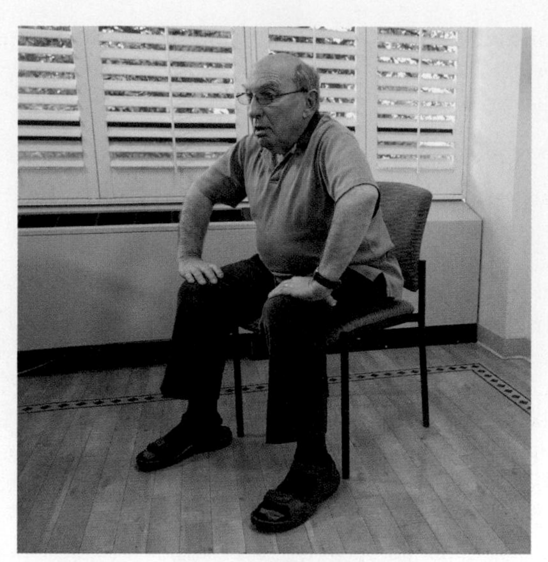

FIGURE 20-26 Patient sitting in tripod position due to shortness of breath.

barely audible near the open mouth or with normal nasal patency. Observe the patient's posture during respiration. The patient should appear relaxed, with the arms comfortably at the sides or with the hands folded in the lap.

Abnormal Assessment Findings

When cerebral palsy, rib fracture, or severe skeletal muscle deformities such as kyphosis are present, movement of the thoracic cage may be limited. This impairment can cause decreased oxygenation or lead to greater susceptibility to infection from pooled secretions or air trapped in the lungs.

In patients with chronic lung disease such as emphysema and chronic obstructive pulmonary disease (COPD), the AP diameter of the chest often is equal to the transverse diameter of the chest, resulting in a "barrel chest" appearance. With this altered anatomy, the ribs become horizontal, losing their downward slope, and the neck muscles undergo hypertrophy from aiding with forced respirations. Chronic lung disease causes hyperinflation of the lungs and forces the patient to adopt a tripod-type posture (leaning forward with the arms braced against the knees, chair, or bed) for the most effective breathing. A tripod posture (Figure 20-26) provides leverage and stability to the patient so that the abdominal, intercostal, and accessory muscles of the neck can assist in expiration. Pursed-lip breathing usually is observed during expiration to slow the patient's rate of breathing and to assist with decreasing respiratory effort.

Unequal excursion of the chest occurs when part of the lung is obstructed or collapsed. This can be due to trauma, infection, or chronic lung disease that causes remodeling of lung tissue. If the patient is experiencing pain in the chest, guarding, splinting (holding an object, such as a pillow, to apply pressure), and grimacing may be seen. Patients with cerebral hypoxia from pulmonary alterations can demonstrate changes in mental status ranging from excessive drowsiness and restlessness to anxiety, irritability, and disorientation.

Palpation of the Chest

Palpate the patient's anterior and posterior thorax to evaluate chest size, shape, and movement. Beginning at the patient's shoulders and moving downward, gently press portions of the thorax with the middle three fingertips of both hands to identify underlying structures. Avoid sliding the hands over the skin or hair on the thorax, to prevent discomfort or abrasions. The chest wall normally is nontender and free of masses or lesions. Note any superficial lumps or masses, increased skin temperature, moisture, or tenderness during palpation. If lesions or masses are present, lightly palpate around the area for size, quality, and shape of the lesion. Avoid deep palpation to tender areas if there is a possibility that the patient has rib fractures. Rib fractures can contain fragments that are easily dislodged into vital organs. Note whether any pain, exudate, or erythema is elicited during palpation.

Tactile fremitus is a palpable vibration transmitted through the chest wall that occurs with the movement of the vocal cords during speech. It normally is symmetric on both sides of the chest and is best felt on the posterior chest. The nurse palpates for tactile fremitus by placing the fingers of one hand on the patient's chest while the patient repeats the words *ninety-nine.* Begin at the top of the lungs, and palpate from one side to the other for comparison. The vibrations should feel the same on each side. Normally, fremitus is more noticeable between the scapulae and around the sternal borders because the major bronchi and bronchioles are more superficial at these sites. Fremitus vibrations commonly decrease with downward palpation, because more tissue and posterior placement of the lungs combine to impede sound transmission. Tactile fremitus is decreased or absent in patients with conditions that obstruct lung tissue, such as pneumothorax, tumors, pleural effusion, or COPD. It can be increased in patients with pneumonia or consolidation close to the chest wall.

Evaluation of the patient's chest excursion, or depth of breathing, is done when there is a concern about chest expansion. Place warmed hands on the posterolateral chest wall, with the thumbs at the approximate level of T9 to T10 on either side of the spine (Figure 20-27). Move the hands toward the spine (medially) to create a small skin fold between the thumbs. Ask the patient to inhale deeply through the mouth, and note thumb movement during inspiration and expiration. The thumbs should move apart symmetrically by approximately 3 to 5 cm (1 to 2 inches). Common causes of decreased or asymmetric chest excursions include pain, musculoskeletal deformity, postural anomalies, lung collapse, obesity, and muscle fatigue or weakness. Chest movement declines with age because of increasing costal cartilage rigidity, atrophy of the diaphragm, and the effects of osteoporosis on the vertebral bodies.

Auscultation of the Lungs

Breath sounds are produced by air moving through the structures of the respiratory tract during inspiration and expiration. They are heard through auscultation with a stethoscope placed directly on the skin. Normal breath sounds are categorized by the airways that transmit them to the chest wall, with the larger airways producing louder and higher-pitched sounds (Table 20-6).

Inspiration normally is longer than expiration in adults. Breath sounds are more difficult to auscultate in obese patients owing to increased tissue mass. Gently moving breast

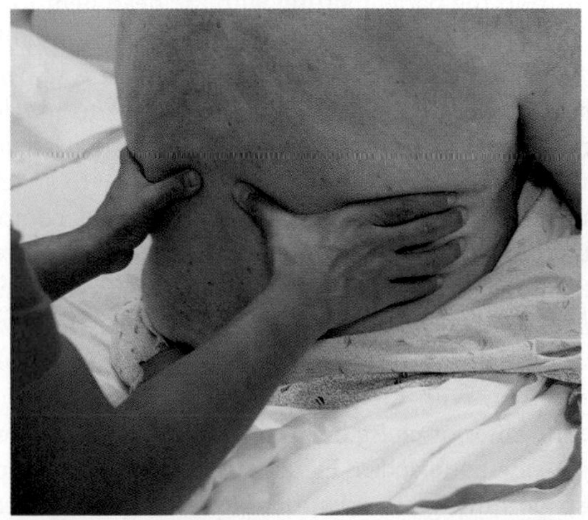

FIGURE 20-27 Assessment of chest excursion.

TABLE 20-6 Normal Breath Sounds

BREATH SOUND	PITCH	QUALITY	AMPLITUDE	DURATION	LOCATION
Tracheal	High	Harsh	Loud		Over the trachea
Bronchial	High	Hollow	Loud	Inspiration < expiration	Over the main bronchi
Bronchovesicular	Medium	Mixed	Medium	Inspiration = expiration	Posterior between the scapulae; anterior around the upper sternum in the first two intercostal spaces
Vesicular	Low	Blowing	Soft	Inspiration > expiration	Over most of the lung fields

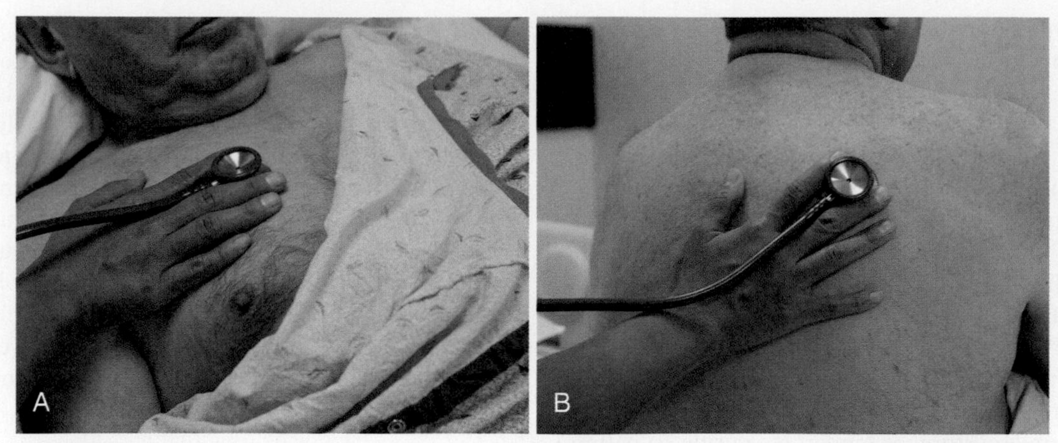

FIGURE 20-28 Placement of the stethoscope for anterior **(A)** and posterior **(B)** auscultation of the chest.

tissue away from the chest wall may be necessary for a more accurate assessment. In children, breath sounds are louder because the chest wall is thinner. When normal lung tissue is displaced by air (emphysema or pneumothorax) or fluid (pleural effusion), breath sounds may be decreased or absent. They may be diminished on auscultation if the patient has **atelectasis** (collapse of all or part of the lung) or absent if the patient has had a lobectomy.

To auscultate posterior breath sounds, stand at the patient's side. Position the patient sitting with the head bent forward. Using the diaphragm of the stethoscope, begin auscultating at the top of the lungs over the posterior chest wall between the ribs at approximately C7. Ask the patient to inhale and exhale through the mouth with slow breaths that are a little deeper than usual. Use a side-to-side sequence to systematically move downward on the posterior chest wall, comparing sounds from one side with those from the other. Auscultate an entire cycle of inspiration and expiration at each location. Auscultate both sides laterally from the axillae down to the seventh or eighth intercostal space, with the patient's arms slightly raised. With the patient sitting or lying supine, auscultate the anterior chest, beginning at the top and following a side-to-side pattern. See Figure 20-28 for placement of the stethoscope during auscultation. Note the quality, location, and characteristics of sounds throughout the thorax. Understanding sounds caused by normal respiration can assist the nurse with better recognition of sounds associated with airway impediment or abnormality.

Abnormal sounds that originate in the lungs and airways are referred to as **adventitious breath sounds**. Such sounds are a result of either airway narrowing or fluid accumulation. Adventitious breath sounds are described in Table 20-7.

CARDIAC AND PERIPHERAL VASCULAR ASSESSMENT

Assessment of the cardiac and peripheral vascular systems builds on information gained while reviewing the respiratory system. Concerns with any one of these systems can have a direct impact on the functioning of the other. The Health Assessment Questions box lists questions that can be used to gather critical information for a patient regarding cardiovascular health.

Assessment of the cardiovascular system requires that the nurse understand the anatomy of the heart and the function of the circulatory system throughout the body. Cardiovascular health is dependent on rhythmic, electrical cardiac impulses and adequate blood supply throughout the body by arteries and veins. Figure 20-29 shows the structure of the heart, which lies under the anterior chest wall. See Chapter 38 for a more detailed description of cardiac function in the context of oxygenation.

Inspection and Palpation of the Heart

Assist the patient into a supine position, or raise the head of the bed 45 degrees. Inspect and palpate following a systematic sequence according to anatomic position. Cardiac function is assessed through the anterior chest wall. The right ventricle composes most of the heart's anterior surface. A portion of the left ventricle is in close proximity to the fourth and fifth intercostal spaces of the anterior chest, medial to the left midclavicular line.

Begin with the base of the heart, and move in the direction of the apex. Inspect and palpate the angle of Louis and sternal ridge. There are anatomic landmarks on the chest wall where heart valve closures are best palpated and auscultated. Find the second intercostal space on the right to locate the first of these landmarks, the aortic area. The second area, the pulmonic region, can be found at the second or third intercostal space on the left. The tricuspid area is found at the fourth or fifth intercostal space, along the sternum. The mitral area is located at the fifth intercostal space, to the left of the sternum, and laterally to the left midclavicular line. The apical impulse, or PMI, is located in the mitral area at the left fifth intercostal space at the midclavicular line. The PMI is felt as a brief pulsation in the area 1 to 2 cm (½ to ¾ inch) around the

TABLE 20-7 **Adventitious Breath Sounds**

SOUND	SITE	CAUSE	CHARACTER
Crackles (formerly called *rales*)	Right and left lung bases	Sudden opening of small airways and alveoli collapsed by fluid or exudate; heard in patients with cystic fibrosis, asthma, COPD, bronchitis, and pulmonary edema from left-sided heart failure	Brief crackling, popping sounds heard when a blocked airway suddenly opens; more common during inspiration; often described as fine, medium, and coarse: *Fine crackles:* Soft, high-pitched, and very brief sounds during late inspiration and not cleared by coughing *Medium crackles:* Lower-pitched, moist sounds best heard at the inspiratory midpoint *Coarse crackles:* Loud, effervescent sounds heard best during inspiration and not relieved after coughing
Rhonchi	Over the trachea and bronchi, but can be referred to all lung fields	Increased secretions in large airways due to pneumonia, increased airway turbulence from mucus or muscle spasm	Low-pitched, snoring sounds heard either during inspiration or expiration and usually cleared with coughing; lower in pitch than wheezes, with a sonorous quality
Wheezing	All lung fields	High-velocity airflow through severely constricted or obstructed airways due to asthma, foreign objects, bronchiectasis, or emphysema	High-pitched, whistling sound heard on inspiration or expiration but most obvious and loudest during expiration; also called *sibilant wheezing*
Stridor	Trachea and large airways	Turbulent airflow in the upper airway; may be indicative of serious airway obstruction from epiglottitis, croup, a foreign body lodged in the airway, or a laryngeal tumor	Intense, high-pitched, and continuous monophonic wheeze or crowing sound, loudest during inspiration when airways collapse owing to lower internal lumen pressure; often heard without the aid of a stethoscope
Pleural friction rub	Anterior lateral thorax	Inflamed pleural surfaces rubbing together during respiration, due to pneumonia or pleuritis	Low-pitched, grating, or creaking sound heard during inspiration or expiration and not cleared by coughing

region of the apex. It is not uncommon to visualize the apical impulse when the patient sits up, because the heart moves closer to the anterior chest wall.

The final anatomic landmark is the epigastric area just below the tip of the sternum. The abdominal aorta is located in the upper midline abdomen, 2 to 3 inches above the umbilicus and below the xiphoid process. It is best palpated by applying gentle, downward pressure with the flattened fingers of both hands to indent the epigastrium toward the spine. Applying firm pressure can dampen aortic pulsations or cause unnecessary discomfort. Ask the patient to completely relax the abdominal muscles. In extremely obese people or in those with very developed abdominal musculature, aortic pulsation may not be detected. Bounding aortic pulsations may indicate an abdominal aortic aneurysm.

The size and stature of the patient are taken into account in performing a heart assessment. People who are tall or have a greater torso-to-leg length often have a heart that is positioned more centrally in the thorax and is suspended more vertically. By contrast, people who are stocky, have shorter torsos, or are short of stature tend to have a heart that sits more horizontally and to the left side of the thoracic cavity.

Auscultation of the Heart

Auscultation of the heart focuses on identifying low-intensity sounds created by heart valve closures. It detects normal heart sounds, murmurs, gallops, and other extra heart sounds. Heart sounds are heard in relation to physiologic activity of the cardiac cycle. On auscultation, two distinct heart sounds known as S1 ("lub") and S2 ("dub") are heard. An entire S1 plus S2 ("lub-dub") cycle constitutes one heartbeat. S1 is the sound of the mitral and tricuspid valves closing and marks the beginning of systole. The S1 sound is dull and low-pitched and is heard best at the apex of the heart. It should coordinate with carotid artery pulsation. S2 is the sound of the aortic

HEALTH ASSESSMENT QUESTIONS

Cardiovascular System

- Are you experiencing chest pain? If so, describe the pain. When was its onset or when did the pain begin? What is its duration or how long have you had this pain? What are the characteristics of the pain (sharp, stabbing, aching, burning, viselike)? Where is the pain? Does the pain radiate? Does anything relieve the pain? Are there any other symptoms associated with the pain?
- Do you have any palpitations or extreme fatigue?
- Do you have any difficulty breathing or difficulty lying flat when sleeping?
- Do you have any past medical history of cardiac surgery or hospitalizations for cardiac events or disorders?
- Have you ever had acute rheumatic fever, swollen or painful joints, or inflammatory rheumatism?
- Do you have any chronic illnesses such as hypertension, hyperlipidemia, diabetes, coronary artery disease, congenital heart defects, or bleeding disorders?
- Do you have a family history of diabetes, heart disease, hypertension, hyperlipidemia, obesity, congenital or acquired heart defects, or sudden death at a young age? If so, include age at the time of diagnosis and death of first-degree relatives.
- Are you on an anticoagulant? Do you have a coagulation disorder?
- Does your employment include physical demands, emotional stress, or environmental hazards such as chemicals, heat, sunlight, or dust?
- Do you use tobacco? If so, at what age did you start? How many packs per day? Have you stopped using it?
- How often do you use alcohol or recreational drugs?
- What is your nutritional status? Have you lost or gained weight recently?
- What do you do to relax?
- Do you exercise? How much and how often?
- Do you have aching, cramping, or pain in the legs while walking or exercising? If so, when did it start, how long have you had it, and what are its characteristics? Does anything relieve the pain?
- Have you ever had loss of consciousness or transient syncope? If so, was the episode associated with any other symptoms?
- Does shortness of breath interfere with your activities of daily living?
- Do you have any tingling, numbness, or coldness in your hands or feet?
- Do you have edema or swelling in your hands, feet, or ankles? If so, what makes it worse? What reduces the edema?
- Have you had any recent change in hair loss or growth on your hands, feet, or ankles?
- Has anything restricted blood flow to your extremities (cast, surgery, trauma, tight clothing)?

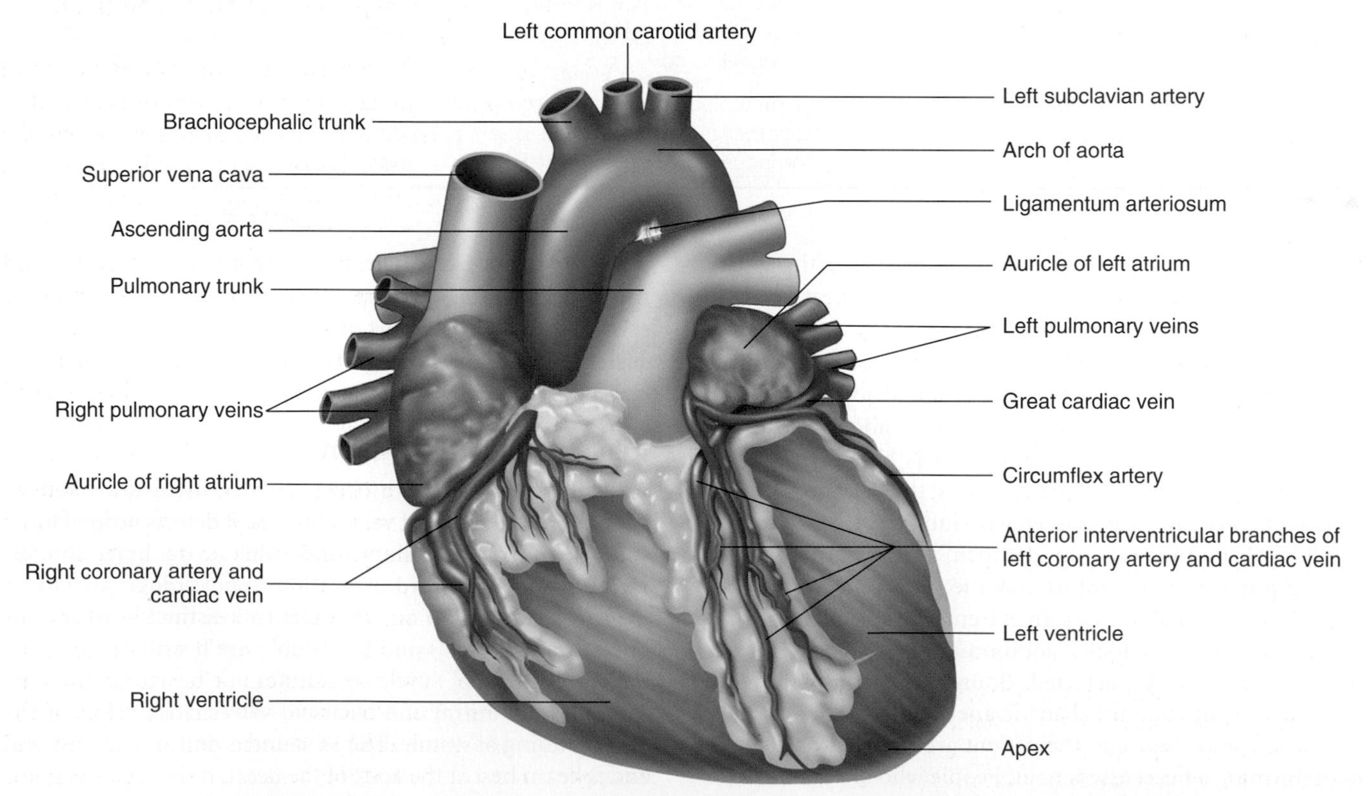

FIGURE 20-29 Structure of the heart. (From Thibodeau GA, Patton KT: *Anatomy and physiology,* ed. 5, St. Louis, 2003, Mosby.)

and pulmonic valves closing and marks the end of systole and the beginning of diastole. It is best heard in the aortic region.

In some cases, rapid ventricular filling creates a third heart sound, S3 ("lub-dub-dub"), which is heard more often in children and adolescent patients. Presence of an S3 sound usually is a benign condition that the affected person outgrows as the cardiac vasculature becomes thicker and stronger. An S3 murmur is considered abnormal in adults older than 25 to 30 years of age. When atria contract to enhance ventricular filling, a fourth heart sound, S4, is created. It is heard just before S1 ("lub-lub-dub"). An S4 heart sound is not a normal finding in adults, but it can be heard in healthy older adults, children, and athletes. Because it may indicate an abnormal condition, the presence of an S4 heart sound should be documented and reported to the patient's health care provider.

! SAFE PRACTICE ALERT

A new onset of S4, a pulse deficit, or extra heart sounds should be reported to the patient's primary care provider for further investigation.

In a quiet environment, auscultate for the complete cycle of heart sounds ("lub-dub"), using the diaphragm first and then the bell of the stethoscope at each of the anatomic locations (Figure 20-30) associated with cardiac valves and blood flow. Take time to isolate each sound, and listen for as many beats as necessary to evaluate the sounds. Glide the stethoscope systematically through each of the anatomic areas in a sequence moving from the base to the apex of the heart. Breast tissue may need to be gently moved to allow heart sounds to be heard more clearly. Use firm pressure with the diaphragm and light pressure with the bell for better auscultation of heart murmurs. Usually, auscultation in all areas is performed with the patient in the supine, sitting, and left lateral recumbent positions if the patient's condition permits.

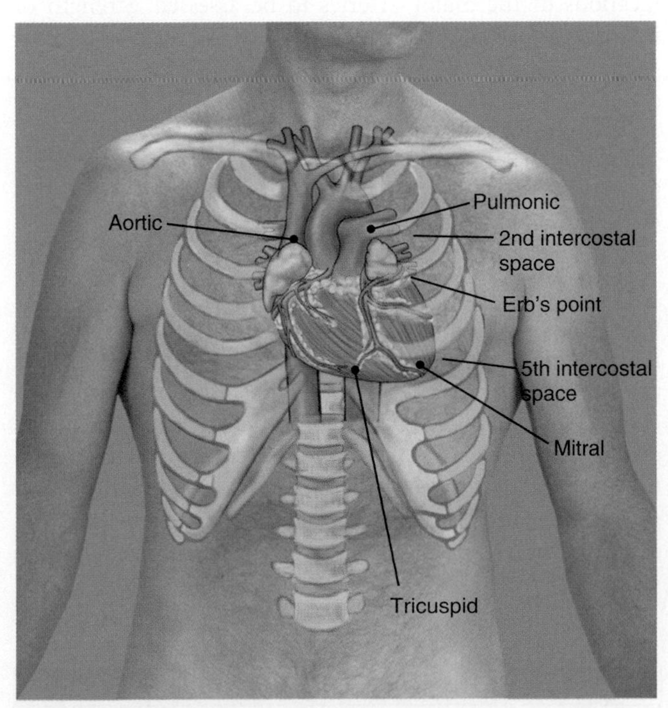

FIGURE 20-30 Anatomic locations for heart auscultation. (In Linton AD: *Introduction to medical-surgical nursing*, ed. 5, St. Louis, 2012, Saunders. From Monahan FD, Drake DT, Neighbors M, eds: *Medical-surgical nursing: Foundations for clinical practice*, ed. 2, Philadelphia, 1998, Saunders.)

To count an apical pulse, listen over the mitral area for 1 full minute. Note the interval between S1 and S2, as well as the interval between S1 and the next S1 cycle. The intervals between each heartbeat should be regular, with a distinct silent pause between S1 and S2. A regular rhythm involves equal intervals of time between each cardiac cycle of heartbeats. Failure of the heart to beat at regular, successive intervals is called **dysrhythmia**. Dysrhythmias can be life-threatening, depending on the portion of the cardiac cycle affected. Dysrhythmia, a disturbance in the normal rhythm of the heart, can prevent the ventricles from effectively pumping blood to the lungs and body. The atrioventricular (AV) node, responsible for the conduction of the heart's electrical impulse from the atria to the ventricles, restricts the number of impulses that can pass through it in a given period. This functional limit prevents the ventricles from contracting at disproportionate or excessive rates when atrial disease produces atypical impulses. The electrical activity of the heart correlates with the heart cycle and can be seen on an electrocardiogram (ECG).

When listening to an irregular heart rhythm, assess apical and radial pulse rates at the same time to determine whether a pulse deficit exists. A **pulse deficit** is present when the patient's radial pulse rate is slower than the apical pulse rate because of cardiac contractions that are weak or ineffective at pumping blood to the peripheral tissues and extremities. A pulse deficit can indicate a serious cardiac event, and the patient's health care provider should be notified immediately.

Assess for extra heart sounds at each cardiac landmark by using the bell of the stethoscope and listening for low-pitched extra heart sounds such as an S3 or S4 gallop, clicks, and rubs. In some patients, extra heart sounds are heard more clearly with position changes. If clicks, snaps, or scratching sounds are heard on auscultation, the primary care provider should be notified so that a determination can be made about referral to a cardiologist.

During auscultation at cardiac landmarks, listen for cardiac murmurs. **Cardiac murmurs** are blowing or swishing sounds heard in systole or diastole. They are caused by increased or abnormal blood flow through the valves of the heart. Heart murmurs tend to be common in children and disappear in adulthood as the cardiac and vascular systems mature. Murmurs may be asymptomatic or benign, with some affected people unaware of the condition throughout life. In other cases, a murmur is a sign of heart disease and can be symptomatic. Documentation of the location, characteristics, and intensity of a murmur will enable the health care provider to determine whether further diagnostic studies are necessary. Assess murmurs for location and radiation to other areas, such as the neck or back. In some instances, a **thrill** (an abnormal vibration felt on palpation) is detected with a murmur. Murmurs are graded according to intensity:

Grade 1: Scarcely audible with a good stethoscope in a quiet room
Grade 2: Quiet but readily audible with a stethoscope
Grade 3: Easily heard with a stethoscope
Grade 4: A loud, obvious murmur with a palpable thrill
Grade 5: Very loud with a palpable thrill; heard over the pericardium and elsewhere in the body (radiates)
Grade 6: Heard with a stethoscope off the chest; thrill palpable and visible

Auscultation for bruits should be performed over the abdominal aorta using the bell of the stethoscope. Abdominal bruits or pulsations can be a sign of an abdominal aortic aneurysm.

Peripheral Vascular Assessment

Inspection and palpation of the peripheral vascular system include assessment of peripheral pulses and blood flow, which the nurse performs while assessing other body systems. A critical aspect of a peripheral vascular examination is assessment of the jugular veins and carotid arteries, which is conducted during examination of the neck (see earlier discussion under Head, Ears, Eyes, Nose, and Throat). Auscultation is performed to obtain a blood pressure reading and to listen for bruits over the peripheral arteries. A Doppler ultrasound unit may be used to assess weak peripheral pulses.

Inspection and Palpation of Peripheral Pulses

A head-to-toe physical examination includes the assessment and documentation of arterial pulses in all superficial locations. While assessing the patient's pulse, the nurse notes its intensity, rate, and rhythm, as well as the existence of blood vessel tenderness, **tortuosity** (bending and twisting), or nodularity. Problem areas identified during inspection of skin and nails may indicate arterial or venous impairment, requiring a more focused assessment.

The rate and rhythm of the radial artery pulse are assessed when vital signs are obtained. Normal pulses are felt at regular intervals from one heartbeat to the next. If an interval is interrupted by an early, late, or missed beat, the pulse is recognized as irregular and should be compared with the carotid artery pulse and apical heart rate for confirmation.

Palpation of the brachial, radial, ulnar, femoral, popliteal, dorsalis pedis, and posterior tibial arteries is done using the fingertips. Peripheral pulses are compared side to side for strength and symmetry. See Figure 20-31 for anatomic locations of the major arteries to be assessed. Strength or intensity of peripheral pulses is graded on a scale of 0 to 4+:

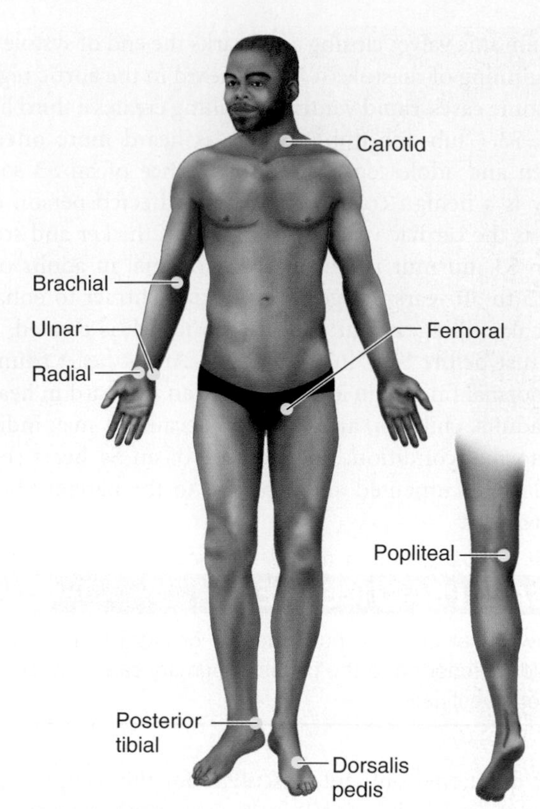

FIGURE 20-31 Anatomic locations of major arteries to be assessed for peripheral pulses.

0	No palpable pulse
1+	Faint but detectable pulse
2+	Normal pulse
3+	Pulse with increased intensity
4+	Bounding pulse

Normal peripheral arteries are palpable and elastic. After palpation of a peripheral pulse, the artery should return to its previous shape immediately. Abnormal findings include arteries that are hard and pulses that are not equal when compared side to side. Either abnormality could indicate an obstruction, peripheral vascular disease, or impaired circulation. Palpation of arterial pulses is performed with the fingertips of the first three fingers. In thinner patients, inspection can assist with pulse location, because arterial pulses may be visible on the skin's surface.

! SAFE PRACTICE ALERT

Always use the fingertips to palpate pulses. Use of the thumb is not recommended because the nurse's own radial pulse might be felt, causing confusion and an erroneous assessment finding.

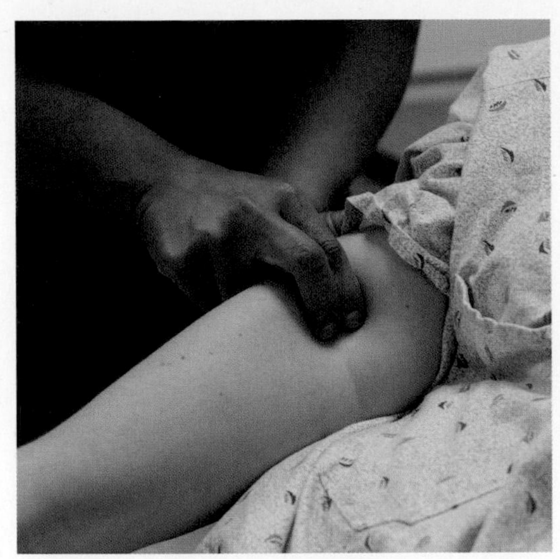

FIGURE 20-32 Locating the brachial pulse is necessary for accurate blood pressure measurement on the upper arm.

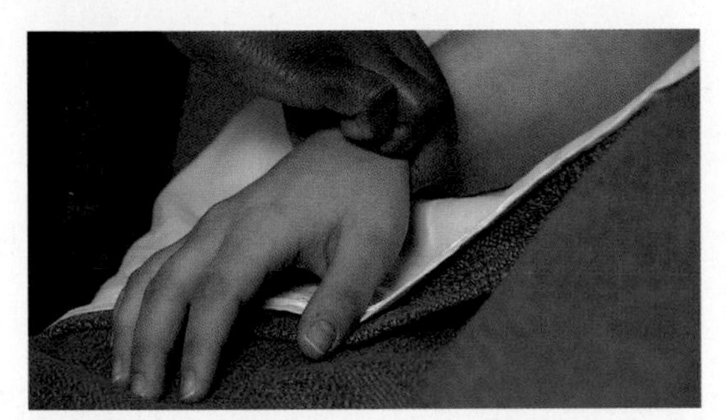

FIGURE 20-33 Assessment of the radial pulse is performed on the thumb side of the wrist.

Brachial Pulses

To assess the brachial pulse (Figure 20-32), support the patient's forearm in an abducted position, with the elbow slightly flexed and the forearm externally rotated. Locate the anterior aspect of the elbow, and palpate along the course of the artery just medial to the biceps tendon. The positions of the hands should be switched when probing the opposite arm.

Radial Pulses

The radial artery (Figure 20-33) is palpated on the inner aspect of the wrist in the groove closer to the thumb. On the opposite side of the wrist, the ulnar artery can be felt. The ulnar pulse is less prominent than the radial pulse and is assessed only in circumstances in which the radial pulse is not palpable. The hand normally is supplied by blood from the ulnar and radial arteries.

The Allen test (Figure 20-34) is used to evaluate for collateral circulation to determine the patency of the arteries of the hand before arterial blood tests. The Allen test is performed by having the patient elevate the extremity and make a fist. The examiner occludes the radial and ulnar arteries,

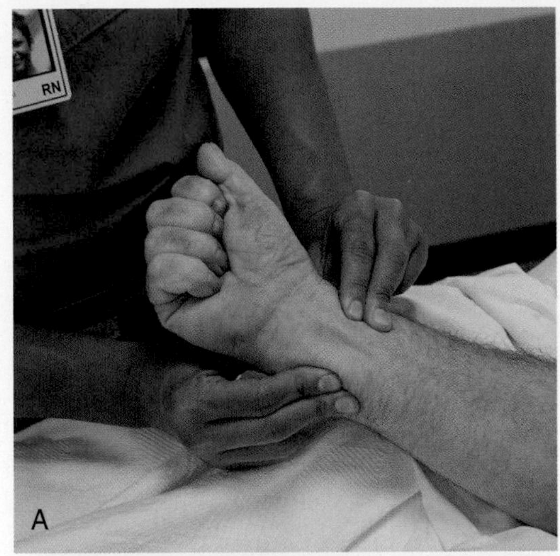

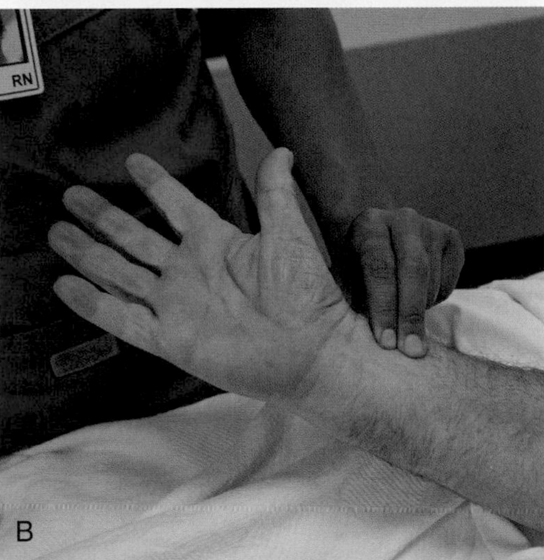

FIGURE 20-34 Conducting the Allen test. **A,** Occlude both the radial and ulnar arteries simultaneously. **B,** Release pressure on the ulnar artery and observe for return of color to the hand.

using pressure. The patient's hand should lose color. The patient then opens the fist, and the pressure is released from the ulnar artery. The normal pink color should return to the hand within 10 seconds, showing good circulation.

Femoral Pulses

The femoral artery (Figure 20-35) surfaces in the upper thigh from beneath the inguinal ligament in the center of the groin. It is best palpated with the nurse standing on the same side as the femoral artery being palpated. The fingertips of the nurse's hand are firmly pressed into the groin area. Auscultation of the femoral arteries is done in the same area, which should be free of bruits.

Popliteal Pulses

The popliteal artery extends vertically through the deep portion of the popliteal space just lateral to the midline of the

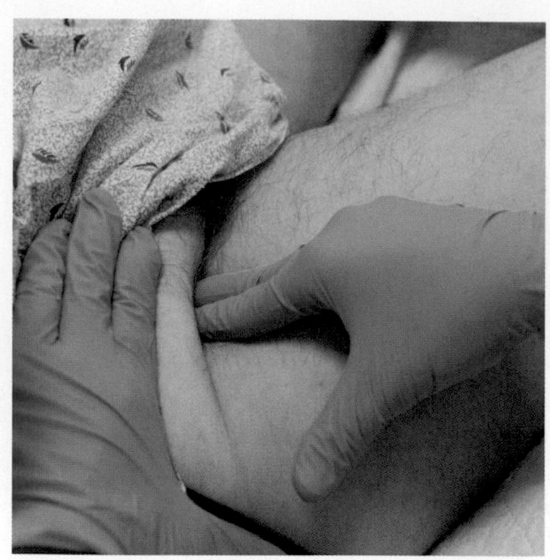
FIGURE 20-35 Femoral pulses are best assessed with the patient in the supine or low Fowler position.

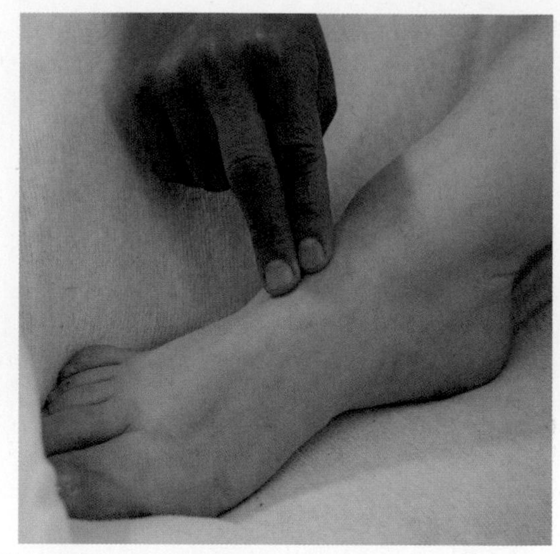
FIGURE 20-37 Assessing the dorsalis pedis pulse.

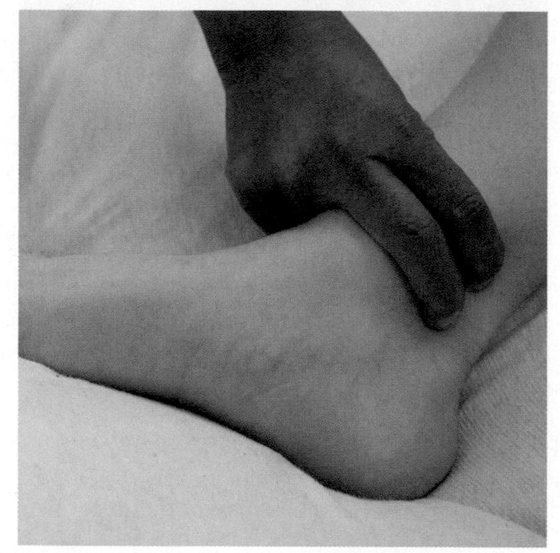
FIGURE 20-36 Assessing the posterior tibial pulse.

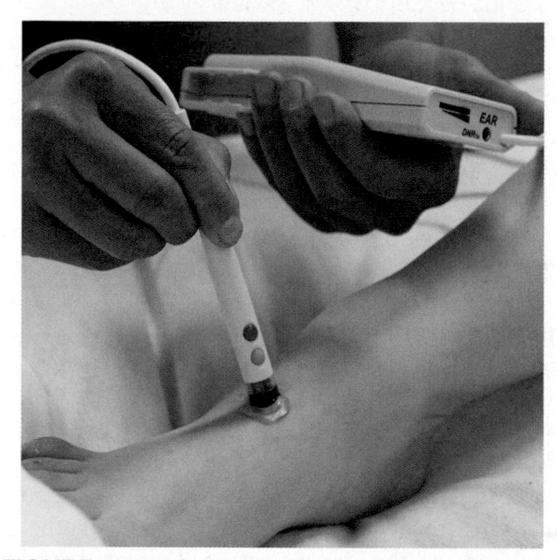

FIGURE 20-38 Assessing a pulse using a Doppler.

area behind the knee. It is difficult to palpate and locate in obese or very muscular people. The popliteal pulse is palpated with the patient in the supine position, and the nurse uses both hands to encircle and support the knee while the patient relaxes the leg. The pulse is detected by pressing deeply into the popliteal space with the fingertips. Popliteal pulses should be assessed if more distal pulses are impalpable or unable to be heard with a Doppler.

Pedal Pulses

One of two pedal pulses is assessed by palpating the posterior tibial artery (Figure 20-36), which lies just behind the medial malleolus of the inner ankle. It can be felt by placing the fingertips around the ankle and gently indenting the soft tissues in the space between the medial malleolus and the Achilles tendon.

The dorsalis pedis artery (Figure 20-37) is the other pedal pulse assessed. The nurse places the fingertips across the top of the forefoot halfway between the toes and the ankle. The artery lies superficially near the center of the long axis of the foot, between the extensor tendons of the great toe and second toe. In some people, it may be in a slightly different location, necessitating palpation across the dorsum of the foot.

Obesity, dehydration, vasoconstriction, diminished cardiac output, edema, genetic abnormalities, or peripheral vascular disease may prevent successful detection of pedal pulses. Doppler assessment can be used to detect weak peripheral pulses (Figure 20-38). A Doppler ultrasound device magnifies sound. When performing a Doppler assessment of a peripheral pulse, place water-soluble transmission gel over the pulse area. Applying very light pressure, place the ultrasound transducer over the pulse site at a 45- to 90-degree angle. The pulse is located by listening for a rhythmic, whooshing sound. Ideally, the sound closely parallels the apical heartbeat.

Assessment for Venous and Arterial Insufficiency

To assess for venous or arterial insufficiency, observe the patient's skin characteristics, especially in the lower extremities, in both sitting and standing positions. Note any swelling, redness, nodules, protruding superficial veins, or peripheral edema. Varicose veins are enlarged superficial veins that may result from pregnancy, obesity, advanced age, or standing for long periods of time.

Dependent edema most often is seen in the lower extremities and usually is caused by venous insufficiency. Gross amounts of swelling in the calves and lower leg can indicate more serious conditions, such as congestive heart failure or liver disease. Assess whether the edema is pitting (see Figure 20-6) or nonpitting by using the procedure discussed in the section on skin assessment, earlier in this chapter. Refer to Box 20-3 for documentation guidelines for pitting edema.

Phlebitis may be noted during assessment of the peripheral vascular system. **Phlebitis** is the inflammation of a vein. It typically is due to irritation, often from intravenous solutions, or infection. Assessment of the area may reveal redness, swelling, warmth, and tenderness. Measurement of the calf may show enlargement on one side of the body. Blood clots may form in areas where phlebitis is present, causing the potentially serious complication of deep vein thrombosis (DVT). In the past, the Homans sign was used to detect phlebitis in the lower extremities. This clinical sign consists of occurrence of pain in the calf on dorsiflexion of the foot. Testing for a Homans sign is now contraindicated owing to its documented unreliability and tendency toward false positives and the possibility of dislodging a clot.

! SAFE PRACTICE ALERT

Never use the Homans sign to assess a patient suspected of having a DVT. Do not massage a reddened area that is a suspected DVT.

Patients with arterial insufficiency often exhibit the five P's of circulation: pain, pallor, pulselessness, **paresthesia** (numbness or tingling), and paralysis. To determine whether distal extremities are receiving adequate blood supply, assess the patient's capillary refill (see Figure 20-7) and document it as either less than or greater than 2 to 3 seconds. Other indicators of circulatory insufficiency include lack of hair growth over distal extremities, recurring ulcers of the feet or lower legs, and brittle, thin skin.

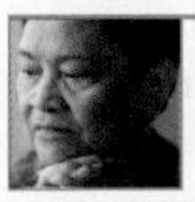

4. Write a minimum of 10 health assessment questions that the nurse would want to ask Mrs. Thatcher that are specific to the purpose of her examination.

MUSCULOSKELETAL ASSESSMENT

Assessment of musculoskeletal function determines the range of joint motion, muscle strength, and associated skeletal stability (Health Assessment Questions box). Determining musculoskeletal health is especially important when the patient reports pain or loss of function in a joint or muscle or has difficulty carrying out activities of daily living.

HEALTH ASSESSMENT QUESTIONS

Musculoskeletal System

- Do you have any pain or stiffness in your joints, muscles, or back? If so, when did it begin? Where is the pain or stiffness? What is its quality? Is the pain burning, aching, shooting, constant, or intermittent? Does anything aggravate or relieve the pain?
- Are you able to perform activities of daily living, such as dressing or preparing meals, without musculoskeletal discomfort?
- Can you climb stairs and walk without limping?
- Do you have numbness or tingling in your extremities?
- Are you able to engage in strenuous activity or exercise?
- Have you experienced any recent trauma to any of your bones, joints, soft tissue, or nerves?
- Do you have any chronic illnesses that may affect the musculoskeletal system, including cancer, osteoporosis, arthritis, and renal or neurologic disorders?
- Do you have any known skeletal deformities or a congenital history that may affect the musculoskeletal system?
- Do you have any family history of arthritis (rheumatoid, osteoarthritis, ankylosing spondylitis), back problems (scoliosis, spina bifida), or genetic disorders (osteogenesis imperfecta, rickets, dwarfing syndrome)?
- Does your diet include adequate calcium and vitamin D?

Disorders that affect the musculoskeletal system arise from injury, disease conditions, metabolic disorders, and neurologic dysfunction. For further information on musculoskeletal functions, see Chapter 28. Muscle strength varies from person to person, depending on the size, strength, and development of skeletal muscle in each individual. A functional and intact neurologic system with innervation to muscles is necessary to maintain the ability of muscular contraction and purposeful movement.

Inspection and Palpation of the Musculoskeletal System

Physical examination of the musculoskeletal system begins by observing the patient's gait. In walking normally, the arms swing freely at the sides with the left arm swinging forward when the right foot takes a step, and vice versa. The function of muscles, joints, and bone alignment is assessed while the patient assumes several positions, including sitting, standing, prone, and supine. During these observations, the nurse notes how the patient walks, sits, changes positions, and rises from a lying or sitting position. Observe the patient in a standing

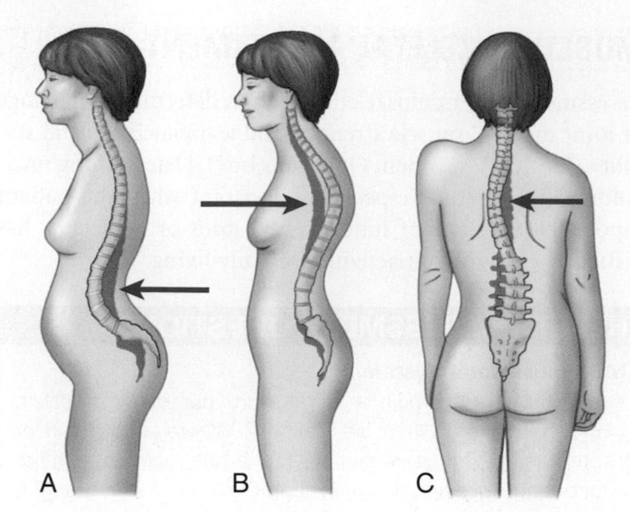

FIGURE 20-39 Abnormal curvatures of the spine: **A,** lordosis; **B,** kyphosis; **C,** scoliosis. (From Thibodeau GA, Patton KT: *The human body in health and disease,* ed. 5, St. Louis, 2010, Mosby.)

position. Normally, the head is held erect, and standing posture is upright, with parallel alignment of the hips and shoulders. The body should appear symmetric when compared side to side. The spine should be aligned, with some gentle curving.

Several postural irregularities can be detected on inspection (Figure 20-39). **Scoliosis** is a sideways or S-shaped curvature of the spine and is always abnormal. **Kyphosis** is an outward curvature of the thoracic spine. **Lordosis** is a condition that causes an increased lumbar curvature just above the buttocks area. Minimal, not exaggerated, kyphotic and lordotic curvature is normal in most patients.

Assess the patient for signs of osteoporosis. Osteoporosis is a condition that causes weakened bones due to mineral loss. It can lead to musculoskeletal abnormalities such as exaggerated kyphosis or pathologic fractures of the spine, hip, or wrist not resulting from trauma. Osteoporosis may affect both males and females of all age groups, including children and adolescents, but it is seen primarily in older adults, especially postmenopausal women. Sudden and severe loss of height and back pain secondary to vertebral fractures often are the first clinical manifestations of osteoporosis.

With the patient in the sitting and then the standing position, evaluate the muscles, cartilage, bones, and joints for overall size, gross deformity, alignment, contour, symmetry, and position. Inspect the muscles for gross hypertrophy or atrophy, spasms, and symmetry of size. Slight differences may be noted, with somewhat increased muscle mass on the patient's dominant side. Occasionally, hands and feet are larger on the dominant side.

Carefully palpate all bones, joints, and muscles. Muscles should feel firm and normally are without masses, pain, or tenderness on palpation. A more detailed focused assessment and range-of-motion evaluation are indicated for any area that is abnormal.

Mobility and Strength

Musculoskeletal examination includes joint range-of-motion assessment (see Chapter 28, Figure 28-5). Ask the patient to move all joints and extremities through their full range of motion. If the patient can achieve independent movement of all four extremities, document that the patient "moves all extremities" (MAE.) If the patient is unable to perform active range of motion, assist the patient, using passive range of motion to assess joint mobility. Normal muscle contraction and relaxation are not painful, and slight resistance to movement through the entire range is expected. Joints usually are free of pain, stiffness, swelling, inflammation, or instability. If abnormalities are detected in any joint, note the surrounding skin color and palpate for warmth and tenderness. If the patient has **hypertonicity**, an increase in muscle tone, greater resistance will be evident on passive-movement range of motion. In **hypotonicity**, a decrease in muscle tone, the muscle feels loose and flaccid during passive range of motion.

Assessment of upper-extremity strength can be completed by having the patient squeeze the nurse's hands and then push and pull against them. Having the patient push and pull each foot against the nurse's hands will provide an evaluation of lower-extremity strength. Document assessment findings, making sure to note any difference in strength from side to side.

Deep Tendon and Cutaneous Reflexes

Deep tendon and cutaneous reflexes can be diminished or absent owing to defects in muscles, sensory neurons, lower motor neurons, and the neuromuscular junction. Acute upper motor neuron lesions and mechanical factors such as joint disease can dampen the impulse of deep tendon reflexes (hyporeflexia). Abnormally increased reflexes (hyperreflexia) are associated with upper motor neuron lesions. Note that reflexes can be influenced by age, metabolic factors (such as thyroid dysfunction or electrolyte abnormalities), and anxiety level of the patient.

Check the deep tendon reflexes by tapping areas using a reflex hammer (Figure 20-40). The limbs should be in a relaxed and slightly stretched position, supported by the examiner, because reflex amplitude cannot be elicited in a contracted muscle group. Assess cutaneous reflexes by stroking the designated area with the handle end of a reflex hammer or the hard end of a cotton-tipped applicator. Table 20-8 describes how some of the most common deep tendon and cutaneous reflexes are assessed. As in muscle strength testing, it is important to compare each reflex side to side so that asymmetric differences can be detected. When reflexes are very brisk, clonus is sometimes seen. **Clonus** is a repetitive vibratory contraction of the muscle that occurs in response to muscle and tendon stretch.

Reflex responses are documented using a subjective scale as follows.

TABLE 20-8 **Deep and Cutaneous Tendon Reflex Assessment**

REFLEX	TECHNIQUE	NORMAL RESPONSE
Biceps	Place your thumb on the base of the biceps tendon in the antecubital fossa of the patient's partially flexed arm. Tap your thumb with a reflex hammer.	Biceps contraction and flexion
Triceps	Hold the upper arm of the patient at a 45-degree angle away from the patient's body, while it is limp, or hold the patient's wrist across the patient's chest for flexion. Tap the triceps tendon just above the elbow.	Extension of the forearm
Quadriceps or Patellar *Knee Jerk*	Allow the patient's leg to dangle freely. Tap the quadriceps tendon just below the patella.	Extension of the leg
Achilles *Ankle Jerk*	Hold the patient's dorsiflexed foot with the leg flexed and the hip externally rotated. Tap the Achilles tendon slightly above and behind the inner heel area.	Plantar flexion of the foot
Plantar	With the patient lying in supine position, stroke the bottom of the patient's foot gently from the heel to the toes, in the shape of an upside down J ending below the big toe.	*Adults and children:* Plantar flexion of the toes and forefoot *Infants:* Dorsiflexion of the big toe and fanning out of the toes (positive Babinski sign)

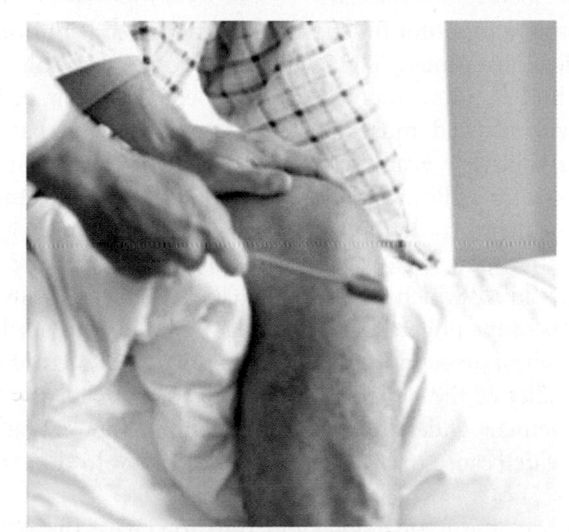

FIGURE 20-40 Assessment of the patellar reflex.

4+ Very brisk, hyperactive with clonus
3+ Brisker than average, slightly hyperactive
2+ Average, normal
1+ Sluggish or diminished
0 No response

Because reflex evaluation is subjective based on the practitioner's perception, it should always be conducted within the context of a thorough neurologic examination.

NEUROLOGIC ASSESSMENT

The nervous system is the axis point for all forms of mental activity, including thought, behavior, learning, and memory. Evaluation of the motor, autonomic, behavioral, sensory, and cognitive elements of neurologic function is one of the most multifaceted segments of the patient's physical assessment (Health Assessment Questions box).

The central nervous system consists of the brain and spinal cord encased in the skull and vertebrae. The peripheral nervous system consists of 31 pairs of spinal nerves that arise from the spinal cord and exit at each vertebral foramen located in the spine. Within the spinal cord, individual spinal nerves separate into ventral and dorsal roots.

A complete neurologic assessment is extensive. Neurologic screening examinations are conducted in all patients as part of the head-to-toe assessment. If abnormal findings are discovered, an in-depth assessment is performed. Knowledge of the function of each area of the brain (Figure 20-41) and of the location of nerves within the spinal cord enables the nurse to determine the area involved when abnormal findings are discovered during an assessment.

Cranial Nerve Assessment

A complete cranial nerve assessment involves testing all 12 of the cranial nerves in their numbered order (Figure 20-42). Dysfunction or irregularity alerts the nurse to an alteration in the pathway of nerve conduction along with the distribution of the cranial nerve. A popular method for remembering the order of cranial nerves is use of the rhyming phrase "On Old Olympic Towering Tops A Finn And German Viewed Some Hops." The first letter of each word in the phrase is the same as the first letter of the name of each cranial nerve listed in Table 20-9.

HEALTH ASSESSMENT QUESTIONS

Nervous System

- Do you have any weakness, tremors, numbness, or tingling in your arms or legs?
- Are you experiencing a loss of balance or difficulty walking?
- How would you describe your mood? Do you ever feel nervous, anxious, depressed, or confused?
- Have you noticed any problems with remembering?
- Have you ever had trauma to the head, spinal cord, or back?
- Do you have a history of meningitis or encephalitis?
- Have you ever had circulatory problems, an aneurysm, or a stroke?
- Do you have a history of seizures or convulsions? If so, when did they first occur? Describe what happens when the seizures occur. Are you on anticonvulsant medications?
- Are you having any pain? If so, where? Describe the pain.
- Do you have headaches? If so, what do they feel like?
- Do you have any dizziness, light-headedness, or fainting spells?
- Do you have any weakness or paresthesias?
- Are you having any problems with coordination or balance?
- Is there a family history of any neurologic disorders?
- Have you ever been diagnosed with a learning disability?
- List any medical or metabolic disturbances such as thyroid disease, diabetes mellitus, and hypertension.
- Do you use alcohol, recreational drugs, or prescription drugs that have mood-altering effects?
- Are you exposed to environmental or occupational hazards such as exposure to lead, insecticides, organic cleaning solvents, arsenic, or other chemicals?

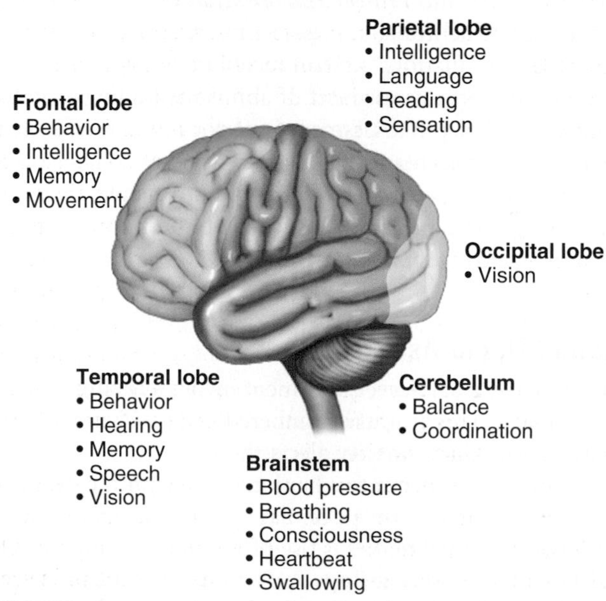

FIGURE 20-41 Functions of each area of the brain. (From Thibodeau GA, Patton KT: *The human body in health and disease*, ed. 5, St. Louis, 2010, Mosby.)

Sensory Nerve Assessment

The central nervous system is composed of sensory pathways that detect and conduct sensations of pain, temperature, vibration, position, and touch. Sensory receptors transmit messages to the spinal cord, from which they then travel to the brain to be interpreted. Screening for sensory nerve dysfunction can be accomplished during other parts of the physical examination, such as during skin assessment. With eyes closed, the patient should feel dull and sharp sensory stimuli equally on both sides of the body. Ask the patient to describe the quality of each stimulus, and note the presence or absence of bilateral symmetry when the stimuli are applied to the patient's extremities and trunk. Compare distal with proximal sensations. Figure 20-43 illustrates the dermatomes of the body associated with each spinal nerve. Knowledge of the dermatomes will help locate problem areas. If any abnormalities are found such as numbness, tingling, or lack of sensation, further assessment should be performed. For example, if numbness is present in the index and middle fingers of either hand or bilaterally, a neurologic lesion or spinal compression of C7 or C8 vertebrae may be the causative factor.

Motor Nerve and Coordination Assessment

Assessment of motor function can be combined with musculoskeletal assessment. The focus of this combined evaluation is the body's motor responses and cerebellar function, including synchronized muscular activity, posture, and balance. Motor skill tests examine the movement of muscles in the body. Motor skills are divided into two groups: gross motor skills, which include the larger movements of arms, legs, or the entire body (e.g., walking, running, jumping), and fine motor skills, which include activities using the smaller muscles of the fingers, hands, or feet and hand-eye coordination. To test gross motor skills during the assessment, assess the quality of the patient's actions for smoothness and ease of movement. Older adults normally exhibit a slower reaction time, which causes movements to be delayed or to appear less fluid.

To test fine motor skills and function, have the patient perform actions such as transferring an object from one hand to the other successfully, picking up and holding two or more objects in the same hand, turning pages one at a time, and writing a signature. To assess the lower extremities for fine motor movement, place a hand just below the toes on the bottom of the patient's foot and have the patient tap the foot in quick, successive, movements. Test each foot to establish symmetry. When testing fine motor movements, understand that the feet do not move as rapidly or as precisely as the hands.

Balance can be assessed using any of several methods. The Romberg test, which is conducted during ear assessment to evaluate equilibrium, is one method (see Figure 20-18). A loss of balance indicates a positive result on Romberg testing and may be due to a cerebellar lesion or dysfunction. Another

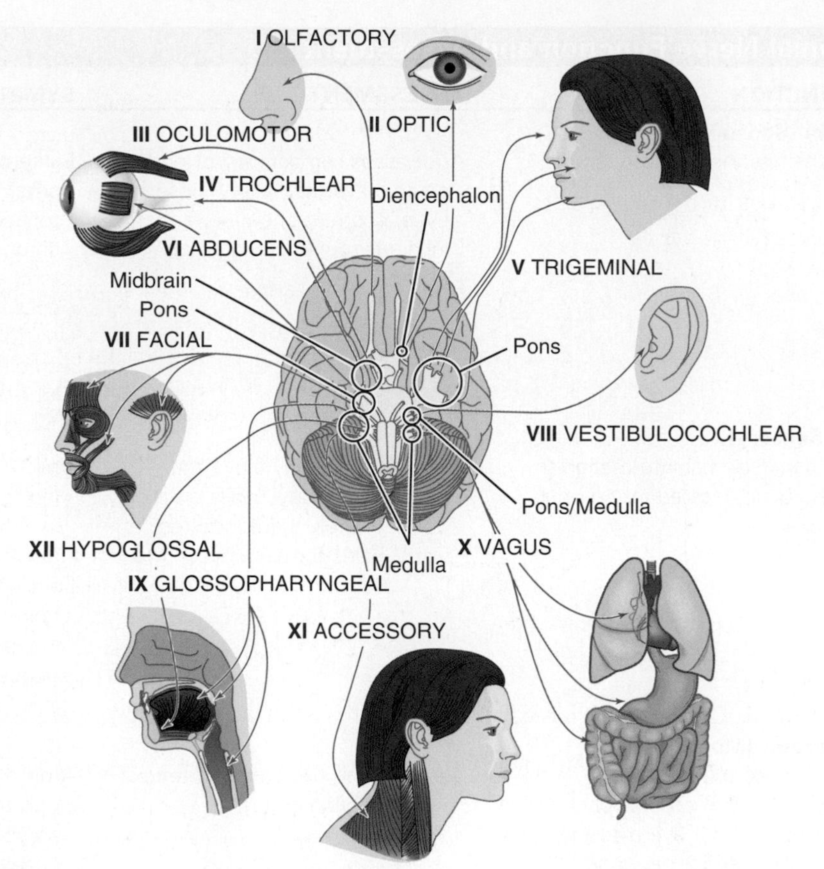

FIGURE 20-42 The cranial nerves are numbered according to the order in which they leave the brain. (Redrawn from McCance KL, Huether SE: *Pathophysiology: The biologic basis for disease in adults and children,* ed. 7, St. Louis, 2014, Mosby.)

method of assessing balance is to ask the patient to close the eyes and stand on one foot and then the other, holding each position for at least 5 seconds. Normally, patients are able to maintain balance for a minimum of 5 seconds with the eyes closed. A third method is to have the patient walk in a straight line (with eyes open) by placing the heel of one foot directly in front of the toes of the other foot while maintaining balance. Normally, patients are able to walk heel to toe without losing balance.

! SAFE PRACTICE ALERT

Always protect the patient from falling by remaining close during balance testing. Instruct patients to open their eyes if they lose their balance or feel that they are going to fall.

Mental Status Assessment

The patient's mental status indicates the level of cerebral function. Obtaining a baseline appraisal of the patient's abilities helps the nurse plan patient education, assess understanding of instruction, and determine the patient's capacity to make decisions. Assessment of mental status evaluates brain function related to intellect, behavior, language, memory, knowledge, judgment, association, attention, level of consciousness, decision making, and abstract thinking.

The Glasgow Coma Scale is an objective assessment tool used to define a person's level of consciousness by assigning a numeric value to the person's level of arousal. The scale is divided into three areas: eye opening, verbal response, and motor response. Each area is scored separately, and a number is assigned to the person's best response. The three numbers are added, and the total score reflects the patient's level of consciousness. A fully alert, normally responsive patient will have a score of 15. Scores from multiple assessments can be plotted on a graph to provide a visual illustration indicating that the patient is stable, improving, or deteriorating. A score of less than 7 reflects a patient who is comatose. Refer to Table 20-10 for the Glasgow Coma Scale.

During initial encounters, the nurse can gather a great deal of information about the patient's cognitive and mental abilities by conversing with the patient. The patient's responses to questions enable the nurse to determine thought processes, knowledge, and behavior. Level of orientation and mental status are assessed by determining the patient's ability to identify person, place, time, and situation.

TABLE 20-9 Cranial Nerve Function and Assessment

ORIGIN	FUNCTION	ASSESSMENT	SYMPTOMS OF DAMAGE
Cranial Nerve I: Olfactory (Sensory)			
Upper nasal passages	Transmits the sense of smell	After assessing patency of both nares, have the patient close the eyes, obstruct one nare, and inhale to identify a common scent.	Bilateral decreased sense of smell occurs with age, tobacco smoking, allergic or chronic rhinitis, overexposure to chemical substances, and cocaine use. Unilateral loss of sense of smell can indicate a frontal lobe lesion.
Cranial Nerve II: Optic (Sensory)			
Eyes	Transmits visual information to the brain; located in the optic canal	Check visual acuity (have the patient read newspaper print or use a Snellen chart), and test visual fields for each eye.	Unilateral blindness can indicate a lesion or pressure in the globe or on the optic nerve. Loss of the same half of visual field in both eyes can indicate a lesion of the opposite-side optic tract, as in a CVA.
Cranial Nerve III: Oculomotor (Motor)			
Midbrain	Innervates four of the six muscles that collectively execute most eye movements; responsible for papillary constriction and dilation	Assess pupil size and light reflex; note direction of gaze.	A unilaterally dilated pupil with unilateral absent light reflex and/or an eye that will not gaze upward can indicate an internal carotid aneurysm or increased intracranial pressure.
Cranial Nerve IV: Trochlear (Motor)			
Midbrain	Innervates muscles responsible for downward and inward gaze of the eyes	Ask the patient to gaze downward, temporally, and nasally. (NOTE: Cranial nerves III, IV, and VI are examined together because they control eyelid elevation, eye movement, and pupillary constriction.)	If the eyes will not move through the inward and downward gazes, the patient may have a fracture of the eye orbit or a brainstem tumor.
Cranial Nerve V: Trigeminal (Sensory and Motor)			
Pons	Is responsible for the corneal reflex; receives sensation from the face and innervates the muscles of mastication	*Motor:* Palpate jaws and temples while patient clenches teeth. *Sensory:* With the patient's eyes closed, gently touch a cotton ball to all areas of the face.	Unilateral deficit is seen with trauma and tumors.
Cranial Nerve VI: Abducens (Motor)			
Pons	Innervates muscles responsible for outward gaze of the eyes	Assess directions of gaze.	Inability to gaze outward may indicate a fracture of an orbit or a brainstem tumor.
Cranial Nerve VII: Facial (Sensory and Motor)			
Pons	Provides motor innervation to the muscles of facial expression; receives the sense of taste from the anterior two thirds of the tongue; provides innervation to the salivary glands (except parotid) and the lacrimal gland	*Motor:* Check symmetry of the face by having the patient frown, close eyes, lift eyebrows, and puff cheeks. *Sensory:* Assess the patient's ability to recognize taste (sugar, salt, lemon juice).	An asymmetric deficit can be found in traumatic injury, Bell's palsy, CVA, tumor, and inflammation.

TABLE 20-9 Cranial Nerve Function and Assessment—cont'd

ORIGIN	FUNCTION	ASSESSMENT	SYMPTOMS OF DAMAGE
Cranial Nerve VIII: Vestibulocochlear or Auditory-Vestibular (Sensory)			
Medulla oblongata	*Vestibular branch:* Carries impulses for equilibrium *Cochlear branch:* Carries impulses for hearing	Assess the patient's ability to hear a spoken and whispered word.	Impairment may result from inflammation or occlusion of the ear canal, infection, drug toxicity, or a possible tumor or may cause vertigo.
Cranial Nerve IX: Glossopharyngeal (Sensory and Motor)			
Medulla oblongata	Receives taste from the posterior third of the tongue; provides innervation to the parotid gland; and provides motor innervation for swallowing	*Sensory:* Assess the patient's ability to taste sour or sweet on last two thirds of tongue. *Motor:* Check for presence of the gag reflex by inserting a tongue blade two-thirds into the pharynx.	Deficits in taste or gag reflex can indicate a brainstem tumor or neck injury.
Cranial Nerve X: Vagus (Sensory and Motor)			
Medulla oblongata	Supplies innervation to the larynx and soft palate responsible for speech and swallowing; provides parasympathetic fibers to nearly all thoracic and abdominal smooth muscles	Depress the tongue with a tongue blade, and have the patient say "ah" or yawn. The uvula and soft palate should rise and be symmetric. Assess speech for hoarseness.	Dysphagia can indicate swallowing problems and the potential for aspiration.
Cranial Nerve XI: Accessory (Motor)			
Medulla oblongata (cranial root) and spinal cord (spinal root)	*Cranial root:* Works with vagus nerve to control the muscles of the soft palate, pharynx, and larynx *Spinal root:* Innervates muscles of the neck and back	Have the patient rotate the head and shrug the shoulders against passive resistance.	If the patient is unable to perform a shoulder shrug or head rotation, this may indicate a neck injury.
Cranial Nerve XII: Hypoglossal (Motor)			
Medulla oblongata	Provides motor innervation to muscles of the tongue not innervated by the vagus nerve and to other glossal muscles; is important for swallowing and speech articulation	Assess tongue control (e.g., have the patient stick out the tongue and move it from side to side).	Inability to stick out the tongue may be associated with swallowing or articulation difficulties.

- *Person:* "What is your name?"
- *Place:* "Where are you?"
- *Time:* "Can you tell me what (day, month, season, or year) it is?"
- *Situation:* "What happened that caused you to come to the hospital?

If a patient is able to respond appropriately to all four questions, the nurse documents that the patient is alert and "oriented × 4." In some cases, hospitalized patients may have difficulty recalling the current date or time but remain completely oriented to person and place, making them alert and "oriented × 2." Assessment of orientation and mental status continues whenever the nurse observes the patient's behavior and ability to concentrate during each interaction.

Assess the patient's short- and long-term memory. Ask the patient to demonstrate short-term memory by having the patient recall three words or numbers chosen by the nurse. Later in the interview, ask the patient to repeat the same three words or numbers used earlier in the assessment. The patient should be able to accurately recite the list. Another way to test patient short-term memory is to ask what occurred earlier in the same day. This can be validated with another staff member or a family member. To assess long-term memory, ask the patient to recall a date or name from the past that can be verified with a family member.

To assess cognitive abilities such as knowledge, decision making, and judgment, ask questions about health status and any chronic or current illnesses. Listening to the patient's description of illness, treatment, and medications enables the nurse to assess language use, patient understanding, and decisions made by the patient concerning health care. On the basis of information shared by the patient during knowledge

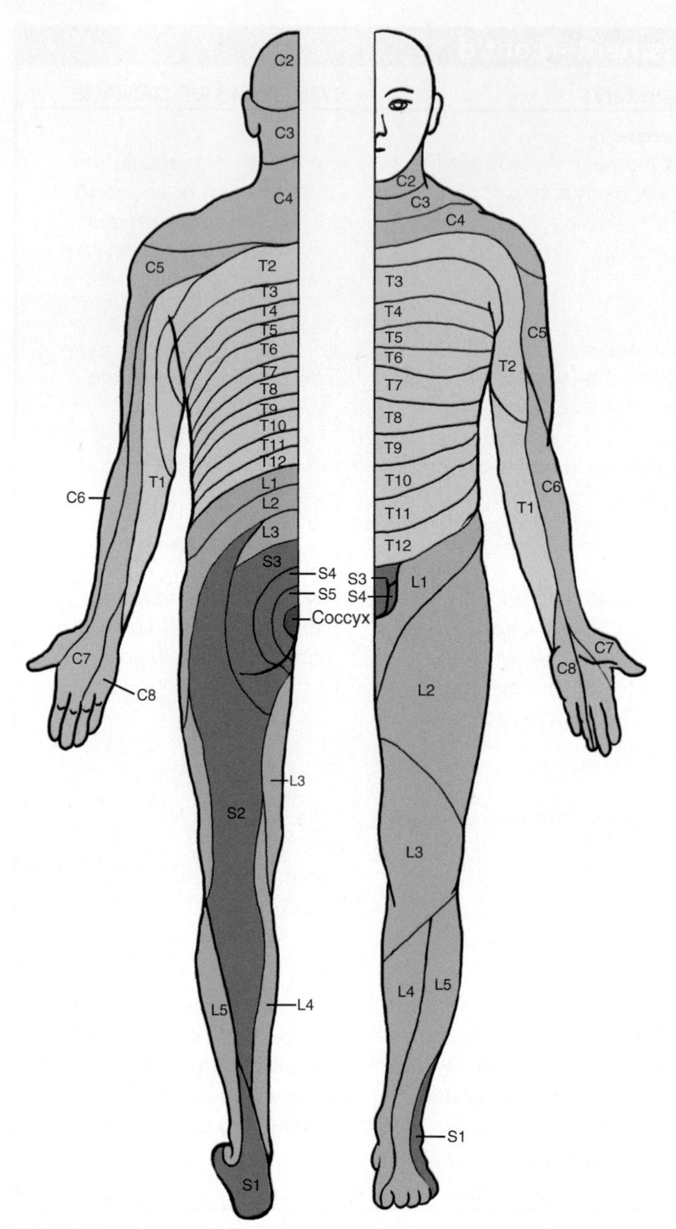

FIGURE 20-43 Dermatomes. (From Linton AD: *Introduction to medical-surgical nursing*, ed. 5, St. Louis, 2012, Saunders.)

assessment, the nurse can interpret the need for patient teaching and reinforce needed information at follow-up visits.

Abstract thinking and association are higher-level cognitive functions. To determine a patient's ability to interpret abstract concepts, ask the patient to explain a common idiom, such as "penny wise and pound foolish." If patients are able to interpret idioms, it is more likely that they will be able to comprehend and apply medication and treatment instructions. Keep in mind that a person whose primary language is different from that of the examiner may be unable to interpret idioms regardless of having intact higher-level cognitive functions. To assess association, ask the patient to relate concepts such as parrot and bird, or guitar and music. Be sure to use simple concepts that are appropriate to the patient's culture and developmental level. If the patient is able to explain idioms and the relationship between associated concepts, higher-level cognitive functions are intact.

TABLE 20-10 Glasgow Coma Scale

RESPONSE	LEVEL OF AROUSAL	SCORING (POINTS)
Eye opening	Spontaneous	4
	To verbal command	3
	To pain	2
	None	1
Verbal	Oriented	5
	Confused but able to answer questions	4
	Inappropriate responses, words discernible	3
	Incomprehensible speech	2
	None	1
Motor	Obeys commands	6
	Purposeful movement to painful stimulus	5
	Withdraws from pain	4
	Abnormal (spastic) flexion, decorticate posture	3
	Extensor (rigid) response, decerebrate posture	2
	None	1
	Possible total score range	**3-15**

Emotional Assessment

The patient's emotional state can quickly be assessed by noting general demeanor and facial expressions, which play a crucial role in interpersonal communication, during interactions with the patient. Assess whether the patient appears calm and comfortable and is at ease with the surroundings. Some discomfort related to the nature of the visit or hospitalization may be evident, but overall the patient should appear relaxed. Note any signs of emotional stress, which may be triggered by a crisis that places the nervous system under severe strain. This could be an event such as losing a loved one, seeing someone die, or experiencing a life-threatening situation. Emotional stress chemically alters how the brain works and can affect the immune system, making the affected person more susceptible to infection or disease. Severe emotional trauma can lead to development of posttraumatic stress disorder.

Emotional stress is not always due to sudden events. It can arise from stressors that accumulate over time to an overwhelming level that prevents the patient from thinking about anything other than problems that appear to have no solution. Emotional stress can lead to detachment, inability to concentrate, fatigue, and memory problems. Assessment of the patient's emotional status is completed throughout the physical examination, with a particular focus on patient reports of the inability to fall asleep and stay asleep at night, decreased or increased appetite, and weight gain or loss.

ABDOMINAL ASSESSMENT

Abdominal assessment focuses on both the gastrointestinal and urinary systems. In seeking information about these systems, however, it is important to broaden the focus to include areas outside of the abdomen (Health Assessment Questions box).

HEALTH ASSESSMENT QUESTIONS

Abdomen

Gastrointestinal Tract

- Do you have any pain or difficulty with swallowing?
- Have you experienced difficulty eating, weight change, or lack of appetite?
- Do you have nausea, vomiting, regurgitation of food, heartburn, indigestion, or bloating? If so, what do you do to relieve the symptoms?
- Are you experiencing abdominal pain? If so, what are the characteristics of the pain? Are there any associated symptoms? Does anything relieve the pain?
- What is your typical 24-hour food intake?
- Have you experienced any changes in bowel habits: diarrhea, constipation, incontinence, or frequent passing of gas?
- Have you noticed any blood in your stool?
- Do you have problems with hemorrhoids?
- Have you ever had abdominal surgery?
- Do you or any family members have a history of abdominal illnesses such as gallbladder disease, cancer, or irritable bowel syndrome?

Urinary Tract

- Are you experiencing any difficulty with urination: frequency or difficulty starting or stopping your stream of urine?
- Do you have a history of urinary tract or kidney infections or kidney stones?
- Is there pain or burning when you urinate?
- Have you noticed a change in your frequency of urination: less often or more often than previously?
- Do you feel that you empty your bladder when you urinate?
- Do you have to get up at night to urinate? If so, how many times?

Abdominal assessment begins with inspection, followed immediately by auscultation, and is completed with palpation and percussion. The nurse performs auscultation before palpation because pressure on the abdomen disturbs the gastrointestinal tract, altering the occurrence and character of bowel sounds. The most common way to assess the abdomen is to visualize dividing it into four quadrants with a horizontal and a vertical line through the umbilicus (Figure 20-44). The upper border of the abdomen is the xiphoid process, and the lower is the symphysis pubis. Knowledge of the location of abdominal cavity organs, including the liver, spleen, pancreas, gallbladder, stomach, urinary tract, and bladder and intestines, enables the nurse to detect normal and abnormal findings during abdominal assessment.

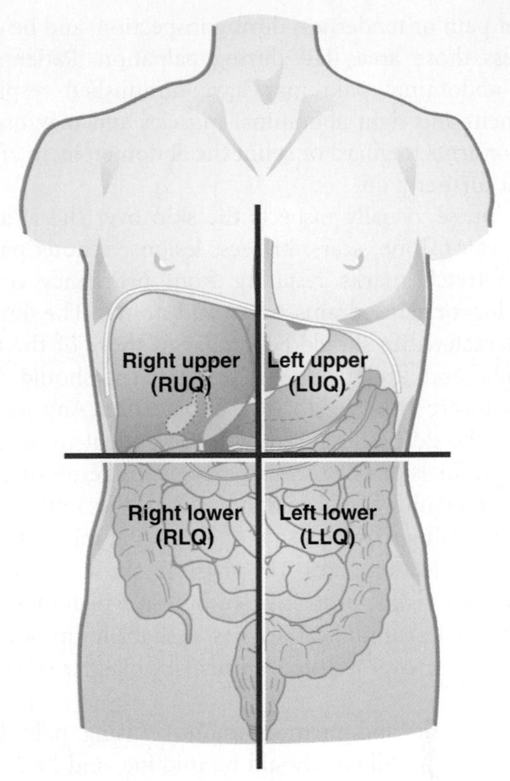

FIGURE 20-44 Abdomen divided into four quadrants at the umbilicus for bowel sound assessment. (From Black JM, Hawks JH: *Medical-surgical nursing: Clinical management for positive outcomes*, ed. 8, St. Louis, 2009, Saunders.)

The gastrointestinal and urinary systems lie within the abdominal cavity and consist of vital organs for energy processing and waste disposal. The organs within the abdominal cavity are surrounded by the peritoneum, a serous membrane that forms the protective cover over the abdominal structures. Bowel elimination is discussed further in Chapter 40. Additional discussion of urinary elimination can be found in Chapter 41.

Abdominal Inspection

The nurse progresses through the examination using a systematic method of assessment to ensure that all abdominal organs are fully evaluated. Visually divide the abdomen into right upper quadrant, left upper quadrant, right lower quadrant, and left lower quadrant, and picture the organs in each quadrant.

Ask the patient to lie supine, in the dorsal recumbent position, with arms at the sides and knees slightly bent. A small pillow may be used to provide support for the knees. Expose only the area of the abdomen between the xiphoid process and the symphysis pubis. Ask the patient to point out any areas of pain or tenderness during inspection, and be careful to assess those areas last during palpation. Patients with severe abdominal pain may have diminished respiratory movement and tight abdominal muscles and may use their hands or arms to guard or splint the abdomen in an effort to prevent further pain.

The nurse visually inspects the skin over the abdomen, noting color, tone, scars, bruises, lesions, venous patterns, **striae** (stretch marks resulting from pregnancy or from weight loss or gain), drains, tubes, and stomas. The skin color and characteristics should be similar to those of the rest of the body, and underlying venous patterns should appear faint. Scars are inspected for keloid formation. Any abnormal findings should be discussed with the patient to determine the origin. Incisions or scarring may be the result of surgery or accidental injury and could indicate changes in the internal organs. Bruising may be a sign of accidental injury, bleeding disorders, injection sites, or physical abuse. Inspect the abdomen for visible protrusion or bulges, which may be due to abdominal or umbilical hernias. A slight lump or protrusion can occur over a distended urinary bladder or loops of bowel.

Normally the abdomen is without bruising, pain, lumps, or scars. The umbilicus should be midline, and hair should be evenly distributed across the abdominal skin surface. Movements or pulsations of the abdomen can indicate an abdominal aortic aneurysm or can be a normal finding in very thin patients. To examine the abdominal musculature, ask the patient to link the hands behind the head or neck; then flex the head forward in a semi-crunch position. This position permits any superficial abdominal wall masses, herniation, and muscle irregularities to become obvious. The abdomen may be flat, concave, or convex, but with all shapes, the abdominal contour should be symmetric and without masses. Obese patients may have a large amount of adipose tissue in the abdominal area, causing a convex appearance.

Symmetric swelling of the abdomen, also known as *distention,* occurs when intestinal gas (flatus), excess fluid, or a tumor is present in the abdominal cavity. The skin over the abdomen may appear stretched and shiny, and the sides (flanks) of the patient's abdomen may bulge, depending on the cause of distention.

Normally the bladder is not visible on inspection. A palpable large, firm area in the lower abdomen above the pubis symphysis often is due to a distended bladder. The inability of the bladder to empty may be caused by a condition called neurogenic bladder (bladder paralysis). In patients with this condition, the bladder is unable to fully contract because of impaired nerve innervation. This deficit causes it to become flaccid and distended, resulting in only partial emptying and continual dribbling of small amounts of urine. Neurogenic bladder can occur at any age, but it is especially common among older patients with chronic disease conditions that directly or indirectly affect the vasculature, innervations, musculature, or output of the bladder. Bladder paralysis is seen in quadriplegic people and some paraplegics, depending on the level of spinal injury or impairment.

Auscultation of the Abdomen

Auscultation of the abdomen is performed for the detection of altered bowel sounds, rubs, or vascular bruits. Normal **peristalsis** (progressive wave action causing movement of contents through the gastrointestinal system) creates bowel sounds that may be altered or absent owing to certain clinical conditions or diseases. Auscultation is performed before palpation or percussion of the abdomen to avoid artificial stimulation of the bowel which may alter bowel sounds. Avoid auscultation of the abdomen immediately before and after meals.

To begin auscultation of the abdomen, position the patient comfortably in the supine position, as just described for inspection. The diaphragm of the stethoscope is placed on the abdomen with gentle pressure, and the nurse listens over each of the four quadrants of the abdomen for the presence of bowel sounds. Normally, as air and fluid move through the intestinal tract, they create soft gurgling sounds that occur in an irregular pattern every 2 to 5 seconds. Sounds can be brief or last a few seconds, depending on bowel stimulation or motility. Under normal circumstances, it takes up to 30 seconds to hear bowel sounds. Bowel sounds can be described as normal, audible, absent, hypoactive (occurring infrequently), hyperactive, or distant. If bowel sounds are not readily audible, listen for 5 minutes in each quadrant to verify a total absence of bowel sounds.

The absence of bowel sounds is an abnormal finding that occurs below a bowel obstruction or in patients with paralytic ileus (paralysis due to lack of peristalsis) or peritonitis. After any type of abdominal surgery or childbirth by cesarean section, intestinal activity frequently is reduced or temporarily inactive, causing bowel sounds to be distant, hypoactive, or absent. As the bowel recovers from surgical stress or manipulation, bowel motility increases and bowel sounds should become active and audible again.

If the intestinal tract is overstimulated or has increased motility, hyperactive bowel sounds, known as **borborygmi**, are heard as a loud "grumbling." Hyperactive sounds can be caused by diarrhea, intestinal inflammation, laxative use, intestinal bleeding, and anxiety. Hyperactive bowel sounds may be audible above the level of a bowel obstruction.

Auscultation for abdominal bruits is the next phase of abdominal examination. Bruits are "swooshing" sounds heard over the major arteries that are caused by **stenosis** (narrowing) of the vessels. Auscultation with the bell of the stethoscope over all four quadrants (renal arteries in the upper quadrants and iliac arteries in the lower quadrants), over the epigastric region (aorta), and in the groin (femoral arteries) can detect bruits. Under normal conditions, no vascular sounds are heard over the aorta or renal, iliac, or femoral arteries. Loud systolic bruits are due to atherosclerotic plaques within the arteries, producing turbulent flow. These plaques are common in the aorta and iliac arteries and less common in the renal arteries.

Palpation of the Abdomen

Ask patients with abdominal pain to point to the area of discomfort so that palpation of that area can be performed last. Palpate each quadrant systematically. When palpating the abdomen, begin with light palpation, using the fingertips of one hand to examine the patient's abdominal wall. Light palpation can detect bladder distention and any irregularities of the abdominal wall such as lipomas or hernias and can reveal tenderness, assess muscle integrity, and identify masses.

When abdominal tenderness is elicited, it should be described according to its location (quadrant), depth of palpation required to elicit it (superficial or deep), and the patient's response (mild or severe). Spasm or rigidity is the involuntary tightening of the abdominal musculature that occurs due to inflammation of underlying abdominal structures. Rigidity can be caused by conditions such as peritoneal inflammation, appendicitis, or acute cholecystitis. Guarding is a voluntary contraction of the abdominal wall musculature to avoid pain. Guarding often can be overcome by having the patient purposely (consciously) relax the muscles.

Rebound tenderness is abdominal pain that occurs immediately following the removal of the examiner's hand after depression of an abdominal area. Palpation for rebound tenderness usually is a difficult skill for the beginning nurse to master. The most common error is removal of the hand too quickly, with an exaggerated motion that surprises the patient. Observe the patient for pain, facial grimace, or spasm of the abdominal wall during palpation. Both tenderness and rebound tenderness can be elicited by palpation in an opposite or different quadrant. Thus palpation of the left lower quadrant may produce tenderness and rebound tenderness in the right lower quadrant in appendicitis. This transfer of the discomfort is called *referred tenderness* or *rebound.*

Palpation is used to evaluate the patient for ascites, an abnormal accumulation of fluid in the peritoneal cavity. A rounded, symmetrical contour of the abdomen that is taut with bulging flanks is seen during inspection of the patient with ascites. Palpation of the abdomen in patients with ascites often yields a wavelike, almost fluctuant sensation. In advanced cases, the abdominal wall is stretched because of distention from excessive fluid. Gas-filled intestines will float to the top of an abdomen filled with fluid.

BREASTS AND GENITALS

Assessment of the male or female patient's breasts and genitals for cancer or tissue abnormalities begins with attention to the patient's safety and privacy, as well as respect for the patient's feelings about preventive care concerning reproductive health. Comfort with the examination for both males and females can be achieved through correct positioning of the patient and the use of a calm and relaxed approach by the nurse. A matter-of-fact approach in asking questions that deal with potentially sensitive issues helps the patient relax and feel safe (Health Assessment Questions box). Remember to take the age of the patient into consideration when preparing to examine the breasts and genitalia.

HEALTH ASSESSMENT QUESTIONS

Breasts and Genitals

Breasts: Male and Female

- Do you do a monthly breast self-examination (BSE)?
- Do you have mammograms done? If so, how often? When was your last mammogram?
- Do you have breast discomfort, masses, or lumps?
- Have you had any nipple discharge or pain?
- Do you or any family members have a history of breast cancer?
- Have you noticed any changes in your breasts?
- Have you ever had surgery on your breasts?

Female Genitals

- When was your last menstrual period? Do you have symptoms associated with your period?
- Have you ever been pregnant? If so, when? Do you have living children? If so, how many?
- Are you sexually active? Do you practice safe sex?
- Do you use contraception?
- Are you having any pain or difficulty associated with intercourse?
- Have you used hormones for contraception or for postmenopausal symptoms?
- Do you drink caffeine or alcohol?
- Have you experienced vaginal discharge, painful lumps or tissue abrasions or tears in the perineal area, or genital warts or lesions?
- Do you have a family history of endometrial, ovarian, or cervical cancer?

Male Genitals

- Have you noticed any changes in urination flow or frequency? Does your urine have an odor?
- Are you sexually active? Do you practice safe sex?
- Do you have any pain, swelling, or discharge from your penis?
- Have you noticed any lumps, enlargement, or pain in your testicles?
- Do you do a monthly self-testicular examination?
- Do you have swelling or any protrusion in your groin? If so, does it get worse when you cough or lift heavy objects?
- Do you have difficulty with achieving or maintaining an erection or with the process of ejaculation?

Breast Assessment

A primary responsibility of the nurse during the breast assessment is to discuss breast self-examination (BSE) with the patient. Because both male and female breast tissue is subject to invasive breast cancer, ask if the patient performs BSE, and review or teach the procedure as needed. For women, the best time for BSE is after the menstrual cycle ends, when the breast tissue is no longer tender or swollen from elevated estrogen levels. Men, postmenopausal women, and pregnant women are advised to perform BSE on the same day each month.

Inspection of the Breasts

Begin breast assessment with the patient standing or sitting with the arms hanging loosely at the sides. Have the patient lower the gown so that both breasts can be compared for symmetry, size, and shape. The breasts normally are almost symmetric in shape and size, with one breast often slightly larger than the other. As a normal sign of aging, the supporting ligaments of the breasts, known as *Cooper's ligaments,* become weak and elongate from the effects of gravity, causing the breasts to sag and the nipples to lower with the surrounding tissue. Even with this elongation, shape and symmetry of the breasts usually are preserved.

Observe breast contour and the skin covering the breast tissue. Note any lumps, masses, flattening, retraction, or dimpling of the breast tissue, as well as any drainage, bruising, or excoriation. The shape of the breast varies from one person to another and can be described as convex, pendulous, conical, or flat. Nipples can be inverted, everted, or flat and should not have any visible drainage unless the patient is a female who is breastfeeding.

To assess the breasts for symmetry, ask the patient to raise the arms above the head, then press the hands against the hips, and then extend the arms straight ahead while sitting and leaning forward. Observe the breasts for any retraction or dimpling that can result from invasion of underlying ligaments and tissues by tumors. If a tumor or malignancy is present, the ligaments of the affected breast will pull the skin and tissues toward the tumor, forming a retraction or dimpled area. Document the location of any abnormalities using a systematic approach that divides the breast into four quadrants extending into the axillary areas (Figure 20-45).

The skin covering the breast can give important clues about the underlying breast tissue. Note the color, venous pattern, and presence of lesions, erythema, dimpling, or inflammation. Lift large or pendulous breasts to observe the underside and the lateral aspects. Patients with large or pendulous breasts or those who wear undergarments that are too tight or conforming can have redness or excoriation on the outer surface of the skin around the breasts, caused by rubbing of the garments or skin-to-skin contact. Patients with excessive moisture from sweat or wet garments can develop a rash or skin excoriations.

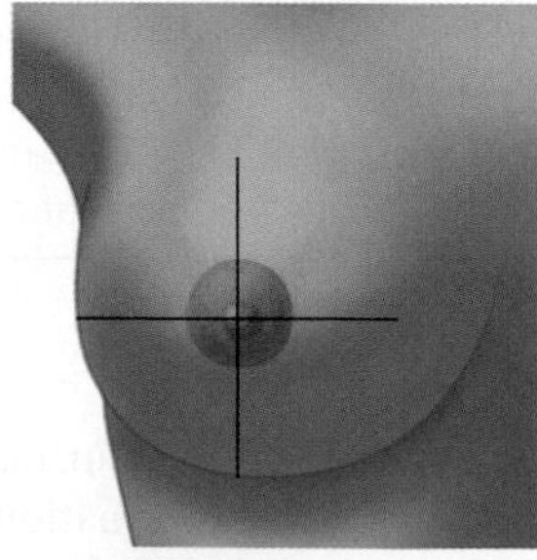

FIGURE 20-45 The breast divided into four quadrants for systematic examination.

Observe the nipples and areolas for size, shape, color, texture, lesions, and discharge. Areolas should be symmetric, pink to dark brown, and round. Nipples normally are everted and point in the same direction relative to the breast. Abnormal findings include dimpling, rashes, or sores anywhere on the breast, extreme asymmetry, and bleeding or discharge from the nipples.

Palpation of the Breasts

Palpation is used to assess the underlying breast tissue and the local lymph nodes. Because of the location of glandular tissue, a large portion of lymphatic drainage from the breasts circulates through the axillary lymph nodes. Metastatic cancers or malignancies can rapidly spread to the axillary lymph nodes and beyond. Therefore, the axilla is palpated bilaterally when doing a breast assessment. To palpate the lymph nodes, ask the patient to sit with the hands and arms relaxed at the sides. Face the patient, and stand on the side that is to be examined. Support the patient's arm in the flexed position, and raise the arm away from the chest wall. Palpate the axillary area using the hand not supporting the patient's arm. Using the fingertips, gently depress the skin surface, and gently roll the soft tissue underneath the fingertips. Examination includes palpating the entire axilla, the pectoralis major and lateral oblique muscles, and the chest wall in the midaxillary line, as well as along the clavicular ridges. Under normal circumstances the lymph nodes are not palpable. If lymph nodes are felt, note their location, consistency, mobility, size, and number. Palpable nodes that are suspect for malignancy are firm, tender, and nonmobile. Repeat the procedure on the patient's other side.

Instruct the patient to lie down in the supine position and raise one arm behind the head. This position causes the breast tissue to flatten against the chest wall. On the side with the arm raised, use the pads of the first three fingers to compress the breast tissue gently against the chest wall, noting the characteristics of the fleshy tissue. Examination of the breast can be methodically performed in several ways, illustrated in Figure 20-46. Instruct the patient to find a systematic pattern of BSE that she or he is comfortable performing, and have the patient demonstrate the chosen technique. Breast malignancies most frequently are located in the upper outer quadrant. Any abnormalities or new findings should be discussed immediately with the patient's health care provider for further diagnostic studies.

The consistency of normal breast tissue can vary across the life span, from person to person, and between genders. The breasts of a younger patient usually are firm and elastic, with denser tissue mass. In older patients, breast tissue feels soft,

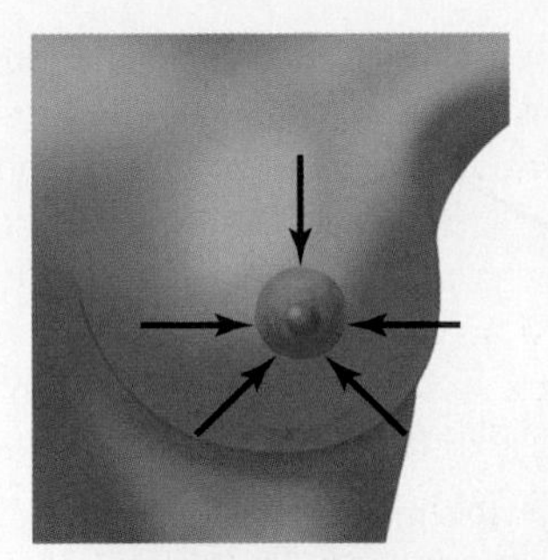
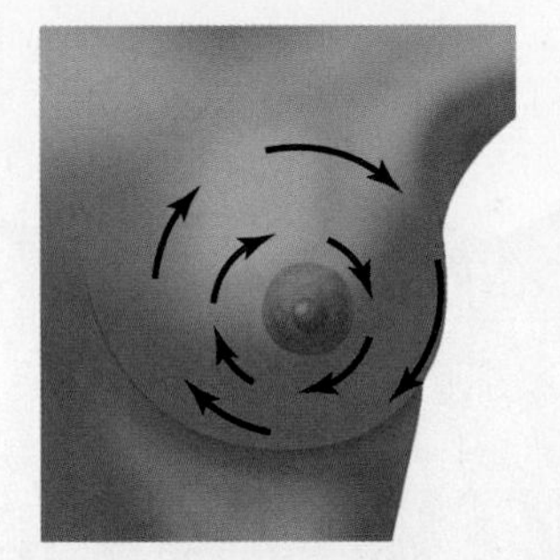
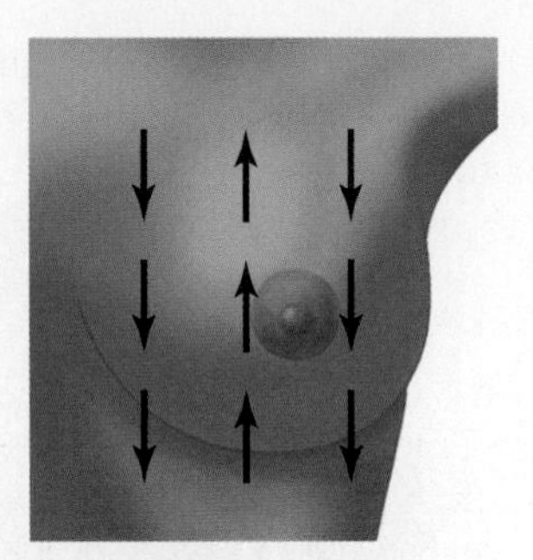

FIGURE 20-46 Different patterns of breast palpation.

nodular, and fibrous. When palpating large or pendulous breasts, support the breast in one hand while using the other hand to gently palpate the breast tissue. Palpation of the breasts should not elicit a pain response. A benign condition, fibrocystic breast disease, typically is characterized by lumpy, unilateral or bilateral cysts that can be painful on palpation. The cysts are more noticeable just before, during, and for a short period after menses, and they can be exacerbated by increased caffeine intake. Cystic breasts contain palpable lumps that are soft and movable and appear in the same area monthly.

When palpating the nipple and areola, note the consistency of the underlying tissue and any color changes that occur with gentle compression. Carefully pinch the nipple, encompassing the surrounding tissue just beneath. Observe for discharge, and palpate for masses. It is not uncommon for malignancies to be located just beneath the nipple as a barely perceptible mass. Encourage patients, both male and female, to demonstrate BSE, and observe the patient's technique. Stress the importance of immediate follow-up evaluation with a primary care provider if any questionable masses or lumps become evident. Although breast cancer is rare in men, those who have a first-degree relative (father, mother, or sister) with a history of breast cancer are at greater risk for developing the disease and need to palpate the breasts at regular intervals. American Cancer Society guidelines for BSE can be found at *www.cancer.org/cancer/breastcancer/moreinformation/breastcancerearlydetection/breast-cancer-early-detection-acs-recs-bse.*

The importance of a healthy lifestyle on breast cancer reduction in women has been the focus of extensive research during the past decade. The Evidence-Based Practice and Informatics box summarizes research findings that address the impact of lifestyle changes on risk reduction. The performance of a physical examination is an excellent time for the nurse to discuss disease prevention strategies with patients.

EVIDENCE-BASED PRACTICE AND INFORMATICS

Breast Cancer Risk Reduction

Several factors have been shown to potentially reduce the risk of breast cancer in women.

- A majority of studies indicate that women who participate in moderate- to high-intensity exercise 30 to 60 minutes per day have a lower incidence of breast cancer. Reported risk reduction varies between 20% and 80%, depending on the study (U.S. Department of Health and Human Services, 2014).
- Research indicates that both premenopausal and postmenopausal women benefit from increased physical activity. Vigorous or moderate physical activity in adolescence appears to be particularly protective (Lee and Oguma, 2006).
- Many studies reveal a relationship between consumption of one to two alcoholic drinks per day by women and a 30% to 50% increase in the incidence of breast cancer. Current recommendations are for women to limit their alcohol intake to less than one drink per day (Terry, Zhang, Kabat, et al, 2006).
- Extensive research has been conducted on the effect of a low-fat diet (with increased consumption of fruits and vegetables) on breast cancer risk. The evidence suggests that the effect of dietary intake on breast cancer risk is much greater during adolescence and young adulthood (Linos and Willett, 2007).

Assessment of the Female Genitalia

Explain the procedure and reasons for genital assessment before the examination. Correct positioning and draping provides privacy and assurance that only the portions of anatomy that need to be exposed are being viewed. Examination includes assessment of the reproductive organs, external genitalia, and anus using inspection and palpation (Figure 20-47). Examination of the internal reproductive organs using a vaginal speculum and digital examination of the rectum are usually performed by an advanced practice nurse or a physician.

! SAFE PRACTICE ALERT

Always wear gloves during assessments that may involve contact with mucous membranes.

Apply clean gloves before beginning the examination. With the patient in the dorsal recumbent position, inspect the outer genitalia for redness, swelling, lesions, masses, or

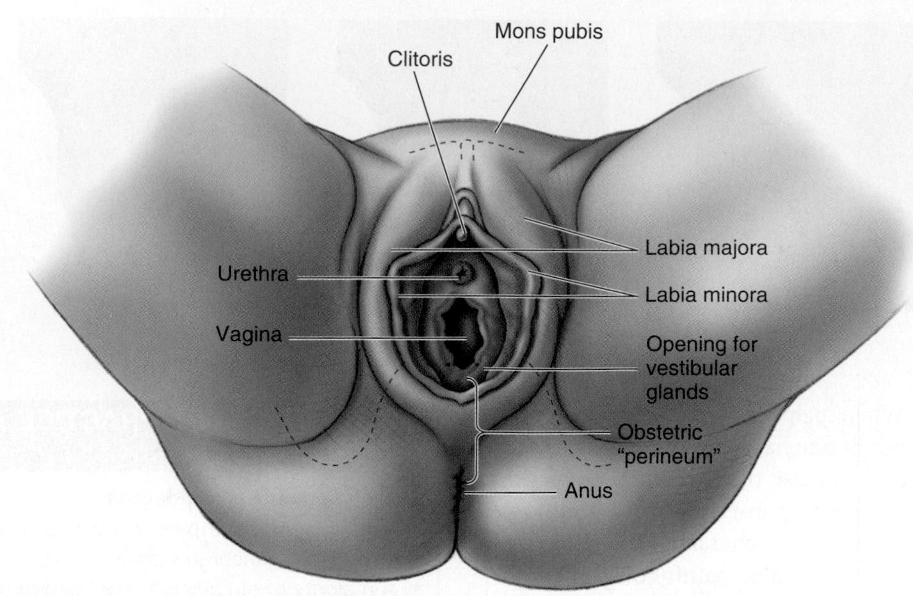

FIGURE 20-47 External female genitalia. (From Herlihy: *The human body in health and illness*, ed. 5, St. Louis, 2014, Saunders.)

infestations. Note the hair growth and distribution in the pelvic area. Preadolescents have no pubic hair; however, adolescents may have sparse hair growth along the labia that becomes darker and coarser toward the mons pubis. In adults, pubic hair, which usually has a curly, coarse texture, grows in a triangular pattern across the mons pubis and perineum and can extend along the inner thigh. Pubic hair thins, lightens, and becomes more sparse with aging.

! SAFE PRACTICE ALERT

Always palpate female genitalia from front to back. This pattern will prevent contamination of the urinary meatus by microorganisms commonly found near the anus.

Palpate the inguinal area for presence of lymph nodes. Carefully separate and palpate the labia majora and minora. Inspect the labia, the folds in between, and the clitoris. Note any redness, swelling, lesions, or discharge. Normally, the skin of the perineum is clean, smooth, and a slightly darker pink color than the skin surrounding it. The mucosal surface should be warm and moist. The labia folds should be symmetric and without lesions. The size of the clitoris can vary from woman to woman; however, it normally does not exceed 2 cm in length and approximately 0.5 cm in width. Note any inflammation, abnormal color, or atrophy. The presence of syphilitic lesions or chancres can be noted during external physical examination of the skin folds. They often appear as small open ulcers with purulent or serous drainage. Note the urethral meatus in relation to the other structures of the perineum. The urethral meatus is anterior to the vaginal orifice and should appear smooth, moist, and pink. Inspect the vaginal orifice for color, smoothness, and moisture.

Inspect the anus, noting any redness, swelling, or hemorrhoids. Palpate the perianal area for lesions or nodules. When examination of the female genitalia is complete, replace the drape or covering. Remove gloves and wash hands, using standard precautions.

Assessment of the Male Genitalia

Assessment of the male genitals includes inspection and palpation of the external genitalia, the inguinal ring, and the inguinal canal (Figure 20-48). It is an essential part of any health maintenance examination for all age groups. The patient can stand or lie supine, appropriately draped for privacy. Clean gloves should be worn by the examiner throughout the assessment.

Explain the parts of the examination before manipulating the genitals, and use efficient examination techniques to avoid causing unnecessary stimulation or discomfort. Note the level of sexual maturity of the patient, and take into consideration any embarrassment or anxiety that is age-sensitive or culturally related.

Begin the assessment with inspection, noting the size and shape of the penis and testes as well as the distribution of pubic hair across the perineal area. Before puberty, in preadolescents, pubic hair is absent in the groin area. With the advent of puberty, the secondary sex characteristics begin to develop, including enlargement and darkening of the testicles, appearance of pubic hair, and lengthening of the penis. Scrotal wrinkling is a normal finding by the end of puberty, and the pubic hair is coarse and thick. The skin in the pubic area should be free of rashes, lesions, masses, and obvious deformity.

When inspecting the penis, note whether the penis is circumcised or uncircumcised and whether the foreskin retracts

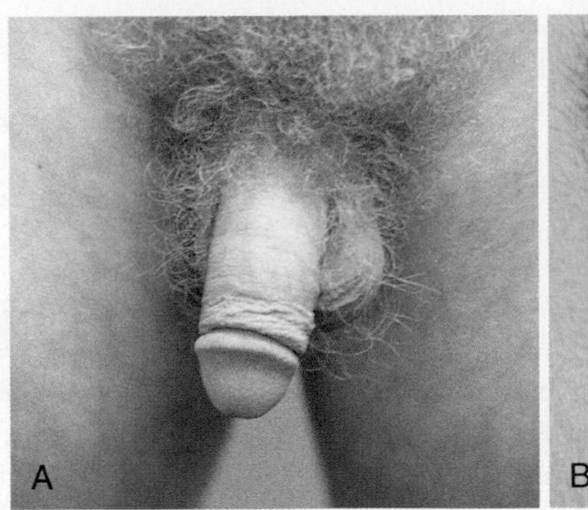

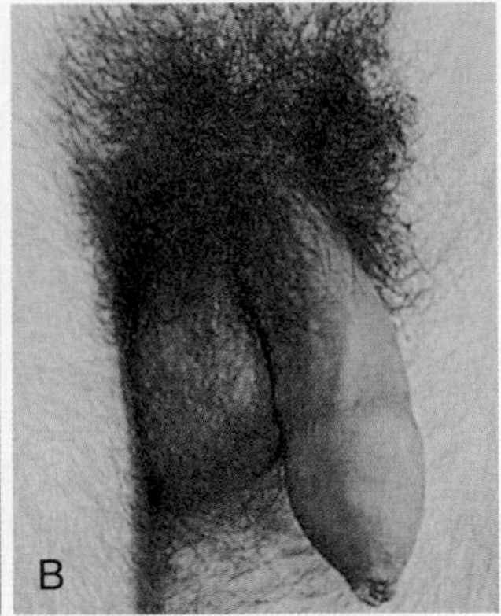

FIGURE 20-48 External male genitals. **A,** Circumcised. **B,** Uncircumcised. (From Ball JW, Dains JE, Flynn JA, et al: *Seidel's guide to physical examination*, ed. 8, St. Louis, 2015, Mosby.)

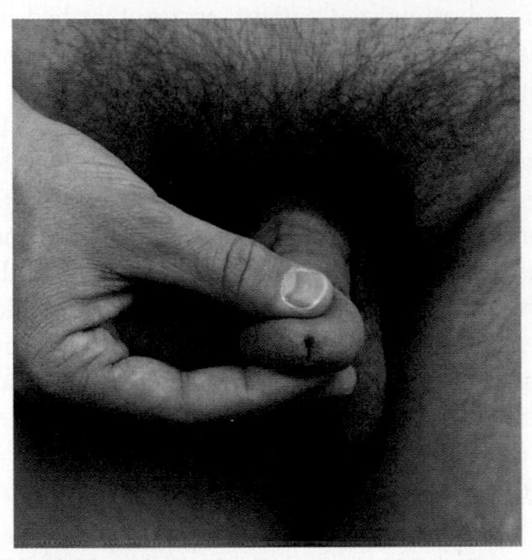

FIGURE 20-49 Self-examination of the penis. (From Ball JW, Dains JE, Flynn JA, et al: *Seidel's guide to physical examination*, ed. 8, St. Louis, 2015, Mosby.)

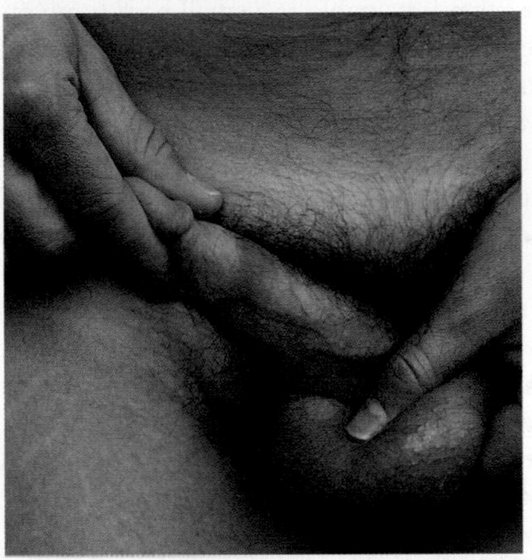

FIGURE 20-50 Self-examination of the testicles. (From Ball JW, Dains JE, Flynn JA, et al: *Seidel's guide to physical examination*, ed. 8, St. Louis, 2015, Mosby.)

easily. Observe for **smegma** (a whitish substance under the foreskin) or abnormal discharge. If discharge or lesions are present, a sample of material from the area should be obtained for culture. Note the appearance of the urethral meatus. It should be located on the ventral surface of the glans, slightly off the tip of the penis. In some patients with congenital defects, the meatus is displaced along the shaft of the penis, and surgery using the foreskin can be performed to correct the condition.

Carefully pinch the glans between the thumb and index finger to open the urethral meatus for examination (Figure 20-49). Normally, the opening appears smooth, glossy, and light pink. Return the foreskin to its original position, and continue by inspecting the entire shaft of the penis, including the posterior surface. Palpation is performed by compressing the shaft of the penis between the thumb and the first two fingers at incremental intervals from the base to the glans. Note any tenderness or pain response elicited during the examination. Document any lesions or scars and swelling or edema noticed during inspection and palpation. Palpate the inguinal area for presence of enlarged lymph nodes.

Examination of the male genitalia includes inspection and palpation of the scrotal sac and testes (Figure 20-50). The scrotal sac should be carefully examined for tenderness, masses, and potential malignant lesions. The scrotum is separated internally into two sections. Each section contains a testicle, vas deferens, and epididymis that are connected by the vas deferens to the inguinal ring. The testes are equal in size; however, when the male is standing, it is normal for the left testicle to be lower than the right within the scrotal sac. Observe the scrotum for any lesions, rashes, or edema. It should be without lesions and symmetric in contour. The scrotal skin usually is darker in color than the surrounding body tissue and has a coarse texture. The skin hangs loose over the testes; however, it may become tightened because of edema. The size of the scrotal sac can change with variation in temperatures, lifting the scrotum toward the body in cold temperatures and relaxing the scrotum to hang away from the body in warmer weather to protect the viability of sperm, which are temperature-sensitive. Continue with the examination by lifting the scrotum to view the posterior surface.

When palpating the scrotum, be cautious because the underlying organs are very sensitive. Severe pain during palpation is not a usual finding. The testes normally are oval in shape and approximately 1 to 2 inches in size. Palpation is performed by gently pressing the testes between the thumb and first two fingers, moving from the base to the distal portion in an incremental manner until the entire surface has been examined. The procedure is then repeated on the other side. The testes should feel smooth and pliable and should be free of nodules. Note the size, shape, and symmetry of the organs as well as any pain or discharge from the penis during testicular palpation. Testicular cancer usually is a painless, solid mass that is palpable as a small hard lump on the anterior aspect of the testes. During assessment of the testicles, assess the patient's knowledge concerning testicular self-examination. The American Cancer Society outlines the procedure for men with risk factors such as previous testicular cancer, undescended testicle, or a family history of testicular cancer to perform a testicular self-examination at *www.cancer.org/cancer/testicularcancer/moreinformation/doihavetesticularcancer/do-i-have-testicular-cancer-self-examination.*

The American Urological Association (AUA) recommends a first-time prostate examination at the age of 50 years for most men, with follow-up testing to be determined on an individual basis. The AUA guidelines call for men at higher risk for prostate cancer—African American men or men with a family history of prostate cancer—to start prostate cancer testing at age 40. The prostate is examined by digital rectal examination, which is done by an advanced practice nurse or a physician.

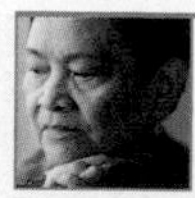

5. What three body systems would be critical to assess during Mrs. Thatcher's physical examination? State a rationale for each. Discuss a minimum of three additional actions that the nurse should take as part of the assessment process.

COMPLETION OF THE PHYSICAL ASSESSMENT LO 20.6

Allow the patient time to dress, and offer supplies necessary for hygiene or personal needs. Return the examination area to its original condition. Use PPE and infection control protocols specific to the facility when disposing of potentially infectious waste and while cleaning or removing soiled instruments or linens. If the physical examination was performed in a hospitalized patient, ensure that bed linens are unsoiled; the bedside table is clean, clear, and accessible; and the call light is within reach.

Record the complete assessment in the patient's EHR in a timely manner. Review the results and documentation for accuracy and attention to detail. Be sure to notify the nurse practitioner or the physician of any serious abnormalities or questionable findings. Document that members of the health care team have been notified. It is the responsibility of the patient's primary care provider to thoroughly investigate suspected medical conditions through diagnostic and lab testing and examination. Document any education provided to the patient or the patient's family related to the physical examination.

SUMMARY OF LEARNING OUTCOMES

LO 20.1 *Apply strategies used to conduct a patient interview, health history, and review of systems:* Controlling the physical environment, preventing interruptions, and limiting the number of people present are essential to conducting a thorough patient interview that protects patient privacy. Various forms of therapeutic communication are used to encourage patient sharing of critical information. Using a structured order for collecting data during the interview process facilitates completion of a thorough patient health history. Data may be collected and organized according to body system, from head to toe, or by Gordon's functional health patterns. Health assessment questions help to identify concerns related to each area of the body during the review of systems.

LO 20.2 *Discuss the environmental and patient care activities that should be completed before and during history taking and physical examination:* Patient safety and comfort are primary concerns during physical examination. Room temperature, drafts, accessibility of the examination table, and availability of blankets and pillows to assist with positioning and comfort are taken into consideration. Physical assessment equipment is collected and organized before initiation of an examination. Patients are gowned and draped as needed to ensure access to assessment areas. Family members or care providers may be present during an examination to assist in positioning and to prevent patient injury from falls. Permission for others to be present during the physical examination is obtained from competent adult patients.

LO 20.3 *Use the four physical assessment techniques when examining each body system:* Inspection, palpation, percussion, and auscultation techniques are used to various degrees in assessing each body system. Auscultation precedes palpation and percussion during abdominal assessment to avoid stimulation of bowel sounds that may cause erroneous assessment findings.

LO 20.4 *Discuss factors for consideration during the general survey:* Special consideration to age, culture preferences, gender concerns, and morphologic issues is required in order to provide safe and patient-centered care. Taking these factors into consideration enhances a patient's experience and results in greater patient satisfaction.

LO 20.5 *Demonstrate a focused and head-to-toe physical assessment, noting opportunities for patient education:* After gathering subjective data during the interview, health history, and review of systems, the nurse initiates the physical examination in an organized manner. A head-to-toe assessment is completed on hospitalized patients at least once per shift, with special attention to areas related to their admitting diagnoses. Focused assessments examine specific areas of concern in emergent and outpatient encounters. A complete head-to-toe examination usually is conducted during an initial patient–primary care provider interaction or referral to a specialist. Patient education focused on prevention, physical care, emotional concerns, stress reduction, nutrition, and exercise can be shared with patients during a physical assessment.

LO 20.6 *Describe the activities and specific documentation that are required at the completion of the physical assessment:* Findings of the assessment must be recorded in the patient's EHR in a timely manner. It is important to review the examination results and documentation for accuracy and attention to detail. The nurse practitioner or the physician should be notified of any serious abnormalities or questionable findings. Documentation is included indicating that members of the health care team have been notified.

Responses to the critical-thinking questions are available at *http://evolve.elsevier.com/YoostCrawford/fundamentals/*.

REVIEW QUESTIONS

1. Objective data can be gathered from the patient during which aspects of the physical assessment process? *(Select all that apply.)*
   a. Patient interview
   b. Health history
   c. General survey
   d. Physical examination
   e. Laboratory testing
2. Which sequence best identifies the order in which the nurse should complete an abdominal assessment?
   a. Inspection, palpation, percussion, auscultation
   b. Auscultation, inspection, palpation, percussion
   c. Auscultation, palpation, percussion, inspection
   d. Inspection, auscultation, palpation, percussion
3. During examination of a patient's neck with the bell of the stethoscope, the nurse identifies a carotid bruit. When are bruits audible in the neck?
   a. When jugular vein distention is present
   b. During normal examination of the neck
   c. When the carotid artery is partially occluded
   d. With complete occlusion of both carotid arteries
4. A nurse is preparing to auscultate a patient's chest. In which area should the nurse listen to evaluate the patient's aortic valve?
   a. Second right intercostal space
   b. Third left intercostal space
   c. Fifth right intercostal space
   d. Fifth left intercostal space along the midclavicular line
5. Which assessment finding would be most important to document in a patient with known liver disease who has a distended, taut abdomen?
   a. Abdominal girth
   b. Dentition condition
   c. Benign cardiac murmurs
   d. Daily ambulatory distance
6. The nurse notes the presence of ptosis when assessing an adult patient's eyes. Which potential cause would be considered of most concern, requiring further evaluation as soon as possible?
   a. Loss of skin elasticity
   b. Levator muscle weakness
   c. Congenital ocular abnormality
   d. Oculomotor cranial nerve III paralysis

7. Which action by a patient with a family history of macular degeneration would demonstrate use of a prevention strategy that has been found to help prevent deterioration of the macula?
   a. Using medicated eye drops
   b. Avoiding the use of sunglasses
   c. Taking vitamin B_6 and B_{12} supplements
   d. Minimizing dietary intake of antioxidants
8. While auscultating a patient's lungs, the nurse notes diminished breath sounds at the base of the right lung. What action should the nurse take next?
   a. Refer the patient for a chest x-ray.
   b. Listen to the base of the patient's left lung.
   c. Notify the patient's primary care provider.
   d. Palpate the patient's lung fields bilaterally.
9. What actions should the nurse take to assess whether a patient with a left above-the-knee amputation has adequate lower extremity circulation to the stump? *(Select all that apply.)*
   a. Palpate the stump for warmth.
   b. Assess pedal pulses bilaterally.
   c. Evaluate the left popliteal pulse rate.
   d. Inspect the stump and right leg for color.
   e. Check the left femoral pulse for strength.
10. Which action by the nurse would be most effective in determining if a patient has muscle hypertonicity?
   a. Watching the patient walk to the bathroom
   b. Asking the patient to squeeze both hands of the nurse
   c. Performing passive range-of-motion exercises with the patient
   d. Checking the patient's spine for the presence of postural irregularities

Answers and rationales for the review questions are available at *http://evolve.elsevier.com/YoostCrawford/fundamentals/.*

REFERENCES

American Academy of Dermatology: Melanoma: Signs and symptoms, 2014. Retrieved from *www.aad.org/dermatology-a-to-z/diseases-and-treatments/m---p/melanoma/signs-symptoms.*

American Dental Association: Antibiotic prophylaxis, 2014. Retrieved from *www.ada.org/2157.aspx.*

Cronenwett L, Sherwood G, Barnsteiner J, et al: Quality and safety education for nurses. *Nurs Outlook* 55(3):122-131, 2007.

Gordon M: *Manual of nursing diagnosis*, ed. 12, Sudbury, Mass, 2011, Jones & Bartlett.

Jun W: Pupil anomalies: Reaction and red flags, 2014. Retrieved from *www.pacificu.edu/optometry/ce/courses/19433/pupilanompg1.cfm.*

Lee I, Oguma Y: Physical activity. In D Schottenfeld, J Fraumeni (Eds): *Cancer epidemiology and prevention*, ed. 3, New York, 2006, Oxford University Press.

Linos E, Willett W: Diet and breast cancer risk. *J Natl Compr Cancer Netw* 5:711-718, 2007.

Terry M, Zhang F, Kabat G, et al: Lifetime alcohol intake and breast cancer risk. *Ann Epidemiol* 16(3):230-240, 2006.

U.S. Department of Health and Human Services: Physical activity guidelines for Americans, 2014. Retrieved from *http://health.gov/paguidelines/report/G7_cancer.aspx#_Toc197843471.*

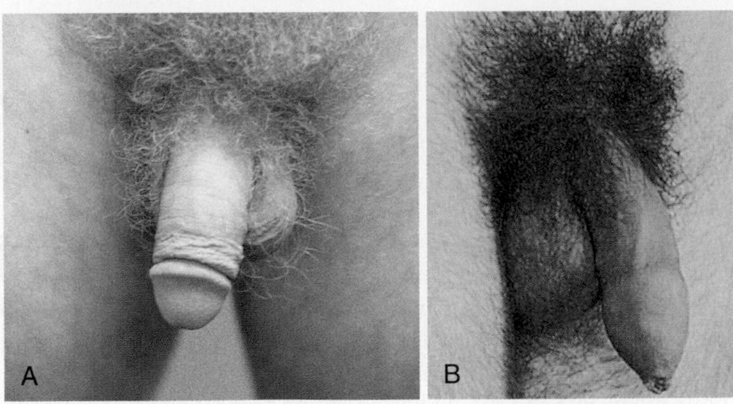

FIGURE 20-48 External male genitals. **A,** Circumcised. **B,** Uncircumcised. (From Ball JW, Dains JE, Flynn JA, et al: *Seidel's guide to physical examination*, ed. 8, St. Louis, 2015, Mosby.)

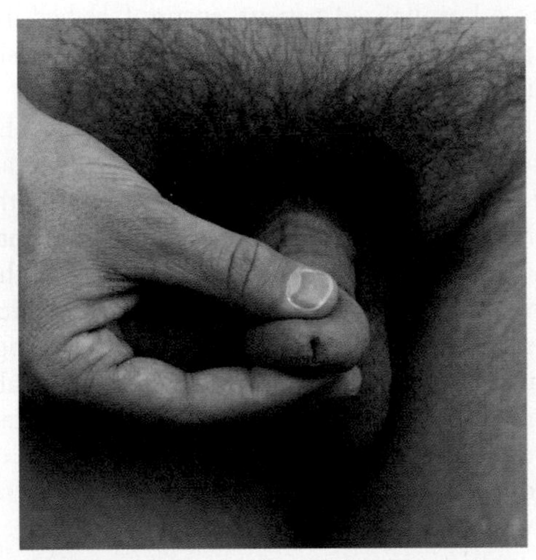

FIGURE 20-49 Self-examination of the penis. (From Ball JW, Dains JE, Flynn JA, et al: *Seidel's guide to physical examination*, ed. 8, St. Louis, 2015, Mosby.)

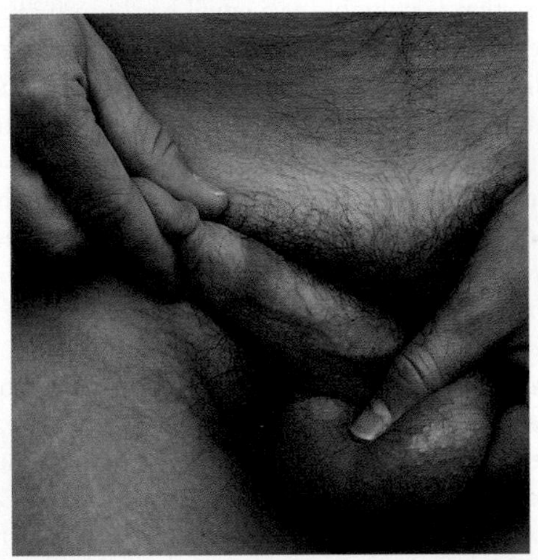

FIGURE 20-50 Self-examination of the testicles. (From Ball JW, Dains JE, Flynn JA, et al: *Seidel's guide to physical examination*, ed. 8, St. Louis, 2015, Mosby.)

easily. Observe for **smegma** (a whitish substance under the foreskin) or abnormal discharge. If discharge or lesions are present, a sample of material from the area should be obtained for culture. Note the appearance of the urethral meatus. It should be located on the ventral surface of the glans, slightly off the tip of the penis. In some patients with congenital defects, the meatus is displaced along the shaft of the penis, and surgery using the foreskin can be performed to correct the condition.

Carefully pinch the glans between the thumb and index finger to open the urethral meatus for examination (Figure 20-49). Normally, the opening appears smooth, glossy, and light pink. Return the foreskin to its original position, and continue by inspecting the entire shaft of the penis, including the posterior surface. Palpation is performed by compressing the shaft of the penis between the thumb and the first two fingers at incremental intervals from the base to the glans. Note any tenderness or pain response elicited during the examination. Document any lesions or scars and swelling or edema noticed during inspection and palpation. Palpate the inguinal area for presence of enlarged lymph nodes.

Examination of the male genitalia includes inspection and palpation of the scrotal sac and testes (Figure 20-50). The scrotal sac should be carefully examined for tenderness, masses, and potential malignant lesions. The scrotum is separated internally into two sections. Each section contains a testicle, vas deferens, and epididymis that are connected by the vas deferens to the inguinal ring. The testes are equal in size; however, when the male is standing, it is normal for the left testicle to be lower than the right within the scrotal sac. Observe the scrotum for any lesions, rashes, or edema. It should be without lesions and symmetric in contour. The scrotal skin usually is darker in color than the surrounding body tissue and has a coarse texture. The skin hangs loose over the testes; however, it may become tightened because of edema. The size of the scrotal sac can change with variation in temperatures, lifting the scrotum toward the body in cold temperatures and relaxing the scrotum to hang away from the body in warmer weather to protect the viability of sperm, which are temperature-sensitive. Continue with the examination by lifting the scrotum to view the posterior surface.

When palpating the scrotum, be cautious because the underlying organs are very sensitive. Severe pain during palpation is not a usual finding. The testes normally are oval in shape and approximately 1 to 2 inches in size. Palpation is performed by gently pressing the testes between the thumb and first two fingers, moving from the base to the distal portion in an incremental manner until the entire surface has been examined. The procedure is then repeated on the other side. The testes should feel smooth and pliable and should be free of nodules. Note the size, shape, and symmetry of the organs as well as any pain or discharge from the penis during testicular palpation. Testicular cancer usually is a painless, solid mass that is palpable as a small hard lump on the anterior aspect of the testes. During assessment of the testicles, assess the patient's knowledge concerning testicular self-examination. The American Cancer Society outlines the procedure for men with risk factors such as previous testicular cancer, undescended testicle, or a family history of testicular cancer to perform a testicular self-examination at *www.cancer.org/cancer/testicularcancer/moreinformation/doihavetesticularcancer/do-i-have-testicular-cancer-self-examination.*

The American Urological Association (AUA) recommends a first-time prostate examination at the age of 50 years for most men, with follow-up testing to be determined on an individual basis. The AUA guidelines call for men at higher risk for prostate cancer—African American men or men with a family history of prostate cancer—to start prostate cancer testing at age 40. The prostate is examined by digital rectal examination, which is done by an advanced practice nurse or a physician.

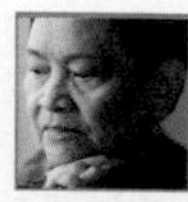

5. What three body systems would be critical to assess during Mrs. Thatcher's physical examination? State a rationale for each. Discuss a minimum of three additional actions that the nurse should take as part of the assessment process.

COMPLETION OF THE PHYSICAL ASSESSMENT LO 20.6

Allow the patient time to dress, and offer supplies necessary for hygiene or personal needs. Return the examination area to its original condition. Use PPE and infection control protocols specific to the facility when disposing of potentially infectious waste and while cleaning or removing soiled instruments or linens. If the physical examination was performed in a hospitalized patient, ensure that bed linens are unsoiled; the bedside table is clean, clear, and accessible; and the call light is within reach.

Record the complete assessment in the patient's EHR in a timely manner. Review the results and documentation for accuracy and attention to detail. Be sure to notify the nurse practitioner or the physician of any serious abnormalities or questionable findings. Document that members of the health care team have been notified. It is the responsibility of the patient's primary care provider to thoroughly investigate suspected medical conditions through diagnostic and lab testing and examination. Document any education provided to the patient or the patient's family related to the physical examination.

SUMMARY OF LEARNING OUTCOMES

LO 20.1 *Apply strategies used to conduct a patient interview, health history, and review of systems:* Controlling the physical environment, preventing interruptions, and limiting the number of people present are essential to conducting a thorough patient interview that protects patient privacy. Various forms of therapeutic communication are used to encourage patient sharing of critical information. Using a structured order for collecting data during the interview process facilitates completion of a thorough patient health history. Data may be collected and organized according to body system, from head to toe, or by Gordon's functional health patterns. Health assessment questions help to identify concerns related to each area of the body during the review of systems.

LO 20.2 *Discuss the environmental and patient care activities that should be completed before and during history taking and physical examination:* Patient safety and comfort are primary concerns during physical examination. Room temperature, drafts, accessibility of the examination table, and availability of blankets and pillows to assist with positioning and comfort are taken into consideration. Physical assessment equipment is collected and organized before initiation of an examination. Patients are gowned and draped as needed to ensure access to assessment areas. Family members or care providers may be present during an examination to assist in positioning and to prevent patient injury from falls. Permission for others to be present during the physical examination is obtained from competent adult patients.

LO 20.3 *Use the four physical assessment techniques when examining each body system:* Inspection, palpation, percussion, and auscultation techniques are used to various degrees in assessing each body system. Auscultation precedes palpation and percussion during abdominal assessment to avoid stimulation of bowel sounds that may cause erroneous assessment findings.

LO 20.4 *Discuss factors for consideration during the general survey:* Special consideration to age, culture preferences, gender concerns, and morphologic issues is required in order to provide safe and patient-centered care. Taking these factors into consideration enhances a patient's experience and results in greater patient satisfaction.

LO 20.5 *Demonstrate a focused and head-to-toe physical assessment, noting opportunities for patient education:* After gathering subjective data during the interview, health history, and review of systems, the nurse initiates the physical examination in an organized manner. A head-to-toe assessment is completed on hospitalized patients at least once per shift, with special attention to areas related to their admitting diagnoses. Focused assessments examine specific areas of concern in emergent and outpatient encounters. A complete head-to-toe examination usually is conducted during an initial patient–primary care provider interaction or referral to a specialist. Patient education focused on prevention, physical care, emotional concerns, stress reduction, nutrition, and exercise can be shared with patients during a physical assessment.

LO 20.6 *Describe the activities and specific documentation that are required at the completion of the physical assessment:* Findings of the assessment must be recorded in the patient's EHR in a timely manner. It is important to review the examination results and documentation for accuracy and attention to detail. The nurse practitioner or the physician should be notified of any serious abnormalities or questionable findings. Documentation is included indicating that members of the health care team have been notified.

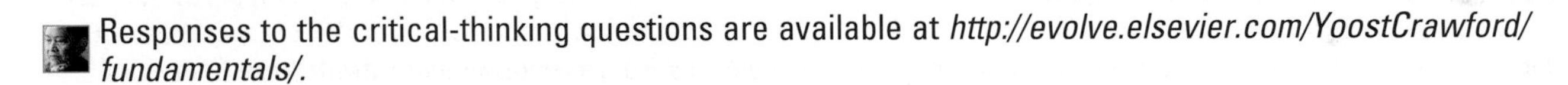

Responses to the critical-thinking questions are available at *http://evolve.elsevier.com/YoostCrawford/fundamentals/.*

REVIEW QUESTIONS

1. Objective data can be gathered from the patient during which aspects of the physical assessment process? *(Select all that apply.)*
   - **a.** Patient interview
   - **b.** Health history
   - **c.** General survey
   - **d.** Physical examination
   - **e.** Laboratory testing
2. Which sequence best identifies the order in which the nurse should complete an abdominal assessment?
   - **a.** Inspection, palpation, percussion, auscultation
   - **b.** Auscultation, inspection, palpation, percussion
   - **c.** Auscultation, palpation, percussion, inspection
   - **d.** Inspection, auscultation, palpation, percussion
3. During examination of a patient's neck with the bell of the stethoscope, the nurse identifies a carotid bruit. When are bruits audible in the neck?
   - **a.** When jugular vein distention is present
   - **b.** During normal examination of the neck
   - **c.** When the carotid artery is partially occluded
   - **d.** With complete occlusion of both carotid arteries
4. A nurse is preparing to auscultate a patient's chest. In which area should the nurse listen to evaluate the patient's aortic valve?
   - **a.** Second right intercostal space
   - **b.** Third left intercostal space
   - **c.** Fifth right intercostal space
   - **d.** Fifth left intercostal space along the midclavicular line
5. Which assessment finding would be most important to document in a patient with known liver disease who has a distended, taut abdomen?
   - **a.** Abdominal girth
   - **b.** Dentition condition
   - **c.** Benign cardiac murmurs
   - **d.** Daily ambulatory distance
6. The nurse notes the presence of ptosis when assessing an adult patient's eyes. Which potential cause would be considered of most concern, requiring further evaluation as soon as possible?
   - **a.** Loss of skin elasticity
   - **b.** Levator muscle weakness
   - **c.** Congenital ocular abnormality
   - **d.** Oculomotor cranial nerve III paralysis

7. Which action by a patient with a family history of macular degeneration would demonstrate use of a prevention strategy that has been found to help prevent deterioration of the macula?
   a. Using medicated eye drops
   b. Avoiding the use of sunglasses
   c. Taking vitamin B_6 and B_{12} supplements
   d. Minimizing dietary intake of antioxidants
8. While auscultating a patient's lungs, the nurse notes diminished breath sounds at the base of the right lung. What action should the nurse take next?
   a. Refer the patient for a chest x-ray.
   b. Listen to the base of the patient's left lung.
   c. Notify the patient's primary care provider.
   d. Palpate the patient's lung fields bilaterally.
9. What actions should the nurse take to assess whether a patient with a left above-the-knee amputation has adequate lower extremity circulation to the stump? *(Select all that apply.)*
   a. Palpate the stump for warmth.
   b. Assess pedal pulses bilaterally.
   c. Evaluate the left popliteal pulse rate.
   d. Inspect the stump and right leg for color.
   e. Check the left femoral pulse for strength.
10. Which action by the nurse would be most effective in determining if a patient has muscle hypertonicity?
    a. Watching the patient walk to the bathroom
    b. Asking the patient to squeeze both hands of the nurse
    c. Performing passive range-of-motion exercises with the patient
    d. Checking the patient's spine for the presence of postural irregularities

Answers and rationales for the review questions are available at *http://evolve.elsevier.com/YoostCrawford/fundamentals/*.

REFERENCES

American Academy of Dermatology: Melanoma: Signs and symptoms, 2014. Retrieved from *www.aad.org/dermatology-a-to-z/diseases-and-treatments/m---p/melanoma/signs-symptoms*.

American Dental Association: Antibiotic prophylaxis, 2014. Retrieved from *www.ada.org/2157.aspx*.

Cronenwett L, Sherwood G, Barnsteiner J, et al: Quality and safety education for nurses. *Nurs Outlook* 55(3):122-131, 2007.

Gordon M: *Manual of nursing diagnosis*, ed. 12, Sudbury, Mass, 2011, Jones & Bartlett.

Jun W: Pupil anomalies: Reaction and red flags, 2014. Retrieved from *www.pacificu.edu/optometry/ce/courses/19433/pupilanompg1.cfm*.

Lee I, Oguma Y: Physical activity. In D Schottenfeld, J Fraumeni (Eds): *Cancer epidemiology and prevention*, ed. 3, New York, 2006, Oxford University Press.

Linos E, Willett W: Diet and breast cancer risk. *J Natl Compr Cancer Netw* 5:711-718, 2007.

Terry M, Zhang F, Kabat G, et al: Lifetime alcohol intake and breast cancer risk. *Ann Epidemiol* 16(3):230-240, 2006.

U.S. Department of Health and Human Services: Physical activity guidelines for Americans, 2014. Retrieved from *http://health.gov/paguidelines/report/G7_cancer.aspx#_Toc197843471*.

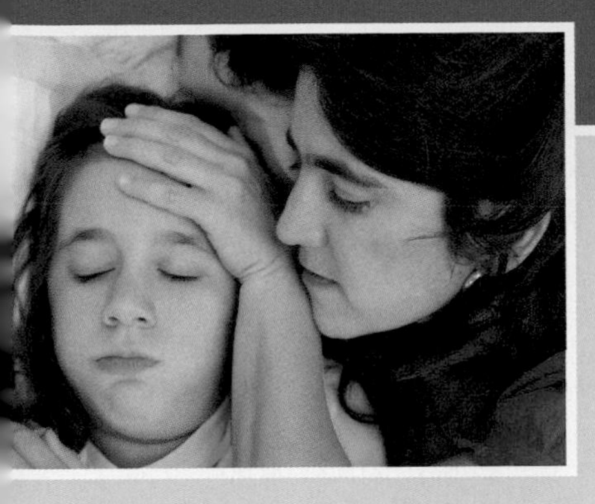

CHAPTER 21

Ethnicity and Cultural Assessment

EVOLVE WEBSITE

http://evolve.elsevier.com/YoostCrawford/fundamentals/

- Additional Evolve-Only Review Questions With Answers
- Answers and Rationales for Text Review Questions
- Answers to Critical-Thinking Questions
- Case Study With Questions
- Glossary

LEARNING OUTCOMES

Comprehension of this chapter's content will provide students with the ability to:

LO 21.1 Compare characteristics of culture and ethnicity.

LO 21.2 Explain cultural concepts that affect a nurse's ability to provide culturally congruent care.

LO 21.3 Identify factors that contribute to cultural identity acquisition.

LO 21.4 Articulate an understanding of transcultural nursing and cultural competence.

LO 21.5 Describe how to develop culturally competent individualized plans of care using cultural assessment tools and the nursing process.

KEY TERMS

acculturation, p. 398
assimilation, p. 398
cultural competence, p. 401
cultural openness, p. 400
cultural sensitivity, p. 400
culturally congruent care, p. 401
culture, p. 395
discrimination, p. 397
emic, p. 400
enculturation, p. 395
ethnicity, p. 395
ethnocentrism, p. 398
etic, p. 400
generalization, p. 396
infrastructure, p. 396
prejudice, p. 397
race, p. 397
racism, p. 397
rituals, p. 399
rule of descent, p. 397
social structure, p. 396
socialization, p. 399
stereotype, p. 396
superstructure, p. 396
symbols, p. 395
transcultural nursing, p. 399

CASE STUDY

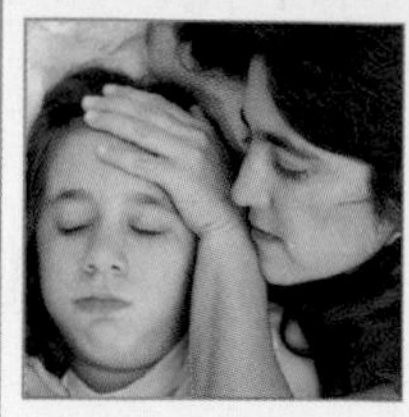

Mrs. Gomez, a 24-year-old Latina, arrives at the community hospital's emergency department with her 4-year-old daughter, Maria. Mrs. Gomez speaks broken English, and none of the nurses who speak Spanish are currently on duty.

The nurse is able to determine that Maria has not been eating for the last several days. Mrs. Gomez says that she has tried to make her daughter drink but Maria refuses. On physical examination, Maria has sluggish skin turgor, is lethargic, and does not communicate with her mother or the nurse. Her vital signs are T 103.3, P 125 and irregular, R 30 and shallow, and BP 86/58. Maria's throat is reddened, and lung auscultation reveals bilateral fine crackles.

When the nurse explains to Mrs. Gomez that an IV line needs to be placed in Maria's arm, Mrs. Gomez says it can't be done until her husband arrives. When Mr. Gomez arrives, he speaks very little English and is skeptical of the need for IV placement. Maria is diagnosed with dehydration, strep throat, and pneumonia, requiring her to be admitted to the hospital.

Refer back to this case study to answer the critical-thinking questions throughout the chapter.

Ethnicity and culture dramatically affect daily life for people throughout the world. Literally thousands of ethnic and cultural groups are recognized globally as well as within entire countries and regions. Statistics from the U.S. Central Intelligence Agency (CIA) *The World Factbook* indicate that Algeria has a population made up of only two primary ethnic groups, whereas the Democratic Republic of the Congo has more than 200 African ethnic groups represented (cited in "People Statistics," 2014). In the United States, the 2010 census identifies a population of more than six different races, not including Hispanics or Latinos of all races, with 2.9% of people identifying with two or more races (U.S. Census Bureau, 2011). Figure 21-1 shows U.S. population statistics by race.

Migration of people creates nations of diverse cultures and ethnicities. Relocation of individuals and families into foreign countries or regions with cultures different from their own causes challenges to both the immigrants or refugees and the health care providers in the area. Research indicates that patient populations experience lower-quality care and poorer outcomes associated with factors such as race, ethnicity, and language (Agency for Healthcare Research and Quality, 2012; Smedley, Stith, and Nelson, 2002). Health care access from culturally sensitive health care providers is a goal of the *Healthy People 2020* initiative (U.S. Department of Health and Human Services, 2014).

Within the past decade, The Joint Commission developed accreditation standards that health care facilities must meet to improve communication and provide culturally competent care (Ethical, Legal, and Professional Practice box). It is imperative that people who are traveling or have relocated from a foreign country have access to health care information and treatment in their own language that is sensitive to cultural norms. Transcultural nursing as a specialty seeks to address the multifaceted aspects of ethnicity and culture (Figure 21-2). All nurses need to achieve increasing levels of cultural competence throughout their careers in order to provide unbiased, holistic care.

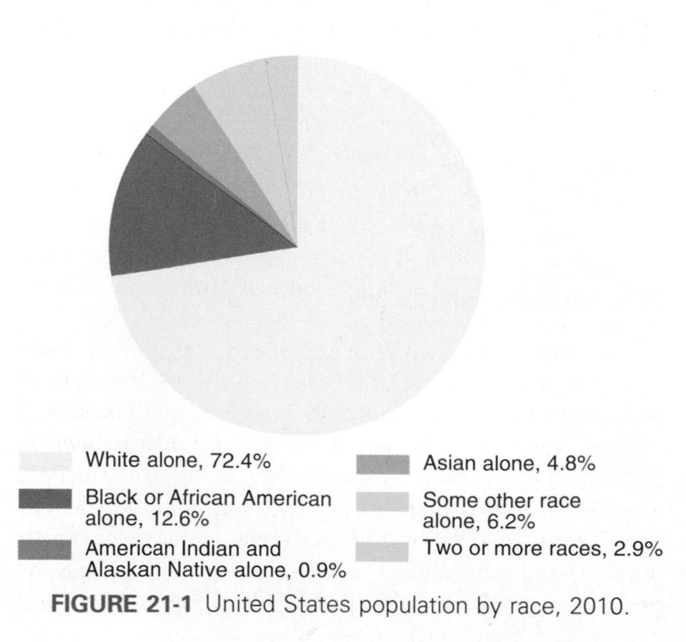

FIGURE 21-1 United States population by race, 2010.

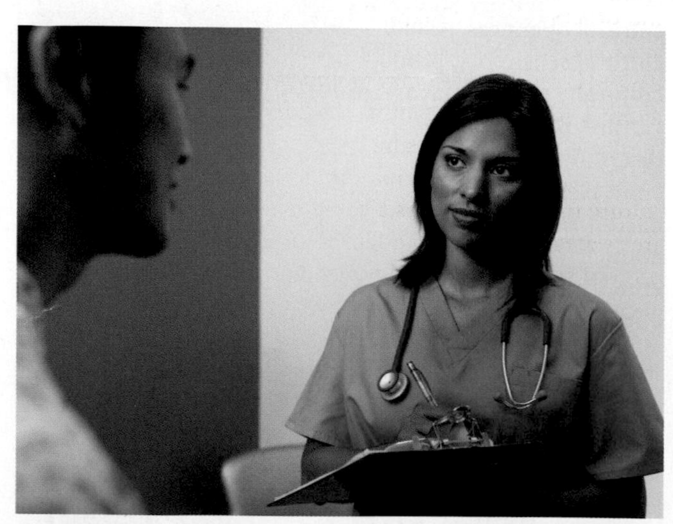

FIGURE 21-2 Nurses are required to collect data regarding the patient's language and ethnic, cultural, spiritual, and dietary preferences when the patient is admitted to a health care facility.

ETHICAL, LEGAL, AND PROFESSIONAL PRACTICE

Enhancing Communication with Cultural Sensitivity

The Joint Commission has identified health care activities within every step of the nursing process to ensure enhanced communication with people of diverse cultures:

- On a patient's admission to a health care facility, patient information regarding language preference; race; ethnicity; cultural, spiritual, and religious beliefs; and dietary needs and restrictions is to be assessed and documented in the electronic health record.
- Throughout treatment, changes in patient communication status, changes in patient dietary needs or restrictions, and accommodations for patient cultural, religious, and spiritual beliefs are to be noted and addressed.
- During discharge planning and community agency referral, patient communication needs are to be met to ensure a smooth transition and enhanced patient outcomes.

From The Joint Commission: A roadmap for hospitals, 2010. Retrieved from *www.jointcommission.org/assets/1/6/ARoadmapforHospitalsfinalversion727.pdf.*

CULTURE AND ETHNICITY LO 21.1

Culture refers to the learned, shared, and transmitted knowledge of values, beliefs, and ways of life of a particular group that generally are transmitted from one generation to another and influence the individual person's thinking, decisions, and actions in patterned or certain ways (Leininger, 1978, 1995). **Ethnicity** is the person's identification with or membership in a particular racial, national, or cultural group and observation of the group's customs, beliefs, and language. Ethnicity is based on cultural similarities and differences within a society or nation. Similarities occur with members of the same group; differences occur between members of the group and others (Kottak, 2012). Ethnicity may include a reference to skin color because group membership often is based on national origin, which may encompass a particular race. Ethnicity is frequently a central consideration in providing culturally appropriate nursing care.

All aspects of behavior can have cultural origins; thus culture may be viewed as a complex whole in which all parts are related. Culture has a family and group component, but it is not transmitted biologically. The values, beliefs, and traditions of a group must be learned by each person within the family and social community. "Culture depends on an underlying social construct that includes knowledge, beliefs, laws, morals, and customs" (Spector, 2012, p. 10).

According to Purnell (2013), culture should be viewed as the "totality of socially transmitted behavioral patterns, art, beliefs, values, customs, ways of life, and all other products of human work and thought characteristics of a population of people that guide their worldview and decision making" (p. 6). Culture involves mostly unconscious thoughts and actions that have a dramatic influence on health and illness. It is imperative that nurses and all health care providers recognize and respect patients' cultural beliefs and make every effort to incorporate these beliefs into their treatment plans. Doing so is a critical skill in providing patient-centered care.

CHARACTERISTICS OF CULTURE

The art, literature, costumes, customs, language, religion, and religious rituals of a particular group of people are manifested by their culture. Thus people and their patterns of life make up the culture of a particular region or country, and cultures vary throughout the world. Such differences extend across geographic boundaries, and this diversity in cultures results in the diversity of people everywhere.

Because culture consists of a system of beliefs held by the people of a region as well as their principles and moral values, behavioral patterns of people from a particular geographic region of the world contribute to the region's culture. Four basic elements of culture are recognized: Culture is (1) learned, (2) symbolic, (3) shared, and (4) integrated.

Culture Is Learned

Culture is learned, and it is not biologically inherited. According to the nineteenth century seminal work of Tylor (1871), culture is passed on through attributes that a person acquires by growing up in a particular society and being exposed to traditions. **Enculturation** is the process whereby a culture is passed from generation to generation. Enculturation begins at birth as parents and other family members begin to teach the child what is expected in terms of familial responsibilities and contributions. This learning process occurs consciously and unconsciously through interactions with other family and community members. Culture can be taught directly, for example, as with a mother teaching her child a family recipe, or indirectly, as occurs when a son observes the behavior of his father and other males in his family. By paying attention to things that happen around them, children modify their behaviors on the basis of the actions of other family members.

Culture Is Symbolic

Culture is based on symbols. Much of human behavior is mediated and moderated by **symbols**—signs, sounds, clothing, tools, customs, beliefs, rituals, and other items that represent meaningful concepts. Language is the most important symbolic aspect of culture. Language represents the most extensive use of symbols in a culture because words are used to represent objects and ideas.

Language is a structure of verbal symbols used to communicate and share cultural beliefs and ideas that can be manipulated and used as tools by individuals and groups to organize their lives. Nonverbal symbols are images, such as flags of countries, that represent shared ideas or beliefs. The American Red Cross uses a single red cross on a field of white on trucks and armbands as a symbol of its relief efforts; many religions use water as a symbol of rebirth through the process of baptism. Cultural symbols are passed on and accepted throughout generations. The mention of certain symbols automatically conjures up images and associations.

Culture Is Shared

Culture is an attribute of essentially all members of a group, not just individuals. People who grow up in a particular culture often have shared values, beliefs, ideals, and expectations. These shared attributes are absorbed and transmitted through generations of teaching and sharing ideas, traditions, and rituals. According to Haviland, Prins, Walrath, and McBride (2013), culture is the "common denominator" that makes the actions of a person intelligible to other group members. One shared element found in all cultures is an understanding of gender roles, the roles that a particular culture assigns to men and women. Although the world is changing, certain values and beliefs regarding gender roles remain unchanged in many cultures.

Culture Is Integrated

Cultures are integrated, patterned systems (Kottak, 2012). According to Haviland and colleagues (2013), the foundation of culture includes three structural elements that work together to keep the culture strong: An **infrastructure** provides the basic necessities of life; a **social structure** determines how people interact with one another; and a **superstructure**, or worldview, provides a belief system that helps people identify themselves, their society, and the world around them. Figure 21-3 visually depicts the three levels of structure within Haviland's Barrel Model of Culture.

As one part of a cultural system changes, other parts of the system change as well. For example, during the 1950s, most American women were stay-at-home mothers and wives; their career was being a housewife. However, the perception of the female role in society changed, and the goal of many women today is to attend college and pursue a professional career. This change is representative of the integration of new beliefs, ideas, attitudes, and behaviors into the previous cultural system.

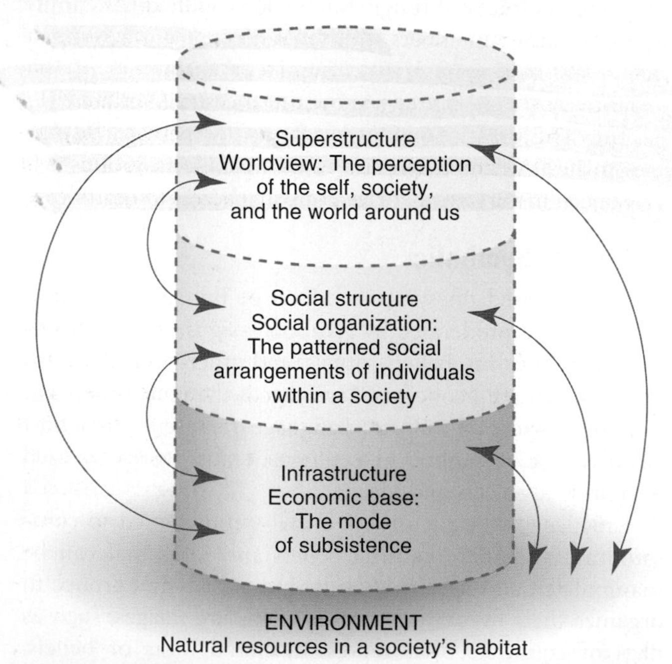

FIGURE 21-3 Haviland's Barrel Model of Culture. (From Haviland W, Prins H, Walrath D, et al: *Cultural anthropology: The human challenge*, ed. 14, Belmont, Calif., 2013, Wadsworth.)

Within the culture of nursing, the nursing cap was a traditional symbol of the nursing profession. However, because of the expanded role of the nurse, the increased numbers of men entering the profession, and the relaxed nature of society as a whole, the cap has been abandoned in most practice settings.

CULTURAL CONCEPTS LO 21.2

To more fully understand the complexities of ethnicity and culture, nurses must be aware of both helpful and detrimental concepts that affect cultural competence. By becoming familiar with these ideas, nurses can better provide culturally sensitive care.

GENERALIZATION

A **generalization** is a statement, idea, or principle that has a broad application. Generalizations typically infer or draw conclusions from many factors. According to Galanti (2008), generalizations are a beginning point; one should gather more information to ascertain whether a generalized statement is appropriately applied to an individual or group. Generalizations tend to be applied broadly in regard to common beliefs, behaviors, and patterns shared by a particular culture.

Generalizations may be applied when traits that are fairly consistent across cultures can be identified within a particular group, but individual differences should never be forgotten. Certain behaviors can be anticipated and understood by using generalizations. However, differences are invariably present among individuals within cultures, and nurses need to consider these differences when providing care.

STEREOTYPES

Kottak (2012) defines **stereotype** as a set of fixed ideas, often unfavorable, about members of a group. Galanti (2008) views stereotypes as an ending point, because no attempt is made to learn whether a perception or belief applies to a particular person. The acceptance of stereotypes ignores the individuality of people within a cultural group. Stereotyping ignores the fact that people belong to many cultural groups, including those based on ethnicity, religion, generational status, educational level, gender, and socioeconomic level.

In the patient-nurse relationship, there is no place for stereotypes, because they are detrimental to providing patients with necessary care. False opinions, perceptions, or beliefs are developed as a consequence of an unwillingness to obtain all of the information necessary to make fair judgments about particular people or situations. In the absence of confirmed knowledge, stereotypes allow people to make unfounded assumptions.

Sometimes society innocently creates and perpetuates stereotypes, but at other times the creation of a stereotype is a deliberate act. Unfavorable stereotypes lead to unfair discrimination and persecution. Stereotyping can have negative results in health care when nurses and other health care professionals assume that all people of a specific culture or ethnicity act in similar ways. For example, if a nurse previously encountered an Asian patient who requested care from only Asian nurses and a new Asian patient is admitted to the unit when no Asian nurses are available to provide care, stereotyping may lead to neglect of the newly admitted patient. In all cases, stereotyping of individual patients should be avoided. The nurse needs to interview and assess each patient with an open mind to obtain accurate information for planning culturally competent care.

PREJUDICE

Prejudice is the process of devaluing an entire group because of assumed behavior, values, or attributes (Kottak, 2012). People demonstrate prejudice when they apply group stereotypes to individuals and assume that all people within a group will act in a predetermined manner. Prejudice includes "labeling" groups or cultures—for example, as lazy or materialistic.

Nurses are guilty of prejudicial thinking if they anticipate certain patient behavior based on a patient's appearance or on previous interactions with people of similar ethnicity or culture. There is no room for prejudice in professional nursing practice. Unchecked stereotyping may lead to discrimination and unequal care of individual patients.

DISCRIMINATION

Discrimination refers to policies and practices that harm a group and its members. According to Kottak (2012), discrimination may be *de facto* (practiced, but not legally sanctioned) or *de jure* (legally sanctioned). An example of de facto discrimination is the harsher treatment that minorities may face from law enforcement agencies or the judicial system. This discrimination is unlawful and illegal but continues to happen. Two examples of discrimination de jure are the once-legal practices of segregation in the United States and apartheid in South Africa. Although these practices are no longer legal, in both instances the unequal treatment of blacks and whites was sanctioned by law. Each group had different rights and privileges, a situation that fostered prejudices and discrimination.

When people are judged on the basis of prejudices or stereotypes and are treated differently, they are victims of discrimination, which can take many forms. Minority groups may face subtle or overt pressures that discourage them from living in certain neighborhoods. Women and minorities often face unequal access to employment, education, and social services. The mentally ill may face this type of discrimination because of an unfounded belief that they will harm others. In the business world, women and minorities often are excluded from upper-management positions. Many social clubs have selective membership policies that, in effect, prevent people of certain religions, races, or genders from joining.

In some cases, civil and criminal justice has not been applied equally to all people as a result of discrimination. In some countries, homosexuals are jailed simply as a result of their sexual orientation. In the United States, some studies indicate that African Americans convicted of first-degree murder have a significantly higher probability of receiving the death penalty than whites (Cohen and Smith, 2010). Race tends to be a more frequent factor in discrimination because of the visible differences between minority races and members of the larger culture.

RACE

Race is thought by many to have a biologic basis. However, this assumption is not true. **Race** is a socially constructed concept that tends to group people by common descent, heredity, or physical characteristics. For example, "In the United States, people acquire their racial identity at birth as an ascribed status not based on biology" (Kottak, 2012, p. 136).

It has been a practice in the United States to use the rule of descent to categorize people by race. The **rule of descent** arbitrarily assigns a race to a person on the basis of a societal dictate that associates social identity with ancestry. For example, in some states, if people have any ancestors of minority descent, they are classified as a member of that minority, no matter how remote the ancestry (Kottak, 2012, p. 136). This practice divides society and perpetuates disparities in health care because it assigns people to groups that have been historically deprived of equal access to health care, wealth, power, and privilege.

Racism

Racism is an unfounded belief that race determines a person's character or ability and that one race is superior or inferior to another. Scientific evidence indicates that no one race is culturally or psychologically superior to another, and past studies that have reached other conclusions have been found to be seriously flawed in their methodology or inherently biased. Despite the preponderance of these scientific findings, some people still maintain that their race is superior to all others. Such people, known collectively as racists, are most likely to engage in discrimination, persecution, and violence against those they deem to be members of inferior races (Grobman, 1990). Health care professionals play a vital role in counteracting racism by providing unbiased, equal access and culturally sensitive care to people of every race and culture.

ACQUISITION OF CULTURAL IDENTITY LO 21.3

People develop and maintain their cultural identity through a variety of methods. When relocating to a new country or region, members of some cultural and ethnic groups choose to integrate into their new cultural environment, whereas others within these groups prefer to retain their traditional patterns of dress and behavior. Recognizing these differences allows nurses to appreciate the needs of culturally diverse patient populations.

ACCULTURATION

Acculturation is a mechanism of cultural change achieved through the exchange of cultural features resulting from firsthand contact between groups (Kottak, 2012). The culture of one or both groups may be changed over the course of time; however, each group remains distinct. Firsthand contact between groups may bring about cultural changes in language, technology, food, clothing, music, and other aspects. Box 21-1 provides an example of language development in acculturation.

ASSIMILATION

Assimilation is the process by which individuals from one cultural group merge with, or blend into, a second group. The concept of assimilation originated in anthropology and generally refers to a group process, although assimilation also can be defined and examined at the individual level. Assimilation involves a transformation in which members of one group, usually the minority group, enter into and become a part of a second group through continuous social interaction. Quite often during this process, the minority group may lose self-identified members of its group and/or aspects of its culture. For centuries, scholars have called the results of assimilation the *melting pot* process and regarded this process as a natural and necessary aspect of immigrant adaptation to life in a new country.

One of the more extreme forms of assimilation involves intergroup marriage (e.g., interracial marriage). Consider, for example, a Chinese-speaking Buddhist woman who immigrates to England and marries an English-speaking Jewish male. If the woman learns English, changes her maiden name, adopts the Jewish religion, and becomes a British citizen, she will have fully assimilated into mainstream English culture while abandoning many of her native cultural ways. Entering into another cultural group via marriage may result in relinquishing important aspects of cultural identity.

People who fully assimilate within a culture different from the one into which they were born undergo psychological changes in cultural orientation (beliefs, attitudes, values) and cultural behaviors (customs, traditions) as well as in personal identity, to the point of losing many of the important aspects of their original native culture. Accordingly, the effect of full assimilation on the psychological and social well-being of human beings may be questioned.

BOX 21-1 Language Development in Acculturation

Pidgin

Pidgin is an example of how language develops during the acculturation process. Pidgin English is the local language in some regions of the world.

- Pidgin is a mixed language that develops to facilitate communication between members of different groups who come in contact with one another.
- It usually develops as a result of trade or colonialism and is a simplified form of English. It blends the basics of English with the grammar and pronunciations of the native language.
- Pidgin English was first used for commerce in Chinese ports and developed in other forms in Papua New Guinea and West Africa (Kottak, 2012).
- Nurses who practice in areas where Pidgin English is spoken need to be fluent in Pidgin and English, although most medical terms sound similar in both dialects.

ETHNOCENTRISM

Ethnocentrism is the belief that one's own culture is superior to that of another while using one's own cultural values as the criteria by which to judge other cultures (Kottak, 2012). One ethnocentric view can be found in Western medicine. Western medical practitioners tend to believe that their approach to health and healing is far superior to that of non-Western practitioners. Many Western practices, especially the use of pharmacologic interventions, can find their roots in the practices of Eastern and Native American cultures, where plants and plant extracts are a mainstay. According to Leininger and McFarland (2006), ethnocentric beliefs lead to cultural imposition, or imposed actions that are based on the dominant culture's view of what works best.

Ethnocentrism poses serious ethical and quality-of-care concerns. Issues of and decisions about care for diverse cultural groups require that nurses and other health care providers be knowledgeable about the principles, concepts, and theoretical frameworks of transcultural care. Being culturally sensitive and culturally competent is important, because preconceived ideas about certain cultures can lead to racial stereotyping of patients, families, and communities by health care providers. Nurses must recognize that their own cultural beliefs are not necessarily superior, and they should refrain from thinking of another person's ideas as ignorant or inferior (Giger and Davidhizar, 2012). The ideas of laypeople and family members may be valid and important and may influence the health care behaviors of patients as well as their health care status.

SOCIALIZATION

Socialization is the process of being reared and nurtured within a culture and acquiring its characteristics. This process can and does occur on many different levels: within families, communities, schools, and spiritual or religious groups. Socialization usually occurs within the structure of a group that influences the health care behaviors and beliefs of its members and can directly and indirectly affect the administration of health care by the nurse.

Family

The family is the basic unit of society in all cultures. From an economic perspective, a family is a social unit that works together to meet material needs. From a sociologic perspective, a family is a social unit that interacts within the larger society. Family also may be viewed as the basic unit in which personality develops and subgroup relationships, such as that between parent and child, are created.

Societal changes in the family unit have created variations of the basic family unit, such as single-parent families, extended families, and blended families. All of these variations will have an impact on how the nurse delivers care to members of these family groups.

Community

Community is defined as a group of people having a common interest or identity. This concept goes beyond the physical environment and includes the physical, social, and symbolic characteristics that connect people within a group. According to Purnell (2012), "The physical concept of community can be defined by such things as mountains, water, rural versus urban, and even railroad tracks can help define a community. Symbolic characteristics of community include sharing a specific dialect or language, lifestyle, history, art, dress or music" (p. 21). Much of the care that nurses deliver today takes place in the community. Therefore the nurse must be cognizant of the cultural influences within the community that can affect the delivery of care.

Delivery of care in the community setting requires that the nurse be comfortable with patients from diverse cultures and socioeconomic levels. Acquiring knowledge about a community's culture begins by conducting a careful assessment of patients and their families in their own environment. The cultural data this assessment yields have implications for the kind of care the nurse will deliver, and the findings should be discussed with the patient and family to develop mutual goals and to meet the desired outcomes for the patient (Andrews and Boyle, 2011).

School

A school is the official place where a generational transmission occurs of a society's accumulated knowledge and skills. Schools are places where a society's cultural values, traditions, and official heritage are taught. The school curriculum can reinforce what is learned in the family, but it also can challenge family socialization. A curriculum is geared toward learning social behaviors that are appropriate for peer groups that are not necessarily friendship groups but become the model for secondary group interactions. In this setting, people learn to communicate or negotiate with, or dominate, peers who are outside their immediate social circle and often are from diverse social backgrounds. In many ways, a social curriculum reinforces and deepens the gender role socialization that starts in the family and continues into the peer group.

Spiritual and Religious Institutions

Spiritual and religious institutions have a profound impact on individual and group socialization. These institutions can greatly influence health beliefs and often provide an entry point for health care access in impoverished communities and less developed countries. Religious practices usually are rooted in culture. Religions may have a set of beliefs that define health and the behaviors that prevent or treat illness. For example, most Jehovah's Witnesses oppose receiving blood transfusions on the basis of their religious beliefs. Nurses caring for known members of the Jehovah's Witness faith community should document patient preferences to ensure compliance with religious beliefs during medical treatment. Refer to Chapter 22 for practices typically associated with specific religious groups.

RITUALS

Rituals are formal, stylized, repetitive, and stereotypical actions performed in special places at special times. These actions convey information about participants and are used to inform others about the beliefs and traditions of a culture. Rituals, through their repetitive nature and generational transmission, translate into enduring messages, values, and sentiments (Kottak, 2012). These repetitive actions include participation in individual and group religious activities, such as praying, baptizing, fasting, singing, meditating, and reading the *Torah*, *Bible*, or *Koran*. All of these activities have implications for the delivery of nursing care. Rituals can sustain and provide support for patients during a time of illness or suffering. In caring for patients, nurses need to be aware of their own beliefs and feelings regarding certain rituals, as well as understand how these rituals may affect their patients and families.

TRANSCULTURAL NURSING LO 21.4

Transcultural nursing focuses on human caring–associated differences and similarities among the beliefs, values, and patterned life ways of cultures to provide culturally congr- ent, meaningful, and beneficial health care (Leininger, 1995). It is both a specialty and a general practice a focuses on worldwide cultures and comparati caring, health, and nursing phenomena. Est

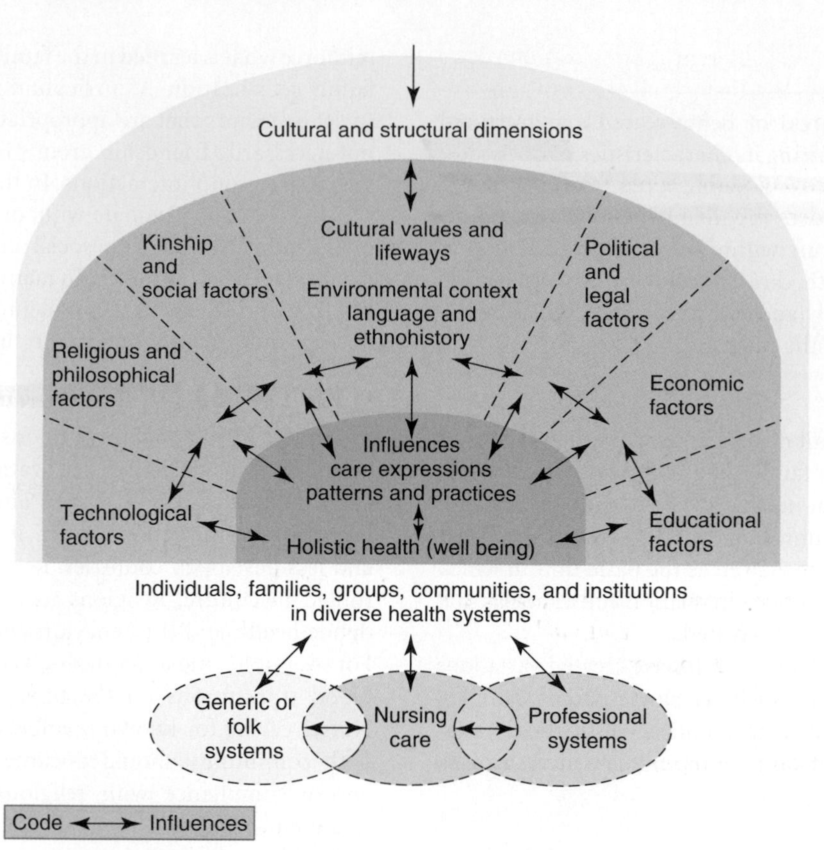

FIGURE 21-4 Leininger's Sunrise Model to depict the Theory of Cultural Care Diversity and Universality. (From Leininger M, McFarland M: *Transcultural nursing: Concepts, theories, research, and practice*, ed. 3, New York, 2002, McGraw-Hill.)

formal area of inquiry and practice in the 1970s, the goal of transcultural nursing is to provide culturally congruent care. The founder and central leader of transcultural nursing is Madeleine Leininger, who, as a graduate clinical nurse specialist in psychiatry, discovered major cultural differences among children and parents in a psychiatric unit. She was among the first to realize the need to address culture as a critical and missing dimension of care.

Transcultural nurses provide knowledgeable, competent, and safe care to people of diverse cultures. Their study encompasses cultural care symbols, expressions, and meanings (Wenger, 1999). Research in transcultural nursing focuses on discovering or explaining largely unknown and vaguely known cultural care and health concerns from two perspectives: The **emic** perspective focuses on the local, indigenous, and insider's culture; the **etic** perspective focuses on the outsider's world, and especially on professional views (Leininger, 2000).

Transcultural nurses are specialists, generalists, and consultants. Functioning in diverse clinical practice settings and in schools of nursing, they assist others to become sensitive to and knowledgeable about diverse cultures. They may identify cultures that are neglected or misunderstood and may help health care systems assess how they serve, or fail to serve, diverse cultures in a community (Seisser, 2002). Whatever the setting, transcultural nurses are committed to **cultural openness**, a lifelong stance that promotes cultural self-awareness and continuing development of transcultural skills (Wenger, 1998, 1999).

Leininger developed the Sunrise Model to depict the essential components of her Theory of Cultural Care Diversity and Universality. A basic tenet of Leininger's theory is that human beings are inseparable from their cultural background and social structure, world view, history, and environmental context. Gender, race, age, and class are embedded within the social structure. Biology, emotions, and other dimensions are studied from a holistic view and are not fragmented or separated. Leininger's work stresses the importance of comprehensive cultural assessment. Figure 21-4 illustrates the Theory of Cultural Care Diversity and Universality and the Sunrise Model.

CULTURAL COMPETENCE LO 21.4

Attaining cultural competence is a lifelong process. It requires intentional effort to more fully understand individuals of different cultures and ethnicities. Nurses use a variety of strategies including cultural sensitivity and culturally congruent care to demonstrate cultural competence in their patient care.

CULTURAL SENSITIVITY

Cultural sensitivity begins with the recognition of the often pronounced differences among cultures. These differences are reflected in the ways that different groups communicate and relate to one another, and they carry over into interactions with health care providers. Cultural sensitivity does not mean, however, that a person need only be *aware* of the differences to interact effectively with people from other cultures. If health care providers and their patients are to interact effectively, they must move beyond both cultural sensitivity and cultural biases that create barriers. Developing this kind of culturally competent attitude is an ongoing process.

CULTURALLY CONGRUENT CARE

A culturally competent clinician realizes the importance of caring for patients as people with unique experiences, beliefs, values, and language. How people perceive health care delivery and respond to diagnoses and treatment depends on a variety of cultural factors. **Culturally congruent care** uses culturally based knowledge in sensitive, creative, safe, and meaningful ways to promote the health and well-being of individual people or groups and improve their ability to face death, disability, or difficult human life conditions (Leininger and McFarland, 2002). Culturally congruent care and culturally competent care are terms that often are used interchangeably.

Cultural Competence

Cultural competence refers to the complex integration of a person's knowledge, attitudes, beliefs, skills, and encounters with those of people from different cultures (Andrews and Boyle, 2011). According to Andrews and Boyle (2011), cultural competence is a process rather than an endpoint, whereby the nurse continuously strives to work effectively within the cultural context of the individual, family, or community. To reach cultural competence, the health care professional has to engage in a cultural self-assessment. This self-assessment will reveal personal cultural beliefs, attitudes, values, biases, and practices that may affect the kind of care the nurse is willing and able to provide for patients from diverse backgrounds and cultures.

Experts have noted that in addition to cultural competence, linguistic competence is needed to offer appropriate care and responses to patients with culturally diverse backgrounds. When health care providers and organizations are culturally and linguistically competent, they can more effectively respond to the needs of the patients and communities they serve. A study conducted among 473 Chinese American immigrants underscores the importance of developing health promotion programs that are both culturally and linguistically appropriate (Evidence-Based Practice and Informatics box). Nurses skilled at cross-cultural communication, including verbal and nonverbal communication, communication dialects, and communication styles within various cultural groups, constitute valuable resources for health care agencies serving highly diverse populations.

National Culturally and Linguistically Appropriate Standards (CLAS) from the U.S. Department of Health and Human Services identify methods for providing culturally competent care and guidelines for their implementation. These standards address language access, organizational support, diverse and culturally competent staff, existing laws, data collection, and information dissemination. The CLAS standards are available at *www.nacddarchive.org/nacdd-initiatives/health-equity/resources-and-publication/clas-standards-1/clas-list-summary/view.*

EVIDENCE-BASED PRACTICE AND INFORMATICS

Cultural Views and Cervical Cancer Screening Among Chinese-American Women

- Cervical cancer is a major health risk in certain female subpopulations, including recent immigrants, Asian American women, and women without health insurance. This is due to lack of regular screening via Pap smear.
- Documented barriers to cervical cancer screening include fear, fatalistic attitudes, lack of health insurance, and language differences.
- Chinese women (aged 50 and older) with traditional Chinese cultural beliefs were less likely to undergo Pap smear testing.
- According to numerous research studies, English proficiency is a significant predictor in whether non–English-speaking minority populations, including Hispanic, French, and Japanese immigrants, receive cervical cancer screening. Other studies indicate that linguistic barriers lead to less-than-optimal health and preventive care overall.
- Research indicates that increasing the availability of culturally and linguistically competent educational materials, programs, and health care professionals to immigrant populations would increase participation in cervical cancer screening.

From Shuang C, Chen M, Sun J, et al: Cultural views, English proficiency and regular cervical cancer screening among older Chinese American women, *Womens Health Issues* 20(4): 272-278, 2010.

QSEN FOCUS!

To provide culturally competent patient-centered care, nurses must recognize personal attitudes related to working with patients from different cultural and ethnic backgrounds and actively seek to overcome prejudices or feelings that might have a negative impact on their nursing practice.

Leininger and McFarland (2002) have outlined 10 steps in the delivery of culturally congruent and culturally competent care (Diversity Considerations box).

Balancing Multiple Cultures

According to Dennis and Small (2003), the cultural competence of a nurse is predicated on an awareness of the interaction of three cultures. Every nurse brings two cultures into a relationship with patients. The first culture is that of the personal self. The qualities and characteristics of the nurse's personal culture are key determinants of personal and

DIVERSITY CONSIDERATIONS

Delivering Culturally Congruent and Culturally Competent Care

Follow these steps to deliver nursing care that is both culturally congruent and culturally competent:

- Gain knowledge of the individual or family culture being assessed from reliable literature and through transcultural nursing courses taught by qualified faculty.
- Be familiar with one's own cultural heritage, patterns, and biases and factors that may interfere with an effective assessment and understanding of the patient.
- Use theory or theoretical perspectives to guide cultural assessment of patients, families, or communities.
- Know some common phrases in the language of the patient to obtain accurate information, and work with qualified interpreters.
- Show respect and a genuine interest in the informant and the culture while remaining an active listener, letting the informant share personal stories, experiences, and ideas.
- Be observant of the environmental context in which assessment and documentation of the patient interaction take place.
- As the patient shares emic or etic data, reflect on and check the meaning of the data with the patient.
- Make the patient an active co-participant in the assessment to obtain credible and accurate data.
- Identify and then recheck specific and general cultural care values, beliefs, and needs related to generic (emic) and professional (etic) data for possible integrated culturally congruent care.
- Use assessment findings in sensitive, knowing, creative, and meaningful ways with the patient so that beneficial and satisfying outcomes are forthcoming. Do a follow-up review with the patient or family to document goal outcomes.

From Leininger M, McFarland M: *Transcultural nursing: Concepts, theories, research, and practice,* ed. 3, New York, 2002, McGraw-Hill.

professional behavior. The second culture, which is equally important, is that of the health care delivery system. The nurse represents the health care system and helps the patient and family to acquire access to this system, which also has its own separate and unique culture. Both of these cultures, that of the nurse and of the health care system, must strike a balance with a third culture, that of the patient.

CULTURAL COMPETENCE AND THE NURSING PROCESS LO 21.5

An understanding of patients from diverse backgrounds begins with a cultural assessment and continues with the development of culturally sensitive individualized care plans. Nurses must understand the specific factors that influence health and illness behaviors within a culture in order to provide culturally competent care.

ASSESSMENT

Some non-nursing models for cultural assessment were used before the development of various transcultural nursing assessment models. Madeleine Leininger's Transcultural Theory and Assessment Model was the first tool developed for nurses to appropriately assess a patient's culture and evaluate the impact of culture on nursing care. Since the development of Leininger's assessment tool, other nursing models have been developed to assist nurses in providing culturally congruent and competent care.

The Giger and Davidhizar Transcultural Assessment Model (2012) is a framework for collecting data related to six cultural domains: communication, space, social orientation, time, environmental control, and biologic variation (Figure 21-5).

The Health Assessment Questions box provides examples of interview questions for assessment of each cultural domain within the Transcultural Assessment Model. Using these questions, and others that are similar, will help to identify and address the cultural needs of patients and families.

Galanti (2008) developed the 4 Cs of Culture, a mnemonic for health care professionals, to aid in providing culturally responsive, patient-centered health assessment and care (Table 21-1). The 4 *C*s stand for *call, caused, cope,* and *concerns.*

Regardless of the format used to conduct a cultural assessment, the nurse needs to be sensitive to several factors that affect how people from culturally diverse backgrounds may interact with others and their environment and how they may view health care. Recognizing the potential impact of these factors will help nurses to develop culturally sensitive treatment plans that meet each patient's individual needs.

Communication

Communication practiced within and among cultural groups dictates how feelings, ideas, decision making, and strategies for exchanging information are expressed both verbally and nonverbally. When a patient and nurse are from different cultures, the chances of misunderstanding one another are greatly increased, which can have a detrimental effect on the nurse-patient relationship and result in negative patient outcomes.

Galanti (2008) provided an example of a verbal misunderstanding between health professionals: A nurse reported that her patient was "getting cold feet" about an upcoming surgical procedure; a Chinese-born physician misinterpreted this expression and ordered vascular studies to rule out circulatory problems. In some cultures, facial expressions, body posture, eye behaviors, and the use of touch can have a multitude of meanings. For example, in some Asian cultures, it is considered disrespectful to make direct eye contact with individuals of authority because doing so implies equality.

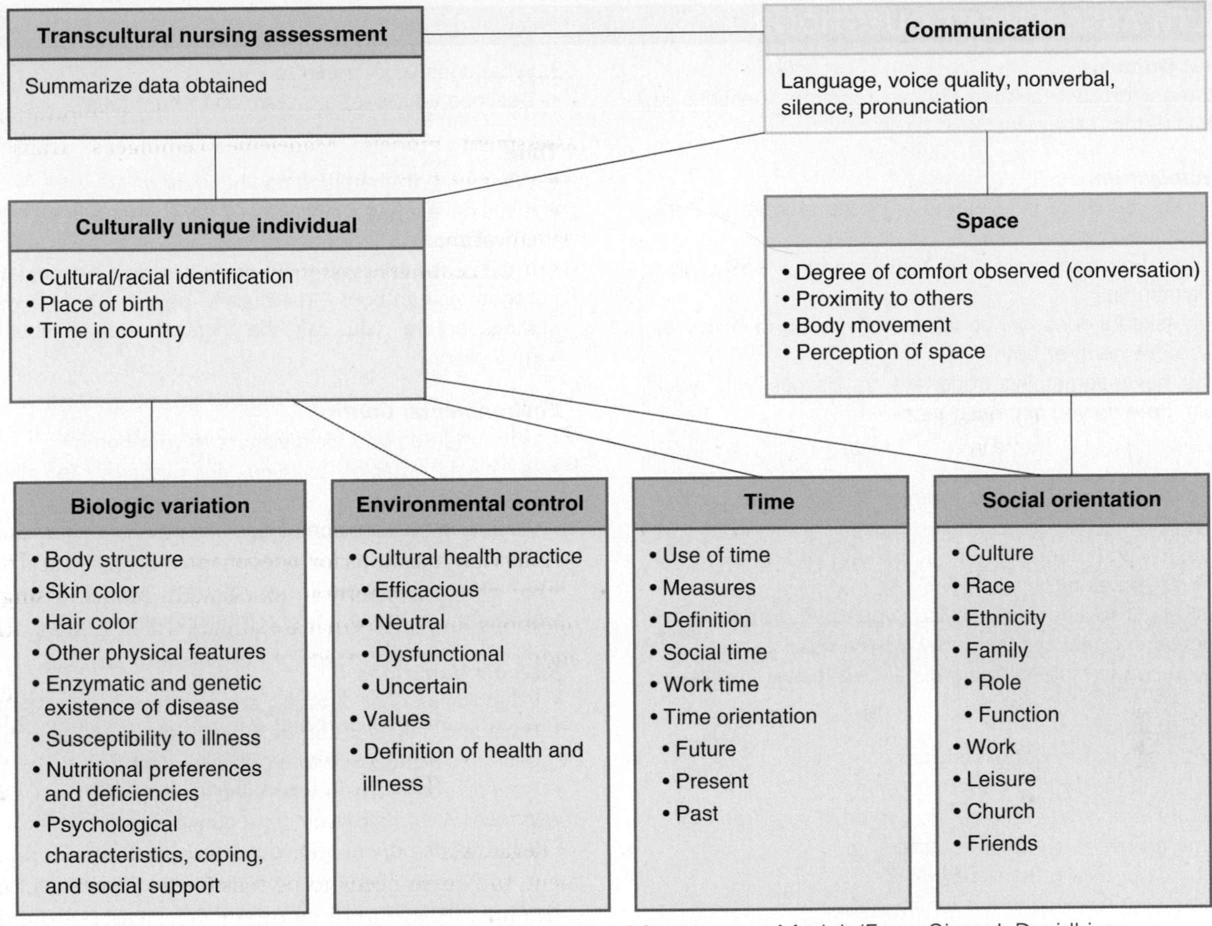

FIGURE 21-5 Giger and Davidhizar's Transcultural Assessment Model. (From Giger J, Davidhizar R: *Transcultural nursing: Assessment and intervention*, ed. 6, St. Louis, 2012, Mosby.)

Some factors that influence communication include the following (Giger and Davidhizar, 2012):

- Physical health and emotional well-being
- The situation being discussed and its meaning to the patient
- Personal needs and interest
- Communication skills
- Knowledge of the subject matter being discussed
- Background, including cultural, social, and philosophical values
- Experiences that relate to the situation
- The senses involved and their functional ability
- Attitudes toward the person and subject being discussed
- The environment in which the communication takes place
- Distractions to the communication process
- The personal tendency to make judgments and to be judgmental

> **! SAFE PRACTICE ALERT**
>
> Use of a professional interpreter is necessary if the nurse and the patient do not speak the same language fluently. Avoid translation of medical information by a patient's family members or friends to ensure privacy and accuracy of essential, personal information.

Skin Color

Skin color probably is the most significant biologic variation nurses encounter in the delivery of culturally competent care. Variations in skin color may be attributable to genetic makeup or may be the result of mutations and environmental factors. The darker a patient's skin is, the more challenging assessment for changes becomes. Procedures used in assessing dark-skinned people are quite different from those used in assessing light-skinned people. Skin color varies in conditions such as jaundice, pallor, and some rashes. In assessing a dark-skinned patient for oxygenation, it is very important to examine the least pigmented areas, such as the buccal mucosa, lips, tongue, nail beds, and palms of the hands. The examiner should not rely on the skin tone alone. A baseline skin color can be established by assessing a patient in direct sunlight or by asking family members who are extremely familiar with the patient's appearance (Purnell, 2013).

HEALTH ASSESSMENT QUESTIONS

Cultural Domains

Assessment of each cultural domain requires questions in several different categories:

Communication

- What do you do to help others understand what you are trying to say?
- Do you like communicating with friends, family, and acquaintances?
- When asked a question, do you usually respond in words, body movement, or both?
- If you have something important to discuss with your family, how do you approach them?

Space

- When you talk with family members, how close do you stand?
- When you communicate with coworkers and others, how close do you stand?
- If a stranger touches you, how do you react or feel?
- If a loved one touches you, how do you react or feel?
- Are you comfortable with the distance between us now?

Social Organization

- How do you define social activities?
- What are some activities that you enjoy?
- What are your hobbies? What do you do in your free time?
- Do you believe in a supreme being?
- What is your role in the family unit?
- What is your function in the family unit?
- When you were younger, who influenced you the most?
- What does work mean to you?
- Describe your past, present, and future jobs.

Time

- What kind of timepiece do you wear daily?
- If you have an appointment at 2 P.M., what is an acceptable arrival time?
- If the nurse tells you that you will receive a medication in "about half an hour," realistically, how much time will you allow before you call the nurses' station about the medication?

Environmental Control

- How often do you have visitors to your home?
- Is it acceptable to you for visitors to drop in unannounced?
- What is your definition of good health?
- What is your definition of poor health?
- What home remedies have you used that worked?
- Will you use these home remedies again?

Biologic Variations

- What illnesses or diseases are common in your family?
- Have any members of your family been told they have a genetic susceptibility to a particular disease?
- How do you respond when you are angry?
- Who or what helps you cope during difficult times?
- What foods do you and your family like?
- Have you ever had any cravings for unusual things such as red or white clay? laundry starch?
- What foods are family favorites or traditional foods?

Adapted from Giger J, Davidhizar R: *Transcultural nursing: Assessment and intervention,* ed. 6, St. Louis, 2012, Mosby.

Gender Roles

Nurses need to be mindful that equalization of genders is predominantly a Western phenomenon, and that many non-Western cultures do not adhere to this cultural ideology. Accommodations must be made to respond to patient preferences in regard to gender. Some patients will require direct care from nurses of the same gender, while others may limit speaking or eye contact with people of the opposite sex.

Gender equality exhibited through shared decision making is a concept not universally accepted in many cultures. For example, some women from Middle Eastern countries are not permitted to make health care decisions for themselves or their children. In some families, decision making is viewed as the responsibility of the men. Nurses should be sensitive when a female patient defers to her husband or father, recognizing that although the woman has the legal right in various parts of the world to consent to a procedure, she may not feel that she has the authority to give consent from a cultural standpoint.

Time Orientation

Time orientation varies by culture. Cultures tend to be oriented to time in the context of past, present, or future events. No single person or culture looks exclusively to the past, present, or future, but different cultures tend to emphasize one period of time over the others (Galanti, 2008). Cultures that are oriented to the past tend to look to traditional approaches to health and healing rather than to new approaches, procedures, and medications. People of these cultures tend to believe that if certain solutions worked for their ancestors, such solutions will work for them. According to Galanti (2008), Australian, British, and Chinese cultures tend to be time-oriented in the past.

Cultures oriented to the present are less likely to embrace preventive health care. The orientation of these cultures is focused on the "here and now," and people in these cultures often use the way they are feeling during the present time to dictate future health practices. For example, if people from present-oriented cultures are diagnosed with a specific disorder but still "feel good," they may reason that prescribed medication is an unnecessary expenditure, because they are not having symptoms. Their orientation is not geared toward preventing the long-term effects of the disorder; rather, they adopt a wait-and-see approach. Nurses also need to be mindful that certain economic pressures can force patients into a present-time orientation. When finances dictate that

TABLE 21-1 The 4 *C*s of Culture: A Mnemonic for Health Care Professionals

QUESTION	RATIONALE
What do you *call* your problem?	• Remember to ask, "What do you think is wrong?" The answer to this question gives the nurse the patient's perception of the problem. (Do *not* literally ask, "What do you call your problem?") • The same symptoms may have very different meanings in different cultures, and this may result in barriers to compliance. Understanding the patient's point of view can help the health care provider address potential barriers to compliance.
What do you think *caused* your problem?	• This question is aimed at discovering the patient's beliefs regarding the source of the problem. Not everyone believes that disease is caused by germs. • In some cultures, disease is thought to be caused by an upset in body balance, a breach of taboos (similar to the idea held by some people that diseases are caused by "sin" and are a punishment from God), or spirit possession. Treatment must be appropriate to the cause; otherwise, patients will not perceive themselves as being cured.
How do you *cope* with your condition?	• This question should be asked to remind the practitioner to ask, "What have you done to try to make it better? Who else have you been to for treatment?" Answers to these questions will provide the health care provider with important information on the use of alternative healers and treatments. • It is important that health care providers ask about traditional remedies in a nonjudgmental manner. Occasionally, a traditional remedy may be dangerous or could lead to a drug interaction with a prescribed medication.
What are your *concerns* regarding the condition and/or recommended treatment?	• This question can take the form of "How serious do you think this is? What potential complications do you fear? How does it interfere with your life or your ability to function? Do you know anyone else who has tried the treatment I've recommended? What was that person's experience?" • The nurse or other health care provider needs to ask these questions to understand the patient's perceptions and fears about the course of the illness so that any concerns can be addressed and misconceptions can be corrected. • Asking about what aspects of the condition pose a problem for the patient may uncover something very different from what the provider expects. • It is important to know the patient's concerns about any treatments that may be prescribed to avoid problems of nonadherence. Some patients do not adhere to treatments due to misplaced concerns that are based on past experiences. By asking questions, the health care provider can correct any misconceptions that can interfere with treatment.

From Galanti A: *Caring for patients from different cultures,* ed. 5, Philadelphia, 2015, University of Pennsylvania Press.

day-to-day survival takes priority over future needs, patients often make choices that are in conflict with the recommendations of nurses and other health care professionals.

According to Giger and Davidhizar (2012), African American and Hispanic cultures tend to think of time in a linear fashion. People in these cultures tend to believe that a particular task or spending time with another has to be accomplished in the "here and now," because that opportunity can never be regained. Some people in these cultures also share the belief that time is flexible and events will begin when they arrive at a destination. This belief has led to a more lenient perception of time, and arriving 30 minutes to an hour late is considered acceptable behavior.

Middle-class Americans, regardless of ethnic or cultural origin, tend to be future-oriented (Giger and Davidhizar, 2012). People in the middle class tend to delay immediate personal gratification if a purchase interferes with their ability to pursue plans for the future, such as buying a home, planning a family, or pursuing higher education. Middle-class people tend to structure time rigidly, adhering to a time-structured schedule as a way of life. The nurse providing care to such patients should be reminded to speak of events in relationship to the future and stick to a schedule of planned events.

! SAFE PRACTICE ALERT

If a patient is late to a scheduled appointment, the nurse should assess the reason for tardiness to determine whether it is due to cultural factors or to reliance on public transportation or other means over which the patient has little control. The nurse will need to decide whether it is appropriate to explain the potential consequences of lateness, such as having to reschedule an appointment or compromise the patient's health. Caution is required to avoid discouraging patients from seeking needed health care.

To give culturally competent care, nurses need to have an understanding of time as it applies to diverse cultural groups. Time orientation and punctuality vary from group to group and from place to place. It is important for the nurse to identify the time orientation of the patient (past, present, future) and realize that nursing care may have to be adapted to the patient's time orientation. This adjustment may seem cumbersome and unnecessary; however, the nurse needs to keep in mind that time orientation dictates many activities in patients' lives and that intolerance of a patient's cultural time perception may have a negative impact on the nurse-patient relationship and affect patient care.

Body Odor

Body odor may result from poor hygiene, the inability to care for oneself, or a cultural acceptance that natural body odors are normal, as is the case in some Middle Eastern populations. In other parts of the world, the fear of offensive natural smells is connected with the concept of attractiveness, and great efforts are made to prevent or mask unpleasant odors. Asian cultures (Filipino, Malaysian, Indonesian, Thai, Indian) stress frequent bathing and often criticize others for not bathing as much as they should. Nurses need to assess a patient's norms associated with body odor and encourage healthy personal hygiene practices that promote health and wellness, but they must do so while demonstrating sensitivity to cultural implications.

Nutritional Needs

Understanding a patient's food patterns is critical to providing culturally congruent dietary counseling. The role of food in a culture, food rituals, common foods and spices, dietary limitations, and nutritional deficiencies are all factors to be assessed by the nurse. For example, nurses may be viewed as culturally incompetent if they attempt to prescribe a diet including pork products to a patient of Middle Eastern background.

Food has a significant role in socialization in a majority of cultures. The celebration of specific holidays often centers on the preparation and sharing of traditional foods with family and friends (Figure 21-6). In addition to cultural influences, socioeconomic status may dictate food selection. Individuals and families with limited financial resources may have to choose between purchasing healthy foods or purchasing economical foods. The inability to afford foods for a healthy diet leads to severe nutritional deficiencies in many cultures. In view of the cross-cultural variation in diets, nurses need to ask about the specific diets and traditional foods of their patients. The Health Assessment Questions box identifies guidelines nurses can use to assess nutrition.

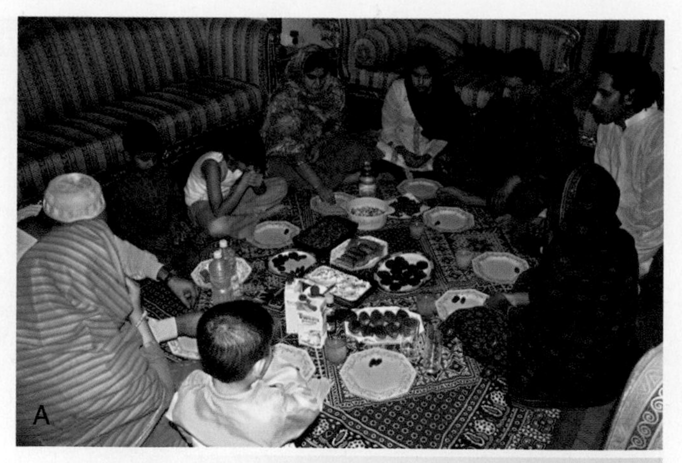

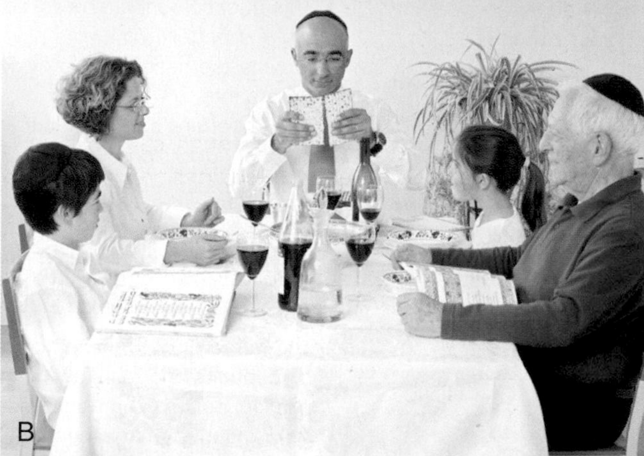

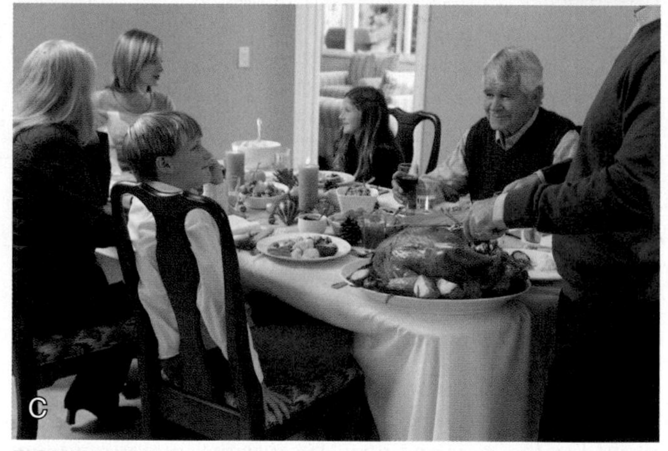

FIGURE 21-6 People from around the world celebrate holidays with traditional foods.

Spirituality and Religious Orientation

Rooted in the culture of groups, spirituality and religious orientation help to define many health beliefs and health practices. Different cultures have differing views of religion; for example, some people view religion as their connection to supernatural beings, whereas others view it as an expression of an instinctual reaction to cosmic forces (Johnstone, 2009). Religion may be viewed as a method of receiving guidance and directional messages from a deity (Giger and Davidhizar, 2012).

Spirituality involves more than the formal beliefs and rituals seen in most religious groups. *Spirituality* refers to behaviors and beliefs that strengthen a person and provide meaning to his or her life. Some people may identify themselves as being spiritual without an affiliation with an organized religious group. Spirituality is a component of health related to the essence of life and is a vital human experience that is shared by most people (Purnell, 2013). Spirituality, for many people, is a stabilizing force between mind, body, and

HEALTH ASSESSMENT QUESTIONS

Nutrition

- What meaning does food have in your life? (Do you eat to satisfy hunger or for other reasons, such as socializing, enjoyment, or boredom?)
- What foods, preparation practices, and major ingredients do you commonly use?
- Do you have any specific food rituals?
- Do you use any dietary practices to promote health or treat illnesses?
- Do you have any enzyme deficiencies or food intolerances?
- Are you aware of having any nutritional deficiencies?
- Is access to any specific foods (e.g., citrus fruits) limited in your area?

From Purnell L: *Transcultural health care: A culturally competent approach,* ed. 4, Philadelphia, 2012, F.A. Davis.

spirit. For a nurse to complete a thorough cultural assessment, the nurse must inquire about religious preferences and determine the extent to which spirituality or religion affects a patient's physical and emotional well-being. In many cases, aspects of religion and spirituality significantly affect patients' ability to cope with adversity and health-related challenges. Refer to Chapter 22 for methods of assessing religious and spiritual needs.

Health Beliefs

Health beliefs vary significantly among and within cultures. It is critical for nurses and all health care professionals to remember that the health beliefs and opinions of people of the same culture vary according to life experience, education, family values, and many other factors. Asking questions to determine the health beliefs of each patient is essential to provide culturally competent care. Some knowledge of traditionally held beliefs can help to guide assessment of health care seeking and treatment options.

African Americans

Some health beliefs of African Americans are derived from their ancestral roots in Africa. As with all cultural groups that are heterogeneous, it is difficult to make blanket statements about the health care beliefs of African Americans. Some African Americans living in the United States believe that illness represents disharmony and conflict in aspects of a person's life, and their beliefs tend to fall into three general categories: impaired relationships, environmental hazards, and divine punishment (Giger and Davidhizar, 2012).

Older African Americans in the U.S. South may have consulted folk medicine practitioners rather than traditional health care providers until much later in their lives. For many in this group, an inherent mistrust of traditional health care providers has developed as a consequence of prior poor treatment of African Americans; others may not seek traditional care because of economic issues. Some, but not all, will seek out traditional health care providers to obtain prescription medications (Giger and Davidhizar, 2012).

Latinos

People of Latino descent may not seek medical care because of a mistrust of the medical establishment, poverty, or problems with immigration status. Traditional healing practices may be preferred. Traditional Latino diagnoses and treatments are categorized as being either "hot" or "cold." For example, hypertension is considered a hot disorder that would be treated with cold therapies, such as passionflower tea (Juckett, 2005). It is important for the nurse to address the patient's understanding of diseases and disorders before the start of treatment.

Asians

Asian cultures span a very large, culturally diverse population that includes, among others, people of Filipino, Chinese, Japanese, Korean, and Vietnamese backgrounds. Each group has its own cultural traditions and practices. Some common Asian cultural values include a strong sense of personal honor, belief in the hierarchical family structure, and emphasis on accommodation as opposed to confrontation (Juckett, 2005). Perceived loss of respect or honor can have devastating effects in people from Asian cultures.

Some health care practices within Asian cultures that nurses should be aware of include coining and cupping; these particular practices can leave bruises on the skin, and may lead the nurse to suspect physical abuse. Mongolian spots are common in both Asian and Latino populations and should not be assumed to be a sign of child abuse. Traditional Chinese medicine is gaining popularity in Western culture. Such types of therapy are based on the concept of balance—keeping the body's *yin* (cold) and *yang* (hot) in balance through lifestyle practices; dietary practices; herbs; and alternative therapies such as acupuncture. Asians, like those in other cultures, have their own interpretation of diseases and disorders. Very few Asians will seek out psychiatric care because of the stigma and sense of shame that mental disorders are perceived to bring to the affected person and the family. Thus certain psychiatric disorders such as somatization may be more prominent in Asian cultures.

Socioeconomic Level

Nurses need to be cognizant of the impact of patients' socioeconomic status on health care. It is important to determine the overall economic factors that influence the patient. Historically, patients from lower socioeconomic levels have poorer health and tend to have shorter life expectancies. Research has suggested that a lack of insurance and access to health care often leads to late diagnosis of disease, when medical intervention is less effective.

Unfortunately, the level of poverty found in minority populations within all cultures is disproportionately higher than that in the nonminority population. Assessment of a patient's employment status, insurance coverage, and educational background can provide data on financial resources that affect access to and compliance with health care. Economic assessment data are helpful in determining interventions and community resources available for treatment.

After gathering, reviewing, and organizing a patient's health assessment data in a culturally competent manner, the nurse is ready to develop a care plan that acknowledges the role of culture in patient-centered care.

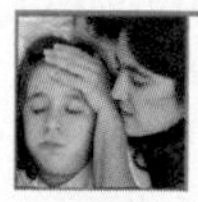

1. List some additional assessment data that should be collected on Maria and her family before her admission to the hospital.

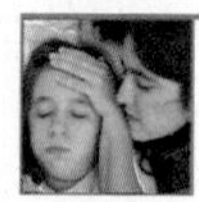

2. List a minimum of four cultural factors, including rationales for each, that the nurse should take into consideration while assessing Maria and planning for her care.

CARE PLAN DEVELOPMENT

No nursing diagnoses address cultural concerns in a unique way. Therefore it is vitally important for the nurse to view patient ethnicity and cultural influences as significant pieces of assessment data, without considering them the only cause of a problem. Just as with any patient, many different nursing diagnoses may be applicable to a patient's situation depending on the health care problem being addressed.

It is particularly important for nurses to avoid cultural bias when identifying potential nursing diagnoses in situations in which the patient and nurse are from dramatically different ethnic and cultural backgrounds. For example, a patient who speaks a language other than that of the nurse does not have *Impaired Verbal Communication;* rather, the patient simply speaks another language. Being familiar with the actual definition of a nursing diagnosis will help to prevent choosing a nursing diagnosis in a culturally insensitive manner.

The culturally competent nurse develops a plan of care by analyzing the assessment data, both subjective and objective, prioritizing needs, and discussing potential goals with patients and their families or support system before formulating a plan of care. Leininger (2002) suggests three types of professional action and decision-making strategies that promote patient-centered care based on a nurse's knowledge of a patient's culture:

- *Cultural maintenance:* Helps people of a particular culture retain and/or preserve relevant care values so that they can maintain their sense of well-being, recover from illness, or face handicaps and/or death
- *Cultural care accommodation or negotiation:* Helps people of diverse cultures adapt to or negotiate with others for beneficial or satisfying health outcomes with professional health care providers
- *Cultural care repatterning or restructuring:* Respects the patients' cultural values and beliefs while helping patients reorder, change, or modify their lives and adopt new, different, and beneficial health care patterns

Each of these strategies may be beneficial in establishing realistic goals or outcome statements for patients from ethnically and culturally diverse backgrounds.

Potential interventions to be included in a plan of care for people of diverse cultures should be discussed with the patient, family, and significant others (e.g., extended family, cultural healers, identified support system) to determine their level of acceptance in advance. Interventions to relieve anxiety for a person who has recently moved to a foreign country and speaks a language other than that of the care providers include the following:

- Arranging for a professional interpreter to be available by phone in challenging situations
- Identifying community agencies that work specifically with people of the patient's culture
- Seeking social service care from a specialist who speaks the patient's language

The more a plan of care reflects patient preferences, the more likely it is to be accepted and successful. If it becomes necessary to revise the plan of care, the nurse must discuss this with the patient and redefine mutual patient-nurse goals. The Diversity Considerations box addresses some cultural tendencies that should be taken into consideration during the planning stage of the nursing process.

Language and Linguistics

An essential aspect of planning interventions for patients from culturally diverse backgrounds involves language and literacy. When the nurse and the patient speak different primary languages, the use of abbreviations and acronyms in speech should be avoided. The nurse should use a slower speech pattern to enhance the patient's ability to comprehend what is being said. Speaking more slowly gives the patient additional time for processing information. The nurse should avoid speaking loudly to the patient. Yelling does not increase a person's ability to understand what is being said. The use of humor, slang, and jargon should be limited. Puns, sarcasm, and colloquialisms are not easily comprehended or interpreted by those who speak a different primary language.

! SAFE PRACTICE ALERT

It is critical that health care providers verify that patients and families understand information. Consistently positive verbal responses from a patient or frequent head nodding may simply indicate that the patient heard the information without comprehending it. Ask questions and seek feedback or a return demonstration from patients to confirm their understanding.

DIVERSITY CONSIDERATIONS

It is critical that nurses seek specific information based on each unique patient care situation to provide culturally competent care.

Family
- In traditional Asian cultures, wives and children take care of a sick husband or father.
- Self-care is valued among most American families.

Gender
- Gender roles differ among cultural groups.
- Women in Latino cultures often adhere to the wife/mother/housewife role.
- Men are the decision makers in traditional Mexican and Indian cultures.

Culture, Ethnicity, and Religion
- Orthodox and some Conservative Jewish patients require a kosher diet.
- Many Jehovah's Witnesses refuse blood transfusions on the basis of scriptural restrictions on consuming blood.
- Seventh Day Adventists regard the body as a temple and typically do not eat meat or consume caffeine, alcohol, or tobacco products.

Morphology
- Asians generally have a smaller body stature than Anglo-Americans, African Americans, and Mexicans.
- African Americans and Latinos may be more comfortable with a higher body mass index than Anglo-Americans and Asians.

Providing written or audiovisual materials that can be comprehended by patients is essential to culturally competent care. Nurses must assess the ability of patients to read and write regardless of their native language. Often, illiterate patients try to hide their inability to read or write by asking others to read to them or by simply agreeing to "read" the pamphlet after the nurse has left the room. The Patient Education and Health Literacy box highlights some of the critical factors necessary to provide appropriate patient education resources to a culturally diverse population.

Individualized Care

A patient's inclusion in care-planning activities is extremely important in the managed care climate, where patient outcomes and satisfaction with the care provided by nurses and others are used as indicators of the provision of quality health care. Nurses need to ensure that the instruments and processes used by health care organizations are culturally appropriate. The feedback obtained from patients from diverse cultures should be used to improve nursing care for people of all cultural backgrounds. Nursing care plans that blend diverse cultural values, beliefs, and health care practices will increase adherence and patient satisfaction. This is clinically essential to avoid nontherapeutic outcomes. Understanding the underlying principles of culturally competent care gives the nurse the ability to see more than one way to achieve the same outcome. For many people of culturally diverse backgrounds, working with community agencies that provide interpretive services and government support is essential.

PATIENT EDUCATION AND HEALTH LITERACY

Assessment Prior to Teaching

Nurses should consider language barriers, the ability of patients to read and write, and their education level when planning patient education interventions.
- Can the patient read and write English, or is another language preferred?
- Are health-related materials available in the patient's primary language?
- What is the patient's highest education level?
- What learning style best suits the patient: written? oral? videos?
- Does the patient's education level affect health behaviors?
- Does the patient's education level affect his or her knowledge level concerning health literacy?
- Does the patient need an interpreter?

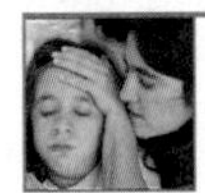

3. Identify the most important nursing intervention to be implemented initially, to ensure culturally competent patient-centered care. Describe ways in which the nurse can implement the intervention identified.

Community Referrals

Collaboration among health care providers, community leaders, and health consumers is required to provide culturally relevant services in the community. A high level of nursing knowledge and skill is needed to help patients from different cultures navigate community services (Collaboration and Delegation box). According to Andrews and Boyle

COLLABORATION AND DELEGATION

Culturally Responsible Hand-offs
- Before patient discharge, nurses must identify community providers that will meet the patient's cultural and linguistic needs.
- Transferring relevant information regarding the patient's language, ethnic, religious, and spiritual needs is critical to ensuring positive patient outcomes.
- Collaboration with patient decision makers, including family members and spiritual advisers, is especially important during end-of-life care. Collaborative palliative care promotes treatment that is sensitive to patient values and personal beliefs.

From The Joint Commission: A roadmap for hospitals, 2010. Retrieved from *www.jointcommission.org/assets/1/6/ARoadmapforHospitalsfinalversion727.pdf.*

(2011), nurses need to understand how to form partnerships with community leaders and health care providers who can meet the needs of patients from culturally diverse backgrounds.

Cultural factors determine whether patients from diverse cultures accept community services. Cultural traditions within a community can dictate the structure of community support systems as well as the types of resources available. Home care considerations are highlighted in the Home Care Considerations box.

HOME CARE CONSIDERATIONS

Considering the Impact of Culture

When formulating a plan of care for a culturally diverse patient in the home setting, be sure to take note of the following:

- Family roles, typical family household and structures, and dynamics in the family, particularly communication patterns.
- Patterns of daily living, including work and leisure activities.
- Health beliefs and practices related to disease causation, treatment of illness, folk practices, and faith healers.
- Extended family kinship and social networks, including friends, neighbors, and significant others, and their influence on health and illness.
- Nutritional practices and how they relate to cultural factors and health.

From Andrews M, Boyle J: *Transcultural concepts in nursing care*, ed. 6, Philadelphia, 2011, Lippincott Williams & Wilkins.

Determining the effectiveness of interventions to address the needs of culturally diverse patient populations requires sensitivity to the norms and expectations of individual patients and their support systems. It is important to refer to mutually agreed-on goals and outcome criteria. The degree to which goals are met should be evaluated on the basis of the patient's perception and the nurse's professional judgment. Input from both sources as well as ideas from community collaborative partners will help to determine the effectiveness of a plan of care and the need to continue, modify, or discontinue treatment interventions.

Nurses need to understand that culture can and does influence how they view patients as well as the quality of care that is delivered. Nurses have to avoid projecting their own cultural worldview onto their patients. To deliver culturally sensitive care, nurses must remember that each individual is unique—the product of experiences, beliefs, and values that have been learned and passed down from generation to generation.

Therefore the culturally competent nurse must be guided by culturally relevant information when assessing, diagnosing, planning, and implementing care for diverse patients. The nurse must carefully examine the fit between the diagnosis and the patient for whom it is intended. The culturally competent nurse is sensitive and flexible while providing outstanding professional care to all patients.

SUMMARY OF LEARNING OUTCOMES

LO 21.1 *Compare characteristics of culture and ethnicity:* Culture is symbolic, learned, shared, and integrated. Culture includes knowledge of values, beliefs, and ways of life of a particular group that are generally transmitted from one generation to another. Culture influences an individual's thinking and decision-making patterns. Ethnicity is expressed by identity with a particular racial, national, or cultural group, including observation of the group's customs, beliefs, and language.

LO 21.2 *Explain cultural concepts that affect a nurse's ability to provide culturally congruent care:* Some cultural concepts such as generalization may be helpful in guiding nursing practice within certain cultural settings. Others, such as stereotyping, discrimination, and racism, have a negative effect on a nurse's ability to provide culturally congruent care.

LO 21.3 *Identify factors that contribute to cultural identity acquisition:* How people choose to identify with or conform to a culture is determined by the extent to which they ascribe to the norms and traditions of the culture.

LO 21.4 *Articulate an understanding of transcultural nursing and cultural competence:* Transcultural nursing focuses on a broad understanding of global health care and the incorporation of culturally sensitive interventions to demonstrate cultural competence.

LO 21.5 *Describe how to develop culturally competent individualized plans of care using cultural assessment tools and the nursing process:* Cultural assessment requires the gathering of data in multiple areas of concern, such as language and traditional health practices. Each aspect of a patient's care plan should be determined after collaboration with patients and should reflect cultural sensitivity to their individual needs.

Responses to the critical-thinking questions are available at *http://evolve.elsevier.com/YoostCrawford/fundamentals/*.

REVIEW QUESTIONS

1. Which statement best serves as a guide for nurses seeking to learn more about ethnicity?
   a. Ethnicity, like culture, generally is based on genetics.
   b. A patient's ethnic background is determined by skin color.
   c. Ethnicity is based on cultural similarities and differences in a society.
   d. Culture and socialization are unrelated to the concept of ethnic origin.
2. Which action taken by a nurse would reflect application of an appropriate generalization in a patient care setting?
   a. Assigning same-gender nurses to all patients admitted to the unit
   b. Sharing with unlicensed assistive personnel that Muslim patients typically do not eat pork
   c. Telling the radiology technician that every Latino family is late for appointments
   d. Assuming that Asians share financial responsibility for medical bills
3. Which statements reflect the practice of transcultural nursing? *(Select all that apply.)*
   a. May be considered a general and specialty practice area
   b. Focuses on the worldview rather than patient needs
   c. Challenges traditional ethnocentric nursing practice
   d. Aims to identify individual patient care preferences
   e. Focuses patient care on the nurse's cultural norms
4. Which questions are appropriate to ask during a transcultural assessment? *(Select all that apply.)*
   a. How do you act when you are angry?
   b. What is your role in your extended family?
   c. Why do you continue to speak German at home?
   d. When communicating with friends, how close do you stand?
   e. What is the purpose of not preparing beef with milk products?
5. How best can a nurse evaluate goal attainment for a patient with a culturally diverse background?
   a. Assume that gender roles will be a challenge to overcome regardless of the patient's ethnicity.
   b. Base decisions on feedback from the patient and the nurse's professional judgment.
   c. Collaborate with future community care providers to determine patient strengths.
   d. Seek input from members of the patient's support system to avoid biased patient responses.
6. What aspect of culture is a full-time employed granddaughter of an elderly Asian woman exhibiting if she asks the social worker to place her grandmother in an extended-care facility against the wishes of her parents?
   a. System change
   b. Gender role
   c. Cultural norms
   d. Shared attributes
7. Culturally competent care would encourage which action by a patient's family?
   a. Asking the family's spiritual advisor to visit the patient
   b. Speaking English to everyone involved in patient care
   c. Adhering to highly publicized restrictive unit visiting hours
   d. Limiting food consumption to items provided by the cafeteria
8. If a patient's primary language differs from that of the health care professionals providing care, which action is most appropriate for the nurse to take?
   a. Use colorful pictures, white boards, and gestures to communicate all important information.
   b. Recognize that continuous affirmative answers by the patient require verification of understanding.
   c. Arrange for a professional language translator to sit with the patient throughout the hospitalization.
   d. Decrease interaction with the patient and family to avoid making them uncomfortable for not understanding.
9. Which nursing diagnosis is most appropriate for a young Middle Eastern immigrant who expresses concern for the safety of his family members who were unable to relocate with him out of a war zone?
   a. *Risk for Spiritual Distress*
   b. *Impaired Role Performance*
   c. *Interrupted Family Processes*
   d. *Ineffective Coping*
10. What is the best method for the nurse to ensure that a Croatian patient's nutritional needs are met during hospitalization?
    a. Preorder a diet that is consistent with the typical Croatian patient's dietary preferences.
    b. Ask a Croatian coworker for ideas on what would be best to order for the patient's meals.
    c. Request that a variety of dietary entrees be provided to the patient to provide options.
    d. Check with the patient on admission to determine dietary limitations and preferences.

Answers and rationales for the review questions are available at *http://evolve.elsevier.com/YoostCrawford/fundamentals/*.

REFERENCES

Agency for Healthcare Research and Quality: *National healthcare disparities report, 2012.* Rockville, Md., 2012, Author. Retrieved from *www.ahrq.gov/research/findings/nhqrdr/nhdr12/index.html.*

Andrews M, Boyle J: *Transcultural concepts in nursing care*, ed. 6, Philadelphia, 2011, Lippincott Williams & Wilkins.

Cohen G, Smith R: The racial geography of the death penalty. *Wash L Rev*, 85:425-492, 2010.

Cronenwett L, Sherwood G, Barnsteiner J, et al: Quality and safety education for nurses. *Nurs Outlook*, 55(3):122-131, 2007.

Dennis B, Small E: Incorporating cultural diversity in nursing care: An action plan. *ABNF J*, 14(1):17-27, 2003.

Galanti A: *Caring for patients from different cultures*, ed. 4, Philadelphia, 2008, University of Pennsylvania Press.

Galanti A: *Caring for patients from different cultures*, ed. 5, Philadelphia, 2015, University of Pennsylvania Press.

Giger J, Davidhizar R: *Transcultural nursing: Assessment and intervention*, ed. 6, St. Louis, 2012, Mosby.

Grobman G: *Stereotypes and prejudices*, 1990. Retrieved from *http://remember.org/guide/History.root.stereotypes.html.*

Haviland W, Prins H, Walrath D, McBride B: *Cultural anthropology: The human challenge*, ed. 14, Belmont, Calif., 2013, Wadsworth.

Johnstone R: *Religion in society: A sociology of religion*, ed. 8, Upper Saddle River, N.J., 2009, Pearson Prentice-Hall.

Juckett G: Cross-cultural medicine. *Am Fam Physician*, 72(11):2267-2273, 2005.

Koffman J: Transcultural and ethical issues at the end of life. In J. Cooper (Ed.), *Stepping into palliative care* (pp. 171-186). Abington, U.K., 2006, Radcliffe Publishing Ltd.

Kottak CP: *Cultural anthropology: Appreciating cultural diversity*, ed. 15, New York, 2012, McGraw-Hill.

Leininger M: *Transcultural nursing: Concepts, theories and practices*, New York, 1978, Wiley.

Leininger M: *Transcultural nursing: Concepts, theories, research and practices*, ed. 2, New York, 1995, McGraw-Hill.

Leininger M: Founder's focus—the third millennium and transcultural nursing. *J Transcult Nurs*, 11(1):69, 2000.

Leininger M, McFarland M: *Transcultural nursing: Concepts, theories, research and practices*, ed. 3, New York, 2002, McGraw-Hill.

Leininger M, McFarland M: *Culture care diversity and universality: A worldwide nursing theory*, ed. 2, Boston, 2006, Jones & Bartlett.

People statistics: Ethnic groups (most recent) by country, 2014. Retrieved from *http://www.nationmaster.com/country-info/stats/People/Ethnic-groups.*

Purnell L: *Transcultural health care: A culturally competent approach*, ed. 4, Philadelphia, 2013, F.A. Davis.

Seisser MA: Interview with a quality leader: Madeleine Leininger on transcultural nursing and culturally competent care. *J Healthc Qual*, 24(Suppl 2):18-21, 2002.

Smedley B, Stith A, Nelson A: *Unequal treatment: Confronting racial and ethnic disparities in health care.* Washington, D.C., 2002, National Academy Press.

Spector R: *Cultural diversity in health and illness*, ed. 8, Upper Saddle River, N.J., 2012, Prentice-Hall Health.

Tylor E: *Primitive culture*, New York, 1871, Harper Torchbooks.

U.S. Census Bureau: 2010 census data, 2011. Retrieved from *www.census.gov/2010census/data.*

U.S. Department of Health and Human Services: *Healthy People 2020*, Washington, D.C., 2014, U.S. Government Printing Office. Retrieved from *www.healthypeople.gov/2020/topicsobjectives2020/overview.aspx?topicId=1.*

Wenger AF: Cultural openness, social justice, global awareness: Promoting transcultural nursing with unity in a diverse world. In P Merilainen, K Vehvilainen-Julkunen (Eds), *The 23rd annual nursing research conference 1997: Transcultural nursing—global unifier of care, facing diversity with unity* (pp. 162-168), Kuopio, Finland, 1998, Kuopio University.

Wenger AF: Cultural openness: Intrinsic to human care. *J Transcult Nurs*, 10(1):10, 1999.

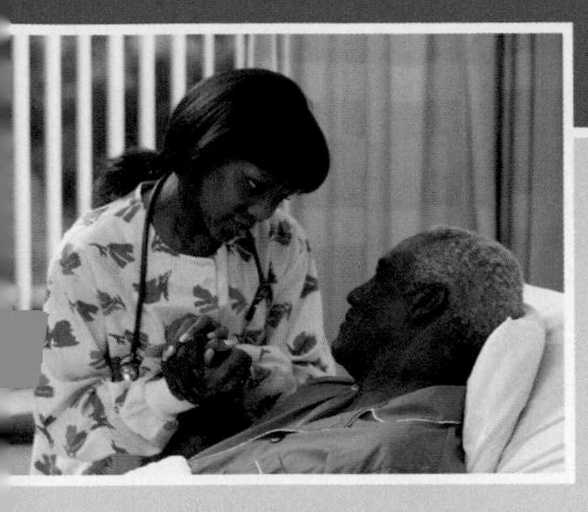

CHAPTER 22

Spiritual Health

EVOLVE WEBSITE

http://evolve.elsevier.com/YoostCrawford/fundamentals/

- Additional Evolve-Only Review Questions with Answers
- Answers and Rationales for Text Review Questions
- Answers to Critical-Thinking Questions
- Case Study with Questions
- Glossary

LEARNING OUTCOMES

Comprehension of this chapter's content will provide students with the ability to:

LO 22.1 Describe spirituality and spiritual practices in which people may engage.
LO 22.2 Discuss religion and religious practices that promote spiritual health.
LO 22.3 Identify ways in which nurses provide spiritual care.
LO 22.4 Explain the use of spiritual assessment frameworks.
LO 22.5 Articulate nursing diagnoses appropriate for the care of patients with spiritual concerns.
LO 22.6 Describe the interdisciplinary aspects of planning when spiritual needs are identified.
LO 22.7 Create a care plan that includes personalized spiritual care interventions and evaluation criteria.

KEY TERMS

agnostic, p. 419
atheist, p. 419
faith, p. 414
hope, p. 414
parish nursing, p. 419
prayer, p. 415
reflection, p. 415
religion, p. 415
spirit, p. 414
spiritual care, p. 416
spiritual distress, p. 420
spirituality, p. 414
transcendence, p. 414

CASE STUDY

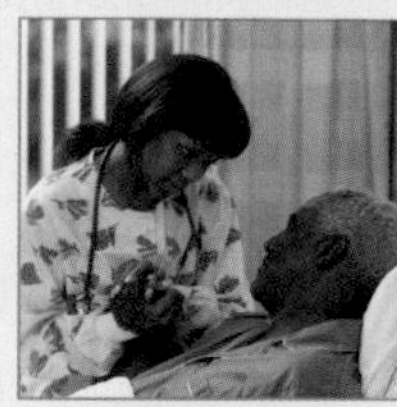

Mr. Gardner is extubated by the nurse who has provided his care for several days. When he begins to talk, he exhibits an easy sense of humor and shares with the nurse how much he misses being at home with his wife, and how much she likes chocolate. He jokingly wonders how he can "sneak out" to buy her a box of candy.

During medical rounds the attending physician walks into Mr. Gardner's room and bluntly, yet gently, tells Mr. Gardner that he has bronchoalveolar carcinoma that is untreatable in its advanced state and that the cancer will lead to his death. The physician suggests that Mr. Gardner start thinking about whether he wants to be intubated or resuscitated in the event of respiratory distress or cardiac arrest. No family members are present when the physician conveys this information, and Mr. Gardner is left to tell his family about his recent diagnosis.

When the physician leaves, the nurse holds Mr. Gardner's hand and expresses sadness regarding his situation. He shares with the nurse that he just wants to go home so that he can die in his own bed. The nurse points out that the doctor did not say that he was going to die right away, and reminds Mr. Gardner that he has a box of chocolates to buy, which makes him laugh. He starts wondering aloud if he should tell his son or his wife first. He begins to talk about his children and grandchildren whom he will "leave behind." The nurse listens to his stories and contributes an occasional joke, noticing that Mr. Gardner responds well to humor, and holds his hand for quite a while because it is evident that he wants company.

Refer back to this case study to answer the critical-thinking questions throughout the chapter.

Nursing has a long history of recognizing and integrating spiritual care into nursing care, beginning with the religious orders in the Middle Ages and continuing with Florence Nightingale in the 1800s to the present. Research has demonstrated that higher levels of spiritual health are associated with increased compliance with treatment regimens, less symptom distress, decreased pain levels, lower anxiety, enhanced quality of life, and lower mortality rates (Etnyre et al, 2006; Kaplar, Wachholt, and O'Brien, 2004; Meraviglia, 2006; Simoni, Frick, and Huang, 2006; World Health Organization, 2006). Particularly in the oncology patient population, higher levels of spiritual well-being are associated with increased levels of general health, hope, coping, social functioning, self-rated health, and quality of life and with less depression, financial strain, and suicidal ideation (Bowie, Sydnor, Granot, and Pargament, 2004; Coleman, 2003; Edward, Welch, and Chater, 2009; Gibson and Parker, 2003; Krause, 2006; McClain, Rosenfeld, and Breitbart, 2003; Meraviglia, 2006; Motyka, Nies, Walker, and Schim, 2010). This research led to The Joint Commission's requirement to provide spiritual care within a multidisciplinary environment in hospitals.

Traditionally, chaplains were the primary providers of spiritual care, but with the adoption of The Joint Commission's requirement, spiritual care became multidisciplinary in focus. Aspects of spiritual care are included in the American Nurses Association (ANA) scope and standards of practice (ANA, 2010a), Social Policy Statement (ANA, 2010b), and Code of Ethics (ANA, 2015). The American Association of Colleges of Nurses (AACN) *Essentials of Baccalaureate Education* (2008) requires registered nurse graduates to be capable of conducting a spiritual assessment and recognizing the impact of spirituality on health care. Integrating spiritual needs into a patient's plan of care is imperative to providing holistic care.

Spirituality and religion are complementary yet distinctly different concepts. *Spirituality* focuses broadly on the meaning of life, death, and existence, whereas *religion* is an organized, structured method of practicing or expressing one's spirituality. Nurses must explore and appreciate the roles both play in people's lives to better understand the attitudes of patients toward health, illness, and medical care.

SPIRITUALITY — LO 22.1

Spirituality is the expression of meaning and purpose in life (Pesut and Thorne, 2007). It is the manifestation of the innermost self. Human beings express spirituality through their unique capability for thought, contemplation, and exploration of meaning and purpose in life. That dimension of self is the **spirit**; the expression of the spirit is spirituality. People have different belief systems defining *spirit.* Some believe the spirit to be the brain, whereas others believe it to be a complex entity or phenomenon that connects with a higher power, or God. Regardless of the belief system, humans are capable of high levels of thought, and this exploration of meaning and purpose in life affects behavior and health. Therefore spirituality is universal among humans and is a central dimension of health, affecting its physical, psychological, and social aspects.

Spirituality involves movement toward growing as a human being throughout life. Such growth happens over time in an ebb-and-flow fashion. **Transcendence** is the process of moving beyond who one is in the moment and toward the person one will become in the future (Pesut and Thorne, 2007). Spirituality requires **faith**, a belief beyond self that is based on trust and life experience rather than scientific data. The ability to have faith allows people to demonstrate **hope** (confident expectation) of a positive outcome in the face of challenging circumstances. Both faith and hope are related to how people practice spirituality.

SPIRITUAL PRACTICES

People search for meaning and purpose by engaging in activities to promote their spirituality (Burkhart and Hogan, 2008). These activities are called *spiritual practices.* Overall, spiritual practices promote three types of activities: connecting with oneself through reflection, connecting with others through relationships, and connecting with a higher power through faith rituals. **Reflection** is the process of contemplating experiences, sometimes even life-changing experiences, and searching for meaning in those events. For example, many nursing students choose to enter nursing school because they have had a life experience that called them into nursing (e.g., a death in the family, observation of nurses in action, a desire to help people). The process of choosing nursing as a career involves engaging in reflection and finding personal meaning in the nursing profession. Not all life experiences require reflection, but those that do often help the person grow spiritually. Many people use methods such as intellectual, artistic, and meditative practices as well as communing with nature to facilitate the process of reflection (Figure 22-1).

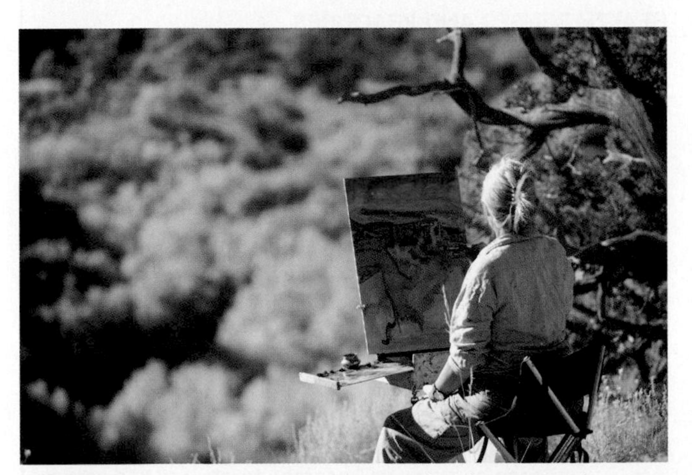

FIGURE 22-1 Artistic endeavors and enjoyment of nature facilitate the process of reflection.

People may express their spirituality within relationships with others. Great meaning can be found in friendships, family relationships, and partner and spouse relationships. These connections with other people can support and contribute to spiritual growth. Nursing students frequently discuss meaningful clinical experiences with other nursing students to search for meaning and purpose in their chosen profession and to help cope with stressful life experiences. This sharing process helps those involved to discern meaning and promote spiritual growth and transcendence.

Some people find meaning in **prayer**, which is spoken or unspoken communication with a higher power. The specific mode of praying often is influenced by the person's religious or faith belief system.

RELIGION LO 22.2

Religion provides a structure for understanding spirituality and involves rites and rituals within a faith community. Many people express their spirituality through religion. Most religions celebrate life events such as birth, marriage, and death with rituals such as baptism, marriage ceremonies, and funerals (Figure 22-2). Religion can provide a process of discerning meaning and purpose during crises, particularly

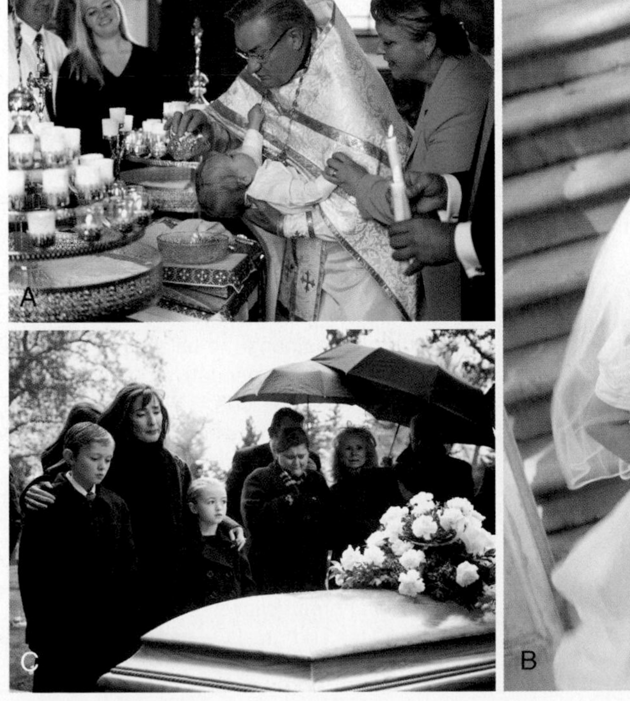

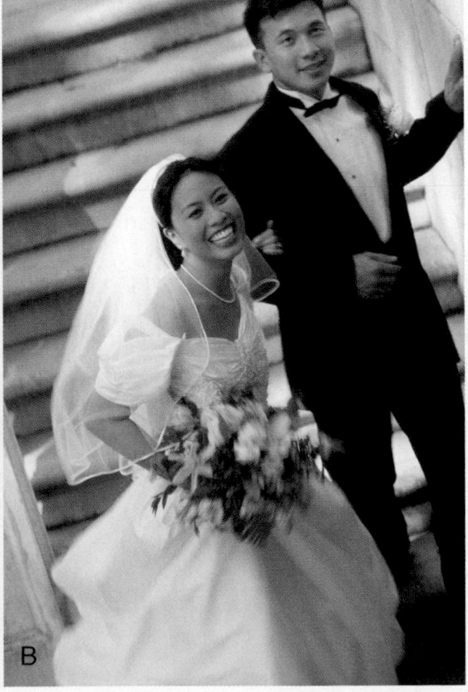

FIGURE 22-2 Religious rituals provide a framework for honoring life events such as birth, marriage, and death.

crises involving health. Therefore religious faith rituals are important in promoting health.

Religious traditions may challenge accepted medical culture, such as when people of the Jehovah's Witness faith refuse lifesaving blood transfusions for themselves or family members. During the assessment process, nurses need to seek information from patients regarding their personal religious practices that may affect medical treatment. An important point in this context is that although some religions are known for specific faith traditions or rituals, not all members of a religious community may subscribe to commonly held beliefs or customs. It is always better for nurses to ask patients about specific spiritual needs or beliefs rather than assume their compliance with those of the general religion to which they belong. Table 22-1 briefly describes the spiritual beliefs of major world religions and summarizes corresponding traditional health beliefs and spiritual practices.

SPIRITUAL CARE LO 22.3

Spiritual care in nursing practice is a mutual, purposeful, interactive process between a nurse and a patient, which

TABLE 22-1 Common World Religions, Health Beliefs, and Spiritual Practices

FOUNDATIONAL BELIEFS	HEALTH BELIEFS AND PRACTICES
Native American Mother Earth and nature are sacred. Relationships to people and nature are valued. Listening, seeing, and peace are central to life. Rituals, ceremonies, and storytelling are central to the religion.	Health is a balance of mind, body, and spirit and is connected to and continually interacting cyclically with nature. Illness is an imbalance. Healing is restoring that balance. Death is the journey to the afterlife. Rituals assist in that journey; the spirit needs to be released. The rituals differ by tribe. The shaman, or medicine man or woman, helps restore the balance between the person and natural forces within a new relationship context. Healing rituals include: • Herbal medicines • Dances, songs, and prayers • Sweat lodge ceremonies (incorporate prayers and sauna conditions in sweat lodge structures) • Storytelling
Hinduism This ancient religion was originally polytheistic and is now monotheistic. Brahma is the ultimate God; different lesser gods are different aspects of the one God: Brahma (creator), Vishnu (preserver), Shiva (destroyer). Basic beliefs include: • Vedas is the law. • Samara is reincarnation. There is a cycle of birth and rebirth. • Karma is consequence. Bad or good experiences are a result of past bad or good behaviors. • Moksha is the path of liberation toward ultimate harmony and occurs through reincarnation. • Dharma is moral conduct. There is a caste system (a hierarchical separation of social groups) that is presently outlawed; however, many of the system's customs and attitudes continue to be practiced.	Health is a harmonic balance of body, mind, and spirit in relation to the environment. Illness is a buildup of toxins. External toxins include pollution and infection. Internal toxins include fear, anger, greed, sorrow, or grief. In death the soul, or atman, is immortal, while the body perishes. Atman is reborn through moksha toward ultimate Brahma. Ayurvedic medicine focuses on cleansing the body of toxins and restoring balance. It includes dietary and elimination patterns. Restoring the balance of mind, body, and spirit includes yoga or meditative practices. Health practices include: • Fasting to remove toxins (hot or cold food and drink also help remove toxins) • Yoga or meditative practices • Preference for modesty and same-sex caregivers • Astrology, which can be part of decision making • Belief that pain and suffering are due to bad karma • Dietary restrictions, prayer, and jewelry, which are part of rites and rituals • Vegetarianism

TABLE 22-1 Common World Religions, Health Beliefs, and Spiritual Practices—cont'd

FOUNDATIONAL BELIEFS	HEALTH BELIEFS AND PRACTICES
Buddhism	
The two different types of Buddhism are Mahayana and Theravada. The four noble truths are: • Life is suffering. • Origin of suffering is want. • Cessation of suffering is to not want (middle path—moderation). • Think right in terms of view, intent, speech, conduct, means of livelihood, endeavor, mindfulness, and meditation. Karma—cause and effect, rebirth—is the concept that what happens in the next life is contingent on how the person lived the previous life. Rebirth occurs until the person reaches nirvana. There is collective karma, which affects social behavior. Thus government should promote health because it is the right thing to do.	Health is a balance of mind, body, emotion, and spirit. Death includes both physical and mental termination. The family stays with the body for 2 hours before it is transferred off the nursing unit. Bodies are cremated. Meditation calms the mind and body.
Chinese*	
Ethical principles and empathy are applied to everyone throughout life, creating a moral social order. Five family relationships represent characteristics that are the basis of a moral, well-ordered, harmonious society: • Gentility/humility (older/younger brothers) • Righteous behavior/obedience (husband/wife) • Consideration/deference (elders/children) • Benevolence/loyalty (ruler/subject) • Chi is life energy manifested in a balance between yin (feminine energy) and yang (masculine energy). Spiritual immortality is achieved through noninterference with and removal of obstructions to the natural flow of chi, creating harmony with Tao, or one's own human nature.	Health is balanced chi. Health practices to restore yin-yang balance include: • Acupuncture • Nutrition • Herb therapy • Exercise (yoga, tai-chi-chuan, chi-kung) • Moxibustion (burning of the mugwort herb to produce heat for promoting circulation) • Cupping (external suction therapy to improve circulation; usually used for pain, respiratory, or digestive problems) • Gua sha therapy (rubbing or scraping oiled skin to produce intentional surface bruising, to treat fever and pain) • Meditation • Inclusion of family in decision making
Sikhism	
The leader, Guru, is more than a teacher and is aligned with divine. Belief focuses on God, equality, truthful living, avoidance of superstition, and study of the teachings of the gurus. Meditation is used to reveal inner light. Five physical symbols, or 5K, are worn by devotees: • Uncut hair • A wooden comb • A steel bracelet • Cotton underwear • A ceremonial sword	Health and disease are a continuum. Health is not viewed only physically. Ceremonies are conducted at birth. Body preparation is completed upon death. Religious leaders and families participate in decision making. Medical care is welcomed along with religious rituals. Religious practices affecting health care include: • Daily bathing • Scripture reading • Shaving restriction • Modesty • Wearing of a turban head covering

Continued

TABLE 22-1 Common World Religions, Health Beliefs, and Spiritual Practices—cont'd

FOUNDATIONAL BELIEFS	HEALTH BELIEFS AND PRACTICES
Islam	
Abrahamic faith (descended from Abraham) Beliefs include that there is one God and that Muhammad is the prophet. Teachings are from the Koran (divine word) and Sunnah (Muhammad's life), for moral imperatives and spiritual values. Rituals include the five pillars of Islam: • Believe in one God. • Pray five times a day, facing Mecca. • Give alms for the less fortunate. • Fast during Ramadan. • Make a pilgrimage to Mecca.	God gave life, and it is the responsibility of people to maintain dignity and to take care of the body. Life on earth is a testing ground for the afterlife. Therefore following rituals is critical at all times. Religious practices affecting health care include: • Privacy for prayer • Preference for modesty and same-sex caregivers • Family involvement in decision making • Imam (religious leader) sometimes involved in decision making • Dietary restrictions (no pork) • No or limited alcohol consumption
Judaism	
Abrahamic religion Beliefs include that there is one God and that God established a covenant with the Jewish people. Life is a gift from God and is precious. There are many sects, with varying levels of observance. The most common are identified by their beliefs and practices: • Orthodox • Conservative • Reform (Progressive) Rites and rituals include specific foods and holiday observance. Sabbath is Friday night to Saturday night.	Everything possible should be done to preserve life. Religious practices affecting health care include: • Kosher diet includes restrictions on pork and shellfish, no mixing of meat and dairy, and consumption only of food that has been designated as kosher. Observance varies. • Holiday observance varies. • A newborn son is circumcised on the eighth day of life in a ritual called a bris. Circumcision is not performed in the hospital. • Restrictions on work during Sabbath may affect health care treatment. Observance varies.
Christianity	
Abrahamic religion Beliefs include that Jesus Christ was incarnate of God and that the Trinity is the Father, Son, and Holy Spirit as one. There are many different denominations of Christianity, with different rituals and sacraments: • Catholic • Orthodox • Anglican • Episcopal • Lutheran • Presbyterian • United Methodist • Baptist • Nondenominational Sacraments practiced in some denominations include baptism, confirmation, matrimony, penance, anointing of the sick, and communion.	Health is viewed as a balance or integrated whole of physical, psychological, social, ethical, and spiritual dimensions at the individual and societal levels. It is important to love God, self, and others within this integrated whole. Providing health care is very important at the individual and global levels. Health care should help relieve both pain and suffering, whether physical, psychosocial, or spiritual. Forgiveness is a major theme. Many Christians believe in prayer as a means of healing. Both proximal and distant intercessory prayers are encouraged.

From Sorajjakool S, Carr MF, Nam JJ: *World religions for healthcare professionals,* New York, 2010, Routledge.
*Chinese religions include Confucianism, Taoism, Buddhism, folk religion, and combinations of all of these.

may include family, to promote the patient's spiritual health (Burkhart and Hogan, 2008). Nurses provide spiritual care when they recognize the interconnectedness of the physical, cultural, and spiritual realms and actively seek to understand and provide for each patient's holistic needs. Interventions to achieve these aims will vary: The nurse may refer a patient to a chaplain or preferred spiritual adviser for support, baptize an at-risk infant in an emergency situation, pray with a patient on request, or facilitate implementation of faith-related rituals for a patient facing a life-changing experience such as birth or death. Spiritual care differs according to the patient's developmental age. Spiritual care needs to be provided in a manner consistent with a patient's own faith developmental level, as further described in the Diversity Considerations box.

DIVERSITY CONSIDERATIONS

Life Span

Fowler's Theory of Faith Development (1981, 2002) describes the developmental phases of faith:

- *Infant (primal faith):* Building trust and loving relationships is fundamental.
- *Toddler/preschool (intuitive projective faith):* With language development comes the ability to find meaning in stories and an understanding of good versus evil.
- *School age (mythic-literal faith):* Spiritual growth happens as a result of finding meaning in social relationships and applying principles of ethical and moral reasoning.
- *Adolescence (synthetic-conventional faith):* Beginning with abstract thinking and the development of self-identity, this is the time of rejecting concrete rules and finding personal meaning in one's own faith beliefs, which may not be thoroughly examined. Some people remain at this stage of faith development throughout adult life.
- *Young adulthood (individuative-reflective faith):* Self-identity is established with a greater understanding of self and appreciation of different perspectives. At this level, decisions are based on a broader world view.
- *Middle adulthood (conjunctive faith):* The person has the ability to accept that multiple interpretations of reality exist. An openness to various religions and faith traditions is exhibited in a person who reaches this stage.
- *Older adult (universalizing faith and the God-grounded self):* The person understands self as part of a universal "whole" of love and justice.

Gender

Gender differences include the following:

- Women more often want communication and reflection with others, along with personal spiritual and religious practices.
- Men typically want facts and information to assist in decision making and participate less in daily spiritual practices than women. (Jacobs-Lawson, Schumacher, Hughes, and Arnold, 2010).

Culture, Ethnicity, and Religion

- Religious traditions differ in spiritual practices. People of various cultural backgrounds, including African Americans and Hispanics, particularly those with chronic illness, find spiritual care to be important to health (Simoni, Frick, and Huang, 2006).
- Life experiences affect the need for spiritual care. People with chronic illness require more spiritual care (Logan, Hackbusch-Pinto, and DeGrasse, 2006).
- Cultural practices surrounding illness and death vary depending on the faith tradition of patients and their families. Nurses must ask about preferences and try to accommodate requests as much as possible.

Disability

- Parents of chronically ill children report "having faith in God" as their most frequent coping resource (Allen and Marshall, 2010).
- Intellectually and developmentally disabled people who participate in bereavement groups after the death of a friend have been found to experience lower rates of depression (Stoddart, Burke, and Temple, 2002).

Research has shown that adult patients want nurses to promote hope, positive perspectives, giving love to others, finding meaning and understanding, and relating to God (Taylor, 2006). Creating an environment of compassion and caring so that patients and families feel comfortable in expressing their spiritual needs is a prerequisite to providing spiritual care. If the patient does not experience compassionate warmth from the nurse, the patient will not accept spiritual care. Patients who describe themselves as being an **atheist** (believing that God or higher powers do not exist) or an **agnostic** (believing that the nature or existence of God is unknowable) require compassionate, nonjudgmental care similar to that for all other patients. It is essential for nurses to respect the personal beliefs of everyone, even if they are dramatically different from their own. If the beliefs of a patient change due to a health crisis, referral to a chaplain, member of the clergy, or a spiritual adviser may become appropriate.

PARISH NURSING

Registered nurses may provide spiritual care through **parish nursing**, an area of nursing practice that originated from the work of the Reverend Dr. Granger Westberg in the mid-1980s. Some roles of a parish nurse are health adviser, health educator, advocate, liaison to faith and community resources, coordinator of volunteers, and developer of support groups. Parish nurses seek to provide holistic care by focusing on the mind, body, and spirit in addition to community wellness. Parish nursing was designated as a specialty by the ANA in 1997. *Faith Community Nursing: Scope and Standards of Practice* (ANA and Health Ministries Association, 2012) defines the parameters of parish nursing. Parish nurses come from many faith traditions; recognized groups include Jewish Congregational Nurses and Muslim Crescent Nurses, as well as registered nurses working within a wide variety of Christian traditions. The International Parish Nurse Resource Center provides educational and resource materials for this specialty in collaboration with the ANA and the Health Ministries Association (Patterson, Wehling, and Mason, 2008).

◆ ASSESSMENT LO 22.4

Spiritual assessment is a process of determining spiritual needs and can take many forms. To comply with The Joint Commission's requirement, many institutions incorporate

HEALTH ASSESSMENT QUESTIONS

Spiritual Health

- Do you have family in the area? (Assess for family importance, relationships, and meaningful experiences at this time.)
- Is there anyone you would like to call?
- How are you handling this hospitalization or illness?
- What faith practices or beliefs will help you cope with this illness or hospitalization?
- Do you belong to a faith community? Do you want the community to be notified? Would you like a chaplain to visit?

initial spirituality-focused questions into the hospital admission process (Health Assessment Questions box). The admissions office or the admitting care provider may ask initial screening questions about the patient's religious tradition, whether the patient's faith community should be notified, and whether care providers need to know of the patient's spiritual or religious needs or practices (Ethical, Legal, and Professional Practice box and Evidence-Based Practice box). Some spiritual assessment frameworks use acronyms to structure this information (Table 22-2).

Nurses assess for spiritual needs on an ongoing basis to determine what holds meaning and purpose in the patient's life. The assessments happen during conversations about family and friends, social supports, employment, or day-to-day life activities outside the health system. Nurses should encourage the patient to lead these conversations and should pay attention to nonverbal cues such as facial expression or tone of voice; for instance, when a patient's eyes light up at the mention of a particular event or person, that subject can be identified as a meaningful aspect of the patient's life.

TABLE 22-2 Formal Spiritual Assessment Frameworks

FRAMEWORK	COMPONENTS
FICA (Puchalski and Romer, 2000)	*F:* Faith and belief *I:* Importance of faith *C:* Faith community involvement *A:* Address spirituality or spiritual practices in care
SPIRIT (Maugans, 1996)	*S:* Spiritual belief system *P:* Personal spirituality *I:* Integration and involvement in a spiritual community *R:* Ritualized practices and restrictions *I:* Implications for medical care *T:* Terminal-events planning (advance directives)
HOPE (Anandarajah and Hight, 2001)	*H:* Sources of hope, meaning, comfort, strength, peace, love, and connection *O:* Organized religion *P:* Personal spirituality and practice *E:* Effects on medical care and end-of-life issues

ETHICAL, LEGAL, AND PROFESSIONAL PRACTICE

Responsibilities Associated With Spiritual Care

- Because of HIPAA requirements, health care providers cannot contact a faith community without the consent of the patient. Therefore most health care institutions ask, as part of the admission process, whether a faith community should be notified.
- Pettigrew (1990) maintains that nursing care that fails to recognize a patient's spiritual needs as a part of holistic care is unethical and defies the ethical concept of fidelity.
- Refusing to provide spiritual care for patients because of a nurse's fear of spiritual vulnerability represents a violation of the nurse's commitment to nonmaleficence (Wright, 1998).
- The International Council of Nurses Code of Ethics for Nurses (2012) urges all nurses to promote environments in which the human rights, customs, spiritual beliefs, and values of individual patients, families, and communities are respected.

EVIDENCE-BASED PRACTICE

Spiritual Assessment Data Accessibility in Electronic Health Records

- Few electronic health records (EHRs) automatically incorporate spiritual assessment and interventions. Health care systems can integrate initial spiritual assessment using the FICA, SPIRIT, or HOPE system and can continually measure spiritual health using a five-point Likert system, as in the Nursing Outcomes Classification system, in flow sheets (Burkhart and Androwich, 2009).
- Because spiritual care is multidisciplinary, spiritual documentation needs to be viewed by all health care providers to ensure integrated, patient-centered care.

Patients are at high risk for **spiritual distress** (belief or value system disruption) in certain health situations that threaten their meaning and sense of purpose in life. For example, patients may have spiritual needs when learning of a life-changing diagnosis or experiencing a health crisis. Patients may require spiritual care when making health care decisions. These types of situations require that patients reflect on meaning and purpose in life, personal values, and the way their decisions affect others. Patients may need assistance during these at-risk times to lessen the degree of their spiritual distress. Nurses must be alert to such situations so that they can intervene appropriately.

Patients exhibit spiritual needs using both verbal and nonverbal cues. In many cases, spiritual distress may be expressed

TABLE 22-3 Spiritual Assessment Cues

PATIENT CUE CATEGORY	EXAMPLES
Verbal	• Asks for prayer or chaplain • Asks if the nurse has time to talk • Talks about topics related to life, death, or purpose • Talks about faith • Uses religious words in conversation • Asks frequent questions about diagnosis; needs to talk • Expresses concerns about family
Nonverbal	• Exhibits neediness • Is angry or noncompliant • Seems depressed or withdrawn • Has emotional outbursts and cries quietly
Environmental	• Has religious books, jewelry, or symbols and/or has prayer objects • Displays family pictures
Situational	• Has a life-threatening diagnosis or life-changing condition • Is facing death • Faces treatment decisions

as anger, depression, neediness, or crying. Nurses need to be attentive to the patient's health situation and behaviors to determine whether spiritual care is needed.

Nurses should be observant of potential religious needs. Religious people often use certain expressions such as in their day-to-day conversations—"God willing" or "blessings." Religious objects in the patient's room, such as holy books, religion-oriented jewelry, or prayer objects, may indicate a religious orientation to spirituality. To promote spiritual health, nurses must be attentive to these verbal, nonverbal, environmental, and situational patient cues indicating a need for spiritual care and must recognize the patient's spiritual or religious orientation. Examples of patient cues are provided in Table 22-3.

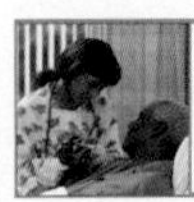

1. What situational and verbal cues in Mr. Gardner's case indicate a need for spiritual care?

NURSING DIAGNOSIS LO 22.5

Multiple nursing diagnoses are available to help address patient concerns related to spirituality. After a thorough spiritual assessment, the nurse can determine which nursing diagnoses are most appropriate for identifying the patient's unique needs. Some nursing diagnoses that may be written for patients exhibiting spiritual needs include:

- *Spiritual Distress* related to chronic illness as evidenced by expressions of hopelessness and statements indicating concern over the recent inability to pray
- *Impaired Religiosity* related to illness as evidenced by difficulty adhering to religious dietary customs and expressions of emotional distress over special diet restrictions
- *Readiness for Enhanced Religiosity* as evidenced by rejecting harmful customs and seeking reconciliation with previously estranged family members
- *Moral Distress* related to cultural conflict between medical treatment and religious beliefs as evidenced by expressions of concern about rejection by religious community and hesitation in accepting blood transfusion
- *Decisional Conflict* related to unclear personal beliefs as evidenced by questioning of personal beliefs while making decisions and delayed decision making

PLANNING LO 22.6

The Joint Commission standards affirm the importance of spirituality and spiritual well-being with regard to improved patient outcomes. On the basis of assessment findings and identified nursing diagnoses, nurses must individualize and prioritize care for every patient (Table 22-4). It is the nurse's responsibility to decide the order in which spiritual concerns and other patient problems need to be addressed.

As appropriate, the spiritual needs component of the care plan should include specific goals or outcome statements, as in the following examples:

- "Patient will report the ability to pray after counsel by the hospital chaplain."
- "After consulting with the dietitian, the patient will identify acceptable ways to blend dietary restrictions with religious customs before discharge."
- "Patient will contact estranged family members to arrange for a combined meeting with a spiritual counselor to reopen lines of communication within 2 weeks."
- "Patient will report acceptance of medical interventions that are consistent with personal religious beliefs and medical necessity within 48 hours."
- "Patient will discuss treatment choices with a trusted confidant to explore acceptable options before beginning treatment next week."

A patient's spiritual adviser, clergy person, rabbi, or imam is an important member of the interdisciplinary health care team. In the absence of a personal spiritual adviser identified by the patient, many medical facilities have interfaith chaplaincy departments to assist in providing appropriate spiritual care. When nursing diagnoses involving spiritual concerns emerge during the assessment process, collaboration with and patient referrals to the hospital chaplain may be indicated (Collaboration and Delegation box).

TABLE 22-4 Care Planning

NANDA-I NURSING DIAGNOSIS LABEL WITH NURSING DIAGNOSIS STATEMENT	NURSING OUTCOME CLASSIFICATION (NOC)	NURSING INTERVENTION CLASSIFICATION (NIC)
Spiritual Distress related to chronic illness as evidenced by expressions of hopelessness and statements indicating concern over the recent inability to pray	*Coping* (1302) Reports increase in psychological comfort (130218)	*Coping enhancement* (5230) Encourage the use of spiritual resources, if desired.

From Bulechek G, Butcher H, Dochterman J, et al (eds): *Nursing interventions classification (NIC)*, ed. 6, St. Louis, 2013, Mosby; Moorhead S, Johnson M, Maas M, et al (eds): *Nursing outcomes classification (NOC)*, ed. 5, St. Louis, 2013, Mosby; NANDA International: *Nursing diagnoses: Definitions and classification, 2012-2014*, West Sussex, England, 2012, Wiley-Blackwell. Reprinted with permission from NANDA International, Inc

COLLABORATION AND DELEGATION

Chaplains as Members of the Health Care Team

- Nurses should make chaplaincy referrals when a patient demonstrates or verbalizes a need for spiritual care, and they should follow up to make sure that patient's spiritual needs are being met. The research of Vanderwerker and colleagues (2008) found that the most common source of referrals to hospital chaplains was nurses (28%). The second most common source was patients themselves (23%), with few referrals coming from physicians or social workers.
- In health care facilities with well-functioning departments of spiritual ministry, frequent communication takes place with the interdisciplinary team that consists of nurses, chaplains, physicians, social workers, case managers, and other care providers.
- Chaplains should be asked to attend care conferences at which they can provide spiritual insight and participate in planning holistic health care for patients.
- Chaplains constitute an excellent resource for providing spiritual counseling for nurses who work on all types of units, especially those that are spiritually challenging, including emergency departments, pediatric burn or oncology units, and hospice or intensive care units, where the patient's spiritual needs often are intense (O'Brien, 2014).

QSEN FOCUS!

Nurses need to value the unique attributes of all members of the health care team, including spiritual advisors and clergy, to provide care that fully addresses the spiritual needs of patients.

IMPLEMENTATION AND EVALUATION LO 22.7

Spiritual care interventions are purposeful actions to promote another person's spirituality. Recognizing a spiritual need and providing spiritual interventions may happen spontaneously. When the nurse recognizes a patient cue, it is important to further determine whether the patient requires assistance that promotes reflection, connections with others, or faith rituals. The nurse may initiate reflective interventions by stating, "This must be a difficult time for you. Much has changed. What are you thinking?" In many cases such discussions involve exploring and searching for meaningful aspects of a situation and the subsequent impact on loved ones. Discussion also may include life plans or health care decision making.

Promoting connectedness with others implies that family and friends are providing the spiritual care; the nurse's role is to encourage that connection and/or to eliminate barriers in the environment that are inhibiting this connectedness. Appropriate interventions can include navigating policies and procedures related to visitation and assisting families to overcome fear related to medical equipment and technology (such as ventilators or cardiac monitors).

To initiate connections with others, the nurse may ask, "Is there someone with whom you would like to talk? Can I call family or friends?" If family is available, the nurse may encourage interaction by saying: "You have much to talk about. Is there anything I can do? Do you need more information? Let me give you privacy so you can talk." Nurses need to individualize their spiritual care based on careful assessment of the environment and recognition of spiritual connections among family members.

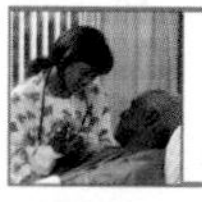

2. What spiritual care was provided by the nurse to Mr. Gardner?

To promote connection with a higher power, nurses frequently offer to call the chaplain for patients. Some nurses offer to pray with patients, but this is contingent on the institution's policies and procedures as well as the nurse's comfort with prayer. If the patient requests prayer and the nurse is uncomfortable participating in this practice, it is best to allow the patient to lead the prayer. Spiritual care includes facilitating religious rituals. Some religious rituals may be contrary to hospital policy (e.g., lighting candles). Nurses need to collaborate with chaplains and administration to maximize religious expression. A variety of nursing interventions can be implemented for patients experiencing spiritual concerns:

- Allow time and opportunity for self-disclosure by the patient.
- Be physically present and actively listen when the patient speaks.
- Support avenues to spiritual growth that are meaningful to the patient, such as praying, meditating, listening to music, viewing or creating art, or reading or writing poetry.
- Arrange for regular visits from religious advisers.
- Monitor and promote supportive social contacts.
- Integrate the family into spiritual practices, as appropriate.
- Avoid sharing personal beliefs that are in direct conflict with those of the patient.
- Refer the patient to or arrange for the patient to engage in a support group or counseling, as appropriate.

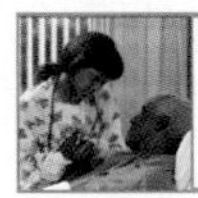

3. List additional spiritual care measures that may be helpful to Mr. Gardner.

IMPACT ON THE NURSE

Although the purpose of providing spiritual care is to promote the patient's spiritual health, providing spiritual care also can affect the nurse. Nurses frequently encounter spiritually distressing situations that may place them at risk for spiritual distress themselves. Nurses who are in spiritual distress may not have the energy to provide spiritual care to their patients. Research has indicated that poor spiritual health can lead to burnout.

To avoid the long-term negative effects of spiritual distress, nurses must attend to their own spiritual health by engaging in spiritual practices that promote their own personal reflection. Because reflection is a time of searching for meaning in a past experience, it can be facilitated by journaling, quiet time, gardening, music, artwork, exercise, or prayer and meditation. Reflecting on a patient-nurse encounter can transform a sad, spiritually distressing encounter (e.g., death of a patient) into a positive spiritual memory, thereby facilitating spiritual growth.

Providing spiritual care, coupled with reflective practice, can help the nurse grow spiritually. Nurses who work in specialties that require frequent spiritual care (e.g., hospice, oncology) typically report that upon reflection, they are able to find meaning and a sense of privilege in this work. Without reflective practice, providing frequent spiritual care in distressing situations can lead to spiritual distress and an inability to provide spiritual care in the future. Research has consistently demonstrated that people in spiritual distress have difficulty providing spiritual care (Baldacchino, 2007; Wallace et al, 2008). Therefore nurses need to attend to their own spiritual health in order to provide spiritual care. Spiritual care is central to nursing practice, is fulfilling, and is one of the reasons that nurses stay in the profession.

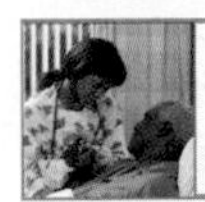

4. What reflective activities did the nurse perform herself while caring for Mr. Gardner?

! SAFE PRACTICE ALERT

Spiritual care is a nursing care requirement. Promoting spiritual health in patients promotes physical, psychological, and social well-being.

EVALUATION

After each intervention designed to help patients meet their spiritual care goals, evaluation of the outcome criteria must be completed.

Merge this paragraph into the paragraph above after the first sentence. Evaluation of goals to address spiritual needs may be difficult to quantify. Nurses should be attentive to physical indications of patient improvement, nonverbal cues, and statements regarding patients' spiritual well-being. Congruency between objective and subjective evaluation data is important to validate goal attainment. After determining the degree to which the patient's spiritual goals were met, the nurse works with the patient to continue, modify, or discontinue the plan of care.

The importance of providing holistic patient care that includes spiritual care cannot be overstated. Nurses must recognize the impact of spirituality on personal health and facilitate the ability of patients to stay connected to their sources of spiritual support during illness or crises.

SUMMARY OF LEARNING OUTCOMES

LO 22.1 *Describe spirituality and spiritual practices in which people may engage:* Spirituality focuses broadly on the meaning of life and existence. Engaging in reflection, connecting with others through relationships, and connecting with a higher power through faith rituals are spiritual practices that enhance spiritual wellness.

LO 22.2 *Discuss religion and religious practices that promote spiritual health:* Religion is an organized, structured method of practicing or expressing one's spirituality. Religious rituals such as ceremonies celebrating births, marriages, and the lives of individuals who have died help people share significant events that bring meaning to life.

LO 22.3 *Identify ways in which nurses provide spiritual care:* Nurses provide spiritual care when they recognize the interconnectedness of the physical, cultural, and spiritual realms and actively seek to understand and provide for a patient's holistic needs. Parish nursing is a professional specialty in which registered nurses practice holistic care within a faith community.

LO 22.4 *Explain the use of spiritual assessment frameworks:* Spiritual assessment frameworks guide nurses in gathering key assessment data such as identification of patient faith and belief systems, valued religious rituals, and implications for medical care.

LO 22.5 *Articulate nursing diagnoses appropriate for the care of patients with spiritual concerns:* Spiritually focused nursing diagnoses include Spiritual Distress, Decisional Conflict, Moral Distress, and Impaired Religiosity.

LO 22.6 *Describe the interdisciplinary aspects of planning when spiritual needs are identified:* Spiritual advisers are an integral part of the interdisciplinary health care team and should be included in care conferences with nurses, physicians, social workers, case managers, and others when spiritual concerns emerge during the assessment process.

LO 22.7 *Create a care plan that includes personalized spiritual care interventions and evaluation criteria:* Spiritual care interventions are purposeful actions to promote another's spirituality that include encouraging conversation on topics of concern, actively listening when spiritual matters are shared, and promoting interaction with support people including spiritual advisers, friends, and family. Evaluation of goals to address spiritual needs may be difficult to quantify. Nurses should be attentive to physical indications of patient improvement, nonverbal cues, and statements regarding the patient's spiritual well-being.

Responses to the critical-thinking questions are available at *http://evolve.elsevier.com/YoostCrawford/fundamentals/*.

REVIEW QUESTIONS

1. The nurse is caring for a 16-year-old boy receiving chemotherapy for testicular cancer. He says that his parents are religious and left a cross next to his bed for "good luck." What is the most appropriate response by the nurse?
   a. "Would you like to talk with a chaplain?"
   b. "Sounds like you are not very religious."
   c. "How well do you get along with your parents?"
   d. "What helps you get through tough times?"
2. A Buddhist patient has end-stage pancreatic cancer. In what spiritual practice would this patient most likely engage?
   a. Reading passages in the Vedas
   b. Visiting with the patient's guru
   c. Practicing tai chi
   d. Meditating on the meaning of life
3. The nurse has been caring for a patient who just died. The patient's daughter is crying uncontrollably, saying, "She was my best friend. I thought she would make it! I don't know what I am going to do." What is the nurse's best response?
   a. Express sympathy, and ask if she would like to talk with a chaplain.
   b. Give the daughter time to cry in her mother's room alone.
   c. Ask the daughter if her father is still living.
   d. Inquire if the daughter would like to pray.

4. A nurse assigned to the neonatal intensive care unit (NICU) has spent most of a day working with a critically ill infant, with the mother standing by. The infant experiences a cardiac arrest and does not survive. The mother spends an hour crying and holding the baby, saying good-bye. Which spiritual care intervention(s) is/are most appropriate for the nurse to implement? *(Select all that apply.)*
   a. If desired, briefly hold the baby to say good-bye after the mother leaves.
   b. Follow procedures to prepare the body for transport to the morgue.
   c. Visit the mother the next day to see how she is doing.
   d. Call the family spiritual adviser or the chaplain.
   e. Ask the mother if you could call a family member or friend to be with her.
5. Which statement by a patient best illustrates reflection on a spiritual need?
   a. "My husband told me what to do about this situation and I'm sure he's right."
   b. "There is little I can do now to change my circumstances. I just need to adapt."
   c. "I need to think a little more about how I feel about undergoing this treatment."
   d. "Whatever the physician wants to do is fine. I don't have much of an option."
6. What is the most important aspect of providing spiritual care in nursing practice?
   a. Call a chaplain.
   b. Complete the FICA spiritual assessment and refer as needed.
   c. Recognize situations and patient behaviors indicating a spiritual need.
   d. Spend some time in self-reflection.
7. When caring for patients who are Jewish, how best can the nurse address their religious needs?
   a. Order a kosher diet.
   b. Allow time for prayer before each meal.
   c. Ask about religious holidays, particularly religious practices around the Sabbath.
   d. Ask about religious practices affecting care.
8. The nurse is caring for a 45-year-old woman who is a breast cancer survivor. What activity associated with her cancer experience will promote this patient's spiritual well-being?
   a. Attending church every week
   b. Ensuring she follows her medication regimen
   c. Genetic testing on family members
   d. Speaking about her cancer experience to increase breast cancer awareness
9. The nurse is caring for a Catholic patient who is going to surgery tomorrow. The patient states that she is afraid and asks the nurse to pray with her, although the nurse is not religious. What is the most appropriate response by the nurse?
   a. "I am not confident praying, but I will think about you tomorrow."
   b. "I need to take care of other patients right now, but I will be back."
   c. "I am uncomfortable praying. May I call the chaplain for you?"
   d. "I don't do that. Nurses are not allowed to do that at our hospital."
10. How do people who participate in organized religion differ from nonreligious people?
   a. Religious people are healthier than spiritual people.
   b. Religious people are more spiritual than nonreligious people.
   c. Religious people express their spirituality through faith traditions.
   d. Religious people have spiritual practices, whereas nonreligious people do not have spiritual practices.

Answers and rationales for the review questions are available at *http://evolve.elsevier.com/YoostCrawford/fundamentals/*.

REFERENCES

Allen D, Marshall E: Spirituality as a coping resource for African American parents of chronically ill children. *Am J Matern Child Nurs*, 35(4):232-237, 2010.

American Association of Colleges of Nurses: *Essentials of baccalaureate education for professional nursing practice*, Washington, D.C., 2008, Author.

American Nurses Association: *Code of ethics for nurses with interpretive statements*, Silver Spring, Md., 2015, Author.

American Nurses Association: *Nursing: Scope and standards of practice*, ed. 2, Silver Spring, Md., 2010a, Author.

American Nurses Association: *Nursing's social policy statement*, ed. 3, Silver Spring, Md., 2010b, Author.

American Nurses Association, Health Ministries Association: *Faith community nursing: Scope and standards of practice*, ed. 2, Silver Spring, Md., 2012, Authors.

Anandarajah, G, Hight, E: Spirituality and medical practice: Using the HOPE questions as a practical tool for spiritual assessment. *Am Fam Physician*, 60:81-89, 2001.

Baldacchino DR: Teaching on the spiritual dimension in care: The perceived impact on undergraduate nursing students. *Nurse Educ Today*, 28:501-512, 2007.

Bowie JV, Sydnor KD, Granot M, Pargament K: Spirituality and coping among survivors of prostate cancer. *J Psychosoc Oncol*, 22(2):41-56, 2004.

Burkhart L, Androwich I: Measuring spiritual care with informatics. *ANS Adv Nurs Sci*, 32(3):200-210, 2009.

Burkhart L, Hogan N: An experiential theory of spiritual care in nursing practice. *Qual Health Res*, 18(7):928-938, 2008.

Coleman CL: Spirituality and sexual orientation: Relationship to mental well-being and functional health status. *J Adv Nurs*, 43(5):457-464, 2003.

Cronenwett L, Sherwood G, Barnsteiner J, et al: Quality and safety education for nurses. *Nurs Outlook*, 55(3):122-131, 2007.

Edward K, Welch A, Chater K: The phenomenon of resilience as described by adults who have experienced mental illness. *J Adv Nurs*, 65(3):587-595, 2009.

Etnyre A, Rauschhuber M, Gilliland I, et al: Cardiovascular risk among older Hispanic women: A pilot study. *AAOHN J*, 54(3):120-128, 2006.

Fowler J: *Stages of faith: The psychology of human development and the quest for meaning*. San Francisco, 1981, Harper & Row.

Fowler J: Faith, selfhood, and the making of meaning. In E Shafranske (Ed), *Religion and the clinical practice of psychology* (pp 165-186), Washington, D.C., 2002, American Psychological Association.

Gibson LM, Parker V: Inner resources as predictors of psychological well-being in middle-income African American breast cancer survivors. *Cancer Control*, 10(5):52-58, 2003.

International Council of Nurses: Code of ethics for nurses, 2012. Retrieved from *www.icn.ch/images/stories/documents/about/icncode_english.pdf*.

Jacobs-Lawson JM, Schumacher MM, Hughes T, Arnold S: Gender differences in psychosocial responses to lung cancer. *Gender Med*, 7(2):137-148, 2010.

Kaplar ME, Wachholt AB, O'Brien WH: The effect of religious and spiritual intervention on biological, psychological, and spiritual outcomes of oncology patients: A meta-analytic review. *J Psychosoc Oncol*, 22(1):39-49, 2004.

Krause N: Exploring the stress-buffering effects of church-based and secular social support on self-rated health in late life. *J Gerontol B Psychol Sci Soc Sci*, B(1):S35-S43, 2006.

Logan J, Hackbusch-Pinto R, De Grasse CE: Women undergoing breast diagnostics: The lived experience of spirituality. *Oncol Nurs Forum*, 33(1):121-126, 2006.

Maugans TA: The SPIRITual history. *Arch Fam Med*, 5(1):11-16, 1996.

McClain CS, Rosenfeld B, Breitbart W: Effect of spiritual well-being on end-of-life despair in terminally-ill cancer patients. *Lancet*, 361:1603-1607, 2003.

Meraviglia M: Effects of spirituality in breast cancer survivors. *Oncol Nurs Forum*, 33(1):E1-E7, 2006.

Motyka CL, Nies MA, Walker D, Schim SM: Improving the quality of life of African Americans receiving palliative care. *Home Health Care Manag Pract*, 22(2):96-103, 2010.

O'Brien MA: *Spirituality in nursing: Standing on holy ground*, ed. 5, Sudbury, Mass., 2014, Jones & Bartlett.

Patterson D, Wehling B, Mason G: Parish nursing: Reclaiming the spiritual dimensions of care. *Am Nurse Today*, 3(10):38-40, 2008.

Pesut B, Thorne S: From private to public: Negotiating professional and personal identities in spiritual care. *J Adv Nurs*, 58(4):396-403, 2007.

Pettigrew J: Intensive nursing care: The ministry of presence. *Crit Care Nurs Clin North Am*, 2(3):503-508, 1990.

Puchalski C, Romer AL: Taking a spiritual history allows clinicians to understand patients more fully. *J Palliat Med*, 3(1):129-137, 2000.

Simoni JM, Frick PA, Huang B: A longitudinal evaluation of a social support model of medication adherence among HIV-positive men and women on antiretroviral therapy. *Health Psychol*, 25(1):74-81, 2006.

Stoddart K, Burke L, Temple V: Outcome evaluation of bereavement groups for adults with intellectual disabilities. *J Appl Res Intellect Disabil*, 15:28-35, 2002.

Taylor EJ: Prevalence and associated factors of spiritual needs among patients with cancer and family caregivers. *Oncol Nurs Forum*, 33(4):729-735, 2006.

Vanderwerker LC, Flannelly KJ, Galek K, et al: What do chaplains really do? III. Referrals in the New York Chaplaincy study. *J Health Care Chaplain*, 14(1):57-73, 2008.

Wallace M, Campbell S, Grossman S, et al: Integrating spirituality into undergraduate nursing curricula. *Int J Nurs Educ Scholarsh*, 5(1):1-13, 2008.

World Health Organization Quality of Life: A cross-cultural study of spirituality, religion, and personal beliefs as components of quality of life. *Soc Sci Med*, 62:1486-1497, 2006.

Wright K: Professional, ethical and legal implications for spiritual care in nursing. *Image J Nurs Scholarsh*, 30(1):81-83, 1998.

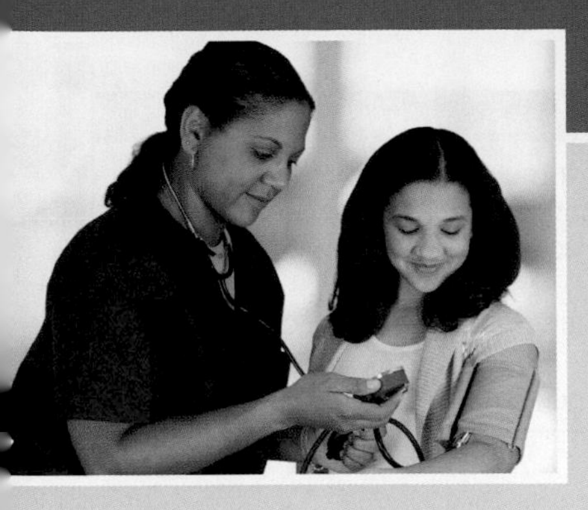

CHAPTER 23

Public Health, Community-Based, and Home Health Care

EVOLVE WEBSITE

http://evolve.elsevier.com/YoostCrawford/fundamentals/

- Additional Evolve-Only Review Questions With Answers
- Answers and Rationales for Text Review Questions
- Answers to Critical-Thinking Questions
- Case Study With Questions
- Glossary

LEARNING OUTCOMES

Comprehension of this chapter's content will provide students with the ability to:

LO 23.1 Describe various types of community health nursing.
LO 23.2 Identify examples of the three levels of prevention.
LO 23.3 Discuss factors affecting the health of a community.
LO 23.4 Articulate an awareness of various target populations, including vulnerable people within a community.
LO 23.5 Complete a community or home health assessment using data collection tools such as the OASIS data set.
LO 23.6 Identify nursing diagnoses for clients or populations of interest.
LO 23.7 Use measurable goals to develop community-based plans of care.
LO 23.8 Implement collaborative interventions to address the needs of the identified target population or client.

KEY TERMS

agents of disease, p. 432
ambulatory care, p. 429
analytic epidemiology, p. 433
case manager, p. 431
community-based nursing, p. 429
descriptive epidemiology, p. 433
early intervention, p. 432
environmental (extrinsic) factors, p. 433
epidemiology, p. 433
etiologic factors, p. 432
home health care nursing, p. 430
hospice care, p. 432
host (intrinsic) factors, p. 433
incidence, p. 428
palliative care, p. 432
prevalence, p. 433
primary prevention, p. 432
public health nursing, p. 428
secondary prevention, p. 432
social determinants of health, p. 428
stakeholders, p. 435
target population (population of interest), p. 428
tertiary prevention, p. 432
vulnerable populations, p. 433
windshield survey, p. 434

CASE STUDY

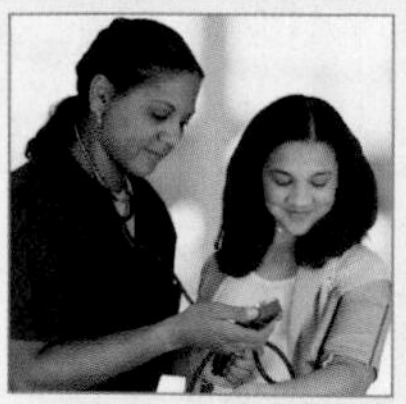

Jean is a certified school nurse working full time at the middle school in a multicultural community. On the weekends Jean provides home care for her elderly father-in-law, who is confined to a hospital bed and enjoys visits from family, including his 3-month-old great-grandchild. In a program implemented in response to a recent national increase in pertussis (whooping cough) cases, Jean is collaborating with the local public health department nurses to develop strategies to educate and vaccinate as many children and adults as possible in her community.

Refer back to this case study to answer the critical-thinking questions throughout the chapter.

This chapter focuses on the last phrase in the American Nurses Association (ANA) definition of *nursing:* "the care of individuals, families, communities, and populations" (ANA, 2014a). The concept of community health takes the nurse out of the acute or ambulatory care setting and places the practice of nursing within a population or in the client's home. Occupational, school, corrections, private-duty, parish, camp, forensic, home, hospice, palliative care, and public health nurses are a few of the many nursing specialists who practice within what is broadly considered the field of community health.

COMMUNITY HEALTH LO 23.1

Community health addresses issues of health, disease, and disability found within a defined group of people (or population) or in a specific person as a member of that community. Community-based nursing provides personal care to individual clients or families. Public health nursing focuses on populations. Population groups may be narrowed or expanded to a particular area or geographic region, such as a neighborhood, school system, city, state, nation, or continent.

PUBLIC HEALTH NURSING

Public health nursing examines the greater community as a whole—the city, county, state, nation, continent, world—and designs collaborative and interdisciplinary strategies to keep the population healthy by preventing or controlling disease and threats to human health (Figure 23-1). In referring to groups of clients within a community (young, elderly, homeless, inmates, or residents of particular cities or other geographic or government-defined areas), the term **target population** or **population of interest** is used. This designation connotes that the plan of care focuses on more than one person and includes groups of people residing within a defined geographic area. Examples of interventions performed by public health nurses are advocating with housing authorities to ensure accessible and safe housing; planning multilingual, culturally based immunization clinics to increase participation; and investigating the **incidence** (occurrence) of foodborne illness.

Scope and Standards of Public Health Nursing Practice

In 1999, the Quad Council of Public Health Organizations convened to develop standards to guide the evolution and development of nursing practice aimed at population-based care. The skills reflected in these standards are similar to those used in acute and ambulatory care settings. The focus of interventions, however, is working with populations rather than just one person or family. Using the nursing process, public health nurses are required to coordinate services, provide health education, promote healthy lifestyles, consult with government officials, and participate in regulatory activities (ANA, 2013). The ANA's *Public Health Nursing: Scope and Standards of Practice* (2013) requires participation in research, responsible resource utilization, ethical behavior, leadership, and advocacy similar to the standards of practice for all nurses.

Social Determinants of Health

Social determinants of health are "the conditions in which people are born, grow, live, work, and age, including the health system" (World Health Organization [WHO], 2012). A specific population's social determinants are affected by distribution of wealth, power, resources, and organizational and government policies. Income, education, health literacy, where people live or work, early childhood development, social exclusion, family structure, the status and role of women, and vaccination compliance are just some of the social determinants of health recognized worldwide. These factors must be assessed and analyzed by public health nurses to determine their potential impact on the health of the populations the nurses serve. Social determinants can cause a population to be healthy or vulnerable to disease and disability. When nurses practice population-based care, they look beyond the individual client to the broader society for interventions and strategies to improve the health of entire groups.

Public Health versus Community Health

In some circumstances, the terms *public health* and *community health* are used interchangeably. Recognition of certain distinctions, however, will enable a more robust and

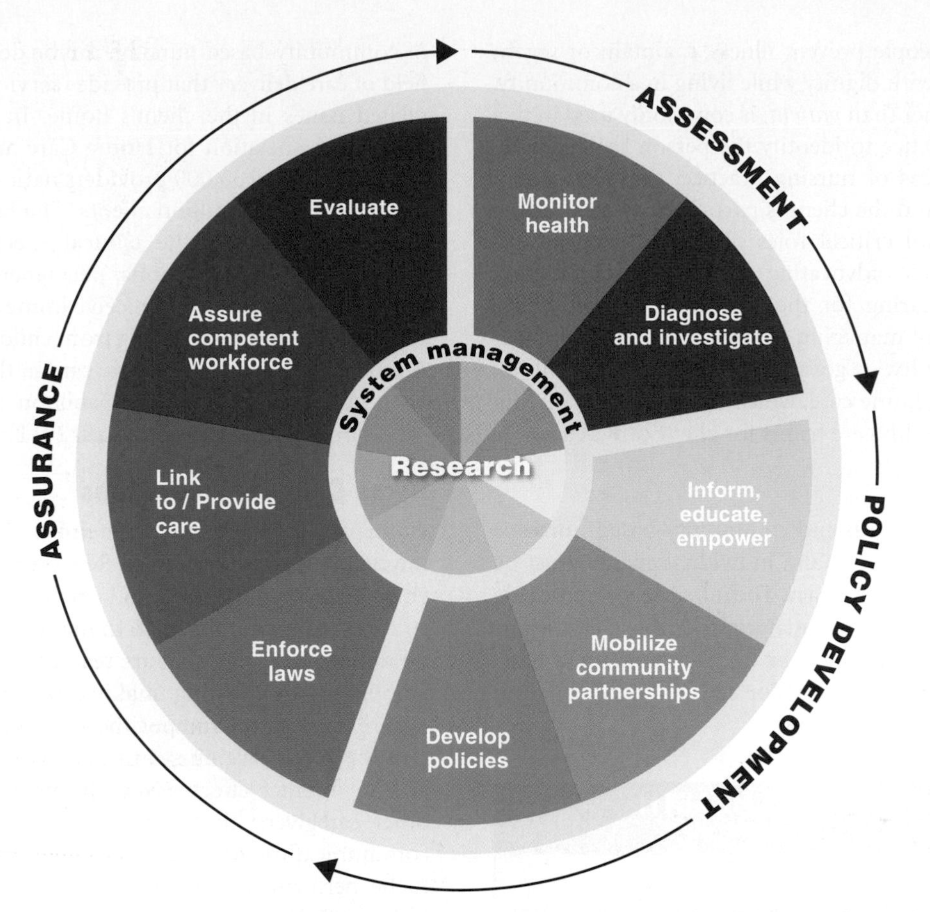

FIGURE 23-1 Essential public health services. (From Centers for Disease Control and Prevention: Essential public health services, 2010. Retrieved from *www.cdc.gov/nphpsp/essentialservices.html*.)

comprehensive understanding of the concepts: According to Stanhope and Lancaster (2012), public health nursing is focused solely on populations. It is not limited to a particular setting but, instead, focuses on disease prevention, health protection, and health promotion within identified populations. Nursing plays a unique role in public health; however, it is not the only health care profession engaged in the practice of improving the health of populations. Medicine, dentistry, dietetics, biostatistics, epidemiology, finance, and health policy makers are a few of the disciplines and collaborative colleagues with which or whom nurses work in assessing, planning, implementing, and evaluating systems of care for target community groups or populations of interest. The goals of their collaboration are to prevent disease and disability and to promote the highest level of wellness that target groups can enjoy.

According to Nies and McEwen (2010), community health encompasses more than public health by including organized community health initiatives of both private and government agencies and groups. Private efforts may include philanthropic health-focused foundations such as the Susan B. Komen Foundation, which is committed to working with providers and researchers to eradicate breast cancer.

What makes nurses ideal community health practitioners is the foundation and preparation for nursing practice, which is grounded in the sciences, liberal arts, and social sciences; the nursing process itself, including evidence-based interventions; and the critical component of evaluating outcomes. It is not uncommon to see nurses leading community planning meetings with other collaborative disciplines as initiatives are developed to improve the health outcomes of a target group, community, or nation. The Institute of Medicine's public health reports and *Healthy People 2020* are examples of science-based plans to (1) reduce targeted illnesses and disabilities, (2) address health care disparity at certain socioeconomic levels, and (3) identify much-needed services. The United Nations–sponsored WHO develops programs to address health concerns globally in response to data collection and analysis conducted worldwide.

COMMUNITY-BASED NURSING

The provision of skilled nursing care outside the traditional acute or **ambulatory care** setting (physician's office or outpatient clinic) is referred to as **community-based nursing**. Community-based nursing focuses on interventions necessary to help people prevent illness, maintain or regain their health, or die with dignity while living in a community. The term *client,* rather than *patient,* is commonly used in this area of nursing practice to identify the person seeking care. As is true in all areas of nursing practice, the relationship between the nurse and the client is participatory and collaborative. Effective and critical roles played by community-based nurses include advocating for clients, conducting routine checkups, caring for the sick or dying, providing client education, and managing chronic client conditions at outpatient, community, or government health care facilities, as well as providing home care, which includes coordinating multidisciplinary health care teams for client care delivery.

Health Literacy

A key role of public health and community-based nurses is education. Both populations and individual clients must be assessed for level of health literacy. The nurse needs to provide information and educational materials in the client's language at a reading level that can be understood (Client Education and Health Literacy box). For additional information on health literacy, see Chapter 14.

CLIENT EDUCATION AND HEALTH LITERACY

Development of Written Resources

When providing health care education, the nurse may develop or provide written materials to introduce or reinforce the presentation of information. For these materials to be effective in educating individual clients or populations about health-related matters, nurses must determine the readability levels of written resources before deciding which clients would best benefit from the information. This can be accomplished through use of specific tools:

- Traditional readability assessment tools, such as the Fry readability formula, which is based on the number of syllables and sentences in 100-word passages
- Online tools that evaluate grammar and word usage

Regardless of how nurses determine the level of readability of written resources, it is imperative that those resources use language familiar to the clients and address their key concerns; otherwise, the resources will not meet the needs of the clients (Osborne, 2013).

HOME HEALTH CARE NURSING

The purpose of **home health care nursing** is to promote, maintain, or restore health at an optimal level of functioning and to reduce the effects of disability and illness for individual clients and their families. Home health care, an alternative to a hospital or a nursing home, is a component of a comprehensive health services system that is provided on a continuum to individuals and families at their place of residence (Centers for Medicare and Medicaid Services, 2010a; Nies and McEwen, 2010). Home health care, an integral part of community-based nursing, can be described as a dynamic field of care delivery that provides services for diverse health-related issues in the client's home. In a recent report, the National Association for Home Care and Hospice (NAHC) (2010) identified 33,000 providers nationwide, with a total of approximately 12 million clients. The health-related services are provided across the clinical spectrum—acute illness, long-term health conditions, permanent disability, and terminal illness. Clients who receive home health care include a variety of age groups, ranging from children to elderly people. Annual expenditures for home care in the United States have been projected to reach $94.5 billion in 2015 (Centers for Medicare and Medicaid Services, 2011).

Home Care Considerations

Home care nurses should remember that they are guests in the client's place of residence. Respect for the client's personal environment, resources, and caregivers must be demonstrated throughout the visit. In many cases, home care nurses do not have supplies that are readily available in the acute or ambulatory care setting, making improvisation necessary to ensure client safety and positive outcomes. It is vitally important for home care nurses to establish trusting relationships and to interact effectively with clients, their families, and other caregivers; these efforts are key to promoting open communication and compliance with procedures that need to be performed routinely when the nurse is not present (Figure 23-2).

Reimbursement for Home Health Care Services

Home health care services are reimbursed by Medicare, Medicaid, and private health insurance. Medicare is a United States federal government–sponsored program. To be eligible as home health services, the care provided must be short-term and skilled. Skilled services are provided or performed by a licensed health care professional. Skilled services may include respiratory ventilation care, intravenous (IV) and

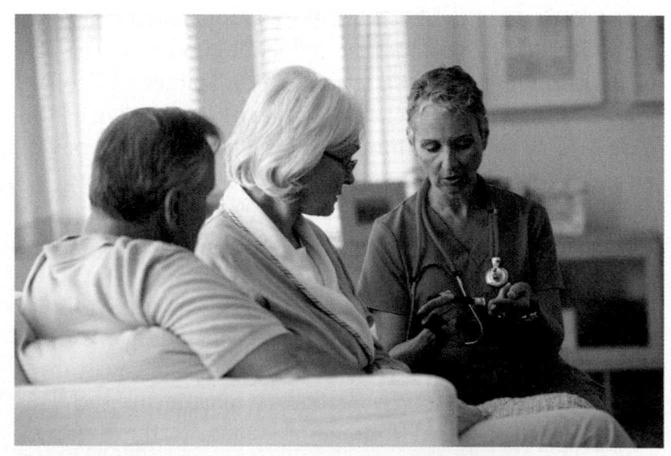

FIGURE 23-2 Home health nurses provide critical services to clients and their families.

peripherally inserted central catheter (PICC) line therapy, chemotherapy, ostomy/wound management, diabetes self-management training, and renal dialysis. Unskilled services include homemaker and personal care tasks, such as meal preparation, cleaning, laundry, bathing, and feeding assistance. Homemaker service is provided by a home care aide and is not reimbursable by Medicare. If, however, a client is receiving a professional skilled service, such as nursing or physical therapy, then the home care aide who provides the unskilled services is reimbursed. Private insurance may cover both skilled and unskilled services, depending on individual plans and the needs of the client (Centers for Medicare and Medicaid Services, 2010a, 2010b; Munchus, Roberts, Rivers, and Gingrich, 1999).

Vital Roles of the Home Care Nurse

The coordination of home health care services most often is provided by the registered nurse, but a multidisciplinary team may be involved, depending on the needs of the client. The team members may include physical therapists, occupational therapists, social workers, pharmacists, registered dietitians, advanced practice nurses, and physicians, as well as unlicensed assistive personnel such as home care aides.

Registered nurses who are employed by a home health care agency may have an associate's degree, a diploma, or a baccalaureate or master's degree. Nurses who have special certifications also may be employed by a home health care agency. The special certifications may be in, for example, diabetes care, wound/ostomy care, or infusion/IV line care. The ANA (2014b) has developed specific standards for home care and defined the unique scope of practice for this specialty (Table 23-1). The role of the registered nurse in home health care is essentially autonomous in that the nurse must be highly proficient in health assessment (physical and psychosocial), be well versed in complex technical and clinical skills, possess strong critical-thinking and clinical reasoning abilities, and demonstrate excellent organizational skills.

Case Management

The home health care nurse serves as a **case manager** (coordinator) of client care, needed services, and needed supplies in the home setting. The nurse must be well versed as a financial resource manager, who needs to be aware of what is or is not covered on the client's insurance plan. If consultation or referral is needed, the home care nurse should be cognizant of community agencies or resources within the client's community, such as the local pharmacy or "Meals on Wheels." The home health care nurse must have strong teaching skills to instruct clients and families about health practices and technical procedures related to their care. The nurse may counsel clients and families, serve as a client advocate, or refer or secure referrals to other disciplines, as needed.

TABLE 23-1 Standards of Care and Professional Performance in Home Care

STANDARDS OF CARE	STANDARDS OF PROFESSIONAL PERFORMANCE
I. **Assessment** Home health nurse collects client data.	I. **Quality of Care** Home care nurse systematically evaluates the quality and effectiveness of nursing practice.
II. **Diagnosis** Home health nurse analyzes the assessment data in determining the nursing diagnosis.	II. **Performance Appraisal** Home health care nurse evaluates his or her own nursing practice in relation to professional practice standards, scientific evidence, and relevant statutes and regulations.
III. **Outcome Identification** Home health nurse identifies expected outcomes customized to the client and the client's environment.	III. **Education** Home health care nurse acquires and maintains current knowledge and competency in nursing practice.
IV. **Planning** Home care nurse develops a plan of care that prescribes interventions to attain expected outcomes.	IV. **Collegiality** Home health nurse interacts with and contributes to the professional development of peers and other health care practitioners.
V. **Implementation** Home care nurse implements the interventions identified in the plan of care.	V. **Ethics** Home health nurse decisions and actions on behalf of clients are determined in an ethical manner.
VI. **Evaluation** Home care nurse evaluates the client's progress toward attainment of outcomes.	VI. **Collaboration** Home health nurse collaborates with the client, family, and other health care practitioners in providing client care.
	VII. **Research** Home health nurse uses research.
	VIII. **Resource Utilization** Home health nurse assists the client and family in becoming informed consumers about the risks, benefits, and costs in planning and delivering client care.

From American Nurses Association: Home health nursing scope and standards of practice, 2007. Retrieved from *www.nursingworld.org.*

Hospice and Palliative Care

Another type of home care nurse is a hospice or palliative care nurse. End-of-life care for the terminally ill is called **hospice care. Palliative care** is comfort care offered to patients at any stage of a serious illness. The goals of hospice nursing are to relieve suffering throughout the illness, to be of support to the client and family, and to work with the family, providing grief support after the death of the client. Hospice and palliative care nurses provide direct care for clients and families in the community setting in their homes, residential facilities, or long-term care facilities. Refer to Chapter 42 for further information on hospice and palliative care nursing.

LEVELS OF HEALTH CARE LO 23.2

Community health care services are designed with a focus on primary, secondary, and tertiary prevention. **Primary prevention** strategies include interventions designed to prevent disease or disability. Examples are employee wellness programs, fitness classes, and nutrition education to increase the consumption of fresh fruits and vegetables in homes, schools, and the community at large.

Secondary prevention focuses on early identification of an illness or phenomenon and limitation of its impact or recurrence through specific interventions, such as blood pressure screening, routine blood sugar testing, or asking patients about their exposure to domestic violence. Secondary interventions to address childhood obesity might be initiated by a school nurse to assess individual student body mass index (BMI), encourage less consumption of processed foods, and promote extended periods of physical activity. Designing **early intervention** programs (strategies introduced at the first detection of a possible health problem) that involve clients, families, and caregivers can change health outcomes for community members of all ages.

Tertiary prevention involves interventions for those already experiencing symptoms of disease or disability. Tertiary care focuses on maintenance or restoration of health, and rehabilitation. Tertiary interventions include patient support groups, pain management counseling, and cardiac rehabilitation programs,. For children already diagnosed with diabetes, the school nurse might be responsible for monitoring blood glucose levels or for administering required insulin injections. In addition to school nurses, public and community-based health nurses work tirelessly to identify, prevent, and treat health issues that compromise the well-being of community members. Figure 23-3 illustrates the three levels of prevention as they relate to cardiovascular disease.

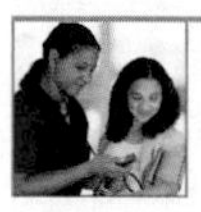

1. List six areas of concern for Jean as a certified school nurse working in the middle school of a multicultural community.

FACTORS AFFECTING COMMUNITY HEALTH LO 23.3

In addition to social determinants of health, many other factors can affect the health of a community, including **agents of disease** and **etiologic factors** (contributors to disease causation) such as excessive or deficient nutritional intake, chemical and airborne agents (such as carbon monoxide or ragweed), physical agents (such as radiation), and infectious

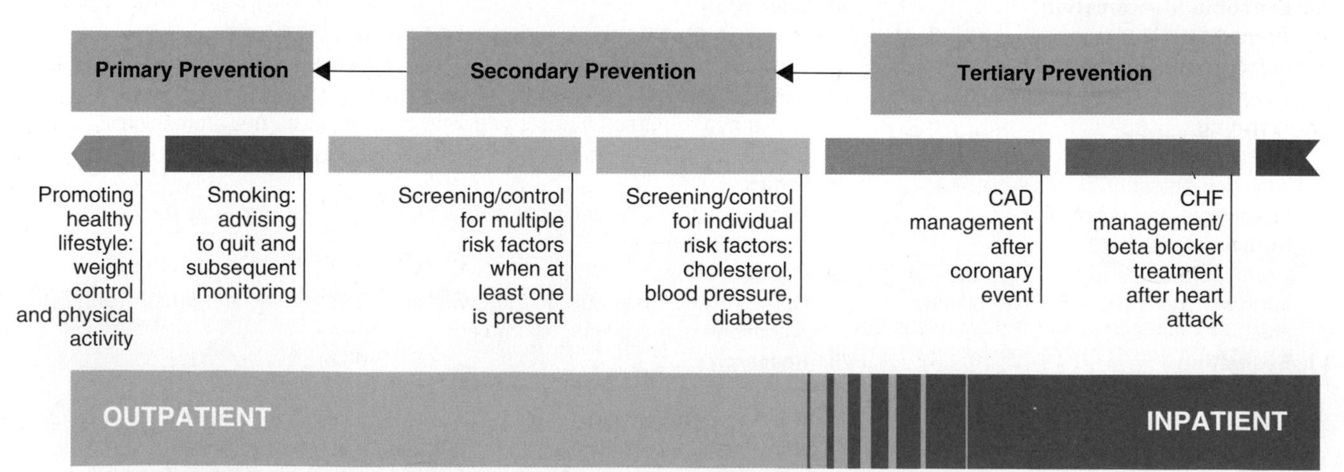

FIGURE 23-3 Cardiovascular care continuum. (*CAD,* Coronary artery disease; *CHF,* congestive heart failure.) Quality Profiles: Focus on cardiovascular disease. (Reproduced with permission from the National Committee for Quality Assurance (NCQA). Retrieved from *www.qualityprofiles.org/leadership_series/cardiovascular_disease/cardiovascular_disease/*.)

agents (such as bacteria and viruses). Clearly, such factors, if left unchecked, can spread through an entire community, with the potential for major impact. **Host**, or **intrinsic, factors** are individual variables such as genetics, age, gender, ethnic group, immunization status, and human behavior. **Environmental factors** or **extrinsic factors** relate to the immediate physical environment, the biologic environment (including food sources and vectors of disease such as animals and insects), and socioeconomic influences such as workplace conditions, or residence in an urban versus a rural setting, and the potential impact of social unrest or disaster on a community. It can be confusing and overwhelming to examine the reams of data and data elements encountered in exploring the health of a community. However, specific tools are available to assist nurses and public health practitioners to understand the factors affecting the health of the community.

Epidemiology is the study of disease incidence and **prevalence** (pervasiveness or extent). Health care professionals who specialize in epidemiology study factors that determine and influence the frequency and distribution of disease, injury, and other health-related events and their causes in a defined human population. The purpose of their work is to establish programs to prevent the development of disease and control its spread.

Descriptive epidemiology consists of studies that are conducted once a disease is evident. Data collected in descriptive epidemiology studies include the time and place of occurrence of the disease and the characteristics of people affected by the disease. In examining a cohort of community members, the nurse would describe the characteristics of those who have a certain disease and those who do not. This analysis would help to determine which variables are most associated with people who have the disease.

Analytic epidemiology generates a hypothesis of why the disease might be occurring in the community and then tests the hypothesis. Considerations in this dual process would include intrinsic factors related to ethnic groups and cultural dietary and health practices. Also included would be environmental, or extrinsic, factors, such as those observed by the nurse during an analysis of pollution levels and community resources, including parks and grocery stores.

TARGETED POPULATIONS IN COMMUNITY HEALTH LO 23.4

Well-recognized target groups within communities include children, adults, teens, elderly people, the homeless, the very wealthy or very poor, single and expectant parents, abused children or adults, and substance abusers. Additional target groups of concern include those in communal living environments in which communicable diseases can spread more easily and quickly, such as prisons, dorms, and extended-care facilities. **Vulnerable populations** (that is, defined groups of people at high risk for health problems) are of particular concern to community health nurses (Box 23-1). For each of these populations, variables to be identified include age, marital status, income, educational level, crime level, and use of illegal or regulated substances (tobacco, alcohol), to name a few. The community nurse can study and plan interventions that pertain to any target population of interest—which is one reason that community-based nursing practice is exciting and seemingly limitless in its potential to improve the health of a community, a nation, or even the world.

BOX 23-1 Vulnerable Populations

People who are at particular risk for compromised health as a result of lack of resources, beliefs, life experiences and circumstances, or dependency include the following:

- Refugees and immigrants
- People who have experienced a natural disaster, such as an earthquake, or a human-caused disaster such as a terrorist attack
- Military personnel and veterans
- Workers exposed to chemicals or radiation
- Homeless people or families
- Minority groups within a larger population, including members of various cultural, racial, religious, age, and gender groups who may be denied equal services based on their differences from the general population
- Mentally ill and disabled people
- Substance abusers or people with severe chronic illnesses
- People who have been emotionally, physically, or sexually abused or neglected
- Age-specific populations such as the very young, adolescents, or elderly people
- International (foreign) travelers

By examining vital statistics records available on the Internet for global, national, state, county, or community regions, nurses can identify the leading causes of disease and death in those areas in regard to noncommunicable diseases, such as heart disease, cancer, hypertension, and diabetes. Reference websites also help community nurses identify the incidence and prevalence of communicable diseases, such as tuberculosis (TB), sexually transmitted infections (STIs), and HIV/AIDS, and the life expectancy of target populations. Useful demographic assessment tools and community health planning resources include the following:

- WHO data and statistics (available at *www.who.int/research/en/*)
- United States Census data *(www.census.gov)*
- State department of health data websites
- Centers for Disease Control and Prevention *(www.cdc.gov)*
- Healthy People 2020 *(www.healthypeople.gov)*
- Occupational Safety and Health Administration *(www.osha.gov)*

Collaboration with public health officials facilitates coordination of care and promotes use of evidence-based interventions to address identified concerns within target populations.

ASSESSMENT LO 23.5

Many assessment tools are available to help the community nurse assess both communities and home clients. As can be seen in the Health Assessment Questions box, some community assessment questions are broad and open-ended to help discern general information, whereas others seek to assess specific concerns within a community, such as nutritional resources or the availability of walking and biking trails. Assessment begins with broad-based collection of data on both communities and individual clients.

HEALTH ASSESSMENT QUESTIONS

Community Focus

- What is the history of the community? Where has the client worked previously, and where does that person work now?
- What sources of information are available to help with identifying key data?
- What are the environmental and sanitation services that protect the water supply, inspect restaurants, and license day care facilities?
- What health promotion and educational services exist, and where are they located? Are there school nurses in each building? Are there public health clinics and health fairs?
- What preventive services are available, where, and to what populations? Are target populations able to gain access to these services where they are located?
- What matters to individual members of the community?
- Who are the stakeholders in the community, and what are their main concerns?

COMMUNITY ASSESSMENT

Various community health assessment instruments have been tested for their usefulness, reliability, and validity. The community or public health nurse may drive or walk through a community and perform a **windshield survey**, observing factors such as the following:

- Whether people are walking or are engaged in physical activity
- Availability of single- or multiple-family private and public housing units
- Availability of health, safety, and social services agencies, located along a bus route or other public transportation line
- Presence of spiritual or religious places of worship, educational institutions, and news and media services, as well as types of open and closed businesses and industries
- Availability of grocery stores
- General appearance and condition of neighborhoods

This process begins the initial needs assessment by collecting data through observation of the community's geography, population, environment, industry, education, recreation, communication, transportation, and public services.

QSEN FOCUS!

Collecting data on the social, cultural, and ethnic traditions that affect community, family, and client values is essential to providing patient-centered care in the community or home setting.

After data are collected on the community, the nursing process is used to (1) diagnose the greatest problems or needs; (2) establish goals; (3) plan interventions on the primary, secondary, and tertiary levels; and (4) evaluate the effectiveness of the interventions in meeting community health care goals. In community and public health nursing, it is especially critical to collaborate with many types of professionals and agencies to attain positive outcomes that can dramatically improve community health (Collaboration and Delegation box).

COLLABORATION AND DELEGATION

Potential Community Intervention Resources

Nurses collaborate with a wide variety of professionals and agencies within the community on planning, implementing, and evaluating community interventions. Such collaborations may involve working with the following:

- Nurse educators
- Exercise physiologists
- Administrators of child and adult day care centers
- Primary health care providers
- Visiting nurse association representatives and leaders
- Public officials, including governors, mayors, and council members
- City parks and recreation department officials
- Community hospital administrators and staff
- Public health department officials
- Media outlets (television, radio, newspaper, and online resources, including social media sites)

HOME CARE ASSESSMENT

In home health care, a comprehensive client assessment tool that encompasses both quality assessment and performance improvement must be completed by nurses working for Medicare-certified home health agencies (Centers for Medicare and Medicaid Services, 2010b). It is known as the Outcome and Assessment Information Set (OASIS). OASIS is a data set of outcome measures for adult home health care clients that is used to track outcome-based quality improvement. Assessment data documented in the OASIS form are summarized in the Home Care Considerations box. For adult clients who receive skilled care, OASIS is used to track the plan of care, note client characteristics, and evaluate and improve the clinical performance of each home health care agency. The OASIS document, which is approximately 24 pages long, is completed by the responsible home health care nurse at the start of care, every 2 months until care is completed, and at discharge. The complete OASIS data assessment document is available at *www.cms.gov*.

HOME CARE CONSIDERATIONS

OASIS Data Set

Nurses use the OASIS data set to assess home care clients in each of the following areas:

- Current and past medical and surgical history
- Influenza and pneumococcal vaccination status
- Living arrangements and activities-of-daily-living capability
- Sensory status and neurologic, emotional, and behavioral status
- Integumentary status
- Respiratory and cardiac status
- Elimination status
- Medication regimen and client and caregiver understanding of required medications and schedule
- Therapy needs and schedule
- Hospitalizations, including admission and discharge plans from inpatient facilities or agencies
- Plan of care management

From Centers for Medicare and Medicaid Services: Home health patient tracking sheet, 2009. Retrieved from *www.cms.gov/Medicare/Quality-Initiatives-Patient-Assessment-Instruments/HomeHealthQualityInits/Downloads/HHQIOASISVerson12-2.pdf*.

During a home care assessment, the nurse focuses on the client's direct health care needs as well as a vast number of environmental factors with potential impact on client safety. These factors include conditions affecting mobility, such as the presence of steps, carpeting or throw rugs, safety railings, and pull bars in the tub or shower. Of concern may be the height of a toilet and the client's ability to ambulate and transfer to the toilet. The nurse notes the client's ability to obtain access to and prepare food or light meals. The client's level of hygiene and ability to groom, dress independently, and bathe are assessed. Living conditions are evaluated for safety and infection control purposes: Is the home relatively clean, with functioning smoke alarms? Is the client able to use the telephone in case of an emergency? As is evident, the role of the home care nurse in assessment is even broader than that of the acute care nurse.

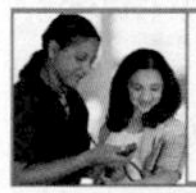

2. Identify a minimum of four areas that Jean should assess while caring for her elderly father-in-law.

NURSING DIAGNOSIS LO 23.6

Identifying nursing diagnoses based on community assessment data is similar to the process used for an individual. A variety of needs may emerge as a result of a thorough community assessment, making it necessary for the nurse to prioritize diagnoses before initiating goals and interventions in collaboration with community partners.

Some nursing diagnoses that may be used to identify community and home care problems are as follows:

- *Deficient Community Health* related to increased risk of pertussis as evidenced by inadequate immunization of children and adults in the community
- *Risk for Injury* with the risk factor of potential chemical exposure
- *Ineffective Community Coping* related to extensive hurricane damage as evidenced by residents expressing powerlessness and lack of financial resources to restore services
- *Caregiver Role Strain* related to 24-hour caregiving responsibilities as evidenced by disturbed sleep and inadequate time to meet personal needs
- *Social Isolation* related to unacceptable social behavior as evidenced by verbalization of hostility when interacting with others and stated preference to be alone
- *Nutrition Imbalance: Less Than Body Requirements* related to inability to obtain access and prepare food as evidenced by 20-lb weight loss in 1 month and inability to drive

PLANNING LO 23.7

Once the greatest concerns of the community or home health client are determined, the nurse can establish goals and desired outcomes to address the needs (Table 23-2). Determining goals for community health must include key **stakeholders** (individuals or groups with an investment or significant interest in a topic). For instance, if the employee health nurse in a large manufacturing plant identifies a risk for injury from inconsistent use of safety goggles by drill press operators, the owners of the company and the workers themselves would be stakeholders. In this case the nurse would want to collaborate with representatives from both groups to establish a safety-related goal acceptable to all parties. This approach would help ensure compliance with agreed-on procedures, thus increasing the likelihood that the best possible outcome, consistent use of safety goggles, would be achieved.

IMPLEMENTATION AND EVALUATION LO 23.8

As is evident, designing interventions and evaluation methods for community-based problems involves a collaborative effort and the assumption of multiple roles by the nurse (Evidence-Based Practice box). An important point in this context is that community-based health nurses coordinate care both as case managers and as home health care nurses. They must be familiar with budget planning and the financial resources available to fund community programs and home care needs. A key intervention by the home health nurse is discharge planning in collaboration with the acute care nurse, a social worker, client caregivers, family and friends, and community resources.

TABLE 23-2 Care Planning

NANDA-I NURSING DIAGNOSIS LABEL WITH NURSING DIAGNOSIS STATEMENT	NURSING OUTCOME CLASSIFICATION (NOC)	NURSING INTERVENTION CLASSIFICATION (NIC)
Deficient Community Health related to increased risk of pertussis as evidenced by inadequate immunization of children and adults in the community	*Community immune status* (2800) Incidence of vaccine-preventable disease at or below recommended national rate (280002)	*Communicable disease management* (8820) Provide vaccine to targeted populations, as available.

From Bulechek G, Butcher H, Dochterman J, et al (eds): *Nursing interventions classification (NIC)*, ed. 6, St. Louis, 2013, Mosby; Moorhead S, Johnson M, Maas M, et al (eds): *Nursing outcomes classification (NOC)*, ed. 5, St. Louis, 2013, Mosby; NANDA International: *Nursing diagnoses: Definitions and classification, 2012–2014*, West Sussex, England, 2012, Wiley-Blackwell. Reprinted with permission from NANDA International, Inc.

EVIDENCE-BASED PRACTICE

The Impact of Collaboration Among Nurses and Unlicensed Community Health Workers

A multicountry study of the effectiveness of expanding the role of nurses and unlicensed community health workers (CHWs) to address treatment for HIV/AIDS in underserved areas identified the following key factors in providing adequate health care:

- Government and political commitment
- Collaborative planning
- Defined scope of practice
- Licensure and certification
- Recruitment and deployment capability
- Mentoring, referral, and supervision
- Adequate equipment and supplies
- Sustainable remuneration
- Evaluation

The study found that employing nurses and well-trained and supervised CHWs improved the quality of HIV health care services and produced better health outcomes and higher levels of client satisfaction. As suggested by the study investigators, the evidence also indicates that use of nurses and CHWs can improve the quality of health care in non-HIV services as well (Celletti et al, 2010).

QSEN FOCUS!

Informatics is critical for communicating with a variety of health care professionals to coordinate client care in the community setting. It is essential that nurses use technology effectively while maintaining patient confidentiality.

One of the most important aspects of a community-based nurse's role is to be familiar with referral agencies. Awareness of the scope of an agency's influence and services helps the community-based nurse to pinpoint which agencies are stakeholders and most capable of addressing specific needs. It is essential that the nurse build relationships with and among agency representatives. Meaningful collaborative relationships facilitate better client care and community cooperation in addressing and evaluating client and program outcomes.

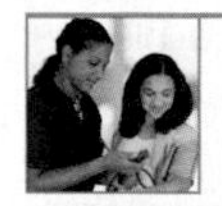

3. Name three public health issues that should be considered before implementation of strategies to reduce pertussis incidence in Jean's community.

EVALUATION

Just as interventions must be collaborative within the community setting, so must evaluation of programs and services. The nurse can lead the evaluation process by designing strategies and tools that will determine whether outcome criteria are met. Data and statistical analysis to support outcome findings is especially significant in working with business owners and government agencies that invest financially in primary-, secondary-, and tertiary-level programs.

QSEN FOCUS!

Seeking care outcome information demonstrates a commitment to quality improvement for populations served within a greater community.

Although the role of the community health nurse is varied and nontraditional in many ways, it is critical to the well-being of people of all ages. Its focus on safety, disease prevalence, health promotion, disability prevention, and collaborative care illustrates the tremendous impact the nurse can have within the life of a community. Making a difference in the lives of millions of people in the world or thousands of people within a community or in the life of one homebound person is what a community health nurse does every day.

SUMMARY OF LEARNING OUTCOMES

LO 23.1 *Describe various types of community health nursing:* Three major types of community health nursing are public health, community-based, and home health care. Public health nursing focuses on addressing the needs of populations in collaboration with interdisciplinary teams. Community-based nursing provides care for individuals within specific areas such as schools, prisons, or businesses. Home health nurses assess and treat homebound clients requiring direct care.

LO 23.2 *Identify examples of the three levels of prevention:* Primary prevention includes activities designed to prevent disease and disability. Secondary prevention focuses on screening and limiting the impact or recurrence of an illness or phenomenon with early interventions. Tertiary prevention is directed at treatment of individuals already diagnosed with a disease or disability.

LO 23.3 *Discuss factors affecting the health of a community:* Factors include disease agents, such as bacteria or viruses, as well as other etiologic factors such as excessive or deficit nutritional intake, chemical agents, physical agents, and socioeconomic factors (e.g., where one works, whether one lives in an urban or rural setting, and the impact that social unrest or disaster can have on the health of a community).

LO 23.4 *Articulate an awareness of various target populations, including vulnerable people within a community:* Target populations include groups of people who have or are at risk for injury, disease, or disability, including those most vulnerable, such as the homeless, infants, elderly people, substance abusers, the mentally ill, and refugees and immigrants.

LO 23.5 *Complete a community or home health assessment using data collection tools such as the OASIS data set:* Demographic and data collection tools for community assessment are available for use and analysis at the international, national, state, and community levels. The OASIS assessment instrument is designed to collect comprehensive data on home health care clients.

LO 23.6 *Identify nursing diagnoses for clients or populations of interest:* Examples of nursing diagnoses used to address the needs of clients in the different types of community nursing are *Risk for Injury, Ineffective Community Coping, Caregiver Role Strain, Social Isolation*, and *Nutrition Imbalance: Less Than Body Requirements.*

LO 23.7 *Use measurable goals to develop community-based plans of care:* Developing measurable goals in community-based nursing may involve collaboration with a variety of health care providers as well as stakeholders who have a significant interest in the outcomes of the goals.

LO 23.8 *Implement collaborative interventions to address the needs of the identified target population or client:* Interventions in community health settings often require referrals and advocacy to help populations and clients successfully reach established goals. It is vital that nurses establish and maintain strong relationships with community agency personnel to enhance cooperation.

Responses to the critical-thinking questions are available at *http://evolve.elsevier.com/YoostCrawford/fundamentals/.*

REVIEW QUESTIONS

1. Which factor(s) should be considered by the public health nurse before scheduling community infant immunization clinics? *(Select all that apply.)*
   a. Individual infant allergies
   b. Transportation availability
   c. Cost of immunization services
   d. Local attitudes toward immunization
   e. Personal feelings about immunization effectiveness
2. Which intervention should the college health clinic nurse implement as a secondary prevention strategy to identify students at risk for diabetes?
   a. Nutrition education about high-protein food availability
   b. Promotion of registration in fitness classes
   c. Blood glucose screening at the health fair
   d. Administration of prescribed insulin
3. What action would be most appropriate for the home care nurse to take if an intrinsic factor appears to be contributing to a client's illness?
   a. Report the presence of multiple insects in the home to the health department.
   b. Document the intrinsic factor in the client's electronic health record.
   c. Explore the possible impact of changing jobs for stress reduction.
   d. Discuss the danger of having multiple throw rugs with the client.

4. When developing treatment plans, which assumption should the nurse make about individual clients in vulnerable populations?
   a. Educational levels are minimal.
   b. Economic resources are strong.
   c. Personal beliefs are important.
   d. Support systems are extensive.
5. When the nurse is establishing goals for a community health initiative, which strategy is most important to incorporate in the planning process?
   a. Collaboration with key stakeholders
   b. Help from professional interpreters
   c. Location of schools and businesses
   d. Gender of primary care providers
6. What is the best method for the public health nurse to determine if community members are involved in outdoor physical activity?
   a. Meet with the parents of high school children.
   b. Complete a windshield survey of the community.
   c. Evaluate the number of community health club members.
   d. Check the local health statistics for the incidence of obesity.
7. Which intrinsic factor(s) would be of major concern to the nurse about when the community has an outbreak of pertussis? *(Select all that apply.)*
   a. Age
   b. Gender
   c. Ethnic group
   d. Cultural background
   e. Immunization status
8. Whom should the school nurse engage in discussion when conducting a needs assessment related to the high incidence of obesity in the school system? *(Select all that apply.)*
   a. Parents
   b. Students
   c. School staff
   d. Community members
   e. Firefighters and police
9. The outpatient clinic nurse develops a plan of care focusing on diet, exercise, and glucose monitoring for a preteen recently diagnosed with early-onset type 2 diabetes. On what type of interventions has the nurse based the client's care plan?
   a. Primary
   b. Progressive
   c. Secondary
   d. Tertiary
10. A client with metastatic cancer shares with the clinic nurse that he has only days or weeks to live. What type of community service would be most appropriate for the nurse to suggest to this client?
   a. Home health care
   b. Hospice care
   c. Forensic care
   d. Acute care

Answers and rationales for the review questions are available at *http://evolve.elsevier.com/YoostCrawford/fundamentals/.*

REFERENCES

American Nurses Association: *Public health nursing: Scope and standards of practice*, ed. 2, Silver Spring, Md., 2013, Author.

American Nurses Association: What is nursing? 2014a. Retrieved from *www.nursingworld.org/especiallyforyou/what-is-nursing.*

American Nurses Association: *Home health nursing: Scope and standards of practice*, ed. 2, Silver Spring, Md., 2014b, Author.

Celletti F, Wright A, Palen J, et al: Can the deployment of community health workers for the delivery of HIV services represent an effective and sustainable response to health workforce shortages? Results of a multicountry study. *AIDS*, 24(1):545-557, 2010.

Centers for Medicare and Medicaid Services: Home health overview, 2010a. Retrieved from *www.cms.hhs.gov/HomeHealthPPS/.*

Centers for Medicare and Medicaid Services: OASIS background, 2010b. Retrieved from *www.cms.hhs.gov/OASIS/02_Background.asp.*

Centers for Medicare and Medicaid Services: National Health expenditure projections 2011–2021, 2011. Retrieved from *www.cms.gov/Research-Statistics-Data-and-Systems/Statistics-Trends-and-Reports/NationalHealthExpendData/Downloads/Proj2011PDF.pdf.*

Cronenwett L, Sherwood G, Barnsteiner J, et al: Quality and safety education for nurses. *Nurs Outlook*, 55(3):122-131, 2007.

Munchus G, Roberts V, Rivers P, Gingrich, B: The U.S. home health care industry: Past, present, and future. *Home Health Care Manage Pract*, 11(4):21-30, 1999.

National Association for Home Care and Hospice: Consumer information: What are my rights as a patient? 2010. Available at *www.nahch.org/consumer/rights.htm.*

Nies M, McEwen M: *Community/public health nursing: Promoting the health of populations*, ed. 5, St. Louis, 2010, Saunders.

Osborne H: *Health literacy from A to Z*, Burlington, Mass., 2013, Jones & Bartlett.

Stanhope M, Lancaster J: *Public health nursing: Population-centered health care in the community*, St. Louis, 2012, Mosby.

World Health Organization: Social determinants of health, 2012. Retrieved from *www.who.int/topics/social_determinants/en/.*

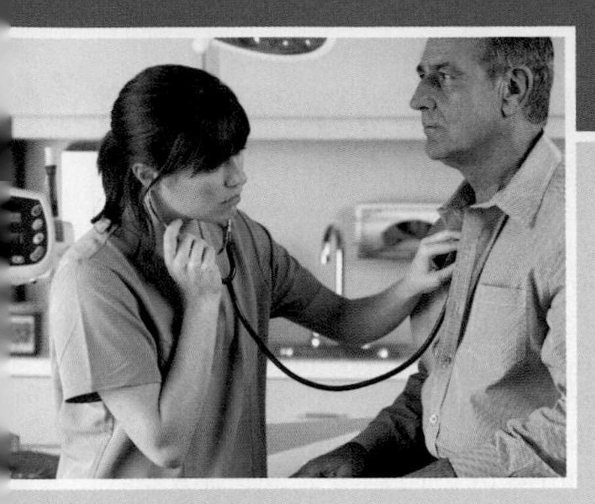

CHAPTER 24

Human Sexuality

EVOLVE WEBSITE

http://evolve.elsevier.com/YoostCrawford/fundamentals/

- Additional Evolve-Only Review Questions With Answers
- Answers and Rationales for Text Review Questions
- Answers to Critical-Thinking Questions
- Case Study With Questions
- Glossary

LEARNING OUTCOMES

Comprehension of this chapter's content will provide students with the ability to:

LO 24.1 Explain sexual development throughout the life cycle.
LO 24.2 Describe the structure and function of the male and female reproductive systems.
LO 24.3 Differentiate among sex, sexuality, and gender identity.
LO 24.4 Describe the sexual response cycles of men and women.
LO 24.5 Identify contraception options.
LO 24.6 Discuss sexually transmitted diseases and their causes and treatments.
LO 24.7 Summarize factors that affect sexuality.
LO 24.8 List factors that affect sexual function.
LO 24.9 Recognize the impact of family dynamics on sexuality.
LO 24.10 Implement a sexual assessment.
LO 24.11 List nursing diagnoses appropriate for the care of patients with potential or identified sexuality concerns.
LO 24.12 Develop a patient-centered care plan designed to address sexuality needs.
LO 24.13 Implement interventions to support enhanced patient sexuality before evaluating their effectiveness.

KEY TERMS

abstinence, p. 446
anorgasmia, p. 445
bisexual, p. 444
circumcision, p. 445
condom, p. 447
contraception, p. 446
detumescence, p. 446
diaphragm, p. 447
dyspareunia, p. 445
erectile dysfunction (ED), p. 446
gay, p. 444
gender identity, p. 444
gender role, p. 444
heterosexual, p. 444
homosexual, p. 444
infertility, p. 440
intrauterine device (IUD), p. 447
lactation, p. 444
lesbian, p. 444
menopause, p. 440
menstruation, p. 443
perimenopause, p. 440
questioning, p. 444
sex, p. 444
sexual orientation, p. 444
sexuality, p. 444
sexually transmitted disease (STD), p. 447
sexually transmitted infection (STI), p. 447
transgendered, p. 444
transsexual, p. 444
transvestite, p. 444
tubal ligation, p. 447
vaginismus, p. 445
vasectomy, p. 447

CASE STUDY

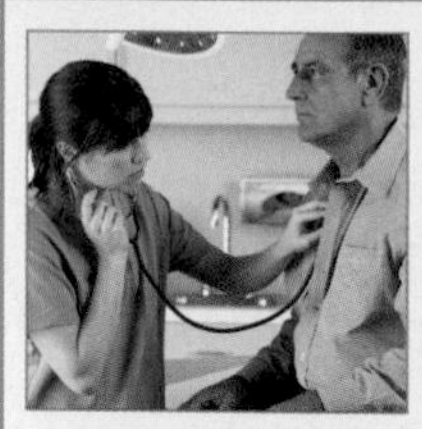

Mr. Wells, a 56-year-old patient with a history of hypertension and mild congestive heart failure (CHF), arrives at the outpatient clinic. While taking his health history and completing his assessment, the nurse notes that Mr. Wells is taking aspirin 325 mg PO daily, a diuretic (furosemide, 20 mg) daily, and an antihypertensive/angiotensin-converting enzyme (ACE) inhibitor (lisinopril 10 mg) bid. He has been married for 30 years, has two grown children, is employed as a teacher, and has no current health restrictions. His current BP is 148/86, and his pulse is 78, regular, and strong. His respirations are 16 and unlabored. In the course of conversation during the assessment, Mr. Wells mentions that he loves his wife and does not understand why he is unable to achieve an erection. The nurse asks him when he first noticed his concern, and offers that his erectile dysfunction (ED) may be caused by the medications he is taking for his elevated blood pressure. He is encouraged to share his concern with the primary care provider (PCP). After examination of the patient, the PCP orders a complete blood count (CBC), prostate-specific antigen (PSA), and urinalysis. Mr. Wells is given a pamphlet on ED and sent home with an appointment to return to the clinic in 1 week for follow-up evaluation.

Refer back to this case study to answer the critical-thinking questions throughout the chapter.

Sexuality is a component of the human experience for all people across the life span and is influenced by many factors. How a person identifies with his or her sexuality influences expression of personality and general well-being. Although sexuality has an impact on every person, both nurses and patients often find the topic uncomfortable to discuss. Gaining information about sexuality and sexual health will help the nurse manage any personal reservations and then be able to advocate for the patient dealing with sexuality issues.

Sexuality encompasses many critical topics, including:

- Sexual health and development across the life span
- Gender identity
- Sexual response
- Contraceptive options
- Sexually transmitted diseases (STDs) or infections (STIs)
- Factors that affect sexuality and sexual function

Sexuality affects family dynamics, including decision making and roles. Depending on the circumstances, the nurse may need to complete a thorough sexual health assessment with special attention to the identification of STDs and instances of sexual abuse or assault. Gathering accurate information aids in the development of a personalized plan of care that includes nursing diagnoses related to sexual concerns as well as appropriate goals and interventions to address those issues. A multidisciplinary approach to treatment may include referral for an in-depth physical examination or sexual counseling. Sexuality influences every aspect of a person's life.

SEXUAL DEVELOPMENT LO 24.1

Sexual development follows the steps of psychological and physical growth and development (Table 24-1). Freud noted that during infancy and early childhood, the first 3 years of life are crucial in gender identification development. This is the period during which trust is developed, setting the groundwork for all future relationships. Self-exploration of the body, including the genitals, is considered to represent normal development at this stage.

During the school-age years, children tend to have same-sex friends and to adopt the behaviors of their biologic gender. At this time, they need accurate and appropriate information concerning their many questions pertaining to the physical and emotional aspects of sex. The Evidence-Based Practice box addresses parents' attitudes concerning the need for sex education for school-age youths.

At puberty, adolescents need factual information regarding sexuality and sexual activity as well as guidance to establish a personal value system to serve as a framework for decision making. Areas of concern for education and parental guidance include contraception, unwanted pregnancy, STDs and human immunodeficiency virus (HIV) infection, sexual abuse, and sexual orientation.

When adolescents reach young adulthood, the focus is on intimacy and sexuality. Areas of concern from adolescence continue as well as the issues of conception and **infertility**, which occurs when a couple has not conceived after 12 months of contraceptive-free intercourse if the female is younger than 34 years or after 6 months of contraceptive-free intercourse if the female is older than 35 years of age.

Middle-adulthood sexual development focuses on social and emotional changes as children leave home to begin their lives, no longer dependent on the parents. The "empty nest" scenario can result in stress because of the perception of no longer being needed, as well as the adjustment of the relationship with a spouse or significant other now that the children are gone. Physical changes and changing appearance due to aging may alter sexuality and sexual function. Areas of concern include **perimenopause** (phase prior to the onset of menopause and the first year after menopause) and **menopause** (permanent cessation of menstrual activity), as well as sexual dysfunction that may result from illness or medication side effects or from injury or aging.

Although the common myth is that elderly people do not engage in or enjoy sexual intimacy, Masters and Johnson (1966) noted that older adults continue to enjoy sexual

TABLE 24-1 Sexual Health Characteristics Across the Life Span

AGE	CHARACTERISTICS	NURSING IMPLICATIONS
Infancy Birth to 12 months	• Gender assignment • Beginning of gender identification • Body exploration	• Sexual self-manipulation is normal. • Teach parents that this is expected behavior for this stage.
Toddler 1 to 3 years	• Continued development of gender identification • Ability to identify own gender	• Toddler needs interaction with both male and female adults. • Self-exploration and manipulation are still normal.
Preschool 3 to 5 years	• Increased self-awareness • Start of asking questions associated with sex • Ability to identify body parts and name them • Exploration of own body parts and those of playmates not uncommon	• Provide simple and direct answers to sex questions. • Do not respond negatively to child's self-exploration. • Identify body parts with appropriate names. • Teach parents the above guidelines.
School Age 6 to 12 years	• Participation in same-sex friendships • Questions about physical and emotional aspects of sex • Development of primary and secondary sexual characteristics possible • Increased modesty • Strong identification with parent of same sex	• Answer sex-related questions honestly. • Provide written information to assist with understanding. • Discuss topics of sex, menses, and reproduction by the time the child is 10 years old. • Respect modesty. • Teach parents the above guidelines.
Adolescence 13 to 18 years	• Value system establishment • Development of primary and secondary sexual characteristics • Opposite-sex relationship development • Risk for pregnancy, STDs, sexual abuse • Exploration of masturbation or homosexual relationships possible	• Recognize the importance of peer group influences. • The adolescent's relationship with the opposite sex sets the stage for future relationships. • Teach pregnancy and STD information.
Young Adult 18 to 40 years	• Active sex life possible • Establishment of values and lifestyle • Sharing of household and finances • Family planning and infertility • Homosexual identity established	• Provide information on pregnancy prevention and STDs. • Partners need open communication to work through issues of being a couple.
Middle Adult 40 to 65 years	• Reduced male and female hormone influences • Perimenopause/menopause • Quality versus quantity of sexual activity now important	• Role adjustment occurs in response to family stressors and physiologic changes.
Older Adult 65 years and older	• Continued interest in sex • Reduced sexual intercourse frequency • *Female:* reduced vaginal secretions and breast atrophy • *Male:* reduced sperm production and need for more time to achieve erection and ejaculation	• Recognize older adults' continued interest in sex. • Teach adaptation techniques to deal with any physical limitations that may interfere with sexual satisfaction.

EVIDENCE-BASED PRACTICE

Support for Comprehensive Sexuality Education

In a study that surveyed 1605 parents of middle school students (with a 63% participation rate) about attitudes toward sexuality education and the grade level at which it should be taught, the results showed that:

- 89.3% of the parents supported education that included both abstinence and more comprehensive sexuality education.
- Parents believed that most topics should first be taught during the middle school years.
  - 34% of adolescents report having intercourse by the ninth grade.
- There was support among all demographic categories of parents of all races, religions, educational levels, incomes, and political parties for multiple sex education strategies for the prevention of pregnancy and sexually transmitted infections, including abstinence and information about condoms and contraceptives.
- There is a significant gap between actual sex education content as currently taught in most schools and parents' opinions or preferences (Eisenberg, Bernat, Bearinger, and Resnick, 2008).

Application to Nursing Practice

- A majority of parents of school-age youths support sex education during the middle school years.
- Sex education should encompass pregnancy and STD prevention, including abstinence and contraception and condom information.
- Parents should be encouraged to speak out for sex education in their school system.
- Nurses should use this evidence to actively advocate for evidence-based sex education in schools.

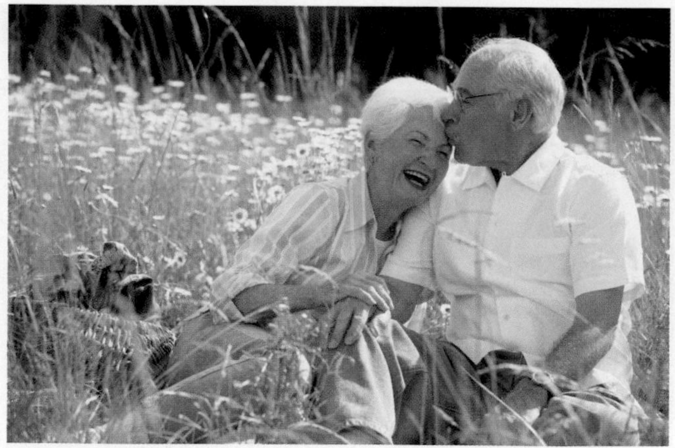

FIGURE 24-1 It is a common myth that elderly people do not engage in or enjoy sexual intimacy.

relationships throughout each decade of their lives. In older adulthood, sexual activity continues if it is not impaired by social, cultural, or physiologic factors (Nusbaum, Lenahan, and Sadovsky, 2005). The male reproductive system gradually changes as age advances. There is a reduction in testosterone levels, sperm production decreases as the testes' size and firmness decrease, and the prostate enlarges. The frequency of intercourse usually decreases, along with the perception of sensation; however, erection attainment speed, ejaculation force, and sexual interest, thoughts, and activity continue through old age (Figure 24-1).

NORMAL STRUCTURE AND FUNCTION OF THE MALE AND FEMALE REPRODUCTIVE SYSTEMS LO 24.2

To gain insight into sexuality and assist patients in achieving sexual health, the nurse is required to have knowledge of sexual development, the normal structure and function of the male and female reproductive systems, male and female sexual response, and gender identity. The reproductive organs are key components of sexual response.

MALE REPRODUCTIVE SYSTEM

The male reproductive system has external and internal organs (Figure 24-2). The external organs are the scrotum and the penis. The scrotum is a loose sac that contains the testes, or male gonads. The testes produce spermatozoa—male sex cells—as well as the male hormone testosterone. The penis is composed of a glans and shaft, which is cylindrical, pendulous, and erectile. Inside the penis is the urethra, which is an outlet for urine from the bladder as well as seminal fluid. The glans is the cone-shaped head of the penis that is covered with the foreskin (prepuce) at birth. If the male is circumcised, the glans is exposed. If the male is uncircumcised, the foreskin needs to be retracted for cleansing and intercourse.

The internal male reproductive organs are the seminal vesicles in the testes and the prostate. Seminal fluid is produced and stored in these organs. Spermatozoa combine with seminal fluid, resulting in semen, which is ejaculated from the erect penis during male orgasm.

FEMALE REPRODUCTIVE SYSTEM

The female reproductive system also has external and internal organs (Figure 24-3). The external female genitalia have several components, known collectively as the *vulva.* These components include the mons pubis, the fatty tissue covering the symphysis pubis; the labia majora, tissue that forms the lateral borders of the vaginal orifice; the labia minora, thinner folds of tissue just inside the labia majora borders; and the clitoris, the female counterpart to the penis, in that it responds to stimulation that can lead to orgasm. Additionally, Skene's

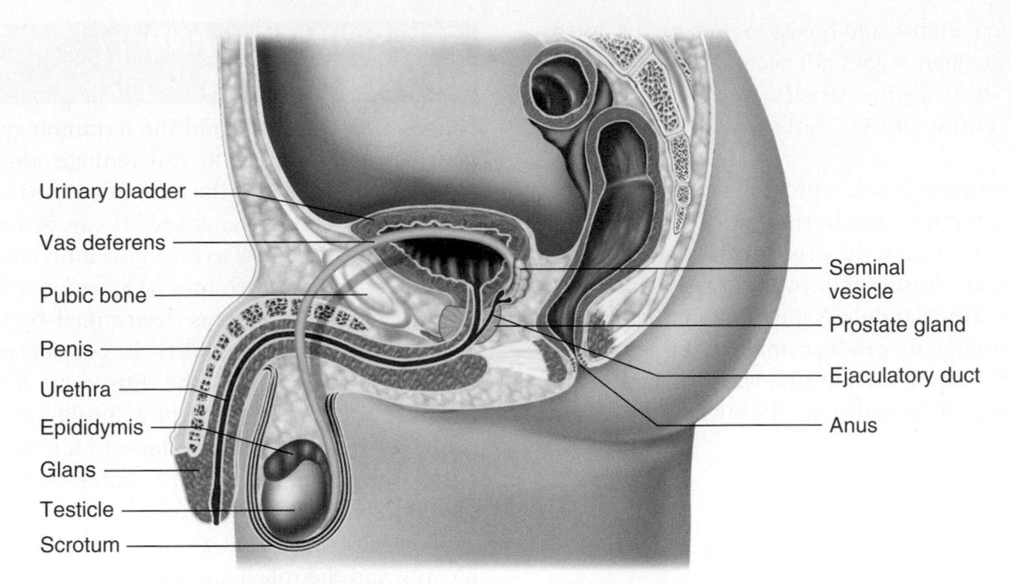

FIGURE 24-2 Male reproductive system.

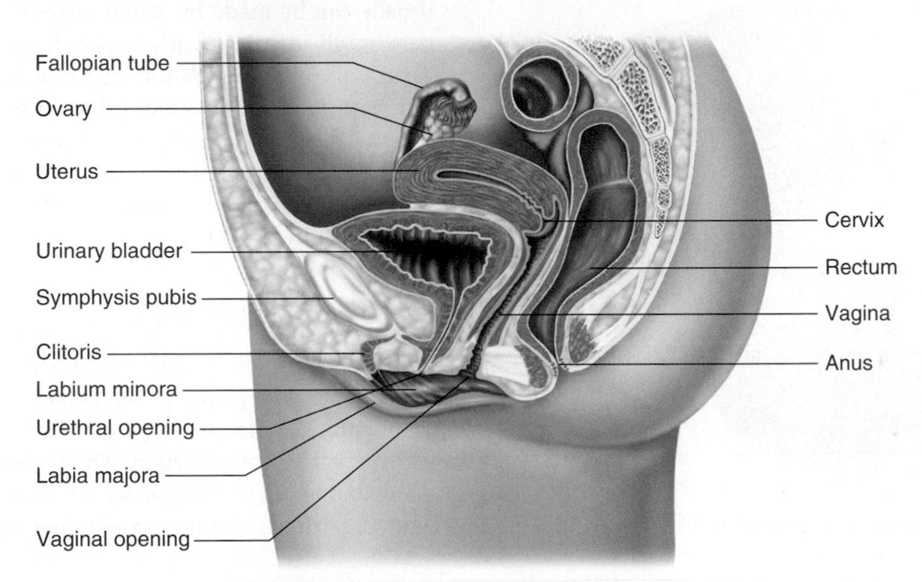

FIGURE 24-3 Female reproductive system.

glands, located inside and posterior in the urethra, and Bartholin's glands, which are small mucous glands in the vaginal vestibule, both produce small amounts of vaginal lubricant during sexual stimulation.

The female internal genitalia include the vagina, uterus, fallopian tubes, and ovaries. The vagina is the connection between the external vulva and the internal uterus. It is composed of muscle and mucous membrane cells and has the ability to expand during intercourse and childbirth. The uterus has three parts: the cervix, which connects the uterus to the vagina; a hollow cavity; and the upper section called the *fundus.* The uterus is pear-shaped and muscular and has the capacity to expand, as in pregnancy. The two fallopian tubes are narrow ducts that extend out the left and right sides of the uterus and end in fingerlike tissue near, but not connected to, the ovaries. The ovaries are two almond-size organs in the left and right sides of the pelvis that contain ova (female reproductive cells) and the female hormones estrogen and progesterone.

Menstruation is the female's cyclic periodic discharge of bodily fluid from the uterus during the reproductive years, encompassing the ages of approximately 12 to 50 years. The cycle is monthly, averaging every 28 days, with a range of 21 to 35 days. This cycle is under hormonal influence from the hypothalamus (gonadotropin-releasing hormone), which stimulates the pituitary (follicle-stimulating hormone [FSH] and luteinizing hormone [LH]). The hormones in turn cause ovarian production of estrogen and progesterone, which stimulate the vagina, uterus, and breast to prepare for potential pregnancy. If pregnancy does not occur, levels of estrogen and progesterone drop, the menstrual cycle (menses, period) occurs, and the entire process restarts via the feedback mechanism.

Breasts are included as female reproductive organs because estrogen and progesterone, the hormones of reproduction, influence them, and they are the organs of **lactation**, which is the production and release of milk by the breasts (mammary glands). They are fatty glandular tissue that contains lobes, which have the ability to produce milk that then drains through ducts to the nipples (Figure 24-4). Touch and stimulation of the breasts can be satisfying during sex.

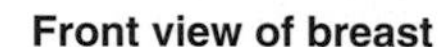

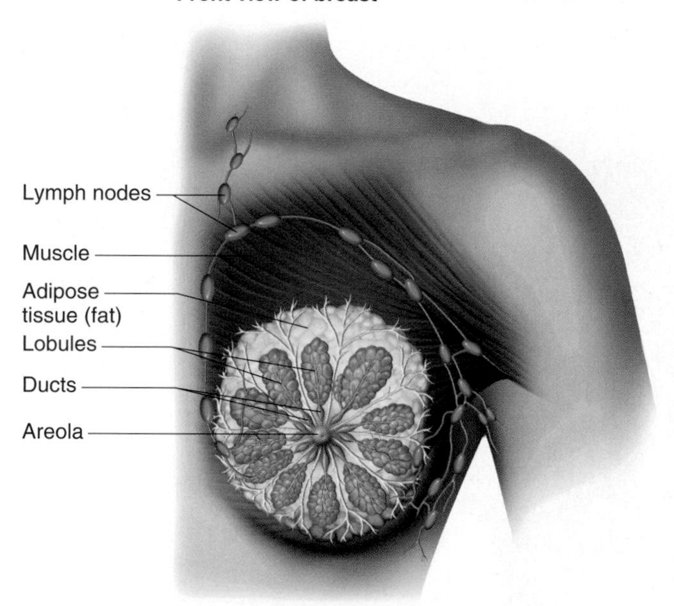

FIGURE 24-4 Breast anatomy.

SEX, SEXUALITY, AND GENDER IDENTITY

LO 24.3

Nurses need to understand the terminology associated with sexuality and be able to differentiate among the various terms' meanings. **Sex** is the term often used to express "sexual intercourse," as in "having sex." It can be further defined in the psychological sense to mean the individual's self-image of his or her gender, which may be at variance with the person's morphological sex (sex as determined by the internal and external genitalia). **Sexuality** is considered the collective characteristics that mark the differences between male and female. Further, it is the nature and life of an individual as related to sex and all that pertains to intimacy, whether associated with sex organs or not. **Gender identity** is the person's self-concept as a male or a female.

It is imperative that the nurse understand that gender identity and the role associated with that identity affects the person's sexuality (Green, 2009). A person's sex is defined by the internal and external genitalia, and this determination usually can be made by visual inspection at birth. How the person self-identifies with respect to gender is affected by a variety of influences. Family experiences and values, association with or lack of a relationship with the same-sex parent, parental identification of gender from birth, self-concept, and confidence about one's sexual identity all influence a person's gender identification. Terms associated with gender identity are defined in Box 24-1.

SEXUAL EXPRESSION

Methods through which individuals express themselves sexually vary depending on social norms and personal preferences. Some people prefer only vaginal intercourse, using a variety of positions. Others engage in oral-genital stimulation, anal intercourse, or masturbation (alone or with a partner). Some people remain celibate, choosing

BOX 24-1 Gender Identity Terminology

- **Gender role** is the set of behaviors of a person as either a male or female and the perception of what constitutes gender-appropriate actions.
- **Sexual orientation** is a person's attraction to his or her own sex, the opposite sex, or both sexes when choosing a sexual partner.
- **Heterosexual** is defined as a person who has sexual interest in or sexual intercourse exclusively with partners of the opposite sex.
- **Homosexual** is defined as a person who has sexual interest in or sexual intercourse exclusively with members of his or her own sex. **Gay** is a term most often associated with male homosexuality, whereas **lesbian** refers exclusively to female homosexuality.
- **Bisexual** describes a person who is emotionally or sexually attracted to people of either sex.
- **Questioning** refers to someone who is unsure or exploring his or her sexual orientation or gender identity.
- **Transgendered** refers to having a gender identity or gender perception different from one's phenotypic gender.
- **Transvestite** is a person who has the desire to dress in the clothes of and be accepted as a member of the opposite sex.
- **Transsexual** is a person who self-identifies as a member of the opposite sex. The sexual anatomy is not consistent with the gender identity. Transsexuals may choose cross-dressing (dressing in the clothing of the other sex) or seek to have their external sex organs changed by transsexual surgery.

DIVERSITY CONSIDERATIONS

Life Span

- Sexual identity changes as a person moves through the stages of life.
- A person moves from friendships with same-sex schoolmates during the school-age years to dating during adolescence.
- Young adults experience a need for intimacy and for establishing a relationship with a significant other to become a couple.
- If parenthood occurs, that person moves from the role of mate to the role of parent. This role may consume the person to the point of losing the sexual identity of being part of a couple for a period of time.
- Middle adults encounter changes that are a result of children's growing up and relying less on the parent, who often needs to reestablish sexual identity with his or her mate. In addition, hormonal changes that occur with age influence sexual performance, and adjustments in expectations may need to occur.
- Older adults may continue to desire the satisfaction of sexual activity but need to make adjustments to accommodate physical and cognitive changes.

Gender

- Gender diversity frequently is noted as sexual orientation, the gender preference of a person in relation to the person's sexual attraction.
- Included in gender diversity are heterosexual, homosexual, bisexual, transvestite, and transsexual.

Culture, Ethnicity, and Religion

- Cultural, ethnic, and religious issues occur in the area of sexual diversity.
- Some Christian religions have a strict doctrine that forbids all forms of sexual expression other than heterosexuality.
- Practices and attitudes regarding contraception, sex education, and sex outside marriage all may be affected by religious teachings.
- **Circumcision**, the surgical removal of the foreskin of the penis, is considered a religious rite for those of the Jewish and Muslim faiths.
- Buddhism followers believe that extremes of modern medicine are to be avoided (some medicines, blood, vaccines). This belief may potentially affect choices for birth control and infertility treatment options.
- Abortion is banned by Catholic doctrine as well as by the Jehovah's Witness faith.
- In the Islamic faith, the husband is present for any informed consent, and women do not make independent decisions. This dynamic can affect choice as well as verbalization of preferences.

Disability

- Disabilities resulting from illnesses, injury, or surgery may alter the sexual experience.
- Physical restrictions from decreased mobility have the potential to reduce sexual function.
- Medication side effects also may have a negative impact on sexual expression.
- Adaptation of positioning during sex, as well as the need for oral or manual stimulation to obtain sexual satisfaction, may be deterrents to sexual activity for those with disabilities.

abstinence as a lifestyle. Sexual expression may vary extensively throughout a person's life span, depending on a variety of factors, some of which are addressed in the Diversity Considerations box.

SEXUAL RESPONSE LO 24.4

FEMALE

Four phases constitute the female sexual response cycle. The phases—excitement, plateau, orgasm, and resolution—consistently occur in this sequence, although the duration of each phase is variable. Arousal typically ends with orgasm or climax, but at times this may not occur. Unlike in males, the response cycle in females does not have a refractory phase, during which sexual response cannot occur, and thus multiple orgasms are possible.

In the female sexual response, two physiologic responses, vasocongestion and myotonia, occur. Vasocongestion of the vagina's blood supply leads to engorgement, increased lubrication, and genital swelling and enlargement, all as a result of sexual stimulation. Myotonia (vaginal muscle spasms) results from muscle tension that leads to both voluntary and involuntary muscle contraction.

Issues of female sexual expression include **dyspareunia** (painful intercourse), **vaginismus** (contraction of the vaginal muscles to the degree that the penis cannot be inserted), and **anorgasmia** (inhibited female orgasm).

MALE

The phases of the male sexual response are stimulation, erection, emission, ejaculation, and detumescence. Both the sympathetic and parasympathetic nervous systems impact the male response. Sexual arousal can be achieved through psychological stimulation, as from sexual thoughts, as well as by genital stimulation. Erection involves the shunting of blood into the penis. Emission causes sperm to move from the epididymis to the urethra. Ejaculation is the expulsion of the sperm from the urethra, which is then followed by **detumescence**, in which the penis is no longer erect. Male orgasm is the period of emission and ejaculation. After the male sexual response, a refractory period occurs, during which there is resistance to muscle or nervous system stimulation.

Issues of male sexual expression include **erectile dysfunction (ED)**, or impotence, which is the inability to achieve or maintain a penile erection for sexual intercourse, and premature ejaculation, which occurs if a male ejaculates before his sex partner achieves orgasm in more than 50% of their sexual encounters (Masters & Johnson, 1966).

CONTRACEPTION OPTIONS LO 24.5

Contraception is the prevention of conception. Contraceptive methods are used for birth control, to prevent pregnancy. Various contraceptive methods are available for males and females, some with and some without the need for a prescription (Table 24-2 and Figure 24-5). Effectiveness of any method is dependent on accuracy and consistency of use. Additionally, contraceptive methods do not necessarily protect against STDs.

Abstinence (going without sexual intercourse), timing of intercourse in connection with the menstrual cycle, and barrier methods are all nonprescriptive contraceptive

TABLE 24-2 Contraception Methods

METHOD	FUNCTION
Abstinence	No sexual intercourse occurs; 100% effective at preventing conception.
Withdrawal of the penis before ejaculation	Semen (sperm) is deposited outside the vagina to reduce the chance of conception.
Timing of sexual intercourse with ovulation and menses (rhythm method)	Intercourse is prohibited during fertile days to reduce the chance of conception.
Male or female condom	Barrier method prevents entry of sperm into the vagina to reduce the chance of conception.
Spermicide (creams, sponges, foams, or jellies)	Agent is inserted into the vagina before intercourse, serving as a barrier to reduce the chance of conception.
Oral contraceptive	Hormonal changes alter the uterine environment and thicken cervical mucus to reduce the chance of conception and stop ovulation. Pills need to be taken daily.
Intrauterine device (IUD)	Device is inserted into the uterus through the cervix by provider. Mechanism of action is not well understood. Various processes are thought to inhibit the ability of either the egg or the sperm or both to unite with one another, so that fertilization does not occur.
Hormonal injection, implant under the skin, or transdermal patch	Hormonal changes alter the uterine environment and thicken cervical mucus to reduce the chance of conception. Prolonged effectiveness of these methods improves compliance.
Diaphragm/cervical cap	Barrier method device is inserted into the vagina and used with spermicidal cream or jelly to reduce the chance of conception.
Vaginal ring/transdermal system	Small, flexible ring is inserted by a woman into her vagina for 3 wk every month and removed for the remaining week; contains the same hormones as in oral contraceptives and is considered easier to use.
Emergency contraception (morning-after pill)	Taken within three days after intercourse to prevent the ovaries from releasing an egg, making pregnancy impossible. Will not abort a fertilized egg. Limited effectiveness in women with BMI > 25.
Hysteroscopic sterilization	Nonsurgical procedure occludes the fallopian tubes with small metal springs. The coils trigger scar tissue growth over time, causing the tubes to be permanently blocked.
Surgical sterilization *Male:* vasectomy *Female:* tubal ligation	This is the most effective contraceptive method other than abstinence. Both vasectomy and tubal ligation are surgical procedures that prevent conception and are considered highly effective.

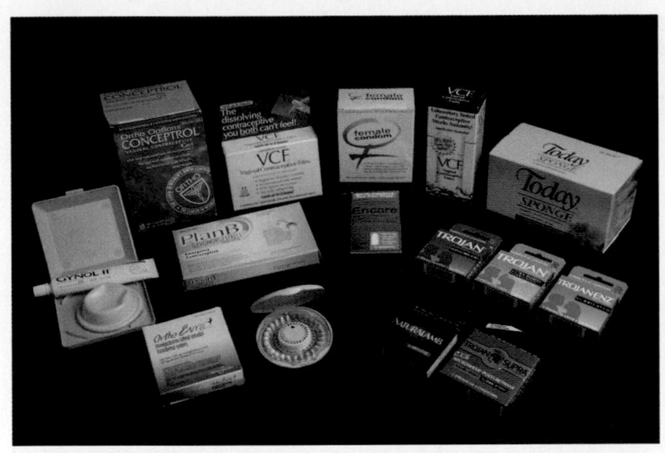

FIGURE 24-5 Types of contraceptive devices.

methods. A **condom**, a thin rubber sheath that covers the penis to prevent sperm from entering the vagina, and spermicidal products (foam, cream, jelly, sponge) are barrier methods. Abstinence currently is the only method that is 100% effective for pregnancy prevention.

The prescription methods of contraception are hormonal contraception; use of a diaphragm, **intrauterine device (IUD)**, or cervical cap; and surgical sterilization. Hormone-based contraception includes oral contraception ("the pill") as well as intramuscular injection, transdermal patch, subdermal implant, vaginal ring, and IUD. Intrauterine devices are placed through the cervix into the uterus and may contain progesterone or copper, which change the uterine lining, thus reducing the chance of implantation.

The **diaphragm**, a flexible, round rubber dome, is used with a spermicidal jelly or cream and inserted into the vagina to cover the entire cervix. The cervical cap functions in the same fashion, but it is smaller and covers only the opening to the cervix.

Sterilization is possible in both genders. Male sterilization (**vasectomy**) is the severing of the vas deferens, which carry sperm out of the testes. When the male ejaculates during sexual intercourse, there are no sperm in the semen. Female sterilization (**tubal ligation**) is the ligation of the fallopian tubes. When the tubes are ligated (tied off or severed), the egg cannot travel through the tube and the sperm cannot get to the egg, thus preventing fertilization. These procedures are the most effective contraceptive methods other than abstinence.

> **! SAFE PRACTICE ALERT**
>
> Teach the patient to use a water-based lubricant with a condom. Oil-based lubricants such as petrolatum (Vaseline) will break down the latex, making the condom ineffective.

SEXUALLY TRANSMITTED DISEASES AND INFECTIONS LO 24.6

A **sexually transmitted disease (STD)** is any disease that may be acquired as a result of sexual intercourse or other intimate contact with an infected person. The term **sexually transmitted infection (STI)** is used if an infection is present without actual signs of disease (Planned Parenthood, 2014). Despite this difference, the terms *STD* and *STI* are often used interchangeably because the designation of "infection" is thought to carry less stigma than "disease."

Identification of an STD can be difficult because symptoms may go unnoticed or be ignored. Common STD symptoms include pain during sex (dyspareunia) or on urination; genital blisters or lesions; discharge from the penis, anus, or vagina; and elevated temperature (Centers for Disease Control and Prevention, 2014). Patients may be embarrassed to admit to having STD symptoms or may find it difficult to discuss sexual practices. Nurses should be nonjudgmental and empathetic in their communication to foster trust and enhance the patient's ability to share personal information.

STDs include conditions caused by bacteria, viruses, protozoa, and fungi. Gonorrhea, syphilis, and chlamydial infection all are caused by bacteria and usually can be treated and cured with antibiotics. The viral diseases, including genital warts (caused by human papillomavirus [HPV]) and genital herpes (due to herpes simplex virus [HSV-1]), can be treated but not cured. All STDs, including HPV infection, can be contracted by both males and females. Table 24-3 presents general information on the symptoms, transmission, and prevention of these relatively common STDs.

> **! SAFE PRACTICE ALERT**
>
> Teach patients taking antibiotics for STDs to take the full course of therapy, even if signs and symptoms decrease or disappear.

HUMAN IMMUNODEFICIENCY VIRUS INFECTION

Human immunodeficiency virus (HIV) infection is caused by a blood-borne virus that may be acquired by sexual contact through exchange of bodily fluids. Risk behaviors include unprotected vaginal and/or oral sex, use of contaminated intravenous (IV) needles, and transfusion of infected blood or blood products. During the initial phase of HIV infection, which lasts approximately 1 month after onset, the patient may have flulike symptoms. The condition then moves into the clinical latency phase, a variable length of time during which the patient has no infection symptoms. In the third phase, symptoms become evident, and HIV infection becomes

TABLE 24-3 Common Sexually Transmitted Diseases

SYMPTOMS	TRANSMISSION	PREVENTION
Chlamydia		
May be totally asymptomatic; flulike symptoms, genital discharge in men or women accompanied by burning with urination	During vaginal, oral, or anal sex or during vaginal delivery	• Abstinence • Monogamous relationship with uninfected partner • Consistent and correct use of latex male condoms • Annual testing of all sexually active women aged 25 or younger, older women with new or multiple sex partners, and all pregnant women
Gonorrhea		
May be asymptomatic; genital discharge, burning, and pain	Contact with the mouth, penis, vagina, or anus	• Abstinence • Monogamous relationship with uninfected partner • Consistent and correct use of latex male condoms
Genital Herpes		
Genital discomfort, sores that heal within 2-4 wk	Contact with sores during an outbreak or with infected skin between periods of outbreak	• Abstinence when lesions or symptoms are present • Use of condoms to reduce risk
Human Papillomavirus (HPV)		
May be totally asymptomatic, especially in males; genital warts with some HPV types, which vary in size and shape; can undergo transformation to various forms of cancer in both men and women	Through vaginal, oral, or anal sex or genital-to-genital contact	• Vaccines *Girls and women:* Cervarix and Gardasil *Boys and men:* Gardasil • Use of condoms, which may lower risk
Syphilis		
Three stages: Begins with sores, advances to a rash with mucous membrane lesions, and ends with a latent, late stage affecting the central nervous system; may lead to blindness, paralysis, and psychosis	Direct contact with syphilis sore (chancre) during vaginal, oral, or anal sex	• Avoidance of alcohol and drugs, because their use may lead to risky sexual behavior • Monogamous relationship with uninfected partner • Consistent and correct use of latex condoms covering infected areas, which may reduce risk

From Centers for Disease Control and Prevention: Sexually transmitted diseases (STDs), 2014. Retrieved from *www.cdc.gov/std/default.htm.*

the acquired immunodeficiency syndrome (AIDS), which is serious and may be fatal. Survival time for patients with AIDS has improved with the use of the multidrug approach of highly active antiretroviral therapy (HAART).

! SAFE PRACTICE ALERT

Strict use of standard precautions including washing hands and wearing clean gloves is imperative for nurses providing care to patients with suspected or verified STDs.

FACTORS AFFECTING SEXUALITY LO 24.7

Sexuality and *sexual function* are not synonymous concepts. Sexual function begins at birth, continues throughout the life span, and involves the physical ability to perform a sex act. Sexuality is more encompassing. It includes the character and life of a person as related to sex along with all the dispositions related to intimacy, whether associated with sex organs or not. Table 24-4 summarizes factors affecting sexuality and nursing implications related to those factors.

TABLE 24-4 **Factors Affecting Sexuality**

FACTOR	SEXUAL HEALTH–RELATED CHARACTERISTICS	IMPACT AND NURSING IMPLICATIONS
Family values and beliefs	• Family constraints on or endorsement of sexuality taught during childhood influence behavior throughout life's stages.	• Explore family influences when gathering a sexual history. • Recognize the impact of various value systems on patients' decisions in relation to their sexuality.
Culture and religion	• Culture and religious beliefs influence family structure, roles within the family, who the dominant figure is within that structure, and how and whether sexuality is displayed. • Guilt and resentment may result from cultural or religious constraints.	• Be knowledgeable about cultural and religious variances and expressions of sexuality. • Remain nonjudgmental. • Teach this information to patients and families.
Self-concept, ego, and body image	• Altered body image, either in reality or by perception, can influence sexuality and sexual expression. • Confidence in sexual expression may be impacted by the perception of altered body image.	• Differentiate reality from perception. • Teach acceptance. • Be nonjudgmental.
Previous experiences and relationships	• Unstable relationships, fear, and power issues can exert a negative impact on one's sexuality.	• Provide a safe environment so that the patient can share past experiences without fear.
Cognition and intellect	• Alterations in cognition or intellect do not equate with alteration of one's sexuality or desire for sexual satisfaction.	• Recognize sexuality regardless of the patient's intellect or cognition level.
Environment	• Privacy may be an essential element for both sexual discussion and sexual activity.	• Comply with all privacy guidelines. • Maintain respect for the patient. • Provide a nonjudgmental environment.
Personal expectations	• Social and peer group interaction may influence personal expectations of sexual experiences.	• Be supportive and nonjudgmental. • Be a resource for education and personal expectations clarification.
Ethics	• Family and religious influences impact ethical decision making as it relates to sexuality. • Ethical differences between partners may lead to denial of experiences or conflict.	• Be aware of the patient's cultural and religious individuality. • Do not impose personal beliefs or value system into interactions with the patient.

FACTORS AFFECTING SEXUAL FUNCTION LO 24.8

Sexual function is affected by many factors, ranging from physical to lifestyle to developmental. Table 24-5 details factors, influences, and outcomes affecting sexual function. Remember: In practice, each scenario is individualized for each person.

Side effects of medications can adversely affect sexual performance by reducing sexual response and satisfaction. When conducting a sexual history with a patient, the nurse should ask about medication use and educate the patient about the potential side effects of medications being used (Patient Education and Health Literacy box). In many cases, if a sexual side effect arises, the patient should be aware that a change in medication may eliminate the sexual function issue.

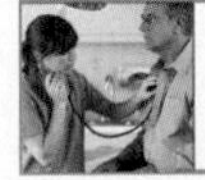

1. In addition to antihypertensive medication, list three potential causes of sexual dysfunction in an adult.

TABLE 24-5 Factors Affecting Sexual Function

FACTOR CATEGORY	INFLUENCES	OUTCOMES
Physical	Minor or chronic illnesses, medications (number or combination), fatigue, pain or discomfort as a result of sex*	Decreased intimacy, personal stress and/or stress with partner, reduction in the frequency of sexual relations
Functional	Diseases that limit sensation or movement (e.g., diabetes, rheumatoid arthritis, multiple sclerosis), acute illnesses, infertility, aging changes† Medications with side effects that may hinder sexual desire or performance (e.g., antidepressants, central nervous system depressants, narcotics, antihypertensives)	Decreased intimacy, personal stress and/or stress with partner, reduction in the frequency or satisfaction of sexual relations
Relationship	Stress, differences in value systems, communication issues, intimacy changes, control issues	Decreased intimacy, personal stress and/or stress with partner, reduction in the frequency or satisfaction of sexual relations
Lifestyle	Work issues, children, family responsibilities, abuse of drugs or alcohol, lack of time or sleep	Fatigue, decreased intimacy, personal stress and/or stress with partner, reduction in the frequency or satisfaction of sexual relations
Developmental	Immature or inappropriate expectations	Personal stress and/or stress with partner, changes in intimacy, changes in frequency and/or satisfaction of sexual relations
Self-concept	Poor body image; altered self-esteem; history of rape, incest, or abuse; negative role models; unrealistic expectations; lack of adequate sex education	Lack of intimacy, personal stress, changes in frequency or satisfaction of sexual relations

*From Gevirtz C: Controlling pain: How chronic pain affects sexuality, *Nursing 2008* 38(1):17, 2008.
†From Fraser C, Mahoney J, McGurl J: Correlates of sexual dysfunction in men and women with multiple sclerosis, *J Neurosci Nurs* 40(5):312-317, 2008.

PATIENT EDUCATION AND HEALTH LITERACY

Potential Side Effects of Medications

- **Anticonvulsants**: Phenytoin (Dilantin, Tegretol) can have a sedating effect and cause a decrease in sexual desire and function.
- **Antidepressants**: Tricyclics, monoamine oxidase inhibitors (MAOIs), and lithium can cause male impotence and some reduction in testosterone levels. Selective serotonin reuptake inhibitors (SSRIs) side effects may include delayed ejaculation, absent or delayed orgasm, and diminished sexual desire.
- **Antihistamines**: The sedative effect can be associated with decreased desire and reduced female vaginal lubrication.
- **Antihypertensives**: ACE inhibitors, alpha and beta blockers, and calcium channel blockers may decrease male and female desire and cause erectile dysfunction.
- **Antipsychotics**: These drugs may reduce desire and cause ED and ejaculation dysfunction.
- **Antispasmodics**: These drugs relax smooth muscle, which may lead to male impotence.
- **Narcotics**: Increased dependence can result in further sexual impairment: ED and ejaculation dysfunction are common; decreased male and female desire and decreased testosterone and semen production are other possible adverse effects.
- **Alcohol (ethyl alcohol)**: A moderate amount reduces inhibition and may improve sexual function. Increased consumption leads to reduced sexual function. Chronic alcoholism results in male impotence, permanent dysfunction, and sterility; in females, reduced desire and orgasmic dysfunction are possible.
- **Marijuana**: Initially, this drug may cause reduced inhibitions and increased sexual function; with chronic use, sexual desire is decreased in both males and females, and male impotence may occur.

FAMILY DYNAMICS LO 24.9

Age, ethnicity, culture, and religion may affect family dynamics when a sexual health issue arises. Communication of a sexual health concern is often impeded due to embarrassment, anxiety, or fear. The value systems specific to age groups within a family may be so different as to block dialogue when a question or problem occurs. Religious teachings may affect the family's choices pertaining to abortion, sterilization, contraception, and sexual preferences. Cultural attitudes and practices may curtail the dynamics between sexual partners, limiting the expression of personal needs or desires. Gender and sexual preference issues may have different impacts within a family, depending on the age of all involved.

In a family where decision making is done unilaterally by one partner instead of by both as a couple, it is possible that the partner who makes the family decisions also may be the one who makes decisions pertaining to intimacy and sexual practices. This inequity may result in resentment, sexual frustration, or anger from the partner who is not the decision maker. In a relationship in which power is shared and roles are equal between the partners instead of dominant and submissive, opportunities for sexual expression and satisfaction are enhanced.

Families dealing with gender identity issues must work to overcome prejudices as well as gain knowledge about the specific gender issue. Personal and public acceptance, along with open communication, should be the family goal. Such acceptance, however, may not be attained because of cultural, religious, or moral constraints.

To meet the needs of such a diverse group as a family, the most appropriate professional often is the home health nurse. The Home Care Considerations box details home care considerations related to sexuality.

HOME CARE CONSIDERATIONS

Sexual Health Foci for the Home Care Nurse

- Patients being monitored by the home health nurse for chronic illness (diabetes, hypertension, heart failure) should be assessed in regard to their sexual health. Any deficit findings should then be correlated with prescribed treatment and medication regimens.
- Patients under postoperative follow-up care (such as after heart surgery, hysterectomy, or knee replacement) should be asked about sexual health concerns during the initial assessment with the home health nurse. Such concerns should be noted and become part of the patient's plan of care.
- The initial home health care visit to new mothers should provide education on contraceptive choices as well as newborn and post-delivery care. Depending on the circumstances, the visit also may include education on STD and HIV/AIDS prevention.
- Home health care visits to the elderly should include assessment and teaching on the subject of sexual health. Education to meet the individualized needs of the aged patient should be provided and routinely reinforced.
- Home health care follow-up for a patient with a reported STD should include education on the signs and symptoms of STDs, HIV/AIDS prevention, avoidance of high-risk behaviors, and treatment methods.

ASSESSMENT LO 24.10

Using a matter-of-fact, organized approach to data collection regarding a patient's sexual health can alleviate anxiety on the part of the patient and unnecessary hesitation on the part of the nurse (Health Assessment Questions box).

HEALTH ASSESSMENT QUESTIONS

Sexual Focus

- How do you feel about the sexual aspect of your life?
- Have you noticed any changes in the way you see yourself (as a man, woman, husband, wife, partner)?
- How has your illness, surgery, or medication affected your sex life?
- Are you active sexually?
- Do you have problems or concerns regarding your sexual abilities, performance, or satisfaction?
- How many sexual partners have you had in your lifetime?
- What are or have been your sexual practices?
- Do you feel safe in your environment?

Research has found that nurses routinely do not inquire about sexual health, and teaching and counseling in this area are at best inconsistent. Reasons include embarrassment, not correlating a sexual issue with the medical problem, fear of legal repercussions from discussion of an inappropriate topic, lack of sexual health expertise, and a mistaken belief that questions about sexuality are an invasion of the patient's privacy (Katz, 2005).

Use of an assessment tool may help the nurse become more comfortable when asking questions dealing with sexual health. One such tool is the PLISSIT model, which provides a format to help the nurse initiate and maintain the discussion of sexuality by asking sequenced open-ended questions (Wallace, 2008). The PLISSIT model is defined as follows:

P: Obtaining *permission* from the patient to initiate sexual discussion

LI: Providing the *limited information* needed to function sexually

SS: Giving *specific suggestions* for the person to proceed with sexual relations

IT: Providing *intensive therapy* surrounding the issues of sexuality for the patient

Using this model, the nurse has a framework for initiating the discussion of sexual issues with the patient and providing guidance for follow-up evaluation or referral.

In addition to recognizing and understanding the patient's current sexual concern, the nurse also should assess the patient's developmental level and then, with that knowledge, gather a sexual health history. The patient's past and current health and sexual practices, as well as medications with a potential impact on sexual function, should be identified. The patient's reproductive history, STD history, sexual dysfunction history, sexual health self-care practices, frequency and technique of breast self-examination (BSE) and/or testicular self-examination (TSE), and sexual identity, self-concept, and self-esteem should be assessed.

When completing a sexual health history, the nurse should incorporate the following steps and attitudes:

- Overcome any prejudices concerning sexuality.
- Be nonjudgmental—nurse approval is not necessary.

- Allow time to discuss and explore patient needs, fears, and feelings.
- Actively listen to the patient.
- Clarify vocabulary as needed.
- Be tolerant, but not permissive.
- Be respectful.
- Watch for nonverbal responses.
- Respect patient privacy.
- Maintain confidentiality.
- Ask questions in a routine, matter-of-fact manner.
- Continue to be an advocate for the patient.

SEXUAL HARASSMENT

Nurses have the right and responsibility to confront patients who display inappropriate sexual behavior. This behavior may be verbal, nonverbal, or physical, from either male or female patients, and may be heterosexual or homosexual in nature. To help end this inappropriate patient behavior, the nurse should implement the guidelines listed in the Ethical, Legal, and Professional Practice box.

ETHICAL, LEGAL, AND PROFESSIONAL PRACTICE

Managing Sexual Harassment in the Workplace

- Be aware of the fact that sexual harassment does occur.
- Be cautious with touching during patient care while maintaining privacy and professionalism.
- Establish a professional relationship with the patient, including minimal sharing of personal information and no sexually oriented conversations or humor.
- Be alert for personal questions of a sexual or suggestive nature from the patient, and do not respond to them. If the inquiries continue, bring in another staff member for any patient contact or conversation.
- Be aware that the patient may deny or defend the behavior if confronted about an inappropriate comment or action.
- If any deliberate physical contact takes place, be assertive so that the action can be curtailed. First, stop the action; second, tell the patient how you feel about the inappropriate behavior.
- Set limits and enforce consequences. Tell the patient that you will not continue to be involved in the patient's care if the behavior continues.
- Acknowledge your own feelings. It is all right to be insulted, angry, or embarrassed by inappropriate patient behavior.
- Educate yourself on the issue of sexual harassment in the workplace.

From Zook R: Handling inappropriate sexual behavior with confidence, *Nursing 1997* 27(4):65, 1997; Zook R: Teaching staff to handle a patient's sexually inappropriate behavior, *J Nurses Staff Dev* 16(4):248, 2000.

Sexual harassment also may occur in the workplace in the form of requests from a supervisor for sexual favors in exchange for employment benefits (quid pro quo) or unwelcomed physical or verbal conduct of a sexual nature by co-workers or nonemployees, resulting in a hostile environment. Nurses are encouraged to work with their employers to develop and enforce policies that support preventive action and workplace environments that protect against sexual harassment of all individuals.

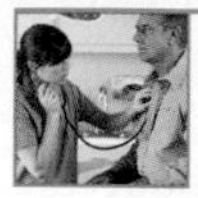

2. Make a list of five assessment questions related to Mr. Wells's concern about erectile dysfunction that the nurse might ask before discussing possible causes during the health history.

NURSING DIAGNOSIS LO 24.11

Nursing diagnoses frequently used to focus on issues of sexuality are *Sexual Dysfunction* and *Ineffective Sexuality Pattern.* NANDA International, Inc. (NANDA-I) (2012) defines *sexual dysfunction* as "the state in which an individual experiences a change in sexual function … that is viewed as unsatisfying, unrewarding, or inadequate" (p. 323). Examples of nursing diagnostic statements are:

- *Sexual Dysfunction* related to altered body structure (surgery) as evidenced by inability to maintain an erection
- *Sexual Dysfunction* related to lack of privacy as evidenced by the patient's stating, "Since the baby arrived we never have any time together"

Ineffective sexuality pattern is defined by NANDA-I (2012) as "expressions of concern regarding [one's] own sexuality" (p. 325). Examples of nursing diagnostic statements are:

- *Ineffective Sexuality Pattern* related to absent role model as evidenced by reporting difficulty with sexual activities
- *Ineffective Sexuality Pattern* related to impaired relationship with significant other as evidenced by the patient's stating, "I can't be a man with my wife"

Other nursing diagnoses related to sexuality are *Rape-Trauma Syndrome, Impaired Parenting, Risk for Impaired Parenting,* and *Readiness for Enhanced Parenting.* Additional nursing diagnoses that may be applicable to sexuality are *Anxiety, Fear, Hopelessness, Ineffective Coping, Interrupted Family Processes, Social Isolation, Powerlessness, Risk for Other-Directed Violence, Risk for Self-Directed Violence,* and *Deficient Knowledge* (contraception/STDs) (NANDA-I, 2012).

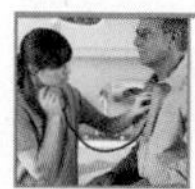

3. Write a primary nursing diagnosis statement for Mr. Wells related to his stated sexual concern. Include the specific related factor identified by the nurse as well as a cluster of supporting data from the case study and the nurses' data collection located on the online conceptual care map.

TABLE 24-6 Care Planning

NANDA-I NURSING DIAGNOSIS LABEL WITH NURSING DIAGNOSIS STATEMENT	NURSING OUTCOME CLASSIFICATION (NOC)	NURSING INTERVENTION CLASSIFICATION (NIC)
Sexual Dysfunction related to altered body structure (surgery) as evidenced by inability to maintain an erection	*Sexual functioning* (0119) Sustains penile erection through orgasm (011902)	*Sexual counseling* (5248) Discuss necessary modifications in sexual activity, as appropriate.

From Bulechek G, Butcher H, Dochterman J, et al (Eds): *Nursing interventions classification (NIC),* ed. 6, St. Louis, 2013, Mosby; Moorhead S, Johnson M, Maas M, et al (Eds): *Nursing outcomes classification (NOC),* ed. 5, St. Louis, 2013, Mosby; NANDA International: *Nursing diagnoses: Definitions and classification, 2012–2014,* West Sussex, England, 2012, Wiley-Blackwell. Reprinted with permission from NANDA International, Inc.

◆ PLANNING LO 24.12

In the planning phase of the nursing process, the nurse should use critical-thinking skills and assimilate information from multiple resources. The patient's individualized plan should evolve using the knowledge the nurse gained when gathering the sexual health history, along with the experience of the nurse in dealing with sexual concerns. Ethical and legal standards associated with sexual issues must be maintained by the nurse during this phase. These include protecting the patient's privacy, giving assurance of confidentiality, and providing unbiased, appropriate assistance. For each nursing diagnosis, an individualized plan of care is developed with realistic goals and measurable outcome criteria (Table 24-6). Setting priorities to address the individual needs of the patient and considering collaboration of care also are components of the planning phase (Collaboration and Delegation box).

COLLABORATION AND DELEGATION

Addressing Patient Sexual Health Needs

- The patient with a sexual health issue will benefit from a multidisciplinary team approach to managing the problem.
- The nurse, primary health care provider, and social worker should collaborate in the care and treatment plan for the patient.
- The sex therapist, psychologist, pharmacist, physical therapist, and dietitian also may provide information and support, depending on the cause of the sexual issue.

The process of developing a care plan is summarized in the following example: A postoperative hospitalized patient has a nursing diagnosis of *Sexual Dysfunction* related to surgical intervention. The nurse works with the patient to develop the goal of improved sexual function within 1 month. Expected outcomes or goals are identified:

- Patient will discuss sexual dysfunction with the primary care provider before discharge from the hospital.
- Patient will report improved sexual function at the 1-month follow-up appointment with the health care provider.

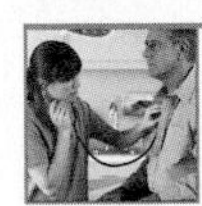

4. Write a short-term goal or outcome statement that would be realistic for Mr. Wells while addressing the identified priority nursing diagnosis.

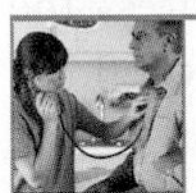

The conceptual care map for Mr. Wells can be found at *http://evolve.elsevier.com/YoostCrawford/fundamentals/*. It is partially completed to indicate how to use the map as a learning tool. Complete the nursing diagnoses using the example conceptual care maps shown in Chapters 8 and 25 to 33.

◆ IMPLEMENTATION AND EVALUATION LO 24.13

The implementation and evaluation of sexual health issues focus on health education, risk prevention, patient counseling, and the outcomes of these endeavors. Interventions to address patient needs are discussed directly with the patient to maximize comfort levels and to ensure compliance.

QSEN FOCUS!

Being sensitive and showing respect for the diversity of patient sexual experiences is essential to providing patient-centered care.

HEALTH EDUCATION

Therapeutic communication skills are a must for the nurse when discussing sexual values, desires, satisfaction, or issues of concern. Teach to the patient's developmental level and in an environment conducive to open communication while maintaining the patient's privacy and ensuring confidentiality. Teach the patient about measures to assess sexual health, including Papanicolaou (Pap) smears to check for cervical abnormalities, BSE and mammograms to assess breast health, monthly TSE starting after the age of 14 years, and prostate examinations (in accordance with American Urological Association guidelines). See Chapter 20 on assessment, and Chapter 41 on urinary elimination for more information on these topics.

RISK PREVENTION

Safe sex practices that prevent risk should be included in any sexual health education discussion. STD recognition and prevention measures include:

- Information regarding the symptoms of STDs
- Need for routine physical examinations with laboratory work for detection of some asymptomatic STDs
- Proper use of condoms
- Avoidance of multiple sex partners, as well as sexual practices that increase risk (e.g., oral or anal sex)

These measures, along with avoiding IV drug use, also help prevent HIV infection.

PATIENT COUNSELING

Counseling by the nurse may be necessary to address the patient's sexual concerns. Therapeutic communication skills, privacy, and confidentiality are essential components. Sexual function associated with chronic illness, sexual desire and performance issues, and sexual abuse are areas for which counseling may occur. The issues of sexual abuse and rape cross all age, ethnic, cultural, and socioeconomic groups, and nurses are likely to care for victims at some time in their practice. Evidence of abuse may be noted on gathering a health history or completing a physical assessment. The nurse should understand the clinical and legal responsibilities involved in dealing with abuse and should have access to a safe environment for the abuse victim (Nursing Care Guideline boxes). Family support and counseling also should be considerations for patients who have been abused.

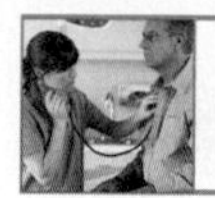

5. Identify at least two nursing interventions to incorporate into Mr. Wells's plan of care.

Nurses who are counseling patients should consider outside resources as sources of additional patient support and education. Community agencies and organizations that work with patients with sexual health issues include:

- Local, state, and federal health departments
- Planned Parenthood, at *www.plannedparenthood.org*

NURSING CARE GUIDELINE

Care for the Victim of Sexual Assault

Background

- An examination of the patient to collect evidence should occur within 72 hours of the assault.
- If possible, a sexual assault nurse examiner (SANE) who is trained and certified as a forensic nurse and who has been designated an expert in evidence collection and legal proceedings should perform the examination.
- A victim advocate for the patient also is needed, because the SANE is an impartial witness. A SANE usually works as a member of a sexual abuse response team (SART) in a facility setting, and the SART usually includes an advocate for the victim.

Procedural Concerns

- The SANE and SART members maintain a professional, nonjudgmental attitude throughout the procedure. They document all procedures and findings, as well as maintain the chain of evidence. Evidence to be collected includes:
  - DNA evidence
  - Seminal fluid evidence
  - Physical injury evidence
  - Blood and urine evidence
  - Genital trauma evidence through colposcopic examination
- The SANE and SART members comfort the patient throughout the examination and provide:
  - Education and information regarding STIs
  - Information on or prophylactic treatment against pregnancy
  - Crisis intervention and information on counseling
- After the examination, the SART provides a place to bathe, supplies clean clothes, and offers to call family or friends for a place to stay or offers information on shelters.

Documentation Concerns

- Accuracy and legibility are essential.
  - Never use the term *alleged sexual assault*.
  - Use the phrase "patient states" or "patient reports."
  - Document both subjective and objective findings.
- Document the following concerns about the patient:
  - Is the patient pregnant?
  - Does the patient have allergies?
  - What is the patient's general appearance?
  - What is the patient's emotional status?
  - What is the patient's response to examination?
  - Does the patient have physical injuries?
  - What are the site and time of the assault?
  - Has the patient performed any self-care activities (bathing, douching, laundering clothes, brushing teeth) since the assault?
  - Was there physical contact by the assailant(s), and if so, how would it be characterized? (Was there actual or attempted penetration? Was a penis or another object involved? Did ejaculation occur? Was a condom used?)
  - What does the patient report about the number of assailants, descriptions, and relationship, if any, to the patient?
  - Were weapons and/or restraints used during the assault?
  - Was there sexual activity 72 hours before and/or since the assault?
  - Has the patient been using tampons or contraception?

Evidence-Based Practice

- Using a SART and a SANE has been shown to increase patient compliance and reporting of crime, decrease emergency department wait time, strengthen chain of evidence collection, improve documentation, increase prosecution rates, and ultimately provide higher-quality patient care (Lewis-O'Connor, 2009; Plichta, Clements, and Houseman, 2007).

NURSING CARE GUIDELINE

Care for the Victim of Domestic Violence

Background

- Domestic violence does not have to be physical violence:
  - It includes a threat or promotion of fear to exert power or control over another person.
  - It can occur through intimidation or isolation or via someone else.
  - It can be emotional, financial, sexual, or physical.
  - It can occur to anyone, by anyone.
- Leaving a domestic violence situation can be just as dangerous as staying.
- Nurses are required to screen for domestic violence by asking questions on admission of the patient to a facility.
- A cycle of violence is common.

Procedural Concerns

- It is imperative to take screening seriously:
  - Provide *total and complete* privacy—no exceptions!
  - Listen without judging.
  - Provide emotional support.
  - Advocate contact with support services.
- Patient and family safety is the top priority.
- Discuss safety plans.
- Victims may refuse to accept printed or written information out of fear. Repeat important information such as:
  - Phone numbers of crisis centers
  - Addresses of shelters
- Reassure the patient that records are confidential and that Health Insurance Portability and Accountability Act (HIPAA) compliance is ensured.

Documentation Concerns

- Accuracy and legibility are essential.
- Use the phrase "patient states" or "patient reports."
- Detail new and old physical injuries. Photograph injuries (with patient consent).
- Document information that is provided both orally and in writing, including patient education and the resources that were suggested or provided.
- Document consultations and referrals.

Evidence-Based Practice

- Rhodes and associates (2007) and Yonaka, Yoder, Darrow, and Sherck (2007) report that victims of domestic violence often may not feel comfortable talking with a health care provider, even though they may want and need assistance. Barriers include the nurse's lack of education on how to approach victims appropriately, a lack of time or privacy, and the nurse's possible own history or biases regarding domestic violence.

- National Infertility Association, at *www.resolve.org*
- Information and support groups for people with particular conditions:
  - American Diabetes Association, at *www.diabetes.org*
  - American Heart Association, at *www.heart.org*
  - American Cancer Society, at *www.cancer.org*
  - American Lung Association, at *www.lung.org*
  - National Multiple Sclerosis Society, at *www.nationalmssociety.org*
- Local support groups and hotlines for sexual abuse
- National Center for Victims of Crime, at *www.ncvc.org*
- Women's Shelters for Physical Abuse, at *www.sheltersforwomen.org*
- Rape, Abuse, and Incest National Network, *www.rainn.org*
- North America Menopause Society, at *www.menopause.org*

EVALUATION

Although patient affect, body language, and nonverbal communication provide some data, the nurse needs direct patient information to evaluate the outcomes of the plan of care dealing with sexual health. The evaluation should include questions on resolution of the issue as well as satisfaction with the outcome. This information will help the nurse determine whether additional actions are necessary to meet the needs of the patient (Alfaro-LeFevre, 2014).

SUMMARY OF LEARNING OUTCOMES

LO 24.1 *Explain sexual development through the life cycle:* Sexual development follows the stages of physical and psychological growth and development.

LO 24.2 *Describe the structure and function of the male and female reproductive systems:* The male external reproductive organs are the scrotum and the penis; the internal reproductive organs are the seminal vesicles in the testes and the prostate. Semen is produced in the internal organs and ejaculated from the penis during orgasm. The female external genitalia, known collectively as the vulva, include the mons pubis, labia majora, labia minora, clitoris, Skene's glands, and Bartholin's glands; the internal genitalia include the vagina, uterus, fallopian tubes, and ovaries. The breasts also are considered female reproductive organs because estrogen and progesterone influence them and because they are the organs of lactation.

LO 24.3 *Differentiate among sex, sexuality, and gender identity:* A person's sex is defined by the internal and external genitalia. Sexuality is defined as the collective characteristics that mark the differences between male and female. Sexuality is associated with every aspect of an individual's life as it relates to sex and intimacy, whether associated with sex organs or not. Gender identity is one's self-concept with respect to being a male or female.

LO 24.4 *Describe the sexual response cycles of men and women:* The four phases in the female sexual response cycle are excitement, plateau, orgasm, and resolution. The phases consistently occur in this sequence, but the duration of each phase varies. The phases of the male sexual response are stimulation, erection, emission, ejaculation, and detumescence. After orgasm, males experience a refractory period during which they are physiologically incapable of having another orgasm. Because females do not have a refractory phase, they can have multiple orgasms.

LO 24.5 *Identify contraception options:* Contraceptive methods with varying degrees of effectiveness are available for males and females. They include abstinence, withdrawal of the penis before ejaculation, rhythm method, male and female condoms, spermicides, oral contraceptives, intrauterine devices, vaginal rings, hormonal injections or transdermal patches, diaphragms, cervical caps, emergency contraception, hysteroscopic sterilization, and surgical sterilization. Some methods require a prescription, whereas others do not.

LO 24.6 *Discuss sexually transmitted diseases and their causes and treatments:* Gonorrhea, syphilis, and chlamydia are caused by bacteria and can usually be treated and cured with antibiotics. Genital warts (caused by HPV) and genital herpes (due to herpes simplex) are caused by viruses; they can be treated but not cured. Human immunodeficiency virus is a blood-borne virus that may be acquired through sexual contact and exchange of bodily fluids; if untreated or unsuccessfully treated, HIV infection progresses to AIDS. The survival time for patients with AIDS has improved with the use of HAART.

LO 24.7 *Summarize factors that affect sexuality:* Family values and beliefs, culture, religion, self-concept, body image, previous experiences, cognition, environment, personal expectations, and ethics all affect a person's acceptance and expression of sexuality.

LO 24.8 *List factors that affect sexual function:* Underlying disease processes and injury can have a negative impact on sexual function, as can medications and relationship issues such as differences in value systems, communication issues, and control issues. Lifestyle factors such as work issues, family responsibilities, lack of time or sleep, and developmental and self-concept concerns are additional stressors that may lead to sexual dysfunction.

LO 24.9 *Recognize the impact of family dynamics on sexuality:* Age, ethnicity, culture, religion, and values affect a family's ability to communicate about sexual issues and the family members' choices regarding abortion, sterilization, contraception, and sexual preferences. The family's decision-making style, whether decisions are made by one partner or by the couple, may affect the partners' sexual practices. Sexual expression and satisfaction are enhanced in relationships in which decision-making power is shared.

LO 24.10 *Implement a sexual assessment:* Sexual health assessment is an integral component of a total health history and physical exam.

LO 24.11 *List nursing diagnoses appropriate for the care of patients with potential or identified sexuality concerns:* Sexual Dysfunction and Ineffective Sexuality Patterns are the most commonly identified nursing diagnoses for concerns arising from sexuality.

LO 24.12 *Develop a patient-centered care plan designed to address sexuality needs:* A patient's individualized plan evolves as the nurse uses the knowledge gained while gathering the patient's sexual health history, along with the experience of the nurse in dealing with sexual concerns. Ethical and legal standards associated with sexual issues must be maintained by the nurse during this phase.

LO 24.13 *Implement interventions to support enhanced patient sexuality before evaluating their effectiveness:* Nurses may provide sexual health teaching on topics such as sex education, safe sex practices, contraceptive use, and self-examination techniques to assist patients in attaining their identified goals and outcomes. Documentation of patient outcomes should be noted in the electronic health record.

Answers to the critical-thinking questions are available at *http://evolve.elsevier.com/YoostCrawford/fundamentals/*.

REVIEW QUESTIONS

1. For which reason are patients unlikely to introduce the topic of sex with health care providers?
   a. Most patients have few, if any, questions or problems relating to this topic.
   b. They are too embarrassed to discuss the topic of sex with a health care provider.
   c. Female patients prefer to discuss problems with female health care providers.
   d. They assume that health care professionals know little about sexual functioning.
2. A patient who had a hysterectomy 3 days ago says to the nurse, "I no longer feel like a real woman." Which response by the nurse would be most appropriate?
   a. "Don't worry about that. The feeling will probably go away."
   b. "You should talk to your doctor about how you feel."
   c. "I don't blame you. I would feel like half a woman also."
   d. "I hear your concern. Tell me more about your feelings."
3. When a patient reports having dyspareunia, which question is it most appropriate for the nurse to ask?
   a. "Have you talked with your partner about this discomfort?"
   b. "Have you had these spasms since you became sexually active?"
   c. "Does the bleeding continue longer than 5 days?"
   d. "Do your breasts swell up large enough for you to need a larger bra?"
4. A 75-year-old male patient reports decreased frequency of sexual intercourse, although he does not express dissatisfaction or difficulty. He seems a little embarrassed by the discussion, but is engaged and asks some questions. Which nursing diagnosis does the nurse determine is most appropriate for this patient?
   a. *Sexual Dysfunction*
   b. *Disturbed Body Image*
   c. *Sedentary Lifestyle*
   d. *Readiness for Enhanced Knowledge*
5. In using the PLISSIT model, what is the first action initiated by the nurse?
   a. Present basic information about sexual functioning.
   b. Ask permission to begin the sexual assessment.
   c. Inquire about any medications the patient is taking.
   d. Ask the patient about sexual activity and practices.
6. Which statement is the best resource for the nurse to use when determining appropriate nursing care for a transsexual patient?
   a. Gender identity is altered by acute psychosis.
   b. Sexual attraction is to people of both genders.
   c. Gonadal gender, internal organs, and external genitals are contradictory.
   d. Anatomy associated with sexual identity is not consistent with gender identity.
7. When a patient is beginning a regimen of an antidepressant medication, which information should the nurse include in the medication teaching as it pertains to sexuality?
   a. "Your partner will be pleased because your sexual functioning is going to improve."
   b. "You may find that your desire for sex will decrease while on this medication."
   c. "Your skin will probably become supersensitive to touch, so you may need to change your activity during sex."
   d. "You will be unable to have an erection while taking your antidepressants."
8. When teaching female reproduction to a group of high school students, the nurse uses what term to indicate the cessation of a woman's menstrual activity?
   a. Menarche
   b. Menopause
   c. Premenstrual syndrome
   d. Menstrual dysfunction
9. When teaching the patient mechanical barriers for birth control, the nurse would include which method?
   a. Diaphragm
   b. Transdermal patch
   c. Hormone injection
   d. Oral contraceptives
10. While performing a physical assessment on a female patient, the nurse finds several bruises on the patient's inner thighs that are in various stages of healing and suspects that the patient may be a victim of sexual abuse. What should be the nurse's first action?
    a. Refer the patient to a sexual counselor.
    b. Tell the patient about the safe house for women.
    c. Ask the patient to describe how she got the bruises.
    d. Report the abuse immediately to the proper authorities.

Answers and rationales for the review questions are available at *http://evolve.elsevier.com/YoostCrawford/fundamentals/*.

REFERENCES

Alfaro-Lefevre R: *Applying nursing process: The foundation for clinical reasoning*, ed. 8, Philadelphia, 2014, Lippincott.

Centers for Disease Control and Prevention: Sexually transmitted diseases (STDs), 2014. Retrieved from *www.cdc.gov/std/default.htm*.

Cronenwett L, Sherwood G, Barnsteiner J, et al: Quality and safety education for nurses. *Nurs Outlook*, 55(3):122-131, 2007.

Eisenberg ME, Bernat DH, Bearinger LH, Resnick MD: Support for comprehensive sexuality education: Perspectives from parents of school-age youth. *J Adolesc Health*, 42:352-359, 2008.

Green R: Gender identity disorders. In B Sadock, V Sadock, P Ruiz (Eds), *Kaplan and Sadock's comprehensive textbook of psychiatry*, ed. 9, Philadelphia, 2009, Lippincott Williams & Wilkins.

Katz A: Do ask, do tell. *Am J Nurs*, 105(7):66-68, 2005.

Lewis-O'Connor A: The evolution of SANE/SART—are there differences? *J ForensNurs* 5(4):220-227, 2009.

Masters W, Johnson V: *Human sexual response*. Philadelphia, 1966, Lippincott Williams & Wilkins.

NANDA International: *Nursing diagnoses: Definitions and classification, 2012–2014*, West Sussex, England, 2012, Wiley-Blackwell.

Nusbaum M, Lenahan P, Sadovsky R: Sexual health in aging men and women: Addressing the physiologic and psychological sexual changes that occur with age. *Geriatrics*, 60(9):18, 2005.

Planned Parenthood: Sexually transmitted diseases (STDs), 2014. Retrieved from *www.plannedparenthood.org/health-topics/stds-hiv-safer-sex-101.htm*.

Plichta S, Clements P, Houseman C: (2007). Why SANEs matter: Models of care for sexual violence victims in the emergency department. *J Forens Nurs*, 3(1):15-23, 2007.

Rhodes K, Frankel R, Levinthal N, et al: Improving patient care. "You're not a victim of domestic violence, are you?" Provider-patient communication about domestic violence. *Ann Intern Med*, 147(9):620-627, 2007.

Wallace, M. (2008). Assessment of sexual health in older adults. *Am J Nurs*, 108(7):52-61, 2008.

Yonaka L, Yoder M, Darrow J, Sherck J: Barriers to screening for domestic violence in the emergency department. *J Contin Educ Nurs*, 38(1):37-45, 2007.

CHAPTER 25

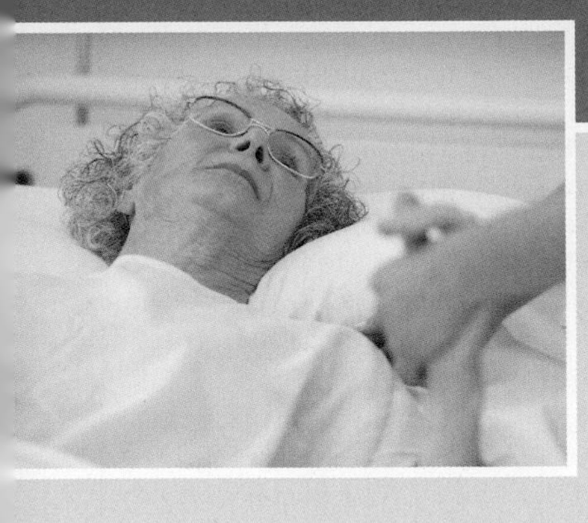

Safety

EVOLVE WEBSITE

http://evolve.elsevier.com/YoostCrawford/fundamentals/

- Additional Evolve-Only Review Questions With Answers
- Answers and Rationales for Text Review Questions
- Answers to Critical-Thinking Questions
- Case Study With Questions
- Video Skills Clips
- Conceptual Care Map Creator
- Skill Checklist
- Glossary

LEARNING OUTCOMES

Comprehension of this chapter's content will provide students with the ability to:

LO 25.1 Discuss safety concerns in the home, community, and health care environments.
LO 25.2 List factors that affect safety.
LO 25.3 Explain situations that alter safety in the home, community, and health care settings.
LO 25.4 Identify safety factors that affect individuals at home, in the community, and in health care settings.
LO 25.5 Choose nursing diagnoses relevant to patient safety–related concerns and issues.
LO 25.6 Prepare nursing care plans that identify interventions to promote patient safety.
LO 25.7 Implement safety measures in the home, community, and health care settings.

KEY TERMS

abuse, p. 465
accidents, p. 461
Ambu bag, p. 476
bioterrorism, p. 466
carbon monoxide, p. 465
Centers for Medicare and Medicaid Services, p. 466
chemical restraint, p. 466
electrical shock, p. 465
falls, p. 476
intentional injuries, p. 461
The Joint Commission, p. 461
lead poisoning, p. 464
physical restraint, p. 466
poisoning, p. 464
RACE, p. 474
safety, p. 460
suffocation, p. 466
toxins, p. 464
unintentional injuries, p. 460
unintentional poisoning, p. 464

CASE STUDY

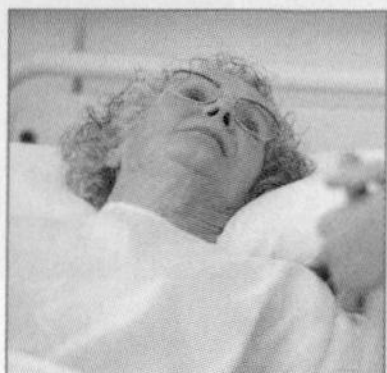

Mrs. Stein is an 88-year-old female who was admitted last night to the hospital from a local nursing home. Her symptoms include fever (T 38.2° C [100.8° F]), increasing confusion, and weakness. Her initial admitting diagnosis was pneumonia with bilateral pulmonary infiltrates. Her medical history includes hypertension and osteoarthritis, and she has fallen twice in the past month at the nursing home. The patient is allergic to heparin and is full-code status.

Mrs. Stein's last vital signs were T 37.4° C (99.3° F), P 85 and regular, R 28 and slightly labored, BP 156/95, O_2 saturation of 95% on 2 L/min of oxygen by nasal cannula. She does not answer when asked if she is in pain. She is oriented to person only and is pleasantly confused and mumbling about her young children. The top side rails are raised to assist in turning and positioning, and her bilateral, untied mitts are in place. No redness or irritation at the mitt site was observed on intermittent release. Her Johns Hopkins Hospital fall risk assessment score is 21, and her Braden Scale score is 17. The evening nurse begins rounds and, on entering the room, finds Mrs. Stein incontinent of loose stool and trying to climb out of bed.

Medication orders are as follows:

- Rocephin: 1 g intravenous piggyback (IVPB) daily for pneumonia
- Albuterol and atrovent nebulizer treatments: q 6 hr for pneumonia
- Guaifenesin: 600 mg PO qid for pneumonia
- Lisinopril: 5 mg PO daily for hypertension
- IV normal saline: 0.9% at 100 mL/hr
- Acetaminophen: 625 mg PO q 6 hr PRN for arthritic or pleuritic chest pain rating of 3 to 6
- Dilaudid: 0.5 to 1.0 mg IVP q 2 hr PRN for pleuritic chest pain rating of 7 to 10
- Ativan: 0.5 to 1.0 mg IVP q 8 hr PRN for agitation

Treatment orders are as follows:

- Vital signs: q 4 hr, including O_2 sat
- Activity: Out of bed (OOB) to chair or bedside commode *only*
- Diet: No added salt
- CBC every morning
- O_2 up to 3 L/min by nasal cannula to keep O_2 sat greater than or equal to 92%
- Incentive spirometry q 1 hr while awake
- Bilateral mitt restraints

Refer back to this case study to answer the critical-thinking exercises throughout the chapter.

Safety, which is the condition of being free from physical or psychological harm and injury, is a global concern. Individuals in every setting and location care about safety. This chapter addresses the environmental safety concerns of individuals in communities and home environments and explores the key principles of maintaining patient safety in health care settings.

Nurses play a critical role in teaching patients and their families how to maintain safety in their homes and communities. In addition to promoting safe delivery of patient care, nurses need to be concerned with their own safety in the working environment. This chapter highlights practical safety concerns in the environment that may exist for nurses who are practicing in a variety of settings. The nursing process provides a framework for the assessment, diagnosis, planning interventions, and evaluation of patient safety goals across settings.

SAFETY IN THE HOME, COMMUNITY, AND HEALTH CARE SETTINGS LO 25.1

The Centers for Disease Control and Prevention (CDC) foster safe and healthful environments by working with partners nationally and worldwide. A branch of the CDC, the National Center for Health Statistics (NCHS), is instrumental in detecting and investigating health problems of the U.S. population. In 2007, the NCHS found that unintentional injuries were the fifth leading cause of death in the U.S. population (Xu, Murphy, Kochanek, et al, 2010), following heart disease, cancer, stroke, and chronic lower respiratory diseases. **Unintentional injuries** result from incidents such as falls, motor vehicle crashes, poisonings, drownings, fire-associated injuries, suffocation by ingested objects, and firearms. Injuries and poisonings can have nonfatal consequences requiring medical care. For example, according to the National Health Interview Survey (NHIS)—a nationwide annual survey of approximately 36,000 households of the noninstitutionalized civilian population conducted by the NCHS and administered by the U.S. Census Bureau—the rate of injuries and poisonings requiring medical attention was 115.7 per 1000 individuals in the U.S. population from 1997 through 2007 (Chen, Warner, Fingerhut, et al, 2009).

In response to the fatal and nonfatal consequences of injuries, the CDC established in 1992 a federal agency called the National Center for Injury Prevention and Control (NCIPC), which works to reduce injury, disability, death, and the costs associated with injuries. The NCIPC studies intentional and unintentional injuries. **Intentional injuries** typically result from deliberate acts of violence or abuse and often have fatal consequences such as suicide and homicide. The risk factors and prevention mechanisms for intentional injuries are better understood than those of unintentional injuries. Unintentional injuries are often referred to as **accidents**, which are incidents that occur at random and may be unavoidable. However, after the study of unintentional injuries for almost two decades, the term *accident* has fallen from favor because the patterns of unintentional injuries are often predictable and, in some cases, preventable.

Beyond the community focus on injury prevention is the large concern about safety in the rapidly changing health care environment. More than a decade ago, *To Err Is Human* introduced the modern patient safety movement and pointed out the problem of medical errors in hospitals (Wachter, 2010). During the past decade, many organizations such as **The Joint Commission** (TJC), an independent, not-for-profit group in the United States that accredits hospitals and other health care–related agencies, have focused on the goal of patient safety. In 2003, TJC developed the first set of performance standards addressing crucial elements of operations related to patient safety. Known as the National Patient Safety Goals (NPSGs), these standards are reevaluated every year. Each goal has specific elements of performance that the health care worker is required to meet. Several NPSGs for 2014 (TJC, 2014) pertain to material in this chapter:

- Identify patients correctly.
- Improve staff communication.
- Use medicines safely.
- Use alarms safely.
- Prevent infection.
- Identify patient safety risks.
- Prevent mistakes in surgery.

QSEN FOCUS!

The nurse demonstrates safety by using strategies to reduce the risk of harm to self and others and by valuing the nurse's role in preventing errors.

The largest proportion of health care workers consists of nurses, and schools of nursing have increasingly emphasized a focus on patient safety in classroom and clinical courses. In 2005, the Robert Wood Johnson Foundation funded the Quality and Safety Education for Nurses (QSEN) project with an overarching goal of preparing nurses of the future with the knowledge, skills, and attitudes needed to advance quality and safety on the job in their health care settings. A definition provided by the QSEN project states that safety "minimizes risk of harm to patients and providers through system effectiveness and individual performance" (Cronenwett, Sherwood, Barnsteiner, et al, 2007).

QSEN FOCUS!

Knowledge, skills, and attitudes concerning safety are demonstrated when the nurse (1) discusses the impact of national patient safety resources, initiatives, and regulations; (2) uses national patient safety resources for professional development and as a means of focusing attention on safety in care settings; and (3) values the relationship between national safety campaigns and implementation in local practice settings.

FACTORS AFFECTING SAFETY LO 25.2

Many factors affect the safety of people, including personal characteristics and those in home, community, and workplace environments, particularly in health care settings. In all settings, reduction of risk and prevention of accidents is the overall goal.

INDIVIDUAL FACTORS

Individual factors that affect personal safety include those related to the functioning of body systems and those associated with an individual's lifestyle. Each person's risk for injury are different based on many internal and external factors.

Body System Integrity

Normal functioning of the musculoskeletal, neurologic, cardiopulmonary, renal, hepatic, and integumentary systems is essential for individual safety. Impairment of any component of the musculoskeletal system can restrict range of motion and diminish strength, producing a loss of balance and an unsteady gait. These changes can affect overall mobility, including the ability to transfer, stand, and walk. Limitations in mobility increase the propensity for falling.

The neurologic system includes cognitive (mental) ability and sensory perception, both of which are critical for safe functioning of individuals and their interactions with the environment. When changes in mental status occur, judgment may become altered, and safety awareness may become compromised. For example, an older adult with loss of short-term memory may forget to turn off the stove, increasing the risk of fire, or may neglect to use an assistive device when dressing or ambulating, escalating the risk of falling. Alterations of the five senses (i.e., vision, hearing, touch, smell, and taste) can produce safety risks. For example, an adult with chronic allergic rhinitis and numerous recurrent sinus infections may have a diminished sense of smell and be unable to recognize that something is burning. Nurses should exercise caution when using heat and cold therapy in patients with altered sensation to prevent burns and tissue damage.

A compromised cardiopulmonary system can impair perfusion, resulting in symptoms such as shortness of breath and chest pain, which can lead to activity intolerance. Inactivity can lead to an unsafe drop in blood pressure with position changes, a condition called *orthostatic hypotension.* Safety concerns arise when the patient has difficulty tolerating or performing routine activities of daily living. For example, depending on the level of cardiopulmonary compromise, an individual may be unable to safely use the toilet, bathe, sit, stand, and walk. A person in this condition may not be able to evacuate a burning building rapidly enough to avoid sustaining burn-related injuries.

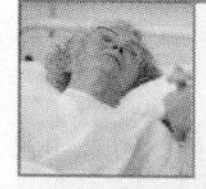

1. Mrs. Stein is at risk for orthostatic hypotension. Describe how to assess her for this condition, and list the nursing interventions for orthostatic hypotension.

Detoxification and excretion of medications occurs in the hepatic and renal systems. Impairment of these systems can lead to symptoms of toxicity, which depend on the drugs but can include cognitive and physical changes. Injury to the integumentary system can make a person more susceptible to infections, because the body's protective barrier has been altered.

Life Span Factors

Age and developmental issues can influence the safety of individuals across the life span. Infants should be placed in a supine position for safe sleeping to decrease the likelihood of sudden infant death syndrome. An infant should never be left unattended. Appropriate rear-facing car seats and carriers should be used correctly. Children older than 1 year of age who outgrow the weight or height limit of the rear-facing seat should ride in forward-facing car seats in the backseat (Parents Central, 2014).

Other safety concerns are discussed in the Diversity Considerations box.

In adulthood, life stressors such as financial concerns, work-related demands, and efforts to balance work with family life are common challenges that can take a physical toll on the body. Individuals should plan relaxation periods or vacations and should schedule annual visits to a health care provider to screen for elevations in blood pressure and cholesterol levels, headaches, depression, and lung disease in smokers.

ENVIRONMENTAL FACTORS

A person's environment includes the home, outdoors, workplace, community, and settings in which care is provided. For individuals to remain safe and healthful in their environment, a variety of factors must be considered and good practices maintained.

Pollution

Pollution is the contamination of air, land, water, and the environment (e.g., noise) by unnatural or harmful substances. Safety concerns are the ill-health effects that result from exposure to pollution. For example, air pollution caused by the release of chemicals or by-products of manufacturing into the atmosphere can increase the risk of chronic lung disease and some cancers. Other forms of air pollution include cigarette smoke and exhaust fumes from vehicles, which can produce allergic symptoms.

Land pollution by the improper disposal of trash or waste can be reduced by reusing and recycling materials and packaging. Land pollution is not limited to littering. Industrial and agricultural waste is associated with birth defects and cancer. Water can become polluted through improper refuse disposal, animal waste, and industrial by-products, resulting in infection and other disease.

Noise pollution from sources such as factories, construction sites, trains, planes, loud music, and cheering in sports stadiums is a real concern. Some of the health effects resulting from noise pollution include hearing loss, stress, and elevated blood pressure.

The best resource for pollution-related concerns and solutions is the Environmental Protection Agency (EPA). The EPA has been in existence since 1970, striving to protect the environment and human health.

Lighting

Inadequate lighting presents safety concerns in home, work, community, and health care environments. For an individual to safely and successfully navigate pathways and perform various activities while avoiding potential obstacles and hazards, the environment must be well illuminated. Well-lit, glare-free halls, stairways, rooms, and work spaces help to reduce the risk of tripping, slipping, and falling. Night-lights reduce the risk of injuries to children, guests, and older adults.

Communicable Diseases

Communicable diseases are transmittable from one individual directly to another, usually through blood or body fluid exposure or through vectors such as insects and spores. Chapter 26 discusses the transmission of communicable diseases. In addition to guidelines that are set on a national level by the CDC, most states have programs for communicable disease surveillance and prevention in their departments of health. For example, the State of Maryland has the Office of Epidemiology and Disease Control Program (EDCP). Usually, a major component of these programs is immunization to prevent disease, such as annual influenza vaccinations.

Workplace Hazards

Some adults spend as much as 40% to 50% of their waking hours at work. As the Baby Boomer generation ages, the population of older adults in the workforce is increasing. Adults and older adults encounter hazards in the workplace and are at risk for injuries that need care in a variety of settings, such as primary care offices, urgent care clinics, and emergency departments. Workplace safety and injury

DIVERSITY CONSIDERATIONS

Life Span

Infants, Toddlers, and Preschoolers

- Parents should be taught to check with the U.S. Consumer Product Safety Commission for information on approved cribs, devices, and toys.
  - Slats on cribs can pose strangulation or entrapment hazards.
  - Paint on toys may cause lead or other chemical poisoning.
- Parents need to childproof the home environment by using child locks for cabinets, childproof caps on medication bottles to prevent poisoning, stairway gates, and safety plugs for electrical outlets; putting padding on or removing furniture with sharp edges and corners; and keeping sharp and dangerous items out of reach.
- Choking or asphyxiation can occur from toys, objects, or foods (e.g., hot dogs, grapes) that block airways. Small objects should be kept out of reach, and food should be cut in small pieces.
- Strangulation is a risk from cords on curtains and blinds. Cord-free window treatments are available and should be used.
- Liquids that are pretty colors and taste sweet, such as fluid medications and antifreeze, should be kept out of reach and secured.
- Swimming pools must be fenced and locked. All children should wear life jackets when near or in lakes and pools.
- Very young children are more sensitive to heat than are adults due to their smaller body surface area, and they can become dehydrated more easily. Adequate fluids should be provided on hot days, and children should *never* be left unattended in vehicles.

School-Age Children

- Drowning is a risk. Children should not be allowed to swim without adult supervision, and they should wear life jackets.
- Trampoline use can cause injury and death. Secure netting is necessary, as is adult supervision. Flips and tricks should not be allowed. Only children 6 years old or older should be permitted on a trampoline.
- Skating and bicycling accidents can cause injuries and deaths. Children should wear appropriately fitted helmets and knee and elbow protectors while skating, skateboarding, sledding, and riding a bike.

Adolescents and Teenagers

- Some teens experiment with the use of nicotine, drugs, and alcohol. Intentional and unintentional poisonings can occur in this group. Parents need to be alert to signs and symptoms of depression, poisoning, and drug use.
- Sexual curiosity and experimentation occur in this population. Conversations about safe sexual practices, including the consequences of unprotected sex, such as pregnancy and sexually transmitted infections, are important.
- Motor vehicle crashes are common. Safety courses, driver's education, use of seatbelts, and avoidance of cell phone use, texting, and other distractions while driving are important.
- Parents should be advised to limit violence exposure from television, the Internet, and movies.

Adults

- Work-related hazards can result in injuries and death (see section on Workplace Hazards).
- Use of illicit substances and overdoses or poisoning from illegal and prescription drugs are a concern. Tobacco use should be avoided.
- Use of drugs or alcohol while driving can result in motor vehicle crashes.
- Unprotected sex and multiple sexual partners may lead to sexually transmitted diseases, including human immunodeficiency virus (HIV) infection.

Older Adults

- The physiologic changes that occur in the body systems with aging put older adults at risk for events such as motor vehicle crashes, falls, and burns.
- Falls are common in the older adult population.
  - Basic strategies, such as removal of obstacles from walking paths indoors and outdoors, including ice from walkways, can help prevent falls.
  - To prevent falls and their subsequent injuries, nurses share many strategies with older adults (see section on Fall Prevention).
- Vision and hearing screenings are recommended for older adults.
- Medication safety precautions (e.g., using pill dispensers and taking medications in a well-lit area) should be employed to prevent incorrect or inadequate dosing and inadvertent overdosing.
- Because older adults may be sensitive to heat and cold, caution should be taken to avoid hypothermia and hyperthermia. Thermometers can be used to check water temperatures in baths and showers to avoid scald burns.
- Driving refresher and safety courses should be explored through the state department of motor vehicles.

prevention are concerns for nursing and other health care professionals.

A unique and sometimes complex set of safety issues exists in each work environment. Depending on the occupation, safety concerns range from work at dangerous heights to exposure to chemicals and hazardous fumes or dust (e.g., asphalt, asbestos) to the ergonomic issues of repetitive motion and heavy lifting. To address safety concerns, the Occupational Safety and Health Administration (OSHA) was established in 1970 to provide employers with guidelines for preventing exposure to hazardous chemicals and hazardous situations and reducing the risk of injury in the workplace. Some workplace settings are particularly hazardous. In 2008, the agriculture, forestry, fishing, and hunting industries topped the death rates with 29 fatalities per 100,000 workers, followed by mining with 21.1, transportation and warehousing with 13, and construction with 8.9 (National Safety Council, 2010). Almost 3 million nonfatal occupational injuries and illnesses occurred in 2012 (Bureau of Labor Statistics, 2013).

In the field of safety science, occupational safety officers work in conjunction with occupational health nurses to promote a healthy, hazard-free workplace. The National Institute for Occupational Safety and Health (NIOSH), a federal agency within the CDC, was established to conduct research and recommend interventions for the prevention of work-related injury and illness.

In the hospital setting, the financial cost of wages lost from employee injuries and safety violations continues to rise (Peled, 2005). In nursing, some well-documented areas of occupational health and safety concerns include needlestick injuries, back and neck injuries resulting from lifting, and patient-on-nurse violence. Factors that contribute to these injuries include lack of appropriate equipment to ensure nurse and patient safety, rising numbers of more acutely ill patients without adequate increases in nurse staffing, an increasingly obese patient population, and lack of staff familiarity with facility safety protocols or a lack of protocols. Long shifts (13 to 15 hr/ day) and workweeks (50 to 60 hr/wk) affect the overall health of nurses and the safety of patients (Trinkoff, Geiger-Brown, Brady, et al, 2006).

PATIENT SAFETY CONCERNS

Concerns related to patient safety in a health care agency are detailed throughout this chapter. Two different examples are fires and the use of restraints. Fires occurring in health care settings usually result from the use of flammable gases, such as anesthetics and oxygen, or electrical equipment, such as heating or cooling devices, respiratory devices, beds, and monitors. The use of physical and chemical restraints in health care settings generates concerns about patient safety and ethical treatment.

ALTERED SAFETY LO 25.3

Nurses are in a position to educate patients about safety issues in inpatient, outpatient, home, and community settings. Prevention of injuries is the overarching goal, and providing patients with safety information gives them the tools needed to ensure their own safety.

ALTERED SAFETY IN THE HOME AND COMMUNITY

Keeping individuals safe in their homes or communities depends on the prevention of illness and injury. A particular concern at home and in the community is food safety, which requires cooking food to appropriate temperatures, carefully monitoring expiration dates, using proper storage methods, and paying attention to food safety recalls announced in the media.

Another concern is the prevention of injuries resulting from motorized and nonmotorized means of transportation and recreation. Available education programs and safety gear are recommended for biking, motorcycling, skating, and driving. Each of these activities has unique environmental factors (e.g., traffic, obstacles, weather) that must be considered for the activity to be undertaken safely.

Equipment in or around the house can present another safety concern. For example, guns should be used only after training and with proper permits; when not in use, they should be locked away, with ammunition removed. Lawn mowers should be operated only while wearing sturdy, laced or Velcro, nonslip shoes and after review of the manufacturer's safety instructions. Specific home and community safety concerns are discussed in the following sections.

Poisoning

Poisoning involves the intentional or unintentional ingestion, inhalation, injection, or absorption through the skin of any substance harmful to the body. This section focuses on **unintentional poisoning**, an act in which the person did not mean to inflict harm by taking or giving the substance; this includes an inadvertent overdose. Unintentional poisoning is a pervasive problem in the United States resulting in emergency department visits and unintentional death. Nurses need to be able to distinguish poisoning from other conditions that it may mimic, such as alcohol intoxication, seizure, stroke, and insulin reaction (Mayo Clinic, 2012).

Toxins

Toxins are substances that can poison or harm individuals or other living organisms through mechanisms such as ingestion, inhalation, and dermatologic exposure. Poisoning is a particular concern because items containing toxins are commonly found in home settings and community environments. Potentially toxic items include medications (i.e., prescription and over-the-counter drugs), illegal drugs, indoor and outdoor plants, pesticides, detergents and other household cleaners, antifreeze, lead, and carbon monoxide.

Lead

Lead poisoning is a public health issue. It occurs when lead levels build up in blood over months or years, and it can affect all body systems. When lead levels are greater than 10 μg of lead/dL of blood, the CDC recommends initiation of public health actions (CDC, 2014b). These blood lead levels are a common occurrence in children 1 to 5 years of age because of exposure to lead-based paint in older buildings and toys. A study by *healthytoys.org* found lead in 20% of the items tested (Colorado Nurses Association, 2009). This finding is of particular concern because lead exposure can irreversibly damage the nervous system and impair development in children.

In addition to lead-based paints in toys, buildings, and ceramic dishes, sources of lead include water from lead pipes or pipes soldered with lead, gasoline or soil contaminated by gasoline, and household dust that may contain paint chips or soil (Mayo Clinic, 2014).

Carbon Monoxide

Carbon monoxide is a colorless, odorless gas that can cause sudden illness and death. It is a leading cause of unintentional poisoning deaths in the United States. Sources of carbon monoxide are combustible fumes produced by automobiles, stoves, gas ranges, portable generators, lanterns, burning charcoal and wood, and heating systems. Carbon monoxide can build up in enclosed spaces, such as in trucks and cars, and in semi-enclosed spaces, such as rooms of houses. Symptoms of carbon monoxide poisoning include dizziness, lightheadedness, and nausea. Death can occur if exposure in an enclosed area is prolonged.

Plants

Although plants used in and around the home and community for decorative purposes can be quite beautiful, some that grow in populated areas are hazards (e.g., philodendron, poison ivy). Because many trees and plants can be poisonous, it is important to keep small children away from them and ensure that children are adequately supervised when encountering them. Resources are available outlining dangerous plants, shrubs, and trees, including lists for specific geographic regions. The safest strategy is to avoid touching or ingesting them unless they are known to be nonpoisonous.

Medications

In the home and community setting, medications present another potential safety hazard that can result in intentional or unintentional poisoning. Medication dosage must be adjusted for children and older adults. Safe medication dosages for children are usually based on the number of milligrams of drug per kilogram of body weight. Children have lower body weights and differences in metabolism and excretion compared with adults. Older adults may have a decline in organ function resulting in slower metabolism and excretion of drugs.

Other important safety considerations include keeping medications secured in child-resistant containers or out of reach. For older adults, pharmacists often recommend "starting low and going slow." Older adults should understand how and when to take medications to avoid underdosing or overdosing. A medication schedule, including reminders, can help. All medications that are old, have been discontinued, or are expired should be properly disposed of and not shared with others.

In the home, the U.S. Food and Drug Administration (FDA) recommends following directions on the medication bottle for disposal or taking unused medications to community take-back programs. If no instructions are on the label and no take-back program is available, most medications can be thrown in the household trash. The drugs should be mixed with an undesirable substance such as coffee grounds or kitty litter to make them less appealing to children and unrecognizable to someone who may go through the trash. The mixture should be placed in a jar, sealable plastic bag, or can, and the container should be put in the trash (FDA, 2013).

In health care facilities, red sharps containers are available in every room for safe disposal of used needles, which prevents needlestick injuries. Some facilities have similar containers in other colors for disposal of other nonhazardous and hazardous medication waste. These color-coded containers facilitate safe disposal of pills, solutions, vials, and patches.

Household Chemicals

Common toxins found in the home include household chemicals such as cleansers (e.g., detergents, ammonia, bleach), adhesives (e.g., glues), hair sprays and dyes, furniture polish, insect repellants, and gasoline. All chemicals should be kept secured and out of reach of children and older adults with cognitive impairment. Household chemicals should be used with care and according to manufacturers' instructions.

Fires and Electrical Hazards

Fire safety is an important concern in residential environments. In the United States in 2011, there were approximately 364,500 fires, resulting in 2450 deaths and 13,900 injuries (U.S. Fire Administration, 2014a). Of fire-related deaths, 80% occur in the home, and smoking is the leading cause. Cooking is another important cause of house fires (Ahrens, 2011). Candles, kerosene heaters, faulty electrical equipment and wiring, and children playing with lighters and matches are other common causes.

An **electrical shock** occurs when a person comes in contact with an energy source and the energy flows through the body or portion of the body to the ground. Exposure to the electrical energy source can result in no injury, burn injuries, contractures, or death from cardiac and respiratory arrest. In the home setting, electrical hazards exist from overloaded electrical circuits, use of appliances near sinks and tubs (i.e., sources of water), and use of lighting or appliances with frayed wires or electrical cords. Open or uncovered electrical outlets are potential hazards for small, curious children.

Abuse

Abuse is anything offensive, harmful, or injurious to an individual that can pose a direct safety threat. The four major types of abuse are physical, psychological or emotional, sexual, and financial. Abuse can occur in all socioeconomic, gender, age, and cultural groups, but some portions of the population are more vulnerable. Abuse is discussed further in Chapters 17 and 18.

Bioterrorism

Before the outbreak of anthrax among U.S. postal workers after the terrorist attacks of September 11, 2001, emergency preparedness in health care and nursing was not the focus that it is today. **Bioterrorism** is the deliberate release of biologic agents such as bacteria, viruses, and other microbes to cause illness or kill people, animals, or plants (CDC, 2007). These biologic agents are dispersed through the air or spread through infection of animals, contamination of food or water supplies, person-to-person contact, or contact with a contaminated object (Federal Emergency Management Agency, 2012). Two common forms of bioterrorism are anthrax and smallpox.

Suffocation and Drowning

Suffocation results when air no longer reaches the lungs and respiration ceases. Common causes of suffocation are smothering, drowning, and choking. In the United States from 2000 through 2006, two thirds of deaths of children younger than 1 year of age were caused by injury resulting from suffocation (Borse, Gilchrist, Dellinger, et al, 2008). The risk of smothering increased by co-sleeping and with the use of pillows and blankets. Curious toddlers are an at-risk group for suffocation due to choking on food (e.g., hot dogs, popcorn), foreign objects lodged in the trachea, and plastic bags placed over the face.

Unintentional deaths also occur as a result of playing the choking game, which has been on the rise among school-age children and teens. This game is a dangerous activity in which individuals choke each other or use a noose to choke themselves to achieve a brief high. From 1995 through 2007, 82 deaths are suspected to have resulted from this activity in the United States in the 6- to- 19-year-old age group (Toblin, Paulozzi, Gilchrist, et al, 2008).

Among older adults, death can occur from choking on food lodged in the trachea as a result of difficulties with chewing and swallowing. Risk factors include ill-fitting dentures and many comorbid conditions such as stroke and dementia.

In the United States between 2000 and 2006, suffocation by drowning was the leading cause of injury-related death of children between 1 and 4 years of age (Borse, Gilchrist, Dellinger, et al, 2008). This age group is at particular risk for drowning due to lack of supervision of children in bathtubs and swimming pools. The risk of drowning is increased among adults who do not use approved life jackets, who swim alone, who swim in hazardous conditions, or who swim under the influence of alcohol.

ALTERED SAFETY IN HEALTH CARE AGENCIES

Falls

Although patient falls have been a safety concern for the past three decades, the lack of financial reimbursement for them has made fall prevention a priority issue for hospitals. The **Centers for Medicare and Medicaid Services** (CMS) no longer makes payments to hospitals for the cost of additional care resulting from patient falls because they are considered reasonably preventable. The CMS is the federal organization that certifies all Medicare- and Medicaid-participating hospitals, which are facilities for acute care, psychiatric and rehabilitation services, and long-term care, as well as children's hospitals and treatment centers for alcohol and chemical dependence.

Restraints

Federal government and accrediting agencies have spent more than two decades working to reduce or eliminate the use of restraints in patient care environments. The Omnibus Budget Reconciliation Act of 1987, enacted in 1990 and revised in 2007, provides guidelines on restraint use for long-term care facilities. When facilities fail to comply with the guidelines for appropriate restraint use, citations and fines may be issued by state quality assurance boards or the CMS. The CMS includes guidelines for restraint use in its final rule on patient's rights (CMS, 2006).

Restraints may be physical or chemical. A **physical restraint** is a mechanical or physical device, such as material or equipment attached or adjacent to the patient's body, used to restrict movement (CMS 2006). Examples of physical restraints are wrist or ankle restraints, a jacket or vest, and side rails. A medication that is administered to a patient to control behavior is a **chemical restraint**.

Although restraints may be used by the nurse with the intent of preventing injury or harm to the patient, the staff, or others, there are inherent risks associated with restraint use. One of the biggest misconceptions is that physical restraints prevent injurious falls. Studies have disproved this belief, finding instead that fall-related injuries have increased with restraint use (Capezuti, Evans, Strumpf, et al, 1996; Capezuti, Strumpf, Evans, et al, 1998; Tinetti, Liu, and Ginter, 1992). Minor to major physiologic harm, including death, is associated with the use of physical restraints. Well-documented negative outcomes for the use of physical restraints include compromised circulation, impaired skin and tissue integrity (e.g., redness, skin tears, abrasions, pressure ulcers), incontinence, mental status changes, difficulty breathing, pneumonia, impaired hydration and nutrition, aspiration, strangulation, entrapment, muscle atrophy, reduced bone mass, contracture, fractures, and death.

Medication Administration Errors

Medication errors occur in many situations. Pronovost and colleagues (2003) found that 46% to 56% of preventable medication errors occur during transfers from nurse to nurse across units as well as across settings.

The lack of interdisciplinary collaboration and communication is a barrier to safe medication administration. Sound-alike or similarly spelled drug names are another area of concern for the safe administration of medication because the drugs often have widely different uses. Examples include Celebrex (arthritis medication) and Celexa (antidepressant), heparin (anticoagulant) and Hespan (plasma volume expander), and vincristine (chemotherapeutic agent) and vinblastine (different chemotherapeutic agent). Interruptions and distractions during medication administration contribute to medication errors.

Medications should be checked and double-checked in accordance with the six Rights of medication administration: the right drug, in the right dose, at the right time, to the right patient, by the right route, and with the right documentation. Chapter 35 discusses errors in medication administration and how to avoid them.

Radiation

Overexposure to radiation or radioactive materials used to diagnose and treat patients is a health hazard of concern for patients and health care professionals. Nurses at risk for radiation exposure are typically those who work with patients receiving radioactive iodine treatments, work in areas where special procedures are performed involving radiation, or are called to diagnostic areas to care for agitated patients during radiographic procedures. Excessive radiation exposure can cause injury to many body systems, including the gastrointestinal tract, skin, and reproductive organs. To prevent overexposure, hospitals and diagnostic imaging centers have detailed policies and procedures in place.

Nurses must be aware of diagnostic procedures that can increase the amount of radiation exposure to themselves and their patients. In addition to x-rays, a potential source of diagnostic radioactive exposure is positron emission tomography (PET), which uses energy released in the breakdown of radiopharmaceutical agents to monitor metabolic activity (Joint Commission Resources, 2007). Another source is computed tomography (CT), which provides incredibly accurate maps, or models, of bone and soft tissue through computer interpretation of multiple-sequenced images gathered by x-ray sensors that rotate around the body (Joint Commission Resources, 2007). PET and CT have been used for approximately 30 years to diagnose pathologic conditions, but only recently have the two been used in conjunction to provide incomparable diagnostic information, which has directed therapeutic treatment with much greater success (Devine and Mawlaw, 2010; Joint Commission Resources, 2007). Combined use of PET and CT creates some special radiation safety issues because each modality is a source of x-ray exposure. Diagnostic centers and hospitals performing PET/CT scanning should have updated policies and procedures to protect health care professionals and patients from overexposure.

Drug-Resistant Microorganisms

Several microorganisms have evolved strains that are resistant to common antibiotics. Methicillin-resistant *Staphylococcus aureus* (MRSA) causes skin and other organ infections, and it is extremely resistant to many antibiotics. It is often spread by contact with the skin of an infected person, or it can be spread by contact with infected objects. A community-associated form of MRSA can infect those who share close living quarters, and skin-to-skin contact is of concern for health care personnel, prison inmates, college dorm residents, team athletes, and military personnel. Resistant microorganisms are discussed in Chapter 26.

Procedural Errors

An example of a procedural error is the failure to properly identify a patient when entering a room to administer medication. Another example is leaving the bed in an elevated position after providing care or performing a procedure on a patient. Other procedural errors that have implications for patient safety are discussed in the section on Reduction of Procedure- and Equipment-Related Events.

◆ ASSESSMENT LO 25.4

Assessment for safety hazards and potential sources of injuries is an important first step in the nursing process. Evaluation includes the collection of subjective information related to the patient's symptoms and chief complaint, history of environmental hazards and exposures, and objective assessment with a focus on affected body systems. The nurse may discover information that provides clues to safety issues. While obtaining the patient's history, the nurse should inquire about causes of prior injuries and probe further into the topic when safety issues are raised. Questions that should be asked in regard to safety in the home and immediate environment are presented in the Health Assessment Questions box. The health history may reveal factors that place the patient at risk for safety concerns, and the physical assessment may reveal issues that should be further investigated.

The assessment of fall risk should be completed on admission to establish a baseline and repeated on a daily basis or with any change in the patient's condition. In any health care setting, assessment of fall risk includes personal factors (e.g., incontinence, unsteady gait) and environmental factors (e.g., tubes or drains, floor surfaces) (Hill, Nguyen, and Shaha, 2009). Many tools exist for the assessment of fall risk. The three most frequently used in hospital settings are the Johns Hopkins Hospital Fall Assessment Tool, the Morse Fall Scale, and the Hendrich II Fall Risk Model.

The Johns Hopkins Hospital Fall Assessment Tool (Figure 25-1) provides a snapshot of overall fall risk. This seven-item tool, which is used nationally and internationally in hospitals, can be completed quickly and easily by the nurse at the bedside. The tool accommodates the influence of advanced age, fall history, specific medication classes, patient care equipment that tethers, and mobility, cognitive, and elimination functions (Poe, Cvach, and Dawson, 2007). After this assessment is completed, an overall summary score is calculated; the higher the score, the greater the patient's risk of

HEALTH ASSESSMENT QUESTIONS

Safety in the Home

Health history and physical assessment should dictate specific safety questions:

- *Activities of daily living:* Do you require human or mechanical assistance with any of the following: walking, toileting, bathing, dressing, grooming, and eating? If yes, please describe the type of assistance you need.
- *Instrumental activities of daily living:* Do you require human or mechanical assistance with any of the following: cooking, cleaning and doing laundry, shopping, driving, and obtaining medications? If yes, please describe the type of assistance you need.
- *Medications:* Do you know how and when to take your medications? Do you know why you take them? Do you take your medications consistently? Have you been experiencing any side effects? If yes, describe them.
- *Health issues:* Do you have any injuries or health issues that place you at risk for falling or for drowsiness? Have you ever had a seizure?
- *Safety issues:* Do you have any safety concerns? Do you have a history of falling? Do you have worries about what you would do in case of a fire? Are you stressed out or tired?
- *Home situation:* Please describe your current living situation. Whom do you live with? Do any elderly people or young children live in the home?

Poisoning

- *Chemicals:* How do you store your household chemicals? Are they out of reach of children and pets?
- *Medications:* Where are your medications stored? Are they out of reach of children, or do they have childproof caps? Are any medications expired?
- *Food:* Are "leftover" foods dated and placed in airtight containers? Is the refrigerator cleared of potentially spoiled items on a weekly basis? Are separate cutting surfaces used for cutting raw fish and meats? Are meats refrigerated during marinating, and is excess marinade discarded before cooking?
- *Carbon monoxide:* Do you experience unexplained headaches, dizziness, drowsiness, nausea, or any other flulike symptoms? Do you have a carbon monoxide detector in your home?

Fire and Electrical Hazards

- Do you have adequate outlets for all of your appliances and electronic devices? If there are children in the home, are all outlets in your home covered?
- Do you check for frays or loose wires on electrical cords, including those of electronic devices such as laptops and cell phones?
- Are your circuit breaker boxes in working order?
- Are your appliances properly grounded?
- Are household appliances, such as irons, hair dryers, and electric razors, used away from sources of water? Are the electrical outlets grounded?
- Do you have smoke detectors? A fire extinguisher? An evacuation plan in case of a fire?
- How do you heat your home?
- Do you use an oven and stove?
- Do you smoke, or does anyone in your home smoke?

Biohazards

- *Needles:* Do you use hypodermic needles? How do you dispose of them?
- *Methicillin-resistant* Staphylococcus aureus *(MRSA):* Do you have any open or inflamed areas on your skin?

Home Temperature Safety

- How do you heat your home? Is it adequate? Do you use space heaters?
- Do you have screens in your windows in the summer?
- Do you have air-conditioning? Fans?

Tripping and Falling Hazards

- Have tripping and falling hazards, such as clutter, toys, and electric cords in walking areas, been removed? Do area rugs have rug pads beneath them?
- Is there adequate lighting in hallways and on the stairs?
- Do you have night-lights?
- If there are children in the house, are gates installed in doorways and at the top and bottom of stairs?
- Are there handrails on the stairs?
- Are there grab bars in the bathroom? Is there a rubber mat in the tub and on the shower floor?

Outside Environment

- Do you have rails on steps?
- Is there adequate outside lighting?
- Do you operate any outside equipment, such as lawn mowers?
- Do you drive? Do you use car seats or safety belts?
- Do you feel safe in your neighborhood?
- What recreational activities do you engage in? Do you use safety equipment?

Work

- What do you do for a living?
- How is your work situation? Do you have any concerns?

falling. From this score, a level of risk is determined, and interventions can be selected from a list of recommended fall prevention strategies (Figure 25-2) to target patient-specific risk factors. The nurse should realize that multiple factors place patients at risk for falling. Because fall risk is multifaceted and often complex in nature, interdisciplinary, comprehensive fall prevention strategies are most effective (Hill, Westmoreland, Soeken, et al, 2002).

The Morse Fall Scale (Figure 25-3) is a fall risk assessment tool that has been widely used nationally and internationally since the late 1980s in acute care and long-term care settings. The tool has been rated by nurses as quick and easy to use,

Fall Risk Factor Category 1	
Scoring not completed for the following reason(s). *(Check any that apply.)* Enter risk category (i.e., Low/High) based on box selected.	
☐ Complete paralysis, or completely immobilized. Implement basic safety (low fall risk) interventions.	
☐ Patient has a history of more than one fall within 6 months before admission. Implement high fall risk interventions throughout hospitalization.	
☐ Patient has experienced a fall during this hospitalization. Implement high fall risk interventions throughout hospitalization.	
☐ Patient is deemed high fall risk per protocol (e.g., seizure precautions). Implement high fall risk interventions per protocol.	
Fall Risk Factor Category 2	
For those patients who are not in the above category, complete the following risk assessment tool and calculate fall risk score. If no box is checked, the score for the category is 0.	
	SCORE
Age *(Select only one)*	
☐ 60-69 years (1 point)	
☐ 70-79 years (2 points)	
☐ 80+ years (3 points)	
Fall history *(Select one)*	
☐ One fall within 6 months before admission (5 points)	
☐ No falls (0 points)	
Elimination, bowel and bladder *(Select one only)*	
☐ No incontinence, urgency, or frequency (0 points)	
☐ Incontinence (2 points)	
☐ Urgency or frequency (2 points)	
☐ Urgency/frequency and incontinence (4 points)	
Medications: Includes PCA/opiates, anticonvulsants, antihypertensives, diuretics, hypnotics, laxatives, sedatives, and psychotropics *(Select one)*	
☐ On one high fall risk drug (3 points)	
☐ On two or more high fall risk drugs (5 points)	
☐ Sedation procedure within past 24 hours (7 points)	
Patient care equipment: Any equipment that tethers the patient (e.g., IV infusion, chest tube, indwelling catheters, SCDs, etc.) *(Select one)*	
☐ One present (1 point)	
☐ Two present (2 points)	
☐ Three or more present (3 points)	
Mobility *(Multiple select, choose all that may apply and add points together)*	
☐ Requires assistance or supervision for mobility, transfer, or ambulation (2 points)	
☐ Unsteady gait (2 points)	
☐ A visual or auditory impairment affecting mobility (2 points)	
Cognition *(Multiple select, choose all that may apply and add points together)*	
☐ Altered awareness of immediate physical environment (1 point)	
☐ Impulsivity/poor safety judgment (2 points)	
☐ Lack of understanding of one's physical and cognitive limitations (4 points)	
Total points scored	
Moderate risk = 6-13 points. High risk = 13+ points.	

Please complete the fall risk assessment tool once every 8 hours or with change in patient's condition.

FIGURE 25-1 Johns Hopkins Hospital Fall Assessment Tool. (Copyright The Johns Hopkins Health System Corporation.)

taking approximately 3 minutes to complete (Morse, 2009). The six items on the scale are weighted and focus on (1) history of falling, (2) existence of a secondary diagnosis, (3) use of an ambulatory aid, (4) use of an intravenous (IV) line or a saline lock, (5) gait, and (6) mental status. The score is totaled for the checked items. If the score is 25 or higher, the patient is considered to be at high risk for falls (Morse, 2009), and fall prevention interventions should be implemented as appropriate.

The Hendrich II Fall Risk Model (Figure 25-4) has been well established and used widely in acute care settings to assess the fall risk of patients. This tool is available in English and Spanish and is being pilot-tested in Italy, Portugal, and Canada (Hendrich, 2007). The tool focuses on eight

LOW FALL RISK	MODERATE FALL RISK	HIGH FALL RISK
Fall risk score: 0-5 points	*Fall risk score:* 6-13 points *Color code:* **YELLOW**	*Fall risk score:* >13 points *Color code:* **RED**
Maintain safe unit environment, including: • Remove excess equipment/supplies/ furniture from rooms and hallways. • Coil and secure excess electrical and telephone wires. • Immediately clean all spills in patient's room or in hallway. Place signage to indicate wet floor danger. • Restrict window openings. The following are examples of basic safety interventions: • Orient patient to surroundings, including bathroom location, use of bed, and location of call light. • Keep bed in lowest position during use unless impractical (as in ICU nursing or specialty beds). • Keep top two side rails up (excludes box beds). In ICU, keep all side rails up. • Secure locks on beds, stretchers, and wheelchairs. • Keep floors free of clutter and obstacles, with attention to path between bed and bathroom or commode. • Place call light and other frequently needed objects within patient's reach. Answer call light promptly. • Encourage patient/family to call for assistance when needed. • Display special instructions for vision and hearing. • Ensure adequate lighting, especially at night. • Use properly fitting nonskid footwear.	Institute flagging system: Yellow card outside room and yellow sticker on medical record, assignment board/ electronic board; Hill ROM flag (if available). Implement measures listed under Low Fall Risk and: • Monitor and assist patient in following daily schedules. • Supervise and/or assist bedside sitting, personal hygiene, and toileting as appropriate. • Reorient confused patients as necessary. • Establish elimination schedule, including use of bedside commode, if appropriate. • Activate bed/chair alarm. Evaluate need for the following: • Physical therapy consultation if patient has a history of fall and/or mobility impairment. • Occupational therapy consultation. • Slip-resistant chair mat (do *not* use on shower chair). • Use of seat belt when in wheelchair. See institution's Med/Surg Restraint policy.	Institute flagging system: Red card outside room and red sticker on medical record, assignment board/electronic board; Hill ROM flag (if available). Implement measures listed under Low and Moderate Fall Risk and: • Remain with patient during toileting. • Observe q 60 min unless patient is on activated bed/chair alarm. • If patient requires an air overlay, use side rail protectors/extenders. • When necessary, transport throughout hospital with assistance of staff or trained caregivers. Consider alternatives (e.g., bedside procedure). Notify receiving area of high fall risk. Evaluate need for the following: • Moving patient to room with best visual access to nursing station. • Activated bed/chair alarm. • Low bed. • Protective devices (e.g., hipsters, helmets). • 24-hr supervision or sitter. • Physical restraint/enclosed bed (only with authorized prescriber order).

FIGURE 25-2 Johns Hopkins Hospital fall prevention intervention guidelines by risk category. *ICU,* Intensive care unit; *OT,* occupational therapy; *ROM,* range of motion. (Copyright The Johns Hopkins Health System Corporation.)

RISK FACTOR	SCALE	SCORE
History of falls	Yes	25
	No	0
Secondary diagnosis	Yes	15
	No	0
Ambulatory aid	Furniture	30
	Crutches/cane/walker	15
	None/bed rest/wheelchair/nurse	0
IV/Heparin lock	Yes	20
	No	0
Gait/transferring	Impaired	20
	Weak	10
	Normal/Bed rest/Immobile	0
Mental status	Forgets limitations	15
	Oriented to own ability	0

To obtain the Morse Fall Score, add the score from each category.

MORSE FALL SCORE	
High risk	45+
Moderate risk	25-44
Low risk	0-24

FIGURE 25-3 Morse Fall Scale. (From Morse JM, Black C, Oberle K, et al: A prospective study to identify the fall-prone patient, *Soc Sci Med* 28(1):81-86, 1989.)

independent risk factors: (1) confusion/disorientation/ impulsivity, (2) symptomatic depression, (3) altered elimination, (4) dizziness/vertigo, (5) male gender, (6) use of antiepileptics, (7) use of benzodiazepines, and (8) performance on the Get Up and Go Test (Hendrich, Bender, and Nyhuis, 2003). On this weighted tool, an item is assigned a zero if it does not apply to the patient. If the total score is 5 or higher on the Hendrich II Fall Risk Model, the patient is at high risk for a fall. As with the other fall assessment tools, when the patient is determined to be at high risk, a care plan with a set of patient-specific fall prevention interventions needs to be implemented.

◆ NURSING DIAGNOSIS LO 25.5

Nursing diagnoses directly associated with safety concerns include *Risk for Injury, Risk for Falls, Risk for Poisoning, Risk for Infection*, and *Risk for Aspiration.* Although these are the most common nursing diagnoses related to safety issues,

COMPLETE 8-HR SHIFT, CHANGED CONDITION, OR TRANSFER			
Confusion/disorientation/impulsiveness	4	4	4
Depression (nursing staff assesses patient, or patient states "depressed")	2	2	2
Altered elimination (leakage of urine or stool, "can't wait," or gets up four or more times per night)	1	1	1
Dizziness/vertigo as reported by patient	1	1	1
Gender (male)	1	1	1
Any antileptic agents: carbamazepine (Tegretol, Carbatrol), divalproex (Depakote), fosphenytoin (Cerebryx injection), gabapentin (Neurontin), lamotrigine (Lamictal), levetiracetam (Kappra), mephobarbital (Mebara), oxcarbazepine (Trileptal), phenobarbital, phenytoin (Dilantin), topiramate (Topamax), valproic acid (Depakene)	2	2	2
Any benzodiazepine medications: alprazolam (Xanax), chlordiazepoxide (Librium, Librax), clonazepam (Klonopin), diazepam (Valium), flurazepam (Dalmane), lorazepam (Ativan), midazolam (Versed), temazepam (Restoril), triazolam (Halcion)	1	1	1
GET-UP-AND-GO TEST *(Select one)*			
Arises in a single movement	0	0	0
Pushes up in one attempt	1	1	1
Multiple attempts, successful	3	3	3
Unable to arise without assistance	4	4	4
ADD TOTAL POINTS (>5 points = High risk)			
Check box if patient is on Fall Prevention Pathway	☐ See Pathway	☐ See Pathway	☐ See Pathway

GET-UP-AND-GO TEST
Instructions: With patient sitting in a chair (preferred location) or on the side of the bed, place hands in lap and ask the patient to stand.

	SCORE
Patient is able to stand and begin stepping in a single movement using only his/her legs.	0
Patient can rise and begin stepping in a single attempt if uses arms or a walker to push up.	1
Patient requires more than one attempt to stand with or without use of hands, arms, and walker.	3
Patient cannot stand without assistance.	4

FIGURE 25-4 Hendrich II Fall Risk Model. (From AHI of Indiana, Inc.

others such as *Impaired Physical Mobility* may apply after a safety-related event such as a fall-related hip fracture. An illness may result in *Acute Confusion,* especially in an older adult, creating safety concerns. Many other nursing diagnoses are related to safety issues directly such those previously described, or indirectly such as illnesses that create safety concerns (e.g., MRSA infection, hypothermia, needlestick-related disease). Some nursing diagnostic statements related to safety are as follows:

- *Risk for Injury* with risk factors of insufficient knowledge of safety precautions and cognitive impairment
- *Risk for Falls* with risk factors of older than age 75 years of age, use of a walker, and confusion
- *Risk for Poisoning* with risk factors of household chemicals present

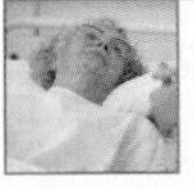

2. Mrs. Stein has *Acute Confusion.* Develop a goal for this nursing diagnosis. List four interventions (not mentioned in Exercise 3) with corresponding rationales that would be appropriate for managing her acute confusion.

◆ PLANNING LO 25.6

Before implementing interventions for the promotion of safety of individuals across settings, the nurse considers critical assessment findings such as the patient's developmental level, cultural background, and baseline understanding of the issue. After taking these considerations into account along with the desires and goals articulated by the patient and

TABLE 25-1 Care Planning

NANDA-I NURSING DIAGNOSIS LABEL WITH NURSING DIAGNOSIS STATEMENT	NURSING OUTCOME CLASSIFICATION (NOC)	NURSING INTERVENTION CLASSIFICATION (NIC)
Risk for Injury with risk factors of insufficient knowledge of safety precautions and cognitive impairment	*Knowledge: Fall prevention* (1828) When to ask for personal assistance (182808)	*Fall prevention* (6490) Instruct patient to call for assistance with movement, as appropriate.

From Bulechek G, Butcher H, Dochterman J, et al (Eds): *Nursing interventions classification (NIC)*, ed. 6, St. Louis, 2013, Mosby; Moorhead S, Johnson M, Maas M, et al (Eds): *Nursing outcomes classification (NOC)*, ed. 5, St. Louis, 2013, Mosby; NANDA International: *Nursing diagnoses: Definitions and classification, 2012-2014*, West Sussex, England, 2012, Wiley-Blackwell. Reprinted with permission from NANDA International, Inc.

family, the nurse can develop individualized, patient-centered interventions and goals (Table 25-1). The following are examples of goals for the three nursing diagnoses previously listed:

- Patient will experience no injuries while hospitalized.
- Patient's risk for falls will be minimized when discharged home.
- Patient will not be exposed to household chemicals when discharged home.

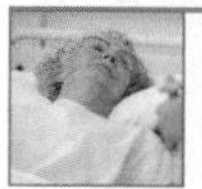

The conceptual care map for Mrs. Stein provided in Figure 25-5 is partially completed to indicate how to use the map as a learning tool. Using it as an example, go to the website at *http://evolve.elsevier.com/YoostCrawford/fundamentals/* to complete Nursing Diagnoses 2 and 3.

IMPLEMENTATION AND EVALUATION LO 25.7

The planning, implementation, and evaluation of interventions to maintain the safety of patients across settings is often best promoted through the use of a multidisciplinary care team. The Collaboration and Delegation box gives examples of how nurses can work with other health care professionals to promote patient safety.

QSEN FOCUS!

Teamwork and collaboration knowledge are demonstrated when the nurse describes examples of the impact of team functioning on safety and quality of care.

COLLABORATION AND DELEGATION

Multidisciplinary Health Care Team

- The nurse collaborates with the pharmacist and physician to identify and implement safe medication alternatives for older adults to minimize side effects such as drowsiness, dizziness, and orthostatic hypotension, which can increase fall risk.
- Occupational therapists evaluate the patient for safe performance of activities of daily living (ADLs) such as bathing, dressing, and grooming, and they make recommendations to enhance safe performance of these activities, such as the use of specialty equipment (e.g., grippers for pants, oversized shoehorns).
- Physical therapists evaluate the patient's ability to perform and maintain balance during routine activities such as sitting, standing, and walking. They make recommendations for assistive devices such as canes and walkers to promote safe performance of these activities.
- The social worker facilitates contact with insurance companies or other agencies to assist with the financing of recommended therapeutic assistive and specialty devices.
- Under the delegation of the registered nurse, unlicensed assistive personnel (UAP) provide hands-on care for patients who require assistance with ADLs, transfers, and ambulation. Registered nurses are responsible for supervising and guiding UAP so that direct care is provided in a safe manner.

For a patient with safety concerns, members of the multidisciplinary team together address the issues associated with safety-related nursing diagnoses. Team members work to accomplish the goals set forth in what is commonly referred to in hospital settings as an interdisciplinary plan of care (IPOC). The nurse may implement several safety interventions:

- Educate the patient and family about the role of protective-equipment use in injury prevention when individuals are engaged in contact sports.
- Collaborate with the social worker to identify community resources for obtaining inexpensive or free protective equipment.
- Educate the patient and family about the importance of removing clutter, throw rugs, cords, and obstacles from the floor and the path of the patient.
- Collaborate with the social worker to identify community resources to install appropriate supportive equipment in the home.
- Educate the patient and family on the importance of and strategies for preventing children from gaining access to household poisons.
- Collaborate with social services for the scheduling of periodic home safety inspections.

Medications

Rocephin 1 g IVPB daily
Albuterol and Atrovent nebulizer treatments q 6 hr
Guaifenesin 600 mg PO qid
Lisinopril 5 mg PO daily for hypertension
Acetaminophen 625 mg PO q 6 hr prn for arthritic or pleuritic chest pain rating 3–6
Dilaudid 0.5-1.0 mg IVP q 2 hr prn for pleuritic chest pain rating 7–10
Ativan 0.5-1.0 mg IVP q 8 hr prn for agitation

Conceptual Care Map

Student name_________ Patient initials Mrs. S_ Date ______
Age 88 Gender F Room # ___ Admission Date _______
CODE Status Full Allergies Heparin
Diet No added salt Activity OOB to chair Braden Score 17
Weight ______ Height _____ Religion ________

Lab Values/Diagnostic Test Results

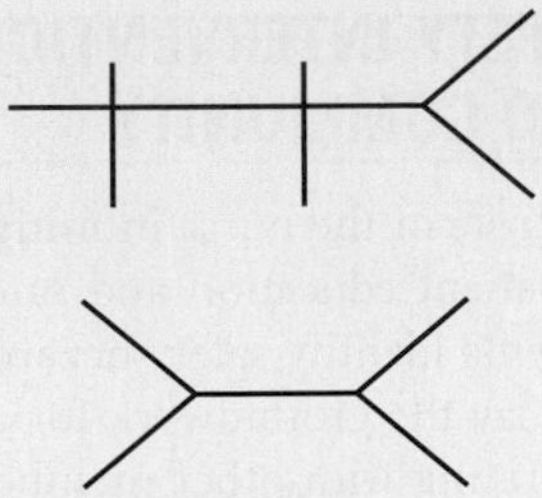

Chest x-ray: bilateral pulmonary infiltrates

Admitting Diagnoses/Chief Complaint
Pneumonia

Fever, T 38.2° C (100.8° F), increasing confusion and weakness

IV Sites/Fluids/Rate

Normal saline 0.9% at 100 mL/hr

Assessment Data

Admitted last night to the hospital from an area nursing home with a fever, T 38.2° C (100.8° F), increasing confusion and weakness.
T 37.4° C (99.3° F), P 85, R 28, BP 156/95, O_2 sat is 95% on O_2 @ 2 L/min nasal cannula. Does not answer when asked if she is in pain
Oriented to person only; pleasantly confused and mumbling about her young children.
Top side rails raised for positioning and turning, and her bilateral untied mitts are in place. No redness or irritation at mitt site noted on intermittent release.
Her Johns Hopkins Hospital (JHH) Fall Score = 21, and her Braden Scale score is 17.
Incontinent of loose stool and trying to climb OOB.

Past Medical/Surgical History

Hypertension
Osteoarthritis
History of falls × 2 in last month

Treatments

VS: q 4 hr with O_2 sat
Out of bed (OOB) to chair or bedside commode ONLY
CBC every morning O_2 up to 3 L/min nasal cannula to keep O_2 sat ≥ 92%
Incentive spirometry q 1 hr while awake
Bilateral mitt restraints

Primary Nursing Diagnosis

Risk for Injury with risk factors of insufficient knowledge of safety precautions and cognitive impairment

Supporting Data

Confusion, oriented to person only
Weakness
JHH score = 21
Hypertension, taking Lisinopril

STG/NOC

Patient will experience no injuries while hospitalized,
NOC: Knowledge: Fall prevention (1828)
When to ask for personal assistance (182808)

Interventions/NIC With Rationale

1. Keep call light within reach at all times, and remind patient to call the nurse for assistance so that the patient does not attempt to getup unassisted.
2. Keep frequently used items in close proximity to the patient to prevent reaching.
3. Place patient in room close to nurse's station for better observation.
4. Place patient on a pressure-sensitive alarm to alert staff to patient's attempt to get out of bed.

NIC: Fall prevention (6490)
Instruct patient to call for assistance with movement, as appropriate.

Rationale Citation/EBP

Yoost BL, Crawford LR: *Fundamentals of nursing: Active learning for collaborative practice*, St. Louis, 2016, Mosby.

Evaluation

- Patient in bed with call light within reach.
- Free from falls and injures during shift.
- Continue plan of care.

Nursing Diagnosis 2

Supporting Data

STG/NOC

Interventions/NIC With Rationale

Rationale Citation/EBP

Evaluation

Nursing Diagnosis 3

Supporting Data

STG/NOC

Interventions/NIC With Rationale

Rationale Citation/EBP

Evaluation

FIGURE 25-5 Partially completed conceptual care map based on Mrs. Stein, the case study patient in this chapter. *CBC*, Complete blood count; *EBP*, evidence-based practice; *JHH*, Johns Hopkins Hospital fall assessment score; *NIC*, Nursing Intervention Classification; *NOC*, Nursing Outcome Classification; *OOB*, out of bed; *STG*, short-term goal; *VS*, vital signs.

SAFETY INTERVENTIONS IN THE HOME AND COMMUNITY

The role of the nurse in mitigating safety risks is largely one of patient education and safety promotion. Nurses helping patients identify safety hazards at home and in the community lay the groundwork for appropriate action. Nurses collaborating with other members of the health care team and with resources in the community can assist patients with arranging to have grab bars installed in the bathroom, improvements made to indoor and outdoor lighting, and increased surveillance inside and outside buildings and in parking lots. In home and community settings, nurses must be aware of specific areas of fall prevention, fire prevention, and poisoning prevention (Patient Education and Health Literacy box).

PATIENT EDUCATION AND HEALTH LITERACY

Fall Prevention at Home

Health teaching for patients discharged to or residing in the home should include environmental interventions for fall prevention:

- Remove obstacles from walking paths (e.g., clutter, throw rugs, cords).
- Ensure adequate lighting in areas such as bathrooms, halls, and stairways.
- Keep assistive devices (e.g., canes, walkers) within reach.
- Use assistive devices consistently and properly when moving.
- Repair loose or uneven floor and stairway surfaces.
- Install and maintain handrails and grab bars.
- Use devices such as long-handled grabbers rather than reaching or stooping.
- Keep frequently used items close by or within reach.
- Maintain floor surfaces that are dry and free of debris.

Following these suggestions can make the patient's environment safer. Patients should be aware of environmental challenges, such as changes in ground slope and unevenness in walking surfaces and curbs. When going out into community settings, patients should be encouraged to take their assistive devices along on all occasions and properly use them. Reminders may be important for those who tend to leave canes or walkers in the car when they are "only going a short distance."

SAFETY INTERVENTIONS IN THE HEALTH CARE ENVIRONMENT

Consistent with the focus of the QSEN project, nurses must possess the knowledge, skills, and attitudes to maintain safety and prevent patient injury across health care settings. For example, a nurse must have adequate knowledge of the variety of risk factors for falls, the skill to select patient-specific interventions to prevent falls, and the attitude that falls can be preventable. When nurses lack the necessary knowledge, skills, and attitudes to care for the population of interest, the delivery of competent care is at risk, and legal issues related to patient safety may result.

Legal Issues Related to Safety

Issues of patient safety can be disputed legally, and nurses must ensure that current and proper standards of care are upheld to avoid lawsuits. Patient safety concerns that have been sources of litigation are listed in the Ethical, Legal, and Professional Practice box. In addition to being guided by the legal issues related to safety, the professional practice of nursing is guided by the American Nurses Association Code of Ethics (see Chapter 11), the individual's internal ethical code of conduct, and the state's nurse practice act.

ETHICAL, LEGAL, AND PROFESSIONAL PRACTICE

Litigation Resulting From Breaches in Patient Safety Standards of Care

- Wrong-side surgeries and amputations
- Wrong-patient errors (i.e., medications given to the wrong patients, diagnostic procedures or treatments performed on the wrong patients)
- Medication dosage errors resulting in organ damage or failure or in death (e.g., not lowering doses for children or geriatric patients)
- Fall-related injuries and death (particularly in older adults)
- Restraint-related injuries and death

Fire

Health care facilities implement several actions to prevent fires and to ensure adequate preparation if one occurs. One example is a no-smoking policy that does not permit smoking on the facility's property or allows it only outside the facility in designated areas. Oxygen is flammable and should not be used near an open fire. Fire evacuation drills and practice in the use of fire extinguishers should be conducted with enough frequency to ensure that health care professionals are prepared to properly respond in the event of a fire. Many health care facilities use the fire emergency response defined by the acronym **RACE**:

R: *Rescue* all patients in immediate danger, and move them to safe areas.

A: Activate the manual-pull station or fire *alarm,* and have someone call 911.

C: *Contain* the fire by closing doors, confining the fire, and preventing the spread of smoke.

E: *Extinguish* the fire if possible after all patients are removed from the area.

Staff members must quickly mobilize to remove or rescue (**R**) patients close to the fire. The fire alarm (**A**) must be sounded and the exact location of the fire reported; 911 is usually called by a facility-wide operator.

HOME CARE CONSIDERATIONS

Fire Prevention

Nurses delivering care in home settings need to assess for fire safety risk factors and should offer strategies for alleviating them:

- Do not use stoves for heating the house.
- Do not use ovens for storing food, such as crackers, cookies, or cereal.
- Do not leave irons face down on the ironing board.
- Do not smoke or have an open flame in a fireplace if oxygen is in use in the home.
- Properly dispose of or recycle trash, and do not allow it to accumulate.
- Install smoke alarms on every floor of the house.
- Change batteries in smoke alarms at least twice per year.
- Establish fire escape plans, and practice them several times each year.
- Ensure that all family members know how and when to call emergency telephone numbers.
- Obtain fire extinguishers, and be sure family members learn how to use them.
- Consider installing fire sprinklers in the home (U.S. Fire Administration, 2014b).

Poisoning Prevention

Nurses offer recommendations for the prevention of poisoning:

- Ensure proper labeling and storage of chemicals and medications in original containers.
- Use alternatives to toxic chemicals, such as baking soda as a deodorizer.
- Store chemicals and medications out of the reach of small children.
- Employ cabinet safeguards and childproof caps to prevent access.
- Take medication in only a well-lit area to ensure correct dosage.
- Verify that medication dosages are appropriate for pediatric and/or geriatric patients.
- Understand potential food and drug interactions associated with the medication.
- Dispose of unused or expired medications; never share medications with others.

If poisoning is suspected, before administering an antidote, call the National Poison Control Center at 1-800-222-1222. Offer first aid for poisoning:

- If a poison has been inhaled, get the individual into fresh air as soon as possible.
- If poison gets in the eyes, flush the eyes immediately with water.
- If poison gets on the skin, remove clothing that was in contact with the poison, and rinse the skin with water for at least 15 minutes.

Be prepared to answer questions from the Poison Control Center:

- How is the person acting, or how does he or she look?
- What and approximately how much was taken?
- When was it taken?

Parents must provide a babysitter with the necessary information in case of poisoning or suspected poisoning of a child in his or her care. They should leave this information in a conspicuous location, such as on the refrigerator or near the telephone, and tell the babysitter that the information is there:

- Phone number of the Poison Control Center (1-800-222-1222)
- Age and weight of the child
- Allergies and medical conditions
- Physician's name and phone number
- Number at which parents can be reached

A medical emergency exists if a person is having seizures, is extremely drowsy, or is unconscious, having difficulty breathing or not breathing, or having any life-threatening symptoms. In such cases, call 911 immediately. While waiting for help, if the person is not breathing, initiate rescue breathing and cardiopulmonary resuscitation (CPR). Take the medication bottle or the container of the ingested substance along to the hospital emergency room. Do not attempt to induce vomiting; do not give syrup of ipecac (Mayo Clinic, 2012).

Lead

Nurses can provide strategies that may minimize lead exposure:

- Scheduling a professional lead inspection and renovation, which may be necessary in older homes; before 1978, lead-based paint was often used
- Doing careful handwashing, especially after gardening and outdoor play
- Washing and peeling vegetables
- Installing a water filter
- Letting water run from the tap for at least 1 minute before use

Carbon Monoxide

The CDC (2014a) recommends the use of several measures in the home or community setting to avoid carbon monoxide poisoning:

- Scheduling annual checks and service of the heating system, water heater, and any other gas-, oil-, or coal-burning devices by a qualified technician
- Installing a battery-operated carbon monoxide detector and checking or replacing the batteries each spring and fall, along with smoke-detector battery checks
- Immediately evacuating and then calling 911 if the carbon monoxide detector alarm goes off
- Seeking medical attention promptly if carbon monoxide poisoning is suspected (i.e., symptoms of nausea, dizziness, light-headedness)
- Using items such as charcoal grills, camp stoves, and generators outside and not inside the garage or basement
- Avoiding running cars or trucks inside a garage attached to the house
- Burning objects or materials only in vented fireplaces or stoves
- Never heating the house with a gas oven

Child Safety

Several measures can promote safety across childhood developmental age groups:

- Using outlet covers in homes with small children to prevent electrical shock
- Keeping household chemicals and medications locked in secure locations
- Ensuring parental supervision of activities such as using trampolines and swimming
- Keeping firearms locked in secure locations with bullets stored in a separate location
- Consistently using seatbelts
- Consistently and appropriately using car seats
- Encouraging teen participation in driver's education courses

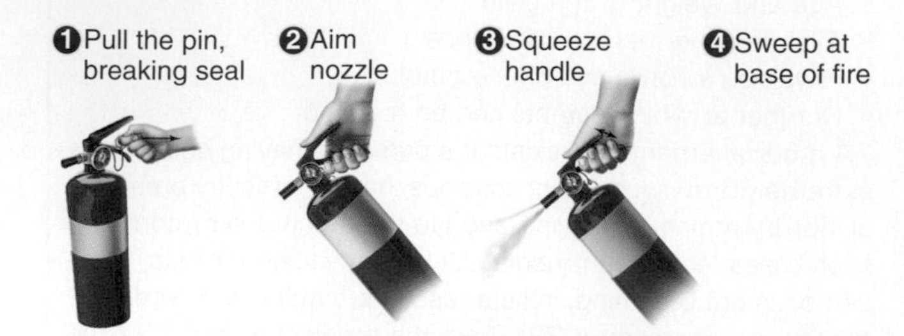

FIGURE 25-6 When using a fire extinguisher, remembering the PASS acronym (i.e., pull, aim, squeeze, and sweep). ensures proper technique.

Measures are taken to contain (C) or prevent the spread of smoke and fire, which include closing doors and turning off oxygen. Patients receiving mechanical ventilation should be disconnected and provided with manual respiration with an Ambu bag. An **Ambu bag** is a resuscitator bag that is used to assist ventilation (see Figure 38-10).

After all patients are removed from the area, an attempt may be made to extinguish (E) the fire if it is small enough. However, an attempt to extinguish a fire should not be made if personal or patient safety would be compromised in the process. Figure 25-6 shows the proper technique for use of a fire extinguisher. When using a fire extinguisher, it is helpful to remember the PASS acronym: pull, aim, squeeze, and sweep.

To enable successful evacuation, patients should be triaged on the basis of their mobility levels. Those who are ambulatory should be directed to a safe area, and those who are immobile must be transported by bed, stretcher, or wheelchair to another area.

Electrical Energy

To ensure fire safety, nurses should regularly check for faulty or loose wiring or anything unusual, and clinical engineers should conduct scheduled checks and routine maintenance of electrical equipment. Patients may be at increased risk for an electric shock because of the multiple electrical devices to which they may be connected for therapeutic purposes, such as bed, IV pump, oxygen, cardiac monitor, and gastrointestinal suction (Figure 25-7).

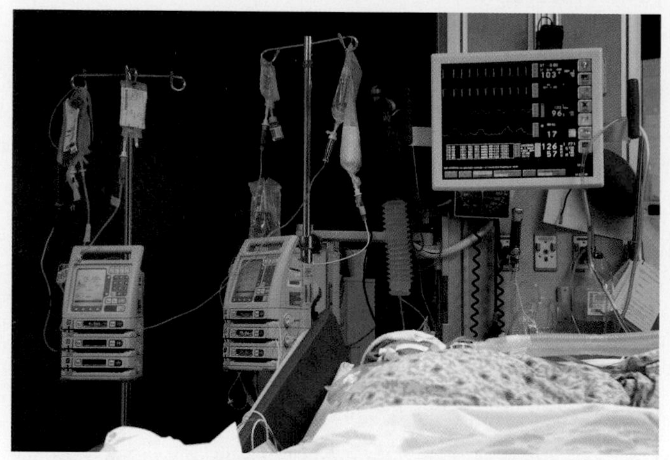

FIGURE 25-7 The risk for an electric shock may be increased for patients who need electrical equipment for therapeutic purposes. The routine use of three-pronged (grounded) outlets and plugs on equipment in health care settings helps to minimize the risk of electrical exposure.

Fall Prevention

Falls are events in which an individual unintentionally and through the force of gravity drops to the ground, floor, or some other lower level. Despite the need for comprehensive fall prevention programs, many interventions are simple and involve manipulation of the environment by the nurse to meet patient needs. For example, the call light should be kept within reach and the patient reminded how to use it with each interaction so that the patient can call for help. Frequently used items should be kept close to the patient to prevent reaching. Making hourly rounds ensures that patient needs are met and reduces patient falls in hospital settings (Meade, Bursell, and Ketelsen, 2006). Patients who are at a high risk for falling should be placed in rooms close to the nurses' station, and pressure-sensitive alarms can be used to alert staff about attempts to get out of bed. Some patients may require a 24-hour sitter for observation.

Nurses can intervene in the care environment to promote patient safety by ensuring that brakes are always applied on beds and that safety locks are employed on wheelchairs (Figure 25-8). Other environmental adaptations that have

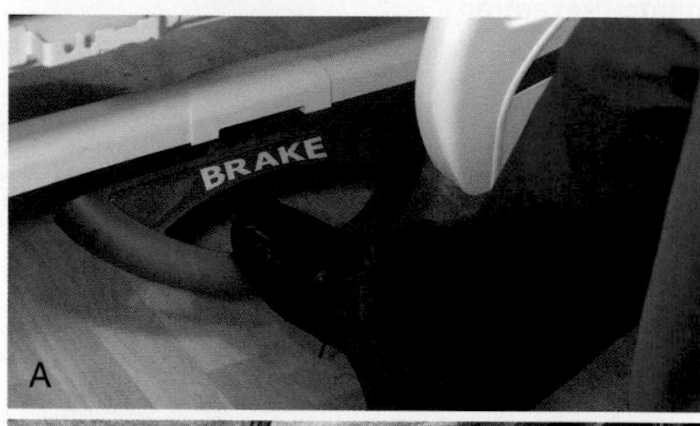

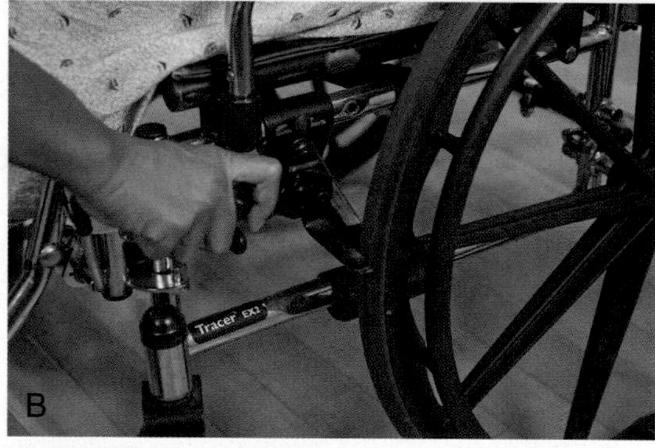

FIGURE 25-8 Nurses contribute to patient safety by ensuring that **(A)** the brakes are applied on beds and **(B)** safety locks are employed on wheelchairs.

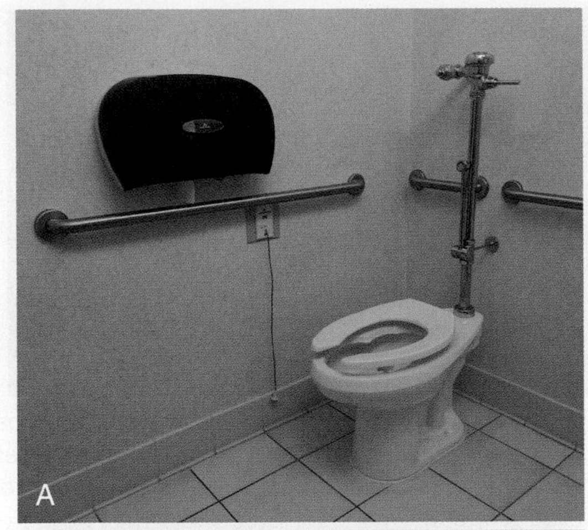

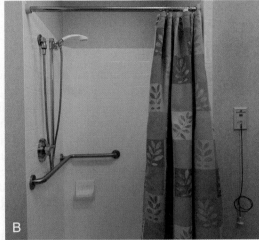

FIGURE 25-9 Grab bars provide a measure of safety for the patient using the toilet and shower.

been made in many health care facilities include the installation of grab bars near toilets and in showers (Figure 25-9).

Seizure Precautions

Special precautions are taken for any patient with a history of seizures. Padding is available for the bed rails to prevent injury in case a seizure occurs. Oxygen and suction equipment is kept at the bedside. During a seizure, a patient should be protected from injury by placing the head on a soft surface and turning it to the side to prevent aspiration and by moving sharp or hard objects out of the way.

Proper Use of Restraints

In light of all of the negative consequences that can result from the use of physical restraints, it is easy to conclude that they may do more harm than good for the patient. Nurses should employ as many restraint-free alternatives (Box 25-1) as possible before requesting orders for and applying a physical restraint (Evidence-Based Practice and Informatics box).

BOX 25-1 Alternatives to Physical Restraints

- Orient the patient to the surroundings, and explain all care-related interventions.
- Relocate the patient to a room near the nurses' station.
- Use pressure-sensitive and motion-sensitive bed and chair alarms consistently. Tabs and Bed-Check alarm systems can be used in the bed or chair.

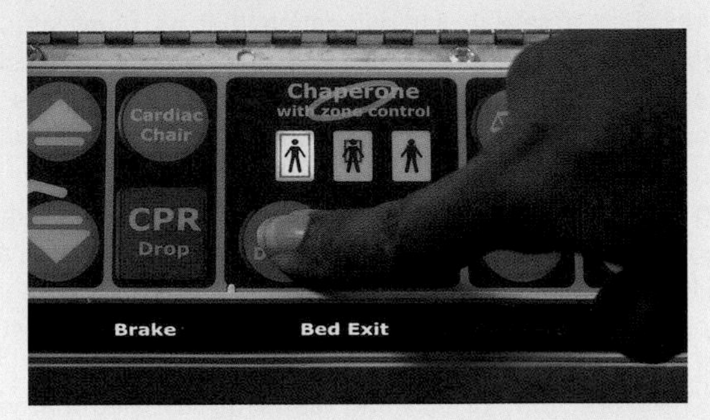

- Ensure that alarms and sensors are properly placed, functioning, and perform battery checks according to facility protocol.
- Encourage the family and significant others to spend time with the patient.
- Minimize environmental stimuli (e.g., noise, bright lights).
- Provide distractions based on patient preferences (e.g., music, television, a doll to hold).
- Promote relaxation through gentle massage.
- Use aromatherapy to relax the patient.
- Assess for sources of agitation, and ensure that the patient's basic needs are met (e.g., food, fluids, toileting, pain or discomfort relief, sleep, ambulation).
- Obtain an order for a 24-hour sitter (i.e., unlicensed assistive personnel [UAP]).
- Cover or disguise tubes or drains with clothing, or wrap IV sites with gauze so that they are kept out of the patient's sight.
- Use untied, cloth-padded protective mitts on the patient's hands to prevent the patient from removing tubes or drains

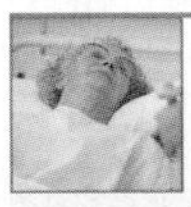

3. After finding Mrs. Stein as described in the case study, list in order four things that the nurse should do and explain why.

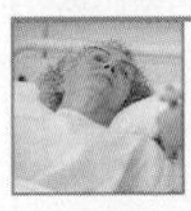

4. Identify at least three restraint-free alternatives that would be appropriate for Mrs. Stein that were not mentioned in an earlier answer.

After all restraint-free alternatives have been exhausted and consultation with other members of the interdisciplinary care team (e.g., geriatrician, geriatric clinical nurse specialist, nurse practitioner) has been unsuccessful in identifying other means of keeping the patient safe, several steps should be carefully followed before restraints are applied.

EVIDENCE-BASED PRACTICE AND INFORMATICS

Restraint Use in Care Settings

- For more than 2 decades, physical restraints, such as safety vests, body holders, and lap and wheelchair belts, have been associated with reports of injuries and deaths due to fractures, burns, entrapment, and strangulation.
- In 1992, the U.S. Food and Drug Administration (FDA) published a safety alert indicating that as many as 100 deaths or injuries each year were associated with physical restraint use. The FDA included recommendations to reduce the incidence of injuries and deaths associated with the use of physical restraints.
- In 1998, a 2-year report by The Joint Commission (which accredits hospitals and other Centers for Medicare and Medicaid Services [CMS] facilities) on 20 cases of death related to the use of physical restraints indicated that 40% of these cases resulted from asphyxiation.
- A hallmark study of falls and restraints revealed that with restraint removal in nursing homes, the risk of falls or injuries did not increase and the risk of minor injuries significantly decreased (Capezuti, Strumpf, Evans, et al, 1998).
- All deaths occurring while a patient is restrained or within 24 hours of physical restraint removal must be reported by phone to the CMS by the close of the next business day after the death (CMS, 2008).
- The Joint Commission (2014) patient safety standards focus on using physical restraints very infrequently and only after the many alternatives to their use have been exhausted.

In the event of an immediate threat of harm to self or others, the nurse can apply a physical restraint without an order from the primary health care provider, but the order must be sought within an hour of application of the restraint. Critical elements for the application and care of a patient requiring physical restraints for a temporary period are described in Skill 25-1. The interventions and their corresponding rationales provide guidance for safe restraint application and measures that can be taken to prevent untoward consequences.

! SAFE PRACTICE ALERT

Frequent checks of the patient under restraint are essential because injuries due to entrapment and death from strangulation or asphyxiation are most likely to result when the patient attempts to escape physical restraint.

! SAFE PRACTICE ALERT

Never tie a restraint in a knot because the knot may prohibit a quick exit in the event of an emergency requiring evacuation. Instead, use quick-release ties or mechanisms such as buckles. Restraints should never be tied to side rails because injuries may result when they are raised or lowered.

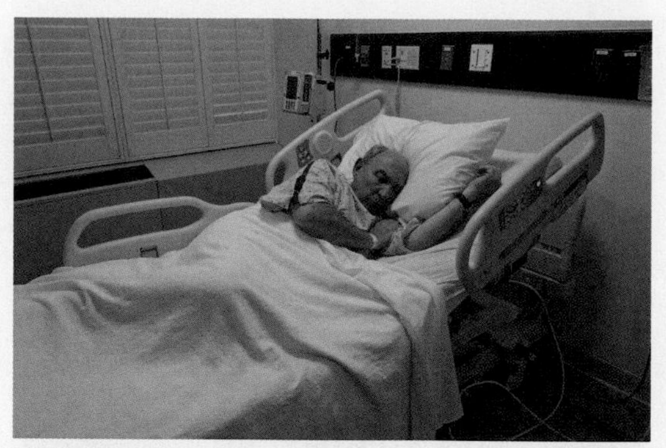

FIGURE 25-10 The top two side rails are used for patient positioning. Use of one of the bottom side rails is necessary in certain patient circumstances. Use of four side rails is considered restraint.

Proper Use of Side Rails

The top two side rails are often used by the patient for turning and positioning. In some circumstances the nurse will raise one of the bottom side rails (Figure 25-10). When all four side rails are raised, it is considered a form of physical restraint, which requires an order from a primary care provider. As with any physical restraint, it is critical to weigh the benefits and risks of the use of side rails. In the United States, there are approximately 2.5 million nursing home and hospital beds. The FDA requires reporting of incidents involving beds with rails. From 1985 through 2013, the FDA (2014) received reports of 901 incidents of patients being trapped, caught, entangled, or strangled in rails, with patient outcomes ranging from death (531 patients) to non-fatal injury (151 patients).

Studies have demonstrated a link between the use of side rails and falls (Capezuti, Maislin, Strumpf, et al, 2002; Capezuti, Talerico, Cochran, et al, 1999). Attempting to escape the bed while navigating the side rails can cause injurious falls. The patient may be attempting to get up and do something purposeful, such as go to the bathroom, which is another high-risk situation for falls. A simple measure to promote patient safety and prevent falls is to make patient rounds hourly to attend to basic needs (Meade, Bursell, and Ketelsen, 2006). The Nursing Care Guideline box outlines safety concerns related to side rail use.

Safe Medication Administration

One of the 2014 National Patient Safety Goals is to improve the safe use of medications (TJC, 2014). The QSEN project focuses on developing nurses' knowledge, skills, and attitudes, each of which is crucial for the safe administration of medication to patients. Page and McKinney (2007) emphasize the importance of theoretical pharmacologic knowledge and implementation of a Medication Safety Day, which focuses on the causes and means of medication errors. Application of the necessary knowledge, skills, and attitudes assists

NURSING CARE GUIDELINE

Side Rail Safety

Background

- Use of four side rails is considered a restraint. Assess the situation carefully before using them.
- Is a specialty mattress in place? If so, use side rails cautiously because functioning of the mattress may be affected by side rails.

Procedural Concerns

- Assessment:
  - Is there a fall risk?
  - Are alternative solutions available?
  - Is the patient confused or at an increased safety risk?
  - Is there a disability or body-positioning requirement? Is an alternative available?
  - Is the patient violent? If so, consider other options, because the patient may hurt himself or herself with rails in place.
  - Will the patient get out of bed without supervision? If so, consider an alternative.
- Reassess the need for all four side rails:
  - When there is a change in the patient's condition
  - At frequent intervals according to facility policy
- Compare the symmetry of the patient's body (i.e., one side of the body compared with the other) for conditions such as hemiparesis or amputations. Asymmetries may compromise patient safety and necessitate the use of safety rails.
- The two top side rails are often used for patient positioning and turning, and their use is not considered a restraint. Many newer beds have controls on the top side rails that the patient can reach only if the top rails are up.

Documentation Concerns

- Follow facility policy and procedures for documentation.
- Important documentation should include both of the following:
  - The reason for using all four side rails
  - Alternatives that have been attempted or considered
- Has a patient been injured with side rail use? If so, follow facility policy and procedure for care and documentation.
- If the patient or patient's family refuse side rail use, document the situation according to facility policy and procedure.

Evidence-Based Practice

- Capezuti and colleagues (2002) found that side rails did not decrease the risk of falls and, considering the high risk of injury and even death, that side rails can be dangerous. Their use must be thoroughly evaluated before employing them with any patient. Side rails are a genuine restraint, and alternatives need to be strongly considered to prevent falls and to assist in controlling behavior.

the entry-level nurse in performing safe medication administration. Practices essential to safely administering medications are discussed in Chapter 35.

Reduction of Pathogen Transmission

Health care–associated infections (HAIs), formerly called *nosocomial infections,* are acquired by patients during the course of treatment for other conditions; pneumonia, gastroenteritis, and urinary tract infections are common examples. To reduce the incidence of HAIs, nurses play a key role in preventing the transmission of pathogens in health care facilities. When determining the best practices for preventing the spread of infection, the nurse should consider the possible routes of transmission.

Key to the prevention of pathogen transmission among patients and health care workers is the use of standard precautions, which are practiced with all patients to avoid exposure to blood and other body fluids (e.g., urine, stool, sputum, gastric fluid), which are all assumed to be infectious. The primary precaution is using proper handwashing or hand-sanitizing techniques before and after each patient contact and procedure. Another important precaution is donning personal protective equipment. Chapter 26 discusses pathogen transmission and methods of prevention.

Reduction of Procedure- and Equipment-Related Events

Infections and injuries may occur in health care facilities as the result of errors in procedures and malfunction of medical equipment. Infections may be caused by improper insertion of therapeutic tubes or drains. A break in sterile technique or contamination of a Foley catheter during insertion may result in a catheter-associated urinary tract infection (UTI). Because of the reimbursement policy changes at the CMS, catheter-associated UTIs are considered to be reasonably preventable errors for which the cost of treatment is no longer covered. Infections can result from placement of a nasogastric tube for temporary tube feedings. If correct placement of the tube is not verified radiologically before administering feedings or the tube becomes dislodged during the course of routine care, aspiration pneumonia may result. To avoid these types of events during procedures, the nurse should carefully follow the steps of facility policy and procedure manuals and adhere closely to sterile technique.

Because injuries can result from improper equipment maintenance or equipment malfunction, several safeguards are in place to prevent them. For example, infusion pumps for IV therapy or patient-controlled analgesia (PCA) often have free-flow protection devices to prevent excessively rapid administration. Routine checks of battery-operated equipment, along with testing and replacement, may be performed by nursing or clinical engineering staff, depending on equipment type. If routine quality-control checks on equipment such as blood glucose meters are not performed, inaccurate readings and inappropriate insulin coverage, with associated hyperglycemia or hypoglycemia, may occur. These examples demonstrate the necessity for thoughtful facility protocols regarding equipment safety checks and maintenance, which must be carefully followed by staff from a variety of disciplines, including nursing, pharmacy, and clinical engineering.

When working with radiation diagnostics or treatments, preventive measures should be followed to avoid exposure. Lead shielding should be used for patients and staff. Staff should be kept as far as possible from the radiation source and the length of exposure limited. Health care professionals working with radiation or radioactive materials should wear a radiation-monitoring device or badge that is periodically checked for cumulative radiation exposure levels to ensure safety.

Bioterrorism

Successful management of a bioterrorist attack depends on the emergency response plans of health care facilities. In addition to nurses' taking part in public health awareness programs, they should be familiar with the disaster management and preparedness programs of the facilities in which they work.

EVALUATION

Evaluation is an ongoing process that involves collaboration with the patient, family, and multiple health care professionals to keep patients safe in health care agencies, community environments, and at home. Nurses develop patient-specific interventions that are continually evaluated to measure the patient's progress toward goal attainment. After evaluation, each patient's safety care plan is updated to reflect changes in his or her condition.

SKILL 25-1 Applying Physical Restraints

PURPOSE

- Physical restraints can be applied only with a physician or health care provider order and only after all reasonable alternatives to restraint use have failed.
- Physical restraints can be applied for either or both of two reasons:
  - Medical necessity
  - Behavioral or mental health issues
- Examples of common reasons for the use of physical restraints are as follows:
  - To immobilize an extremity
  - To prevent harmful patient behavior
  - To allow treatments or procedures to proceed without patient interference

RESOURCES

- Cloth restraint of correct size for the patient, situation, or site
- Soft cloth or foam (for padding)

COLLABORATION AND DELEGATION

- Most facilities require restraints to be applied by a registered nurse or licensed practical nurse.
- Assistance with applying and monitoring a physical restraint may be delegated to unlicensed assistive personnel (UAP) after the initial assessment of the patient.
- UAP should report any of the following to the nurse:
  - Skin changes (e.g., sores, wounds, irritations, lesions) in the area where the restraint is to be applied
  - Patient complaints related to restraint application, especially tightness, numbness, tingling, or pain
  - Changes in basic assessments that can be delegated to UAP, such as changes in vital signs
  - Patient communications of an unusual nature and any unusual concerns
- UAP should be instructed in the following:
  - Appropriate placement of restraints and reason for applying restraints
  - Appropriate use and type of restraint equipment
  - Appropriate assessment and documentation in accordance with institution policy
  - Ethical standards and basic therapeutic communication

EVIDENCE-BASED PRACTICE

- Restraint use has caused negative health outcomes, such as deterioration in the ability to walk, in cognitive abilities, and in performing activities of daily living (Engberg, Castle, and McCaffrey, 2008).
- Waist restraints or lap restraints are as harmful and restrictive as vest restraints, and they have just as many adverse events attributed them. All other alternatives must be implemented before initiating any type of restraint (Capezuti, Brush, Won, et al, 2008).
- Proper training and education of staff can reduce the use of restraints. Education includes understanding alternative options, de-escalation techniques, regulatory standards, barriers to change and overcoming resistance, and issues of violence, aggression, and power (Curran, 2007; Huizing, Hamers, Gulpers, et al, 2009; Kontio, Välimäki, Putkonen, et al, 2009; Paterson and Duxbury, 2007).
- Ethical considerations do not preclude the use of restraints, but alternatives should be implemented before restraint initiation to avoid further physical, mental, ethical, and social harm (Gastmans and Milisen, 2006).
- During application of a restraint, the primary nurse should be calm and reassure the patient that it is not a punishment. Focus must remain on the emotional and social health of the patient, or the situation may escalate for the patient and staff (Curran, 2007).

SPECIAL CIRCUMSTANCES

1. **Assess:** What are the possible causes of harmful patient behavior?
   Intervention: Document alternatives to restraints that have been tried and failed (to justify the use of restraints). Exhaust other treatment options (e.g., patient sitters, frequent toileting, monitoring, medications, proper positioning, treatment of pain, assessment and treatment of infections) that may underlie the patient's behavior before applying restraints.
2. **Assess:** What is the condition of the skin at the site of restraint application?
   Intervention: If wounds, irritations, or sores occur, use an alternative to the restraint. If bony prominences are involved, pad them with a soft cloth or foam. Perform frequent circulation, movement, and sensation checks, and document the results.
3. **Assess:** What is the least restrictive restraint choice?
   Intervention: Exhaust other treatment choices first. Do not restrain the entire body if only one limb needs to be restrained. May need to consider a waist or vest restraint instead of bilateral wrist restraints. In some circumstance bilateral wrist restraints may cause increased agitation because the patient cannot use the upper extremities.
4. **Assess:** Has the primary care provider (PCP) been notified?
   Intervention: Obtain the PCP order (including time frame for restraints) and patient or guardian informed consent before applying restraints. If a significant risk exists, apply restraints before contacting the PCP and obtaining an order for the restraints, and notify the PCP immediately after application.
5. **Assess:** Does the patient have abdominal or chest incisions or devices?
   Intervention: Do not use vest or body restraints; use an alternative restraint.

PREPROCEDURE

I. Check PCP orders and the patient care plan.
Knowledge of patient-specific orders is critical for safe patient care.

II. Gather supplies and equipment.
Preparing for the patient encounter saves time and promotes patient trust.

III. Perform hand hygiene.
Frequent hand hygiene prevents the spread of microorganisms.

IV. Maintain standard precautions.
Use of the correct personal protective equipment (PPE) is required whenever contact with bodily fluids is possible, to reduce the transfer of pathogens.

V. Introduce yourself.
Initial communication establishes the role of the nurse and begins a professional relationship.

VI. Provide for patient privacy.
It is important to maintain patient dignity.

VII. Identify the patient, using two identifiers.
Identifying a patient involves scanning barcodes or comparing the patient's stated name and birthdate to information on the patient's wristband or health record. The correct person must receive the correct treatment.

VIII. Explain the procedure to the patient.
The nurse has a responsibility to inform a patient before initiating care. Information may ease patient anxiety and facilitate cooperation.

PROCEDURE

Use of Restraints

Follow preprocedure steps I through VIII.

1. Obtain the correct restraint for the situation:
   a. Lap belt
   Keeps the patient from standing up or sliding or falling out of the wheelchair.
   b. Limb (wrist or ankle) restraint
   Keeps the patient from pulling at tubes or thrashing limbs.
   c. Mitt restraint
   May be used just to restrain a hand or restrict finger movement; keeps the patient from interfering with medical devices, removing dressings, and pulling at tubes or scratching skin.
   d. Vest restraint
   Keeps the patient in the bed or wheelchair; prevents the patient from fully sitting up in bed or bending over far in the wheelchair.
   e. Roll belt
   Keeps the patient from falling out of bed; permits side-to-side movement in bed.

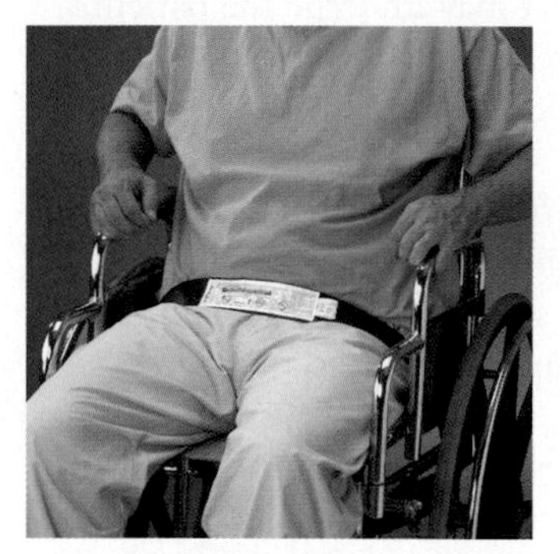

STEP 1a
(Courtesy Posey Company, Arcadia, Calif.)

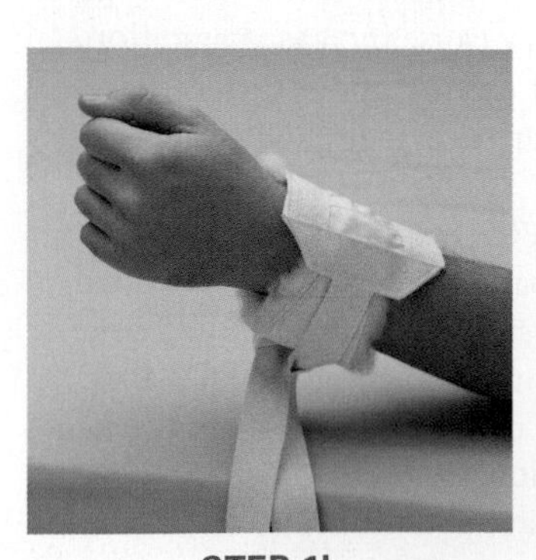

STEP 1b
(Courtesy Posey Company, Arcadia, Calif.)

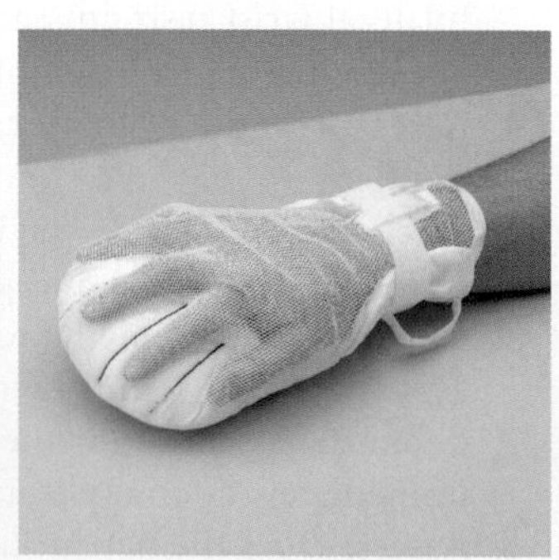

STEP 1c
(Courtesy Posey Company, Arcadia, Calif.)

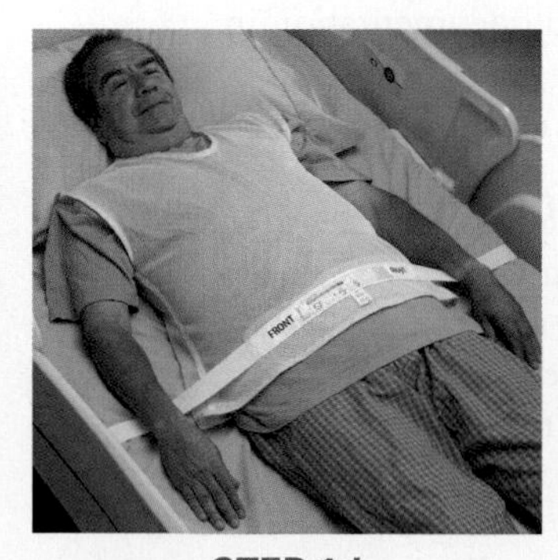

STEP 1d
(Courtesy Posey Company, Arcadia, Calif.)

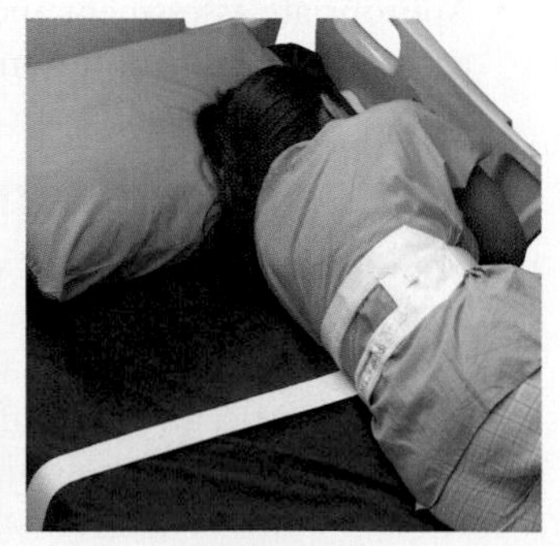

STEP 1e
(Courtesy Posey Company, Arcadia, Calif.)

2. Place the padded side of the restraint toward the skin.
   Prevents skin breakdown.
3. Wrap the strap to ensure that two fingers, side by side, fit between the restraint and the skin.
   Allows proper circulation.
4. Secure the strap in a loop or buckle.
   Prevents removal by patient.
5. Tie the end of the strap to the appropriate location, using a quick-release knot.
   Allows emergency release; some manufacturers provide quick releases in buckle devices.
   a. Bed: Tie to a part of the bed frame that moves with the patient, not to the side rails.
      Permits position changes (a safety concern).
   b. Wheelchair: Cross-tie to the frame.
      Permits wheels to roll (a safety concern).
6. Assess the patient every hour or more often. Consult agency policy because some require assessment of the patient every 15 minutes for behavioral health reasons or every 30 minutes for medical reasons. Place the call bell within reach.
   Ensures safety, enables determination of when to discontinue restraint use, provides patient stimulation, reassures the patient, and allows care plan update and other interventions to be made.
7. Remove the restraint. Assess skin, range of motion, and activities of daily living every 2 hours or more often, according to facility policy.
   Ensures safety, health, and comfort; ensures compliance with regulations and standards.

Follow postprocedure steps I through VI.

POSTPROCEDURE

I. Return the bed to its lowest position, raise the top side rails, and verify that the call light is within reach for the patient.
   Precautions are taken to maintain patient safety. Top side rails aid in positioning and turning. Raising four side rails is considered a restraint.
II. Assess for additional patient needs and state the time of your expected return.
   Meeting patient needs and offering self promote patient satisfaction and build trust.
III. Properly dispose of PPE.
   Gloves, gowns, and masks must be appropriately discarded to prevent the spread of microorganisms.
IV. Clean equipment if it was in contact with the patient; see specific manufacturer instructions.
   Disinfection eliminates most microorganisms from inanimate objects.
V. Perform hand hygiene.
   Frequent hand hygiene prevents the spread of infection.
VI. Document the date, time, assessment, procedure, and patient's response to the procedure.
   Accurate documentation is essential to communicate patient care and to provide legal evidence of care.

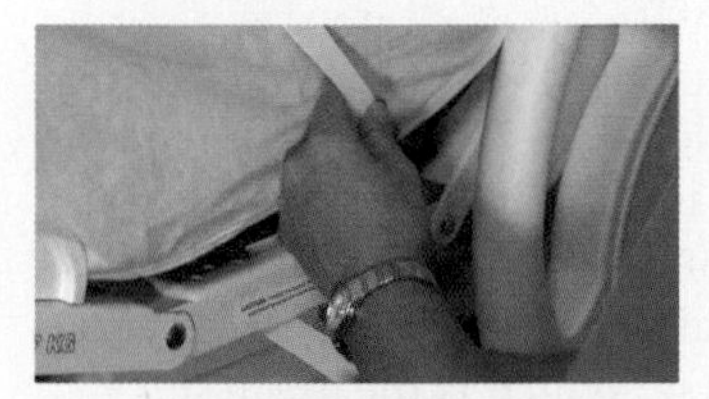

STEP 5a

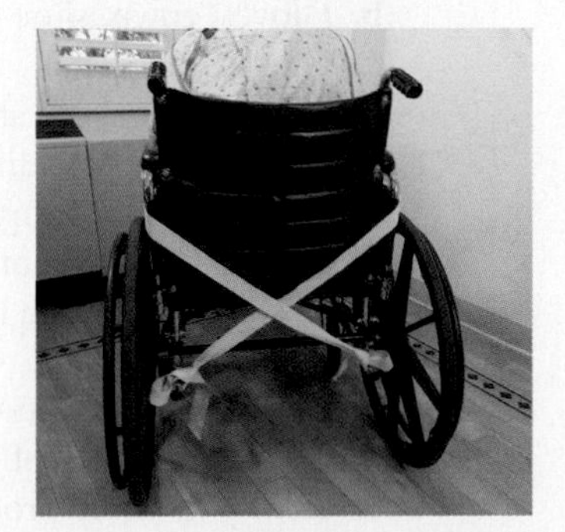

STEP 5b

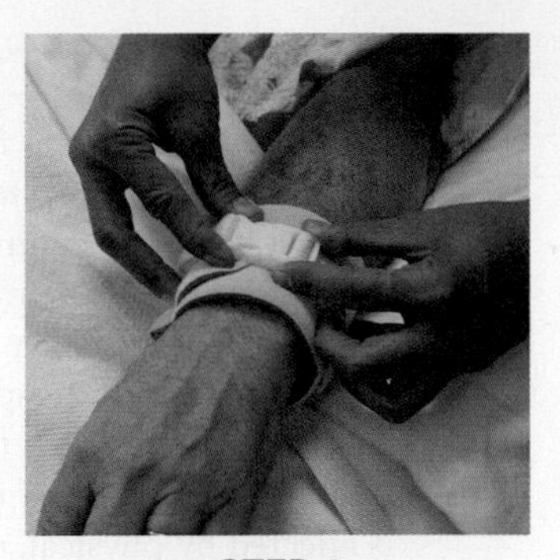

STEP 4

How to tie the posey quick-release tie

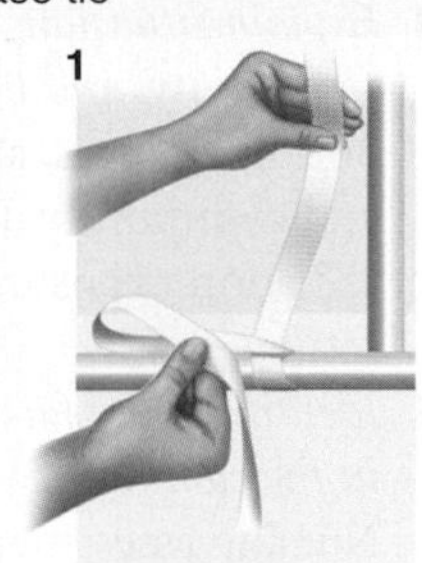

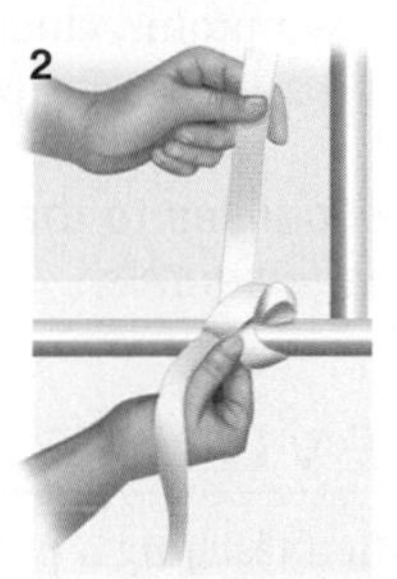

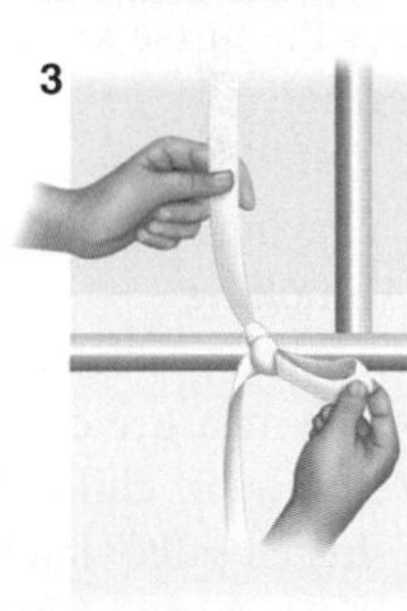

1. Wrap the strap once around a movable part of the bed frame leaving at least an 8" (20 cm) tail. Fold the loose end in half to create a loop and cross it over the other end.
2. Insert the folded strap where the straps cross over each other, as if tying a shoelace.
3. Pull on the loop to tighten. Test to make sure strap is secure and will not slide in any direction.
4. Repeat on other side. Practice quick-release ties to ensure the knot releases with one pull on the loose end of the strap.

STEP 5

(Courtesy Posey Company, Arcadia, Calif.)

SUMMARY OF LEARNING OUTCOMES

LO 25.1 *Discuss safety concerns in the home, community, and health care environments:* Major safety concerns in the home and community are unintentional injuries. The Joint Commission has developed National Patient Safety Goals to highlight areas of critical concern in hospital, long-term care, home care, and outpatient settings.

LO 25.2 *List factors that affect safety:* An individual's safety is affected by physical, mental, and cognitive health; age; environmental factors; and workplace hazards.

LO 25.3 *Explain situations that alter safety in the home, community, and health care settings:* Injuries, poisoning, fires, and biohazards exist in the home and community. Falls, injuries from restraints, and radiation exposure are risks in the health care setting.

LO 25.4 *Identify safety factors that affect individuals at home, in the community, and in health care settings:* Nursing assessment includes the collection of subjective information about the patient's symptoms, chief complaint, and environmental hazards and exposures and a corresponding objective assessment. Information in the patient's history may provide clues about safety issues. The physical assessment may reveal issues that should be further investigated.

LO 25.5 *Choose nursing diagnoses relevant to patient safety–related concerns and issues:* Some NANDA nursing diagnoses related to patient safety include Risk for Injury, Risk for Falls, and Risk for Poisoning.

LO 26.6 *Prepare nursing care plans that identify interventions to promote patient safety:* Numerous nursing interventions specific to safety promotion are individualized to prevent the negative influence that untoward events can have on patient outcomes.

LO 25.7 *Implement safety measures in the home, community, and health care settings:* The nurse provides patient education and safety promotion for patients to minimize safety risks in the home and community. Through the use of fall assessment tools, the nurse decreases the risk of injury from falls by implementing safety measures according to each patient's risk. Keeping patients and staff safe from the risks of electrical hazards, fire, radiation exposure, and infections is part of the nurse's role.

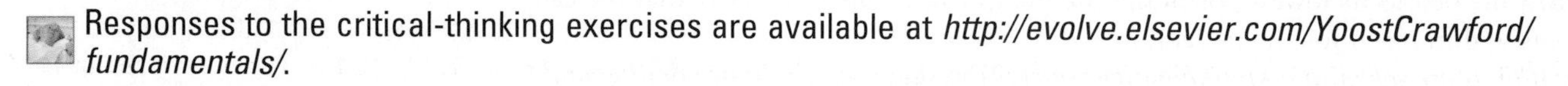
Responses to the critical-thinking exercises are available at *http://evolve.elsevier.com/YoostCrawford/fundamentals/*.

REVIEW QUESTIONS

1. When teaching a patient about fire safety, which activity does the nurse know is the leading cause of fire-related death?
   a. Cooking
   b. Playing with matches
   c. Smoking
   d. Heating with kerosene heaters
2. Which measure can the nurse teach to prevent poisoning of children? *(Select all that apply.)*
   a. Install safety latches on reachable cabinets.
   b. Keep syrup of ipecac on hand.
   c. Use childproof caps on medications.
   d. Use a plunger rather than a chemical drain cleaner.
   e. Keep cleaning supplies under the kitchen sink.
3. Which restraint-free alternative is best for the nurse to use for an 84-year-old patient after hip replacement who has acute confusion and incontinence?
   a. A room near the nurses' station and decreased sensory stimuli
   b. A pressure sensor alarm and a room near the nurses' station
   c. Side rails up and decreased sensory stimuli
   d. A 24-hour sitter and the patient's favorite TV program
4. The nurse is performing a fall risk assessment on a newly admitted patient. Which finding is a known risk factor for falls?
   a. Medications
   b. Urinary incontinence
   c. Multiple comorbidities
   d. Malnutrition
5. A patient is ordered to have a urine culture to rule out methicillin-resistant *Staphylococcus aureus* (MRSA). When obtaining this specimen, which personal protective equipment (PPE) should the nurse don?
   a. Gloves, mask, eye shield
   b. Gloves, gown, shoe covers
   c. Gloves, mask, hat
   d. Gloves, gown, eye shield
6. An elderly client residing in the community with cardiopulmonary compromise and impaired ability to perform activities of daily living (ADLs) presents safety concerns to the nurse. Which is the greatest concern?
   a. Ability to obtain and take medications correctly
   b. Ability to safely get on and off a toilet
   c. Ability to safely procure food and prepare meals
   d. Ability to safely eat without choking

7. What other health care professional should the nurse consult when a patient has difficulty with activities of daily living (ADLs) and why?
   a. Occupational therapist to evaluate the ability to perform ADLs
   b. Physical therapist to evaluate the patient's need for assistive devices
   c. Social worker to arrange for needed assistive devices
   d. Area agency on aging to arrange for Meals on Wheels
8. A 56-year-old man who has been staying at a cabin while hunting arrives at the emergency department with complaints of dizziness, light-headedness, and nausea. What does the nurse initially suspect?
   a. Carbon monoxide poisoning
   b. Lead poisoning
   c. Radon exposure
   d. Food poisoning
9. Which activity would be most appropriate for the registered nurse (RN) to delegate to unlicensed assistive personnel (UAP)?
   a. Assessing the patient for fall risk and complications of restraint use
   b. Evaluating the patient's ability to perform activities of daily living (ADLs)
   c. Assisting with or performing the patient's ADLs
   d. Teaching the patient use of assistive devices
10. When working with radiation diagnostics or treatments, which preventive measure should be followed to avoid exposure? *(Select all that apply.)*
   a. Using lead shielding of patients and staff
   b. Keeping staff at the farthest distance possible from the radiation source
   c. Limiting the length of exposure
   d. Wearing a badge to monitor the length of exposure
   e. Following procedures and safety checks

Answers and rationales to the review questions are available at *http://evolve.elsevier.com/YoostCrawford/fundamentals/*.

REFERENCES

Ahrens M: Home structure fires (National Fire Protection Agency), 2011. Retrieved from *www.nfpa.org/assets/files/PDF/OS.Homes.pdf*.

Borse NN, Gilchrist J, Dellinger AM, et al.: *CDC childhood injury report: Patterns of unintentional injuries among 0–19 year olds in the United States, 2000–2006*, Atlanta, 2008, Centers for Disease Control and Prevention, pp. 1-116.

Bureau of Labor Statistics: *Workplace injuries and illnesses 2012*, Washington, D.C., 2013, Author.

Capezuti E, Brush BL, Won RM, et al.: Least restrictive or least understood? Waist restraints, provider practices, and risk of harm. *J Aging Soc Policy*, 20(3):305-322, 2008.

Capezuti E, Evans L, Strumpf N, Maislin G: Physical restraint use and falls in nursing home residents. *J Am Geriatr Soc*, 44(6):627-633, 1996.

Capezuti E, Maislin G, Strumpf N, Evans LK: Side rail use and bed-related fall outcomes among nursing home residents. *J Am Geriatr Soc*, 50(1):90-96, 2002.

Capezuti E, Strumpf NE, Evans LK, et al.: The relationship between physical restraint removal and falls and injuries among nursing home residents. *J Gerontol A Biol Sci Med Sci*, 53(1):M47-M52, 1998.

Capezuti E, Talerico KA, Cochran I, et al: Individualized interventions to prevent bed-related falls and reduce siderail use. *J Gerontol Nurs*, 25(11):26-34, 1999.

Centers for Disease Control and Prevention (CDC): Bioterrorism, 2007. Retrieved from *http://emergency.cdc.gov/bioterrorism/*.

Centers for Disease Control and Prevention (CDC): Carbon monoxide poisoning, 2014a. Retrieved from *www.cdc.gov/co/default.htm/*.

Centers for Disease Control and Prevention (CDC): Lead, 2014b. Retrieved from *www.cdc.gov/nceh/lead/*.

Centers for Medicare and Medicaid Services (CMS): Medicare and Medicaid programs; hospital conditions of participation: Patients' rights—Final rule. *Fed Regist*, 71(236):71377-71428, 2006.

Centers for Medicare & Medicaid Services (CMS): Update of state operations manual (SOM): Release of person-identifiable data related to restraint/seclusion deaths to protection and advocacy organizations, 2008. Retrieved from *https://www.cms.gov/Medicare/Provider-Enrollment-and-Certification/SurveyCertificationGenInfo/downloads/SCLetter09-12.pdf*.

Chen LH, Warner M, Fingerhut L, Makuc D: Injury episodes and circumstances: National Health Interview Survey, 1997–2007. *Vital Health Stat*, 10(241):1-55, 2009.

Colorado Nurses Association: The American Nurses Association joins environmental health groups in urging the phase out of harmful chemicals in toys and other products. *Colo Nurse*, 109(1):24, 2009.

Cronenwett L, Sherwood G, Barnsteiner J, et al: Quality and safety education for nurses. *Nurs Outlook*, 55(3):122-131, 2007.

Curran SS: Staff resistance to restraint reduction: Identifying & overcoming barriers. *J Psychosoc Nurs Ment Health Serv*, 45(5):45-50, 2007.

Devine CE, Mawlawi O: Radiation safety with positron emission tomography and computed tomography. *Semin Ultrasound CT MRI*, 31(1):39-45, 2010.

Engberg J, Castle NG, McCaffrey D: Physical restraint initiation in nursing homes and subsequent resident health. *Gerontologist*, 48(4):442-452, 2008.

Federal Emergency Management Agency (FEMA): Biological threats, 2012. Retrieved from *www.ready.gov/biological-threats*.

Food and Drug Administration (FDA): FDA safety alert: Potential hazards with restraint devices, 1992. Retrieved from *www.fda.gov/MedicalDevices/Safety/AlertsandNotices/PublicHealthNotifications/ucm242670.htm*.

Food and Drug Administration (FDA): How to dipose of unused medicines, 2013. Retrieved from *www.fda.gov/forconsumers/consumerupdates/ucm101653.htm.*

Food and Drug Administration (FDA): Hospital beds, 2014. Retrieved from *www.fda.gov/MedicalDevices/ProductsandMedicalProcedures/GeneralHospitalDevicesandSupplies/HospitalBeds/ucm2018117.htm.*

Gastmans C, Milisen K: Use of physical restraint in nursing homes: Clinical-ethical considerations. *J Med Ethics,* 32:148-152, 2006.

Hendrich A: How to try this: Predicting patient falls: Using the Hendrich II Fall Risk Model in clinical practice. *Am J Nurs,* 107(11):50-58, 2007.

Hendrich AL, Bender PS, Nyhuis A: Validation of the Hendrich II Fall Risk Model: A large concurrent case/control study of hospitalized patients. *Appl Nurs Res,* 16(1):9-21, 2003.

Hill EE, Nguyen TH, Shaha M, et al: Person-environment interactions contributing to nursing home resident falls. *Res Gerontol Nurs,* 2(4):287-296, 2009.

Hill-Westmoreland EE, Soeken K, Spellbring AM: A meta-analysis of fall prevention programs for the elderly: How effective are they? *Nurs Res,* 51(1):1-8, 2002.

Huizing AR, Hamers JP, Gulpers MJ, Berger MP: Preventing the use of physical restraints on residents newly admitted to psycho-geriatric nursing home wards: A cluster-randomized trial. *Int J Nurs Stud,* 46(4):459-469, 2009.

Joint Commission Resources: PET/CT and patient safety. *Jt Comm J Qual Patient Saf,* 7(10):5-6, 2007.

Kontio R, Välimäki M, Putkonen H, et al.: Nurses' and physicians' educational needs in seclusion and restraint practices. *Perspect Psychiatr Care,* 45(3):198-207, 2009.

Mayo Clinic: Poisoning: First aid, 2012. Retrieved from *www.mayoclinic.org/first-aid/first-aid-poisoning/basics/art-20056657.*

Mayo Clinic: Lead poisoning, 2014. Retrieved from *www.mayoclinic.org/diseases-conditions/lead-poisoning/basics/definition/con-20035487.*

Meade CM, Bursell AL, Ketelsen L: Effects of nursing rounds: On patients' call light use, satisfaction, and safety. *Am J Nurs,* 106(9):58-70, 2006.

Morse JM: *Preventing patient falls: Establishing a fall intervention program,* ed. 2, New York, 2009, Springer.

National Safety Council: Injury facts, 2010. Retrieved from *www.nsc.org/Pages/UnderstandtheLatestInjuryTrendsInjuryFacts2010Edition.aspx.*

Page K, McKinney AA: Addressing medication errors—The role of undergraduate nurse education. *Nurse Educ Today,* 27(3):219-224, 2007.

Parents Central: Car seat recommendations for children, 2014. Retrieved from *www.safercar.gov/parents/RightSeat.htm.*

Paterson B, Duxbury J: Restraint and the question of validity. *Nurs Ethics,* 14(4):535-545, 2007.

Peled K: Workplace safety assessment and injury prevention in hospital settings. *Work,* 25(3):273-277, 2005.

Poe SS, Cvach M, Dawson PB., et al: The Johns Hopkins Fall Risk Assessment Tool: Postimplementation evaluation. *J Nurs Care Qual,* 22(4):293-298, 2007.

Pronovost P, Weast B, Schwarz M, et al: Medication reconciliation: A practical tool to reduce the risk of medication errors. *J Crit Care,* 18(4):201-205, 2003.

The Joint Commission: Preventing restraint deaths, 1998. Retrieved from *www.jointcommission.org/assets/1/18/SEA_8.pdf.*

The Joint Commission (TJC): National patient safety goals, 2014. Retrieved from *www.jointcommission.org/assets/1/6/HAP_NPSG_Chapter_2014.pdf.*

Tinetti ME, Liu WL, Ginter SF: Mechanical restraint use and fall-related injuries among residents of skilled nursing facilities. *Ann Intern Med,* 116(5):369-374, 1992.

Toblin RL, Paulozzi LJ, Gilchrist J, Russell PJ: Unintentional strangulation deaths from the "choking game" among youths aged 6-19 years: United States, 1995-2007. *MMWR Morb Mortal Wkly Rep,* 57(6):141-144, 2008.

Trinkoff A, Geiger-Brown J, Brady B, et al: How long and how much are nurses now working? *Am J Nurs,* 106(4):60-71, 2006.

U.S. Fire Administration: Residential and nonresidential building fire estimates, 2014a. Retrieved from *www.usfa.fema.gov/statistics/estimates/index.shtm*

U.S. Fire Administration: Home fire sprinkler outreach materials, 2014b. Retrieved from *www.usfa.fema.gov/citizens/home_fire_prev/sprinklers/.*

Wachter RM: Patient safety at ten: Unmistakable progress, troubling gaps. *Health Aff (Millwood),* 29(1):165-173, 2010.

Xu JQ, Murphy SL, Kochanek KD, Tejada-Vera B: Deaths: Final data for 2007. *Natl Vital Stat Rep,* 58(19):2010.

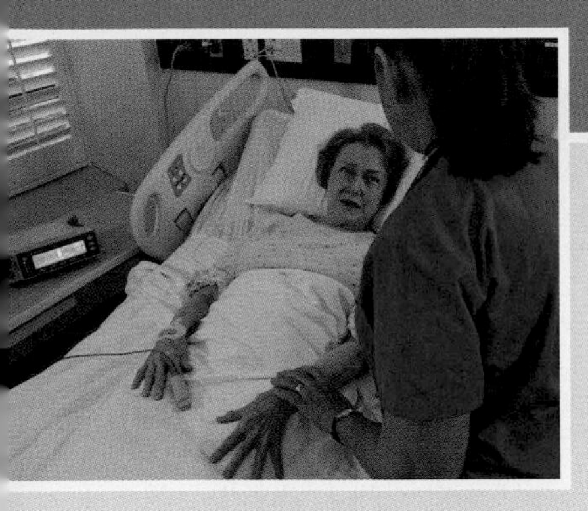

CHAPTER 26

Asepsis and Infection Control

EVOLVE WEBSITE

http://evolve.elsevier.com/YoostCrawford/fundamentals/

- Additional Evolve-Only Review Questions With Answers
- Answers and Rationales for Text Review Questions
- Answers to Critical-Thinking Questions
- Case Study With Questions
- Video Skills Clips
- Conceptual Care Map Creator
- Animations
- Skill Checklists
- Glossary

LEARNING OUTCOMES

Comprehension of this chapter's content will provide students with the ability to:

LO 26.1 Summarize the body's defense system.
LO 26.2 Explain the links of the chain of infection.
LO 26.3 Outline techniques of assessing for infection or risk of infection.
LO 26.4 Identify nursing diagnoses for patients with infection or at risk for infection.
LO 26.5 Use measurable goals for patients with complications from infection.
LO 26.6 Carry out interventions to decrease the risk of infection and reverse the negative effects of infection.

KEY TERMS

airborne transmission, p. 491
antibodies, p. 489
antigen, p. 489
asepsis, p. 488
bacteria, p. 490
cellular immunity, p. 489
contact, p. 491
disinfection, p. 501
droplet transmission, p. 491
fungi, p. 491
health care–associated infections, p. 492
host, p. 491
humoral immunity, p. 489
immune response, p. 489
immunization, p. 500
infection, p. 488
inflammatory response, p. 488
medical asepsis, p. 500
mode of transmission, p. 491
normal flora, p. 488
parasites, p. 491
pathogen, p. 490
personal protective equipment, p. 500
portal of entry, p. 491
portal of exit, p. 491
replication, p. 490
reservoir, p. 491
sterilization, p. 501
surgical asepsis, p. 500
susceptible host, p. 492
vectors, p. 491
viruses, p. 491

CASE STUDY

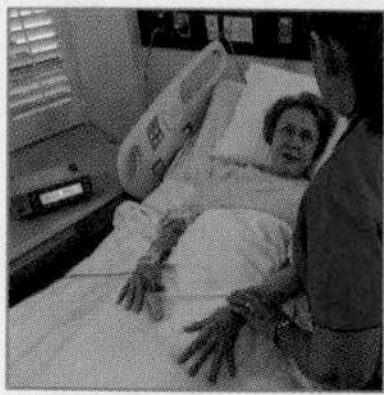

Mrs. Payne is a 76-year-old female who was admitted to the hospital 2 days earlier with complaints of right lower quadrant abdominal pain. Her medical history includes type 2 diabetes mellitus. She was evaluated in the emergency room and sent to the operating room for an appendectomy 8 hours after coming to the hospital.

Mrs. Payne's vital signs are temp 38.4°C (101.2°F), P 96 and regular, R 22 and unlabored, BP 130/72, and pulse oximetry of 96% on room air (RA). She rates pain in her right lower abdomen as 3 of 10, but with movement, the pain level increases to 8 of 10. She reports sharp, stabbing pain in the abdominal area around her incision site. Pain medication and position change relieve the pain. The skin around the incision is warm and red, and the area is tender to the touch. Laboratory results are WBC 20,000, Hgb 16, Hct 47, BUN 25, creatinine 0.8, K 4.0, and Na 142.

Treatment orders are as follows:

- Vital signs q 4 hr and as needed (PRN)
- Regular diet with supplements twice daily
- Intake and output (I&O)
- Activity: up with assist of one
- Right abdominal dressing: dry sterile dressing, change q 8 hr
- Turn, cough, and deep breathe q 4 hr while awake
- Incentive spirometry q 2 hr while awake
- Antiembolism stockings while out of bed
- Sequential compression devices (SCDs) while in bed
- Complete blood count every morning
- Fall precautions
- Physical therapy (PT) for ambulation daily

Medication orders are as follows:

- Continuous intravenous (IV) 5% dextrose in 0.45% normal saline (D_5/0.45 NS) at 50 mL/hr
- Enoxaparin 40 mg subcutaneously daily
- Metformin 500 mg PO twice daily
- Hydrocodone 5 mg and acetaminophen 500 mg PO q 4 hr PRN for pain
- Cefuroxime 750 mg IV q 8 hr

Refer back to this case study to answer the critical-thinking questions throughout the chapter.

Nurses are responsible for understanding their role in preventing the transmission of infectious agents. Infection control practices are essential for providing a safe health care environment for patients and the clinicians who care for them. During the past several years, the number of health care–associated infections (HAIs) has increased significantly, endangering everyone in the health care environment. This chapter explores the basic aseptic technique and infection control measures necessary to protect patients and the community from the spread of potentially harmful microorganisms.

NORMAL STRUCTURE AND FUNCTION OF THE BODY'S DEFENSE SYSTEM LO 26.1

An **infection** is the establishment of a pathogen in a susceptible host; a disease state is caused by the infectious agent. Many microorganisms are contagious and can cause serious illness. Nurses cannot be familiar with every microorganism, but they can prevent the spread of infection through aseptic interventions. **Asepsis** refers to freedom from and prevention of disease-causing contamination.

The body has many defenses against microorganisms that can cause illness. The three main defenses are normal flora, the inflammatory response, and the immune response.

NORMAL FLORA

Normal flora is a group of non–disease-causing microorganisms (e.g., bacteria, fungi, protozoa) that live in or on the body. These benign microorganisms are found in and on the skin, eyes, nose, mouth, upper throat, lower urethra, small intestine, and large intestine. The normal flora constitutes the body's first line of defense against infection because it inhibits pathogenic microorganisms from colonizing healthy individuals (Abedon, 2009).

INFLAMMATORY RESPONSE

The second line of defense is the **inflammatory response.** Inflammation is a local response to cellular injury or infection that includes capillary dilation and leukocyte infiltration. This response produces redness, heat, pain, and swelling. The leukocytes release a chemical that increases the temperature in the area. The dilation, infiltration, and increase in temperature are protective mechanisms that help the body neutralize, control, and eliminate invading pathogens, preventing them from surviving and multiplying. If inflammation becomes systemic, signs include fever (caused by prostaglandins acting on the hypothalamus), chills, malaise, and altered mental status. Inflammation causes the body to mount the third defense, which is the immune response. The animation "Inflammation" shows this process.

IMMUNE RESPONSE

Inflammation activates the **immune response**, which is the body's attempt to protect itself from foreign and harmful substances. The immune response is initiated by recognition of antigens. An **antigen** is any substance that provokes an adaptive immune response. Antigens include protein molecules on the surface of pathogens and nonliving substances such as toxins, chemicals, drugs, or particles. The immune system recognizes and destroys substances that contain foreign antigens.

Most people are born with innate (nonspecific) immunity (Goronzy and Weyand, 2012). The adaptive mechanisms of direct (active) and indirect (passive) immunologic memory determine how a person's immune system recognizes antigens. This can be seen in the animations "Active Immunity" and "Passive Immunity."

Innate Immunity

The innate (nonspecific) immune system provides immediate defense against foreign antigens. The skin, cough reflex, mucus, enzymes on the skin and in tears, and acid in the gastrointestinal tract prohibit harmful substances from entering the body. In addition to acting as a barrier to infectious agents, the innate immune system produces chemical mediators that fight infection, remove foreign substances, and activate the adaptive immune system.

Adaptive Immunity

The adaptive (acquired or specific) component of the immune system provides long-term immunity when the body is exposed to an antigen. Humoral (antibody-mediated) and cellular (cell-mediated) immunity are two types of adaptive immunity.

Humoral Immunity

Humoral immunity is a defense system that involves white blood cells (B lymphocytes) that produce antibodies in response to antigens or pathogens circulating in the lymph and blood. **Antibodies** are immunoglobulin molecules that recognize foreign invaders. The antigen-antibody reaction initiates a complex chain of events to protect the body from the invading microorganism.

Humoral immunity enables production of inflammatory molecules such as interferon and interleukin-1, which cause fever. If a pathogen gets past the innate response, it is attacked by the adaptive immune system, which generates antigen-specific antibodies and lymphocytes (Goronzy and Weyand, 2012).

Cellular Immunity

Cellular immunity involves defense by white blood cells against any microorganisms that the body does not recognize as its own. T lymphocytes, such as cytotoxic T cells, directly attack cells displaying nonself antigens (e.g., infected cells). Helper T cells release interleukins and other substances that stimulate antibody production by B cells and antigen destruction by other cells (e.g., macrophages).

Immunologic Memory

Adaptive immunity is antigen specific and involves active, long-term immunologic memory. As B cells and T cells develop, they learn to differentiate between the body's tissues and substances that are not normally found in the body. Some cells are sensitized by interaction with a specific antigen and become memory cells. Subsequent exposure to the antigen produces a stronger and faster immune response by these memory cells, which can ease or prevent later illness in many cases. Long-term active immunity can be artificially acquired by immunization with vaccines.

Passive immunity occurs when a person receives an antibody produced in another body. Passive immunization provides immediate but short-term protection against antigens. Infants acquire passive immunity naturally in utero or through breast milk, and these antibodies disappear between the ages of 6 and 12 months. Passive immunity can be acquired artificially when antibodies are transferred from one person to another by injection of an antibody-rich serum (e.g., immune globulin).

OTHER BODY SYSTEMS

The integumentary, respiratory, and gastrointestinal systems have roles in fighting infection. Skin is a barrier that is impermeable to most infectious microorganisms. Any break in the skin can create a portal of entry or exit for pathogens. The skin contains squamous epithelial cells, which help to remove microorganisms and other infectious agents. Sweat decreases the likelihood of infection because its low pH inhibits bacterial growth (Mayer, 2009).

The respiratory system plays a role in helping the body fight infection. The respiratory system contains cilia and mucus, which move or trap foreign bodies and therefore decrease the risk for infection. The respiratory system is equipped with proteins that have antimicrobial properties and promote phagocytosis (Mayer, 2009).

The gastrointestinal system plays an active role in helping the body fight infection. The flora and low pH of the gastrointestinal tract prevent the colonization of pathogenic microorganisms by secreting toxic substances or competing with the microorganism for the nutrients needed to make it thrive (Mayer, 2009).

ALTERED STRUCTURE AND FUNCTION OF THE BODY'S DEFENSE SYSTEM LO 26.2

To understand how to prevent the spread of potentially harmful microorganisms, nurses must understand the chain of infection.

CHAIN OF INFECTION

The chain of infection has six main components: the infectious agent, the source of infection, the portal of exit, the mode of transmission, the portal of entry, and the susceptible host (Figure 26-1). Infectious agents are the first link of the chain of infection that is necessary to spread disease-causing organisms.

Infectious Agents

Any infectious agent that causes disease is referred to as a **pathogen**. Pathogens include bacteria, viruses, fungi, and parasites.

Bacteria are single-cell organisms. Bacteria live as normal flora on and in the skin, eyes, nose, mouth, upper throat, lower urethra, lower intestine, and large intestine. They are capable of causing disease in the human population when they overgrow due to immune system compromise or when they enter different areas of the body. Bacteria have different sizes, shapes, growth patterns, and means of **replication**, which is a term used to describe bacterial reproduction or duplication. They are named according to their shape and are classified by their ability to live with or without oxygen (i.e., aerobic or anaerobic) and their staining qualities (i.e., gram positive or gram negative). Bacteria reproduce by dividing;

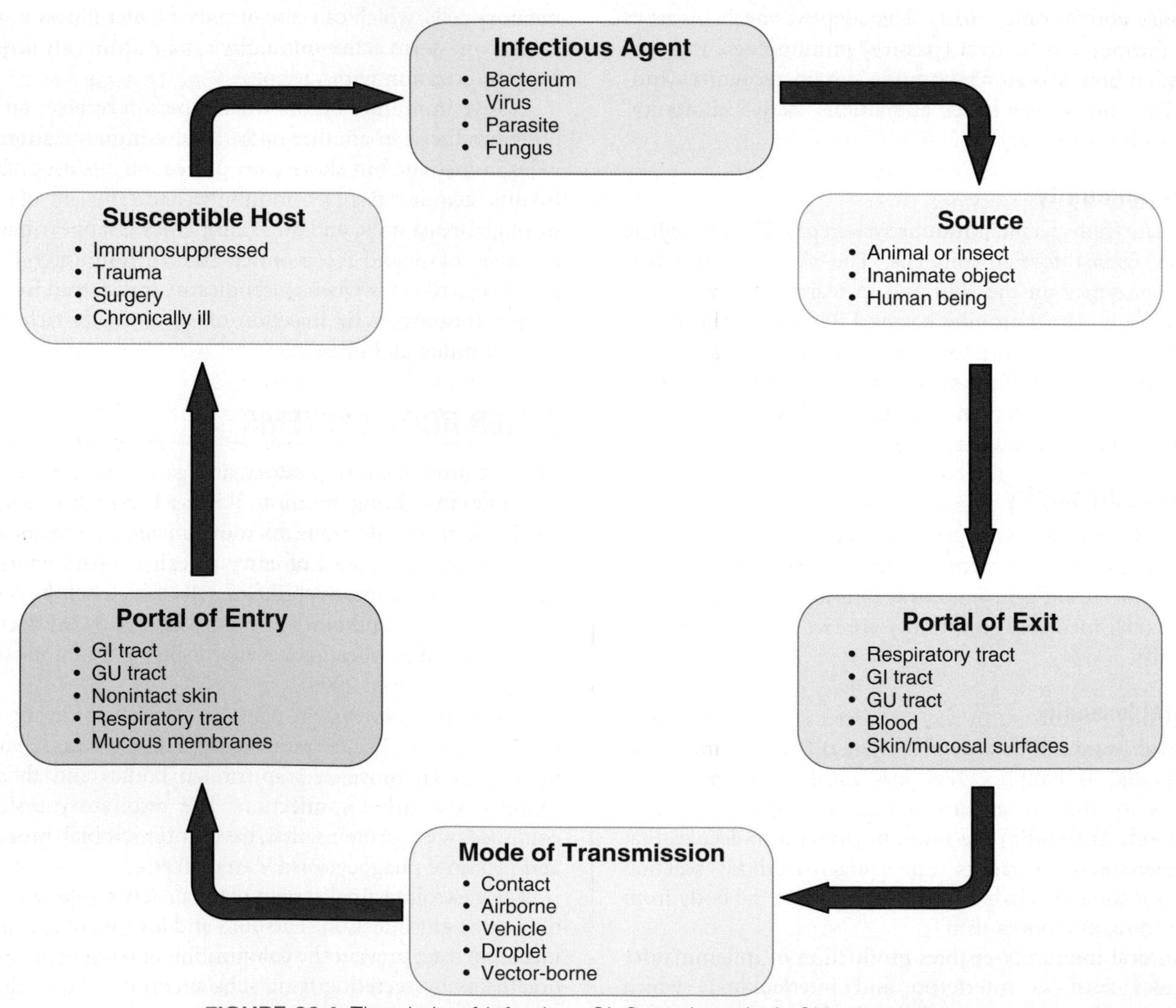

FIGURE 26-1 The chain of infection. *GI,* Gastrointestinal; *GU,* genitourinary.

one cell becomes two identical cells. Bacteria are identified when a sample taken from the body is cultured, and exact antibiotic sensitivity is tested so that appropriate antibiotics are prescribed.

Viruses are the smallest microorganisms. Viruses reproduce inside living cells of the host and are responsible for causing many different types of disease. Illnesses range from the common cold to acquired immune deficiency syndrome (AIDS). Viruses cannot be killed by antibiotics. Certain antiviral medications are used to manage the symptoms of a viral infection. These medications, if given during the early phases of illness, can decrease the amount of time that the patient has viral symptoms.

Fungi, like bacteria, are single-cell organisms that can cause infection. Molds and yeast are examples of common fungi. Fungi are present in the air, the soil, and water and are responsible for conditions such as athlete's foot, ringworm, and yeast infections. Infections that are caused by fungi are treated with antifungal medications.

Parasites are organisms that live on or in other organisms. Examples of these organisms include protozoa, helminths, and arthropods. Parasites are typically transmitted by sexual contact, insects, and domestic animals. They cause many diseases in humans. Protozoa cause malaria, helminths are responsible for intestinal worm infestations, and arthropods are responsible for transmitting many skin and systemic diseases such as ringworm and malaria.

Source of Infection

The second link of the chain is the source of infection, also called a **reservoir** or **host**. Reservoirs can be inanimate objects such as surfaces, equipment, medication, air, food, and water on which microorganisms can find nourishment and survive. Human sources of infection are health care personnel, family, friends, and patients. Animals such as insects, rats, birds, pigs, and cows spread disease and have been the reservoirs for many epidemics in the past and for current diseases such as avian flu and mad cow disease (Centers for Disease Control and Prevention [CDC], 2012a).

Portal of Exit

Infection spread requires a **portal of exit**, which is the means by which the pathogen escapes from the reservoir of infection. Microorganisms escape through emesis, sputum, urine, stool, blood, genital secretions, and wound drainage.

Mode of Transmission

The microorganism must have a way to travel from the source to the susceptible host. The form of transportation is referred to as the **mode of transmission**. Modes of transmission include contact, airborne, vehicle (e.g., food, water, contaminated objects), droplet, and vector-borne (e.g., insects, animals).

Most microorganisms are transmitted by **contact**, which is when body surfaces touch surfaces of other bodies or objects. Direct contact involves a physical transfer of the microorganism from the infected individual to a susceptible host. Indirect contact occurs when the microorganism is transferred by of a contaminated object, such as a dressing, needle, or surgical instrument such as a retractor or scalpel. In the health care setting, the most common means of transmission are contaminated hands (CDC, 2012b).

Some microorganisms can be transmitted through the air. **Airborne transmission** occurs when microorganisms are dispersed by air currents and inhaled or deposited on the skin of a susceptible host. Examples of illnesses transmitted through the air include tuberculosis, measles, and chickenpox.

Some microorganisms are transmitted by droplets. **Droplet transmission** occurs when the mucous membranes of the respiratory tract (i.e., nose, mouth, or conjunctiva) are exposed to the secretions of an infected individual. Droplets cannot remain suspended in the air for long periods and seldom travel more than 3 feet. Examples of illnesses transmitted by droplets are influenza and respiratory syncytial virus (RSV) infection (Siegel, Rhinehart, Jackson, et al., 2007).

Airborne transmission and droplet transmission are often hard to differentiate. Microorganisms travel through the air in both cases, but the difference between the two modes is the size of the microorganism. Because smaller microorganisms can travel longer distances and can remain suspended for longer periods, they are considered to be transmissible by air. Larger microorganisms cannot travel long distances and usually require closer contact for transmission; they are considered to be transmissible by droplet.

Special precautions have been written by the CDC for certain diseases such as Ebola. See the CDC website for specifics on these special types of isolation.

Vectors carry the pathogens from one host to another. Vectors often are invertebrate animals such as ticks, but they can also be vertebrate animals such as raccoons, which can transmit rabies by biting. Vector-borne diseases include Lyme disease, Rocky Mountain spotted fever, West Nile virus, and viral encephalitis.

Portal of Entry

For the chain of infection to continue and the microorganism to be successfully transmitted from a primary host to a susceptible host, there must be a **portal of entry**, which is the means by which the microorganism enters the susceptible host. There are many portals of entry: the gastrointestinal tract by ingestion, the genitourinary tract by contact with mucous membranes, the respiratory tract by inhalation, the integumentary system by breaks in the skin, and the urinary tract by introduction through the urethra. Individuals who are hospitalized are at increased risk for infection because of greater exposure to infectious agents and because many of the invasive procedures that are performed access the portals of entry.

The nurse can take steps at any link in the chain to halt the spread of infection. Standard precautions are used with all patients to limit direct exposure to blood and body fluids. Bodily discharges are disposed of immediately and properly to prevent spreading potentially harmful microorganisms. Handwashing destroys microorganisms so that others are not infected. Patients with contagious illnesses are isolated and personal protective equipment (PPE) is used when entering the room so that a removable barrier is formed between the health care worker and the patient. These and other interventions practiced to break the chain of infection are discussed later in the chapter.

Susceptible Host

After the pathogen exits the reservoir, it must be transported to a susceptible host for the chain to be completed. A **susceptible host** is someone exposed to an infectious disease who is likely to contract the disease. Increased susceptibility is associated with people at the extremes of age, those who are nutritionally compromised, and those who have had recent trauma or surgery. Those who are immunocompromised because of chemotherapy, radiation treatments, long-term use of steroids, or transplantation have lower resistance to infection. Patients with chronic illnesses, such as heart or lung disease, diabetes, liver or kidney disease, and human immunodeficiency virus (HIV) infection or AIDS also have lower resistance to infection.

HEALTH CARE–ASSOCIATED INFECTIONS

Health care–associated infections (HAIs), formerly referred to as *nosocomial infections,* are infections acquired while the patient is receiving treatment in a health care facility such as a hospital, long-term care facility, clinic, or primary care office. HAIs cost $28.4 billion to $38.8 billion annually (CDC, 2014). Their impact includes delays in recovery, treatment, and discharge; longer hospital stays; permanent disability; increased costs associated with prescriptions; loss of earnings; disruption of family routine; anxiety; pain; and death (Hart, 2007). Data about HAIs are collected by the CDC in an effort to improve the infection-control methods used by health care providers.

HAIs are associated with the use of medical devices such as catheters and ventilators, complications after a surgical procedure, contagious transmission between patients and health care workers, and the overuse of antibiotics (CDC, 2014). HAIs may be caused by drug-resistant microorganisms such as methicillin-resistant *Staphylococcus aureus* (MRSA); vancomycin-resistant *S. aureus* (VRSA); vancomycin-resistant enterococci (VRE); blood-borne pathogens such as hepatitis B, hepatitis C, and HIV; and *Clostridium difficile* (C. diff) and other microorganisms that affect the gastrointestinal tract (CDC, 2014).

! SAFE PRACTICE ALERT

Handwashing is the most effective method for preventing hospital-acquired infections.

RESISTANT ORGANISMS

Microorganisms adapt to their environment to compete for survival. As early as the 1940s, there were documented cases of microorganisms developing resistance to medications that had been previously successful at treating the infection. This phenomenon is known as *drug resistance* (CDC, 2014). A microorganism is considered resistant if replication cannot be stopped by two or more antibiotics sequentially or simultaneously (Tarrac, 2008).

Resistance is observed for community- and hospital-acquired infections. Community-acquired microorganisms that have developed drug resistance include *Enterobacteriaceae (Salmonella* and *Shigella), Mycobacterium tuberculosis, Staphylococcus aureus, Streptococcus pneumoniae, Haemophilus influenzae,* and *Neisseria gonorrhoeae.* Microorganisms that have developed resistance in the hospital setting include MRSA, VRSA, VRE, and C-Diff (CDC, 2014).

Many factors contribute to resistance, including overprescribing of antibiotics for nonbacterial infections, use of inappropriate antibiotics for the infecting microorganism, and incomplete courses of antibiotics. Infections are becoming increasingly hard to treat, and some microorganisms cannot be effectively destroyed by any known antibiotic.

Until recently, new drugs have been provided in time to treat bacteria that had become resistant to older antibiotics. This is no longer the case because the cost of developing new antibiotics is astronomical, and the development of new antibiotics has slowed (CDC, 2014).

SAFE PRACTICE ALERT

Drug-resistant microorganisms pose a considerable health risk for the general population and health care workers. Appropriate use of PPE and handwashing can decrease the risk of transmission.

BLOOD-BORNE PATHOGENS

Several blood-borne pathogens can put patients and health care providers at risk for infection. They include hepatitis B virus, hepatitis C virus, and HIV. Exposure occurs through contact with contaminated blood or body fluids. Exposure does not necessarily mean disease development. Exposure and disease development can be decreased with the appropriate precautions and barriers (CDC, 2011).

If exposure occurs, several steps can be taken to decrease the risk of developing disease. These steps vary by individual institution, but anyone who is exposed to a blood-borne pathogen should have baseline laboratory work completed to check for HIV and hepatitis. If the patient source is known, the patient is tested. Subsequent testing and medical prophylaxis may also be warranted (CDC, 2011).

SIGNS AND SYMPTOMS OF INFECTION

The type and location of the infection determine the specific signs and symptoms observed during assessment. Infections are classified as localized or systemic. Localized infections can cause redness, swelling, warmth, pain, tenderness, drainage, numbness or tingling, and loss of function to the affected area. Systemic infections (i.e., infections that infiltrate the bloodstream) can cause fever, increases in heart and respiratory rates, lethargy, anorexia, and tenderness or enlargement of lymph nodes.

Many factors can cause an individual to be more susceptible to infections (Diversity Considerations box).

ASSESSMENT LO 26.3

HEALTH HISTORY

During assessment, a history is obtained before observation. A vigilant nursing assessment considers the patient's susceptibility and clinical appearance and the effectiveness of the patient's defenses against disease (Health Assessment Questions box).

HEALTH ASSESSMENT QUESTIONS

Infection Assessment

The nurse observes the patient's general appearance to detect infection. Specific questions can help to determine whether the patient already has or is at risk for an infection:

- Do you feel tired or fatigued?
- Do you feel short of breath?
- Do you often feel chilled and require a blanket when others in the room are comfortable?
- How is your appetite?
- Do you have any areas of pain, redness, swelling, and warmth?
- Do you have any rashes, breaks in the skin, or reddened areas?
- Do you have swollen lymph nodes?
- Do you feel that you empty your bladder when you go to the bathroom?
- Do you have a cough or difficulty swallowing?
- Have you had a fever?
- What medications are you on? Have you taken an antibiotic recently?
- Are your immunizations up to date?

DIVERSITY CONSIDERATIONS

Life Span

- Extremes in age cause an individual to be more susceptible to infection. Infants and the elderly are at the greatest risk for infection.
- Infants are more susceptible to infection because they have immature immune systems and have not been immunized against communicable diseases.
- As people age, the immune system becomes less effective due to decreased numbers of macrophages and other white blood cells.
- The elderly are at an increased risk for respiratory, urinary, and skin infections. Respiratory infections are increased due to decreased cough reflex, decreased elastic recoil of the lungs, decreased activity of the cilia, and abnormal swallowing reflex. Urinary tract infections (UTIs) in the elderly are caused by incomplete emptying of the bladder, decreased sphincter control, bladder outlet obstruction due to an enlarged prostate gland, pelvic floor relaxation because of estrogen depletion, and reduced renal blood flow.
- The elderly are at an increased risk for skin infections due to loss of elasticity, increased dryness, thinning of the epidermis, slowing of cell replacement, and decreased vascular supply.

Gender

- Females are at greater risk for UTIs because of the anatomy of the genitourinary system.
- Males with an enlarged prostate may have incomplete emptying of the bladder, leaving them vulnerable to UTIs.

Culture, Ethnicity, and Religion

- Various cultural, ethnic, and religious factors may influence a patient's ability or desire to seek medical assistance, which can increase the risk of developing or maintaining an infection.

Disability

- Disabilities causing immobility can increase the risk for respiratory, skin, and urinary tract infections.

Morphology

- Obesity has been linked to an increased risk of certain skin infections in the skin folds.

EFFECTS OF INFECTION ON THE BODY'S DEFENSE SYSTEM

Infections are classified as acute or chronic. Acute infections develop and run their course rapidly. Examples of acute infections include coughs, colds, and ear infections, which last 10 to 14 days. Chronic infections, such as infectious mononucleosis, may persist for months, as may wound and bone infections. Infectious diseases such as hepatitis and AIDS may last for years.

Some patients with an infectious disease may have no visible symptoms at presentation, whereas others can have a varied clinical picture, depending on the specific infection. Signs and symptoms of infection that may be observed are fever, chills, malaise, altered mental status, headache, and fatigue. Confusion is a common presentation in the elderly and is often the first indication of an infection such as pneumonia or a UTI.

Assessment of Vital Signs

Altered vital signs can indicate an infection. Temperature elevates slightly as the infection process begins. This is one of the body's defense mechanisms. As time passes and no interventions are initiated, the temperature continues to increase, and other symptoms occur. As the infection progresses, the blood pressure rises, and pulse and respiratory rates increase. Some patients with a severe infection such as sepsis may have damage to the body's organs and may be hypothermic. Decreased blood pressure is a late sign of infection, indicating septicemia and shock.

Nutritional Assessment

Adequate nutrition is important in the body's defense against infection. Infection depletes proteins, vitamins, minerals, and water in the body. These nutrients must be replaced to ensure adequate functioning of the body's defense mechanisms. During the physical assessment, the nurse assesses the patient's skin, mucous membranes, and overall appearance in addition to asking the patient about dietary intake.

Risk Assessment

Nurses must be aware of the many conditions that place patients at increased risk for infection. Chronic diseases, alterations in the immune system, medications such as chemotherapeutic drugs, alterations in skin integrity, malnutrition, indwelling medical devices such as urinary catheters, lack of proper immunizations, and other conditions can cause a patient to develop an infectious disease when exposed to certain microorganisms. During the physical assessment, the nurse assesses the patient's skin and dietary intake and the integrity of invasive catheters to detect any subtle signs of infection.

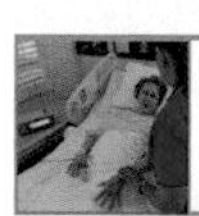

1. List the techniques necessary to assess Mrs. Payne's possible infection.

Laboratory and Diagnostic Tests

The nurse monitors several laboratory tests when assessing for infection. Tests include a complete blood count (CBC) and a differential white blood cell (WBC) count. The normal WBC count for adults is 4500 to 10,500 cells/mm^3. The differential WBC count is the proportion of each type of WBC in a sample of 100 WBCs. It helps to determine whether the body is mounting an immune response to an infection. A shift to the left (i.e., relative increase in immature forms of blood cells) with a higher percentage of neutrophils than normal indicates an infection.

Culture and sensitivity testing of the blood, urine, stool, or wound drainage may be indicated. Culture of a specimen determines which microorganism is causing an infection, and sensitivity testing determines which antibiotics, if any, can be used to treat the infection. The presence of pathogens in a specimen is a positive result.

Another laboratory test that is useful is assessing infection is the erythrocyte sedimentation rate (ESR). The ESR measures the degree of inflammation in the body, and the result can be an indicator of infection. An ESR that remains elevated indicates a poor response to current therapy, whereas an ESR that decreases indicates a good response. An ESR test is performed by timing how fast red blood cells settle to the bottom of a tube of whole blood; they settle faster when inflammation is present. Chapter 34 provides CBC and differential WBC count values.

◆ NURSING DIAGNOSIS LO 26.4

Nursing diagnoses are developed on the basis of patient data collected by the nurse. Nursing diagnoses clearly identify patient problems for which a nursing intervention is required and nursing care plans are developed. Many appropriate nursing diagnoses can be used for a patient with an infection. The following examples of nursing diagnoses with diagnostic statements are applicable to infectious diseases:

- *Risk for Infection* with risk factors of break in skin integrity and chronic disease
- *Knowledge Deficit* related to lack of knowledge about what causes infection as evidenced by patient not washing hands after toileting or before meals
- *Impaired Skin Integrity* related to prolonged bed rest and improper diet as evidenced by an open area on the coccyx
- *Imbalanced Nutrition: Less than Body Requirements* related to medication therapy as evidenced by decreased serum albumin and patient's refusal to eat meals or take supplements

Nursing diagnoses based on the effects of infection on various body systems also may be appropriate.

◆ PLANNING LO 26.5

The planning stage of the nursing process involves prioritizing identified nursing diagnoses, evaluating patient abilities and resources, and setting goals. The nurse carefully considers the importance of each nursing diagnosis and addresses the most critical ones first in the nursing care plan (Table 26-1). Maslow's hierarchy of needs is a helpful resource for ranking nursing diagnoses.

Reviewing data collected during the assessment process helps the nurse set realistic outcome criteria based on identified patient capabilities. Goals take into consideration the economic, psychosocial, physical, and other resources available in individual situations.

Collaboration with patients and families and with members of the health care team is imperative to identify

TABLE 26-1 Care Planning

NANDA-I NURSING DIAGNOSIS LABEL WITH NURSING DIAGNOSIS STATEMENT	NURSING OUTCOME CLASSIFICATION (NOC)	NURSING INTERVENTION CLASSIFICATION (NIC)
Risk for Infection with risk factors of break in skin integrity and chronic disease	*Tissue integrity: Skin and mucous membranes* (1101) Erythema (110121)	*Incision site care* (3440) Monitor incision for signs and symptoms of infection.

From Bulechek G, Butcher H, Dochterman J, et al (Eds): *Nursing interventions classification (NIC)*, ed. 6, St. Louis, 2013, Mosby; Moorhead S, Johnson M, Maas M, et al (Eds): *Nursing outcomes classification (NOC)*, ed. 5, St. Louis, 2013, Mosby; NANDA International: *Nursing diagnoses: Definitions and classification, 2012–2014*, West Sussex, England, 2012, Wiley-Blackwell. Reprinted with permission from NANDA International, Inc.

desired patient outcomes and set mutually acceptable goals. Goals are directed at alleviating the specific problems identified in each nursing diagnosis, are patient centered, and are measurable.

From each nursing diagnosis, the nurse develops specific goals for the patient who has or is at risk for an infection. Examples of goal and outcome statements follow:

- Patient's incision will remain infection free during hospitalization.
- Patient will maintain good personal hygiene by the end of day 3 after admission.
- Patient's open area on the coccyx will decrease in size by the end of day 4 after admission.
- Patient will consume 50% of all meals and supplements by the end of the week.

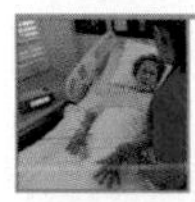

2. Write a goal for the nursing diagnosis of *Risk for Infection* with risk factors of break in skin integrity and chronic disease.

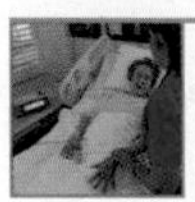

The conceptual care map for Mrs. Payne provided in Figure 26-2 is partially completed to indicate how to use the map as a learning tool. Using it as an example, go to the website at *http://evolve.elsevier.com/YoostCrawford/fundamentals/* to complete Nursing Diagnoses 2 and 3.

IMPLEMENTATION AND EVALUATION LO 26.6

The nurse plays an important role in infection control. The nurse must be proficient in aseptic technique to reduce the patient's risk for an HAI.

INFECTION CONTROL AND ASEPTIC INTERVENTIONS

Nurses can implement many interventions to decrease the risk of infectious illness (Table 26-2). Diligence in performing these interventions decreases the likelihood of spreading infections from one patient to another in a health care facility.

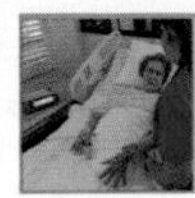

3. List at least three actions with rationales for Mrs. Payne on her second postoperative day to prevent respiratory complications.

Hand Hygiene

Hand hygiene includes handwashing with soap and water, the use of an alcohol-based sanitizer, or use of a surgical hand scrub. It is one of the most important acts that a nurse can perform to protect the patient, self, and other patients from the spread of infection (Evidence-Based Practices and Informatics box). Hand hygiene (Skill 26-1) breaks the chain of infection by interrupting the mode of transmission.

EVIDENCE-BASED PRACTICE AND INFORMATICS

Infection Control

All nursing practice should be guided by research. Infection control measures are constantly updated so that the best and most evidence-based practices can be accessed and used. Keeping abreast of these changes can be challenging to the nurse who is busy with day-to-day clinical practice. Evidence-based practices can be found at the following websites:

- Centers for Disease Control and Prevention (CDC) at *www.cdc.gov* provide information to promote health and healthy decisions and focus on disease prevention and control, especially infectious diseases.
- National Guideline Clearinghouse (NGC) at *www.ngc.gov* serves as a public resource for evidence-based clinical practice guidelines.
- National Institute for Health and Clinical Excellence (NICE) at *www.nice.org.uk* provides access to authoritative health and social care evidence and best practice.
- National Resource for Infection Control at *www.nric.org.uk* provides access to resources regarding infection control.
- The Cochrane Collaboration at *www.cochrane.org* provides access to evidence for best practice.

A surgical hand scrub must be performed before all surgical procedures and before other procedures as necessary. This type of hand hygiene is performed with an antiseptic agent. A disposable sponge is used to scrub the hands, fingers, and wrists to reduce the number of microorganisms on intact

Medications

Enoxaparin 40 mg subcutaneously daily
Metformin 500 mg PO twice daily
Hydrocodone 5 mg/acetaminophen 500 mg po q 4 hr prn for pain
Cefuroxime 750 mg IV q 8 hr

IV Sites/Fluids/Rate
D5.45 NS at 50 ml/hr

Conceptual Care Map

Student name______ Patient Initials Mrs. P Date ______
Age 76 Gender F Room # ___ Admission date 2 days ago
CODE Status ______ Allergies ______ Braden score ______
Diet Reg with supplements bid Activity up with assist of one
Weight ______ Height ______ Religion ______

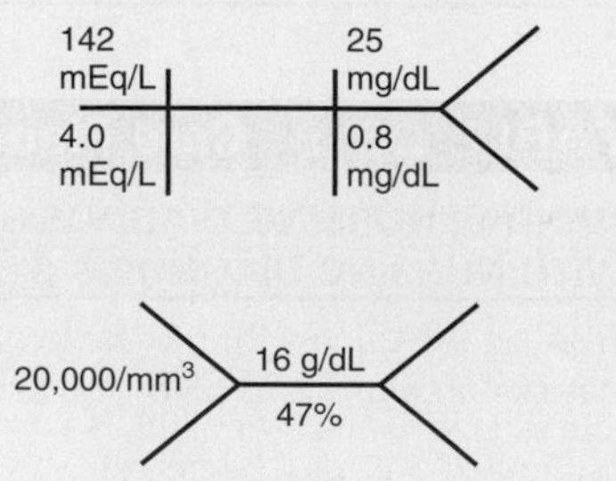

Admitting Diagnoses/Chief Complaint

RLQ abdominal pain

Lab Values/Diagnostic Test Results

142 mEq/L | 25 mg/dL
4.0 mEq/L | 0.8 mg/dL

20,000/mm^3 — 16 g/dL — 47%

Assessment Data

2 days post-op appendectomy.
Vital signs are T 38.4 °C (101.2 °F), P 96 and regular, R 22 nonlabored, BP 130/72, and pulse oximetry 96% on room air (RA).
Patient states that her pain is 3 of 10 but with movement the pain level increases to 8 of 10. She reports sharp, stabbing pain in the abdominal area around her incision site.
She has relief with pain medication and position change.
RLQ incision: Skin around the incision is warm and red, and the area is tender to the touch.

Treatments

VS q 4 hr and PRN
I&O
Right abdominal dry sterile dressing, change q 8 hr
Turn, cough, and deep-breath q 4 hr while awake
Incentive spirometry q 2 hr while awake
Antiembolism stockings while out of bed
Sequential compression devices (SCDs) while in bed
CBC every morning
Fall precautions
Physical therapy (PT) for ambulation daily

Past Medical/Surgical History

Diabetes mellitus

Primary Nursing Diagnosis

Risk for Infection with risk factors of break in skin integrity and chronic disease

Supporting Data

RLQ incision: Skin around the incision is warm and red, and the area is tender to the touch.
Diabetes mellitus

STG/NOC

Patient's incision will remain infection-free during hospitalization.

NOC: Tissue integrity and mucous membranes (1101)

Erythema (110121)

Interventions/NIC With Rationale

1. Change dressing q 8 hr or when soiled to remove soiled dressing that could be a medium for bacterial growth.
2. Cleanse area around dressing with sterile saline during dressing changes to remove exudate and organisms present on skin.
3. Use sterile technique with dressing changes to minimize exposure to microorganisms.
4. Use hand hygiene before and after dressing changes and with direct care to decrease number of microorganisms on hands.
5. Administer antibiotic as ordered to destroy microorganisms that are present in the wound.

NIC: Incision site care (3440)
Monitor incision for signs and symptoms of infection.

Rationale Citation/EBP

Yoost BL, Crawford LR: *Fundamentals of nursing: Active learning for collaborative practice*, St. Louis, 2016, Mosby.

Evaluation

During evening dressing change, sutures intact, incision dry and well approximated, slightly pink around edges, no exudate. Continue plan of care.

Nursing Diagnosis 2

Supporting Data

STG/NOC

Interventions/NIC With Rationale

Rationale Citation/EBP

Evaluation

Nursing Diagnosis 3

Supporting Data

STG/NOC

Interventions/NIC With Rationale

Rationale Citation/EBP

Evaluation

FIGURE 26-2 Partially completed conceptual care map based on Mrs. Payne, the case study patient in this chapter. *CBC*, Complete blood count; *EBP*, evidence-based practice; *NIC*, Nursing Interventions Classification; *NOC*, Nursing Outcomes Classification; *RLQ*, right lower quadrant; *STG*, short-term goal; *VS*, vital signs.

TABLE 26-2 Prevention of Infection

INTERVENTION	RATIONALE
Wash hands before and after giving care to each patient.	Washing hands is the single best way to avoid spreading infection. This process interrupts the infection cycle.
Educate patients regarding handwashing techniques, factors that increase the risk of infection, and the signs and symptoms of infection.	Patients can participate in their care, and this helps to establish and maintain a healthy lifestyle.
Wear gloves to maintain asepsis during any direct patient care when there is a risk of exposure to blood or other body fluids.	Gloves offer a barrier of protection.
Monitor the patient's temperature q 4 hr.	A temperature that is elevated after surgery or a diagnostic procedure may indicate the start of an infection.
Monitor the white blood cell (WBC) count as ordered.	An elevated total WBC count indicates infection.
Assist the patient with oral hygiene q 4 hr.	Oral hygiene helps to prevent colonization of bacteria.
Use strict aseptic technique when inserting an intravenous (IV) or Foley catheter and when performing suctioning of the lower airway.	Sterile technique helps to prevent the spread of pathogens.
Change IV tubing, and give site care q 24-48 hr or in accordance with hospital or facility policy.	Changing the tubing helps to keep pathogens out of the body.
Rotate the IV catheter q 48-72 hr or in accordance with hospital or facility policy.	Rotating the IV catheter reduces the chance of infection at the site by decreasing the time that the vein is compromised.
Have the patient perform cough and deep-breathing exercises q 4 hr.	Cough and deep-breathing exercises help remove secretions and prevent respiratory complications.
Turn the patient q 2 hr, and perform skin care, especially over bony prominences.	Turning helps to prevent skin breakdown, which can lead to pathogens entering the open tissue.
Ensure optimal nutrition by offering high-protein supplements unless contraindicated.	Optimal nutrition assists in stabilizing the patient's weight, aids in wound healing, and improves muscle tone and mass.

skin. Chapter 37 provides more detailed information on the surgical scrub.

Precautions and Isolation

Use of standard, airborne, droplet, and contact precautions reduces the transmission of pathogens. Standard precautions are used with every patient. They are the practices that prevent the spread of infectious diseases by minimizing the risk of transmission or exposure (Nursing Care Guideline: Standard Precautions box). Because it is not possible to identify patients who may or may not be infectious at any given time, the nurse practices standard precautions in dealing with every patient to protect other patients, visitors, and staff from exposures (Siegel, Rhinehart, Jackson, et al, 2007).

Patients who are immunocompromised (i.e., neutrophil count less than 500/mm^3) may be placed in protective isolation. This type of isolation protects susceptible patients, who may not be able to fight infection, from microorganisms in the environment. Patients who are undergoing chemotherapy, irradiation, or bone marrow transplantation and patients with severe burns may be placed in protective isolation.

Transmission precautions (i.e., airborne, droplet, and contact) are used in addition to standard precautions to decrease the transfer of highly transmissible pathogens (Nursing Care Guideline: Contact, Airborne, and Droplet Precautions and Protective Isolation box). Each transmission-based precaution requires the use of specific PPE to prevent the spread of a communicable illness.

QSEN FOCUS!

The nurse creates a culture of safety when standard and transmission-based precautions are followed and when education is provided to patients, families, and the health care team about the hazards of not following specific precautions.

Patients and their families can become partners in preventing the spread of infectious illnesses. It is important to educate them on how they can play a role in reducing the spread of infectious illnesses (Patient Education and Health Literacy box).

NURSING CARE GUIDELINE

Standard Precautions

Background

The use of standard precautions (i.e., basic aseptic techniques) prevents and controls the spread of microorganisms among patients and providers.

Procedural Concerns

- Use standard precautions for all patients when contact with potentially infectious bodily materials is possible.
- Use standard precautions during contact or potential contact with the following:
  - Blood and bodily fluids (except perspiration), secretions, and excretions; precautions *must* be used whether blood is visible or not
  - Nonintact skin
  - Mucous membranes
  - Other potentially infectious material
- Use gloves routinely with any patient care where blood or body fluid might be present. If splashing is possible, use conservative judgment about whether other PPE is necessary:
  - Eyewear
  - Mask
  - Gown
- Practice good hand hygiene:
  - Good hand hygiene (see Skill 26-1) is essential at all points of a procedure:
    - Before and after a procedure
    - Before applying and after removing gloves
  - When hands are visibly soiled, they must be washed. If hands are not visibly soiled, alcohol-based hand sanitizer may be used.
  - Is there possible contact with *Clostridium difficile?* If so, use soap and water to disinfect hands because alcohol-based hand sanitizers are ineffective against *C. difficile.*
- Clean or discard equipment after use.
- Follow special precautions when using needles (sharps):
  - Discard needles in sharps containers.
  - Use safety needles.
  - Needleless systems are preferred when their use is feasible.
- Educate patients and staff regarding the procedure to be performed on the patient.

Documentation Concerns

- Standard precautions themselves do not require documentation.
- Patient and family education regarding standard precautions should be documented.

Evidence-Based Practice

Siegel and colleagues and the Healthcare Control Practices Advisory Committee (2007) added respiratory etiquette as a part of standard precautions. This includes covering the mouth and nose with a tissue when sneezing or coughing and disposing of the tissue immediately, washing hands promptly thereafter, wearing a mask if infected, posting signs and educating patients and staff regarding etiquette, and remaining more than 3 feet away from another person. These simple steps have reduced transmission of many organisms and prevented infections in health care facilities.

NURSING CARE GUIDELINE

Contact, Airborne, and Droplet Precautions and Protective Isolation

Background

- Basic standard precaution principles apply to all patients (see Nursing Care Guideline: Standard Precautions box).
- PPE and supplies are usually found on an isolation cart outside the room (in an anteroom).

Contact Precautions

Contact precautions are used when a known or suspected contagious disease may be present.

- Transmission of a contagious disease may occur through several routes:
  - Direct transmission (contact with the patient).
  - Indirect transmission (contact with equipment or items in the patient's environment).
- The following are typical diseases and conditions requiring use of contact precautions:
  - Multidrug-resistant organisms (MDROs), including vancomycin-resistant enterococci, methicillin-resistant *Staphylococcus aureus, Clostridium difficile,* respiratory syncytial virus, and hepatitis A
  - Scabies and herpes simplex virus (HSV)
  - Draining wounds in which certain organisms have been cultured

Airborne Precautions

Airborne precautions are used when known or suspected contagious diseases can be transmitted by means of small droplets or particles that can remain suspended in the air for prolonged periods of time. Small droplets or particles can cause disease transmission over a greater distance and longer time than larger droplets (see section on Droplet Precautions).

Precautions include the following:

- A negative-pressure room with a high-efficiency particulate air (HEPA) filtration system is necessary.

NURSING CARE GUIDELINE—cont'd

- A special N95 respirator mask is required. Medical evaluation and measurement for the wearer are required before obtaining the respirator. It must be fit-tested by the facility.

Typical diseases and pathogens include the following:

- Varicella or disseminated varicella zoster (chickenpox)
- Rubeola (measles)
- *Mycobacterium tuberculosis* (pulmonary or laryngeal tuberculosis)

Droplet Precautions

Droplet precautions are used when known or suspected contagious diseases can be transmitted through large droplets suspended in the air.

- Droplets may be generated when an infected patient coughs, sneezes, or talks.
- Droplets may be produced during medical procedures such as suctioning, endotracheal intubation, cardiopulmonary resuscitation (CPR), or chest physiotherapy.

Typical diseases include the following:

- Pharyngeal diphtheria
- Mumps, rubella, and pertussis
- Streptococcal pharyngitis and scarlet fever
- Pneumonias (streptococcal, mycoplasmal, meningococcal)
- Pneumonic plague
- Meningococcal sepsis
- Influenza

Protective Isolation

Protective isolation is used for patients who have compromised immune systems. This type of isolation protects the patient from microorganisms in the environment. Protective isolation varies according to the reason that the patient's immune system is compromised, and a variety of protective precautions may be used:

- A positive-pressure room with a HEPA filtration system may be required.
- A mask is required for anyone entering the room or for the patient if leaving the room.
- Meticulous handwashing is essential.
- The patient must be assessed carefully for signs and symptoms of infection.
- No live plants, fresh flowers, fresh raw fruit or vegetables, sushi, or blue cheese may be brought into the room because they may harbor bacteria and fungi.

Several conditions require protective precautions:

- Allogeneic hematopoietic stem cell transplantation
- Chemotherapy
- Certain diseases or disorders in which medications have caused immunosuppression, including leukemia, myelodysplastic syndrome, aplastic anemia, systemic lupus erythematosus (SLE), rheumatoid arthritis (RA), human immunodeficiency virus (HIV) infection, and severe sepsis

Procedural Concerns

- Address room concerns.
  - A private room is preferred for a patient who has a contagious disease or who needs protective isolation.
  - Cluster care to avoid multiple trips in and out of the patient's room.
- Address equipment concerns:
  - Keep some equipment in the patient's room, including a thermometer, a stethoscope, and a blood pressure cuff.
  - Thoroughly clean all equipment with an alcohol-based cleaning agent after each use.
- Avoid contamination by donning and removing PPE in a prescribed sequence (see Skill 26-3).
- Place used linens from the patient's room into special isolation linen bags to prevent spread of microorganisms. A second "clean" person outside the room may be needed to double-bag items to prevent contamination outside the patient's room.
- Assemble all equipment and supplies for use in the patient's room before entering the room. If additional items are needed while in the room, do the following:
  - Have another staff member retrieve the needed items.
  - Perform a hand-off (by having a clean person outside the room assemble the needed equipment and pass it into the isolation room) to avoid leaving the room if possible.
- To transport a patient on isolation precautions, apply these guidelines:
  - The patient should wear PPE.
  - The receiving department should be notified before transport of the patient so that all necessary arrangements can be made at the patient's destination.
  - Transport should occur only when absolutely necessary.

Documentation Concerns

- Document isolation when it is begun and discontinued.
- Document patient and family education concerning the proper procedures.
- Mark "Isolation Precautions Required" on the chart.
- Place signs in clear view on the door: "Visitors should report to the nurses' station before entering the room."
- If isolation is broken, refer to institutional policy and procedures.

PATIENT EDUCATION AND HEALTH LITERACY

Standard Precautions

Teach patients and their families the importance of the following on admission to the health care facility:

- Appropriate hand hygiene
- Respiratory hygiene and cough etiquette
- Importance of vaccinations (especially against influenza)

Transmission-Based Precautions

If a patient is diagnosed with a transmission-based illness and requires precautions, educate the patient and the family:

- Provide fact sheets or pamphlets on the illness.
- Provide rationales for the new precautions.
- Explain any risk to family members.
- Explain the personal PPE being used and provide directions for its use by the family.
- Be available to explain and ask questions as necessary.

From Siegel J, Rhinehart E, Jackson M, et al.: *2007 Guidelines for isolation precautions: Preventing transmission of infectious agents in healthcare settings.* Retrieved from *www.cdc.gov/hicpac/2007IP/2007isolationPrecautions.html.*

! SAFE PRACTICE ALERT

Never recap a dirty or used needle because doing so increases the risk of exposure to blood-borne pathogens.

Personal Protective Equipment

Personal protective equipment (PPE) is the equipment that health care personnel use to protect against the spread of infection. Gloves, masks, goggles, face shields, gowns, caps, and shoe coverings are examples. Clean, nonsterile gloves are used when direct contact with body secretions is possible. Sterile gloves (Skill 26-2) are needed during sterile procedures, such as urinary catheter insertion. Gloves decrease the risk of transferring organisms from one individual to another. Gloves are changed if they become soiled and are always changed between patients. Proper use of PPE is essential to stop the spread of microorganisms (Skill 26-3).

QSEN FOCUS!

The nurse demonstrates effective use of strategies to reduce the risk of harm to self or others by properly using PPE.

SAFE PRACTICE ALERT

When abrasions or skin breakdown is noticed, be sure to wear gloves during patient care.

Masks protect against the transmission of infectious agents through the air. The individual is protected against large particles that travel only a short distance (usually less than 3 feet) and small particles that can remain suspended in the air and can travel much farther. The effectiveness of masks is decreased when they get wet or are worn for long periods. Special particulate respirators (e.g., N95 masks) are used when a patient is suspected of having or has a contagious airborne disease such as tuberculosis. These special masks look like regular masks but fit securely against the face. The nurse is fitted to determine which mask size to use. The nurse who works in high-risk communities should have a particulate respirator on hand at all times.

Waterproof gowns are used when there is a possibility that the health care provider's clothes will become soiled. Gowns are used only once and are discarded or cleaned after each use. Some health care facilities use disposable gowns.

Caps are used to cover the individual's hair, and shoe covers are used to protect the shoes. They are used in areas where there is a high risk for contamination, such as in the labor and delivery room and the operating room.

Immunization

Immunization is the process by which an individual develops immunity against a specific agent; it is important in preventing the spread of communicable diseases. Immunizations can be acquired through various techniques, the most common of which is vaccination.

Immunizations provided by vaccination protect an individual against a particular communicable disease. Although vaccine-preventable diseases are at an all-time low, there is still an issue with underimmunized children, adolescents, and adults. The CDC has recommended schedules for immunizations for children and adults. Schedules can be accessed at *www.cdc.gov/vaccines/schedules/index.html.* This information is regularly updated, and the nurse must remain vigilant about educating patients to decrease the spread of preventable contagious diseases.

SAFE PRACTICE ALERT

All women of childbearing age should be up to date on immunizations according to CDC recommendations. Urge women trying to conceive to avoid exposure to infectious diseases.

Medical Asepsis and Surgical Asepsis

Medical asepsis and surgical asepsis are techniques used to prevent infection or to break the chain of infection (Box 26-1). **Medical asepsis** is often referred to as *clean technique.* Medical aseptic procedures include handwashing, wearing gloves, gowning, and disinfecting. **Surgical asepsis**, or sterile technique, is used to prevent the introduction of microorganisms from the environment to the patient. Surgical asepsis is used for surgical procedures, invasive procedures such as catheterization, procedures that invade the

BOX 26-1 Medical Asepsis versus Surgical Asepsis

MEDICAL ASEPSIS

- Perform diligent hand hygiene to assist in interrupting the chain of infection.
- Avoid allowing soiled items such as linen to touch clothing to decrease the chance of spreading infectious material to other patients.
- Keep soiled items off the floor to decrease the chance of contamination.
- Teach patients the proper use of tissues to cover sneezes and coughs. Prevent patients from coughing, sneezing, or breathing directly on others.
- Avoid shaking linens to decrease the chance of infectious particles becoming airborne.
- Clean from less soiled to more soiled areas to avoid increasing contamination.
- Place items that are moist from body fluids in the appropriate receptacle immediately. Wrap heavily soiled items in plastic to prevent direct contact with the substance by others.
- Pour liquids (e.g., bath water, mouthwash) directly into the drain to avoid splashing.
- Sterilize items suspected of being contaminated.
- Maintain personal hygiene. Keep fingernails short, keep hair short or pulled back, and avoid wearing rings with grooves or stones, which can harbor microorganisms.
- Follow agency guidelines for standard and transmission-based precautions carefully.

SURGICAL ASEPSIS

- Perform hand hygiene before sterile procedures.
- Ensure that sterile objects touch only other sterile objects to maintain a sterile environment.
- Open a sterile package away from the body to avoid contamination.
- Keep sterile surfaces dry. Avoid spilling liquids on a cloth or paper that is used as a sterile field. Fluids give organisms a means of transportation.
- Keep all sterile items above the waistline to ensure the sterile object is kept in sight.
- Avoid coughing, talking, sneezing, or reaching across the sterile field.
- Face the sterile field. Never turn your back on or walk away from a sterile field.
- Keep items sterile that are used to enter a normally sterile environment (e.g., those that penetrate the skin or body). This includes dressings, needles, and catheter tubes.
- Use dry, sterile forceps when necessary.
- Remember that the outer 1-inch edge of a sterile field is contaminated.
- Consider an object contaminated rather than sterile if there is any doubt.

bloodstream or break the skin, dressing changes, and wound care (Skill 26-4).

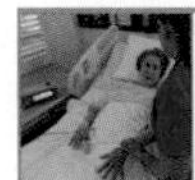

4. Identify a minimum of three nursing interventions for the goal designed to prevent complications.

Disinfection and Sterilization

Disinfection and sterilization are used to remove potentially harmful microorganisms and to eliminate microorganisms as potential sources of infection. **Disinfection** is the removal of pathogenic microorganisms; it typically destroys all pathogenic microorganisms except spores from inanimate objects. Germicidal agents are used to disinfect objects, and antiseptic agents are used to disinfect skin. Examples of chemical disinfectants include alcohol and chlorhexidine (Rutala, Weber, and HICPAC, 2008).

Sterilization is a process used to destroy all microorganisms, including their spores. Sterilization is used on equipment that is entering a sterile body cavity. Many items are purchased as sterile or can be sterilized through physical or chemical means. The nurse should always check the expiration on the package before use. If the date on the package has expired, the contents are no longer considered sterile. Physical sterilization occurs through steam, boiling water, dry heat, or radiation. Chemical sterilization occurs through the use of gases such as ethylene oxide gas or solutions (Rutala, Weber, and HICPAC, 2008).

INFECTION CONTROL AND ASEPTIC INTERVENTIONS IN THE HOME

Asepsis in the home environment requires educating patients and their families or caregivers about the mode of transmission of pathogens and the means of prevention. Many aseptic procedures that are performed in the health care environment can be performed in the home with some modifications. The nurse must know what these modifications are and how to teach patients and their families the necessary skills before discharge (Home Care Considerations box).

EVALUATION

Evaluation is an ongoing portion of the nursing process. It allows the nurse to determine whether the patient has met his or her treatment goals. Evaluation is also an analysis that determines the effectiveness of the nursing interventions. The evaluation process typically brings the nurse back to an assessment, in which the whole nursing process begins again. Evaluation may allow trends in infection control in the health care environment to be observed and acted on.

HOME CARE CONSIDERATIONS

Infection Control

- Teach proper hand hygiene (before handling foods, before eating, after toileting, before and after required home care treatment, and after touching body substances such as wound drainage) and related hygienic measures for all family members.
- Instruct the patient and family not to share personal care items, such as toothbrushes, washcloths, and towels. Infections can be transmitted from shared personal items.
- Discuss antimicrobial soaps and effective disinfectants.
- Instruct about cleaning reusable equipment and supplies: Use soap and water, and disinfect with a chlorine bleach solution.
- Teach the patient and family members the signs and symptoms of infection, how to avoid infections, and when to contact a health care provider.
- Remind them to avoid coughing, sneezing, or breathing directly on others and to cover the mouth and the nose to prevent the transmission of airborne microorganisms.
- Emphasize the need for proper immunizations of all family members.
- For patients with wound care
  - Teach the patient and family the signs of wound healing and wound infections.
  - Explain the proper technique for changing dressings and disposing of the soiled ones. Reinforce the need to place contaminated dressings and other disposable items containing body fluids in moisture-proof plastic bags.
  - Have the patient and family repeat instructions and demonstrate skills.
- If self-injections are required, advise the patient to put used needles in a puncture-resistant container with a screw-top lid and to label the container so that it will not be discarded in the garbage.

SKILL 26-1 Hand Hygiene

PURPOSE

- Hand hygiene is essential to prevent the spread of microorganisms.
- It is standard practice for patient care.

RESOURCES

- Soap
- Warm running water
- Paper towels
- Alcohol-based hand sanitizer

COLLABORATION AND DELEGATION

- Hand hygiene is mandatory for all health care workers who come in contact with patients or their belongings; it is not delegated. Hand hygiene is mandated for all patients.
- It is important for the nurse to speak up when observing anyone not following required hand hygiene.

EVIDENCE-BASED PRACTICE

- Alcohol-based products and sanitizers should not be used when one or both hands are visibly soiled (CDC, 2012b; Gould and Drey, 2008; Hossein and Sajjad, 2009).
- Natural fingernails should be kept short and be trimmed often (CDC, 2012b).
- Health care providers do not wash their hands in accordance with the CDC's guidelines, which leads to an increased rate of hospital-acquired infections. The rate of handwashing can be increased and the rate of infections decreased by implementing an educational model aimed at increasing the behavior of handwashing; this may be as simple as getting health care providers to speak up when they see another provider not washing his or her hands (CDC, 2012b; Creedon, 2006; Gould and Drey, 2008; Kovach, 2005).

SPECIAL CIRCUMSTANCES

1. **Assess:** Are there any cuts, open sores, or breaks in the skin around cuticles, including hangnails?
   Intervention: Cover the injuries with appropriate dressing after washing; wear gloves; or delegate the assignment or request a different one.
2. **Assess:** Are fingernails long or do they have artificial nails or nail polish?
   Intervention: File nails, remove artificial nails, and remove nail polish.
3. **Assess:** Is the handwasher wearing jewelry?
   Intervention: Remove jewelry; a plain wedding band, thoroughly washed and dried, is permitted.
4. **Assess:** Is the handwasher wearing a watch or long sleeves?
   Intervention: Push the watch and sleeves above the wrist.
5. **Assess:** Is there visible soiling or dirt on the hands?
   Intervention: Soap and water must be used to thoroughly clean hands if there is any visible soiling or dirt; otherwise, an alcohol-based hand sanitizer may be substituted.

SPECIAL CIRCUMSTANCES DURING THE PROCEDURE

1. **Assess:** Did hands (skin) directly touch any individual or surface (e.g., sink, clothing) when washing them?
   Intervention: Body, clothing, sink, and other surfaces are considered contaminated. Start handwashing again.
2. **Assess:** Did hands (skin) touch any other surface when retrieving paper towels?
   Intervention: Body, clothing, sink, and other surfaces are considered contaminated. Start handwashing again.

PROCEDURE

Handwashing: Soap and Water Method

1. Introduce self and educate the patient regarding handwashing if procedure is taking place within a patient room.
   Builds a trusting, professional relationship; eases patient anxiety; facilitates cooperation.
2. Turn on warm water at a medium flow.
   Warm water removes dirt and microorganisms but, unlike hot water, does not remove protective skin oils; medium flow prevents splashing.

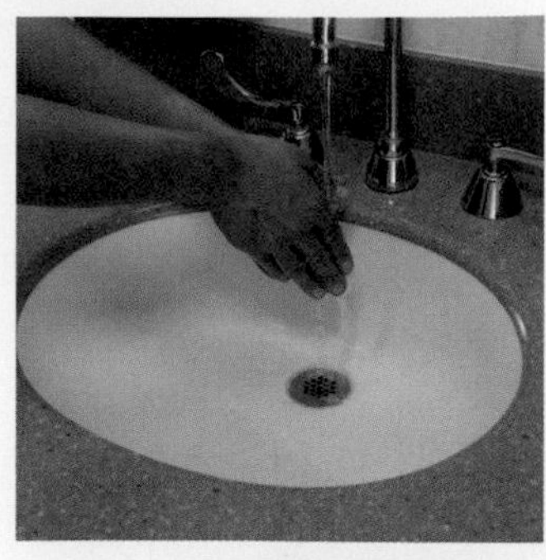
STEP 3

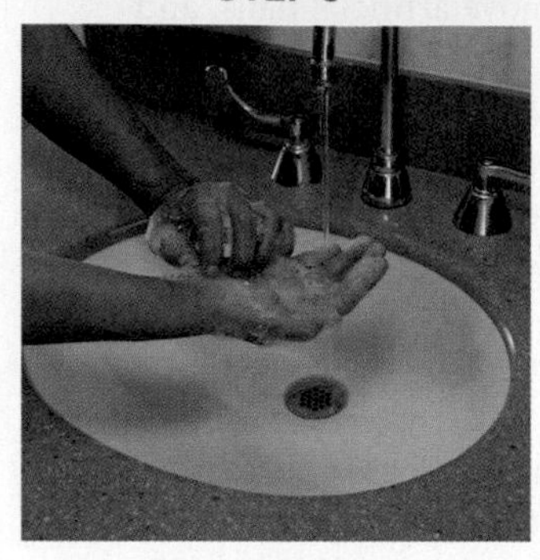
STEP 5a

3. Wet the wrists and hands; with fingers pointing downward.
   Washing should be done from the least contaminated to the most contaminated area (i.e., from the area of fewer microorganisms to the area of more microorganisms).
4. Apply soap.
   Soap removes microorganisms.
5. Lather; rub using a circular movement; wash for 15 to 20 seconds in this order:
   a. Palms of hands with fingertips
   b. Backs (dorsum) of hands
   c. Wrists
   d. Between fingers (interlaced, including thumbs)
   e. Fingers
   f. Fingertips; clean under nails
   Friction helps remove microorganisms; lather indicates friction has occurred.
6. Rinse from wrist to fingertips, keeping hands with fingers pointing downward.
   Prevents spread of microorganisms.
7. Using clean paper towels, dry thoroughly in the same order (from wrists to fingers) using a patting motion.
   Prevents spread of microorganisms, which like dampness; patting (rather than rubbing) dry prevents injury to the skin.
8. Throw the paper towels in an appropriate receptacle.
   Prevents spread of microorganisms.
9. Turn off the water by holding the faucet with a clean, dry paper towel.
   Prevents spread of microorganisms back to hands.
10. Throw the paper towel in an appropriate receptacle.
    Prevents spread of microorganisms.

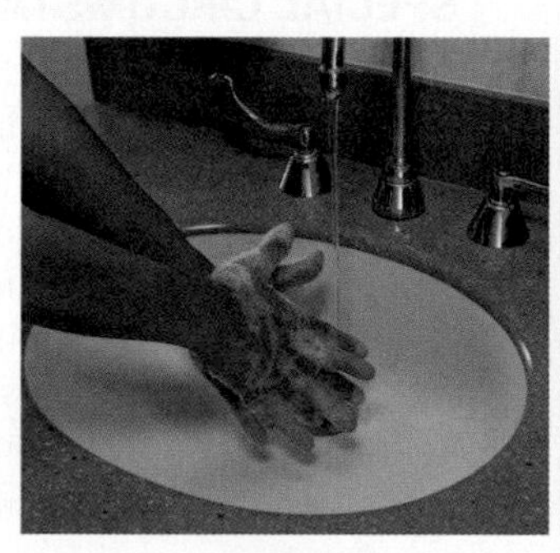
STEP 5d

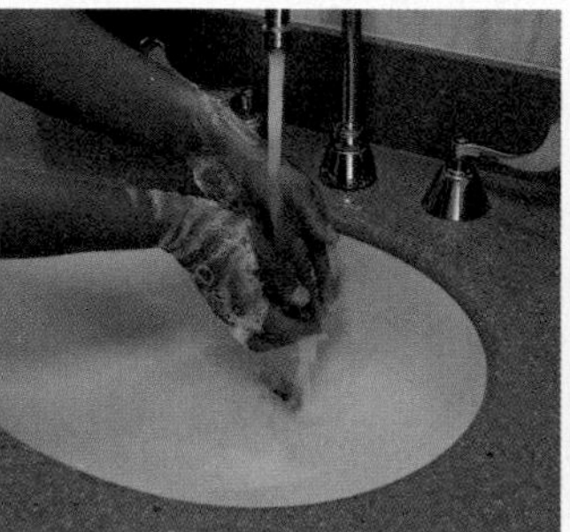
STEP 6

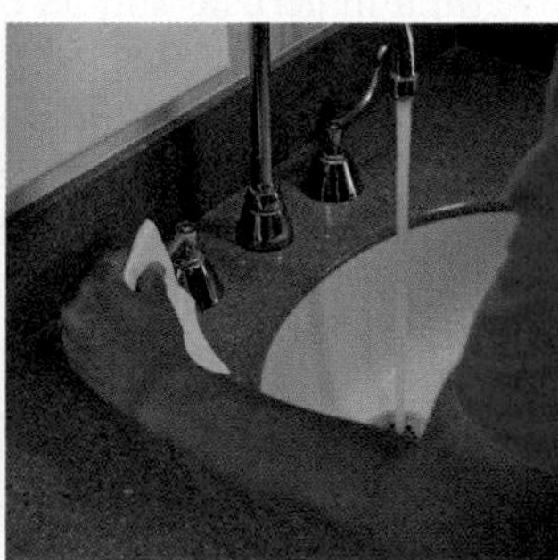
STEP 9

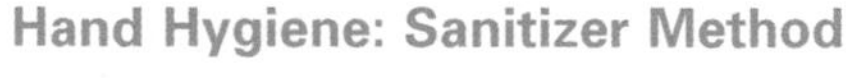

Hand Hygiene: Sanitizer Method

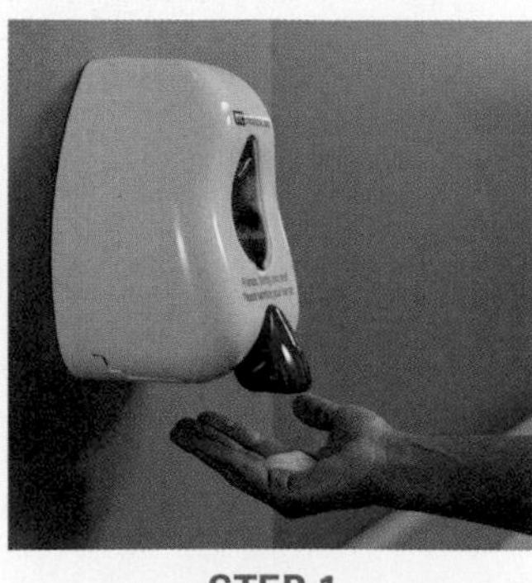
STEP 1

1. Apply an appropriate amount of hand sanitizer into the palm of one hand.
   Soap and water must be used to thoroughly clean hands if there is any visible soiling or dirt and with certain infections such as Clostridium difficile *and vancomycin-resistant enterococci when preparing for a sterile or surgical procedure, before and after eating, and after using the restroom. In all other situations, a hand sanitizer is as effective as soap and water.*
2. Rub hands together using a circular motion, spreading sanitizer over palms and backs of both hands then the wrist; continue until dry.
   Friction from rubbing helps to remove microorganisms; the sanitizer is not effective until dry.
3. Gloves should not be applied until hands are dry.
   Moisture inside gloves may contribute to skin breakdown, and gloves will be easier to apply on dry hands.

SKILL 26-2 Sterile Gloving

PURPOSE

- Sterile gloving technique protects highly susceptible patients, open wounds, and sterile objects from the transfer of microorganisms.
- Sterile gloving technique is required in most procedures requiring sterile technique.

RESOURCES

- Sterile gloves of correct size
- A flat, clean, dry work surface above waist height near the location of the procedure

COLLABORATION AND DELEGATION

- Sterile gloving is mandated for any health care provider who is participating in a procedure that requires sterile technique; it is not delegated.
- Sterile gloving may be performed by unlicensed assistive personnel (UAP) who are assisting in a procedure and have been trained in the proper application. The nurse must make sure that sterile technique is maintained. The nurse should verify facility policy before involving UAP in sterile procedures.

SPECIAL CIRCUMSTANCES

1. **Assess:** Are there breaks in the skin or around cuticles, cuts, open sores, or hangnails?
   Intervention: Cover the injuries with appropriate dressing after washing; request a different assignment.
2. **Assess:** Are fingernails long or do they have artificial nails or nail polish?
   Intervention: File nails; remove artificial nails; remove nail polish.
3. **Assess:** Is jewelry being worn?
   Intervention: Remove all jewelry for sterile gloving to avoid the possibility of tearing and contaminating the gloves.
4. **Assess:** Is the glove package damaged or past its expiration date?
   Intervention: Acquire a new pair of sterile gloves.
5. **Assess:** Is the work surface below waist level?
   Intervention: Work surfaces below waist level are considered contaminated; gloved hands are considered contaminated if they fall below waist level. Raise the work surface or find a new surface to use when applying sterile gloves.
6. **Assess:** Did skin touch a sterile part of the glove or the sterile field? Did the glove touch skin or anything outside the sterile field? Did the patient touch the gloves?
   Intervention: Any contact between a sterile glove or item from a sterile field and skin or a nonsterile item outside the sterile field is considered contamination. Acquire a new pair of gloves; start the gloving process again.
7. **Assess:** Was the glover's back turned on the gloves or sterile area?
   Intervention: Acquire a new pair of gloves; start over.
8. **Assess:** Did the gloves tear or were they punctured during the procedure?
   Intervention: Acquire a new pair of gloves; start over.

PROCEDURE

Applying Sterile Gloves

1. If gloving is taking place in a patient room, introduce self; explain the procedure.
   Builds a trusting, professional relationship; eases patient anxiety; facilitates cooperation.
2. Perform hand hygiene (see Skill 26-1).
   Prevents spread of microorganisms.
3. Peel open the glove package using a slow, smooth motion.
   Prevents inner package from being inadvertently opened and the gloves becoming contaminated.

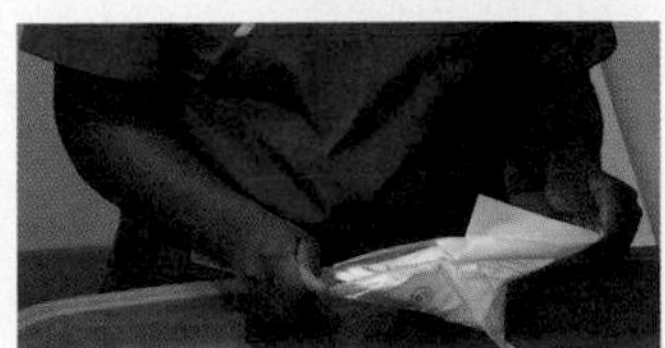

STEP 3

4. Put the inner glove package on the working surface. The working surface must be above waist level; the side of the package marked "cuff" must be closest to the person who is to glove.
   Below the waist is considered contaminated. The cuff marking on the packaging ensures correct placement of the gloves so that it will not be necessary to reach over the gloves to pick them up after the inner package is opened (gloves must be picked up using the cuff side).

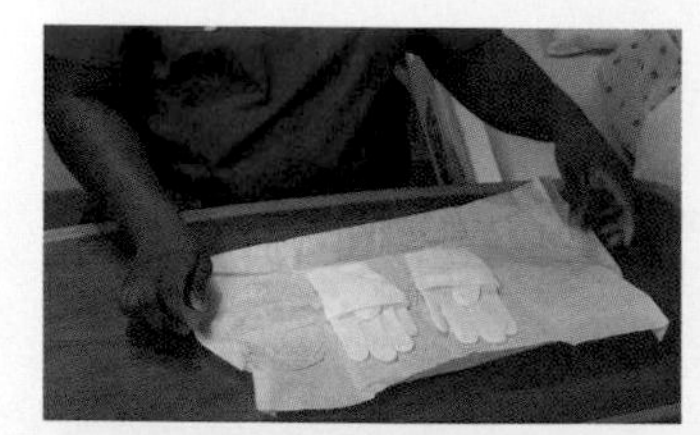

STEP 5

5. Open the inner package, using thumbs and index fingers to gently pull the package edges apart.
   The outer 1-inch margin of the inside package is not sterile.
6. With the thumb and two fingers of the nondominant hand, grasp the inside edge of the cuff of the glove for the dominant hand.
   The cuff is folded over; the inner edge of the cuff will lie against skin and therefore is not sterile, so it can be touched without contaminating it.

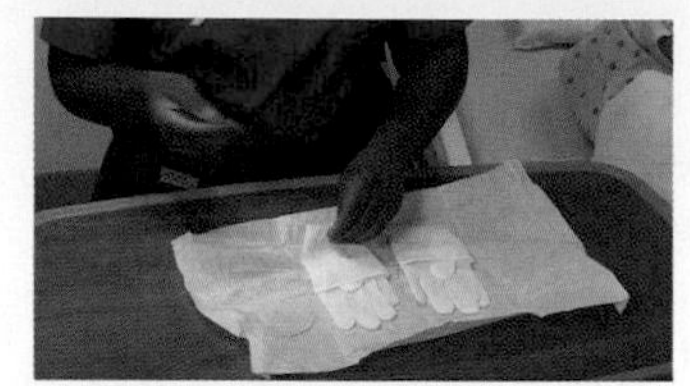

STEP 6

7. Pull the glove onto the dominant hand, with both hands held above the waist and over the sterile field.
   Moving hands away from the sterile field increases the risk of contamination.

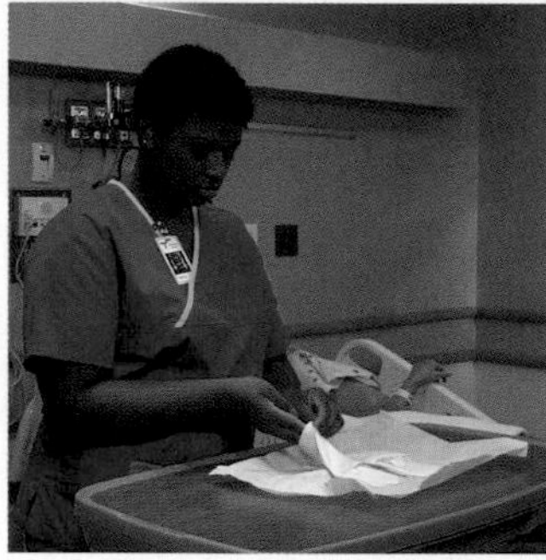

STEP 7

8. Slide all gloved fingers underneath the cuff of the remaining glove (sterile gloved hand to sterile outer glove); hold the gloved thumb apart.
   The sterile glove on the dominant hand touches only the sterile part of the other glove; holding the thumb away from the nongloved hand avoids risk of contamination.
9. Pull the glove onto the nondominant hand, with hands held above the waist and over the sterile field; keep the gloved thumb apart. Do not use the sterile-gloved thumb to help pull on the second glove.
   Avoids risk of contamination.
10. Adjust the gloves to fit correctly by carefully pinching and shifting each glove with the other hand. Do not "snap" the gloves to adjust them.
    Sometimes gloves do not go on correctly and must be adjusted; the fit can be corrected without contamination. Snapping may cause contamination.
11. Hold both hands together and interlock the fingers; hold hands above the waist and away from the body.
    Avoids risk of contamination before the procedure.

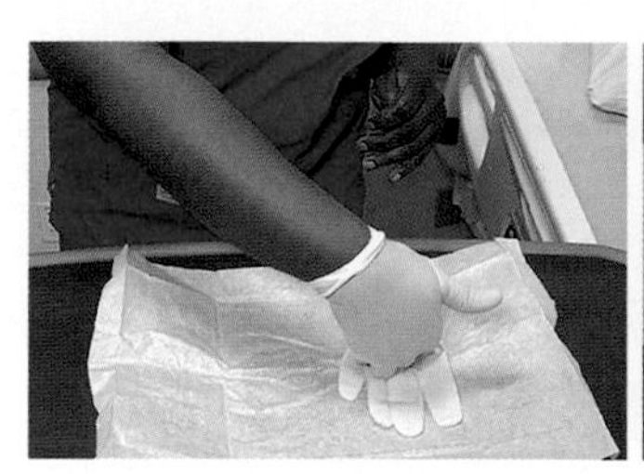

STEP 8

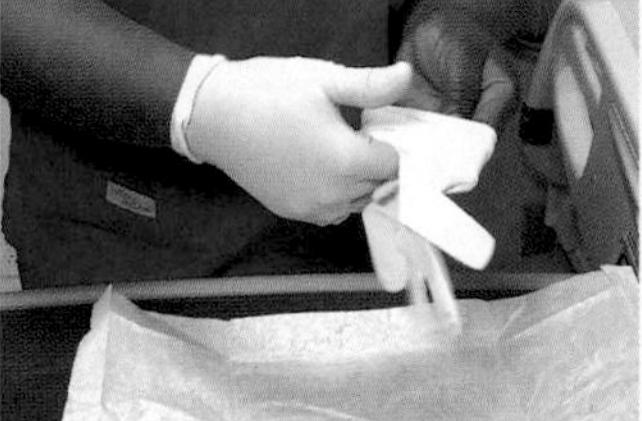

STEP 9

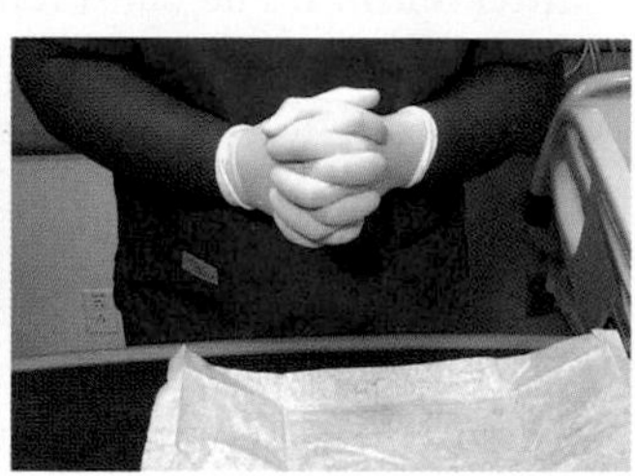

STEP 11

Removing Sterile Gloves

1. With the dominant hand, grasp the surface of the glove from the nondominant hand right below the base of the thumb; pull off without touching exposed skin.
   Prevents spread of microorganisms.
2. Keep the removed glove crumpled in the hand that is still gloved.
   Prevents spread of microorganisms.
3. Slide a finger or thumb of the gloveless hand under the cuff of the glove on the other hand (skin to skin); the remaining fingers of the ungloved hand should avoid touching the glove.
   Prevents spread of microorganisms; the fingers of the ungloved hand do not touch the contaminated surface of the glove.
4. Peel off the second glove, turning it inside out and encasing the first glove inside the second glove.
   Prevents spread of microorganisms.
5. Discard the gloves in an appropriate receptacle.
   Prevents spread of microorganisms.
6. Perform hand hygiene.
   Prevents spread of microorganisms.

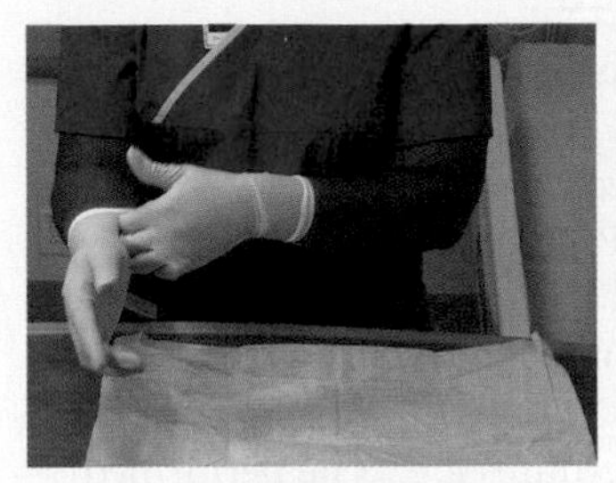
STEP 1

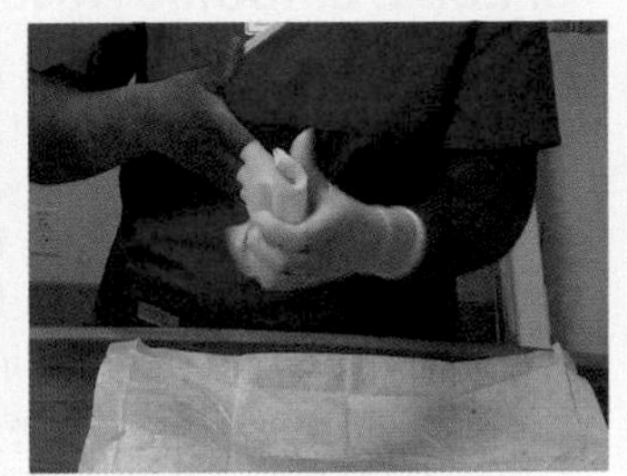
STEP 2

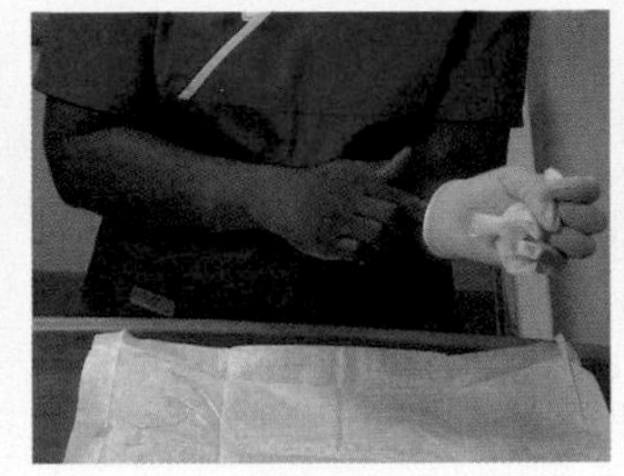
STEP 3

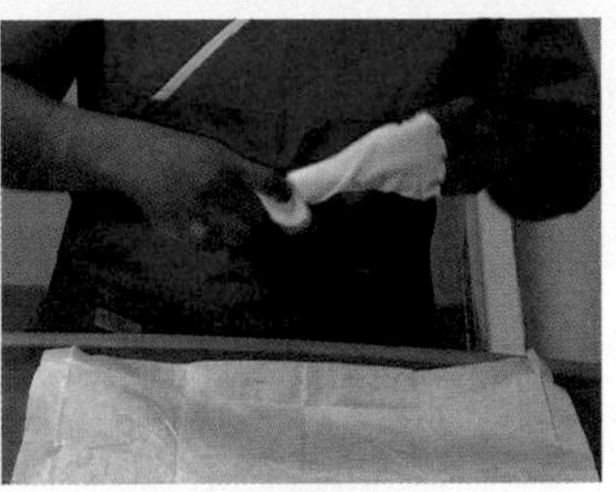
STEP 4

SKILL 26-3 Personal Protective Equipment

PURPOSE

- Use of personal protective equipment (PPE) prevents the spread of microorganisms.
- PPE may be required for specialized procedures.
- Use of PPE protects self and others when:
  - Caring for patients on isolation precautions.
  - Caring for patients when any contact with blood or body fluids may be expected.

RESOURCES

- Surgical mask with ties or ear loop; face shield; N95 respirator
- Long-sleeved, nonsterile isolation gown
- Goggles or protective eyewear (if a face shield is not facility protocol)
- Nonsterile gloves
- Laundry receptacle (provided inside the room by the facility)
- Container or receptacle for eyewear (if not disposable; provided inside the room by the facility)

COLLABORATION AND DELEGATION

- PPE is mandated for all health care workers who come in contact with patients on isolation or are in situations in which contact with blood or body fluids may be expected; it is not delegated.
- It is important to speak up when you see anyone not following appropriate and prescribed PPE requirements. Not following PPE requirements may cause harm to the health care worker and the patient.
- UAP care for patients under these conditions. UAP should report any of the following to the nurse:
  - Any need for further patient education regarding use of PPE
  - Personnel or visitors not following required PPE guidelines
  - Concerns regarding care of patients when PPE is required
- UAP should be instructed in the following:
  - Appropriate technique and PPE equipment required for patient care
  - Appropriate donning and removal of PPE
  - Appropriate communication techniques for discussing the need for PPE with the patient

EVIDENCE-BASED PRACTICE

- The order of donning and removing PPE is important in preventing contamination. Equipment is put on in order, starting with whatever part of the body is considered most contaminated and moving to the cleanest. Removing PPE should occur in an isolation anteroom, if available, or just inside the patient's door before leaving the room (CDC, 2014; Siegel, Rhinehart, Jackson, et al, 2007).
- The mask is removed last because it prevents airborne particles from other garments from entering the respiratory system (CDC, 2014).

SPECIAL CIRCUMSTANCES

1. **Assess:** What type of PPE is needed?
   Intervention: Check chart, orders, care plan, symptoms, facility policy, laboratory work, and diagnoses to ensure that the most appropriate PPE is used.
2. **Assess:** What is the state of the PPE? Is it torn, soiled, mispackaged, past expiration date, or damaged?
   Intervention: Acquire new PPE.
3. **Assess:** What care and procedures are to be performed while in the patient room?
   Intervention: Gather all equipment needed before entering the room; decide whether all PPE is necessary.
4. **Assess:** Has the PPE become wet, soiled, damaged, or torn during the procedure?
   Intervention: Stop patient care as soon as possible; remove equipment; wash hands; inspect self; start over; report the incident and document as needed in accordance with facility policy.
5. **Assess:** What should be done if a needed item has been left outside the room?
   Intervention: Ring the call bell for assistance. Ask another staff member to acquire any needed supplies.

PROCEDURE

Applying PPE

1. Wash hands (see Skill 26-1).
2. Put on a gown.
   Tie at the neck, tie at the waist, and pull sleeves to wrists. Ensures protection and correct fit.
3. Put on a mask.
   a. *For a surgical mask with ties, tie the top strings above ears; tie bottom strings around neck; adjust the metal nose bridge (if applicable).*
   Ensures protection and correct fit.
   b. *For a surgical mask with ear loops, loop around ears; adjust the metal nose bridge (if applicable).*
   Ensures protection and correct fit.
4. Put on eyewear, which fits over the mask if not connected to the mask.
   Ensures protection from microorganisms and prevents fogging. Some manufacturers provide a splashguard for the eyes that is attached to the mask.
5. Put on gloves, and pull cuffs over the gown.
   Ensures protection from microorganisms.
6. Introduce self, and explain the procedure and the need for PPE.
   Creates a professional relationship and trust; promotes comfort of the patient; eases fear of PPE.

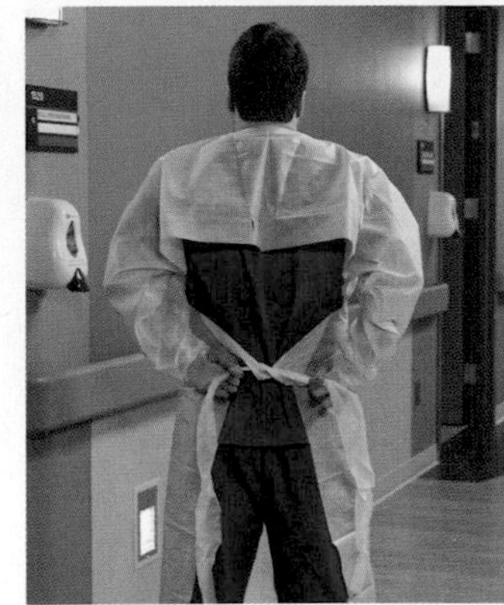

STEP 2

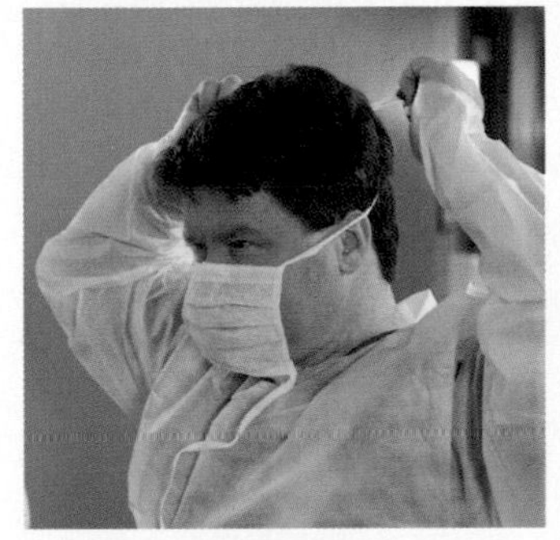

STEP 3a

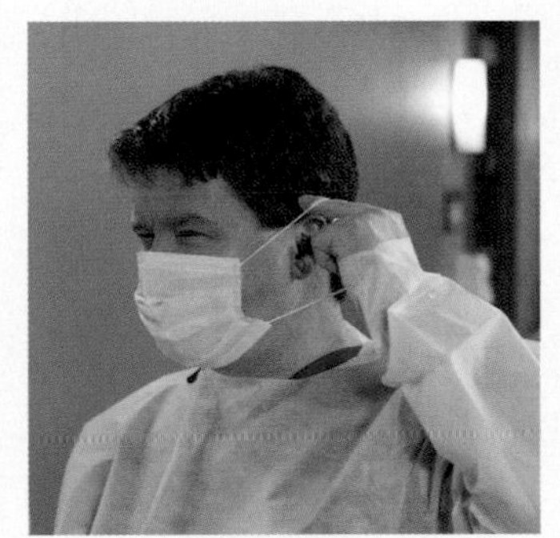

STEP 3b

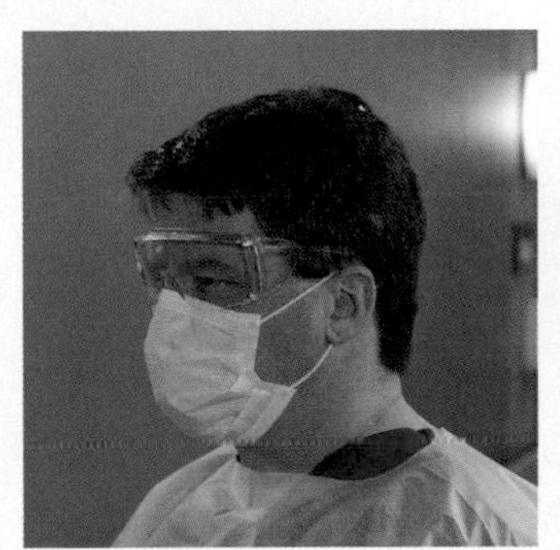

STEP 4

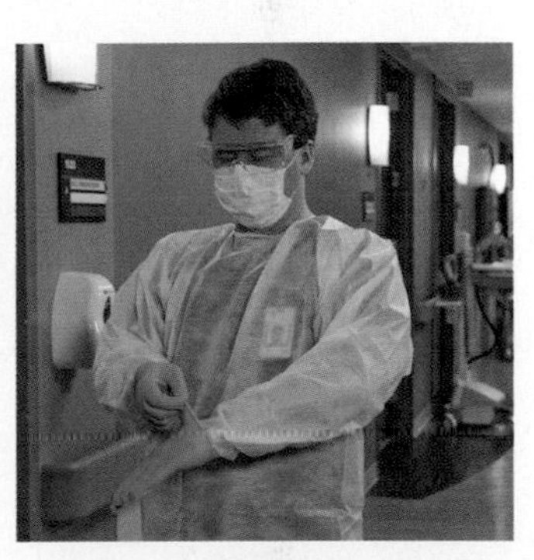

STEP 5

Removing PPE

1. Remove gloves (see Skill 26-2).
   Gloves are contaminated; removing gloves first prevents contamination of the face and eyes during removal of the mask and prevents spread of microorganisms.
2. Remove eyewear (if separate from mask): Handle by the earpieces, and lift away from the face.
   The outside of eyewear is contaminated; holding eyewear by the earpieces lessens the chance of contaminating hands.
3. Put eyewear into an appropriate receptacle for disposal or cleaning.
   Prevents spread of microorganisms.
4. Remove gown: Untie at the waist, untie at the neck, and grasp the gown on the inside of the neck in back and pull it down from the shoulders, pulling it off inside out and rolling it into a ball.
   The front of the gown and the sleeves are contaminated; touching only the inside with bare hands prevents spread of microorganisms.
5. Put the gown into an appropriate receptacle for disposal or cleaning.
   Prevents spread of microorganisms.

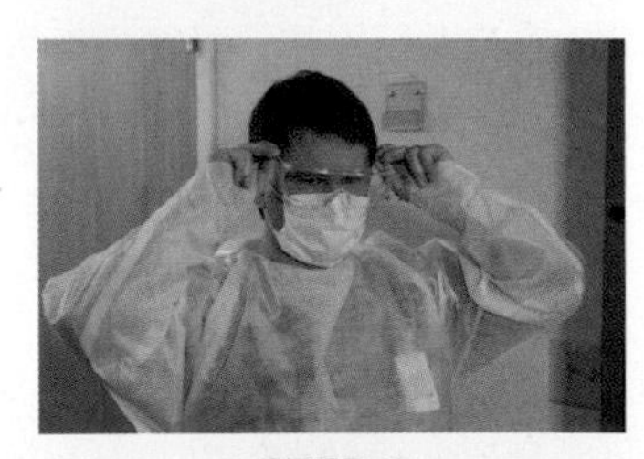

STEP 2

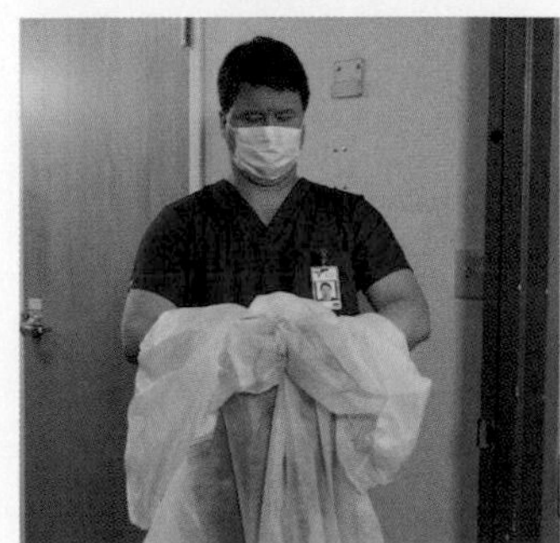

STEP 4

6. Remove mask: Untie at the bottom, and then untie at the top or slide ear loops over ears while holding onto the ties or loops; pull away from the face without touching the outside of the mask.
   Holding onto the ties or loops keeps the mask from falling and causing contamination; removing the mask last prevents spread of respiratory microorganisms.
7. Throw the mask into an appropriate receptacle.
   Prevents spread of microorganisms.
8. Perform hand hygiene (see Skill 26-1).

SKILL 26-4 Sterile Fields

PURPOSE

- Use of a sterile field prevents the spread of microorganisms.
- A sterile field is used in procedures requiring sterile technique.

RESOURCES

- Sterile procedural kit
- Sterile disposable drape
- Flat, clean, dry work surface above waist height near the location of the procedure

COLLABORATION AND DELEGATION

- Preparing a sterile field may not be delegated to UAP without special training to work in areas such as surgical units or possibly the emergency room.
- Check facility policy before considering delegation.

SPECIAL CIRCUMSTANCES

1. **Assess:** Does the sterile kit contain all needed items?
   Intervention: Acquire all items needed according to facility policy.
2. **Assess:** Are extra gloves and sterile drapes included?
   Intervention: To avoid having to restart the entire process if contamination occurs during the procedure, bring extra gloves and sterile drapes into the room.
3. **Assess:** Is the sterile kit damaged, wet, or past its expiration date?
   Intervention: Acquire a new sterile kit.
4. **Assess:** Is the work surface below waist level?
   Intervention: Work surfaces below the waist level are considered contaminated. Raise the work surface or find a new surface to prepare the sterile field.
5. **Assess:** Did skin touch the sterile field? Did the patient touch the sterile field?
   Intervention: Any contact between the sterile field and skin or a nonsterile item outside the sterile field is considered contamination. Acquire a new sterile drape or kit, and start over.
6. **Assess:** Did the preparer turn his or her back toward the sterile field?
   Intervention: Acquire a new sterile drape or kit, and start over.
7. **Assess:** Did the sterile drape tear during the procedure?
   Intervention: Acquire a new sterile drape or kit, and start over.

PROCEDURE

Preparing an Individually Wrapped Sterile Drape

1. If procedure is taking place in a patient room, introduce self; explain the procedure and the need for special handling.
   Builds a trusting, professional relationship; eases patient anxiety; facilitates cooperation.
2. Wash hands (see Skill 26-1).
   Prevents spread of microorganisms.
3. Open the packaging.
4. With the thumb and index finger, lift the drape out of its cover by the corner.
   Do not reach across the kit; reach around it to grasp the drape. Reaching across the field contaminates it.
5. Hold the drape above the waist and away from the body. With the thumb and index finger of the other hand, grasp the other corner and let the drape unfold.
   Below the waist is considered contaminated. The outer 1-inch margin is not sterile. Holding the drape this way allows for positioning on the work surface and maintains sterility of the field.
6. Place the lower section of the drape on the work surface farthest from you; then place the upper section onto the surface closest to you.
   Reaching across the field contaminates it.

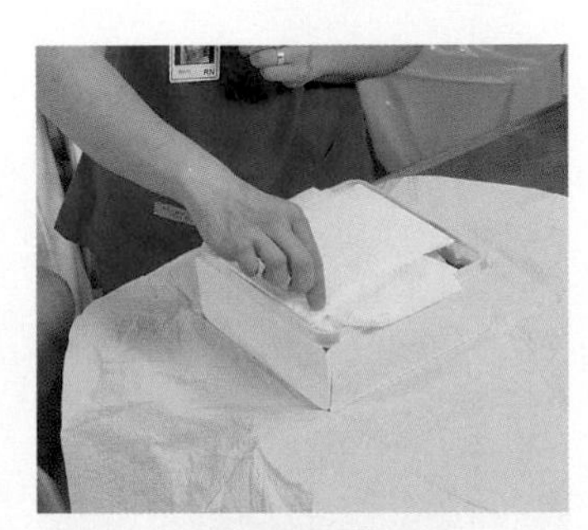

STEP 4

7. To place items that were not included in the kit onto the sterile field (see the section on Adding Sterile Supplies to a Sterile Field).
   The procedure may require additional items, which must be accessible in a sterile manner.

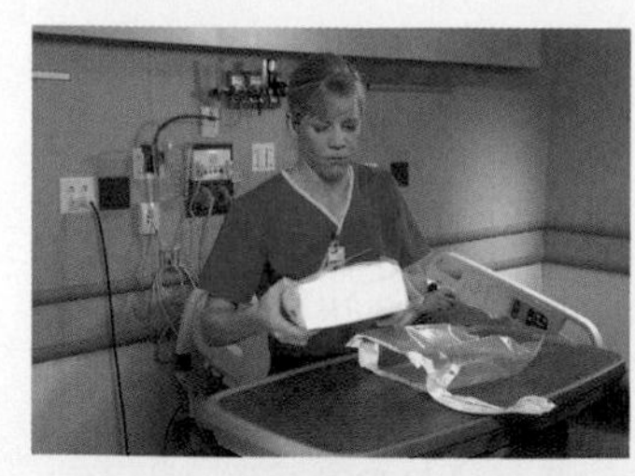

STEP 3

Preparing a Sterile Field Using a Commercial Procedural Kit

Some commercial kits contain a sterile drape for establishing a sterile work field near the patient or over the body.

1. If procedure is taking place in a patient room, introduce self; explain the procedure and the need for special handling.
   Builds a trusting, professional relationship; eases patient anxiety; facilitates cooperation.
2. Wash hands (see Skill 26-1).
   Prevents spread of microorganisms.
3. Open the outer packaging, and remove the procedural kit; place it on the work surface.
   The outer packaging protects the inner package from opening and becoming contaminated; the inside covering opens to become the sterile field.

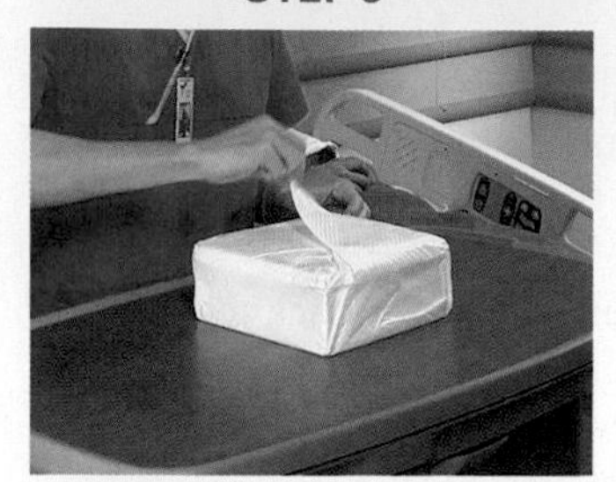

STEP 4a

4. With the thumb and index finger, grasp the outer 1 inch of the cover, first unfolding the flap away from you to open. Do not reach across the kit; reach around it to open.
   The 1-inch outer margin of the covering is not sterile. Grasping the outside eliminates the possibility of touching beyond this 1-inch field; reaching across the field contaminates it.
5. Continue opening the cover by opening the first side flap keeping the hand and arm to the side of the field; then the second side flap.
   The outer margin of the covering is not sterile; grasping the outside eliminates the possibility of touching the sterile field.

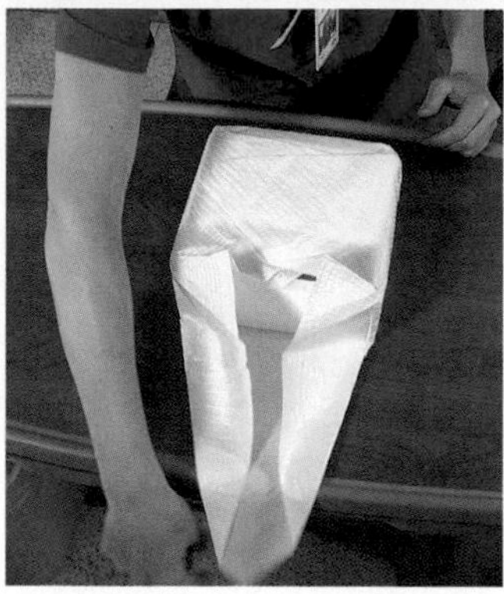

STEP 4b

6. Finish opening the sterile packaging by unfolding the last flap toward you; stand back, and let it fall flat on the work surface. Do not let it touch you or your clothing.
   The order used in opening the cover maintains sterility of the field.
7. To place items that were not included in the kit onto the sterile field (see the section on Adding Sterile Supplies to a Sterile Field).
   The procedure may require additional items, which must be accessible in a sterile manner.
8. Apply sterile gloves (see Skill 26-2).
   All items in the kit are sterile; they cannot be touched until sterile gloves have been donned.
9. Place items included in the kit onto the field; do not place them on the outer edge.
   The outer 1-inch border on the inside covering of the sterile field is not sterile.

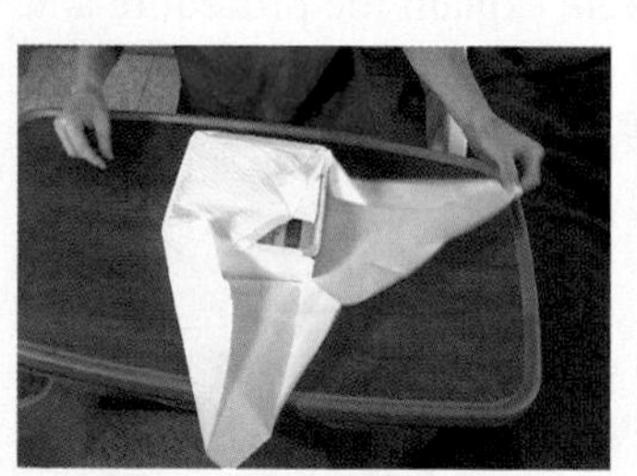

STEP 5

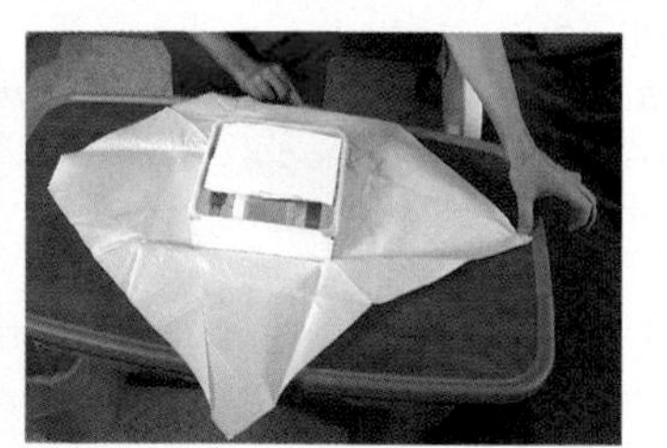

STEP 6

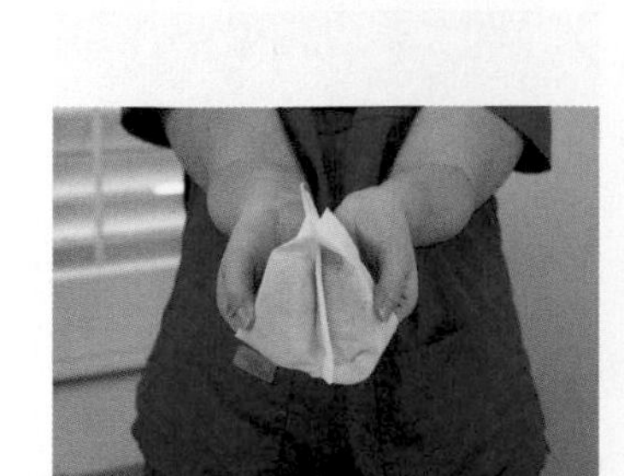

STEP 2

Adding Sterile Supplies to a Sterile Field

1. The hands are not yet gloved.
   Items are sterile inside the package; the outside wrapper is not sterile.
2. Following the package instructions, open each individually wrapped sterile item while holding it away from the body. Drop the item from a height of 10 inches onto the center of the sterile field. Do not hold the arm across the sterile field; approach from the side of the field.
   Prevents contamination; prevents reaching across field, which contaminates it.

3. To open a large, sterile item, hold it in the nondominant hand, and peel away the packaging with the dominant hand. Let the outer (nonsterile) side of the wrapping cover the nondominant hand while dropping or placing the item in the center of the field. Do not hold the arm across the sterile field; approach from the side of the field.
Prevents contamination of the sterile item.
4. To pour liquid into a sterile container within the sterile field, hold the lid of the bottle in the nondominant hand with the inside facing up. Hold the bottle in the dominant hand and pour the liquid slowly into the sterile container. Place the bottle on a nonsterile surface, and replace the lid.
The inside of the sterile liquid bottle is not contaminated, and putting the lid down risks contamination. Pouring slowly prevents splashing and possible contamination.

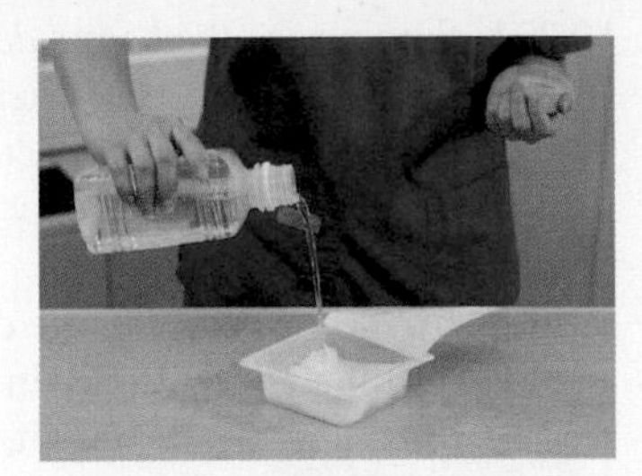

STEP 4

SUMMARY OF LEARNING OUTCOMES

LO 26.1 *Summarize the body's defense system:* The risk of infection decreases when the three main defenses of the body are kept intact. These defenses are normal flora, the inflammatory response, and the immune response.

LO 26.2 *Explain the links of the chain of infection:* The chain of infection includes an infectious host, source of infection, portal of exit, mode of transmission, portal of entry, and susceptible host.

LO 26.3 *Outline techniques of assessing for infection or risk of infection:* The nurse assesses the patient's risk factors, general appearance, vital signs, skin, laboratory results, and nutritional status to determine the patient's risk of infection or presence of an infection.

LO 26.4 *Identify nursing diagnoses for patients with infection or at risk for infection:* Examples of nursing diagnoses related to asepsis and infection control are *Risk for Infection, Knowledge Deficit, Impaired Skin Integrity,* and *Imbalanced Nutrition: Less than Body Requirements.*

LO 26.5 *Use measurable goals for patients with complications from infection:* The planning of care is designed around and involves prioritizing identified nursing diagnoses related to asepsis and infection control, evaluating the patient and the resources available, and setting patient-centered, measurable goals.

LO 26.6 *Carry out interventions to decrease the risk of infection and reverse the negative effects of infection:* Specific nursing interventions and patient activities can enhance the body's natural defense mechanisms. Some of them are handwashing and hand hygiene, precautions (i.e., standard, airborne, droplet, and contact), personal protective equipment, immunizations, asepsis, and disinfection and sterilization.

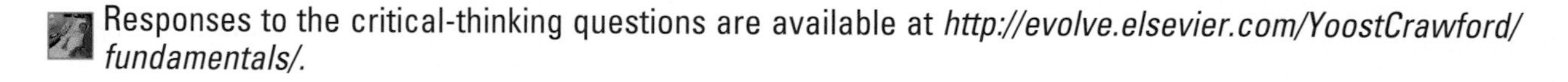
Responses to the critical-thinking questions are available at *http://evolve.elsevier.com/YoostCrawford/fundamentals/.*

REVIEW QUESTIONS

1. The nurse is caring for a patient who has been diagnosed with methicillin-resistant *Staphylococcus aureus* located in her incision. What transmission-based precautions will the nurse implement for the patient?
   a. Private room
   b. Private, negative-airflow room
   c. Mask worn by the staff when entering the room
   d. Mask worn by the staff and the patient when leaving the patient's room
2. A new patient is admitted to a medical unit with *Clostridium difficile.* Which type of precautions or isolation does the nurse know is appropriate for this patient?
   a. Airborne Precautions
   b. Droplet Precautions
   c. Contact Precautions
   d. Protective isolation
3. In which situations does the nurse wear clean gloves as part of standard precautions? *(Select all that apply.)*
   a. In the care of a patient diagnosed with an infectious process
   b. When the patient is diaphoretic
   c. During care of each individual under treatment in the facility
   d. In the presence of urine or stool
   e. When taking the patient's blood pressure
4. The nurse is providing patient education on infection prevention. Which definition of an infection does the nurse use as a teaching point?
   a. An illness resulting from living in an unclean environment
   b. A result of lack of knowledge about food preparation
   c. A disease resulting from pathogens in or on the body
   d. An acute or chronic illness resulting from traumatic injury
5. The nurse is caring for a patient who had abdominal surgery and has developed an infection in the wound while hospitalized. Which agent is most likely the cause of the infection?
   a. Virus
   b. Bacterium
   c. Fungus
   d. Spore
6. A nurse is preparing to change a sterile dressing and has donned two sterile gloves. To maintain surgical asepsis, what else must the nurse do?
   a. Keep the amount of splashes on the sterile field to a minimum
   b. If a sneeze is imminent, cover the nose and mouth with a gloved hand
   c. With a moist saline sponge, use the dominant hand to clean the wound and then apply a dry dressing
   d. Regard the outer 1 inch of the sterile field as contaminated

7. What is the proper order of removal of soiled personal protective equipment (PPE) when the nurse leaves the patient's room?
   a. Gown, goggles, mask, gloves, and exit the room
   b. Gloves, wash hands, remove gown, mask, and wash hands
   c. Gloves, goggles, gown, mask, and wash hands
   d. Goggles, mask, gloves, gown, and wash hands
8. Which hospitalized patient is most at risk for acquiring a health care–associated infection?
   a. 60-year-old who smokes two packs of cigarettes per day
   b. 40-year-old who has an indwelling urinary catheter in place
   c. 65-year-old who is a vegetarian and slightly underweight
   d. 60-year-old who has a white blood cell count of 6000
9. A patient develops food poisoning from contaminated food. What is the means of transmission for the infectious organism?
   a. Direct contact
   b. Vector
   c. Vehicle
   d. Airborne
10. Which assessment findings indicate to a nurse that a patient has a surgical site infection? *(Select all that apply.)*
   a. Thick, white drainage in the Jackson-Pratt tubing
   b. Redness or warmth at the affected site
   c. Purulent drainage at the incision site
   d. Temperature 38° C (100.4° F)
   e. Tenderness and localized pain
   f. Wound with well-approximated edges
   g. Purulent drainage at the incision site

Answers and rationales for the review questions are available at *http://evolve.elsevier.com/YoostCrawford/fundamentals/*.

REFERENCES

Abedon S: Supplemental lecture: Normal flora, 2009. Retrieved from *www.mansfield.ohio-state.edu/~sabedon/biol2035.htm*.

Centers for Disease Control and Prevention (CDC): Bloodborne infectious diseases: HIV/AIDS, hepatitis B, hepatitis, 2011. Retrieved from *www.cdc.gov/niosh/topics/bbp/genres.html*.

Centers for Disease Control and Prevention (CDC). CDC resources for pandemic flu, 2012a. Retrieved from *www.cdc.gov/flu/pandemic-resources/*.

Centers for Disease Control and Prevention (CDC): Handwashing: Clean hands save lives, 2012b. Retrieved from *www.cdc.gov/handwashing/*.

Centers for Disease Control and Prevention (CDC): Healthcare-associated infections, 2014. Retrieved from *www.cdc.gov/hai/*.

Creedon SA: Health care workers' hand decontamination practices: An Irish study. *Clin Nurs Res,* 15(1):6-26, 2006.

Cronenwett L, Sherwood G, Barnsteiner J, et al: Quality and safety education for nurses. *Nurs Outlook,* 55(3):122-131, 2007.

Goronzy J, Weyand C: The innate and adaptive immune systems. In L Goldman, A Schafer (eds), *Goldman's Cecil medicine*, ed. 24, Philadelphia, 2012, Saunders.

Gould D, Drey N: Hand hygiene technique. *Nurs Stand,* 22(34): 42-46, 2008.

Hart S: Using an aseptic technique to reduce the risk of infection. *Nursing Standard,* 21(47):43-48, 2007.

Hossein S, Sajjad R: Hand washing versus hand hygiene in intensive care unit: A clinical trial. *J Crit Care,* 24(3):15-17, 2009.

Kovach TL: Freedom from the chain of septic flow: Hand washing in infection control. *J Pract Nurs,* 55(4):10-15, 2005.

Mayer G: Innate (non-specific) immunity, 2009. Retrieved from *http://pathmicro.med.sc.edu/ghaffar/innate.htm*.

Rutala W, Weber D, Healthcare Infection Control Practices Advisory Committee (HICPAC): Guideline for disinfection and sterilization in healthcare facilities, 2008. Retrieved from *www.cdc.gov/hicpac/Disinfection_Sterilization/acknowledg.html*.

Siegel J, Rhinehart E, Jackson M, Chiarello L, Healthcare Infection Control Practices Advisory Committee (HICPAC): 2007 Guideline for isolation precautions: Preventing transmission of infectious agents in healthcare settings. Retrieved from *www.cdc.gov/hicpac/2007IP/2007isolationPrecautions.html*.

Tarrac S: Application of the updated CDC isolation guidelines for health care facilities. *AORN J,* 87(3):534-546, 2008.

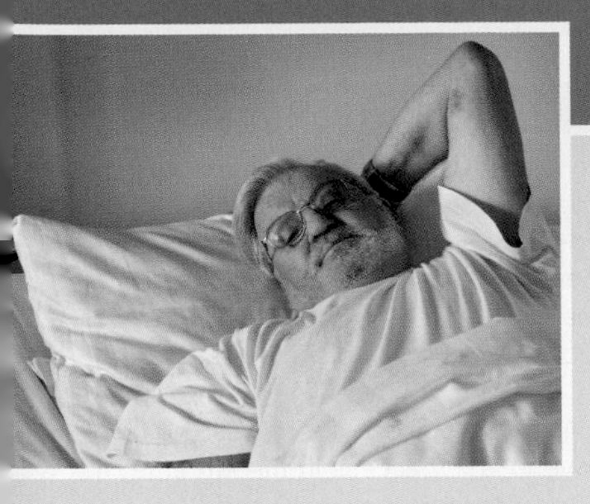

CHAPTER 27

Hygiene and Personal Care

EVOLVE WEBSITE

http://evolve.elsevier.com/YoostCrawford/fundamentals/

- Additional Evolve-Only Review Questions With Answers
- Answers and Rationales for Text Review Questions
- Answers to Critical-Thinking Questions
- Case Study With Questions
- Video Skills Clips
- Conceptual Care Map Creator
- Skills Checklist
- Glossary

LEARNING OUTCOMES

Comprehension of this chapter's content will provide students with the ability to:

LO 27.1 Describe the importance of hygiene related to skin, hair, nails, and mucous membranes.

LO 27.2 Identify how alterations in skin, hair, nails, and mucous membranes affect hygienic care.

LO 27.3 Determine patients' hygiene status and need for assistance with care.

LO 27.4 Select nursing diagnoses for patients who need assistance with hygiene or are experiencing alterations in self-care abilities.

LO 27.5 Establish measurable, patient-centered goals for patients with hygiene concerns and self-care alterations.

LO 27.6 Implement nursing care plans that include interventions to address the hygienic needs of patients.

KEY TERMS

activities of daily living, p. 521
alopecia, p. 518
axilla, p. 519
cerumen, p. 528
chafing, p. 520
cilia, p. 519
dandruff, p. 521
dentures, p. 527
effleurage, p. 526
epithelial tissue, p. 518
excoriation, p. 519
gingivae, p. 519
gingivitis, p. 520
halitosis, p. 520
hygiene, p. 518
integumentary system, p. 518
maceration, p. 524
mastication, p. 519
mucous membranes, p. 519
mucus, p. 519
nits, p. 526
pediculosis, p. 519
perineal care, p. 518
pétrissage, p. 526
prosthetic, p. 528
salivary glands, p. 519
sebaceous glands, p. 518
Sitz baths, p. 525
tapotement, p. 526
toothette, p. 527

CASE STUDY

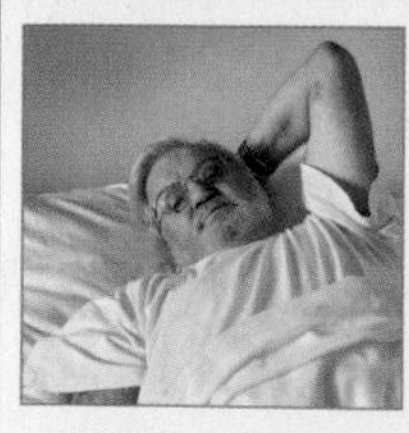

Mr. Randall is a 78-year-old widowed father of four and grandfather of seven who has a history of hypertension and chronic obstructive pulmonary disease (COPD). Mr. Randall was admitted the previous night for worsening of COPD symptoms. He is allergic to sulfa drugs. He has a history of a two-pack-per-day (ppd) smoking habit, which he quit 10 years ago. His surgical history includes removal of his appendix 30 years ago and a total right knee replacement 8 years ago. He states that his "left knee is bad, but I can't get it replaced because of my lungs." A chest x-ray, complete blood cell (CBC) count, and basic metabolic panel (chem 7 blood tests) were performed on admission, and results are pending.

Mr. Randall's vital signs are T 38.8° C (101.8° F), P 82 and regular, R 26 and labored, BP 136/84, with a pulse oximetry reading of 88% on room air (RA). His pain level is 2 of 10, with pain in the chest when coughing. The intravenous (IV) access in the left antecubital space has no redness or swelling. He exhibits shortness of breath (SOB) with activity. His Braden score is 20 and Morse Fall score is 45. Mr. Randall admits that he is not able to take care of himself "like he used to." He states that it is difficult for him to get in and out of the tub shower at home, and he often just "washes up by the sink." His hair is unkempt and shaggy. His face shows a few days' growth of a beard. He has strong body odor.

Treatment orders are as follows:

- Vital signs q 4 hr
- Oxygen by nasal cannula at 2 L/min
- No-added-salt diet
- Intravenous access saline lock
- Bathroom privileges with assistance
- Intake and output
- Daily weights

Medication orders are as follows:

- Lisinopril 20 mg daily
- Ipratropium multidose inhaler (MDI), 2 puffs four times daily
- Albuterol MDI, 2 puffs q 4 hr PRN for wheezing
- Acetaminophen 650 mg q 4 hr PRN for pain or temperature higher than 38° C (101.4° F)

Refer back to this case study to answer the critical-thinking questions throughout the chapter.

Assisting patients with **hygiene** (practices such as cleanliness that promote and preserve health) is an essential part of patient care. The hospitalized patient may depend on the nurse for basic care that is usually completed independently at home. Hygienic practices include bathing, oral care, **perineal care** (cleansing the genital area, urinary meatus, and anus), foot care, and shaving. These practices vary according to personal habits, cultural beliefs, ethnic customs, and age. The nurse assesses patients' backgrounds and provides hygienic care in a manner that is sensitive to their differences in habits and customs. During patient care, the nurse communicates with the patient, assesses the skin, and observes for any abnormalities. Bathing cleans the skin, removes organisms that can cause infection and odor, provides comfort, and contributes to the patient's health and well-being.

STRUCTURE AND FUNCTION OF SKIN, HAIR, AND NAILS LO 27.1

While performing hygienic care, the nurse observes the entire integumentary system and aspects of the respiratory, gastrointestinal, and genitourinary systems. Healthy skin, hair, nails, and mucous membranes contribute to the overall health and well-being of patients. The nurse has the opportunity to assess all of these areas during bathing.

SKIN, HAIR, AND NAILS

Skin, nails, hair, sweat glands, and sebaceous (oil) glands form the **integumentary system**. Skin is the body's vulnerable barrier to the outside world, but it is strong, self-renewing, and easily cleaned. Mucous membranes of the lips, nostrils, anus, urethra, and vagina join seamlessly with the skin (McKinley and O'Loughlin, 2012). Chapter 29 provides a detailed description of the skin and its structure and functions.

Sweat glands are an accessory organ of the skin and produce a water-like substance. These glands are activated by heat, nervousness, or stress. Sweat can produce a foul-smelling body odor. During hygienic care, the nurse cleanses all areas of the integumentary system to maintain healthy tissue, reduce body odor, and enhance comfort. Cleansing rids the skin of microorganisms that can cause infection and odor.

Hair follicles, sebaceous glands, nails, and sweat glands are accessory organs of the skin. Hair follicles arise from the dermis, are made up of **epithelial tissue** (tissue that lines tubes and cavities and the surface of the skin), and generate hair. When hair follicles go into a resting cycle, hair may fall out. The hair follicle begins a growing cycle again and produces a new hair. When hair follicles completely die, **alopecia** (absence or loss of hair) develops. Located in the dermis, **sebaceous glands** secrete an oily substance that keeps the hair and skin soft. If left unwashed, hair becomes oily as a result of these secretions (Booth, Wyman, and Stoia, 2012).

Nails arise from the epidermis and are composed of keratinized epithelial cells. They grow from the nail matrix, which is the actively growing portion of the nail. Nails protect the ends of fingers and toes. Unlike skin, nails do not slough off and must be cut (Booth, Wyman, and Stoia, 2012). Normal nails are smooth and pink (see Chapter 20, Figure 20-7).

NOSE, MOUTH, AND ORAL CAVITY

Mucous membranes are surfaces that line the passages and cavities of the body, such as nasal, oral, vaginal, urethral, and anal areas. The outer layer of mucous membranes is composed of epithelial cells. **Mucus** (fluid secreted by mucous membranes) traps particles in the nose, and **cilia** (tiny hairs lining the nasal passages) help move the trapped particles to the throat, where they are swallowed.

The **salivary glands** in the mouth secrete mucus, enzymes, and a watery fluid, which mix to form saliva. This fluid begins chemical digestion of food and keeps the oral cavity moist. Teeth begin mechanical digestion through **mastication**, or chewing (McKinley and O'Loughlin, 2012). The roots of the teeth are surrounded by **gingivae** (gums), which are composed of connective tissue and epithelial cells. The ability to ingest and chew food depends on the health of all parts of the oral cavity (see Chapter 20, Figure 20-20).

ALTERATIONS IN STRUCTURE AND FUNCTION AFFECTING HYGIENIC CARE LO 27.2

Many alterations of the skin and mucous membranes affect the nurse's decisions about hygienic care. Knowledge of how these alterations change the normal structure and function enables the nurse to plan interventions specific to each patient.

ULCERS, INCISIONS, AND WOUNDS

Many hospitalized patients have openings in the layers of skin caused by wounds, incisions, or ulcers. Any interruption in the skin, which is the body's first line of defense, may lead to infection. Excessively dry skin can lead to cracks and openings in the integumentary system. **Excoriation** (red, scaly areas with surface loss of skin tissue) occurs in patients whose skin is exposed to bodily fluids such as stool, urine, or gastric juices. Excoriation also occurs in areas where skin rests on skin, such as in the **axilla** (armpit); under large, pendulous breasts; or in abdominal folds.

DECREASED SENSATION

Damage to peripheral nerves occurs for a variety of reasons. Patients with neurologic deficits, such as peripheral neuropathy due to diabetes, may not be able to identify extremes of hot and cold. The nurse should monitor the temperature of bath water for patients with decreased sensation. Burns may result if skin is exposed to extremely hot water during bathing.

ALOPECIA

Patients may have alopecia due to hereditary factors, certain illnesses, or the effects of drugs such as those used in chemotherapy. This condition may affect the patient's self-esteem. Collaboration with a beautician or barber may be needed if a patient is actively losing hair as a result of treatment. Special care should be given to the scalp. The Patient Education and Health Literacy box outlines some education suggestions for patients with alopecia.

PATIENT EDUCATION AND HEALTH LITERACY

Alopecia

- Educate patients undergoing treatments (e.g., chemotherapy) that cause alopecia about when hair loss will occur, special care of the scalp, and protection of the skin.
- Arrange referrals to in-house beauticians or barbers for patients who want to have their hair cut shorter before hair loss begins.
- Provide resources such as where the patient can obtain a wig or find a support group.
- Make available to patients information on community agencies that may be helpful in providing care during chemotherapy.

PEDICULOSIS

A contagious scalp infection, **pediculosis**, is caused by *Pediculus humanus capitis.* This disorder is more commonly known as *head lice* (Figure 27-1). Transmission occurs through contact with infested personal items such as combs, hats, or linens. Symptoms of pediculosis are itching and redness of the scalp. If the condition is untreated, secondary bacterial infections can occur.

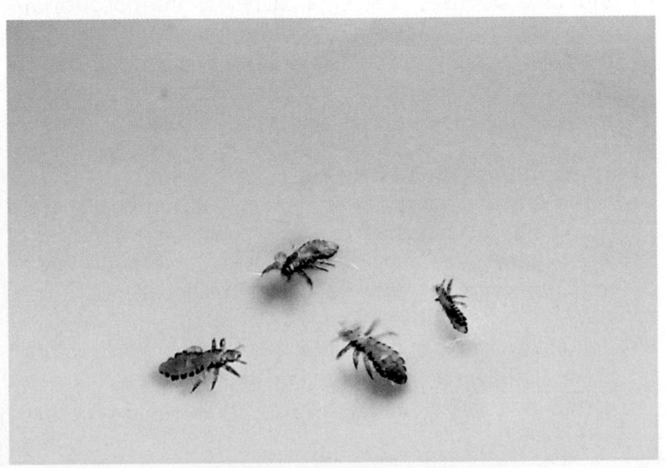

FIGURE 27-1 Head lice.

NAILS

Fungal, bacterial, and viral infections of the fingernails and toenails occur that cause discoloration and thickening of the nails. Some patients have a decreased ability to heal due to poor circulation. Any cut in the skin can lead to an ulcer in these patients. An order from the primary care provider (PCP) may be necessary for nail trimming, or a podiatrist may be consulted.

ORAL CAVITY

Alterations in the health of the oral cavity can affect the patient's ability to chew or overall health. Sores anywhere in the oral cavity, **gingivitis** (inflammation of the gums), and broken or missing teeth create problems with chewing. Certain medications cause the mouth to be dry, creating discomfort for the patient. **Halitosis** (unpleasant breath odor) may result from poor dental hygiene, fungal or bacterial infections, and complications of medical conditions such as diabetic ketoacidosis or renal failure. Oral health depends on diligent oral hygiene.

SELF-CARE ALTERATIONS

Many hospitalized patients have alterations in self-care abilities due to illness, recent surgery, immobility, and cognitive dysfunction. Assessing the patient's level of ability to perform skills such as self-bathing helps the nurse devise an appropriate plan of care and assist the patient when needed. Some diversity considerations related to hygiene are outlined in the Diversity Considerations box.

QSEN FOCUS!

Patient-centered care requires the nurse to understand how diverse cultural, ethnic, and social backgrounds function as sources of patient, family, and community values. The nurse provides hygienic care with sensitivity and respect for the diversity of human experience and supports care for individuals and groups whose values differ from those of the nurse.

ASSESSMENT — LO 27.3

During patient care the nurse has an opportunity to establish a therapeutic relationship with the patient and assess cognitive functioning, range of motion, condition of the skin, and hygienic practices. Good hygiene directly impacts the health of the integumentary system. Gathering subjective and objective data about the effects of hygienic practices helps the nurse decide on a specific care plan for the patient (Health Assessment Questions box).

DIVERSITY CONSIDERATIONS

Life Span

- Infants and young children depend on others to care for their hygienic needs.
- Skin becomes thinner, drier, and less elastic with age, making older adults more susceptible to skin breakdown.

Gender

- Proper perineal care is an important step in preventing urinary tract infections, especially in women. The female urethra is shorter than the male urethra and is closer to the anus.
- Providing perineal care for a patient of the opposite sex should be done with sensitivity to the patient's feelings. If the nurse approaches personal care with a professional attitude and communicates the importance of the procedure, the patient's comfort level is likely to increase.

Culture, Ethnicity, and Religion

- In Hispanic and Arab cultures, male nurses may be prohibited from performing perineal care or examining private areas of a female patient's body. Similar cultural restrictions may be true for a female nurse caring for male patients (Pullen, 2007).
- Cultural traditions and religious beliefs affect hygienic practices. North American and many other cultures consider it common to shower or bathe daily. In other cultures, bathing weekly is the norm.
- A beard in certain religions or cultures indicates that a man is married.
- Women of some cultures shave their axillae (armpits) and legs. In other regions of the world, women do not shave these areas. The nurse should always consult with the patient or family before shaving or cutting a patient's hair.
- People of African descent tend to have hair that is drier and does not require frequent washing.

Disability

- Patients with disabilities that affect mobility and range of motion may depend on the nurse for bathing, hygiene, and personal care.

Morphology

- Obesity creates unique concerns for the nurse providing hygienic care. Areas on the body where skin touches skin, such as in abdominal folds, under breasts, and in the groin area, are prone to accumulation of moisture and **chafing** (inflammation due to friction). This can lead to skin breakdown and bacterial or fungal infections.
- It may be difficult for the nurse to move and position obese patients for bathing and care. Use of mechanical lift equipment is necessary to ensure patient safety.

HEALTH ASSESSMENT QUESTIONS

Self-Care Focus

- Are you able to bathe yourself?
- How often do you bathe or shower?
- Has there been a change in your ability to care for yourself?
- Can you reach your feet and legs when you bathe or shower?
- Are you ever incontinent of urine or stool?
- Do you become short of breath during your bath?
- Can you raise your arms up to brush your teeth?
- Are you able to shampoo and comb your hair?

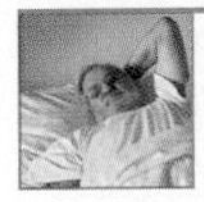

1. Write at least five assessment questions that the nurse should ask Mr. Randall about his personal hygiene habits at home.

ASSESS SKIN, HAIR, NAILS, AND ORAL CAVITY

Assessment of the skin occurs before and during hygienic care. Before care, the nurse asks if the patient has noticed dry skin, rashes, skin changes, or sores. The nurse observes the condition of the exposed skin and notices body odors. During a complete bed bath, the nurse has the opportunity to objectively assess the skin for changes, performing inspection and palpation to note the color, texture, warmth, and intactness of the skin and related structures. After inspection, the nurse documents the skin assessment and calculates the Braden score to document the patient's risk for impaired skin integrity. Chapter 29 provides more information.

While gathering the health history, the nurse observes the patient's hair for cleanliness and grooming. Poor hygienic practices or self-care deficits are indicated by oily, matted, or tangled hair. Inspection of a patient's hair may reveal **dandruff** (scaling and flaking of scalp skin) or head lice.

While assessing the patient's peripheral vascular status, the nurse observes the condition of the fingernails and toenails. The nails are assessed for color, thickness, cracking, odor, and capillary refill.

Inspection of the oral mucosa and teeth is part of a complete head-to-toe assessment. By inspecting the condition of the patient's mouth, the nurse assesses oral hygiene. Broken or missing teeth, red gums, halitosis, and open sores are all indications of altered oral health and poor oral hygiene. The nurse assesses for excessive dryness, color of the oral mucosa, and presence of any sores.

ASSESS SELF-CARE ABILITIES

The patient's self-care ability related to hygiene needs affects the nursing care plan. If a patient is unable to care for basic needs, the nurse assists the patient during hospitalization and refers the patient to appropriate community resources for assistance after discharge. The patient's self-care abilities are assessed during the health history by asking questions about home care and by observing for any odors or signs of poor hygiene. The nurse must observe the patient's abilities to complete **activities of daily living** (ADLs), which include bathing, mouth care, grooming, toileting, dressing, and eating.

HYGIENE AND INFECTION

The presence of skin, scalp, or oral infections may indicate poor hygiene. The nurse observes for signs of infection on the skin by looking for redness, swelling, or drainage. Infections, redness, itching, or sores on the scalp may indicate poor hygiene or exposure to an infestation, as in pediculosis. Red, swollen gums or sores in the oral cavity may be signs of poor oral hygiene. The nurse assesses patients for signs of infection due to poor hygienic practices during the initial interview and while giving care. Patient education may be needed to change the patient's view of hygiene and its relation to health.

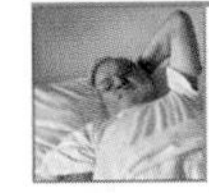

2. List three focused assessments related to hygiene that the nurse should perform on Mr. Randall. Give rationales for each.

◆ NURSING DIAGNOSIS LO 27.4

Nursing diagnoses related to hygiene and patient care are formulated after assessing patient hygienic practices and self-care abilities using subjective and objective data. Some common nursing diagnoses associated with hygiene and self-care are *Bathing Self-Care Deficit, Dressing Self-Care Deficit, Readiness for Enhanced Self-Care, Ineffective Health Maintenance,* and *Disturbed Body Image.* Patients may have nursing diagnoses based on self-care abilities and hygiene. Examples of nursing diagnostic statements related to hygiene are listed:

- *Hygiene Self-Care Deficit* related to weakness due to decreased tissue perfusion as evidenced by strong body odor and unkempt hair
- *Readiness for Enhanced Self-Care* as evidenced by patient expressing a desire to be independent in ADLs
- *Ineffective Health Maintenance* related to impaired ability to understand due to cognitive changes as evidenced by poor hygiene, unkempt appearance, and halitosis

◆ PLANNING LO 27.5

During the planning stage of the nursing process, the nurse prioritizes identified hygiene-related nursing diagnoses based on patient needs and recognized risks. Nursing care plans are developed for each nursing diagnosis after considering the patient's self-care abilities, available resources, and family involvement. Setting realistic goals helps the nurse develop a plan of care that will enable the patient to meet goals (Table 27-1). These goals must take into consideration the patient's

TABLE 27-1 Care Planning

NANDA-I NURSING DIAGNOSIS LABEL WITH NURSING DIAGNOSIS STATEMENT	NURSING OUTCOME CLASSIFICATION (NOC)	NURSING INTERVENTION CLASSIFICATION (NIC)
Hygiene Self-Care Deficit related to weakness due to decreased tissue perfusion as evidenced by strong body odor and unkempt hair	*Self-care: Hygiene* (0305) Shampoos hair (030508)	*Bathing* (1610) Wash hair as needed and desired.

From Bulechek G, Butcher H, Dochterman J, et al (Eds): *Nursing interventions classification (NIC)*, ed. 6, St. Louis, 2013, Mosby; Moorhead S, Johnson M, Maas M, et al (Eds): *Nursing outcomes classification (NOC)*, ed. 5, St. Louis, 2013, Mosby; NANDA International: *Nursing diagnoses: Definitions and classification, 2012-2014*, West Sussex, England, 2012, Wiley-Blackwell. Reprinted with permission from NANDA International, Inc.

self-care abilities, family involvement, living situation, extent of hospital stay, and available resources.

Collaboration with other health care professionals, patients, and families is necessary when setting long- and short-term goals (Collaboration and Delegation box). Each identified nursing diagnosis must have goal statements that are intended to address the specific problem. Examples of goals or outcome statements follow:

- Patient will accept assistance with hygiene within 24 hours.
- Patient will begin to perform 50% of her ADLs within 24 hours.
- Patient will remain free of body odors during hospitalization.

COLLABORATION AND DELEGATION

Hygienic Care

- Collaboration with colleagues is necessary when a patient requires a caregiver of the same sex for personal care because of cultural or religious reasons or personal preference.
- Family members or friends need to be involved in goal setting if the patient needs assistance with self-care activities after discharge from the hospital.
- Some aspects of personal care and hygiene may be delegated to unlicensed assistive personnel after assessment of the patient and specific instruction. The Skill features in this chapter provide delegation guidelines.
- Collaboration with physical therapists for assessment of the patient's motor abilities and with occupational therapists for evaluation of the patient's ADLs may be necessary.

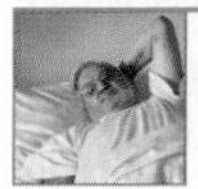

The conceptual care map for Mr. Randall provided in Figure 27-2 is partially completed to indicate how to use the map as a learning tool. Using it as an example, go to the website at *http://evolve.elsevier.com/YoostCrawford/fundamentals/* to complete Nursing Diagnoses 2 and 3.

3. Write a goal for this nursing diagnosis: *Bathing Self-Care Deficit* related to weakness due to decreased tissue perfusion as evidenced by the following: Mr. Randall admits that he is not able to take care of himself "like he used to." He states that it is difficult for him to get in and out of the tub shower at home and that he often "washes up by the sink." His hair is unkempt and shaggy. His face shows a few days' growth of a beard.

IMPLEMENTATION AND EVALUATION LO 27.6

Hygiene is a fundamental nursing activity (Ethical, Legal, and Professional Practice box). Implementing evidence-based oral care, bathing, and incontinence management helps to prevent health care–acquired pneumonia, pressure ulcers, and other skin problems (Vollman, Garcia, and Miller, 2005). Interaction with the patient during bathing and personal care helps in the development of a therapeutic relationship and provides comfort for the patient. Evaluation of hygiene and personal care is ongoing.

ETHICAL, LEGAL, AND PROFESSIONAL PRACTICE

Respect, Competence, and Compassion

- A provision in the American Nurses Association (ANA) Code of Ethics for Nurses states that the principle underlying nursing practice is respect for the dignity, worth, and human rights of each person (see Chapter 11).
- Showing respect for a patient's dignity is apparent when the nurse cares for the patient's basic needs for cleanliness and hygiene.
- A nurse's ethical response to patients who are unable to care for themselves is to provide care with competence and compassion.

INTERVENTIONS

Nursing care plans for hygiene-oriented nursing diagnoses are tailored to the patients' specific needs. Plans contain

Medications
Lisinopril 20 mg daily
Ipratropium multidose inhaler (MDI), 2 puffs four times daily
Albuterol MDI, 2 puffs q 4-6 hr prn for wheezing
Acetaminophen 650 mg q 4 hr prn for pain or temperature >38° C (101.4° F)

IV Sites/Fluids/Rate
IV access left antecubital: saline lock

Conceptual Care Map
Student name ________ Patient initials Mr. R Date ________
Age 78 Gender M Room # ___ Admission date last night
CODE Status ______ Allergies Sulfa drugs Braden score 20
Diet no added salt Activity bathroom privileges with assistance
Weight ______ Height ______ Religion ________

Admitting Diagnoses/Chief Complaint
Worsening of COPD symptoms

Assessment Data
Widowed, father of 4, grandfather of 7.
Vital signs: T 38.8° C (101.8° F), P 82 regular, R 26 and labored, BP 136/84, with a pulse oximetry reading of 88% on room air (RA). Pain level is 2 out of 10, with pain in chest when coughing.
IV access, left antecubital, without redness or swelling.
Shortness of breath (SOB) with activity. Morse Fall Scale score is 45.
Admits that he is not able to take care of himself "like he used to." States that his "left knee is bad but I can't get it replaced because of my lungs." States that it is difficult for him to get in and out of the tub shower at home and he often just "washes up by the sink."
Hair is unkempt and shaggy. Face shows a few days' growth of a beard. Strong body odor present.

Lab Values/Diagnostic Test Results
CBC, chem 7 pending
Chest x-ray pending

Treatments
Vital signs q 4 hr
Oxygen via nasal cannula at 2 L/min
Intake and output
Daily weights

Past Medical/Surgical History
Hypertension and COPD
Right knee replacement 8 years ago
Appendectomy 30 years ago
History of 2-ppd smoking habit; quit 10 years ago

Primary Nursing Diagnosis
Hygiene Self-Care Deficit related to weakness secondary to decreased tissue perfusion as evidenced by strong body odor and unkempt hair.

Supporting Data
Admits that he is not able to take care of himself "like he used to." States that "left knee is bad but I can't get it replaced because of my lungs." States that it is difficult to get in and out of the tub shower at home and he often just "washes up by the sink." Hair is unkempt and shaggy. Face shows a few days' growth of a beard. Body odor present.

STG/NOC
Patient will accept assistance with hygiene within 24 hours.
NOC: Self-care: Hygiene (0305)
Shampoos hair (030508)

Interventions/NIC With Rationale
1. Offer assistance with one part of ADLs at a time because patient may tire if too much is done at once.
2. Have UAP give complete bed bath and shampoo, giving breaks between care to allow patient to rest.
3. Offer sips or water or ice chips and oral and nasal care at least every 2 hours due to the drying nature of oxygen therapy.
4. Assess patient and family for home care considerations to establish whether patient needs adaptive equipment or assistance in the home.

NIC: Bathing (1610)
Wash hair as needed and desired.

Rationale Citation/EBP
Yoost BL, Crawford LR: *Fundamentals of nursing: Active learning for collaborative practice*, St. Louis, 2016, Mosby.

Evaluation
During morning care patient had a complete bed bath and shampoo and was able to assist with 20% of the bath. Continue plan of care.

Nursing Diagnosis 2

Supporting Data

STG/NOC

Interventions/NIC With Rationale

Rationale Citation/EBP

Evaluation

Nursing Diagnosis 3

Supporting Data

STG/NOC

Interventions/NIC With Rationale

Rationale Citation/EBP

Evaluation

FIGURE 27-2 Partially completed conceptual care map based on Mr. Randall, the case study patient in this chapter. *ADLs,* Activities of daily living; CBC, complete blood count; *COPD,* chronic obstructive pulmonary disease; EBP, Evidence-based practice; *IV,* intravenous; *NIC,* Nursing Interventions Classification; *NOC,* Nursing Outcomes Classification; *ppd,* packs per day; *STG,* short-term goal; *UAP,* unlicensed assistive personnel.

interventions focused on cleanliness, comfort, and prevention of injury or infection. Side benefits of assisting patients with their personal care include the opportunity to thoroughly assess the patient's skin and communicate with the patient in a therapeutic manner. Patient and family education regarding proper hygiene practices and assessment of the patient's home situation (Home Care Considerations box) occur during this time.

HOME CARE CONSIDERATIONS

Self-Care Deficits in Patients Discharged to Home

Patients with self-care deficits who are being discharged to home require special considerations to ensure that hygienic care continues:

- What are the patient's self-care deficits?
- Will there be caregivers in the home to help the patient with hygienic needs?
- Is there a bathroom that will be accessible to the patient?
- Does the patient need equipment to facilitate care in the home such as a shower stool or stabilizing bars in the bathroom?
- Are referrals to community agencies necessary to meet the patient's needs in the home?

Patients may be able to return home if the proper aids are used or installed. They include handrails near stairs and in the bathroom, raised toilet seats, extension grabbers, and other adaptive tools.

Bathing and Skin Care

Bathing and skin care are essential components of patient care. The amount of assistance patients need depends on their self-care abilities. Hygiene teaching can be incorporated throughout care. There are many methods of bathing a patient, depending on the setting and the equipment available. Individual bathing preferences should be taken into account when planning bathing care.

QSEN FOCUS!

Patient-centered hygienic care integrates an understanding of patient and family preferences and values, coordination of care, and provision of physical comfort and emotional support. The nurse elicits the patient's values and preferences when planning care.

Bathing removes dead skin, bacteria, and body fluids that build up on the skin. Keeping the skin clean and dry can help to prevent problems caused by breakdown of the skin. Bathing is a comfort and therapeutic intervention; it provides relaxation and skin benefits such as prevention of **maceration** (breakdown of the skin caused by fluid) and infection caused by breeding microorganisms. After the bath, the nurse documents the type of care performed, date and time, skin assessment, and the patient's current position, ability to assist, and response to bathing.

! SAFE PRACTICE ALERT

Avoid massaging reddened areas on the skin during the bath. Further tissue breakdown can occur if reddened areas are massaged.

Complete Bed Bath

A complete bed bath is performed for patients who are bedridden or depend totally on others for care. Skill 27-1 outlines the steps for portion of the bath, which the nurse can adapt for patient's individual needs. Nurses or unlicensed assistive personnel (UAP) wash the patient and perform passive range-of-motion exercises as appropriate. Assessment of the patient's tolerance of this activity is essential before the bath.

Equipment used during the bath is facility specific and tailored to patient needs. Some facilities use bath basins, washcloths, towels, and soap or skin cleanser, whereas others use prepackaged bath cloths (Figure 27-3). The packages contain several premoistened, disposable, no-rinse cloths that can be used instead of soap and water.

Partial Bed Bath

A partial bed bath is performed when only part of the body is washed. Some patients want to wash their hands and face before breakfast. Others need perineal care after using the bedpan. Many patients can independently perform parts of the bath but need help with washing their back and feet.

After assessment, the nurse may decide to do a partial bath if a patient has extremely dry skin. Many older adults find that a complete bath daily causes excessive drying of their skin. If a patient cannot tolerate a complete bed bath because of weakness or activity intolerance, the nurse washes only the areas where skin problems could develop or are causing discomfort.

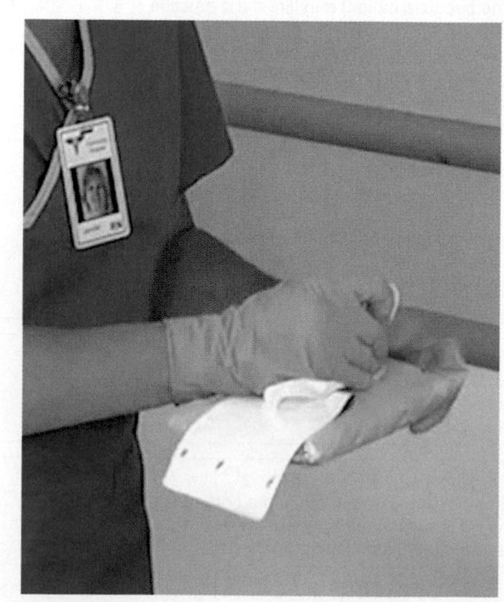

FIGURE 27-3 Pack of disposable bath cloths.

Sink Bath

Patients who are ambulatory may prefer to wash while standing or sitting in front of a bath basin or sink. Patients may still need assistance with their legs, feet, and back. Assessment of the patient's ability to ambulate and wash independently is necessary.

Shower

Some hospital rooms or units are equipped with stand-up showers for patients who are strong enough to shower independently. The nurse assesses the patient and checks health care provider orders to determine whether it is safe for a patient to shower.

! SAFE PRACTICE ALERT

Patients with peripheral neuropathy may not be able to feel the water temperature on their extremities. It is the nurse's responsibility to adjust the bath or shower water to a comfortably warm temperature: 40.5° to 43.3° C (105° to 110° F).

Chair Shower

Some long-term care patients are washed in the shower while sitting in a shower chair. A shower chair is durable, waterproof, and easily disinfected. It allows nurses or UAP to wash patients in the shower who are physically dependent or cognitively impaired. Shower chairs have an open seat so that perineal care can be completed. Some shower chairs have hydraulic lifts, making it easier for the caregiver to clean all areas of the body. Showering is a more efficient method of cleansing and is usually completed on a scheduled basis for dependent patients in long-term care.

For patients with dementia or other cognitive impairments, an individualized bathing routine must take into account their former bathing preferences, current abilities and limitations, and responses to environmental stimuli. Adapting the routine to the patient helps maintain a calm environment. A soft voice, soothing music, and a warm room help the patient relax.

! SAFE PRACTICE ALERT

An individualized bathing routine should be established for patients with dementia or other cognitive impairments.

SAFE PRACTICE ALERT

Always keep the top-half side rails up and the bed in its lowest position with the wheels locked when not at the bedside.

Perineal Care

Perineal care, or personal care, involves cleaning the genital area, urinary meatus, and anus (Skill 27-2). This care is particularly important for patients who are dependent or incontinent or those who have a urinary catheter. The caregiver always wears gloves to provide perineal care due to the risk of exposure to body fluids. Patients recovering from perineal or genital surgery and women who are menstruating require diligent care to prevent infections and odors. **Sitz baths** (baths for soaking a patient's perineal area) are sometimes used therapeutically after perineal surgery or childbirth to cleanse the area. Patients who can perform personal care independently should be allowed to do so after the nurse assesses their abilities and risks of complications.

Perineal care is provided during a bath or shower but may be necessary more frequently, especially for incontinent patients. Patients are sometimes embarrassed to depend on others for personal care. A professional approach and caring attitude can allay patients' anxiety.

Documentation after personal care includes the type of procedure performed, the date and time, skin-related issues, incontinence, drainage or odors, catheters or dressings, and the patient's self-care abilities and response to the procedure. This documentation is included even if personal care was done as part of a complete bath.

Male Perineal Care

Male personal care is an important part of hygiene. It can be provided during a bath or after an incontinence episode. A caregiver of either gender can provide male perineal care, but in some cultures, it is taboo for an unrelated female to touch male genitals. If the patient or family requests a caregiver of the same gender, this request should be honored.

A male patient may have an erection during care, which is a normal response to tactile stimulation. The care provider can ignore the erection and continue with the procedure or return later to complete the care, depending on the comfort level and the situation. Documentation is part of hygienic care. Document any redness, drainage, odor, edema, or skin changes.

Female Perineal Care

Personal care for females is always performed by cleansing from the front to the back of the perineal area. This essential component of good hygienic practice is completed as often as necessary to keep the patient clean, dry, and odor free. Providing privacy is an important aspect of personal care.

Some female patients request that a female caregiver perform their personal care. This may be a cultural tradition or may be personal preference. Staffing in most hospitals allows the nurse to honor this request. Documentation after care should include noting any odor or areas of redness, drainage, or swelling.

! SAFE PRACTICE ALERT

Always wash the female patient from the urinary meatus back to the anus to prevent introducing organisms into the urinary tract.

Foot and Hand Care

Care of the hands and feet is part of the bathing routine or can be completed separately (Skill 27-3). Feet and hands are soaked briefly during the bath if this is not contraindicated by the patient's condition. Diligent foot care provides comfort while preventing odors and skin breakdown. Assessment of the patient's self-care abilities and patient education on care of the feet and hands are accomplished during the procedure.

Some patients require specialized care of the hands, feet, and nails. If the patient has decreased sensation in the lower extremities, the feet are inspected for redness, sores, and dry areas. Patients with peripheral neuropathy should not soak their feet due to drying of the tissue and the risk of infection. Care is taken to avoid nicks or cuts in the skin when cutting toenails of a patient with circulatory impairment in the lower extremities due to the decreased ability to heal. In some care settings, a health care provider order is necessary before trimming toenails, or patients are referred to a podiatrist for this procedure.

> **! SAFE PRACTICE ALERT**
>
> Soaking the feet of a diabetic patient is contraindicated. Diabetic patients have a decreased ability to heal, and soaking their feet may lead to skin breakdown.

Documentation of hand and foot care includes the procedure performed, date and time, problems observed during the procedure such as sores and skin breakdown, odors, and the patient's response to the procedure. This important documentation is included even if the care was done as part of a complete bath.

Massage

Massage provides relaxation and comfort, increases circulation, and promotes sleep. Areas of the body that can be massaged are arms, hands, legs, feet, neck, and back.

A back massage may be given as part of a complete bed bath or at any time of the day (Skill 27-4). A variety of techniques are used during the back massage. **Effleurage** is a massage technique that employs long hand movements along the length of the back muscles. The nurse's hands move in a continuous, firm motion, forming a circle near the shoulders, running down the length of the spine, and forming another circle on the lower back. This cycle is repeated several times. **Pétrissage** is performed by using a kneading motion with the fingers and thumb along the patient's back and shoulders. This technique provides stimulation to the deep muscle tissue. A third technique, called **tapotement**, involves a tapping or percussion motion with the palm or ulnar side of the hand. This technique stimulates the skin but should not be used over the kidney area. The nurse may use one or all of these techniques during a back massage, making sure to continually assess the patient's tolerance of the procedure.

Documentation includes the date, time, and duration of the massage. The patient's response and any areas of tenderness should also be noted.

Hair Care

Shampooing a patient's hair and cleansing the scalp increases comfort and provides a sense of well-being. Patients who are weak or debilitated may be unable to follow their usual grooming routine, and their hair may become oily and matted. Routinely combing or brushing a patient's hair during morning and evening care helps prevent tangling.

Shampooing can be accomplished during a shower for patients who use a stand-up shower or shower chair. For bedridden patients, a variety of shampooing methods exist, depending on the equipment available in each facility. The nurse can pad the bed with waterproof pads or use a shampoo basin. Some facilities have no-rinse shampoos, which are lathered in and toweled dry. Others have shampoo caps (Figure 27-4) that have a shampoo solution in them. The cap is applied and the hair is lathered under the cap and then dried with a towel. Skill 27-5 lists the steps for shampooing a patient's hair in bed.

Special shampoos called *pediculicidal shampoos* are sometimes used when a patient has head lice. These shampoos can be toxic and may cause central nervous system side effects such as headache, dizziness, and seizures. They are contraindicated for patients with a history of seizures, pregnant women, and young children. The nurse uses personal protective equipment when bathing and providing care for patients with pediculosis to avoid spreading the infestation. Combing the patient's hair with a fine-tooth comb before and after application of the shampoo helps to remove the lice and their eggs (**nits**).

Documentation of hair care includes the assessment of the patient's scalp and tolerance of the procedure. If the patient

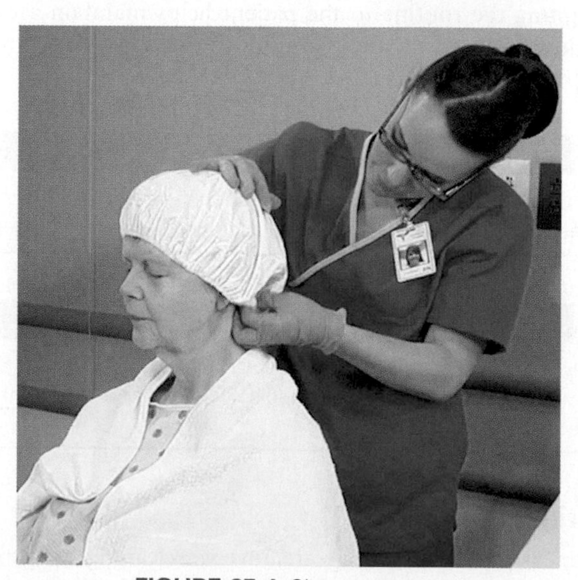

FIGURE 27-4 Shampoo cap.

is being treated for pediculosis, the medicated shampoo may be documented on the medication administration record.

Oral Care

Oral care is an essential nursing intervention that provides patient comfort, removes plaque and bacteria, reduces the risk of tooth decay, and decreases halitosis. Oral care includes brushing the teeth and tongue, flossing, rinsing the mouth, and cleaning dentures. When helping a dependent patient with oral care, the UAP or nurse always wears gloves.

Teeth should be brushed several times daily using fluoride toothpaste. Encourage patients to floss their teeth daily at home. Patients should perform oral hygiene independently if possible. If patients have a difficult time grasping or maneuvering the toothbrush, adaptive equipment such as a large-handle toothbrush may be necessary. The patient may find that using an electric toothbrush at home makes brushing easier. Performing oral care for patients who are dependent cleans the teeth and moistens the oral mucosa (Skill 27-6). Documentation of oral care includes the procedure, date, time, patient's tolerance, and findings of unusual sores, bleeding, or tenderness.

Dentures

Care of **dentures** (artificial teeth) should be performed at least every morning and evening (see Skill 27-6). The nurse or UAP performs this procedure for patients who cannot clean their own dentures. Denture care is performed wearing gloves.

Patients With Special Needs

Patients who are to receive nothing by mouth (NPO) or are receiving oxygen are susceptible to drying of the oral mucosa. Unconscious or intubated patients may not be able to swallow their own saliva. Oral care should be provided every 2 hours for these patients by using a toothbrush and a small amount of water or a moistened **toothette**, which is a disposable foam swab that is used for oral care (Figure 27-5). Unconscious patients are at risk for aspiration, and the oral care procedure is modified for them (see Skill 27-6). Patients who have undergone chemotherapy for cancer have special oral care needs (Evidence-Based Practice and Informatics box).

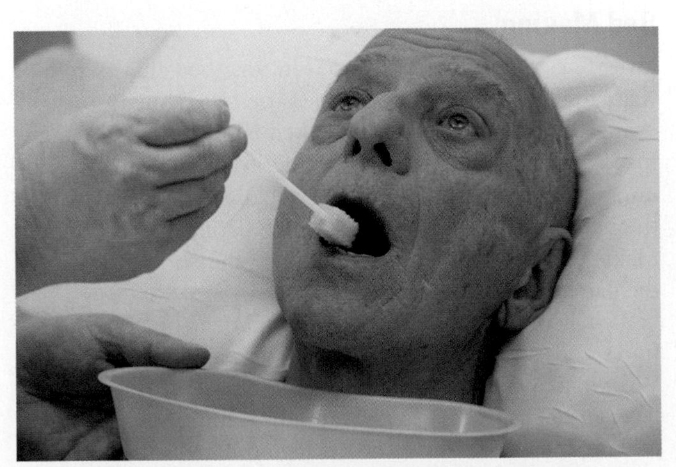

FIGURE 27-5 Use of a toothette for oral care.

EVIDENCE-BASED PRACTICE AND INFORMATICS

Oral Care During Cancer Therapy

Routine oral hygiene reduces the severity and incidence of oral problems during cancer therapy. Patients should tell the primary care provider or oncologist if they have the following:

- Changes in taste or smell
- Dry mouth
- Pain when eating hot or cold foods
- Trouble eating or swallowing
- White spots in the mouth
- Sores on the lips or in the mouth

Basic guidelines include the following:

- Brushing with a soft-bristle brush and baking soda or fluoride toothpaste after meals and before bedtime
- Rinsing the oral cavity frequently with a baking soda, salt, and water mixture
- Applying a lip balm to keep the lips from drying
- Taking frequent sips of water or sucking on ice cubes to keep oral mucosa moist

These strategies reduce the risk of oral soft tissue infection in patients undergoing cancer therapy. Preventing dryness of the lips reduces the risk for tissue injury.

From National Cancer Institute: Managing chemotherapy side effects: Mouth and throat changes, 2012. Retrieved from *www.cancer.gov/cancertopics/coping/chemo-side-effects/mouth-and-throat.pdf*.

! SAFE PRACTICE ALERT

Patients on anticoagulants should use a soft-bristle toothbrush.

! SAFE PRACTICE ALERT

Always have suction equipment at the bedside of comatose patients or patients with decreased gag reflex during oral care.

Eye Care

Eye care is part of the bathing routine. Eyes are washed with plain water from the inner to the outer canthus, using a different part of the washcloth for each eye. If the patient has dry, crusty drainage around the eyes or on the eyelids, a washcloth moistened with warm water or gauze moistened with saline can be applied. For patients whose eyes do not totally close at night, an eye patch and prescribed eyedrops may be necessary to prevent corneal drying.

Visual Aids

Patients who need glasses or contact lenses should be encouraged to use them in the health care setting. Nurses help patients keep their glasses clean during hospitalization using the technique that the patient uses at home (Nursing Care Guideline: Care of Contact Lenses and Glasses box). Glass lenses can be cleaned with water and dried with a soft cloth. Plastic lenses scratch easier and should be cleaned with an appropriate solution and dried with a lens cloth. Glasses are stored in a glass case when not worn and are labeled with the patient's name.

If a patient wears contact lenses, it is important for the nurse to know the type of lens. Some contact lenses are disposable; others are made of a more rigid plastic and are cleaned after wearing. Each type of contact lens should be cleaned with the appropriate cleaning solution. If the lenses are to be worn again, store them in an appropriately marked container with the correct lenses in the right and left sides of the storage cup.

Prosthetic Eye

A **prosthetic**, or artificial, eye may be a permanent implant or one that is removed for cleaning. Most patients care for their own prosthesis. If the patient requires assistance, the eye can be removed by pulling down on the lower lid with a gloved hand and exerting pressure on the lower edge of the artificial eye. This breaks the suction that holds the eye in the socket. The prosthesis and the socket can be cleaned with saline.

Nose Care

Some patients need specialized care of the nose. The nurse may have to remove mucus or secretions from the nares of patients who are unable to blow into a tissue. Removing moist secretions is accomplished by using suction. Removing dried mucus is performed using a moistened, cotton-tipped applicator. The applicator should never be inserted into the nostril further than the depth of the cotton tip. If a patient is on oxygen by a nasal cannula, the nasal passages may become dry. Humidifying the oxygen can help alleviate this problem.

Patients with nasogastric feeding or suction tubes may have crusting around the tube. The crusting may be gently removed using saline on gauze or a cotton-tipped applicator. If tape is being used to hold the tube in place, the tape should be removed daily during cleaning of the area.

Ear Care

Routine ear care is accomplished during bathing. Washing the ear with a washcloth and soap is sufficient for most patients. If the patient has a buildup of wax, or **cerumen**, the health care provider may order special oil drops to soften the wax before irrigating the ear canal. Do not try to remove the wax using a cotton-tipped applicator because it can push the wax farther into the ear canal.

! SAFE PRACTICE ALERT

Caution patients to never insert anything sharp, such as bobby pins, into the ear. Sharp objects can rupture the tympanic membrane.

Many patients wear hearing aids to amplify sound. These small electronic devices are expensive and must be kept dry. Handle hearing aids carefully, and clean them with a dry cloth (Nursing Care Guideline: Care of Hearing Aids box). When not in use, they are stored in a container labeled with the patient's name.

Shaving a Patient

Shaving a patient may be part of hygienic care. Many men shave their faces daily. Some women shave their legs and axillae during bathing or showering. Many older women have facial hair that they prefer to shave. The nurse or UAP can provide assistance with this grooming task when the patient is weak or debilitated. Some patients have their own electric razor, or an inexpensive hospital-supplied electric razor can be used. Razors should not be shared. If the patient's condition permits, shaving can be accomplished with a disposable razor (Skill 27-7). Having a clean-shaven face or legs boosts the patient's self-esteem. Document the date, time, body part shaved, type of razor, and skin issues observed during or after shaving.

! SAFE PRACTICE ALERT

Patients on anticoagulants should use an electric razor for shaving.

Beards or mustaches should not be shaved off without the consent of the patient or the family. Grooming of beards and mustaches is a part of daily hygienic care. These areas can be washed with soap and water and rinsed well during the bath. If the hair is long, it can be combed out to remove tangles.

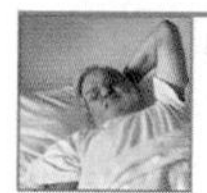

4. Identify at least five nursing interventions for Mr. Randall designed to meet the goals written in question 3.

Bed Making

Providing the patient with a clean, dry bed that is free of wrinkles is a basic nursing measure. Bed linens may be changed after a bed bath. If the bed is not soiled, the nurse may wait until the patient is sitting in a chair or off of the nursing unit for testing. A lift may be used to temporarily lift the patient off the bed surface if the patient is on bed rest. Making an unoccupied bed is easier on the nurse or UAP and the patient.

If it is not possible to move the patient out of bed, the nurse can change the linens with the patient lying in bed. When making an occupied bed (Skill 27-8), the nurse should have all linens in the room before beginning the procedure. Making the bed can be done during or after the bath or after perineal care for incontinence.

NURSING CARE GUIDELINE

Care of Contact Lenses and Glasses

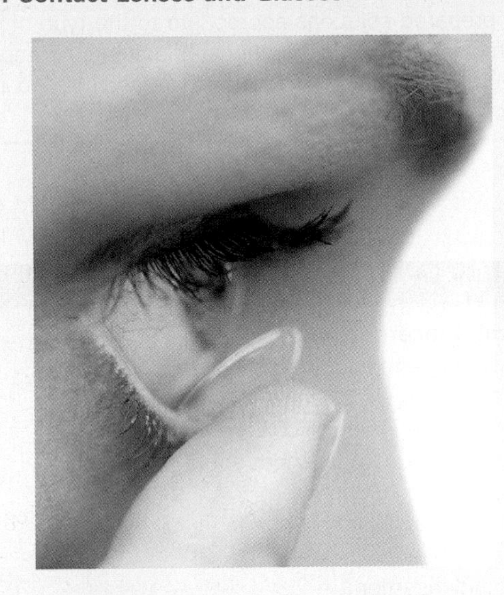

Background

- Contact lenses fit on the cornea directly over the pupil. They improve vision by correcting:
  - Shape abnormalities
  - Refractive errors
- There are three types of corrections:
  - Single vision
  - Bifocal
  - Alternative bifocal (i.e., one contact corrects for near vision and the other for far vision)
- Contacts are made to be worn under one of three wear conditions:
  - Daily-wear contact lenses
    - Inserted and removed daily
    - Not discarded until a new prescription is issued
  - Extended-wear contact lenses
    - Worn for up to 1 week (including overnight use)
    - Not discarded until a new prescription is issued
  - Disposable-wear contact lenses
    - Used for daily or extended wear
    - Discarded daily, weekly, or monthly, based on the prescription
- Glasses are worn by many patients and are necessary for vision correction.
  - Clean glasses with a soft cloth.
  - If extremely soiled, glasses can be cleaned with liquid soap and water and dried with a soft cloth.

Procedural Concerns for Contact Lenses

- Start with the same eye for insertion and removal.
  - This prevents inserting a lens into the wrong eye.
  - Some lenses are manufactured with a small mark on the right lens to avoid confusing which lens is for which eye.
- Clean lenses immediately after removing them.
- Store the lenses in a manufacturer-recommended lens solution until they are reinserted.
- Store each lens in its own compartment that is clearly labeled to indicate the eye (right or left) in which the lens should be inserted.
- Never reuse the lens solution.
- After reinserting the lenses, thoroughly clean the storage container.
- Air-dry the container to prevent contamination by microorganisms.
- If a lens is dropped, do the following:
  - Moisten a finger with the lens solution, and then gently touch the lens with the moistened finger to pick it up.
  - Clean, rinse, and disinfect the lens to avoid a potential eye infection from microorganisms that might have adhered to the lens.
- If the patient is able to insert and remove contact lenses independently, allow the patient to continue to use the contact lenses. If not, have the patient return to wearing glasses.
- If eyedrops must be instilled, remove the patient's contact lenses.
- If emergency removal of contact lenses is necessary:
  - For soft lenses, pull down the lower lid, and have the patient look up. Use the thumb and forefinger to pinch the edges of the contact lens together. Squeeze the lens, and remove it from the eye.
  - For hard lenses, place a gloved thumb below the patient's lower eyelid and an index finger on the upper lid. Separate the lids, and have the patient blink. The lens should pop out.
  - Place the lenses in sterile normal saline solution in a sterile closed container, and label the container with the patient's name and room number.

Documentation Concerns

- Record the type of lens worn by the patient, including when and how often the lenses are worn.
- Record the typical cleaning and storage of the lenses.
- Document patient complaints and signs and symptoms associated with contact lens wear.
- Complaints may include dryness, tearing, redness, irritation, swelling, and burning, which may be caused by overwear.
- Signs and symptoms may include redness, sensitivity, vision problems, and pain (RSVP); these are reasons to contact the ophthalmologist for an examination of the patient.

Evidence-Based Practice

Noncompliance with care of contact lenses is one of the largest contributors to microbial keratitis, a potentially dangerous infection of the eye that can cause loss of vision and most often results from contact lens wear. Health care providers and patients must adhere to all instructions regarding care to prevent these infections, and health care providers need to educate their patients and stress the importance of this matter.

Cohen (2009) found that noncompliant and typically compliant patients failed to effectively follow manufacturer instructions

Continued

NURSING CARE GUIDELINE—cont'd

regarding cleaning solutions, causing microorganisms to remain on the lenses and transfer to the eye on the next insertion, despite soaking overnight. Keay, Edwards, and Stapleton (2009) reported similar findings related to care of the case and length of time the lens was worn. Watt and Swarbrick (2007) agree with the need for education and stress the need to use commercially prepared solutions appropriate to the type of contact lens worn, thereby eliminating nonsterile solutions, tap water, and homemade remedies from the care regimen to prevent infections.

NURSING CARE GUIDELINE

Care of Hearing Aids

Background

Hearing aids are used for mild, moderate, severe, or profound hearing loss. They range from simple amplifiers, in which sound comes into the device and enters the ear with a higher volume, to complex, computerized aids that reduce background noise and adjust tone, pitch, and amplitude.

- Hearing aids are available in three basic types:
  - In-the-canal (ITC) hearing aids are the smallest of the three types. ITC hearing aids fit entirely inside the ear canal, which may improve comfort and be cosmetically desirable. They require special fitting.
  - In-the-ear (ITE), or intra-aural, hearing aids are an intermediate size. No part of the device is outside the ear; it fits snugly into the external ear canal. This type is more noticeable than the ITC hearing aid but can accommodate more hearing adjustments.
  - Behind-the-ear (BTE) hearing aids are the largest type. Plastic tubing goes in the ear canal, and a receiver fits behind the ear. It is very noticeable because of its size and is used for the most profound cases of hearing loss.
- Battery life depends on the model. Placement and removal may be delegated to unlicensed assistive personnel (UAP), but they must be instructed and trained in proper procedural care and concerns related to the specific hearing aid device for an individual patient.
- A cochlear implant is a specialty hearing device:
  - Use of a cochlear implant is indicated for patients with severe to profound hearing loss after a multidisciplinary assessment and after a 3-month trial of hearing aids has failed to demonstrate appropriate improvement.
  - The plastic earpiece contains a tiny microphone, and a sound transmitter fits behind the ear. This electronic device can be removed for bathing. It should be kept away from water.
  - The receiver, which is surgically implanted behind the mastoid bone, stimulates nerve fibers to simulate hearing.

Procedural Concerns

- Assess the hearing aid before insertion:
  - Is the hearing aid clean?
  - Are the batteries charged and inserted?
  - Is the battery compartment shut?
  - Is the cord or tubing intact?
  - Are the dials clean and rotating easily?
  - Is static absent?
- Hearing aid insertion:
  - Place the hearing aid in the patient's ear.
  - Turn the hearing aid on and to one-third volume, slowly increasing it to one-half volume.
  - Ensure that the volume is properly adjusted: The patient should be able to hear a normal speaking voice at a distance of 3 feet.
  - If the patient complains of whistling, check for possible causes:
    - An improper fit
    - Cerumen in the auditory canal or device
    - Fluid in the ear
    - Improper insertion into the canal
    - Volume turned too high
- Observe precautions:
  - Avoid getting the device wet.
  - Avoid exposing it to extreme temperatures.
  - Avoid spraying products such as hair spray or perfume around the hearing aid.
- Clean with a dry soft cloth.
- Follow the manufacturer's instructions.

Documentation Concerns

- Document which ear (left, right, or both) requires the device.
- Include the following specifics about the hearing aid:
  - The type of hearing aid and the batteries required
  - The procedure to turn on the hearing aid, adjust its volume, and change batteries
  - Typical storage and cleaning instructions
- Note patient complaints about an inability to hear or discomfort.

EVALUATION

Evaluation of hygiene and personal care patient goals is ongoing. The nurse observes the patient during care to assess the attainment of self-care goals. When goals are reached, new ones are established that may be longer-term goals. Noticeable improvement in the patient's hygienic practices shows the nurse that the patient understood teaching regarding hygiene. Patients who are able to do more of their own care on a daily basis are showing increased self-care abilities. Goal attainment sometimes is slower, and the nurse continues the same plan of care or revises it to include more assistance.

Goal statements and outcome criteria related to hygiene guide care. Most strive for the patient to become more independent. Diligent nursing care is needed for the dependent patient. The focus of the care plan is on helping the patient gain self-care abilities and move toward independence.

SKILL 27-1 Bathing a Patient in Bed

PURPOSE

- Bathing a patient serves many functions:
  - Provides routine hygienic care
  - Reduces body odor
  - Promotes circulation and blood flow
  - Prevents skin breakdown
  - Provides range of motion
  - Provides comfort and relaxation
  - Strengthens a general feeling of health and wellness

RESOURCES

- Bath basin
- Bath blanket
- Drawsheet
- Laundry bag
- Personal protective equipment (PPE) when appropriate
- Skin cleanser, soap, or disposable bath cloths
- Towels
- Warm running water
- Washcloths
- Clean hospital gown
- Deodorant
- Shampoo
- Body lotion
- Prescribed skin care products

COLLABORATION AND DELEGATION

- Bathing a patient may be delegated to unlicensed assistive personnel (UAP) after the initial assessment of the patient.
- UAP should report the following to the nurse:
  - Sores, wounds, irritations, lesions, redness, or rashes on the patient
  - Concerns regarding the procedure or patient
  - Any portion of the bath not completed
- UAP should be instructed in the following:
  - The type and time of bath for the patient
  - Special hygienic care that should be performed with the bath, such as foot and hand care or shampoo
  - Never soak the feet or trim toenails of a patient when contraindicated
  - Appropriate encouragement of the patient's abilities to assist with the procedure
  - Positioning concerns specific to the patient
  - Do not massage reddened areas on the patient's skin
  - Appropriate care and positioning of specialized medical interventions for the patient during the procedure (e.g., a Foley catheter, IV catheter, casts, traction)
  - Appropriate documentation according to facility policy
- Occupational therapists, physical therapists, or hospice aids and nurses may want to assist with or perform bathing for a patient to whom they are assigned. Consider timing and the needs of these collaborative caregivers when planning this procedure.
- Family members may want to assist with bathing.

EVIDENCE-BASED PRACTICE

- Nurses are accountable for all components of hygiene care, even when they are delegated. Bittner and Gravlin (2009) found that care is often not completed in its entirety, resulting in poor patient satisfaction. Because basic hygiene procedures prevent the spread of microorganisms and increase the sense of health and well-being, omission may result in poor patient outcomes. These factors must be considered when performing and delegating hygiene procedures.
- Some cultural beliefs restrict touching between nonrelatives of the opposite sex. In such situations, it is prudent to thoroughly explain the purpose of the care you are about to provide and to ask for permission before touching the patient (Pullen, 2007).

SPECIAL CIRCUMSTANCES

1. **Assess:** Is the patient able to assist?
   Intervention: Allow the patient to perform as many steps as possible to promote independence.
2. **Assess:** Considering the patient diagnosis, are there pain concerns?
   Intervention: Consider pain medication in accordance with orders before performing the procedure to prevent discomfort.
3. **Assess:** Are disposable bath cloths available?
   Intervention: Warm the bath cloths if possible, using a new cloth for each step.
4. **Assess:** What is the room temperature?
   Intervention: Adjust the room temperature if possible so that the patient is comfortable; otherwise, add blankets, using warmed blankets if available.
5. **Assess:** Has the patient had recent blood clots?
   Intervention: Lightly wash the patient's legs and pat them dry instead of using firm strokes.
6. **Assess:** What is the assessment of the patient's skin determined by the thorough evaluation performed during bathing?
   Intervention: Gently wash any reddened or swollen areas, and pat them dry. Use clean, nonsterile gloves as needed to comply with standard precautions. Do not apply lotion or powder to any open areas. Document the findings from the assessment.

7. **Assess:** Is the patient able to move his or her limbs?
   Intervention: Provide passive or active range-of-motion exercises (see Chapter 28).
8. **Assess:** Is the bathwater dirty or cold?
   Intervention: Change the bathwater.
9. **Assess:** Does the patient wear hearing aids?
   Intervention: Remove the hearing aids while washing the patient's ears and neck, and then replace the hearing aids.
10. **Assess:** Does the patient wear contact lenses?
    Intervention: Carefully wash around the eyes, or remove the contact lenses.
11. **Assess:** Is there crusting around the eyes?
    Intervention: Place a warm washcloth over the patient's eyes to soak the crust before washing for easier removal.

PREPROCEDURE

I. Check PCP orders and the patient care plan.
Knowledge of patient-specific orders is critical for safe patient care.

II. Gather supplies and equipment.
Preparing for the patient encounter saves time and promotes patient trust.

III. Perform hand hygiene.
Frequent hand hygiene prevents the spread of microorganisms.

IV. Maintain standard precautions.
Use of the correct personal protective equipment (PPE) is required whenever contact with bodily fluids is possible, to reduce the transfer of pathogens.

V. Introduce yourself.
Initial communication establishes the role of the nurse and begins a professional relationship.

VI. Provide for patient privacy.
It is important to maintain patient dignity.

VII. Identify the patient by using two identifiers.
Identifying a patient involves scanning barcodes or comparing the patient's stated name and birthdate to information on the patient's wristband or health record. The correct person must receive the correct treatment.

VIII. Explain the procedure to the patient.
The nurse has a responsibility to inform a patient before initiating care. Information may ease patient anxiety and facilitate cooperation.

PROCEDURE

Bathing a Patient

Follow preprocedure steps I through VIII.

1. Prepare supplies on the bedside table. Offer the bedpan or urinal.
   Preparing supplies and providing for elimination before the procedure avoid interruptions during the procedure.
2. Follow the steps in Skill 27-6 as needed.
   Routine hygienic care is ideally performed with bathing.
3. Raise the bed to working height; lower the top side rail and the head of the bed if tolerated by the patient.
   The bed should be at a height that does not require the provider to stretch or bend unnecessarily to prevent discomfort and possible injury. A flat bed, if tolerated, provides for patient comfort during turning.
4. Cover the patient with a bath blanket or linens for comfort. Pull the bed blanket and top sheet toward the bottom of the bed and remove. Place the soiled sheet and blanket in the linen bag. Remove the patient's gown sufficiently to expose only the body part currently being bathed, and do so throughout the procedure. If the patient has an intravenous line, an injury, or reduced mobility on one side, begin from the unaffected side.
   Proper positioning of the bath blanket, bed linens, and patient gown provide warmth, comfort, and privacy while protecting the linens and gown from becoming dirty or wet.

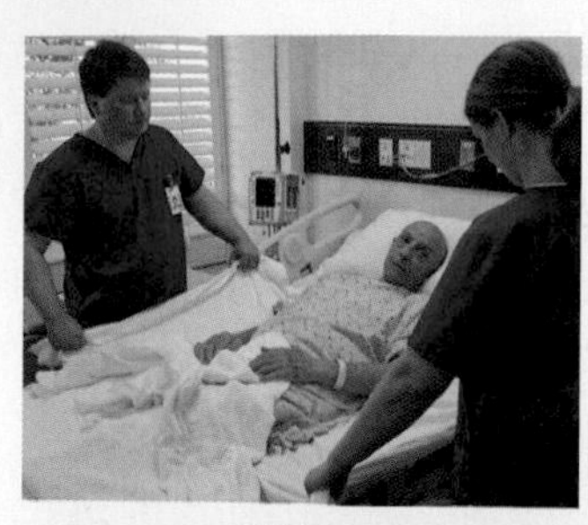
STEP 5

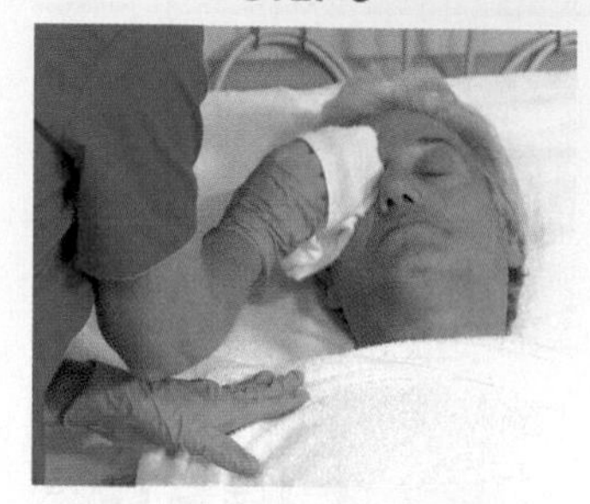
STEP 6

5. If the patient is unable to assist or roll (see Skill 28-1), place a drawsheet. Seek assistance from another health care provider if needed.
Minimize provider discomfort and possible injury by following the proper procedure. Use of a drawsheet reduces the force necessary to roll the patient and prevents possible injury to the patient. Having enough help provides for patient safety.
6. Place a towel over the pillow and under the patient's head. Place another towel across the patient's chest. Don nonsterile gloves for any portion of the bath in which there may be exposure to mucous membranes or open sores. Using a washcloth and warm water without soap, wash the patient's eyes, wiping from the inner to outer canthus. Use a different part of the cloth for each eye.
Properly placed towels protect the linens from becoming dirty or wet. Gloves prevent the spread of microorganisms. Avoid the spread of microorganisms by wiping from the inner to outer canthus (i.e., less contaminated to more contaminated region) and using a fresh surface of the cloth for each eye. Warm water is typically the most comfortable for the patient. Avoid using soap to prevent stinging, burning, and irritating the eyes.
7. Assess the skin thoroughly throughout the bath.
Bathing is an opportune time for skin assessment because all areas are visible.
8. Wash the face with warm water and soap if the patient prefers. Wash the ears and neck with soap and water. Rinse and dry the face, ears, and neck. Remove the towel. Use soap sparingly, and change the water frequently during the bath. Ask a male patient if he wishes to be shaved (see Skill 27-7).
Soap can dry the skin on the face. Giving patients a choice enables them to have some control over their care. Soap can be difficult to rinse off the skin. Keeping water clean and warm provides for patient safety and comfort.

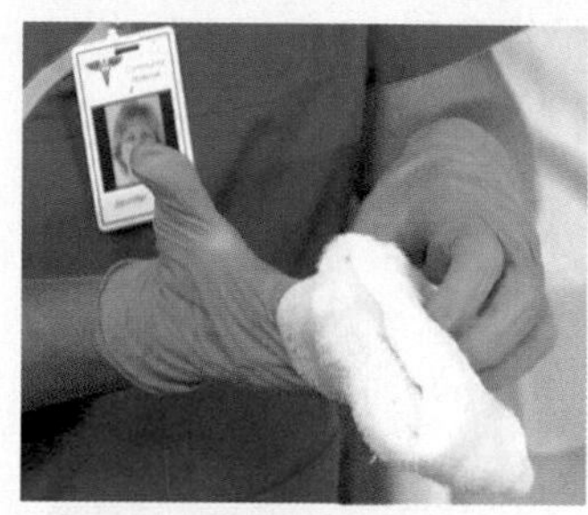
STEP 9

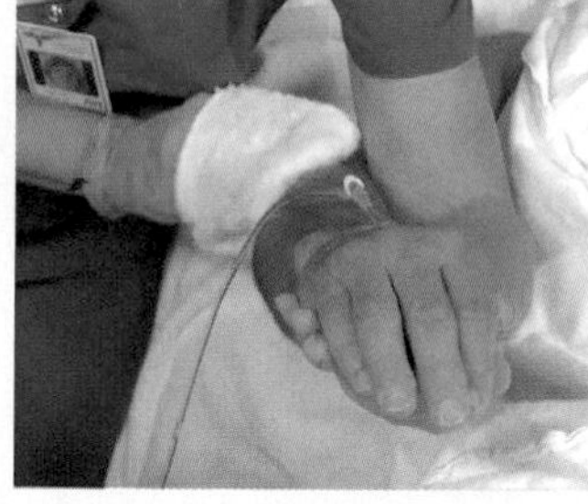
STEP 10

9. Wrap the washcloth around the dominant hand, or continue to use new cloths from the packet of disposable bath cloths throughout the bath if available.
Wrapping a washcloth around the hand maintains heat and water in the cloth and prevents the washcloth from touching surfaces. Using clean cloths from the packet helps prevent the spread of microorganisms.
10. Lower the top side rail. Uncover the closest arm, and place a towel under the arm. Wash, rinse, and dry the arm, moving from fingers to shoulder. Provide passive range of motion of the fingers, hand, wrist, elbow, and shoulder during care if the patient is unable to perform active range of motion. See Skill 27-3 for hand care specifics.
Lowering the rail prevents provider discomfort and possible injury, and the towel prevents the sheets from becoming dirty or wet. Washing from distal to proximal promotes circulation and blood return. Range-of-motion exercise maintains joint flexibility.
11. Apply deodorant and lotion if preferred by the patient. Remove the towel.
Routine hygienic care prevents body odor and dry skin. Asking the patient about his or her preferences allows the patient to have some control and facilitates cooperation.
12. Raise the side rail of the bed.
Precautions must be taken to maintain patient safety.
13. Repeat steps 10 through 12 on the opposite side of the patient.
Moving to the other side of the bed facilitates provider safety.
14. Lower the side rail on the side from which the work will be done. Fold down the bath blanket, and place a towel over the patient's chest.
This provides the patient with warmth, comfort, and privacy.

15. Lift the towel with one hand; wash, rinse, and dry the chest and abdomen with the other hand, taking care to include the areas under skin folds. Check the water temperature after washing the chest and abdomen, and change the water if necessary.
This continues to provide warmth and privacy. Cleansing and drying under the skin folds prevent skin breakdown from excessive moisture.

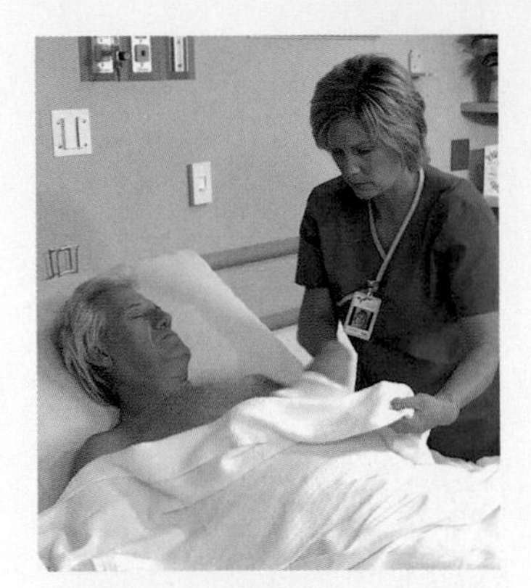
STEP 15

16. Remove the towel, put a new gown on the patient, and cover the patient with a bath blanket. Raise the side rail.
This provides the patient with warmth, comfort, and privacy, while ensuring that safety needs are met.
17. Uncover the closest leg, and place a towel under the leg. Wash, rinse, and dry the leg, working from the ankle to the knee and then from the knee to the thigh. Next wash the patient's foot, making sure to dry thoroughly between the toes. See Skill 27-3 for foot care specifics.
The towel prevents the sheets from becoming dirty or wet. Washing from distal to proximal promotes circulation and blood return. Ensuring that skin between the toes and under skin folds is dry helps to prevent breakdown.

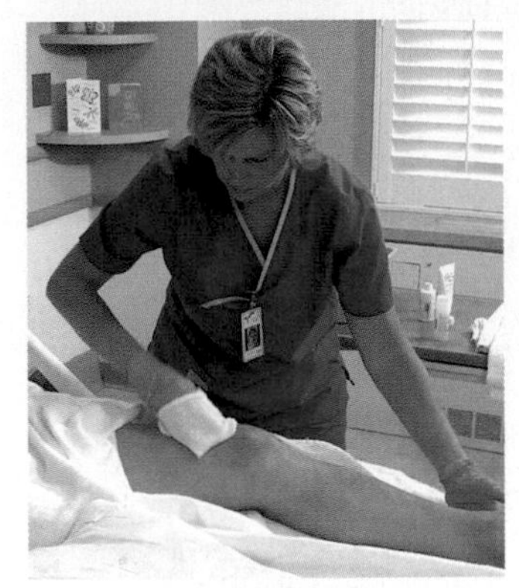
STEP 17

18. Apply lotion if preferred by the patient. Remove the towel.
Using lotion prevents dry skin. Asking the patient about his or her preferences allows the patient some control and facilitates cooperation.
19. Repeat steps 17 and 18 on the patient's opposite side.
20. Follow the steps for perineal care in Skill 27-2.
21. Change gloves and obtain clean water and a fresh washcloth when they are soiled.
This helps to prevent the spread of microorganisms.
22. Lower the side rail, and assist the patient onto his or her side, facing away from you. Use a drawsheet if necessary (see Skill 28-1). Expose the patient's entire back if possible.
Lowering the rail prevents provider discomfort and possible injury while preparing the patient for having his or her back washed. One goal is to minimize the exertion and activity required from the patient.
23. Place a towel lengthwise next to the patient's back. Wash, rinse, and dry the back, progressing from the neck to the buttocks.
Proper positioning of the towel prevents the sheets from becoming dirty or wet. Washing from the neck to the buttocks promotes circulation and relaxation.

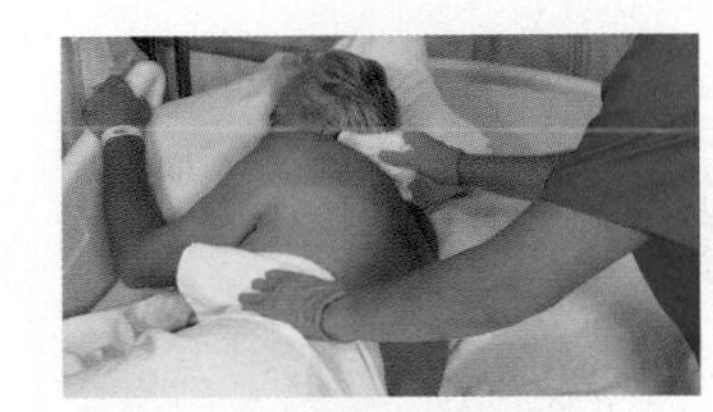
STEP 23

24. Wearing gloves, wash, rinse, and dry the buttocks and anus. Cover the patient. Remove and discard the gloves, and raise the side rail.
Covering the patient provides warmth, comfort, and privacy. Using and properly disposing of gloves prevents the spread of microorganisms. Raised side rails ensure safety.
25. Provide a back massage if desired by the patient (see Skill 27-4).
Massage promotes relaxation; asking the patient about his or her preferences allows the patient some control and facilitates cooperation.
26. Discard the water, clean the bedside table, place dirty linens in a laundry bag, and remove the bag from the room. Raise the head of the bed.
Removal of potentially contaminated items reduces the spread of microorganisms. The bed position ideally should promote patient comfort.
27. Comb the patient's hair, unless shampooing is to be done (see Skill 27-5). Ask for the patient's input on the desired hair styling.
Routine hygienic care is ideally performed with bathing. Combing the hair removes tangles, and asking about styling preferences allows the patient to have some control and facilitates cooperation.
28. Follow the steps in Skill 27-8 if the linens need to be changed.
Linen changes are performed after the bed bath to provide a clean, dry surface for the patient.

Follow postprocedure steps I through VI.

POSTPROCEDURE

I. Return the bed to its lowest position, raise the top side rails, and verify that the call light is within reach for the patient.
Precautions are taken to maintain patient safety. Top side rails aid in positioning and turning. Raising four side rails is considered a restraint.

II. Assess for additional patient needs and state the time of your expected return.
Meeting patient needs and offering self promote patient satisfaction and build trust.

III. Properly dispose of PPE.
Gloves, gowns, and masks must be appropriately discarded to prevent the spread of microorganisms.

IV. Clean equipment if it was in contact with the patient; see specific manufacturer instructions.
Disinfection eliminates most microorganisms from inanimate objects.

V. Perform hand hygiene.
Frequent hand hygiene prevents the spread of infection.

VI. Document the date, time, assessment, procedure, and patient's response to the procedure.
Accurate documentation is essential to communicate patient care and to provide legal evidence of care.

SKILL 27-2 Perineal Care

PURPOSE

- Prevents infection
- Prevents skin breakdown
- Provides routine hygienic care
- Removes buildup of secretions
- Prevents odor
- Provides comfort
- Strengthens a general feeling of health and wellness

RESOURCES

- Bath basin
- Peri-bottle (optional for females)
- Bath blanket
- Clean, nonsterile gloves
- Bed protector
- Laundry bag
- Personal protective equipment, if appropriate
- Skin cleanser, soap, or disposable bath cloths
- Towels
- Warm water
- Washcloths
- Bedpan
- Clean linens, if needed
- Barrier creams or other prescribed special perineal care products

COLLABORATION AND DELEGATION

- Perineal care may be delegated to unlicensed assistive personnel (UAP) after assessment of the patient.
- UAP should report the following to the nurse:
  - Sores, wounds, irritations, lesions, redness, or rashes on the patient
  - Episodes of incontinence (urinary or fecal), including quantity and unusual characteristics
  - Patient discomfort reported during the procedure
- UAP should be instructed in the following:
  - Positioning concerns specific to the patient
  - Appropriate techniques for the procedure
  - Cultural, privacy, and ethical concerns
  - Appropriate documentation

SPECIAL CIRCUMSTANCES

1. **Assess:** Has the patient had recent surgery, or are there wounds, sores, or drains in the perineal area?
   Intervention: Do not delegate the procedure; refer to Chapter 29 for specific care.
2. **Assess:** Does the patient have a urinary catheter?
   Intervention: Chapter 41 describes catheter care.
3. **Assess:** Is the foreskin difficult to retract on a male patient?
   Intervention: Wash the penis with soap and water, which may lubricate the foreskin; if the foreskin still is not easily retracted after washing, repeat the washing procedure. Do *not* force the skin. Check the patient's chart for notations about previous concerns, notify the primary care provider, and document the findings.
4. **Assess:** What should be done if the patient has fecal incontinence?
   Intervention: Clean the feces from the area, restart the perineal cleansing procedure from the beginning, and document the intervention.

PREPROCEDURE

I. Check PCP orders and the patient care plan.
Knowledge of patient-specific orders is critical for safe patient care.

II. Gather supplies and equipment.
Preparing for the patient encounter saves time and promotes patient trust.

III. Perform hand hygiene.
Frequent hand hygiene prevents the spread of microorganisms.

IV. Maintain standard precautions.
Use of the correct personal protective equipment (PPE) is required whenever contact with bodily fluids is possible, to reduce the transfer of pathogens.

V. Introduce yourself.
Initial communication establishes the role of the nurse and begins a professional relationship.

VI. Provide for patient privacy.
It is important to maintain patient dignity.

VII. Identify the patient by using two identifiers.
Identifying a patient involves scanning barcodes or comparing the patient's stated name and birthdate to information on the patient's wristband or health record. The correct person must receive the correct treatment.

VIII. Explain the procedure to the patient.
The nurse has a responsibility to inform a patient before initiating care. Information may ease patient anxiety and facilitate cooperation.

PROCEDURE

Male Perineal Care

Follow preprocedure steps I through VIII.

1. If performing a bed bath (see Skill 27-1), proceed to step 2; if not, prepare supplies on the bedside table. Raise the bed to working height, and lower the top side rail. Lower the head of the bed if tolerated by the patient.
Preparing supplies avoids unnecessary interruption of the procedure. Setting the bed at the correct working height for the provider prevents provider discomfort and possible injury. A flat bed provides for patient positioning, if tolerated.
2. Put on nonsterile gloves. The patient should be in the supine position. Fold down the bath blanket or bed sheets, raise the patient's gown, and cover the remainder of the body with a bath blanket or towel. Place a towel on the bed close to the buttocks.
Using gloves reduces the spread of microorganisms. Keeping the patient covered provides the patient with comfort and privacy. The towel protects the linens from becoming dirty or wet.
3. Wash, rinse, and dry the patient's thighs. Gently hold the shaft of the penis; if the patient is uncircumcised, retract the foreskin by gently pushing it toward the body. Starting at the urinary meatus, wash the tip of the penis with soap, using a circular motion; wash the shaft of the penis using downward strokes.
Proper cleansing prevents infection and the buildup of secretions.

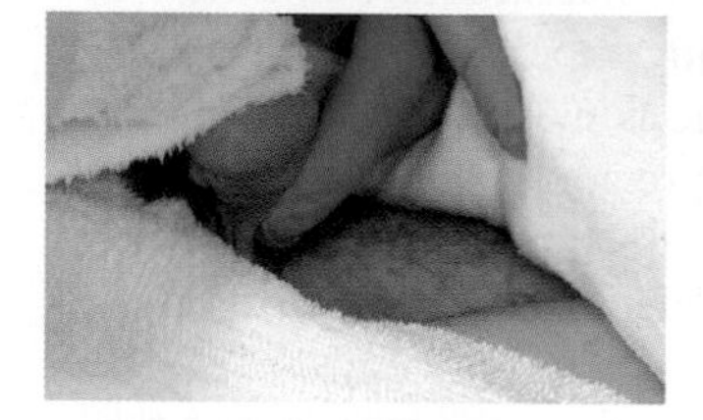
STEP 3

4. Rinse and dry the penis. Reposition the foreskin in uncircumcised patients by gently pushing the skin toward the tip of the penis.
The foreskin must be in its normal position to prevent contraction and swelling.
5. Using a clean area of the washcloth, wash, rinse, and dry from the scrotal area to the buttocks, including all skin folds.
Proper cleaning should be used to prevent the spread of microorganisms. Thorough drying prevents skin irritation.
6. If performing a bed bath, return to Skill 27-1; if not, proceed to the next instruction.
This avoids unnecessary interruption of the procedure.

Follow postprocedure steps I through VI.

Female Perineal Care

Follow preprocedure steps I through VIII.

1. If performing a bed bath (see Skill 27-1), proceed to step 3; if not, prepare supplies on the bedside table. Raise the bed to working height, and lower the top side rail. Lower the head of the bed if tolerated by the patient.
Preparing supplies in advance avoids interruption during the procedure. Setting the bed at the correct working height for the provider prevents provider discomfort and possible injury. A flat bed provides for patient positioning if tolerated.
2. Put on nonsterile gloves. Place the patient in the supine or dorsal recumbent position. Fold down the bath blanket or bed sheets; raise the patient's gown, and cover the remainder of the body with a bath blanket or towel. Place a towel on the bed close to the buttocks.
Using gloves reduces the spread of microorganisms. Keeping the patient covered provides the patient with comfort and privacy. The towel protects the linens from becoming dirty or wet.

3. Wash, rinse, and dry the upper thighs. Using your nondominant hand, gently separate the labia. Clean the pubic area by using downward strokes toward the anus. Use a different part of the washcloth for each stroke. Repeat until the area is clean. Rinse and dry the area. Continue to clean thoroughly around the labia minora, clitoris, urinary meatus, and vaginal orifice. If the patient uses a bedpan, you can rinse by pouring warm water from a peri-bottle over the perineal area. Then dry the area thoroughly, again working from front to back.
Proper cleansing prevents infection and the buildup of secretions. Wiping from front to back and using a clean washcloth surface each time prevents microorganisms from entering the urinary tract. Thorough drying prevents skin irritation.

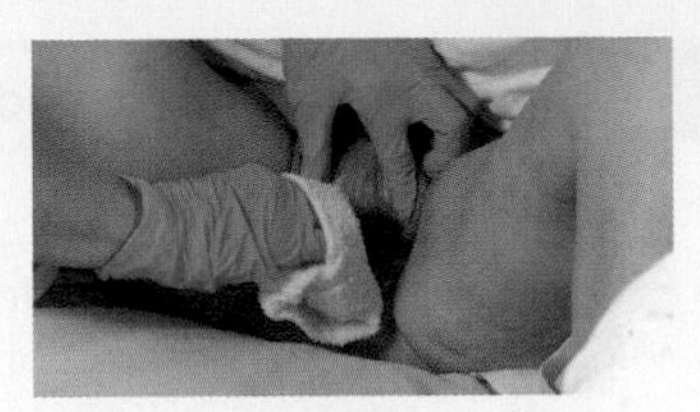
STEP 3

4. If performing a bed bath, see Skill 27-1; if not, proceed to the instruction below.
Avoids unnecessary interruption of the procedure.

Follow throughout steps I through VI.

POSTPROCEDURE

I. Return the bed to its lowest position, raise the top side rails, and verify that the call light is within reach for the patient.
Precautions are taken to maintain patient safety. Top side rails aid in positioning and turning. Raising four side rails is considered a restraint.

II. Assess for additional patient needs and state the time of your expected return.
Meeting patient needs and offering self promote patient satisfaction and build trust.

III. Properly dispose of PPE.
Gloves, gowns, and masks must be appropriately discarded to prevent the spread of microorganisms.

IV. Clean equipment if it was in contact with the patient; see specific manufacturer instructions.
Disinfection eliminates most microorganisms from inanimate objects.

V. Perform hand hygiene.
Frequent hand hygiene prevents the spread of infection.

VI. Document the date, time, assessment, procedure, and patient's response to the procedure.
Accurate documentation is essential to communicate patient care and to provide legal evidence of care.

SKILL 27-3 Foot and Hand Care

PURPOSE

- Provides routine hygienic care
- Removes buildup of secretions and oils on the feet and hands
- Prevents foot odor
- Promotes circulation and blood flow
- Prevents infection
- Softens rough skin and calluses
- Removes buildup of dirt and dead-skin cells under the nails
- Provides comfort and relaxation

RESOURCES

- Bath basin or emesis basin (can be used for soaking hands)
- Bath blanket
- Laundry bag
- Personal protective equipment (PPE), when appropriate
- Skin cleanser, soap, or disposable bath cloths
- Towels
- Warm water
- Washcloths
- Lotion
- Nail clippers (if facility policy allows)
- Nail file or emery board (if facility policy allows)
- Cuticle stick (if facility policy allows)

COLLABORATION AND DELEGATION

- A patient diagnosed with diabetes is usually seen by a podiatrist or diabetic specialist for foot care. Appropriate collaboration should be planned for these patients.
- Foot care may be delegated to unlicensed assistive personnel (UAP) after assessment of the patient, provided the patient does not have diabetes.
- Hand care may be delegated to UAP after assessment of the patient.
- UAP should report the following to the nurse:
  - Sores, wounds, irritations, lesions, redness, or rashes on the patient
  - Nails that are thick, yellowed, or otherwise unusual
  - Concerns regarding the procedure or patient
- UAP should be instructed in the following:
  - Appropriate care, including trimming and filing of nails, if allowed by facility policy
  - Positioning concerns specific to the patient
  - Appropriate documentation
- Hospice aids and nurses may want to assist with or perform foot and hand care for a patient to whom they are assigned. Consider timing and the needs of these collaborative caregivers when planning this procedure.

EVIDENCE-BASED PRACTICE

- Neglecting to file and trim fingernails and toenails can result in trauma to the skin through inadvertent scratches. Long nails can get caught on medical paraphernalia in the hospital setting, causing the nail to tear from the nail bed.
- Nurses often omit nail care, especially for patients with diabetes. This can result in increased rates of infection and poor hygiene. The registered nurse is trained to perform proper nail care, seeking collaboration with podiatry as necessary. The nurse should not omit the skill, thinking it is not within the scope of practice (Malkin and Berridge, 2009).

SPECIAL CIRCUMSTANCES

1. **Assess:** Does the patient have peripheral vascular disease or cardiovascular disease?
   Intervention: Do not soak the feet; this may cause skin breakdown or infection.
2. **Assess:** Does the patient have diabetes or peripheral neuropathy?
   Intervention: Do not soak hands or feet; this may cause skin breakdown or infection. Seek referral to a podiatrist or diabetic foot care specialist.
3. **Assess:** Does the patient have thick, brittle nails?
   Intervention: Soak longer for easier filing and trimming.
4. **Assess:** Is clipping nails contraindicated by the patient's diagnosis, condition, or medications or by facility policy?
   Intervention: Do not proceed. Document the need for intervention, but allow the primary care provider to attend to trimming of nails.

PREPROCEDURE

I. Check PCP orders and the patient care plan.
Knowledge of patient-specific orders is critical for safe patient care.

II. Gather supplies and equipment.
Preparing for the patient encounter saves time and promotes patient trust.

III. Perform hand hygiene.
Frequent hand hygiene prevents the spread of microorganisms.

IV. Maintain standard precautions.
Use of the correct personal protective equipment (PPE) is required whenever contact with bodily fluids is possible, to reduce the transfer of pathogens.

V. Introduce yourself.
Initial communication establishes the role of the nurse and begins a professional relationship.

VI. Provide for patient privacy.
It is important to maintain patient dignity.

VII. Identify the patient by using two identifiers.
Identifying a patient involves scanning barcodes or comparing the patient's stated name and birthdate to information on the patient's wristband or health record. The correct person must receive the correct treatment.

VIII. Explain the procedure to the patient.
The nurse has a responsibility to inform a patient before initiating care. Information may ease patient anxiety and facilitate cooperation.

PROCEDURE

Follow preprocedure steps I through VIII.

1. If performing a bed bath (see Skill 27-1), proceed to step 2; if not, prepare supplies on the bedside table. Raise the bed to working height, and lower the top side rail.
Preparing supplies in advance avoids interruption during the procedure. Setting the bed at the correct working height for the provider prevents provider discomfort and possible injury.

2. Place a towel or waterproof pad on the bed; place a basin of warm water on the towel or pad, and pad the edge of the basin with a towel. Soak the hand or foot for about 10 minutes. If the patient is unable to sit in a chair and foot care is being performed in bed, support the patient's knees with pillows as needed.
Raising the knees with a pillow reduces pressure on the skin on the back of the leg and increases patient comfort. Soaking loosens dirt, softens skin and nails, and promotes relaxation.

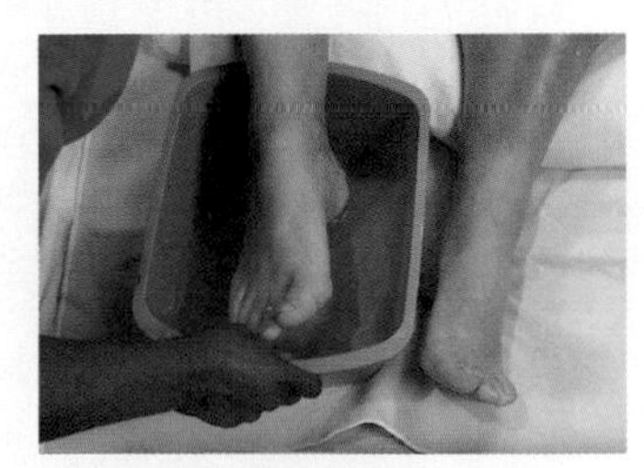

STEP 2

3. Remove the hand or foot from the water. Wash with soap, rinse, and dry, working especially between the fingers or toes.
Thorough washing prevents infection and reduces odor. Thorough drying prevents skin irritation.

4. Inspect the fingernails or toenails. File or trim the nails at the level of the finger or toe (straight across) if within facility policy. When finished, use a new disposable emery board to round off any sharp corners.
Inspection is part of a thorough assessment procedure. Filing straight across helps avoid injury to the cuticles and skin surrounding the nails. Following facility policy ensures that the caregiver is practicing within the scope and standards of the facility.

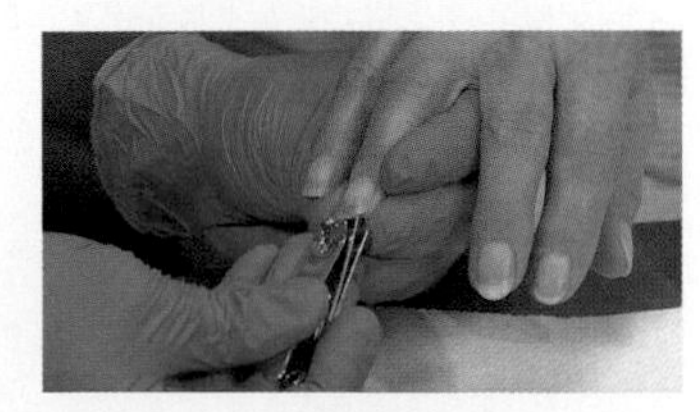

STEP 4

5. Gently clean debris from beneath the patient's nails with the cuticle stick if doing so is not contraindicated.
Keeping fingernails clean helps prevent the spread of microorganisms.

6. Apply lotion if desired by the patient.
Lotion prevents dry skin.

7. Repeat steps 2 through 6 as needed for each hand or foot.

8. If foot or hand care is part of the procedure for bathing a patient, see Skill 27-1, procedure step 11 after the hand care is completed, or procedure step 20 after the foot care is completed. Otherwise, proceed to the next instruction.
Avoids unnecessary interruption of the procedure.

Follow postprocedure steps I through VI.

POSTPROCEDURE

I. Return the bed to its lowest position, raise the top side rails, and verify that the call light is within reach for the patient.
Precautions are taken to maintain patient safety. Top side rails aid in positioning and turning. Raising four side rails is considered a restraint.

II. Assess for additional patient needs and state the time of your expected return.
Meeting patient needs and offering self promote patient satisfaction and build trust.

III. Properly dispose of PPE.
Gloves, gowns, and masks must be appropriately discarded to prevent the spread of microorganisms.

IV. Clean equipment if it was in contact with the patient; see specific manufacturer instructions.
Disinfection eliminates most microorganisms from inanimate objects.

V. Perform hand hygiene.
Frequent hand hygiene prevents the spread of infection.

VI. Document the date, time, assessment, procedure, and patient's response to the procedure.
Accurate documentation is essential to communicate patient care and to provide legal evidence of care.

SKILL 27-4 Therapeutic Massage

PURPOSE

- Decreases tension in muscles
- Decreases pain
- Stimulates blood flow to the skin, helping to prevent skin breakdown
- Induces feelings of sleep and relaxation
- Strengthens general feeling of health and wellness

RESOURCES

- Lotion
- Towels
- Bath blanket
- Nonsterile gloves if needed for standard precautions

COLLABORATION AND DELEGATION

- Back massage may be delegated to unlicensed assistive personnel (UAP) after assessment and consent of the patient. Nurses should encourage UAP to incorporate back massage into patient care routines.
- UAP should report the following to the nurse:
  - Sores, wounds, irritations, lesions, redness, or rashes on the patient
  - Patient discomfort reported during the procedure
- UAP should be instructed in the following:
  - Positioning concerns specific to the patient
  - Appropriate techniques for the procedure (e.g., effleurage, pétrissage, tapotement)
  - Avoidance of pressure over bony prominences
  - Appropriate documentation
- Hospice aides and nurses may want to perform a back massage for a patient to whom they are assigned. Consider timing and the needs of these collaborative caregivers when planning this procedure.
- Licensed massage therapists may provide therapeutic massage as part of care for some patients.

EVIDENCE-BASED PRACTICE

- Massage provides an alternative to pain relievers in the elderly adult who may have pharmacokinetic concerns about traditional pain medications, especially narcotics (Baumann, 2009).
- Massage reduces pain and depression for up to 48 hours (Gulick, Hasledalen, and Wesa, 2008).
- Agitation in dementia patients has been shown to decrease with the intervention of simple massage (Cohen-Mansfield, Libin, and Marx, 2007).

SPECIAL CIRCUMSTANCES

1. **Assess:** Are there musculoskeletal concerns related to the neck, back, or spinal cord?
   Intervention: Do not perform the procedure.
2. **Assess:** Is the patient unable to position himself or herself on one side or prone?
   Intervention: Assist the patient with pillows, adjust a bath blanket to keep the patient covered, and expose only the back and buttocks.
3. **Assess:** Does the patient have any open lesions or rashes?
   Intervention: Wear nonsterile gloves for the procedure, and avoid massaging any skin areas that are open.
4. **Assess:** Using a pain scale, what is the patient's level of pain?
   Intervention: Using a pain scale pre and post procedure will determine effectiveness of massage as a means to reduce pain.

PREPROCEDURE

I. Check PCP orders and the patient care plan.
Knowledge of patient-specific orders is critical for safe patient care.

II. Gather supplies and equipment.
Preparing for the patient encounter saves time and promotes patient trust.

III. Perform hand hygiene.
Frequent hand hygiene prevents the spread of microorganisms.

IV. Maintain standard precautions.
Use of the correct personal protective equipment (PPE) is required whenever contact with bodily fluids is possible, to reduce the transfer of pathogens.

V. Introduce yourself.
Initial communication establishes the role of the nurse and begins a professional relationship.

VI. Provide for patient privacy.
It is important to maintain patient dignity.

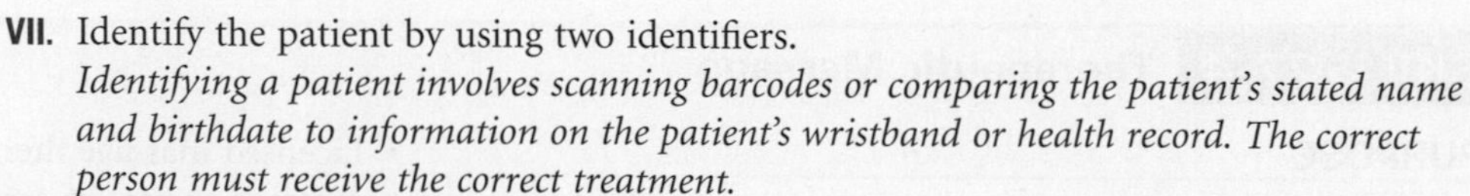

VII. Identify the patient by using two identifiers.
Identifying a patient involves scanning barcodes or comparing the patient's stated name and birthdate to information on the patient's wristband or health record. The correct person must receive the correct treatment.

VIII. Explain the procedure to the patient.
The nurse has a responsibility to inform a patient before initiating care. Information may ease patient anxiety and facilitate cooperation.

PROCEDURE

Follow preprocedure steps I through VIII.

1. If performing a bed bath (see Skill 27-1), proceed to step 4; if not, prepare supplies on the bedside table.
   Preparing supplies in advance avoids interruption during the procedure.
2. Raise the bed to a comfortable working height, with the side rail lowered.
   The bed should be at a height that does not require the provider to stretch or bend unnecessarily; this prevents provider discomfort and possible injury.
3. The patient should be on his or her side, facing away from you, or be put in the prone position, using the drawsheet if necessary.
   The patient must be in the proper position for the procedure; either of these positions minimizes exertion and activity for the patient.
4. Untie the patient's gown; expose the entire back and buttocks if possible. Cover the rest of the patient with the bath blanket.
   This provides the patient with warmth, comfort, and privacy.
5. Pour lotion in your hands, and rub them together.
   Lotion provides lubricant for the massage and prevents injury to the patient's skin. The friction from rubbing the hands together warms the lotion.

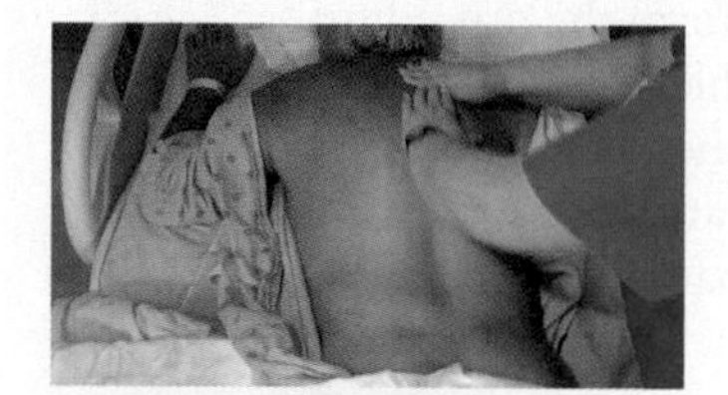

STEP 6

6. Massage from the buttocks to the shoulders and then back to the buttocks, using long, firm strokes (i.e., effleurage technique) for several minutes.
   Effleurage prevents tickling, promotes relaxation, promotes trust, and imparts a sense of caring.

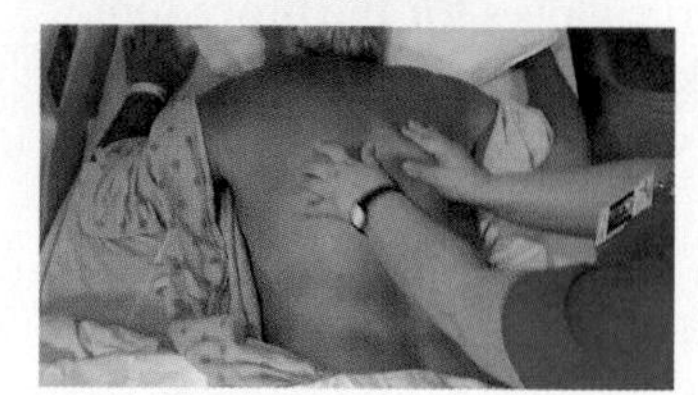

STEP 7

7. If specific muscles are tense, apply pressure with your palm. Knead the muscle or rub it if indicated (i.e., pétrissage technique).
   Pétrissage promotes specific muscle relaxation. It may be contraindicated for or disliked by some patients.

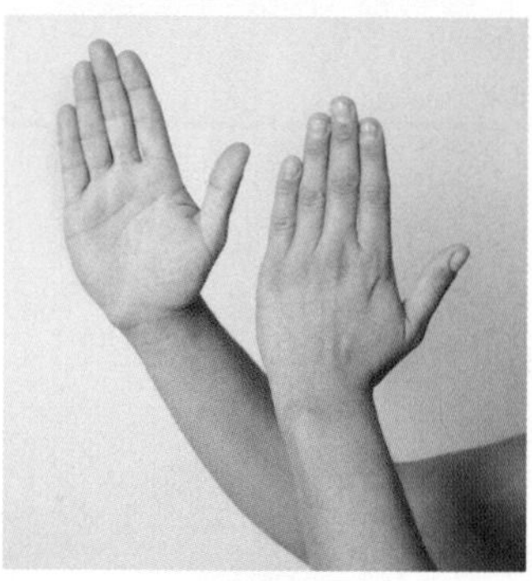

STEP 8

8. If tolerated and preferred by the patient, tap with the sides of the palm or ulnar surface of the hand up and down the patient's back, avoiding the lower back and kidneys (i.e., tapotement technique).
   Tapotement promotes circulation, respiratory function, and relaxation. It may not be tolerated by some patients; tapping over the kidneys may cause injury.
9. Friction is accomplished by performing strong circular strokes. Apply strong circular strokes going from the buttocks to the neck. End the massage with long stroking effleurage movements.
   Friction also promotes circulation and relaxation.
10. Wipe excess lotion off the back with a towel.
    Removal of excess lotion promotes patient comfort.
11. If performing a bed bath, see Skill 27-1; if not, proceed to the next instruction.
    Avoids interruption during the procedure.

Follow postprocedure steps I through VI.

POSTPROCEDURE

I. Return the bed to its lowest position, raise the top side rails, and verify that the call light is within reach for the patient.
Precautions are taken to maintain patient safety. Top side rails aid in positioning and turning. Raising four side rails is considered a restraint.

II. Assess for additional patient needs and state the time of your expected return.
Meeting patient needs and offering self promote patient satisfaction and build trust.

III. Properly dispose of PPE.
Gloves, gowns, and masks must be appropriately discarded to prevent the spread of microorganisms.

IV. Clean equipment if it was in contact with the patient; see specific manufacturer instructions.
Disinfection eliminates most microorganisms from inanimate objects.

V. Perform hand hygiene.
Frequent hand hygiene prevents the spread of infection.

VI. Document the date, time, assessment, procedure, and patient's response to the procedure.
Accurate documentation is essential to communicate patient care and to provide legal evidence of care.

SKILL 27-5 Hair Care

PURPOSE

- Provides routine hygienic care
- Promotes circulation and blood flow
- Provides comfort and relaxation
- Strengthens a general feeling of health, wellness, and self-esteem

RESOURCES

- Shampoo basin
- Bath basin for drainage, if required
- Shampoo
- Conditioner, if desired
- Comb or hair brush
- Graduated cylinder or other container for water
- Laundry bag
- Gloves
- Blow dryer
- Towels
- Washcloth
- Waterproof pads
- Warm water
- Shampoo cap or dry shampoo

COLLABORATION AND DELEGATION

- Shampooing a patient's hair in bed may be delegated to unlicensed assistive personnel (UAP) after assessment of the patient.
- UAP should report the following to the nurse:
  - Sores, wounds, irritations, lesions, redness, or rashes on the patient
  - Patient complaints regarding neck or back discomfort
  - Provider concerns regarding the procedure or patient
  - Completion of the procedure
- UAP should be instructed in the following:
  - The type of shampoo for the patient and the appropriate time for hair care
  - The patient's abilities to assist with the procedure, such as combing and styling
  - Positioning concerns specific to the patient
  - Appropriate care and positioning of specialized medical devices needed by the patient during the procedure (e.g., hearing aid)
  - Ethnic hair variations and specific interventions (e.g., use of a wide-tooth comb)
  - Appropriate documentation
- Hospice aids and nurses may want to assist with or provide shampooing for a patient to whom they are assigned. Consider timing and the needs of these collaborative caregivers when planning this procedure.
- Long-term care facilities often have a barber or hairdresser for patients. Before performing a shampoo, determine whether the patient has other appointments, and coordinate the care accordingly.

SPECIAL CIRCUMSTANCES

1. **Assess:** Does the patient wear hearing aids?
   Intervention: Remove hearing aids from the ears before shampooing with water.
2. **Assess:** Are there musculoskeletal concerns related to the patient's neck, back, or spinal cord?
   Intervention: Use an alternative dry or no-rinse method (e.g., shampoo cap), or defer the procedure. Document the intervention.
3. **Assess:** Does the patient's hair have tangles?
   Intervention: Apply warm water and a conditioner or a detangler if available to release tangles and avoid injury to the scalp. Use a comb or fingers to work through the tangles individually before shampooing.
4. **Assess:** Does the patient have matted blood in the hair?
   Intervention: Mix a solution of 25% hydrogen peroxide and 75% saline, and apply the solution to the matted area with cotton balls to dissolve the mats. Use a comb or gloved fingers to work through the matted tangles individually before shampooing.
5. **Assess:** What should be done if the patient is unable to lie flat in the supine position?
   Intervention: Use an alternative dry or no-rinse method (e.g., shampoo cap), or defer the procedure. Document the intervention.
6. **Assess:** Does the patient have sores on the scalp?
   Intervention: Use nonsterile gloves when washing the patient's hair.

PREPROCEDURE

I. Check PCP orders and the patient care plan.
Knowledge of patient-specific orders is critical for safe patient care.

II. Gather supplies and equipment.
Preparing for the patient encounter saves time and promotes patient trust.

III. Perform hand hygiene.
Frequent hand hygiene prevents the spread of microorganisms.

IV. Maintain standard precautions.
Use of the correct personal protective equipment (PPE) is required whenever contact with bodily fluids is possible, to reduce the transfer of pathogens.

V. Introduce yourself.
Initial communication establishes the role of the nurse and begins a professional relationship.

VI. Provide for patient privacy.
It is important to maintain patient dignity.

VII. Identify the patient by using two identifiers.
Identifying a patient involves scanning barcodes or comparing the patient's stated name and birthdate to information on the patient's wristband or health record. The correct person must receive the correct treatment.

VIII. Explain the procedure to the patient.
The nurse has a responsibility to inform a patient before initiating care. Information may ease patient anxiety and facilitate cooperation.

PROCEDURE

Follow preprocedure steps I through VIII.

1. If performing a bed bath (see Skill 27-1), proceed to step 2; if not, prepare the supplies on the bedside table. Raise the bed to working height, lower the top side rail, and lower the head of the bed.
Preparing supplies avoids unnecessary interruption of the procedure. Setting the bed at the correct working height for the provider prevents provider discomfort and possible injury. The procedure requires supine positioning.

2. Remove the pillow; place towels or waterproof pads under the patient's head; and place a towel across the chest.
This protects the linens from becoming dirty or wet, and keeps the patient dry.

3. Place the shampoo basin under the patient's head, with the spout directed over the edge of the bed. Pad the edge of the basin and the shoulder area with towels. *Comb the patient's hair.* Offer a washcloth to the patient to hold over the eyes. Wet the hair with warm water. (If a shampoo cap is used, pad the bed with towels, and omit the shampoo basin.)
Water must be drained appropriately. Padding the basin provides comfort and prevents unnecessary pressure on the skin and neck. Combing removes tangles before beginning the procedure. Using a washcloth protects the patient's eyes from water and shampoo, and it will stay on the face without the patient straining to hold it. Asking the patient for preferences allows the patient some control and facilitates cooperation.

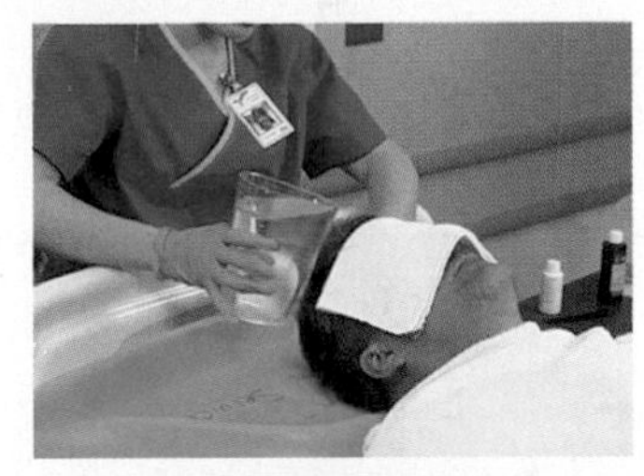

STEP 3

4. Apply shampoo, lather, massage, and rinse. (If a shampoo cap is used, apply the cap, and massage to lather.)
The process removes the buildup of oily secretions and promotes relaxation.

5. Remove the shampoo basin and the top layer of wet linen.
Provides the patient with warmth and comfort.

6. Dry the hair, and massage the scalp with a towel.
Both processes provide warmth. Massage promotes relaxation, circulation, and blood flow.

7. Comb and style the patient's hair; ask for patient input on style.
Combing removes tangles. Asking about style preferences allows the patient some control and facilitates cooperation.

8. If performing a bed bath, see Skill 27-1; if not, proceed to the instruction below.
Avoids unnecessary interruption of the procedure.

Follow postprocedure steps I through VI.

POSTPROCEDURE

I. Return the bed to its lowest position, raise the top side rails, and verify that the call light is within reach for the patient.
Precautions are taken to maintain patient safety. Top side rails aid in positioning and turning. Raising four side rails is considered a restraint.

II. Assess for additional patient needs and state the time of your expected return.
Meeting patient needs and offering self promote patient satisfaction and build trust.

III. Properly dispose of PPE.
Gloves, gowns, and masks must be appropriately discarded to prevent the spread of microorganisms.

IV. Clean equipment if it was in contact with the patient; see specific manufacturer instructions.
Disinfection eliminates most microorganisms from inanimate objects.

V. Perform hand hygiene.
Frequent hand hygiene prevents the spread of infection.

VI. Document the date, time, assessment, procedure, and patient's response to the procedure.
Accurate documentation is essential to communicate patient care and to provide legal evidence of care.

SKILL 27-6 Oral Hygiene

PURPOSE

- Provides routine hygienic care
- Removes tartar, plaque, and food particles from, around, and between teeth
- Prevents infection and irritation of teeth and the oral cavity
- Prevents halitosis
- Strengthens general feelings of health and wellness

RESOURCES

- Toothbrush, toothpaste, dental floss
- Disposable oral swabs or toothettes
- Paper cups and water
- Straw, if not contraindicated
- Mouthwash, as desired
- Emesis basin
- Towels
- Paper towels
- Nonsterile gloves
- 4 × 4 gauze pad, if required
- Water-soluble lubricant for lips, if required

COLLABORATION AND DELEGATION

- Oral care may be delegated to unlicensed assistive personnel (UAP) after the initial assessment of the patient.
- UAP should report the following to the nurse:
  - Coughing or choking symptoms (report immediately)
  - Sores, wounds, irritations, lesions, or bleeding in and around the mouth
  - Complaints of discomfort related to teeth, such as sensitivities that may indicate cavities or other dental concerns
  - Discomfort or refusal related to denture wear or any damage noted to dentures
  - Lost or missing dentures
  - Obvious tooth decay or dental problems
  - Difficulties during the procedure
- UAP should be instructed in the following:
  - Appropriate adaptations and emergency care for patients at risk for choking
  - Appropriate encouragement of the patient's abilities to assist with the procedure
  - Positioning concerns specific to the patient
  - Appropriate care and positioning of specialized dental devices for the patient during the procedure, such as braces, full or partial dentures, or retainers
  - Appropriate documentation, as required
- Hospice aids and nurses may want to assist with or provide oral care for a patient to whom they are assigned. Consider timing and the needs of collaborative caregivers when planning this procedure.

EVIDENCE-BASED PRACTICE

- To reduce the risk of infection and associated dental and oral complications, oral care routines should be performed twice daily using a soft toothbrush (AACN, 2006).
- It is important to review the medications and thoroughly assess the oral cavity while performing oral care. Many medications prescribed for common chronic conditions prevent the normal secretion of saliva, especially in the geriatric population. This can lead to dental complications (e.g., cavities) and affect the oral mucosa (e.g., sores, lesions) (DePaola, Curro, and Zero, 2008; Ettinger, 2007; Jayasakara, 2009).
- Daily use of an antimicrobial mouthwash can prevent the risk or slow the progression of periodontal disease (Lamster, 2006).

SPECIAL CIRCUMSTANCES

1. **Assess:** Has the patient had anticoagulant therapy or bleeding disorders?
   Intervention: Using a soft-bristle toothbrush, make gentle brushing strokes to clean the teeth and gums. Do not floss. Assess carefully for bleeding. Notify the primary care provider if excessive bleeding occurs. Document assessment findings.
2. **Assess:** Does the patient cough or gag during the cleaning procedure?
   Intervention: Remove any equipment from the patient's mouth; assist the patient as needed; and document the occurrence.
3. **Assess:** Is the toothbrush frayed?
   Intervention: Supply a new toothbrush.

SPECIAL RESOURCES AND CIRCUMSTANCES FOR SPECIFIC PATIENT POPULATIONS

Conscious Patient

Special Circumstances

1. **Assess:** Is the patient complaining of tooth sensitivities or showing overt signs of cavities or other tooth decay?
   Intervention: Notify the primary care provider or dentist, and document.
2. **Assess:** Has the caregiver inadvertently been bitten during the procedure?
   Intervention: Stop the procedure; clean the wound; report and document the injury according to facility policy.
3. **Assess:** Does the patient have orthodontic braces, retainers, mouth guards, or other specialized dental devices?
   Intervention: Clean the devices appropriately, referring to the patient's chart for specific recommendations, and document.

Patient With Dentures

Special Resources

- Denture cup
- Denture adhesive, if required

Special Circumstances

1. **Assess:** Is the patient unable to remove the dentures?
   Intervention: Use a gentle side-to-side rocking motion to release suction, and remove the dentures.
2. **Assess:** Are there cracks or breaks in the dentures?
   Intervention: Notify the primary care provider and dentist; do not place the dentures in the patient's mouth if sharp edges are present. Document the problem.

Unconscious Patient

Special Resources

- Towels
- Yankauer suction catheter and suction equipment
- Irrigation kit (i.e., cylinder with piston or bulb syringe) or oral syringe
- Bite block or oral airway, if required

Special Circumstances

1. **Assess:** Has the patient demonstrated a gag reflex?
   Intervention: Carefully consider whether to delegate oral care to UAP; check facility policy for delegation in this situation. If the procedure is delegated, UAP must be carefully trained and instructed on positioning and suctioning techniques.
2. **Assess:** Are there positioning concerns, such as the patient's being unable to lie flat?
   Intervention: Lower the head of the bed as appropriate. Turn the patient's head toward the side facing you, and place a towel on the pillow with an emesis basin on top of the towel, as appropriate. Have suction equipment turned on and easily available.

PREPROCEDURE

I. Check PCP orders and the patient care plan.
Knowledge of patient-specific orders is critical for safe patient care.

II. Gather supplies and equipment.
Preparing for the patient encounter saves time and promotes patient trust.

III. Perform hand hygiene.
Frequent hand hygiene prevents the spread of microorganisms.

IV. Maintain standard precautions.
Use of the correct personal protective equipment (PPE) is required whenever contact with bodily fluids is possible, to reduce the transfer of pathogens.

V. Introduce yourself.
Initial communication establishes the role of the nurse and begins a professional relationship.

VI. Provide for patient privacy.
It is important to maintain patient dignity.

VII. Identify the patient by using two identifiers.
Identifying a patient involves scanning barcodes or comparing the patient's stated name and birthdate to information on the patient's wristband or health record. The correct person must receive the correct treatment.

VIII. Explain the procedure to the patient.
The nurse has a responsibility to inform a patient before initiating care. Information may ease patient anxiety and facilitate cooperation.

PROCEDURE

Conscious Patient

Follow preprocedure steps I through VIII.

1. Prepare supplies on the bedside table. Place paper towels under the emesis basin.
   Preparing materials before beginning the procedure avoids interruption during the procedure. Placing paper towels under the emesis basin keeps the work area clean.
2. Raise the bed to a comfortable working height, and lower the top side rail. Raise the head of the bed. Place a towel across the patient's chest, and put on nonsterile gloves.
   Proper bed position prevents provider discomfort and possible injury. Raising the head of the bed reduces the risk of choking. A properly placed towel can prevent the bed linens and patient's gown from becoming dirty or wet. The use of nonsterile gloves complies with standard precautions.
3. Apply water and toothpaste to the toothbrush.
   Toothpaste helps clean teeth and freshen breath.
4. Brush the teeth, gums, and tongue using short, gentle strokes.
   Brushing removes tartar, plaque, microorganisms, and food or loose particles.
   a. *Front teeth:* Brush the upper and then the lower teeth, working on the outside surfaces of the teeth and then the inside surfaces. Use the entire brush surface of the toothbrush, and brush starting at the gum line.
   b. *Outside of side teeth:* Hold the toothbrush at a 45-degree angle, and brush the upper and then the lower teeth, rolling the brush away from the gum line.
   c. *Inside of side teeth:* Brush the upper and then the lower teeth, rolling the brush away from the gums.
   d. *Chewing surface of teeth:* Brush the upper and then lower teeth using a back-and-forth motion.
   e. *Tongue:* Brush gently from front to back; use a 4 × 4 gauze pad to hold the tongue if needed. Care must be taken to prevent triggering the gag reflex and to reduce the risk of aspiration.

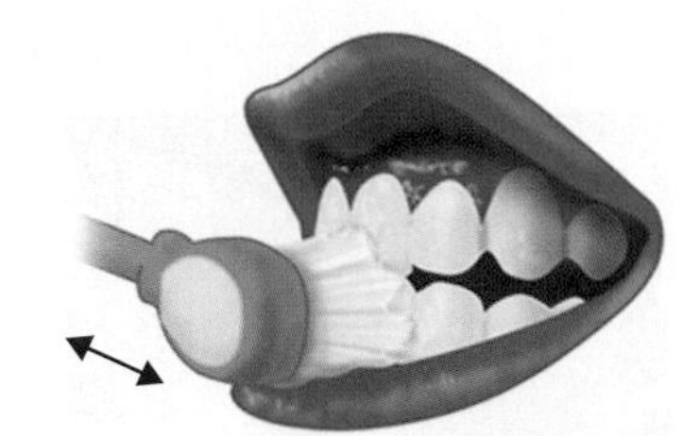

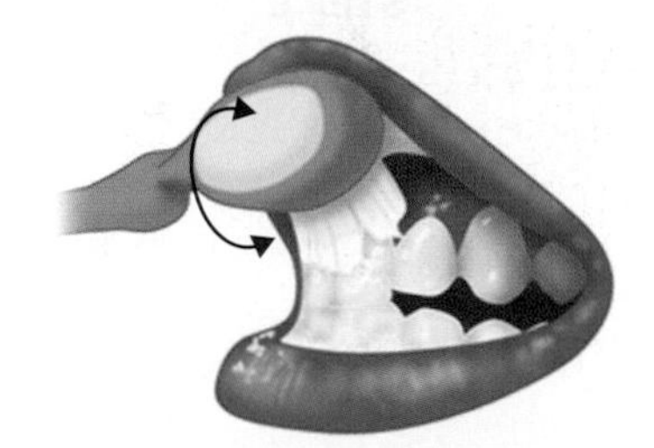

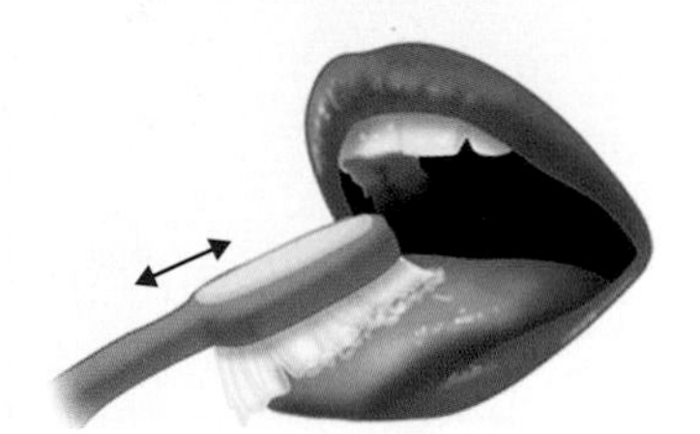

STEP 4a

5. Give the patient water. Have the patient rinse the mouth and spit into the emesis basin; repeat the rinse and spit.
   Using a water rinse removes loosened particles.
6. Provide time for the patient to floss.
   Flossing removes plaque from between the teeth.
7. Give the patient water. Have the patient rinse the mouth and spit into the emesis basin; repeat the rinse and spit.
   Using a water rinse removes loosened particles.
8. Offer mouthwash. Instruct the patient to swish the mouthwash inside the mouth, gargle (if desired), and spit into the emesis basin.
   Mouthwash freshens breath; asking about preferences allows for patient control and facilitates cooperation.
9. Dry the patient's mouth; offer lubricant for the lips.
   Drying the mouth promotes comfort. Lubricant prevents drying and cracking of tissues, and asking about preferences allows for patient control and facilitates cooperation.
10. If performing a bed bath, see Skill 27-1; if not, proceed to the instruction below.
    Avoids unnecessary interruption of the procedure.

Follow postprocedure steps I through VI.

Patient With Dentures

Follow preprocedure steps I through VIII.

1. Follow procedure steps 1 and 2 in the Conscious Patient section.
   Preparing materials before beginning the procedure avoids interruption during the procedure. The positioning and setup for the procedure are unchanged for a patient with dentures. Proper use of personal protective equipment (PPE) prevents the spread of microorganisms.

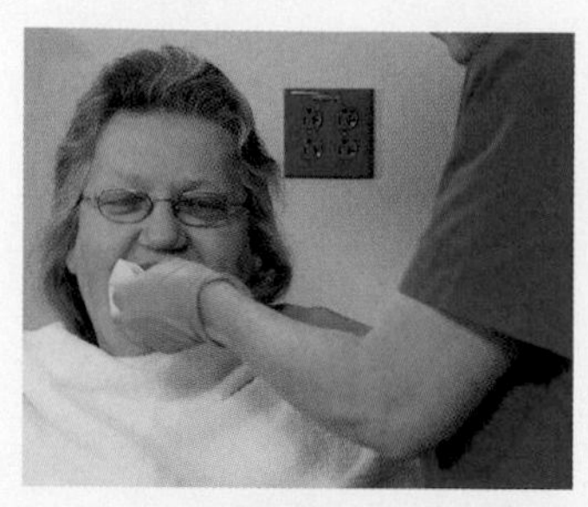
STEP 2

2. Partially fill a denture cup with water; remove the lower and then upper dentures with 4 × 4 gauze pad; and place the dentures in the denture cup.
   Soaking dentures in water allows easier removal of debris. A 4 × 4 gauze pad provides a more secure grip on the dentures than fingers alone. Lower dentures are easier to remove because upper dentures have stronger suction. Using the water-filled denture cup prevents damage to dentures during the cleaning procedure or while carrying them to the sink.
3. Follow procedure steps 3 through 5 in the Conscious Patient section to brush the gums and oral mucosa.
4. Raise the side rail.
   Proper side rail positioning ensures patient safety.
5. Place a towel in the sink, and fill the sink with about an inch of water. Brush the dentures over the towel. Follow procedure steps 4a through 4d in the Conscious Patient section to clean the dentures. Rinse the dentures using warm water
   The towel prevents damage to the dentures during the cleaning procedure if the dentures are dropped. The brushing technique used with dentures is the same as that used with teeth; it removes tartar, plaque, microorganisms, and food or loose particles.

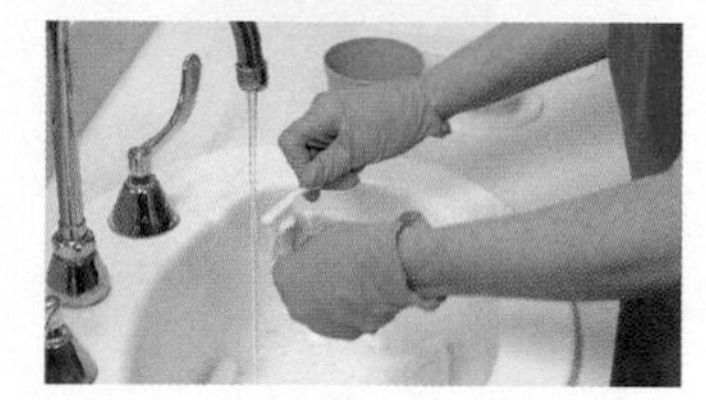
STEP 6

6. Brush the remaining surfaces of the dentures, and rinse the patient's mouth. Place the dentures into the denture cup.
   Loosened particles must be removed; using fresh water prevents the spread of microorganisms.
7. Lower the side rail. Offer the patient mouthwash. Instruct the patient to swish the mouthwash, gargle, and spit into the emesis basin. Apply denture adhesive (if used), and using 4 × 4 gauze, insert the upper plate first and then the lower plate. Offer water for the patient to drink or rinse. (The patient may prefer to store the dentures. If so, store them in warm water in a denture cup labeled with the patient's name.)
   Mouthwash freshens breath; asking about preferences allows for patient control and facilitates cooperation. The 4 × 4 gauze pad provides a better grip than fingers alone and prevents damage to the dentures during the procedure. Although lower dentures are easier to insert, the upper dentures are easier to insert without lower dentures in place.
8. Dry the patient's mouth; offer lubricant for lips.
   Drying the mouth promotes comfort. Lubricant prevents drying and cracking of tissues, and asking about preferences allows for patient control and facilitates cooperation.
9. If performing a bed bath, see Skill 27-1; if not, proceed to the next instruction.
   Avoid unnecessary interruption of the procedure.

Follow postprocedure steps I through VI.

Unconscious Patient

Follow preprocedure steps I through VIII.

1. If performing a bed bath (see Skill 27-1), proceed to step 2; if not, prepare supplies on the bedside table. Raise the bed to working height and lower the top side rail. Apply clean gloves and assess for a gag reflex. Use a tongue blade and a pen light to inspect the condition of the oral cavity. Remove and dispose of your gloves. If suctioning is needed, connect the tubing to the suction, turn on the machine, and test the suction catheter.
   Preparing materials before beginning the procedure avoids interruption during the procedure. Proper bed position prevents provider discomfort and possible injury. Assessment before the procedure helps the nurse decide how to proceed.
2. Lower the head of the bed to 30 degrees or less, if tolerated by the patient. Using a drawsheet, place the patient on his or her side, facing you (see Skill 28-1) if not contraindicated by a head or neck injury or other condition. Place a towel on the bed along the side of the patient's face, and place an emesis basin along the side of the patient's mouth. Put on nonsterile gloves.
   If tolerated, a flat bed provides for patient comfort. Turning the patient's head to the side facing you allows fluid to drain from the side of the mouth and reduces the risk of choking. A properly placed towel prevents linens from becoming dirty or wet. Proper use of PPE prevents the spread of microorganisms.

3. Follow procedure steps 3 and 4a through 4d in the Conscious Patient section. Use a bite block or an oral airway to keep the patient's mouth open. Suction any accumulated secretions.
A bite block or an oral airway prevents inadvertent injury to the care provider because the normal reflex of oral stimulation is to bite down.

4. Use a toothbrush moistened with water. Apply toothpaste or an antibacterial solution to the toothbrush and use it to loosen any crusts. Disposable oral swabs dipped in water to clean oral tissues (i.e., cheeks, roof of mouth, bottom of mouth, tongue) may be used if a toothbrush is contraindicated. Use a new swab for each area.
Using disposable swabs that are frequently replaced prevents the spread of microorganisms. Swabs remove excess debris and dead tissue; the water keeps oral tissues moist.

5. Use a bulb syringe or Yankauer suction catheter to remove excess water from the oral cavity.
A Yankauer catheter is designed for oral suctioning; water that is not suctioned may be aspirated after the patient is repositioned.

6. Dry the patient's mouth with a towel, and lubricate the lips if needed.
Drying the mouth promotes comfort. Lubricant prevents drying and cracking of tissues.

7. If performing a bed bath, see Skill 27-1; if not, proceed to the next instruction.
Avoids unnecessary interruption of the procedure.

Follow postprocedure steps I through VI.

POSTPROCEDURE

I. Return the bed to its lowest position, raise the top side rails, and verify that the call light is within reach for the patient.
Precautions are taken to maintain patient safety. Top side rails aid in positioning and turning. Raising four side rails is considered a restraint.

II. Assess for additional patient needs and state the time of your expected return.
Meeting patient needs and offering self promote patient satisfaction and build trust.

III. Properly dispose of PPE.
Gloves, gowns, and masks must be appropriately discarded to prevent the spread of microorganisms.

IV. Clean equipment if it was in contact with the patient; see specific manufacturer instructions.
Disinfection eliminates most microorganisms from inanimate objects.

V. Perform hand hygiene.
Frequent hand hygiene prevents the spread of infection.

VI. Document the date, time, assessment, procedure, and patient's response to the procedure.
Accurate documentation is essential to communicate patient care and to provide legal evidence of care.

SKILL 27-7 Shaving a Male Patient

PURPOSE

- Provides routine hygienic care
- Removes unwanted hair
- Strengthens a general feeling of health and wellness

RESOURCES

- Disposable safety razor or electric razor, as appropriate
- Bath basin
- Shaving cream or soap
- Towels
- Warm water
- Washcloths
- Nonsterile gloves
- Aftershave lotion or powder, if desired
- Mirror

COLLABORATION AND DELEGATION

- Shaving a patient may be delegated to unlicensed assistive personnel (UAP) after assessment of the patient.
- UAP should report the following to a nurse:
  - Any nicks or cuts that occur during the procedure
  - Sores, wounds, irritations, lesions, redness, or rashes on the patient
  - Difficulties in performing the procedure
- UAP should be instructed in the following:
  - Appropriate equipment and training for the procedure
  - Conditions specific to the patient (e.g., bleeding tendencies) and training for interventions and reporting concerns
  - Appropriate positioning specific to the patient and diagnosis
  - Ethnic and cultural variations and concerns, such as differences in hair texture
  - Consent for and desires regarding care of the mustache and beard
  - Appropriate documentation
- Hospice aids and nurses may want to assist with shaving or shave patients to whom they are assigned. Consider timing and the needs of these collaborative caregivers when planning this procedure.

SPECIAL CIRCUMSTANCES: ALL METHODS

1. **Assess:** Does the patient have a mustache or beard?
   Intervention: Do not shave the patient unless consent is obtained; wash and comb the facial hair instead.
2. **Assess:** Does the patient have any bleeding disorder, or is the patient being treated with anticoagulant therapy?
   Intervention: Use an electric razor.
3. **Assess:** Does the patient have very sensitive skin, or is the patient prone to ingrown hairs in the shaved area?
   Intervention: Shave the patient first in the direction of hair growth; then shave again against the direction of hair growth. Shaving against the direction of hair growth gives a closer shave but may nick the patient's skin easier and may cause ingrown hairs because the hair is shaved off at a level closer to the skin surface.

PREPROCEDURE

I. Check PCP orders and the patient care plan.
Knowledge of patient-specific orders is critical for safe patient care.

II. Gather supplies and equipment.
Preparing for the patient encounter saves time and promotes patient trust.

III. Perform hand hygiene.
Frequent hand hygiene prevents the spread of microorganisms.

IV. Maintain standard precautions.
Use of the correct personal protective equipment (PPE) is required whenever contact with bodily fluids is possible, to reduce the transfer of pathogens.

V. Introduce yourself.
Initial communication establishes the role of the nurse and begins a professional relationship.

VI. Provide for patient privacy.
It is important to maintain patient dignity.

VII. Identify the patient by using two identifiers.
Identifying a patient involves scanning barcodes or comparing the patient's stated name and birthdate to information on the patient's wristband or health record. The correct person must receive the correct treatment.

VIII. Explain the procedure to the patient.
The nurse has a responsibility to inform a patient before initiating care. Information may ease patient anxiety and facilitate cooperation.

PROCEDURE

Follow preprocedure steps I through VIII.

1. If performing a bed bath, proceed to step 2; if not, prepare supplies on the bedside table. Raise the bed to working height, raise the head of the bed, and lower the top side rail.
   Preparing supplies in advance avoids interruption during the procedure. Setting the bed at the correct working height for the provider prevents provider discomfort and possible injury. Raising the head of the bed promotes patient comfort.
2. Place a towel around the patient's neck and across his chest. Put on nonsterile gloves.
   Using a towel prevents the bed linens and patient's gown from becoming dirty or wet. Gloves are required to comply with standard precautions in case a cut occurs.
3. Apply warm water to the patient's face with a washcloth for several seconds.
   Moist warmth softens the hair for easier removal and lowers the risk of nicks.
4. Put the shaving cream in your hands or lather soap in your hands, rub hands together, and apply the cream or soap over the hair on the patient's face and neck that is to be removed. The patient should be given the choice between shaving cream and soap.
   Friction warms the cream or soap and provides comfort, and the lather lubricates the skin and protects it from injury. Allowing the patient to make choices about care gives the patient a sense of empowerment.
5. Hold the skin taut; shave one side of the face using long, firm strokes in the direction in which the hair grows. Use short strokes around the chin and lips. Rinse the razor with warm water after each stroke.
   Taut skin provides a smooth surface and prevents injury to the skin. Shaving in the direction of hair growth is better for sensitive skin and prevents ingrown hairs. Using warm water cleans the razor and softens the hair, easing its removal.

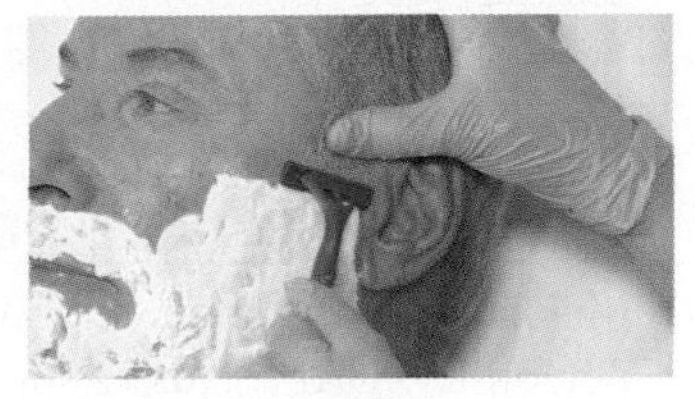

STEP 5

6. Dispose of the used razor in the sharps container. Rinse excess shaving cream or soap from the patient's face with warm water.
   Proper disposal protects the patient and staff from injury. Removing residual cream or soap prevents drying of the skin and irritation.
7. Offer aftershave or lotion. If the patient wants either, apply it with a patting motion of the fingertips.
   Using aftershave or lotion promotes comfort and prevents skin irritation. Asking about preferences allows the patient some control and facilitates cooperation.
8. If performing a bed bath, see Skill 27-1; if not, proceed to the next instruction.
   Avoids unnecessary interruption of the procedure.

Follow postprocedure steps I through VI.

POSTPROCEDURE

I. Return the bed to its lowest position, raise the top side rails, and verify that the call light is within reach for the patient.
Precautions are taken to maintain patient safety. Top side rails aid in positioning and turning. Raising four side rails is considered a restraint.

II. Assess for additional patient needs and state the time of your expected return.
Meeting patient needs and offering self promote patient satisfaction and build trust.

III. Properly dispose of PPE.
Gloves, gowns, and masks must be appropriately discarded to prevent the spread of microorganisms.

IV. Clean equipment if it was in contact with the patient; see specific manufacturer instructions.
Disinfection eliminates most microorganisms from inanimate objects.

V. Perform hand hygiene.
Frequent hand hygiene prevents the spread of infection.

VI. Document the date, time, assessment, procedure, and patient's response to the procedure.
Accurate documentation is essential to communicate patient care and to provide legal evidence of care.

SKILL 27-8 Making an Occupied or Unoccupied Bed

PURPOSE

- Provides routine hygienic care
- Prevents skin irritations
- Helps prevent the spread of infection
- Provides comfort and relaxation
- Reduces body odor
- Strengthens a general feeling of health and wellness

RESOURCES

- Flat or fitted bottom sheet
- Top sheet
- Blanket and/or bedspread
- Pillowcases
- Drawsheet
- Bed protector or waterproof pad, if required
- Laundry bag
- Bath blanket (if the bed is occupied)
- Clean, nonsterile gloves

COLLABORATION AND DELEGATION

- Making a bed is often delegated to unlicensed assistive personnel (UAP). Nurses should encourage UAP to incorporate bed making into routine care duties.
- UAP should report the following to the nurse:
  - Injury or potential injury (e.g., dislodged medical devices or dressings) that may occur while making an occupied bed
  - Medications found in bed linens
  - Difficulties in performing the procedure
- UAP should be instructed in the following:
  - Appropriate activity level of the patient and type of bed-making procedure (occupied or unoccupied) required
  - Procedure for handling clean and soiled linens
  - Importance of checking for personal items left in the bed linens (e.g., eyeglasses, jewelry, dentures)
  - Appropriate assistance required for moving the patient into and out of bed
  - Necessity of keeping the call bell within reach of the patient when the patient is out of bed
  - Restraint and safety policies regarding side rails and over-bed tables
  - Appropriate documentation of the patient's tolerance and experience of the procedure

SPECIAL CIRCUMSTANCES: UNOCCUPIED OR OCCUPIED BED

1. **Assess:** Will the linens, such as bedspread or top sheet, be reused for the patient?
   Intervention: Remove and fold the linens before starting the procedure. Fold the bedspread or top sheet down in half, and then fold it from side to side. Place the linens on the bedside table or chair. Cover the patient with a bath blanket if removing the top linens.
2. **Assess:** Does the patient require additional space in the foot area to accommodate his or her diagnosis or concerns (e.g., space for a cast)?
   Intervention: Apply a horizontal toe pleat to the top sheet of the bed for all patients while making it:
   - Pinch 2 to 4 inches of the sheet together near the foot of the bed.
   - Fold this pinched pleat neatly over itself.
   - Do not complete procedure step 9e of the mitered corner in the Unoccupied Bed section.
   - Continue to make the bed according to the skill procedure steps 10 through 13.

SPECIAL CIRCUMSTANCES: OCCUPIED BED ONLY

1. **Assess:** Does the patient diagnosis include pain concerns if the patient is moved?
   Intervention: Consider pain medication according to orders before performing the procedure to prevent discomfort.
2. **Assess:** Are there positioning concerns such that the patient is unable to lie flat?
   Intervention: Lower the head of the bed as appropriate.
3. **Assess:** Are there musculoskeletal concerns?
   Intervention: Obtain appropriate assistance (personnel or mechanical) before repositioning the patient. Check the patient's chart and orders regarding proper positioning, and use pillows if needed to assist or elevate.
4. **Assess:** Are the dirty linens wet and soiled?
   Intervention: Place an extra sheet or towel around them to absorb additional moisture. Clean the mattress before applying a clean bottom sheet.

PREPROCEDURE

I. Check PCP orders and the patient care plan.
Knowledge of patient-specific orders is critical for safe patient care.

II. Gather supplies and equipment.
Preparing for the patient encounter saves time and promotes patient trust.

III. Perform hand hygiene.
Frequent hand hygiene prevents the spread of microorganisms.

IV. Maintain standard precautions.
Use of the correct personal protective equipment (PPE) is required whenever contact with bodily fluids is possible, to reduce the transfer of pathogens.

V. Introduce yourself.
Initial communication establishes the role of the nurse and begins a professional relationship.

VI. Provide for patient privacy.
It is important to maintain patient dignity.

VII. Identify the patient by using two identifiers.
Identifying a patient involves scanning barcodes or comparing the patient's stated name and birthdate to information on the patient's wristband or health record. The correct person must receive the correct treatment.

VIII. Explain the procedure to the patient.
The nurse has a responsibility to inform a patient before initiating care. Information may ease patient anxiety and facilitate cooperation.

PROCEDURE

Unoccupied Bed

Follow preprocedure steps I through VIII.

1. Check around the bed for spills. Check that the bed is locked. Prepare supplies on the bedside table or chair; do *not* use another patient's bed. Raise the bed to the appropriate working height, lower all side rails, and lower the head and foot of the bed. Wear nonsterile gloves when there is potential for coming into contact with soiled linens or body fluids.
Checking for spills prevents injury to the staff. Using a table or chair prevents the spread of microorganisms between patient beds. Setting the bed at the correct working height for the provider prevents provider discomfort and possible injury. A flat bed provides for proper fit of linens. Wearing gloves prevents the spread of microorganisms.

2. Remove the dirty linens.

a. Slide the pillowcase off the pillow and place the pillowcase in the center of the bed. Place the pillow on the bedside table or chair.
Proper temporary storage of bedding is used to prevent the spread of microorganisms.

b. Systematically loosen the linens at the foot of the bed. Remove the bedspread and blankets separately. If they are soiled place them in the linen bag. If they are to be reused, fold them into a square and place them in a chair. Walk around the bed and loosen the linens at the head of the bed.
Walking around the bed prevents provider discomfort and possible injury from stretching and reaching.

c. Roll the linens toward the center of the bed.
Rolling the dirty side of the sheets inside prevents the spread of microorganisms.

d. Hold the dirty linens away from you and place them in a laundry bag.
Avoids spreading microorganisms by contact with the caregiver's clothing.

e. Position and align the mattress to fit the bed frame, and wipe down the mattress with an appropriate solution if needed.
The mattress may slip toward the foot of the frame if the head of the bed is elevated. Alignment of the mattress with the bed frame provides patient safety and comfort and restores foot space that was affected by a slipping mattress. Proper cleaning prevents the spread of microorganisms.

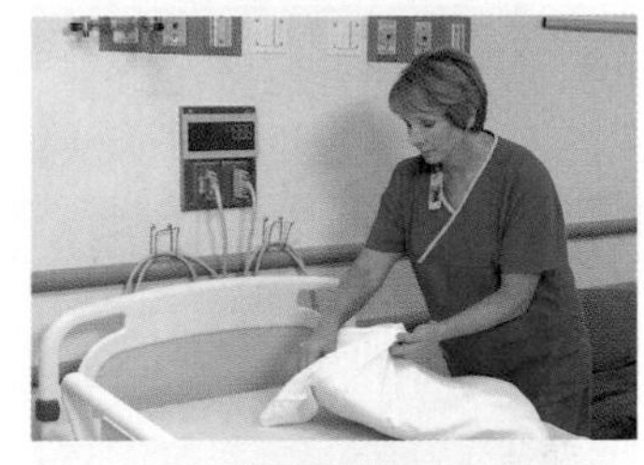
STEP 2a

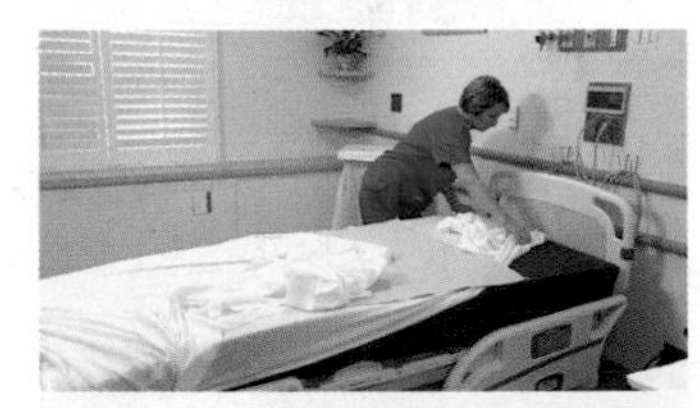
STEP 2b

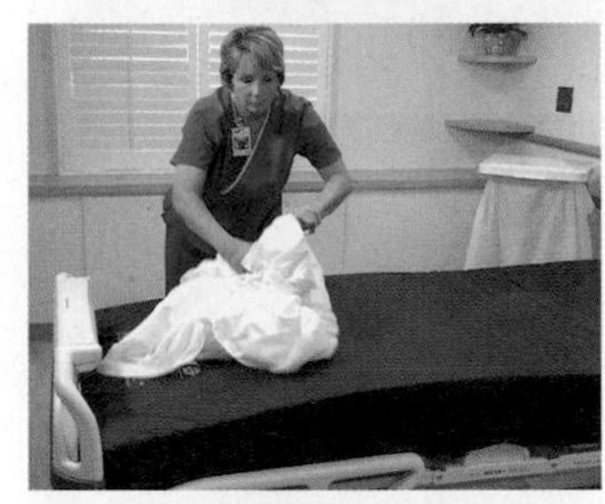
STEP 2c

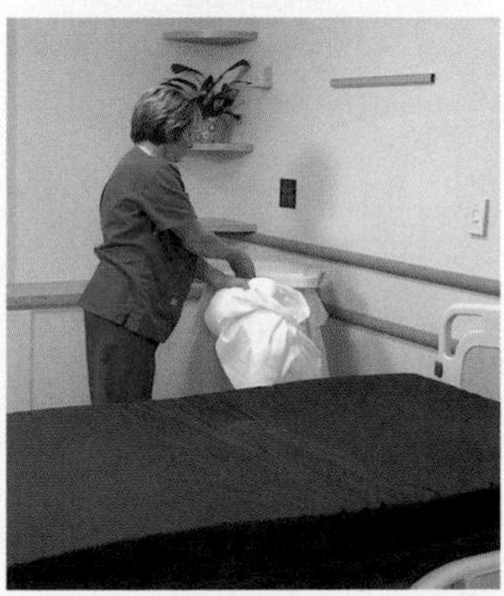
STEP 2d

3. Wash hands and apply clean gloves if needed.
   Washing hands and changing gloves after handling the dirty sheets prevents the spread of microorganisms from dirty sheets to clean sheets.
4. For all linen applications, fold the sheets out on the bed, opening them from side to center and center to side. Do *not* shake the sheets.
   Shaking sheets spreads microorganisms into the air. Holding linens up and out to shake them can cause provider discomfort and possible injury.
5. Apply the bottom fitted sheet, or use a flat sheet and miter the top corners; walk around the bed to do so.
   Walking around the bed prevents provider discomfort and possible injury from stretching and reaching.

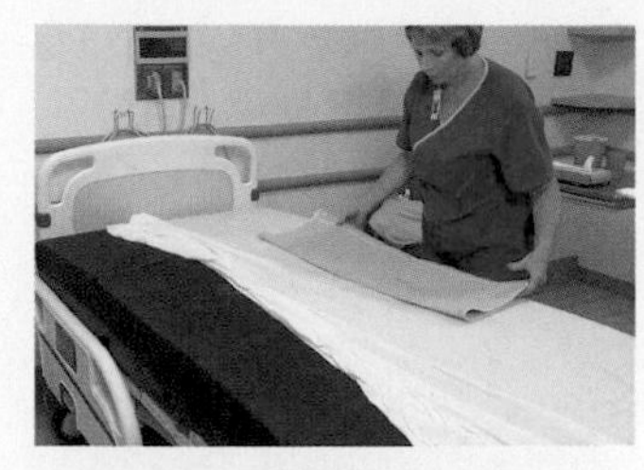

STEP 6

6. If the patient is incontinent, apply a waterproof pad. If the patient requires assistance with movement in bed, apply a drawsheet.
   A waterproof pad protects the bed linens from becoming soiled and/or wet. A drawsheet prevents injury if the patient needs to be moved.
7. Apply the top sheet with the hems facing up, and apply the blanket and bedspread with the hems facing down. The top blanket or bedspread should be 6-8 inches down from the top of the top sheet.
   Keeping the rough edges of bed linens away from the patient's skin prevents skin irritation. The top sheet can be folded down to have a clean and neat appearance (see procedure step 10).

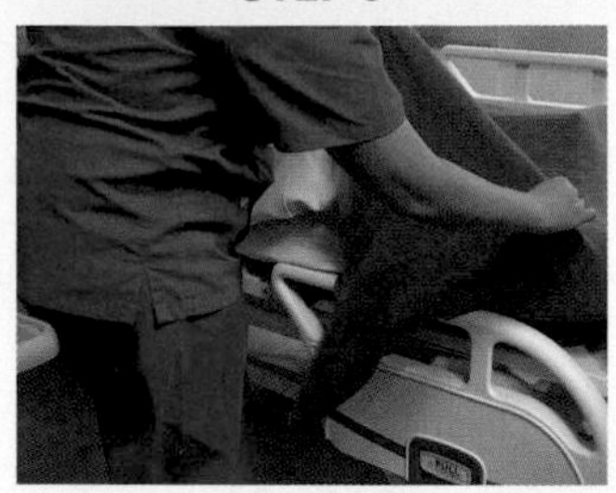

STEP 8c

8. Use mitered corners at the bottom of the bed. Tuck the top sheet and blanket (or bedspread) together.
   a. Mitered corners secure linens on the bed while providing a clean and neat appearance.
   b. Tuck in the linens across the foot of the bed.
   c. Pull up the side of the linens near the bottom edge of the sheet to form a triangle, with equal amounts of sheet above and below the mattress.
   d. Tuck in the linens at the bottom part of the triangle in line with the bottom of the mattress.
   e. Fold down the top corner of the triangle over the mattress.

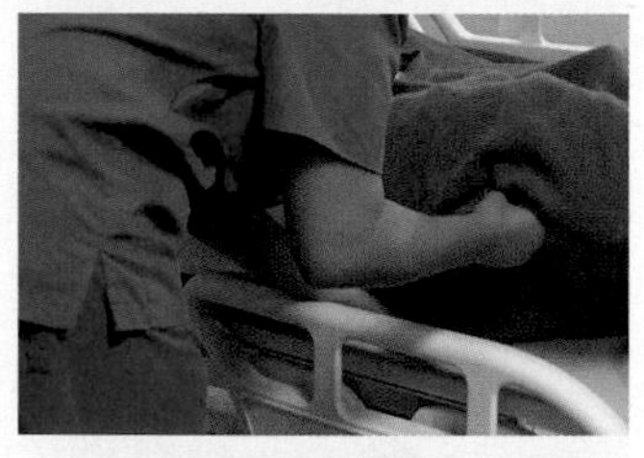

STEP 8d

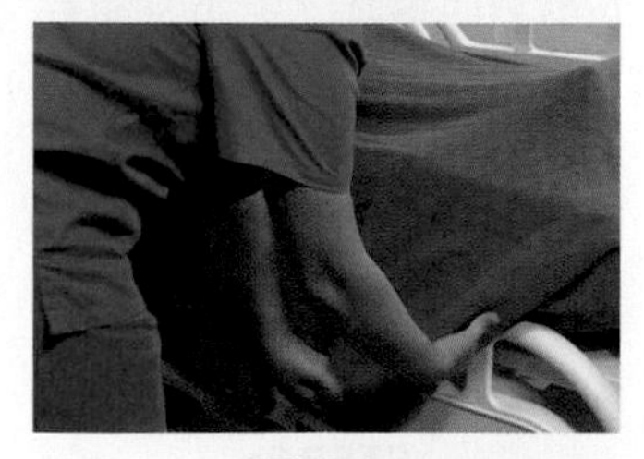

STEP 8e

9. Make a cuff by turning down the top sheet over the top edge of the blanket or bedspread.
   The cuff is easy for a patient to grab to pull up the sheets, and it provides a clean and neat appearance.
10. Make a horizontal toe pleat. At the foot of the bed fanfold the sheet 5 to 10 cm (2 to 4 inches) across the bed. Pull the sheet up from the bottom to make a fold about 15 cm (6 inches) from the bottom of the mattress.
    Allows room for the patient's feet.
11. Apply the pillowcase.
    a. Grasp the center of the outside hem of the closed end of the pillowcase with your dominant hand; use the other hand to pull the pillowcase inside out over your dominant hand.
    This approach prevents shaking of the pillow or case.
    b. Grasp the center of the edge of the pillow with the same hand.
    c. Slide the pillowcase around the pillow using your nondominant hand.

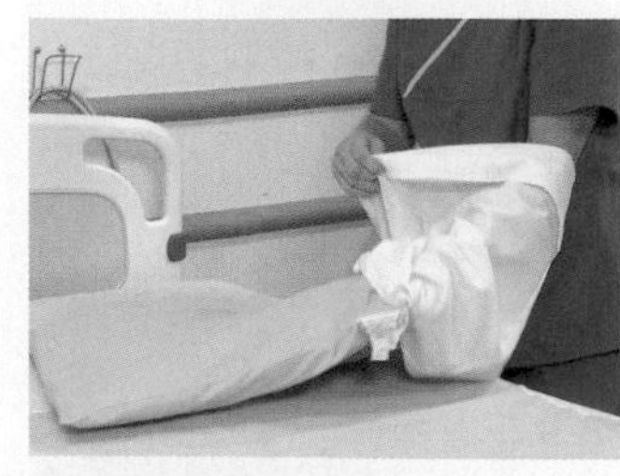

STEP 11

12. Place the pillow on the bed with the open end of the pillowcase away from the door.
    The overall appearance of the room should be clean and neat.
13. If the patient is not in the room, place the call light on the bed; if the patient is in the room and wants to get back into the bed, provide assistance, and then proceed to the next instruction. Remove the soiled linen from the patient's room.
    This avoids unnecessary interruption of the procedure or prepares the bed for the patient's return.

Follow postprocedure steps I through VI.

Occupied Bed

Follow preprocedure steps I through VIII.

1. If performing a bed bath (see Skill 27-1), proceed to procedure step 3; if not, prepare supplies on the bedside table, raise the bed to working height, and lower the top side rail.
   Preparing supplies avoids unnecessary interruption of the procedure. Setting the bed at the correct working height for the provider prevents provider discomfort and possible injury.
2. Lower the head and foot of the bed. Put on clean gloves. Untuck the top sheet at the foot of the bed. Remove the bed spread and blanket separately. If they are soiled place them in the linen bag. If either is to be reused, fold the item into a square and place them on the back of a chair. Place a bath blanket over the top sheet on the patient.
   The bed should be flat to reduce provider discomfort and possible injury and to allow for proper fit of linens. The bath blanket provides warmth, comfort, and privacy for the patient during the linen change.
3. Remove the top sheet by reaching under the bath blanket, grasping the top of the sheet, and pulling it down to the foot of the bed. Hold the linens away from you, and place them in a laundry bag.
   Proper removal prevents spread of microorganisms.
4. Assist the patient onto the side facing away from you keeping that side rail up for safety. Loosen the four corners of the bottom sheet, and roll the sheet on the working side (i.e., along the patient's back) in toward the patient.
   Make one side of the bed at a time. Loosening all four corners at once minimizes the time that the patient must be on his or her side.

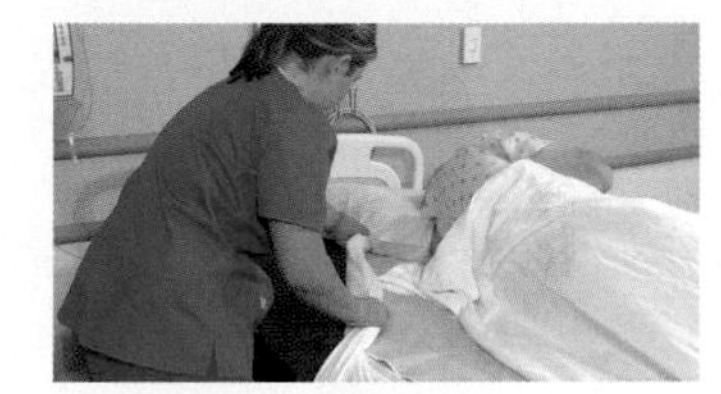

STEP 4

5. With assistance, reposition the mattress to align with the bed frame. Clean the mattress if appropriate. Remove gloves and perform hand hygiene.
   The mattress may slip toward the foot of the frame if the head of the bed is elevated. Alignment of the mattress with the bed frame provides patient safety and comfort and restores foot space that was affected by a slipping mattress. Cleaning the mattress reduces the risk of nosocomial infections.
6. Apply a fitted sheet (or use a flat sheet as the bottom sheet) to one side of the bed by unfolding it lengthwise from the center of the bed and tucking in the corners. Wearing clean gloves, fan-fold the remaining half of the clean sheet, and tuck it under the cleaner underside of the dirty linens.
   The side of the dirty sheet that was exposed to patient contact is rolled into itself so that only the cleaner underside contacts the clean sheets; this reduces the spread of microorganisms.

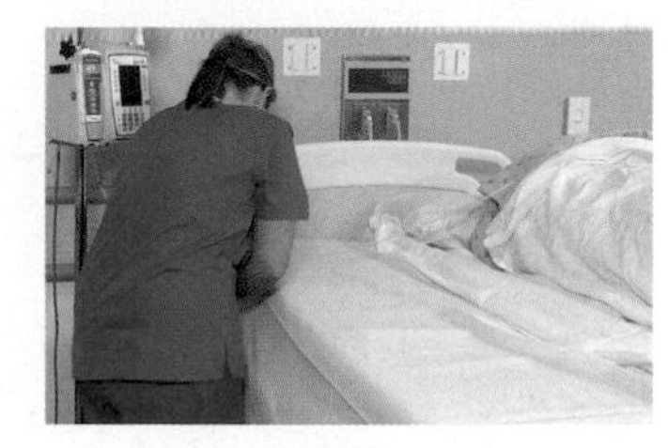

STEP 6

7. Follow step 6 in the Unoccupied Bed section for applying a waterproof pad or drawsheet if required.
   A waterproof pad protects the bed linens from becoming soiled and wet. A drawsheet prevents injury to the patient if he or she needs to be moved.
8. Raise the top side rail; roll the patient over the roll of bedding onto the opposite side to face toward you. Walk around the bed.
   Precautions must be taken to maintain patient safety while you make the other side of the bed.
9. Lower the top side rail. Fold the dirty linens inward into a bundle, and remove it from the bed. Hold the linens away from you, and place them in a laundry bag. Remove dirty gloves and wash hands.
   The bed rail is positioned to prevent provider discomfort and possible injury. Proper handling of dirty linens and frequent handwashing prevent the spread of microorganisms.
10. Unfold and smooth the bottom sheet, waterproof pad, and drawsheet from under the patient.
    Removing wrinkles from the bedding avoids skin irritation and patient discomfort.

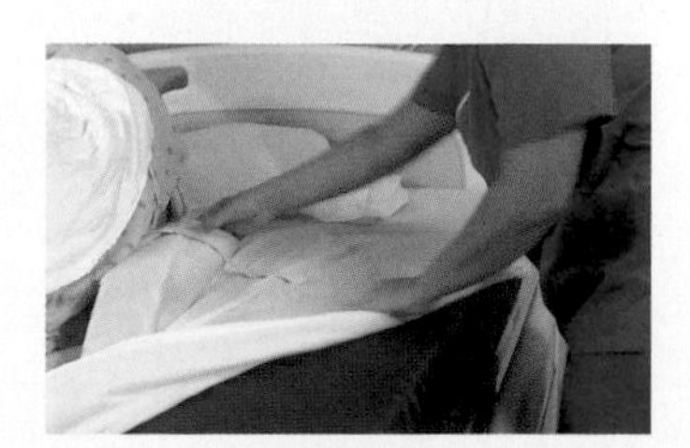

STEP 10

11. Tuck in the corners of the fitted sheet (or miter the top corners of a flat sheet used as a bottom sheet), and tuck the drawsheet under the mattress.
    This secures the bedding to complete the application of the bottom sheets of the bed.
12. Raise the top side rail, and roll the patient onto his or her back.
    This ensures patient safety and provides a position of comfort for the patient.
13. Place the top sheet over the patient with the hems facing up, remove the bath blanket by sliding it out from under the top sheet, and place the blanket or bedspread with the hems facing down.
    Keep the rough edges of bed linens away from the patient's skin to prevent skin irritation.
14. Follow procedure steps 8 through 12 in the Unoccupied Bed section.
    Linens are secured on the bed, providing a clean and neat appearance.

Follow postprocedure steps I through VI.

POSTPROCEDURE

I. Return the bed to its lowest position, raise the top side rails, and verify that the call light is within reach for the patient.
   Precautions are taken to maintain patient safety. Top side rails aid in positioning and turning. Raising four side rails is considered a restraint.
II. Assess for additional patient needs and state the time of your expected return.
   Meeting patient needs and offering self promote patient satisfaction and build trust.
III. Properly dispose of PPE.
   Gloves, gowns, and masks must be appropriately discarded to prevent the spread of microorganisms.
IV. Clean equipment if it was in contact with the patient; see specific manufacturer instructions.
   Disinfection eliminates most microorganisms from inanimate objects.
V. Perform hand hygiene.
   Frequent hand hygiene prevents the spread of infection.
VI. Document the date, time, assessment, procedure, and patient's response to the procedure.
   Accurate documentation is essential to communicate patient care and to provide legal evidence of care.

SUMMARY OF LEARNING OUTCOMES

LO 27.1 *Describe the importance of hygiene related to skin, hair, nails, and mucous membranes:* Caring for patients' basic needs of cleanliness and hygiene is at the core of nursing care. Diligent hygienic care provides patient comfort and prevents infections and odors.

LO 27.2 *Identify how alterations in skin, hair, nails, and mucous membranes affect hygienic care:* Alterations in skin, hair, nails and mucous membranes affect the care plan. Care is taken to minimize and heal existing problems and prevent new alterations from developing.

LO 27.3 *Determine patients' hygiene status and need for assistance with care:* Self-care deficits lead to open skin lesions, infection, body odor, and halitosis, which are evident during assessment. Assessment determines the level of assistance needed for the patient's hygienic care while in a care facility or after discharge.

LO 27.4 *Select nursing diagnoses for patients who need assistance with hygiene or are experiencing alterations in self-care abilities:* Some nursing diagnoses related to hygiene are *Bathing Self-Care Deficit, Dressing Self-Care Deficit, Readiness for Enhanced Self-Care, Ineffective Health Maintenance,* and *Disturbed Body Image.*

LO 27.5 *Establish measurable, patient-centered goals for patients with hygiene concerns and self-care alterations:* The planning phase of the nursing process involves prioritizing hygiene-related nursing diagnoses, evaluating patient self-care abilities and resources, and setting realistic goals and outcomes.

LO 27.6 *Implement nursing care plans that include interventions to address the hygienic needs of patients:* Specific nursing interventions are designed to provide thorough hygienic care for patients who cannot care for themselves and to encourage self-care by patients who are able to attend to some of their own hygiene needs.

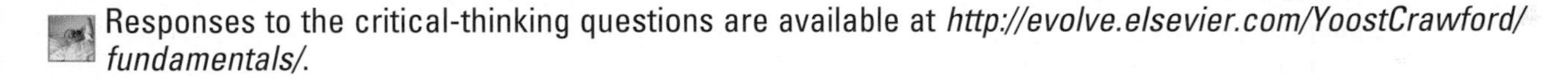
Responses to the critical-thinking questions are available at *http://evolve.elsevier.com/YoostCrawford/fundamentals/.*

REVIEW QUESTIONS

1. An ambulatory diabetic patient states that she is unable to reach her feet to clip her toenails. The patient's toenails are long and thick. What is the next step the nurse should take?
   a. Soak the patient's feet, and trim her toenails using clippers.
   b. Delegate foot care of this patient to the unlicensed assistive personnel (UAP).
   c. Assess the patient's self-care status.
   d. Ask for a referral to a podiatrist.
2. An alert and oriented elderly male patient has been admitted to the hospital with a diagnosis of chronic obstructive pulmonary disease (COPD). He is unshaven, has unkempt hair, and has a foul body odor. Asking which hygiene-related assessment question is a priority for the nurse?
   a. "Do you have friends or family nearby?"
   b. "Can you raise your arms up to brush your teeth?"
   c. "Do you become short of breath during your shower?"
   d. "Are you able to get in and out of your bed at home?"
3. Which action by a female patient lets the nurse know that the patient has understood perineal care teaching?
   a. The patient washes her perineum with a circular motion beginning at the urinary meatus.
   b. The patient washes her perineum from front to back using a clean washcloth.
   c. The patient washes her perineum from back to front with long, firm strokes.
   d. The patient washes her perineum lightly to prevent tissue damage.
4. What should the nurse do before leaving a patient's room after giving a complete bed bath?
   a. Place the call light within reach, and leave the bed as it was during the bath.
   b. Lower the bed to its lowest position, raise all four side rails so that the patient does not fall out of bed, and place the call light within reach.
   c. Lower the bed to its lowest position, raise the top two side rails to assist the patient in turning and positioning, and place the call light within reach.
   d. Leave the bed in a position that is comfortable for the caregiver because more care will be needed, raise the top two side rails, and place the call light within reach.

5. Which actions by the nurse concerning oral care on an unconscious patient are considered safe? *(Select all that apply.)*
   a. Performing oral care with the patient in a supine position
   b. Performing oral care with the patient turned to the side
   c. Installing suction equipment at the bedside
   d. Providing oral care every 2 hours
   e. Using a hard-bristle toothbrush
6. Which safety precaution is a priority for the nurse when bathing a patient with peripheral neuropathy?
   a. Keeping the top two side rails up during the bath
   b. Checking the bath water temperature before the bath
   c. Encouraging independence with perineal care during the bath
   d. Facilitating range-of-motion exercises and dangling before the bath
7. Which nursing diagnosis is a priority for a patient who needs assistance with activities of daily living?
   a. *Self-Care Deficit*
   b. *Deficient Knowledge*
   c. *Risk for Activity Intolerance*
   d. *Readiness for Enhanced Self-Care*
8. Which statements are true regarding back massage? *(Select all that apply.)*
   a. Only a licensed massage therapist can perform back massage.
   b. Back massage may stimulate the deep muscles.
   c. Massage provides relaxation and comfort.
   d. Tapotement stimulates the skin.
   e. A massage may promote sleep.
9. A patient diagnosed with head lice has an order for pediculicidal shampoo. Which statement is true about this shampoo?
   a. It can be used only on patients with the ability to stand in the shower.
   b. It can cause central nervous system side effects, including dizziness.
   c. It is used by pregnant women and young children.
   d. It is safe for patients with seizures.
10. Which statement indicates an understanding by the UAP of eye care during a patient's bath using washcloths and a bath basin?
    a. "The eyes are washed with soap and water from the inner canthus to the outer canthus."
    b. "The eyes should always be washed using sterile normal saline and a gauze sponge."
    c. "The eyes are washed from the outer canthus to the inner canthus using water only."
    d. "The eyes are washed with water using a clean part of the washcloth for each eye."

Answers and rationales for the review questions are available at *http://evolve.elsevier.com/YoostCrawford/fundamentals/*.

REFERENCES

American Association of Critical-Care Nurses (AACN): Practice alert: Oral care in the critically ill, *AACN News,* 23(8), 2006. Retrieved from *www.aacn.org/WD/AACNNews/Content/2006/aug-practice.content?menu=Practice.*

Baumann S: A nursing approach to pain in older adults, *Med Surg Nurs,* 18(2):77-82, 2009.

Bittner NP, Gravlin G: Critical thinking, delegation, and missed care in nursing practice, *J Nurs Admin,* 39(3):142-146, 2009.

Booth KA, Wyman TD, Stoia V: *Anatomy, physiology and disease for health professions,* ed. 3, Boston, 2012, McGraw-Hill.

Cohen EJ: Contact lens solutions: Part of the problem, *Arch Ophthalmol,* 127(11):1544-1546, 2009.

Cohen-Mansfield J, Libin A, Marx MS: Nonpharmacological treatment of agitation: A controlled trial of systematic individualized intervention. *J Gerontol Med Sci,* 62A(8):908-916, 2007.

Cronenwett L, Sherwood G, Barnsteiner J, et al: Quality and safety education for nurses, *Nurs Outlook,* 55(3):122-131, 2007.

DePaola DP, Curro FA, Zero DT: Saliva: The precious body fluid, *J Am Dental Assoc,* 139:5S-10S, 2008.

Ettinger RL: Oral health and the aging population, *J Am Dental Assoc,* 138:5S-6S, 2007.

Gulick M, Hasledalen G, Wesa KM: Massage, meditation, and music become tools, *Hospice Manage Advisor, December,* 137-140, 2008.

Jayasakara R: *Dementia: Oral hygiene care* (Evidence Summaries Report). Adelaide, South Australia, 2009, Joanna Briggs Institute.

Keay L, Edwards K, Stapleton F: An evidenced-based brochure to educate contact lens wearers about safe contact lens wear, *Clin Exp Optom,* 92(5):407-409, 2009.

Lamster IB: Antimicrobial mouth rinses and the management of periodontal disease: Introduction to the supplement, *J Am Dental Assoc,* 137(11):5S-9S, 2006.

Malkin B, Berridge P: Guidance on maintaining personal hygiene in nail care, *Nurs Stand,* 23(41):35-38, 2009.

McKinley M, O'Laughlin VD: *Human anatomy,* ed. 3, Boston, 2012, McGraw-Hill.

Pullen RL: Tips for communicating with a patient from another culture, *Nursing,* 37(10):48-49, 2007.

Vollman K, Garcia R, Miller L: Interventional patient hygiene: Proactive (hygiene) strategies to improve patients' outcomes, *AACN News,* 22(8):12-16, 2005.

Watt KG, Swarbrick HA: Trends in microbial keratitis associated with orthokeratology, *Eye Contact Lens,* 36(6):373-377, 2007.

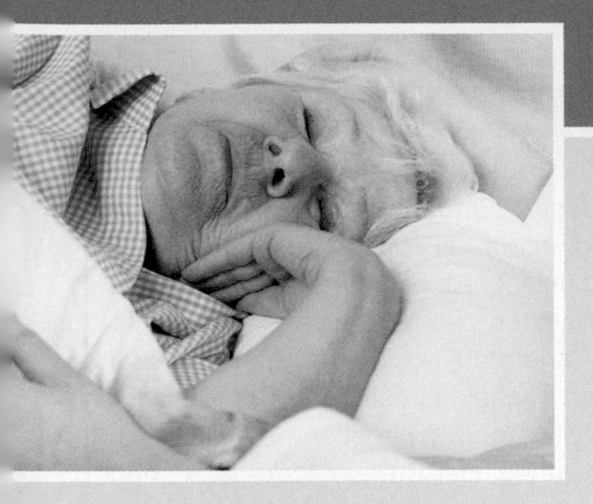

CHAPTER 28

Activity, Immobility, and Safe Movement

EVOLVE WEBSITE

http://evolve.elsevier.com/YoostCrawford/fundamentals/

- Additional Evolve-Only Review Questions With Answers
- Answers and Rationales for Text Review Questions
- Answers to Critical-Thinking Questions
- Case Study With Questions
- Glossary
- Video Skills Clips
- Conceptual Care Map Creator
- Skills Checklists
- Animations

LEARNING OUTCOMES

Comprehension of this chapter's content will provide students with the ability to:

LO 28.1 Describe the function of the musculoskeletal, neurologic, and cardiopulmonary systems in normal activity and movement.

LO 28.2 Identify changes in the musculoskeletal, neurologic, and cardiopulmonary systems that cause alterations in activity and movement throughout the life span.

LO 28.3 Assess the effects of decreased activity and immobility on multiple body systems.

LO 28.4 Discuss nursing diagnoses for patients experiencing immobility and impaired levels of activity.

LO 28.5 Generate nursing care goals and outcome criteria for patients with complications from inactivity or immobility.

LO 28.6 List interventions to enhance patient activity, promote safety, and reverse negative effects of immobility that can be evaluated after implementation.

KEY TERMS

active range of motion, p. 569
aerobic exercise, p. 573
anaerobic exercise, p. 573
atrophy, p. 568
contracture, p. 568
dangling, p. 569
disuse osteoporosis, p. 568
equilibrium, p. 566
flaccidity, p. 567
footdrop, p. 568
friction, p. 588
gait, p. 569
hemiparesis, p. 567
hemiplegia, p. 567
hypertonicity, p. 567
hypotonicity, p. 567
ischemia, p. 567
isometric exercise, p. 573
isotonic exercise, p. 573
logrolling, p. 575
necrosis, p. 571
paraplegia, p. 567
passive range of motion, p. 569
pathologic bone fractures, p. 568
pressure ulcers, p. 571
proprioception, p. 566
quadriplegia, p. 567
range of motion, p. 569
spasticity, p. 567
trapeze, p. 578

CASE STUDY

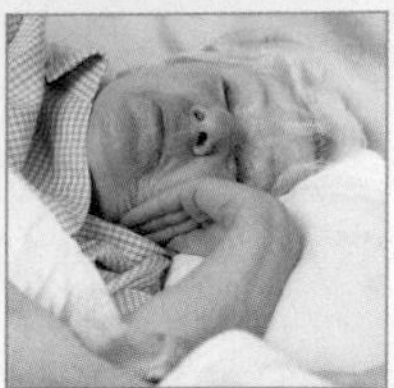

Mrs. Ryan is a 75-year-old female who was admitted to the hospital 72 hours earlier because of a right hip fracture sustained while walking her dog. She is currently 36 hours status post (S/P) total right-hip replacement. She has a medical history of hypertension, no known drug allergies (NKDA), and a full code status.

Mrs. Ryan's vital signs are T 36.6° C (97.9° F), P 84 and regular, R 20 and unlabored, BP 164/90, with a pulse oximetry reading of 99% on room air (RA). She rates her pain as 8 of 10, located primarily at the surgical site when she moves in bed or tries to get up to go to the chair or bathroom. She states, "The pain is sharp and shooting from my hip to midcalf when I move too fast." She grimaces when changing position and is reluctant to move. The right hip incision is well approximated, with slight redness at the edges, no swelling, and minimal serosanguineous drainage on the dressing. Mrs. Ryan complains of weakness and fatigue while bathing or ambulating. Her Braden score is 20, and her Morse Falls Risk score is 80. Her hemoglobin and hematocrit are 10.5 and 36.9, respectively.

Treatment orders are as follows:

- Vital signs q 4 hr, including neurovascular checks
- Adult regular diet
- Intravenous (IV) access saline lock
- Bathroom privileges (BRP) and ambulation with assistance
- Dry, sterile dressing to incision site, change q 8 hr
- Intake and output (I&O)
- Encourage coughing and deep breathing (C&DB)
- Incentive spirometry q 1 hr while awake
- Knee-high antiembolism stockings
- Sequential compression devices (SCDs) while awake and in bed
- Complete blood count (CBC) every morning

Medication orders are as follows:

- Morphine sulfate: 4 mg intravenous piggyback q 4 hr PRN for severe pain
- Lovenox: 60 mg subcutaneously q 12 hr for deep vein thrombus prophylaxis
- Metoprolol: 50 mg PO bid for hypertension

Refer back to this case study to answer the critical-thinking exercises throughout the chapter.

The ability to move has a tremendous impact on the physical health and psychological well-being of individuals. Activity and immobility influence many body systems. Although the methods of safely moving patients have changed significantly in the past decade, the impact of lack of activity and immobility has remained constant. Patients must be encouraged and supported by nurses to achieve or maintain their highest level of independent function. Knowing the effects of activity, immobility, and safe movement is essential to nursing practice.

NORMAL STRUCTURE AND FUNCTION OF MOVEMENT LO 28.1

Movement depends on many body systems. The musculoskeletal, neurologic, and cardiopulmonary systems work together to ensure a person's ability to move and maintain posture, alignment, and balance.

MUSCULOSKELETAL SYSTEM

The musculoskeletal system provides the framework for movement. Five types of bones in conjunction with muscles, tendons, ligaments, cartilage, and joints provide the essential components of this system. Bones are classified by their shape: long (femur), short (carpal), flat (skull), irregular (vertebrae), and sesamoid or round (patella) (Shier, Butler, and Lewis, 2012). Bones such as the rib cage protect critical organs in the body. Bones assist in the maintenance of calcium and phosphorus balance and the production of blood cells.

Skeletal muscles consist of contractile tissue. They provide stability and facilitate posture and movement. Ligaments connect bones and cartilage to bones, and tendons connect muscles to bones. Joints can be classified according to their ability to move or by tissue type: fibrous (immobile), cartilaginous (slightly movable), and synovial (movable). View the animation on action potential and muscle contraction for further information.

NERVOUS SYSTEM

The nervous system controls voluntary movement, posture, balance, and gait (Figure 28-1). The cerebral cortex regulates motor activity, with coordination primarily controlled by the cerebellum. Motor activity on the right side of the body is controlled by the motor fibers on the left side of the brain, and motor activity on the left side of the body is controlled by the motor fibers on the right side of the brain.

Neurotransmitters communicate electrical impulses from nerves to muscles, facilitating movement. The nervous system controls posture and gait through **proprioception** (awareness of posture and movement) and balance. **Equilibrium** (balance) depends on the cerebellum and inner ear. Inner ear fluid

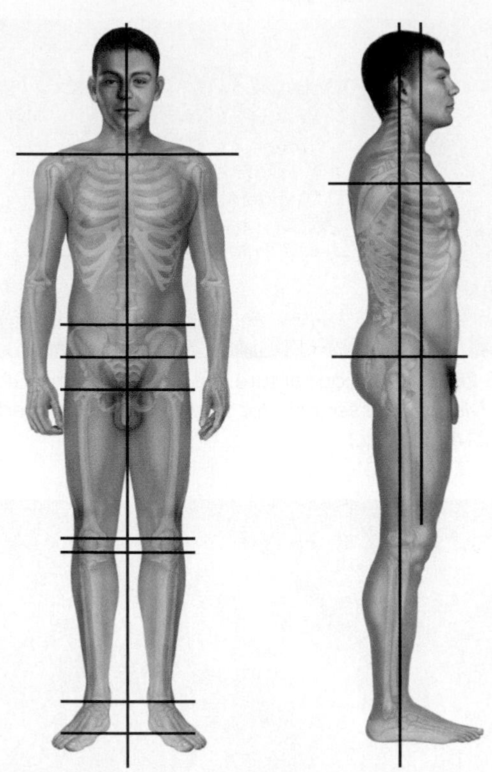

FIGURE 28-1 Correct upright body alignment.

remaining stationary when the head moves quickly allows a person to maintain balance.

CARDIOPULMONARY SYSTEM

The cardiopulmonary system provides oxygen and circulates nutrients to body tissues. Blood circulates throughout the body, supplying bones, muscles, and organ tissues with oxygen, chemicals, and fluids that are essential for normal cell function. Adequate circulation and oxygenation are needed for movement and exercise.

ALTERED STRUCTURE AND FUNCTION OF MOVEMENT LO 28.2

The musculoskeletal, nervous, and cardiopulmonary systems coordinate to facilitate normal body movement. Alterations in any of these systems may lead to impaired mobility or decreased capacity for exercise. Impaired mobility has serious implications for patient well-being and treatment outcomes.

MUSCULOSKELETAL SYSTEM

Impairment or injury of any component of the musculoskeletal system affects the body's ability to move. Inadequate dietary intake of calcium and vitamin D or impaired calcium metabolism may result in osteoporosis, which increases bone fragility and may lead to fractures. The animation "Osteoporosis" provides additional information on this common disease in older adults. Decreased physical exercise and lack of weight bearing exercise also contribute to bone fragility, deterioration, and loss of strength. **Flaccidity** or **hypotonicity** (lack of muscle tone) may result from lack of physical activity, injury, or neurologic impairment.

Many factors cause alterations that affect the musculoskeletal system (Diversity Considerations box). Rheumatoid arthritis and osteoarthritis cause inflammation of joints, resulting in pain and limited joint mobility. View the animation "Osteoarthritis and Rheumatoid Arthritis" for more information on these disease processes. Genetic disorders such as muscular dystrophy result in muscle weakness and gradual muscle wasting, causing difficulty with maintaining posture and impairing mobility.

DIVERSITY CONSIDERATIONS

Life Span

- Children with developmental disorders such as cerebral palsy or genetic disorders such as spina bifida may have limited mobility. Assessment may reveal **spasticity** or **hypertonicity** (increased muscle tone), which results in reduced range of motion and abnormal movement patterns. Flaccidity may also affect movement.
- Osteoporosis (loss of bone mass) and osteoarthritis (deterioration of joint cartilage) are two diseases prevalent in the older adult population that cause reduced mobility. Bones deteriorate in osteoporosis, and joint tenderness results from cartilage breakdown in osteoarthritis.

Gender, Culture, and Morphology

- Small-framed individuals and Caucasian and Asian women are at greatest risk for osteoporosis (Schiff, 2012).
- In midlife, loss of bone mineral density usually increases in men and women (National Osteoporosis Foundation, 2014).

NERVOUS SYSTEM

Damage to the cerebrum or cerebellum and spinal cord injury impair a person's ability to ambulate and control movement. **Ischemia** (reduced blood flow) or brain injury to the right side of the brain results in left-sided **hemiparesis** (weakness on one side of the body) or **hemiplegia** (paralysis of one side of the body). Left-sided brain injury results in right-sided hemiparesis or hemiplegia. These types of limitations can be caused by strokes (i.e., cerebrovascular accidents [CVAs]) and traumatic brain injuries. The level and severity of a spinal cord injury determines the limitations associated with movement. **Paraplegia** (lower body paralysis) and loss of sensation are most commonly associated with lower spinal cord trauma. Cervical spinal cord injuries may result in **quadriplegia** (inability to move all four extremities) and cause difficulty with breathing.

CARDIOPULMONARY SYSTEM

Compromised cardiac function, decreased tissue perfusion, and diminished respiratory capacity directly affect a person's ability to perform activities of daily living (ADLs) and exercise. Congestive heart failure (CHF), peripheral vascular disease, and chronic obstructive pulmonary disease (COPD) decrease the body's ability to deliver oxygen and nutrients to body organs and tissues. Without these essential components, normal cell function is impaired, resulting in diminished capacity for exercise.

ASSESSMENT LO 28.3

Assessment of a person's level of activity and the possible effects of immobility begins with observation and continues by asking a variety of questions (Health Assessment Question box). Answers to these questions provide data about body systems that are affected by a person's activity and agility.

HEALTH ASSESSMENT QUESTIONS

Immobility Focus

- Are you experiencing any stiffness, joint discomfort, or pain with movement?
- How far do you walk each day? Do you ever use any assistive devices such as a walker or cane?
- Have you noticed any dizziness or difficulty with balance?
- Do you require help with your activities of daily living (ADLs)?
- Do you become short of breath or easily fatigued when completing your ADLs?
- How is your appetite? What is your typical dietary intake in a day?
- What is the frequency of your bowel movements?
- Describe your normal sleep pattern.

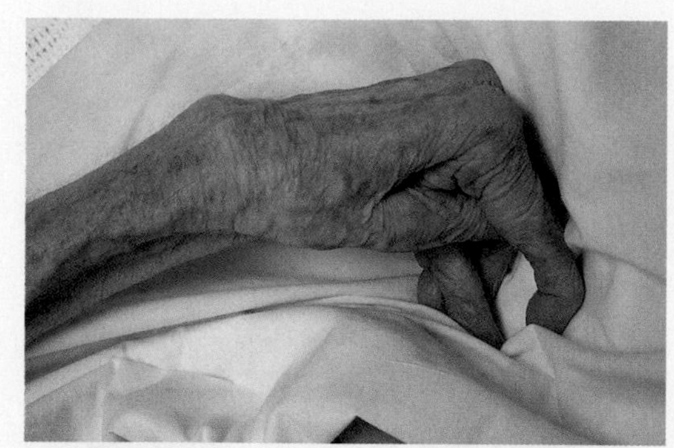

FIGURE 28-2 Joint contracture. (From Sorrentino SA, Remmert L: *Mosby's essentials for nursing assistants,* ed. 5, St. Louis, 2014, Mosby.)

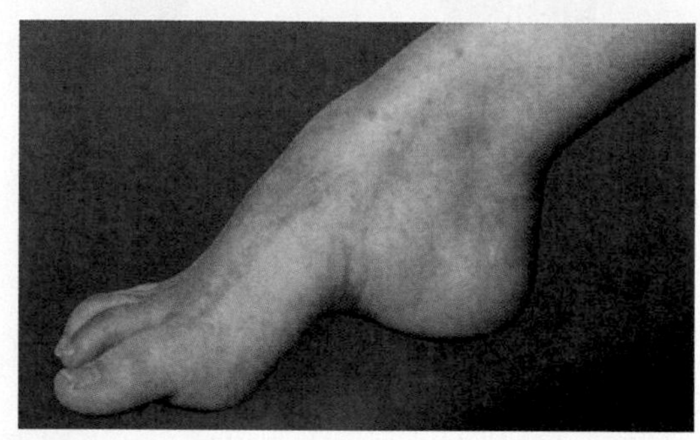

FIGURE 28-3 Footdrop. (From Rosenberg RN: *Atlas of clinical neurology,* ed 2, Current Medicine Group, 2009, Springer Science and Business Media.)

EFFECTS OF IMMOBILITY

Immobility may cause weakness, instability, anorexia, elimination alterations, decreased muscle tone, circulatory stasis, and skin breakdown. Knowing the effects of immobility on various body systems allows the nurse to quickly assess a patient's risk and recognize signs of impending complications.

Musculoskeletal System

Immobility predisposes a person to weakness, decreased muscle tone, decreased bone and muscle mass, muscle **atrophy** (wasting), and **contracture** (permanent fixation of a joint) (Figure 28-2).

Joint contractures can begin within hours of disuse (Fletcher, 2005). The ability of a patient to fully extend the knee joint may be diminished by 15% after only 2 weeks of bed rest (Brower, 2009). **Footdrop** (Figure 28-3), one of the more common contractures, results in permanent plantar flexion. Unused muscles may decrease in mass by half in a few months (Shier, Butler, and Lewis, 2012). Studies indicate that muscle mass diminishes at a rate of 1.5% to 2% daily during the first 14 to 21 days of bed rest (Brower, 2009).

Sustained lack of activity may lead to resorption of bone, causing bones to become less dense and calcium to be released into the bloodstream. Excess calcium is excreted through the kidneys and intestinal tract. Reduced bone density can lead to **disuse osteoporosis** (loss of bone mass due to lack of activity) and **pathologic bone fractures** (spontaneous breaks without trauma).

Joint stiffness and pain with movement, which result from immobility, discourage activity and exercise. The pain scale should be used with particular attention to the behavioral effects of patients' pain and the observed and reported activity tolerance. Lack of muscle tone and weakness increase the incidence of falls, contribute to poor posture, and result in unsteady gait. These musculoskeletal impairments require careful assessment by nurses.

Initial assessment of mobility and patient activity includes observation (i.e., inspection) of the patient's gait and coordination. Observe the patient's position and body alignment standing or lying in bed. Lack of proper body alignment may indicate musculoskeletal abnormalities and lead to increased pain or an unsteady gait.

A fall risk assessment should be completed on all patients at least daily (Nursing Care Guideline box). The Morse Fall Risk Scale and the St. Thomas Risk Assessment Tool in Falling Elderly Inpatients (STRATIFY) (Perell, Nelson, Goldman, et al, 2001) are examples of resources available to nurses (see Chapter 25, Figure 25-3). Nurses should familiarize themselves with facility- or institution-specific guidelines.

NURSING CARE GUIDELINE

Fall Precautions

Background

- Fall risk assessment
  - An initial fall risk assessment must be performed on every patient admitted to any facility.
  - Assessment must be repeated at least daily and more often, as needed, in acute care settings.
- Fall reduction programs
  - Fall reduction is part of The Joint Commission's National Patient Safety Goals.
  - Programs for reducing the number of falls should be outlined in every facility's policies and procedures.

Procedural Concerns

- On the basis of the fall risk assessment score and institutional policy and procedure, implement specialized fall precautions:
  - Frequently observing the patient
  - Placing the patient in a room near the nurses' station
  - Using a low bed
  - Using a mattress or wheelchair seat with pressure alarms
  - Using side rails (use of four side rails is considered a restraint)
- Implement generalized fall precautions:
  - Always return the bed to its lowest position.
  - Keep the call bell within reach of the patient.
    - Remind the patient about how to use the call bell.
    - Immediately answer the call bell if it is sounded.
  - Keep the wheels of any wheeled device (e.g., bed, wheelchair) in the locked position.
  - Leave lights on or off at night, depending on the patient's cognitive status and personal preference.
  - Keep patient belongings (e.g., tissues, water, urinals, personal items) within the patient's reach.
  - Frequently orient and reorient the patient.
  - If the patient is ambulatory, require the use of nonskid footwear.
  - Clear potential obstructions from the walking areas.
  - Ensure that the patient's clothing fits properly; improper fit can cause tripping.

Documentation Concerns

- Document the fall risk assessment and reassessment scores (e.g., Morse Fall Risk score).
- In the general assessment, include the patient's medical history, subjective and objective data, medication review, musculoskeletal status, and history of falls.
- List the use of ambulatory assistive devices.
- Include interventions implemented (specific and general), nursing diagnosis, outcomes, and plan of care.
- Thoroughly document a fall or reported fall:
  - Document the primary concern: nursing care and intervention.
  - Document the fall in accordance with institutional guidelines.
- Include patient and family education.

Evidence-Based Practice

- The Joint Commission (2014) Long Term National Patient Safety Goals seek to prevent falls, especially in the long-term care environment.
- "Falls account for a significant portion of injuries in hospitalized patients, long term care residents, and home care recipients. Organizations should evaluate the resident's risk for falls and take action to reduce the risk of falling as well as the risk of injury, should a fall occur. This evaluation could include a resident's fall history; review of medications and alcohol consumption; gait and balance screening; assessment of walking aids, assistive technologies, and protective devices; and environmental assessments" (The Joint Commission, 2014, p. 6).
- Using palpation, nurses identify muscle strength, muscle tone, and joint **range of motion** (degrees of movement). Muscle strength is measured by asking the patient to squeeze the nurse's hands and having the patient plantar-flex the feet against resistance by the nurse's hands. Nurses must evaluate muscle symmetry by comparing one side of the patient's body with the other. Decreased muscle tone may indicate muscle wasting or atrophy.
- To assess joint range of motion, the nurse asks the patient to actively demonstrate full movement of each joint (**active range of motion**), or the nurse passively moves each joint to the point of resistance while evaluating patient comfort level (**passive range of motion**) (Figure 28-4).

! SAFE PRACTICE ALERT

Stop range-of-motion exercises if the patient begins to complain of pain or if resistance to movement is experienced. Never hyperextend or flex a patient's joints beyond the position of comfort.

Nervous System

The patient's ability to actively perform range of motion may be significantly affected by neurologic alterations. After a prolonged period of immobility, proprioception and equilibrium can be altered. The nurse should assist the patient who is getting out of bed for the first time. **Dangling**, in which the patient sits on the side of the bed before standing, is important to prevent injury to previously nonambulatory patients.

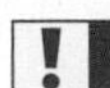

SAFE PRACTICE ALERT

Assess patients for dizziness and their ability to stand unassisted before allowing ambulation.

Observe the patient's **gait** (manner of walking), posture, and balance after a period of bed rest. Problems with

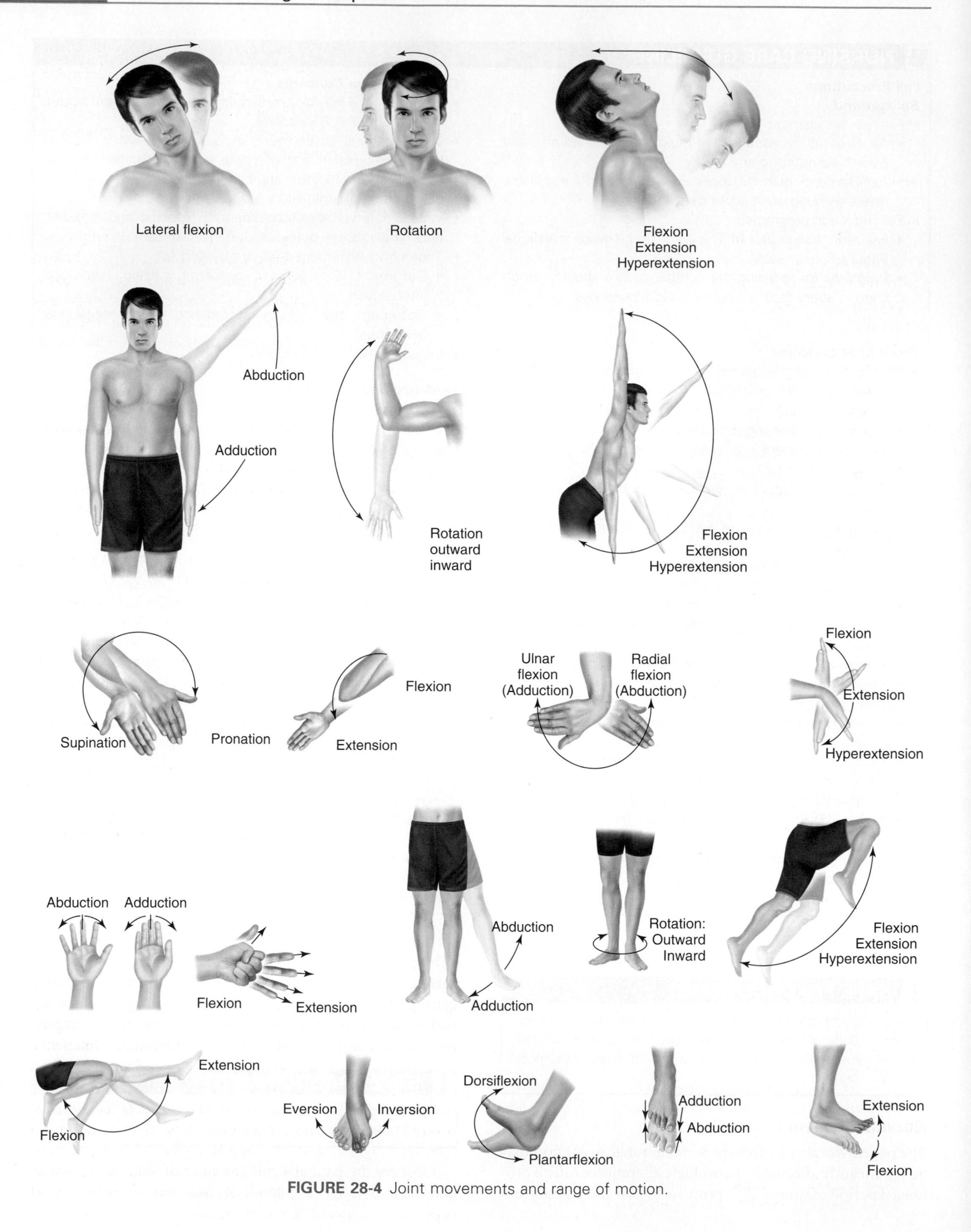

FIGURE 28-4 Joint movements and range of motion.

equilibrium and posture are magnified in patients with cerebellar problems.

Cardiopulmonary System

Bed rest has profound effects on the cardiopulmonary system. The cardiac workload is increased when the body is in the supine position due to increased venous return to the heart. Lung expansion is decreased because the body's weight against the bed puts pressure on the rib cage. The diaphragm has less room to expand than in an upright position due to pressure from abdominal organs. Decreased lung expansion and dependent positioning of areas of the lungs can lead to pooling of secretions in the lungs, pneumonia, or atelectasis.

Circulatory stasis occurs as the heart works harder to pump the circulating blood. The pooled blood combined with weakened calf muscles can lead to deep vein thrombosis (DVT) especially in the lower extremities. When a patient has been immobile, changes in position can result in postural or orthostatic hypotension due to pooling of blood in the lower extremities and lack of vasoconstriction. The heart suddenly has less blood to pump, leading to a drop in blood pressure.

Apical and peripheral pulses and baseline vital signs should be routinely assessed by the nurse for patients who are immobile. It is especially important to monitor blood pressure and pulse when a patient changes position from lying or sitting to standing for the first time. A drop in systolic blood pressure of 20 mm Hg, an increase in heart rate of 20 beats/min, or a drop of diastolic blood pressure of 10 mm Hg when a patient stands is classified as orthostatic hypotension.

Completing a thorough peripheral vascular assessment is essential to identify potential deep vein thromboses and weak pedal pulses due to decreased circulation in the lower extremities (Evidence-Based Practice box). If an area of warmth, redness, swelling, or pain is observed in an extremity, an ultrasound examination may be needed to rule out DVT. Edema may develop from decreased peripheral circulation. Determine whether the edema is nonpitting or pitting, and assess pitting depth by following the guidelines outlined in Chapter 20.

EVIDENCE-BASED PRACTICE

Pulmonary Embolism and Deep Vein Thromboses

- One of the most life-threatening side effects of immobility is a pulmonary embolism (PE). A PE may develop as a result of untreated deep vein thrombosis (DVT).
- Traditionally, Homans sign (calf pain with flexion of the knee and dorsiflexion of the foot) was used in the assessment and diagnosis of DVT.
- Years of research found that Homans sign was an inaccurate method for DVT assessment and potentially dangerous because of possible clot dislodgment.
- Nurses should no longer use Homans sign to assess for DVT.
- More information on the significance of the Homans sign is available at *www.ncbi.nlm.nih.gov/pubmed/10526599*.

Activity intolerance may also develop as a result of bed rest. Observing patients while they complete their ADLs provides insight into the level of activity intolerance. Signs of shortness of breath (SOB) or dyspnea on exertion (DOE) or patient reports of fatigue with minimal activity indicate the significant impact of bed rest.

Nutrition

Diminished activity reduces the basal metabolic rate (BMR). When the BMR decreases, the body begins breaking down muscle protein (i.e., catabolic activity) for energy. Catabolism of protein leads to a negative nitrogen balance in the body if dietary protein is insufficient. Continued immobility may lead to anorexia (decreased appetite) and nausea due to the body's lower nutritional demands. Assess patients for nutritional intake, and monitor serum albumin levels.

Elimination

Immobility has a significant impact on urinary elimination. Urinary stasis may develop due to the dependent position of the bladder when patients are supine. Stagnant urine trapped in the bladder provides a breeding ground for urinary tract infections (UTIs). A combination of urinary stasis and excess calcium excretion due to bone reabsorption associated with disuse osteoporosis increases the risk of renal calculi (i.e., kidney stones) formation. Carefully assess intake and output, the concentration and odor of urine, and the frequency of urination.

Inactivity, decreased appetite, and decreased fluid intake cause hypomotility of the gastrointestinal tract. This is manifested by decreased bowel sounds on auscultation and by constipation. Complete a thorough abdominal assessment by auscultating bowel sounds in all four quadrants and palpating the abdomen for distention and discomfort. Patients' dietary intake should be monitored for adequate fiber and fluid volume while on bed rest. Observe and record the frequency of bowel movements to avoid a potential fecal impaction (buildup of hardened feces in the lower intestine).

Skin

The impact of immobility on skin integrity is potentially catastrophic. Pressure on bony prominences can cause tissue ischemia. Prolonged tissue ischemia may lead to **necrosis** (death of cells, tissues, or organs) and destruction of all layers of the skin, muscle, and fat. **Pressure ulcers** (pressure sores, bedsores, or decubitus ulcers) may develop on areas damaged due to tissue ischemia caused by compression and inactivity. Areas most at risk for pressure ulcers include the buttocks, coccyx, heels, hips, shoulders, elbows, and ears.

Assessment of the skin includes overall observation of color, texture, warmth, and intactness. Special attention should be given to areas that appear darkened in tone or reddened. Assess for tissue blanching and normal reactive hyperemia (increased blood flow after restoration of the blood supply). A standardized skin assessment tool such as the

Braden Scale should be used to identify patients at risk for compromised skin integrity (see Chapter 29, Figure 29-14).

Psychosocial Impact

Isolation may result from inactivity and bed rest, causing a variety of psychosocial challenges for patients. With limited ability to ambulate or interact with people outside their immediate space, immobile patients may become lonely, anxious, angry, depressed, or confused. Sensory deprivation (lack of external stimuli) may result from decreased interaction with others. A patient's self-concept may be altered by the inability to interact with the environment. Traditional coping strategies may not be effective, causing irregular patterns of behavior.

Sleep and rest patterns may be disturbed because of inactivity, environmental noise, constant disruptions for direct care and treatments, and frequent napping throughout the day. Anxiety related to medical diagnoses or concerns may also contribute to dyssomnia (difficulty sleeping).

Observe patients for mood, behavior, and sleep patterns. Interviewing patients regarding their typical hours and nature of sleep is important to establish a baseline. Watch for subtle changes in mood or behavior that may indicate concern related to immobility or isolation.

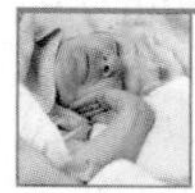

1. List focused assessments with rationales that should be completed on Mrs. Ryan during her second postoperative day.

◆ NURSING DIAGNOSIS LO 28.4

Common nursing diagnoses directly associated with immobility are *Impaired Physical Mobility, Impaired Bed Mobility, Impaired Walking, Impaired Wheelchair Mobility,* and *Impaired Transfer Ability.* Patients also have nursing diagnoses based on the specific effects of immobility on various body systems. Examples of nursing diagnostic statements follow:

Impaired Physical Mobility related to postoperative status after hip fracture as evidenced by inability to ambulate independently, pain with movement, and limited range of motion

Risk for Falls with risk factor of altered mobility secondary to cerebrovascular accident

Activity Intolerance related to the deconditioning effects of bed rest as evidenced by shortness of breath, oxygen saturation below 90%, and pulse rate above 100 with activity

Imbalanced Nutrition: Less than Body Requirements related to decreased desire to eat as evidenced by dietary intake of less than 30%; patient stating, "I just don't feel like eating"; muscle weakness; and weight loss

Constipation related to decreased peristalsis secondary to immobility as evidenced by patient report of no bowel movement for 3 days, abdominal distention, and hypoactive bowel sounds

Impaired Skin Integrity related to ischemia as evidenced by reddened area on left heel, softened left heel tissue, and bed rest restriction

Social Isolation related to therapeutic treatment as evidenced by patient stating, "I feel lonely. No one comes to visit, and I can't get out of bed"; patient appearing anxious; and patient being unable to complete ADLs independently

◆ PLANNING LO 28.5

Carefully consider the importance of each identified nursing diagnosis and address the most critical ones first in the nursing care plan (Table 28-1). Collaboration with patients, families, and members of the health care team is imperative when addressing problems associated with mobility (Collaboration and Delegation box). Short-term and long-term goals must be directed at alleviating the specific problems identified in each nursing diagnosis.

Examples of goals or outcome statements follow:

- Patient will ambulate with the assist of one caregiver within 24 hours.
- Patient will experience no falls during hospitalization.
- Patient's pulse oximetry reading will remain above 92% with activity by the end of the shift.
- Patient will consume 50% of the diet each day.
- Patient will have daily bowel movements.

TABLE 28-1 Care Planning

NANDA-I NURSING DIAGNOSIS LABEL WITH NURSING DIAGNOSIS STATEMENT	NURSING OUTCOME CLASSIFICATION (NOC)	NURSING INTERVENTION CLASSIFICATION (NIC)
Impaired Physical Mobility related to postoperative status following hip fracture as evidenced by inability to ambulate independently, pain with movement, and limited range of motion	*Ambulation* (0200) Walks at slow pace (020003)	*Exercise therapy: Ambulation* (0221) Assist patient to stand and ambulate specified distance with specified number of staff.

From Bulechek G, Butcher H, Dochterman J, et al (Eds): *Nursing interventions classification (NIC),* ed. 6, St. Louis, 2013, Mosby; Moorhead S, Johnson M, Maas M, et al (Eds): *Nursing outcomes classification (NOC),* ed. 5, St. Louis, 2013, Mosby; NANDA International: *Nursing diagnoses: Definitions and classification, 2012–2014,* West Sussex, England, 2012, Wiley-Blackwell. Reprinted with permission from NANDA International, Inc.

- Patient's heels will remain intact without further breakdown for the remainder of the hospital stay.
- Patient's family will visit or call at least every other day during hospitalization and rehabilitation.

COLLABORATION AND DELEGATION

Multidisciplinary Strategy for Care of the Immobilized Patient

- Nurses use a multidisciplinary approach when planning care for immobilized patients to ensure maximal recovery.
- Physical therapists, occupational therapists, and social workers provide ambulation support, assistive devices, activities, and psychosocial resources.
- Dietitians address nutritional concerns.
- Speech therapists evaluate patients' ability to chew and swallow.
- Unlicensed assistive personnel (UAP) provide hands-on care for immobilized patients under the direct supervision of registered nurses. Turning and positioning of patients, range-of-motion exercises, transfers, and assistance with ambulation may be delegated to properly trained UAP.

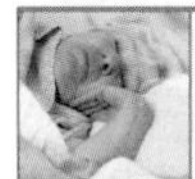

The conceptual care map for Mrs. Ryan provided in Figure 28-5 is partially completed to indicate how to use the map as a learning tool. Using it as an example, go to the website at *http://evolve.elsevier.com/YoostCrawford/fundamentals/* to complete Nursing Diagnoses 2 and 3.

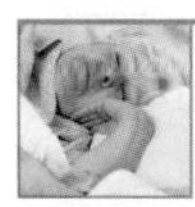

2. Write a short-term and long-term goal for this nursing diagnosis: *Impaired Physical Mobility* related to postoperative limitations as evidenced by a pain rating of 8 of 10, grimacing with movement, and reluctance to move.

IMPLEMENTATION AND EVALUATION LO 28.6

Interventions to address activity and mobility concerns are designed to respond to individual patient needs. Various interventions assist patients with multisystem issues. Critically evaluating interventions and patient outcomes is essential before determining whether the patient's plan of care should be modified, continued, or discontinued.

MUSCULOSKELETAL AND NERVOUS SYSTEM INTERVENTIONS

Exercise is essential to prevent the negative impact of immobility on patients, and it should be encouraged. Early ambulation after injury, illness, or surgery promotes muscle strength, retains joint flexibility, minimizes joint pain and stiffness, and arrests bone reabsorption. Exercises are defined by muscle status (i.e., isotonic or isometric exercise) or by energy source (i.e., aerobic or anaerobic exercise).

- **Isotonic exercise** involves active movement with constant muscle contraction. Examples include walking, turning in bed, and self-feeding.
- **Isometric exercise** requires tension and relaxation of muscles without joint movement. An example is tension and relaxation of pelvic floor muscles (i.e., Kegel exercise).
- **Aerobic exercise** requires oxygen metabolism to produce energy. Patients may engage in rigorous walking or repeated stair climbing to achieve the positive effects of aerobic exercise.
- **Anaerobic exercise** builds power and body mass. Without oxygen to produce energy for activity, anaerobic exercise takes place. Heavy weight lifting is an example of anaerobic exercise.

If patients are restricted to bed rest, active or passive range-of-motion exercises must be employed to prevent joint contractures (see Figure 28-2). It is important to educate patients on the steps they can take to ensure continued mobility (Patient Education and Health Literacy box).

PATIENT EDUCATION AND HEALTH LITERACY

Activity

- Teach patients to actively move each joint to its fullest extent at least four times each day to ensure continued mobility.
- Ask patients to verbalize an understanding of the importance of continued joint movement and demonstrate range of motion of each joint.

Pain is assessed by the nurse during each patient interaction. Nonsteroidal antiinflammatory drugs are used for mild to moderate pain relief and are particularly beneficial for patients with inflammatory disease of the joints. Narcotic analgesics are administered for moderate to severe pain. Medicating patients for pain before activity or positioning enhances the patient's ability to move.

! SAFE PRACTICE ALERT

Monitor the patient's vital signs and stability with position changes when narcotic analgesics are prescribed for pain relief. Potential adverse side effects of narcotics include respiratory depression, hypotension, confusion, sedation, constipation, and dizziness.

Positioning devices help to maintain proper body alignment and positioning of joints. Pillows are used for positioning patients. Placing a pillow between the legs and arms of a side-lying patient helps to prevent pressure on the bony prominences of the knees and elbows. This pillow position is also used when rolling a patient after hip surgery to prevent movement of the femur. A pillow positioned under the calves of a supine patient

Medications
Morphine sulfate 4 mg IVP q 4 hr prn for pain
Lovenox 60 mg SQ q 12 hr
Metoprolol 50 mg PO bid

Conceptual Care Map
Student name________ Patient initials Mrs. R Date ______
Age 75 Gender F Room # ___ Admission date ______
CODE Status Full Allergies NKDA
Diet Adult Regular Activity BRP Braden score 20
Weight ______ Height ______ Religion ______

Lab Values/Diagnostic Test Results
10.5
36.9%
Hemoglobin: 10.5
Norm-women: 12-16 g/dL
Hematocrit: 36.9%
Norm-women: 38%-47%
Preoperative hip x-ray: shattered R femoral head

Admitting Diagnoses/Chief Complaint
R hip fracture; status post (S/P) total right hip replacement

IV Sites/Fluids/Rate
IV saline lock L forearm

Assessment Data
T 36.6, P 84 reg, R 20, B/P 164/90, O_2 saturation 99% on RA, pain 8 of 10 with movement.
Patient states, "The pain is sharp and shooting from my hip to midcalf when I move too fast." Grimaces with movement, reluctant to move.
Right-hip incision is well approximated, with slight redness at edges, no swelling, and minimal serosanguinous drainage on dressing.
C/o weakness and fatigue while bathing or ambulating.
Morse Falls Risk Score is 80.

Past Medical/Surgical History
Hypertension

Treatments
VS q 4 hr, neurovascular checks
Dry sterile dressing to incision site, change q 8 hr
I&O
C&DB, incentive spirometry q 1 hr while awake
Knee-high TED hose
SCDs while awake and in bed
CBC q am
Ambulate with assistance

Primary Nursing Diagnosis
Impaired Physical Mobility related to postoperative status following hip fracture as evidenced by inability to ambulate independently, pain with movement, and limited range of motion.

Supporting Data
Pain rating of 8 of 10. Grimacing with movement. Reluctant to move.

STG/NOC
Patient will ambulate with the assist of one within 24 hr.
NOC: Ambulation (0200)
Walks at slow pace (020003)

Interventions/NIC With Rationale
1. Medicate patient regularly or at least 1 hour prior to planned ambulation to moderate pain level and reduce muscle spasms and tension.
2. Encourage patient to participate in physical therapy and range-of-motion exercises, as prescribed, to strengthen muscles.
3. Encourage participation in ADLs to promote independence and patient control of progress.
4. Provide encouragement for patient efforts to boost confidence and promote psychological well-being.

NIC: Exercise therapy: Ambulation (0221)
Assist patient to stand and ambulate specified distance with specified number of staff

Rationale Citation/EBP
Yoost BL, Crawford LR: *Fundamentals of nursing: Active learning for collaborative practice,* St. Louis, 2016, Mosby.

Evaluation
Patient walking with assistance of two within 24 hr. Expressing pain level of 5 following preambulation analgesia administration. Continue plan of care.

Nursing Diagnosis 2

Supporting Data

STG/NOC

Interventions/NIC With Rationale

Rationale Citation/EBP

Evaluation

Nursing Diagnosis 3

Supporting Data

STG/NOC

Interventions/NIC With Rationale

Rationale Citation/EBP

Evaluation

FIGURE 28-5 Partially completed conceptual care map based on Mrs. Ryan, the case study patient in this chapter.

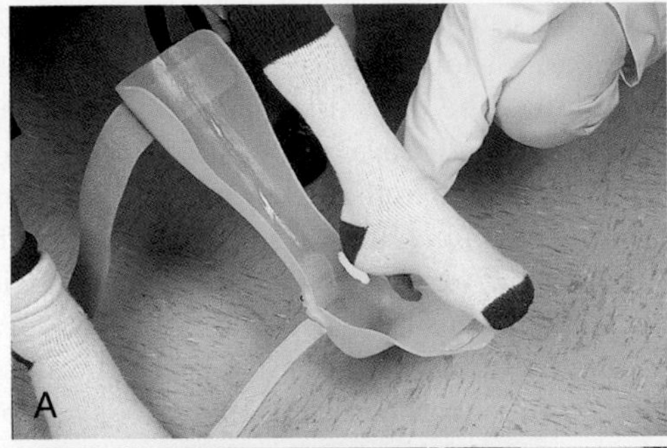

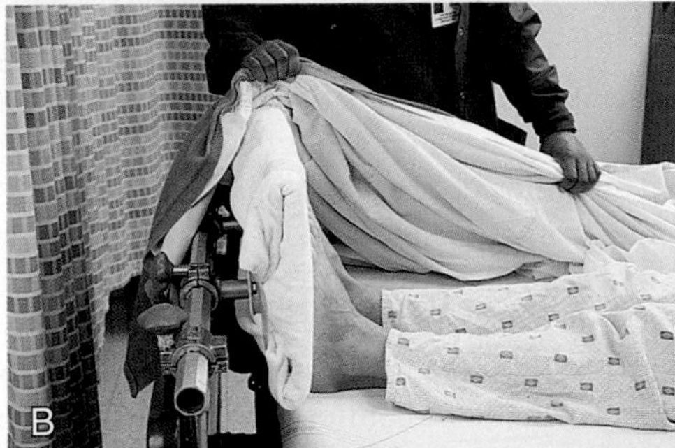

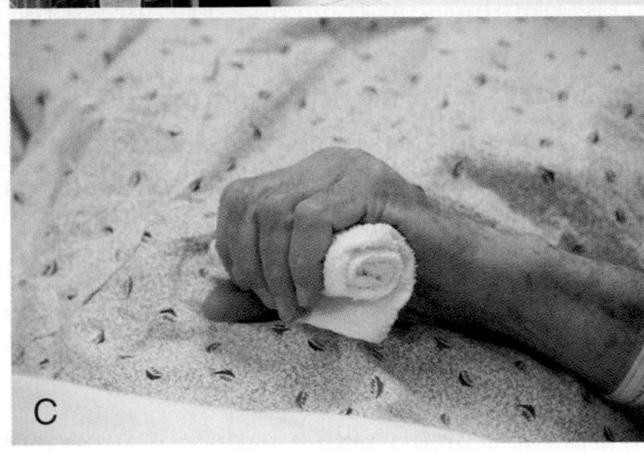

FIGURE 28-6 Splints and braces are used on extremities to keep joints in functional positions. **A,** Ankle-foot orthotic. **B,** Foot board. **C,** Hand roll. (**A** and **B** from Sorrentino SA, Remmert L: *Mosby's textbook for nursing assistants*, ed. 8, St. Louis, 2012, Mosby.)

alleviates pressure on the heels but should not impede circulation in the calves. Pillows can also be used to support a body part in a functional position or to elevate an injured extremity.

Splints and braces are used on extremities to keep joints in functional positions (Figure 28-6). An ankle-foot orthotic (AFO) is a brace or splint that holds the foot at a right angle to the leg. This device is used to prevent footdrop. A footboard at the end of the bed or high-top tennis shoes can have the same effect. Custom-made splints for the upper extremities can maintain proper alignment of the hand and wrist. Hand rolls may be used to keep the hand in a functional position and prevent contractures on a short-term basis. Long-term use of hand rolls should not be employed to prevent the stimulation of flexion. Hand rolls can be specially made, or a washcloth can be rolled and placed in the patient's palm.

Trochanter rolls are used to keep the hip from externally rotating when the patient is in the supine position. One can be made by rolling a large towel or bath blanket and placing

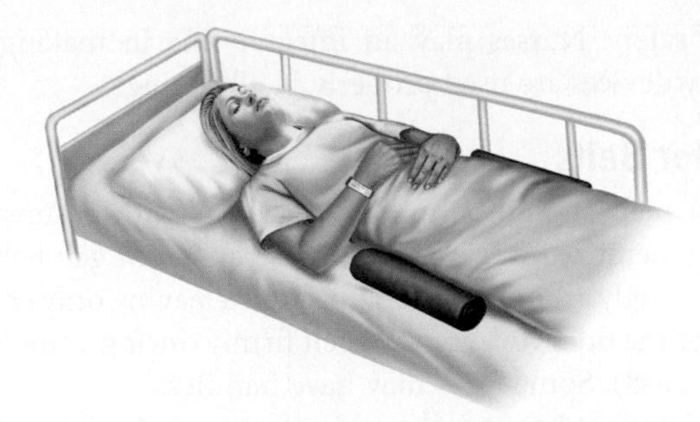

FIGURE 28-7 Trochanter roll positioned next to the patient.

it alongside the patient's hip joint (Figure 28-7). This type of positioning aid is often used after hip surgery.

Patients with spinal cord injuries or after surgery may require **logrolling** (moving the whole body as a unit) during positioning (Skill 28-1). The assistance of at least one or two caregivers in addition to the nurse is required. The nurse must ensure that the patient's spine remains aligned during repositioning. A pillow is placed between the patient's legs during logrolling and may remain there if the patient is in the side-lying position.

! SAFE PRACTICE ALERT

Smooth movement that maintains straight and stabilized alignment of the patient's spine prevents possible injury.

Fall prevention is a high priority for patients with unsteady gait, poor posture, or balance concerns. Encourage patients who have been immobile to call for assistance before ambulation. The importance of allowing a previously nonambulatory patient to dangle on the side of the bed before ambulation to prevent injury cannot be overstated.

A variety of nursing interventions can provide support to ensure patient safety. Observe patients' rooms for physical obstacles, including electrical and call light cords, intravenous and oxygen tubing, drains and catheters, phone cords, and other potential tripping hazards. Keep linens off the floor. Clean up spills immediately. Provide nonskid slippers and barrier-free access to the bathroom.

! SAFE PRACTICE ALERT

Assisting patients to ambulate who have intravenous therapy, nasogastric tubes, or urinary catheters helps to prevent falls.

Position needed items within reach of the patient, including the call light and over-the-bed table. Patients at risk for falls should be assigned to rooms close to the nurses' station. Sitters or family members at the bedside may be helpful in situations that require constant monitoring.

Ambulation aids such as transfer (ambulation or gait) belts, crutches, canes, walkers, or mobile ambulation devices should be used to promote safety for weak or unsteady patients. Each device has specific procedures associated with its use to ensure patient safety. Nurses play an integral role in making sure mobility devices are used properly in all settings.

Transfer Belts

Transfer belts should be used for patients with an unsteady gait or generalized weakness. Canvas transfer or gait belts are applied snugly around the patient's waist, leaving only enough room for the nurse to grasp the belt firmly during ambulation (Figure 28-8). Some belts may have handles.

If the patient has a weaker side, the nurse should stand on that side and hold the gait belt firmly at the back of the patient's waist while ambulating (Skill 28-2).

Canes

Patients who need additional support when walking due to balance problems or weakness may use a cane. Canes may be straight, wooden or metal, and have one point of support on the ground or four points of support (quad cane). Figure 28-9 shows types of canes.

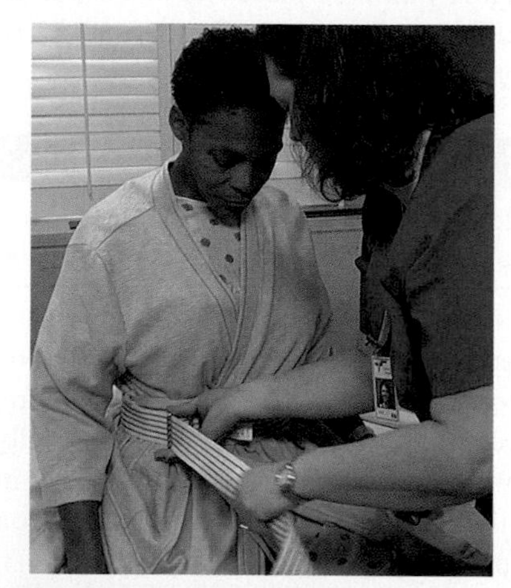

FIGURE 28-8 Placing a gait belt on a patient.

The top of the cane should be level with the hip joint, and the patient's arm should be comfortably bent when the patient is walking. The patient should hold the cane on his or her stronger side and move the cane forward first, followed by the weaker leg and then the stronger leg. This ensures that another point of support is always on the ground when the weaker leg is bearing weight and gives the patient a wide base of support. A patient using a cane should be encouraged to stand up straight and look forward. Leaning to one side or looking down can jeopardize safety and cause poor posture.

Crutches

Crutches facilitate increased patient mobility. Different types of crutches may be used on a short-term or long-term basis for patients with lower extremity injury or paralysis (Figure 28-10). Underarm crutches should be fitted to allow approximately 2 inches or three finger widths of space between the top of the crutch and the axilla when the crutch is placed slightly in front of and 6 inches to the side of the foot. The patient's elbow should be comfortably bent to avoid pressure on the nerve running into the axilla. Encourage the patient to immediately report tingling in the hands. Forearm or Lofstrand crutches are traditionally used for patients with long-term or permanent impairment. Forearm crutches are designed with a handgrip and a metal cuff that partially or completely surrounds the lower arm.

Patients need to possess adequate upper body strength and coordination when using all types of crutches. The crutch-walking pattern employed depends on the extent and nature of the patient's disability.

The two-point crutch-walking pattern is used by patients who can bear partial weight on either or both lower extremities. This method provides stability and support for ambulation. Patients move one crutch forward simultaneously with the opposite leg, providing a wide base of support.

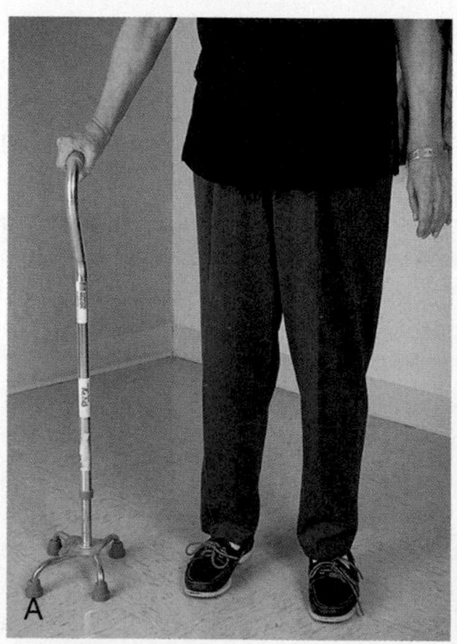

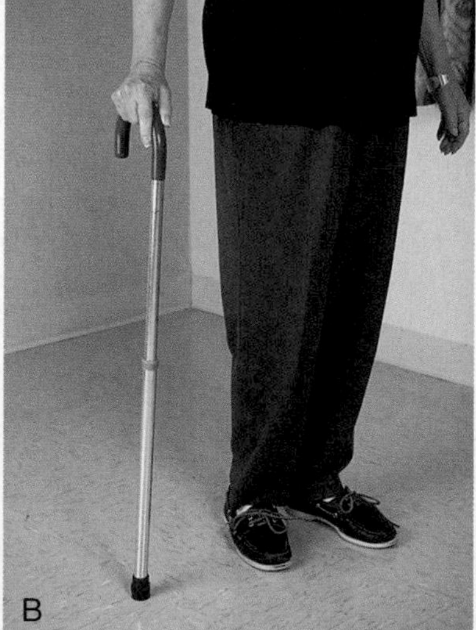

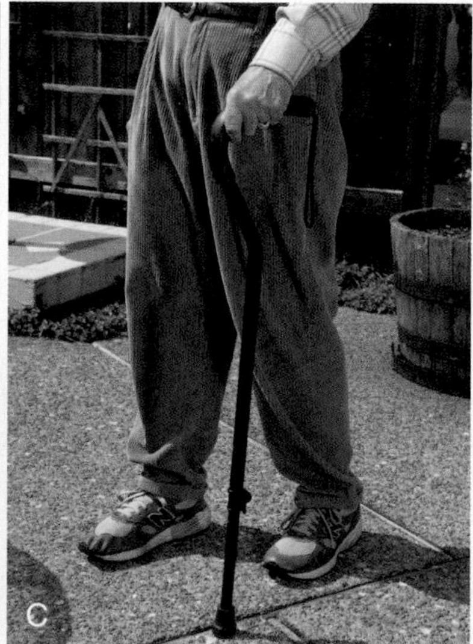

FIGURE 28-9 Types of canes. **A,** Quad cane. **B,** Curved-handle aluminum cane. **C,** Offset-handle cane. (**A** and **B** from Sorrentino SA, Remmert L: *Mosby's textbook for nursing assistants*, ed. 8, St. Louis, 2012, Mosby; **C** from Birchenall JM: *Mosby's textbook for the home care aide*, ed. 3, St. Louis, 2013, Mosby.)

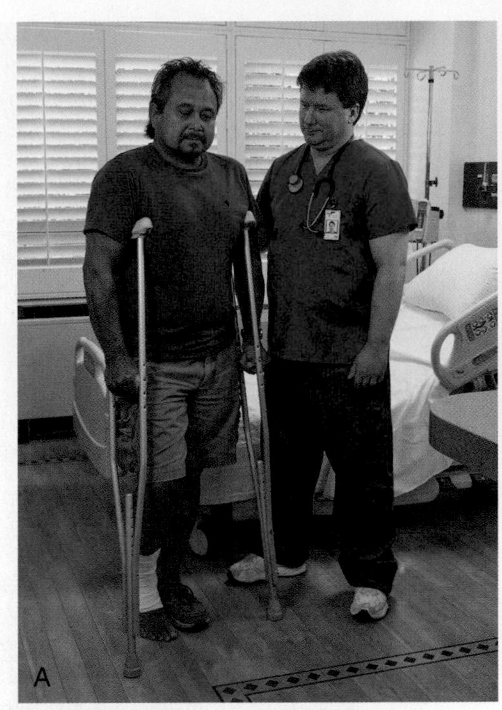
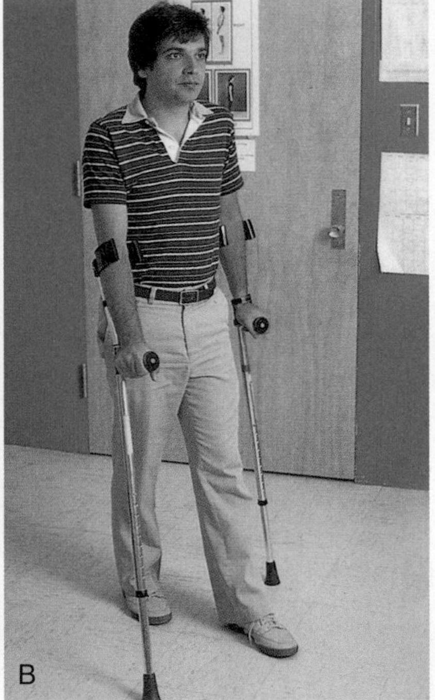

FIGURE 28-10 Types of crutches. **A,** Underarm. **B,** Forearm. (**B** from Sorrentino SA, Remmert L: *Mosby's textbook for nursing assistants*, ed. 8, St. Louis, 2012, Mosby.)

Three-point crutch walking is employed by patients who have injury to one leg. To begin this gait pattern, both crutches are placed forward, and patients swing their legs through, bearing weight on only the uninjured leg. A similar pattern, commonly referred to as a *swing-through gait*, is used by paraplegics. In this method, patients place the crutches forward and then swing their lower extremities simultaneously through the crutches to facilitate forward movement.

The four-point crutch gait requires partial weight bearing on both lower extremities. This provides more stability than the two-point pattern, because only one of four points of support is lifted off the floor at any time. In this ambulation technique, the patient moves one crutch forward, followed by the opposing leg, and repeats the pattern by moving the opposite crutch and then the leg forward. Skill 28-3 illustrates the different crutch-walking patterns.

Figure 28-11 shows a patient with crutches ascending stairs. A gait belt is in place, and a caregiver is spotting. The patient transfers weight from the crutches to the unaffected leg on the stairs. The crutches are then brought up onto the stair and aligned with the unaffected leg. In descending stairs (Figure 28-12), body weight is transferred from the unaffected leg to the crutches. The unaffected leg is then brought down onto the stair and aligned with the crutches.

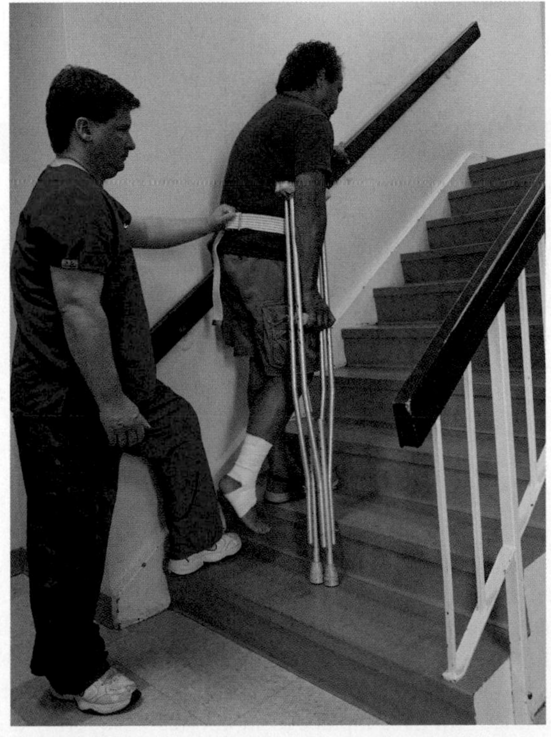

FIGURE 28-11 Use of crutches to ascend stairs.

Walkers

Walkers are metal ambulation aids that come with and without wheels. They provide more support than a cane and can be used for patients who have weakness or balance problems or who are recovering from back or leg injuries. Walkers should be waist high and slightly wider than the patient.

A walker without wheels is used in a manner similar to crutches. While standing in the walker, the patient lifts the walker forward one step, plants it on the ground, and then steps into the walker. This type of device can be used in the same manner as a three-point crutch walk: The patient lifts the walker forward one step and then swings both legs into it. Caution

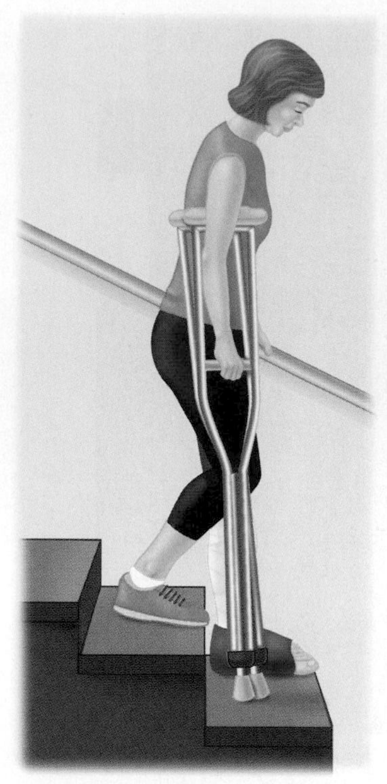

FIGURE 28-12 Use of crutches to descend stairs.

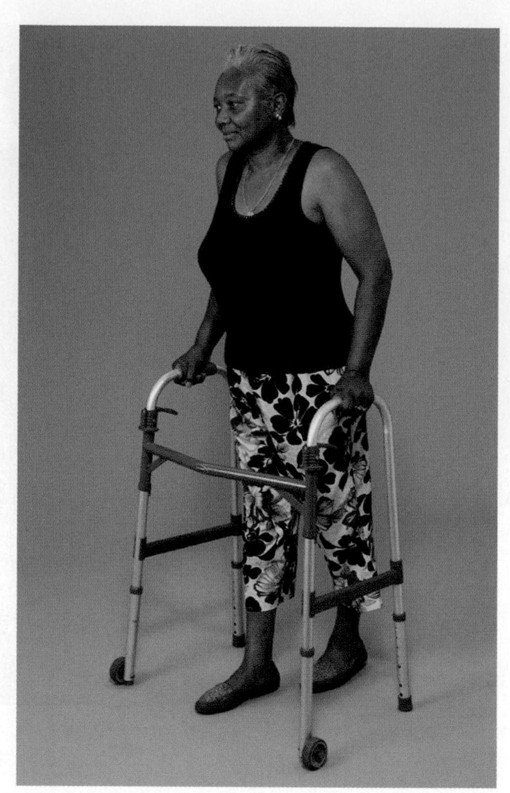

FIGURE 28-13 Ambulation with a front wheel walker. (From Sorrentino SA, Remmert L: *Mosby's textbook for nursing assistants*, ed. 8, St. Louis, 2012, Mosby.)

must be taken to prevent loss of balance. A home assessment should be conducted for the patient being discharged with an assistive device (Home Care Considerations box).

HOME CARE CONSIDERATIONS

Home Assessment Before Discharge

Patients being discharged with assistive devices such as canes, walkers, and crutches should have a home assessment to ensure safety during ambulation.

- Are the patient's living quarters on one floor?
- Are there throw rugs that pose a tripping hazard?
- Are nonskid mats in place in front of sinks, tubs, and showers?
- Is there a clear way to exit in case of emergency?

Front-wheel walkers are used for patients who need support when walking but do not have the strength to pick up a walker and move it forward. The patient must be able to bear weight on both legs to use a front-wheel walker. The patient pushes the walker ahead while ambulating. Three- and four-wheel walkers with seats, baskets, and brakes are available. They can be used for patients who have activity intolerance and need a place to sit and rest frequently during ambulation. Figure 28-13 shows a front wheel walker.

Mechanical Lifts

Mechanical lifts and lift teams are preferred transfer methods to decrease the incidence of patient and staff injuries. Mobile mechanical lift devices and some overhead lifts can be used for ambulation when equipped with a special harness. The patient is placed in the harness and lifted to a point where the feet are just touching the ground. The patient walks holding onto the lift device. This is an extremely safe method for ambulating an unsteady patient because the patient's weight is supported by the lift device. If the patient becomes unsteady, the mechanical lift prevents falls and injuries (Nursing Care Guideline box).

Safe Patient Movement

Nurses have a history of injuries from moving and lifting patients. Maximizing patient assistance in movement and proper use of lift equipment when needed can drastically reduce injuries to nurses (Nelson, 2006).

If patients on bed rest have some mobility, the nurse should teach them to shift their position every 15 minutes while awake. Top side rails should be left up to aid in positioning. Patients with upper body strength can use a **trapeze** (triangular device suspended above the bed) to facilitate repositioning and transfers.

As with many of the complications of bed rest, early ambulation can greatly diminish problems with skin integrity. Patients who lack upper body strength or the ability to move independently may require the assistance of specialized positioning equipment (Nursing Care Guideline box).

The first step in safely moving patients is to assess their ability to assist. A useful assessment tool for safe patient handling and movement (SPHM) is shown in Figure 28-14.

NURSING CARE GUIDELINE

Mechanical Lift Devices

Background

- The National Institute for Occupational Safety and Health (NIOSH) and the American Nurses Association (ANA) support the Safe Patient Handling and Movement Guidelines released in March 2010. Under these guidelines and position statements, manual lifting should be used in a few extreme situations instead of using mechanical lift devices, such as the following:
  - Life-threatening situations
  - For pediatric or small patients
  - For patients who mostly are bearing their own weight
- Mechanical lift devices
  - Are hand operated or electrically operated
  - Are used to prevent injury to caregivers when transferring patients

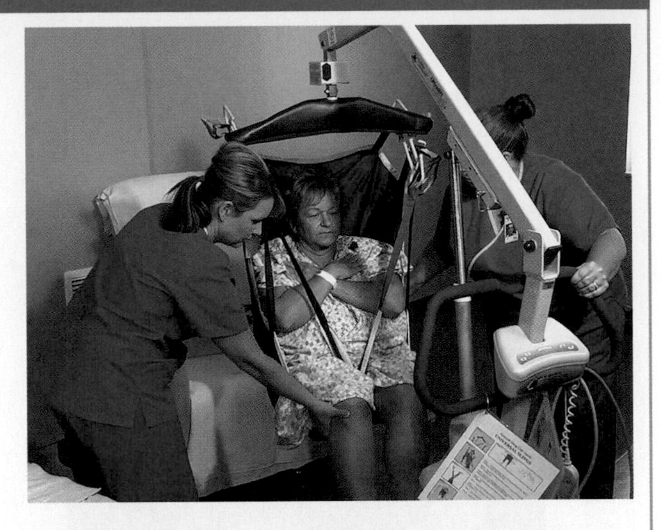

Procedural Concerns

- Facility- and equipment-specific training is required before use of mechanical lift devices.
- Devices should be checked for operational status before use.
- The proper and safe use of all mechanical lift devices requires at least two health care professionals or unlicensed assistive personnel (UAP), but it is recommended that at least three caregivers carry out the procedure.
- There are algorithms for determining the appropriate lift device and number of caregivers needed to move a patient:
  - The algorithms were created by the Department of Veterans Affairs and are recommended by the ANA and NIOSH.
  - Nurses should refer to facility-specific policies and procedures to determine the proper lifting choices.
- Each mechanical lift has a weight limit assigned to it by the manufacturer of the device. This can usually be found on the device or in the operator's manual. Know the patient's weight and the weight limit of the device to avoid exceeding the weight limit, which risks injury to the patient or staff.
- The following are specific types of mechanical lift devices:
  - *Hydraulic lifts* are also known as *Hoyer lifts* or *powered full-body lifts.* They have independently mounted sling devices for non–weight-bearing or immobile patients.
  - *Ceiling lifts* have a ceiling-mounted track sling and stay in the patient's room, which helps maintain infection control standards.
  - *Stand-up assist lifts* use a hydraulic sling lift for partial-weight-bearing and cooperative patients, and they promote independence.

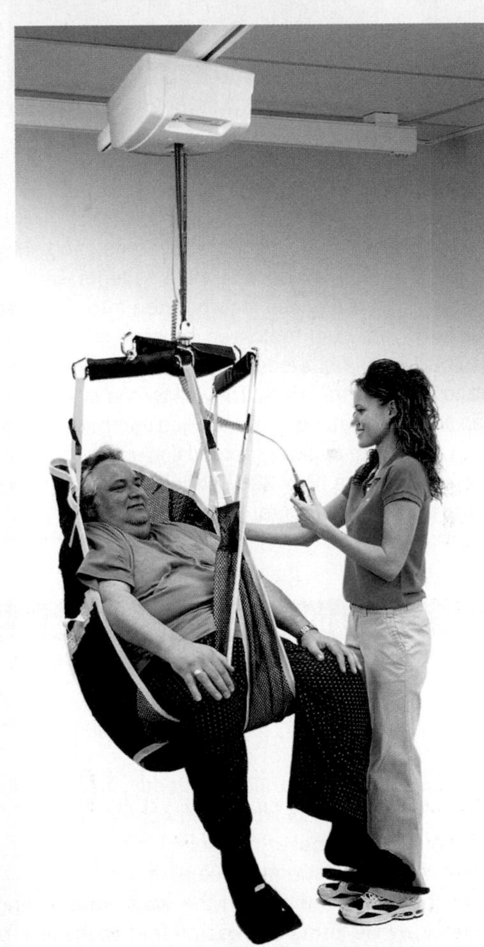

(Courtesy MedCare Products, Burnsville, Minn.)

Continued

NURSING CARE GUIDELINE

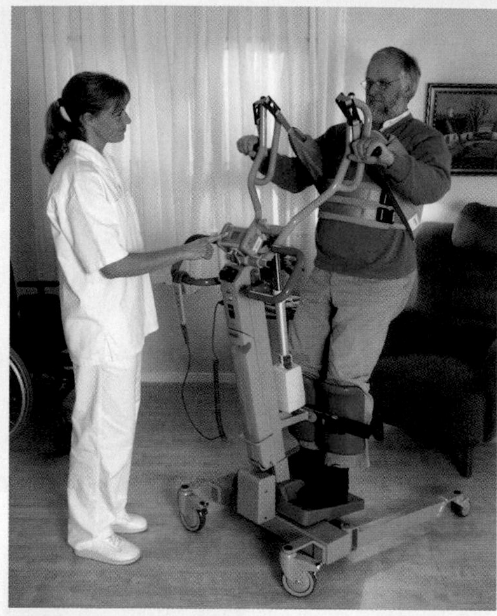

(From Sorrentino SA, Remmert L: *Mosby's essentials for nursing assistants*, ed. 5, St. Louis, 2014, Mosby.)

Mechanical Lift Devices—cont'd

- *Transfer chairs* are convertible chair-stretcher devices for non–weight-bearing or immobile patients, and they are useful for confused or uncooperative patients. Many types have lateral assist devices incorporated into the design.
- *Lateral assist lifts* are motorized or hand-cranked transfer devices built onto a stretcher for immobile patients who are unable to assist in transfers. They allow the space between the bed and the stretcher to be bridged without the caregiver reaching or pulling, avoiding potential injuries.

- Basic body mechanics (Box 28-1) should be used during a lift to prevent injury to the nurse.
- Ensure that the lift device works correctly before using it with a patient. Remove the device from service if any parts are missing or damaged.

Documentation Concerns

- Document any repositioning or transfer that occurred, the reason, and the new position.
- Include the weight-bearing status and the use of a caregiver to assist in the transfer, and identify which routine lift device was used.
- Itemize any difficulties that arose during the transfer.
- Note the patient response to the repositioning or transfer, including musculoskeletal strength assessment and the patient's assistance and cooperation.
- Specify the need to collaborate with or refer the patient to a physical or occupational therapist.
- Document the patient and family education that was provided.

Evidence-Based Practice

- The ANA (2008) reports that "performing manual patient handling places nurses at increased risk for musculoskeletal disorders ... [that] can be attributed to several factors, including weight of load, patient characteristics, awkward posture and positioning, and environmental factors" (p. 2).
- Although manual lifting is sometimes necessary, through commitment of the facility and education of the staff, it can be almost eliminated, increasing safety for staff and patients.
- Many states have already passed or are in the process of passing legislation requiring lift teams or specifying other mechanical lift device requirements in facilities (Cohen, Nelson, Green, et al, 2010). It is imperative to check with your state board of nursing and facility for specific policies and procedures before attempting lift techniques.

BOX 28-1 Principles of Body Mechanics

- Keep the spine in natural alignment while lifting or transferring.
- Elevate work surfaces to approximately elbow height, close to the body's center of gravity.
- Never lift more than 35 lb independently; use additional caregivers and mechanical lifts when appropriate.
- Work with gravity whenever possible.
- Push rather than pull patients or objects.
- Bend from the knees rather than the waist when lifting.
- Avoid twisting while lifting by keeping feet apart, with one foot placed in the direction of transfer.
- Keep patients or objects close to the body to minimize reach.
- Diminish friction and shear by using friction-reducing devices during transfers and having patients lay their arms across the chest during repositioning.
- Use safe patient-handling and movement algorithms for decision making in all patient transfers.

Safe patient-handling and movement algorithms were developed by the Veterans Integrated Services Network 8, Patient Safety Center, in Tampa, Florida, to assist nurses in promoting safe patient positioning and transfers (U.S. Department of Veterans Affairs, 2014). These algorithms are designed to keep nurses and patients safe. Algorithms essential to caring for the immobilized patient are shown in Figures 28-15 through 28-17.

Additional algorithms are available for other patient care situations. Special bariatric patient care algorithms have been developed for this growing population.

QSEN FOCUS!

Referencing guidelines on mechanical lift devices from national patient safety resources demonstrates an appreciation for the values of research and interventions designed to prevent patient and caregiver injury.

I. Patient's level of assistance

_____ *Independent*: Patient performs task safely, with or without staff assistance, with or without assistive devices.

_____ *Partial assist*: Patient requires no more help than stand by, cueing or coaxing, or caregiver is required to lift no more than 35 lb of the patient's weight.

_____ *Dependent*: Patient requires nurse to lift more than 35 lb of the patient's weight, or patients is unpredictable in the amount of assistance offered; assistive devices should be used.

An assessment should be made before each task if the patient has varying levels of ability to assist because of medical reasons, fatigue, or medications. When in doubt, assume the patient cannot assist with the transfer/repositioning.

II. Weight-bearing capability

_____ Full
_____ Partial
_____ None

III. Bilateral upper-extremity strength

_____ Yes
_____ No

IV. Patient's level of cooperation and comprehension

_____ *Cooperative*: May need prompting; able to follow simple commands.

_____ *Unpredictable* or *varies* (patient whose behavior changes frequently should be considered as "unpredictable"): Not cooperative or unable to follow simple commands.

V. Weight _________ **Height** _________

Body mass index (BMI)* (needed if patient's weight is over 300 lb) _____

If BMI exceeds 50, institute bariatric algorithms.

The presence of the following conditions is likely to affect the transfer/repositioning process and should be considered when identifying equipment and technique needed to move the patient.

VI. Check applicable conditions likely to affect transfer/repositioning techniques

_____ Amputation
_____ Contractures/spasms
_____ Fractures
_____ Hip/knee/shoulder replacement
_____ History of falls
_____ Paralysis/paresis
_____ Postural hypotension
_____ Respiratory/cardiac compromise
_____ Severe edema
_____ Severe osteoporosis
_____ Severe pain/discomfort
_____ Splints/traction
_____ Tubes (IV, chest, etc.)
_____ Unstable spine
_____ Urinary/fecal stoma
_____ Very fragile skin
_____ Wounds affecting transfer/positioning

Comments:

____
____
____

VII. Care plan:

Algorithm	Task	Equipment/Assistive device	# Staff
1	Transfer to and from bed to chair, chair to toilet, chair to chair, or car to chair		
2	Lateral transfer to and from bed to stretcher, trolley		
3	Transfer to and from chair to stretcher or chair to examination table		
4	Reposition in bed: side-to-side, up in bed		
5	Reposition in chair: wheelchair and dependency chair		
6	Transfer patient up from the floor		
Bariatric 1	Bariatric transfer to and from bed to chair, chair to toilet, or chair to chair		
Bariatric 2	Bariatric lateral transfer to and from bed to stretcher or trolley		
Bariatric 3	Bariatric reposition in bed: side-to-side, up in bed		
Bariatric 4	Bariatric reposition in chair: wheelchair, chair, or dependency chair		
Bariatric 5	Patient-handling tasks requiring access to body parts (limb, abdominal mass, gluteal area)		
Bariatric 6	Bariatric transporting (stretcher)		
Bariatric 7	Bariatric toileting tasks		

Sling type: Seated _____ Seated (Amputation) _____ Standing _____ Supine _____ Ambulation _____ Limb Support _____________

Sling size: _____________

Signature: ______________________ **Date:** ______________________

*If patient's weight is over 300 lb, the BMI is needed. For online BMI table and calculator go to *www.nhlbi.nih.gov/guidelines/obesity/bmi_tbl.htm.*

FIGURE 28-14 Safe patient handling and movement (SPHM) assessment criteria and care plan. (Courtesy U.S. Department of Veterans Affairs: Safe patient handling and movement algorithms, 2014. Retrieved from *www.visn8.va.gov/visn8/patientsafetycenter/safePtHandling/default.asp.*)

NURSING CARE GUIDELINE

Specialized Transfer and Positioning Equipment

Background

Special Mattress

- Special mattresses or beds are designed to minimize transfer and repositioning. Several types are available:
  - A surface redesign mattress has rotating surfaces that eliminate the need to move the patient (bed surface moves instead) and has an air cushion that eliminates friction during movement.
  - A Gatch bed has a frame that is made in three sections, which permits raising the head, foot, and middle of the bed; for example, raising the middle of the bed helps to prevent the patient from sliding down in bed.
  - A foam mattress reduces pressure to avoid or alleviate decubitus ulcers.
  - A foam or gel combination mattress reduces pressure.
  - A low-air-loss bed uses multiple air-filled cushions and various amounts of air, can support a wide range of patient weights, and reduces pressure to avoid or alleviate decubitus ulcers.
  - An air-fluidized bed uses airflow to move silicone particles in the bed, creating a watery, fluid-like movement and resulting in lower pressure to avoid or alleviate decubitus ulcers.

Trapeze Bar

- A trapeze bar fastens to an overhead bar that is attached to the bed frame.
- It is used for patients with equal bilateral upper extremity strength.
- Patients can use a trapeze bar to assist with repositioning.
- Use of the bar decreases the risk of shearing.
- Musculoskeletal strength increases because the bar accommodates upper extremity exercises.
- Having a trapeze bar available to the patient promotes independence.

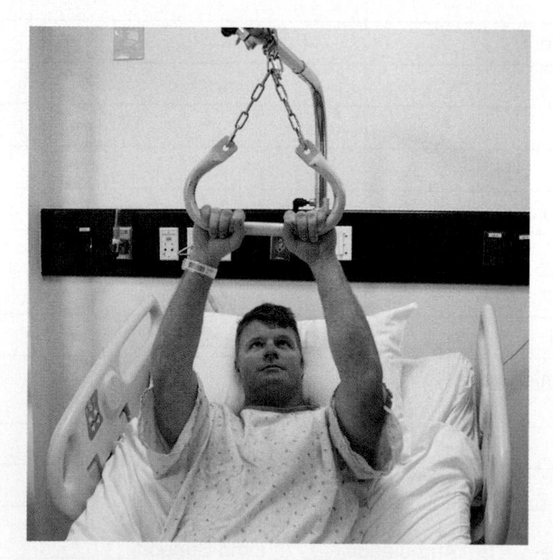

Transfer or Slide Board

- A transfer or slide board is made of plastic-like material that reduces friction.
- Linens easily slide over the board, facilitating bed linen changes.
- Patients can be repositioned or transferred with a minimum of force required.

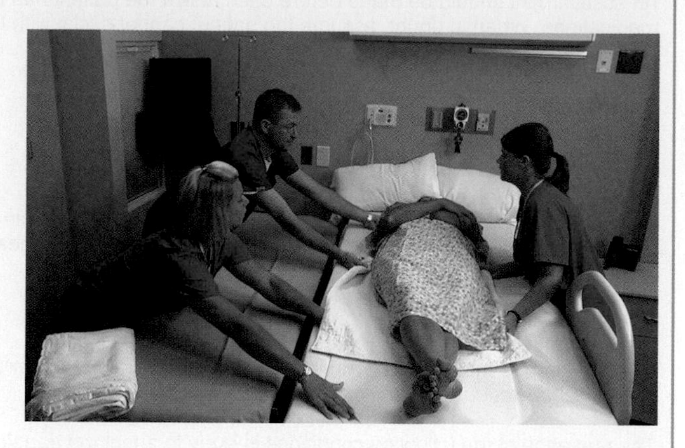

Friction-Reducing Sheet

- Friction-reducing sheets are somewhat similar to transfer or slide boards:
  - They are made of a specialized material that reduces shear and friction.
  - When placed under a patient, the sheet minimizes the force required for repositioning or transfer.

Trochanter Roll

- A trochanter roll prevents outward rolling of the hip when a patient is lying on his or her back.

Procedural Concerns

- Devices are available from many different manufacturers.
  - Follow the guidelines for the specific brands being used.
  - Follow institution policy and procedures for the use and cleaning of special mattresses, transfer or slide boards, and friction-reducing sheets.
- Trapeze bar
  - The patient grabs the bar with one or two hands and pulls the upper body off the bed.
  - The bar assists in repositioning, transferring, or performing basic hygienic care.
- Trochanter roll
  - A blanket or sandbag may be substituted for a trochanter roll.
  - When the device is placed correctly next to the patient's thigh, the patella faces directly up.

Documentation Concerns

- Explain if repositioning or transfer occurred, the reason for it, and the new position.
- Note the patient's weight-bearing status, the need for caregiver assistance in the transfer, and use of a lift or specialized device.
- Document the patient's response to repositioning or transfer, including musculoskeletal strength and integumentary assessment and the patient's assistance and cooperation.
- Indicate the need to collaborate with or refer the patient to a physical or occupational therapist.

NURSING CARE GUIDELINE

- Note the patient and family education that was provided.
- Specify difficulties that occurred during the transfer.

Evidence-Based Practice

- "Friction or shear injuries can occur during the positioning of patients in the bed, during the placement of a bedpan, during a transfer to another bed surface or wheelchair, and when moving patients up in bed" increasing the potential for pressure ulcer development (Hanson, Langemo, Anderson, et al, 2010, p. 21).
- Research indicates that proper body mechanics are not adequate to prevent injury during patient transfers.
- A recommended 35-lb maximum weight limit for patient lifting makes it imperative that nurses and UAP use assistive transfer devices to prevent injury to their backs during patient transfers (Waters, 2007).
- Studies reveal that implementation of safe patient movement programs and use of specialized positioning equipment does not negatively affect functional outcomes in patients (Arnold, Radawiec, Campo, et al, 2011).

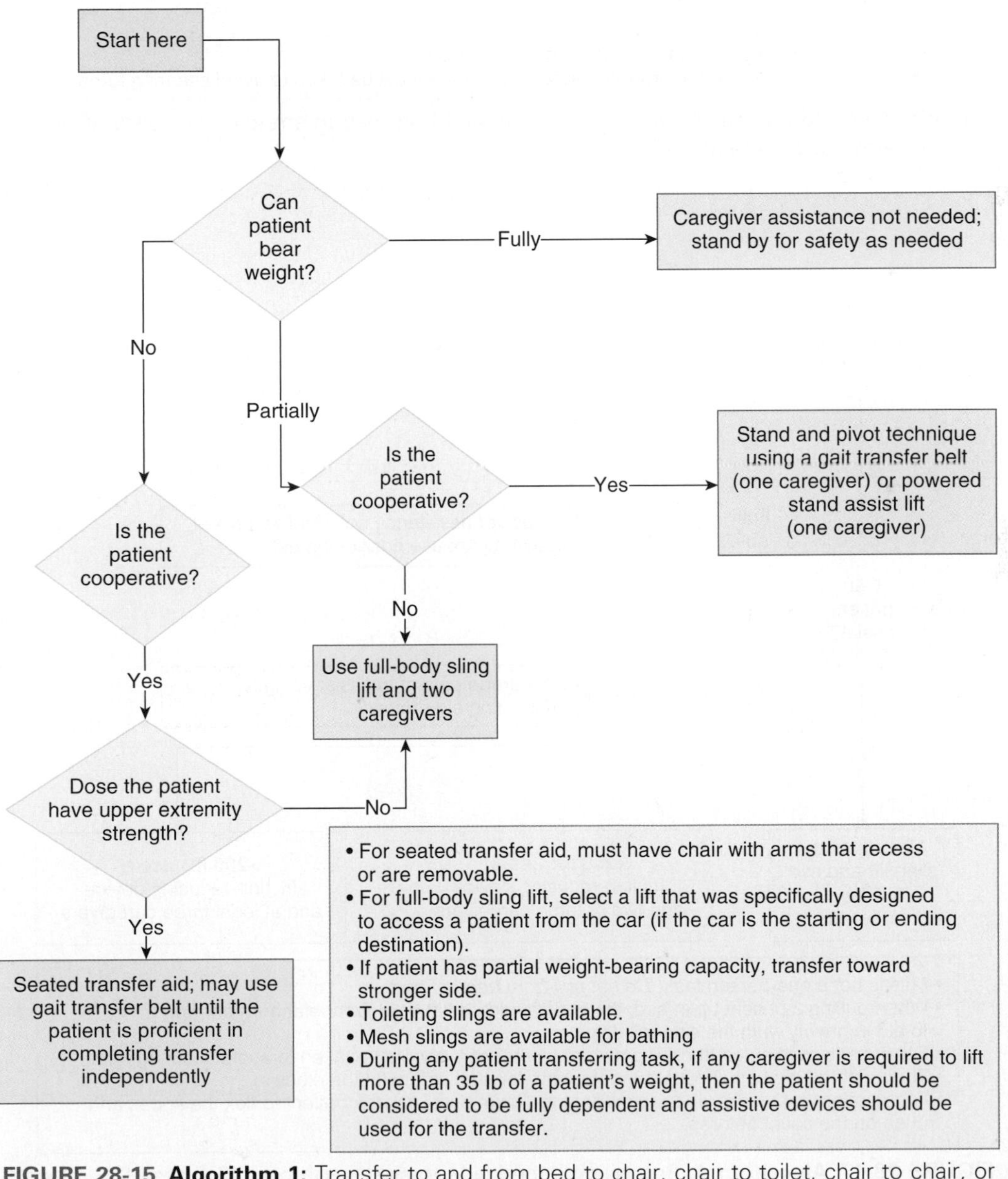

FIGURE 28-15 Algorithm 1: Transfer to and from bed to chair, chair to toilet, chair to chair, or car to chair. (Courtesy U.S. Department of Veterans Affairs.)

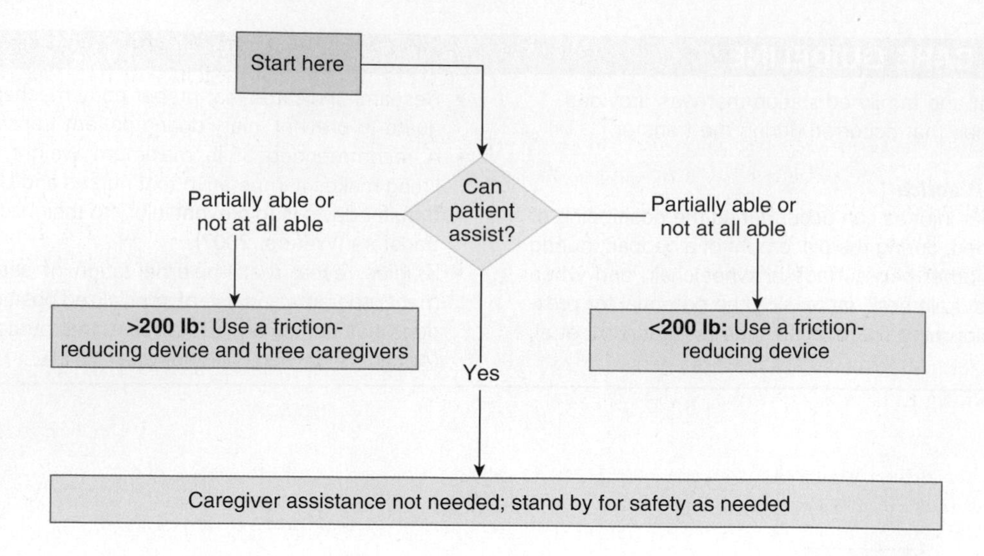

FIGURE 28-16 Algorithm 2: Lateral transfer to and from bed to stretcher or trolley. (Courtesy U.S. Department of Veterans Affairs.)

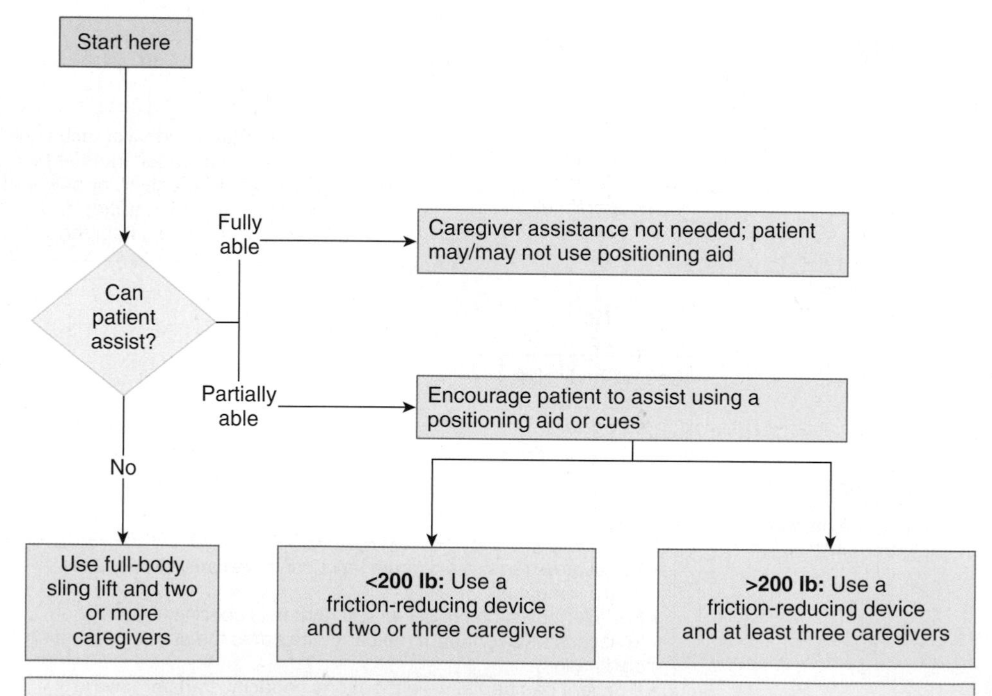

FIGURE 28-17 Algorithm 4: Reposition in bed side to side, up in bed. (Courtesy U.S. Department of Veterans Affairs.)

CARDIOPULMONARY SYSTEM INTERVENTIONS

Every effort should be made to keep the lungs expanded in an immobile patient. If the patient's condition permits, raising the head of the bed can enhance lung expansion by relieving pressure on the diaphragm and chest wall. Routine coughing and deep-breathing exercises and the use of an incentive spirometer aid in lung expansion. Turning and repositioning the immobilized patient, incentive spirometry, and chest physiotherapy decrease the likelihood of pulmonary secretions pooling in dependent areas of the lungs.

Several nursing interventions can help to prevent deep vein thromboses in patients on bed rest. Teach the patient to perform leg, ankle, and foot exercises, or perform passive range of motion if the patient is unable to exercise without assistance (Nursing Care Guideline box). Two means of applying pressure to the calf to promote venous return are antiembolism hose (Skill 28-4), which are tightly fitting elastic stockings (e.g., TED hose), and sequential compression devices (SCDs), which are plastic or cloth sleeves that fit over the patient's legs and are intermittently inflated and deflated with an electric air pump (Skill 28-5).

NURSING CARE GUIDELINE

Active, Active Assistive, and Passive Range of Motion

Background

- Range of motion (ROM) is the distance a joint can move in any direction that is considered normal for the patient (see Figure 28-4).
- There are three types of ROM:
  - *Active ROM:* The patient has full independent movement of all joints; this is also known as *isotonic exercise*.
  - *Active assistive ROM:* The caregiver minimally assists the patient or the patient minimally assists himself or herself in the movement of joints through a full motion.
  - *Passive ROM:* The caregiver moves the patient's joints through a full motion. This exercise does not maintain or improve strength but maintains flexibility and prevents contractures and atrophy.
- ROM activities have several goals:
  - To maintain or improve functioning of the musculoskeletal system
  - To ultimately improve the patient's abilities to perform activities of daily living
- Coordination of care can be done while performing ROM activities:
  - The caregiver can perform a full assessment of the integumentary system while performing ROM activities.
  - The caregiver can coordinate ROM activities with hygienic care.
- ROM activities can be delegated to unlicensed assistive personnel (UAP):
  - UAP must receive proper instruction regarding the procedure and must know when to notify a nurse for assistance.
  - UAP may not perform an assessment of the integumentary system but should notify the nurse if skin issues are noticed.

Procedural Concerns

- Have the patient wear comfortable, loose-fitting clothing.
- Encourage the patient to perform ROM exercises as independently as possible to achieve his or her highest level of function.
- Exercises usually should be performed consistently:
  - Two times per day
  - Three to five times per joint
- Move the joints smoothly and slowly until resistance is met, and stop before pain begins.
- Prevent injury by supporting the joint during exercise. Support may be in one of three forms:
  - A cup is provided when one hand holds the joint while the other hand exercises the extremity.
  - A cradle is provided when one hand holds the joint while the other arm supports the rest of the extremity.
  - Support is provided when one hand holds the muscles above the joint while the other holds the muscles below the joint and moves the extremity.
- Stop an exercise if the patient's condition warrants a professional opinion and assessment.
- Perform the exercises in the same order or sequence, and move from head to toe to avoid omitting any joints.

Documentation Concerns

- Include ROM on the care plan, clearly specifying achievable, measurable goals.
- Document the following patient responses to exercises if they occur:
  - Patient assistance needed with exercises
  - Patient compliance with the activity
  - Pain or discomfort
  - Resistance or contractures
- Note joints that did achieve full ROM, the degree of motion achieved, and the movement that was being attempted.
- Include the frequency and times that ROMs were performed.
- Add observations regarding the need to collaborate with or refer the patient to a physical or occupational therapist.
- Describe the patient and family education that has occurred.

Evidence-Based Practice

- Studies have indicated that active range of motion is the best method of exercise for intensive care patients to prevent the development of DVT (Palamone, Brunovsky, Groth, et al, 2011).
- Exercises performed twice daily have been shown to reduce muscle spasticity and improve functional ability in debilitated patients (Arbesman and Sheard, 2014).
- Range of motion exercises diminish the incidence of skin breakdown and prevent joint contractures in bedridden patients (Bowyer and Glover, 2010).

Anticoagulation therapy may be prescribed for patients with decreased mobility. Heparin, low-molecular-weight heparin such as enoxaparin, or warfarin is given to prevent DVT and pulmonary embolism. Postoperative patients or those on bed rest are most likely to be prescribed prophylactic anticoagulants. Monitor coagulation laboratory values before administering anticoagulants to ensure patient safety.

! SAFE PRACTICE ALERT

Assess patients who are receiving anticoagulation therapy for bruising or hemorrhage. Patients may be placed on bleeding precautions which include the use of electric shavers and soft-bristle toothbrushes to avoid bleeding.

Position immobilized patients so that there are no areas of pressure on the lower extremities or under the knees to prevent occlusion of blood flow (Nursing Care Guideline box). Caution patients against crossing their legs or ankles because these positions can occlude blood flow. Ambulation as soon as possible is an important preventive measure.

Allow the patient to participate in ADLs, and plan for frequent rest periods between activities. Gradually increase the amount of activity that the patient performs independently so that activity intolerance is minimized.

Dangling can prevent a previously nonambulatory patient from being injured. Raise the head of the bed slowly, and assist the patient to a sitting position. Ease the patient's legs over the side of the bed, and have the patient place the feet on the floor. Postural hypotension and syncope (i.e., fainting) may be prevented by allowing patients to sit with their legs in a dependent position for a few minutes before standing (Figure 28-18). Monitor vital signs before, during,

NURSING CARE GUIDELINE

Positioning in a Bed

Background

- The patient's position in a bed is important to maintain proper respiratory status and body alignment, prevent skin breakdown, and provide comfort for a patient who is unable to reposition himself or herself.
- Coordination of care may be performed while the patient is being repositioned.
  - The caregiver can perform a full assessment of the integumentary system.
  - The caregiver can perform a full assessment of the musculoskeletal system.
- Repositioning a patient can be delegated to unlicensed assistive personnel (UAP):
  - Provide proper instruction regarding specific positioning techniques, individualized patient concerns, and circumstances that require notifying a nurse.
  - UAP may not perform assessments but should notify the nurse about any skin or musculoskeletal issues.
  - UAP should report difficulties with the procedure.

Procedural Concerns

- Determine whether mechanical lift devices or other specialized devices are needed (see Nursing Care Guideline: Mechanical Lift Devices and Nursing Care Guideline: Other Specialized Mobility and Safety Equipment) and how many caregiver assists are necessary.
- Assess the patient's medical history and current diagnoses to determine whether there are contraindications to the procedure.
- Assess the medical equipment in the room to determine whether the patient needs to be repositioned to optimize equipment function.
- When changing the patient's position, complete the following:
  - Lower the head of the bed to reduce resistance to gravity during repositioning, as tolerated and permitted by the patient's condition.
  - Raise the bed to waist height of the nurse or UAP assisting in positioning, to avoid back injury.
  - Use bed side rails or lift equipment to assist the patient during repositioning, as appropriate.
  - Align the patient's spine in the center of the bed.
  - Place pillows or supportive devices such as trochanter rolls for comfort, to prevent skin breakdown on boney prominences, and to assist the patient in maintaining the new position.
  - Raise two or three side rails and lower and lock the bed to provide for patient safety following repositioning.

Documentation Concerns

- Include repositioning of the patient on the care plan.
- Include a systematic schedule of positions.
- Document the patient's response to positioning changes, including any of the following that apply:
  - Patient's assistance with positioning
  - Patient's compliance with and tolerance of the activity
  - Pain or discomfort experienced by the patient
- Document the times when repositioning was performed, current position, body alignment, and support devices used.
- Explain the need to collaborate with or refer the patient to a physical or occupational therapist.
- Document the patient and family education that was provided.

Evidence-Based Practice

- Muscle strength has been found to decrease by 10% in healthy individuals confined to bed rest for 1 week (Hopkins, Spuhler, Thomsen, 2007).
- Repositioning helps prevent the complications of immobility including atelectasis, pneumonia, PE, DVT, orthostatic hypotension, constipation, ileus, urinary stasis, hyperglycemia, insulin resistance, muscle atrophy, bone demineralization, contractures, decubitus ulcers, and depression (Palamone, Brunovsky, Groth, et al, 2011).

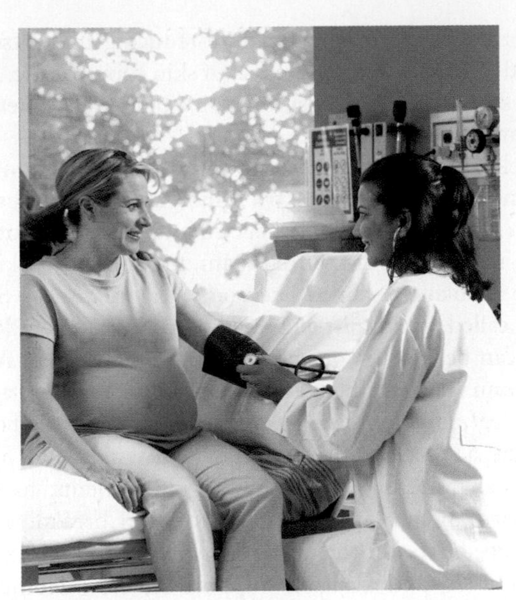

FIGURE 28-18 Patient dangling on side of bed.

and after dangling and ambulation to assess for orthostatic hypotension.

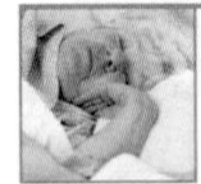

3. Identify at least four actions with rationales that should be taken to provide for Mrs. Ryan's safety and prevent her from falling.

NUTRITION INTERVENTIONS

Patients on prolonged bed rest need adequate protein intake to prevent negative nitrogen balance. Patients should be offered meals that include lean protein. Because immobilized patients often have a decreased appetite, offer smaller, more frequent meals. Involving patients in dietary choices and increasing patient activity as tolerated may also increase appetite.

Adequate fluid intake is an essential component in preventing many complications of immobility, including DVT, urinary tract infections, thickened pulmonary secretions, and constipation. The nurse should encourage intake of at least 2 liters of fluid in 24 hours unless contraindicated. Before discharging a patient with mobility issues, the nurse should consider the patient's dietary needs (Home Care Considerations box). Chapter 30 provides more information on nutritional support.

ELIMINATION INTERVENTIONS

Adequate fluid intake prevents some of the urinary and bowel complications associated with bed rest. When encouraging patients to drink 2 liters of fluids each day, the nurse should plan to offer at least half of the fluid intake during the day shift, when the patient is most alert and active. Position changes, toileting programs, a bedside commode, and provision of a bedpan for immobile patients at regular intervals help to prevent urinary stasis.

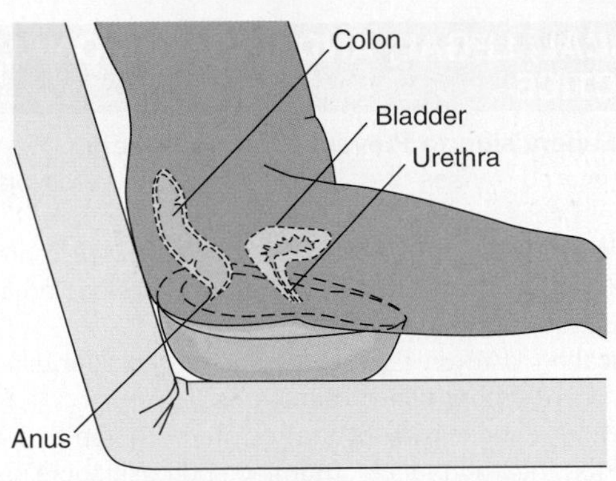

FIGURE 28-19 Proper positioning on a bedpan. (From Sorrentino SA, Remmert L: *Mosby's textbook for nursing assistants*, ed. 8, St. Louis, 2012, Mosby.)

HOME CARE CONSIDERATIONS

Nutritional Concerns for Patients Living Alone

- Consider the dietary needs of patients discharged to home who live independently.
  - How will the patient prepare or receive well-balanced, nutritious meals necessary to promote wound healing?
  - Is the patient able to grocery shop, or have arrangements been made with a supportive person to bring food or meals to the patient's home?
  - Is the patient's water supply adequate and safe for drinking and food preparation?
  - Has the patient verbalized an understanding of the necessity of adequate fluid intake to prevent significant urinary, bowel, and circulatory complications?

Increasing the fiber in a patient's diet helps to prevent constipation. A diet rich in whole grains, fruits, and vegetables helps to soften and increase the mass of stools, making it easier for the patient to defecate (i.e., evacuate the bowels). Assisting patients to sit upright on a bedpan can aid in elimination (Figure 28-19).

Because activity and exercise contribute to healthy bowel patterns, early ambulation is desirable. If a patient is having difficulty with constipation, a doctor's order may be required for a stool softener, laxative, or enema.

SKIN INTERVENTIONS

After at-risk patients are identified by using a skin assessment tool, interventions should be initiated to prevent skin breakdown. Turn immobile patients at least every 2 hours. A more frequent turning schedule should be employed for patients who have other risk factors, such as poor nutrition, fragile skin, lack of adipose tissue, or incontinence. Nurses should direct and supervise assistive personnel to whom patient turning and positioning responsibilities have been be delegated (Ethical, Legal, and Professional Practice box).

ETHICAL, LEGAL, AND PROFESSIONAL PRACTICE

UAP Supervision to Prevent Pressure Ulcers

- Registered nurses are legally responsible for planning patient care related to pressure sore prevention.
- Unlicensed assistive personnel (UAP) provide more than 20% of direct patient care according to Needleman and colleagues (2002).
- Educating UAP on the importance of thorough skin care can prevent poor patient outcomes.
- It is the responsibility of the registered nurse to educate UAP on the importance of turning and positioning patients on bed rest, thorough skin care, and the use of moisture barriers and skin protectants (Howe, 2008).

! SAFE PRACTICE ALERT

Position patients so that pressure is minimized on all bony prominences.

Pressure-relieving and pressure-reducing mattresses can be used to further reduce the risk of skin compromise. Figure 28-20 shows different positions with pillow placement and positioning devices.

Heel and elbow protectors are used to cushion bony prominences and prevent **friction** (rubbing) between the patient's skin and the bed sheets. These types of protectors can be made of cloth-covered foam, foam, or sheepskin and can be tubular or shaped like boots (Figure 28-21). Special AFOs called pressure-relief ankle-foot orthotic (PRAFO) boots can be used to prevent pressure on the heels. A rigid aluminum frame lined in sheepskin is applied to the lower leg and foot using Velcro straps. PRAFO boots have the added benefit of keeping the ankle and foot in proper alignment. Before discharging patients to home who have an increased potential for skin breakdown, the nurse needs to thoroughly assess the patient's mobility, environment, and available support services (Home Care Considerations box).

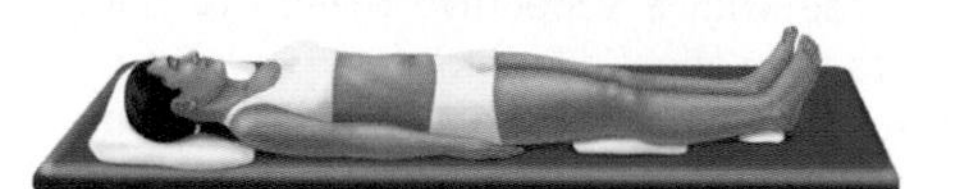

Supine: Patient lies flat on back

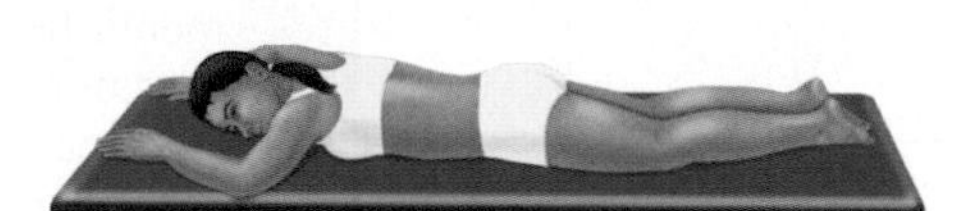

Prone: Patient lies face-down

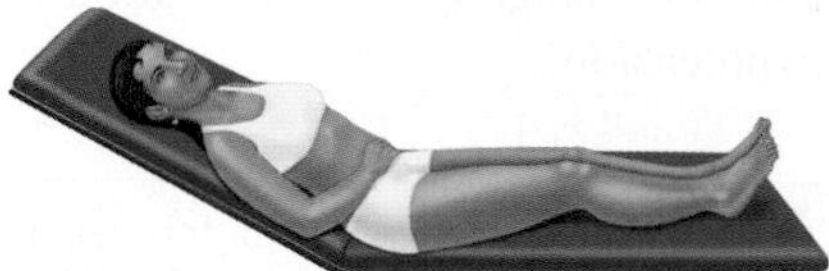

Semi-Fowler: Patient semisitting with head elevated

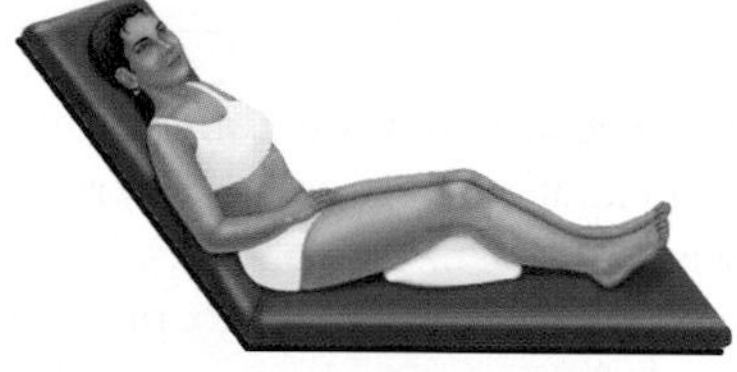

Fowler: Patient in sitting position with pillow supporting thigh and legs

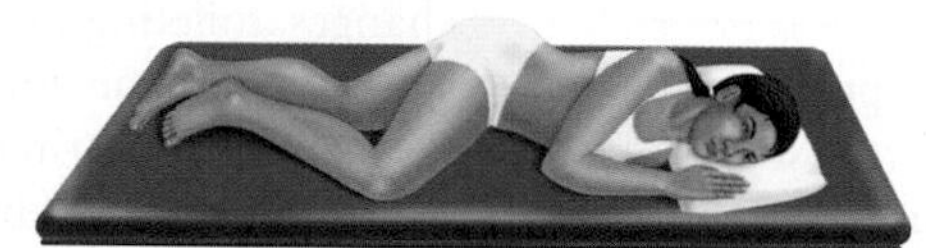

Sim's: Patient in semiprone position lying on the left side

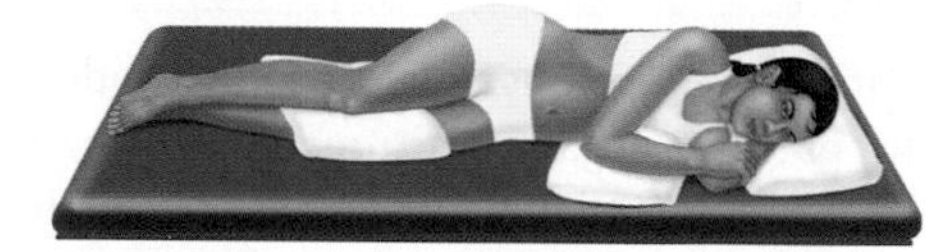

Side-lying: Patient lying on side

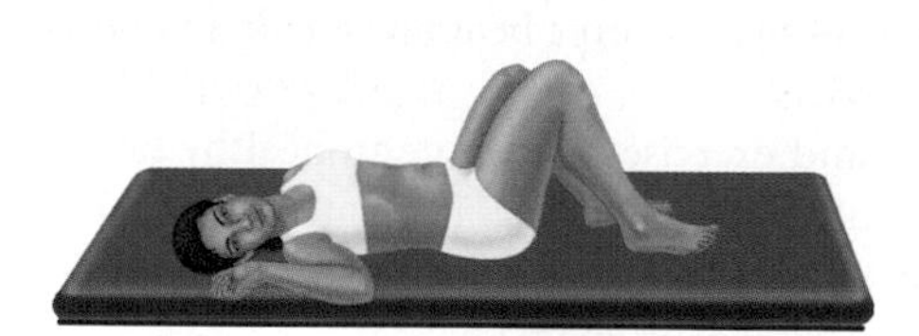

Dorsal recumbent: Patient lying supine with legs bent

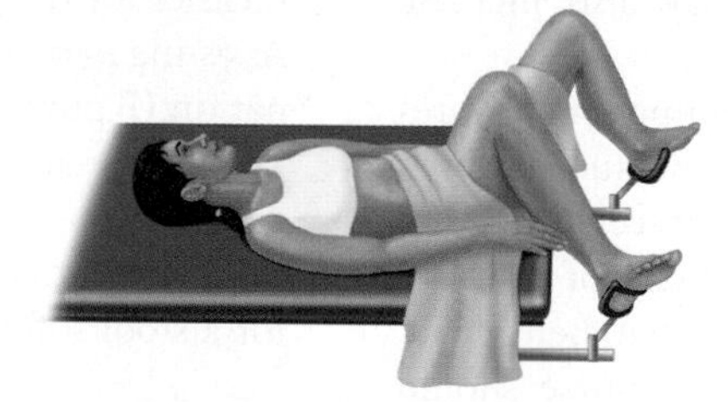

Lithotomy: Patient lying supine

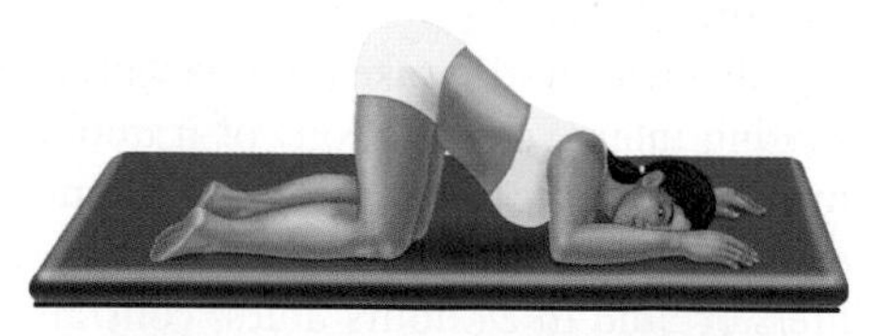

Knee-chest: Patient lying in prone position with buttocks and knees drawn to the chest

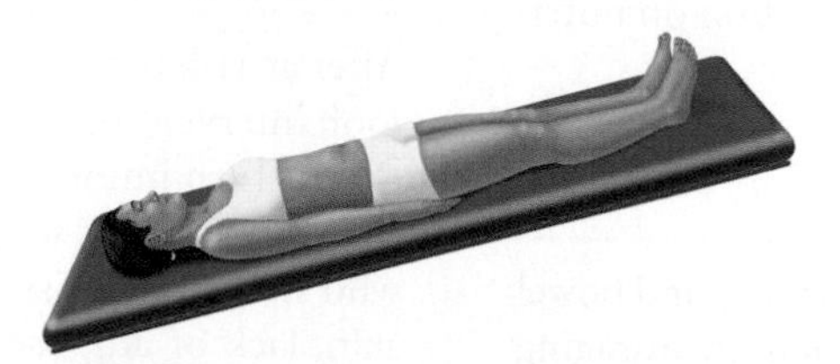

Trendelenburg's: Patient lying supine with legs elevated higher than head

FIGURE 28-20 Patient positioning.

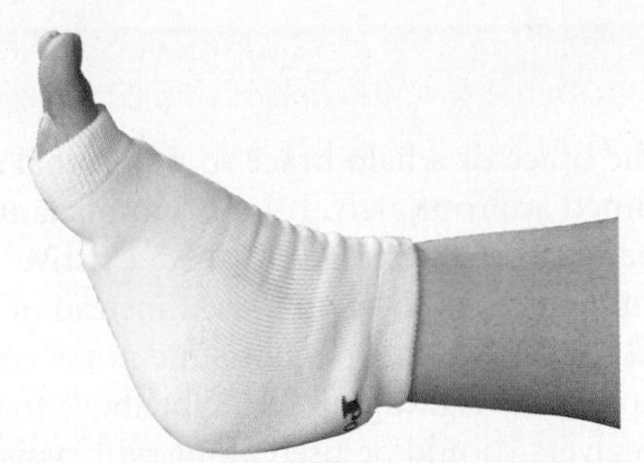

FIGURE 28-21 Heel protectors provide protection against skin breakdown. (Courtesy Posey Company, Arcadia, CA.)

HOME CARE CONSIDERATIONS

Assessing Potential Immobility Concerns for Discharged Patients

When patients are discharged to home, their activity and exercise need to continue to prevent significant skin breakdown and psychosocial isolation.

- Is the patient able to move independently, or is it necessary for a caregiver to reposition the patient on a scheduled frequency?
- Are preventive skin care measures in place for patients confined to bed?
- Does a pressure-reducing mattress need to be ordered for the patient's home convalescence?
- How often are caregivers or other support people visiting or scheduled to visit and provide diversional activities for the home-bound patient?
- Are referrals to community agencies in place to support the home-bound patient?

PSYCHOSOCIAL INTERVENTIONS

Preventing social isolation of immobilized patients can be challenging. Include patients in planning and implementing care so that they have some control over their environment. Patients should be encouraged to have contact with their family and friends through visits, phone calls, or email. Provide spiritual support as needed.

During hospitalization, disruption of sleep and rest patterns should be minimized. Nursing care should be planned to limit the number of times patients are awakened at night. Noise and light from the hallway should be kept at a minimum. During the day, open window blinds to provide the sunlight needed to maintain sleep-wake cycles.

The nurse should always talk with the patient and explain all procedures. Knowing what is going to happen in advance allows patients to assist in their care when possible and helps them cope with uncomfortable procedures.

Reality orientation is important. Patients should be able to see a clock and a calendar. Access to television or radio may help to prevent sensory deprivation and boredom. Occupational therapists may assist in providing patient activities. If the immobilized patient is a child, specialized play therapists (i.e., child life specialists) can be valuable in providing therapeutic activities.

Mobilization of the patient's support system is especially important if a long recovery period is anticipated. Referrals to community resources such as transportation assistance and outpatient therapy may be necessary for some patients. Early involvement of social services is beneficial. If the nurse notices changes in a patient's behavior, referral to a counselor may be necessary.

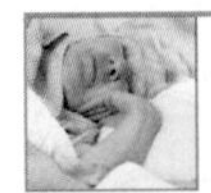

4. Identify a minimum of five nursing interventions necessary to prevent postoperative complications of immobility.

EVALUATION

To evaluate treatment interventions for patients who have limited mobility or are confined to bed rest, pay particular attention to nursing care plan goals and outcome criteria. Nurses must continually evaluate the effectiveness of interventions on the basis of attainment of short- and long-term goals. Evaluation is a dynamic aspect of the nursing process that determines the need for revision of patients' individualized plans of care.

SKILL 28-1 Manual Logrolling

- If the patient is to be rolled using a special bed adaptation or mechanical device, refer to facility policy and training for the specific manufacturer's device. The procedure described here should be used only if a mechanical device is not used.
- Safe patient-handling recommendations include bed assistive devices for patients weighing more than 78 lb (Gonzalez, Howe, Waters, et al, 2009; Nelson and Baptiste, 2006; Sedlak, Doheny, Nelson, et al, 2009).

PURPOSE

- To maintain the patient's spinal alignment through special repositioning
- To maintain skin integrity
- To prevent pressure ulcers
- To promote patient comfort
- As needed to provide basic hygiene (e.g., changing linens, bathing)

RESOURCES

- Appropriate staffing numbers
- Pillows
- Drawsheet

COLLABORATION AND DELEGATION

- Logrolling a patient may be delegated to unlicensed assistive personnel (UAP) without a nurse's assistance after the initial assessment of the patient, provided a spinal cord injury is stabilized (at the nurse's discretion).
- UAP should report the following:
  - Pain before, during, or after the procedure
  - Sores, wounds, irritations, and lesions
  - Difficulties in performing the procedure
- UAP should be instructed in the following:
  - Appropriate number of staff required to safely perform the procedure
  - Appropriate procedure and timing
  - Appropriate documentation
- Collaborate with the physical therapist if he or she would like assistance in assessing the patient's abilities.
- Collaborate and coordinate the procedure with the primary care provider (PCP) or surgeon rounds if dressings or surgical implementation must be examined or changed.

EVIDENCE-BASED PRACTICE

- The current recommendation is that at least three nurses should be involved when turning patients who have an orthopedic brace or a halo brace so that spinal alignment is maintained appropriately. It is also important to determine whether mechanical or bed assistive repositioning devices should be used instead of nursing personnel for turning the patient. One nurse can safely logroll a patient weighing up to 78 lb; above that, two or more caregivers should be used along with assistive mechanical devices (Gonzalez, Howe, Waters, et al, 2009; Nelson and Baptiste, 2006; Sedlak, Doheny, Nelson, et al, 2009).
- Safe patient-handling recommendations are consistent with decreasing caregiver injuries. The top three interventions included mechanical assistive devices, a no-lift policy, and a lift team with a lead or resource nurse (Nelson and Baptiste, 2006).
- Patient weight and lack of cooperation are two of the most important contributors to caregiver injuries when repositioning or assisting with mobility, and they must be considered when planning the best method of assistance for moving the patient (Gonzalez, Howe, Waters, et al, 2009; Nelson and Baptiste, 2006; Sedlak, Doheny, Nelson, et al, 2009).

SPECIAL CIRCUMSTANCES

1. **Assess:** Is the patient experiencing pain?
   Intervention: Determine whether the pain is new or preexisting.
   - Anticipate whether the procedure will produce pain and therefore require pain medication before moving the patient.
   - Stop the procedure if the patient complains of new pain.
   - Medicate or premedicate according to orders.
   - Notify the PCP if no orders exist for pain medication.
2. **Assess:** What is the most appropriate assistance for the specific patient situation?
   Intervention: Identify the patient's weight and level of cooperation, medical interventions, orthopedic interventions, and facility policies.
   - Use a lift team, mechanical assistive device, or multiple staff members to move the patient.
   - One additional staff member may be needed for each orthopedic intervention (e.g., cast, brace), depending on the appliance and the patient's ability to assist.
   - Before the other staff arrives, arrange medical interventions (e.g., IV lines, tubing) to avoid twisting or other complications.

PREPROCEDURE

I. Check PCP orders and the patient care plan.
Knowledge of patient-specific orders is critical for safe patient care.

II. Gather supplies and equipment.
Preparing for the patient encounter saves time and promotes patient trust.

III. Perform hand hygiene.
Frequent hand hygiene prevents the spread of microorganisms.

IV. Maintain standard precautions.
Use of the correct personal protective equipment (PPE) is required whenever contact with bodily fluids is possible, to reduce the transfer of pathogens.

V. Introduce yourself.
Initial communication establishes the role of the nurse and begins a professional relationship.

VI. Provide for patient privacy.
It is important to maintain patient dignity.

VII. Identify the patient, using two identifiers.
Identifying a patient involves scanning barcodes or comparing the patient's stated name and birthdate to information on the patient's wristband or health record. The correct person must receive the correct treatment.

VIII. Explain the procedure to the patient.
The nurse has a responsibility to inform a patient before initiating care. Information may ease patient anxiety and facilitate cooperation.

PROCEDURE

Logrolling

Follow preprocedure steps I through VIII.

1. Raise the bed to a working height, lower the side rails as appropriate and safe, and ensure that the bed wheels are locked.
   Proper positioning of equipment prevents provider discomfort and reduces the chance of possible injury.
2. Place the drawsheet.
   Using a drawsheet helps to avoid friction or shearing injuries to the patient that may accompany movement and prevents provider discomfort and possible injury by facilitating the movement of the patient.
3. Place pillows
   a. Between the patient's knees
   b. Move pillow to the side of the patient's head
   Appropriately placed pillows help to maintain spinal alignment during movement.
4. Position the patient's arms across his or her chest.
   Proper arm position prevents twisting of the extremities during movement and reduces the risk of injury to the patient.
5. Nurses may assume various positions in preparation for turning the patient:
   a. At the head of the bed to support the patient's head and neck alignment
   b. At the patient's back or chest to support back alignment
   c. At the legs to support hip and leg alignment
   d. Where needed to watch tube placement and beside casts or braces, which require one nurse for each device
   Proper position of personnel around the patient ensures patient safety by maintaining spinal alignment and prevents provider discomfort and possible injury by ensuring there is enough assistance to minimize injury to providers during the lift.
6. Make sure side rails are raised on the side of the bed opposite the nurses. On the count of three, pull the patient toward the nurses' side of the bed. The nurse at the head of the bed should initiate the count.
   Starting with the patient on one side of the bed allows room for the patient to be turned safely throughout the roll.

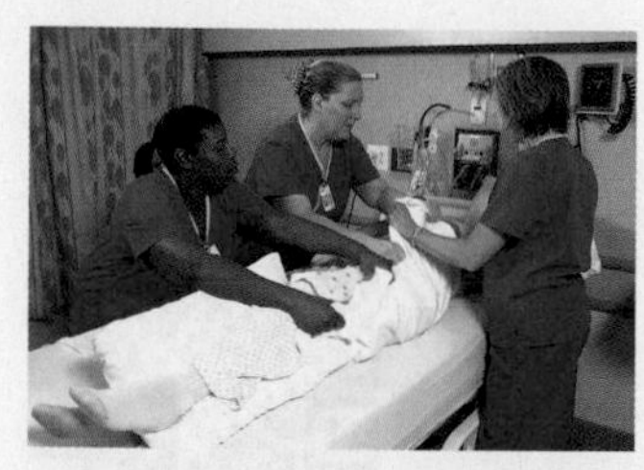

STEP 7(1)

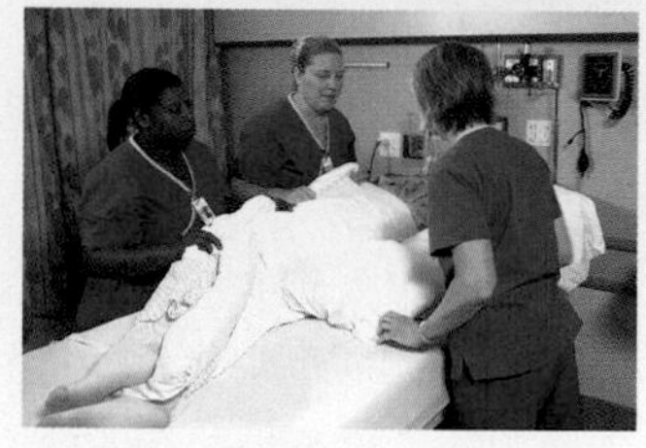

STEP 7(2)

7. On a second count of three, roll the patient, and then place pillows behind the patient to support him or her in the new position.
Counting allows the staff to coordinate their actions and move the patient as a team, which gives the best opportunity to maintain spinal alignment.

Follow postprocedure steps I through VI.

POSTPROCEDURE

I. Return the bed to its lowest position, raise the top side rails, and verify that the call light is within reach for the patient.
Precautions are taken to maintain patient safety. Top side rails aid in positioning and turning. Raising four side rails is considered a restraint.

II. Assess for additional patient needs and state the time of your expected return.
Meeting patient needs and offering self promote patient satisfaction and build trust.

III. Properly dispose of PPE.
Gloves, gowns, and masks must be appropriately discarded to prevent the spread of microorganisms.

IV. Clean equipment if it was in contact with the patient; see specific manufacturer instructions.
Disinfection eliminates most microorganisms from inanimate objects.

V. Perform hand hygiene.
Frequent hand hygiene prevents the spread of infection.

VI. Document the date, time, assessment, procedure, and patient's response to the procedure.
Accurate documentation is essential to communicate patient care and to provide legal evidence of care.

SKILL 28-2 Ambulation With Assistive Devices

PURPOSE

- Increases patient activity level
- Promotes independence
- Promotes self-esteem
- Prevents complications of immobility
- Increases muscle strength
- Promotes safety
- Decreases risk of further injury

RESOURCES: ALL METHODS

- Appropriate assistive device (e.g., gait belt, cane, walker), as prescribed.
- Sturdy shoes with nonskid soles.

COLLABORATION AND DELEGATION: ALL METHODS

- Educating patients on how to walk with assistive devices may not be delegated to unlicensed assistive personnel (UAP).
- Ambulation of a patient may be delegated to UAP only if the patient's musculoskeletal strength is stable.
- UAP may assist the nurse so that adequate staff can prevent injury to the patient or staff members.
- UAP should report any of the following:
  - Noticeable incorrect usage or fit of assistive devices
  - Complaints of soreness or weakness
  - Difficulties involving balance or strength
  - Difficulties in performing the procedure or other concerns verbalized by the patient
- UAP should be instructed in the following:
  - Appropriate ambulation assistive techniques
  - Appropriate equipment usage
  - Appropriate documentation
- Physical therapists (PTs) work with patients for rehabilitation. Collaborate with these specialists.
- Check the primary care provider (PCP) orders to ensure that duplication of activity for the patient is not occurring.
- A PT may ambulate the patients on the unit and assist as appropriate to ensure safety for all involved.
- Orthopedic specialists may change dressings or assess patient outcomes. Attempt to coordinate ambulation with visits by the orthopedic specialists, as appropriate.
- Home health workers ensure safety in the home. They should be aware of assistive devices and the home layout.

EVIDENCE-BASED PRACTICE

- Mechanical assistive ambulation devices (e.g., sit-to-stand lifts, ambulation assists, ceiling-mounted walking slings) should be considered when ambulating any patient to prevent injury to the caregiver and the patient (Radawiec, Howe, Gonzalez, et al, 2009).
- Assistive ambulation for rehabilitative patients is often a progression from maximal supportive devices to least supportive devices. Various tools have been developed, such as the Timed Up and Go (TUG) test, to determine and predict maximal functional mobility for these patients. It is important to determine whether facility policy has implemented any such scoring system and, if so, to use it for patient safety (Kristensen, Bandholm, Holm, et al, 2009).
- Staff should assist with ambulation only if the patient is stable or if a mechanical device is not available. Safe patient-handling recommendations include the use of mechanical devices, specialized patient teams, and special ambulation and lift policies. Facility policies and safe patient-handling recommendations should be followed for the safety of the patient and staff.
- One caregiver working alone should never ambulate a patient with a gait belt. There is conflicting evidence on whether a back belt prevents injury to staff. Three caregivers are a minimum recommendation for a lift, and the recommendation should be followed if there is any chance of having to lift the patient during ambulation (Nelson, 2006; Radawiec, Howe, Gonzalez, et al, 2009; Sedlak, Doheny, Nelson, et al, 2009).

SPECIAL CIRCUMSTANCES: ALL METHODS

1. **Assess:** Is the patient in pain?
   Intervention: Determine whether the pain is new or preexisting.
   - Anticipate whether ambulating will produce pain and whether there is a need for pain medication.
   - Stop the procedure if the complaint is for a new pain.
   - Medicate or premedicate the patient according to the PCP orders.
   - Notify the PCP if no orders exist for pain medication.
2. **Assess:** Is the patient on a medication regimen?
   Intervention: Determine whether any of the medications may cause issues with balance, coordination, or alertness.
   - Stop the procedure if any adverse medication side effects are evident.
   - Notify the PCP.
3. **Assess:** During the musculoskeletal assessment, was there any indication of difficulty with balance, weakness (unilateral versus bilateral), upper or lower extremity strength, weight bearing, injuries, or range of motion?
   Intervention: Ensure that the appropriate assistive device and the prescribed walking technique can be used.
   - If the patient can raise the legs 1 inch off the bed, the patient has enough strength to begin ambulation.
   - If the patient is weak, place chairs along the intended route at appropriate unobtrusive areas so that the patient may safely rest if necessary.

- If the patient is severely weak or this is the first opportunity to ambulate, ensure that a staff member is available to follow with a wheelchair.
- Cane use:
  - To fit properly, a cane should come to the hip of the patient.
  - Canes should be held on the stronger side.
  - Quad canes, with four points of support, should be used by patients with a poor sense of balance.
  - Straight-handle canes are not recommended for patients with poor balance.
  - Curved-handle canes provide minimal support.

4. **Assess:** Is the patient wearing sturdy, nonskid footwear with low or no heels?
   Intervention: Educate the patient, and obtain nonskid shoes or slippers to provide the necessary support and reduce the risk of falling with ambulation.
5. **Assess:** Are appropriate numbers of staff available to assist?
   Intervention: Do not proceed until adequate staff are available; otherwise, staff and patient may be injured.
6. **Assess:** Is the intended ambulatory route clear of obstacles?
   Intervention: Remove any items that may impede the staff or patient from walking appropriately.
7. **Assess:** Is the assistive device sturdy and intact (e.g., tips intact, aluminum not bent, wood not cracked, padding intact, tips dry)?
   Intervention: For safety reasons, replace any portion of the device that has wear and tear. Dry any portion of the device that is wet. Educate the patient on appropriate inspection and safety techniques.
8. **Assess:** Do the patient's normal routines require modifications at home?
   Intervention: Educate the patient.
   - Further assistive devices may be needed (e.g., book bags, "reachers").
   - Instruct the patient to check for furniture in the household that may be creating a safety issue.
   - Instruct the patient to check for the availability of stairs and elevators at home and work.
9. **Assess:** Does the patient have a diagnosis of osteoporosis?
   Intervention: Do not use a gait belt. It may cause vertebral compression fractures due to pressure.

PREPROCEDURE

I. Check PCP orders and the patient care plan.
Knowledge of patient-specific orders is critical for safe patient care.

II. Gather supplies and equipment.
Preparing for the patient encounter saves time and promotes patient trust.

III. Perform hand hygiene.
Frequent hand hygiene prevents the spread of microorganisms.

IV. Maintain standard precautions.
Use of the correct personal protective equipment (PPE) is required whenever contact with bodily fluids is possible, to reduce the transfer of pathogens.

V. Introduce yourself.
Initial communication establishes the role of the nurse and begins a professional relationship.

VI. Provide for patient privacy.
It is important to maintain patient dignity.

VII. Identify the patient, using two identifiers.
Identifying a patient involves scanning barcodes or comparing the patient's stated name and birthdate to information on the patient's wristband or health record. The correct person must receive the correct treatment.

VIII. Explain the procedure to the patient.
The nurse has a responsibility to inform a patient before initiating care. Information may ease patient anxiety and facilitate cooperation.

PROCEDURE

Gait Belt: One Nurse, Independent Ambulation

Follow preprocedure steps I through VIII.

1. Fit the gait belt around the patient's waist; ensure that it is securely fastened and fits snugly.
   Precautions must be taken to maintain patient safety.
2. Stand behind the patient on the patient's weaker side, and grasp the belt at the patient's back; ambulate at the patient's pace.
   Caregiver position should be such that it promotes patient safety.

Follow postprocedure steps I through VI.

Gait Belt: One Nurse, Minimal Assist

Follow preprocedure steps I through VIII.

1. Fit the gait belt around the patient's waist; ensure that it is securely fastened and fits snugly.
   Precautions must be taken to maintain patient safety.
2. Stand on the patient's weaker side. Using an underhand grasp, hold the gait belt at the patient's back, and walk with the patient at the patient's pace.
   Caregiver position should be such that it promotes patient safety.

Follow postprocedure steps I through VI.

Gait Belt: One Nurse, Moderate Assist

Follow preprocedure steps I through VIII.

1. Fit the gait belt around the patient's waist; ensure that it is securely fastened and fits snugly.
   Precautions must be taken to maintain patient safety.
2. Stand on the patient's weaker side; interlock your forearm with the patient's forearm, and ambulate with the patient at the patient's pace.
   Caregiver position should be such that it promotes patient safety. The gait belt can be reached easily if needed.

Follow postprocedure steps I through VI.

Gait Belt: One Nurse, Maximum Assist

Follow preprocedure steps I through VIII.

1. Fit the gait belt around the patient's waist; ensure that it is securely fastened and fits snugly.
   Precautions must be taken to maintain patient safety.
2. Stand on the patient's weaker side. Hold the gait belt with the arm closest to the patient, and support the patient's elbow with your outside arm. Ambulate with the patient at the patient's pace.
   Caregiver position should be such that it promotes patient safety.

Follow postprocedure steps I through VI.

Gait Belt: Two Nurses, Minimal Assist

Follow preprocedure steps I through VIII.

1. Fit the gait belt around the patient's waist, and ensure that it is securely fastened and fits snugly.
   Precautions must be taken to maintain patient safety.
2. One nurse stands on each side and slightly behind the patient. The nurses support the patient under the axillae and ambulate with the patient at the patient's pace.
   Caregiver position should be such that it promotes patient safety. The nurses should be able to easily reach the gait belt if needed.

Follow postprocedure steps I through VI.

Gait Belt: Two Nurses, Maximum Assist

Follow preprocedure steps I through VIII.

1. Fit the gait belt around the patient's waist; ensure that it is securely fastened and fits snugly.
   Precautions must be taken to maintain patient safety.
2. One nurse stands on each side of the patient, with the arm closest to the patient holding the gait belt. Each nurse supports the patient's arm with the nurse's outside arm and ambulates with the patient at the patient's pace.
   Caregiver position should be such that it promotes patient safety.

Follow postprocedure steps I through VI.

Cane Walking: Maximum Support

Follow preprocedure steps I through VIII.

1. The patient holds the cane on his or her stronger side.
   Using the patient's stronger side promotes optimal alignment of the body while ambulating and promotes optimal support.
2. The patient moves the cane forward 6 inches in front and 6 inches to the side of the strong leg, with the elbow flexed 30 degrees.
3. The patient moves the weak foot forward to the cane.
4. The patient moves the strong leg past the cane.
5. Repeat procedure steps 2 through 4.

Follow postprocedure steps I through VI.

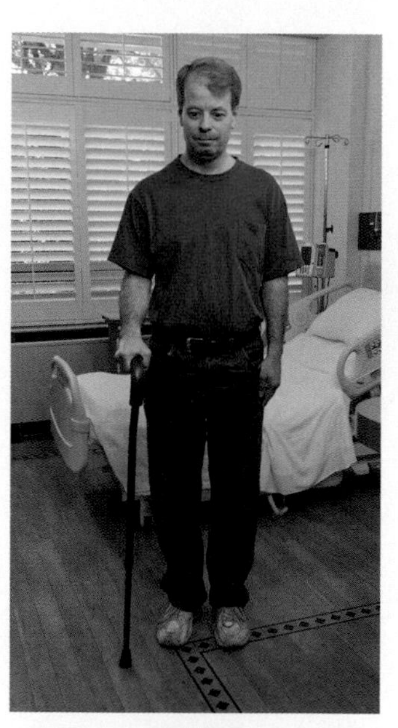

STEP 2

Cane Walking: Minimal Support

Follow preprocedure steps I through VIII.

1. The patient holds the cane on his or her stronger side.
   Using the patient's stronger side promotes optimal alignment of the body while ambulating and promotes optimal support.
2. The patient moves the cane and the weak leg forward at the same time.
3. The patient moves the strong leg past the cane.
4. The patient repeats steps 2 and 3 (i.e., mimics walking).

Follow postprocedure steps I through VI.

Rising from a Chair to a Walker

Follow preprocedure steps I through VIII.

1. The patient moves to the edge of the chair.
   Positioning the patient on the edge of the chair eases the patient's burden of lifting the body out of the chair.
2. The patient positions his or her legs close to the chair and slightly apart. The patient's hands are placed on the armrests of the chair, and the walker is in front of the chair.
   This position provides the strongest base of support to facilitate lifting the body and standing.
3. The patient pushes off the chair and balances.
   Taking the time to balance more fully ensures patient safety before moving and reduces the risk of falls.
4. The patient moves his or her hands, one at a time, to the walker.
   The patient should always have one hand grasping an arm of the chair or the walker to ensure safety before moving. This reduces the risk of falls.
5. Proceed to the Walker: Maximal Support or Walker: One Leg Weaker section.

Follow postprocedure steps I through VI.

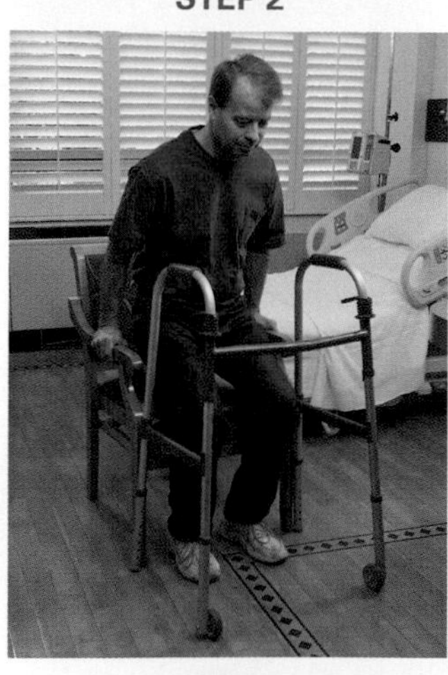

STEP 2

Walker: Maximum Support

Follow preprocedure steps I through VIII and procedure steps 1 through 4 in the Rising from a Chair to a Walker section.

1. The patient moves the walker 6 to 8 inches forward.
2. The patient moves the right foot forward.
3. The patient moves the left foot forward.
4. Repeat procedure steps 1 through 3.

Follow postprocedure steps I through VI.

Walker: One-Leg Weaker

Follow preprocedure steps I through VIII and procedure steps 1 through 4 in the Rising from a Chair to a Walker section.

1. The patient moves the walker and the weak leg forward at the same time.
2. The patient moves the strong leg forward.
3. Repeat procedure steps 1 and 2.

Follow postprocedure steps I through VI.

POSTPROCEDURE

I. Return the bed to its lowest position, raise the top side rails, and verify that the call light is within reach for the patient.
Precautions are taken to maintain patient safety. Top side rails aid in positioning and turning. Raising four side rails is considered a restraint.

II. Assess for additional patient needs and state the time of your expected return.
Meeting patient needs and offering self promote patient satisfaction and build trust.

III. Properly dispose of PPE.
Gloves, gowns, and masks must be appropriately discarded to prevent the spread of microorganisms.

IV. Clean equipment if it was in contact with the patient; see specific manufacturer instructions.
Disinfection eliminates most microorganisms from inanimate objects.

V. Perform hand hygiene.
Frequent hand hygiene prevents the spread of infection.

VI. Document the date, time, assessment, procedure, and patient's response to the procedure.
Accurate documentation is essential to communicate patient care and to provide legal evidence of care.

SKILL 28-3 Walking With Crutches

PURPOSE

- To increase activity level
- To promote independence
- To promote safety
- To decrease risk of further injury
- To limit weight bearing on the affected extremity, as ordered

RESOURCES

- Appropriate crutches as prescribed by the primary care provider (PCP) or physical therapist: underarm (axillary), Lofstrand, or platform
- Sturdy shoes with nonskid soles

COLLABORATION AND DELEGATION

- Education on how to walk with crutches may not be delegated to unlicensed assistive personnel (UAP).
- Ambulation of a patient who is crutch walking may be delegated to UAP, provided the patient is experienced and stable on the crutches.
- UAP should report any of the following:
  - Noticeable incorrect usage or fit of crutches
  - Complaints of soreness or weakness
  - Difficulties with balance or strength
  - Difficulties with the procedure or other concerns verbalized by the patient
- UAP should be instructed in the following:
  - Appropriate ambulation assistive techniques
  - Appropriate equipment usage
  - Appropriate documentation
- Physical therapists (PTs) work with patients for rehabilitation. Collaborate with these specialists.
- Check the orders to make sure that duplication of activity for the patient is not occurring.
- A PT may ambulate the patient on the unit and assist as appropriate to ensure safety for all persons involved.
- Orthopedic specialists may change dressings or assess patient outcomes. Attempt to coordinate ambulation with orthopedic visits as appropriate.
- Home health workers ensure the patient's safety in the home. They should be aware of assistive devices and the home layout.
- If the patient is an inpatient, stair climbing should be taught by a PT because the physical therapy department has appropriate safety stairs on which the patient can practice. If the patient is in the emergency department, it is important to review the basics of stair climbing with the patient, who should indicate comprehension.

EVIDENCE-BASED PRACTICE

- Spring-loaded crutches are a better choice for patients because they assist in the biomechanics of the patient's gait for all gait methods, ultimately reducing injuries that occur from crutch walking (Segura and Piazza, 2007).
- Mechanical assistive ambulation devices (e.g., sit-to-stand lifts, ambulation assists, ceiling-mounted walking slings) should be considered when ambulating a patient to prevent injury to the caregiver and the patient (Radawiec, Howe, Gonzalez, et al, 2009).
- Crutch walking may be a progressive ambulation technique for patients who originally started their rehabilitation with more supportive devices. Various tools have been developed, such as the Timed Up and Go (TUG) test, to determine and predict maximal functional mobility for patients on assistive devices. It is important to determine whether the facility policy has implemented such a scoring system and, if so, to use it for patient safety (Kristensen, Bandholm, Holm, et al, 2009).

SPECIAL CIRCUMSTANCES

1. **Assess:** Is the patient experiencing pain?
   Intervention: Determine whether the pain is new or preexisting.
   - Anticipate whether ambulation will produce pain and require pain medication.
   - Stop the procedure if the patient complains of new pain.
   - Medicate or premedicate the patient for pain according to orders.
   - Notify the PCP if no order exists for pain medication.
2. **Assess:** In a musculoskeletal assessment, does the patient show any difficulty with balance, weakness (unilateral or bilateral), or upper extremity strength?
   Intervention: Ensure that the patient is using the appropriate crutches and the prescribed walking technique.
   - Evaluate the size of crutches for the patient. There should be three finger widths between the axilla and axillary piece when the patient is standing erect, with elbow flexion of 30 degrees for the handbar when supporting weight.
   - Stress the importance of compliance with exercises that are intended to increase upper extremity strength.
   - There are five crutch-walking techniques:
     1. *Two-point:* Both feet bear partial weight.
     2. *Three-point:* One foot bears weight, and the other foot can be used for balance.
     3. *Four-point:* Both feet bear weight.
     4. *Swing-to:* Both feet are able to bear weight, but there is hip and leg paralysis and weaker upper body strength.
     5. *Swing-through:* Both feet bear weight; there is hip and leg paralysis, but the patient has stronger upper body strength.

3. **Assess:** Is the patient wearing sturdy, nonskid shoes with low or no heels?
   Intervention: Educate the patient, and obtain nonskid shoes or slippers to provide the necessary support and reduce the risk of falling with ambulation.
4. **Assess:** Are the crutches sturdy and intact (e.g., crutch tips are intact, aluminum is not bent, wood is not cracked, padding is intact, crutch tips are dry)?
   Intervention: Replace any portion of the crutch that is indicating wear and tear for safety; dry any portion that is wet; and educate the patient on appropriate inspection and safety techniques.
5. **Assess:** Do the normal routines require modifications?
   Intervention: Educate the patient with regard to further assistive devices that may be needed (e.g., book bags, reachers), household furniture that may create a safety issue, and stairs and elevators at home or work.

PREPROCEDURE

I. Check PCP orders and the patient care plan.
Knowledge of patient-specific orders is critical for safe patient care.
II. Gather supplies and equipment.
Preparing for the patient encounter saves time and promotes patient trust.
III. Perform hand hygiene.
Frequent hand hygiene prevents the spread of microorganisms.
IV. Maintain standard precautions.
Use of the correct personal protective equipment (PPE) is required whenever contact with bodily fluids is possible, to reduce the transfer of pathogens.
V. Introduce yourself.
Initial communication establishes the role of the nurse and begins a professional relationship.
VI. Provide for patient privacy.
It is important to maintain patient dignity.
VII. Identify the patient, using two identifiers.
Identifying a patient involves scanning barcodes or comparing the patient's stated name and birthdate to information on the patient's wristband or health record. The correct person must receive the correct treatment.
VIII. Explain the procedure to the patient.
The nurse has a responsibility to inform a patient before initiating care. Information may ease patient anxiety and facilitate cooperation.

PROCEDURE

Rising From a Chair by Using Crutches

Follow preprocedure steps I through VIII.

1. The patient moves to the front edge of the chair. Check that the chair is secure. If it is a wheelchair, make sure that the wheels are locked.
   By starting close to the edge of the chair, the patient eases the burden of lifting the body out of the chair.
2. The patient's strongest leg should be close to the chair. The patient's hand on the weak side holds the handbar of the crutches, and the hand on the patient's strong side holds onto the armrest of the chair.
   This position provides the strongest base of support to facilitate lifting the body and standing.
3. The patient pushes up and off the chair and then balances.
   Taking the time to balance properly ensures patient safety before moving and reduces the risk of falls.
4. The patient moves the crutches to a tripod position (i.e., starting point for a gait). Crutches are held 6 inches in front of the patient and 6 inches to the side of each foot.
   The stable tripod position ensures the patient's safety before moving and reduces the risk of falls.
5. Proceed to the Two-Point Gait, Three-Point Gait, Four-Point Gait, Swing-To Gait, Swing-Through Gait, or Sitting onto a Chair section.

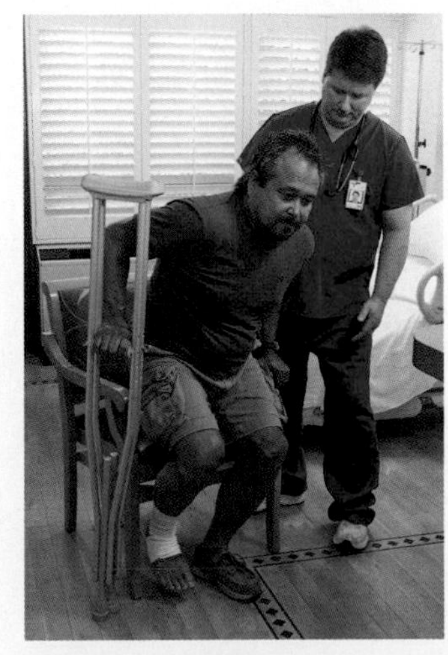
STEP 2

Two-Point Gait

Follow preprocedure steps I through VIII and procedure steps 2 through 4 in the Rising from a Chair Using Crutches section.

1. The patient starts in the tripod position.
   The tripod position is relatively stable, and it ensures the patient's safety before moving and reduces the risk of falls.
2. The patient moves the right crutch and right foot forward at the same time.
3. The patient moves the left crutch and left foot forward at the same time.
4. Repeat procedure steps 2 and 3 to mimic walking.
5. The patient ends in the tripod position.
   The tripod position is relatively stable, and it ensures the patient's safety before moving and reduces the risk of falls.

Follow postprocedure steps I through VI.

Three-Point Gait

Follow preprocedure steps I through VIII and procedure steps 2 through 4 in the Rising from a Chair Using Crutches section.

1. The patient starts in the tripod position.
   The tripod position is relatively stable, and it ensures the patient's safety before moving and reduces the risk of falls.
2. The patient moves both crutches and the weak foot forward at the same time.
3. The patient moves the strong foot forward.
4. Repeat procedure steps 2 and 3.
5. The patient ends in the tripod position.
   The tripod position is relatively stable, and it ensures the patient's safety before moving and reduces the risk of falls.

Follow postprocedure steps I through VI.

Four-Point Gait

Follow preprocedure steps I through VIII and procedure steps 2 through 4 in the Rising from a Chair section.

1. The patient starts in the tripod position.
   The tripod position is relatively stable, and it ensures the patient's safety before moving and reduces the risk of falls.
2. The patient moves the right crutch forward.
3. The patient moves the left foot forward.
4. The patient moves the left crutch forward.
5. The patient moves the right foot forward.
6. Repeat procedure steps 3 through 5.
7. The patient ends in the tripod position.
   The tripod position is relatively stable, and it ensures the patient's safety before moving and reduces the risk of falls.

Follow postprocedure steps I through VI.

Swing-To Gait

Follow preprocedure steps I through VIII and procedure steps 2 through 4 in the Rising from a Chair Using Crutches section.

1. The patient starts in the tripod position.
   The tripod position is relatively stable, and it ensures the patient's safety before moving and reduces the risk of falls.
2. The patient moves both crutches forward at the same time.
3. The patient lifts the body and swings both legs to the crutches.
4. Repeat procedure steps 2 and 3.

5. The patient ends in the tripod position.
   The tripod position is relatively stable, and it ensures the patient's safety before moving and reduces the risk of falls.

Follow postprocedure steps I through VI.

Swing-Through Gait

Follow preprocedure steps I through VIII and procedure steps 2 through 4 in the Rising from a Chair Using Crutches section.

1. The patient starts in the tripod position.
   The tripod position is relatively stable, so it ensures the patient's safety before moving and reduces the risk of falls.
2. The patient moves both crutches forward at the same time.
3. The patient lifts the body and swings both leg past the crutches.
4. Repeat steps 2 and 3.
5. The patient ends in the tripod position.
   The tripod position is relatively stable, and it ensures the patient's safety before moving and reduces the risk of falls.

Follow postprocedure steps I through VI.

Sitting Down on a Chair While Using Crutches

Follow preprocedure steps I through VIII.

1. The patient backs up to a chair that has armrests and stands in the tripod position.
   The tripod position is relatively stable, and it ensures the patient's safety before moving and reduces the risk of falls.
2. The patient makes sure that the stronger leg is against the back of the secure chair or locked wheelchair, balances, and then moves the crutches to the affected side, holding on to the handbars.
   This position ensures patient safety while the patient is preparing to sit and reduces the risk of falls.
3. The patient reaches for the armrest of the chair with the arm on his or her stronger side and sits down.
   Using the stronger arm ensures safety and reduces the risk of falls.

Follow postprocedure steps I through VI.

POSTPROCEDURE

I. Return the bed to its lowest position, raise the top side rails, and verify that the call light is within reach for the patient.
   Precautions are taken to maintain patient safety. Top side rails aid in positioning and turning. Raising four side rails is considered a restraint.

II. Assess for additional patient needs and state the time of your expected return.
   Meeting patient needs and offering self promote patient satisfaction and build trust.

III. Properly dispose of PPE.
   Gloves, gowns, and masks must be appropriately discarded to prevent the spread of microorganisms.

IV. Clean equipment if it was in contact with the patient; see specific manufacturer instructions.
   Disinfection eliminates most microorganisms from inanimate objects.

V. Perform hand hygiene.
   Frequent hand hygiene prevents the spread of infection.

VI. Document the date, time, assessment, procedure, and patient's response to the procedure.
   Accurate documentation is essential to communicate patient care and to provide legal evidence of care.

SKILL 28-4 Antiembolism Hose

PURPOSE

- Prevent edema to lower extremities
- Prevent deep vein thrombosis and venous stasis
- Promote blood flow of venous return
- Ultimately, prevent pulmonary emboli

RESOURCES

- Antiembolism hose (knee length or thigh length)
- Tape measure

COLLABORATION AND DELEGATION

- Applying, removing, and cleaning antiembolism hose may be delegated to unlicensed assistive personnel (UAP) after proper fitting and skin assessment by the nurse.
- UAP should report any of the following:
  - Complaints related to pain, application, or fit
  - Sores, wounds, irritations, lesions, edema, redness, or localized warmth in the lower extremities
  - Difficulties in performing the procedure
- UAP should be instructed in the following:
  - Appropriate application methods
  - Appropriate cleaning methods
  - Appropriate documentation

EVIDENCE-BASED PRACTICE

- Compared with thigh-length antiembolism hose, the use of knee-length antiembolism hose facilitates patient compliance and improves patient outcomes due to greater comfort, easier application, lower cost, and less risk of bunching and constricting blood flow (Brady, Raingruber, Peterson, et al, 2007; Roman, 2005).
- Homans sign should not be performed or relied on as evidence of deep vein thrombosis (DVT). More than 50% of diagnosed cases of DVT are asymptomatic. Homans sign is positive for less than 50% of patients with diagnosed DVT, and false positives are numerous. The procedure can cause a clot to dislodge, resulting in harm and negative patient outcomes (Agudelo, Morgan, and Smith, 2005; Beck, 2006; Roman, 2005; Shifaza, 2007).

SPECIAL CIRCUMSTANCES

1. **Assess:** Did the initial fitting of hose and measurements fall outside the range listed in the manufacturer's size charts?
   Intervention: Notify the primary care provider (PCP). Alternative compression devices, such as sequential compression devices (see Skill 28-5) or ACE bandages, may be needed.
2. **Assess:** Has the patient been out of bed before hose application?
   Intervention: Have the patient elevate the legs or lie down for 15 to 30 minutes. Having the legs in a dependent position promotes edema; if edema exists when the hose are applied, the desired outcome will not be achieved.
3. **Assess:** Is there pain, redness, or soreness in the patient's legs?
   Intervention: Determine whether the pain is new or a preexisting problem.
   - Stop the procedure if the complaint is new, and assess for possible DVT or an incorrect fit.
   - Notify the PCP.
4. **Assess:** What is the patient's neurovascular status at baseline? Check for the following:
   - Toes are warm and pink.
   - The posterior tibial and/or dorsalis pedal pulses are palpable or audible with a doppler.
   - Assess for edema or distended veins.

   Intervention: Determine whether any unusual neurovascular symptoms are new or preexisting.
   - Stop the procedure if the symptom is new, and assess for possible DVT.
   - Notify the PCP.
5. **Assess:** Does the patient have incisions or open wounds?
   Intervention: Determine whether they are new or preexisting.
   - If an incision or wound is draining, cover it with a bandage to avoid the spread of microorganisms to the hose.
   - Carefully apply the stocking over this area to avoid causing further trauma or injury.
   - If the wound is new, notify the PCP.
6. **Assess:** Do the hose apply easily?
   Intervention: Determine whether they are the correct fit and size, and ensure that the legs are dry:
   - Resize the patient.
   - Ensure that the hose were dried flat after washing; hanging hose to dry may cause stretching.
   - Discard the hose, and obtain a new pair.
   - Determine whether the legs are wet or damp. If they are, application of the hose will be difficult, possibly causing trauma to the skin. Ensure that the legs are dry.
   - Ensure that the hose are washed frequently; the recommendation is every 3 days. Having two pairs of hose allows for the use of one pair while the other is being laundered.

PREPROCEDURE

I. Check PCP orders and the patient care plan.
Knowledge of patient-specific orders is critical for safe patient care.
II. Gather supplies and equipment.
Preparing for the patient encounter saves time and promotes patient trust.
III. Perform hand hygiene.
Frequent hand hygiene prevents the spread of microorganisms.
IV. Maintain standard precautions.
Use of the correct personal protective equipment (PPE) is required whenever contact with bodily fluids is possible, to reduce the transfer of pathogens.
V. Introduce yourself.
Initial communication establishes the role of the nurse and begins a professional relationship.
VI. Provide for patient privacy.
It is important to maintain patient dignity.
VII. Identify the patient, using two identifiers.
Identifying a patient involves scanning barcodes or comparing the patient's stated name and birthdate to information on the patient's wristband or health record. The correct person must receive the correct treatment.
VIII. Explain the procedure to the patient.
The nurse has a responsibility to inform a patient before initiating care. Information may ease patient anxiety and facilitate cooperation.

PROCEDURE

Fitting: Knee-High Hose

Follow preprocedure steps I through VIII.

1. Measure from the heel to the popliteal space (behind the knee).
This measurement is required for manufacturers' sizing charts. Accurate measurements ensure the correct fit, avoiding patient harm that can occur from estimating sizes.
2. Measure around the widest part of the calf.
This measurement is required for manufacturers' sizing charts. Accurate measurements ensure the correct fit, avoiding patient harm that can occur from estimating sizes.
3. Compare these measurements with the manufacturer's sizing charts. If a patient's measurements fall between two sizes on the charts, take both sizes of hose, and try them on the patient to see which has the better fit.
It is essential to have the correct fit to ensure positive patient outcomes. If a stocking is too small, it will constrict blood flow; if it is too large, it can cause skin irritation and will not promote venous return of blood.
4. Proceed to the Application: Knee-High Hose section.

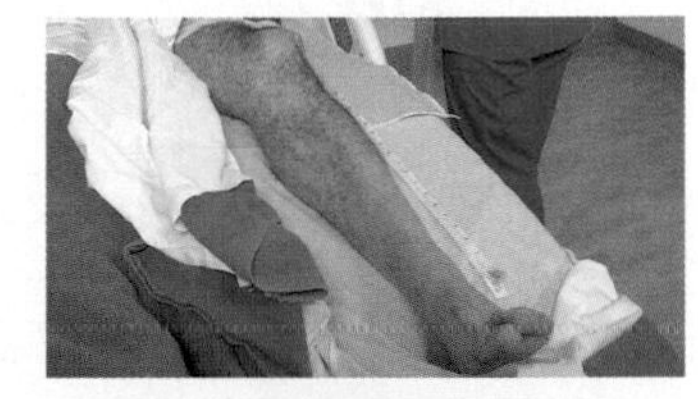

STEP 1

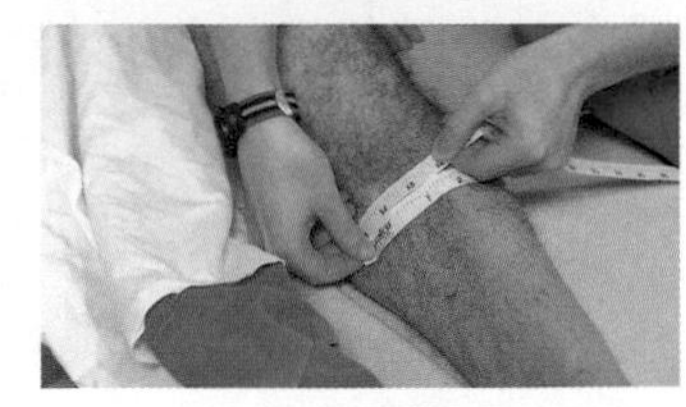

STEP 2

Fitting: Thigh-High Hose

Follow preprocedure steps I through VIII.

1. Measure from the heel to the gluteal fold below the buttocks.
2. Measure around the widest part of the calf.
3. Measure around the widest part of the thigh.
4. Compare these measurements with the manufacturer's sizing charts. If a patient's measurements fall between two sizes on the charts, take both sizes of hose and try them on the patient to see which has the better fit.
5. Proceed to the Application: Thigh-High Hose section.

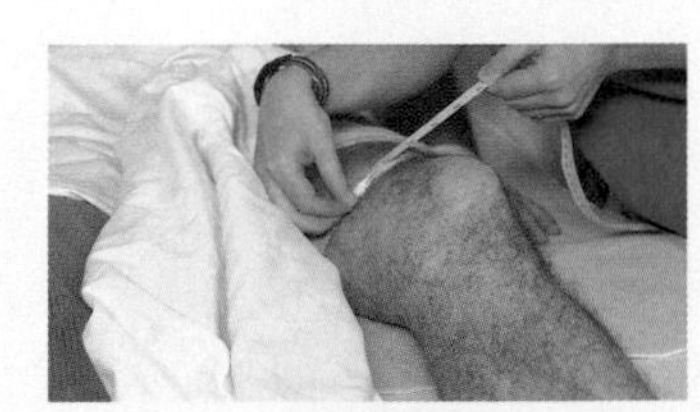

STEP 3

Application: Knee-High Hose

Follow preprocedure steps I through VIII.

1. Raise the bed to working height.
Setting the bed at the correct working height for the provider prevents provider discomfort and possible injury.

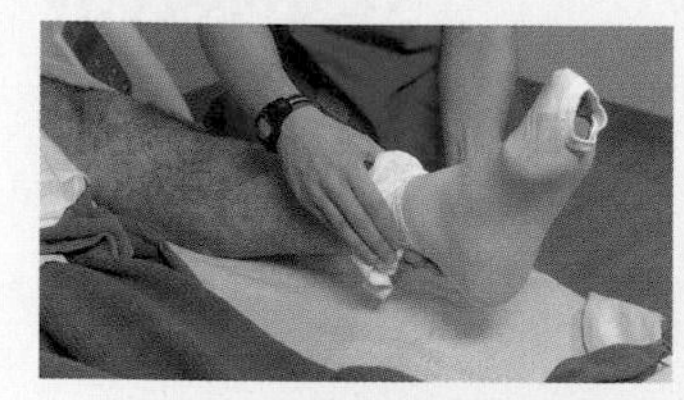
STEP 3

2. Roll the hose inside out around hands; the leg of the hose will be inside out, covering the foot of the hose.
   Rolling the hose in this way allows easy application and prevents possible trauma to the skin during application.
3. Have the patient point the toes; put each stocking over the toes and heel, and smooth wrinkles away from the foot.
   Pointing the toes allows easy application of the hose; wrinkles and bunching of the hose can cause trauma to the skin and constrict blood flow, preventing venous return.
4. Unroll the remainder of each stocking over the leg, smoothing wrinkles as the hose are unrolled.
   Wrinkles and bunching of the hose can cause trauma to the skin and constrict blood flow, preventing venous return.
5. Ensure that the top of each stocking is 1 to 2 inches below the knee.
   Correctly fit hose do not apply excessive pressure to the area or interfere with circulation.

Follow postprocedure steps I through VI.

Application: Thigh-High Hose

Follow preprocedure steps I through VIII.

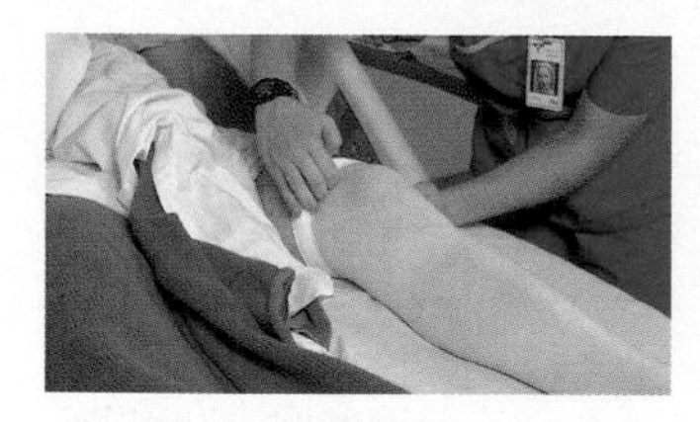
STEP 2

1. Follow procedure steps 1 through 4 in the Application: Knee-High Hose section.
2. Have the patient bend the knee. Unroll each stocking over the knee, and have the patient straighten the knee. Smooth wrinkles.
   Bending the knee allows easy application of the hose and prevents possible trauma to the skin during application. Wrinkles and bunching of the hose can cause trauma to the skin and constrict blood flow, preventing venous return.
3. Unroll the remainder of each stocking on the upper leg, smoothing wrinkles.
   Wrinkles and bunching of the hose can cause trauma to the skin and constrict blood flow, preventing venous return.
4. Ensure that the top of each stocking is 1 to 3 inches below the buttock.
   Correctly fit hose; do not apply excessive pressure to the area or interfere with circulation.

Follow postprocedure steps I through VI.

POSTPROCEDURE

I. Return the bed to its lowest position, raise the top side rails, and verify that the call light is within reach for the patient.
   Precautions are taken to maintain patient safety. Top side rails aid in positioning and turning. Raising four side rails is considered a restraint.

II. Assess for additional patient needs and state the time of your expected return.
   Meeting patient needs and offering self promote patient satisfaction and build trust.

III. Properly dispose of PPE.
   Gloves, gowns, and masks must be appropriately discarded to prevent the spread of microorganisms.

IV. Clean equipment if it was in contact with the patient; see specific manufacturer instructions.
   Disinfection eliminates most microorganisms from inanimate objects.

V. Perform hand hygiene.
   Frequent hand hygiene prevents the spread of infection.

VI. Document the date, time, assessment, procedure, and patient's response to the procedure.
   Accurate documentation is essential to communicate patient care and to provide legal evidence of care.

SKILL 28-5 Sequential Compression Devices (SCDs)

PURPOSE

- To prevent edema to the lower extremities
- To prevent deep vein thrombosis (DVT) and venous stasis
- To promote venous blood flow
- To prevent pulmonary emboli

RESOURCES

- Sequential compression device (SCD)
- SCD sleeves (knee length or thigh length)
- Tape measure

COLLABORATION AND DELEGATION

- Applying and removing SCDs may be delegated to unlicensed assistive personnel (UAP) after the nurse has verified proper fitting, completed skin assessment, and ensured proper device function. These checks by the nurse must be performed at least once per shift.
- UAP should report any of the following:
  - Complaints related to pain, application, or fit of the sleeves
  - Sores, wounds, irritations, lesions, edema, redness, or localized warmth in the lower extremities
  - Difficulties in performing the procedure
- UAP should be provided instructions about the following:
  - Appropriate application methods
  - Proper use of the mechanical device, tube connections, alarm settings, and inflation sequencing
  - Restrictions on removal of SCD sleeves (i.e., SCD sleeves should not be removed for long periods of time).
  - Appropriate documentation

EVIDENCE-BASED PRACTICE

- SCDs and other external compression devices are not effective in preventing DVT or pulmonary emboli in trauma patients if used alone. Evidence reveals that pharmacologic intervention should be ordered in conjunction with this treatment modality (Agudelo, Morgan, and Smith, 2005; Kakkos, Griffin, Geroulakos, et al, 2005; Roman, 2005).
- Patients and nursing staff require reminders regarding compliance for use of SCDs after hygienic care or other therapeutic activities. A major reason for failure of these devices to promote optimal outcomes in the prevention of DVT is noncompliance or improper use by patients and staff (Beck, 2006; Bockheim, McAllen, Baker, et al, 2009; Brady, Raingruber, Peterson, et al, 2007; Kakkos, Griffin, Geroulakos, et al, 2005; Roman, 2005).

SPECIAL CIRCUMSTANCES

1. **Assess:** Did the initial fitting of sleeves and measurements fall outside the range listed in the manufacturer's size charts?
   Intervention: Notify the primary care provider (PCP); alternative compression devices may be needed.
2. **Assess:** Is there pain, redness, or soreness?
   Intervention: Determine whether the sign is new or preexisting.
   - Stop the procedure if the sign is new, and assess for possible DVT or incorrect fit.
   - If the patient has a known DVT, do not apply SCDs.
   - Notify the PCP.
3. **Assess:** What is the patient's neurovascular status at baseline? Check for the following:
   - Toes are warm and pink.
   - The posterior tibial and dorsalis pedal pulses are palpable.
   - Assess for edema or distended veins.

   Intervention: Determine whether any unusual neurovascular symptoms are new or preexisting.
   - Stop the procedure if the symptom is new, and assess for a possible DVT or incorrect fit.
   - If a DVT is detected, discontinue the evaluation, and notify the PCP.
   - Two fingers should fit under the sleeve when it is not inflated; reapply the sleeve if it is too tight or too loose.
   - If the sleeve is thigh length, remeasure and determine the correct fit.
4. **Assess:** Does the patient have incisions or open wounds?
   Intervention: Determine whether they are new or preexisting.
   - If the incision or wound is draining, cover it with a bandage to avoid the spread of microorganisms to the SCD sleeves.
   - If the wound is new, notify the PCP.
5. **Assess:** Has only one SCD sleeve been ordered (i.e., for one leg)?
   Intervention: Keep the other sleeve in the package and attached to the machine for proper inflation and functioning of the device.
6. **Assess:** Has the patient complained of warmth, or is there overt perspiration on the leg?
   Intervention: Ensure that the cooling control on the device is activated (i.e., it resets to *off* each time the device is turned off). Place a stockinette on the leg to absorb perspiration if antiembolism hose were not ordered in conjunction with the SCDs.
7. **Assess:** Is an alarm sounding?
   Intervention: Ensure that the ankle pressure on the device is set at 35 to 55 mm Hg. Check that all tubing is connected and that the tubing has the arrows correctly aligned with the arrows on the machine at connection. If only one sleeve is being used, verify that the other sleeve is connected and remains in an enclosed space so that it can inflate against something.

PREPROCEDURE

I. Check PCP orders and the patient care plan.
Knowledge of patient-specific orders is critical for safe patient care.

II. Gather supplies and equipment.
Preparing for the patient encounter saves time and promotes patient trust.

III. Perform hand hygiene.
Frequent hand hygiene prevents the spread of microorganisms.

IV. Maintain standard precautions.
Use of the correct personal protective equipment (PPE) is required whenever contact with bodily fluids is possible, to reduce the transfer of pathogens.

V. Introduce yourself.
Initial communication establishes the role of the nurse and begins a professional relationship.

VI. Provide for patient privacy.
It is important to maintain patient dignity.

VII. Identify the patient, using two identifiers.
Identifying a patient involves scanning barcodes or comparing the patient's stated name and birthdate to information on the patient's wristband or health record. The correct person must receive the correct treatment.

VIII. Explain the procedure to the patient.
The nurse has a responsibility to inform a patient before initiating care. Information may ease patient anxiety and facilitate cooperation.

PROCEDURE

Fitting and Application: Knee-High SCD Sleeves

Follow preprocedure steps I through VIII.

1. Raise the bed to working height.
Setting the bed at the correct working height for the provider prevents provider discomfort and possible injury.

2. Place the device on the foot of the bed.
The manufacturer's design prevents possible provider and patient injury.

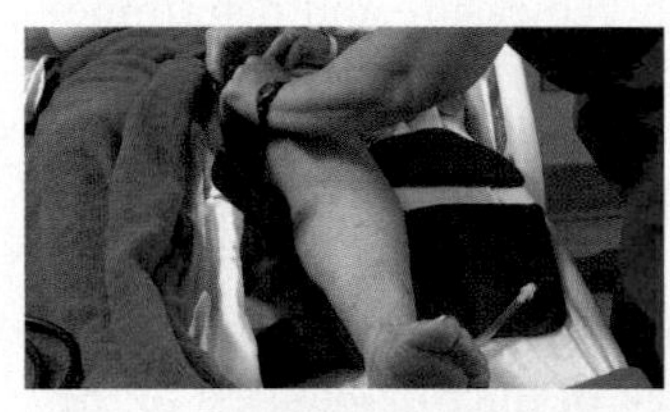
STEP 3

3. Place the sleeve of the SCD under the patient's leg, with the leg resting in the center of the sleeve.
Proper positioning of the SCD sleeve allows proper fit and application, which decreases the risk of constricting the blood flow or diminishing optimal outcomes.

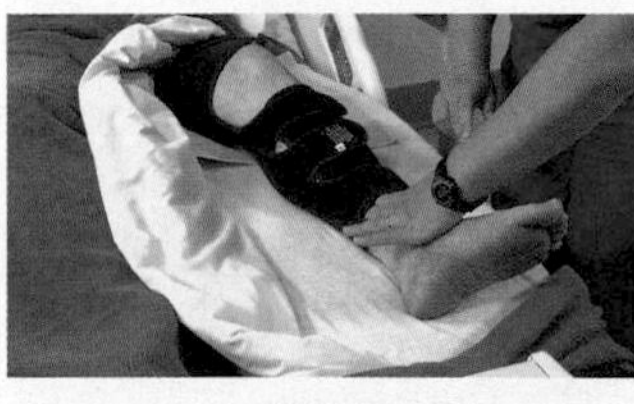
STEP 4

4. Wrap the sleeve around the leg, and fasten it with Velcro straps. Verify that two fingers fit between the leg and the sleeve when the sleeve is not inflated.
The proper fit is necessary when the sleeve is inflated to maximize optimal outcomes and decrease the risk of constricting blood flow.

5. Repeat on the other leg if ordered. If a sleeve has been ordered for only one leg, leave the other sleeve in the package.
The proper fit is necessary when the sleeve is inflated to maximize optimal outcomes and decrease the risk of constricting blood flow.

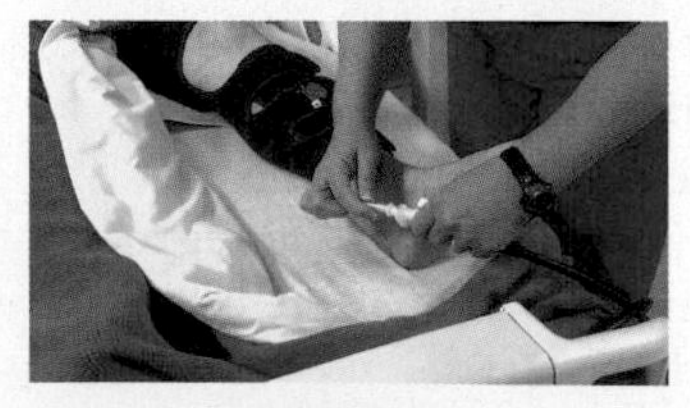
STEP 6

6. Connect the sleeve tubing for both sleeves to the device. Verify that there are no kinks in the tubing and that the arrows on the tubing align with the arrows on the machine.
Proper connections are needed for the device to function correctly.

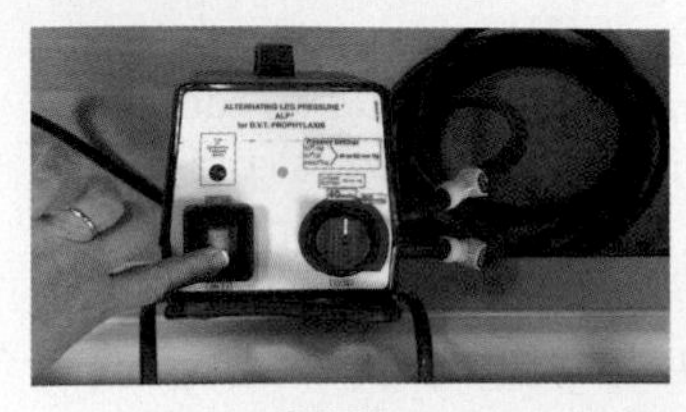
STEP 7

7. Turn on the device. Set the cooling control to *on*, and set the alarm to *on*. Ensure that the ankle pressure is 35 to 55 mm Hg.
The cooling control feature ensures patient comfort and decreases skin irritation and breakdown caused by excess perspiration. The alarm provides safety notification in the event of malfunction.

8. Ensure that sequential inflation is occurring and that the machine is functioning properly.
Proper function of the device optimizes patient outcomes.

Follow postprocedure steps I through VI.

Fitting: Thigh-High SCD Sleeves

Follow preprocedure steps I through VIII.

1. Measure around the thigh at the gluteal fold below the buttocks.
   This measurement is required for manufacturers' sizing charts. Accurate measurements ensure the correct fit, avoiding patient harm that can occur from estimating sizes.
2. Compare the measurements to the manufacturer's sizing charts. If a patient's measurements fall between two sizes on the charts, take both sizes of sleeves, and put them on the patient to see which has the better fit.
   The correct fit ensures positive patient outcomes. If a sleeve is too small, it will constrict blood flow; if it is too large, it can cause skin irritation and will not promote venous blood return.
3. Proceed to the Application: Thigh-High SCD Sleeves section.

Application: Thigh-High SCD Sleeves

Follow preprocedure steps I through VIII and procedure steps 1 and 2 in the Fitting: Thigh-High SCD Sleeves section.

1. Follow procedure steps 2 through 5 in the Fitting and Application: Knee-High SCD Sleeves section.
2. Verify that the knee is seen through the opening in the sleeve.
   Proper application and fit of the sleeve are needed to decrease the risk of constricting blood flow or diminishing optimal outcomes.
3. Follow procedure steps 6 through 9 in the Fitting and Application: Knee-High SCD Sleeves section.

Follow postprocedure steps I through VI.

POSTPROCEDURE

I. Return the bed to its lowest position, raise the top side rails, and verify that the call light is within reach for the patient.
Precautions are taken to maintain patient safety. Top side rails aid in positioning and turning. Raising four side rails is considered a restraint.

II. Assess for additional patient needs and state the time of your expected return.
Meeting patient needs and offering self promote patient satisfaction and build trust.

III. Properly dispose of PPE.
Gloves, gowns, and masks must be appropriately discarded to prevent the spread of microorganisms.

IV. Clean equipment if it was in contact with the patient; see specific manufacturer instructions.
Disinfection eliminates most microorganisms from inanimate objects.

V. Perform hand hygiene.
Frequent hand hygiene prevents the spread of infection.

VI. Document the date, time, assessment, procedure, and patient's response to the procedure.
Accurate documentation is essential to communicate patient care and to provide legal evidence of care.

SUMMARY OF LEARNING OUTCOMES

LO 28.1 *Describe the function of the musculoskeletal, neurologic, and cardiopulmonary systems in normal activity and movement:* The musculoskeletal, nervous, and cardiopulmonary systems work together to ensure a person's ability to move and maintain posture, alignment, and balance.

LO 28.2 *Identify changes in the musculoskeletal, neurologic, and cardiopulmonary systems that cause alterations in activity and movement throughout the life span:* Impairment or injury of any component of the musculoskeletal, nervous, or cardiopulmonary system affects the body's ability to move. Immobility predisposes a person to weakness, decreased muscle tone, decreased bone and muscle mass, muscle atrophy, contractures, increased cardiac workload, decreased lung expansion, urinary stasis, and constipation.

LO 28.3 *Assess the effects of decreased activity and immobility on multiple body systems:* Initial assessment of mobility and patient activity includes observation (i.e., inspection) of the patient's gait and coordination. A fall risk assessment helps to ensure patient safety. Neurologic, cardiovascular, nutritional, skin, and psychosocial assessment data as they relate to activity and mobility concerns must be collected.

LO 28.4 *Discuss nursing diagnoses for patients experiencing immobility and impaired levels of activity:* NANDA-I nursing diagnoses related to activity, immobility, and safe patient movement include *Impaired Physical Mobility, Risk for Falls, Activity Intolerance, Imbalanced Nutrition: Less than Body Requirements, Constipation, Impaired Skin Integrity,* and *Social Isolation.*

LO 28.5 *Generate nursing care goals and outcome criteria for patients with complications from inactivity or immobility:* Nursing care plans should be developed in collaboration with patients and other health care professionals to prevent potential complications of immobility.

LO 28.6 *List interventions to enhance patient activity, promote safety, and reverse negative effects of immobility that can be evaluated after implementation:* Specific nursing interventions to encourage exercise, promote safety, enhance lung expansion, prevent deep vein thrombosis, provide adequate nutrition and fluid, maintain skin integrity, and prevent social isolation are necessary to prevent the negative impact of immobility on patients. Safe patient-handling and movement algorithms have been developed to assist the nurse in promoting safe patient positioning and transfers. Evaluation of treatment interventions for patients who have limited mobility or are confined to bed rest must be based on the attainment of goals and be an ongoing process.

Responses to the critical-thinking exercises are available at *http://evolve.elsevier.com/YoostCrawford/fundamentals/.*

REVIEW QUESTIONS

1. An uncooperative 70-year-old male with right-sided paralysis from a recent cerebrovascular accident (CVA) has to be transferred from the bed to a wheelchair. Which action indicates the best method to transfer this patient?
   a. A two-person lift is performed, with one person on each side of the patient.
   b. The patient is steadied under the arms and pivoted on his left leg.
   c. A full-body sling lift is used with the help of unlicensed assistive personnel (UAP).
   d. A stand assist lift is used with the help of another nurse.

2. After instruction, which action by a patient who can bear weight on both feet indicates an understanding of the proper use of crutches?
   a. Adjusting the crutches so that they rest directly under the axilla
   b. Moving the opposing crutch and leg together for a two-point crutch walk
   c. Using a four-point crutch walk when not weight bearing on the left leg
   d. Placing the crutches 28 inches forward and then swinging both legs forward when using a three-point crutch walk

3. What bony prominences are at greatest risk for skin breakdown on a patient who is restricted to bed rest and placed in the side-lying position? *(Select all that apply.)*
   a. Sternum
   b. Ears
   c. Elbows
   d. Hips
   e. Coccyx
4. Which area of the central nervous system has most likely sustained damage if a patient exhibits a lack of coordination and an unsteady gait after a traumatic head injury?
   a. Medulla oblongata
   b. Articular disk
   c. Brainstem
   d. Cerebellum
5. A nurse is providing patient education on the prevention of osteoporosis. Which important fact should the nurse include in the teaching care plan?
   a. Calcium should be taken with vitamin D to increase calcium absorption.
   b. African American women are more prone to developing osteoporosis than are Asian American women.
   c. Increased phosphorus metabolism may lead to bone fragility.
   d. Aerobic exercise is more advantageous than weight-bearing exercise in preventing osteoporosis.
6. What nursing intervention would be most effective in preventing flaccidity in a hospitalized patient?
   a. Early ambulation after surgery
   b. Administering calcium with vitamin D
   c. Coughing and deep breathing exercises
   d. Referring the patient to occupational therapy
7. Identify all nursing interventions that are necessary when caring for a quadriplegic patient injured 2 years earlier in a motor vehicle accident. *(Select all that apply.)*
   a. Monitoring respiratory status and breathing difficulties
   b. Assisting with feeding and activities of daily living (ADLs)
   c. Developing a care plan with the patient's power of attorney
   d. Using mechanical lifts to assist with transferring the patient
   e. Placing a gait belt around the patient's waist before ambulation
8. Which discovery found during an admission assessment of a patient transferred from a long-term care facility does the nurse recognize as the result of immobility?
   a. Bilateral elbow contractures
   b. Increased muscle tone
   c. Decreased cardiac workload
   d. Orthostatic hypertension
9. Which nursing diagnosis label is most appropriate for a patient who is experiencing sensory deprivation due to a lack of interaction with others?
   a. *Impaired Verbal Communication*
   b. *Sedentary Lifestyle*
   c. *Social Isolation*
   d. *Disturbed Personal Identity*
10. After application of sequential compression devices (SCDs) on a patient, what assessment finding is essential for the nurse to include in documentation?
   a. Warmth of bilateral upper extremities
   b. Lower extremity circulatory status
   c. Circumoral cyanosis
   d. Bowel sounds

Answers and rationales to the review questions are available at *http://evolve.elsevier.com/YoostCrawford/fundamentals/*.

REFERENCES

Agudelo JF, Morgan SJ, Smith WR: Venous thromboembolism in orthopedic trauma patients, *Orthopedics,* 28(10), 1164, 2005.

American Nurses Association (ANA): Elimination of manual patient handling to prevent work-related musculoskeletal disorders. Position statement, 2008. Retrieved from *www.nursingworld.org/position/practice/handling.aspx.*

Arbesman M, Sheard K: Systematic review of the effectiveness of occupational therapy-related interventions for people with amyotrophic lateral sclerosis, *Am J Occup Ther,* 68(1):20-26, 2014.

Arnold M, Radawiec S, Campo M, Wright LR: Changes in functional independence measure ratings associated with a safe patient handling and movement program, *Rehabil Nurs,* 36:138-144, 2011.

Beck DM: Venous thromboembolism (VTE) prophylaxis: Implications for medical-surgical nurses, *Med Surg Nurs,* 15(5):282, 2006.

Bockheim HM, McAllen KJ, Baker R, Barletta JF: Mechanical prophylaxis to prevent venous thromboembolism in surgical patients: A prospective trial evaluating compliance, *J Crit Care,* 24(2):192-196, 2009.

Bowyer H, Glover M: Guillain-Barre syndrome: Management and treatment options for patients with moderate to severe progression, *J Neurosci Nurs,* 42(5):288-293, 2010.

Brady D, Raingruber B, Peterson J, et al: The use of knee-length versus thigh-length compression stockings and sequential compression devices, *Cri Care Nurs Q,* 30(3):255-262, 2007.

Brower R: Consequences of bed rest, *Cri Care Med,* 37(10): S422-S428, 2009.

Cohen MH, Nelson GG, Green DA, et al: *Patient handling and movement assessments: A white paper.* Dallas, 2010, Faculty Guidelines Institute.

Cronenwett L, Sherwood G, Barnsteiner J, et al: Quality and safety education for nurses. *Nurs Outlook,* 55(3):122-131, 2007.

Fletcher K: Immobility: geriatric self-learning module, *Med Surg Nurs,* 14(1):35, 2005.

Gonzalez CM, Howe CM., Waters TR, Nelson A: Recommendations for turning patients with orthopaedic impairments, *Orthop Nurs,* 28(2):S9-S12, 2009.

Hanson D, Langemo D, Anderson J, Thompson P, Hunter S: Friction and shear considerations in pressure ulcer development, *Adv Skin Wound Care,* 23(1):21-24, 2010.

Hopkins R, Spuhler V, Thomsen G: Transforming ICU culture to facilitate early mobility, *Crit Care Clin,* 23(1):81-96, 2007.

Howe L: Education and empowerment of the nursing assistant: Validating their important role in skin care and pressure ulcer prevention, and demonstrating productivity enhancement and cost savings, *Adv Skin Wound Care,* 21(6):275-281, 2008.

The Joint Commission: Long term care national patient safety goals, 2014. Retrieved from *www.jointcommission.org/assets/1/6/LT2_NPSG_Chapter_2014.pdf.*

Kakkos SK, Griffin M, Geroulakos G, Nicolaides AN: The efficacy of a new portable sequential compression device (SCD express) in preventing venous stasis, *J Vasc Surg,* 42(2):296-303, 2005.

Kristensen MT, Bandholm T, Holm B, et al: Timed Up & Go test score in patients with hip fracture is related to the type of walking aid. *Arch Phys Med Rehabil,* 90(10):1760-1765, 2009.

National Osteoporosis Foundation: *Bone basics,* 2014. Retrieved from *http://nof.org/learn/bonebasics.*

Needleman J, Buerhaus P, Mattke S, et al: Nurse-staffing levels and the quality of care in hospitals, *N Engl J Med,* 346:1715-1722, 2002.

Nelson A (ed): *Safe patient handling and movement: A practical guide for healthcare professionals.* New York, 2006, Springer.

Nelson A, Baptiste AS: Evidence-based practices for safe patient handling and movement, *Orthop Nurs,* 25(6):366, 2006.

Palamone J, Brunovsky S, Groth M, Morris L, Kwasny, M: "Tap and twist": Preventing deep vein thrombosis in neuroscience patients through foot and ankle range-of-motion exercises, *J Neurosci Nurs,* 43(6):308-314, 2011.

Perell K, Nelson A, Goldman R, et al: Fall risk assessment measures, an analytic review, *J Gerontol A Biol Sci Med Sci,* 56:M761-M766, 2001.

Radawiec S, Howe C, Gonzalez C, Waters T, Nelson A: Safe ambulation of an orthopaedic patient, *Orthop Nurs,* 28(2):S24, 2009.

Roman M: Deep vein thrombosis: An overview, *Med Surg Matters,* 14(1):1, 2005.

Schiff W: *Nutrition for healthy living,* ed. 3, Boston, 2012, McGraw-Hill.

Sedlak C, Doheny M, Nelson A, Waters T: Development of the National Association of Orthopaedic Nurses guidance statement on safe patient handling and movement in the orthopaedic setting, *Orthop Nurs,* 28(2):S2, 2009.

Segura A, Piazza SJ: Mechanics of ambulation with standard and spring-loaded crutches, *Arch Phys Med Rehabil,* 88(9): 1159-1163, 2007.

Shier DN, Butler JL, Lewis R: *Hole's essentials of human anatomy & physiology,* ed. 11, Boston, 2012, McGraw-Hill.

Shifaza F: *Deep venous thrombosis: Clinician information (evidence summaries report),* Adelaide, South Australia, 2007, Joanna Briggs Institute.

U.S. Department of Veterans Affairs. Algorithms for safe patient handling and movement, 2014. Retrieved from *www.tampavaref.org/safe-patient-handling.htm.*

Waters TR: When is it safe to manually lift a patient? *Am J Nurs,* 107(8):53-58, 2007.

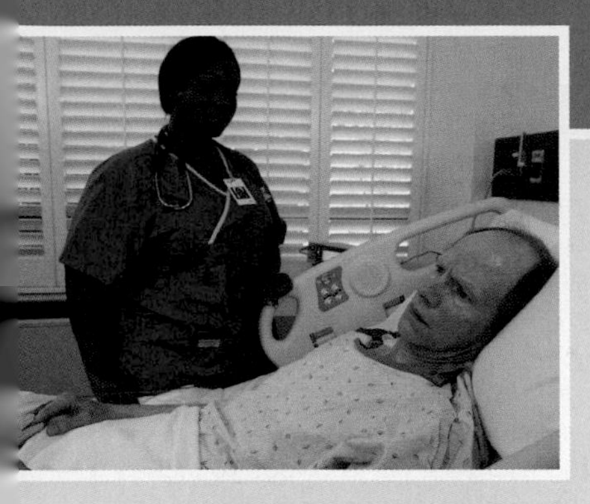

CHAPTER 29

Skin Integrity and Wound Care

EVOLVE WEBSITE

http://evolve.elsevier.com/YoostCrawford/fundamentals/

- Additional Evolve-Only Review Questions With Answers
- Answers and Rationales for Text Review Questions
- Answers to Critical-Thinking Questions
- Case Study With Questions
- Video Skills Clips
- Conceptual Care Map
- Animations
- Skills Checklists
- Glossary

LEARNING OUTCOMES

Comprehension of this chapter's content will provide students with the ability to:

LO 29.1 Describe the normal structure and function of skin.
LO 29.2 Review the factors that alter the skin's structure and function.
LO 29.3 Discuss the components of a focused skin and wound assessment, including the use of risk assessment tools.
LO 29.4 Identify appropriate nursing diagnoses for the patient with impaired skin integrity.
LO 29.5 Develop measurable patient-centered goals for patients with impaired skin integrity.
LO 29.6 Select interventions to prevent and treat impaired skin integrity.

KEY TERMS

abnormal reactive hyperemia, p. 620
acute wound, p. 615
approximated, p. 615
bioburden, p. 634
capillary closing pressure, p. 619
chronic wound, p. 615
clean contaminated wound, p. 615
clean wound, p. 615
closed wound, p. 615
colonized wound, p. 615
contaminated wound, p. 615
critical closing pressure, p. 619
debridement, p. 633
dehiscence, p. 617
dermis, p. 613
epidermis, p. 613
eschar, p. 621
evisceration, p. 617
fistulas, p. 617
friction, p. 619
full-thickness wound, p. 615
granulation tissue, p. 616
healing ridge, p. 617
Hemovac drain, p. 635
infected wound, p. 615
infection, p. 614
inflammatory phase, p. 616
Jackson-Pratt drain, p. 635
maceration, p. 620
maturation phase, p. 616
open wound, p. 614
papillary dermis, p. 613
partial-thickness wound, p. 615
Penrose drain, p. 635
pressure ulcer, p. 618
primary intention, p. 615
proliferative phase, p. 616
rete ridges, p. 613
sanguineous, p. 627
scar tissue, p. 616
secondary intention, p. 615
serosanguineous, p. 627
serous, p. 627
shear, p. 619
sinus tract, p. 621
stage I pressure ulcer, p. 620
stage II pressure ulcer, p. 620
stage III pressure ulcer, p. 621
stage IV pressure ulcer, p. 621
stratum corneum, p. 613
stratum germinativum, p. 613
subcutaneous layer, p. 613
superficial wound, p. 615
suspected deep tissue injury, p. 621
sutures, p. 635
tertiary intention, p. 615
tunnel, p. 621
undermining, p. 621
unstageable pressure ulcer, p. 621
wounds, p. 614

CASE STUDY

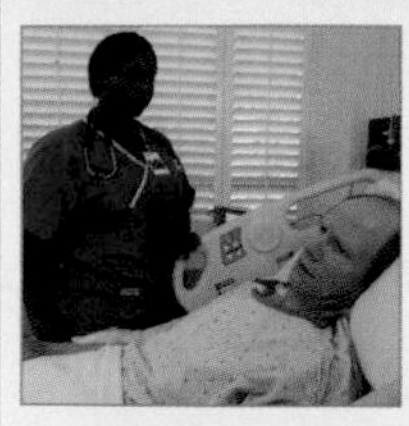

Mr. Joseph is a 64-year-old male with a 30-year history of multiple sclerosis (MS). He worked as a high school math teacher until 8 years ago, when his deteriorating health necessitated early retirement. His wife has taken a part-time job to supplement their income from his pension. Mr. Joseph is alert and oriented ×3 and able to move all extremities, but weakly. He is incontinent of urine and stool and using adult briefs. He is able to sit on a chair but requires assistance from his wife or adult son, who lives nearby, and tends to slide down in the chair. He requires assistance with meals, tires easily, and rarely finishes 50% of a meal. Mr. Joseph expressed sadness over his declining health and the "burden" that it has placed on his family, both physically and financially.

He is admitted to the unit with the diagnosis of a urinary tract infection. He has no known drug allergies. He is 5 feet 10 inches tall and weighs 132 pounds. His albumin is 2.5 g/dL, and his prealbumin is 20 mg/dL. During his admission assessment his vital signs are T 38.3° C (101° F), P 110 regular and thready, R 28 and labored, and BP 110/60, with a pulse oximetry reading of 94% on room air. Physical assessment reveals a wound on Mr. Joseph's right hip that measures 5.5 cm in length and 5 cm in width, with bone palpable along the medial edge. The periwound skin is intact. The wound has been treated at home with normal saline-moistened gauze that is changed once or twice a day. Mr. Joseph states that the wound has been present for more than 3 months and "it just doesn't get better." The gauze dressings are saturated by exudate in 3 hours, with a slight foul odor. A 2 cm by 2 cm area of redness also is present on his left heel that does not blanch when pressure is applied.

Mr. Joseph is diaphoretic and appears anxious. He states, "I can't turn myself! Who will take care of me here? I hurt all over but especially my hip!" He rates his pain at 6 of 10 in the right hip.

Treatment orders are as follows:

- Turn q 2 hr
- Regular adult diet
- Up in chair twice daily
- VS q 4 hr
- Dietary consult

Medication orders are as follows:

- IV infusion of D_5 0.45%NS at 125 mL/hr
- Ceftriaxone 1 g q 24 hr via intravenous piggyback (IVPB)
- Acetaminophen 650 mg PO q 6 hr as needed for a temperature >38° C (101° F) or mild pain

Refer back to this case study to answer the critical-thinking exercises throughout the chapter.

Knowledge and understanding of the structure and function of the skin and wound healing, as well as the factors that influence the processes involved, are essential for the nurse. Alterations in skin integrity can have a tremendous impact on the physical and psychological well-being of the affected person. Although some changes to the skin structure are inevitable secondary to the aging process, the patient and the health care provider can implement measures to protect the skin from harm and to promote wound healing in the event of injury.

NORMAL STRUCTURE AND FUNCTION OF SKIN LO 29.1

Skin is a part of the body that many take for granted, yet it is a complex and vital organ. The skin, the largest organ of the body, weighing more than 6 pounds, has many important functions that are essential for overall health. It is involved in thermoregulation through its ability to dilate and constrict blood vessels, allowing for heat to be released or retained by the body. This ability of the skin to change the size of blood vessels and produce perspiration in response to changes in internal and external temperatures assists in the maintenance of a steady body temperature. The skin has a major role in sensation, giving tactile feedback from the surrounding environment. The sensitivity of the skin as a sensory organ allows us to feel something as personal as the touch of a loved one and identify objects without the aid of sight. The skin alerts us to potential danger through its ability to transmit the sensations of pressure, pain, and temperature extremes. The skin is involved in the production of vitamin D in the presence of sunlight, works to rid the body of waste products, and is essential in fluid and electrolyte regulation. Intact skin serves as an effective barrier to environmental hazards such as ultraviolet light, chemicals, and the microbes or pathogens commonly on the skin surface, preventing them from entering the body. The skin's normally acidic pH provides a protective mechanism against pathogens. In addition to its physiologic functions, the skin is part of each person's self-perception and is intricately connected to personal and cultural identity, body image, and self-expression.

It is important to understand the normal anatomy of the skin. The skin is composed of three main layers: the epidermis, the dermis, and the subcutaneous layer (Figure 29-1). Each layer has its own functions, its own unique characteristics.

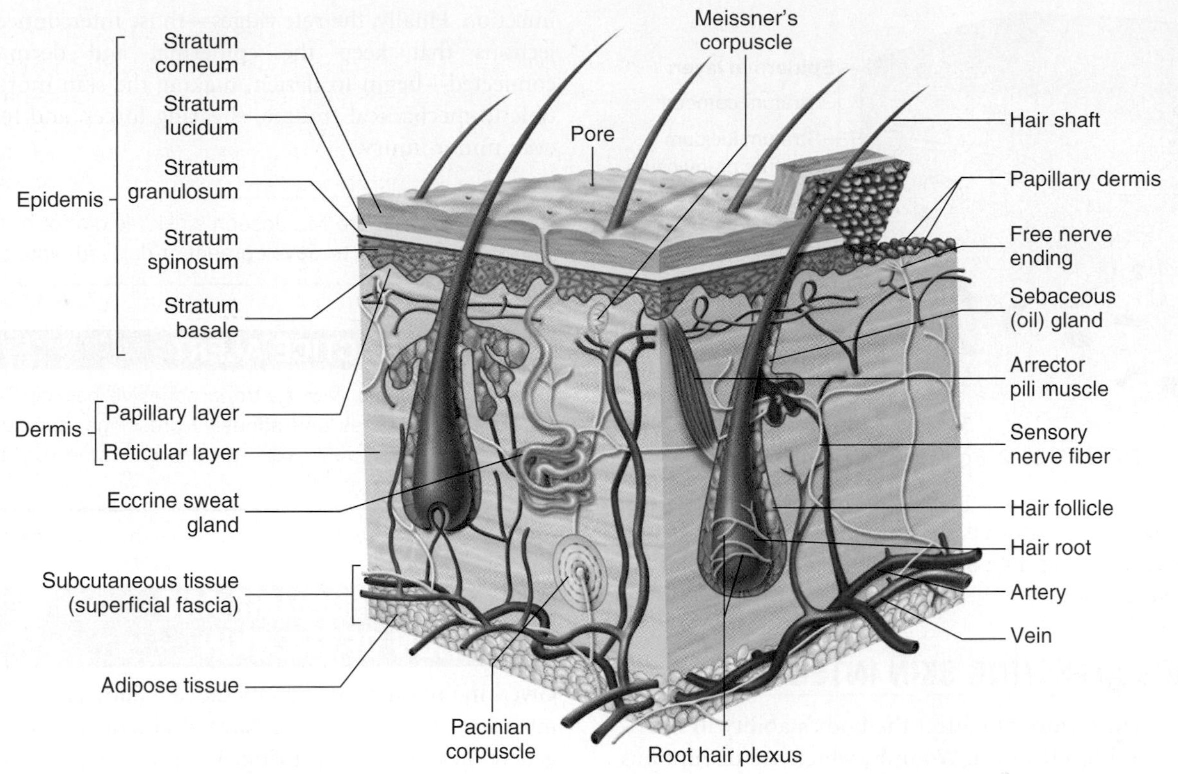

FIGURE 29-1 Cross section of the layers and structures of the skin.

EPIDERMIS

The **epidermis** is the outermost layer of the skin and the thinnest of the layers. Despite its lack of a blood supply, it has the ability to regenerate every 4 to 6 weeks. The epidermis can be subdivided into five more layers: the stratum corneum, stratum lucidum, stratum granulosum, stratum spinosum, and stratum germinativum or basale.

The outermost of the epidermal layers is the **stratum corneum**, which is made up of flattened dead cells. These are the flakes of skin that are seen being removed during normal bathing or with rubbing. Even though the cells themselves are dead, this layer is very important to the skin's roles of providing protection from outside dangers and regulating fluids and electrolytes. The middle three layers, each of which is one to five cells thick, provide for a transition from the stratum germinativum to the stratum corneum and help in the reduction of friction and shear. The innermost layer, the **stratum germinativum**, also called the *basal layer,* is only a single layer of cells but is very active. This layer constantly produces new cells that are pushed upward through the other layers of the epidermis toward the stratum corneum, where they flatten, die, and are eventually sloughed off and replaced by new cells. The protein keratin is synthesized in the stratum germinativum and is found throughout the layers of the epidermis as the cells migrate outward. Keratin gives the skin strength and flexibility and allows the skin to repair itself. Melanin, which gives the skin its distinctive and unique color and provides protection from ultraviolet light, and Langerhans cells, which are involved in the digestion of bacteria and in the immune system's response to foreign materials, are also found in the epidermis.

DERMIS

The **dermis**, lying between the epidermis and the deeper subcutaneous layer, is much thicker than the epidermis, although this thickness varies depending on the part of the body. For example, the skin on the soles of the feet is thicker than that on the fingertip or eyelid. The epidermal and dermal layers are joined to each other by the basal membrane. Extending up from the dermis are irregular, interconnected projections that link with the epidermis above (Figure 29-2). These projections, known as **rete ridges**, or the **papillary dermis**, provide the "stick" that anchors these layers of the skin together, preventing them from sliding back and forth. The connective tissue contained in the dermis, with its elastin and collagen fibers, provides strength and elasticity that is characteristic of the skin, while its abundant vascular system provides the necessary oxygen and blood. Embedded in the dermis are sebaceous glands, sweat glands, hair and nail follicles, nerves, and lymphatics.

SUBCUTANEOUS LAYER

The **subcutaneous layer** is a layer of adipose tissue, or fat, that, in addition to attaching the dermis to the underlying muscles and bone, delivers the blood supply to the dermis,

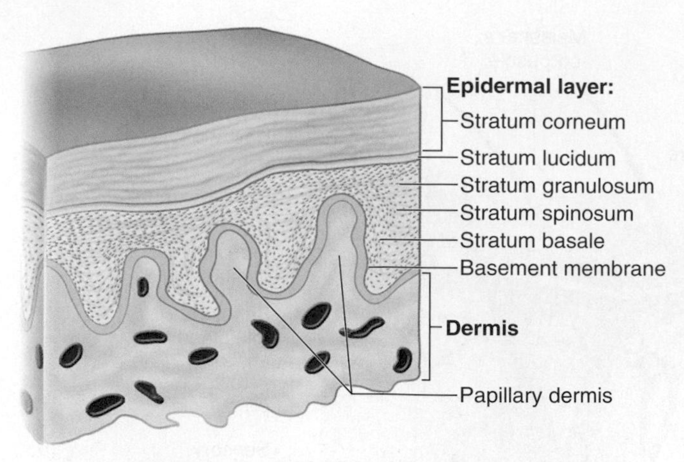

FIGURE 29-2 Epidermis and dermis.

provides insulation, and has a cushioning effect. The size of this layer varies depending on the body location and person's weight, sex, and age.

FACTORS AFFECTING SKIN INTEGRITY

Many different factors can affect the body's ability to maintain intact and healthy skin. **Wounds**, which are disruptions that may occur in the skin's integrity, lead to a loss of the skin's normal functioning. Other factors contribute to the development of wounds and lead to delays in wound healing. Examples are comorbid conditions such as vascular disease, which impairs the skin's ability to obtain required oxygen and nutrients, and diabetes, which adversely affects not only the microvasculature but also the skin's normally acidic pH; malnutrition involving inadequate proteins, cholesterol and fatty acids, vitamins, and minerals; medications such as steroids, nonsteroidal antiinflammatory drugs, and anticoagulants; excessive moisture; and external forces such as pressure, shear, and friction.

One significant factor influencing skin integrity and wound healing is the aging process. As people age, it is more likely that they will have some comorbidity such as diabetes or cardiovascular disease, take medications that affect the skin, and exhibit damage to skin from ultraviolet light exposure over the years. Additionally, aging dramatically affects the appearance and functioning of the skin. Aging is associated with thinning of the epidermis, dermis, and subcutaneous layers, with a resultant reduction in elastin, collagen fibers, sweat glands, and sebaceous glands. These changes lead to sagging or wrinkling of the skin and to the dry, paper-thin appearance of skin often seen in elderly people. It contributes to a reduction in the skin's ability to serve as both insulation and cushioning, thereby increasing vulnerability to trauma and temperature extremes characteristic of this population. A loss of melanocytes after age 40 leads to the graying of hair and an increased susceptibility to the development of skin cancers. With the decrease in number of Langerhans cells with aging, a corresponding decrease occurs in resistance to infection. Finally, the rete ridges—those interconnected projections that keep the epidermal and dermal layers connected—begin to flatten, making the skin more susceptible to mechanical trauma, shearing forces, and tears from even minor injury.

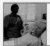

1. What are Mr. Joseph's risk factors for further pressure ulcer development or delayed wound healing?

! SAFE PRACTICE ALERT

Remove products with a strong adhesive backing, such as that found in tapes and adhesive dressings, carefully from the elderly person's skin to prevent stripping off the epidermis.

ALTERED STRUCTURE AND FUNCTION OF THE SKIN LO 29.2

Given the many functions of the skin, any alteration in the integrity of the skin can have dramatic implications for general health and well-being. The nurse is in a unique position to assess skin, implement interventions designed to promote the integrity of the skin, and carry out actions to promote the healing of any wounds. If a wound is identified, an additional assessment of the wound takes place. It is important to understand the different ways in which wounds are classified and the normal phases of the wound healing process.

WOUND CLASSIFICATION

There are many ways to classify wounds. They can be labeled according to the underlying cause; for example, the terms *diabetic ulcer, arterial ulcer,* and *pressure ulcer* are used to describe wounds. The same wounds could be classified more broadly by a basic description of the integrity of the skin and referred to as either *open* or *closed* wounds. Wounds are also classified on the basis of wound depth and are termed *superficial,* or *partial thickness,* versus *deep,* or *full thickness.* The presence of **infection** or contamination in the wound, or the length of time that it is taking for the wound to heal, results in the terms *chronic* and *acute.* For the nurse, it is important to understand what these terms mean and to see where they overlap to better communicate both with the patients and with other members of the health care team.

Skin Integrity

An **open wound** is characterized by an actual break in the skin's surface. For example, an abrasion, a puncture wound, and a surgical incision are types of open wounds. Some chronic wounds, like those frequently seen resulting from pressure or vascular diseases, can be open wounds. In a closed wound, as seen with bruising, the skin is still intact. Although any wound that is open puts the patient at greater risk for infection from outside organisms, a closed wound does not necessarily indicate a more benign condition. Some injuries first occur below the level of the skin, such as pressure-related injuries or fractured bones, and the integrity of the skin is not a good indicator of the severity of the underlying tissue damage.

Wound Depth

A superficial wound involves only the epidermis, whereas a partial-thickness wound involves the epidermis and the dermis but does not extend through the dermis to the subcutaneous layer. These wounds tend to heal quickly, leaving no scar, unless other outside factors delay the normal healing process. A deeper wound, or full-thickness wound, extends through the dermis to the subcutaneous layer and may extend farther, to the muscle, bone, or other underlying structures. Full-thickness wounds tend to heal slowly and leave scarring, and they are more likely to become chronic in nature.

BURNS

Burns are tissue injuries to the skin caused by heat, electricity, chemicals, radiation, extreme cold, or friction. Burns can be superficial, causing damage to only the epidermis, with resulting pain and erythema. Partial-thickness burns destroy the epidermis and part or all of the dermis, causing blistering and pain. Full-thickness burns destroy the epidermis, dermis, and part of the subcutaneous tissue. These severe burns cause the area to be white or brown, charred, and without sensation. They cannot heal without surgery. When burns occur over a large percentage of the body, the patient is at risk for severe fluid and electrolyte disturbances. These disturbances are considered further in Chapter 39.

Amount of Contamination

On the basis of the degree of contamination, wounds can be classified as clean, clean contaminated, contaminated, infected, or colonized. A clean wound is one in which there is no infection and the risk for development of an infection is low. For example, a closed surgical incision made in the controlled, sterile environment of the operating room that does not involve bacteria-containing organ systems would be considered a clean wound. A clean contaminated wound is similar to a clean wound, but because the surgery involves organ systems that are likely to contain bacteria, the risk for infection is greater. Contaminated wounds result from a break in sterile technique during surgery; from the perforation of an organ such as the colon, small bowel, or appendix before surgery, which allows for spillage of bacteria-laden material into the wound; or from certain types of trauma or accidents, such as penetrating trauma or a fall. These wounds have a higher risk of infection than clean contaminated wounds. An infected wound shows clinical signs of infection,

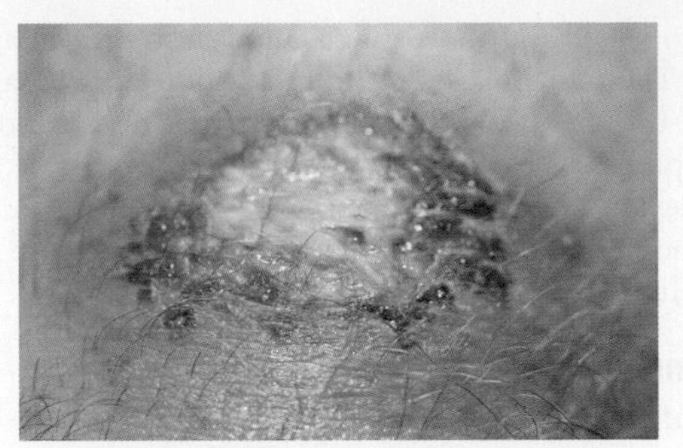

FIGURE 29-3 An infected wound.

including redness, warmth, and increased drainage that may or may not be purulent (contain pus), and has a bacterial count in the tissue of at least 10^5 per gram of tissue sampled when cultured (Figure 29-3). In a colonized wound, one or more organisms are present *on the surface* of the wound when a swab culture is obtained but there is no overt sign of an infection in the tissue below the surface. Colonization is common in chronic wounds and may contribute to delayed wound healing.

Healing Process

A wound that progresses through the phases of wound healing in a rapid, uncomplicated manner is an acute wound. Wounds such as surgical incisions or traumatic wounds in which the edges of the wound can be approximated (brought together) to heal are examples of acute wounds. This type of wound is said to heal by primary intention. Wounds that heal by primary intention tend to heal quickly and result in minimal scar formation. By contrast, a chronic wound fails to progress to healing in a timely manner, often remaining open for an extended period of time. Chronic wounds commonly heal by secondary intention. When a wound heals by secondary intention, new tissue must fill in from the bottom and sides of the wound until the wound bed is filled with new tissue. Such wounds are often associated with disease processes such as diabetes or vascular disease or with other factors that have inhibited proper wound healing.

In some situations it is necessary to initially leave a wound open for a period of time after an injury. For example, if contamination occurs during surgery, as can happen in surgeries involving the gastrointestinal tract, the wound may at first be left open to allow for observation and better wound drainage. Later, when the danger of infection is judged to be less, the edges of the wound may be pulled together to achieve closure. When a delay occurs between injury and closure, the wound healing is said happen by tertiary intention.

PHASES OF WOUND HEALING

The classification of a wound is important in selecting an appropriate treatment regime and in educating the patient on ways to better heal an existing wound or to prevent a recurrence. The actual phases of wound healing are the same for all full-thickness wounds regardless of type or causation. The three phases of healing are the inflammatory phase, which includes the process of homeostasis; the proliferative phase; and the maturation phase. These phases are shown in the animation "Wound Healing."

Inflammatory Phase

The **inflammatory phase** of healing begins with the body's initial response to wounding of the skin and lasts about 3 days. With the initial injury to the skin, bleeding occurs, which triggers what is known as the *coagulation cascade* and the formation of a clot to stop the bleeding. This process is an important way of preventing blood loss because of the release of numerous growth factors by the platelets involved in clot formation. These growth factors, along with cytokines, which are released during the inflammatory phase, play an important role in wound healing. During the inflammatory phase, there is an increase in pain, redness, warmth, and swelling in the injured area as the blood vessels dilate and leak fluid to the tissue surrounding the injury. Macrophages and neutrophils are drawn to the site of injury and begin the process of cleaning the wound of bacteria and debris. At the end of this phase, the wound bed is clean and ready to begin the actual repair process.

Proliferative Phase

The events of the **proliferative phase** of healing are repair of the defect, filling in the wound bed with new tissue (called *granulation tissue*), and resurfacing the wound with skin. This phase usually lasts several weeks, but it can be shorter with a surgically closed wound—healing by primary intention—or significantly longer if the wound is large or left to heal by secondary intention. The proliferative phase involves the development of new blood vessels (a process known as *angiogenesis*) that are needed to support the new tissue, collagen synthesis, wound contraction, and epithelialization. The key cells in this phase of wound healing are the fibroblasts, which produce growth factors, synthesize the collagen and proteins needed to form granulation tissue, promote angiogenesis, and are thought to work to contract the edges of the wound, thereby reducing the amount of granulation that needs to be produced. **Granulation tissue**, the new tissue created to fill the wound, is beefy red in appearance because of the many newly created blood vessels. This new tissue bleeds easily and has a granular, or "bumpy," texture (Figure 29-4). It consists of an immature type of collagen, the strength of which is only about 20% of that of mature collagen, making it more susceptible to injury. Finally, in this phase, epithelial cells proliferate and migrate laterally from the edges of the wound, across the moist granulation tissue, until the wound has been resurfaced with epithelial cells and the normal layers of the skin are reestablished. The need of epithelial cells to migrate across a moist, vascular wound bed is the basis for many of the moist wound dressings used today to support and promote wound healing.

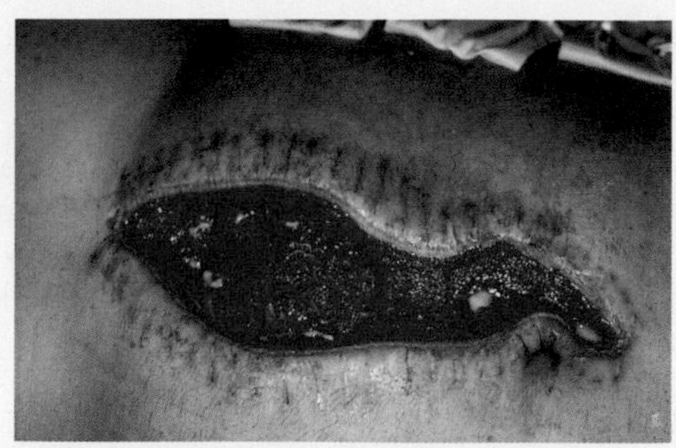

FIGURE 29-4 Granulation tissue. (From Bryant RA, Nix DP: *Acute and chronic wounds,* ed. 4, St. Louis, 2012, Mosby.)

Maturation Phase

The last phase of wound healing, the **maturation phase**, is known as the *remodeling phase* and can last up to a year. During this time collagen continues to be deposited and remodeled, and scar tissue is formed and strengthens. **Scar tissue** is an avascular mass of collagen that gives strength to the repaired wound. However, the strength of the scar is never equal to that of unwounded tissue, achieving only about 80% of its previous tensile strength.

FACTORS AFFECTING WOUND HEALING

As stated earlier, many of the same factors that affect overall skin integrity will significantly affect the ability of the skin to heal once injured. Factors include disease processes, age, infections, and nutrition.

Oxygenation and Tissue Perfusion

All cells in the body need oxygen to function properly. Specifically, chronic tissue hypoxia is associated with a reduction in collagen formation, a decrease in the action and proliferation of fibroblasts, a reduction in leukocytes, and an impairment of the cell's ability to migrate. Any condition that affects the body's ability to perfuse the tissue with an adequate amount of oxygen will adversely affect wound healing. Therefore, comorbid conditions such as heart disease, peripheral vascular disease, and pulmonary disease can lead to a prolongation of the healing process. Smoking, even before lung damage has occurred, is a huge risk to successful wound healing. Smoking impairs the hemoglobin's ability to carry oxygen. The nicotine in cigarettes causes vasoconstriction and increased coagulability of the blood, reducing the body's ability to circulate oxygen.

Diabetes

According to the American Diabetes Association (2014), in 2012 diabetes mellitus affected more than 21 million people in the United States alone. An additional 86 million

Americans were termed prediabetic, and an estimated 8.1 million had diabetes but had not yet been diagnosed. In view of the impact of diabetes on wound healing, this is a significant factor to consider in assessing a patient with a wound. Diabetes causes changes in the microvascular and macrovascular systems, leading to a thickening of the vessel wall and occlusion of blood flow with decreased supply of needed nutrients and oxygen. For a patient with diabetes, the presence of a wound is accompanied by a reduction in collagen synthesis, a decrease in the strength of that collagen, impaired functioning of leukocytes, and a reduction in the number and action of macrophages.

Nutrition

Adequate nutrition is essential for wound healing to occur. With any injury, including any surgical procedure, the body requires additional energy to recover and heal from the injury. While overall caloric needs increase, sometimes by more than 100%, depending on the severity of the injury, the need for protein increases disproportionately. Protein is needed by the fibroblasts for the purpose of synthesizing collagen. In addition, deficiencies in vitamins C and A and the trace minerals zinc and copper have been found to have a significant impact on wound healing. Many patients enter the health care system in a malnourished state; others become depleted nutritionally because of illness, surgery, or medical treatments. An adequate, ongoing assessment of the patient's nutritional status is an essential component of the overall plan for wound healing. See Chapter 30 for more information on this factor in healing.

Age

Although the older person can heal from wounds, the aging process affects all phases of wound healing. With increasing age, the entire inflammatory response is decreased or delayed; the action of the macrophages and fibroblasts is reduced, resulting in a decrease in collagen synthesis and a slowing of the epithelialization of the wound. These physiologic factors, in addition to the frequent presence in the older patient of comorbidity such as diabetes and the use of medications that affect wound healing, contribute to the older patient's risk for poor wound healing.

Infection

Infection is both a cause of delayed wound healing and a complication of impaired wound healing. A wound that is left open or is contaminated is at increased risk for invasion by infective agents. (The signs of an infected wound are discussed earlier, under "Amount of Contamination.") Once a wound is infected, the infection causes a prolongation of the inflammatory phase, delays collagen synthesis, prevents epithelialization, and can lead to additional tissue destruction. Infection contributes to failure of the wound to progress through the normal phases of healing, and to the development of chronic wounds. Any wound that shows no progress toward healing despite appropriate treatment should be assessed for an underlying infection and treated aggressively for the infection if present.

COMPLICATIONS OF WOUND HEALING

Complications of wound healing, in addition to the failure to heal in a timely manner, include dehiscence, evisceration, and fistula formation. These complications lead to an increased length of stay in a health care setting, additional costs for both the health care system and the affected patient, and increased pain and suffering.

Dehiscence and Evisceration

Dehiscence, which usually occurs in connection with surgical incisions, is the partial or complete separation of the tissue layers during the healing process. **Evisceration** is the total separation of the tissue layers, allowing the protrusion of visceral organs through the incision. People at risk for these complications are the same patients who are at risk for delayed or impaired wound healing. In addition, coughing, vomiting, or straining puts additional stress on the healing tissue, increasing the risk of dehiscence and evisceration. These complications usually occur 5 to 9 days after surgery and are related to a delay in collagen synthesis. If a wound is healing properly, a 1-cm-wide ridge, or area of induration, can be palpated next to the incision line. This ridge is indicative of the new collagen being laid down in the wound. If this "**healing ridge**" is not felt, the wound is at increased risk for dehiscence and evisceration. Symptoms include a "popping" sensation accompanied by an increase in drainage from the wound. Sutures and staples may be applied to keep the wound closed, and nursing interventions include teaching the patient to "splint" the incision with a pillow or folded blanket or to use an abdominal binder for comfort while coughing and deep breathing and during movement (Figure 29-5). If dehiscence or evisceration occurs, cover the wound with gauze moistened with a sterile normal saline, and notify the physician immediately. Although small areas of dehiscence can sometimes be treated without additional surgery, large dehiscent wounds and eviscerations can require emergency surgery.

Fistula Formation

Fistulas are abnormal connections between two internal organs or between an internal organ and, through the skin, the outside of the body. The organs involved can be identified by the name of the fistula. For example, an enterovaginal fistula involves an opening between the intestine (entero) and the vagina, allowing intestinal content to drain into the vagina. An enterocutaneous fistula is an opening between the intestine (entero) and the skin (cutaneous). Fistulas usually are the result of a specific disease process such as that in certain cancers and Crohn's disease, treatment modalities such as radiation, or any of the factors implicated in poor wound healing. Fistulas predispose the affected person to fluid and electrolyte loss, nutritional deficits, and alterations in skin integrity. This is particularly true if the fistula is draining material that is naturally destructive to the skin's surface. For example, exposure to the digestive enzymes normally found in fluids from the small intestine or pancreas can cause extensive damage to the skin in a short time.

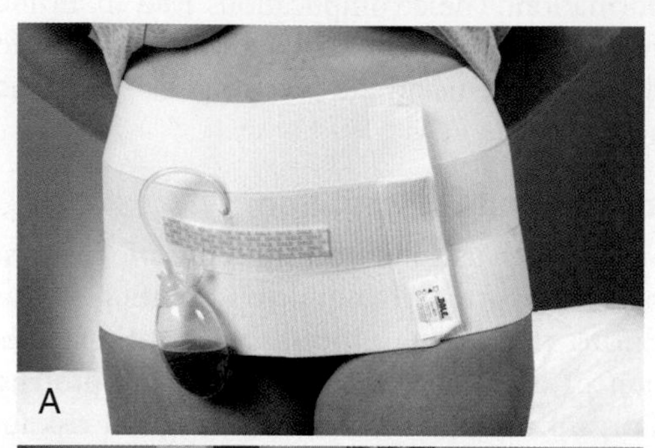

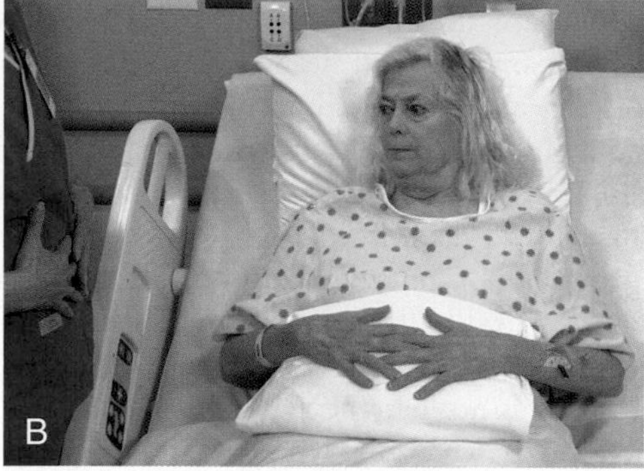

FIGURE 29-5 **A,** Abdominal binder. **B,** Splinting. (**A,** Courtesy Dale Medical Products, Plainville, Mass.)

PRESSURE ULCERS

It is estimated that every year, between 1 million and 3 million people in the United States develop a pressure ulcer in acute care and long-term care facilities, with a total cost of $9 billion to $15 billion (Dorner, Posthauer, and Thomas, 2009). In addition to the pain and suffering incurred by affected patients, the ulcers contribute to an estimated 60,000 deaths. In 2008, Medicare stopped reimbursing many hospitals and other health care facilities at higher reimbursement levels for conditions deemed "reasonably preventable" on the basis of existing evidence-based guidelines. One such condition is hospital-acquired pressure ulcers. These facts are an impetus for developing effective prevention and treatment protocols. The development and implementation of these protocols are of great concern to nursing. Nursing plays a critical role in the identification of patients at risk for this complication, and many independent nursing actions have a direct impact on the prevention of pressure ulcers and their ultimate resolution.

Pressure ulcers are sometimes referred to as *bedsores* or *decubitus ulcers*. However, the term *pressure ulcer* more closely reflects the underlying etiology of the wound. A **pressure ulcer** is a "localized injury to the skin and/or underlying tissue usually over a bony prominence, as a result of pressure, or pressure in combination with shear" (European Pressure Ulcer Advisory Panel and National Pressure Ulcer Advisory Panel, 2009). Although these lesions most commonly occur over bony prominences such as the sacrum, ischium, trochanter, and heel, any part of the body that is subjected to pressure can be affected, including the areas under casts and wraps (Figure 29-6).

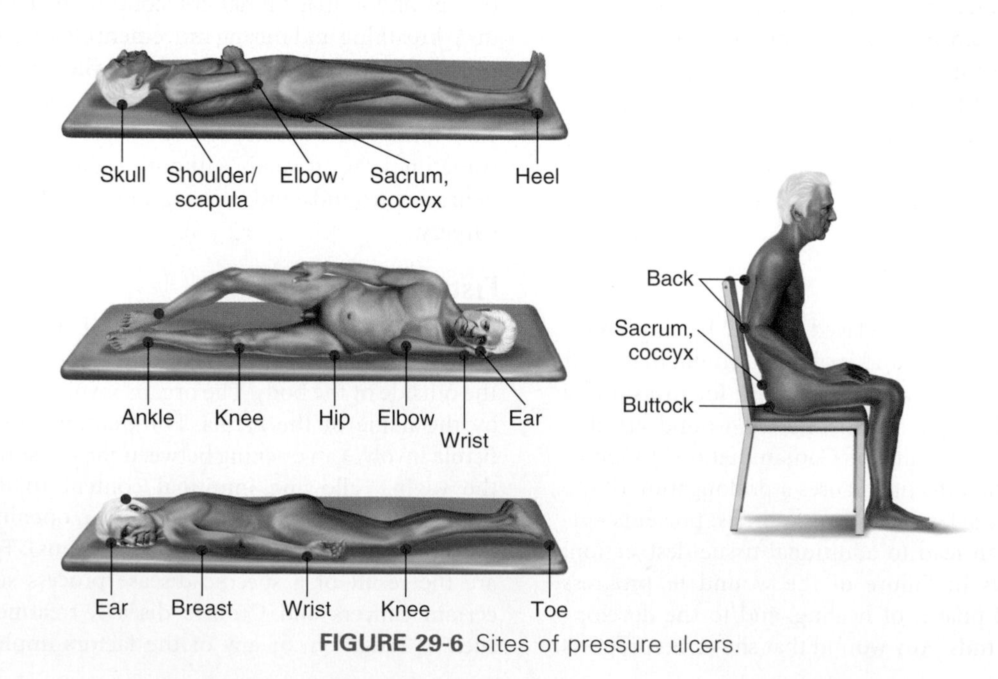

FIGURE 29-6 Sites of pressure ulcers.

The primary cause of pressure ulcers is, as the name suggests, pressure. The injury mechanism is more than just pressure, however; specific factors include the intensity of the pressure, the length of time that the tissue is subjected to the pressure, and intrinsic and extrinsic factors that affect the tissue's ability to withstand or tolerate that pressure.

Intensity of Pressure

The terms **capillary closing pressure** and **critical closing pressure** refer to the minimum pressure required to collapse a capillary. With the collapse of the capillary walls, blood flow to the tissue is impaired, leading to tissue hypoxia and cell death. Although the measurement of capillary closing pressure is difficult to achieve, it generally is accepted to be 12 to 32 mm Hg. This value usually is exceeded in anyone seated in a chair or lying on a hard surface, yet there is no tissue damage. Normally, pain is felt when tissue ischemia occurs, and this pain prompts a position shift, relieving the pressure and restoring the flow through the capillaries. If the pressure is not relieved, because the person is either unable to move or unable to sense the warning signal of pain, the ischemia leads to tissue damage and the development of an actual pressure ulcer. It has been found that subcutaneous and muscle tissues are more susceptible to the effects of pressure than other tissues, including the epidermis and dermis (European Pressure Ulcer Advisory Panel and National Pressure Ulcer Advisory Panel, 2009; Kottner, Balzer, Dassen, and Heinze, 2009). With pressure-related injuries, the damage occurs first in the subcutaneous and muscle layers, and the degree of damage may not be readily observable on initial assessment of the skin condition.

Duration of Pressure

It has been found that low levels of pressure over long periods of time can be as damaging to the skin and underlying tissue as high levels of pressure over a short period of time. Pressure seems to have a cumulative effect on the tissue. Thus, once a tissue has been exposed to pressure, even if the pressure is then removed, later reexposure of that tissue to the same or even less pressure may result in considerable damage.

Friction and Shear

Friction is the rubbing together of two surfaces—in this case, the skin and the bed or some other surface that the skin is in contact with. Friction by itself damages the epidermal layer but does not cause damage to the deeper structures (Kottner, Balzer, Dassen, and Heinze, 2009). The real danger of friction comes from the relationship between friction and gravity and the resultant phenomenon of **shear**. The classic example of friction that results in shear is the clinical scenario in which a patient "slides" down in bed as the head of the bed is elevated. The friction encountered by the skin as it slides over the bed surface leads to a "sticking" of the skin to the bed linens while the body's weight continues to pull the person downward (Figure 29-7) These opposing stresses on the skin result in hyperangulation and stretching of the blood vessels, damaging them and their ability to transport blood. Shear is thought to significantly contribute to the development of pressure ulcers, particularly in areas routinely subjected to both pressure and shear: the sacrum and coccyx. Use of mechanical lifts to move immobile patients, discussed in Chapter 28, helps to reduce injuries due to friction and shear.

Sensory Loss or Immobility

Patients who are unable to feel pain (the warning sign of tissue ischemia), unable to respond appropriately, or limited in their ability to move or maintain their position independently are at increased risk for the development of pressure ulcers. This risk group includes patients with neurologic conditions such as spinal cord injury or advanced multiple sclerosis; those with chronic conditions that lead to neuropathies, as seen in diabetes; patients with dementia or brain injury; and those who, because of medical interventions such as the use of traction and restraints, are unable to reposition themselves independently.

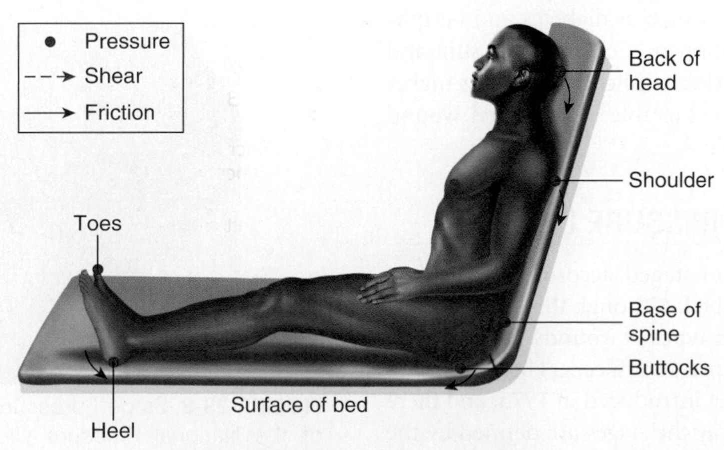

FIGURE 29-7 Friction and shear.

Moisture

Incontinence is thought to contribute to the development of pressure ulcers because of the effects of **maceration**, a condition in which excessive moisture causes a softening of the skin. However, more recent studies show that while the skin may become macerated, and the enzymes found in stool can lead to perineal inflammation and dermatitis, the damage from moisture is confined to the more superficial layers (Kottner, Balzer, Dassen, and Heinze, 2009; Pieper, Langemo, and Cuddigan, 2009).

Nutrition

Proper nutrition, as already discussed, is essential for wound healing. Inadequate nutrition is implicated in the development of pressure ulcers. Patients at risk for nutritional deficits include those who are unable or unwilling to feed themselves or to take in enough nutrients to meet their metabolic requirements. When inadequate nutrition results in an unintentional weight loss of 5% or more; a low body mass index (BMI); deficiencies in vitamins A, C, and E and the minerals zinc and copper; and protein-calorie malnutrition, the ability of the tissue to withstand the forces of pressure and shear and to combat infectious agents is compromised (Dorner, Posthauer, and Thomas 2009). A thorough nutritional assessment including an evaluation of weight and recent changes in weight, BMI, diet history, and pertinent laboratory findings (including serum albumin, serum prealbumin, nitrogen balance, and other measures) is an essential first step in preventing the development of pressure ulcers while promoting healing of those already present. Collaboration with a registered dietitian and other members of the health care team, as well as the patient and family members, is needed in the development of a plan to address the nutritional needs of the at-risk patient. This plan must be consistent with the overall plan of care and the wishes of the patient and family.

For all of the reasons already discussed, the elderly population is at increased risk for developing pressure ulcers, and such lesions, if they occur, will be slower to heal. The combination of comorbid conditions such as diabetes and peripheral vascular disease, medication use, exposure to sun, and the changes in skin characteristics inherent in aging makes the elder population highly vulnerable to impaired wound healing.

CLASSIFICATION OF PRESSURE ULCERS

Pressure ulcers are classified, or staged, according to the type of tissue visible in the wound bed. Although this classification system has been used for other types of wounds, it is designed for use in the description of pressure ulcers. The system has been modified since it was first introduced in 1975, and there are slight differences in the way the stages are defined by the European Pressure Ulcer Advisory Panel (EPUAP) and by the National Pressure Ulcer Advisory Panel (NPUAP). The ulcer classification system requires knowledge of the different tissue types seen in a wound and the ability to accurately identify those tissue types. Because this knowledge often is lacking in health care practitioners, confusion and disagreement may arise regarding the stage of the wound being evaluated. If the wound is filled with necrotic tissue, accurate identification of the underlying tissue type is not possible, so the wound cannot be staged. Questions also can arise about the underlying etiology of a wound. For example, it can be difficult to differentiate a superficial wound resulting from a tape tear, friction, or incontinence from a stage II ulcer secondary to pressure. Despite these limitations, staging of pressure ulcers is the accepted method for describing pressure ulcers.

Stage I

A **stage I pressure ulcer** is characterized by *intact,* nonblistered skin with nonblanchable erythema, or persistent redness, in the area that has been exposed to pressure (Figure 29-8). The redness is called **abnormal reactive hyperemia** and is due to excessive vasodilation caused by pressure. When the area is pressed lightly with a finger, it does not blanch but instead remains red. When the redness blanches, or turns white, with gentle fingertip pressure, normal reactive hyperemia is occurring owing to vasodilation, and the redness will disappear. Such changes can be difficult to see in darkly pigmented skin, so the definition was expanded to include an area that is painful and differs in firmness (either softer or firmer) or in temperature (warmer or cooler) from the surrounding tissue (EPUAP and NPUAP, 2009).

Stage II

A partial-thickness wound that involves the epidermis and/or dermis but does not extend below the level of the dermis is called a **stage II pressure ulcer**. It is shallow and superficial, with a pink wound bed (Figure 29-9). Intact or ruptured blisters that are the result of pressure also are considered to be stage II ulcers.

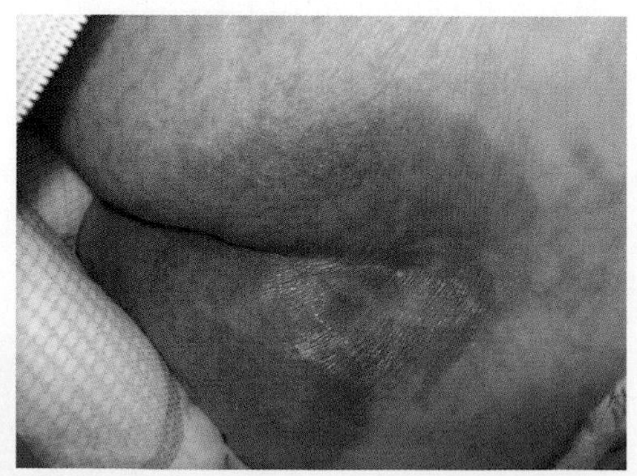

FIGURE 29-8 Stage I pressure ulcer. (Used with permission of the National Pressure Ulcer Advisory Panel. Copyright NPUAP.)

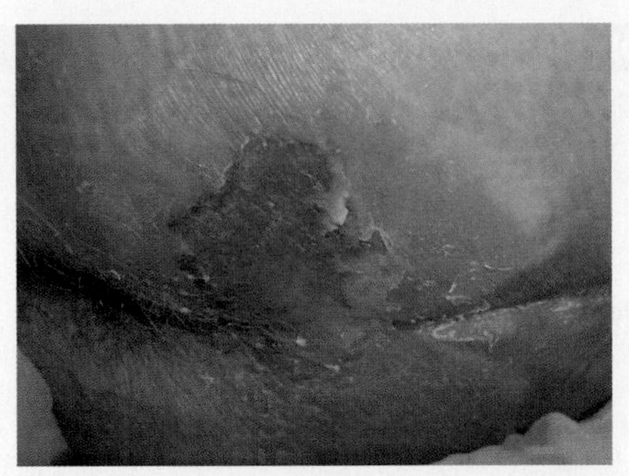

FIGURE 29-9 Stage II pressure ulcer. (Used with permission of the National Pressure Ulcer Advisory Panel. Copyright NPUAP.)

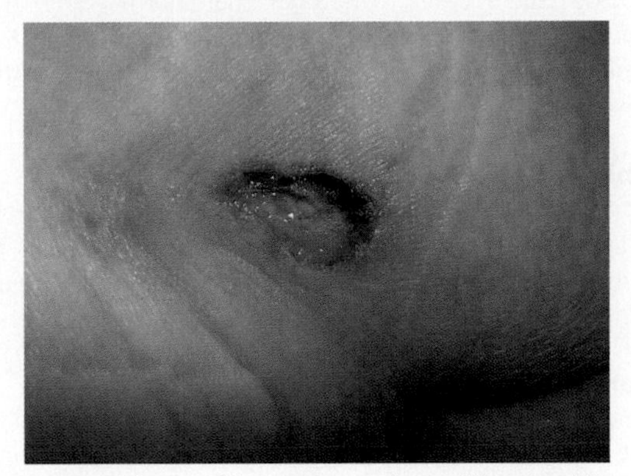

FIGURE 29-10 Stage III pressure ulcer. (Used with permission of the National Pressure Ulcer Advisory Panel. Copyright NPUAP.)

Stage III

Stage III pressure ulcers are full-thickness wounds that extend into the subcutaneous tissue but do not extend through the fascia to muscle, bone, or connective tissue (Figure 29-10). There may be undermining or tunneling present in the wound. Undermining is an area of tissue loss present under intact skin, usually along the edges of the wound, forming a "lip" around the wound. A tunnel or sinus tract is similar to an undermining but is a narrower passageway extending outward from the edge of the wound. Although a stage III pressure ulcer is described as a deeper wound than a stage II ulcer, the degree of depth is dependent on the location of the wound and the amount of subcutaneous tissue present. For example, far less subcutaneous tissue is present on the heel or back of the head than on the hip or shoulder.

Stage IV

Another full-thickness wound is a stage IV pressure ulcer. This wound is deeper than a stage III pressure ulcer and involves exposure of muscle, bone, or connective tissue such as tendons or cartilage. The considerable depth of the wound, particularly if the bone is palpable, makes osteomyelitis, or an infection of the bone, likely (Figure 29-11).

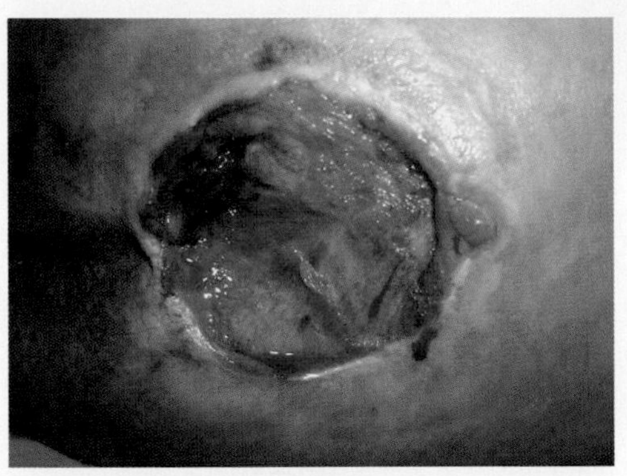

FIGURE 29-11 Stage IV pressure ulcer. (Used with permission of the National Pressure Ulcer Advisory Panel. Copyright NPUAP.)

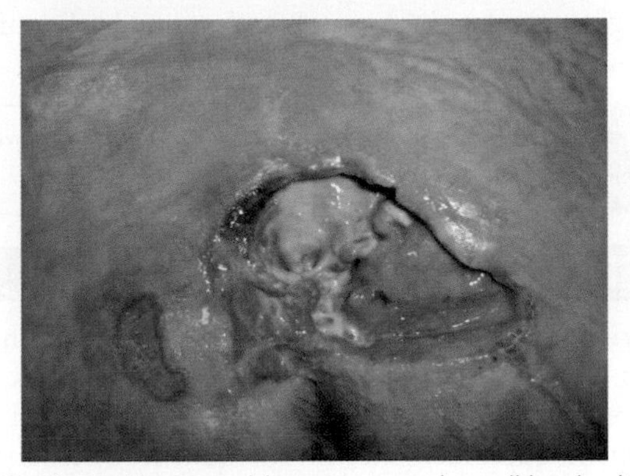

FIGURE 29-12 Unstageable pressure ulcer. (Used with permission of the National Pressure Ulcer Advisory Panel. Copyright NPUAP.)

Unstageable

An unstageable pressure ulcer is a full-thickness wound in which the amount of necrotic tissue, or eschar, in the wound bed makes it impossible to assess the depth of the wound or the involvement of underlying structures (Figure 29-12). Even if it is suspected that a wound is a stage III or IV based on location and other characteristics, the wound cannot be staged until the necrotic tissue is removed, or debrided.

Suspected Deep Tissue Injury

Suspected deep tissue injury, a category of classification added in 2007, is seen as an area of intact skin that is purple or maroon or a blood-filled blister (Figure 29-13). Like stage I ulcers, suspected deep tissue injuries may be difficult to detect in darker-skinned patients. The true depth of tissue damage is not readily apparent on initial inspection; however, these injuries can progress rapidly, exposing deeper layers of tissue even if treated quickly and appropriately.

As a pressure ulcer heals, it does not travel in reverse in terms of staging; that is, a stage IV pressure ulcer does not go from stage IV to stage III to stage II to stage I. Because the tissue will never be the same as it was before injury, the wound should be referred to as a *healed stage IV.* Some

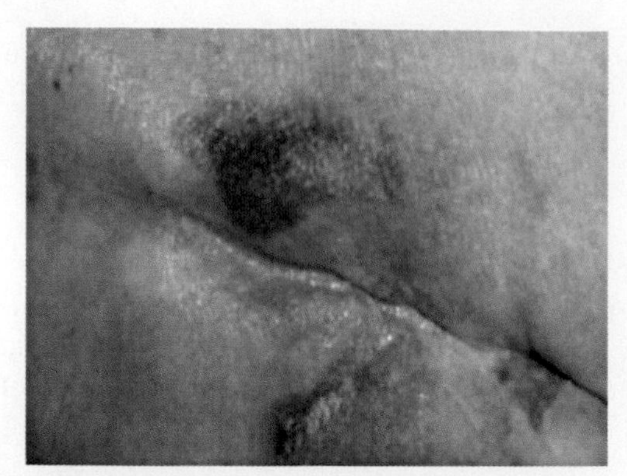

FIGURE 29-13 Suspected deep tissue injury. (Used with permission of the National Pressure Ulcer Advisory Panel. Copyright NPUAP.)

nursing issues related to wounds and wound healing are outlined in the Diversity Considerations box.

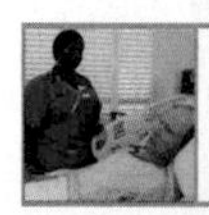

2. Stage Mr. Joseph's right hip and left heel wounds.

ASSESSMENT LO 29.3

A thorough assessment of the skin is performed on every patient in both acute- and long-term care facilities, as well as those receiving home care. It should include focused health assessment questions (Health Assessment Questions box) and an assessment of the skin's temperature, overall color and local variations in that color, presence of excessive moisture or dryness, odor, texture, turgor, and integrity (see Chapter 20). The presence of risk factors associated with skin breakdown or impaired wound healing, and any actual wounds present, are included in the assessment. After a baseline is obtained, regular reassessments should occur as indicated by the patient's risk factors, the presence and characteristics of wounds, and the clinical setting.

DIVERSITY CONSIDERATIONS

Life Span

- Chronic wounds can result in an inability to work and a loss of independence in people of all ages. A significant financial burden may be incurred from costs associated with treatment of chronic wounds.

Ethnicity

- Full-thickness wounds, especially those allowed to heal by secondary intention, as with stage III and IV pressure ulcers, demonstrate a loss of certain epidermal structures including hair follicles, sweat glands, and melanocytes. This loss can be permanent. For a person of African American heritage, local loss of skin pigment leads to a change in color at the wound site.
- Keloids (scars that grow larger than normal and have a smooth, rubbery appearance) and areas of hypo- and hyperpigmentation are more common in African Americans.

Disability

- Patients with disabilities that cause difficulty with mobility or sensory perception are at risk for development of pressure ulcers. Such disabilities include spinal cord injuries, peripheral neuropathies, and neuromuscular disorders.

Morphology

- Obesity is a risk factor for poor wound healing. Weight is not a good indicator of protein stores or nutritional health, so the obese patient can be deficient in the nutrients essential to wound healing. In addition, adipose tissue is poorly vascularized, compared with the epidermis and dermis, and therefore at greater risk for tissue ischemia. Because of the increase in mechanical forces that can be exerted on the edges of a healing wound, possible reduction in the ability to reposition oneself due to size, and common comorbid conditions such as heart disease and diabetes in this population, obesity increases the risk of chronic wounds and poor wound healing.

HEALTH ASSESSMENT QUESTIONS

Skin

General Skin Assessment Questions

- How would you describe your overall skin condition?
- Have you ever had problems with your skin? What kind of problems? Location? When?
- Describe your usual skin care regime.
- Describe your usual diet. Have you experienced any recent unintended weight loss?
- Are you ever incontinent of urine or stool?
- Have you been told that you have diabetes or problems with your circulation?
- Do you smoke?
- Have you noticed any numbness or tingling in your feet?
- Has it seemed to take a long time for a wound to heal in the past?

Focused Wound Assessment

- How long has this wound been present? What do you think caused this wound? Have you ever had a wound like this before?
- What are you doing for this wound at home? What are you using to clean the wound? What have you put on it?
- Have you noticed any changes in the appearance of the wound or the skin around it?
- How much wound drainage is there? Has the amount, color, or odor of the drainage changed? How often do you need to change the bandage at home?
- Do you live alone? Do you have anyone who helps you at home?
- Is the cost of caring for this wound difficult for you to manage?

If a wound is present, an accurate and detailed assessment is conducted to determine the most appropriate treatment, monitor healing progress, and adjust the treatment plan as needed. It includes close inspection of the wound, determination of the suspected etiology of the wound, a thorough patient history, and a head-to-toe physical examination. Additional testing may be required, such as vascular studies to assess arterial and venous status, blood work to evaluate chronic diseases such as diabetes or malnutrition, or biopsy of the wound to rule out infection or malignancy.

RISK ASSESSMENT FOR PRESSURE ULCERS

Several tools have been developed specifically to assist in the identification of patients at risk for the development of pressure ulcers. Although risk assessment tools may not directly reduce the number of pressure ulcers acquired, accurate and timely assessment of at-risk patients serves as a guide to the need for implementation of preventive strategies. Early identification of each person's risk factors allows health care facilities to focus available resources on the patients at greatest risk for breakdown. Two available tools are the Braden Scale (Figure 29-14) and the Norton Scale (Figure 29-15). Each tool ranks certain risk factors, the number of which varies, and the summation of the individual rankings determines the overall risk score. With both the Braden and Norton scales, the lower the score, the greater the overall risk.

The most valuable tool would be one that predicts with 100% precision those patients who will or will not develop a pressure ulcer. When comparing the predictive abilities of the Braden and Norton scales, researchers found them to be similar, with both scales overpredicting the risk of pressure ulcer development (Balzer, Pohl, Dassen, and Halfens, 2007). While this means that some people who will not develop pressure ulcers receive unnecessary preventive interventions, it is thought that this is preferable to failing to intervene and having a pressure ulcer subsequently develop.

With each of these tools, it is essential to understand the definitions of the different categories in order to accurately arrive at a risk score that is reflective of actual risk. Too often, the risk score becomes just another number on a flow sheet instead of something that serves to guide practice. Although the overall risk score is important and may be the assessment finding that initiates prevention protocols, the scores in each of the tool's individual categories can help the nurse in the selection of interventions. By reducing the impact of these contributing risk factors, it is possible to reduce the person's overall risk for pressure ulcers. The Braden Scale ranks the patient on the risk categories of sensory perception, moisture, activity, mobility, nutrition, and friction and shear. A score lower than 18 places the person at risk for pressure ulcer development. If, on assessing that score, the nurse notes that the patient scored particularly low in one or more of the categories, preventive strategies can be directed more precisely at those specific areas as a way to decrease overall risk.

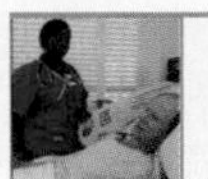

3. On the basis of the information in the case study, calculate Mr. Joseph's score on the Braden scale.

WOUND ASSESSMENT

A focused wound assessment includes an evaluation of the wound's location, size, and color; presence of drainage; condition of the wound edges; characteristics of the wound bed; and patient's response to the wound or wound treatment.

Location

The location of the wound is described using clear, anatomic terminology whenever possible. For example, referring to the left outer malleolus instead of the left ankle clarifies for those subsequently assessing the wound exactly where the wound is located. This distinction becomes more important if more than one wound is present. The use of anatomic diagrams to illustrate wound locations is now widely practiced in documentation. Wound care is documented in the electronic health record (Figure 29-16).

Size

The nurse assesses the size of the wound. With the healing process, the edges of an open wound contract and the wound bed fills with new tissue. Consistency in wound measurements is important in accurately monitoring progression toward healing (Nursing Care Guideline: Measuring a Wound box).

! SAFE PRACTICE ALERT

The nurse should be cautious when palpating inside a wound with a sterile gloved finger. Exposed bone, if present, can be sharp, resulting in a cut in the glove and finger. Only wound care nurse specialists and those with special training in wound assessment should attempt palpation of a deep wound.

Presence of Undermining or Tunneling

Undermining can be present around the entire wound or only part of the wound and can vary in its depth. Undermining is often seen when the wound is a result of pressure and shear forces, and is often present in sacral ulcers. The presence and location of undermining are determined by exploring the edge of the wound with a cotton-tipped applicator. The undermined area is part of the wound and is included in the treatment plan for the wound. Tunnels increase the actual size of the wound, are a part of the wound, and must be treated appropriately. Because wounds heal from the edges inward and from the bottom up, tunneled wounds usually are packed lightly with gauze or other dressing materials so that they can heal along with the rest of the wound, instead of prematurely closing, which would result in pockets of dead space. Such

BRADEN SCALE FOR PREDICTING PRESSURE SORE RISK

Patient's name________________ Evaluator's name________________ Date of assessment

SENSORY PERCEPTION Ability to respond meaningfully to pressure-related discomfort	**1. Completely Limited** Unresponsive (does not moan, flinch, or gasp) to painful stimuli due to diminished level of consciousness or sedation. OR Limited ability to feel pain over most of body.	**2. Very Limited** Responds only to painful stimuli. Cannot communicate discomfort except by moaning or restlessness. OR Has a sensory impairment that limits the ability to feel pain or discomfort over ½ of body.	**3. Slightly Limited** Responds to verbal commands, but cannot always communicate discomfort or the need to be turned. OR Has some sensory impairment that limits ability to feel pain or discomfort in 1 or 2 extremities.	**4. No Impairment** Responds to verbal commands. Has no sensory deficit that would limit ability to feel or voice pain and discomfort.				
MOISTURE Degree to which skin is exposed to moisture	**1. Constantly Moist** Skin is kept moist almost constantly by perspiration, urine, etc. Dampness is detected every time patient is moved or turned.	**2. Very Moist** Skin is often, but not always moist. Linen must be changed at least once a shift.	**3. Occasionally Moist** Skin is occasionally moist, requiring an extra linen change approximately once a day.	**4. Rarely Moist** Skin is usually dry; linen only requires changing at routine intervals.				
ACTIVITY Degree of physical activity	**1. Bedfast** Confined to bed.	**2. Chairfast** Ability to walk severely limited or non-existent. Cannot bear own weight and/or must be assisted into chair or wheelchair.	**3. Walks Occasionally** Walks occasionally during day, but for very short distances, with or without assistance. Spends majority of each shift in bed or chair.	**4. Walks Frequently** Walks outside room at least twice a day and inside room at least once every 2 hours during waking hours.				
MOBILITY Ability to change and control body position	**1. Completely Immobile** Dose not make even slight changes in body or extremity position without assistance.	**2. Very Limited** Makes occasional slight changes in body or extremity position, but unable to make frequent or significant changes independently.	**3. Slightly Limited** Makes frequent though slight changes in body or extermity position independently.	**4. No Limitation** Makes major and frequent changes in position without assistance.				
NUTRITION Usual food intake pattern	**1. Very Poor** Never eats a complete meal. Rarely eats more than ⅓ of food offered. Eats 2 servings or less of protein (meat or dairy products) per day. Takes fluids poorly. Does not take a liquid detary supplement. OR Is NPO and/or maintained on clear liquids or/IVs for more than 5 days.	**2. Probably Inadequate** Rarely eats a complete meal and generally eats only about ½ of any food offered. Protein intake includes only 3 servings of meat or dairy products per day. Occasionally will take a dietary supplement. OR Receives less than optimum amount of liquid diet or tube feeding.	**3. Adequate** Eats over half of most meals. Eats a total of 4 servings of protein (meat, dairy products) per day. Occasionally will refuse a meal, but will usually take a supplement when offered. OR Is on a tube feeding or TPN regimen that probably meets most of nutritional needs.	**4. Excellent** Eats most of every meal. Never refuses a meal. Usually eats a total of 4 or more servings of meal and dairy products. Occasionally eats between meals. Does not require supplementation.				
FRICTION and SHEAR	**1. Problem** Requires moderate to maximum assistance in moving. Complete lifting without sliding against sheets is impossible. Frequently slides down in bed or chair, requiring frequent repositioning with maximum assistance. Spasticity, contractures, or agitation leads to almost constant friction.	**2. Potential Problem** Moves feebly or requires minimum assistance. During a move, skin probably slides to some extent against sheets, chair restraints, or other devices. Maintains relatively good position in chair or bed most of the time but occasionally slides down.	**3. No Apparent Problem** Moves in bed and in chair independently and has sufficient muscle strength to lift up completely during move. Maintains good position in bed or chair.					
				Total score				

FIGURE 29-14 The Braden scale for predicting pressure sore risk. (Copyright Barbara Braden and Nancy Bergstrom, 1988. All rights reserved.)

NORTON PRESSURE ULCER SCALE

Resident's name: ______________________

Parameter	Score	Resident's condition	DATE ⇨
PHYSICAL CONDITION	4	Good	
	3	Fair	
	2	Poor	
	1	Bad	
MENTAL STATE	4	Alert	
	3	Apathetic	
	2	Confused	
	1	Stupor	
ACTIVITY	4	Ambulant	
	3	Walks with assistance	
	2	Chairbound	
	1	Bedrest – bedbound	
MOBILITY	4	Fully mobile	
	3	Slightly limited	
	2	Very limited	
	1	Immobile	
CONTINENCE	4	Continent	
	3	Occasionally incontinence	
	2	Usually incontinent of urine	
	1	Incontinent of bowel and bladder	
		NORTON TOTAL ⇨	1

Scores: ***16-30*, Low risk; *11-15*, moderate risk; *10 or below*, high risk.**

FIGURE 29-15 Norton Scale. (Adapted from Norton, D: *Calculating the risk: Reflections on the Norton Scale,* Decubitus 2:24, 1989.)

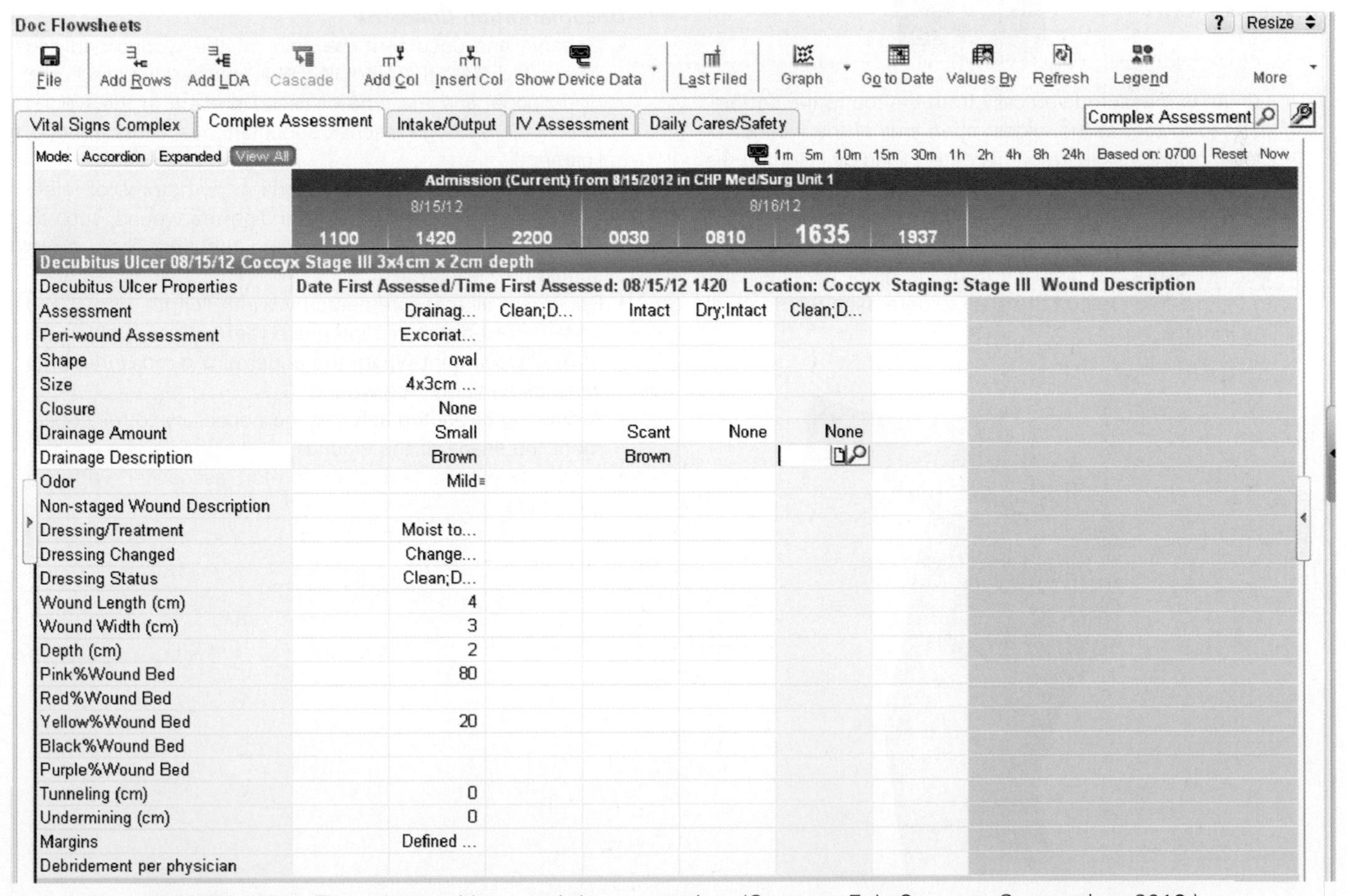

	8/15/12 1100	8/15/12 1420	8/15/12 2200	8/16/12 0030	8/16/12 0810	8/16/12 1635	8/16/12 1937
Assessment		Drainag...	Clean;D...	Intact	Dry;Intact	Clean;D...	
Peri-wound Assessment		Excoriat...					
Shape		oval					
Size		4x3cm ...					
Closure		None					
Drainage Amount		Small		Scant	None	None	
Drainage Description		Brown		Brown			
Odor		Mild					
Non-staged Wound Description							
Dressing/Treatment		Moist to...					
Dressing Changed		Change...					
Dressing Status		Clean;D...					
Wound Length (cm)		4					
Wound Width (cm)		3					
Depth (cm)		2					
Pink%Wound Bed		80					
Red%Wound Bed							
Yellow%Wound Bed		20					
Black%Wound Bed							
Purple%Wound Bed							
Tunneling (cm)		0					
Undermining (cm)		0					
Margins		Defined ...					
Debridement per physician							

FIGURE 29-16 Flow sheet with wound documentation. (Courtesy Epic Systems Corporation, 2012.)

NURSING CARE GUIDELINE

Measuring a Wound

Background

- Wound size changes over time, and size can indicate healing or negative progression.
- Measuring a wound is considered assessment and therefore cannot be delegated to unlicensed assistive personnel (UAP).
- Measurement is performed using the metric system with a facility-provided ruler that has increments in centimeters or millimeters. Sterile cotton-tipped applicators can be used to measure the depth of a wound.

Procedural Concerns

- Always wear clean or sterile gloves, depending on the type of wound and dressing-change orders.
- Take measurements in the following manner:
  - Width is measured laterally from the left to right sides at the widest open area of the wound.

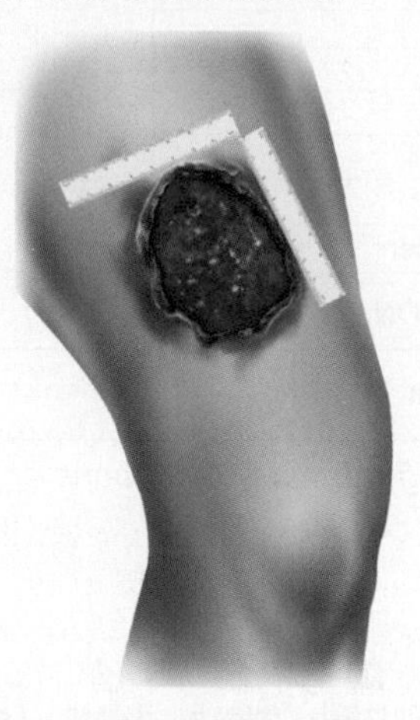

  - Length is measured vertically from the top to the bottom, or head to toe, at the widest open area of the wound.
  - Depth of the visible wound is determined by inserting the tip of a sterile cotton-tipped applicator straight down into the deepest part of the wound. Mark the area on the stick portion of the applicator that is even with the level of the skin. Measure the distance from the tip of the applicator to the marked area on the stick to determine the depth of the wound.

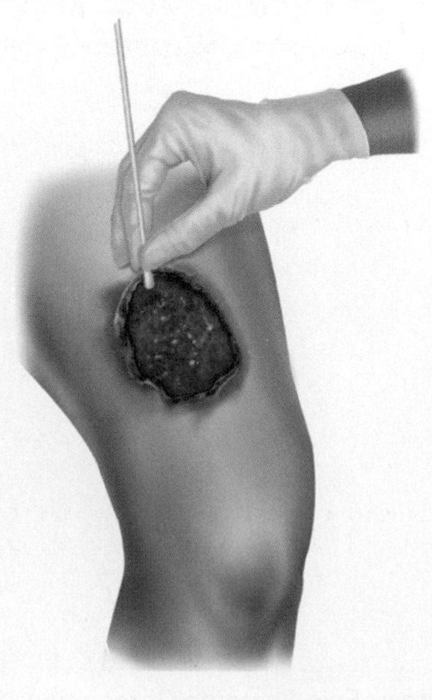

  - Depth of undermining is determined by laterally inserting the tip of a sterile cotton-tipped applicator into the widest section of the undermining. Mark the area on the stick end of the applicator that is even with the edges of the skin, and measure the distance from the tip of the applicator to the marked area to determine the depth of the undermining.

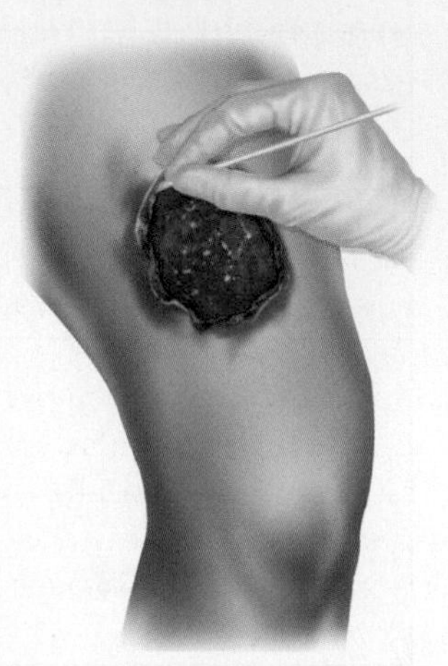

  - Tunneling is measured using the same procedure as that for with undermining.
- When measuring depth, be sure to insert the sterile cotton-tipped applicator gently. The patient may require pain medication before the procedure.

Documentation Concerns

- Observe and document the color of the wound bed and periwound area; the amount, color, consistency, and odor of drainage; and the type of tissue present in the wound (granulation, slough, eschar, subcutaneous, muscle, bone, ligament).
- Observe and document any signs or symptoms of infection. Changes in the skin surrounding the wound, such as redness or breakdown, can indicate infection. These areas should be measured.
- Document all measurements by width, length, depth, and undermining depth in appropriate metric units such as *cm* or *mm*. Document where the undermining measurements were taken within the wound.
- A drawing or photograph may be necessary to fully document the shape of the wound.
- Note any patient pain or discomfort associated with the procedure.

pockets can predispose the patient to the development of an abscess or infection.

Drainage

During wound assessment, note whether drainage is present, the amount of drainage, and its color, consistency, and odor. **Serous** drainage contains clear, watery fluid from plasma. **Serosanguineous** drainage is pink to pale red and contains a mix of serous fluid and red, bloody fluid. **Sanguineous** drainage usually indicates bleeding and is bright red. Purulent drainage usually is thick and indicates infection. It can be yellow, greenish, or beige. The amount of drainage (small, moderate, or large) from a wound is difficult to ascertain and is determined somewhat subjectively by evaluators. Usually, knowledge of the exact amount of drainage is not required. Increases in the amount of drainage and the presence of purulence or a foul odor can indicate infection or the presence of a fistula. In cases in which infection is suspected, the nurse can seek an order for a wound culture. Common organisms causing wound infections include *Staphylococcus aureus* and *Streptococcus pyogenes.* Infectious organisms are discussed in Chapter 26.

An important point to remember is that the production of drainage requires energy, and the drainage may have a high protein content. Therefore excessive drainage can exacerbate the nutritional deficiencies that are common in this patient population.

Conditions of Wound Edges and Surrounding Tissue

Because wounds heal from the edges inward, wound edges should be examined for regeneration of epithelial tissue. A lack of epithelial tissue is an indication that something is preventing the wound from healing so reassessment is needed to determine the cause. The surrounding tissue is inspected for maceration, which appears as pale, soft, or wrinkled skin; signs of infection (redness, warmth, induration); and further tissue breakdown or the development of new wounds. Maceration (Figure 29-17) can provide a clue to the amount of drainage produced by a wound, serve as an indicator of an incorrectly applied dressing that allowed contact of a moist dressing with intact skin, or indicate the need for more frequent dressing changes or a more absorbent dressing.

The development of new wounds, or the expansion of old ones, may mean that the underlying cause of or associated risk factors for the wound have not been adequately addressed, allowing additional tissue damage to occur. For example, a sacral pressure ulcer with nonblanching tissue or bruising around the ulcer warns of the presence of additional tissue damage.

Wound Bed

In addition to determining the type of tissue in the wound bed (granulation tissue, necrotic tissue, subcutaneous tissue, muscle, or bone), the nurse assesses the color of the wound. The wound bed should be beefy red and shiny or moist in appearance. A wound that is pale or dry (Figure 29-18) may be reflective of conditions that are not optimal for wound healing, such as anemia, poor vascular status, nutritional deficiencies, or dehydration. Wounds are examined for the presence of foreign bodies, particularly in the case of traumatic injuries, because foreign bodies can serve as a source of infection and delayed wound healing.

Patient Response

Wounds cause pain. This holds true for acute and chronic wounds, deep and superficial wounds, and wounds occurring in the young and the old, regardless of race or gender. Yet the pain associated with wounds, especially chronic wounds, often is not considered or treated appropriately. The skin is full of sensory nerves; therefore damage to the skin, and the presence of inflammation and infection in the wound, can cause intense pain. This pain affects the patient's self-image and ability to perform customary societal roles, decreases perceived quality of life, decreases appetite, and activates the stress response, which causes vasoconstriction and a reduction in wound healing.

Treatments used in the care of wounds can be additional sources of pain and anxiety, with reported pain levels ranging from mild to excruciating during dressing changes (Pieper, Langemo, and Cuddigan, 2009). The patient's report of the level of pain or distress is the most reliable indicator of the

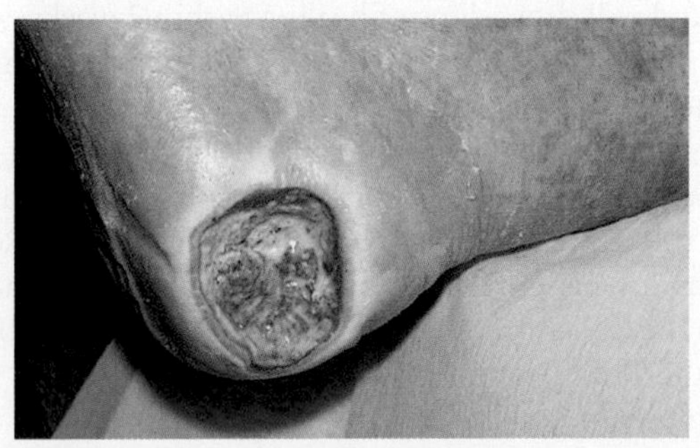

FIGURE 29-17 Wounds with maceration. (From Bryant RA, Nix DP: *Acute and chronic wounds,* ed. 4, St. Louis, 2012, Mosby.)

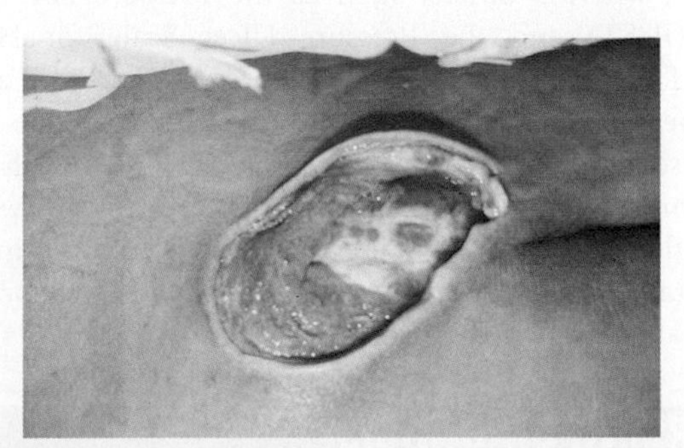

FIGURE 29-18 Pale wound bed. (From Bryant RA, Nix DP: *Acute and chronic wounds,* ed. 4, St. Louis, 2012, Mosby.)

presence of pain in wounds or during dressing changes and needs to be acknowledged as real and assessed frequently. Although some studies have looked at the value of various topical, systemic, and alternative treatment modalities, additional research is needed to determine the most effective ways to manage the pain found in different types of wounds and across diverse patient populations (Pieper, Langemo, and Cuddigan, 2009). Some recommendations regarding the management of wound-related pain include the appropriate selection of dressings; protection of surrounding tissue from irritating wound drainage or dressing materials; aggressive treatment of infection, which is known to increase the presence of inflammation and pain; positioning of the patient in a way that avoids pressure over the wound; use of binders or other devices to splint the wound edges; and premedication before turning, dressing changes, and debridement (Krasner, Shapshak, and Hopf, 2012). In 2009, the NPUAP and the EPUAP included the management of pain in their guidelines for patients with pressure ulcers, emphasizing that these wounds cause pain both during procedures and at rest and that this pain adversely affects quality of life. Additional suggestions for the management of acute and chronic pain can be found in Chapter 36.

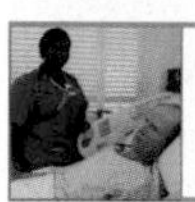

4. What other major areas of clinical concern should the nurse address for Mr. Joseph?

QSEN FOCUS!

Patient-centered care is demonstrated when the nurse assesses for and treats the patient's pain before procedures such as dressing changes, thereby integrating understanding of multiple dimensions of care such as physical comfort and emotional support.

Tools for the Assessment of Wound Healing

Although the assessment and documentation of wound characteristics monitor progression toward healing, specific tools are used both in the clinical setting and in research to track wound healing over time. Some, such as the Wound Characteristic Instrument, are used to assess any open wound, whereas others, such as the Pressure Sore Status Tool (PSST) and the Pressure Ulcer Scale for Healing (PUSH), are specific for pressure ulcers. The PSST assigns a numerical score based on 13 wound attributes; the PUSH tool's score is based on 3 characteristics. With both tools, the scores obtained from the serial observations of wounds allow the health care provider to track wound healing and more rapidly identify trends that may be positively or negatively affecting wound healing.

NURSING DIAGNOSIS LO 29.4

Many nursing diagnoses may be applicable for a patient with a wound. Identifying appropriate diagnoses is based on the assessment data obtained from a thorough history and physical examination, including an assessment of the risk factors associated with impaired wound healing and a focused assessment of the actual wound. Examples of nursing diagnoses related to skin integrity are:

- *Impaired Skin Integrity* related to compromised nutritional status and immobility as evidenced by pressure ulcers on the hip and heel
- *Impaired Physical Mobility* related to pain during position changes as evidenced by the patient's grimacing when turned in bed
- *Impaired Tissue Integrity* related to pressure secondary to immobility as evidenced by a stage III pressure ulcer on the coccyx
- *Acute Pain* related to trauma as evidenced by pain in the area of the wound rated by the patient at 8 of 10
- *Imbalanced Nutrition: Less Than Body Requirement* related to increased demand secondary to healing wounds as evidenced by continued weight loss
- *Risk for Infection* with risk factors of open wound site and imbalanced nutrition
- *Disturbed Body Image* related to change in appearance secondary to surgical incision as evidenced by patient refusal to look at the incision
- *Ineffective Coping* related to change in body image as evidenced by inability to follow wound care directions
- *Deficient Knowledge* related to lack of familiarity with resources as evidenced by improper wound care

PLANNING LO 29.5

Goals, or the desired outcomes for the nursing diagnoses chosen for a patient, are determined after collaboration with the patient and other members of the health care team. These goals or desired outcomes are the driving force behind the selection of the interventions that will aid in the achievement of the goals. Goals include specific evaluation criteria on which to base the patient's response to care and achievement of the stated goal (Table 29-1). For example, the overarching goal for the nursing diagnosis *Impaired Skin Integrity* may be complete healing of the wound. However, a more complete goal statement for an alteration in skin integrity related to a pressure ulcer is:

- Wound will show signs of healing within 2 weeks, with no new ulcers, as evidenced by the presence of granulation tissue in the wound, a decrease in size and depth, and no new pressure ulcers on assessment.

This statement includes a stated period for reevaluation as well as the criteria needed to meet the stated goal. Relevant concerns for patients with impaired skin integrity are outlined in the Collaboration and Delegation box and the Ethical, Legal, and Professional Practice box.

Examples of goal statements are:

- Patient will ingest 75% of each meal during hospitalization.
- Patient will be able to participate in position changes within 24 hours.

TABLE 29-1 Care Planning

NANDA-I NURSING DIAGNOSIS LABEL WITH NURSING DIAGNOSIS STATEMENT	NURSING OUTCOME CLASSIFICATION (NOC)	NURSING INTERVENTION CLASSIFICATION (NIC)
Impaired Skin Integrity related to compromised nutritional status and immobility, as evidenced by pressure ulcers on hip and heel	*Nutritional status: Nutrient intake* (1009) Caloric intake (100901)	*Nutrition therapy* (1120) Monitor food and fluid ingested, and calculate daily caloric intake, as appropriate

From Bulechek G, Butcher H, Dochterman J, et al (Eds): *Nursing interventions classification (NIC),* ed. 6, St. Louis, 2013, Mosby; Moorhead S, Johnson M, Maas M, et al (Eds): *Nursing outcomes classification (NOC),* ed. 5, St. Louis, 2013, Mosby; NANDA International: *Nursing diagnoses: Definitions and classification, 2012–2014,* West Sussex, England, 2012, Wiley-Blackwell. Reprinted with permission from NANDA International, Inc.

COLLABORATION AND DELEGATION

Patients With Wounds

- Assessment and evaluation of a patient's skin and wounds, and the effectiveness of the treatment plan, are the nurse's responsibility and cannot be delegated to unlicensed assistive personnel (UAP). UAP should report to the nurse any changes in skin condition or integrity, elevation in temperature, complaints of pain, increased wound drainage or incontinence, and observed changes in dietary intake.
- Depending on the setting and treatment, some dressing changes can be performed by a UAP. For example, application of nonsterile dressings for chronic wounds with an established treatment plan may be delegated in some situations. The nurse retains responsibility for the delegated task and must supervise the UAP. Care is taken to follow the policies of the facility and stay within the scope of practice.
- In view of the complexity of the patient with a chronic wound, collaboration among specialists in the fields of surgery, infectious disease, physical and occupational therapy, social work and discharge planning, nutrition, and nursing is essential for achieving optimal wound outcomes.
- Collaboration with a specialist in wound care and incontinence should be considered in caring for an at-risk patient.
- A nursing representative is an important member of the purchasing committee charged with the selection of skin and wound care products. Effectiveness, as well as unit cost, must be considered in the selection process, making the role of nursing in product selection essential.
- Families should be included in the purchasing of supplies for home wound care because the selection of products on the basis of insurance coverage may ease financial concerns.

- Patient will show signs of wound healing as evidenced by presence of granulation tissue in the wound within 1 week.
- Patient will report that the pain management regime relieves pain to a level of 3 of 10 or less within the shift.
- Patient will consume nutrition adequate to meet the nutritional requirement within 1 week.
- Patient will remain free of infection during hospitalization.

ETHICAL, LEGAL, AND PROFESSIONAL PRACTICE

Wound Care

- The development of a pressure ulcer often is seen as an indicator of neglect and inadequate care that reflects badly on the facility in which the care took place and on the personnel providing that care. Such wounds cause great pain and suffering for the patient and family and often result in litigation that is costly to all involved. Documentation of initial and ongoing assessments, including a risk assessment, initiation of appropriate prevention and treatment interventions, and the involvement of any specialty services needed to improve wound healing, is critical.
- As with all decisions regarding health care, how aggressively chronic wounds should be treated is a choice that needs to be made by the patient in collaboration with the family and health care providers. It is important for all to remember that the whole patient is the focus of care, not just the wound.
- Potential barriers to good wound care are many and may include a lack of knowledge, lack of access to consistent health care, lifestyle choices, and fiscal constraints at both the patient and facility levels. Many wound-related treatments, as well as the availability of acute, long-term, and home care, are dependent on financial resources. This creates great disparities in wound care among affected patients and in the outcomes of that care.

- Patient will show acceptance of the change in body image by helping with dressing change within 48 hours.
- Patient will verbalize the ability to cope with changes in body image during home care.
- Patient will be able to state strategies to promote wound healing during patient education sessions.

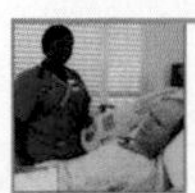

The conceptual care map for Mr. Joseph provided in Figure 29-19 is partially completed to indicate how to use the map as a learning tool. Using it as an example, go to the website at *http://evolve.elsevier.com/YoostCrawford/fundamentals/* to complete Nursing Diagnoses 2 and 3.

Medications

Ceftriaxone 1 g q 24 hr IVPB
Acetaminophen 650 mg PO q 6 hr as needed for a T>38°C (101°F) or mild pain

IV Sites/Fluids/Rate

IV of D_5 0.45NS at 125 mL/hr

Conceptual Care Map

Student name____ Patient initials Mr. J Date ____
Age 64 Gender M Room # ___ Admission date Today
CODE Status ____ Allergies NKDA
Diet Reg adult Braden score ____
Weight 132 Height 5′10″ Religion ____

Admitting Diagnoses/Chief Complaint

Urinary tract infection

Lab Values/Diagnostic Test Results

Albumin 2.5 g/dL
Prealbumin 20 mg/dL

Past Medical/Surgical History

Multiple sclerosis x 30 yr

Assessment Data

Admission: T 38.3°C (101°F), P 110 reg & thready, R 28 & labored, BP 110/60, with pulse oximetry of 94% on RA. Pain 6 of 10, right hip.
A&O x3, MAE weak. Incontinent of urine and stool, adult briefs.
Rt hip wound 5- × 5 cm, bone palpable along medial edge. Periwound skin intact. Wound treated at home with normal saline-moistened gauze, changed once or twice a day. Patient states has had wound for more than 3 months and "it just doesn't get better." Gauze dressings are saturated in 3 hours, foul odor is present.
A 2- × 2-cm area of redness on his left heel does not blanch when pressure is applied.
Sits in a chair but requires assistance from wife or adult son; tends to slide down in the chair.
Requires assistance with meals, tires easily, and rarely finishes 50% of a meal.
Mrs. J works part-time to supplement their income. Mr. J expressed sadness over his declining health and the "burden" that it has placed on his family, both physically and financially. Worked as a high school math teacher until 8 years ago, when his deteriorating health necessitated his early retirement.
Diaphoretic and anxious, he states, "I can't turn myself! Who will take care of me here? I hurt all over but especially my hip!"

Treatments

Turn q 2 hr
Up in chair twice daily
VS q 4 hr
Dietary consult

Primary Nursing Diagnosis

Impaired Skin Integrity related to compromised nutritional status and immobility as evidenced by pressure ulcers on hip and heel.

Supporting Data

Albumin 2.5 g/dL
Right-hip and left-heel pressure wounds
Requires assistance to move from bed to chair

STG/NOC

Patient will ingest 75% of each meal during hospitalization.
NOC: Nutritional status: Nutrient intake (1009)
Caloric intake (100901)

Interventions/NIC With Rationale

1. Document food and fluids ingested with each meal and in between meals so that appropriate calorie counts can be obtained.
2. Consult a registered dietitian so that a diet high in proteins; calories; vitamins A, C, and E; and minerals zinc and copper is provided to promote healing.
3. Plan diet and snacks with patient input to increase likelihood of patient ingesting more of food offered.
4. Provide assistance with meals so that patient is offered entire meal to increase chance of patient eating more.
5. Offer breaks during the meal so that patient does not tire as easily to increase ability to consume enough calories

NIC: Nutrition therapy (1120)
Monitor food and fluid ingested and calculate daily caloric intake, as appropriate.

Rationale Citation/EBP

Yoost BL, Crawford LR: *Fundamentals of nursing: Active learning for collaborative practice*, St. Louis, 2016, Mosby.

Evaluation

Patient ate 75% of breakfast and lunch during day shift. Continue plan of care.

Nursing Diagnosis 2

Supporting Data

STG/NOC

Interventions/NIC With Rationale

Rationale Citation/EBP

Evaluation

Nursing Diagnosis 3

Supporting Data

STG/NOC

Interventions/NIC With Rationale

Rationale Citation/EBP

Evaluation

FIGURE 29-19 Partially completed conceptual care map based on Mr. Joseph, the case study patient in this chapter.

IMPLEMENTATION AND EVALUATION LO 29.6

Nursing care of all patients is aimed at protecting intact skin and promoting healing of existing wounds. Many devices exist to relieve and reduce pressure. Any of the numerous available forms of treatment for wounds may be used, depending on the type of wound and resources available.

INTERVENTIONS TO PRESERVE SKIN INTEGRITY

Interventions are selected to meet the related goals of promoting healing in existing wounds and preventing the development of additional wounds. Nurses, along with other health care providers, must provide care based on a critical appraisal of the most current available information and research using evidence-based practice (Evidence-Based Practice and Informatics box).

EVIDENCE-BASED PRACTICE AND INFORMATICS

Resources for Wound Care

Providers base the selection of interventions on the strength of available evidence. Although the discussion of interventions presented in this text reflects evidentiary guidelines, research continues to produce new knowledge and new recommendations for treatments and products. Nurses have a responsibility to scrutinize the effectiveness of their practice, analyze research findings, use research-based guidelines whenever possible, and actively participate in the development and implementation of guidelines. Some resources for current wound care are:

- Guidelines developed by the National Pressure Ulcer Advisory Panel *(www.npuap.org)*
- Resources provided by groups such as the Joanna Briggs Institute *(www.joannabriggs.edu.au)*
- Research from the Agency for Healthcare Research and Quality *(www.ahrq.gov)*
- The Cochrane Library *(www.cochrane.org)*

Turning and Positioning

The 2009 Pressure Ulcer Prevention and Treatment Guidelines, developed by the NPUAP and the EPUAP, recommend frequent position changes as a way of relieving the duration of pressure to which tissue is subjected, thereby reducing the development of pressure-related wounds. The current recommendations are to change the patient's position at least every 2 hours and to elevate the head of the bed no more than 30 degrees to reduce the effects of shear. When side-lying, patients should be positioned at 30 degrees (Figure 29-20), as opposed to 90 degrees, to avoid direct pressure on bony prominences such as the head of the trochanter. Folded towels, blankets, or a pillow are used to keep bony prominences from exerting pressure against each other, such as to keep the inner knees from pressing against each other in a side-lying position. Use of a posted turning schedule is helpful for the patient, family, and health care worker and serves as a visual reminder of the need to change the patient's position regularly. Despite the need to reposition the patient frequently and reduce the impact of shear forces, it is important to consider the patient's overall medical condition and related health concerns, ability to be turned, support surface, and comfort level. A review of the literature related to the recommendations for position changes revealed that although position changes are important, more research is needed to better understand what frequency and type of positioning are most effective in the prevention of pressure ulcers in different populations (Krapfl and Gray, 2008).

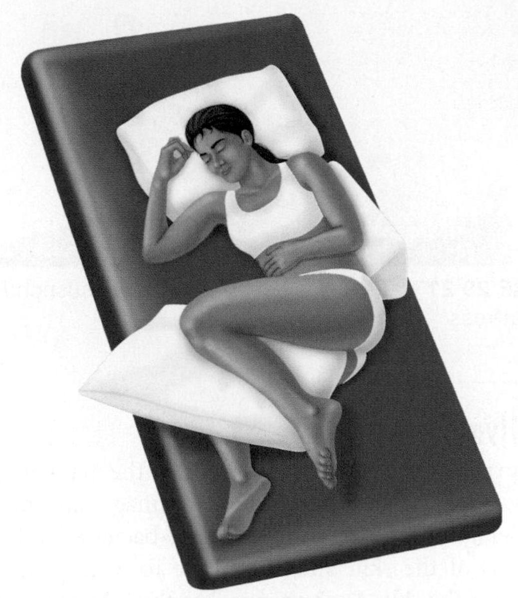

FIGURE 29-20 Patient in a 30-degree side-lying position.

The skin over the heels is at a particularly high risk for breakdown because of the small surface area involved, the lack of a subcutaneous "cushion," and the relatively large amount of underlying bone. Any discussion of proper positioning to relieve pressure must address the heels. Although many products designed to address the prevention of heel ulcers are on the market, little evidence at this time indicates that they are more effective than positioning the leg with pillows so that the heel "floats" clear of the mattress surface, thereby relieving pressure (Junkin and Gray, 2009) (Figure 29-21).

It is important to remember that the recommendations for frequent position changes also apply to the seated person. Patients who are seated in a chair for long periods and who are unable to sense the need to shift their weight or unable to do so independently need assistance in altering their postion while seated. The amount of time spent in a chair without pressure relief should be limited to 2 hours or less (EPUAP and NPUAP, 2009).

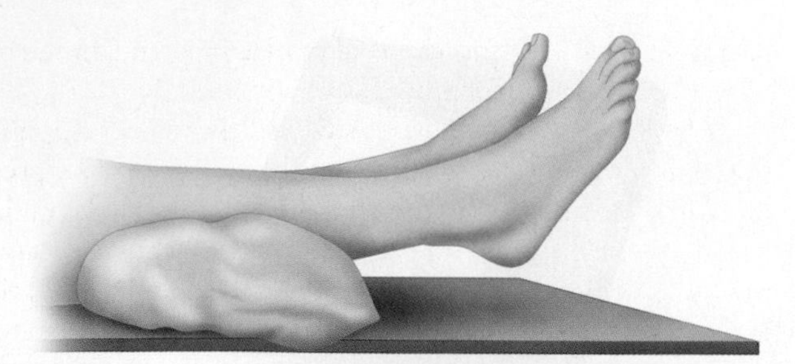

FIGURE 29-21 Patient positioned with heels suspended off the mattress.

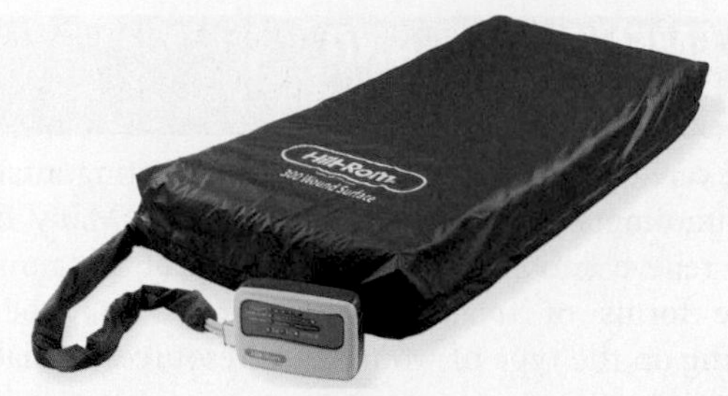

FIGURE 29-22 Pressure-reducing or pressure-relieving support surfaces. (Copyright Hill-Rom Services PTE. Reprinted with permission. All rights reserved.)

Skin Hygiene

Appropriate skin hygiene is important in the maintenance of healthy skin. Incontinence, wound drainage, and moisture from perspiration increase the risk of bacterial and fungal infections of the skin and contribute to a decrease in the strength of the skin. Such changes are thought to be a factor in skin tears, perineal injuries, and abrasions. The specific content of wound drainage may increase the severity of the damage to the skin. Regular cleansing of the skin with timely response to episodes of incontinence is an important component of nursing care. Use of soap and hot water can remove the oils from the skin, leading to excessive dryness. Overuse of many soaps, including antibacterial soaps, can change the skin's normally acidic pH and decrease its natural protective antimicrobial action. Some cleansers are marketed specifically for bathing and incontinence care, and use of any of several mild, pH-neutral soaps also may be appropriate. It is important to choose a product that preserves the normal pH of the skin and does not result in overly dry skin. One that combines a moisturizer with a cleanser is a good choice for cleansing and should be used with warm water as opposed to hot water. In the case of incontinence and wound drainage, the skin can be further protected after cleansing through the correct use of a moisture barrier ointment (EPUAP and NPUAP, 2009; Wysocki, 2012). Knowledge of the specific characteristics of different classifications of skin cleansers and barrier ointments aids in the selection of a suitable product.

PRESSURE-REDUCING MATTRESSES AND SUPPORT SURFACES

Many mattresses and seat cushions are specifically designed to reduce or relieve pressure and especially to decrease the risk for development of pressure ulcers (Figure 29-22). The selection of a suitable support surface is only one component of a prevention and treatment plan. It is critical to recognize that none of the specialty surfaces eliminates the need for a thorough assessment, identification and modification of known risk factors, and regular position changes. The erroneous belief that a specialty support surface eliminates the need for position changes is a common one, with potentially serious consequences for the patient.

All support surfaces work to reduce pressure by redistributing or "spreading out" the body's weight over a greater surface area. By doing so, the resulting intensity and magnitude of the pressure on a given body surface area are decreased. Many different materials and technologies are used in support surfaces. They are made of foams or gels, can be fluid- or air-filled, and can be dynamic or static. Available as overlays, replacement mattresses, or specialty beds, they are designed for adults, children, or the obese and specifically for beds, chairs, operating room tables, and stretchers, as well as certain risk areas (e.g., heels). Although an in-depth discussion of the available support surfaces and their underlying technologies is beyond the scope of this textbook, it is important to recognize that different advantages, disadvantages, and costs are associated with each. These considerations and the need to use available resources judiciously have necessitated that health care facilities and insurers develop guidelines for the use of specialty support surfaces and that the users of these surfaces understand the indications for their use as well as their strengths and limitations.

INTERVENTIONS RELATED TO WOUND CARE

Wound care depends on the type of wound, amount of drainage, presence of infection, and resources available. Wounds are assessed on an ongoing basis, because changes occur during the healing process. The type of wound care may change as the wound heals.

Wound Cleansing and Irrigation

Wound cleansing is important in removing surface contaminants or debris that can become a reservoir for bacteria, thereby allowing the bacteria to adhere to the wound and invade deeper tissue. The selected cleansing agent and method of cleansing must provide for balance between the need to clean the wound and the need to minimize further damage or trauma to the wound bed and allow wound healing to occur. For example, antiseptic solutions such as Dakin's solution, povidone-iodine, acetic acid, and hydrogen peroxide, although cytotoxic to bacteria, are harmful to the cells needed for wound healing, and their use can actually delay wound healing. Although numerous wound cleansers are commercially available, 0.9% normal saline solution is an adequate wound cleanser and is readily available in most health care settings. Cold irrigation solutions (cooler than room temperature) decrease the activity of leukocytes and other cells for hours after irrigation, again delaying the ability of these cells to perform their necessary roles in wound healing. In irrigating a wound, the force of the irrigation must be sufficient to actually remove the surface contaminants yet not so strong that it damages the delicate new tissue of the healing wound (Skill 29-1).

QSEN FOCUS!

Safety requires that the nurse demonstrate effective use of strategies, such as use of personal protective equipment (PPE), that reduce the risk of harm to self or others when wound care may result in exposure to potentially infectious drainage.

! SAFE PRACTICE ALERT

Wound irrigation can result in splashing of the fluid and debris; therefore, the use of PPE such as gowns, masks, and goggles is required.

Debridement

Debridement is the removal of necrotic tissue, which would otherwise prolong the inflammatory phase of wound healing and provide a reservoir for bacteria. The removal of necrotic tissue is necessary for the wound to be assessed adequately for viable tissue and staged in the case of pressure ulcers. For some types of wounds, such as those on heels, debridement is not usually recommended if the necrotic tissue is dry and stable, with no evidence of infection. This is the exception, however. Several types of debridement may be used: sharp, mechanical, enzymatic, autolytic, and biologic. The selection of the type of debridement is based on an assessment of the wound, the patient's other health conditions, available resources, and the patient's concerns.

Sharp debridement is the use of a sharp instrument (scalpel, curette, or scissors), by health care personnel with appropriate training, to remove necrotic tissue. It is the fastest way of removing nonviable tissue and is the method of choice if an underlying infection is suspected or if a large amount of necrotic tissue needs to be removed rapidly. Caution is used in patients with bleeding disorders.

Mechanical debridement is a nonselective form of debridement in that it not only removes the necrotic tissue but also can remove or disturb exposed viable tissue that may be in the wound. The main forms of mechanical debridement are wet/damp-to-dry dressings and whirlpools. Wet/damp-to-dry dressings usually are saline-moistened dressing materials that are allowed to dry to the wound and are then removed, pulling the surface layer off the wound bed (Skill 29-2). Mechanical debridement often is painful for the patient, is harmful to viable tissue, can lead to bleeding, and, in the case of wet/damp-to-dry dressings, is labor-intensive.

Enzymatic debridement is achieved through the application of topical agents containing enzymes that work by breaking down the fibrin, collagen, or elastin present in devitalized tissue, thus allowing for its removal. Although a slower method of debridement than mechanical or sharp, it is selective for nonviable tissue and is quite effective when used appropriately. The various enzymatic agents on the market differ in terms of action, application, and potential complications. Some examples are Santyl, Panafil, and Accuzyme.

Occlusive dressings such as hydrocolloids and transparent films are used for autolytic debridement, as are hydrogels. Autolytic debridement is based on the principle that wounds have an innate ability to clean themselves of debris and necrotic tissue through the action of the body's own enzymes and phagocytic cells. Because it is a normal part of the wound healing process, it requires a moist wound environment and the optimization of the other factors important for wound healing in order to be successful. This type of debridement is the slowest, and it is contraindicated in infected wounds. It is the most comfortable form of debridement for the patient.

Biologic debridement involves the use of sterile, medicinal larvae from green bottle flies (maggots), which secrete proteolytic enzymes that break down necrotic tissue, digest bacteria, and stimulate the formation of granulation tissue. The use of maggots may cause pain, and the patient may find both the sight and sensation of the maggots to be disturbing. However, maggot therapy is an effective form of debridement in certain types of wounds.

Dressings

Dressings have multiple purposes: They are intended to keep the wound free of contamination, absorb drainage yet prevent overdrying of the wound bed, protect the periwound tissue, treat infection, and aid in the debridement of the wound. When selecting a dressing for a wound, the nurse must keep in mind the differences inherent in the various classifications of dressings, the assessment of the wound and surrounding tissue, and the goal of treatment (see Skill 29-2). No single dressing type is ideal for all wounds, and it is essential to match the wound to the dressing in order to select the best treatment. Reassessment of the wound as it heals may necessitate a change in the type of dressing used. Although many wound care products are available, there are certain broad classifications of dressings with which the nurse should be familiar: gauze dressings, transparent dressings, hydrocolloids, foams, alginates, and gels. The development of these dressing types, with the exception of dry gauze dressings, is based on the pioneering work of Dr. George D. Winter in the 1960s. He demonstrated in animal models that wounds heal faster in a moist skin environment than if allowed to become dry (Doughty, 2012). This discovery represented a radical departure from earlier beliefs about wound healing.

Many of these dressings are available impregnated or otherwise treated with antimicrobial agents such as silver to reduce the bacterial load, or **bioburden,** in the wound and thereby improve wound healing. For wounds with signs of infection or chronic wounds that are not responding to appropriate treatment, use of this type of dressing may be indicated after a wound culture is obtained (Skill 29-3).

Gauze dressings are the oldest category of dressings, and both patients and health care workers are familiar with their use. Gauze comes in many forms, shapes, and sizes, which makes it a versatile dressing. Although it is one of the most commonly used dressings, gauze as a primary dressing has many disadvantages: It is not an effective barrier to infection, particularly when moist; its removal often results in pain and inadvertent damage to the healing wound bed; fibers can be left in the wound; and its use is time-consuming and labor-intensive. The greatest disadvantage is its inability to maintain the moist wound environment required for healing even if moistened before being placed in the wound. Because of these disadvantages, its use often delays wound healing, thereby increasing overall costs. Despite this limitation, gauze remains a commonly used wound dressing and is preferable to allowing the wound to become dry (Doughty, 2012; EPUAP and NPUAP, 2009). Gauze comes in many configurations and may be impregnated with antibiotics, petrolatum, or other materials. It is therefore useful as packing in all types of wounds, as a cover dressing, and for absorbing exudate from a heavily draining wound.

QSEN FOCUS!

Evidence-based practice demonstrates knowledge of basic scientific methods and processes. When selecting appropriate wound dressings, the nurse values the concept of evidence-based practice as an integral factor in determining best clinical practice.

Transparent films are made of adhesive-backed polyurethane that sticks to the periwound skin but not to the actual wound bed. Because polyurethane has no absorbent capability, this type of dressing is inappropriate for wounds with more than a minimal amount of drainage. The films prevent bacteria and fluids from entering the wound but allow oxygen and water vapor to move through the dressing. They imitate the action of a blister by keeping the body's own wound fluid next to the wound bed, thus maintaining a moist environment. Transparent films come in a variety of shapes and sizes and can be used as a primary or secondary dressing. Their use is appropriate for autolytic debridement of a minimally draining wound that has no sign of infection.

Hydrocolloids are occlusive, adhesive dressings composed of gelling agents and carboxymethylcellulose. They absorb a small to moderate amount of drainage over a 3- to 7-day period, forming a gel as drainage is absorbed. This gel is sometimes mistaken for the purulent drainage suggestive of infection when the dressing is removed, so it is important to cleanse the wound before reassessment. Hydrocolloids provide a moist wound environment, and their absorbent capabilities prevent the wound bed and surrounding tissue from becoming too wet. Because of their occlusive properties and long wear time, they generally are not recommended for wounds suspected of being infected. Hydrocolloids are versatile dressings available in multiple shapes, sizes, and thicknesses and are appropriate for use with clean, uninfected wounds with small to moderate amounts of drainage.

Foams are able to pull fluid away from the wound bed yet maintain a moist wound environment. They are used for wounds producing moderate to heavy amounts of exudates and should not be used for wounds with only a small amount of drainage. They can be used over enzymatic debriding agents or gels, although the absorptive nature of the foam may cause these other materials to be absorbed into the foam dressing. Like transparent films and hydrocolloids, foams are available in a wide variety of sizes, shapes, and configurations, including sheets, rolls, and "pillows" designed to fill cavities. Although they sometimes are used as padding, important points are that they do not relieve pressure; this type of usage is not covered by insurers in the home care setting; and many less costly and more appropriate materials are available for this purpose (Home Care Considerations box).

HOME CARE CONSIDERATIONS

Wound Care Supplies in the Home

- The cost of wound care supplies in the home can be significant, and coverage for these supplies by insurers is not universal. If they are covered, the amount of the product provided is based on the documented assessment of the wound and the recommended usage of the product.
- Sterile supplies usually are not needed, and other, more readily available and sometimes more affordable products are utilized. For example, the use of sanitary napkins and disposable diapers as absorptive dressings can be acceptable on the basis of the assessment of the wound. Although further research is needed on the possible effects of these products on wound healing, their use remains common for many chronic wounds in the home care setting.
- A saline solution can be prepared in the home setting by boiling a quart of water for 5 minutes and then dissolving 2 teaspoons of salt in the water. Once the water has cooled, it can be used for wound cleansing or in dressing changes.
- The solution can be kept for 1 week at room temperature if stored in a tightly closed container.

Like foams, alginates are useful in the highly exudative wound. They are made from brown seaweed fibers and are highly absorbent, capable of absorbing up to 20 times their weight. They are nonadhesive, nonocclusive, and usable in a variety of wounds. They can be combined with a foam or another dressing type to increase the dressing's overall absorbent capabilities and decrease the frequency of dressing changes. Like foams, alginates should be avoided in dry wounds. They have a homeostatic property, meaning they have the ability to stop bleeding, so they are useful in bleeding wounds.

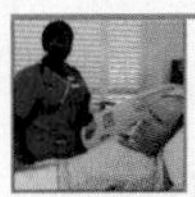

5. What type of dressings might be appropriate for Mr. Joseph's wounds? State the rationale for your answer.

Gels, made in both tube and sheet versions, are used to add moisture to a wound, thus creating a moist environment and allowing autolytic debridement and wound healing to occur. Because of their high moisture content, they absorb very little wound drainage and thus are inappropriate for a highly exudative wound, and they can cause maceration of the periwound skin if used incorrectly.

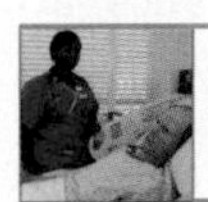

6. What nursing interventions would be appropriate to address Mr. Joseph's risk factors?

Drains

The placement of drains in or around surgical sites is thought to reduce the chance of infection by preventing excess blood, serum, or pus from collecting in the surgical area. The nurse is responsible for understanding the different types of drains and the care required by the patient with a drain. The amount, color, consistency, and odor of the drainage are assessed on a regular basis, with changes noted and reported to the physician or other health care provider. The skin around the drain is assessed for signs of infection (increasing warmth, drainage, erythema, pain) or damage from the drainage. Drainage from the small intestine, gallbladder, stomach, and pancreas is damaging to the skin, and protective action is taken in areas exposed to drainage from these sources. Effective strategies to prevent chemical damage to the skin from drainage include the use of barrier ointments designed for incontinence together with frequent dressing changes and the use of pouches similar to those used for ostomy management.

Drains can be closed or open systems and may or may not be sutured into place. Closed drainage systems (Nursing Care Guideline: Closed-Wound Drainage System box) such as **Jackson-Pratt (JP) drains** and **Hemovac drains** are soft drains attached to a bulblike (JP) or springlike (Hemovac) suction device. When the drain is compressed and plugged, it provides suction by pulling drainage from the wound as it reexpands. Although many closed drainage systems are placed during surgery, they can be inserted into fluid collections using ultrasound or CT guidance.

Closed drainage systems allow for a more accurate assessment of the drainage and prevent bacteria on the dressing from tracking up the drainage tube. Like open drains, closed drains often are removed before hospital discharge, but they can still be in place in a patient discharged to the home setting.

The **Penrose drain**, an open drain that is a flexible piece of tubing, usually is not sutured into place (Nursing Care Guideline: Open-Wound Drainage System box). Care is taken to not inadvertently remove the drain during dressing changes. This type of drain usually is removed over a period of several days before discharge.

Negative-Pressure Wound Therapy

Negative-pressure wound therapy (NPWT), or vacuum-assisted closure (VAC), uses negative pressure to remove excess wound fluid, stabilize the wound edges, and stimulate granulation tissue (Skill 29-4). In some studies, this management technique has been shown to reduce the bacteria count in the wound. Although specific features vary among brands, application of the negative-pressure system generally consists of placing a foam sponge or other dressing into the wound, covering this dressing with a transparent adhesive drape, and applying a controlled amount of suction to the wound through the drape. The dressing usually is changed every 3 days but can be changed more frequently, depending on the wound assessment. It is used on acute and chronic wounds, including dehiscent wounds and fasciotomies, pressure ulcers, venous stasis ulcers, and skin flaps, to promote wound healing. Although the cost of this device is absorbed by the prospective payment received from insurance in the acute care setting, it may not be fully covered in the home care setting.

Suture Care

Sutures are used to bring the edges of a wound together in order to speed wound healing and reduce scar formation (Nursing Care Guideline: Suture Care box). The sutures can be threads or metal staples. Some are located deep within the tissue, usually dissolving over time; others are visible from the skin surface and need to be removed later (Figure 29-23). The timing of suture removal will vary, depending on the type of surgery and patient factors that might affect wound healing, but sutures generally are removed 7 to 14 days after insertion, when the formation of the healing ridge indicates that collagen synthesis has taken place. Special tapes, such as Steri-Strips, although not providing as strong a closure as with sutures, sometimes are used to close superficial or partially healed wounds.

Nursing care for the patient with sutures includes an assessment of the incision line and the tissue around each individual suture for changes in drainage, warmth, erythema, and pain. Although some erythema is a normal reaction to the presence of a foreign body, increasing redness, particularly when accompanied by an increase in pain, warmth, or drainage, can be an indication of infection.

NURSING CARE GUIDELINE

Closed-Wound Drainage System: Hemovac and Jackson-Pratt

Background

- Closed-wound drainage most commonly is used for orthopedic and abdominal surgical patients.
- The system drains extra fluid from inside the surgical wound to the outside of the body and into a reservoir, or collection device, at the end of the tubing by maintaining constant mild to moderate suction.
- The system promotes healing because granulation tissue (healing cells) can adhere to the surgical site when the wound is drained.
- The number of microorganisms entering the wound is reduced, because the system is closed (i.e., it has no open ends), and the drain usually is sutured in place in the sterile environment during surgery.
- The drain usually is disconnected by the PCP 3 to 5 days after surgery.

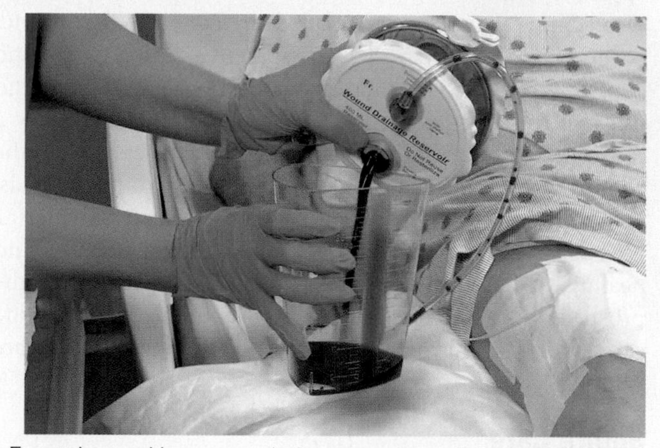

Emptying a Hemovac drainage system into a graduated cylinder.

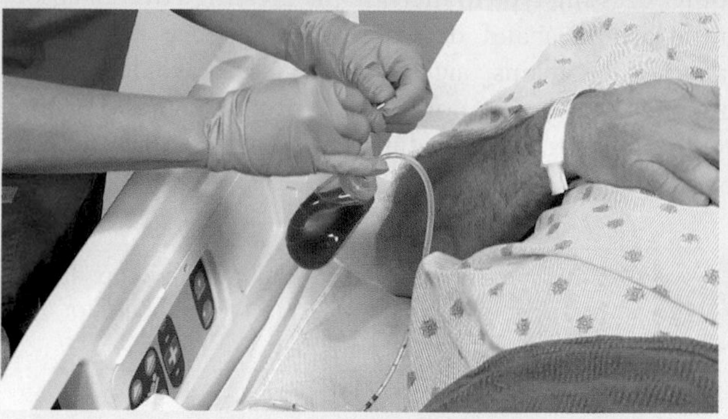

Opening the plug on a Jackson-Pratt drainage system.

Procedural Concerns

- Always wear gloves, and do not touch the port or plug when emptying the reservoir.
- Use a marked, graduated measuring device to collect the drainage when emptying the reservoir to facilitate accurate measurement of the drainage. (A graduated cylinder or specimen cup can be used to drain a Hemovac device; a 30-mL plastic medication cup usually is used to drain a Jackson-Pratt device.)
- Empty the reservoir every 4 to 8 hours, depending on PCP orders and the amount of drainage.
- After emptying, recompress the device to maintain suction: With the port open, squeeze the reservoir, wipe the port and plug with an alcohol wipe, and close the port. The container should remain compressed to ensure that suction is applied.
- Secure the container(s) to the patient's hospital gown below the level of the wound, avoiding tension on the tubing.

Documentation Concerns

- Observe and document the amount, color, type (serous, serosanguineous, sanguineous), odor, and consistency of the drainage.
- Observe and document any signs of infection at the opening for the tubing or in the drainage.
- If multiple drains are in place, label them and document observations by the drain label.
- If no drainage is seen, check the tubing for kinks or blockage; make sure that the tubing is not dislodged. Notify the PCP of any problems.

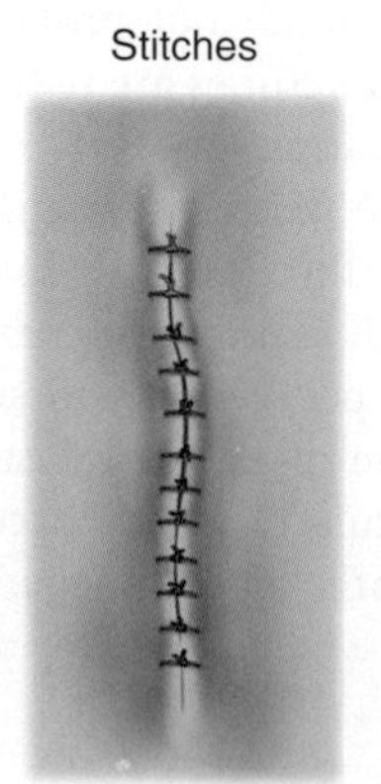

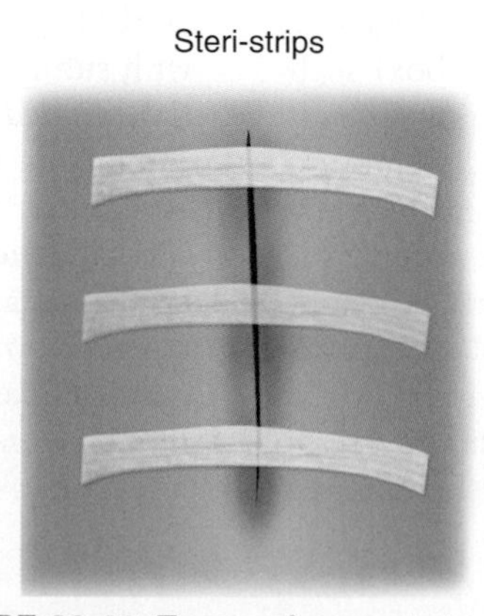

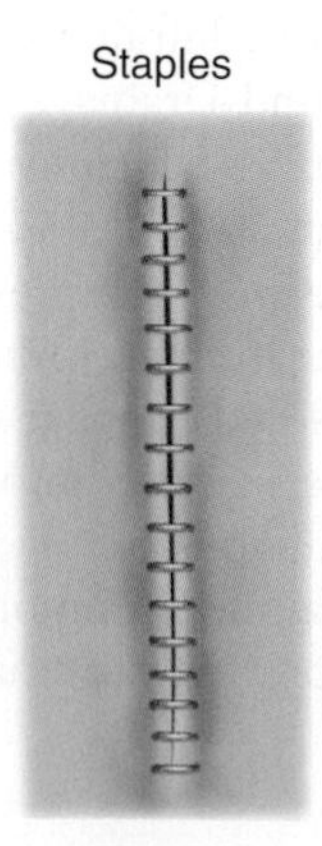

FIGURE 29-23 Types of wound closures.

NURSING CARE GUIDELINE

Open-Wound Drainage System: T-Tubes and Penrose Drains

Background

- Open-wound drainage is most commonly used in patients who have had abdominal surgery, particularly after incision and drainage procedures, gallbladder surgery, or other operative procedures involving the common bile duct.
- The system drains excess fluid through a passage created from an internal wound to the outside of the body and onto a wound dressing. The pressure inside the wound is greater than the pressure outside the body; therefore the drainage flows out of the tube onto the dressing.
- The drains typically are inserted through stab wounds a few centimeters away from the surgical incision line, to prevent any interference with healing of the main surgical site.

Procedural Concerns

- To prevent infection, always wear sterile gloves, and avoid touching the opening except with sterile forceps.
- Penrose drains are not sutured in place.

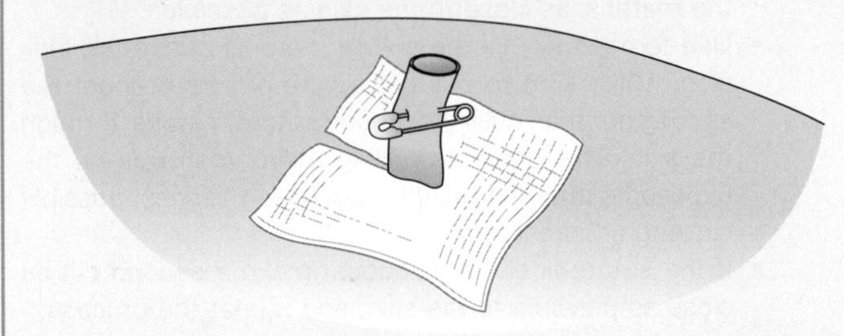

Penrose drains are not sutured in place. (From deWit SC, O'Neill PA: *Fundamental concepts and skills for nursing*, ed. 4, St. Louis, 2014, Saunders.)

  - A sterile safety pin is placed through the portion of the drain outside the body during surgery, to prevent the tube from slipping inside the wound.
  - Care must be taken when changing dressings to keep the drain from becoming dislodged and to prevent the tube from being compressed
- T-tubes or biliary draining tubes are T shaped tubes. The top of the T is inserted into the bile duct during surgery with the straight end exiting the skin similar to a penrose drane. They may or may not be sutured in place.
  - A T-tube may remain connected to the drainage bag for approximately 1 week, at which time the bag may be disconnected and the tube tied or capped. The tube may be left in place for up to 6 weeks.
  - Care should be taken to prevent drainage from coming into contact with the skin around the site, because the drainage is highly irritating to skin.
- Cleansing an open-wound drainage system is performed in a circular motion, working from the site of the drain outward and away from the drain. Drain sponges are applied after cleansing, and then sterile 4 × 4 gauze pads and an absorbent abdominal (ABD) pad are applied to absorb drainage.

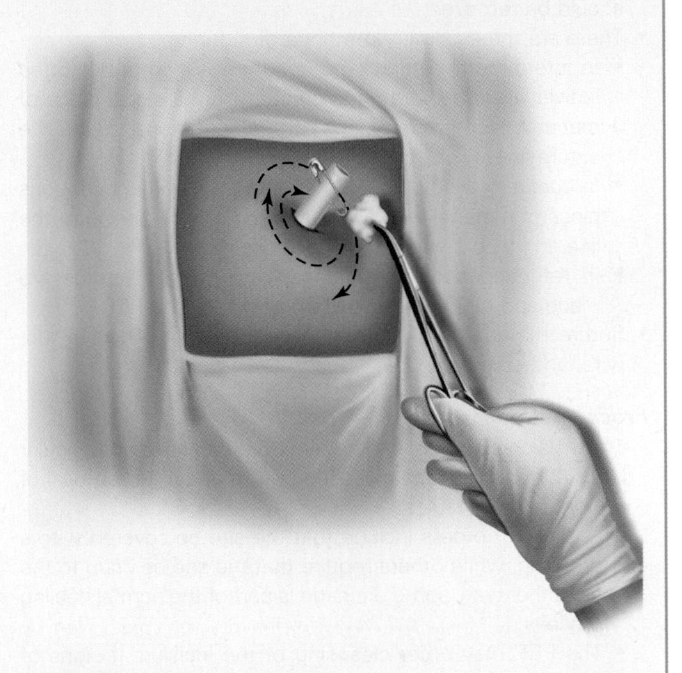

Documentation Concerns

- Observe and document the amount, color, type (serous, serosanguineous, sanguineous), odor, and consistency of drainage.
- Observe and document any signs of infection at the opening for the tubing or in the drainage.
- If multiple drains are in place, label them and document observations by drain label.
- If no drainage is seen, check the tubing for kinks or blockage; make sure that the tubing is not dislodged. Notify the PCP of any problems; for example, an abscess can be a common complication with this type of drainage system.

Bandages and Binders

Bandages and binders are placed over wound dressings to secure a dressing or splint, to provide support and protection to the healing wound, to apply pressure to reduce bleeding, or to immobilize a body part (Skill 29-5). They come in many shapes, sizes, and compositions and may be intended for a single use, as in the case of rolls of gauze, or for multiple uses, as with elastic bandages, slings, and binders. An additional reason for their use is to reduce the amount of tape required during dressing changes by securing the underlying dressing with a bandage or binder. Use of this means of wound support reduces the incidence of skin tears due to tape. The bandage or binder is wrapped so that the underlying circulation is adequate and the patient is comfortable. Adjustments of the bandage or binder may be necessary after application. When a bandage is applied to an extremity, the nurse assesses the five *P*s of circulation—*p*ain, *p*allor, *p*ulselessness, *p*aresthesia, and *p*aralysis—within 30 minutes of application. If any of the

NURSING CARE GUIDELINE

Suture Care

Background

- Wounds may be closed with Steri-Strips, Dermabond glue, sutures, or staples. The choice is made by the PCP, with the main goal of decreasing infection and minimizing scarring.
- Policies vary among facilities regarding whether the nurse is allowed to remove sutures and staples. If the nurse is allowed to remove them, an order from the PCP is required. This order should specify how many days after application the removal should occur and whether all staples or sutures should be removed.
- There are three primary methods of suturing:
  - In intermittent suturing, each suture is tied and knotted individually. Each suture is created from a single piece of material. Numerous pieces of suture material create the suture line.
  - In continuous suturing, the suture line is one continuous piece of material with a tie or knot at the beginning of the line and a second tie or knot at the end.
  - In retention suturing, stronger and deeper sutures are made and typically must be removed by the PCP.
- Suture materials include silk, cotton, Dacron, linen, nylon, wire, and steel.

Procedural Concerns

- The incision may or may not have to be cleansed on a regular basis, but it should be cleansed before and after removal of the sutures or staples.
  - Some PCP orders include that the site be covered with a dressing, while others require that the site be open to the air. Either way, some drainage is part of the normal healing process.
  - The PCP may order cleansing of the incision. If signs of infection are noted, cleansing of the suture line may be required.
  - Cleansing is always performed from the least contaminated area to the most contaminated area:
    - Clean from the suture line outward (first on one side of the incision and then on the other).
    - Alternatively, clean directly down the suture line and then to either side.
    - For each cleansing stroke, use a new sterile gauze pad with the ordered cleansing solution applied.
    - See Skill 29-2 (Changing a Sterile Dressing: Dry, Wet/Damp-to-Dry), for further information.
- Sutures and staples typically are removed 7 to 14 days after insertion, depending on the PCP's order. Retention sutures are left in place longer (typically 14 to 21 days).
  - Use sterile technique.
  - When removing sutures or staples, skip every other one. This is a precaution to ensure that the incision is healed and the edges are approximated before completely removing all sutures or staples.
  - To remove sutures:
    - Put on sterile gloves. To avoid sliding the scissors under the skin, use forceps to lift the suture material away from the skin. Then, using curved suture scissors, cut the material as close to the skin as possible.
    - Use forceps to pull the suture material out of the incision. Make sure to pull the suture out from under the skin, rather than pulling exposed suture material through the skin. This prevents pulling microorganisms on the exposed suture material through clean tissues, possibly causing an infection.
    - If the suture line is continuous, make a second cut as close as possible to the skin, and repeat the process.

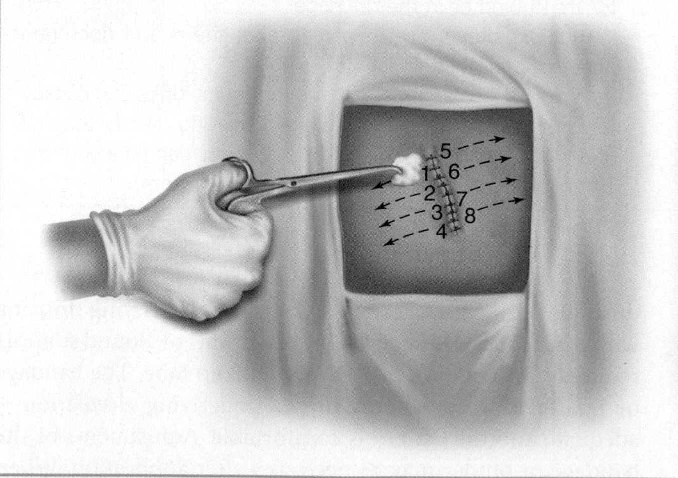

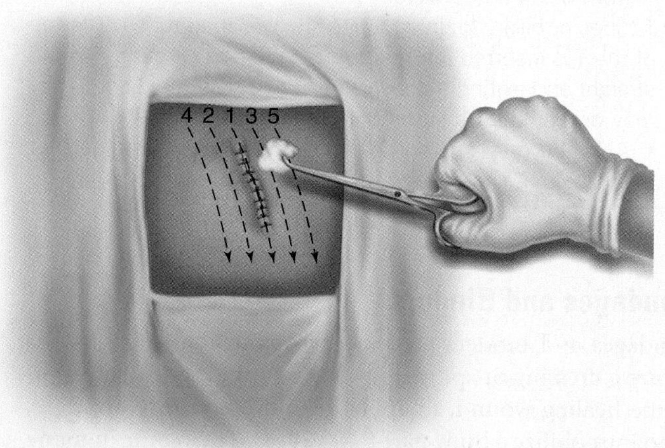

NURSING CARE GUIDELINE—cont'd

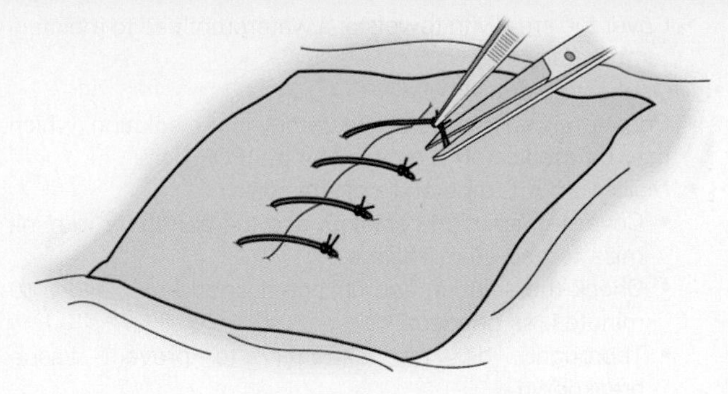

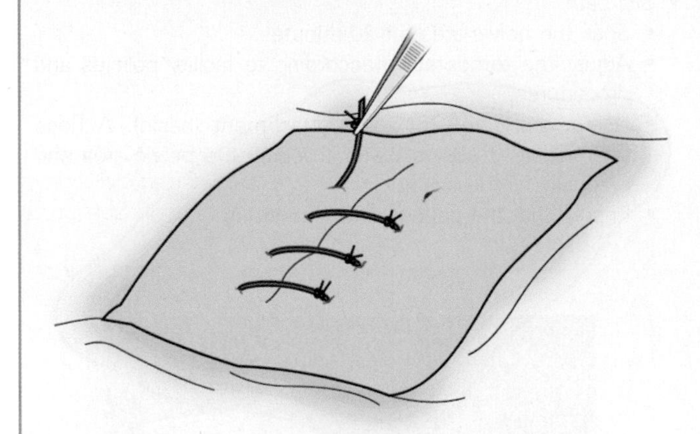

(From deWit SC, O'Neill PA: *Fundamental concepts and skills for nursing,* ed. 4, St. Louis, 2014, Saunders.)

- To remove staples:
  - Use a medical staple remover. It is important to recognize that removal of staples may be more painful for the patient than removal of sutures.
  - Slide the tip of the staple remover under the center of each staple, and slowly squeeze the handles to bend the staple. The staple should not break.
  - Free the staple from the skin and incision line. If necessary, use forceps to gently remove the staple.
  - Discard removed staples in a sharps disposal container.
- Steri-Strips may be applied after suture or staple removal to support wound approximation and minimize scarring.

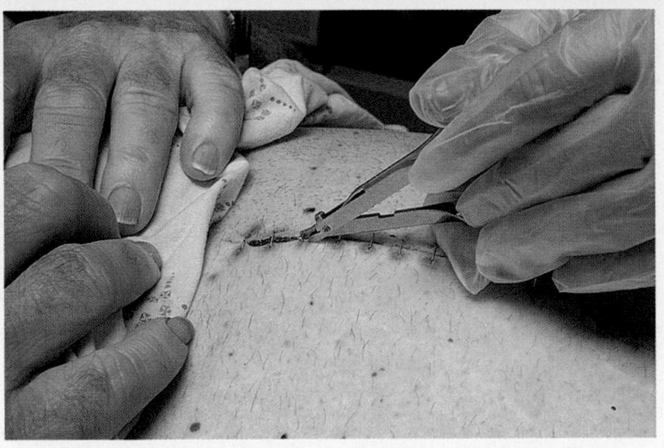

(From deWit SC, O'Neill PA: *Fundamental concepts and skills for nursing,* ed. 4, St. Louis, 2014, Saunders.)

Documentation Concerns
- Observe and document the amount, color, type, odor, and consistency of any drainage at the incision site or on the dressing.
- Observe and document any signs of infection at or around the incision site or in the drainage.
- Document the type of suture line, material, and number of sutures, as well as any problems with the procedure and patient tolerance.
- Document the number of staples, as well as the ease of removal and patient tolerance.
- Notify the PCP before removing sutures or staples if there are signs of infection. Notify the PCP if the wound edges separate after removing the sutures or staples.

Evidence-Based Practice
- Current guidelines strongly recommend that incisions be covered with a sterile dressing for 24 to 48 hours, but the evidence is inconclusive as to whether the incision should remain covered or be left open to the air after this time frame to avoid infection. It is clear, however, that hand hygiene and the utilization of sterile technique when changing the dressing are imperative to prevent infection at the site (Betsy Lehman Center for Patient Safety and Medical Error Reduction, 2008).

Ps are present, the bandage is removed and rewrapped so that it is less constricting.

Montgomery straps may be used instead of a binder. Montgomery straps are adhesive, multiholed straps placed on the skin on opposite sides of a wound. Gauze ties are then placed connecting the opposite holes of each piece of the paired tapes. This provides a means of securing a bandage, and subsequently changing it, without having to replace tape each time, thereby helping to reduce the incidence of skin tears. See Chapter 37 for more information.

HEAT AND COLD APPLICATION

The therapeutic application of heat or cold has been used for years to reduce pain, improve circulation, and reduce swelling. In many cases the use of these therapies requires a doctor's order, because serious complications related to their use have been documented. The order should specify the type of application, the length of the treatment, and its frequency, as well as the body part to be treated (Nursing Care Guideline: Application of Heat and Cold Therapies box).

NURSING CARE GUIDELINE

Application of Heat and Cold Therapies

Background

- Heat causes vasodilation, improving blood flow and bringing oxygen, nutrients, and leukocytes to the area; it decreases edema, promotes muscle relaxation and decreases stiffness, helps to debride wounds, and can be soothing for the patient. It can be applied through moist heat in compresses, soaks, or baths; through dry heat delivered using electric heating pads, disposable hot packs, or pads through which warm water is circulated; or through radiant heat from a heat lamp.
- Cold causes vasoconstriction, reducing the oxygen demands of the tissue; it decreases pain, decreases swelling, decreases blood flow, prevents edema, provides anesthesia, and relieves muscle spasms. It can be applied through the use of ice bags, cool compresses, cool soaks or baths, or pads through which cool water is circulated.

Procedural Concerns

Assessments

- Examine the baseline integumentary status in the area designated for application of heat or cold.
- Assess for sensory changes in the area to be treated. Assess for neuropathies.
- Check the condition of equipment: Do not use any equipment if there are questionable safety conditions.
- Assess extremity circulation. If circulation is impaired, do not apply cold; notify the PCP.

Patient Position

- Patient must never lie on a heat therapy device. Pressure intensifies the effects of heat, increasing the risk for burns.

Contraindications

- Heat should not be used in the presence of:
  - Bleeding (heat promotes vasodilation, so bleeding will continue)
  - Cardiovascular pathophysiology (heat should not be applied to large areas of skin because it disrupts blood flow to organs)
  - Local abscess, because rupture could occur
- Cold should not be used if any of the following is present:
  - Edema (cold application slows reabsorption of the fluid)
  - Circulatory pathophysiology (cold application causes vasoconstriction, further reducing circulation to the area)
  - Shivering (this is a comfort concern)
- Application of heat or cold in the following situations results in altered sensory abilities and, ultimately, tissue damage. Frequent assessment of the patient is needed if treatment is applied under conditions of:
  - Neuropathy
  - Altered level of consciousness
  - Advanced age (skin thickness is a concern)

Specific Orders

- Application time for heat is as stated in the PCP order; for cold, it is a maximum of 20 to 30 minutes.
- Moist heat/cold compress:
  - With this type of compress, sterile gauze or linens soaked with sterile solution typically are applied over the wound.
  - Cover the area with towels or a waterproof pad to maintain temperature.
- Moist heat/cold soak:
  - Completely submerge the extremity in the solution, which may be medicated if ordered by the PCP.
  - Maintain the temperature of the soak:
    - Cover the solution container and the extremity to minimize temperature change.
    - Check the solution and change it or add to it every 10 minutes, as needed.
    - Thoroughly dry the extremity to prevent tissue breakdown.
- Sitz bath:
  - Soak the pelvic area for 20 minutes.
  - Adjust the temperature according to facility policies and procedures.
  - Use a chair, tub, or toilet attachment (basin). A hose attached to it allows water to spray the pelvic area and gradually fill the basin.
  - Ensure that the patient is able to sit up.

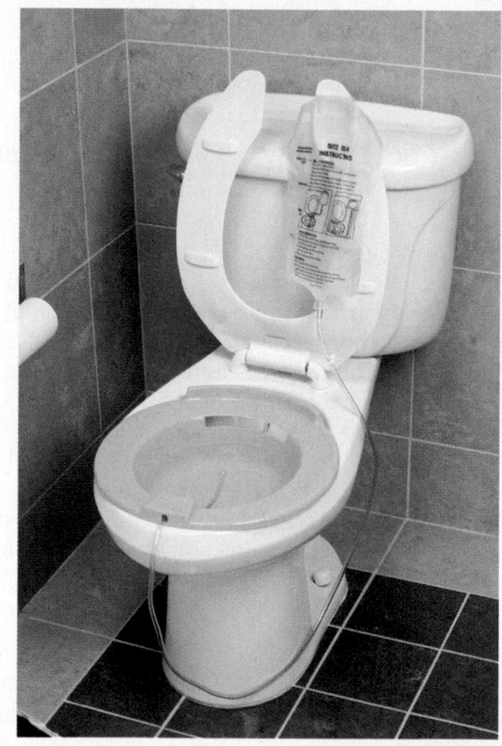

(From Theratherm, Chattanooga, Tenn., a DJO company.)

- Aquathermia (Aqua-K) pads (hot or cold):
  - Each pad contains a control unit that regulates water flow and temperature through the channels in the pad.
  - Use only distilled water.
  - Place a towel between the patient's skin and the pad to prevent burns.
  - Place the pad on top of the area being treated.

NURSING CARE GUIDELINE—cont'd

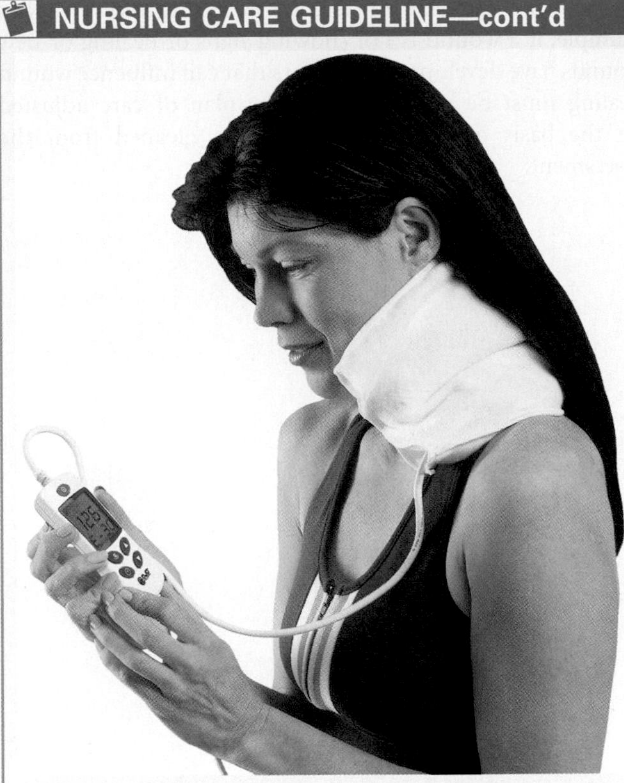

(Courtesy Briggs Healthcare, West Des Moines, Iowa.)

- Commercial hot/cold packs: Follow the manufacturer's instructions.
- Ice bags:
  - Fill with water.
  - Fill only two-thirds full if using crushed ice.
  - Release air from the bag before sealing.

Documentation Concerns

- Document the equipment used and patient assessments.
- Assess and document any signs of infection at the site of application on the patient's skin or in the drainage.
- Note the time of application and application frequency. Document skin assessments throughout treatments.
- Treat and document adverse effects in accordance with facility policy and procedure. Note patient concerns and complaints, as well as interventions. Document patient education.

Evidence-Based Practice

- Heat and cold therapies have been shown to be safe adjuncts, after effective education, for treating and managing pain in pediatric patients (Lane and Latham, 2009).
- Cold applications had a positive impact on postcardiac patients for pain relief from coughing when applied to the sternal incision in the form of a gel pack (Chailler, Ellis, Stolarik, and Woodend, 2010).

The most serious complication that can result from the application of heat or cold arises secondary to the body's loss of its normally protective ability to sense temperature extremes through its adaptation to the change in temperature. With such deficits, after an initial sense of a change in temperature, the body then adapts and, within a short time, no longer senses the temperature as being unusually hot or cold. Damage to tissue, from either temperature extreme, can result. The nurse assesses the patient's age and ability to sense temperature and pain, the integrity of the skin, and the specific area to be treated and its size before applying either heat or cold. Patients who are more at risk for injury are the very young or very old; those with a history of cardiovascular or peripheral vascular disease, peripheral neuropathies, sensory changes, or open wounds; and those in whom a large area of tissue requires treatment. The skin of the neck, the inner aspect of the forearm, and the perineal area are less tolerant of temperature extremes and should be monitored carefully for changes (Patient Education and Health Literacy box).

With both heat and cold therapies, it is important to have the patient report any pain or changes in sensation, to monitor the time that the tissue is exposed to the heat or cold source, to assess the skin before and after treatment, and to follow facility and manufacturer guidelines.

PATIENT EDUCATION AND HEALTH LITERACY

Heat and Cold Therapy

- Use of heat and cold therapies in the home requires patient and family education to maximize patient safety.
- Written instructions, photos, demonstration of the equipment needed, and videos all enhance the use of equipment for providing heat and cold therapies.
- A return demonstration by the patient or family member ensures understanding of the principles of safe use of these therapies.
- Patient education includes coordination with the social worker or the discharge planner to ensure that the teaching accomplished in the health care setting about all of the issues related to skin and wound problems can realistically translate to the home environment.

! SAFE PRACTICE ALERT

Warm compresses and water for soaks should not be heated in the microwave unless the product and microwave are specifically designed for this type of heating. The uneven heating and inability to measure the resultant temperature can result in serious burns to the patient.

EVALUATION

It is essential to evaluate whether the patient has achieved the agreed-on goals. Although this often is considered the last step in the nursing process, it is really an integral part of an ongoing process whereby the effectiveness of interventions is assessed and the plan of care is revised as necessary. For example, if a wound is not showing signs of healing or new wounds have developed, the factors that can influence wound healing must be reassessed and the plan of care adjusted on the basis of the new information gleaned from the assessment.

SKILL 29-1 Irrigating a Wound

PURPOSE

Wound irrigation is used to:
- Clean a wound.
- Apply heat, which promotes healing.
- Apply medication such as antibiotics.
- Remove debris and exudates.
- Remove bacterial colonizations.
- Prevent skin from healing over a deeper wound that must remain open.

RESOURCES

- Solutions (may be warmed):
  - Sterile normal saline solution
  - Lactated Ringer's solution
  - Ordered antibiotic solution
- Irrigation delivery system:
  - Deep wound: 30- to 50-mL piston syringe with an 18-gauge Angiocath
  - Oral waterjet system
  - Sterile catheter
- Sterile irrigation set.
- Personal protective equipment (PPE):
  - Goggles
  - Gown
  - Mask
- Sterile drape
- Sterile gloves
- Sterile gauze pads
- Waterproof pads or towels
- Sterile basin
- Clean emesis basin

COLLABORATION AND DELEGATION

- Irrigating a wound may not be delegated to unlicensed assistive personnel (UAP), but UAP can assist in the following tasks:
  - Transporting specimens
  - Positioning, comfort, and support of the patient
- Collaboration with the following professionals might occur before, during, and after wound irrigation:
  - A wound care nurse specialist:
    - May perform the procedure.
    - Coordinates assessment and timing of this procedure with other procedures.
  - An infection control nurse:
    - Documents any confirmed infection.
    - Places the patient on appropriate isolation precautions.
    - Consults with the primary care provider (PCP) for appropriate actions.
- The PCP provides appropriate orders, which are carried out by the nurse and other personnel.

EVIDENCE-BASED PRACTICE

- The irrigation solution is delivered to the wound bed using a 30- to 50-mL syringe and an 18-gauge catheter. Unlike the 1 pound per square inch (psi) of pressure or less that is delivered by a standard bulb syringe, the use of a 30- to 50-mL syringe and an 18-gauge catheter has been shown to achieve an irrigation force that falls within the recommended 4 to 15 psi (Rodeheaver and Ratcliff, 2007).
- Cleansing a wound with tap water has not been shown to increase infection rates as long as the water is drinkable. Some evidence has shown that tap water has been just as effective as sterile water or normal saline solutions in cleansing wounds. This has important implications for home care and emergency situations, because tap water is much more cost-effective and more readily available than other solutions (Fernandez and Griffiths, 2012).

SPECIAL CIRCUMSTANCES

1. **Assess:** Does the patient have signs of a systemic infection, such as fever and elevated heart rate?
   Intervention: Notify the PCP; obtain orders for cultures; and document.
2. **Assess:** Is the patient in pain?
   Intervention: Determine whether the pain is new or preexisting:
   - Stop the procedure if the pain is a new complaint. Medicate the patient, and wait ½ hour before resuming the procedure.
   - With known discomfort, premedicate the patient ½ hour before the procedure.
   - Notify the PCP, if needed, and document as appropriate.
3. **Assess:** Was there bleeding during the procedure?
   Intervention: Determine whether the bleeding is new or happened previously.
   - Stop the procedure if new bleeding is evident. Assess the wound, and notify the PCP as appropriate.
   - Document.
4. **Assess:** What should be done if there is a bulb syringe in the irrigation kit?
   Intervention: Obtain a piston syringe instead. Only limited control can be achieved with a bulb syringe, and it is not appropriate for wound irrigation.

PREPROCEDURE

I. Check PCP orders and the patient care plan.
Knowledge of patient-specific orders is critical for safe patient care.

II. Gather supplies and equipment.
Preparing for the patient encounter saves time and promotes patient trust.

III. Perform hand hygiene.
Frequent hand hygiene prevents the spread of microorganisms.

IV. Maintain standard precautions.
Use of the correct personal protective equipment (PPE) is required whenever contact with bodily fluids is possible, to reduce the transfer of pathogens.

V. Introduce yourself.
Initial communication establishes the role of the nurse and begins a professional relationship.

VI. Provide for patient privacy.
It is important to maintain patient dignity.

VII. Identify the patient, using two identifiers.
Identifying a patient involves scanning barcodes or comparing the patient's stated name and birthdate to information on the patient's wristband or health record. The correct person must receive the correct treatment.

VIII. Explain the procedure to the patient.
The nurse has a responsibility to inform a patient before initiating care. Information may ease patient anxiety and facilitate cooperation.

PROCEDURE

Wound Irrigation

Follow preprocedure steps I through VIII.

1. Follow the steps in Skill 29-2 under "Positioning/Preparation."
2. Follow the steps in Skill 29-2 under "Removing Old Dressing."
3. Place a waterproof pad and the clean basin beneath the wound.
   Use the pad and basin to protect the bed linens from irrigation fluids.
4. Prepare a sterile field (see Chapter 26, Skill 26-4). There are several variations for this skill:
   a. Be aware that supplies vary depending on the wound type and assessment and on the PCP orders.
   b. Place the sterile solution container on a clean work field. Do *not* touch the inside of the container.
   c. Pour sterile normal saline solution or the PCP-ordered solution into the sterile basin (see step 4 in the *Adding Sterile Supplies to a Sterile Field* section of Skill 26-4).
   d. Drop other sterile items (such as gauze rolls, 2 × 2 pads, 4 × 4 pads, or foam) from their packages onto the sterile field (see step 17 in Skill 26-4).
   e. Put on sterile gloves (see Chapter 26, Skill 26-2).
   The sterile field and proper glove use reduce the number of microorganisms, thereby preventing or reducing further infection. Preparation of the field before the procedure provides organization to facilitate the procedure.
5. Fill the syringe with solution.
   Avoids unnecessary interruption of the procedure once it has begun.
6. Irrigate the wound from the least contaminated area to the most contaminated.
   a. If a syringe is used, keep it 1 inch above the wound.
   b. If a catheter is used, gently insert it until it meets resistance.
   Irrigation should be from the least contaminated to the most contaminated area to prevent the spread of microorganisms from more contaminated areas.

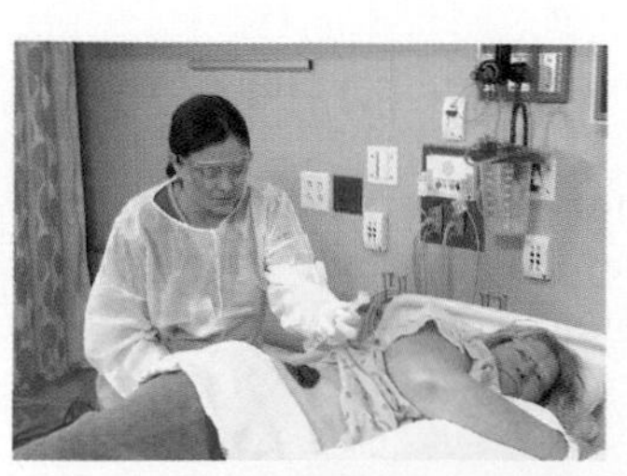

STEP 6

7. If you run out of solution before completing the wound irrigation, pinch the catheter, remove the syringe, refill it with fresh solution, reattach the syringe to the catheter, and continue.
   Maintains sterile procedure.
8. Stop when the solution flow is clear or the ordered amount has been administered.
9. Thoroughly dry the periwound area using sterile gauze and a patting motion; do *not* rub the wound to dry it. Dispose of gauze and waterproof pads in appropriate containers.
   Proper drying prevents further skin breakdown from moisture. Patting (rather than rubbing) prevents healthy tissue from being removed and reduces trauma to the wound.
10. Re-dress the wound (see Skill 29-2 or Skill 29-4.)

Follow postprocedure steps I through VI.

POSTPROCEDURE

I. Return the bed to its lowest position, raise the top side rails, and verify that the call light is within reach of the patient.
   Precautions must be taken to maintain patient safety. Top side rails aid in positioning and turning. Raising four side rails is considered a restraint.

II. Assess for additional patient needs, and state the time of your expected return.
   Meeting patient needs and offering self promote patient satisfaction and build trust.

III. Properly dispose of PPE.
   Gloves, gowns, and masks must be appropriately discarded to prevent the spread of microorganisms.

IV. Clean equipment that was in contact with the patient; see specific manufacturer instructions.
   Disinfection eliminates most microorganisms from inanimate objects.

V. Perform hand hygiene.
   Frequent hand hygiene prevents the spread of infection.

VI. Document the date, time, assessment, procedure, and patient's response to the procedure.
   Accurate documentation is essential to communicate patient care and to provide legal evidence of care.

SKILL 29-2 Changing a Sterile Dressing: Dry, Wet/Damp-to-Dry

PURPOSE

Sterile dressings are required for:
- Preventing infection
- Protecting a wound from injury
- Promoting wound healing

Sterile dressings may be removed to:
- Clean a wound
- Debride unhealthy tissue
- Apply a clean dressing
- Apply a new treatment
- Observe or assess wound healing
- Leave a wound open to the air

RESOURCES

- Sterile normal saline solution
- Goggles
- Gown
- Sterile gloves
- Clean nonsterile gloves
- Waterproof pads or towels
- Sterile basin
- Waterproof trash bag or biohazard bag
- Sterile gauze pads:
  - The size of the gauze depends on the wound size
  - Wet-to-dry dressings also may require a gauze roll
- Large, absorbent outer dressing or abdominal (ABD) pad
- Sterile cotton-tipped applicators
- Sterile forceps
- Tape
- Skin protectant
- Metric ruler
- Acetone-free adhesive remover, if appropriate

COLLABORATION AND DELEGATION

- If allowed by facility policy, simple nonacute wound dressing changes may be delegated to unlicensed assistive personnel (UAP) without a nurse's assistance after assessment of the wound.
- UAP should report the following to the nurse:
  - Patient pain before, during, or after the procedure
  - Difficulties encountered while performing the procedure
- UAP should be instructed in:
  - Appropriate procedure and appropriate time to complete the procedure
  - Appropriate documentation
- Coordinate the procedure with a physical therapist if other wound debridement or stimulation treatments are required (such as whirlpool or electrical stimulation).
- Collaborate with the primary care provider (PCP) or the surgeon, and coordinate the procedure with the physician's rounds if the wound needs to be examined.
- It is important for health care providers at the next level of care to be aware of the wound care treatment plan before patient transfer or discharge to home or another facility. It may be necessary to order supplies and equipment for home or the next facility before discharging the patient from the acute care facility.

EVIDENCE-BASED PRACTICE

- Promoting a moist wound environment has been shown to improve wound healing. In a wet/damp-to-dry dressing, the moistened gauze dries out, adhering to the surface of the wound. When the dressings are removed, debridement of the surface tissues occurs. However, wet/damp-to-dry gauze dressings are not selective, so they may remove healthy tissues, causing further damage to the wound bed. Wet/damp-to-dry dressings may be appropriate for short-term use for debridement; however, other types of debridement should be considered (Snyder, 2008).

SPECIAL CIRCUMSTANCES

1. **Assess:** Is the patient complaining of pain?
   Intervention: Determine whether the pain is new or preexisting.
   - Stop the procedure if the complaint of pain is new.
   - Medicate or premedicate the patient, according to orders.
   - Notify the PCP if no orders exist for wound pain.
2. **Assess:** Does the patient show signs or symptoms of infection?
   Intervention: Consider culturing the wound (see Skill 29-3).
   - Consult with a wound care nurse specialist or the health care team.
   - Notify the PCP.
3. **Assess:** Is the patient knowledgeable about the wound care procedures?
   Intervention: Educate the patient and the patient's family. Include:
   - The purpose of the treatment
   - An explanation of who will be changing the dressings and when
   - The procedure for dressing changes and their frequency
   - The signs and symptoms of infection or other complications, and guidance on when to notify the PCP if they occur
   - The appropriate disposal of soiled dressings
   - Have the patient or caregiver perform a return demonstration.

4. **Assess:** Is assistance required for performing the procedure?
   Intervention: Obtain assistance, if needed, from UAP or through collaboration with the wound care specialist or physical therapist. Consider the following when making this decision:
   - The patient's ability to cooperate
   - The complexity of the required interventions
   - The support systems available
   - The facility policies, procedures, and requirements
5. **Assess:** Is the gauze sticking to the wound as the old dressing is being removed?
   Intervention: Assess the type of dressing involved.
   - If it is a wet/damp-to-dry dressing, do *not* moisten the dressing. Warn the patient of the discomfort, and continue to remove the dressing. The purpose is to debride the wound, so moistening the gauze would defeat this purpose.
   - If it is a dry dressing, moisten the dressing with normal saline solution and gently attempt to remove the gauze; this prevents further trauma to the wound.
6. **Assess:** What is a safe way to dispose of a small dressing?
   Intervention: Fold the dressing inside the gloves as they are removed using the technique described in Skill 26-2.
   - Dispose of the gloves with the dressing in an appropriate trash receptacle.
   - Keeping the dirty dressing inside gloves for disposal further reduces the spread of microorganisms.
7. **Assess:** Is an additional dressing needed on top of the dry dressing?
   - An additional dressing can absorb excess drainage from a wound.
   - An additional dressing can ensure that the dressing is secure.

   Intervention: Place an ABD pad or another dressing material on top of the sterile gauze, and tape it in place.
8. **Assess:** Did bleeding occur during the dressing change?
   Intervention: Observe, monitor, treat, and document as appropriate.
   - The wound may require pressure to stop the bleeding.
   - Notify the PCP if bleeding is excessive.

PREPROCEDURE

I. Check PCP orders and the patient care plan.
Knowledge of patient-specific orders is critical for safe patient care.

II. Gather supplies and equipment.
Preparing for the patient encounter saves time and promotes patient trust.

III. Perform hand hygiene.
Frequent hand hygiene prevents the spread of microorganisms.

IV. Maintain standard precautions.
Use of the correct personal protective equipment (PPE) is required whenever contact with body fluids is possible in order to reduce the transfer of pathogens.

V. Introduce yourself.
Initial communication establishes the role of the nurse and begins a professional relationship.

VI. Provide for patient privacy.
It is important to maintain patient dignity.

VII. Identify the patient, using two identifiers.
Identifying a patient involves scanning barcodes or comparing the patient's stated name and birthdate to information on the patient's wristband or health record. The correct person must receive the correct treatment.

VIII. Explain the procedure to the patient.
The nurse has a responsibility to inform a patient before initiating care. Information may ease patient anxiety and facilitate cooperation.

PROCEDURE

Positioning/Preparation

Follow preprocedure steps I through VIII.

1. Raise the bed to working height and lower the side rails as appropriate and safe.
   Setting the bed at the correct working height prevents provider discomfort and possible injury. Positioning should expose the wound but provide privacy and prevent overexposure.
2. Expose the wound, and position the patient appropriately:
   a. Treatments/solutions should flow from the least infected area to the most infected area.
   b. Towels and a waterproof pad must be under the patient/wound area before beginning the procedure.
   Washing should proceed from the least contaminated to the most contaminated area to prevent the spread of microorganisms, and use of the proper solution should reduce the number of microorganisms and prevent infection. Towels and a pad protect linens and clothing. Preparing supplies in advance avoids interruption during the procedure, promotes organization that facilitates the procedure, prevents patient discomfort due to repositioning, and ensures optimal care and dressing placement.
3. Place a waterproof trash bag or biohazard bag on the bed; fold the top of the bag over to make a cuff that will keep the bag open, and place the bag within reach.
   Proper disposal of waste reduces the spread of microorganisms, protects linens, and provides organization to facilitate the procedure. Preparing supplies in advance avoids interruption of the procedure.

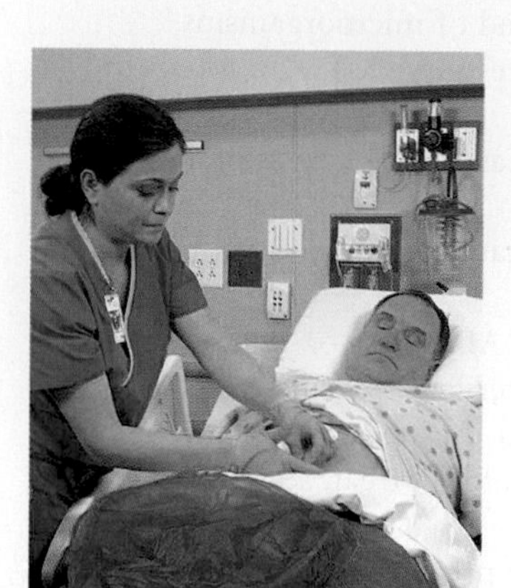
STEP 3

Removing an Old Dressing

Follow preprocedure steps I through VIII.

1. Follow steps 1 to 3 under Positioning/Preparation, above.
2. Apply clean nonsterile gloves.
   Using clean gloves reduces the spread of microorganisms.
3. Remove the old dressing:
   a. Remove the tape by holding the skin taut and pulling the tape toward the dressing.
   b. Gently remove one layer at a time of the gauze/packing/foam while observing the drainage on the dressing for color, quantity, and type.
   c. Dispose of the dressing by folding it in on itself (soiled side of the dressing should be on the inside), and place it in the trash or biohazard bag.
   Careful tape removal reduces irritation of the wound edges. Removing layers of the dressing one at a time reduces the risk of infection and allows assessment of drainage and wound healing. Proper disposal of waste prevents the spread of microorganisms.

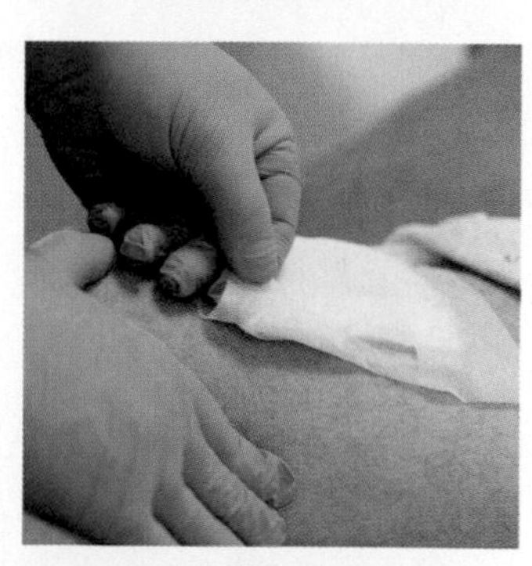
STEP 3a

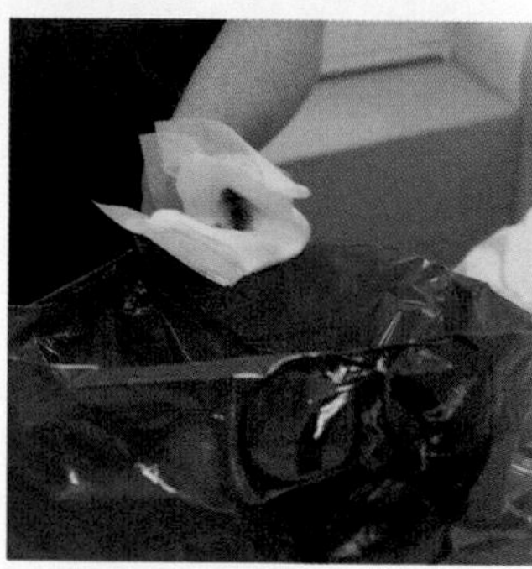
STEP 3c

4. Remove excess adhesive on the patient's skin with an acetone-free adhesive remover.
   Removing excess adhesive, if present, with each dressing change prevents build-up of adhesive, decreases skin irritation, and increases adherence of the new dressing.
5. Assess the wound:
   a. Observe for color, and tissue type in the wound base.
   b. Observe the tissues around the wound.
   c. Measure the wound (see Nursing Care Guideline: Measuring a Wound box).
   d. Observe the drainage characteristics, including the amount visible.
   e. Assess the wound for signs and symptoms of infection.
   The initial assessment provides a baseline that can be used to assist in determining whether the wound is healing, the need for any additional supplies, the best dressing type, and whether any changes are needed in the treatment plan concerning supplies or orders. If signs or symptoms of infection are noted, action taken at this time can prevent further infection and deterioration.
6. Remove the gloves, and dispose of them properly in the trash or biohazard bag. Perform hand hygiene.
   Proper disposal of gloves and hand hygiene prevent the spread of microorganisms.

Follow postprocedure steps I through VI.

Dressing Change: Dry Sterile Dressing

Follow preprocedure steps I through VIII.

1. Follow steps 1 to 6 under "Removing an Old Dressing," above.
2. Prepare a sterile field (see Skill 26-4). Variations for this skill are as follows:
   a. Be aware that supplies vary depending on the type and assessment of the wound and on PCP orders.
   b. The sterile solution container should be placed on a clean work field. Do *not* touch the inside of the container.
   c. Pour sterile normal saline solution into a sterile basin (see step 4 in the Adding Sterile Supplies to a Sterile Field section of Skill 26-4).
   d. Drop other sterile items (such as gauze rolls, 2 × 2 pads, 4 × 4 pads, or foam) from packages onto the sterile field (see step 2 in the Adding Sterile Supplies to a Sterile Field section of Skill 26-4).
   e. Put on sterile gloves (see Skill 26-2).

   Using a sterile field reduces the spread of microorganisms and prevents or reduces further infection. Preparation of the sterile field in advance of the procedure provides organization to facilitate the procedure.
3. Determine whether specific cleansing solutions or medications are indicated to treat the wound:
   a. If specific products were ordered, follow the manufacturer instructions on the proper use of the product. You must comply with the Six Rights of Medication Administration (see Chapter 35, Nursing Care Guideline: Six Rights of Medication Administration box) before proceeding to step 5 below).
   b. If specific products were not ordered, proceed to step 5.

   Cleansing products remove excess drainage, reduce the spread of microorganisms, and prevent adverse events. Medications may be applied to a wound to debride or to prevent infection.
4. Determine whether irrigation of the wound was ordered:
   a. If irrigation was ordered, see Skill 29-1.
   b. If irrigation was not ordered, proceed to step 5.

   Irrigation removes excess drainage and reduces the spread of microorganisms.
5. Clean the wound with sterile normal saline solution:
   a. Depending on the size of the wound, use either a sterile cotton-tipped applicator (for small wounds) or gauze pads (for large wounds; use with sterile forceps, if needed).
   b. Direction of cleaning should progress from the center of the wound toward the edges; cleaning should be performed using full- or half-circle motions.
   c. Use a new applicator or gauze pad for each circle.

   Proper application of sterile saline solution keeps the area of least contamination clean. Using a prescribed pattern ensures that all areas are cleaned. Frequent changes to new applicators or gauze pads will reduce the spread of microorganisms.
6. Clean the area around the wound (periwound area):
   a. Use sterile normal saline solution.
   b. Clean to at least 1 inch beyond the edges of the dressing.

   Cleansing the area with sterile normal saline solution keeps the area clean, prevents infection, and reduces the spread of microorganisms.
7. Thoroughly dry the wound and periwound areas using sterile gauze and a patting motion; do not rub these areas.

   Proper drying prevents further skin breakdown from moisture. Patting, rather than rubbing, prevents healthy tissue from being removed and reduces trauma to the wound.

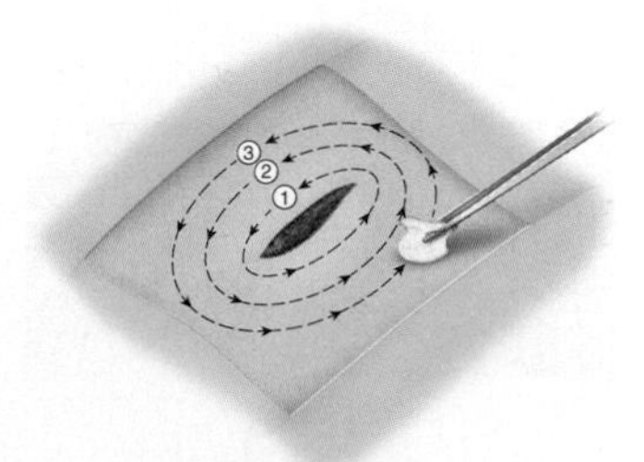

STEP 6

8. Apply the dressing: Use an appropriate-size sterile gauze pad to cover the wound.
   A dressing protects the wound from trauma and exposure to microorganisms.

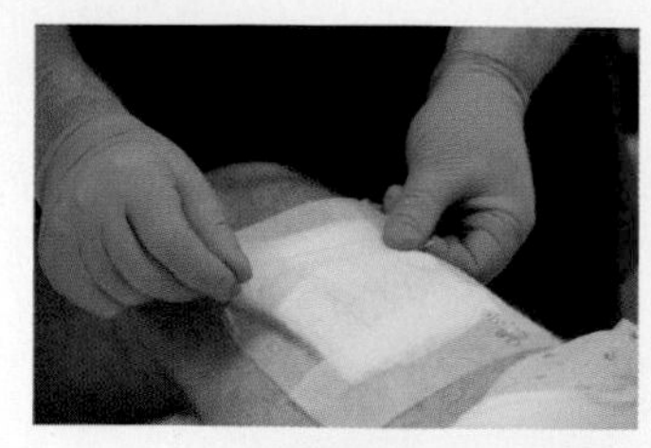
STEP 9

9. Secure the dressing with the least amount of tape needed.
   Removal of tape can cause skin damage; using less decreases the likelihood of tears when removing the tape.
10. Remove gloves, and dispose of them properly in the trash or biohazard bag. Perform hand hygiene.
    Proper disposal of waste and hand hygiene reduce the spread of microorganisms.

Follow postprocedure steps I through VI.

Dressing Change: Wet/Damp-to-Dry Dressing

Follow preprocedure steps I through VIII.

1. Follow steps 1 to 6 under "Dressing Change: Dry Sterile Dressing," above.
2. Thoroughly dry the periwound area; pat the wound dry with sterile gauze (do not rub the wound); and apply skin protectant.
   Dry the wound to prevent further skin breakdown from moisture and protect healthy tissue. Patting the wound and using a skin protectant prevents trauma to the skin and wound edges.
3. Prepare packing gauze:
   a. Use the ordered solution and packing material, or use sterile normal saline solution and gauze.
   b. Saturate the sterile gauze.
   c. Squeeze excess solution from the gauze.
   d. Open the gauze pads, or unravel the gauze rolls.
   e. "Fluff" the gauze by separating the layers.
   Wet/damp-to-dry dressings should not be dripping wet; they should be moist. Squeezing out excess moisture ensures that gauze is completely dry at the next dressing change. Proper preparation of the packing allows the gauze to absorb drainage.

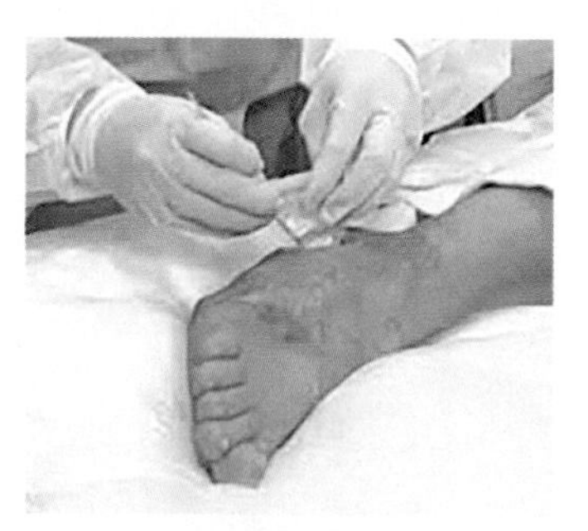
STEP 4a

4. Pack the wound:
   a. Pack the gauze gently and loosely into the wound to fill it.
   b. Use sterile forceps to insert the packing in most wounds.
   c. Use a sterile cotton-tipped applicator to insert the gauze or gauze strip if the wound is tunneled.
   d. Do not allow gauze to cover the wound edges.
   e. Use sterile scissors to cut the gauze roll, if used.
   Packing too tightly increases pressure on the wound, leading to wound damage. Loose packing allows the wound drainage to soak into the gauze or wick. Using forceps or an applicator reduces the spread of microorganisms. Avoiding moist gauze on healthy tissue prevents further skin breakdown from moisture.
5. Apply the primary dressing:
   a. Use an appropriate size of sterile gauze.
   b. Cover the wound.
   A dressing protects the wound from trauma and exposure to microorganisms.

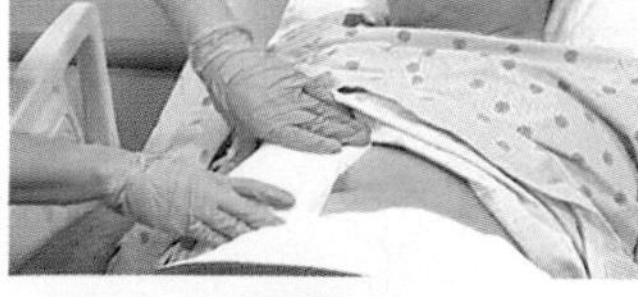
STEP 6

6. Apply a large, absorbent secondary dressing or ABD pad over the gauze.
   A second layer of absorbent dressing absorbs excess drainage, promotes more secure dressing, and better protects the wound.
7. Secure all sides of the dressing with tape.
8. Remove gloves, and dispose of them properly in the trash or biohazard bag. Perform hand hygiene.
   Proper disposal of waste and hand hygiene reduce the spread of microorganisms.

Follow postprocedure steps I through VI.

POSTPROCEDURE

I. Return the bed to its lowest position, raise the top side rails, and verify that the call light is within reach of the patient.
Precautions must be taken to maintain patient safety. Top side rails aid in positioning and turning. Raising four side rails is considered a restraint.

II. Assess for additional patient needs, and state the time of your expected return.
Meeting patient needs and offering self promote patient satisfaction and build trust.

III. Properly dispose of PPE.
Gloves, gowns, and masks must be appropriately discarded to prevent the spread of microorganisms.

IV. Clean equipment that was in contact with the patient; see specific manufacturer instructions.
Disinfection eliminates most microorganisms from inanimate objects.

V. Perform hand hygiene.
Frequent hand hygiene prevents the spread of infection.

VI. Document the date, time, assessment, procedure, and patient's response to the procedure.
Accurate documentation is essential to communicate patient care and to provide legal evidence of care.

SKILL 29-3 Obtaining a Wound Culture Specimen

PURPOSE

Wound cultures are performed to:
- Determine whether infection exists
- Determine appropriate treatment for infection (by testing the sensitivity of the cultures to various medications)
- Evaluate the effectiveness of treatment for infection

RESOURCES

- Sterile culturette swabs
- Waterproof trash bags
- Patient labels
- Laboratory requisitions
- Clean or sterile gloves, depending on the wound
- Sterile normal saline solution
- Irrigation syringe
- Personal protective equipment, as needed

COLLABORATION AND DELEGATION

- Collecting a wound culture may not be delegated to unlicensed assistive personnel (UAP), but UAP can assist in the following tasks:
  - Transporting specimens
  - Patient positioning, comfort, and support
- Collaboration with the following professionals might occur before, during, and after collection of a wound culture:
  - A wound care nurse specialist:
    - May note signs or symptoms of infection
    - May note improvement or deterioration of the wound
    - May request or collect a culture
    - Must ensure that appropriate cultures are obtained
  - An infection control nurse:
    - Documents any confirmed infection
    - Places the patient on appropriate isolation precautions
    - Consults with the PCP for appropriate actions
  - The PCP:
    - Provides appropriate orders, which are carried out by the nurse and other personnel
    - Consults with the nurse for any changes in medications based on the results of the culture

EVIDENCE-BASED PRACTICE

- Many health care providers are not educated regarding the proper techniques of collecting swab cultures of a wound, which is the specimen type that gives the least accurate results of wound culture (the gold standard is a tissue biopsy). It is imperative that nurses follow the facility's guidelines, based on standardized protocols, to collect a wound culture specimen via swab. This prevents unnecessary testing and/or treatment (Bonham, 2009).
- In addition to understanding the assessment of signs and symptoms of localized and systemic infection, the nurse must recognize that patients with chronic wounds may not exhibit these clinical manifestations. The nurse needs to assess for foul-smelling drainage and pus, delayed healing, and increased wound breakdown; increased localized pain, warmth, redness, and swelling; and granulation tissue discoloration (Ayello, Baranoski, and Salati, 2006).

SPECIAL CIRCUMSTANCES

1. **Assess:** Is the patient complaining of pain?
   Intervention: If the patient has pain at the wound site:
   - Medicate the patient 30 minutes before the procedure.
   - Document the pain assessment and intervention.

PREPROCEDURE

I. Check PCP orders and the patient care plan.
Knowledge of patient-specific orders is critical for safe patient care.

II. Gather supplies and equipment.
Preparing for the patient encounter saves time and promotes patient trust.

III. Perform hand hygiene.
Frequent hand hygiene prevents the spread of microorganisms.

IV. Maintain standard precautions.
Use of the correct personal protective equipment (PPE) is required whenever contact with bodily fluids is possible in order to reduce the transfer of pathogens.

V. Introduce yourself.
Initial communication establishes the role of the nurse and begins a professional relationship.

VI. Provide for patient privacy.
It is important to maintain patient dignity.

VII. Identify the patient, using two identifiers.
Identifying a patient involves scanning barcodes or comparing the patient's stated name and birthdate to information on the patient's wristband or health record. The correct person must receive the correct treatment.

VIII. Explain the procedure to the patient.
The nurse has a responsibility to inform a patient before initiating care. Information may ease patient anxiety and facilitate cooperation.

PROCEDURE

Aerobic Culture: Swab

Aerobic means "needing or giving oxygen"; an aerobic culture would be available from a surface wound.

Follow preprocedure steps I through VIII.

1. Remove the dressing (see Skill 29-2).
2. Cleanse or irrigate the wound (see Skill 29-1):
   a. Use only sterile normal saline solution.
   b. Ensure that exudates (drainage) are removed.
   Irrigation removes noninfectious microorganisms (normal flora), as well as potentially infectious microorganisms; the exudate is considered contaminated because it contains microorganisms, whether they are infectious or not.
3. Collect the wound drainage sample:
   a. Open the aerobic swab collection tube, while ensuring that the swab does not touch anything.
   b. Apply clean gloves.
   c. Moisten the swab with sterile normal saline solution.
   d. Insert the swab into actively draining tissue, *not* into necrotic tissue.
   e. Cover the swab with drainage material by rotating the swab and applying pressure.
   f. Reinsert the swab in the culturette tube making sure nothing touches the swab as it is replaced into the tube.
   g. Secure the tubing top.
   Using clean gloves prevents the spread of microorganisms and protects the provider from infection. Sterile gloves are used for irrigation and for sterile dressing changes and would be used to obtain a culture specimen only if the nurse needed to touch the wound area to obtain the culture. Proper preparation of the swab prevents contamination of the specimen, and covering the swab with exudate ensures the accuracy of the test by providing a sufficient quantity of sample for testing. Applying pressure produces wound fluid for sampling.

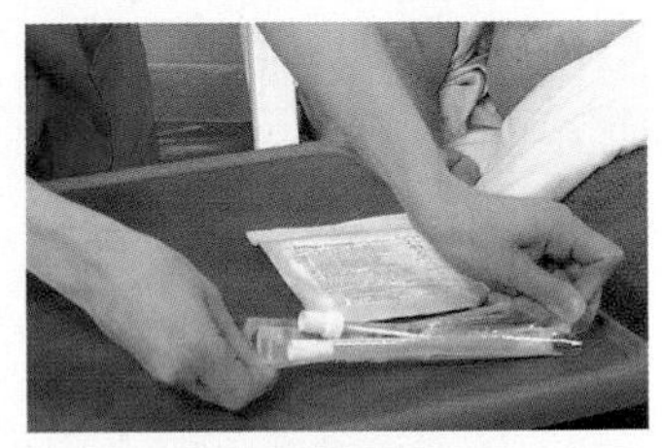
STEP 3a

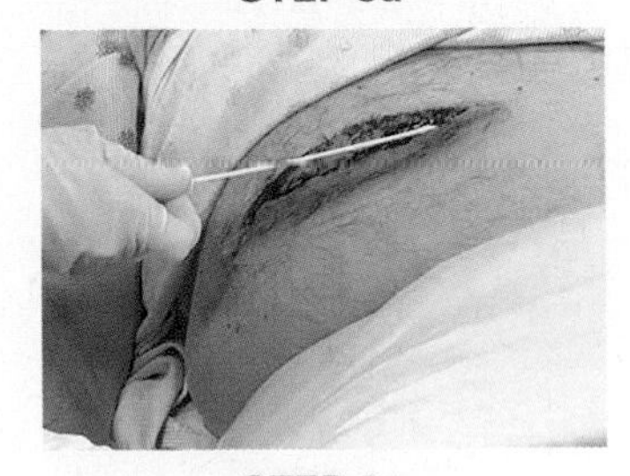
STEP 3e

4. Crush an ampule of the collection medium within the culturette tube if required by the manufacturer's instructions.
   The ampule contains a chemical to preserve the specimen; such a medium is provided with most culture tubes.
5. Label the tube in accordance with facility policy and procedure; include the specific site from which the culture was drawn.
   Proper labeling of samples prevents adverse events and medical errors.
6. Re-dress the wound (see Skill 29-2, or Skill 29-4).
7. Place the tube in the resealable plastic bag or an appropriate transportation container.
   Proper transport of specimens reduces the spread of microorganisms and protects providers from possible infections.
8. Transport the specimen to the laboratory.
   Many tests are time- or temperature-sensitive, so avoid unnecessary delays.

Follow postprocedure steps I through VI.

Anaerobic Culture: Swab

Follow preprocedure steps I through VIII.

1. Follow steps 1 through 3e under "Aerobic Culture: Swab," above. Ensure that the special anaerobic culture swab is used.
   Anaerobic *means "without oxygen"; an anaerobic culture would be obtained from locations such as deep within a tunneling wound.*
2. Quickly remove the swab from the wound, and place it in the culturette tube.
   Minimize exposure of the sample to the air to ensure accurate results.
3. Label the tube in accordance with facility policy and procedure; include the specific site from which the culture was drawn.
   Proper labeling of samples prevents adverse events and medical errors.
4. Place the tube in the resealable plastic bag or an appropriate transportation container, and transport it immediately to the laboratory.
   Proper transport of specimens reduces the spread of microorganisms. Many tests are time- or temperature-sensitive, so avoid unnecessary delays.
5. Re-dress the wound (see Skill 29-2, or Skill 29-4.)

Follow postprocedure steps I through VI.

POSTPROCEDURE

I. Return the bed to its lowest position, raise the top side rails, and verify that the call light is within reach of the patient.
   Precautions must be taken to maintain patient safety. Top side rails aid in positioning and turning. Raising four side rails is considered a restraint.

II. Assess for additional patient needs, and state the time of your expected return.
   Meeting patient needs and offering self promote patient satisfaction and build trust.

III. Properly dispose of PPE.
   Gloves, gowns, and masks must be appropriately discarded to prevent the spread of microorganisms.

IV. Clean equipment that was in contact with the patient; see specific manufacturer instructions.
   Disinfection eliminates most microorganisms from inanimate objects.

V. Perform hand hygiene.
   Frequent hand hygiene prevents the spread of infection.

VI. Document the date, time, assessment, procedure, and patient's response to the procedure.
   Accurate documentation is essential to communicate patient care and to provide legal evidence of care.

SKILL 29-4 Negative-Pressure Wound Therapy, or Vacuum-Assisted Closure

PURPOSE

Negative-pressure wound therapy (NPWT):
- Promotes wound healing
- Provides a moist wound-healing environment
- Assists in development of granulation tissue
- Removes excess fluid
- Removes infectious materials

RESOURCES

- Vacuum unit
- Evacuation canister
- Suction tubing
- Foam dressing
- Transparent occlusive dressing
- Sterile irrigation solution
- Normal saline solution
- Irrigation syringe
- Sterile scissors
- Sterile gloves
- Clean gloves
- Goggles
- Gown
- Waterproof pads or towels
- Waterproof trash bag or biohazard bag
- Skin protectant

COLLABORATION AND DELEGATION

- The system setup for NPWT dressing changes and vacuum-assisted closure (VAC) therapy cannot be delegated to unlicensed assistive personnel (UAP). UAP may gather supplies and assist by handing the nurse supplies during dressing changes. UAP may assist with patient comfort, support, and positioning during and after the procedure at the nurse's discretion.
- UAP should report any of the following:
  - Fever or a change in vital signs
  - Mechanical problems with the VAC unit
  - Loose dressings or alterations in the dressing
  - Patient pain, discomfort, complaints, or concerns
- UAP should be instructed in appropriate:
  - Hygienic care for patients on VAC therapy
  - Equipment usage
  - Documentation
- Collaborate with the wound care specialist who may be responsible for dressing and system changes:
  - Check the primary care provider (PCP) orders to make sure that correct supplies are readily available
  - Ensure that the vacuum setting matches the PCP order
  - Ensure that the vacuum is not disconnected for longer than 2 hours a day
- Coordinate dressing changes with PCP or surgeon rounds if possible. The PCP or the surgeon may want to assess the wound bed when the dressing is removed.
- It is important for health care providers at the next level of care to be aware of the wound care treatment plan. It may be necessary to order supplies and equipment for the patient to take home or for the next facility before discharging the patient from the acute care facility.

EVIDENCE-BASED PRACTICE

- Vacuum-assisted closure (VAC) therapy is used for acute and traumatic wounds, dehiscent wounds, partial-thickness burns, pressure ulcers, and chronic open wounds, such as diabetic ulcers, meshed grafts, and skin flaps. Localized subatmospheric pressure draws wound edges toward the center of the wound, leading to reduced edema and bacterial colonization and promotion of granulation tissue formation in the wound (Andros, Armstrong, Attinger, et al, 2006).
- VAC can be beneficial to both the nurse and the patient. For the nurse, VAC therapy requires fewer dressing changes. For the patient, VAC therapy has been shown to speed healing time, decrease expenses in terms of supplies and care, and shorten hospital stays (Speding, 2008).

SPECIAL CIRCUMSTANCES

1. **Assess:** Are there any contraindications to VAC therapy?
   Intervention:
   - Do *not* proceed with therapy; contact the PCP for:
     - Wound tunneling (fistulas) that involve organs or body cavities
     - Necrotic tissue covered with eschar
     - Untreated infection of the bone (osteomyelitis)
     - Malignant wounds
     - Wounds with exposed arteries and veins
   - Use VAC cautiously in patients who:
     - Have active bleeding
     - Are on anticoagulant therapy
     - Have wounds with recurrent bleeding problems
2. **Assess:** Is the patient experiencing pain?
   Intervention: Determine whether the pain is new or preexisting:
   - Nonpainful stinging is common on the initiation of therapy.
   - Stop the procedure if the pain is a new complaint.
   - Medicate or premedicate the patient, according to orders.
   - Notify the PCP if specific orders to address patient pain are lacking.
3. **Assess:** Does the patient show any signs or symptoms of infection?

Intervention: Contact the PCP for signs and symptoms of local or systemic infection.

4. **Assess:** Does the patient have knowledge of the VAC treatment modality?
   Intervention: Educate the patient and family regarding the following:
   - Purpose of treatment
   - Who will be changing the dressings and when
   - Not to change vacuum settings
   - Not to remove the dressing unless directed
   - Not to disconnect the vacuum for longer than 2 hours a day
   - How to troubleshoot alarms
5. **Assess:** Are the canister and vacuum system functioning appropriately?
   Intervention: Educate the patient on appropriate inspection and safety techniques.
6. **Assess:** Do the normal routines require modifications?
   Intervention: Educate the patient on:
   - How to disconnect and reconnect the system for showering and bathing
   - How to monitor tubing, canister, and plug placement to minimize the risk of falls
   - How to appropriately dispose of soiled dressings
7. **Assess:** Is an alarm sounding during treatment with a VAC?
   Intervention: Troubleshoot the most common problems:
   - The canister has tipped more than 45 degrees.
   - The canister has been dislodged.
   - The canister is full, requiring change.
   - There is an air leak in the dressing.

PREPROCEDURE

I. Check PCP orders and the patient care plan.
Knowledge of patient-specific orders is critical for safe patient care.

II. Gather supplies and equipment.
Preparing for the patient encounter saves time and promotes patient trust.

III. Perform hand hygiene.
Frequent hand hygiene prevents the spread of microorganisms.

IV. Maintain standard precautions.
Use of the correct personal protective equipment (PPE) is required whenever contact with bodily fluids is possible in order to reduce the transfer of pathogens.

V. Introduce yourself.
Initial communication establishes the role of the nurse and begins a professional relationship

VI. Provide for patient privacy.
It is important to maintain patient dignity.

VII. Identify the patient, using two identifiers.
Identifying a patient involves scanning barcodes or comparing the patient's stated name and birthdate to information on the patient's wristband or health record. The correct person must receive the correct treatment.

VIII. Explain the procedure to the patient.
The nurse has a responsibility to inform a patient before initiating care. Information may ease patient anxiety and facilitate cooperation.

PROCEDURE

VAC Device Preparation

Follow preprocedure steps I through VIII.

1. Assemble a VAC device at the patient's bedside, following the manufacturer instructions.
   The VAC setup varies according to different manufacturer specifications.
2. Set the negative-pressure setting according to the PCP order (usually 25 to 200 mm Hg).
   Having the caregiver set the machine ensures compliance with the PCP order. The VAC setting range promotes optimal, safe, high-quality patient care and prevents inadvertent errors.
3. Warm the irrigating solution to 90° to 95°F (32° to 35° C).
   Use a temperature range that promotes patient comfort and prevents tissue damage.
4. Proceed to "VAC Dressing Change," next.

VAC Dressing Change

1. Refer to Skill 29-2, and follow steps 1 through 6 under "Dressing Change: Dry Sterile Dressing."
2. Thoroughly pat the wound dry with sterile gauze, dry the periwound area, and apply skin protectant.
   Proper drying prevents further skin breakdown from moisture. Patting (rather than rubbing) prevents healthy tissue from being removed and reduces trauma to the wound.
3. Prepare the foam: Use sterile scissors to cut the appropriate type and size of foam material. More than one piece may be required.
   Maintain sterile procedure to prevent the spread of microorganisms and reduce infection. Foam comes in a variety of types and shapes; the appropriate size depends on the size of the wound and treatment goals.
4. Place the foam in the wound.
   Foam placement prepares the wound for a VAC dressing.
5. Place the transparent occlusive dressing over the foam, also covering 2 inches of intact skin around the wound. If the dressing supplied does not have a hole in the center, cut a hole with sterile scissors.
   A proper seal is required to ensure that negative pressure is established.
6. Place the suction tubing in the center of the hole. *Note*: Tubing should not touch the wound bed. Place a second transparent dressing over the tubing and first dressing.
   The suction tubing provides negative pressure to the wound, so it must be positioned properly.
7. Connect the other end of the suction tubing to the evacuation canister.
   Once all tubing is in place, the system setup is complete.

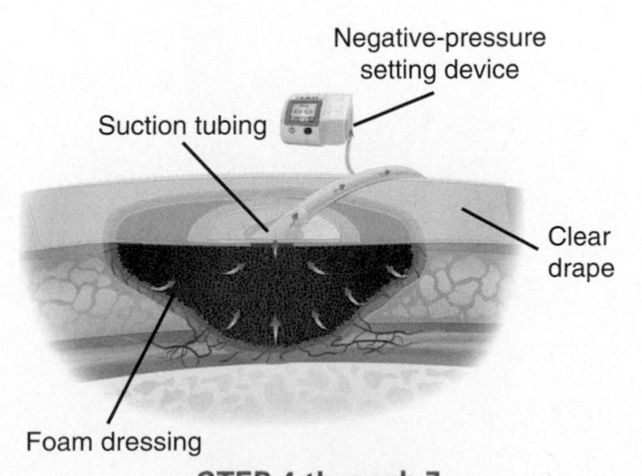

STEP 4 through 7

(Courtesy KCI, an Acelity Company. Used with permission.)

8. Remove gloves, and dispose of them properly in the trash or biohazard bag; perform hand hygiene.
   Proper disposal of waste and frequent hand washing reduce the spread of microorganisms.
9. Turn on the vacuum unit to start the negative pressure; the transparent dressing should shrink and conform to the foam and skin.
   Therapy begins once negative pressure is established. Shrinkage and conformation of the dressing to the foam and skin ensure a proper seal with no air leaks.
10. Maintain the unit by:
    a. Measuring the drainage amount every shift
    b. Changing the canister once a week or more frequently if it is full (follow facility policies and procedures)
    c. Changing the dressing every 48 to 72 hours
    Proper equipment maintenance provides optimal, safe, quality patient care.

Follow postprocedure steps I through VI.

POSTPROCEDURE

I. Return the bed to its lowest position, raise the top side rails, and verify that the call light is within reach of the patient.
   Precautions must be taken to maintain patient safety. Top side rails aid in positioning and turning. Raising four side rails is considered a restraint.
II. Assess for additional patient needs, and state the time of your expected return.
   Meeting patient needs and offering self promote patient satisfaction and build trust.
III. Properly dispose of PPE.
   Gloves, gowns, and masks must be appropriately discarded to prevent the spread of microorganisms.
IV. Clean equipment that was in contact with the patient; see specific manufacturer instructions.
   Disinfection eliminates most microorganisms from inanimate objects.
V. Perform hand hygiene.
   Frequent hand hygiene prevents the spread of infection.
VI. Document the date, time, assessment, procedure, and patient's response to the procedure.
   Accurate documentation is essential to communicate patient care and to provide legal evidence of care.

SKILL 29-5 Applying Wraps and Bandages

PURPOSE

The use of wraps, bandages, and binders:

- Promotes independence
- Secures dressings
- Promotes safety
- Decreases the risk of contamination
- Decreases the risk of further injury

RESOURCES

- Appropriate-size wrap, bandage, or binder, as prescribed
- Tape measure
- Clean gloves
- Goggles
- Gown
- Mask
- Tape, pins, or self-closure devices (avoid metal clips)
- Gauze pads

COLLABORATION AND DELEGATION

- Application of wraps, bandages, or binders may be delegated to unlicensed assistive personnel (UAP) without a nurse's assistance after assessment of the patient and any existing wounds, if allowed by facility policy and at the nurse's discretion.
- UAP should report any of the following:
  - Pain before, during, or after the procedure
  - Staining of underlying dressings
  - Difficulties in performing the procedure
- UAP should be instructed in:
  - Appropriate procedure and timing
  - Appropriate documentation
- Collaboration with the following professionals might occur before, during, and after the application:
  - A wound care nurse specialist:
    - May perform the procedure
    - Coordinates assessment and timing with other procedures
  - An infection control nurse:
    - Documents any confirmed infection
    - Places the patient on appropriate isolation precautions
    - Consults with the primary care provider (PCP) for appropriate actions
  - Coordinate the procedure with a physical therapist if other wound debridement or stimulation treatments, such as whirlpool or e-stimulation, are required.
  - Collaborate with the PCP or the surgeon and coordinate the procedure with the physician's rounds if the wound needs to be examined.
- It is important for health care providers at the next level of care to be aware of the wound care treatment plan. It may be necessary to order supplies and equipment for the patient to take home or for the next facility before the patient is discharged from the acute care facility.

EVIDENCE-BASED PRACTICE

- Wraps, bandages, and binders apply gentle, evenly distributed compression on a body part. Benefits include promoting venous return, decreasing blood pooling in lower extremities, increasing hemostatic pressure, and maintaining dressing placement.
- Patient compliance with bandages and wraps can be an issue that delays healing and well-being. The nurse needs to be aware of issues that promote noncompliance, such as pain, cost, discomfort related to heat or movement, and the patient's belief that the appliances do not help with underlying pathophysiology. The use of bandages and wraps is a proven best practice, and expertise in this modality will help the nurse provide effective patient education and encouragement. A wound care specialist may be of assistance (Annells, O'Neill, and Flowers, 2008).

SPECIAL CIRCUMSTANCES

1. **Assess:** Is the patient experiencing pain?
   Intervention: Determine whether the pain is new or preexisting:
   - Stop the procedure if the pain is a new complaint.
   - Medicate or premedicate the patient, according to orders.
   - Notify the PCP if no orders exist to address patient pain.
2. **Assess:** Are there signs or symptoms of infection or overcompression?
   Intervention: Immediately remove any wrap, bandage, or binder.
   - Contact the PCP if there are signs and symptoms of local or systemic infection or any other complication.
   - Perform complete circulation checks of the distal portion of the affected limb to ensure presence of adequate circulation.
   - Never wrap the toes unless it is absolutely necessary.
3. **Assess:** Is the patient knowledgeable about wound care procedures?
   Intervention: Educate the patient and the family. Include:
   - The purpose of the treatment
   - An explanation of who will be changing the dressings and when
   - The procedure and frequency of dressing changes

- Signs and symptoms of infection or other complications (and when to notify the PCP if they occur)
- The cleaning, care, storage, and appropriate disposal of wraps, bandages, and binders

4. **Assess:** Is assistance required for performing the procedure?
Intervention: Obtain assistance, if needed, from UAP or through collaboration with the wound care specialist or physical therapist. Consider the following when making this decision:
   - Identify the patient's ability to cooperate.
   - Determine the complexity of the required medical interventions.
   - Determine the support systems available.
   - Follow the facility's policies, procedures, and requirements.

PREPROCEDURE

I. Check PCP orders and the patient care plan.
Knowledge of patient-specific orders is critical for safe patient care.

II. Gather supplies and equipment.
Preparing for the patient encounter saves time and promotes patient trust.

III. Perform hand hygiene.
Frequent hand hygiene prevents the spread of microorganisms.

IV. Maintain standard precautions.
Use of the correct personal protective equipment (PPE) is required whenever contact with bodily fluids is possible in order to reduce the transfer of pathogens.

V. Introduce yourself.
Initial communication establishes the role of the nurse and begins a professional relationship.

VI. Provide for patient privacy.
It is important to maintain patient dignity.

VII. Identify the patient, using two identifiers.
Identifying a patient involves scanning barcodes or comparing the patient's stated name and birthdate to information on the patient's wristband or health record. The correct person must receive the correct treatment.

VIII. Explain the procedure to the patient.
The nurse has a responsibility to inform a patient before initiating care. Information may ease patient anxiety and facilitate cooperation.

PROCEDURE

Wraps and Bandages

Follow preprocedure steps I through VIII.

1. Use a wrap or bandage that is an appropriate size for the body part—for example, narrower widths for the lower leg and wider widths for the upper leg.
Using the correct-size wrap or bandage promotes the appropriate distribution of pressure.
2. Ensure that the wrap or bandage is clean and rolled.
Cleanliness decreases the spread of microorganisms. Using a rolled wrap or bandage facilitates easy application.
3. Raise the bed to working height, and lower the side rails as appropriate and safe.
Setting the bed at the correct working height for the provider prevents discomfort and possible injury.

4. Expose the wound appropriately while maintaining the limb in a functional position. Ensure that the extremity is elevated for 15 to 30 minutes before applying the wrap or bandage.
Prepares the wound and limb to facilitate the procedure and prevent interruption of the procedure; prevents patient discomfort by avoiding repositioning. Proper limb position prevents complications. Elevation promotes venous return and reduces edema.
5. Assess the area to be wrapped or bandaged:
   a. If a wound is noted, assess the wound (see Skill 29-2, step 5 under "Removing an Old Dressing").
   b. Assess for signs and symptoms of infection.
   c. Note any other skin lesion or abnormality.
   d. Check circulation.
   e. Apply a sterile dressing over the wound, if applicable (see Skill 29-2).
The initial assessment provides a baseline that can be used to assist in determining the progress of wound healing, the need for any additional supplies, and the best dressing type, as well as whether any changes are needed in the treatment plan concerning supplies or orders. Early detection and treatment of infection and lesions prevents further infection and deterioration and prevents injury.
6. Place gauze or cotton between the skin surfaces of toes and fingers.
Padding between the digits prevents injury and pressure ulcers.
7. Apply the wrap:
   a. Begin at the distal portion of the limb, and wrap around the limb twice.
   b. Wrap up the limb from distal to proximal.
   c. Directions of wrappings are spiral or reverse spiral for extremities, figure eight for joints, or recurrent wrap for the head or an amputated limb.

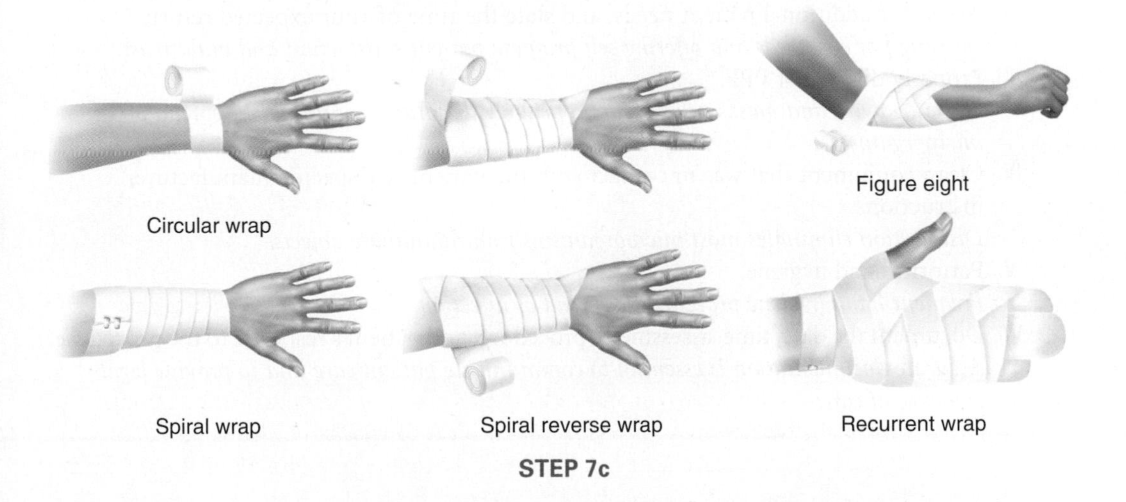

STEP 7c

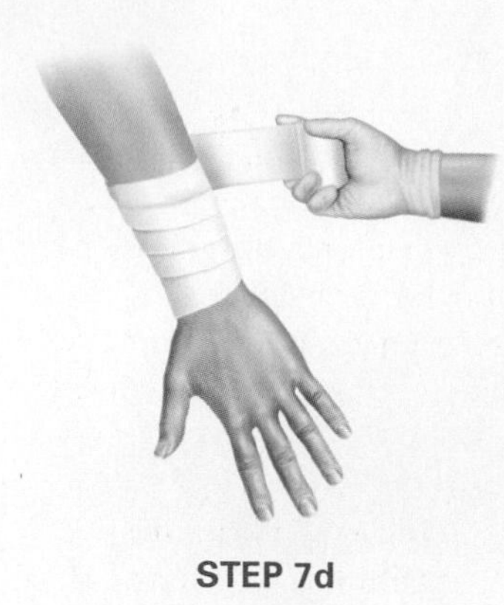

STEP 7d

d. Overlap each wrap by half of the bandage.
A double circular wrap anchors the bandage. Proper wrapping promotes venous return and even compression.

8. Secure the wrap or bandage; ensure safety when applying tape, pins, or self-closure devices.
Securing the wrap maintains compression and anchors the bandage or wrap.

9. Elevate the extremity for 15 to 30 minutes.
Elevation promotes venous return and reduces edema.

10. Assess circulation:
a. Check the distal pulses.
b. Check for tingling, numbness, pain, and itching.
c. Loosen the bandage or wrap if a circulation problem is noted.
Assessing circulation prevents injury or other adverse events and promotes optimal, safe, quality patient care.

11. Maintain the bandage or wrap:
a. Remove every 8 hours.
b. Use a clean bandage or wrap daily or as needed (e.g., if it is soiled).
Removing the bandage or wrap facilitates skin assessment and skin care, allows maintenance of adequate compression, and prevents infection.

Follow postprocedure steps I through VI.

POSTPROCEDURE

I. Return the bed to its lowest position, raise the top side rails, and verify that the call light is within reach of the patient.
Precautions must be taken to maintain patient safety. Top side rails aid in positioning and turning. Raising four side rails is considered a restraint.

II. Assess for additional patient needs, and state the time of your expected return.
Meeting patient needs and offering self promote patient satisfaction and build trust.

III. Properly dispose of PPE.
Gloves, gowns, and masks must be appropriately discarded to prevent the spread of microorganisms.

IV. Clean equipment that was in contact with the patient; see specific manufacturer instructions.
Disinfection eliminates most microorganisms from inanimate objects.

V. Perform hand hygiene.
Frequent hand hygiene prevents the spread of infection.

VI. Document the date, time, assessment, procedure, and patient's response to the procedure.
Accurate documentation is essential to communicate patient care and to provide legal evidence of care.

SUMMARY OF LEARNING OUTCOMES

LO 29.1 *Describe the normal structure and function of skin:* The skin is composed of the epidermis, dermis, and subcutaneous layers, each of which has its own role.

LO 29.2 *Review the factors that alter the skin's structure and function:* The functionality of the skin is affected by other disease processes, nutrition, the use of medications, external forces such as pressure and shear, and aging. Alterations of skin integrity and complications of wound healing can occur as a consequence of many of these factors.

LO 29.3 *Discuss the components of a focused skin and wound assessment, including the use of risk assessment tools:* A focused skin and wound assessment includes an assessment of the overall integrity of the skin and risk factors for impaired skin integrity, as well as an assessment of the wound's location, size, and tissue type; the condition of the periwound skin; the presence of drainage, undermining, and tracts; and the patient's response to wound assessment and care. Risk assessment tools include the Braden Scale and Norton Scale.

LO 29.4 *Identify appropriate nursing diagnoses for the patient with impaired skin integrity:* Many nursing diagnoses are applicable for patients who have wounds or who are at risk for developing or incurring wounds. A determination of appropriate diagnoses must be based on a thorough assessment of the patient.

LO 29.5 *Develop measurable patient-centered goals for patients with impaired skin integrity:* Goals are developed in collaboration with the patient and other health care providers to prevent development of wounds or promote wound healing, and they include measurable evaluation criteria and a time frame for completion.

LO 29.6 *Select interventions to prevent and treat impaired skin integrity:* Interventions include those aimed at prevention (such as turning, pressure relief, nutritional support, and attention to moisture, friction, and shear) and those designed to promote wound healing (e.g., a variety of treatments and dressings).

Responses to the critical-thinking exercises are available at *http://evolve.elsevier.com/YoostCrawford/fundamentals/.*

REVIEW QUESTIONS

1. On initial assessment of a patient, the nurse notices an area of redness over the right trochanter that, when pressed lightly, does not blanch. What does this assessment finding indicate to the nurse?
   a. The presence of an infection in the area
   b. The presence of a stage I pressure ulcer
   c. An allergic reaction to the sheets
   d. The need to apply a cold compress to reduce inflammation
2. Four days after abdominal surgery, the patient is getting out of bed and feels something "pop" in his abdominal wound. An increase in amount of drainage from the wound is seen, and further examination shows that the sutured incision is now partially open, with tissue protruding from the wound. What is the nurse's next action?
   a. Apply Steri-Strips to close the wound edges.
   b. Cover the wound with saline-moistened gauze, and notify the physician.
   c. Assure the patient that this is common, and document the findings.
   d. Apply a binder to pull the wound edges together and provide support to the edges.
3. Which features are characteristic of a closed drainage system such as a Jackson-Pratt (JP) drain? *(Select all that apply.)*
   a. Works by gravity
   b. Provides for early discharge
   c. Usually is inserted at surgery
   d. Reduces the amount of antibiotics required
   e. Allows for accurate measurement of wound drainage
   f. Allows bacteria to migrate up the drain from the surrounding dressing
4. Which intervention should be initiated by the nurse caring for a patient with urinary or fecal incontinence?
   a. Using a heat lamp to dry the skin
   b. Changing the adult brief every 8 hours
   c. Frequently cleansing with hot water and a strong soap
   d. Using an incontinence cleanser and a moisture barrier ointment

5. Based on knowledge of areas at greatest risk for development of a pressure ulcer in the bedridden patient, the nurse identifies which position to minimize this risk?
   a. 30-degree side-lying
   b. Sitting with the head of the bed elevated 75 degrees
   c. 90-degree side-lying
   d. Lying supine with the bed flat at all times
6. A patient who has suffered a stroke is unable to maintain his position in a chair without sliding down. His physician has ordered him to be up in a chair for part of the day. What does the nurse recognize as the patient's greatest risk factor for development of pressure ulcers?
   a. Moisture from incontinence
   b. Nutritional deficiencies
   c. Pressure and shear
   d. Aging
7. A patient has a stage III pressure ulcer on the coccyx. Which food will be most beneficial in improving the healing process?
   a. Foods high in vitamin D
   b. Whole-grain carbohydrates
   c. High-calorie, high-protein drink
   d. Foods high in fat and water content
8. Which technique is used to collect an aerobic culture specimen from a wound?
   a. Collect the specimen immediately after removing the old dressing.
   b. Apply sterile gloves; then open the culture tube.
   c. Always be sure to culture any necrotic tissue.
   d. Irrigate the wound before collecting the culture material.
9. Which patient is at highest risk for impaired wound healing?
   a. 22-year-old involved in a motor vehicle accident with a pelvic fracture
   b. 49-year-old with a history of smoking 2 packs a day who just had abdominal surgery
   c. 72-year-old with diabetes and cardiovascular disease who had surgical repair of a broken hip
   d. 90-year-old with no chronic health conditions with a small blistered burn on her hand
10. Which statement best describes the healing process for a surgical wound that has been closed with the use of sutures?
   a. The edges of the wound are approximated.
   b. New tissue fills the sides and base of the wound.
   c. The proliferate phase is longer with surgical wounds.
   d. Debridement aids in the surgical healing process.

ⓔ Answers and rationales for review questions are available at *http://evolve.elsevier.com/YoostCrawford/fundamentals/.*

REFERENCES

American Diabetes Association. Diabetes statistics, 2014. Retrieved from *www.diabetes.org/diabetes-basics/statistics/?loc=db-slabnav.*

Andros G, Armstrong DG, Attinger C, et al: Consensus statement on negative pressure wound therapy (V.A.C.® therapy) for the management of diabetic foot wounds, *Ostomy Wound Manag* 52(Suppl):1-32, 2006.

Annells MA, O'Neill J, Flowers C: Compression bandaging for venous leg ulcers: The essentialness of a willing patient, *J Clin Nurs* 17(3):350-359, 2008.

Ayello EA, Baranoski S, Salati DS: Best practices in wound care prevention and treatment, *Nurs Manage* 37(9):42-48, 2006.

Balzer K, Pohl C, Dassen T, Halfens R: The Norton, Waterlow, Braden and care dependency scales: Comparing their validity when identifying patients' pressure sore risk, *J Wound Ostomy Continence Nurs* 34(4):389-398, 2007.

Betsy Lehman Center for Patient Safety and Medical Error Reduction: Prevention of surgical site infections. In Prevention and control of healthcare-associated infections in Massachusetts [National Guidelines Clearinghouse], Boston, 2008, Massachusetts Department of Public Health. Retrieved from *http://guidelines.gov/content.aspx?id=12921.*

Bonham PA: Swab cultures for diagnosing wound infections: A literature review and clinical guideline, *J Wound Ostomy Continence Nurs* 36(4):389-395, 2009.

Chailler M, Ellis J, Stolarik A, Woodend K: Cold therapy for the management of pain associated with deep breathing and coughing post-cardiac surgery, *Can J Cardiovasc Nurs* 20(2):18-24, 2010.

Cronenwett L, Sherwood G, Barnsteiner J, et al: Quality and safety education for nurses, *Nurs Outlook* 55(3):122-131, 2007.

Dorner B, Posthauer ME, Thomas D: The role of nutrition in pressure ulcer prevention and treatment: National Pressure Ulcer Advisory Panel White Paper, 2009. Retrieved from *www.npuap.org/.*

Doughty D, Sparks-DeFriese B: Wound healing physiology. In R Bryant, D Nix (Eds), *Acute and chronic wounds: Current management concepts*, ed. 4, St. Louis, 2012, Mosby, pp 56-81.

European Pressure Ulcer Advisory Panel and National Pressure Ulcer Advisory Panel: *Pressure ulcer prevention and treatment: Clinical practice guideline*, Washington, DC, 2009, National Pressure Ulcer Advisory Panel.

Fernandez R, Griffiths, R: Water for wound cleansing, *Cochrane Database Syst Rev* (5):CD003861, 2012.

Junkin J, Gray M: Are pressure redistribution surfaces or heel protection devices effective for preventing heel pressure ulcers? *J Wound Ostomy Continence Nurs* 36(6):602-608, 2009.

Kottner J, Balzer K, Dassen T, Heinze S: Pressure ulcers: A critical review of definitions and classifications, *Ostomy Wound Manage* 55(9):22-29, 2009.

Krapfl L, Gray M: Does regular repositioning prevent pressure ulcers? *J Wound Ostomy Continence Nurs* 35(6):571-577, 2008.

Krasner D, Shapshak D, Hopf H: Managing wound pain. In R Bryant, D Nix (Eds), *Acute and chronic wounds: Current management concepts*, ed. 4, St. Louis, 2012, Mosby, pp 539-565.

Lane E, Latham T: Managing pain using heat and cold therapy, *Paediatr Nurs* 21(6):14-18, 2009.

Pieper B, Langemo D, Cuddigan J: Pressure ulcer pain: A systematic literature review and National Pressure Ulcer Advisory Panel White Paper, *Ostomy Wound Manage* 55(2):16-31, 2009.

Rodeheaver G, Ratcliff C: Wound cleansing, wound irrigation, wound disinfection. In D Krasner, G Rodeheaver, R Sibbald (Eds), *Chronic wound care: A clinical source book for healthcare professionals*, Malvern, Pa., 2007, HMP Communications.

Snyder L: Wound basics: Types, treatment, and care, *Reg Nurse* 71(8):32-36, 2008.

Speding I: Management of a patient using VAC therapy, *J Commun Nurs* 22(7):14-16, 2008.

Wysocki A: Anatomy and physiology of skin and soft tissue. In R Bryant, D Nix (Eds), *Acute and chronic wounds: Current management concepts*, ed. 4, St. Louis, 2012, Mosby, pp 39-55.

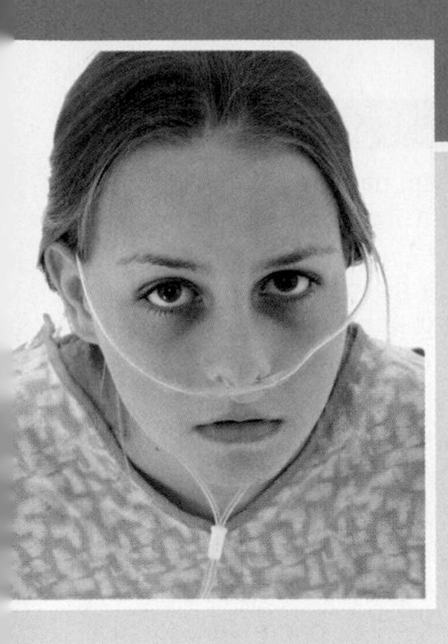

CHAPTER 30

Nutrition

EVOLVE WEBSITE

http://evolve.elsevier.com/YoostCrawford/fundamentals/

- Additional Evolve-Only Review Questions With Answers
- Answers and Rationales for Text Review Questions
- Answers to Critical-Thinking Questions
- Case Study With Questions
- Video Skills Clips
- Conceptual Care Map
- Animations
- Skill Checklists
- Glossary

LEARNING OUTCOMES

Comprehension of this chapter's content will provide students with the ability to:

LO 30.1 Describe the role of nutrition and food metabolism in achieving and maintaining normal body structure and function.

LO 30.2 Identify nutritional imbalances that can result in physical alterations, psychological disturbances, and the development of disease.

LO 30.3 Discuss critical aspects of a thorough nutritional assessment.

LO 30.4 Identify nursing diagnoses for patients experiencing an alteration in nutrition.

LO 30.5 Determine nursing care goals and outcome criteria for patients experiencing complications from an alteration in nutrition.

LO 30.6 Explain the implementation and evaluation of interventions designed to address nutritional needs.

KEY TERMS

absorption, p. 675
amino acids, p. 671
anabolism, p. 669
anorexia, p. 680
anorexia nervosa, p. 680
anthropometry, p. 683
aspiration, p. 684
basal metabolic rate (BMR), p. 668
bingeing, p. 680
body mass index (BMI), p. 679
bulimia nervosa, p. 680
cachexia, p. 682
carbohydrates, p. 669
catabolism, p. 669
cholesterol, p. 670
chyme, p. 675
digestion, p. 674
dysphagia, p. 678
enteral feeding, p. 677
enzymes, p. 672
fat-soluble vitamins, p. 672
fiber, p. 669
free radicals, p. 672
hyperlipidemia, p. 679
ketones, p. 675
kilocalorie, p. 669
kwashiorkor, p. 678
lipids, p. 670
macronutrients, p. 669
malabsorption, p. 678
malnutrition, p. 668
marasmus, p. 678
metabolism, p. 668
micronutrients, p. 669
minerals, p. 669
monounsaturated fatty acids, p. 670
nutrients, p. 668
nutrition, p. 668
obesity, p. 669
osmolality, p. 677
peristalsis, p. 675
polyunsaturated fatty acids, p. 670
purging, p. 680
saturated fatty acids, p. 670
total parenteral nutrition (TPN), p. 692
***trans* fatty acids, p. 670**
triglycerides, p. 670
vitamins, p. 669
water-soluble vitamins, p. 672

CASE STUDY

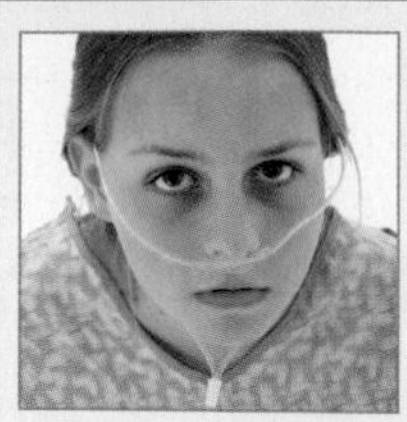

Amy is a 17-year-old high school student admitted to the hospital for severe weight loss, nausea, vomiting, and blood-tinged emesis. She has a medical history of anorexia nervosa since the age of 15 and a surgical history of appendectomy at 11 years of age. She has no known drug allergies (NKDA).

Amy's vital signs are T 97.2°F (36.2°C), P 90 and regular, R 16 and unlabored, and BP 98/68, with a pulse oximetry reading of 93% on 2L of oxygen. She reports abdominal pain at a level of 2 to 3 on a 0-to-10 scale when vomiting. Her height is 5 feet 6 inches and her weight is 98 lb, with a 40 lb weight loss in the past 6 months. Her Braden score is 19. She denies use of alcohol or recreational drugs.

Assessment reveals cachectic appearance; lungs are clear to auscultation, with prominent scapulae and clavicles. Skin is cool to touch, with poor turgor. Hair is dull, dry, and thin. Pallor is evident, with dark circles under the eyes and pale oral mucous membranes. Bowel sounds are hypoactive, and the abdomen is distended; the patient reports that her last BM was "3 or 4 days ago" and that she has an increasing problem with constipation. The patient's mother reports, "Amy refuses to eat and is losing too much weight." The mother also reports that her daughter is obsessed with exercising: "She exercises before and after meals and is exercising when I get up in the morning and when I go to bed." Amy states, "I don't exercise that much—I just don't want to be fat any longer!" Denies bingeing and purging but does admit to drinking 12 to 15 glasses of water and diet soda a day.

Refer back to this case study to answer the critical-thinking questions throughout the chapter.

Nutrition is the body's intake and use of adequate amounts of necessary nutrients for tissue growth and energy production. **Nutrients** are the necessary substances obtained from ingested food that supply the body with energy; build and maintain bones, muscles, and skin; and aid in the normal growth and function of each body system.

Nutritional balance has a significant impact on the normal growth, development, function, and maintenance of the body. Health care professionals must be cognizant of the concepts of proper nutrition and be able to apply them in practice to enhance wellness, promote healthy lifestyle choices, and reverse negative effects of improper nutritional habits. Research conducted by the National Institute on Aging (Boyd, Ritchie, Tipton, et al, 2008) reveals that improper nutrition may result in the onset of specific diseases of the endocrine, cardiovascular, gastrointestinal, and musculoskeletal systems, such as type 2 diabetes, atherosclerosis, diverticulosis, osteoporosis, and some cancers.

With the prominence of fad diets and false advertising in the media claiming "quick weight loss," the public needs accurate information for making nutritional decisions. Many people suffer from **malnutrition** (an imbalance in the amount of nutrient intake and the body's needs). Among them are those who are overweight or undernourished, lacking important nutrients due to poor food choices. To improve public health, health care professionals need to teach health care consumers how to do more than simply count calories. Choosing nutrient-rich foods helps people get the most benefit from calories ingested, resulting in better nutritional intake and fewer calories consumed. The U.S. Department of Health and Human Services (2014) has published *Healthy People 2020* topics and objectives, which focus on promotion of healthy lifestyles and decreasing the health variances across all cultures, races, and ethnic and socioeconomic groups. When patients and families are provided with dietary information and are educated to take a positive approach that focuses on the total nutritional quality of foods without calorie overconsumption, people can achieve better health.

NORMAL STRUCTURE AND FUNCTION LO 30.1

Overall health is dependent on a combination of appropriate nutritional intake, adequate exercise, weight management, and rest. Neglect of or improper emphasis on any of these factors places the person at risk for developing life-threatening conditions or premature death. Poor nutrition, lack of exercise, obesity, and stress contribute to health issues such as heart disease, some cancers, strokes, hypertension, and diabetes or kidney disease. A strong relationship is recognized between infection and malnutrition. People who practice proper dietary habits have stronger immune systems, less illness, and better health. Healthy children learn more effectively. Healthy people are stronger, more industrious, and able to achieve a better quality of life.

METABOLISM

Metabolism is the process of chemically changing nutrients, such as fats and proteins, into end products that are used to meet the energy needs of the body or stored for future use, thereby helping to maintain homeostasis in the body. Body processes such as repair and replacement of cells, elimination of waste through the kidneys, and functioning of the brain to maintain a pulse rate and respirations are the results of metabolism. The **basal metabolic rate (BMR)** is the minimum amount of energy required to maintain body functions in the resting, awake state. Even during rest or sleep, the body requires a certain amount of calories to support critical processes such as cardiac function and breathing.

Metabolism is necessary to maintain life and is composed of two major biochemical processes: **anabolism** (the use of energy to change simple materials into complex body substances and tissue) and **catabolism** (the breaking down of substances from complex to simple, resulting in a release of energy). These two processes can be thought of as constructive and destructive, respectively. Anabolism permits cell growth, such as the mineralization of bone or development of muscle mass. An example of catabolism is the breaking down of proteins and their subsequent conversion into amino acids, which creates glucose for use by the body as fuel.

Metabolism is a continuous process within the body and is dependent on the intake of proper nutrients. The essential nature of each nutrient and its functions underscores the importance of nutritional balance and its impact on a healthy, proper functioning body. A deficiency of any major nutrient has an overwhelming effect on more than just one organ.

NUTRIENTS

The major nutrients, often referred to as **macronutrients** (nutrients that are needed in large amounts), include carbohydrates (sugar, starches, and dietary fiber), which provide energy for cells, tissues, and organs; fats, which are major sources of energy and promote the absorption of vitamins; and proteins, which build, maintain, and repair muscles and tissue. Water also is a macronutrient, in that it is essential for proper functioning as well as for assisting the body with metabolic processes (metabolism). The animation "Food Absorption" shows this process.

Minerals (chemicals needed for energy, muscle building, nerve conduction, blood clotting, and immunity to diseases) and **vitamins** (organic compounds responsible for regulation of body processes, reproduction, and growth) are referred to as **micronutrients** (nutrients needed by the body in limited amounts). Failure of the body to properly use nutrients can result in diseases and other conditions such as heart and kidney disease, renal disorders, diabetes, malnutrition, and obesity. **Obesity** is the result of the person's energy intake consistently exceeding energy use. The consequence is the excessive accumulation of body fat, which affects overall health.

Carbohydrates

Carbohydrates are chemical substances composed of carbon, hydrogen, and oxygen molecules. Carbohydrates supply the body with 4 kilocalories (kcal) per gram. A **kilocalorie** is the amount of heat energy it takes to raise the temperature of 1000 grams of water 1 degree Celsius. Carbohydrates are major suppliers of energy and include sugars, starches, and fiber. They keep the body from using valuable proteins for energy, prevent ketosis, and enhance memory and learning capabilities. Carbohydrates are further classified as simple or complex. Simple carbohydrates are broken down and absorbed quickly, providing a quick source of energy. Examples are sugars such as those derived from fruit (fructose), table sugar (sucrose), milk products (lactose), and blood sugar (glucose). Complex carbohydrates are composed of starches, glycogen, and fiber. They take longer to break down before absorption and use by the body's cells. Proper functioning of the brain and other tissues depends on a sufficient supply of carbohydrates in the form of glycogen. During physical activity, the need for carbohydrates is increased to meet the energy demands of the muscles. A major portion of the glycogen from complex carbohydrates that is necessary for functioning is derived from stored "fuel." Muscles store glycogen and use it during strenuous exercise. If glycogen supplies become depleted, the person may suffer from extreme fatigue.

Complex carbohydrates also provide the body with vitamins and minerals. Food sources include bread; rice; pasta; legumes such as dried beans, peas, and lentils; and starchy vegetables such as corn, pumpkin, green peas, and potatoes. It is recommended that adults consume approximately 50% of their calories from carbohydrates. People should be observant of overall nutritional content when selecting foods containing carbohydrates. Foods containing highly processed sugars, such as cakes, pies, and other pastries, should be avoided because they contain little or no nutrient value, adding only calories to the diet.

Fiber

Fiber is a complex carbohydrate and is classified as soluble or insoluble. *Solubility* refers to the disposition of the fiber when mixed with another substance such as water. Soluble fiber mixes with water and forms a gel like substance, which results in slower digestion. Insoluble fiber does not retain water but allows formation of bulk, resulting in the accelerated passage of the end products of food through the intestines and a slowing of starch absorption. Research studies have discovered certain benefits of adequate soluble fiber intake, including promotion of cardiovascular health by lowering serum cholesterol levels, assistance in weight control, improvement of glycemic control in people with diabetes, and improvement of regularity.

Emerging research indicates that the intake of certain soluble fibers enhances immune function in humans. Psyllium is a natural product that is packaged without chemical modification. Psyllium is the only fiber supplement that has clearly documented cholesterol-lowering properties and has a health claim with respect to heart disease. Psyllium and other soluble fiber supplements have also been associated with reduced blood pressure (Anderson, 2009). The lack of fiber can lead to bowel-related conditions such as constipation, hemorrhoids, and formation of diverticula, which are protrusions of the intestinal membrane through the muscular layer of the intestine, most often in the large colon. The presence of these protrusions is referred to as *diverticulosis.* Older children, adolescents, and adults should consume 20 to 35 grams of fiber a day. Food sources include whole grains,

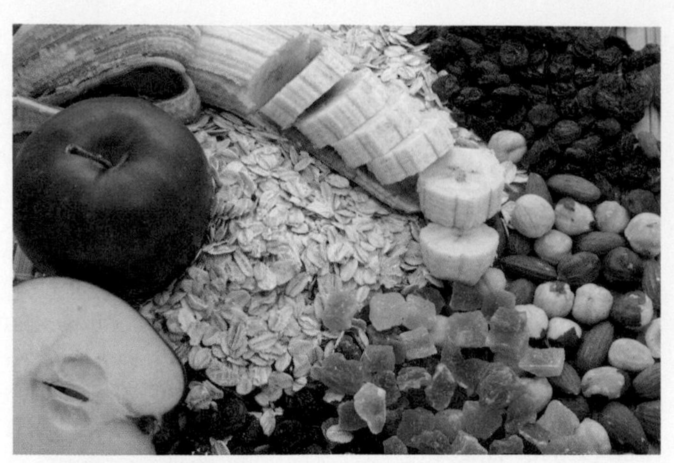

FIGURE 30-1 Soluble and nonsoluble fiber foods.

wheat bran, cereals, fresh fruits, vegetables, and legumes (Figure 30-1).

Fats

Fats are composed of carbon, hydrogen, and oxygen and yield 9 kilocalories per gram when metabolized within the body. **Lipid** refers to any fat found within the body, including true fats and oils such as fatty acids, cholesterol, and phospholipids. Total fat intake, as recommended by the American Heart Association (2012a), should be between 25% and 35% of caloric intake each day. Ideally, less than 7% should be from saturated fat. Dietary fat takes longer to digest than other major nutrients and requires the presence of carbohydrates to associate with oxygen and produce energy for the body's use. **Triglycerides** are the most abundant lipids in food. An important point is that although the intake of a limited amount of triglycerides is important, an excess can be unhealthy, contributing to health problems such as coronary artery disease and obesity. Benefits of fat in the body include energy production, support and insulation of major organs and nerve fibers, energy storage of adipose tissue, lubrication for body tissues, vitamin absorption, and transportation of fat-soluble vitamins A, D, E, and K, and fat has a role in the development of the cell membrane structure.

Fats are composed of one (monoglyceride) to three (triglyceride) fatty acids, which consist of chains primarily made up of carbon and hydrogen atoms. The number of fatty acids contained in a fat has dietary and health implications. **Saturated fatty acids** contain as many hydrogen atoms as the carbon atoms can bond with and no double carbon bonds. **Monounsaturated fatty acids** have only one double bond between carbon atoms, whereas **polyunsaturated fatty acids** have multiple pairs of double carbon bonds.

Monounsaturated fat sources include canola, olive, and peanut oils, as well as almonds, sesame seeds, avocados, and cashews. Polyunsaturated sources include corn, safflower, sesame, soybean, and sunflower seed oils. Fish such as halibut, herring, mackerel, salmon, sardines, fresh tuna, trout, and whitefish are known sources of polyunsaturated fats. Saturated fats are found in hard margarines, vegetable shortenings, pastries, crackers, fried foods, cheese, ice cream, and other processed foods. Foods from animal sources, especially beef, lamb, and processed meat, remain major sources of total fat, saturated fat, and cholesterol in dietary intake. Typically, patients are encouraged to increase their intake of monounsaturated fats (which also contribute fiber and antioxidants to the diet), while decreasing intake of polyunsaturated and saturated fats.

Trans fats (***trans* fatty acids**), composed of partially hydrogenated fatty acids, and saturated fats are known to raise the body's total **cholesterol**, a waxy, fatlike substance that is found in all cells of the body. Approximately 75% of cholesterol is produced by the liver and intestines; the remaining 25% is obtained from dietary intake (American Heart Association, 2012a). Cholesterol is an essential component of cell membranes; is necessary for the production of some hormones such as adrenaline, estrogen and testosterone, and cortisone; and aids in digestion as a component of bile salts. See Chapter 34 for an extensive discussion of cholesterol levels in the body.

Omega-3 (linolenic acid) and omega-6 (linoleic acid) are referred to as unsaturated "essential" fatty acids that need to be included in the diet, because human metabolism cannot produce them. They are necessary for a number of functions including blood clotting and normal brain and nervous system functioning. They help to prevent atherosclerosis and lower triglyceride levels. Omega-3 fatty acids are believed to improve learning ability in children, enhance immune function, and relieve arthritis symptoms. Consuming one to two servings a week of fish, particularly fish that is rich in omega-3 fatty acids, appears to reduce the risk of heart disease, particularly sudden cardiac death. Dietary sources include fatty fish, such as salmon, tuna, mackerel, and lake trout, and nuts, seeds, and oils; flaxseed oil contains the highest amount of total omega-3 fatty acids. Linoleic acid plays an important role in lowering cholesterol levels. Omega-6 fatty acid is an unsaturated fat found in various types of seeds, nuts, and vegetable oils (Mayo Clinic, 2011). It is recommended that people learn to read nutrition labels and to avoid intake of *trans* fatty acids and saturated fats to minimize their adverse effects (Patient Education and Health Literacy box).

Protein

Proteins are active participants in the development, maintenance, and repair of the body's tissues, organs, and cells. Hemoglobin, the part of erythrocytes (red blood cells) responsible for transporting oxygen throughout the body, is one type of protein critical to regulating body function, as is prothrombin, the protein necessary for clotting blood. Proteins are involved in many other tasks throughout the body, including the production of hair and nails, muscle movement, nerve conduction, digestion, and defense against

PATIENT EDUCATION AND HEALTH LITERACY

Interpreting the Language of Food Labels

- Uniform nutrition labeling for packaged food was introduced in the United States in 1994, as part of the Nutrition Labeling and Education Act (NLEA), to increase consumer awareness about the nutritional content of food and to improve dietary practices (Wojcicki and Heyman, 2012).
- Evidence indicates a consistent link between eating healthier foods and reading nutrition labels (Campos, Doxey, and Hammond, 2011).
- Studies indicate that the use of food labels to guide food selection is significantly lower among children, adolescents, older adults, ethnic minorities, and people of lower socioeconomic status (Campos, Doxey, and Hammond, 2011).
- Patients should be asked if they read food labels when shopping for groceries or food products. Evaluate their understanding of the main elements of a nutrient label (i.e., calories, fats, carbohydrates, sugar, and serving size).
- Assess patient understanding of the percentages of recommended daily allowances of fats, proteins, and carbohydrates listed on food labels.
- Assist patients with planning strategies for eating a well-balanced diet based on knowledge of caloric intake and nutrient content.

bacteria and viruses. They consist of organic compounds called **amino acids**, which often are referred to as the "building blocks" of proteins. Unlike fat and carbohydrates, amino acids must be consumed in food every day, because the human body does not produce or store excess amino acids for later use. When the accumulation of protein exceeds the need for growth and repair of tissues, the protein is removed and excreted by the kidneys in urea. If the production of fat or carbohydrates is deficient, protein may assume the role of providing energy. This demand on protein stores can lead to a deficiency of protein in the body. The Dietary Guidelines for Americans (U.S. Department of Agriculture, 2014) recommend that the daily allowance of protein be 0.8 gram per kilogram of ideal body weight. Like carbohydrates, proteins supply 4 kilocalories of energy per gram while supplying 15% of the total energy intake. The animation "Protein Synthesis" shows the process.

Proteins often are referred to as complete or incomplete. *Complete* proteins contain all essential amino acids. Sources of complete protein include animal-based foods such as milk, eggs, cheese, fish, meat, and poultry. The only plant protein considered to be a complete protein is found in soybeans. *Incomplete* proteins lack one or more essential amino acids. Sources of incomplete protein include beans, peas, nuts, seeds, fruits, vegetables, bread, and bread products. The combination of two or more plant proteins can form a complete protein and provide all of the essential amino acids. Examples of this type of combination are pasta and broccoli, rice and beans, and peanut butter and whole wheat bread.

Water

Water plays a major role in the body and is necessary for processes such as helping to control body temperature, maintaining acid-base balance, regulating fluid and electrolytes, and transporting nutrient and waste products from the kidneys. Water is a component of intracellular and extracellular fluids within the body. Two thirds of the body's fluids are contained within the cells (intracellular). The extracellular fluids are components of the blood, of the interstitial fluid between the cells, and within certain structures. When water loss continues without replacement, blood volume is diminished. When this happens, ample oxygen and nutrients cannot be furnished to body cells, and carbon dioxide and waste products cannot be efficiently removed. Every organ of the body is affected, including the brain and central nervous system. More important, water makes up approximately 60% of body weight; if it is not replaced after being lost through breathing, sweating, urine, and the intestines, the ability of the body to function properly is affected. Some water may be obtained through most food sources or may be added in the preparation of foods.

Thirst is an indication that the body needs water or fluids. Even a slight decrease in water in the body, failure to meet the body's hydration needs, or loss of a disproportionate amount through excessive sweating, diarrhea, or vomiting can result in dehydration. Physical symptoms may include headaches and loss of concentration.

By contrast, excessive water intake or failure to excrete adequate amounts of urine, as seen in some renal conditions, can lead to water intoxication. Excessive amounts of fluid intake can dilute the amount of sodium in the body and cause hyponatremia. The Food and Nutrition Board of the Institute of Medicine recommends that healthy adult men drink approximately 3.7 liters a day of water and healthy adult women drink 2.7 liters a day (Institute of Medicine, 2013). Fluid intake needs to be monitored closely in patients experiencing fluid overload, congestive heart failure, or a renal disease in which fluid intake is limited.

Vitamins

Vitamins are organic compounds that contribute to important metabolic and physiologic functions within the body. Vitamins are regarded as indispensable in proper dietary intake. Other characteristics include the body's inability to manufacture them or, often, limitation of production by environmental factors. They do not produce energy; however, they are crucial in chemical reactions within the body from nutrients such as fats, carbohydrates, and proteins. They typically are categorized according to their solubility in fat or water and their absorption, transportation, and storage processes within the body.

Fat-Soluble Vitamins

Fat is necessary in the diet to assist with the absorption of the fat-soluble vitamins A, D, E, and K. Excess fat-soluble vitamins are stored in the liver and fat tissue and are not excreted by the kidneys. Because of this storage, if an excessive amount of these vitamins is taken, toxicity may result, especially with vitamins A and D.

Vitamin A

Vitamin A is important for its ability to increase the resistance to infection, promote night vision through the development of normal visual pigment, develop and maintain normal function of epithelial tissue, and aid in the development of normal bones and teeth. Vitamin A and compounds created by its metabolism are responsible for maintaining the integrity and function of skin and mucosal cells, which are the body's first line of defense against infection (Linus Pauling Institute, 2011). Hemoglobin receives stored iron with the assistance of vitamin A. Deficiencies in vitamin A may cause night blindness (because of the inability of the cornea to adapt to darkness), poor appetite, decreased immunity to infections, and impaired growth and development. Foods rich in vitamin A include liver, milk, egg yolk, and dark, leafy green vegetables. Yellow and orange vegetables and fruits such as sweet potatoes, pumpkin, carrots, and apricots also are good sources.

Vitamin D

Vitamin D has long been referred to as the "sunshine vitamin" because it is synthesized in the skin when exposed to sunlight. It is not found in most foods. Vitamin D is important for the development of bone and tissue formation because of its collaborative efforts with minerals such as calcium and phosphorus to develop and strengthen bones. It is recommended that people be exposed to direct sunlight for 15 minutes several times a week to promote the manufacture and storage of vitamin D, which assists in the development of collagen, a constituent of bone that aids in the bone strengthening. Dietary sources of vitamin D include dairy products, eggs, fortified food products, liver, and fatty fish (salmon and mackerel).

Vitamin E

Vitamin E is an antioxidant that protects cells from injury from free radicals (by-products that result when the body transforms food into energy). The accumulation of these by-products over time is mainly responsible for the aging process and can contribute to the development of numerous health conditions, such as cancer, heart disease, and various inflammatory conditions. Risk factors associated with formation of harmful oxygen free radicals include cigarette smoking, extensive exposure to the sun, and air pollution, which may result in damage to cells, tissues, and organs. Vitamin E is effective in maintaining a healthy immune system. Dietary sources may include nuts, seeds, and soybean, canola, corn, and other vegetable oils.

Vitamin K

Vitamin K is synthesized in the body by bacteria that are found in the large intestine. It is essential for the synthesis of proteins that promote the clotting, or coagulation, of blood. The liver produces a protein known as prothrombin and is dependent on vitamin K for this process. Deficiency of this vitamin can result in bruising and bleeding. Dietary resources include dark-green leafy vegetables such as broccoli, spinach, Brussels sprouts, and cabbage.

Water-Soluble Vitamins

Water-soluble vitamins dissolve in the body and are excreted in the urine. They are easily destroyed by air, light, and heat (cooking). Water-soluble vitamins must be ingested daily through dietary sources or supplements because they are not stored in the body.

Vitamin C

Vitamin C (ascorbic acid) is considered to be one of the most important vitamins because it plays a major role in promoting a healthy body. Among its functions is the synthesizing of the protein collagen. Collagen is important in connective tissue, wound healing, and repair and maintenance of cartilage, bones, and teeth. Vitamin C is effective as an antioxidant that guards against cellular damage from toxic chemicals and pollutants in the environment. Vitamin C contributes to the development of a strong immune system by producing antibodies that fight bacteria and viruses to protect against infections and illnesses. Dietary sources include fresh yellow and orange fruits, papaya, kiwi, broccoli, and sweet and white potatoes.

Vitamin B Complex

The vitamin B complex contains eight principal water-soluble vitamins. The B vitamins help to form red blood cells and act in part as *coenzymes,* small molecules that combine with an enzyme to make it active. They facilitate energy production in the body. Enzymes are proteins responsible for catalyzing most chemical reactions in the body, such as digesting food and synthesizing new compounds.

Vitamin B_1 (thiamine) is essential for the metabolism of protein, fat, and carbohydrates including sugar to produce energy for the body's cells. It is important for normal growth and development and promotes normal heart, muscle, and nervous system functions. It also is necessary for the production of hydrochloric acid (which is necessary for proper digestion). Dietary sources include egg yolk, fruits, organ meat, lean pork, legumes, nuts, vegetables, and whole grains.

Vitamin B_2 (riboflavin) assists in the metabolism of protein and the function of other B vitamins such as vitamin B_3 (niacin) and vitamin B_6 (pyridoxine). It assists in promoting visual adaptation to light and maintaining healthy skin.

Dietary food sources include milk and dairy products, whole grains, enriched bread and cereals, legumes, dark-green vegetables (collard greens, spinach, and broccoli), and organ meats.

Vitamin B_3 (niacin), referred to as *nicotinic acid* or *nicotinamide,* is a coenzyme for energy production. It also has a critical role in the formation of fatty acids. Dietary sources are meats, poultry, fortified breads and cereals, brewer's yeast, fish (swordfish and salmon), mushrooms, whole grains, green leafy vegetables, dried beans, and peanuts. Coffee contains a significant amount of niacin, which helps to prevent deficiencies in cultures that consume little protein and large amounts of coffee.

Pantothenic acid and biotin are two B vitamins that are used by the body to produce energy. Biotin is necessary to form purines, which are essential components of DNA and RNA. It is found in liver, legumes, tomatoes, and egg yolk. Pantothenic acid, also known as vitamin B_5, is necessary for the metabolism of carbohydrates, fats, and protein as well as the synthesis of acetylcholine. High amounts of pantothenic acid are found in whole-grain cereals, potatoes, legumes, broccoli, and egg yolks.

Vitamin B_6 (pyridoxine) assists as a coenzyme in the synthesis and catabolism of amino acids. Vitamin B_{12} (cyanocobalamin) is essential for the production of red blood cells. It facilitates the entrance of folate into cells and maintains the protective sheath (myelin) that surrounds nerve fibers. It is necessary to make DNA, the genetic material in all cells. Vitamin B_{12} is found in animal products including meat, eggs, and dairy products.

Folic acid (vitamin B_9) is a water-soluble vitamin that must be provided in the diet or supplemented because it is not produced in the body. It is necessary for the synthesis of DNA (which controls heredity) and is used in red blood cell formation. Folic acid is especially critical to the formation of rapidly growing cells, such as those in blood and in fetal and gastrointestinal tissue. Its absorption may be affected by certain drugs such as oral contraceptives and antibiotics. Folic acid supplements taken before and during pregnancy have been a major factor in the decline of neural tube defects (NTDs) in newborns. Dietary sources of folic acid include leafy green vegetables (kale, spinach, Brussels sprouts), oranges, strawberries, dried beans, peas and nuts, and enriched breads and cereals and other fortified grain products.

Additional information on vitamins and drug interactions may be found at the Linus Pauling Institute website *(http://lpi.oregonstate.edu/infocenter/contentnuts.html).*

Minerals

Minerals are considered to be micronutrients and are classified as macrominerals or microminerals, depending on their daily dietary requirements. Potassium, sodium, and chloride play a critical role in maintaining fluid balance in the body. They are important in nerve conduction and muscle contraction. If the body is able to maintain an adequate level of these nutrients, muscle tissue, including that of the heart, can function properly. Dietary sources of potassium include milk, bananas, legumes, green leafy vegetables, and orange juice, tomatoes, vegetable juice, avocados, and cantaloupe. Dietary sources of sodium include table salt, smoked meat, fish, olives, and pickled foods. Sources of chloride include tomatoes, celery, seaweed, and olives.

Calcium, phosphorus, and magnesium are minerals that are important in the production and maintenance of bone tissue. Most of the body's calcium is found in the bones and teeth, with approximately 1% found in the blood (Lutz, 2010). Calcium is required for nerve conduction, muscle contraction, blood vessel expansion and contraction, and the secretion of hormones and enzymes. Dietary sources of calcium include milk and milk products, salmon with bones, spinach, kale, fortified whole wheat bread, tofu, and orange juice. Phosphorus, like calcium, plays a major role in the development of bone. It aids in the contraction of muscles, kidney function, nerve conduction, and maintenance of a regular heartbeat. It also plays an important role in the body's use of other major nutrients such as carbohydrates, fats, and proteins, all of which are crucial in the maintenance and repair of cells and tissues. Intake of phosphorus is considered adequate if intake of milk and meat products is sufficient.

Magnesium works in conjunction with calcium to promote structural support. The remaining amount is involved in a large number of chemical reactions, such as energy production and bone formation. Magnesium combined with calcium regulates blood pressure and maintains a regular heartbeat and nerve and muscle function. This nutrient is associated with the production of dopamine, norepinephrine (noradrenaline), and epinephrine (adrenaline). Increasing research focuses on the use of magnesium to treat conditions such as asthma, diabetes, cardiovascular disease, and attention deficit disorder in children. The mineral stimulates the production of the neurotransmitter gamma-aminobutyric acid (GABA), which is believed to produce a calming effect (Challem, 2014). Magnesium deficiency may result from a dietary intake with little or no nutritional value, including additives, refined sugars, and foods high in calories and low in protein, vitamins, and minerals. An excessive amount of zinc intake may lower magnesium levels. Dietary sources of magnesium include halibut, seeds, nuts, tofu, Swiss chard, spinach, whole-grain wheat, brewer's yeast, and molasses. For more information on electrolytes, see Chapter 39.

Antioxidants

Antioxidants are substances that may protect body cells against the effects of free radicals. Free radicals are molecules produced when the body breaks down food or is subjected to environmental exposures to potential toxins such as tobacco smoke and radiation. Antioxidants work by significantly slowing or preventing the oxidative process—or damage from oxygen—caused by free radicals, which can lead to cell dysfunction and the onset of problems such as heart disease, cancer, diabetes, and other diseases. Antioxidants also may improve immune function and perhaps lower the risk for infection and cancer. Antioxidants include beta carotene, lutein, lycopene, selenium, and vitamins A, C, and E. Food sources of antioxidants are listed in Table 30-1.

TABLE 30-1 Antioxidant Food Sources

ANTIOXIDANT	FOOD SOURCES
Beta carotene	Dark-orange, red, yellow, and green vegetables and fruits, including red and yellow peppers, spinach, kale, sweet potatoes, carrots, broccoli, apricots, mangos, and cantaloupes
Selenium	Most vegetables and oatmeal, brown rice, chicken, dairy products, garlic, onions, seafood (salmon and tuna in particular), and whole grains
Vitamin C	Citrus fruits, dark-green vegetables and tomatoes, red and yellow peppers, pineapples, cantaloupes, guavas, and berries
Vitamin E	Olive, soybean, and corn oil; nuts, seeds, whole grains, legumes, and dark leafy vegetables

DIGESTION

The body is ultimately dependent on the digestive system for the processing of food and fluid taken in for nutritional purposes (Figure 30-2). The body's metabolic processes rely on the *ingestion* or consumption of food. **Digestion** (the breaking down of food into smaller particles of nutrients) is dependent on physiologic and chemical changes within the body. These changes are necessary for the body to receive the nutritional benefits of food or fluid intake. As food enters the mouth, it becomes the target for enzymes. These are substances that chemically break down the food so that it can be

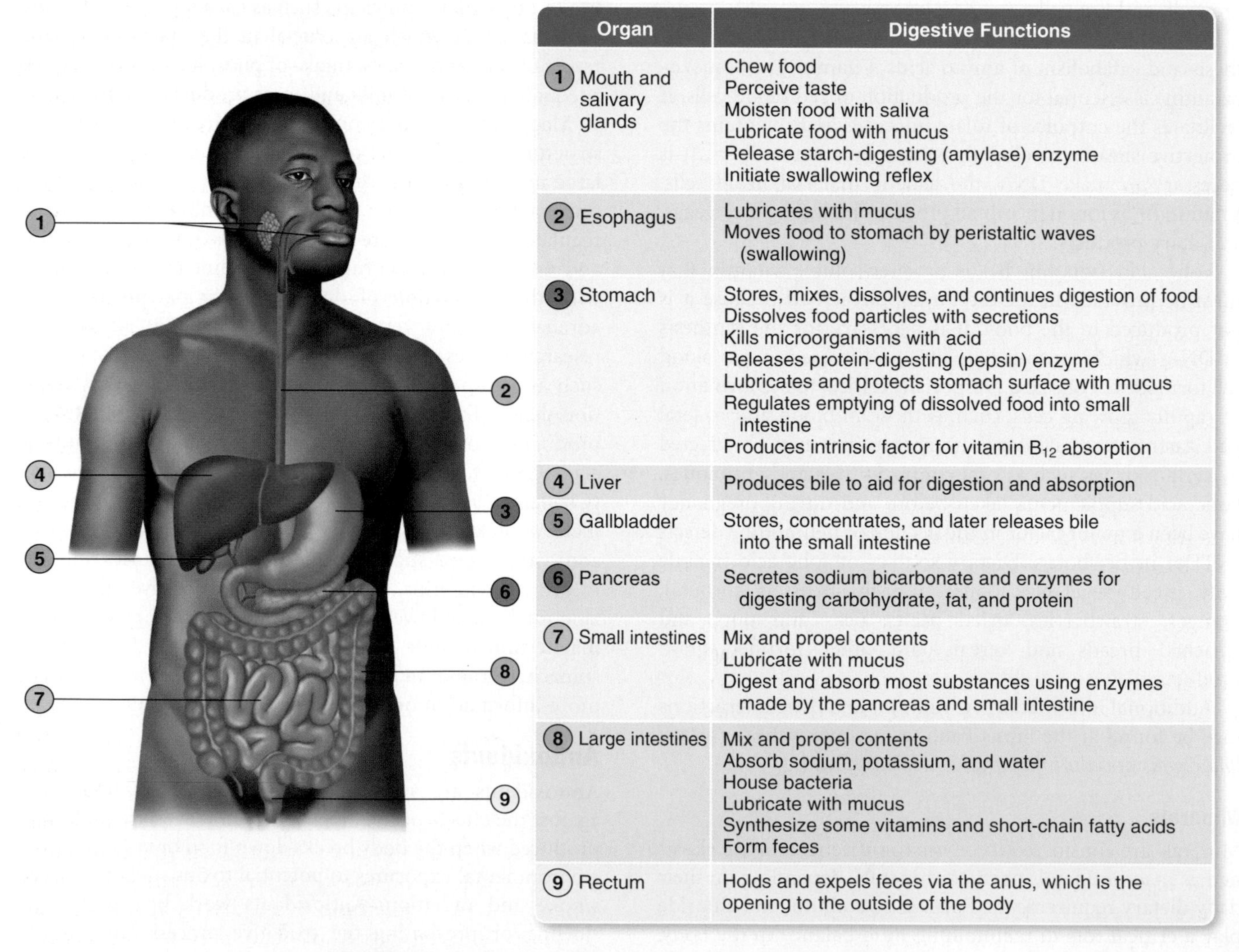

Organ	Digestive Functions
(1) Mouth and salivary glands	Chew food Perceive taste Moisten food with saliva Lubricate food with mucus Release starch-digesting (amylase) enzyme Initiate swallowing reflex
(2) Esophagus	Lubricates with mucus Moves food to stomach by peristaltic waves (swallowing)
(3) Stomach	Stores, mixes, dissolves, and continues digestion of food Dissolves food particles with secretions Kills microorganisms with acid Releases protein-digesting (pepsin) enzyme Lubricates and protects stomach surface with mucus Regulates emptying of dissolved food into small intestine Produces intrinsic factor for vitamin B_{12} absorption
(4) Liver	Produces bile to aid for digestion and absorption
(5) Gallbladder	Stores, concentrates, and later releases bile into the small intestine
(6) Pancreas	Secretes sodium bicarbonate and enzymes for digesting carbohydrate, fat, and protein
(7) Small intestines	Mix and propel contents Lubricate with mucus Digest and absorb most substances using enzymes made by the pancreas and small intestine
(8) Large intestines	Mix and propel contents Absorb sodium, potassium, and water House bacteria Lubricate with mucus Synthesize some vitamins and short-chain fatty acids Form feces
(9) Rectum	Holds and expels feces via the anus, which is the opening to the outside of the body

FIGURE 30-2 Essential components of the digestive system.

used to build and nourish cells and provide energy. Enzymes are classified according to the type of chemical reaction they trigger, and they are reactive to temperature and the pH condition of the food (acid or alkaline). The first stage of digestion is performed by the salivary glands as food enters the mouth and chewing takes place. These glands secrete specific enzymes that break down certain components of the food. For example, salivary amylase (ptyalin) breaks down carbohydrates (starch) into maltose, which is then further broken down by enzymes in secretions from the pancreas and the lining of the small intestine. The enzyme in the lining of the small intestine splits the maltose into glucose molecules as **absorption** (movement of the smaller elements through the walls of the digestive tract and into the blood) takes place. Glucose is then carried through the bloodstream to the liver, where it is stored or used to provide energy for the work of the body. As the food is being digested, it becomes a semiliquid mass as it travels through the intestines; this mass is referred to as **chyme**. The waste products are then propelled through the rest of the intestines, the rectum, and the anus by **peristalsis** (a wavelike muscular movement) for elimination to occur.

Ingestion, digestion of food, absorption of nutrients, and elimination of waste are the primary functions of the gastrointestinal system. When digestion and absorption are completely undeterred, the necessary amounts of nutrients are delivered to the cells, tissues, and organs. During digestion, ingested foods are physically or chemically converted into a form that can be absorbed through the membranes of the intestines and enter the bloodstream. This process is known as *catabolism*, during which the body receives nutrients needed to provide energy for physical activity. These nutrients, such as proteins, carbohydrates, calories, and fat, are energy sources and substances needed to build and repair muscle. As the body uses this energy to build tissues, it is in a state of anabolism. Another instance of the need for energy is the metabolism of fat. For fat to be adequately utilized by the body, the body has to have a sufficient supply of carbohydrates. If carbohydrate levels are deficient, an excessive amount of fat is rapidly metabolized for energy. This imbalance results in the production of **ketones** (from incomplete fat oxidation when carbohydrates are not available). Chewing and moistening of the food with saliva produce a bolus of food that is swallowed and pushed along the esophagus by peristalsis into the stomach. In the stomach, the food is mixed with gastric juices to form chyme. As the food is pushed into the intestine by the peristaltic waves, the digested food makes contact with the intestinal mucosa, thus facilitating absorption and moving the food along the remainder of the digestive tract. Once the remaining contents are propelled into the sigmoid colon and rectum, elimination occurs. The actions of the digestive system promote health, prevent disease, and reduce preventable deaths and disabilities. The digestive system can be regarded as a major transportation system dependent on each structure to accomplish specific tasks.

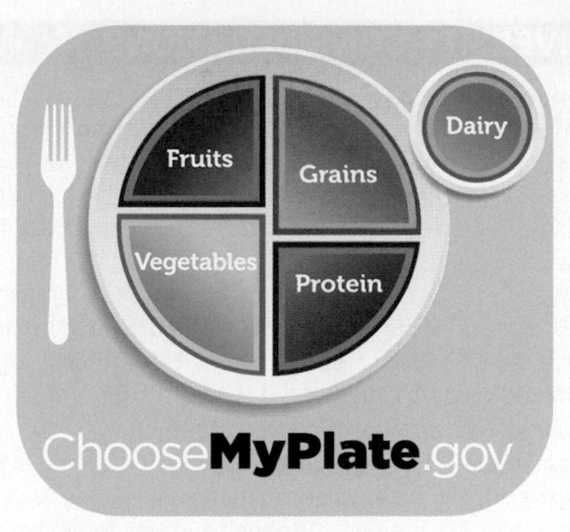

FIGURE 30-3 MyPlate Dietary Guidelines. (From U.S. Department of Agriculture: Dietary Guidelines for Americans, 2014. Retrieved from *www.choosemyplate.gov/food-groups/*.)

DIETARY GUIDELINES

The Dietary Guidelines are updated routinely by the U.S. Department of Agriculture (USDA) in collaboration with other federal agencies. These guidelines constitute a reliable resource and provide guidance for the intake of proper nutrients and the development of healthy dietary habits, which can promote health and reduce risk for major chronic diseases. According to the 2011 Dietary Guidelines, a healthy diet is one that:

- Emphasizes fruits, vegetables, whole grains, and fat-free or low-fat milk and milk products
- Includes lean meats, poultry, fish, beans, eggs, and nuts
- Is low in saturated fats, trans fats, cholesterol, salt (sodium), and added sugars

People are encouraged to eat smaller portions and to drink water rather than sugary beverages. Serving sizes of fruits and vegetables are to cover half of a plate, as illustrated in Figure 30-3. The MyPlate guide is intended for healthy people, not for those on a prescribed or specialized diet. Factors related to diet and nutrition are discussed in the Diversity Considerations box.

ALTERED STRUCTURE AND FUNCTION LO 30.2

Poor nutritional intake, inadequate exercise, and lack of rest can result in improper growth and development in children and adolescents and serious health concerns in the adult. Alterations in the musculoskeletal, neurologic, cardiopulmonary, and digestive systems and disturbances in metabolism and in psychological well-being can adversely affect nutritional status and contribute to the development of disease processes and conditions that may decrease the patient's ability to lead an active and productive life.

DIVERSITY CONSIDERATIONS

Life Span

- The longer a woman breastfeeds her child, the lower her risk for serious diseases such as diabetes, heart disease, and breast cancer and the lower the child's risk for infections, obesity, diabetes, and other diseases and conditions. Medical experts agree with the U.S. Department of Health and Human Services in recommending exclusive breastfeeding for 6 months and continued breastfeeding for the first year of life and beyond. Recent health care reform legislation promotes breastfeeding in the workplace. For more information, visit *http://usbreastfeeding.org.*
- Breastfeeding is not always an option. Some mothers do not breastfeed or choose to combine breastfeeding with supplemental formula feeding. Although formula-fed babies do not get all the complex nutrients or immune system benefits that are in breast milk, they do receive sufficient nutrients for growth and development.
- Some babies have milk allergies or significant medical conditions that impair normal digestion. For these infants, soy-based formulas and formulas with hydrolyzed (predigested) proteins are available. The content of infant formulas is regulated and is sometimes modified by the manufacturer with the intent to improve the overall health benefit to the consuming infant. The U.S. Food and Drug Administration (FDA) regulates formula companies to ensure that they provide all of the known necessary nutrients (including vitamin D) in their formulas.
- Infants require more essential nutrients than do adults to meet the demands of rapid growth. Infants typically double their birth weight at 5 to 6 months and triple it by the age of 1 year. Adolescents need additional calcium to meet the body's demand for mineralization of bone. Adolescent boys require an increase in iron to aid in the development of lean body mass; adolescent girls need to replenish iron lost during menstruation.
- Pregnant women and women of childbearing age are at high risk for development of iron deficiency anemia.
- Older adults are at risk for development of osteoporosis as a consequence of increased bone loss and low calcium intake in this age group (see Chapter 28 for additional information on osteoporosis).
- Aging results in decreased functioning of all major organs. This creates the need for increased amounts of some vitamins and minerals such as vitamin D, calcium, and phosphorus.
- Specific concerns regarding the nutritional status of elderly people are well recognized. Calorie needs change owing to more body fat and less lean muscle. Less activity further decreases calorie requirements. Older adults may experience a decrease in the sense of smell or taste, difficulty chewing, impaired mobility, decreased motivation to cook for themselves, and financial limitations. Nurses should recommend including a variety of colors and textures of fruits and vegetables, adding whole-grain breads and cereals, and decreasing the amount of saturated fatty foods in the diet. The addition of spices and herbs may enhance the taste of foods.
- The challenge for older adults is to choose foods that are **nutrient-dense.** These foods are high in nutrients in relation to their calories. For example, an apple has approximately 80 calories plus vitamins and fiber. The fiber and water in the apple will fill the stomach. By contrast, a doughnut has more than 200 calories, contains less fiber, does not promote satisfaction, and usually does not satisfy hunger, leading to the consumption of additional food. Foods that are high in calories but have very few nutrients, such as colas, chips, cookies, and alcohol, should be avoided.
- Food selection by older adults also affects digestion. Eating whole-grain foods and a variety of fruits and vegetables and drinking water may minimize the risk of constipation.
- People with food allergies are advised to avoid the offending food, because the symptoms can be triggered any and every time a small amount of the food is consumed.
- Food intolerances are often related to the amount consumed. Symptoms are related to the quantity consumed and the frequency of consumption. For example, a person with fructose intolerance may be able to drink a single glass of fruit juice or regular soda but will become ill if several glasses are consumed.
- People who have symptoms after ingestion of certain foods should seek medical care to determine whether the cause is an allergy or intolerance and to establish a plan to help control the symptoms.
- Health care providers should determine the need for patient education on safe food handling and storage to promote the older adult's health. Some older adults are homebound and must rely on delivered food. For educational resources visit *www.foodsafety.gov/blog/blog.html.*
- According to the Meals On Wheels Association of America (MOWAA) (2010), statistics relevant to hunger among the older American population indicate that "nearly 8.3 million seniors face the threat of hunger every day in America." MOWAA plays a major role in investigating the causes and consequences of nutrient-related deficiencies and other health outcomes among older adults. For additional information, visit *http://mowaa.org.*

Gender

- Optimal caloric intake for both men and women depends on their level of exercise and body size.
- Women and men should avoid excess protein intake, to decrease calcium loss and help to prevent osteoporosis and kidney stones.
- Excess calcium intake in men has been identified as a possible factor in the development of advanced prostate cancer *(www.health.harvard.edu/fhg/updates/update0906b.shtml).*

Culture, Ethnicity, and Religion

- Culture, ethnic background, and religion affect individual food preferences. It is important that health care providers take this into consideration when selecting foods for someone who is incapable of making food decisions.
- Culture consists of all learned patterns of behavior passed down from one generation to the next. The patient's religious

DIVERSITY CONSIDERATIONS—cont'd

beliefs, language, communication skills or language barriers, traditions, and values influence the delivery of nursing care.

- Foods traditionally consumed by various ethnic groups may contribute to the development of chronic illnesses. People who consume large amounts of salted pork products may be prone to hypertension, whereas ethnic groups whose diet includes high levels of carbohydrates may experience an increased incidence of obesity and/or diabetes.
- Religious beliefs are individualized and may often affect patients' acceptance or refusal of traditional medical treatments. Health care providers should be cognizant of these differences and integrate them into the delivery of health care or assist patients to understand the impact of the decisions on their health status.

Disability

- **Enteral feeding**, or tube feeding, as the only method of nutritional support poses certain challenges:
  - Selection of an appropriate formula to meet specific patient needs is based on the variables of nutritional adequacy, digestibility, viscosity, **osmolality** (ionic concentration), ease of use, and cost.
  - Patient-specific variables are current disease state, nutritional and hydration status, renal function, medication therapy, and digestive tract function. Existing chronic illnesses and factors that increase metabolic demands on the body, such as stress or fever, must be considered if the patient's fluid and dietary needs are to be met.
  - Patients with disabilities are often limited in the amount or degree to which they can participate in physical exercise, and this can lead to obesity. Nurses should encourage patients to exercise within their capabilities. Regular physical activity provides important health benefits for people with disabilities. The benefits include improved cardiovascular and muscle fitness, improved mental health, and better ability to do tasks of daily life. For more information on the Physical Activity Guidelines for Americans, visit *www.health.gov/PAGuidelines.*

Morphology

- Patients who have had surgery to help with their obesity, such as gastric bypass and banding, are at risk of nutritional deficiencies due to the altered state of digestion and absorption. Supplemental nutrients are necessary to minimize the effects of vitamin and mineral deficiencies.
- The challenge of adequate nutritional intake in patients with anorexia nervosa often is compounded by a patient's distorted self-perception and internal physical sensations. For example, patients with anorexia nervosa do not perceive hunger as hunger, or after eating a small amount of food, they report a feeling of fullness. Absence of internal physical sensations also may result in excessive, strenuous exercising without an awareness of fatigue.
- Nurses may be instrumental in helping anorexic patients overcome their nutritional deficiencies by contracting with the patient for the intake of a certain amount of food each day, establishing a target weight, and having the patient discuss any fears related to weight gain and loss of control.
- Exercise should be limited in people who are underweight as a result of an eating disorder. Excessive physical exercise can result in decreased estrogen levels and consequent thinning of bones, which are then easily broken.

MUSCULOSKELETAL ALTERATIONS

Poor nutritional intake affects the musculoskeletal system by placing the person at risk for bone defects as a result of an imbalance of vitamins, particularly vitamins A and D. One of these defects is a softening of the bone due to vitamin D deficiency, referred to as *osteomalacia.* Poor absorption of calcium, which is facilitated by vitamin D, may lead to osteopenia or osteoporosis, in which bone mass density decreases and bone tissue deteriorates. Decreased bone mass density increases bone fragility, which increases the risk of fractures.

Deficiencies of minerals such as calcium, phosphorus, and magnesium also affect bone mass density. According to Notelovitz (2008), when adequate calcium is consumed, absorption is higher in children versus adults, providing better protective benefits. Decreased muscle size and strength (atrophy) limit the protection afforded to connective tissue and bones as well as the ability of the body to produce heat.

NEUROLOGIC ALTERATIONS

Nutritional intake has an impact on physical, emotional, and cognitive behavior. Poor nutrition may result in increased or decreased body fat, slower mental problem solving, decreased alertness, and slower muscle response time. Excess dietary intake of sodium is of particular concern because of its role in hypertension, which can lead to an increased incidence of stroke (cerebrovascular accident [CVA]). Stroke ranks fourth after heart disease, cancer, and chronic lower respiratory diseases as a major cause of death in the United States. This condition killed more than 129,000 Americans in 2010 (Murphy, Xu, and Kochanek, , 2013). The Evidence-Based Practice box highlights the importance of limited sodium intake.

A deficiency of folate contributes to the incidence of macrocytic or megaloblastic anemia. Folic acid deficiencies in the adult patient may be evident in symptoms such as depression, mental confusion, glossitis (inflamed tongue), loose stools, and a decrease in nerve function. Folic acid and some of the

EVIDENCE-BASED PRACTICE

Sodium Intake and Its Effect on Health

- On average, Americans consume more than double the recommended intake of sodium. The American Heart Association (2012b) recommends that sodium intake should not exceed 1500 mg per day. This restriction can be accomplished by choosing foods that are prepared with little or no salt.
- In the United States, hypertension is the major cause of cardiovascular disease; it is responsible for 62% of strokes and 49% of cases of coronary heart disease.
- Numerous health conditions such as left ventricular hypertrophy, renal disease, obesity from excessive soft drink consumption, renal calculi, asthma, and stomach cancer are linked to high salt intake.
- Salt reduction is one of the most cost-effective strategies to combat the epidemic of hypertension and associated cardiovascular disease and improve population health.
- The American Heart Association has joined with federal agencies to assist Americans to lower their consumption of sodium through strategies such as:
  - Reducing the amount of sodium in the food supply.
  - Making more healthy foods available (e.g., more fruits and vegetables).
  - Providing consumers with education and decision-making tools to help them make better choices.

other B vitamins have been researched for the treatment of memory loss and Alzheimer disease, a neurologic disorder that affects cognitive, memory, and functional ability (Linus Pauling Institute, 2011).

CARDIOPULMONARY ALTERATIONS

Imbalanced nutrition has significant effects on the cardiopulmonary system. Substances secreted from fat cells produce most of the pathologic changes that result in conditions such as atherosclerotic heart disease (ASHD). Cholesterol and lipids combine with other substances and have the propensity to attach themselves to the walls of the arteries, leading to multiple forms of coronary artery disease. In atherosclerosis, blood flow to a part of the heart is occluded due to the presence of plaque or a piece of plaque that has broken off and entered the arteries. This condition may lead to cardiac damage as a result of an acute myocardial infarction (AMI), or heart attack, due to the lack of blood flow to the heart tissue.

DIGESTIVE SYSTEM ALTERATIONS

Conditions that alter the digestive system affect the body's ability to metabolize and absorb nutrients. For digestion and absorption to occur properly, the ability to consume adequate amounts of food must be present. **Dysphagia** (difficulty in swallowing) may result from the presence of an obstruction from a mass or tumor, residual effects of a cerebrovascular accident (CVA), neurologic damage, or psychological disorders. **Malabsorption** (problematic or inadequate absorption of nutrients in the intestinal tract) may cause weight loss, fatigue, gastrointestinal upset (as seen in celiac disease or gluten-sensitive enteropathy), and vitamin and mineral deficiencies such as rickets (vitamin D deficiency) and scurvy (a deficiency of vitamin C). Deficiencies of vitamin C interfere with normal tissue synthesis and may result in gingivitis, which produces swollen and bleeding gums with loosened teeth, and painful, stiff joints. Other problems associated with malabsorption include anemia (a deficiency of red blood cells), excessive bleeding, petechiae (bleeding under the skin), poor wound healing, and neural tube defects. According to the World Health Organization (2013), approximately 30% of the more than 7.6 million deaths of children younger than 5 years of age worldwide are attributed to malnutrition secondary to conditions such as **marasmus**, resulting from both protein and calorie deficiency, and **kwashiorkor**, a lack of protein accompanied by fluid retention (Figure 30-4). Although these conditions primarily affect children in developing countries, they may be seen in vulnerable populations anywhere, including abused or neglected children or older adults.

Failure of the body to break down and properly use other nutrients may result in conditions such as phenylketonuria, a condition in which an infant's body fails to metabolize the amino acid phenylalanine. This inborn error of metabolism may result in impaired brain development, progressive cognitive delays, and irreversible damage. With any obstruction in the esophagus or gastrointestinal tract, nausea, vomiting, constipation, diarrhea, and severe pain may occur. Inflammatory bowel diseases such as Crohn's disease, diverticulitis, and ulcerative colitis can have a significant impact on nutritional

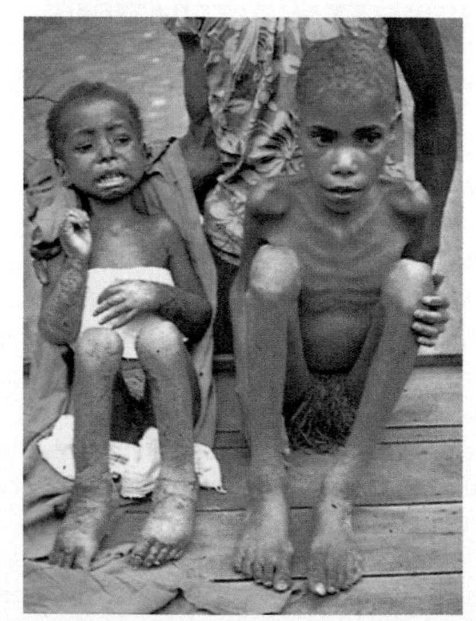

FIGURE 30-4 Children with malnutrition-related conditions: *left,* marasmus; *right,* kwashiorkor. (From Forbes C, Jackson W: *Color atlas and text of clinical medicine,* ed. 2, St. Louis, 2003, Mosby.)

health. For additional information on conditions that contribute to malabsorption or elimination problems, see Chapter 40.

METABOLIC ALTERATIONS

The body's metabolism typically works effectively without a conscious awareness of the processes taking place. If metabolism is altered by an imbalance of enzymes or hormones or their malfunction, the subsequent excess or deficiency may lead to serious illness. Symptoms of metabolic alterations vary depending on the enzyme or hormone imbalance involved.

Diabetes Mellitus

Controlling excessive amounts of circulating glucose in the body is one of the responsibilities of the pancreas. The pancreas has a major role in producing insulin. Insulin aids in regulating the use and storage of glucose, the end product of carbohydrate metabolism. Failure of the pancreas to produce adequate insulin to regulate glucose levels allows the accumulation of glucose in the circulatory system and its decreased diffusion, or entry, into the cells. This results in a condition known as *diabetes mellitus.* The two common types of diabetes are insulin-dependent (IDDM), or type 1, and non–insulin-dependent (NIDDM), or type 2. Replacement of insulin through injections is necessary for the proper metabolism of glucose in patients with type 1 diabetes. Although injectable insulin used to be derived from the pancreas of pigs or cattle, it is now biosynthetic, eliminating concerns for people who do not consume pork or beef. Oral antiglycemic agents, diet, and exercise are most frequently effective in controlling glucose levels in type 2 diabetics. Patients with diabetes are at high risk for developing blindness (because of retinal changes), renal failure, neuropathy (loss of sensation in the lower extremities), and poor wound healing.

Allergies and Intolerances

Patients may have allergies or intolerances to various foods or dietary supplements that should be noted. Food allergies are a response of the immune system that occurs when the body erroneously identifies an ingredient or food product as harmful and produces antibodies to fight it. The most common food allergens include peanuts, fish, shellfish, tree nuts such as pecans or almonds, and wheat.

Food intolerances trigger a digestive system response, resulting in the irritation of the digestive tract or the inability to digest or break down food. Lactose intolerance, which may occur after consuming dairy products, is the most common food intolerance. Whereas food intolerance causes discomfort, food allergies are potentially life-threatening.

Obesity

Obesity in adults is defined as a **body mass index (BMI)** of 30 or higher. Obesity is prevalent throughout the world. According to the U.S. Department of Health and Human Services (2011), obesity is "epidemic." The following statistics support that health concern:

- Two thirds of adults and nearly one third of children are overweight or obese.
- Approximately 70% of American Indian and Alaskan Native adults are overweight or obese.
- The prevalence of obesity in the United States more than doubled (from 15% to 34%) among adults and more than tripled (from 5% to 17%) among children and adolescents from 1980 to 2008.
- Compared with a nonobese teenager, an obese teenager has more than a 70% greater risk of becoming an obese adult.
- Obesity is more common among non-Hispanic black teenagers (29%) than Hispanic teenagers (17.5%) or non-Hispanic white teenagers (14.5%).

Individuals are classified as morbidly obese when their BMI is greater than 40 or they are more than 50% above their ideal body weight. Morbid obesity is known to interfere with the normal activities of daily living. Overweight (BMI between 25 and 29.9) and obesity contribute to an increased incidence of health-related conditions such as diabetes, hypertension, heart disease, and other chronic diseases.

BMI is a helpful tool for determining the extent of obesity and its potential health complications. According to the National Institutes of Health, as BMI levels rise, blood pressure and cholesterol levels also rise, and the average high-density lipoprotein (HDL), or good, cholesterol levels decrease. Men with a high BMI (above 31.3) are at greater risk for hypertension, hyperlipidemia, or both compared with men of normal weight. **Hyperlipidemia** (elevation of plasma cholesterol, triglycerides, or both) or low HDL levels contribute to the development of atherosclerosis (buildup of fat deposits on arterial vessel walls). Women with an elevated BMI (above 32.3) have four times the risk for development of either or both of these conditions. Nutrition and weight status objectives from *Healthy People 2020* are outlined in Box 30-1.

Malnutrition

Just as obesity is seen worldwide, so is malnutrition. Malnutrition may result from absorption or digestive problems, illness, or an inadequate or imbalanced intake of calories. Sadly, although plenty of food is available to feed everyone on earth, it most often is a problem with distribution or access that leads to many cases of malnutrition. Malnutrition may be mild and cause few or no symptoms, or it also may lead to starvation and death. As discussed earlier, the lack of just one vitamin can cause an individual to be malnourished. Children are especially vulnerable to malnutrition. Poverty, government discord, and natural disasters such as drought may lead to famines or epidemics of malnutrition.

BOX 30-1 Nutrition and Weight Status Objectives From *Healthy People 2020*

Healthier Food Access

- Increase the number of states with nutrition standards for foods and beverages provided to preschool-age children in child care.
- Increase the proportion of schools that offer nutritious foods and beverages outside school meals.
- Increase the number of states that have state-level policies that incentivize food retail outlets to provide foods that are encouraged by the Dietary Guidelines for Americans.
- Increase the proportion of Americans who have access to a food retail outlet that sells a variety of foods that are encouraged by the Dietary Guidelines for Americans.

Health Care and Work Site Settings

- Increase the proportion of primary care physicians who regularly measure the BMI of their patients.
- Increase the proportion of physician office visits that include counseling or education related to nutrition or weight.
- Increase the proportion of work sites that offer nutrition or weight management classes or counseling.

Weight Status

- Increase the proportion of adults who are at a healthy weight.
- Reduce the proportion of adults who are obese.
- Reduce the proportion of children and adolescents who are considered obese. Prevent inappropriate weight gain in youths and adults.

Food Insecurity

- Eliminate very low food security among children.
- Reduce household food insecurity and, in doing so, reduce hunger.

Food and Nutrient Consumption

- Increase the contribution of fruits to the diets of the population age 2 years and older.
- Increase the variety and contribution of vegetables to the diets of the population age 2 years and older.
- Increase the contribution of whole grains to the diets of the population age 2 years and older. Increase the contribution of whole grains to the diets of the population age 2 years and older
- Reduce consumption of calories from solid fats and added sugars in the population age 2 years and older.
- Reduce consumption of saturated fat in the population age 2 years and older.
- Reduce consumption of sodium in the population age 2 years and older.
- Increase consumption of calcium in the population age 2 years and older.

Iron Deficiency

- Reduce iron deficiency among young children and females of childbearing age.
- Reduce iron deficiency among pregnant females.

From U.S. Department of Health and Human Services: *Healthy People 2020,* 2014. Retrieved from *www.healthypeople.gov/2020/topicsobjectives2020/objectiveslist.aspx?topicId=29.*

PSYCHOLOGICAL ALTERATIONS

The term **anorexia** refers to a loss of appetite in patients experiencing illness or side effects from allergies, medications, or treatments, such as chemotherapy, that suppress the desire to eat. These symptoms typically dissipate after resolution of the illness or treatment. Two major psychological alterations, however, are linked to improper nutritional intake, lack of absorption, and metabolism of nutrients: anorexia nervosa and bulimia.

Anorexia Nervosa

Anorexia nervosa is a serious disorder in which the person exhibits life-threatening practices as a result of an altered mental state. This disorder may be used to gain some sense of control, especially when diagnosed in adolescents and young adults. Adolescents and young adults may feel as though they have no control over their lives; they may experience hopelessness in establishing relationships or dealing with family conflicts. Strict dietary intake regulation seen in anorexia nervosa may be used as a means of gaining control. The disorder may begin as a result of the desire to be thin through strict dieting and then the desire becomes more of an obsession. There is a distortion of body image, with an intense fear of gaining weight or being viewed as "fat," despite the fact that the individual's weight is less than healthy or normal, according to the National Association for Anorexia Nervosa and Associated Disorders (ANAD) (2012).

Many factors contribute to the eating disorder, such as limited caloric intake, omission of healthy foods, excessive exercise routines, and obsessive behaviors. These behaviors may include excessive use of laxatives or diuretics, self-induced vomiting, and refusal to socialize with friends or family when food is involved. According to ANAD, it is estimated that approximately 15% of people diagnosed with anorexia will die from malnutrition complications such as cardiac arrhythmias, anemia, kidney dysfunction, decreased immune system, infections, muscle and bone injuries, or suicide (2012). The Ethical, Legal, and Professional Practice box addresses some of the concerns associated with caring for adolescents suffering from anorexia nervosa.

Bulimia Nervosa

Bulimia nervosa is another common eating disorder. This illness involves an obsession with **bingeing** (the intake of excessive amounts of food), as many as 2000 to 3000 calories at one time, followed by **purging** (vomiting). In an effort not to gain weight from the excessive amount of food eaten, the person may use self-induced vomiting or excessive exercise. Bulimia may also result from the abuse of laxatives or

ETHICAL, LEGAL, AND PROFESSIONAL PRACTICE

Treatment of Adolescents With Eating Disorders

The issue of how best to treat adolescents suffering from eating disorders is a challenging one for health care professionals. Certain bioethical concepts must guide the decision making of nurses participating in and guiding patient care. This is especially true in cases of forced hospitalization.

- Involving adolescents in decisions about their care reinforces the ethical principle of autonomy.
  - This becomes especially challenging when issues of competency arise regarding the young adolescent's ability to make sound treatment decisions.
- Determining the extent to which adolescents suffering from eating disorders may harm themselves must be a factor in deciding plans of care. This approach supports the ethical principle of beneficence, or doing no harm.
- Health care insurance policies that do not cover specialized inpatient treatment may be a challenge to the ethical concept of justice, or equity, of social and medical resources.
  - Although most adolescents with eating disorders can be treated on an outpatient basis, those who exhibit severe depression, extreme physical complications secondary to electrolyte imbalances, or suicidal tendencies may require extensive inpatient treatment.
- Research indicates that although forced hospitalization is indicated in some cases of anorexia, compulsory tube feedings are not always the best option.
- Highly skilled nursing care with hospitalization is preferred before BMI drops below 13 kg/m^2.
- Ultimately, the decision on how best to ethically treat an adolescent suffering from an eating disorder needs to be one of collaboration among the child's physician, nurse, counselor, spiritual adviser, parents, and other concerned adults.
- All treatment decisions must be considered within the legal context of the country and/or state in which the child resides.
  - Related issues include the age of consent, the age limit up to which parents are required to be informed of a child's medical issues, and the age limit up to which parents are permitted to access confidential information about a child.

From Michaud P, Berd-Kelly K, Macfarlane A, et al: Ethics and adolescent care: An international perspective, *Curr Opin Pediatr* 22(4):418-422, 2010.

diuretics. It is not known specifically what causes this eating disorder, but it is thought to be a combination of psychological, biologic, and sociocultural factors. Complications from bulimia nervosa may vary, ranging from tooth decay or mild gastrointestinal symptoms to more serious ones such as electrolyte imbalance, cardiac dysrhythmias, heart failure, and death. Identification of these problems is extremely important, and treatment must be expeditiously initiated to obtain a favorable patient outcome.

Early identification of people with the predisposition for such behaviors is essential to minimize the long-term effects of eating disorders. Assessing adolescents and understanding the vulnerability of this age group promote early intervention. Recognizing relationship pressures from peers or family is imperative. Each aspect of the person's life has to be assessed to determine the underlying factors that contribute to the disordered eating behavior. When providing patient education, the health care professional should focus on body weight, nutrition, and exercise while stressing the importance of avoiding behaviors that could result in eating disorders. The health care professional also should recognize the family's role in collaborating with the physician, psychologist, family therapist, and registered dietitian in clinical management of the person suffering from an eating disorder.

◆ ASSESSMENT LO 30.3

Assessment of a patient's nutritional status includes observation of the patient's general health and completion of a health history followed by physical assessment (Health Assessment Questions box). The process is time-consuming, yet it is essential for determining dietary needs and nutritional status.

HEALTH ASSESSMENT QUESTIONS

Nutrition Focus

- What was your dietary intake for the past 24 hours?
- Have you noticed any changes in appetite or food intake?
- Have you gained or lost weight in the past month?
- While eating, do you experience any difficulty chewing or swallowing?
- Are you taking any prescribed or over-the-counter (OTC) medication that may be affecting your sense of taste or smell?
- Do you experience any gastric distress after eating, such as nausea, vomiting, heartburn, increased flatulence (gas), or changes in your bowel pattern (e.g., loose stools or constipation)?
- Are you allergic to or unable to tolerate any foods, such as milk or other dairy products?
- When looking in a mirror, what parts of your body do you think are your best or worst features, and why?
- How do you feel about your weight?
- How often do you weigh yourself?
- Have you ever used diet pills, laxatives, diuretics (water pills), or vomiting to lose weight?
- Do you ever feel that your eating is out of control?

NUTRITION HISTORY

The nurse should conduct a nutrition history, noting dietary intake and any changes in weight or appetite reported by the patient. Collection of a diet history allows the nurse to analyze data regarding the type and quantity of foods consumed, establish baseline values for identifying any health problems that may adversely affect the patient's nutritional status, and identify the need for nursing interventions. When collecting data, the nurse should take into consideration the patient's culture and ethnicity. Recognizing these influences on the patient's nutritional intake allows the nurse to make informed decisions. The data analysis may reveal the need to refer the patient to a registered dietitian for further evaluation of nutritional status. The registered dietitian performs additional assessments that result in recommendations for an individualized program of exercise, diet, and behavior modifications designed to meet the patient's nutritional needs.

Two common practices for obtaining information regarding the patient's dietary patterns are the 24-hour recall and the food diary. The 24-hour recall is dependent on the ability of the patient to remember consumption of foods and their quantities from the previous day. It is vital to remember that the patient's recall may not be factual and the intake may not be that of a typical day. The other means of assessing a patient's usual dietary pattern is to have the patient keep a written journal of food intake for a certain amount of time. The food diary should encompass entries for 3 to 5 days and include dietary intake for a typical weekend. The patient should be encouraged to include the type and amount of food and how the food was prepared (i.e., fried, grilled, with gravies or sauces). The nurse reviewing the journal entries or discussing the patient's recall of foods eaten should be nonjudgmental to motivate the person to better understand and use the information in ways that will promote and maintain good health. With the evaluation of the dietary history and a collaborative approach, the needs of the patient are met holistically.

A full nutritional assessment may be performed on admission if the nurse suspects eating disorders or an altered nutritional status. It is important to recognize that altered nutritional states may include a variety of problems associated with physiologic, psychological, socioeconomic, cultural, and religious factors, among other health-related issues. All patients should be asked about their typical dietary intake, food preferences, and allergies.

Screening for Malnutrition in Older Adults

Nurses must be sure to consider the effects of nutrition on older adults. Assessment of the older adult (age 65 years of age and older) must include close attention to the mouth, teeth, and gums. Consideration must be given to the decrease in sense organ function related to aging, such as changes in the ability to smell, taste, chew, and digest food. Other physiologic changes may include increased fat stores, limited activity, decreased bone mass, decreased kidney function, and a decline in the immune system. These changes place the older person at risk for obesity, poor tolerance of activity, fractures, renal failure, and increased susceptibility to infection. Tools such as the Mini Nutritional Assessment (MNA) or the DETERMINE self-assessment are helpful in screening for malnutrition in older adults. The acronym *DETERMINE* stands for "disease, eating poorly, tooth loss, economic hardship, reduced social contact, multiple meds, involuntary weight loss, needs assistance in self-care, and elderly above age 80" (Duffy, 2012).

PHYSICAL ASSESSMENT

A thorough physical assessment with a focus on nutritional status includes height and weight measurements, determination of BMI, evaluation of laboratory values, notation of any adverse signs and symptoms typical of malnourished people (poor dentition, poor skin turgor, or dull, thinning hair), and recognition of any existing physical and psychological illness. Assessment of the person's waist circumference, vital signs, past medical history, current medications, and activity level is essential in identifying the potential risk factors for cardiovascular diseases related to imbalanced nutrition (Box 30-2).

Morphology

Determining the patient's BMI is helpful to establish the presence of obesity, malnutrition, or cachexia (Nursing Care Guideline box). **Cachexia** (physical wasting) often is seen in patient suffering from terminal illnesses who are unable to consume an adequate intake of food; the effects of the disease are evident in weight loss and the loss of muscle mass. Malnutrition may result as a consequence of eating disorders, dysphagia (difficulty swallowing), irritable bowel syndrome, chronic alcoholism, celiac disease, and intestinal damage from radiation therapy. It also may result from unmet

BOX 30-2 Waist Circumference and Risks for Cardiovascular Disease

- Abdominal fat (waist circumference) has a higher risk associated with it than overall fatness as reflected by BMI results.
- BMI uses the weight-for-height standard and is a convenient tool for determining whether a person is overweight or underweight and obesity level.
- The risks for cardiovascular disease increase as the BMI rises.
- An apparent correlation has been found between waist-to-hip ratio and the development of specific disease conditions.
- People with "apple-shaped" bodies, with more fat deposited around the waist, are more likely to develop cardiovascular and pulmonary diseases, such as irregular cardiac rhythms, hypertension, and sleep apnea, as well as breast cancer and diabetes. People with "pear-shaped" bodies store most of the accumulated fat below the waist, in the buttocks and thighs, and are more likely to develop varicose veins and bone disorders such as osteoporosis (Klein et al, 2007).
- In North America, a waist size of 88 cm (35 inches) for women and 102 cm (40 inches) for men puts them in the high-risk category for heart disease.

increased metabolic needs in patients with infection, sepsis, burn injury, or cancer.

Anthropometric Measurements

Nurses often use **anthropometry** (the study of measurements of the human body) when performing nutritional or growth and development assessments of infants and children. The measurements include height, weight, length (used in infants and toddlers because they are unable to stand), and head circumference. These measurements must be accurate to be valid.

Anthropometric measurements used for adults usually include height, weight, BMI, and waist-to-hip ratio. These findings are compared against reference standards to assess weight status (underweight, ideal weight, overweight) and the risk for various diseases.

The distribution of body fat is significant in determining health risk potential. A strong relationship is recognized between obesity and cardiovascular health. Waist circumference can be used as a strong diagnostic criterion for metabolic syndrome, which is a cluster of medical conditions characterized by insulin resistance and the presence of obesity, significant abdominal fat, elevated blood glucose and serum triglycerides and cholesterol, and hypertension. The increasing number of people with this condition is linked to the rise in obesity rates among adults. In the future, metabolic syndrome may overtake smoking as the leading risk factor for heart disease (National Heart, Lung, and Blood Institute, 2011).

Skinfold measurements are one means of determining a person's body composition and body fat percentage. The percentage of body fat is estimated by measuring skinfold thickness, using calipers, at specific locations on the body. The thickness of the folds is a measure of the fat under the skin, also called *subcutaneous adipose tissue.* Skinfold thickness results rely on formulas that convert the numbers into an estimate of body fat stores and nutritional status for the person's age and gender.

NURSING CARE GUIDELINE

Height and Weight Assessment and Body Mass Index Calculation

Background

- Height, weight, and BMI assessment is used to track weight trends, which can be an indicator of disease processes.
- BMI is not an independent diagnostic assessment. It is part of a full assessment of various body systems.

Procedural Concerns

Height

- Is the patient capable of weight bearing?
  - Instruct the patient to remove his or her shoes and stand erect.
  - Use a tape measure or scale measure.
  - Make sure there is a 90-degree angle from the top of the head to the measurement device for accuracy.
- Is the patient not capable of weight bearing?
  - Instruct the patient to remove his or her shoes; assist if needed.
  - Position the top of the patient's head against the headboard or measuring device for accuracy.
  - Instruct the patient to straighten the body and legs; assist if needed. Measure from the top of the head to the bottom of the heel; some measuring devices have movable footboards.

Weight

- When repeated measurements of the patient's weight are needed, make sure the patient is weighed at the same time of day, on the same scale, and in the same clothing (if possible) for each measurement.
- Instruct the patient to remove his or her shoes; assist if needed.
- Follow the manufacturer's directions for the scale used (electronic, platform, stretcher, chair, bed).

Body Mass Index

- Standard BMI calculations are assessed for patients older than 20 years of age. Specific BMI charts are available for patients younger than 20 years.
- Calculation is the weight in kilograms/(height in meters)^2.
- Interpretations of BMI calculations are:
  - Less than 18.5 kg/m^2 = Underweight
  - 18.5 kg/m^2 to 24.9 kg/m^2 = Normal weight
  - 25.0 kg/m^2 to 29.9 kg/m^2 = Overweight
  - 30.0 kg/m^2 to 34.9 kg/m^2 = Obese (class 1)
  - 35.0 kg/m^2 to 39.9 kg/m^2 = Obese (class 2)
  - More than 39.9 kg/m^2 = Extreme obesity (class 3)

Documentation Concerns

- Document and graph the patient's height, weight, and BMI in accordance with facility policy and procedure.
- Notify the primary care provider (PCP) of unusual or unexpected changes in height or weight.

Evidence-Based Practice

- It is important to calculate and document a patient's BMI and educate the patient regarding the interpretation. Patients who do not perceive themselves as overweight are not likely to participate in weight-control behaviors. Education may begin to change this perception (Bak-Sosnowska and Zahorska-Markiewicz, 2009; Foti and Lowry, 2010).
- There has been discussion on whether BMI is truly a reliable and valid instrument to determine weight-related health risks. Gelber, Kurth, Manson, et al (2007) performed a study of approximately 100,000 adult males that consistently found an increased risk of mortality when the BMI was not within the normal weight range.

Skin and Hair

The influence of improper nutrition on the skin is evident during the physical assessment. Poor nutrition is reflected by the presence of thinning hair that has a dry, stiff texture and lack of shine. In severe cases of malnutrition, hair may totally lose its color and appear pale. The lips can have a deep red appearance with open lesions and deep cracks in the corners of the mouth. The oral mucosa may be a darker red than normal, with oral lesions, and/or the tongue may reveal white irregular areas. In conditions such as pernicious anemia, a characteristic finding is a sore, smooth-surfaced, beefy-red tongue; the soreness may interfere with the person's ability to chew certain foods.

A dry, rough appearance of the skin, pallor, and changes in the pigmentation of the skin may be noted. Skin may be easily bruised or have small pinpoint hemorrhages under the skin (petechiae). Skin changes in the more severely malnourished person may range from loose, wrinkled skin (due to loss of underlying fat tissue) to deep wounds that will not heal.

Skin turgor is an indication of the patient's level of hydration. In dehydration, when the skin is pinched, the skin takes on the appearance of a tent and returns to its original position very slowly. See Chapter 29 for further information on skin integrity and the use of skin assessment tools.

Dentition

Older adults can retain their teeth with proper care. Normal wear and tear occurs with the aging process, resulting in the loss of tooth integrity: decreased amount of enamel, shrinkage of the gum tissue, and lengthening of the teeth, with the diminished ability of the teeth to cut and chew efficiently. However, a high prevalence of tooth loss also has been documented in the older adult population. Loss of natural dentition affects nutrient consumption and may result in the increased development of cardiovascular disease. Edentulous people have been found to have significantly higher BMI values (Oral Care Report, 2007). The increase in BMI appears to occur from increased consumption of high-calorie foods with low-level nutrients, such as soft, sweet foods that promote obesity. Nutritional intake and chewing efficiency often are not significantly compensated in people with partial or complete dentures.

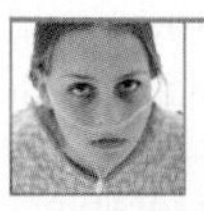

1. Identify three pieces of data that would be essential for the nurse to document while caring for Amy on the nursing unit.

Swallow Studies

People who have residual effects of stroke or other injury may experience dysphagia or choking during meals. People who have difficulty swallowing are also at risk of aspirating food and fluids into their lungs. Inhaling oral secretions or stomach contents may result in complications that vary from aspiration pneumonia to respiratory distress to death. Factors responsible for these complications are the amount and the character of the aspirated contents.

Individuals at risk for **aspiration** (inhalation of fluid or foreign matter into the lungs and bronchi) should be monitored closely for coughing, wheezing, dyspnea, apnea, bradycardia, and hypotension. Depending on the patient's condition—level of consciousness, recent sedation, ability to reposition self, limited mobility, and/or restrictions—and if the patient has been intubated for a long period of time, aspiration precaution measures should be established (Palmer, 2008) (Nursing Care Guideline box). People with these risk factors may need a swallow study or dysphagia screening. Swallow studies are normally conducted by a speech therapist. A registered dietitian will help to determine the most appropriate food textures and means of hydration. If the person is unable to take nutrition and hydration orally, the dietitian may make a recommendation to the patient's PCP for a nonoral route, such as an enteral feeding tube, total parenteral nutrition (TPN), or nasogastric tube (for short-term therapy).

QSEN FOCUS!

Recognizing the value of contributions from other members of the health care team demonstrates an understanding of each person's unique professional role in helping patients achieve their health care goals.

LABORATORY STUDIES

Laboratory tests add objectivity to the nutritional assessment. No single laboratory value will specifically predict nutritional risk or measure the presence or degree of malnutrition or the response to nutritional intervention therapy. However, some levels, such as serum protein or prealbumin levels, are affected by factors such as fluid balance, liver and renal function, acute stress, and colloid administration. Normal values for tests performed vary with institutions, testing facilities, and authors. It is important that nurses monitor laboratory results ordered by the PCP, to complement information obtained in a complete assessment of the patient.

Prealbumin

Prealbumin levels are a measure of the amount of protein contained in the internal organs. Protein is synthesized in the liver and broken down by the kidneys. Prealbumin assays are valuable for determining recent nutritional status. Prealbumin levels below 11 mg/dL indicate the presence of malnutrition (Table 30-2). Decreased prealbumin levels may result from stress, inflammation, surgery, and renal failure.

Albumin

Assessment of plasma protein levels such as albumin often is used to determine liver function. Albumin is synthesized in the liver and accounts for almost half of the total serum

NURSING CARE GUIDELINE

Aspiration Precautions

Background

- Aspiration precautions are taken to prevent the following materials from entering the lungs of at-risk patients instead of being swallowed:
  - Food
  - Fluid
  - Saliva
  - Other foreign objects
- To determine whether there is a risk of aspiration, do any or all of the following:
  - Consult the nutritional therapist.
  - Consult the speech therapist.
  - Have a swallow study done on the patient.
- Conditions that place patients at risk include:
  - Seizures
  - Cerebrovascular accidents
  - Dementia
  - Gastroesophageal reflux disease (GERD)
  - Cerebral palsy, muscular dystrophy, multiple sclerosis, Parkinson disease, and other diseases affecting mobility
  - Endoscopy procedures
  - Medications with a sedative or muscle relaxant effect, including anesthesia
  - Feeding of the patient by another person or an eating pattern that is too fast

Procedural Concerns

- Follow orders for dietary consistencies and textures.
- Follow the manufacturer's instructions and facility policies and procedures for thickening of liquids as ordered.
- Elevate the head of the bed to 45 degrees or higher during eating and tor a minimum of 45 minutes after eating.
- Keep the head of the bed elevated to 30 degrees at all other times, including during enteral feeding.
- Encourage slow eating patterns.
- Instruct the patient to avoid eating or drinking for 2 to 3 hours before sleep.
- Administer gastrointestinal medications as ordered.
- Inspect the patient's mouth for pocketing of food.
- Observe the patient for swallowing between bites of food and fluids.
- Instruct the patient to alternate between bites of food and sips of fluids to facilitate swallowing.
- Maintain patient NPO status after procedures in which the throat was anesthetized, until return of a gag reflex has been verified.

Documentation Concerns

- Document any gagging, choking, and/or coughing during meals.
- Monitor respiratory status.
- Note any intermittent fevers that may occur.
- Record hesitance or fear of eating.
- Include occurrences of nausea, vomiting, regurgitation, and/or reflux symptoms.
- Document any dehydration and/or weight loss.
- Describe the aspiration protocol and plan of care expectations and guidelines.

Evidence-Based Practice

- Nurses often are the first health care provider to notice signs or symptoms of aspiration pneumonia. Although aspiration pneumonia is actually a rare occurrence, when it does happen, it has a high mortality rate. As a result, it is imperative that nurses implement all precautions possible to decrease the risk of aspiration. It also is necessary to recognize that complete elimination of this risk is not possible (Goodwin, 2009; Hines, Wallace, Crowe, et al, 2011).

TABLE 30-2 Laboratory Values Indicating Degrees of Malnutrition

TEST	HALF-LIFE (DAYS)	NORMAL	MILD	MODERATE	SEVERE
Prealbumin (mg/dL)	2	16-30	10-15	5-10	<5
Albumin (g/dL)	21	3.5-5.0	2.8-3.5	2.1-2.7	<2.1
Transferrin (mg/dL)	8-9	200-400	150-200	100-150	<100

From Dawodu S: Nutritional management in the rehabilitation setting, 2013. Retrieved from *http://emedicine.medscape.com/article/318180-overview*.

protein in the human body. Albumin levels should be included on the initial chemistry profile for nutritional screening purposes and monitored during hospitalization to determine the presence of an ample supply of protein over an extended period of time. The synthesis of protein may be affected by nonnutritional factors such as cirrhosis, acute stress, congestive heart failure, and hypoxia. Decreased levels may be caused by renal and liver disorders, altered fluid status, medications, chronic diseases, and malnutrition. Elevated levels may result from decreased fluid balance (dehydration), exercise, or medications.

Transferrin

Transferrin transports iron in the body and is sensitive to a decrease in protein and iron stores, as seen in iron deficiency anemia and kwashiorkor. Transferrin levels may be elevated in acute fasting, chronic infection, inflammation, burns, or pernicious anemia. Transferrin levels become elevated as the deficiency worsens and decrease as the iron level responds to treatment and returns to within an acceptable range. See Table 30-2 for key prealbumin, albumin, and transferrin levels.

Hemoglobin and Hematocrit

Hemoglobin and hematocrit laboratory values are used to identify the number and percentage of circulating erythrocytes, their ability to provide oxygen to the cells, and the body's iron store status. Iron is an essential portion of hemoglobin. It assists in gas exchange within the lungs and helps meet the oxygen demands of the body. If iron stores are depleted, less oxygen is available to meet the demands of the body, resulting in signs and symptoms such as fatigue, pallor, shortness of breath, and rapid respirations. Iron deficiency anemia indicated by low hemoglobin levels usually is treated by providing iron in the form of oral supplements or intramuscular injections. People with low hemoglobin should be encouraged to increase their intake of foods that are high in iron such as liver, dark-green leafy vegetables, seafood, and bran.

The hematocrit indicates the number and size of the red blood cells found in whole blood and are expressed as the percentage of total blood volume occupied by the erythrocytes. A low hematocrit is indicative of anemia. The size and shape of the red blood cell can be related to the type of anemia from which a person is suffering.

Blood Urea Nitrogen and Creatinine

Blood urea nitrogen (BUN) and serum creatinine assays (tests) commonly are ordered together as part of a basic or comprehensive metabolic profile. These two tests are used primarily to evaluate kidney function in people with disease processes known to affect the kidneys, such as diabetes or hypertension. BUN and serum creatinine levels determine the extent of kidney dysfunction, its progression, and the effectiveness of treatment. Elevated levels may be a result of dehydration, atherosclerosis, or injury to the kidneys from infection or trauma. For further information on diagnostic tests and normal values, see Chapter 34.

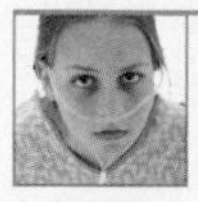

2. List three laboratory values (and give a rationale for each) that the nurse needs to monitor in relation to Amy's nutritional status.

ELIMINATION PATTERNS

A thorough abdominal assessment should be performed, including attention to the presence of bowel sounds; bowel pattern; color, amount, and character of stools; and use of laxatives.

Good or poor nutrition can have a drastic impact on bowel elimination. Constipation (hard stools) results from the slow progression of digested food through the gastrointestinal tract. Lack of fluids or fiber can create dry, hardened feces and make evacuation of the bowel difficult. Patients should be instructed to increase their intake of fluids and add foods with high insoluble fiber content to the diet unless contraindicated by conditions such as diverticulitis.

Excessive bowel elimination, referred to as *diarrhea,* may be a result of high fat intake, use of artificial sweeteners, or excessive intake of insoluble fibers. Increasing the amount of soluble fiber, which absorbs excess water and firms the stools, aids in delaying gastric emptying and, as a result, eases the diarrhea. Loss of fluids through diarrhea or vomiting may result in fluid and electrolyte imbalance, as may overuse of laxatives. Accurate documentation of a patient's elimination patterns is an essential aspect of nutritional assessment.

◆ NURSING DIAGNOSIS LO 30.4

Once patient information and assessment data (subjective and objective) are collected and the patient's problems are identified and grouped together, the nurse develops nursing diagnostic statements based on the findings. These statements are the foundation on which the patient's care plan will be developed.

Common nursing diagnoses directly related to altered nutritional intake are:

- *Imbalanced Nutrition: More/Less than Body Requirements*
- *Impaired Swallowing*
- *Risk for Aspiration*
- *Feeding: Self-Care Deficit*
- *Readiness for Enhanced Nutrition*

Additional nursing diagnoses related to specific body systems may also be relevant for the individual patient.

Examples of nursing diagnostic statements are:

- *Imbalanced Nutrition: Less than Body Requirements* related to inadequate dietary intake, as evidenced by cachectic appearance and 40-lb weight loss in past 6 months

- *Impaired Swallowing* related to residual effects of neurologic damage secondary to cerebrovascular accident, as evidenced by gagging and choking with oral intake attempts
- *Imbalanced Nutrition: More than Body Requirements* related to daily intake of excessive number of calories, as evidenced by weight gain of 5 lb over a week
- *Risk for Aspiration* with risk factor of difficulty swallowing secondary to facial paralysis
- *Feeding: Self-Care Deficit* related to sensory and motor deficits secondary to spinal cord injury, as evidenced by bilateral upper-extremity paralysis and an inability to self-feed
- *Readiness for Enhanced Nutrition* related to expression of desire for a balanced, healthy dietary intake and verbalization of American Diabetic Association nutritional guidelines

PLANNING LO 30.5

After prioritization of the patient's needs, appropriate goals or outcomes are identified, and decisions are made to perform specific nursing actions aimed at helping the patient achieve the identified goals or outcomes. Collaboration with the patient and with other members of the health care team is crucial to attain the best possible outcomes (Collaboration and Delegation box).

Goals may be short- or long-term and should be realistic and measurable. As nurses initiate the planning portion of the patient's plan of care (Table 30-3), they need to have specific objectives in mind for the patient to accomplish as a result of the individualized nursing care being delivered. Consideration must be given to the possible need for home care, referrals to community resources, or assistive devices upon discharge.

Examples of goals or outcome statements are:

- Patient will gain 1 to 2 lb each week until weight is within normal range.
- Patient will not exhibit any signs or symptoms of aspiration during this hospitalization (e.g., lungs clear, respiratory rate within normal range for patient).

COLLABORATION AND DELEGATION

Providing Comprehensive Nutritional Care

- A registered dietitian is helpful in providing nutritional education and services that may address the psychosocial and economic factors that affect patient care.
- Case managers are responsible for coordinating timely, cost-effective inpatient and outpatient services such as provision of durable medical equipment, infusion therapy, and transportation for patients and follow-up after discharge to promote quality care.
- Collaboration with a speech therapist is needed for patients who have impaired swallowing and/or require restorative therapy.
- Collaboration with a board-certified psychologist may be necessary if psychological factors might have an impact on the patient's recovery.
- Assistance with feeding can be delegated to unlicensed assistive personnel (UAP).

- Patient will identify factors related to obesity before discharge.
- Patient will demonstrate the ability to use assistive devices for self-feeding before discharge.
- Patient will be able to restate the side effects of newly prescribed medication before the end of the shift.
- Patient will explain the disease process (anorexia) and need for prescribed treatment (total parenteral nutrition) by the end of the day.

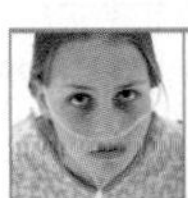

The conceptual care map for Amy provided in Figure 30-5 is partially completed to indicate how to use the map as a learning tool. Using it as an example, go to the website at *http://evolve.elsevier.com/YoostCrawford/fundamentals/* to complete Nursing Diagnoses 2 and 3.

IMPLEMENTATION AND EVALUATION LO 30.6

Proper nutrition is necessary to prevent the adverse effects associated with excessive or minimal intake of the proper

TABLE 30-3 Care Planning

NANDA-I NURSING DIAGNOSIS LABEL WITH NURSING DIAGNOSIS STATEMENT	NURSING OUTCOME CLASSIFICATION (NOC)	NURSING INTERVENTION CLASSIFICATION (NIC)
Imbalanced Nutrition: Less than Body Requirements related to inadequate dietary intake as evidenced by cachectic appearance and 40-lb weight loss in past 6 months	*Nutritional status: Food and fluid intake* (1008) Oral food intake (100801)	*Eating disorders management* (1030) Monitor patient for behaviors related to eating, weight loss, and weight gain.

From Bulechek G, Butcher H, Dochterman J, et al (Eds): *Nursing interventions classification (NIC),* ed. 6, St. Louis, 2013, Mosby; Moorhead S, Johnson M, Maas M, et al (Eds): *Nursing outcomes classification (NOC),* ed. 5, St. Louis, 2013, Mosby; NANDA International: *Nursing diagnoses: Definitions and classification, 2012–2014,* West Sussex, England, 2012, Wiley-Blackwell. Reprinted with permission from NANDA International, Inc.

Medications

IV Sites/Fluids/Rate

Conceptual Care Map

Student name__________ Patient initials A Date __________

Age 17 Gender F Room # ___ Admission date __________

CODE Status Full Allergies NKDA

Diet High-calorie adult general Activity BRP Braden score 19

Weight 98 lb Height 5′ 6″ Religion Roman Catholic

Admitting Diagnoses/Chief Complaint

Severe weight loss; nausea, vomiting, and blood-tinged emesis

Assessment Data

T 36.2° C (97.2° F); P 90, regular; R 16, unlabored and regular; BP 98/68; O_2 saturation 93% on 2L of oxygen; pain 2-3 of 10 when vomiting.

Cachectic appearance with 40-lb weight loss in past 6 months; lungs clear, with prominent scapulas and clavicles; skin cool to touch, with poor skin turgor; hair dry, dull, and thin. Pallor present, with dark circles under eyes and pale oral mucous membranes.

Bowel sounds are hypoactive. Abdomen is distended. Patient reports last BM 3 or 4 days ago and increasing problem with constipation.

Mother states, "Amy refuses to eat and is losing too much weight. She is obsessed with exercising; she exercises before and after meals and is exercising when I get up in the morning and when I go to bed."

Patient states, "I don't exercise that much. I just don't want to be fat any longer!" Patient denies bingeing and purging but does admit to drinking 12-15 glasses of water and diet soda a day.

Lab Values/Diagnostic Test Results

Treatments

VS q 4 hr
I&O q shift

Past Medical/Surgical History

Anorexia nervosa since age 15
Appendectomy at age 11

Primary Nursing Diagnosis

Imbalanced Nutrition: Less than Body Requirements related to inadequate dietary intake as evidenced by cachetic appearance and 40-lb weight loss in past 6 months

Supporting Data

Cachetic appearance with 40-lb weight loss in 6 months. "Amy refuses to eat and is losing too much weight."

STG/NOC

Patient will gain 1-2 lb per week until weight is within normal range.

NOC: Nutritional status: Food and fluid intake (1008) Oral food intake (100801)

Interventions/NIC With Rationale

1. Discuss a minimum weight goal with patient to promote compliance with treatment.
2. Sit with patient while she is eating to monitor intake; avoid making negative comments and build trust without coercion.
3. Provide small, frequent meals to prevent abdominal pain and vomiting due to too much intake at one time.
4. Provide a limited high-calorie menu from which the patient can select food choices to allow patient control of high-calorie, healthy intake.
5. Maintain a regular schedule for weighing the patient to accurately monitor weight gain or loss.

NIC: Eating disorders management (1030) Monitor patient for behaviors related to eating, weight loss, and weight gain.

Rationale Citation/EBP

Yoost BL, Crawford LR: *Fundamentals of nursing: Active learning for collaborative practice,* St. Louis, 2016, Mosby.

Evaluation

Patient gained 1 lb during 2-week hospitalization. Appears reluctant to limit exercise. Monitor frequency of walking on unit. Continue plan of care.

Nursing Diagnosis 2

Supporting Data

STG/NOC

Interventions/NIC With Rationale

Rationale Citation/EBP

Evaluation

Nursing Diagnosis 3

Supporting Data

STG/NOC

Interventions/NIC With Rationale

Rationale Citation/EBP

Evaluation

FIGURE 30-5 Partially completed conceptual care map based on Amy, the case study patient in this chapter.

nutrients. Patients suffering from physical and psychological diseases often require an alteration in their dietary intake, including an increase or decrease in calories, a specialized diet, or a change in fluid or food consistency (e.g., no added salt [NAS], low cholesterol, 1800-calorie American Diabetic Association [ADA], thickened liquids). Such diets often are used to control or minimize the effects of acute and chronic disease and promote health.

DIETARY PREFERENCES

Vegetarian diets and the reasons people may choose to follow them vary widely. Vegetarian diets and lifestyle have been associated with improved health outcomes. Vegans do not consume any animal products, whereas lacto-ovo vegetarians consume milk and eggs. Although not strict vegetarians, many people choose to consume only small or minimal amounts of animal products. Vegetarian and vegan diets need to include food sources that provide protein, iron, calcium, and zinc. By including cereals, dried beans and peas, and a variety of vegetables to their daily intake, vegetarians are able to acquire the daily essential amino acids necessary for growth and development. Vegans are at risk for development of pernicious anemia and should supplement the diet with vitamin B_{12} to minimize this risk.

FOOD PATTERNS BASED ON RELIGION OR CULTURE

Some people choose to follow dietary restrictions such as kosher or vegetarian diets based on religious traditions. It is important for nurses to be aware of these customs, while remembering that not all people of a particular culture or religion adhere to similar dietary traditions. Patient-centered plans of care are best developed when the nurse asks about the patient's individual dietary preferences and demonstrates respect for cultural and religious nutritional needs.

For people adhering to a kosher diet, the consumption of pork, shellfish, rare meats, and blood is prohibited, as is the combining of milk or dairy products with meat. There are strict kosher food preparation laws, as well as cooking restrictions on the Sabbath. Certain Jewish holidays require eating only unleavened bread or fasting. Catholics observe holy days with fasting, especially on Fridays during the season of Lent.

Islamic tradition prohibits the consumption of alcohol, pork, and caffeine, and halal food preparation rules share similarities with kosher laws. The month-long holy season of Ramadan requires abstaining from food and drink until sundown. Similarly, those of Mormon tradition avoid the use of alcohol, tobacco, and caffeine. Seventh-day Adventists encourage a vegetarian diet and exclusion of alcohol. Some cultural traditions identify foods as "hot" or "cold" on the basis of their healing quality, not their temperature or degree of spiciness.

Most devout Buddhists avoid the consumption of meat and meat by-products and follow vegetarian dietary guidelines, as do many Hindus. The cow is sacred to Hindus, so no beef is consumed; however, other products from the cow, such as milk, yogurt, and butter, are not prohibited.

In faith traditions where fasting is stressed, it typically is prohibited for young children and for older children and adults whose health status would be negatively affected by a decreased dietary intake. It is important to ask patients about dietary restrictions before administration of alcohol-based medications such as antitussives (cough syrups).

The foods typically consumed by some ethnic groups may include items high in fat, sodium, or carbohydrates. These dietary preferences present a challenge when nutritional intervention is needed to avoid serious health complications.

QSEN FOCUS!

Patient-centered care is exhibited when nurses respect the dietary needs of people with cultural or religious traditions different from their own.

SPECIAL DIETS

Collaboration with a registered dietitian is helpful when the nurse is providing nutritional support while addressing medical or surgical conditions such as hypertension, dysphagia, cardiac disease, diabetes, or recovery after gastrointestinal surgery. The PCP typically orders a special diet for the patient. Advancement from one level of special diet to the next may be at the discretion of the nurse; however, provisions for this are included in the patient's orders. Examples of special diets to address specific patient needs are:

- *Clear liquid* has limited nutrients and is used only for a short period of time. Clear juices that do not contain pulp, such as apple or cranberry juice, gelatin, popsicles, and clear broths, are examples of clear liquids. Clear-liquid diets most commonly are ordered for patients with gastrointestinal problems, before surgery (preoperatively) and after surgery (postoperatively), and before some diagnostic tests.
- *Full-liquid* diets consist of foods that are or may become liquid at room or body temperature. Full-liquid diets include juices with and without pulp, milk and milk products, yogurt, strained cream soups, and liquid dietary supplements. Such diets are often used to advance patients who have gastrointestinal disturbances, who have just had dental work performed, or who cannot tolerate solid food.
- *Pureed* diets, often referred to as *blended,* consist of food that is placed into a blender and made into a pulplike mixture. This type of diet is used for individuals who cannot safely chew or swallow solid food. The addition of raw eggs, nuts, and seeds should be avoided.

- *Mechanical soft* diets include food consistencies that have been modified, such as ground meat or soft-cooked foods. They are used for those who have difficulty chewing effectively.
- *Thickened liquids* are used for patients who have difficulty swallowing and are at risk for aspiration. Liquids can be thickened by adding a commercially prepared thickening agent. Nuts, seeds, and other hard or raw foods should be avoided, to decrease the risk of aspiration.
- *Regular diets,* or *general diets,* are commonly referred to as *diet as tolerated.* There are no dietary restrictions, but foods should supply patients with a balanced diet of essential nutrients.
- *Diabetic* (ADA) diets are prescribed to control the amount of calories by controlling the carbohydrate intake. Foods that have a high glycemic index and rapidly raise the body's blood glucose concentration should be avoided. High-fiber complex carbohydrates from vegetables and fruits are preferred to simple carbohydrates, sugars, and starchy foods such as bread or pie.
- *Cardiac* diets are used to control the dietary intake of foods that contribute to conditions affecting the cardiovascular system. They typically consist of low-cholesterol and low-sodium dietary items. Cardiac diets minimize the intake of animal products, which contain cholesterol, and soups and processed foods such as pickles and lunchmeats, which are high in sodium. Patients with hypertension, high cholesterol, atherosclerosis, chronic renal failure, or similar diseases may be placed on some type of cardiac (low-cholesterol, low-sodium) diet.
- *Renal* diets restrict potassium, sodium, protein, and phosphorus intake. Fresh fruits (except bananas) and vegetables are excellent dietary choices for people on a renal diet. Meats, processed foods, and peanut butter, cheese, nuts, caramels, ice cream, and colas typically are allowed in limited quantities or contraindicated.

ASSISTANCE WITH FEEDING

Patients who have limited mobility of their hands or arms, poor tolerance of activity, or a poor cognitive or physical state may require assistance with feeding (Nursing Care Guideline box). If patients are confined to bed and require assistance with feeding, it is extremely important to elevate the head of the bed at least 30 to 45 degrees (unless contraindicated), closely observe the patient's ability to swallow, and watch for signs and symptoms of dysphagia. Signs may include coughing, incomplete lip closure, poor tongue control, excessive chewing, gagging before swallowing or failure to swallow, holding foods in the cheek (pocketing), or refusal to eat. Patients who normally must be maintained in a flat position should be logrolled to side-lying for meals to aid in swallowing and aspiration prevention.

The task of feeding patients who are unable to feed themselves can be delegated to unlicensed assistive personnel. The nurse is responsible for advising UAP of any pertinent infor-

NURSING CARE GUIDELINE

Assisting an Adult With Feeding

Background

- Assisting an adult with feeding should never be rushed, or aspiration may occur (see Nursing Care Guideline, Aspiration Precautions).
- Delegation to unlicensed assistive personnel (UAP) is appropriate, but UAP should be instructed on proper techniques and dietary restrictions to avoid complications.
- Follow any dietary and nutritional orders, including food texture and use of thickening agents.
- Find food that the patient likes: Check the patient's chart, and ask the patient or family members about food preferences.

Procedural Concerns

- Provide oral care before and after feeding.
- If the patient has dentures, ensure that they are in place and well fitted (see Skill 27-6, Oral Hygiene).
- The patient's head should be elevated at least 30 to 45 degrees unless contraindicated.
- Special caution should be taken if the patient has impaired swallowing:
  - If the patient has one-sided muscle weakness, have the patient turn the head to the affected side to assist in airway protection.
  - Chin-tucking may help to prevent aspiration.
- If assistive devices are in use, follow the occupational or nutrition therapy guidelines or the manufacturer's instructions for use.
- Position yourself so that the patient can see you.
  - Allow at least 30 minutes for each meal. Offer small bites (½ to 1 teaspoon).
  - Wait at least 10 seconds between bites.
  - Alternate food with fluids.
  - Avoid unnecessary use of straws to prevent air ingestion.
- Observe for the rise and fall of the patient's larynx to verify swallowing.
- Check the patient's mouth frequently to prevent retention of food in the cheeks (pocketing).

Documentation Concerns

- Note the intake of food (percentage of food eaten) and liquids (in milliliters).
- Document any aspiration symptoms (see Nursing Care Guideline: Aspiration Precautions) and/or patient or caregiver difficulties with the feeding procedure.

> **! SAFE PRACTICE ALERT**
>
> Do not attempt to feed a patient food or liquids in the supine position. The head of the bed must be elevated 30 to 45 degrees, with the patient in an upright position, to minimize the risk for aspiration. Logroll the patient into side-lying position if semi-Fowler position is contraindicated. Have a suction machine at the bedside at all times.

mation, such as risk factors for aspiration or indications that the patient is experiencing difficulty in chewing or swallowing.

PATIENTS WITH NPO ORDERS

Patients who are NPO cannot receive anything by mouth. This requirement often is in place before and after surgery, to allow the intestinal tract to rest and decrease the stimulation of nerves that can lead to vomiting of stomach contents. Conditions such as gastrointestinal bleeding or intestinal blockage may warrant the patient's not receiving anything by mouth. When patients are on NPO status, mouth care is an important nursing intervention, to help keep the oral mucosa moist and aid in swallowing. Oral care should include brushing the teeth, flossing to remove plaque, and using mouthwash. Patients who are unconscious require special attention to their oral care, as well. It is important to place the patient in a position such as on the side to allow the drainage of secretions from the mouth. A padded tongue blade can be used to aid in holding the mouth open and allow the toothbrush to reach inside the cheeks and lips.

ENTERAL FEEDING TUBES

Enteral feeding tubes are used to provide short-term nutritional support for patients who have a functional gastrointestinal tract but cannot swallow, refuse to eat, or need additional nutrients to meet the body's needs. Nasogastric feeding tubes are placed through one of the nares and into the stomach and are also used for short-term nutritional therapy and bowel decompression. Percutaneous endoscopic gastrostomy (PEG) tubes are surgically placed through an incision in the upper-left quadrant of the abdomen (Evidence-Based Practice box). This placement is for long-term nutritional therapy and is indicated in patients who are neurologically impaired (e.g., after a CVA,) or have a condition that affects the stomach and its normal function. Patients who have had esophageal cancer or traumatic injury to the nose and mouth may be candidates for this type of nutritional support (Skills 30-1 and 30-2).

If the patient is being discharged to home with a feeding tube, the role of the nurse is to assess the patient's understanding of this type of nutritional support, determine patient needs (Home Care Considerations box), share information, and instruct the patient or caregiver in the proper manner of administering enteral feedings or formula. Return demonstrations by the patient or caregiver allow the nurse to reinforce information regarding preparation, including the safe handling of the equipment (Nursing Care Guideline box, Percutaneous Endogastric Tube Care). Instructions may include how to check for residual as well as how to administer medication through the tube and how to prevent occluding the tube. The nurse should inform the patient of signs and symptoms to report that could indicate adverse effects of the formula, such as diarrhea, nausea and vomiting, and abdominal cramps.

> **EVIDENCE-BASED PRACTICE**
>
> **Confirming Enteral Tube Placement**
>
> - Studies support the use of radiographic confirmation as the only reliable method to date of confirming enteral tube placement.
> - Using only pH and the appearance of aspirate from the newly inserted tube is not a safe method of verifying proper gastric tube placement, especially in patients receiving antacid medications.
> - Auscultation of an air bolus to assess tube placement is no longer recognized as a reliable source in determining gastric tube placement.

From Lemyze M: The placement of nasogastric tubes, *Can Med Assoc J*, 2010. Retrieved from *www.cmaj.ca/content/182/8/802.full.pdf.*

> **! SAFE PRACTICE ALERT**
>
> Always check to make sure that tube feedings are properly connected to enteral tubes only! Accidently hooking up an enteral feeding tube to a patient's intravenous line can be fatal. Take the extra time necessary to ensure safe practice by following each tube from its point of origin to its destination before initiating intravenous or enteral therapy.

> **HOME CARE CONSIDERATIONS**
>
> **Addressing Enteral Feeding Concerns**
>
> The need for dietary education and assistance with nutritional planning is important when enteral feeding continues after patients are discharged to home. Questions that need to be considered include:
>
> - Is the patient cognitively and physically able to perform the feeding independently, or is it necessary for a caregiver to provide the feeding on a predetermined schedule?
> - Is the patient at risk of skin breakdown due to bed confinement?
> - Has the patient or caregiver received instructions to minimize the risk of infection at the tube insertion site?
> - Does a suction machine need to be ordered for the patient's home setting?
> - Are referrals to community agencies or support groups in place?

NURSING CARE GUIDELINE

Percutaneous Endogastric Tube Care

Background

- The percutaneous endogastric (PEG) tube is used to infuse food directly into the stomach. This method:
  - Bypasses the mouth.
  - Bypasses the swallowing mechanisms.
- The PEG tube is placed in the stomach (or stomach and small intestine) through the abdominal wall.
- It is placed as a long-term feeding option.
- Several types of PEG tubes are available:
  - Traditional gastrostomy (G) tube placed in the stomach
  - Double-lumen gastrojejunostomy (GJ) tube:
    - One lumen—the gastrostomy, or G, tube—is placed in the stomach for feeding.
    - The other lumen—the jejunostomy, or J, tube—is placed in the jejunum for decompression.
  - Low-profile MIC-KEY gastrostomy feeding tube
  - Low-profile MIC transgastric-jejunal feeding tube

Procedural Concerns

- Use surgical asepsis if PEG tubes are newly inserted.
- Clean the site with warm water and mild soap:
  - Occasional use of hydrogen peroxide or normal saline solution is permitted.
  - Cleansing should be based on the patient's routine and facility policy and procedure.
- Dry the site thoroughly to prevent skin breakdown.
- A split-drain dressing may be applied to provide comfort and to prevent or treat skin breakdown.
- If the tube becomes occluded, flush it with a small amount of air. If this is unsuccessful in removing the occlusion, flush the tube using a 50- to 60-mL syringe and 20 to 30 mL of warm water. If flushing the tube with water is ineffective, try carbonated beverages or pineapple juice if not contraindicated.

Documentation Concerns

- Document results of the skin assessment.
- Include notes on patency of the tube.
- Record patient tolerance of feedings.
- Document patient and family teaching related to PEG tube care and maintenance.

SAFE PRACTICE ALERT

Monitor the patient's skin around the PEG tube insertion site for signs of skin breakdown or infection, including increased warmth, redness, edema, and drainage.

Medication Administration via Enteral Tube

Special care should be taken in administering medications by way of an enteral tube. Compatibility, medication solubility, and possible reduction in effectiveness or increase in toxicity must be considered. Medications are never added directly to a tube feeding; rather, they are given in liquid form or ground into powder (as permitted, depending on the medication) and dissolved in 15 to 30 mL of sterile water before instillation into the tube. The enteral tube placement is verified, the tube is flushed with a minimum of 15 mL of sterile water, and the diluted medication is then allowed to flow into the tube by gravity or pushed in gently by plunger, followed by 15 to 30 mL of sterile water to flush the tube after medication administration. Tube feeding may continue immediately unless the contents would interfere with absorption of the medication, in which case the feeding is delayed for a designated time period, determined by medication administration guidelines, before it is resumed.

TOTAL PARENTERAL NUTRITION

Total parenteral nutrition (TPN) may be given through a peripherally inserted central catheter (PICC) line or central venous catheter (CVC) by means of an infusion pump. Typically, infusions with greater than 10% dextrose concentration require a CVC rather than a peripheral intravenous site for infusion. TPN may be the only feasible option for patients who do not have a functioning gastrointestinal (GI) tract, or it may be given when patients are unable to ingest, digest, or absorb essential nutrients due to conditions such as some stages of Crohn's disease or ulcerative gastritis, gastrointestinal obstruction, diarrhea unresponsive to treatment, abdominal trauma, or postoperative status. The disadvantage of TPN is that it should not be used routinely in patients with an intact GI tract. Compared with enteral nutrition, it causes more complications, does not preserve GI tract structure and function as well, and is more expensive. TPN formula is individualized to meet the patient's needs, and its composition often has to be recalculated until the patient's nutritional status improves and stabilizes. This adjustment requires collaboration of the interdisciplinary team responsible for the patient's care, most likely consisting of physicians, dietitians, nurses, and pharmacists.

Monitoring the patient's progress and documenting the patient's assessment should be done consistently and communicated to all members of the health care team. Assessment of patients receiving TPN should include weight, complete blood count (CBC), electrolytes, and BUN (i.e., daily for inpatients). Measurement of plasma glucose and electrolytes helps determine tolerance to the solution. Glucose levels should be checked at least every 6 hours or more frequently until they stabilize. Fluid intake and output should be monitored continuously. When patients become stable, blood tests can be done much less often (Thomas, 2013). The TPN administration system should be monitored regularly to prevent complications. The formula and the tubing should be assessed daily for evidence of contamination. Tubing should be marked and clearly identified so that no other solution is infused through it. Tubing should be changed every 24 hours, with aseptic technique used to minimize the risk of contamination, and the dressing over the site should be changed every 48 hours, with assessment for signs and symptoms of infection (redness, swelling, or drainage).

Numerous potential complications may result from parenteral nutrition, including site infections, air embolism, catheter-related infections, and dislodgment or occlusion of tubing. Metabolic complications can range from common glucose abnormalities to adverse reactions to the lipid formula, liver dysfunction, metabolic bone disease, gallbladder dysfunction (cholelithiasis, cholecystitis), and other metabolic abnormalities (Thomas, 2013).

Nurses unfamiliar with the administration and monitoring of TPN should review the facility policies and procedures before assuming care of patients receiving parenteral nutritional support.

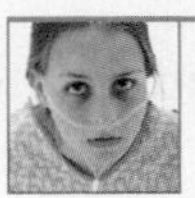

3. Describe at least four nursing interventions necessary to prevent Amy from experiencing further complications from inadequate nutritional intake.

EVALUATION

During the last phase of the nursing process, nurses should clearly evaluate whether or not patients have achieved short- and long-term goals and met established outcome criteria. Evaluation of the patient experiencing nutritional concerns should focus on the patient's response to the nursing interventions. Nutrition is a complex aspect of patient care that must be addressed on an individual basis. Assessing patient dietary needs and providing meals that meet the medical, surgical, cultural, and spiritual concerns of each patient are critical aspects of patient-centered care designed to promote positive patient outcomes.

SKILL 30-1 Insertion, Placement, and Removal of Nasogastric and Nasojejunal Tubes

PURPOSE

Nasogastric (NG) and nasojejunal (NJ) tubes:

- Provide a short-term feeding method for nutritional intake and hydration
- Facilitate suction of stomach contents, which can be used to monitor gastrointestinal disorders
- Allow irrigation of the stomach
- Decompress the stomach
- Permit the gastrointestinal system to rest
- Promote healing

RESOURCES

- NG or NJ tube: 8 to 12 French (Fr)
- Water-soluble lubricant
- Irrigation kit:
  - 60-mL syringe
  - Graduated container
- Tap water or sterile normal saline solution for irrigation
- 1-inch tape or tube fixation device with clamp
- Skin prep and/or skin adhesive
- Emesis basin
- Towels and/or paper towels
- Tissues
- Penlight
- Suction equipment
- Pulse oximeter
- Water and straw (if the patient is able to swallow)
- Permanent marker
- pH test strips, if required
- Waste container
- Clean gloves and other PPE, as needed

COLLABORATION AND DELEGATION

- Insertion of an NG or NJ tube may not be delegated to unlicensed assistive personnel (UAP). UAP may assist with patient comfort, support, and positioning during and after the procedure, at the nurse's discretion.
- UAP should report any of the following to the nurse:
  - Patient complaints of difficulty breathing
  - Fever or change in vital signs
  - Tube displacement
  - Vomiting
  - Loose tape or a loose tube fixation device
  - Any other patient complaints or concerns
- UAP should be instructed in:
  - Essential oral care for patients with NG or NJ tubes
  - Appropriate use of equipment if the patient is connected to a suction or feeding pump
  - Required documentation
- Collaborate with the primary care provider and/or surgeon on appropriate tube choice.
- Collaborate with appropriate radiology department staff to verify tube placement before the initial feeding with an NG or NJ tube.

EVIDENCE-BASED PRACTICE

- Auscultation was previously taught as the standard for checking and verifying placement of an NG tube. This practice is extremely unreliable and should be discontinued. The gold standard for tube placement is radiology verification before the initial feeding. This may be combined with testing aspirated secretions for pH levels and consistently verifying measurement placement markings (Bourgault and Halm, 2009; Goodwin, 2009; Metheny, 2010).
- The fact that a patient has a cuffed tracheostomy tube is not a reliable guarantee that the NG or NJ tube will not enter the airway during insertion. A tracheostomy tube with a cuff is not sufficient to protect the airway because the cuff may deflate slightly throughout placement, leaving room for the tube, especially a small-bore feeding tube, to enter the airway (Goodwin, 2009).
- Capnography (measuring the carbon dioxide level) has been shown to have promise as an effective secondary measure for tube verification but should not be used as an independent placement verification method (Metheny, 2010; Bourgault and Halm, 2009).

SPECIAL CIRCUMSTANCES

1. **Assess:** Was resistance encountered during the insertion of the tube?
   Intervention: Stop the procedure.
   - Rotate the tube, because this may enable easier insertion.
   - Ensure that the patient is swallowing when the tube is being inserted.
   - Ensure proper positioning of the patient and the tube.
   - Withdraw the tube, and reapply water-soluble lubricant.
   - Attempt insertion in the other naris.
   - If indicated, the tube may be placed orally.
   - Notify the PCP if the tube cannot be placed properly.
2. **Assess:** Is the patient gagging with insertion of a tube?
   Intervention: Stop briefly.
   - Do not immediately remove the tube completely; withdraw it until the nasopharynx (back of the throat) is reached.
   - Support and encourage the patient.
   - Provide water for swallowing if the patient is able to swallow and allowed oral intake.

- Use a penlight to inspect the tube in the back of the throat:
  - If the tube is coiled, withdraw it until it straightens or withdraw it completely and start again.
  - If the tube is straight, reassure the patient and proceed with the insertion.
- If the patient is showing signs of respiratory distress, withdraw the tube and start again.
- If necessary, use an anesthetic or analgesic spray. An order may need to be obtained from the PCP; check facility policy and procedure.

3. **Assess:** Has verification of placement been done by appropriate radiology evaluation?
Intervention: Ensure that radiology staff have verified proper tube placement.
4. **Assess:** Does the tube have a vent lumen, such as that found in a double-lumen (Salem sump) tube?
Intervention: Secure the vent above the level of the stomach.
   - Do not use a safety pin because of the risk of injury.
   - Tape the vent lumen to the patient's gown.
     - Leaving some slack in the tube allows for patient movement.
     - Securing the vent lumen prevents accidental displacement or dislodgment.
5. **Assess:** Are you unable to obtain an aspirate for pH level testing?
Intervention: Try again 30 minutes after placing the patient in the side-lying position.
   - Check the measurement marking; if the mark is outside the naris, advance the tube to the mark.
   - If there is no aspirate after *two* attempts:
     - Assume that the tube position is incorrect.
     - Do not use the tube for any procedures.
     - Notify the PCP.
     - Obtain an x-ray order to recheck the tube placement.

PREPROCEDURE

I. Check PCP orders and the patient care plan.
Knowledge of patient-specific orders is critical for safe patient care.

II. Gather supplies and equipment.
Preparing for the patient encounter saves time and promotes patient trust.

III. Perform hand hygiene.
Frequent hand hygiene prevents the spread of microorganisms.

IV. Maintain standard precautions.
Use of the correct personal protective equipment (PPE) is required whenever contact with bodily fluids is possible in order to reduce the transfer of pathogens.

V. Introduce yourself.
Initial communication establishes the role of the nurse and begins a professional relationship.

VI. Provide for patient privacy.
It is important to maintain patient dignity.

VII. Identify the patient, using two identifiers.
Identifying a patient involves scanning barcodes or comparing the patient's stated name and birthdate to information on the patient's wristband or health record. The correct person must receive the correct treatment.

VIII. Explain the procedure to the patient.
The nurse has a responsibility to inform a patient before initiating care. Information may ease patient anxiety and facilitate cooperation.

PROCEDURE

Insertion

Follow preprocedure steps I through VIII.

1. Raise the bed to working height, and lower the side rails as appropriate and safe.
Setting the bed at the correct working height for the provider prevents provider discomfort and possible injury.
2. Assess the patient's cough and gag reflexes. Raise the head of the bed to the high-Fowler position (or as far as the patient can tolerate up to that position). Affix a pulse oximeter and check the patient's vital signs.
Assessing the patient's ability to swallow before insertion of the tube and monitoring vital signs throughout the procedure helps to ensure patient safety. Raising the head of the bed allows gravity to assist with proper insertion and decreases patient discomfort during the procedure.

3. Choose a naris on the basis of which one is most intact and has the greatest airflow; try to avoid placement in a naris that has undergone previous surgery or injury. As a safeguard tell the patient to raise a finger to let you know if he is gagging or feels uncomfortable during the procedure.
   a. Examine skin and tissue integrity with a penlight; note any breaks in the skin or tissue.
   b. Verify nares patency by closing one naris, asking the patient to sniff, and repeating the process with the other naris.

   Skin and tissue integrity issues can worsen with placement of a tube. Eliminate difficulties with placement by detecting obstructions or septal defects before insertion of the tube. Establishing a method to communicate during the procedure will help decrease patient anxiety.
4. Prepare the bedside setup.
   a. Prepare the setup on whichever side of the bed allows the dominant hand to be closest to the patient.
   b. Place a towel over the patient's chest.
   c. Ensure that the patient can reach tissues, the emesis basin, and a cup of drinking water (if allowed).
   d. Place the following on the bedside table: NG or NJ tube, water-soluble lubricant packet, tape or tube fixation device, and skin prep or skin adhesive (if needed).

   Preparing supplies in advance facilitates efficient actions, avoids interruptions during the procedure, and thus promotes patient comfort. Tube insertion may cause natural tearing and trigger the gag reflex; drinking through a straw during insertion facilitates accurate placement and patient comfort. Skin prep or adhesive may be needed to ensure adhesion and prevent tube dislodgment.
5. Prepare the NG or NJ tube:
   a. Open the package.
   b. For an NG tube, measure the length of tube needed for the patient by placing the tip of the tube at the tip of the patient's nose and extending it to the patient's earlobe and then to the patient's xiphoid process.
   c. For an NJ tube, follow step B, above, but add another 20 to 30 cm.
   d. Document the length of the tube to be used if the tube has a preprinted measurement scale. For any tube (with or without a preprinted scale), mark the measurement on the tube using a small piece of tape or indelible ink to ensure proper placement of the tube; fold the ends of the tape for easy removal.
   e. Continue preparing your supplies. Set up your syringe with water. Squeeze the water soluble lubricant out for the tubing. Apply clean gloves and inject 10 mL of water into the tube using a 30 to 60 mL irrigation syringe. If there is a stylet, ensure that it is properly fitted. If the tube has a surface lubricant, dip the tube into a glass of room temperature water to activate it.
   f. Lubricate 4 inches of the tube tip with a water-soluble lubricant.

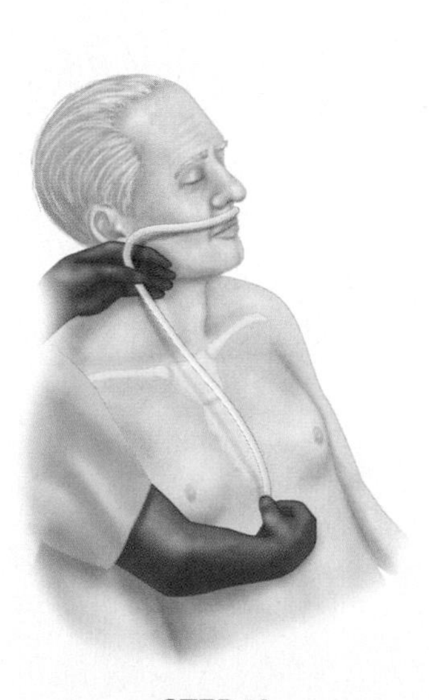

STEP 5b

This measuring technique estimates the insertion length appropriately; placing tape at the marker provides a visual reminder of the measurement that is used during insertion to promote safety (avoiding overinsertion or underinsertion). Use of a permanent marker provides a line that may be incorrect once the placement is verified by radiology; having multiple incorrect marks on the tube leads to potential errors. Lubricant facilitates insertion and promotes patient comfort; it also prevents trauma to the nasal and pharyngeal passages, and, because it is water-soluble, it dissolves and will not harm the lungs if the lubricated tube tip is inadvertently inserted into a lung.

Correct patient position promotes facilitation of insertion, as does following the nasal passage direction and rotating the tubing. Careful insertion of the tubing reduces patient discomfort and prevents mucosal trauma; swallowing helps occlude the trachea, so it reduces the likelihood of inserting the tube into a lung.

6. Prepare the tape or tube fixation device:
   a. Using 1-inch-wide tape, cut a piece of tape 4 inches long and then cut 2 inches of that piece lengthwise; fold the ends of the two pieces created by the lengthwise cut; keep the tape within reach.
   b. The tube fixation device is usually a winged adhesive bandage with a connection clamp: Unwrap the patch, but do not remove the backing; ensure that the clamp is open. (If using another type of fixation device, follow the manufacturer's instructions.)

   Prevent interruption of the procedure by ensuring that all resources are ready before beginning the procedure itself. Prior preparation of the tube fixation device allows it to be applied quickly once the tube is in place; thereafter, the device prevents displacement of the tube.
7. Insert the tube. Do not force it.
   a. The patient's neck should be hyperextended.
   b. Direct the tube down and back.
   c. When the tube has reached the nasopharynx (back of the throat), have the patient tilt the chin forward to rest on the chest.
   d. Advance the tube while the patient is swallowing; provide water to the patient (if the patient is able to swallow and allowed to drink fluids).
   e. Encourage the patient to mouth-breathe.
   f. Advance the tube as gently, quickly, and calmly as possible, rotating the tube if needed and stopping when the tape marking is at the naris. Once the tube has been advanced 25 to 30 cm, stop and listen for air escaping from the tubing. The presence of air indicates the tube might be in the trachea rather than the esophagus. If air is present, withdraw the tube and start again. If there is no air, continue to advance the tube to the distance marker.

   Correct patient position promotes facilitation of insertion, as does following the nasal passage direction and rotating the tubing. Careful insertion of the tubing reduces patient discomfort and prevents mucosal trauma; swallowing helps occlude the trachea, so it reduces the likelihood of inserting the tube into a lung.
8. Secure the tube.
   a. If using tape, apply a skin prep or adhesive if needed. Attach one end of the prepared piece of tape at a time to secure the ends of the tape on the bridge of the nose, forming a sling for the tube. Secure the tube away from nasal mucosa by wrapping each of the split ends in opposite directions where it exits the nose.
   b. If using a tube fixation device (a winged adhesive bandage is described here), apply a skin prep or adhesive if needed; remove the backing from the Band-Aid, and place it over the bridge of the nose. If using a membrane dressing to secure the tube, apply tincture of benzoin or another skin adhesive to the patient's cheek and to the section of the tube you wish to secure. Place the tube against the patient's cheek and use the membrane dressing to anchor it out of the patient's line of sight. Insert the tube into the clamp of the fixation device, and close the clamp. Fasten the end of the tube to the patient's gown using a clip or piece of tape. Do not use a safety pin to fasten the tube to the patient's gown.

   Securing the tube appropriately prevents displacement or inadvertent dislodgment; securing it away from the nasal mucosa prevents trauma to tissues from pressure. If the skin is oily, using a skin preparation or adhesive ensures adherence.
9. Keep the tube clamped until placement of the tube is verified.

   To prevent aspiration or other adverse events, the tube should not be used until placement is verified by radiology.
10. Check the initial tube placement with an x-ray; checking pH may be permitted to confirm correct placement after verification by x-ray. See Intermittent Placement Verification: pH Testing on next page.

    Radiology is the only reliable method of determining accurate placement; however, the placement may be re-verified with an alternative method.

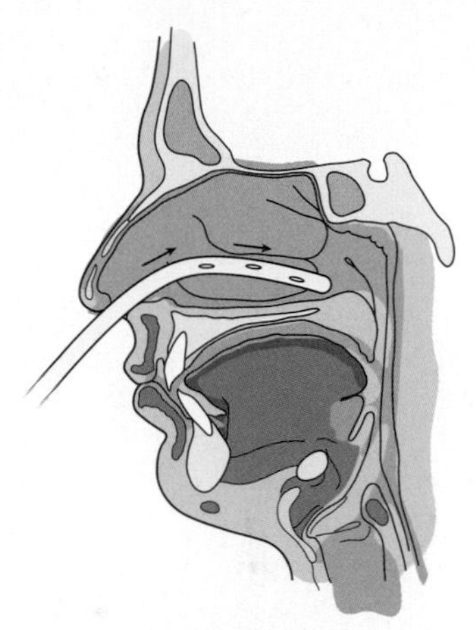

STEP 7b

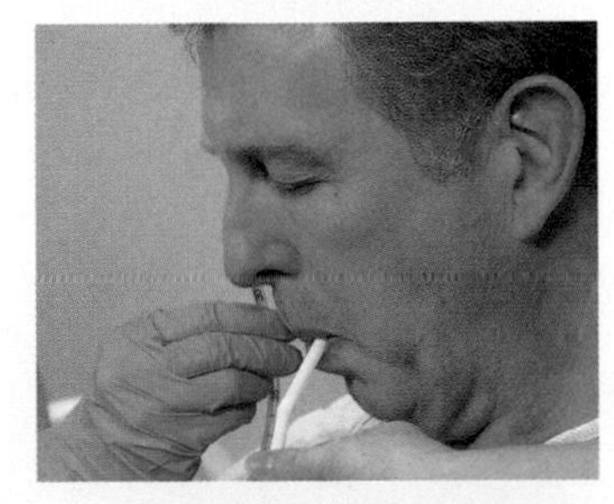

STEP 7d

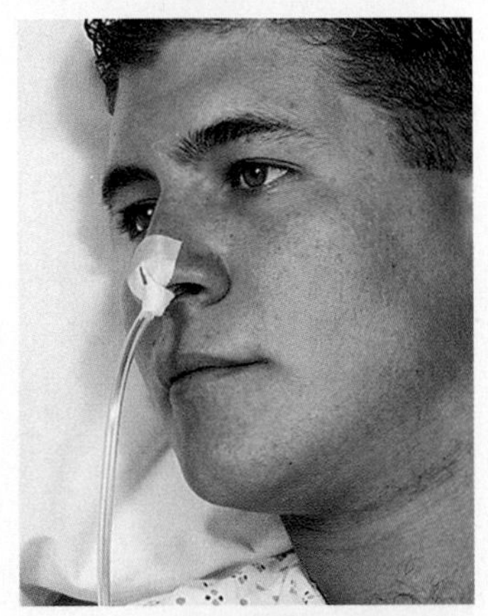

STEP 8b

(From Lilley, et al, 2014.)

11. Placement verification:
    a. If placement of the tube is incorrect, remove the tube, obtain new equipment, and begin the procedure again.
    b. If placement of the tube is correct, remove the measurement marking tape, mark the measurement designation on the tube with a permanent marker, and proceed with the ordered treatment.

    The tube should not be used until placement is verified. This prevents aspiration and other adverse events.
12. Provide oral hygiene.

Follow postprocedure steps I through VI.

Intermittent Placement Verification: pH Testing

Follow preprocedure steps I through VIII.

1. Raise the bed to working height, and lower the side rails as appropriate and safe.
   Setting the bed at the correct working height for the provider prevents provider discomfort and possible injury.
2. Raise the head of the bed to the semi-Fowler or high Fowler position, as tolerated by the patient. Place the patient in the side-lying position.
   Allow gravity/positioning to aid aspiration of fluid.
3. Check placement via pH levels just before intermittent feedings, as indicated. If the patient is on continuous feedings and is not experiencing any difficulties, x-ray evaluation has confirmed tube placement, and the tube measurement marking is stable, continuous feedings may run without interruption for pH testing. Testing pH levels may need to be delayed following medication administration orally or via tube.
   Nutritional feedings and medication administration will interfere with pH levels, if testing is required.
4. Prepare the bedside setup:
   a. Place a towel or disposable sheet over the patient's chest, under the tube connection.
   b. Place the following on the bedside table: irrigation kit, the pH test paper (placed on a paper towel), and the pH color results chart (available on the bottle or in the box that the test paper came in). Check the expiration date for the test paper, and verify that the paper is *not* litmus paper.

   Preparing supplies in advance facilitates efficient actions, avoids interruptions during the procedure, and thus promotes patient comfort. Towels protect the bed linens and gown and prevent the spread of microorganisms.
5. Assess measurement marking:
   a. Verify that the measurement marking has been made in permanent ink *and* is at the naris. If the mark is present and correctly located, continue with the procedure.
   b. If the mark is not there or is not at the naris, stop the procedure and order an x-ray to verify tube location.

   This is the primary check for verification of placement before beginning the procedure with an NG or NJ tube. Proceeding without verification can cause trauma, aspiration, and other adverse events.
6. Withdraw aspirate:
   a. Apply clean gloves.
   b. Draw up 30 mL of air into a 60-mL syringe. Attach the syringe to the NG or NT tube. Flush the tube with 30 mL of air before attempting to aspirate stomach contents.
   c. Slowly pull the plunger back to obtain at least 1 mL of aspirate (5 to 10 mL is ideal).

   Using gloves prevents the spread of microorganisms. Using a large syringe allows sufficient negative pressure to withdraw aspirate. Most pH test papers need at least 1 mL of aspirate for testing.

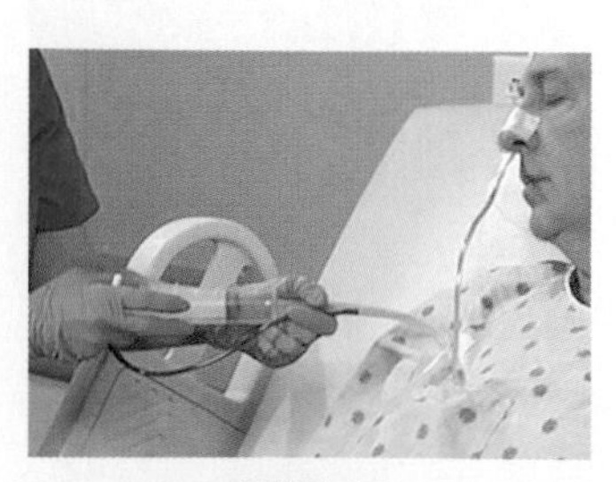
STEP 6c

7. Complete the basic steps to test the pH level of aspirate. Follow the manufacturer's instructions for the test paper strip.
  a. Apply a drop of aspirate to the pH test paper, following the manufacturer's instructions:
    i. While ejecting the aspirate from the syringe into a 30-mL plastic medication cup, allow the pH test paper to become covered with aspirate.
    ii. If not enough aspirate covers the pH test paper, the paper should be dipped into the 30-mL plastic medication cup.
  b. Compare the color on the test strip to the color chart provided by the manufacturer.
  c. After checking gastric pH, irrigate the tubing with 30 mL of water. Remove gloves, and dispose of supplies properly.
  - *The pH level is one means of verifying correct tube placement.*
    Correct placement of the tube in the stomach is verified if the pH is lower than 5.
    If the tube has been inadvertently placed in a lung or the intestines, the aspirate pH is 6 or higher.
  - *Owing to the high risk of adverse events, a pH above 6 is reason to stop the procedure and again verify placement through radiologic methods.*
  - *Aspirate pH may be altered because of medications or feedings (pH value of 4.5 to 6). If other indicators verify correct placement, waiting and retesting is recommended, rather than radiologic exposure.*

Follow postprocedure steps I through VI.

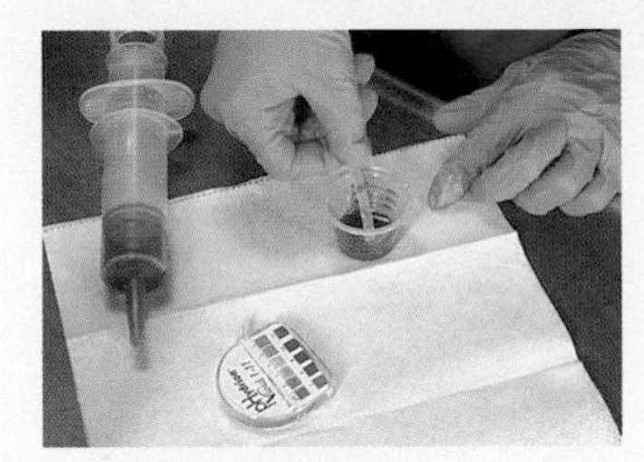
STEP 7aii

Removal

Follow preprocedure steps I through VIII.

1. Raise the bed to working height, and lower the side rails as appropriate and safe. Raise the head of the bed to the high Fowler position unless contraindicated.
Setting the bed at the correct working height for the provider prevents provider discomfort and possible injury.

2. Prepare the bedside setup:
  a. Place a towel over the patient's chest.
  b. Ensure that the patient can reach tissues, an emesis basin, and a cup of drinking water with a straw (if allowed).
Preparing supplies in advance facilitates efficient actions, avoids interruptions during the procedure, and thus promotes patient comfort. Tube removal may cause natural tearing and trigger the gag reflex.

3. Disconnect the tube from the pump or wall suction, if connected:
  a. Apply clean gloves.
  b. If feedings are running (see Skill 30-2, Enteral Feedings via Nasogastric, Nasojejunal, and Percutaneous Endoscopic Gastrostomy Tubes), stop the flow, flush the tube, and then disconnect *and* clamp the tube.
  c. Stop wall suction, if connected, and then disconnect, flush, *and* clamp the tube.
The tube must be disconnected in order to be removed. Clamping the tube ensures that secretions do not reenter the tube.

4. Apply clean gloves and remove any tape securing the tube to the patient's gown, and remove the tape from the patient's nose.
Removing the tape facilitates easy removal of the tube and avoids interruption of the procedure.

5. To remove the tube, instruct the patient to take a deep breath and hold it; pinch the tube, and pull it out smoothly and quickly. Immediately dispose of the tube, and remove and discard gloves.
The risk of having gastric secretions from the tube enter the respiratory tract is removed by having the patient hold his or her breath and the caregiver pinch the tube. Smooth, quick removal facilitates patient comfort and reduces the spread of microorganisms.

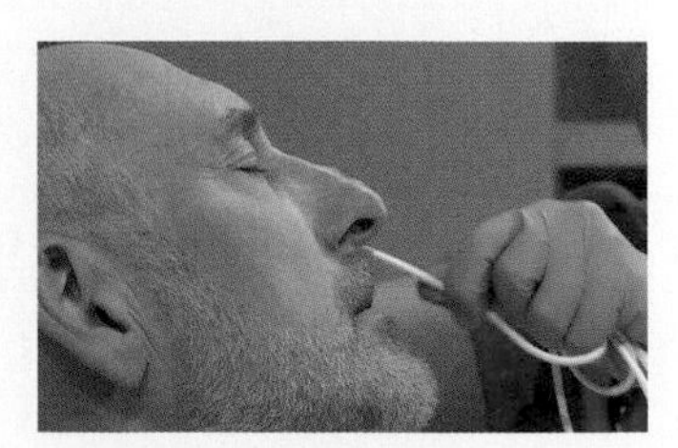
STEP 5

6. Provide mouth care for the patient. Offer the patient a drink (if allowed) and tissues. Use soap and water or adhesive remover to clean the bridge of the patient's nose.
   Promotes patient comfort: Mouth care clears mucous secretions or inadvertent gastric secretions from the tube, while a drink soothes the throat. Tissues assist with nasal secretion removal. The bridge of the nose may be sticky from tape or a tube fixation device.

Follow postprocedure steps I to VI.

POSTPROCEDURE

I. Return the bed to its lowest position, raise the top side rails, and verify that the call light is within reach for the patient.
   Precautions are taken to maintain patient safety. Top side rails aid in positioning and turning. Raising four side rails is considered a restraint.

II. Assess for additional patient needs, and state the time of your expected return.
   Meeting patient needs and offering self promote patient satisfaction and build trust.

III. Properly dispose of PPE.
   Gloves, gowns, and masks must be appropriately discarded to prevent the spread of microorganisms.

IV. Clean equipment if it was in contact with the patient; see specific manufacturer instructions.
   Disinfection eliminates most microorganisms from inanimate objects.

V. Perform hand hygiene.
   Frequent hand hygiene prevents the spread of infection.

VI. Document the date, time, assessment, procedure, and patient's response to the procedure.
   Accurate documentation is essential to communicate patient care and to provide legal evidence of care.

SKILL 30-2 Enteral Feedings via Nasogastric, Nasojejunal, and Percutaneous Endoscopic Gastrostomy Tubes

PURPOSE

Enteral feedings are indicated for patients who are unable or not permitted to ingest oral feedings because of their level of consciousness, inability to swallow, or esophageal obstruction.

Enteral feedings may be used to:

- Provide sole nutritional intake
- Provide supplemental nutritional intake
- Ensure adequate hydration

RESOURCES

- Irrigation kit:
  - 50- to 60-mL catheter-tip syringe
  - Graduated container
- Tap water or sterile normal saline solution for irrigation
- Feeding pump
- Feeding bag and tubing
- Appropriate labels for bag and tubing
- Prescribed enteral formula
- Alcohol swabs
- Graduated container
- pH test strips
- Waste container
- Clean gloves and other PPE, as needed

COLLABORATION AND DELEGATION

- Administering an enteral feeding may be delegated, at the nurse's discretion, to unlicensed assistive personnel (UAP) in accordance with state regulations and facility policies and procedures.
- The nurse should verify tube placement and assess the patient before delegating this procedure.
- UAP should report any of the following to the nurse:
  - Patient complaints of difficulty breathing
  - Fever or change in vital signs
  - Tube displacement
  - Vomiting
  - Loose tape or a loose tube fixation device
  - Other patient complaints or concerns
- UAP should be instructed in:
  - Essential oral care for patients with NG or NJ tubes
  - Appropriate use of equipment
  - Required documentation
- UAP should understand:
  - The ordered nutritional supplement
  - Ways to reduce medication errors
  - The rights of medication administration (see the Six Rights of Medication Administration Nursing Care Guideline found in Chapter 35)
- Collaborate with the primary care provider and/or the surgeon on the appropriate nutritional choice.

EVIDENCE-BASED PRACTICE

- Throughout continuous feedings, and before intermittent feedings, it is imperative that aspirated secretions be tested for pH levels. In addition, routine aspiration precautions should include strict adherence to standard practices such as residual volume checks, elevated head of bed during feedings, and verification of tube measurement markings (Bourgault, Ipe, Weaver, et al 2007; Goodwin, 2009; Nichols, Taylor, Varnholt, and Williams, 2006).
- The feeding tube should be flushed with 30 mL of water at least every 4 hours to ensure that the tube remains patent, unless contraindicated by fluid restrictions (Bourgault, Ipe, Weaver, et al, 2007).

SPECIAL CIRCUMSTANCES

1. **Assess:** Is the feeding solution for the facility in a prefilled bottle?
   Intervention: Replace the original cap on the prefilled bottle with a new, prepackaged cap with the special tubing that is required for the procedure (see step 6 under Procedure).
2. **Assess:** Was bolus gravity feeding ordered?
   Intervention: Feeding is administered without tubing or a pump (see step 6 under Procedure).
   - A syringe without a plunger is connected to the tube.
   - The syringe is held slightly above the patient's stomach level to allow the feeding solution to flow slowly through the tubing by means of gravity.
   - Pour the feeding solution into the syringe while avoiding overflow; add solution to the syringe as the fluid level decreases.
   - Gravity allows the feeding solution to flow through the tube and into the stomach.
   - If the patient is not to receive the complete contents of the feeding bottle or can, refrigerate any unused portion for up to 24 hours.
3. **Assess:** Does the patient have discomfort or cramping with feeding?
   Intervention: Slow or stop the feeding. If necessary, check the amount of residual gastric content (stomach contents remaining from the preceding feeding).
   - Follow the facility policy or PCP orders regarding residual volume.
4. **Assess:** Is there a PEG/gastrostomy/MIC-KEY button?
   Intervention: An extension may have to be placed for intermittent feedings to connect to the pump tubing or syringe.

5. **Assess:** Are any special precautions indicated if the patient is on intermittent feedings?
   Intervention: Clean the tubing and bag thoroughly after feeding to prevent growth of microorganisms.
   - Use warm water only.
   - Use a new feeding set every 24 hours.
6. **Assess:** Is the patient showing signs or symptoms of dumping syndrome? Look for:
   - Nausea, vomiting, and/or diarrhea
   - Pallor and sweat
   - Heart palpitations and/or increased heart rate
   - Abdominal cramping
   - Fainting

   Intervention: Notify the PCP if these signs or symptoms occur during jejunostomy feedings.
   - They may be due to distention of the jejunum.
   - The ordered nutritional therapy may need to be changed.
7. **Assess:** What if there is no clamp on the tubing?
   Intervention: Pinch the tubing instead.
8. **Assess:** Are there any assessments that should be made to monitor for hydration status?
   Intervention: Monitor patient intake and output to assess hydration status.
9. **Assess:** What specific laboratory values should be monitored for a patient on enteral feedings?
   Intervention: Monitor glucose, blood chemistries, and electrolytes as ordered; enteral feedings can cause electrolyte and fluid imbalance.
10. **Assess:** Are there any special precautions that must be taken if the patient is on continuous feeding?
    Intervention: Check residual gastric content every 4 to 6 hours, as ordered or in accordance with facility policy.

PREPROCEDURE

I. Check PCP orders and the patient care plan.
Knowledge of patient-specific orders is critical for safe patient care.

II. Gather supplies and equipment.
Preparing for the patient encounter saves time and promotes patient trust.

III. Perform hand hygiene.
Frequent hand hygiene prevents the spread of microorganisms.

IV. Maintain standard precautions.
Use of the correct personal protective equipment (PPE) is required whenever contact with bodily fluids is possible in order to reduce the transfer of pathogens.

V. Introduce yourself.
Initial communication establishes the role of the nurse and begins a professional relationship.

VI. Provide for patient privacy.
It is important to maintain patient dignity.

VII. Identify the patient by using two identifiers.
Identifying a patient involves scanning barcodes or comparing the patient's stated name and birthdate to information on the patient's wristband or health record. The correct person must receive the correct treatment.

VIII. Explain the procedure to the patient.
The nurse has a responsibility to inform a patient before initiating care. Information may ease patient anxiety and facilitate cooperation.

PROCEDURE

Administering a Tube Feeding

Follow preprocedure steps I through VIII.

1. Raise the bed to working height, and lower the side rails as appropriate and safe. Apply clean gloves. Auscultate for bowel sounds and assess the patient's abdomen.
   Setting the bed at the correct working height for the provider prevents provider discomfort and possible injury. Conducting an abdominal assessment determines the patient's ability to tolerate the tube feeding,
2. Raise the head of the bed at least 30 degrees and preferably to 45 degrees for continuous feeding; the bed must be raised to a similar degree during and for at least 1 hour after bolus or intermittent feedings. If the patient must remain supine, place the patient in the reverse Trendelenburg position.
   Elevation of the patient's head prevents aspiration and promotes the flow of the feeding solution via gravity into the stomach.

3. Prepare an irrigation kit:
   a. Fill the graduated container with tap water or sterile normal saline solution as specified in the order or the facility policy and procedure for irrigation.
   b. Ensure that the syringe and tube are compatible.
   c. Ensure that the syringe is functioning correctly.
   An adaptor may be needed if the syringe and tube locks are not compatible (Luer-Lok versus catheter tip). Preparing supplies in advance and verifying that they are functioning avoids interruption during the procedure.
4. Verify tube placement (see Intermittent Placement Verification: pH Testing in Skill 30-1).
5. For tubes placed in the stomach and used for bolus or intermittent feeding, checking residual volume (stomach contents remaining from the preceding feeding) may be required. If facility policy or PCP orders require checking residual volume:
   a. Use a 50- to 60-mL or larger syringe. Draw up 30 mL of air.
   b. Connect the syringe to the feeding tube.
   c. Unclamp the tube. Inject the air into the feeding tube.
   d. Pull back the plunger of the syringe.
   e. Continue aspirating until the fluid stops.
   f. Typically, if the residual amount is less than 250 mL or half the amount of the last feed, proceed with the new feeding. Do not feed the patient if any single gastric residual volume (GVR) measurement exceeds 500 mL or if two consecutive measurements taken 1 hour apart each exceed 250 mL.
   g. Instill the fluid that was aspirated back into the tube.
   h. Instill 30 mL of tap water or ordered irrigation solution into the tube.
   i. Remove the syringe.
   j. Clamp the tube.
   Note that this procedure does not ever apply to intestinal placement; that content cannot be aspirated. New evidence indicates that checking residual volume may not be necessary, nor is it a true reflection of the patient's tolerance of the feeding. Replacing the aspirated fluid maintains homeostasis because the stomach contents also contain electrolytes and other chemicals.
6. Prepare for feeding:
   a. Ensure that the nutritional feeding solution is as ordered. Check the expiration date. (Follow the principles given in Chapter 35, Nursing Care Guideline: Six Rights of Medication Administration.)
   b. Ensure that the feeding solution is room temperature. Shake the container thoroughly and clean the top of the can with an alcohol swab before opening it.
   c. Measure the feeding amount: For continuous feeding, use not more than the amount required for 4 hours plus the amount needed for priming the tubing. For intermittent feeding, use the ordered amount plus the amount needed for priming the tubing.
   d. Open the pump tube and bag package.
   e. Close all clamps on the pump tubing.
   f. Open the cap on the top of the bag.
   g. Pour the appropriate amount of feeding solution into the bag.
   h. Reapply the cap to the top of the bag.
   i. Hang the bag on the feeding pump pole.
   Knowledge of patient-specific orders is critical for safe patient care. Cold solutions can cause cramping.
7. Squeeze the drip chamber, if present, and allow the suction to fill it one-third to one-half full with irrigation solution.
   Squeezing the drip chamber prevents air in tubing and creates suction.

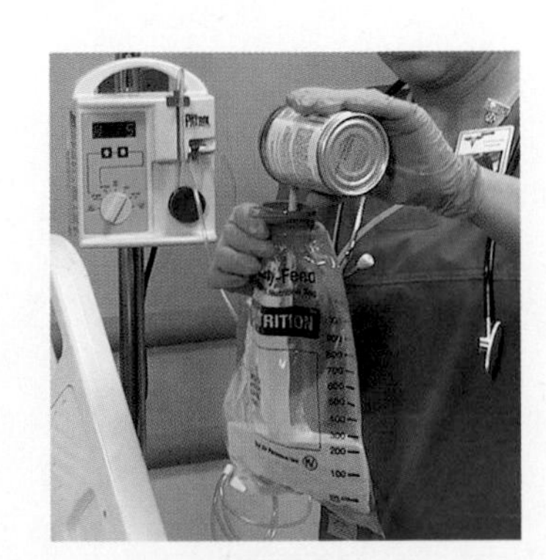

STEP 6g

8. Fill the pump tubing with irrigation solution to prime the tubing. (Note: Some pumps prime the tubing automatically when the tubing is placed in the pump; follow the manufacturer's instructions.)
   a. Remove the cap on the end of the tubing but do *not* discard it; place the end of the tubing over the sink.
   b. Open the clamp slowly.
   c. Allow the solution to run through the tubing.
   d. Close the clamp when the tubing is full.
   e. Replace the cap on the tubing.
   Use proper procedure to prevent contamination and prevent air from entering the tubing. Clamping prevents loss of irrigation solution.
9. Flush the tubing with irrigation fluid before initiating feeding:
   a. Draw 15 to 30 mL of irrigation solution into the syringe.
   b. Connect the syringe to the feeding tube.
   c. Unclamp the feeding tube.
   d. Instill the irrigation solution.
   e. Clamp the feeding tube.
   f. Disconnect the syringe.
   Instilling irrigation fluid through the tube ensures that the feeding tube is patent, prevents air from entering the tubing, prevents loss of solution, and provides hydration for the patient.
10. Label the administration set "Tube feeding only." Label the bag with the type, strength, and amount of the tube feeding. Mark the date, time, and your initials on the label, per facility policy. A new set should be used every 24 hours.
    Correct labeling prevents adverse events and promotes safety. Frequent replacement of equipment prevents contamination and the spread of microorganisms.
11. Attach the pump tubing and bag to the pump, following the manufacturer's instructions.
    Proper use of equipment prevents adverse events and promotes safety.
12. Connect the pump tubing to the feeding tube, and start the feeding via the pump:
    a. Make sure the feeding and pump tubes are securely connected.
    b. Unclamp the pump tubing.
    c. Unclamp the feeding tube.
    d. Start the pump, following the manufacturer's instructions and the PCP order.
    e. Ensure that the feeding solution is flowing appropriately.
    Proper use of clamps prevents adverse events and promotes safety.
13. When feeding is to be stopped, it should be stopped by means of the pump:
    a. Stop the pump; follow the manufacturer's instructions and the PCP order.
    b. Clamp the feeding tube.
    c. Clamp the pump tubing.
    Prevents adverse events; promotes safety.
14. Disconnect the pump tubing and the feeding tube:
    a. Disconnect the feeding tube from the pump tube.
    b. Recap the pump tubing.
    Disconnecting the feeding tube ensures that it remains patent.
15. Flush the feeding tube:
    a. Draw 15 to 30 mL of irrigation solution into the syringe.
    b. Connect the syringe to the feeding tube.
    c. Unclamp the feeding tube.
    d. Instill the irrigation solution.
    e. Clamp the feeding tube.
    f. Disconnect the syringe.
    The irrigation solution prevents obstruction of the feeding tube by any residual nutritional feeding solution and provides hydration.

Follow postprocedure steps I through VI.

POSTPROCEDURE

I. Return the bed to its lowest position, raise the top side rails, and verify that the call light is within reach for the patient.
Precautions are taken to maintain patient safety. Top side rails aid in positioning and turning. Raising four side rails is considered a restraint.

II. Assess for additional patient needs, and state the time of your expected return.
Meeting patient needs and offering self promote patient satisfaction and build trust.

III. Properly dispose of PPE.
Gloves, gowns, and masks must be appropriately discarded to prevent the spread of microorganisms.

IV. Clean equipment if it was in contact with the patient; see specific manufacturer instructions.
Disinfection eliminates most microorganisms from inanimate objects.

V. Perform hand hygiene.
Frequent hand hygiene prevents the spread of infection.

VI. Document the date, time, assessment, procedure, and patient's response to the procedure.
Accurate documentation is essential to communicate patient care and to provide legal evidence of care.

SUMMARY OF LEARNING OUTCOMES

LO 30.1 *Describe the role of nutrition and food metabolism in achieving and maintaining normal body structure and function:* Normal body structure and function are dependent on the adequate intake of nutrients, their metabolism, and their absorption.

LO 30.2 *Identify nutritional imbalances that can result in physical alterations, psychological disturbances, and the development of disease:* Various vitamin deficiencies contribute to the development of diseases such as osteoporosis, scurvy, and rickets. Malnutrition may occur as a consequence of lack of protein or inadequate dietary intake and may lead to diseases such as kwashiorkor, marasmus, and anorexia nervosa. Imbalanced or excess intake of certain foods may promote development of coronary artery disease, hypertension, or diabetes.

LO 30.3 *Discuss critical aspects of a thorough nutritional assessment:* Assessment of nutritional status includes observation of the patient's general health and completion of a health history followed by physical assessment. The process is time-consuming yet essential in determining dietary needs and nutritional status.

LO 30.4 *Identify nursing diagnoses for patients experiencing an alteration in nutrition:* Alterations in nutrition are described most frequently by the NANDA-I nursing diagnosis labels of *Imbalanced Nutrition: More or Less than Body Requirements, Impaired Swallowing, Risk for Constipation, Ineffective Health Maintenance, Ineffective Tissue Perfusion,* and *Disturbed Body Image.*

LO 30.5 *Determine nursing care goals and outcome criteria for patients experiencing complications from an alteration in nutrition:* Goals and outcomes should focus on alleviating nutritional deficiencies or excesses and be formulated in collaboration with the patient, PCP, and others directly involved in the patient's care.

LO 30.6 *Explain the implementation and evaluation of interventions designed to address nutritional needs:* Specific nursing interventions to encourage the intake of essential nutrients and fluid, prevent food-nutrient-drug interactions, and manage impaired swallowing are necessary to enhance wellness. Evaluation focuses on patient progress made toward attaining the agreed-on goals and outcomes.

Responses to the critical-thinking questions are available at *http://evolve.elsevier.com/YoostCrawford/fundamentals/.*

REVIEW QUESTIONS

1. What snack choice would be the best suggestion by the nurse for a patient on a renal diet?
   a. Peanut butter
   b. Bananas
   c. Diet cola
   d. Carrot sticks
2. A patient recovering from major abdominal surgery is to progress from a clear liquid diet to the next diet level. Which statement by the nurse would be most appropriate in this circumstance?
   a. "You will progress from a clear liquid diet to a mechanical soft diet."
   b. "If you can tolerate the clear liquid diet, your next meal will be a full liquid."
   c. "You will receive a regular diet tray with anything you want at the next meal."
   d. "It is important that you eat a pureed diet after you are able to tolerate the clear liquids."
3. What nursing intervention would be most beneficial to implement in an effort to prevent aspiration by a patient receiving tube feedings?
   a. Check the pH of stomach contents before starting each feeding.
   b. Hold prescribed medications until after each feeding.
   c. Elevate the head of the patient's bed at least 45 degrees.
   d. Slow the delivery of the tube feeding to 15 mL/hour.
4. Which action should the nurse take when caring for a patient receiving a continuous enteral feeding through a percutaneous endoscopic gastrostomy (PEG) tube if the feeding tube becomes occluded?
   a. Use 15 mL of cranberry juice in a 30-mL syringe to clear the tubing.
   b. Ask to have the PEG tube replaced to prevent rupture of the gastrostomy.
   c. Flush the PEG tube with 60 mL of cold tap water, using gravity.
   d. Try using cola if a 20- to 30-mL warm-water flush is ineffective.

5. The nurse is caring for an elderly patient who has residual weakness on the right side as the result of a cerebrovascular accident (stroke). The nurse is correct in reporting dysphagia when the patient exhibits which symptom(s)? *(Select all that apply.)*
   a. Incomplete lip closure
   b. Presence of a normal gag reflex
   c. A change in voice quality after eating
   d. Difficulty speaking, with a slow, weak voice
   e. Abnormal movements of the mouth, tongue, and lips
6. A young adult female is considering becoming pregnant and is not taking any multivitamins. Which instruction would best help reduce the potential for development of neural tube defects in the fetus?
   a. Discuss taking selenium supplements with meals.
   b. Stress the importance of prenatal exercise.
   c. Recommend folic acid dietary supplements.
   d. Inquire about the patient's diet and birth control method.
7. A patient tells the nurse that he needs to increase his intake of potassium because he has been taking large doses of diuretics. To minimize complications from hypokalemia, the nurse should instruct the patient to include which foods as a part of his diet?
   a. Cheese and crackers
   b. Peanut butter and jelly sandwich
   c. Tomatoes and spinach
   d. Apples and grapes
8. A Jewish patient who adheres to a kosher diet is diagnosed with type 1 diabetes. What would be the best response of the nurse when the patient refuses to take insulin, stating, "Insulin contains pork and I do not eat pork"?
   a. "There is only a tiny amount of pork by-product in insulin."
   b. "All of the insulin used today is made synthetically."
   c. "I will notify your physician to change the insulin order."
   d. "You really do not have the option of not taking insulin."
9. A female Muslim patient is admitted to the hospital and informs the nurse that it is the month of Ramadan. Which action by the nurse is most appropriate in caring for this patient?
   a. Provide a vegetarian diet for the patient on Friday throughout her hospitalization.
   b. Ask the dietitian to visit the patient to ensure that fruit and cheese are not combined.
   c. Check on the potential effect fasting until sundown will have on the patient's condition.
   d. Document that milk and milk products cannot be prepared with meat or meat products.
10. A 15-year-old female gymnast is hospitalized with the diagnosis of bulimia nervosa. Which data would the nurse anticipate finding in the patient's admission history and physical assessment?
   a. Excessive intake of food, self-induced vomiting, and use of laxatives
   b. Refusal to eat, body image disturbance, constipation, and amenorrhea
   c. Excessive exercise, refusal to eat, poor muscle tone, and social isolation
   d. Hair loss, BMI of 27, occasional use of diuretics, calorie intake 2200/day

ⓔ **Answers and rationales for the review questions are available at *http://evolve.elsevier.com/YoostCrawford/fundamentals/*.**

REFERENCES

American Heart Association: Know your fats, 2012a. Retrieved from *www.heart.org/HEARTORG/Conditions/Cholesterol/PreventionTreatmentofHighCholesterol/Know-Your-Fats_UCM_305628_Article.jsp*.

American Heart Association: Sodium (salt or sodium chloride), 2012b. Retrieved from *www.heart.org/HEARTORG/GettingHealthy/NutritionCenter/HealthyDietGoals/Sodium-Salt-or-Sodium-Chloride_UCM_303290_Article.jsp*.

Anderson JB: Health benefits of dietary fiber, *Nutr Rev* 67(4):188-205, 2009.

Bak-Sosnowska M, Zahorska-Markiewicz B: The image of one's own body and the effectiveness of weight loss therapy, *Wiad Lek* 62(2):104-110, 2009.

Bourgault AM, Halm MA: Feeding tube placement in adults: Safe verification method for blindly inserted tubes, *Am J Crit Care* 18(1):73-76, 2009.

Bourgault AM, Ipe L, Weaver J, et al: Development of evidence-based guidelines and critical care nurses' knowledge of enteral feeding, *Critic Care Nurse* 27(4):17-29, 2007.

Boyd C, Ritchie C, Tipton E, et al: From bedside to bench: Summary from the American Geriatrics Society/National Institute on Aging Research Conference on Comorbidity and Multiple Morbidity in Older Adults, *Aging Clin Exp Re* 20(3):181-188, 2008.

Campos S, Doxey J, Hammond D: Nutrition labels on pre-packaged foods: A systematic review, *Public Health Nutr* 14(8):1496-1506, 2011.

Challem J: Stressed out, 2014. Retrieved from *www.alive.com/articles/view/19084/stressed_out.*

Cronenwett L, Sherwood G, Barnsteiner J, et al: Quality and safety education for nurses, *Nurs Outlook* 55(3):122-131, 2007.

Duffy E: Malnutrition in older adults: Deciphering a complex syndrome, *Advance for NPs & PAs*, 2012. Retrieved from *http://nurse-practitioners-and-physician-assistants.advanceweb.com/article/malnutrition-in-older-adults.aspx?CP=2.*

Foti K, Lowry R: Trends in perceived overweight status among overweight and non-overweight adolescents, *Arch Pediatr Adolesc Med* 164(7):636-642, 2010.

Gelber RP, Kurth T, Manson JE, et al: Body mass index and mortality in men: Evaluating the shape of the association, *Int J Obes (Lond)* 31(8):1240-1247, 2007.

Goodwin RS: Prevention of aspiration pneumonia: A research-based protocol, 2009. Retrieved from *www.pspinformation.com/disease/aspiration/pneu.shtml.*

Hines S, Wallace K, Crowe L, et al: Identification and nursing management of dysphagia in individuals with acute neurological impairment (update), *Int J Evid Based Healthc* 9(2):148-150, 2011.

Institute of Medicine: Dietary reference intakes: Water, potassium, sodium, chloride, and sulfate, 2013. Retrieved from *www.iom.edu/Reports/2004/Dietary-Reference-Intakes-Water-Potassium-Sodium-Chloride-and-Sulfate.aspx.*

Klein S, Allison D, Heymsfield S, et al: Waist circumference and cardiometabolic risk: a consensus statement from Shaping America's Health: Association for Weight Management and Obesity Prevention; NAASO, The Obesity Society; the American Society for Nutrition; and the American Diabetes Association, *Am J Clin Nutr* 85:1197-1202, 2007.

Lilley LL, Collins, SR, Snyder JS: Pharmacology and the nursing process, ed 7, St. Louis, 2014, Mosby.

Linus Pauling Institute: Micronutrient information center, 2011. Retrieved from *http://lpi.oregonstate.edu/infocenter/vitamins/fa/.*

Lutz CP: *Nutrition and diet therapy: Evidence-based applications*, ed. 5, Philadelphia, 2010, FA Davis.

Mayo Clinic: What are omega-6 fatty acids? Can eating omega-6 fatty acids cause heart disease? 2011. Retrieved from *www.mayoclinic.com/health/omega-6/AN02030.*

Meals On Wheels Association of America: About senior hunger, 2010. Retrieved from *www.mowaa.org/page.aspx?pid=281.*

Metheny N: Verification of feeding tube placement [Practice Alert], 2010. Retrieved from *www.aacn.org/WD/Practice/Docs/PracticeAlerts/Verification_of_Feeding_Tube_Placement_05-2005.pdf.*

Murphy, SL, Xu J, Kochanek KD: Deaths: Final data for 2010, *Natl Vital Stat Rep* 61(4):1-118, 2013.

National Association of Anorexia Nervosa and Associated Disorders: Anorexia nervosa, 2012. Retrieved from *www.anad.org/get-information/get-informationanorexia-nervosa/.*

National Heart, Lung, and Blood Institute: What is metabolic syndrome? 2011. Retrieved from *www.nhlbi.nih.gov/health/health-topics/topics/ms/.*

Nichols JH, Taylor D, Varnholt, H, Williams L: *pH testing: Laboratory medicine practice guidelines: Evidence based practice for point-of-care testing*, Washington, DC, 2006, National Academy of Clinical Biochemistry, pp 120-125. Retrieved from *www.guideline.gov/summary/summary.aspx?ss=15&doc_id=10821&string.*

Notelovitz M: *Osteoporosis: Prevention, diagnosis, and management*, ed. 5, West Islip, NY, 2008, Professional Communications, Inc.

Oral care report: Tooth loss and systemic health, 2007. Retrieved from *www.medfielddentist.com/your-oral-health/tooth-loss/tooth-loss-and-systemic-health/.*

Palmer JM: Preventing aspiration in older adults with dysphagia, *Am J Nurs* 108(2):40-48, 2008.

Pfenninger JL, Fowler GC: *Pfenninger and Fowler's procedures for primary care*, ed 3, St. Louis, 2011, Saunders.

Thomas D: Total parenteral nutrition (TPN), 2013. Retrieved from *www.merck.com/mmpe/sec01/ch003/ch003c.html.*

U.S. Department of Agriculture: Dietary guidelines for Americans, 2014. Retrieved from *www.choosemyplate.gov/food-groups/.*

U.S. Department of Health and Human Services: HHS secretary and surgeon general join First Lady to announce plans to combat overweight and obesity and support healthy choices, 2011. Retrieved from *www.hhs.gov/news/press/2010pres/01/20100128c.html.*

U.S. Department of Health and Human Services: *Healthy People 2020*, 2014. Retrieved from *www.healthypeople.gov/2020/topicsobjectives2020/default.aspx* .

Wojcicki J, Heyman M: Adolescent nutritional awareness and use of food labels: Results from the national nutrition health and examination survey, *BMC Pediatr* 12(55):1471-1479, 2012.

World Health Organization: Children: Reducing mortality, 2013. Retrieved from *www.who.int/mediacentre/factsheets/fs178/en/.*

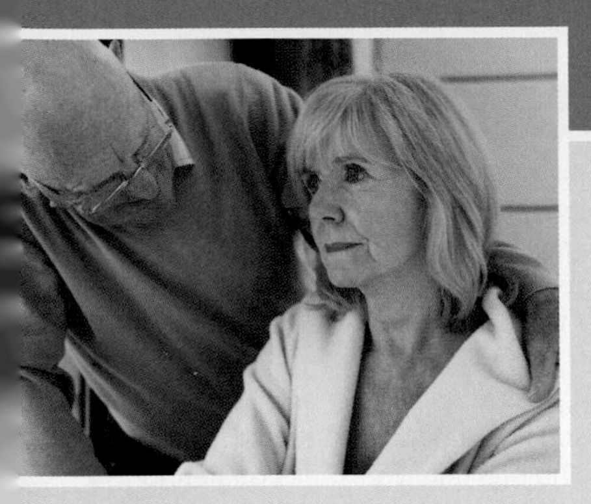

CHAPTER 31

Cognitive and Sensory Alterations

EVOLVE WEBSITE

http://evolve.elsevier.com/YoostCrawford/fundamentals/

- Additional Evolve-Only Review Questions With Answers
- Answers and Rationales for Text Review Questions
- Answers to Critical-Thinking Questions
- Case Study With Questions
- Conceptual Care Map Creator
- Animations
- Glossary

LEARNING OUTCOMES

Comprehension of this chapter's content will provide students with the ability to:

LO 31.1 Describe the normal structure and function of brain and body regions involved in cognition and sensation.

LO 31.2 Identify how alterations in structure and function associated with impaired cognition and sensation affect patients' abilities.

LO 31.3 Perform assessments of patients' cognitive and sensory function.

LO 31.4 Choose nursing diagnoses for patients who need assistance or modifications in care because of cognitive or sensory deficits.

LO 31.5 Articulate goals for patients with cognitive or sensory alterations.

LO 31.6 Carry out nursing care plans that include interventions to enhance patients' cognitive and sensory function.

KEY TERMS

Alzheimer disease, p. 713
amyloid plaques, p. 713
anosmia, p. 714
aphasia, p. 714
atrophy, p. 713
auricle, p. 712
cataract, p. 715
cerebrovascular accident (CVA), p. 713
chemoreceptors, p. 712
cognition, p. 710
cones, p. 712
decussate, p. 711
delirium, p. 713
dementia, p. 713
depression, p. 713
diabetic retinopathy, p. 715
equilibrium, p. 712
glaucoma, p. 715
gustation, p. 712
labyrinths, p. 712
macular degeneration, p. 715
myopia, p. 714
neurofibrillary tangles, p. 713
olfaction, p. 712
ossicles, p. 712
perception, p. 711
peripheral neuropathy, p. 714
presbycusis, p. 714
presbyopia, p. 715
retina, p. 712
rods, p. 712
semicircular canal, p. 712
sensation, p. 710
sensory adaptation, p. 711
sensory deprivation, p. 713
sensory overload, p. 715
stimulus, p. 711
sundowning, p. 713
tactile, p. 711
telecommunications device for the deaf (TDD), p. 725
tinnitus, p. 714
vertigo, p. 714

CASE STUDY

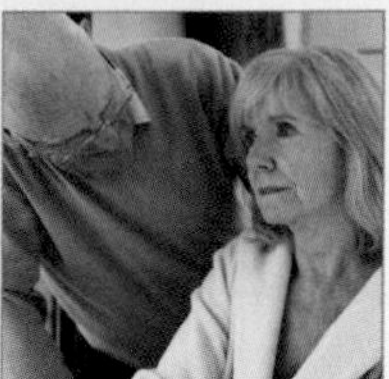

Mrs. Matson is a 67-year-old married mother of three and grandmother of five. She was admitted 2 days ago with symptoms of slurred speech and weakness on her right side. An MRI study, done in the emergency department, showed a clot in her left frontal lobe. She was given a clot-dissolving drug, alteplase. Mrs. Matson's condition has been improving since she was hospitalized. She has no allergies. She has a history of hypercholesterolemia and moderate hearing deficits, which have been worsening over the past 5 years. She is a full code. Her Braden score is 21.

Mrs. Matson's vital signs are T 36.7°C (98.1°F), P 68 regular and strong, R 18 and unlabored, and BP 128/76, with a pulse oximetry reading of 96% on room air. She is alert and oriented to person but confused about place and time. Her lungs are clear. Her abdomen is soft and nontender, with bowel sounds present ×4. She denies pain. She has mild weakness on her right side and is slightly unsteady on her feet, requiring the assistance of one person. The IV access site in the left antecubital space is without redness or swelling. She demonstrates mild difficulty finding some words but has been able to express her needs. Since admission, Mrs. Matson's speech has become clearer, and the strength on the right side of her body has improved. She has slight difficulty hearing when spoken to in a conversational tone but does not wear a hearing aid. In her laboratory results today, CBC showed hemoglobin 13.2 g/dL and hematocrit 39%, and PT/INR was 23.4/2.1. All other laboratory values were within normal limits.

Mrs. Matson's husband visits daily and spends most of the day with her. He appears to be alert and oriented and has no obvious physical problems. Two of their children live out of state, but a daughter who lives locally has been in to visit.

Treatment orders are as follows:

- Vital signs q 4 hr
- Low-cholesterol diet
- IV access saline lock
- Up with assistance
- Intake and output
- Physical therapy
- Speech therapy
- Fall precautions

Medication orders are as follows:

- Warfarin; call physician with PT/INR results daily for dosage
- Atorvastatin 10 mg daily
- Acetaminophen 650 mg q 4 hr PRN for pain

Refer back to this case study to answer the critical-thinking questions throughout the chapter.

Sensory input and cognitive ability allow humans to react to their environment. When alterations occur in any of the cognitive areas or sensory pathways of the central nervous system, the person's ability to respond is affected. Alterations are caused by a variety of factors, including traumatic injuries, illnesses, metabolic imbalances, and aging. Patients may come to the health care setting with previously known alterations in cognition or sensation, or they may develop changes due to a current illness or injury.

NORMAL STRUCTURE AND FUNCTION OF BRAIN AND BODY REGIONS INVOLVED IN COGNITION AND SENSATION LO 31.1

Knowledge of the normal structure and function of the brain and nervous system helps the nurse to recognize alterations in cognition and sensation when they occur. Helping patients with deficits deal with the unfamiliar health care environment is an essential nursing responsibility.

Cognition is knowing influenced by awareness and judgment; it is composed of skills that include language, calculation, memory, attention, reasoning, learning, problem solving, and decision making. **Sensation** is a feeling, within or outside the body, of conditions resulting from stimulation of sensory receptors. Areas of the cerebrum are responsible for both cognition and the processing and integration of information from sensory input (McKinley and O'Loughlin, 2012).

COGNITION

Each hemisphere of the cerebrum is divided into four main lobes: frontal, parietal, temporal, and occipital. The frontal lobes of the cerebrum are the areas of the brain responsible for voluntary motor function, concentration, communication, decision making, and personality. The parietal lobes are responsible for the sense of touch, distinguishing the shape and texture of objects. The temporal lobes are concerned with the senses of hearing and smell. The occipital lobes process visual information. A fifth, smaller lobe called the *insula* lies beneath the temporal lobe and is thought to be involved with memory and taste (McKinley and O'Loughlin, 2012). See Chapter 20 for further information on and illustrations of the

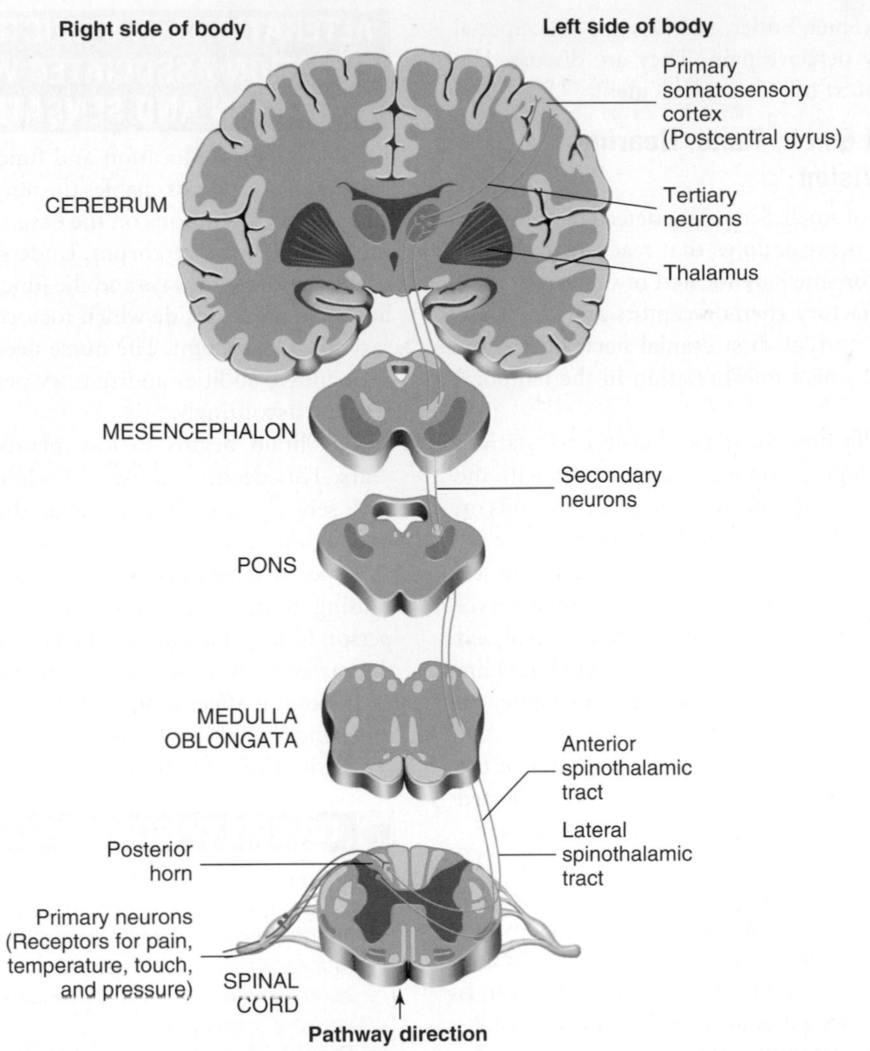

FIGURE 31-1 Sensory pathways ascend the spinal cord and cross to the other side of the body before reaching the brain.

structure and function of the central nervous system and cranial nerves.

SENSATION

When a **stimulus**, which is a change in the environment sufficient to evoke a response, occurs, sensory receptors trigger a response, which results in nerve impulses ascending sensory pathways to the central nervous system for processing. The way the brain perceives the information is called **perception**. The person must be in a state of alertness to recognize and respond to stimuli. The area of the brain that controls alertness and attention is the reticular activating system (RAS). During times of alertness, some impulses are ignored by the brain because they are not assigned priority as more important than others. This process is called **sensory adaptation**.

Two main types of sensory receptors are recognized. One type is found throughout the body in the skin and deeper tissue; these receptors detect the somatic senses of touch, pressure, temperature, and pain. As these impulses travel through sensory pathways up the spinal cord, they cross over, or **decussate**, to the other side of the body before reaching the brain (Figure 31-1). The second type of receptor is found in specialized sensory organs and detects the senses of smell, taste, hearing, equilibrium and vision (Shier, Butler, and Lewis, 2012).

General Senses of Touch, Pressure, Temperature, and Pain

Tactile receptors, or those detectable by touch, are located in the dermis and subcutaneous tissue. These nerve fibers supply the brain with information regarding touch and pressure by way of sensory pathways.

Two types of nerve endings supply the brain with information regarding temperature: warm receptors and cold receptors. These skin receptors respond to moderately warm (more than 35°C or 77°F) or cold (10° to 20° C or 50° to 68°F) temperature changes (Shier, Butler, and Lewis, 2012). Special receptors in the body perceive pain. They are discussed in Chapter 36 in the context of pain management.

Special Senses of Smell, Taste, Hearing, Equilibrium, and Vision

Olfaction is the sense of smell. Scents are detected by **chemoreceptors**, or sensory nerve endings that react to chemicals. The chemoreceptors for smell are located in the upper nasal passages. Once the olfactory chemoreceptors are stimulated by an odor, the right and left first cranial nerves carry the impulses to the brain, where interpretation in the temporal lobe takes place.

Closely related to olfaction, the sense of taste, or **gustation**, requires that chemoreceptors come in direct contact with the stimulus. These sensory receptors are located in taste buds on the tongue, the roof of the mouth, and the throat. They are stimulated by food when it is consumed. The right and left seventh cranial nerves and right and left ninth cranial nerves transfer taste information to the brain, where it is analyzed in the insula lobe of the cerebrum (McKinley and O'Loughlin, 2012). All of the cranial nerves are discussed in Chapter 20 in the context of physical assessment.

The sense of hearing occurs through the workings of the outer, middle, and inner ears. Sound waves are collected by the outer ear, or **auricle**, causing the eardrum (the membrane dividing the outer and middle ears) to vibrate. The vibrations of the eardrum cause the three small bones, or **ossicles**, in the middle ear to vibrate. This vibration transmits the sound to the fluid-filled inner ear via a membrane-covered opening called the *oval window*. The inner ear is composed of a complicated set of **labyrinths**, which are intricate communicating passageways. Receptor cells pick up the sound waves and send messages to the brain by way of the right and left eighth cranial nerves, the vestibulocochlear nerves. Auditory impulses are interpreted in the temporal lobe of the cerebrum.

A second set of labyrinths in the inner ear, the **semicircular canal**, has receptor cells that interpret the head's position and maintain **equilibrium**, or state of balance. Different receptors detect when the head is still and when it is in motion. This information is sent to the brain via the vestibulocochlear nerves.

The eye is the sense organ of vision. Light stimuli enter the eye through the cornea and then go through the lens. Photoreceptors in the **retina** (innermost layer of the eye) detect visual images by perceiving light waves, which are different lengths for different colors. Two types of photoreceptors, rods and cones, are present in the retina. **Rods** are more sensitive to light and so can provide vision in dim light. **Cones** detect sharp, color images (Shier, Butler, and Lewis, 2012). Visual impulses travel from the receptors on the retina to the brain by way of the right and left second cranial nerves, the optic nerves, to the occipital lobes of the cerebrum.

ALTERATIONS IN STRUCTURE AND FUNCTION ASSOCIATED WITH IMPAIRED COGNITION AND SENSATION LO 31.2

Knowledge of the location and function of the lobes of the cerebral hemispheres enables the nurse to anticipate cognitive and sensory alterations on the basis of the location of disease or damage in the cerebrum. Understanding the mechanism of the sensory pathways and the function of the special senses helps the nurse decide which focused assessments are necessary for each patient. The nurse needs to be alert to changes in cognitive abilities and sensory perception in patients and respond accordingly.

The brain begins to lose neurons after the age of 30 years. This decrease causes a decline in the ability to interpret sensory stimuli that reach the brain (McKinley and O'Loughlin, 2012). As aging progresses, changes in the tactile and special senses occur. Loss of neurons affects cognition, causing response times to be slower. Aging may cause a person to forget a word or the last place where he or she put the car keys. In most people, however, the change is gradual and does not affect judgment, language, or the ability to live independently. Many factors affect cognition and sensation (Diversity Considerations box).

DIVERSITY CONSIDERATIONS

Life Span

- Children are more prone to otitis media because of the shorter, more horizontal eustachian tube in this age group.
- Infants who are not touched and cuddled or who do not bond with a caregiver often suffer from the effects of sensory deprivation.
- Each newborn's hearing is tested, before the infant leaves the hospital, for early assessment and intervention.
- Hearing alterations with aging lead to social isolation in many patients. The person with a hearing deficit often feels embarrassed by the impairment, which draws unwanted attention and prevents easy interaction with others.
- Sensory perceptual changes with aging may lead to less discriminating taste and smell or to problems with equilibrium in older adults.
- The risk of dementia increases with age.

Gender

- Postmenopausal women receiving hormone replacement therapy are at increased risk for cerebrovascular accidents caused by clots.

Disability

- Sensory deprivation can occur in patients who have sensory deficits, especially those with visual or auditory impairment.

Morphology

- Obesity predisposes patients to development of hypertension, putting them at a higher risk for cerebrovascular accidents.

COGNITIVE ALTERATION

Symptoms of cognitive impairment include disorientation, loss of language and/or simple arithmetic skills, poor judgment, and memory loss. If the patient exhibits these symptoms, further investigation is needed. Although some decline in cognitive ability occurs with aging, these symptoms are not a normal part of aging.

Delirium

Delirium is a reversible state of acute confusion. It is characterized by a disturbance in consciousness or a change in cognition that develops over 1 to 2 days and is caused by a medical condition. Fluctuating awareness, impairment of memory and attention, disorganized thinking, hallucinations, and disturbances of sleep-wake cycles are signs and symptoms (U.S. National Library of Medicine, 2014a). Some causes are drug or alcohol use, the side effects of medication, infections, fluid and electrolyte imbalances, low oxygen level, and pain. Delirium may occur in patients in the intensive care unit because of sensory overload. Once the underlying cause of delirium is identified and treated, the confusion subsides.

Depression

Depression is a mood disorder characterized by a sense of hopelessness and persistent unhappiness. Signs and symptoms of depression are loss of interest, sadness for an extended period of time, decreased self-esteem, sleeping too much or insomnia, and changes in eating patterns. Depression that is triggered by life situations, such as illness or loss, is called *situational* or *exogenous depression.* Major depression that is intrinsic, or *endogenous,* is believed to be caused by chemical changes in the brain. With both types of depression, the symptoms interfere with daily living (U.S. National Library of Medicine, 2014b).

Patients taking a variety of medications may experience drug side effects that mimic depression. Social circumstances often trigger depression, especially in elderly people who are isolated from activity because of their living situations. **Sensory deprivation** (decreased stimulation from the environment) from lack of contact with others can lead to depression. Depression usually has a rapid onset, and the affected person's mood typically is constant. It usually is reversible with treatment either by eliminating the underlying cause, providing counseling, or prescribing antidepressive agents.

Dementia

Dementia, which is a permanent decline in mental function, has a subtle onset. It is characterized by the decline in many cognitive abilities, including reasoning, use of language, memory, computation, judgment, and learning. Dementia is not reversible and worsens over time. Although the percentage of people with dementia increases with increasing age, it is not a normal part of aging. However, up to half of people

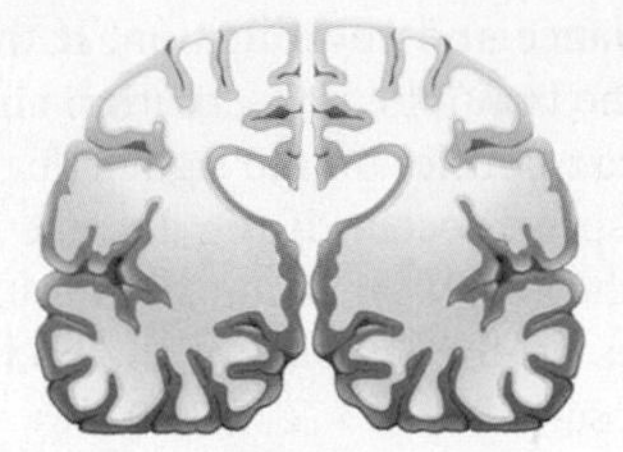

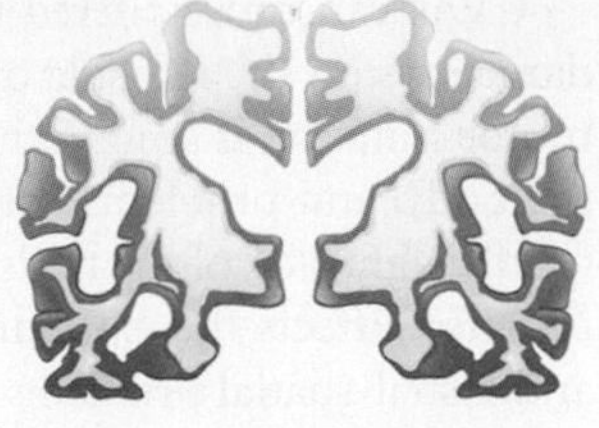

FIGURE 31-2 MRI cross-sectional appearance. **A,** Normal brain. **B,** Marked atrophy of the brain associated with Alzheimer disease.

age 85 and older may have some signs of dementia (National Institutes of Health [NIH] News in Health, 2014).

The most common type of dementia is **Alzheimer disease**, which has specific pathologic findings. In Alzheimer disease, protein fragments called **amyloid plaques** build up between the nerve cells of the brain, blocking electrical and chemical connections between neurons. Another change that occurs is the development of **neurofibrillary tangles**, which are twisted fragments of protein that clog the nerve cells. This interrupts nutrient delivery to brain cells. These changes cause problems within the cells that lead to diminished nerve conduction and cell death (National Institute of Neurologic Disorders and Stroke, 2014). The brain of a person with Alzheimer disease shows marked cerebral **atrophy**, a decrease in size (Figure 31-2). All of these changes interfere with the communication between nerve cells, causing the person with Alzheimer disease to lose cognitive function and, eventually, basic functions such as breathing. Although genetics and environment both are believed to play a role in Alzheimer disease, no specific cause has been identified. The animation "Alzheimer Disease" further explains the pathophysiology of this disorder.

Behavioral problems that arise in dementia patients include wandering; agitation; repetitive behaviors; **sundowning**, or worsening of agitation and confusion in the evening; and verbal or physical outbursts. These behaviors can result from frustration, confusion, fear, anxiety, or lack of control.

Brain Injuries and Illnesses

Traumatic brain injuries and infections such as meningitis impair cognitive and sensory functioning. Other infections can cause delirium and affect cognition. A **cerebrovascular accident (CVA)**, which occurs when an area of the brain is deprived of blood flow and also is called a *stroke,* causes damage to an area of the brain. The resulting impairment depends on the area of the cerebrum involved. CVAs are of three types: (1) ischemic stroke in which a clot forms, narrowing a blood vessel and blocking blood flow; (2) ischemic stroke in which an embolus breaks from a clot in the systemic circulation and lodges in a small cerebral blood vessel, blocking blood flow; and (3) hemorrhagic stroke, with bleeding in the brain from a burst aneurysm or traumatic injury. Any of these events can cause temporary or permanent damage. More information is presented in the animation "Stroke."

CVAs can cause altered balance and coordination. If the damage is on the left side of the brain, loss of sensation and motor function is seen in the extremities on the right side of the body, and problems with speech occur. If the damage is on the right side of the brain, the loss of sensation and motor function affects the extremities on the left side of the body, and visual-spatial problems occur.

Some speech problems that occur after a stroke or other traumatic brain injury include different types of **aphasia**, or speech or language impairment. The patient with receptive aphasia, also known as *Wernicke's aphasia* (named for the area of the temporal lobe that interprets language), cannot comprehend written or spoken language. The auditory pathway is intact, but words do not make sense. In expressive aphasia, or *Broca's aphasia,* the damage is to the motor speech area of the frontal lobe. In this type of aphasia, patients understand language but are unable to answer questions, name common objects, or express simple ideas.

Meningitis is an infection of the lining of the brain caused by a virus or bacteria. In addition to signs of infection, meningitis can cause mental changes. Other infections, especially in elderly people, can cause changes in cognitive abilities that are temporary. When the patient exhibits sudden or rapid changes in behavior or cognition, a urinary tract infection and pneumonia are possible causes. The patient's cognitive ability will revert back to the preinfection level after successful treatment of the underlying condition.

SENSORY DEFICITS

Patients with sensory deficits have difficulty interacting with the environment. Hospitalized patients with any alterations in sensory reception or perception depend on the nurse to provide a safe environment, which adapts to each patient's special needs.

Tactile

Damage to sensory nerve fibers in the arms and legs leads to **peripheral neuropathy**, nerve damage away from the center of the body. Patients may not be able to feel sharp objects or discern extreme hot and cold temperatures, leaving them vulnerable to injury. Peripheral neuropathy occurs in patients with diabetes mellitus and renal disease.

Smell

Olfactory chemoreceptors decline in number and lose their sensitivity with age, causing a decreased ability to detect odors. Infections, smoking, and cocaine use can damage chemoreceptors and cause a decline in or loss of the ability to smell. **Anosmia** is the complete loss of the sense of smell.

Taste

The number of gustatory cells declines after the age of 50 years, resulting in a decreased ability to distinguish taste in later life. Upper dentures, if present, cover part of the roof of the mouth, making detection of some tastes difficult. Injury to the tongue, cheeks, or roof of the mouth, or exposure to extremely hot or cold food can temporarily damage taste buds.

Hearing

Partial or complete hearing loss can occur at any age. Congenital hearing loss is due to genetic factors in more than one half of all cases. Other causes of congenital hearing loss are maternal diseases, such as rubella or diabetes, and lack of oxygen at birth.

Otitis media may cause temporary hearing loss from a buildup of fluid behind the eardrum. In cases of repetitive or chronic infection, permanent damage to the eardrum or ossicles can occur. A buildup of cerumen, which blocks sound in the outer-ear canal, also may cause temporary hearing loss. Both simple otitis media and blockage with cerumen cause a type of hearing deficit called *conductive hearing loss,* because the problem occurs in the portion of the ear that conducts sound waves. Another type of hearing loss is sensorineural, or damage to the receptor nerves or nerve pathways. Potential causes include: loud noises, adverse reaction to ototoxic drugs, head injuries, or certain types of infection.

Age-related hearing loss is called **presbycusis.** It usually comes on slowly and affects the hearing in both ears. It seems to exhibit a familial pattern (National Institute on Aging, 2013). Loss does not occur at the same rate with all people, or even in both ears in the same person.

Equilibrium

Motion sickness is a common equilibrium problem associated with mixed signals that the brain is receiving. If a person is in motion in an airplane, boat, or car, for example, and views only stationary objects, such as the seat in front of the person, the eye is seeing stillness while the inner ear is detecting movement. Signs and symptoms are dizziness, nausea, and vomiting. It is unknown why some people experience this problem whereas others do not.

Ménière's disease is associated with **vertigo**, or the sensation that objects are moving around the person; **tinnitus**, or a ringing or other abnormal sound in the ear; and progressive hearing loss. It is caused by excess fluid accumulation in the labyrinth in the inner ear. Patients with fluid buildup or infections of the inner ear may describe dizziness, lightheadedness, unsteadiness, or vertigo. The symptoms disappear if the underlying cause is successfully treated.

Vision

Many changes in the structure and function of the eye and related structures cause problems with vision. Some of these problems are easily corrected with lenses, whereas others lead to permanent damage. **Myopia**, or nearsightedness, causes the affected person to be able to see clearly only a short distance. This is because the image is focused in front of the retina instead of on the retina. In most cases, the eye is

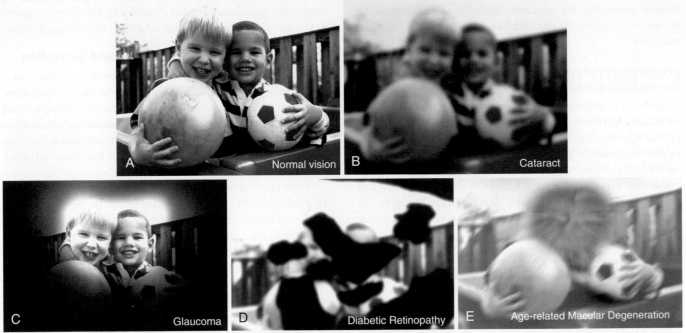

FIGURE 31-3 A, Normal vision. Loss of visual fields in **(B)** cataracts, **(C)** glaucoma, **(D)** diabetic retinopathy, and **(E)** macular degeneration. (Courtesy National Eye Institute, National Institutes of Health.)

elongated, but the cause of the elongation is unknown. Myopia is corrected with use of a concave lens (eyeglasses or contact lenses) or through refractive surgery.

Presbyopia, manifesting as farsightedness, is an age-related decrease in the ability to focus on near objects. This loss of near vision occurs gradually, usually beginning after the age of 40 years. The cause is unknown, but the lens of the eye appears to become less flexible and lose its ability to change shape in order to focus. Reading lenses are worn to correct presbyopia.

Clouding of the lens of the eye is called a **cataract**. Cataracts cause blurring of vision and usually occur with aging. The visual deficit can be corrected with surgery, which usually is performed only if vision is severely affected. The clouded lens is removed, and a new lens is placed in the eye.

Glaucoma is a serious medical condition of the eye. It causes increased intraocular pressure, which puts pressure on the optic nerve, leading to loss of peripheral visual fields and possibly blindness. Because there are no early symptoms of glaucoma, screening is done during routine eye examinations.

Diabetic retinopathy is a complication of diabetes mellitus in which the blood vessels of the retina become damaged. Because the retina is the area of the eye that contains the photoreceptors, destruction of these cells leads to loss of vision. Usually, visual loss starts with distortion of the image, but the condition can lead to blindness.

The macula is the area of the retina that provides central vision. **Macular degeneration** is the leading cause of visual defects in the United States. It typically begins after the age of 50 years; loss of vision occurs in the central visual fields. Visual acuity is diminished. Causes include diabetes, genetics, smoking, and hypertension; however, some affected patients do not have these risk factors.

Figure 31-3 depicts changes in vision associated with cataracts, glaucoma, diabetic retinopathy, and macular degeneration.

SENSORY DEPRIVATION

Any of the sensory alterations discussed can lead to sensory deprivation. A person who cannot see, hear, feel, or respond to the environment may feel socially isolated. Sensory deprivation is a concern in the acute care setting because of decreased sensory input, lack of stimuli or ability to receive stimuli, and decreased meaning of stimuli due to the strange environment. Restrictions within the environment, such as isolation precautions, contribute to deprivation. The patient may appear bored, restless, and disinterested and complain of a decreased ability to think.

SENSORY OVERLOAD

The best example of **sensory overload** in a hospitalized patient is that encountered in the environment of the intensive care unit. The cause is an overabundance of stimuli—noise from machines, pressure from tubes, frequent interactions with health care personnel throughout a 24-hour day, constant lighting, and pain. When the brain is overly stimulated, it ceases to make sense of the incoming stimuli.

Susceptibility to sensory overload varies from person to person, depending on tolerance levels. Signs and symptoms of sensory overload are anxiety, attention deficit, and confusion.

◆ ASSESSMENT LO 31.3

Cognitive and sensory alterations can cause problems with socializing, performing activities of daily living (ADLs) independently, working, or driving. The nurse's assessment helps to identify patients who are at risk for alterations, are experiencing alterations, or need special interventions for managing deficits (Health Assessment Questions box). Knowing the causes of cognitive and sensory deficits helps the nurse to quickly assess areas that are possible problems for individual patients.

HEALTH ASSESSMENT QUESTIONS

Cognitive Focus

When the patient has cognitive problems, the nurse may need to obtain the health history from a family member or other reliable person.

- Do you have trouble sleeping or do you sleep too much?
- Have you noticed difficulty adding numbers or doing your banking?
- Are you able to have conversations with others, either in person or on the phone?
- Are you able to drive to the store or do errands?
- Do you ever feel sad?
- Do you read the newspaper?
- Do you live with anyone? If so, with whom?
- What medication do you take every day?

Sensory Focus

- Can you feel the difference between hot and cold water?
- Have you ever had a sore on your leg or foot that wouldn't heal?
- Do you have any pain, numbness, or tingling in your hands, legs, or feet?
- Are you able to smell different foods?
- Can you taste salty foods? sweet? sour?
- Have you noticed changes in your hearing?
- Have you ever had a hearing examination?
- Do you wear hearing aids?
- Do you ever lose your balance or feel like the room is spinning?
- When was your last eye examination?
- Do you wear glasses or contacts?
- Can you see to read the newspaper?
- Can you see objects to the your left and to your right?
- Is your vision blurry?

HEALTH HISTORY

A thorough history and physical assessment of the patient with cognitive or sensory deficits is essential to determine the extent and cause of the deficit. The nurse starts by asking general questions about the patient's health history, followed by specific questions aimed at discovering whether the patient is at risk for or is experiencing cognitive or sensory deficits.

Effects of Lifestyle on Cognition and Sensation

Certain lifestyle choices put patients at higher risk for cognitive or sensory problems. Smoking, obesity, a high-cholesterol diet, and excessive alcohol use can cause hypertension and drastically increase the risk of stroke. Cocaine use can destroy olfactory receptors in the nasal passages, causing a decrease in the sense of smell. Smoking decreases the senses of smell and taste.

High stress levels in a patient's life can lead to alterations in a patient's physical status. Stress is one of the risks associated with hypertension, which can cause dizziness and stroke. In patients experiencing extremely high levels of stress, symptoms such as anxiety and confusion can be similar to those of sensory overload. The patient is interviewed regarding family, work, and personal stressors, including recent job loss, divorce, death of a loved one, illness in the family, and pressure to succeed at work.

Metabolic syndrome consists of a group of specific risk factors that together are associated with a greatly increased risk for development of coronary artery disease, stroke, and diabetes mellitus type 2. If three or more of the defining features are documented, metabolic syndrome is considered to be present, and the patient is at a higher risk for developing the sensory deficits associated with the associated diseases. The features of metabolic syndrome are (U.S. National Library of Medicine, 2014c):

- High blood pressure
- High blood glucose
- Excess fat around the waist
- Low levels of high-density lipoprotein (HDL) cholesterol
- High levels of triglycerides

Lack of sleep may cause problems with concentration, judgment, and mental abilities, as well as blurred vision and decreased response to auditory stimuli. The nurse obtains a thorough sleep history from any patient with a change in cognitive or sensory awareness. For more information on sleep deprivation, see Chapter 33.

Effects of Environment on Cognition and Sensation

Exposure to environmental toxins poses a variety of health risks, including damage to some of the special sense organs. Hearing is adversely affected if loud noises have been a part of the patient's environment. Excessive exposure to ultraviolet light contributes to cataract development and other visual problems in some patients.

Safety in the home and hospital environments is a concern in patients who have sensory alterations. Home assessment can be accomplished through questioning the patient and family about the home environment, with referral to home health agencies when necessary.

Effects of Medical Conditions on Cognition and Sensation

Knowledge of the patient's past and current medical conditions is essential for the nurse who is planning patient care. Certain illnesses and infections cause sensory or cognitive changes. Diligence in monitoring the patient's condition decreases the detrimental effects of these changes. For example, the patient with diabetes is at risk for eye problems such as diabetic retinopathy, glaucoma, and cataracts, which can lead to visual loss and blindness. Yearly dilated-eye examinations are essential to monitor these conditions. Keeping weight, blood sugar, and cholesterol levels under control will decrease the complications of diabetes.

Effects of Medications on Cognition and Sensation

Certain over-the-counter, prescription, and street drugs have side effects that alter sensory or cognitive status, and some symptoms are traced back to medication use. For example, aspirin can cause tinnitus. Narcotics and some street drugs can cause confusion, dizziness, and hallucinations. Pupils may be dilated from medication used to view the retina or from other drugs. The nurse asks the patient about all medications, including prescription drugs and over-the-counter medications such as herbal preparations and alternative medications, vitamins, and minerals.

PHYSICAL ASSESSMENT

A thorough physical assessment is necessary for all patients exhibiting a change in cognitive or sensory status. The nurse obtains vital signs and performs a complete head-to-toe assessment to determine the extent of sensory or cognitive alterations as well as problems that could lead to deficits.

Vital Signs

The nurse monitors the patient's vital signs on a regular basis and notes changes or abnormal findings. Hypertension is a leading cause of stroke. If orthostatic hypotension is present, dizziness and loss of consciousness may occur when the patient changes position too quickly. Cognitive changes such as confusion or disorientation may be effects of a high fever. Hypoxia leads to dizziness and changes in levels of cognition and consciousness. For more information on normal vital signs, see Chapter 19.

Neurologic Assessment

A neurologic assessment is completed for any patient experiencing changes in cognitive or sensory awareness. The patient's orientation is assessed during the health history. While talking with patients, the nurse assesses their cognitive abilities, such as reasoning, judgment, and language. For patients with suspected deficits in cognition, the nurse can use a screening tool such as the Mini-Mental State Examination (MMSE) developed by Folstein, Folstein, and McHugh (1975). This examination is simple and quick to administer and tests the patient's cognitive orientation, attention, calculation, recall, language, and spatial orientation. Periodic reassessment is necessary for patients who have been diagnosed with dementia, to determine further cognitive impairment over time.

Cranial nerves are assessed if problems with the special senses are suspected. Assessing only the cranial nerve or nerves involved in the sensory alteration is acceptable. For a complete description of cranial nerve assessment, see Chapter 20.

Laboratory Tests

Screening blood work is obtained for patients with complaints indicating sensory or cognitive changes. A complete blood count should be performed in any patient who exhibits a sudden change in behavior, to rule out infection.

Electrolytes, such as sodium, potassium, chloride, calcium, and magnesium, are monitored. Both high and low levels of certain electrolytes in the body can cause problems with level of consciousness, cognition, and sensation. Patients with either hypernatremia and hyponatremia have central nervous system-related symptoms. Tactile disturbances, such as tingling and numbness around the mouth and in the fingers, are signs of hypocalcemia. Mental changes are associated with both hypercalcemia and hypocalcemia. For a complete description of electrolyte disturbances and related signs and symptoms, see Chapter 39.

Blood glucose levels are monitored as part of routine blood work, and in patients with diabetes they are monitored several times daily. Patients experiencing hypoglycemia may exhibit symptoms of irritability and have difficulty concentrating. If the level of glucose in the blood becomes extremely low, loss of consciousness, coma, and even death can occur. If glucose levels are extremely high, diabetic ketoacidosis or diabetic coma may develop. Close monitoring of glucose levels in diabetic patients helps to prevent complications of hyperglycemia that may contribute to cognitive and sensory deficits, such as diabetic retinopathy, peripheral neuropathy, and stroke.

A urinalysis with culture and sensitivity testing is obtained for any patient exhibiting a change in cognition, to rule out a urinary tract infection. Presence of bacteria, nitrates, and white blood cells in the urine indicates an infection. Culture and sensitivity results specify the type of bacteria and indicate which antibiotics can be used to treat the infection. When the infection is treated successfully, behavior should return to the patient's baseline level.

EFFECTS OF AGE, ILLNESS, STRESS, AND TRAUMA ON COGNITION AND SENSATION

The nurse's knowledge of symptoms of cognitive and sensory alterations caused by age, illness, and trauma enables appropriate assessment of patients. These alterations cause changes in the patient's ability to function independently, communicate, and carry out ADLs.

Mental Status and Cognitive Function

The normal aging process causes neurons to decrease in numbers, and loss of neurons causes a decrease in the number of synapses in the brain, leading to a decreased ability to identify sensations such as pain, touch, pressure, and postural changes. As aging occurs, the person's ability to sense harmful stimuli in the environment, such as a hot stove or a noxious odor, is reduced. In some people, arteries become narrowed from a buildup of plaque, causing a diminished nutrient supply. All of these changes impair cognitive abilities and response to sensory stimuli (McKinley and O'Loughlin, 2012).

> **QSEN FOCUS!**
>
> Safety is maximized when the nurse uses strategies to reduce the risk of harm to self or others, especially in patients who have cognitive and sensory impairments. The nurse notes the cognitive and physical limits of each patient.

Any illness or trauma that involves the central nervous system can alter mental status and cognition. Brain injuries, as well as any damage to cranial nerves, inhibit stimuli from reaching the proper part of the brain and being interpreted correctly. The nurse's thorough assessment of the nervous system, including cranial nerve assessment if indicated, localizes the impairment and discovers its extent. To assess cognitive abilities, the nurse asks the patient to add simple numbers. Having the patient draw the face of a clock gives the nurse information about spatial perception and cognitive function.

> **! SAFE PRACTICE ALERT**
>
> Assess the patient's ability to stand and walk independently before permitting activities such as ambulation or transferring.

Ability to Communicate

The patient's ability to communicate affects all aspects of care. If a brain insult has caused expressive aphasia, the patient will understand the spoken or written word but will not be able to respond correctly to questions or statements. The nurse assesses the patient daily to monitor for changes and improvements in language expression. If the brain deficit results in receptive aphasia, the nurse continues to assess the patient's ability to understand simple directions.

Communication can be a challenge in patients with degenerative brain disorders such as dementia. The patient's ability to communicate is assessed using simple conversation and directions. Testing communication skills is part of the Mini-Mental State Examination discussed earlier, which screens for communication difficulties and shows progression of problems over time.

Hearing, Vision, Touch, Smell, and Taste

Hearing ability can be determined by observing the patient's conversation and responses and by talking with the patient in a normal conversational tone while standing slightly behind the patient. If the patient does not respond appropriately, a hearing impairment may exist. The nurse questions the patient about previous hearing examinations and the use of hearing aids. If the nurse suspects a hearing impairment, hearing acuity is assessed (see Chapter 20).

In the decade between the ages of 40 and 50 years, most people begin to exhibit presbyopia. The affected patient needs to hold reading materials at a distance or becomes unable to read normal-size or small print. Other age-related vision changes that can occur, such as cataracts, macular degeneration, and diabetic retinopathy, cause the patient to be unable to see in certain visual fields or to have blurred vision. Visual ability is assessed by testing vision in central and peripheral visual fields.

> **! SAFE PRACTICE ALERT**
>
> The nurse ensures the safety of a hospitalized patient who has visual changes by describing the room environment and identifying the location of needed objects. As with all patients, it is imperative that a call light be within reach.

Detection of touch and pressure stimuli diminishes with age. In some patients this change is insignificant; in others the change is more severe. Diseases such as diabetic neuropathy decrease the patient's ability to discern touch, especially in the lower extremities. The nurse assesses the patient's ability to feel light touch and pressure by touching the patient's legs and feet (Figure 31-4). A complete peripheral sensory assessment is completed in any patient who exhibits diminished sensation in the extremities.

The special senses of smell and taste decline with age, altering the taste of food. Patients with diminished smell and taste either prefer a bland diet or add too much salt or seasoning to foods. Some lose interest in food, leading to poor nutritional status. The nurse facilitates provision of appealing, nutritious meals by determining the patient's food preferences and eating patterns while the patient is in the hospital or long-term care facility.

Ability to Perform ADLs

The nurse assesses the patient's understanding of and ability to perform ADLs. Patients who have damage to the brain due

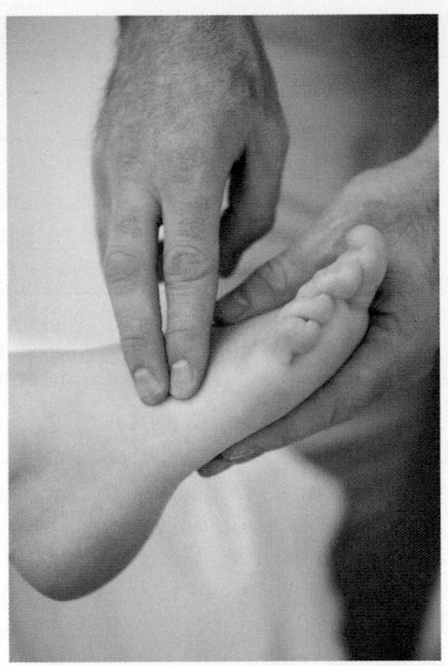

FIGURE 31-4 Assessment of the lower extremities for light-touch and light-pressure sensations.

to illness or trauma may have decreased motor functions. The patient who has had a CVA or a head injury may have weakness or paralysis on one side of the body, making it difficult to ambulate or perform tasks of self-hygiene or toileting. Observing the patient's abilities during care and assisting the patient with tasks that cannot be performed independently help the nurse determine the plan of care.

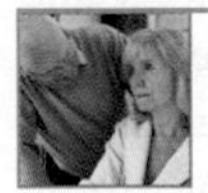

1. List two focused assessments that the nurse should perform for Mrs. Matson. Give rationales for each.

NURSING DIAGNOSIS LO 31.4

Nursing diagnoses related to cognitive and sensory alterations are numerous, and the diagnoses identified for a particular patient depend on the specific deficit. A thorough assessment is conducted, and diagnoses are based on the objective and subjective data that are collected. They are chosen to coincide with patient problems for which nursing interventions can be outlined. Unique patient care plans are written that are intended to address specific patient goals. Some common nursing diagnoses associated with cognition are *Acute Confusion, Chronic Confusion,* and *Disturbed Thought Processes.* Sensory nursing diagnoses include those associated with the special senses as well as tactile alterations.

The following are some examples of nursing diagnostic statements:

- *Acute Confusion* related to cerebral hypoxia secondary to a clot in the cerebral artery as evidenced by being oriented to person and confused about place and time
- *Chronic Confusion* related to progressive brain degeneration secondary to Alzheimer disease as evidenced by poor judgment, wandering, loss of ability to compute numbers, memory loss, and change in personality
- *Impaired Verbal Communication* related to alterations of the central nervous system secondary to cerebrovascular accident as evidenced by inability to recognize words or understand questions
- *Impaired Memory* related to central nervous system changes as evidenced by inability to recall address or daughter's name; does not remember medical history
- *Risk for Falls* with risk factors of lack of awareness of environmental hazards and confusion
- *Impaired Social Interactions* related to communication deficits secondary to hearing impairment as evidenced by quiet and withdrawn behavior, avoidance of social situations, and the statement "It is too hard to hear people talking"
- *Disturbed Thought Processes* related to degenerative brain disorder as evidenced by inaccurate history and memory deficit
- *Social Isolation* related to alterations in mental status secondary to dementia as evidenced by sad affect and the statement "I feel so alone"

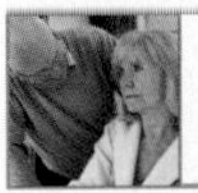

2. Identify three cognitive, sensory, and psychosocial nursing diagnoses for Mrs. Matson.

PLANNING LO 31.5

The third phase of the nursing process is the planning phase. After nursing diagnoses are identified and prioritized for the patient, desired outcomes and patient-centered goals are established. Nursing care plans are developed for each nursing diagnosis, with interventions aimed at meeting the patient goals. Careful consideration is given to the patient's abilities, the resources available, and the time frame for goal attainment.

For patients with cognitive and sensory alterations, collaboration with families or significant others is imperative. Often, other health care providers also are consulted to ensure continuity of care and maximization of cognitive and sensory function for the patient (Collaboration and Delegation box).

After identifying specific nursing diagnoses, the nurse writes goal statements that are patient-centered, set measurable goals, and include a time frame (Table 31-1). The

TABLE 31-1 Care Planning

NANDA-I NURSING DIAGNOSIS LABEL WITH NURSING DIAGNOSIS STATEMENT	NURSING OUTCOME CLASSIFICATION (NOC)	NURSING INTERVENTION CLASSIFICATION (NIC)
Acute Confusion related to cerebral hypoxia secondary to clot in cerebral artery as evidenced by being oriented to person and confused about place and time	*Cognitive orientation* (0901) Identifies current place (090103)	*Reality orientation* (4820) Engage patient in concrete "here and now" activities, which focus on something outside self that is concrete and reality-oriented.

From Bulechek G, Butcher H, Dochterman J, et al (Eds): *Nursing interventions classification (NIC),* ed. 6, St. Louis, 2013, Mosby; Moorhead S, Johnson M, Maas M, et al (Eds): *Nursing outcomes classification (NOC),* ed. 5, St. Louis, 2013, Mosby; NANDA International: *Nursing diagnoses: Definitions and classification, 2012–2014,* West Sussex, England, 2012, Wiley-Blackwell. Reprinted with permission from NANDA International, Inc.

COLLABORATION AND DELEGATION

Patients With Cognitive or Sensory Alterations

- Family and friends of the patient with dementia will be involved in the day-to-day care of the affected person and therefore need to be included in the planning process.
- Ensure that full-time caregivers have a support system, to avoid caregiver burnout.
- The patient with cognitive alterations needs an interdisciplinary team to assess deficits and provide ongoing treatment.
- A speech therapist is consulted for patients with hearing deficits or aphasia.
- A patient who has had a stroke benefits from consultation with an occupational therapist for adaptations necessary to maintain ADLs and with a physical therapist for ambulation training.
- For the patient with cognitive or sensory alterations, care may be delegated to unlicensed assistive personnel after assessment by the nurse.
- Consultation with social services to arrange home care specialists may be needed for patients with cognitive or sensory alterations that preclude safe self-medication.

following are some examples of goal statements that coincide with each of the nursing diagnoses listed in the previous section:

- Patient will respond appropriately to questions about place and time within 48 hours.
- Patient will remain within the unit while in long-term care.
- Patient will communicate basic needs through the use of photos within 1 week.
- Patient will use a calendar, a clock, and written notes to remember pertinent information daily.
- Patient will use the call light before getting out of bed while in the hospital.
- Patient will express increased satisfaction with her social situation after being fitted with a hearing aid.
- Patient will participate in cognitive exercises and reality orientation during hospitalization.
- Patient will interact with other nursing home residents during planned activities.

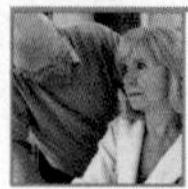

3. Write a short-term goal for this nursing diagnosis: *Impaired Verbal Communication* related to alterations of the central nervous system secondary to cerebrovascular accident as evidenced by mild difficulty finding some words while retaining the ability to express needs.

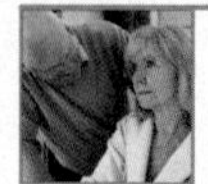

The conceptual care map for Mrs. Matson provided in Figure 31-5 is partially completed to indicate how to use the map as a learning tool. Using it as an example, go to the website at *http://evolve.elsevier.com/YoostCrawford/fundamentals/* to complete Nursing Diagnoses 2 and 3.

◆ IMPLEMENTATION AND EVALUATION LO 31.6

The final two steps in the nursing process are dynamic. The nurse delivers care through appropriate interventions and continuously evaluates the effects of that care. Patients who have experienced a change in cognitive or sensory status need ongoing reevaluation and adjustment of the plan of care to maximize their functional potential.

INTERVENTIONS

Nursing care plans for patients with cognitive or sensory alterations are individualized, depending on the clinical problem and the nursing diagnosis. Patient-centered care plans specify interventions focused on maximizing the patient's capabilities.

Patients With Cognitive Alterations

The nurse ensures that any patient with cognitive changes has had a thorough workup, including a history, physical, blood work, urinalysis, and other diagnostic studies as necessary. Ruling out the presence of infection and differentiating among dementia, delirium, and depression are important diagnostic steps. The nurse functions as an advocate for the patient during the diagnostic process and collaborates with other specialists as needed.

Medications

Warfarin: Call health care provider with PT/INR results daily for dose

Atorvastatin: 10 mg daily

Acetaminophen: 650 mg q 4 hr prn for pain

IV Sites/Fluids/Rate

Intravenous (IV) access saline lock

Past Medical/Surgical History

Hypercholesterolemia
Moderate hearing deficit worsening over the past 5 years

Conceptual Care Map

Student name__________ Patient initials Mrs. M Date __________

Age 67 Gender F Room # ___ Admission date 2 days ago

CODE Status Full Allergies NKDA Braden score 19

Diet Low-cholesterol diet Activity Up with assistance

Weight __________ Height __________ Religion __________

Admitting Diagnoses/Chief Complaint

Symptoms of slurred speech and weakness on right side/CVA

Assessment Data

T 36.7° C (98.1° F); P 68, regular and strong; R 18, unlabored and regular; BP 128/76; pulse oximetry 96% on RA; denies pain.
Abdomen soft and nontender; bowel sounds present × 4. Mild weakness on right side and slightly unsteady on her feet, requiring assistance of one person.
IV access in left antecubital space is without redness or swelling. Having mild difficulty finding some words but has been able to express her needs.
Speech has become clearer and her strength on the right side of her body has improved since admission. Slight difficulty hearing when spoken to in conversational tone but does not wear a hearing aid.
Married mother of three and grandmother of five. Mr. M visits daily and spends most of the day with his wife. He is alert and oriented and has no obvious physical problems. Two of their children live out of state, but a daughter who lives locally has been in to visit.

Laboratory Values/ Diagnostic Test Results

13.2 g/dL
39%

PT/INR 23.4/2.1

All other lab values were within normal limits.

MRI done in the ED showed a clot in left frontal lobe.

Treatments

VS q 4 hr
I&O q shift
Physical therapy
Speech therapy
Fall precautions

Primary Nursing Diagnosis

Acute Confusion related to cerebral hypoxia, secondary to clot in cerebral artery as evidenced by being oriented to person and confused about place and time.

Supporting Data

MRI done in ED showed a clot in left frontal lobe.
Chief complaint: Symptoms of slurred speech and weakness on right side.
Alert and oriented to person but confused about place and time.

STG/NOC

Patient will respond appropriately regarding place and time within 48 hours.
NOC: Cognitive orientation (0901)
Identifies current place (090103)

Interventions/NIC With Rationale

1. Use a clock, calendar, and statements about the name and location of the hospital to help orient the patient.
2. Keep the patient's environment stable to avoid confusing the patient.
3. Place familiar objects such as photos in the patient's room to help with orientation.
4. Open blinds in the morning to let natural light in to help patient with day-night orientation.

NIC: Reality orientation (4820)
Engage patient in concrete "here and now" activities focusing on something outside of self that is concrete and reality oriented.

Rationale Citation/EBP

Yoost BL, Crawford LR: *Fundamentals of nursing: Active learning for collaborative practice,* St. Louis, 2016, Mosby.

Evaluation

Patient able to state that she is in the hospital and the appropriate day of the week on day 3 of admission. Continue plan of care.

Nursing Diagnosis 2

Supporting Data

STG/NOC

Interventions/NIC With Rationale

Rationale Citation/EBP

Evaluation

Nursing Diagnosis 3

Supporting Data

STG/NOC

Interventions/NIC With Rationale

Rationale Citation/EBP

Evaluation

FIGURE 31-5 Partially completed conceptual care map based on Mrs. Matson, the case study patient in this chapter.

! SAFE PRACTICE ALERT

When the patient is in bed, leave the bed in the lowest position and the top two side rails up. The side rails are a reminder to the patient that he or she is near the edge of the bed. Check facility policy regarding use of side rails.

The hospitalized patient with cognitive alterations is oriented by use of a clock, a calendar, and statements about the location or name of the hospital. Monitoring orientation to person, place, and time is ongoing. Staff members always identify themselves by name, both verbally and nonverbally (with a name tag). The patient's environment is kept as consistent as possible, and moving the patient from room to room is avoided. Some familiar objects, such as a family photo, are placed near the patient if the hospital stay is longer than a few days. The environment is kept free of distractions such as loud noises and bright lights. Natural lighting to provide the patient with orientation to time of day can be accomplished by opening blinds or curtains during the day and darkening the room at night. The nurse talks with the patient while completing the assessment and care and explains all changes and procedures in simple terms. If a family member or significant other has a health care power of attorney, involve that person in decisions about care.

QSEN FOCUS!

Through patient-centered care, the nurse understands the importance of involvement of family and friends. The nurse communicates patient values, preferences, and expressed needs to other members of the health care team.

! SAFE PRACTICE ALERT

The nurse always reminds the patient about the location and proper use of the call light each time the patient will be left alone.

Maintaining a safe environment is essential for patients who are confused. Floors are kept dry and free of cords and tubes. The call light is placed within reach of the patient. The room should be lit so that the patient can see the surroundings. Patients who are unable to use the call light are checked frequently. Pressure-sensitive alarms may be used to alert the nurse of patient attempts to get out of bed.

! SAFE PRACTICE ALERT

The nurse checks the room for clutter and makes sure the floor is clear, clean, and dry. Nonskid footwear is provided for all patients.

Caring for the patient with dementia poses special challenges. Communication needs to be kept clear and simple. If negative behavior occurs, the patient is redirected or distracted. Reminiscing about the past provides a distraction. The patient often remembers details from many years ago even when he or she cannot remember what just occurred. The nurse must be flexible and creative when planning care for the patient with dementia. A gentle, caring approach shows the patient that the nurse is there to help.

If the patient has damage to the speech centers of the brain, special communication methods are needed. The nurse uses simple phrases and questions and speaks clearly without shouting. If the patient has expressive aphasia, asking questions that can be answered with yes or no and using a communication board with pictures may be beneficial. For patients with receptive aphasia, the nurse can point to pictures that represent basic needs such as food, drink, or use of the bathroom. In dealing with patients who have either type of aphasia, the nurse is patient and unrushed. The environment is without distractions, and the nurse should stand or sit somewhere that enables the patient to watch facial expressions. Gestures, facial expressions, and other cues help the patient to understand what is being said. A notepad or whiteboard may enhance communication.

! SAFE PRACTICE ALERT

Communication is key to all nursing interactions. Modifications are made for patients with deficits to enable meaningful communication.

The patient may be able to physically perform self-care but may need to be reminded to take a bath or brush the teeth. If the patient has motor damage that makes self-care difficult or if the patient's cognitive status is such that self-care cannot be completed independently, assistance with hygiene, toileting, and ambulation may be necessary. After doing a thorough assessment, the nurse may delegate some care to unlicensed assistive personnel. Patients with cognitive deficits depend on the nurse for reminders to eat and drink adequate amounts. Caffeine is discouraged because it can contribute to sleeplessness. Regular exercise helps decrease restlessness and wandering.

Social interaction is important for the patient with cognitive changes. The nurse facilitates interaction with family members and friends in person or by phone. Reading newspapers or magazines of interest, or engaging in other activities that stimulate the brain, is encouraged.

Patient education is needed to ensure a safe home environment and adaptation within the community for patients with cognitive alterations. Safety is a primary concern with discharge of the patient to home. Providing adequate social interaction is another priority.

The dementia patient needs a simple environment and a consistent routine. The environment is adapted to the patient. Adequate nutrition and rest are important. Harmful substances, such as chemicals and medications, are kept under

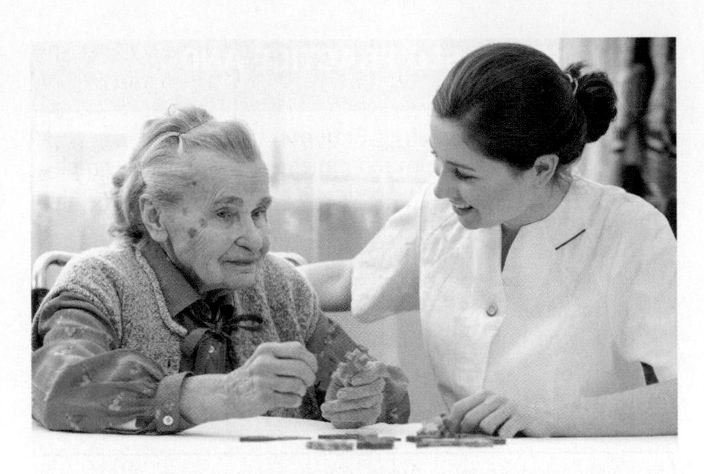

FIGURE 31-6 Talking with a patient with dementia about the past can help make the person feel loved and accepted.

lock. The patient is supervised, to minimize the chance of wandering. Activities that are enjoyable are made available to the patient. Reality orientation involves helping the patient stay as aware as possible of his or her circumstances, through use of clocks, calendars, notes, and other reminders, thereby minimizing confusion. Providing activities that the patient enjoys can help prevent boredom and deter negative behavior (Figure 31-6).

Because patients with dementia gradually lose the ability to reason and make decisions, a guardian often is necessary. A loving family member or friend typically fills this role to protect the patient from injury and abuse. If no one is available, the court will appoint a guardian (Ethical, Legal, and Professional Practice box).

ETHICAL, LEGAL, AND PROFESSIONAL PRACTICE

Patients With Dementia

- If no legal guardian has been established for the patient with dementia during the early stages of the disease when the patient can still reason and make decisions, in the later stages the court can declare a patient incompetent and appoint a guardian or authorize a person through a health care power of attorney to make health care decisions for the patient. Often the person appointed or authorized is a family member.
- Ethical issues arise for patients with dementia, such as how much they should be told about their illness and who should make care decisions if no one has been appointed.

Patient and family education about dementia is an ongoing process. Educating family members on how to relate to their loved one reduces caregiver frustration and burnout. Resources available for caregivers include respite care, household help, support groups, books, and workshops. Caregivers should manage their own stress through relaxation, exercise and pursuit of hobbies, and care for their health needs with regular doctor visits (Robinson, Wayne, and Segal, 2014).

Patients With Tactile Alterations

Numerous safety concerns are recognized for the patient with tactile deficits. The nurse tests the temperature of bath water to reduce the risk of burns in patients who cannot feel differences in temperature. Frequent monitoring of the extremities is indicated. Any changes indicating decreasing sensation or circulation are reported to the primary care provider. If the patient can move the affected extremities, active range-of-motion exercise is encouraged to stimulate circulation.

The patient who is unable to move in bed independently should be turned and repositioned at least every 2 hours to prevent damage to tissue from unrelieved pressure. Sharp objects such as pins and clips are kept away from the affected extremity or area and are not used to hold bandages. The patient who has limited sensation may not feel skin stress leading to development of a pressure ulcer or damage to tissue from a sharp object.

Patients With Olfactory and Gustatory Alterations

Some patients have a decreased sense of smell and taste because of aging, smoking, or infections. The nurse encourages intake of a well-balanced diet during hospitalization while taking into account the patient's specific dietary preferences. Serving highly aromatic foods stimulates the sense of smell. Enhancing the flavor and smell of foods to make them more appealing encourages intake. Diligent oral hygiene at least twice per day to keep the oral cavity pleasant tasting and hydrated has a positive impact on appetite.

The environment is kept clean, and noxious odors are eliminated as quickly as possible. Stimulation with pleasant odors such as fresh flowers or room deodorizer enhances the sense of smell.

The patient is encouraged to eat a variety of foods and to enhance the flavor with spices and herbs. Different flavors appeal to different patients depending on specific deficits. Nutrition education encourages healthy lifestyles. Other health promotion interventions are outlined in the Patient Education and Health Literacy box.

PATIENT EDUCATION AND HEALTH LITERACY

Health Promotion

- Promoting healthier lifestyles to older adults is an important nursing consideration. Hearing and vision examinations are part of health promotion.
- Interventions to encourage healthy lifestyles include education regarding nutrition, exercise, smoking cessation, and the importance of health screening.
- Byam-Williams and Salyer (2010) found that older adults with a higher level of self-efficacy, or interest in their own welfare, had healthier lifestyles. Older women reported healthier lifestyles than did older men.
- Health education and promotion of healthy lifestyles in older adults should be a key nursing intervention in the inpatient setting as well as in the outpatient and community settings.

Patients With Auditory Alterations

Many hospitalized patients have hearing impairments. If the patient uses an assistive device such as a hearing aid at home, its use in the hospital is encouraged. Care is taken to keep the hearing aid in good working order and prevent it from getting lost. See Chapter 27 for a discussion on the use and care of hearing aids. Communication is facilitated when the nurse is positioned so that the patient can see the nurse's mouth, because many hearing-impaired patients read lips and watch facial expressions to assist hearing. The nurse speaks clearly and slowly without shouting. Background noise is kept to a minimum. Hearing loss may not be equal in both ears. Ask the patient if hearing is better in one ear than the other, and stand on the patient's stronger-hearing side to converse. If the patient is cognitively and visually able to read, the use of written instructions and information is helpful. Paper and pencil, a whiteboard, or a computer can be kept at the bedside. A sign language interpreter is used when a patient communicates through sign language.

Closed captioning on television for the patient with hearing impairment provides a way to keep up with current events and a means of distraction while hospitalized. A light on the telephone that signals an incoming call and an amplified receiver will enable the patient to use the phone to make and receive calls.

Patients With Equilibrium Alterations

The patient with equilibrium alterations is instructed to call for assistance when ambulating to prevent injury. If the patient is experiencing nausea or vomiting, a basin is kept on the bedside stand within easy reach. Keeping the lights dim and noise at a minimum may relieve some of the symptoms. Balance and coordination diminish with age, so obstacles are kept off the floor to prevent tripping and falls.

> **! SAFE PRACTICE ALERT**
>
> Patients experiencing problems with equilibrium or those taking over-the-counter medication to combat motion sickness should not drive.

Patients With Visual Alterations

The patient with a visual alteration is oriented to the placement of items in the hospital room. It is best to limit the amount of change in the environment. Furniture is kept in the same place. Items that the patient needs are left within easy reach, and the nurse confirms that the patient knows the location. The call light is placed within reach so that the patient can call for assistance with ambulation, especially in the first few days of hospitalization. If eyeglasses or other visual assistive devices, such as contact lenses, are used, they should be kept in good working order and be available on the bedside table. For information about the care of these devices, see Chapter 27. Adequate lighting without glare is provided if the patient needs to read print (Evidence-Based Practice and Informatics box).

> **EVIDENCE-BASED PRACTICE AND INFORMATICS**
>
> **Care for Visually Impaired Patients**
>
> Care for the visually impaired patient involves some simple steps that can enhance the patient's experience and facilitate the nurse-patient relationship:
>
> - Maintain adequate lighting, and minimize glare.
> - Make sure the patient is wearing eyeglasses or contact lenses if prescribed.
> - Use large print or clear handwriting when giving written instructions.
> - Use photos, pictures, diagrams, or audiotaped instructions if necessary.

From National Institute on Aging: Aging and your eyes, 2011. Retrieved from *www.nia.nih.gov/health/publication/aging-and-your-eyes*.

When a visually impaired patient is served a meal tray, the nurse describes the placement of food on the tray in terms of the numbers on a clock (Figure 31-7). For example, the nurse may say, "Your carrots are at the 2 o'clock position." The Home Care Considerations box outlines considerations for patients with cognitive or sensory deficits.

Patients With Sensory Deprivation

Any hospitalized patient who has a cognitive or sensory deficit, especially auditory or visual, is at risk for sensory deprivation. Providing social interaction for the hospitalized patient with a sensory deficit prevents feelings of isolation. Engaging in meaningful interactions with the patient and encouraging enjoyable activities (e.g., watching television, doing crossword puzzles, reading) are ways to avoid sensory deprivation. For the visually impaired patient, listening to audiobooks or music is stimulating and provides diversion.

Tactile stimulation is provided when the nurse touches the patient. Giving a backrub during the bath, holding the patient's hand while conversing, or gently touching the

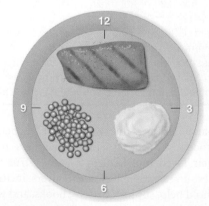

FIGURE 31-7 The nurse identifies position of food on the patient's plate or tray by referring to the numbers on a clock face.

HOME CARE CONSIDERATIONS

Patient With Cognitive Alterations

- If 24-hour supervision and assistance with care are needed, provisions are made with loved ones or a day care service, or placement in a long-term care facility is arranged.
- If the patient is cared for at home, information on day care and respite care is provided.
- Simple, calm environments help to optimize function in the patient with dementia.
- Use of door locks that require a key may be necessary if the patient wanders.
- The environment is kept free of hazards such as sharp objects.
- Referral to home health agencies is made if assistance with care is needed.

Patient With Tactile Alterations

- A simple kitchen thermometer is used to verify that bath water temperature is approximately 37.8° C (100° F).
- Hot water heaters are set so that scalding is not possible.
- The patient is instructed not to use heat or cold therapy on an affected extremity or region.
- Wearing gloves in the winter to prevent frostbite is especially important in patients with decreased sensation in the fingers.
- Sturdy shoes can prevent foot injuries when the patient has decreased sensation in the lower extremities.
- Any decrease in sensation, change in the color of the skin, and wounds or other lesions are reported to the health care provider.

Patient With Olfactory and Gustatory Alterations

- The patient may not be able to smell noxious odors such as from gas or spoiled food. The home should be checked for safety of gas stoves, hot water heaters, and furnaces.
- The patient is reminded to use other senses to detect spoiled food.
- Smoke detectors need to be in good working order.
- Use of noxious cleaning and other chemicals is avoided because the patient is at risk for being overcome by fumes.

Patient With Auditory Alterations

- The patient is instructed on the use and care of hearing aids and encouraged to wear them in the home environment.
- Family members are given communication tips such as speaking in a slow, distinct voice and standing in good lighting 3 to 5 feet in front of the hearing-impaired person.
- If the patient uses sign language, family members are encouraged to become proficient in this modality.
- Smoke detectors, doorbells, and telephones should have visual signals for a severely hearing-impaired person or amplification for the patient with some hearing.
- An amplified telephone or a **telecommunications device for the deaf (TDD)**—an electronic device that sends text communications through a telephone line—is a helpful adaptive tool.
- Computer communication such as email or texting helps keep the patient in touch with loved ones.

Patient With Equilibrium Alterations

- The patient experiencing dizziness or vertigo should change positions slowly and cautiously.
- Installation of a secure grab bar in the tub or shower at home gives the patient stability when getting in and out of the tub.
- Use of a tub chair may be necessary.
- Keeping rooms well lighted and instructing the patient to focus ahead when walking will help with equilibrium.
- Use of a cane or walker to provide further stability is advised, especially when the patient is walking in unfamiliar areas.
- Anyone with a current symptom of dizziness or vertigo is cautioned not to drive or operate machinery.
- The patient suffering from motion sickness should ride in the front seat of the car and look far ahead through the car windshield. Over-the-counter motion sickness medications, such as dimenhydrinate and meclizine, are available. These medications inhibit vestibular stimulation but may cause drowsiness and dizziness.

Patient With Visual Alterations

- If the patient is living independently, care is taken to rid the home of safety hazards. Furniture is placed to allow wide passageways. Throw rugs, which are a tripping hazard, are removed. Nonskid mats are used in bathrooms and kitchens. Grab bars placed in the tub or shower and stair railings are kept in good repair.
- Bright lighting in hallways and stairways prevents falls by the patient who has limited vision.
- The patient is oriented to the environment and the location of specific items.
- If vision is severely limited, use of a cane or walking stick held slightly in front helps the patient feel objects in his or her path.
- The patient with severe visual impairment may use Braille or voice recognition equipment in the home.
- The patient may use a seeing-eye dog.

Patient With Sensory Deprivation

- The patient who is discharged with sensory alterations is at risk for sensory deprivation.
- Use of sensory aids such as glasses and hearing aids promotes social interactions.
- Information on support groups and public transportation helps the patient maintain independence.
- Activities that the patient enjoys are encouraged.
- Referral to community agencies or use of home health aides may be necessary if the patient needs assistance with ADLs.

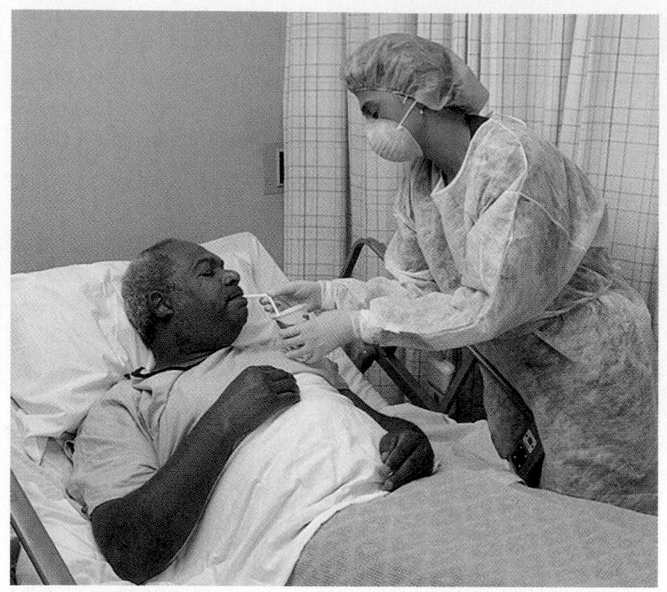

FIGURE 31-8 The nurse provides emotional support for a patient in isolation. (From deWit SC, O'Neill PA: Fundamental concepts and skills for nursing, ed 4, St. Louis, 2014, Saunders.)

shoulder conveys a caring attitude. Patients who are ambulatory and not at risk for falling are encouraged to walk in the hospital room or in the hallway.

The patient in isolation for medical reasons is at risk for sensory deprivation due to the restricted environment. The nurse uses proper personal protective equipment and enters the room as often as necessary to provide patient care, including emotional support. Family can visit the patient as long as proper protocol for the type of isolation is followed (Figure 31-8).

Patients With Sensory Overload

Sensory overload is common in intensive care patients. To prevent or alleviate overload, the nurse reduces sensory stimuli, dimming unnecessary lights and turning the sound down on alarms if possible. Nursing care is planned so that the patient is not constantly disturbed. Internal stimuli such as pain and nausea can contribute to sensory overload. Pain medication decreases unpleasant stimuli for the patient. Nursing interventions such as soothing music or a backrub help some patients. For other patients, these interventions may add to the overload. Visits from family members serve as reality orientation and provide a soothing, recognizable presence for some patients experiencing overload.

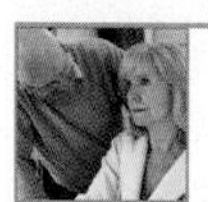

4. Identify at least four nursing interventions for Mrs. Matson designed to meet the short-term goal written for critical-thinking question 3.

EVALUATION

Ongoing evaluation of short- and long-term goal attainment is necessary to document patient progress. Changes in the patient's condition and goal attainment require updating the care plan and setting new goals. Improvement in sensory or cognitive abilities enables the patient to perform more self-care. A decline in the patient's condition necessitates more assistance from the nursing staff.

Goal statements are patient-centered and identify ways to move the patient toward independence, if possible. Evaluation of the plan of care includes information gathered from the patient and family.

SUMMARY OF LEARNING OUTCOMES

LO 31.1 *Describe the normal structure and function of brain and body regions involved in cognition and sensation:* Cognitive abilities and nervous system interpretation of sensory input enable individuals to respond to their environment.

LO 31.2 *Identify how alterations in structure and function associated with impaired cognition and sensation affect patients' abilities:* Illness, trauma, stress, and aging may cause alterations in cognitive and sensory function. When alterations occur, thought processes may be affected and sensory loss may occur.

LO 31.3 *Perform assessments of patients' cognitive and sensory function:* A thorough assessment is crucial for all patients at risk for or experiencing cognitive or sensory alterations.

LO 31.4 *Choose nursing diagnoses for patients who need assistance or modifications in care because of cognitive or sensory deficits:* Nursing diagnoses are based on the specific deficit and may include *Confusion, Impaired Verbal Communication,* and *Impaired Social Interaction.*

LO 31.5 *Articulate goals for patients with cognitive or sensory alterations:* When planning care for patients with cognitive or sensory alterations, the nurse establishes goals that are aimed at the patient's reaching his or her full potential. The patient's abilities and specific deficits are taken into consideration when the nurse establishes outcome criteria.

LO 31.6 *Carry out nursing care plans that include interventions to enhance patients' cognitive and sensory function:* Nursing care plans are individualized for patients with specific cognitive or sensory alterations to maximize each patient's capabilities.

Responses to the critical-thinking questions are available at *http://evolve.elsevier.com/YoostCrawford/fundamentals/.*

REVIEW QUESTIONS

1. A visually impaired diabetic patient states that he has lost the call light. What is the next step the nurse should take?
   - **a.** Clip the call light closer to the patient.
   - **b.** Tell the patient that the call light is clipped to the bed.
   - **c.** Describe the call light location, and take the patient's hand and guide it to that location.
   - **d.** Instruct the patient to verbally call for a staff member because "someone is always nearby."
2. When caring for a hearing-impaired patient, use of which technique by the nurse would facilitate communication?
   - **a.** Speaking clearly with distinct words
   - **b.** Talking slowly to facilitate understanding
   - **c.** Sitting behind the patient to decrease distractions
   - **d.** Standing near the patient's affected ear to balance sound
3. The nurse is caring for a patient with decreased sensation in the lower extremities. Which precaution does the nurse advise the patient to take?
   - **a.** The patient should use heat to warm hands during cold weather.
   - **b.** The patient should go barefoot at home to prevent blisters from shoes.
   - **c.** The patient should soak feet in cold water daily to decrease swelling.
   - **d.** The patient should test the bath water temperature to prevent burning injuries.
4. Which statement by the patient with vertigo lets the nurse know that the patient has understood the home-going instructions?
   - **a.** "I will buy a visual signal for my smoke detectors."
   - **b.** "I will have grab bars installed in my bathtub."
   - **c.** "I will change positions quickly to avoid vertigo."
   - **d.** "I will get a home phone with amplified sound."
5. Which nursing intervention is appropriate for a patient with sensory overload?
   - **a.** Dimming the lights
   - **b.** Performing care a little at a time
   - **c.** Leaving the patient's door open
   - **d.** Rushing to get care done quickly
6. Which recommendation in the home-going instructions is appropriate for a patient with damage to the chemoreceptors of the upper nasal passages?
   - **a.** Arranging for lighted signals on doorbells and telephones
   - **b.** Obtaining a thermometer for testing bath water temperature
   - **c.** Installing amplification devices on televisions, doorbells, and telephones
   - **d.** Scheduling yearly safety checks of gas hot water heaters and furnaces
7. When caring for an elderly patient who presents with acute confusion of sudden onset, which test would the nurse expect to be ordered?
   - **a.** Urine culture and sensitivity testing
   - **b.** Mini-Mental State Examination
   - **c.** Swallow evaluation
   - **d.** MRI with contrast
8. Which nursing diagnosis is the highest priority for a patient with presbycusis?
   - **a.** *Impaired Social Interaction*
   - **b.** *Disturbed Thought Processes*
   - **c.** *Disturbed Sensory Perception*
   - **d.** *Impaired Physical Mobility*
9. Which nursing interventions would be necessary in caring for a patient with cognitive alterations who is hospitalized? *(Select all that apply.)*
   - **a.** Apply wrist restraints for combativeness.
   - **b.** Place a clock in the room for orientation.
   - **c.** Keep floor free of clutter for safety.
   - **d.** Identify staff with each interaction.
   - **e.** Play loud music for distraction.
10. Which goal statement is appropriate for a patient with the nursing diagnosis of *Impaired Memory*?
    - **a.** Patient will remember nurse's name.
    - **b.** Nurse will remind patient of his/her name each shift.
    - **c.** Patient will state name and date with each nursing encounter.
    - **d.** Nurse will remind patient of name and date with each nursing encounter.

Answers and rationales for the review questions are available at http://evolve.elsevier.com/YoostCrawford/fundamentals/.

REFERENCES

Byam-Williams J, Salyer J: Factors influencing the health-related lifestyle of community dwelling older adults, *Home Healthc Nurse* 28(2):115-121, 2010.

Cronenwett L, Sherwood G, Barnsteiner J, et al: Quality and safety education for nurses, *Nurs Outlook* 55(3):122-131, 2007.

Folstein MF, Folstein SE, McHugh PR: Mini-mental state: A practical method for grading the cognitive state of patients for the clinician, *J Psychiatr Res* 12:189-198, 1975.

McKinley M, O'Loughlin VD: *Human anatomy*, ed. 3, Boston, 2012, McGraw-Hill.

National Institute on Aging: Hearing loss, 2013. Retrieved from *www.nia.nih.gov/health/publication/hearing-loss.*

National Institute of Neurologic Disorders and Stroke: NINDS Alzheimer's disease information page, 2014. Retrieved from *www.ninds.nih.gov/disorders/alzheimersdisease/alzheimersdisease.htm.*

National Institutes of Health News in Health: Dealing with dementia: When thinking and behavior decline, 2014. Retrieved from *http://newsinhealth.nih.gov/issue/Jan2014/Feature1.*

Robinson L, Wayne MS, Segal J: Support for Alzheimer's & dementia caregivers, 2014. Retrieved from *www.helpguide.org/elder/alzheimers_disease_dementia_support_caregiver.htm.*

Shier DN, Butler JL, Lewis R: *Hole's essentials of human anatomy & physiology*, ed. 11, Boston, 2012, McGraw-Hill.

U.S. National Library of Medicine: Delirium, 2014a. Retrieved from *www.nlm.nih.gov/medlineplus/delirium.html.*

U.S. National Library of Medicine: Depression, 2014b. Retrieved from *www.nlm.nih.gov/medlineplus/depression.html.*

U.S. National Library of Medicine: Metabolic syndrome, 2014c. Retrieved from *www.nlm.nih.gov/medlineplus/metabolicsyndrome.html.*

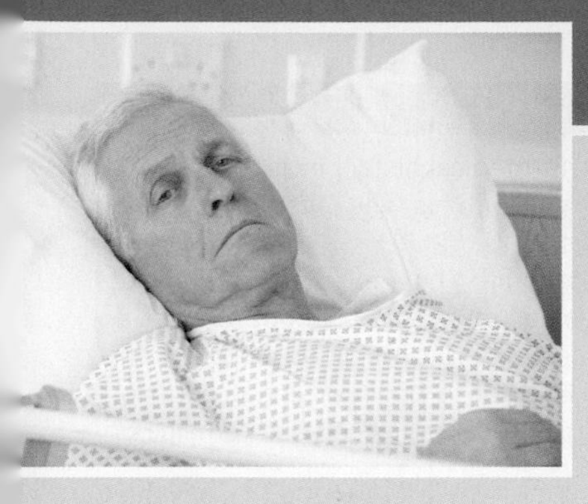

CHAPTER 32

Stress and Coping

EVOLVE WEBSITE

http://evolve.elsevier.com/YoostCrawford/fundamentals/

- Additional Evolve-Only Review Questions With Answers
- Answers and Rationales for Text Review Questions
- Answers to Critical-Thinking Questions
- Case Study With Questions
- Conceptual Care Map Creator
- Glossary

LEARNING OUTCOMES

Comprehension of this chapter's content will provide students with the ability to:

LO 32.1 Identify the key concepts associated with the body's physiologic and psychological responses to stress.

LO 32.2 Describe psychological and physiologic responses of the nervous, endocrine, and immune systems to stress.

LO 32.3 Describe the effects of stress on health.

LO 32.4 Demonstrate assessment techniques for recognizing signs and symptoms of stress.

LO 32.5 Identify stress-related nursing diagnosis labels.

LO 32.6 Articulate stress reduction goals and patient outcomes.

LO 32.7 Develop patient-centered care plans with interventions designed to address stress-related conditions.

LO 32.8 Discuss the potential impact of stress on nurses.

KEY TERMS

allostasis, p. 731
anger, p. 735
anxiety, p. 735
burnout, p. 744
coping, p. 732
crisis intervention, p. 743
defense mechanisms, p. 732
depression, p. 735
distress, p. 731
eustress, p. 731
fight-or-flight response, p. 730
general adaptation syndrome (GAS), p. 730
generalized anxiety disorder, p. 735
homeostasis, p. 730
local adaptation syndrome (LAS), p. 731
post-traumatic stress disorder (PTSD), p. 735
sense of coherence (SOC), p. 732
stress, p. 730
stress appraisal, p. 730
stressor, p. 730

CASE STUDY

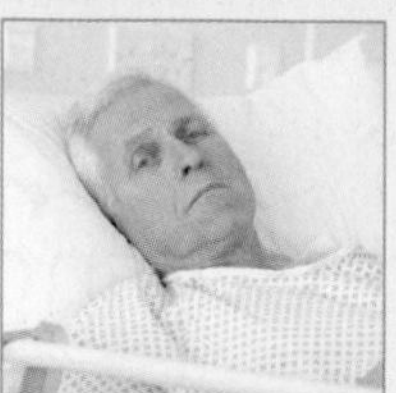

Mr. Hastings is a 60-year-old retired architect who is financially comfortable. His medical history includes a heart attack 5 years ago and a second heart attack just 4 weeks ago. Mr. Hastings lives with his wife in their two-story home, which they own. The bedrooms and bathroom are upstairs.

During the intake interview at his first clinic visit, Mr. Hastings states that his wife "hovers" over him, taking care of him physically and seeing that he does not overexert himself. He denies any chest pain but mentions that he occasionally experiences slight shortness of breath when climbing the stairs. Mr. Hastings looks downcast and somewhat depressed, despite being given permission by the cardiologist to begin driving again. He states, "I am going to die from this heart condition, so why treat it?" He states that he has difficulty falling asleep and remaining asleep because he feels anxious and jittery.

The nurse takes Mrs. Hastings aside and asks how she is feeling. Mrs. Hastings states that she is afraid her husband will have another heart attack if he exerts himself doing routine daily tasks and feels that she must take on his responsibilities. She knows that he is frustrated and stressed, and she does not know what to do to help him.

Refer back to this case study to answer the critical-thinking questions throughout the chapter.

Stress is ever-present in life, affecting every person regardless of socioeconomic status, age, gender, lifestyle, education, or occupation. Unrelieved stress has a negative impact on health. The stress response can directly cause damage to body tissues by increasing heart rate and blood pressure and causing the release of powerful stress hormones. Nurses need to recognize stress in their patients and themselves to facilitate appropriate and effective interventions to ameliorate these responses.

Stress is a complex concept that has been identified historically in several ways. Physiologic stress is the body's potentially harmful reaction to a stimulus (Selye, 1976). Psychological stress comprises the emotional and cognitive factors involved in the appraisal of threat (Lazarus, 1966). When the affected person interprets an event as a threat, the physiologic stress response is activated. A third form of stress, sociocultural stress, occurs when social systems are challenged by factors such as racism, economic hardship, or political upheaval. All three types may interact and are related.

The term **stress** is defined by Kasl (1992) as a demand from the internal or external environment that exceeds the person's immediately available resources or ability to respond. Selye (1956) defines stress as "a nonspecific response of the body to any demand made upon it." *Stress* may refer to the physiologic response pattern itself. A **stressor** is an event or stimulus that disrupts the person's sense of equilibrium. People react to stress in different ways, which are determined by their appraisal of the stressful event and their self-perceived ability to respond to the stressor. **Stress appraisal** is the process by which the person interprets a stressor as either a threat or a challenge (Folkman, Lazarus, Dunkle-Schetter, et al, 1986). The way a person responds to stress determines its impact on the person's attitude and physiologic response. Stress may lead to creative changes that enhance the person's life and well-being. Stress also may trigger dermatologic and gastrointestinal problems, heart problems, and autoimmune diseases such as rheumatoid arthritis (Stojanovich and Marisavljevich, 2008).

Knowledge of stress, coping, and adaptation is important for health care personnel because of the link between health and stress. The stress and coping components of this knowledge base are especially relevant for nurses because of their primary concern with the human responses to stressful conditions. The negative effect of stressful circumstances may be minimized if the stress is recognized early, resources for coping are identified, and appropriate interventions are implemented.

Sister Callista Roy's Adaptation Model (1970) provides a solid theoretical foundation for nursing care of patients facing stressful situations. In Roy's theory, people adapt to stress by meeting their physiologic needs, developing a positive identity, performing social role functions, and balancing dependence and independence. Stressors disrupt the person's equilibrium, resulting in illness. Nursing care is directed at altering stimuli that are stressors to the patient. In Roy's model, the nurse's role is to help patients adapt to illness or develop positive adaptive behaviors.

SCIENTIFIC FOUNDATION LO 32.1

The concept of **homeostasis**, the body's regulation of systems to maintain a steady state, was first described by Walter Cannon in 1932. Seventeen years earlier, Cannon (1915) identified the **fight-or-flight response** to excitement or threat. This physiologic response to stress, whether physical or psychological, is activation of the autonomic nervous system, resulting in an increase in heart rate, blood pressure, and respirations along with pupil dilation and a decrease in gastric motility and blood flow to the skin (Figure 32-1). When experiencing the fight-or-flight response, people report symptoms of rapid heartbeats, palpitations, nausea, and anxious feelings.

GENERAL ADAPTATION SYNDROME

Hans Selye (1976) named the physical response to stress the **general adaptation syndrome (GAS)**. He noted that the body responds in the same way to any demand, whether it be

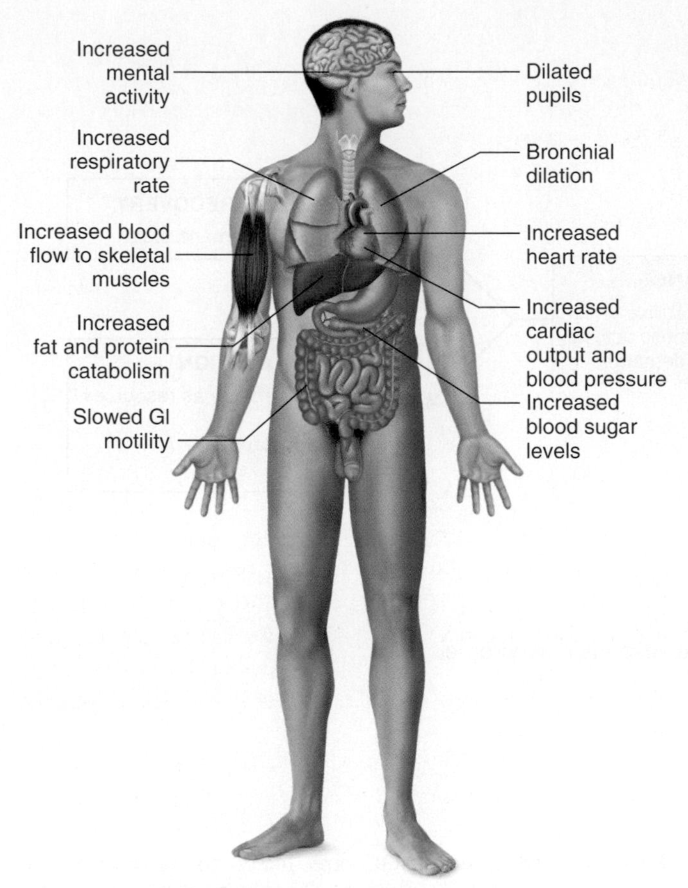

FIGURE 32-1 Fight-or-flight response.

physical, emotional, pleasant, or unpleasant. The GAS is evoked when the stimulation or stressor is strong enough to activate the autonomic nervous branch of the central nervous system, eliciting an adaptive response. Selye referred to the demands that produce the adaptive response as *stressors* and noted that stress is unavoidable. He labeled negative stress as **distress** (stress that is beyond the ability of the affected person to cope with or adapt to effectively), which can cause physical illness or emotional dysfunction. He identified positive stress as **eustress** (motivational stress), which is associated with effective coping and adaptation. Eustress is thought to be essential for normal growth and development.

The GAS consists of three stages: alarm reaction, resistance, and exhaustion. Most stressful events involve only the first two, but some ongoing demands can exceed the body's resources and lead to the final stage of exhaustion (Figure 32-2).

When the level of stress from a stressor reaches a threshold that threatens homeostasis, it is strong enough to activate the *alarm* stage of the stress response. In the alarm stage, the hypothalamic-pituitary-adrenal and autonomic nervous systems are activated, successively triggering responses in the sympathetic nervous system and the endocrine and immune systems. In the *resistance* stage, the body attempts to adapt to the stressor, and some of the initial responses are attenuated as the parasympathetic nervous system reverses the sympathetic stimulation and stabilization occurs. The body begins to repair damage and restore resources. However, if the stress is not relieved or the resources are inadequate to meet persistent demands, the body advances to the third stage, *exhaustion*.

When resources are depleted and the body is unable to continue the efforts of adaptation, the body cannot maintain physical function and death may result at a cellular or systemic level. This stage may be reversed by augmentation of the body's resources from the outside, such as through medication, nutritional support, or other therapies. Chronic, prolonged, unrelieved stress, such as that typical of the exhaustion stage, may cause disease. Such illnesses are recognized as stress-related diseases.

Local Adaptation Syndrome

Selye noted that tissues of the body more directly affected by stress demonstrate a **local adaptation syndrome (LAS)**, which may manifest as inflammation, reflexive response to pain, or hypoxia secondary to catecholamine release. Hypoxia can negatively affect wound healing as well as the ability to think clearly at times of severe anxiety. The GAS and the LAS are closely related, but the effects of the LAS are most notably manifested by activities in the immune system.

ALLOSTASIS

McEwan and Lasley proposed *allostasis* as an alternate term for the stress response. According to these researchers, **allostasis** is the means by which homeostasis is reestablished, and the purpose of allostasis is to assist the body in maintaining stability (McEwan and Lasley, 2002). A sustained stress response is potentially damaging. Allostatic responses (such as the fight-or-flight response) should terminate when no longer needed, reducing the allostatic load. The physiologic responses caused by physical and psychological stress are adaptive in the short term, but the body does not tolerate prolonged periods of sympathetic arousal. Chronic, high levels of stress have been shown to produce atrophic changes in the brain (McEwan, 2000).

STRESS APPRAISAL

Richard Lazarus and his colleagues developed a theory of cognitive mediation within emotion. An important concept within that theory is *appraisal*, or the automatic, often unconscious assessment of a demand or stressor. This evaluation of threat occurs in two stages, which may occur almost simultaneously. In the first stage, the immediacy of the threat and the degree of ambiguity of the threat are factors. The person measures what is at stake in the stressful encounter. In the second stage, coping options are evaluated. Primary

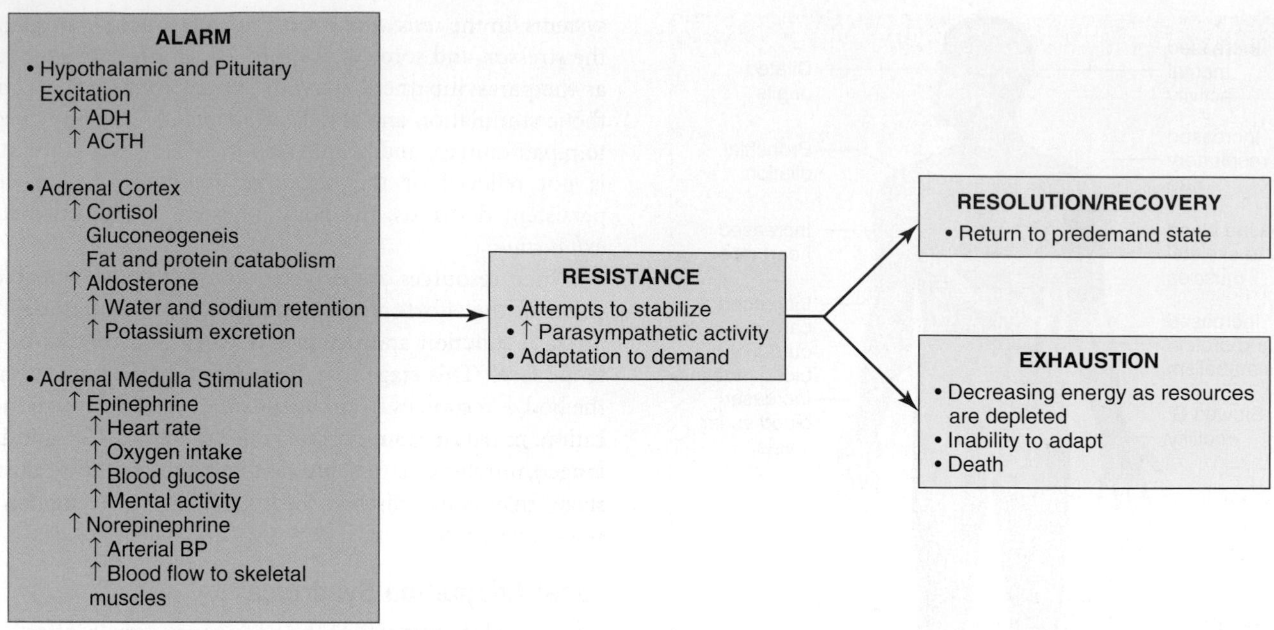

FIGURE 32-2 The general adaptation syndrome.

and secondary appraisals determine whether the stressful situation or transaction is a threat or a challenge. A threat invokes the possibility of harm or loss, whereas a challenge holds forth the possibility of benefit (Folkman, Lazarus, Dunkle-Schetter, et al, 1986). Current related research is focused on the concepts of conscientiousness and responsibility as they relate to the appraisal of daily stressors (Gartland, O'Connor, and Lawton, 2012).

SENSE OF COHERENCE

The fact that some people experience considerable stress but do not develop physical illness or prolonged emotional distress was of interest to stress researchers after World War II. In studying the survivors of concentration camps, they noted that personality factors, cultural and other support systems, and the timing and clustering of events affected the person's response to life events. Antonovsky (1979) developed the concept of sense of coherence to help explain this variation in response to stress.

Sense of coherence (SOC) is a characteristic of personality that references one's perception of the world as comprehensible, manageable, and meaningful. *Comprehensible* means that the demands of the internal and external environments are understandable and predictable; *manageable* means that the person recognizes resources that are available to meet these demands; and *meaningful* is the person's interpretation of the demands as worthy of engagement. Persons with strong SOC are likely to recognize and utilize resources in a stressful situation, while those with low SOC are likely to be overwhelmed and have difficulty coping.

COPING

Coping has been defined as the dynamic cognitive and behavioral efforts to manage demands (internal or external) that are appraised as exceeding immediately available resources (Lazarus and Folkman, 1984). Coping is recognized as a dynamic process that changes over time and does not guarantee success or healthy behavior. Some coping responses may have little or no effect, and some may be damaging to health, especially if used inappropriately. Examples of potentially damaging responses are defense mechanisms such as denial and suppression or the excessive use of alcohol and other drugs.

Defense Mechanisms

Defense mechanisms are predominantly unconscious, protective coping methods that people may apply in response to a perceived threat. Use of defense mechanisms on a short-term basis initially may prevent harm to the person in distress. However, long-term coping strategies that are based on defense mechanisms can prevent healthy growth and development. Examples of defense mechanisms are presented in Table 32-1.

TABLE 32-1 Defense Mechanisms

MECHANISM	DESCRIPTION
Compensation	Focusing on strengths rather than perceived weaknesses
Denial	Ignoring aspects of reality that induce anxiety or contribute to a loss of self-esteem
Displacement	Redirecting negative emotions perceived as unacceptable or threatening to a safer focus
Intellectualization	Overthinking a challenging situation or impulse to avoid dealing with the emotions it elicits
Projection	Attributing one's own motives, values, desires, situational responses, and personality traits to another person
Rationalization	Explaining personal actions in a way that enhances one's own self-image
Regression	Reverting to behavior associated with an earlier stage of development when challenged by thoughts and stressors
Repression	Blocking unacceptable thoughts and feelings from consciousness
Reaction formation	Responding to negative thoughts or feelings by demonstrating opposite emotions and actions
Sublimation	Channeling unacceptable emotions or impulses into acceptable actions or responses

Coping Strategies

Problem-focused coping techniques are aimed at altering or removing the stressor. In circumstances in which the problem may not have a solution, emotion-focused coping strategies work to ease the emotional distress associated with a stressful condition. For example, a person with a new diagnosis of diabetes may use strategies such as information gathering (seeking information about diabetes) and direct action (learning how to manage diet and medications), which are problem-focused. For another person, a new diagnosis of diabetes may be overwhelming, leading to feelings of helplessness or despair. That person may use avoidance or other emotion-focused strategies to relieve the stress associated with what is perceived to be a threat.

Studies have shown that successful coping usually involves both problem-focused and emotion-focused efforts. Coping strategies may be chosen on the basis of personal experience of success with various mechanisms, the degree of threat, and the availability of social resources. Persons who are able to apply different strategies in varying stressful situations generally are found to cope more effectively (Folkman, Lazarus, Dunkle-Schetter, et al, 1986).

NORMAL STRUCTURE AND FUNCTION — LO 32.2

The physiologic responses to stress may be understood if the responses of the three major systems of the body are recognized. The nervous, endocrine, and immune functions of an individual are all interrelated and affected by stress, and the stress response may activate other physiologic systems indirectly. Because all systems are connected, a stressor has the potential to affect any or many body systems.

NERVOUS SYSTEM RESPONSES TO STRESS

The physical signs of stress are those of sympathetic nervous system stimulation. When a demand is perceived, a stimulus in the form of sensory impulses from any of the sensory organs, such as the skin, eyes, or ears, is transmitted along spinothalamic pathways in the peripheral nervous system. These afferent impulses activate the reticular formation located in the brainstem, relaying the stimulus to the thalamus. The reticular activating system (RAS) and the thalamus are a primitive part of the brain that functions to maintain alertness.

From the thalamus the impulses are sent to the cerebral cortex, the seat of higher brain functions, including conscious thought and reasoning. The cerebral cortex interprets the somatic, auditory, visual, and other sensory input. In the frontal areas of the cerebral cortex, the brain evaluates the information, considering past experience and future implications. The temporal areas of the cerebral cortex, when stimulated, produce a sensation recognized as fear. Fear can modify the perception of a stressor.

The hypothalamus, located superior to the pituitary gland, has many functions useful in the adaptation to stress. Baroreceptors in the carotid sinuses transmit information to the hypothalamus about blood pressure. Emotional stimuli activating the limbic system also may activate the hypothalamus and the sympathetic nervous system. Corticotropin-releasing hormone (CRH) released by the hypothalamus stimulates the pituitary to release adrenocorticotropic hormone (ACTH).

These hormones increase the heart rate, resulting in increased cardiac output and elevated blood pressure. There is an increase in the flow of blood to muscles at the expense of the digestive and other systems not immediately needed in the fight-or-flight response. Smooth muscle in the bronchi relax and dilate the bronchi and smaller airways, and the respiratory rate increases, allowing for an enhanced flow of well-oxygenated blood to muscles and other organs. The motility of the digestive tract is decreased, slowing digestive processes, but glucose and fatty acids are mobilized from the liver and other stores to support increased mental activities (alertness) and skeletal muscle function. Pupillary dilation produces a larger visual field. Some of these changes result from direct nervous system stimulation and some from the secretion of hormones and other neurotransmitters such as cortisol, ACTH, aldosterone, testosterone, and catecholamines stimulated by the autonomic system activation. These changes occur within the first minutes of exposure to a stressor and may be experienced as the sensations of palpitations, light-headedness, nausea, and anxiety.

IMMUNE SYSTEM RESPONSES TO STRESS

The immune system coordinates the body's defense against infection and injury. This system's white blood cells, created in bone marrow and circulated by the bloodstream, determine what is healthy body, or "self," and what is foreign, or "not self." Foreign cells or proteins are destroyed.

The first immune response to infection or injury is pain, a signal to the brain that something is wrong. Immune cells at the local site of the injury trigger changes in adjacent blood vessels that cause redness (vasodilation) and swelling (increased capillary permeability). Phagocytes and macrophages migrate to the area and ingest the infecting agents. Other white blood cells, the T and B lymphocytes, are aggressively cytotoxic to infected cells. If the local responses cannot neutralize the invader, the hypothalamus is signaled and a general response is triggered.

ENDOCRINE SYSTEM RESPONSES TO STRESS

A consequence of hypothalamic activation is sympathetic stimulation, which triggers epinephrine and norepinephrine release from the adrenal medulla. The combined effect of these catecholamines is known as the *sympathoadrenal response.* Psychological as well as physiologic stressors can activate the hypothalamic-pituitary-adrenal complex. The secretion of CRH by the hypothalamus initiates release of a precursor of ACTH and a neuropeptide, beta-endorphin. Endorphins are known to act as analgesics, reducing the sensation of pain. ACTH stimulates the secretion of corticosteroids and aldosterone.

Corticosteroids are important in the stress response, because they increase serum glucose levels and inhibit the inflammatory response. Catecholamines also have an effect on blood vessels. Alterations in blood flow include the shunting of blood flow to muscles, at the expense of some internal organs, and increased clotting time functions that protect circulation to vital organs when blood loss occurs. Inhibition of the stress response by corticosteroids can mediate the negative effects of a prolonged stress response.

Stress-induced hyperglycemia may result from various stressors. Gestational diabetes during pregnancy, hyperglycemia experienced after acute myocardial infarction, and postoperative hyperglycemia must be addressed to avoid serious complications. Increased infection rates and poor wound healing, similar to those seen in patients with type 1 diabetes mellitus, are associated with untreated stress-induced hyperglycemia.

PSYCHOLOGICAL RESPONSES TO STRESS

Although research initially focused on the physiologic changes caused by stress, specific factors including age, nutritional status, and genetic inheritance were identified to affect a person's response, and great variation among individual responses to the same stressor was recognized. Stress appraisal, the affected person's attribution of meaning to a stressful event, also influences the expression of this stress response and reflects the complex psychological processing involved.

One perspective suggests that the frequency and intensity of stress exposure account for differences in adaptive responses, explaining why some people appear to be more resistant to stress-related illness. Holmes and Rahe (1967) developed a measure called the Social Readjustment Rating Scale to identify stressors and estimate the degree of stress. Major stressors are assigned a numeric value, and a person's total score may be used to predict the likelihood of illness. Similar measures are the Everyday Hassles Scale of Lazarus and Folkman (1989) and the Stress Audit developed by Miller, Smith, and Mehler (1991). All of these tools have been criticized as insensitive to age, gender, or sociocultural differences, but they can be useful if these limitations are taken into account.

Another point of view is that personality factors such as resilience, hardiness, and sense of coherence can buffer the impact of stress, reducing the negative consequences. Resilience is flexibility or resourcefulness in problem solving (Wagnild and Young, 1993). Resilient people bend but do not break under stress and use a variety of coping strategies. Hardy people have clear personal values and goals, a sense of meaningfulness, and an internal locus of control, and they exhibit lively interaction with the environment (Ford-Gilboe and Cohen, 2000).

Coping style refers to a pattern of measures taken to relieve stress. Effective coping is validated when adaptive mechanisms maintain stress within manageable limits, enhance physical recovery, and preserve psychological well-being. How well each person copes will vary and may be influenced by the number of and intensity of stressors, the duration of exposure, past experiences, personality factors, and availability of resources.

Anxiety

Anxiety is a response to stress that causes apprehension or uncertainty. It differs from fear, which has an identifiable source of impending danger. Anxiety may manifest as vague nervousness or as a feeling of dread. Various levels and types of anxiety have been identified.

Mild anxiety can be motivational, foster creativity, and actually increase the ability to think clearly. For example, a person who experiences mild performance anxiety when acting in a play may have a heightened ability to remember lines or cues, which keeps the person at top performance level. *Moderate* anxiety narrows focus, dulls perception, and may challenge the person to pay attention or use appropriate problem-solving skills. Both mild and moderate anxiety are considered normal and are experienced by everyone on a regular basis.

Severe anxiety results in the inability to make decisions or solve problems, whereas *panic* (the highest level of anxiety) is associated with a multitude of physiologic changes as well as subjective feelings of extreme dread or terror. Panic causes the affected person to become immobilized, unable to concentrate, communicate, or think in a rational manner. Panic attacks may be manifested as physical signs such as diaphoresis, chest pain, difficulty breathing, and palpitations.

Many types of anxiety are recognized, including generalized anxiety disorder, social anxiety disorder, obsessive-compulsive disorder, and post-traumatic stress disorder. **Generalized anxiety disorder** (GAD) is characterized by unrealistic levels of worry and tension with or without an identifiable cause. Social anxiety involves fear of being judged by others and overwhelming self-consciousness in social situations. Obsessive-compulsive disorder can be immobilizing or interfere with daily activities by causing the affected person to repeat ritualistic behaviors in an effort to avert unrealistic concerns about harm. **Post-traumatic stress disorder (PTSD)** is a very serious mental health condition characterized by flashbacks and erratic behaviors that results from exposure to a horrifying experience. PTSD may develop when the person's ability to cope is exceeded by the trauma that was experienced.

Anger

Anger is an emotion that involves antagonism toward another person or situation. It is evoked by a feeling of being wronged in some way. Anger actually prepares the affected person to "attack," physically or otherwise. Healthy people seek ways to effectively channel or resolve feelings of anger through conflict resolution strategies, counseling, or active exercise. Unresolved anger may be expressed through violent, abusive behavior, whereas chronically suppressed anger may lead to physiologic changes, such as high blood pressure and gastrointestinal upset, or depression.

Depression

Depression sometimes is described as "anger turned inward." Typically, depression results from an experience of loss—loss of a loved one, relationship, or job; failure of a professional goal; or diminished physical health or appearance. People experiencing depression may feel worthless, guilty, or hopeless. A depressed person may have difficulty getting out of bed, experience insomnia, lack energy for activities of daily living, display a flat affect, act chronically tired or withdrawn, or appear disheveled. If initial feelings of depression are not addressed, clinical depression may develop, leading to suicide attempts or loss of life. Psychotherapy and medication are recommended methods of treatment for people experiencing any form of depression. Ideally, feelings of depression serve as a motivator for change, leading to a healthier, happier lifestyle.

ALTERED STRUCTURE AND FUNCTION LO 32.3

Prolonged or severe stress can have significantly detrimental physical effects on the body. In certain stressful situations, parasympathetic, rather than sympathetic, stimulation is the primary event. In these circumstances, increased gastrointestinal motility and bronchial constriction may occur, resulting in stress-induced conditions such as irritable bowel syndrome or asthma.

The ability of the body's immune system to respond to infections is significantly altered by stress. Lymphocytes are created in response to particular infective agents after initial exposure; this is the principle behind the formation of antibodies and vaccinations. If exposed to those same infectious agents at a later time, antibodies recognize and react to the agent as foreign. However, antibody concentrations in vaccinated people and animals have been found to be lower under conditions of stress (Herbert and Cohen, 1993); stress decreases the activity of some lymphocytes (Welsh, Bustamonte, Nayak, et al, 2004). Stress has accelerated the progression of HIV infection toward active AIDS (Leserman, Whetten, Lowe, et al, 2005), and stress has a positive correlation with high viral loads, making highly active antiretroviral therapy (HAART) less effective.

High stress levels are known to exacerbate multiple sclerosis and other autoimmune diseases. Herpes simplex and zoster viruses have the ability to become latent within an infected cell and show an affinity for neurons. Periodic reactivation of herpes infections commonly occurs with stress, especially with herpes simplex virus type 1 and type 2 (HSV-1 and HSV-2) infections, producing skin lesions on the mouth or genital areas.

The unrelieved exposure to some stress hormones can lead to organ failure. Aldosterone secretion increases sodium reabsorption in the kidney, and stimulation of the posterior pituitary in stress results in increased secretion of antidiuretic hormone (ADH); both contribute to increased extracellular volume. These hormonal stress responses result in retention of sodium and loss of potassium and calcium from the body.

Measurement of cortisol, found in the blood, urine, and saliva, is the standard for laboratory assessment of physiologic stress. Testosterone levels are known to rise in physically stressful conditions in males. The hormonal milieu for females is more complicated before menopause, but studies have demonstrated that stress can delay ovulation and suppress menstruation (Edozien, 2006). The Diversity Considerations box highlights the impact of stress on males and females of various ages and cultural backgrounds.

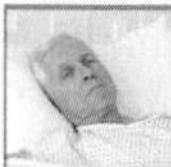

1. List a minimum of three factors that are contributing to Mr. Hastings's stress level.

ASSESSMENT LO 32.4

A trusting relationship permits the nurse to pursue assessment of personal and sensitive information regarding stress and the coping skills used by patients. The use of open-ended questions assists in obtaining accurate information regarding specific stressors and coping skills (Health Assessment Questions box). Identifying the ability of the patient to successfully use problem-focused (changing or removing a stressor) and emotion-focused (modifying one's reaction to a stressor) coping skills assists in planning appropriate interventions. Coping strategies can be individually tailored on the basis of past successful use.

Cultural competence of the nurse is essential in assessing patients from other cultures for stress. With patients from cultural backgrounds different from that of the nurse, the nurse needs to obtain a knowledge base for each patient's culture as well as to identify health beliefs and cultural values

DIVERSITY CONSIDERATIONS

Each person responds to stress slightly differently. However, some commonalities have been noted in research that assist health care providers in adapting care to meet the unique needs of specific populations.

Life Span*

Children

- Studies suggest that most children can successfully cope with a single stressful event, but developmental difficulties may emerge with prolonged or chronic stress.
- All studies consider the importance of assessing childhood stress within the context of the family. The most important modulating factor in stress is the relationship of the mother and the child, but other strong influences are the supportiveness of the parent-child relationship, the child's social support outside the family, and the child's individual coping strategies.
- Stressors that are significant for children include child abuse, maternal stress and lack of social support, divorce and family dissolution, temperament, and life changes such as the arrival of a sibling.
- Childhood stress related to the school experience centers on competition, goal achievement, and test anxiety.

***Adults*†**

- People of all ages are susceptible to stress under predisposing conditions.
- Job stress, family stress, and health, economic, political, and cultural stressors significantly impact the level of anxiety experienced by adults.
- Research indicates that younger adults experience more interpersonal stressors and are more reactive to them than are older adults.
- Studies have shown that younger adults, people with a poor self-concept, and those with a perceived lack of situational control demonstrate greater reactivity to stress.

***Older Adults*‡**

- Stress is as much a fact of life for elderly people as it is for younger persons, but there are differences in the amount of stress and the nature of their stressors. Most stressors for older adults involve loss and grieving. The changes of aging reflect a loss or decrease in physical function, which may be distressing in and of itself, as well as represent a potential loss of independence and dignity.
- The allostatic load in the older adult may be overwhelming because of diminished physical capabilities. Loss of appetite, sleep disturbances, and depression may be symptoms of stress in the older adult.
- Cognitive changes may affect the older adult's ability to cope. Anger or withdrawal as a coping strategy may be used more frequently than in the past.

Culture, Ethnicity, and Religion§

- Personal beliefs and culture will have an impact on the patient's conceptualization of health and illness, willingness to seek health care assistance, and compliance with therapies.
- Religious practices such as prayer, attendance at services, liturgy, and pastoral visits are reported as very important to chronically ill patients facing an uncertain future. Spiritual concerns complicate the patient's ability to cope and manage stressors.
- Cultural factors that affect health care include language and communication, social and family organization, perceptions of environmental control, and spatial and time orientation.

*Brobek, Marklund, Haraldsson, and Berntsson, 2007; Humphrey, 2005; Sharrer and Ryan-Wenger, 2002.
†Hay and Diehl, 2010; Neupert, Almeida, and Charles, 2007.
‡Kuwert, Brahler, Glaesner, et al, 2010.
§Elliott, Gessert, Larson, and Russ, 2012; Johnson, Thompson, and Downs, 2009.

HEALTH ASSESSMENT QUESTIONS

Present Stressors
- What personal stress are you currently experiencing?
- Have you experienced any changes in your life recently?
- Have you experienced changes in your stress level due to these changes?

Coping Skills
- How have you dealt with stressful situations in the past?
- Were these techniques of handling stress effective?
- Whom can you ask for assistance during stressful times?

Symptoms of Stressors
- Are you experiencing feelings of anxiety or nervousness?
- Are you experiencing feelings of depression, irritability, or anger?
- Are you experiencing your heart racing and pounding?
- Have you experienced episodes of hyperventilating?
- Does stress cause you to experience muscle tension in your neck, back, and head?
- Do you experience migraine headaches when you are under stress?
- Have you experienced diarrhea or constipation during stressful times?
- Are you experiencing difficulty sleeping?
- Have you had any changes in weight?

Adults
- Have you recently experienced any social, physical, emotional, or financial losses?
- Do you suffer from physical illnesses?
- Have there been any major changes in your life recently?

Children
- What has been bothering you lately?
- How does this make you feel?

Support Network
- Whom do you turn to when you need help?
- Whom do you talk to about your feelings and problems?

Additional Considerations
- Does your cultural or spiritual background provide you with certain beliefs that are helpful in times of stress?
- Do you see someone other than a doctor or nurse for health care, such as a psychologist, social worker, faith healer, folk healer, or medicine man?

Observations During the Assessment
- How would you describe the patient's physical appearance, facial expression, behavior, and mood?
- What are the patient's posture and gait?
- Can the patient sit still? Is the patient experiencing tremors or muscle tension?
- Does the patient appear to be depressed or withdrawn?
- Is the patient agitated, aggressive, or angry?

Physical Assessment
- What are the patient's vital signs? Are the patient's heart rate and blood pressure elevated? Are the patient's respirations shallow? Does the patient report any pain?
- Is the patient experiencing any shortness of breath, dry mouth, or gastrointestinal upset?

from that patient's world view. The patient's world view provides insight into how illness is interpreted and possibly treated. In such situations, the nurse may need to conduct a cultural assessment. For more information on the many cultural and spiritual aspects of health care, refer to Chapters 21 and 22, respectively.

Stress can be manifested both physically and psychologically, and assessment should include appropriate questions to address both spheres. The nurse needs to closely observe the verbal responses as well as the nonverbal behaviors exhibited by the patient. Nonverbal behaviors such as irritability, agitation, anxiety, and poor eye contact may prove more revealing than verbal responses. Lack of congruence between nonverbal behavior and verbal responses requires further exploration. See Chapter 3 for additional information on congruence.

Stress may be caused by the loss of a job, the death of a family member or friend, the diagnosis of an illness, finances, and relationships. Many adults are in the "sandwich generation," which means they are caring for their own children as well as their parents. Meeting the daily needs of their children as well as those of ill or aging parents while holding down full-time employment creates both physical and psychological stressors. Caregivers experience stress while providing assistance to others. The nurse should observe caregivers for symptoms of stress to determine the strength of patient support systems.

Symptoms of stress are manifested in multiple ways. Stressors may be exhibited as physical or psychosocial symptoms or through denial. Identifying the stressors and finding resolution will facilitate the patient's recovery. Stressors for one person are not necessarily stressors for another. A stressor for one hospitalized patient may be concern that a pet is not receiving daily care. For another, absence from work may mean no income while hospitalized, with corresponding concern about food for the family.

The coping skills of the patient will determine whether positive or negative responses occur in these situations. Ineffective coping skills may lead to physical or psychological responses in reaction to the stressor and be manifested as symptoms in the nervous system, immune system, or endocrine system. It is necessary to assess for cardiovascular, respiratory, neurologic, musculoskeletal, gastrointestinal, urinary, cognitive, and emotional signs of stress.

Stress assessment tools, such as the Holmes-Rahe Social Readjustment Rating Scale (Figure 32-3), are available for

Social Readjustment Rating Scale (SRRS)

Event	Value
1. Death of a spouse	100
2. Divorce	73
3. Marital separation	65
4. Jail term	63
5. Death of a close family member	63
6. Personal injury or illness	53
7. Marriage	50
8. Fired at work	47
9. Marital reconciliation	45
10. Retirement	45
11. Change in health of family member	44
12. Pregnancy	40
13. Sex difficulties	39
14. Gain of a new family member	39
15. Business readjustments	39
16. Change in financial state	38
17. Death of a close friend	37
18 Change to different line of work	36
19. Change in no. of arguments with spouse	35
20. Mortgage over $50,000	31
21. Foreclosure of mortgage	30
22. Change in responsibilities at work	29
23. Son or daughter leaving home	29
24. Trouble with in-laws	29
25. Outstanding personal achievements	28
26. Wife begins or stops work	26
27. Begin or end school	26
28. Change in living conditions	25
29. Revision of personal habits	24
30. Trouble with boss	23
31. Change in work hours or conditions	20
32. Change in residence	20
33. Change in school	20
34. Change in recreation	19
35. Change in religious activities	19
36. Change in social activities	18
37. Loan less than $50,000	17
38. Change in sleeping habits	16
39. Change in no. of family get-togethers	15
40. Change in eating habits	15
41. Vacation	13
42. Holidays	12
43. Minor violation of laws	11

SCORING

Each event should be considered if it has taken place in the last 12 months. Add values to the right of each item to obtain the total score.
Your susceptibility to illness and mental health problems:
Low <149 Mild 150–200 Moderate 200–299 Major >300

FIGURE 32-3 Holmes-Rahe Social Readjustment Rating Scale. (From Holmes TH, Rahe RH: The Social Readjustment Rating Scale, *J Psychosom Rese* 11(2):213-218, 1967.)

identifying stressors in the daily lives of patients. The nurse also needs to examine stress assessment tools for cultural appropriateness before use.

! SAFE PRACTICE ALERT

Verbalization of suicidal ideation or a suicide plan must be taken seriously. In the case of a hospitalized patient, one-on-one observation should be implemented to ensure patient safety, and referral to psychiatric services also should be implemented. Do not leave the patient alone.

◆ NURSING DIAGNOSIS LO 32.5

People use coping skills to deal with stressors that threaten their physical and mental well-being. If people have poor or no coping skills, they generally respond to "life challenges with denial and avoidance" (Kleinke, 2002, p. 305).

Possible nursing diagnoses for stress and coping include:

- *Ineffective Coping* related to lack of confidence in ability to cope as evidenced by reports of fatigue, lack of sleep, and anxiety and negative attitude toward recovery
- *Anxiety* related to a change in health status as evidenced by fatigue and difficulty concentrating
- *Caregiver Role Strain* related to complexity of activities as evidenced by fatigue, gastrointestinal upset, and weight change
- *Readiness for Enhanced Coping* as evidenced by defining stressors as manageable and verbalizing the need for social support
- *Stress Overload* related to family violence as evidenced by reports of increased feelings of anger and difficulty making decisions

◆ PLANNING LO 32.6

Once the assessment data are analyzed, nursing diagnoses are identified and ranked in order of priority. Highest-priority nursing diagnoses are those of a life-threatening nature.

Examples of goals that address concerns related to stress and coping are:

- Patient will discuss possible coping strategies during weekly office visits.
- Patient will report increased ability to concentrate on care instructions before discharge.
- Caregiver will use respite care for his loved one once a week for the next month.
- Patient will attend a support group on a weekly basis.
- Patient will discuss strategies for coping with family violence with a social worker within 24 hours.

Collaboration among members of the health care team often is incorporated into the plan of care (Table 32-2) for a patient experiencing stress. Depending on the patient's situation, consultation with professionals from various health care and other specialties may be appropriate (Collaboration and Delegation box).

Addressing the needs of patients experiencing extreme levels of stress requires interventions by health care professionals as well as family members, significant others, and friends who can play a vital role in assisting patients with coping skills. Nurses and other members of the patient's support system provide social support and encouragement, which prevents the patient from giving up or failing to try potential coping strategies. Encouragement from others prevents discouragement if there are relapses. Including patients in the development of their own individualized plans of care promotes the best chance of achieving positive outcomes.

TABLE 32-2 Care Planning

NANDA-I NURSING DIAGNOSIS LABEL WITH NURSING DIAGNOSIS STATEMENT	NURSING OUTCOME CLASSIFICATION (NOC)	NURSING INTERVENTION CLASSIFICATION (NIC)
Ineffective Coping related to lack of confidence in ability to cope as evidenced by reports of fatigue, lack of sleep, and anxiety and negative attitude toward recovery	*Coping* (1302) Identifies multiple coping strategies (130211)	*Coping enhancement* (5230) Encourage the patient to identify own strengths and abilities.

From Bulechek G, Butcher H, Dochterman J, et al (Eds): *Nursing interventions classification (NIC)*, ed. 6, St. Louis, 2013, Mosby; Moorhead S, Johnson M, Maas M, et al (Eds): *Nursing outcomes classification (NOC)*, ed. 5, St. Louis, 2013, Mosby; NANDA International: *Nursing diagnoses: Definitions and classification, 2012–2014*, West Sussex, England, 2012, Wiley-Blackwell. Reprinted with permission from NANDA International, Inc.

COLLABORATION AND DELEGATION

Approaching Stress-Related Concerns Holistically

- A dietitian can be consulted to assess the patient's nutritional needs and develop a nutritional plan.
- To identify appropriate services and resources, a social worker is incorporated into the plan of care.
- Family members and assistive personnel may be involved in care planning to ensure a comprehensive approach.
- Pastoral care plays a significant role in addressing stress and anxiety issues when the patient has a preferred religion or strong faith background.
- If coordination of care between multiple health care disciplines is needed, a case manager is used.
- Patients with mental health issues related to current health problems or with chronic mental health or psychiatric issues need referral to a psychologist, psychiatrist, or advanced practice psychiatric nurse.

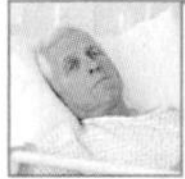

The conceptual care map for Mr. Hastings provided in Figure 32-4 is partially completed to indicate how to use the map as a learning tool. Using it as an example, go to the website at *http://evolve.elsevier.com/YoostCrawford/fundamentals/* to complete Nursing Diagnoses 2 and 3.

Nurses play a vital role in alleviating the potential damage that stress can cause to a person's physical and emotional health.

◆ IMPLEMENTATION AND EVALUATION LO 32.7

Interventions for stress management focus on decreasing stressors and improving or mobilizing coping strategies. Interventions need to be agreed on by the patient and the nurse to achieve the desired outcomes. Social support and emotional support from family members, significant others, or friends have been found to decrease stress (Ross, Zeller, Srisaeng, et al, 2005) and influence adaptation to stressful situations (Glanz and Schwartz, 2008). Psychosocial and physical symptoms of stress decrease with social support. Social support interventions also may focus on the family and community.

Managing stress and developing coping skills involves identification of both internal and external strategies. Internal strategies address the person's feelings associated with stress. External strategies seek to provide relief through social networking and mobilization of support systems. Working with patients, families, and communities to identify their general resistance resources when they are faced with stressors helps people use sources of support that already exist. Antonovsky (1979) identified general resistance resources as physiologic, tangible, emotional, attitudinal, interpersonal, and relational, as well as cultural, in nature. Examples of general resistance resources are the body's fight-or-flight response, money, health insurance, a positive attitude, hope for the future, adaptability, family, and social service agencies.

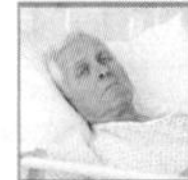

2. Identify five general resistance resources that Mr. Hastings has as sources of support.

STRESS MANAGEMENT

Stress management is a holistic approach to stress reduction that incorporates a variety of individualized interventions to address specific sources of stress and complementary and alternative therapies, including relaxation therapies and mind-body therapy, to address the negative emotional and physiologic effects of stress. Integrating relaxation and mind-body techniques into one's daily routine has been found to decrease pain, decrease blood pressure, increase a sense of well-being, improve quality of life, and increase the sense of coherence (Esmonde and Long, 2008; Lafferty, Downey, McCarty, et al, 2006).

Strategies for stress management must focus on the principles of balance, relaxation, and nutrition. To maximize the

Medications

Conceptual Care Map

Student name__________ Patient initials Mr. H Date ________

Age 60 Gender M Room # __ Admission date ________

CODE Status Full ________ Allergies NKDA ________

Diet ________ Activity ________ Braden score ________

Weight ______ Height ______ Religion ________

Laboratory Values/ Diagnostic Test Results

Admitting Diagnoses/Chief Complaint

Follow-up visit 4 weeks after myocardial infarction

Assessment Data

Retired architect owns home, financially stable.

Recovering from second heart attack in the past 5 years.

Lives in a two-story home with his wife; states that his wife "hovers" over him, taking care of him physically and protecting him from overexertion.

Denies chest pain; notes minimal shortness of breath when climbing stairs.

Appears downcast and somewhat depressed, and states, "I am going to die from this heart condition, so why treat it?"

Complains of difficulty falling asleep and remaining asleep due to feeling anxious and jittery.

Wife notes that her husband is stressed and frustrated; shares that she feels like she must take on her husband's responsibilities to avoid his overexerting himself and having another heart attack.

IV Sites/Fluids/Rate

Treatments

May resume all normal activities, including driving

Cardiac rehabilitation three times a week

Past Medical/Surgical History

Myocardial infarction 4½ years ago

Primary Nursing Diagnosis

Ineffective Coping related to lack of confidence in ability to cope as evidenced by reports of fatigue, lack of sleep, anxiety, and negative attitude toward recovery.

Supporting Data

Patient states that his wife takes care of him physically and protects him from overexertion.

Complains of difficulty falling asleep and remaining asleep due to feeling anxious and jittery.

States, "I am going to die from this heart condition, so why treat it?"

STG/NOC

Patient will identify a minimum of three activities that he will take responsibility for immediately without his wife's assistance.

NOC: Coping (1302)

Identifies multiple coping strategies (130211)

Interventions/NIC With Rationale

1. Assess patient's level of activity before the myocardial infarction to provide a baseline for establishing realistic rehabilitation goals.
2. Discuss physical, psychological, and sleep benefits of increased exercise to encourage active participation in rehabilitation and address identified patient stressors.
3. Establish gradual rehabilitation goals that the patient views as attainable to promote success and progressive improvement.

NIC: Coping enhancement (5230)

Encourage patient to identify own strengths and abilities.

Rationale Citation/EBP

Yoost BL, Crawford LR: *Fundamentals of nursing: Active learning for collaborative practice*, St. Louis, 2016, Mosby.

Evaluation

Goal met. Patient described four activities, such as driving himself to cardiac rehab appoinments, that he will begin doing without assistance. Revise plan of care to reflect patient progress.

Nursing Diagnosis 2

Supporting Data

STG/NOC

Interventions/NIC With Rationale

Rationale Citation/EBP

Evaluation

Nursing Diagnosis 3

Supporting Data

STG/NOC

Interventions/NIC With Rationale

Rationale Citation/EBP

Evaluation

FIGURE 32-4 Partially completed conceptual care map based on Mr. Hastings, the case study patient in this chapter.

effectiveness of these strategies, a balance must exist between activity and rest. An imbalance of activity and rest contributes to further physiologic and physical signs of stress. The attainment of relaxation is accomplished through interventions such as active and passive activity, exercise, yoga, biofeedback, and guided imagery. An optimal state of nutrition provides adequate nutrients for body functioning.

Time Management

When stress results from overwhelming perceived work and/or personal responsibilities, time management may be an effective intervention to help people address identified issues. Multitasking facilitated by technology has been identified as a significant source of stress that actually increases the time required to complete a task by as much as 25% (Schwartz, 2012). Research over the past two decades suggests that switching from task to task may reduce worker productivity as much as 40% and reduce cognitive ability (Ophir, Nass, and Wagner, 2009; Rubinstein, Meyer, and Evans, 2001). Strategies such as prioritizing tasks, setting goals, increasing concentration skills, decreasing distractions, avoiding procrastination, setting boundaries, and maintaining self-discipline are time management interventions that people may use to address certain types of stressors.

Anger Management

Anger management strategies can help people deal with anger in a positive way, thereby reducing stress and potentially destructive actions and emotions that lead to compromised health and fractured relationships. Some anger management interventions include expressing feelings in a calm and non-confrontational manner, exercising, identifying potential solutions, taking a time-out, forgiving, diffusing the situation with humor, "owning" the negative feelings, and doing deep-breathing exercises (Mayo Clinic, 2011). These strategies may require appropriate training or counseling for effective application. People whose stress is exacerbated by feelings of anger should be encouraged to enroll in anger management classes or to seek professional counseling to identify and address concerns.

Nutrition

Research has revealed that stress often leads to unhealthy food choices that affect mood and impact a person's response to inflammation. Stress puts people at a greater risk for infection and delayed wound healing (Kiecolt-Glaser, 2010). Because inflammation plays a role in diseases such as cancer, diabetes, depression, and cardiovascular disease, encouraging people to eat a balanced diet can facilitate stress reduction and improve physical well-being. Increasing the intake of fruit, vegetables, legumes, fish, poultry, and whole grains can enhance both psychological and physical responses to stress. Stress reduction also may be facilitated by taking multivitamins and herbal supplements (Harris, Kirk, Rowsell, et al, 2011). Collaboration among the patient, the PCP, and a registered dietitian should be implemented by the nurse to identify a diet that will promote stress reduction while adhering to limitations, such as food exclusion, as required by specific health problems.

Support Groups

For some people, attending a support group is an effective intervention to reduce stress related to specific life circumstances. Patients who share a common disease process or loss often find solace in knowing they are not alone in their struggle. Nurses should consult with the patient's PCP to discuss the possibility of referral to a community- or facility-based support group. Often, the patient's assigned social worker can suggest available support groups in the person's local area.

More recently, online support services have become increasingly popular. If patients choose to become involved in online support groups, the nurse should provide guidance on how to evaluate the legitimacy of an online group. Support groups facilitated through national agencies such as the American Cancer Society, research and health care institutions such as the Cleveland Clinic and the Mayo Clinic, or professionals directly affiliated with health care or academic institutions should take priority over informally lead or configured groups.

Complementary and Alternative Therapies

Complementary therapies frequently are used in conjunction with medical therapies. Alternative therapies are used in place of medical treatment. These types of interventions are useful when patients are experiencing physiologic and psychological responses to stress such as increased heart rate, increased respiratory rate, and gastrointestinal symptoms. When coping mechanisms are ineffective or nonexistent, stress-related illnesses such as gastrointestinal problems, pain, and heart disease may occur. Relaxation techniques decrease the physiologic response by decreasing heart rate, respiratory rate, and gastrointestinal motility. Psychological responses to relaxation techniques include an increased sense of well-being and a decrease in depression and anxiety.

Some complementary and alternative therapies such as therapeutic touch, Reiki, biofeedback, and massage therapy require additional certification and training, whereas muscle relaxation and guided imagery do not (Evidence-Based Practice box). Benefits of mind-body therapies include improved sleep, relaxation, and decreased pain (Esmonde and Long, 2008; Lafferty, Downey, McCarty, et al, 2006).

Relaxation Therapy

Relaxation therapy incorporates the use of nonpharmacologic techniques to reduce psychological or physiologic distress. The development of cognitive skills for use in stressful situations provides patients with the ability to recognize potential stressors and initiate relaxation techniques. Relaxation therapy increases awareness of muscle tension and incorporates interventions to decrease tension.

EVIDENCE-BASED PRACTICE

Effect of Alternative Stress Reduction Modalities

- Progressive relaxation and guided imagery have been shown to significantly:
  - Reduce pain as reported by patients
  - Improve scores on anxiety and stress scales
  - Promote sleep
- Many studies have indicated that progressive relaxation is effectively used to treat:
  - Nausea and vomiting
  - Pain
  - Depression and anxiety
  - Sleep disturbance
- Individual training sessions and use of CD recordings to allow additional practice of the techniques were found to be effective methods for instructing patients in both progressive relaxation and guided imagery.

From Chen Y, Francis A: Relaxation and imagery for chronic, nonmalignant pain: Effects on pain symptoms, quality of life, and mental health, *Pain Manage Nurs* 11(3):159-168, 2010.

Progressive relaxation is implemented by having patients focus on muscles that are tensed and then intentionally relax those muscle groups. Typically, relaxation progresses from head to toe. With practice the patient visualizes an image of the relaxed muscles and will be able to relax muscles from the mental image (Snyder, Pestka, and Bly, 2006). This technique should be done daily.

Exercise

Exercise has been found to decrease stress level and cortisol levels and increase a sense of well-being in patients of all ages (Starkweather, 2007). Other benefits of exercise include improved muscle tone, weight management, and improvement of cardiovascular and pulmonary functioning (Starkweather, 2007; Treat-Jacobson and Lindquist, 2007). Increasing daily exercise may decrease the risk of physiologic as well as psychological issues, such as depression (Nabkasorn, Miyai, Sootmongkol, et al, 2006). Exercise does not need to be formal. Increasing exercise can begin as a daily walking program.

Sleep

Sleep is essential to engage in activities of daily living. Sleep is a restful state during which metabolism is reduced. Sleep disturbances resulting from stress and worry may be seen as difficulty falling asleep and/or remaining asleep; poor quality of sleep; frequent night awakenings; difficulty awakening; and daytime tiredness (Rausch, Baker, and Boonmee, 2007). Disturbances in sleep patterns can lead to irritability, fatigue, depression, tiredness, decreased ability to concentrate, and immunosuppression (Lai and Good, 2006). Lai and Good (2006) found that quiet music played at bedtime for older adults improves perceived sleep quality and daytime functioning. Nurses can implement interventions to facilitate sleep, including limiting interruptions during the night and controlling the environment, such as lighting, noise, and room temperature.

Guided Imagery

Guided imagery focuses on positive external images, such as a patient's favorite vacation spot, to create a relaxed state. Guided imagery is a verbal form of instruction by the nurse or another clinician that directs the patient's attention away from upsetting thoughts. Well-conducted guided imagery improves physiologic functions such as heart rate, respiratory rate, blood pressure, gastrointestinal motility, and hormonal levels (Fontaine, 2005). Guided imagery can be incorporated into care to boost the immune system, decrease pain, and develop positive feelings.

Meditation

Meditation involves relaxing the body and quieting the mind by directing one's focus on a specific word, sound, or image. During meditation, breathing is deep, slowed, and relaxed. Meditation can be used to decrease stress and anxiety in adults and by children as young as 10 years of age (Humphrey, 2005). Meditation affects the sympathetic nervous system by creating a state of relaxation, thereby lowering blood pressure, heart rate, breathing, metabolism, and blood flow to the muscles (Fontaine, 2005).

Mindfulness

Mindfulness-based stress reduction has become increasing popular in recent years, especially within the medical community. It is a form of therapy that helps people become more aware of their thoughts, emotions, and motivating behaviors; this awareness often results in reduced levels of anxiety, chronic pain, insomnia, and depression (Lawson, 2011). Mindfulness combines the practices of meditation, body scan (progressive attention to various areas of the body), and yoga.

Yoga

Yoga has been defined as a "journey of the body, mind, and spirit on a path toward unity" (Fontaine, 2005, p. 267). The practice of yoga includes physical exercises, breathing, and meditating to strengthen the body, mind, and soul. Engaging in yoga increases flexibility, improves endurance, decreases blood pressure, enhances breathing, promotes relaxation, and reduces stress (Fontaine, 2005). The benefits of yoga are attainable by patients across the life span, from children to older adults (Figure 32-5).

Biofeedback

Biofeedback involves the use of electronic devices to help the patient develop a learned awareness of the body's physiologic responses to unconscious, involuntary stressors. The learned awareness enables the patient to engage in voluntary actions to decrease the stress response. The patient learns the

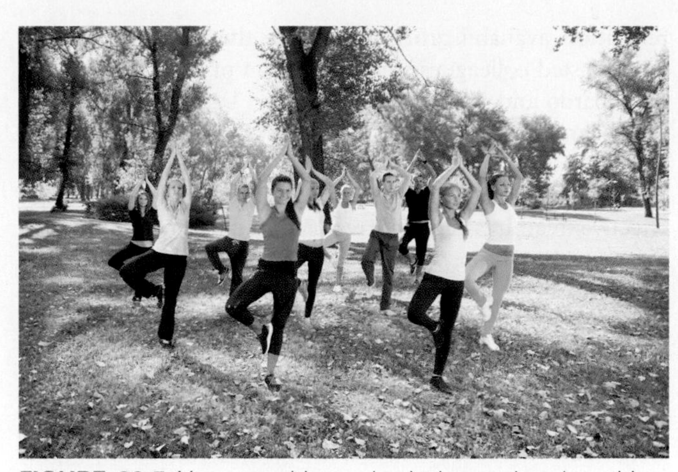

FIGURE 32-5 Yoga combines physical exercise, breathing, and meditation to promote relaxation and reduce stress.

correlation between feelings, thoughts, and physiologic responses to stressors. Biofeedback requires a referral. Techniques are taught under the guidance of a biofeedback therapist with specialized training. It generally requires 8 to 10 sessions to master these skills. Biofeedback is used to treat problems such as stress, addictions, and back pain.

Energy Therapy

Energy therapy uses the hands of the practitioner as a conduit to manipulate the negative energy fields of the patient and move the congestion or obstruction of the negative energy away from the energy field. Energy therapy has been shown to decrease stress, anxiety, and acute and chronic pain and to promote a sense of well-being. This technique enhances and promotes comfort in children, older adults, cancer patients, and dying patients (Umbreit, 2006). Therapeutic touch and Reiki are types of energy therapy, both of which require training.

- **Reiki**: The hands of the practitioner transfer energy from the practitioner to the patient, thus restoring balance and harmony to the body during times of health issues.
- **Therapeutic touch**: The use of touch through hand motions enhances energy fields to promote healing. Therapeutic touch decreases pain and anxiety, increases the sense of well-being, enhances the functioning of the immune system (Snyder, Pestka, and Bly, 2006), promotes relaxation, and reduces depressive symptoms.

Eastern Medicine

Traditional Chinese medicine (TCM) originated more than 2000 years ago and is based on the balance of harmony and equilibrium of humans as they exist within a continually changing environment (Fontaine, 2005). In TCM, health is a balance of yin and yang (two opposite forces of nature). Imbalance between yin and yang causes illness and disease. Herbal medicine, massage, acupuncture, and feng shui are several of the many TCM modalities.

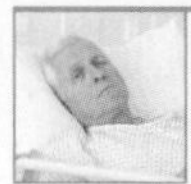

3. Name three stress management therapies that could benefit Mr. Hastings. Discuss the best way to incorporate these therapies into Mr. Hastings's plan of care.

Crisis Intervention

Crisis intervention is short-term assistance provided at a time of physical or emotional upheaval with the goal of helping the person in distress to regain equilibrium. Crisis intervention involves immediate action to help reduce the impact of a traumatic event in the affected person's life. When people are overwhelmed by the circumstances confronting them, crisis intervention strategies can help them adapt and restore their ability to function. Crisis intervention involves simple, innovative, accessible, practical, and immediate actions that ensure a person's safety and mental well-being, such as providing counselors for school students after the sudden death of a classmate or encouraging a person to drive as soon as possible after involvement in a fatal accident that took the life of a friend. Nurses, doctors, clergy, counselors, and community workers such as firefighters and police often are called on to provide crisis intervention at times of natural disasters, tragic accidents, or unexpected loss. Lack of appropriate assistance for a person in crisis to help reestablish a sense of equilibrium may lead to development of mental illness. Crises should be approached by professionals as teachable moments in which people have great openness to change and growth.

QSEN FOCUS!

Implementing strategies that empower patients and their families to make healthy decisions to address identified stressors is central to patient-centered care.

EVALUATION

It is the nurse's responsibility to evaluate the outcome of interventions that are implemented into a patient's plan of care. A point to keep in mind is that situations of acute stress resolve more quickly than those of chronic stress. Once stress decreases, patients typically report feeling better, sleeping more soundly, and feeling less anxious. It is important to observe patient behaviors and compare them with self-reported accounts. Patients should be reminded to continue using stress reduction techniques to maintain a feeling of well-being. Patients may require continued care for stress management after discharge from a health care setting. Because modification of coping skills for stress management is a slow process, sometimes requiring months or years, referrals may need to be made for long-term follow-up assessment and treatment.

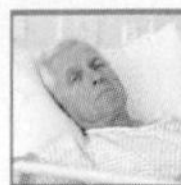

4. What suggestions should the nurse make to Mr. Hastings's wife regarding her husband's care?

STRESS AND NURSING LO 32.8

The profession of nursing requires a constant vigilance to the needs of others. The demands of workplace stress can lead to depression, compassion fatigue, **burnout** (mental or physical exhaustion due to constant stress or activity), and decreased job satisfaction (Aiken, Clarke, Sloane, et al, 2002; Fisher and Abrahamson, 2002; Shapiro, Astin, Bishop, and Cordova, 2005). Researchers note that nurse burnout increases through a cycle of "exhaustion, cynicism, and lack of civility" in the workplace (Sapatkin, 2012). Research has raised concerns about the impact of nursing burnout on patient safety (Cimiotti, Aiken, Sloane, and Wu, 2012).

Compassion fatigue occurs when deeply caring and empathetic nurses become overwhelmed by the constant needs of patients and families. Reported manifestations include mood swings, avoidance of working with some patients, frequent sick days, irritability, reduced memory, poor concentration, and a decreased ability to show empathy. Physical signs of compassion fatigue are similar to those exhibited by nurses experiencing burnout, including headaches, digestive upset, muscle tension, fatigue, and in some cases chest pain or palpitations. Interventions designed specifically to prevent nurse burnout and address compassion fatigue include mentoring programs, availability of quiet areas on the nursing unit for relaxation, availability of pastoral care, the sharing of feelings with trusted colleagues, and promotion of work-life balance (Lombardo and Erye, 2011).

To care most effectively for others, nurses must first take time to care for themselves. Many of the stress reduction interventions incorporated into patient care plans can be effective in addressing the stressors faced by nurses. Exercise, balanced nutrition, and mindfulness therapy have been shown to help health care professionals in coping with the demands of patient care (Lawson, 2011). Some hospital systems offer worksite fitness facilities or health club memberships and Employer Assistance Programs, that include counseling services, to help their employees cope with work stress. In an effort to promote self-care and reduce the impact of stress on nurses, Kent State University College of Nursing has established the Interprofessional Institute for Self-Care to encourage research and practices that enhance the well-being of nurses and promote patient safety. For more information, visit *https://nursing.kent.edu/iisc.*

Reducing daily stressors through the use of healthy coping strategies promotes wellness and emotional stability that enhance a nurse's ability to care. In situations in which stressors may become overwhelming, such as the occurrence of multiple patient deaths on a unit within a short period of time, it is important for nurses to collaborate with their professional counseling colleagues, who can help guide the healing process. Taking the time to cope effectively with stress will ultimately strengthen the nurse's ability to provide empathetic patient care and thrive in the stressful health care environment.

SUMMARY OF LEARNING OUTCOMES

LO 32.1 *Identify the key concepts associated with the body's physiologic and psychological responses to stress:* The fight-or-flight response is a physiologic response to physical or psychological stress that activates the autonomic nervous system. The body's GAS consists of three stages: alarm reaction, resistance, and exhaustion. Allostasis is the means by which homeostasis is reestablished. Stress appraisal, SOC, and general resistance resources all contribute to a person's response to stress.

LO 32.2 *Describe psychological and physiologic responses of the nervous, endocrine, and immune systems to stress:* Stress appraisal influences the unique response of each person and reflects the complex psychological processing in the stress response. Increased cardiac output, elevated blood pressure, and increased blood flow to muscles result from direct nervous system stimulation and from the secretion of hormones during stress. Endocrine responses to stress include alterations in blood flow to muscles, at the expense of some internal organs, and increased clotting time to protect circulation to vital organs when blood loss occurs. The LAC, or inflammation, is the most notable response to stress by the immune system.

LO 32.3 *Describe the effects of stress on health:* In certain stressful situations, parasympathetic, rather than sympathetic, stimulation is the primary event. In such circumstances, increased gastrointestinal motility and bronchial constriction may occur, resulting in serious stress-induced physical conditions.

LO 32.4 *Demonstrate assessment techniques for recognizing signs and symptoms of stress:* Interviewing patients and observing for nonverbal signs of stress are critical assessment strategies that the nurse can implement during the assessment phase. The use of stress assessment tools adapted for specific populations may also be helpful.

LO 32.5 *Identify stress-related nursing diagnosis labels: Ineffective Coping, Anxiety, Caregiver Role Strain, Readiness for Enhanced Coping,* and *Stress Overload,* as well as *Fear, Hopelessness, Situational Low Self-Esteem,* and *Family Coping* are all nursing diagnoses that may be used in addressing patient needs associated with stress.

LO 32.6 *Articulate stress reduction goals and patient outcomes:* Goals for stress reduction should include realistic and measurable patient outcomes that reflect increased patient control of situational stress.

LO 32.7 *Develop patient-centered care plans with interventions designed to address stress-related conditions:* Including interventions such as exercise, improved dietary intake, and a variety of stress management strategies in stress-related care plans is most effective when patients have major input in choosing which treatments should be implemented.

LO 32.8 *Discuss the potential impact of stress on nurses:* The demands of workplace stress can lead to depression, compassion fatigue, burnout, and decreased job satisfaction.

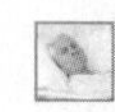

Responses to the critical-thinking questions are available at *http://evolve.elsevier.com/YoostCrawford/fundamentals/*.

REVIEW QUESTIONS

1. The nurse has been assigned the same patients for the past 4 days. Two of the patients demand a great deal of attention, and the nurse feels anxious and angry about being given this assignment again. What action would demonstrate the most effective way for the nurse to cope with the patient care assignment?
   - **a.** Share complaints about the assignment with the nurse manager.
   - **b.** Prioritize the patients' needs, and identify a specific time period for care of each patient.
   - **c.** Talk with the patients, and explain that they cannot expect so much personal attention.
   - **d.** Trade assignments with another nurse who is unaware of the concerns regarding the patient assignment.
2. A patient is newly diagnosed with diabetes and requires insulin injections. He requests information about classes offered by the diabetes educator. Which type of coping technique is this patient using?
   - **a.** Emotion-focused
   - **b.** Problem-focused
   - **c.** Avoidance
   - **d.** Denial
3. Which statements by a patient would indicate the use of effective coping strategies? *(Select all that apply.)*
   - **a.** "Each month, my wife and I attend a support group for parents of children with autism."
   - **b.** "Talking with my spiritual adviser may challenge my thinking as to how best to handle this situation."
   - **c.** "I've invited my son to join me for drinks at the bar each night on his way home from work so we can spend more time together."
   - **d.** "We are looking into joining the new health club facility in our neighborhood."
   - **e.** "After working all day, I eat dinner in front of the television while my family sits at the kitchen table."
4. When using a stress assessment tool with a patient from another culture, what factors must the nurse take into consideration? *(Select all that apply.)*
   - **a.** Specific methods of managing stress are revealed in using stress assessment tools.
   - **b.** Stress assessment tools should be used only for persons living in North America.
   - **c.** Stress assessment tools may not be appropriate for all persons of all ages.
   - **d.** Resistance resources become evident when stress assessment tools are analyzed.
   - **e.** Adaptations may need to be made to the assessment tool based on circumstances.
5. Two adult siblings are caring for their ill mother, who requires 24-hour care. She needs assistance with feeding, bathing, and toileting. One of the siblings takes time to exercise after work, whereas the other goes directly to the mother's home before and after work each day. The nurse recognizes that people may react differently to the same stressors depending on which factors? *(Select all that apply.)*
   - **a.** Individual coping skills
   - **b.** Type of identified stressor
   - **c.** Amount of perceived stress
   - **d.** Personal appraisal of the stressor
   - **e.** Hair color, gender, and skin type
6. A patient is told that he may have colon cancer. Which response by the patient best indicates that his initial appraisal of the situation is primarily a challenge to be met?
   - **a.** Requesting information on various treatment options
   - **b.** Demanding to see another physician immediately
   - **c.** Storming out of the gastroenterologist's office
   - **d.** Yelling at the nurse who is scheduling his colonoscopy

7. A 25-year-old patient demands that her mother or father be present during all blood testing. Which defense mechanism could the nurse document as being used by this patient?
   a. Sublimation
   b. Repression
   c. Projection
   d. Regression
8. In the immediate postoperative period after open heart surgery, a patient who is not a diabetic has elevated blood glucose levels. What physiological stress response best describes the rationale for the patient's increased blood sugar?
   a. Release of epinephrine
   b. Secretion of CRH
   c. Circulation of endorphins
   d. Increase of corticosteroids
9. Which short-term goal would be most appropriate for a patient with the nursing diagnosis *Anxiety* related to upcoming diagnostic tests, as evidenced by expressions of concern and pacing around the room?
   a. Patient will discuss specific aspects of concern.
   b. Nurse will administer prescribed anti-anxiety medication.
   c. Patient will understand diagnostic test procedures.
   d. Nurse will describe test procedures in detail to allay concerns.
10. Which intervention would be most appropriate for the nurse to include in the care plan for a patient who is experiencing constipation and increased heart and respiratory rates?
    a. Time management
    b. Decreased grain intake
    c. Relaxation therapy
    d. Regimented exercise

Answers and rationales for the review questions are available at *http://evolve.elsevier.com/YoostCrawford/fundamentals/*.

REFERENCES

Aiken L, Clarke S, Sloane D, et al: Hospital nurse staffing and patient mortality, nurse burnout, and job dissatisfaction, *JAMA* 288(16):1987-1993, 2002.

Antonovsky A: *Health, stress and coping,* San Francisco, 1979, Jossey-Bass.

Brobek E, Marklund B, Haraldsson K, Berntsson L: Stress in children: How fifth year pupils experience stress in everyday life, *Scand J Caring Sci* 1:3-9, 2007.

Cannon WB: *Bodily changes in pain, hunger, fear and rage: An account of recent researches into the function of emotional excitement,* New York, 1915, Appleton.

Cimiotti JP, Aiken LH, Sloane DM, Wu ES: Nurse staffing, burnout, and health care–associated infection, *Am J Infect Control* 40(6):486-490, 2012.

Cronenwett L, Sherwood G, Barnsteiner J, et al: Quality and safety education for nurses, *Nurs Outlook* 55(3):122-131, 2007.

Edozien C: Mind over matter: Psychological factors and the menstrual cycle, *Curr Opin Obstet Gynecol* 18(4):452-456, 2006.

Elliott B, Gessert C, Larson P, Russ T: Religious beliefs and practices in end-stage renal disease: Implications for clinicians, *J Pain Sympt Manage* 44(3):400-409, 2012.

Esmonde L, Long A: Complementary therapy use by persons with multiple sclerosis: Benefits and research priorities, *Complement Ther Clin Pract* 14:176-184, 2008.

Fisher P, Abrahamson K: *When working hurts: Stress, burnout, and trauma in human, emergency, and health services,* Victoria, B.C., 2002, Spectrum Press.

Folkman S, Lazarus R, Dunkle-Schetter C, et al: Dynamics of a stressful encounter: Cognitive appraisal, coping and encounter outcomes, *J Personal Soc Psychol* 50(5):992-1003, 1986.

Fontaine KL: *Complementary and alternative therapies for nursing practice,* ed. 2, Upper Saddle River, N.J., 2005, Pearson/Prentice Hall.

Ford-Gilboe M, Cohen JA: Hardiness: A model of commitment, challenge and control. In VH Rice (Ed), *Stress, coping and health,* Thousand Oaks, Calif., 2000, Sage.

Gartland N, O'Connor D, Lawton R: The effects of conscientiousness on the appraisals of daily stressors, *Stress Health* 28(1):80-86, 2012.

Glanz K, Schwartz, MD: Stress, coping, and health behavior. In K Glanz, BK Rimer, K Viswanath (Eds), *Health behavior and health education: Theory, research, and practice,* pp 211-236, San Francisco, 2008, Jossey-Bass.

Harris E, Kirk J, Rowsell R, et al: The effect of multivitamin supplementation on mood and stress in healthy older men, *Hum Psychopharmacol Clin Exp* 26(8):560-567, 2011.

Hay E, Diehl M: Reactivity to daily stressors in adulthood: The importance of stressor type in characterizing risk factors, *Psychol Aging* 25(1):118-131, 2010.

Herbert T B, Cohen S: Stress and immunity in humans: A meta-analytic review, *Psychosom Med* 55:364-379, 1993.

Holmes TH, Rahe RH: The social readjustment rating scale, *J Psychosom Res* 11(2):213-218, 1967.

Humphrey JH: *Anthology of stress revisited,* New York, 2005, Nova Science Publishers.

Johnson H, Thompson A, Downs M: Non-Western interpreters' experiences of trauma: The protective role of culture following exposure to oppression, *Ethn Health* 4:407-418, 2009.

Kasl SV: Stress and health among the elderly: An overview of issues. In M Winkle, E Kahana, J Kowal (Eds), *Stress and health among the elderly,* New York, 1992, Springer.

Kiecolt-Glaser JK: Stress, food, and inflammation: Psychoneuroimmunology and nutrition at the cutting edge, *Psychosom Med* 72(4):365-369, 2010.

Kleinke C: *Coping with life challenges,* ed. 2, Long Grove, Ill., 2002, Waveland Press.

Kuwert P, Brahler E, Glaesner H, et al: PTSD in older bereaved people, *Aging Mental Health* 14(3):310-318, 2010.
Lafferty W, Downey L, McCarty R, et al: Evaluating CAM treatment at the end of life: A review of clinical trials for massage and meditation, *Complement Ther Med* 14:100-112, 2006.
Lai H, Good M: Music improves sleep quality in older adults, *J Adv Nurs* 53(1):134-144, 2006.
Lawson K: Demystifying mindfulness, *Minn Med* 94(1):37-39, 2011.
Lazarus R: *Psychological stress and the coping process,* New York, 1966, McGraw-Hill.
Lazarus R, Folkman S: *Stress, appraisal and coping,* New York, 1984, Springer.
Lazarus R, Folkman S: *Manual for the hassles and uplifts scales,* res ed., Palo Alto, Calif., 1989, Consulting Psychologists Press.
Leserman J, Whetten K, Lowe K, et al: How trauma, recent stress events and PTSD affect functional health status and health utilization in HIV-infected patients in the south, *Psychosom Med* 67:500-507, 2005.
Lombardo B, Eyre C: Compassion fatigue: A nurse's primer, *Online J Issues Nurs* 16(1), 2011. Retrieved from *www.nursingworld.org/MainMenuCategories/ANAMarketplace/ANAPeriodicals/OJIN/TableofContents/Vol-16-2011/No1-Jan-2011/Compassion-Fatigue-A-Nurses-Primer.html.*
Mayo Clinic: Anger management: 10 tips to tame your temper, 2011. Retrieved from *www.mayoclinic.com/health/anger-management/MH00102.*
McEwan BS: Effects of adverse experiences for brain structure and function, *Biol Psychol* 48:721, 2000.
McEwan BS, Lasley EN: *The end of stress as we know it,* Washington, D.C., 2002, Joseph Henry Press.
Miller L, Smith A, Mehler B: The stress audit, *Annu Rev Neurosci* 24:1161-1192, 1991.
Nabkasorn C, Miyai N, Sootmongkol A, et al: Effects of physical exercise on depression, neuroendocrine stress hormones and physiological fitness in adolescent females with depressive symptoms, *Eur J Public Health* 16(2):179-184, 2006.
Neupert S, Almeida D, Charles S: Age differences in reactivity to daily stressors: The role of personal control, *J Gerontol Psychol Sci* 62B:216-225, 2007.
Ophir E, Nass C, Wagner AD: Cognitive control in media multitaskers, *Proc Natl Acad Sci Ud Sf A* 106(37):15583-15587, 2009.
Rausch S, Baker K, Boonmee J: Sleep disturbances in caregivers of patients with end-stage congestive heart failure: Part II—assess and intervene, *Progr Cardiovasc Nurs* 22(2):93-96, 2007.
Ross R, Zeller R, Srisaeng P, et al: Depression, stress, emotional support, and self-esteem among baccalaureate nursing students in Thailand, *Int J Nurs Educ Scholarsh* 3:Article 21, 2006. Retrieved from *www.bepress.com/ijnes.*
Roy C: Adaptation: A conceptual framework for nursing, *Nurs Outlook* 18:42-45, 1970.
Rubinstein J, Meyer D, Evans J: Executive control of cognitive processes in task switching. *J Exp Psychol Hum Percept Perform* 27(4):763-797, 2001.
Sapatkin D: Penn study examines link between nurse burnout and care, 2012. Retrieved from *http://articles.philly.com/2012-07-31/news/32943021_1_infection-data-infection-control-center-for-health-outcomes/3.*
Schwartz T: The magic of doing one thing at a time, *Harvard Bus Rev* 2012. Retrieved from *http://blogs.hbr.org/schwartz/2012/03/the-magic-of-doing-one-thing-a.html.*
Selye H: *The stress of life,* New York, 1956, McGraw-Hill.
Selye H: *The stress of life,* rev ed., New York, 1976, McGraw-Hill.
Shapiro S, Astin J, Bishop S, Cordova M: Mindfulness-based stress reduction for health care professionals: Results from a randomized trial, *Int J Stress Manage* 12(2):164-176, 2005.
Sharrer VW, Ryan-Wenger NA: School age children's self-reported stress symptoms, *Pediatr Nurse* 28:21-27, 2002.
Snyder M, Pestka E, Bly C: Muscle relaxation techniques. In M Snyder, R Lindquist (Eds), *Complementary/alternative therapies in nursing,* ed. 5, pp 323-334, New York, 2006, Springer.
Starkweather A: The effects of exercise on perceived stress and IL-6 levels among older adults, *Biol Res Nurs* 8(3):186-194, 2007.
Stojanovich L, Marisavljevich D: Stress as a trigger of autoimmune disease, *Autoimmun Rev* 7:209-213, 2008.
Treat-Jacobson D, Lindquist R: Exercise, quality of life, and symptoms in men and women five to six years after coronary artery bypass graft surgery, *Heart Lung* 36(6): 387-397, 2007.
Umbreit AW: Healing touch. In M Snyder, R Lindquist (Eds), *Complementary/ alternative therapies in nursing,* ed. 5, pp 203-224, New York, 2006, Springer.
Wagnild G, Young H: Development and psychometric evaluation of the Resilience Scale, *J Nurs Meas* 1:165ff, 1993.
Welsh CJ, Bustamonte L, Nayak M, et al: The effects of restraint stress on the neuropathogenesis of Theilers virus infection II: NK cell function and cytokine levels in acute disease, *Brain Behav Immunity* 18:166-174, 2004.

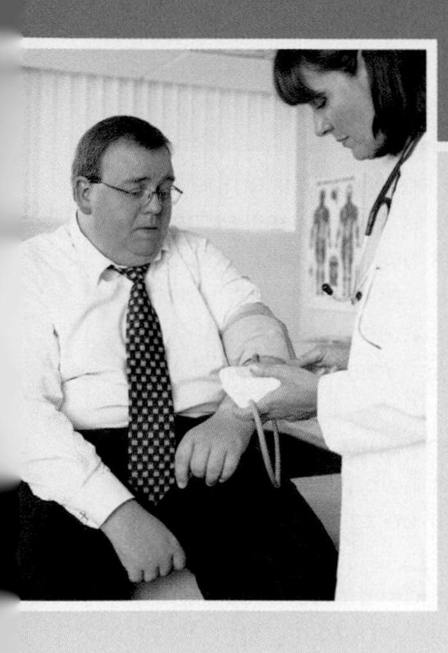

CHAPTER 33

Sleep

EVOLVE WEBSITE

http://evolve.elsevier.com/YoostCrawford/fundamentals/

- Additional Evolve-Only Review Questions With Answers
- Answers and Rationales for Text Review Questions
- Answers to Critical-Thinking Questions
- Case Study With Questions
- Conceptual Care Map Creator
- Glossary

LEARNING OUTCOMES

Comprehension of this chapter's content will provide students with the ability to:

LO 33.1 Explain the physiology and functions involved in sleep.
LO 33.2 Discuss characteristics of common sleep disorders.
LO 33.3 Summarize assessment techniques for determining sleep patterns.
LO 33.4 Identify nursing diagnoses for patients with sleep disturbances.
LO 33.5 Determine patient goals based on specific sleep problems.
LO 33.6 Implement interventions that promote sleep.

KEY TERMS

bruxism, p. 756
cataplexy, p. 755
circadian rhythms, p. 751
dyssomnias, p. 753
hypersomnia, p. 755
hypnotics, p. 764
insomnia, p. 754
narcolepsy, p. 754
nocturnal enuresis, p. 756
non–rapid eye movement (NREM) sleep, p. 750
obstructive sleep apnea (OSA), p. 755
parasomnias, p. 756
polysomnography, p. 751
rapid eye movement (REM) sleep, p. 750
restless legs syndrome, p. 756
secondary sleep disorders, p. 757
sleep, p. 750
sleep apnea, p. 755
sleep deprivation, p. 756
somnambulism, p. 756

CASE STUDY

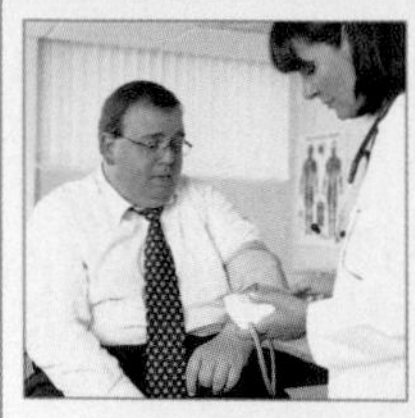

Mr. Barnes is a 51-year-old male who owns a small business. All of his employees are family members. He recently had to lay off two of his five employees and increase his own working hours. The stress of dealing with the financial losses and laying off of family members has caused a change in his overall health and sleep habits. His day-to-day work involves managing all aspects of the business and employees, and handling customer relations. He drinks approximately six cups of coffee a day, smokes two packs of cigarettes a day, has three or four alcoholic drinks at night to "relax," and has gained more than 30 pounds in the last year. He arrives at the clinic, accompanied by his wife, requesting "something to help me sleep."

Assessment data for Mr. Barnes reveal a man who looks older than his stated age, has dark circles around puffy eyes, and yawns frequently during the assessment. His height is 5 feet 11 inches and his weight is 259 lb. Vital signs are T 36.3°C (97.4° F), P 96 and regular and steady, R 26 and slightly labored, and BP 174/96, with a pulse oximetry reading of 90% on room air. He has no complaints of pain or discomfort at this time.

Mr. Barnes reports daytime sleepiness, trouble getting to sleep, headache when awakening in the mornings, difficulty concentrating, and two recent car accidents. His wife states that he is irritable, goes to bed late, sleeps for only 4 or 5 hours at night, is very restless in bed, and has periods of not breathing followed by periods of loud snoring. He currently is taking no prescription medications.

Refer back to this case study to answer the critical-thinking questions throughout the chapter.

Sleep is a naturally occurring altered state of consciousness regulated by the central nervous system. Without healthy sleep, concentration and judgment become impaired, and participation in daily activities decreases. People who experience an acute or chronic illness often need more rest and sleep. To promote adequate sleep and rest for patients, the nurse needs to understand the characteristics of sleep, factors that influence sleep, the way to assess for sleep disorders, and the use of interventions to support the practice of good sleep habits, known as sleep hygiene, for patients of all age groups.

NORMAL STRUCTURE AND FUNCTION INVOLVED IN SLEEP LO 33.1

Physical and emotional health depend on proper nutrition, adequate exercise, and the right type and amount of sleep and rest. Sleep is a universal human need. According to the National Heart, Lung, and Blood Institute's Sleep Disorder Research Plan (2011), 25% to 30% of Americans have sleep disorders.

During sleep, both awareness of and reaction to the environment are decreased. Historically, it was thought that sleep was a period of time during which the body was at complete rest and activity was dormant. It is now known that sleep has stages that cycle through the night, each with vital tasks to help the person feel rested and maintain health and function (National Institutes of Health [NIH], 2011).

PHYSIOLOGIC AND PSYCHOLOGICAL CHANGES SURROUNDING THE SLEEP CYCLE

Although the effects of sleep on the body are not well understood, well-recognized physiologic and psychological changes occur with adequate sleep. The heart beats 10 to 20 fewer times per minute when sleeping, and respirations, blood pressure, and muscle tone all decrease during sleep (McCance and Huether, 2006). **Rapid eye movement (REM) sleep** occurs during deep sleep and is manifested by quick scanning movements of the eyes that are associated with dreaming. REM sleep is associated with memory storage, learning, increased cerebral blood flow, and epinephrine release (McCance and Huether, 2006). During **non–rapid eye movement (NREM) sleep**, in which REM does not occur, growth hormone is released to repair epithelial and brain cells, cell division for skin and bone marrow renewal occurs, and energy is conserved (Izac, 2006). The effect of sleep on psychological well-being is best illustrated by the diminished mental functioning associated with sleep deprivation. People with too little sleep have difficulty making decisions, experience decreased concentration, and become emotionally irritable. Accidents and injuries are common in people who drive or operate heavy machinery while sleep-deprived.

Many physiologic rhythms fluctuate in preparation for activity or rest. Body temperature, cortisol, and melatonin levels change in preparation for waking or sleeping. For example, in anticipation of daytime activity, cortisol levels increase around 4 A.M. and peak around 6 A.M. Core body temperature, which typically is coupled closely with activity rhythm, starts to increase after the minimum core temperature level is reached between 2 and 4 A.M., in anticipation of activity. Activity and core temperature peak at approximately 4 P.M. Conversely, a rapid decline in core temperature normally occurs approximately 2 hours before sleep onset. Melatonin is the hormone believed to induce sleep in humans. Although core temperature and cortisol levels decrease with the onset of darkness, melatonin levels increase. Eight hours of uninterrupted sleep are more easily achieved when sleep begins approximately 6 hours before the minimum temperature is reached (Berger and Hobbs, 2006).

NEUROTRANSMITTERS AND THE RETICULAR ACTIVATING SYSTEM

Sleep is a complex process regulated by the reticular activating system (RAS) and neurotransmitter interactions. The RAS receives sensory impulses from the spinal cord and relays motor impulses to the thalamus and all parts of the cerebral cortex. As messengers of the nervous system, neurotransmitters provide communication between neurons. The neurotransmitters acetylcholine and norepinephrine influence REM sleep; the neurotransmitters serotonin and gamma aminobutyric acid (GABA) affect NREM sleep.

CIRCADIAN RHYTHMS

Biologic rhythms exist in plants, animals, and humans. In humans, these biorhythms, along with internal and external factors, affect sleep. The most familiar rhythm is the day-night, 24-hour circadian rhythm cycle. **Circadian rhythms** influence patterns of biologic and behavioral functions. Some creatures are diurnal, or primarily active during the day, while others are nocturnal, with most of their activity during the night.

Nerve cells within the hypothalamus control the 24-hour circadian rhythms, which affect body temperature, endocrine functions, blood pressure, sleep, and other functions. Factors such as daily routines, work schedules, social commitments, alarm clocks, and noise affect the circadian rhythm and sleep-wake cycle. Melatonin, synthesized in the pineal gland, regulates the circadian phase of sleep and is closely related to light conditions. The sleep-wake circadian rhythm is further affected by the light-dark cycle of the natural environment as input of surroundings is received by the retina of the eyes (Izac, 2006).

SLEEP CYCLES

Humans spend approximately one third of their lives asleep. At night, an adult normally falls asleep within 10 minutes and then goes through a sequence of five sleep stages. **Polysomnography** is the recording of brain waves and other physiologic variables, such as muscle activity and eye movements, during sleep. A normal polysomnograph shows a sleep sequence of four NREM stages and one REM stage. NREM sleep alternates with REM sleep in time intervals of approximately 90 minutes, and a normal sleep pattern consists of three to five cycles of sleep each night (Table 33-1). Quality of sleep is affected by frequent wakening, pain, and shortened REM stage of sleep.

SLEEP RHYTHMS

Polysomnography recordings of sleep show recurring patterns of sleep lasting approximately 90 minutes. The usual

TABLE 33-1 Sleep Stages

STAGE IN SLEEP CYCLE	DESCRIPTION
NREM 1	• Lightest level of sleep, between sleep and wakefulness • Vital signs and metabolism begin to decrease/slow down • Easy arousal by external stimuli, such as noise • Feeling of drowsiness • Lasts a few minutes • May occur during the day as "resting my eyes"
NREM 2	• Relaxation increases • Sleep becomes deeper • Snoring may occur • Relatively easy arousal • Physiologic functions continue to slow • Accompanied by occasional small muscle jerks • Lasts 10-20 min
NREM 3	• Initial stage of deep sleep • More difficult arousal and rare movement • Muscles relaxed • Vital signs decrease, but regular rhythms/patterns maintained • Restorative processes such as the release of growth hormone occur • Lasts 15-30 min
NREM 4	• Deepest stage of sleep • Strong stimuli needed for arousal • Vital signs decreased much more than during wake time • Restorative processes continue • Somnambulism and nocturnal enuresis may occur • May be lengthy period of sleep if sleep deprivation has occurred • Lasts 15-30 min
REM	• Occurrence of vivid, colorful dreaming (less vivid dreaming may occur in other stages) • Starts approximately 90 min after sleep is initiated • Autonomous response causes rapid eye movements, fluctuating heart rate and respirations, and increased blood pressure • Muscle tone decreased • Gastric secretions increased • Very difficult arousal • Duration of REM sleep increases with each sleep cycle and averages 20 min

sleep sequence for a person is a fairly rapid progression through NREM stages 1 through 4, back through NREM stages 3 and 2, and then into REM sleep (Figure 33-1). During the early hours of sleep, NREM stages 3 and 4 are longer; in the later hours of sleep, REM sleep may last as long as 45 minutes of the cycle. If someone is fully awakened and goes back to sleep, the cycle begins again with NREM stage 1.

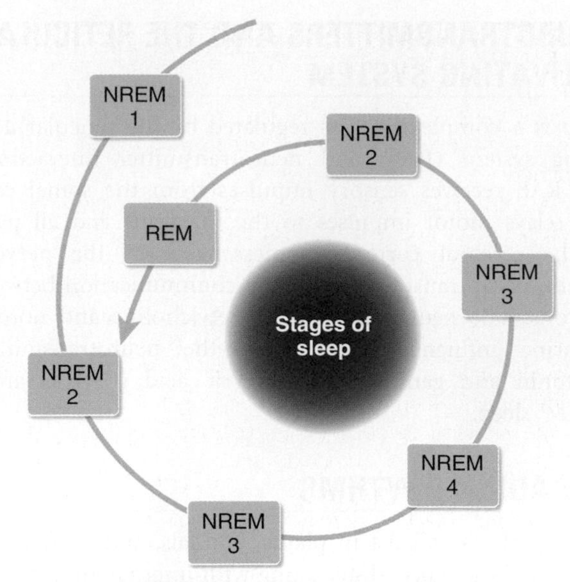

FIGURE 33-1 The sleep cycle.

PATTERNS OF SLEEP THROUGHOUT THE LIFE CYCLE

The overall amount of time spent sleeping and the amount of time spent in each stage of sleep vary among people, especially with age. Although sleep is affected by several variables, sleep changes follow a predictable age-related pattern (Diversity Considerations box). Newborns require the most sleep of all age groups, and elderly people require the least sleep.

DIVERSITY CONSIDERATIONS

Life Span

Newborn

- Newborns should sleep in 2- to 4-hour blocks between feedings.
- Teach parents to position newborns and infants on the back for sleeping, to decrease the risk of sudden infant death syndrome or (SIDS) (Evidence-Based Practice and Informatics box).

Infant

- Infants sleep 10 to 12 hours at night, with naps during the day.
- Half of their sleep is in lighter stages.
- Sleep patterns are unique for each child. The general pattern consists of sleeping, awakening to eat, and sleeping again.
- Caution against using blankets, pillows, and bumpers in cribs, to decrease suffocation risk.
- Teach that eye movements, grimacing, and body movement are normal features of sleep at this age.
- Encourage parents to have infants sleep in their own cribs. According to the American Academy of Pediatrics 2011 revised guidelines on SIDS, the infant may sleep in the parents' room if the infant sleeps in his or her own crib and not with parents or siblings.
- Older infants may safely roll to their stomachs during sleep because they have developed good head control.

Toddler and Preschooler

- Children in this group sleep 10 to 12 hours a day.
- The sleep-wake cycle usually is established by the age of 2 to 3 years.
- Sleep needs fluctuate with growth spurts.
- A nap during the day can restore energy.
- Toddlers and preschoolers may exhibit resistance to going to bed.
- They may be moved out of the crib to a bed at approximately 2 years of age.
- Bedtime rituals are important. Teach parents to establish a regular bedtime routine and consistently follow it.
- Address safety needs that arise when children are able to get out of bed. For example, a safety gate across a doorway may be needed to protect a child from stairs or other hazards should the child get up.
- Educate parents on how to address a child's fear of the dark (by using a nightlight) or nightmares (by soothing the child but allowing the child to return to sleep).

School-Age Child

- School-age children sleep 8 to 12 hours a night. Naps are rare.
- The occurrence of nightmares decreases with age.
- The stress of starting school may disrupt the sleep pattern.
- Less sleep is needed by the age of 11 to 12 years, so bedtime may be extended.
- The bedtime routine is still important.

Adolescent

- Adolescents need 8 to10 hours of sleep each night.
- Sleep patterns may change to wakening later in the morning, with occasional naps.
- Males may experience nocturnal emissions ("wet dreams").
- Adolescents who drink caffeinated beverages and use technology late into the night, may experience daytime sleepiness with impaired alertness and functioning (Calamaro, Mason, and Ratcliffe, 2009).
- Complaints of tiredness or poor school performance may be related to inadequate sleep.

DIVERSITY CONSIDERATIONS—cont'd

Adult

- Adults sleep 6 to 8 hours a night.
- They tend to continue sleep patterns established when younger.
- They may begin to have more night awakenings.
- Teach adults about sleep hygiene and nonpharmacologic measures (especially stress reduction) to enhance sleep patterns.
- Discourage the long-term use of sleep medications.

Older Adult

- Older adults sleep approximately 6 hours a night.
- Stage 4 sleep is decreased, resulting in less restorative sleep.
- The first REM stage is longer.
- Older adults awaken more at night and take longer to go back to sleep.
- A decline in health or the use of medications may interfere with sleep.
- Encourage older adults to maintain the usual bedtime and routines as much as possible.
- Older adults should exercise caution when using sleep medications.
- When hospitalized, an environment that is warm and safe (night light, call light) encourages relaxation for the older adult.
- Resolving underlying health issues, if possible, will enhance sleep.

Gender

- Adult males are at higher risk for development of obstructive sleep apnea. Children and adult females are at lower risk for the disorder.

Culture and Ethnicity

- In some cultures, a family bed in which children sleep with parents is common. Instruct families about the dangers of infants sleeping with adults.

Morphology

- People who sleep less than average are more likely to be overweight, develop diabetes, and eat a high-calorie, high-carbohydrate diet (NIH, 2011).
- Obesity predisposes affected people to obstructive sleep apnea.

EVIDENCE-BASED PRACTICE AND INFORMATICS

Sudden Infant Death Syndrome

Sudden infant death syndrome (SIDS) was first formally defined in 1969 as the sudden unexpected death of an infant younger than 1 year of age that remains unexplained after a thorough postmortem investigation.

- SIDS is the second most common cause of death among infants 1 to 12 months of age.
- It has a devastating impact on surviving family members.
- The etiology remains largely unknown.
- Risk factors include the infant's sleeping on the stomach, being exposed to cigarette smoke, and/or sleeping in the same bed as the parents, as well as premature and multiple-birth babies, soft bedding in cribs, a sibling with SIDS, poor or no prenatal care, and drinking and drug use during pregnancy (National Institute of Child Health and Human Development, 2013).
- The most important modifiable SIDS risk factor appears to be prone sleeping.
- Dramatic decreases in SIDS rates (reaching 50%) have been observed in countries that actively discourage prone sleeping and emphasize the supine (back) sleeping position.
- Instructions from health care providers about prone sleeping are essential.
- Parent and caregiver information, "About SIDS and Safe Infant Sleep," is available from the National Institutes of Health (NIH) at *www.nichd.nih.gov/sts/about/Pages/default.aspx* (2013).

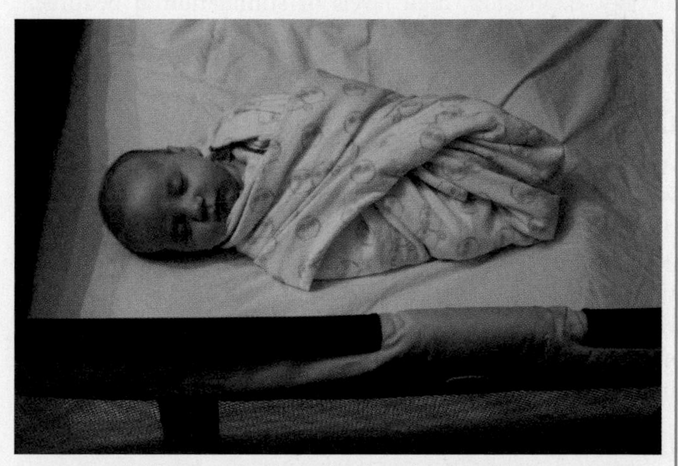

Infant supine in safe sleeping position.

ALTERED SLEEP LO 33.2

Sleep alterations, if left unaddressed, can cause disturbed sleep, resulting in insomnia, abnormal movements or sensations during sleep, or excessive daytime sleepiness. People deprived of REM sleep become agitated and impulsive; deprivation of NREM sleep results in withdrawal and vague physical complaints. Sleep disorders are classified into dyssomnias, parasomnias, and secondary sleep disorders on the basis of their underlying cause (Table 33-2).

DYSSOMNIAS

Dyssomnias are disorders associated with getting to sleep, staying asleep, or being excessively sleepy. Decreases in the amount or changes in the timing of sleep result in daytime

TABLE 33-2 Sleep and Sleep-Related Disorders

CATEGORY	SPECIFIC DISORDER/UNDERLYING CAUSE
Dyssomnias	• Insomnia • Obstructive sleep apnea • Shift-work sleep disorder • Time zone change (jet lag) • Hypersomnia • Restless legs syndrome • Narcolepsy • Sleep deprivation
Parasomnias	• Nocturnal enuresis • Somnambulism • Sleep terrors • Bruxism

Secondary sleep disorders	• Physiologic effect of medical conditions: heart failure, chronic obstructive pulmonary disease, pain, or gastric reflux disease
	• Hospitalization with a serious illness
	• Mental health disorders:
	  • Depression
	  • Anxiety
	  • Fear

sleepiness, poor concentration, and a feeling of not being rested. Causes of dyssomnias include too much napping, anxiety, depression, high levels of stimulation at bedtime, medication use, shift work, and hyperthyroidism (Sleep Disorders Guide, 2012).

Circadian Rhythm Sleep Disorders

A disruption of the normal circadian sleep pattern occurs when the person cannot sleep when sleep is wanted, needed, or expected. This disorder is common in shift work and time zone change (jet lag) situations (Ethical, Legal, and Professional Practice box). The potential consequences of circadian rhythm disturbances include depression, sexual dysfunction, memory difficulties, high blood pressure, obesity, and an increased risk for accidents.

Insomnia

Insomnia is the most common dyssomnia and is characterized by difficulty in falling asleep or staying asleep, sleep that is too light, or early-morning awakenings. Concern with the problems related to not getting enough sleep further interferes with sleep, contributing to an ongoing cycle of sleep disturbance. The occurrence of insomnia increases with age, and the disorder affects more women than men (National Institute of Neurological Disorders and Stroke [NINDS], 2014a). Short-term insomnia usually can be traced to acute stress or lifestyle changes and often is self-limiting. Insomnia can lead to symptoms of sleep deprivation and daytime fatigue, which can cause impairment in work, social, and other areas of functioning. Medications for insomnia do not deal with the cause of the sleep problem, and prolonged use can create drug dependency.

ETHICAL, LEGAL, AND PROFESSIONAL PRACTICE

Effects of Shift Work on Safety

Shift work generally is defined as work hours that are other than the day shift. The definition includes lengthy (e.g., 12-hour) and extended shifts.

Since the 1960s, scientists have been examining the effect of conditions such as air travel and shift work on biological functions, activity, and rest. The body's internal clock is cued by the light-dark cycle, and shift work disrupts the pattern. Possible results may include sleep disturbances, increased accidents and injuries, and social isolation. For example, after a 12-hour nursing shift, the risk of making a medication error or incurring a needlestick can be double that associated with an 8-hour shift.

Nurses working various shifts can adopt countermeasures such as taking power naps, eliminating overtime on 12-hour shifts, and completing challenging tasks early in the shift to reduce patient care errors. Other strategies that can help adaptation to shift work include:

- Take responsibility for obtaining a minimum of 6 hours of sleep each 24-hour period.
- Maintain a regular sleep schedule when working and on nights off.
- Include a 4-hour "anchor" sleep time during which sleep is scheduled whether on or off work. For example, after working, sleep from 8:30 A.M. to 4:30 P.M., and on days off, sleep from 4:30 A.M. to 12:30 P.M. The anchor sleep time is from 8:30 A.M. to 12:30 P.M.
- Wear dark glasses that block blue light when driving home after night work.
- Seek exposure to bright light (sunlight is best) as soon as possible after waking.
- Before the first night shift, power-nap 30 to 90 minutes before leaving for work.

Adapted from Berger AM, Hobbs BB: Impact of shift work on the health and safety of nurses and patients, *Clin J Oncol Nurs* 10(4):465-471, 2006.

Narcolepsy

Narcolepsy is a chronic neurologic disorder caused by the brain's inability to regulate the sleep-wake cycle normally, resulting in an uncontrollable desire to sleep. This sleep starts with the REM phase. At various times throughout the day, people with narcolepsy experience overwhelming sleepiness and fall asleep for periods of seconds to several minutes. These sleep episodes can occur at any time; accordingly, the disorder can be very disabling. People may involuntarily fall asleep while at work or at school, or when having a conversation, playing a game, eating a meal, or, most dangerously, driving an automobile or operating other types of potentially hazardous machinery. In addition to daytime sleepiness, three other major symptoms frequently characterize narcolepsy: cataplexy, or the sudden loss of voluntary muscle tone; vivid hallucinations during sleep onset or on awakening; and brief episodes of total paralysis at the beginning or end of sleep.

Scientists now believe that narcolepsy results from disease processes affecting brain mechanisms that regulate REM sleep. For normal sleepers, a typical sleep cycle begins with NREM sleep and undergoes transition to REM sleep. People with narcolepsy frequently enter REM sleep within a few minutes of falling asleep. The diagnosis of narcolepsy is confirmed by sleep diagnostic tests: the polysomnogram and the multiple sleep latency test.

Hypersomnia

Hypersomnia is excessive daytime sleepiness lasting at least 1 month that causes impairment in the ability to function in occupational or other areas of the affected person's life. Even after 8 to 12 hours of sleep each night, the person still experiences trouble awakening in the morning. Hypersomnia can be caused by medical conditions such as some kidney or liver disorders, diabetic acidosis, central nervous system damage, or hypothyroidism.

Sleep Apnea

Sleep apnea is a condition in which the person experiences the absence of breathing (apnea) or diminished breathing during sleep between snoring intervals. It is characterized by a lack of airflow through the mouth and nose for at least 10 seconds, lasting up to 2 minutes, during sleep. The most common type is obstructive sleep apnea (OSA), which affects 12 million to 18 million people in the United States.

OSA involves collapse of the upper airway despite respiratory effort (Figure 33-2). The affected person continues to try to breathe, evidenced by chest and abdominal movements with loud snoring or snorting sounds. Diaphragmatic movements become stronger until the obstruction is relieved. Increased carbon dioxide levels in the blood that accumulate during the apneic episodes cause the person to awaken, and these awakenings can occur hundreds of times each night. Prolonged sleep apnea can cause an increase in blood pressure, leading to cardiac arrest. Cardiac arrhythmias, pulmonary hypertension, and left-sided heart failure can result from prolonged sleep apnea. The affected person's sleep partner's sleep may be disrupted by the snoring or by the abrupt cessation of breathing occurring with periods of apnea. Sleep partners often report staying awake to be sure the patient starts breathing again after each apnea period.

> **QSEN FOCUS!**
>
> Through patient-centered care, the nurse values an active partnership with patients, their families, or designated surrogates in planning, implementation, and evaluation of care. This approach is especially important in assessing the patient's sleep, because the significant other or family member often can describe what is happening with the patient during sleep.

Risk factors for OSA include obesity, large neck circumference, smoking, alcohol use, and a family history of OSA. Structural abnormalities such as a recessed chin, abnormal upper airway structures, deviated septum, nasal polyps, or enlarged tonsils can predispose the affected person to OSA (Dugan, 2007). The disorder is more common in adult males, but it can affect adult females and children as well (Mendez and Olson, 2006). The diagnosis of OSA is confirmed with polysomnography to measure respirations, heart rate, and muscle movements.

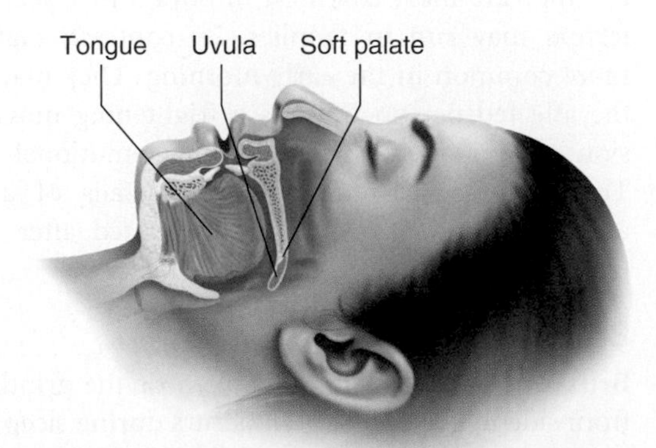

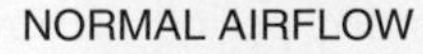

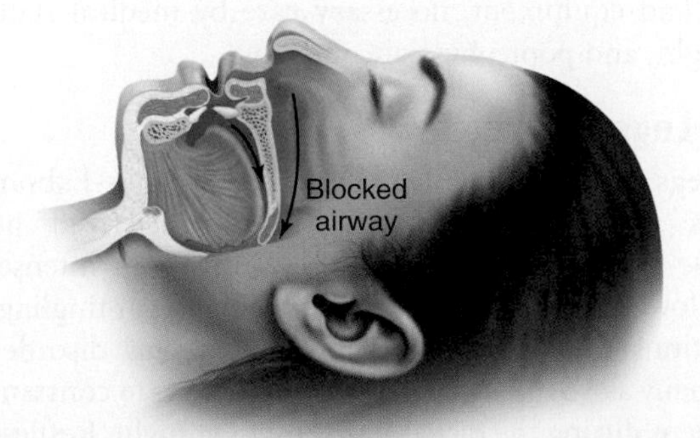

FIGURE 33-2 Changes occurring in obstructive sleep apnea.

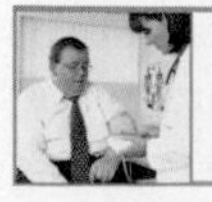

1. What signs and symptoms does Mr. Barnes exhibit that are indicative of obstructive sleep apnea?

! SAFE PRACTICE ALERT

OSA can cause fragmented sleep and low blood oxygen levels to the body, including the heart, leading to hypoxia, acidosis, and hypercapnia (increased carbon dioxide).

Sleep Deprivation

Sleep deprivation occurs from prolonged lack of sleep of good quality and adequate quantity. Disturbances of sleep leading to deprivation can be associated with aging or may result from hospitalization, drug and substance abuse, emotional stress, medications, factors in the environmental (e.g., noise, light), and disruption of normal sleep patterns such as with shift rotations or changes in lifestyle patterns. Sleep deprivation can cause symptoms of fatigue, headache, nausea, increased sensitivity to pain, decreased neuromuscular coordination, irritability, and difficulty concentrating. Eventually, disorientation and hallucinations may occur. Sleep deprivation can have negative health effects on blood pressure (hypertension), glucose metabolism, and hormone regulation and leading to inflammation, increased frequency of seizures in patients with seizure disorders, and increased weight gain contributing to obesity (Jones, Johnson, and Harvey-Berino, 2008; Kotagal and Yardi, 2008; Mullington, Haack, Toth, et al, 2009). Florence Nightingale's nursing theory work discussed environmental adaptation with appropriate noise, hygiene, light, comfort, socialization, hope, nutrition, and conservation of patient energy. Many of these adaptations have been found to promote sleep and rest. See Chapter 1 for more on Nightingale's theory. People respond variably to sleep deprivation. The most effective treatment is correction of the factors interrupting the sleep patterns.

Hospitalization, especially in acute care units such as intensive care or cardiac care units, puts patients at risk for sleep deprivation. This is secondary to the unfamiliar noises from staff and equipment, necessary care by medical staff, constant light, and poor physical condition.

Restless Legs Syndrome

Restless legs syndrome (also known as Willis-Ekbom disease) is a familial sleep disorder characterized by disagreeable-feeling leg movements resulting from intense, abnormal, lower-extremity sensations of crawling or tingling. The sensations cause delay in sleep onset. This disorder affects as many as 12 million Americans and leads to constant leg movement during the day and insomnia at night. Restless legs syndrome can occur at any age but is more common in elderly people.

PARASOMNIAS

Parasomnias are disorders associated with abnormal sleep behaviors, rather than disorders of sleep itself. The behaviors come from activation of the autonomic nervous system, motor system, or cognitive processes during sleep or during the transitions between sleep and wakefulness. These disorders are more common in children and adolescents. Attempts to awaken the person from a parasomnia should be discouraged. Although safety needs must be met, help should be given to the extent the person will accept it, which includes encouraging the person to return to sleep as the event ends.

Somnambulism

Somnambulism, or "sleepwalking," affects up to 4% of adults and constitutes one of the leading causes of self-injury and sleep-related violence, which may include injury of others and even homicide (Zadra, Pilon, and Montplaisir, 2008). Sleepers may sit up with glassy eyes and get up and walk around; generally, they will avoid anyone who attempts to talk to them.

Nocturnal Enuresis

Nocturnal enuresis (bedwetting at night) is a socially disruptive and stressful condition that is common in childhood. Bed alarms are the treatment that currently appears to work best in the long term. These alarms sound when moisture is present, waking the child. Behavioral therapy may be used either alone or in conjunction with a bed alarm (Glazener, Evans, and Peto, 2008).

Sleep Terrors

Sleep terrors, or night terrors, are a parasomnia in which a person quickly awakens from sleep in a terrified state. Sleep terrors occur during deep sleep, usually during the first third of the night. The cause is unknown, but they may be triggered by fever, lack of sleep, use of alcohol, or periods of emotional stress or conflict. Night terrors are fairly common in children age 3 to 7 years of age, but they are most common in boys 5 to 7 years old. Night terrors may run in families. By contrast, nightmares are more common in the early morning. They may occur after the affected person watches a frightening movie or television program or has a strong emotional experience. The person may remember the details of a dream on awakening and will not be disoriented after the episode (NIH, 2014).

Bruxism

Bruxism is the clenching of teeth or the grinding of teeth from side to side. This often occurs during sleep and may be due to stress. Pain can result if the clenching is tight or occurs over an extended period of time (U.S. National Library of Medicine, 2014).

SECONDARY SLEEP DISORDERS

Secondary sleep disorders can be disabling symptoms of underlying medical or psychiatric disorders. The physiologic effect of medical conditions affects the sleep-wake cycle. For example, heart failure, chronic obstructive pulmonary disease, pain, and gastric reflux disease all may affect sleep. Mental health disorders cause changes in sleep-wake regulation. Up to 90% of patients with depression report disturbed sleep. Anxiety, which is common in people who are hospitalized or who have a serious illness, also interferes with sleep.

FACTORS CAUSING SLEEP ALTERATIONS

Many factors in a person's life can alter sleep patterns. Some of these factors are within a person's control such as diet and exercise. Others are outside factors that the person cannot control such as an illness or hospitalization.

Lifestyle

A work schedule that does not match the person's biologic rhythms (as can occur with rotating shifts or periodic assignment to a night shift) frequently interferes with sleep. Younger adults may adjust to shift work more easily than older adults who are more set in sleep patterns. Accumulated sleep loss may affect decision making as well as patient safety in health care. The stress of a fast-paced life with multiple demands can prevent a person from relaxing and falling easily to sleep.

Diet and Exercise

The type and amount of food and liquid consumed both are recognized to affect sleep. Highly caffeinated substances such as coffee, cola, and chocolate are central nervous system stimulants that can disrupt the sleep cycle. Going to bed hungry or eating a large, heavy, or spicy meal just before going to bed can interfere with sleep. Bedtime snacks that contain complex carbohydrates are recommended to promote calmness and relaxation.

Sleep and rest are important in addressing the rise in obesity in the United States. Both children and adults who sleep less than the recommended number of hours each night are more likely to be overweight (NIH, 2011). Exercise can assist with weight loss efforts and promote relaxation, but excessive exercise, especially in the evening, interferes with sleep.

Smoking

Nicotine has a stimulating effect, and smokers may have more trouble falling asleep and arouse more easily once asleep. Long-term smoking can lead to permanent lung damage, which in turn is associated with hypoxia, requiring an increased need for rest. People who quit smoking usually report improved sleep, although temporary sleep disturbance may occur immediately after complete withdrawal from nicotine.

Alcohol

Small amounts of alcohol may help some people fall asleep, but alcohol increases wakefulness in the last half of the night. Ingesting large quantities of alcohol creates difficulty falling asleep and limits REM sleep. These effects may cause a restless sleep, contributing to any "hangover" experienced on arising. Alcohol ingested when taking sleeping pills can cause dangerous side effects.

Stimulants and Other Medications

Many prescription and over-the-counter medications can affect the quality of sleep, causing sleepiness, restlessness, or insomnia. Medications that decrease REM sleep include barbiturates, amphetamines, and some antidepressants. Other medications that affect sleep patterns include diuretics, antiparkinsonian medications, antihypertensives, steroids, decongestants, and asthma drugs. Beta blockers have been reported to cause nightmares and insomnia. Narcotics suppress REM sleep, cause frequent awakening, and may cause excessive daytime sleepiness.

Short-term use of medications such as zaleplon (Sonata) and zolpidem (Ambien) may be indicated to improve sleep patterns. Eszopiclone (Lunesta) has been approved by the U.S. Food and Drug Administration (FDA) for longer-term treatment of insomnia.

Environmental Factors

People tend to sleep best in familiar settings where they feel comfortable and secure. Sleeping in new environments influences both NREM and REM sleep stages. People accustomed to the noise associated with living in a city may not rest well in country locales, whereas those accustomed to the quiet of the country may find it difficult to sleep in a city. Temperature and light are other variables that affect the ability to sleep.

Illness and Hospitalization

Illness and hospitalization are both physiologic and psychological stressors that influence sleep. Any illness that results in pain, discomfort, or mood changes can result in sleep problems. Sleep disturbances are more common with certain illnesses (Box 33-1).

Hospitalization is a stressor that disrupts sleep. Hospitals and residential care facilities usually do not adapt care routines to the person's sleep-wake cycle. When possible, health care providers should cluster care activities to provide 90- to 120-minute blocks of uninterrupted sleep time. This schedule allows for completion of all sleep stages. Maintaining a regular routine as much as possible enhances sleep for the hospitalized patient. When the sleep-wake cycle is disrupted, the patient may experience anxiety, restlessness, impaired judgment, and irritability, along with other negative effects on overall health. During a hospitalization, factors that affect sleep include unfamiliar surroundings, sounds, and smells; proximity to other patients; lack of privacy; increased light

BOX 33-1 Sleep Disturbances Associated With Illnesses

- Peptic ulcers cause pain at night, which may be related to the normal increase in gastric secretions during REM sleep. Antacids that neutralize gastric acidity may relieve the pain and help sleep patterns.
- Pain associated with coronary artery disease is more likely to occur during REM sleep.
- Hypertension often causes early morning awakening and fatigue.
- Epileptic seizures are more likely in NREM sleep stages.
- Hypothyroidism tends to decrease the amount of NREM sleep.
- Hyperthyroidism makes it difficult for a person to fall asleep.
- Low estrogen levels in women cause daytime fatigue, hot flashes, or night sweats, any of which may interfere with sleep.
- End-stage renal disease disrupts sleep and leads to daytime sleepiness.
- Shortness of breath impairs the ability to sleep, and sinus drainage may cause difficulty breathing.
- Any illness or injury associated with pain may disrupt sleep.
- Anxiety, fear, or stress may cause problems with falling and staying asleep

levels; medical technology; and underlying medical illnesses.

Anxiety and Stress

Psychological stress decreases REM sleep and can prevent a person from getting enough sleep. Anxiety, including the stress associated with work, finances, illness, and family, can cause intrusive thoughts, muscular tension, and increased norepinephrine levels, all of which may interfere with being able to go to sleep and stay asleep.

Relationships

New parents often report sleep disturbance as they adjust to the parenting role and associated frequent nightly awakenings. The sleep disturbance may become chronic if young children in the home do not establish regular sleep patterns or have ongoing care needs. Similarly, caregivers of persons with chronic illnesses living at home may become sleep-deprived.

People whose primary relationships are disrupted often suffer from sleep disorders. A person going through the grieving process after a loss commonly may have difficulties sleeping; children away from home and suffering from homesickness often have trouble sleeping as well. Marital problems contribute to sleep disorders in both the involved adults and the children in the home. Sleep also is disrupted for those with a partner who has a sleep disorder. This can lead to sleep deprivation consequences for both partners.

◆ ASSESSMENT LO 33.3

All patients should be assessed periodically for the presence of sleep disturbances. Assessment can occur during regular health checks or on admission to a health care facility. A sleep history starts with asking the patient to describe his or her usual sleeping pattern, sleeping and waking times, typical hours of sleep, and satisfaction with sleep. Bedtime routines, the use of sleep medications and other medications, the normal sleep environment, and any recent changes in sleep patterns should be assessed. An introductory assessment question could be "How have you been sleeping?" followed by "Do you feel rested when you arise in the morning, and do you have enough energy to do your expected tasks during the day?" If the patient does not identify any sleep difficulties, this history may be brief, allowing time for reinforcement of good sleep practices. If any sleep difficulties are identified, further questioning will help the nurse identify specific issues related to the patient's sleep (Health Assessment Questions box).

HEALTH ASSESSMENT QUESTIONS

Sleep

- How have you been sleeping?
- Do you have any bedtime routines?
- What time do you usually go to bed?
- What time do you usually awaken?
- Do you feel rested when you awaken?
- How long does it take for you to go to sleep?
- Do you awaken during the night? how often? what do you do?
- Do you have enough energy to complete your tasks during the day?
- Do you take naps during the day? for how long?
- What is your normal eating pattern?
- Do you drink beverages with caffeine, such as colas, coffee, or tea?
- Does your sleep partner comment about your sleep? snoring? pauses in breathing?
- What do you do to help yourself sleep? use of over-the-counter meds? prescription meds?

HEALTH HISTORY

A sleep assessment should be completed when a patient is admitted to a health facility. The nurse assesses the patient's usual sleeping and waking times, medications, illnesses, bedtime routines, and sleeping environment preferences and incorporates the information into the plan of care when possible. The nurse also should assess current life events and emotional status. Sleep instruments that can be used as part

BOX 33-2 Focused Health Assessment Questions

Sleep Disorders
- Why do you think you are having sleep problems?
- Have you recently had any changes at home or at work?
- Have you started any new medications?
- Is there anyone else at home who does not sleep well?

Insomnia
- How long does it take you to go to sleep?
- How often do you have trouble falling asleep?
- Do you have trouble staying asleep? waking up early and not getting back to sleep?
- What time do you wake up in the morning? Do you use an alarm clock?
- What do you do to prepare for sleep?
- What have you tried to improve your sleep?

Sleep Apnea
- Has anyone told you that you snore loudly or stop breathing while you sleep?
- Do you have headaches when you wake up?
- Do you have trouble staying awake during the day?
- Do you feel tired all the time?

Narcolepsy
- Do you fall asleep unexpectedly at random times? (Family or coworkers may report such episodes.)
- Do you have episodes of weakness, causing you to fall to the floor?
- Do you have vivid dreams when falling asleep?

of the sleep assessment include the Epworth Sleepiness Scale, a self-reported 8-item questionnaire that can differentiate between sleep disorders and sleep deprivation; the Pittsburgh Sleep Quality Index, a self-reported 19-item instrument that assesses sleep quality and sleep disturbance over a 1-month period; and the Sleep Hygiene Index, a 13-item self-reported assessment that examines sleep hygiene behaviors (Dugan, 2007; Smyth, 2008).

A more focused assessment may need to be done if sleep problems are identified (Box 33-2). Information that should be obtained if a sleep disturbance is present includes:

- The type of problem
- Any potential causes
- Identified signs and symptoms
- When the disturbance started
- The effect on daily roles and activities
- How the patient copes with the problem
- The ability of the nurse to treat the problem or the need for a referral to another professional

PHYSICAL ASSESSMENT

Findings from a physical assessment can be used to validate the presence or absence of sleep disturbances. Key assessment findings include an adequate energy level for tasks, physical weakness, fatigue, lethargy, decreased affect, and behavioral signs such as yawning or slow speech. Physical signs that may indicate potential sleep problems include obesity, thick neck, nasal polyps or deviated septum, or shortness of breath. Other signs that can be assessed during hospitalization include the presence of muscle contractions and jerks that arouse the patient from sleep, snoring, sleep apnea, or the irregular periods of silence followed by an abrupt snort indicative of OSA.

DIAGNOSTIC TESTS

Objective data regarding sleep characteristics are obtained in a sleep disorder laboratory and are interpreted by a sleep specialist. Polysomnography records eye movements, muscle movement and activity, heart and respiratory rates, oxygen levels, airflow, and brain activity while the patient sleeps. The results of polysomnography include the apnea-hypopnea index, or the number of apneic or hypopneic episodes per hour. The normal number of these episodes for an adult is fewer than 5 per hour; mild OSA ranges from 5 to 15 episodes per hour; moderate OSA ranges from 15 to 30 episodes per hour; and severe OSA is more than 30 apneic or hypopneic episodes per hour (Berry, 2008).

Another test is the multiple sleep latency test. The patient is monitored for brain waves, heartbeat, and eye movement during several 20-minute naps during the day. This test is used for patients suspected of having narcolepsy, and it shows whether they enter REM sleep shortly after falling asleep.

◆ NURSING DIAGNOSIS LO 33.4

When a sleep problem is identified that is amenable to nursing interventions, it is labeled *Disturbed Sleep Pattern* if the problem is time-limited (e.g., present only since admission to the hospital) or *Sleep Deprivation* if the problem is more prolonged. These and additional nursing diagnoses related to sleep disturbances and based on data clustered for each patient are shown in the diagnostic statements below:

- *Sleep Deprivation* related to lifestyle factors and sleep apnea as evidenced by poor sleep patterns, daytime sleepiness, and snoring
- *Disturbed Sleep Pattern* related to lighting and noise in the hospital as evidenced by reports of being awakened at night and by changes in normal sleep pattern
- *Fatigue* related to sleep deprivation as evidenced by daytime drowsiness
- *Insomnia* related to anxiety as evidenced by difficulty falling asleep
- *Anxiety* related to inability to fall asleep as evidenced by inability to concentrate

TABLE 33-3 Care Planning

NANDA-I NURSING DIAGNOSIS LABEL WITH NURSING DIAGNOSIS STATEMENT	NURSING OUTCOME CLASSIFICATION (NOC)	NURSING INTERVENTION CLASSIFICATION (NIC)
Sleep Deprivation related to lifestyle factors and sleep apnea as evidenced by poor sleep patterns, daytime sleepiness, and snoring	*Sleep* (0004) Hours of sleep (000401)	*Sleep enhancement* (1850) Encourage the patient to establish a bedtime routine to facilitate transition from wakefulness to sleep

From Bulechek G, Butcher H, Dochterman J, et al (Eds): *Nursing interventions classification (NIC),* ed. 6, St. Louis, 2013, Mosby; Moorhead S, Johnson M, Maas M, et al (Eds): *Nursing outcomes classification (NOC),* ed. 5, St. Louis, 2013, Mosby; NANDA International: *Nursing diagnoses: Definitions and classification, 2012–2014,* West Sussex, England, 2012, Wiley-Blackwell. Reprinted with permission from NANDA International, Inc.

- *Disturbed Thought Processes* related to chronic insomnia as evidenced by inability to understand instructions
- *Compromised Family Coping* related to frequent awakening of infant as evidenced by parent complaints of lack of sleep
- *Risk for Injury* with risk factor of sleepwalking

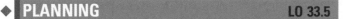

PLANNING LO 33.5

The major goal for a patient with a sleep disorder is to develop and maintain sleeping patterns that provide appropriate energy for daily activities. Care planning and outcomes for patients with a sleep disorder need to be individualized (Table 33-3). Interventions and outcomes should be identified in collaboration with the patient to increase success in implementation.

GOALS AND OUTCOME STATEMENTS

The primary goal for the patient with a sleep disorder is to improve the quality and quantity of sleep. It should be recognized that it may take weeks to achieve outcomes for sleep problems.

Potential goals that support the nursing diagnoses related to sleep and rest include the following:

- Patient will remain asleep for 6 to 7 hours consistently within 1 month.
- Patient will sleep for at least 90 minutes at a time during hospitalization.
- Patient will take two 20-minute naps daily.
- Patient will fall asleep within 15 minutes of going to bed within 2 weeks.
- Patient will report the ability to concentrate during the workday within 1 week.
- Patient will repeat medication instructions upon discharge.
- Parents will keep a sleep journal showing increased periods of sleep nightly at the next well-child visit.
- Patient will remain injury-free during hospitalization.

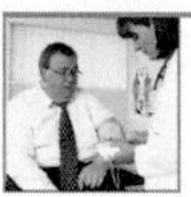

2. Write a short-term goal for the nursing diagnosis *Sleep Deprivation* related to lifestyle factors and sleep apnea as evidenced by poor sleep patterns, daytime sleepiness, and snoring.

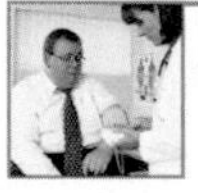

The conceptual care map for Mr. Barnes provided in Figure 33-3 is partially completed to indicate how to use the map as a learning tool. Using it as an example, go to the website at *http://evolve.elsevier.com/YoostCrawford/fundamentals/* to complete Nursing Diagnoses 2 and 3.

IMPLEMENTATION AND EVALUATION LO 33.6

Nursing interventions to improve sleep quality are based on health-promotion principles. During illness, sleep is important for recovery. The nurse should have a caring attitude when implementing strategies to improve sleep. Addressing the sleep environment, maintaining sleep routines, providing light snacks if allowed, instituting relaxation measures, and carefully using medications can enhance sleep in both hospital and home settings. Medications do not reset the circadian rhythms. These rhythms can be adjusted by progressing through shift rotation in a forward motion (days to evenings to nights), implementing sleep hygiene practices (evening routine diet, alcohol, tobacco, and activity restrictions), and arising at the same time each day.

INTERVENTIONS FOR SPECIFIC SLEEP DISORDERS

Treatment for insomnia should include interventions such as stimulus control (using the bedroom for only sleep and sex), sleep restriction (staying in bed only if asleep), sleep hygiene, and cognitive therapy (relaxing and changing thought patterns). A combination of nonpharmacological methods is often necessary to change sleep patterns.

Medications

IV Sites/Fluids/Rate

Conceptual Care Map

Student name__________ Patient initials Mr. B Date ________

Age 51 Gender M Room # ______ Admission date ________

CODE Status ____________ Allergies ____________

Diet ____________ Braden score ____________

Weight 259 lb Height 5′11″ Religion ____________

Admitting Diagnoses/Chief Complaint

Requesting "something to help me sleep"

Laboratory Values/ Diagnostic Test Results

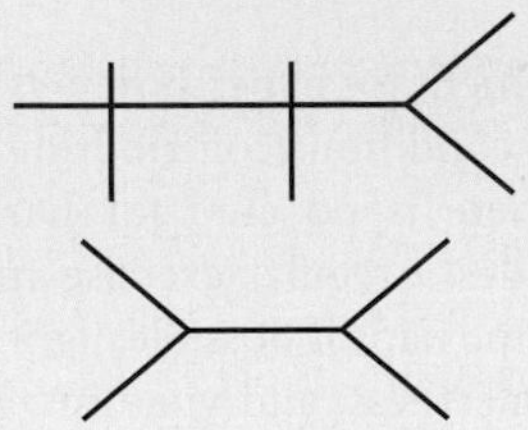

Assessment Data

Owns a small business and all employees are family members. Recently laid off two employees and increased his own working hours. The stress of the financial losses and laying off family members changed his overall health and sleep habits. Manages all aspects of the business and employees, and handles customer relations.

Drinks approximately six cups of coffee a day, smokes two packs of cigarettes a day, has three or four alcoholic drinks at night to "relax."

Has gained over 30 lb in the last year.

Looks older than his stated age, has dark circles around puffy eyes, and yawns frequently during the assessment.

Vital signs are T 36.3°C (97.4° F), P 96, regular and steady; R 26, slightly labored; BP 174/96; and SaO_2 90% on room air; no complaints of pain or discomfort at this time.

Reports daytime sleepiness, trouble getting to sleep, headache on waking, difficulty concentrating, and two recent car accidents.

Wife states that he is irritable, goes to bed late, sleeps only 4-5 hours, restless in bed, and has periods of not breathing and periods of loud snoring. He is currently on no prescription medications.

Treatments

Past Medical/Surgical History

Primary Nursing Diagnosis

Sleep Depivation related to lifestyle factors and sleep apnea as evidenced by poor sleep patterns, daytime sleepiness, and snoring.

Supporting Data

Patient drinks six cups of coffee per day, smokes two packs of cigarettes per day, has three or four alcoholic drinks at night, ≥30-lb weight gain over last year.

Daytime sleepiness, trouble getting to sleep at night, headache when waking, difficulty concentrating, two car accidents.

Wife states he is irritable, goes to bed late, is restless, and has periods of not breathing followed by periods of loud snoring.

STG/NOC

Patient will remain asleep for 6 to 7 hours consistently within 1 month.

NOC: Sleep (0004)

Hours of sleep (000401)

Interventions/NIC with Rationale

1. Encourage the patient to limit coffee, food, and alcohol intake in the evening to reduce stimulants.
2. Establish a routine before bedtime that includes a quiet environment, soothing music, and a relaxing activity to promote relaxation and transition into sleep.
3. Instruct wife in backrub techniques to promote relaxation.
4. Reduce noise and light at bedtime to provide a comfortable environment conducive to sleep.

NIC: Sleep enhancement (1850)

Encourage the patient to establish a bedtime routine to facilitate transition from wakefulness to sleep.

Rationale Citation/EBP

Yoost BL, Crawford LR: *Fundamentals of nursing: Active learning for collaborative practice*, St. Louis, 2016, Mosby.

Evaluation

At next clinic visit patient states that he is sleeping 6 hours a night. Continue plan of care.

Nursing Diagnosis 2

Supporting Data

STG/NOC

Interventions/NIC with Rationale

Rationale Citation/EBP

Evaluation

Nursing Diagnosis 3

Supporting Data

STG/NOC

Interventions/NIC with Rationale

Rationale Citation/EBP

Evaluation

FIGURE 33-3 Partially completed conceptual care map based on Mr. Barnes, the case study patient in this chapter. *NIC*, Nursing Intervention Classification; *NOC*, Nursing Outcome Classification; *STG*, short-term goal.

Treatment for hypersomnia is aimed at correcting any underlying conditions contributing to the hypersomnia.

There is no cure for narcolepsy at present. Treatment includes a regular exercise routine, a regular sleep routine, daytime naps if possible, light meals high in protein to maintain alertness, and vitamins. Avoiding alcohol, heavy meals, long-distance driving, and long periods of sitting is helpful. Medications for narcolepsy include central nervous system stimulants, the nonamphetamine wake-promoting drug modafinil, and tricyclic and selective serotonin reuptake inhibitor antidepressants. In 2002, the FDA approved Xyrem, which is the trade name for gamma hydroxybutyrate (GHB), for treating people with narcolepsy who experience episodes of cataplexy (NINDS, 2014b).

Treatments for OSA include lifestyle changes for good sleep practices, decreased alcohol use, no use of tobacco products, and weight loss (Mendez and Olson, 2006). Additional treatment consists of surgical procedures to correct abnormalities of the soft tissue or bone structure that is obstructing the patient's airway, use of an oral appliance while sleeping to keep the airway open, or continuous positive airway pressure (CPAP). CPAP is noninvasive and consists of a face or nasal mask, connected to an air pump, that is worn during sleep and maintains pressure to hold the airway open (Figure 33-4). Some patients report discomfort, skin irritation, or claustrophobia sensations; however, continued use of CPAP should be encouraged.

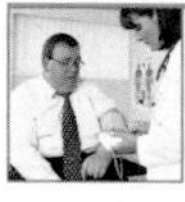

3. A sleep study with polysomnography is performed, and it verifies the diagnosis of obstructive sleep apnea. After discussing treatment options with his primary care provider, Mr. Barnes decides to try continuous positive airway pressure (CPAP). How would the nurse explain the function of CPAP to Mr. Barnes and his wife?

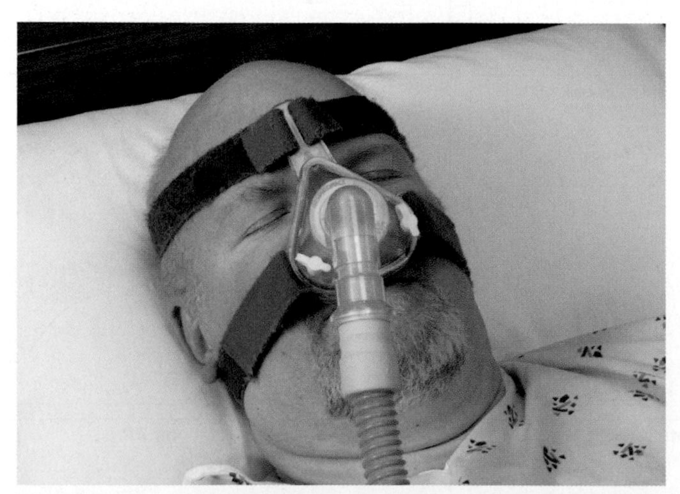

FIGURE 33-4 Patient with continuous positive airway pressure device. (From Black JM, Hawks JH: *Medical-surgical nursing: Clinical management for positive outcomes,* ed. 8, St. Louis, 2009, Saunders.)

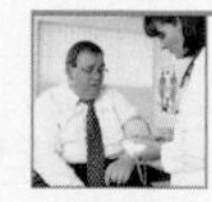

4. The nurse plans to counsel Mr. Barnes regarding lifestyle factors that affect sleep in general. Identify at least four lifestyle factors that Mr. Barnes might work on to improve his sleep patterns.

Treatment for restless legs syndrome includes lifestyle changes of decreased caffeine, alcohol, and tobacco use, as well as maintaining a regular sleep pattern. Massaging the legs, walking, or doing deep knee bends may temporarily relieve symptoms. Supplements to correct deficiencies in iron, folate, and magnesium may be helpful. No one medication is effective for restless legs syndrome, but drugs such as dopaminergic agents (largely used to treat Parkinson's disease), ropinirole (Requip), benzodiazepines, opioids, and anticonvulsants may be prescribed (Cuellar, 2009; NINDS, 2013).

NONPHARMACOLOGIC INTERVENTIONS

Feeling comfortable and safe when attempting to sleep is important. A comfortable bed with linens that are not wrinkled and allow freedom of movement helps promote relaxation. Body alignment should prevent muscle strain and discomfort. A quiet, darkened room with privacy is helpful for most people, but a night light may be needed in unfamiliar surroundings. Infants and older adults may sleep best in softly lit rooms, but not with light shining directly in their eyes. Noise is a common sleep disrupter in the hospital; equipment sounds and staff conversations should be modified, as possible, to decrease noise (Box 33-3). Room temperature and the use of extra clothing or blankets should be at the discretion of the patient.

BOX 33-3 Ways to Control Noise in the Hospital

- Provide visual cues to decrease noise by dimming lights and closing curtains, but provide a night light for safety.
- Provide privacy by drawing curtains between patients or closing room doors, if possible.
- Negotiate times to mute television, radios, and music on hospital units.
- Limit overhead pages to emergencies only at night.
- Lower volume of telephone ringtones.
- Limit staff conversations in hallways and at nursing stations.
- Conduct shift reports in areas away from patient rooms, unless the facility requires bedside reporting. If the patient is asleep during change-of-shift rounds, the nurses can check the patient and then step away and speak in soft voices.
- Move equipment quietly, without hitting other objects.
- Monitor equipment frequently to prevent alarm tones as much as possible.

It is not unusual for hospitalized patients to be awakened for sleeping pills or long before it is time for a meal or procedure. When possible, treatments and care should be scheduled for when a patient normally is awake. Scheduling of medications and treatments that can disrupt sleep (e.g., nebulizer treatments) should be carefully considered. It is best to reserve at least 90 to 120 minutes of "sleep windows," to allow progression through all stages of sleep.

Bedtime Routines

Bedtime routines relax patients in preparation for sleep (Collaboration and Delegation box). The nurse should make every effort to allow the patient to follow his or her regular sleep schedule. Normal daytime nap patterns that do not interfere with nighttime sleep should be considered in planning and administering care.

Most people follow a bedtime routine. Such routines are important in promoting relaxation and mental preparation for sleep (Box 33-4). Reading, watching the news, praying, meditating, and doing physical hygiene procedures such as washing the face, bathing, and brushing teeth are common components of bedtime routines. Some children and adults have a light snack as part of their bedtime ritual. Children may have a very specific routine that includes bathing, stories, music, *good-nights* to everyone, prayers, and presence of a specific toy or blanket for sleep time.

COLLABORATION AND DELEGATION

Care of Patients Before Bedtime

Evening care, or h.s. ("hour of sleep"—at bedtime) care, is provided to prepare the patient for an uninterrupted period of sleep. Activities to prepare for sleep that the nurse may delegate to unlicensed assistive personnel (UAP) include:

- Providing oral care
- Doing partial bathing, to cleanse the face and hands
- Providing skin care
- Giving a backrub
- Straightening or changing bed linen
- Offering the opportunity for toileting
- Offering a snack or water

BOX 33-4 Bedtime Routines That Promote Sleep

- Take a warm bath.
- Eat a light snack that contains carbohydrates.
- Drink warm milk.
- Avoid caffeine, tobacco, and excessive alcohol.
- Get a back massage.
- Relax using aromatherapy and music therapy.
- Adjust the environment for temperature, noise, and light.
- Elevate the head of the bed for patients diagnosed with gastroesophageal reflux disease (GERD).
- Avoid large meals and certain medications in the evening.

Bedtime Snacks

Going to bed hungry or eating a large, heavy, or spicy meal just before going to bed can interfere with sleep. A snack with complex carbohydrates seems to promote sleep for some people, so a piece of toast, crackers, or a glass of juice may help initiate sleep if allowed in the patient's plan of care. Tryptophan, an amino acid found in milk, stimulates the production of serotonin, which promotes sleep. Alcohol after dinner may help some people sleep, but in general it interferes with sleep cycles and should be avoided. Likewise, caffeine in foods (such as chocolate) and drinks should be avoided for several hours before bedtime owing to its central nervous system stimulation. Fluids may be decreased in the evening if the person often awakens during the night with the need to void. Large, heavy, or spicy meals close to bedtime should be avoided because they can lead to discomfort and increase the likelihood of GERD.

Exercise

Physical activity can promote fatigue and relaxation and can increase both NREM and REM sleep. Vigorous exercise within 2 hours of normal sleep time, however, can hamper sleep and should be avoided. Excessive exercise and exhaustion can hinder normal sleep.

Relaxation

Sleep rarely occurs until a person feels relaxed. Coping mechanisms that decrease stress include enlisting the help of friends, family, or clergy to deal with problems, learning to deal with problems only at certain times of the day, and using relaxation techniques. Aromatherapy, music therapy, and spiritual supportive measures, when correctly used, can be especially effective for patients experiencing stress or anxiety that contributes to sleep disorders. A backrub, warm shower or bath, oral care, and face wash help most patients relax. Adequate clothing or bedding prevents feeling cold and increases relaxation, especially in children and elderly people. Pain, which commonly occurs in illness or with surgery, is a major deterrent to sleep. Measures to relieve pain can include administering medication as appropriate, staying with a frightened child or adult, providing a warmed blanket, or offering a backrub. For other methods of treating pain, see Chapter 36.

QSEN FOCUS!

Patient-centered care requires that the nurse provide physical comfort and emotional support. When addressing sleep disturbances, the nurse elicits the patient's preferences and expressed needs as part of the clinical interview, implementation of the care plan, and evaluation of care.

A backrub provides the comfort of human touch, promotes relaxation, decreases pain, and stimulates the immune system. The use of the therapeutic massage in nursing practice has declined through the years in favor of high-tech interventions, yet it is one of the simplest ways to improve patient sleep patterns (see Skill 27-4). The time spent on giving a backrub can be simultaneously used to reinforce goals reached by the patient during the day, activities accomplished, visits from friends and families, or positive thoughts of other events of the day that will help calm the patient's mind in preparation for sleep.

SLEEP MEDICATIONS

After nonpharmacologic methods have been tried, medications to assist with sleep are prescribed for some patients with chronic, ongoing sleep disturbances that interfere with daily life. For medications prescribed on an as-needed basis, the nurse must assess the need for medication and understand how the drug works. Nonpharmacologic measures, including patient teaching, should be used as appropriate in addition to any prescribed medications to assist with the initiation of sleep.

Antianxiety medications reduce anxiety and tension, but they can cause physical and psychological dependence. Antihistamines such as diphenhydramine (Benadryl) have mild sedative effects that can promote sleep. Tricyclic antidepressants, such as amitriptyline (Elavil) or doxepin (Sinequan), or trazodone may be prescribed at a lower dose than that needed to alleviate depression, for their beneficial effect on sleep patterns. Sedative-**hypnotics** induce sleep, but it is an unnatural sleep that is associated with disturbances in REM and NREM sleep patterns. With this group of agents, tolerance may develop after several days, and the patient may then increase the dose of medication to obtain the same effect, which creates specific safety concerns. Withdrawal symptoms (weakness, tremors, restlessness, insomnia, increased pulse rate, and death) can occur if barbiturate sedative-hypnotics are stopped abruptly. Some medications have adverse effects in elderly people and must be used with caution in this population.

Medications used to induce sleep can cause daytime drowsiness. Long-term use of antianxiety, sedative, or hypnotic medications further disrupts sleep and may cause additional problems. In 2007, the FDA mandated that the product labels of sleep medications include new safety warnings that provide information related to potential severe allergic reactions, severe facial swelling, and complex sleep behaviors such as sleep-driving or preparing and eating food while asleep.

SAFE PRACTICE ALERT

When administering medications that affect sleep, be sure beds are in the low position, night lights are on, and call lights are within reach to help prevent patient falls. No alcohol products should be ingested with sleeping medications.

HOME CARE CONSIDERATIONS

Patients may underestimate their need for rest while recuperating from illness or surgery. Discharge planning should include recommendations for rest and activity. Patients should be taught about normal variations in sleep patterns along with common measures to promote relaxation and sleep when at home (Home Care Considerations box). Caregivers also should receive education on how they can best meet their own energy and sleep needs, so that they are able

HOME CARE CONSIDERATIONS

Sleep Hygiene Practices for Home

Activity

- Activity promotes sleep. Find physical activity that can be done daily, such as walking, swimming, or exercising.
- Relaxation is difficult after vigorous exercise. Avoid exercise within 2 hours of bedtime.
- Multiple interventions increase sleep success by promoting physical and mental relaxation. Implement complementary relaxation strategies before attempting sleep, including music, massage, or aromatherapy.

Diet

- Carbohydrates affect serotonin levels in the brain, inducing relaxation. Therefore eat a light bedtime snack with carbohydrates if hungry in the evening.
- Heavy meals interfere with sleep. Avoid heavy meals within 3 hours of bedtime.
- Central nervous system stimulants interfere with sleep. Limit caffeine, alcohol, and tobacco use, especially in the evening.

Sleep Pattern

- Using the bedroom only for sleep and sex helps the mind associate the room with these activities. Use the bedroom for sleep and sex only; do not watch television, read, study, or eat in this space.
- Getting out of bed if unable to sleep trains the mind to sleep when in bed. If unable to fall asleep within 20 minutes, get out of bed and engage in a relaxing activity such as reading or listening to music until sleepy.
- Maintaining a regular sleep pattern helps maintain circadian rhythms. Continue the regular sleep pattern on weekends and on holidays.
- A consistent bedtime routine signals to the mind and body that it is time to go to sleep. Follow a consistent routine.
- Identify lifestyle factors (e.g., long work hours, late meals, family stress) that may interfere with sleep, and change those factors.

Environment

- Comfort and security, along with decreased sensory input, promote sleep. Adjust the environment to enhance sleep: Darken the room; decrease noise or wear earplugs; adjust the temperature to a comfortable level; and wear loose, comfortable clothing.

to provide the necessary care for the patient in addition to meeting self-care needs.

Interventions to enhance sleep in the home are similar to those used in the hospital. Patients may be taught to keep a sleep diary to record sleep patterns at home: The patient records data over the course of several days and nights, including information about sleep quality, sleep patterns, and interventions to improve sleep (Patient Education and Health Literacy box). If the sleep diary adds to the stress of trying to improve the quality of sleep, the diary should be discontinued and the data obtained by interview.

PATIENT EDUCATION AND HEALTH LITERACY

Sleep Diary

Information to be recorded daily in the sleep diary includes:

- Activities and food within 2 hours of going to bed
- Time of retiring
- Time of awakening
- Required time to fall asleep
- Number of times aroused during the night
- Length of time awake if aroused during the night
- Degree of restfulness in the morning
- Use or nonuse of an alarm
- General comments regarding sleep

EVALUATION

The effectiveness of the plan of care to promote sleep is evaluated by determining whether the identified outcomes have been reached. Outcomes are likely to be achieved if the patient is able to:

- Rest in an environment that promotes sleep
- Follow bedtime rituals as much as possible
- Report feeling rested after sleeping
- Maintain adequate energy and mental alertness to complete necessary tasks
- Identify factors that interfere with sleep and measures to improve sleep habits
- Use a variety of techniques to promote sleep

Follow-up assessment of the effectiveness of the interventions is an important step in ensuring healthy sleep patterns for patients in hospital and home settings.

SUMMARY OF LEARNING OUTCOMES

LO 33.1 *Explain the physiology and functions involved in sleep:* Sleep is a reversible and naturally occurring altered state of consciousness during which awareness, responsiveness, and perception of the environment are decreased. It is restorative, protective, and necessary for optimal health. Sleep occurs in a predictable cycle of specific stages.

LO 33.2 *Discuss characteristics of common sleep disorders:* Common sleep disorders fall into the major categories of dyssomnias (insomnia, OSA, narcolepsy, restless legs syndrome, circadian rhythm disorders), parasomnias (sleepwalking, nightmares), and secondary sleep disorders resulting from underlying medical or psychiatric illnesses.

LO 33.3 *Summarize assessment techniques for determining sleep patterns:* Assessment of sleep may be brief if no problems are discovered or more extensive if issues surrounding the patient's sleep patterns are identified. A detailed history, physical examination, and specialized tests will help determine the nature of the sleep problem.

LO 33.4 *Identify nursing diagnoses for patients with sleep disturbances:* Nursing diagnoses for patients with sleep problems may be directly related to the problem, such as *Sleep Deprivation* and *Disturbed Sleep Pattern,* or may pertain to a side effect of the particular sleep disturbance, such as *Anxiety* and *Risk for Injury.*

LO 33.5 *Determine patient goals based on specific sleep problems:* Goals are individualized in accordance with the specific sleep disturbance and its effects on the patient's daily life.

LO 33.6 *Implement interventions that promote sleep:* Nursing interventions that promote sleep include pharmacologic measures, such as the use of hypnotics, and nonpharmacologic measures to improve sleep habits, or sleep hygiene (bedtime rituals, relaxation, regular exercise, and diet changes). Nursing interventions for promoting sleep in the hospitalized patient include reducing noise and lighting, ensuring a period of uninterrupted sleep, and controlling pain.

Responses to the critical-thinking questions are available at *http://evolve.elsevier.com/YoostCrawford/fundamentals/.*

REVIEW QUESTIONS

1. An elderly, tense patient is having trouble relaxing enough to sleep. Which measures should be implemented by the nurse to help promote sleep? *(Select all that apply.)*
   a. Give the patient a backrub.
   b. Take the patient for a brisk walk right before bedtime.
   c. Provide a warm, quiet environment.
   d. Encourage the patient to eat a large meal in the evening.
   e. Give the patient a diet cola.
   f. Play soft music during the 30 minutes before bedtime.
2. A nurse who was hired to work in a sleep lab understands that the most common type of sleep apnea is caused by which factor?
   a. Airway collapse
   b. Lack of exercise
   c. Dietary factors
   d. Medication use
3. A patient has been referred for polysomnography to confirm a diagnosis of narcolepsy. What behavior would the nurse expect the patient to be exhibiting?
   a. Excessive use of sleeping medications
   b. A lack of dreaming during sleep
   c. Consistent use of relaxation techniques
   d. Unexpected daytime sleeping episodes
4. A mother brings her toddler for a well-child checkup and mentions that she is having a lot of trouble getting the child to go to bed. Which intervention can the nurse teach the mother to help her toddler establish good sleep habits?
   a. Establish and maintain a consistent bedtime routine.
   b. Put the child to bed immediately after the evening meal.
   c. Allow the child to stay up as long as desired to increase sleepiness.
   d. Allow the child to sleep with the parents until the child is older.
5. An elderly patient complains of difficulty sleeping after the death of his spouse of 56 years. What would be an appropriate assessment for this patient?
   a. Assess the patient for possible use of sedatives.
   b. Obtain a health history regarding sleep hygiene.
   c. Assess the patient's weight over the past year.
   d. Request a sleep study to rule out sleep apnea.
6. The nurse is completing a sleep assessment for a newly admitted patient. Which data reported by the patient would cause the nurse to suspect obstructive sleep apnea? *(Select all that apply.)*
   a. Morning headaches
   b. Sudden weight loss
   c. Loud snoring during sleep
   d. Daytime sleepiness
   e. Deep sleep during the night
   f. Increased blood pressure problems
7. A patient complains of not being able to sleep while in the hospital. What action would be a priority for the nurse to implement?
   a. Administer a sleeping medication with the evening meal.
   b. Restrict visitors for the patient in the evening.
   c. Decrease noise around the patient during the night.
   d. Offer a hot drink of regular tea at bedtime.
8. A patient reports that the prescribed sleeping medication is no longer effective. What information would be appropriate for the nurse to recommend to the patient? *(Select all that apply.)*
   a. Take the medication with an alcoholic drink.
   b. Use relaxation techniques before sleep.
   c. Do not study in the bedroom before bedtime.
   d. Adjust sleep temperature for comfort.
   e. Sleep in a different room of the home.
9. A nurse is working a night shift after several months of working day shift. What action does the nurse take to protect patient safety?
   a. Take a meal break at midnight.
   b. Plan critical tasks for early in the shift.
   c. Ask another nurse to administer all medications.
   d. Turn up lights on the unit to maintain alertness.
10. At a routine clinic visit, an athlete training for a major sports event reports difficulty sleeping that is affecting the training schedule. What would be the best recommendation by the nurse for this patient?
    a. Increase the use of electrolyte-enriched drinks to increase stamina.
    b. Obtain a short-term prescription for sleeping medications.
    c. Plan to arise later in the morning to accommodate sleep changes.
    d. Avoid vigorous exercise for at least 2 hours before bedtime.

ⓔ Answers and rationales for the review questions are available at *http://evolve.elsevier.com/YoostCrawford/fundamentals/*.

REFERENCES

American Academy of Pediatrics: AAP Expands Guidelines for Infant Sleep Safety and SIDS Risk Reduction, 2011. Retrieved from *http://www.aap.org/en-us/about-the-aap/aap-press-room/Pages/AAP-Expands-Guidelines-for-Infant-Sleep-Safety-and-SIDS-Risk-Reduction.aspx.*

Berger AM, Hobbs BB: Impact of shift work on the health and safety of nurses and patients, *Clin J Oncol Nurs* 10(4):465-471, 2006.

Berry D: Case study: Obstructive sleep apnea, *Medsurg Nurs* 17(1):11-16, 2008.

Calamaro CJ, Mason TB, Ratcliffe SJ: Adolescents living the 24/7 lifestyle: Effects of caffeine and technology on sleep duration and daytime functioning, *Pediatrics* 123(6):e1005-e1010, 2009.

Cronenwett L, Sherwood G, Barnsteiner J, et al: Quality and safety education for nurses, *Nurs Outlook* 55(3):122-131, 2007.

Cuellar N: Restless legs syndrome: FAQs you can use, *Am Nurse Today*, 2009. Retrieved from *www.americannursetoday.com/restless-legs-syndrome-faqs-you-can-use/.*

Dugan M: A tale of sleep apnea, *Nurs Made Incred Easy!* May/June:28-38, 2007.

Glazener CM, Evans JH, Peto RE: Complex behavioural and educational interventions for nocturnal enuresis in children, *Cochrane Database Syst Rev* (1):CD004668, 2008. Retrieved from *www.cochrane.org/reviews/en/ab004668.html.*

HealthNews.org: Sleep disorders guide, 2012. Retrieved from *www.SleepDisordersGuide.com.*

Izac SM: Basic anatomy and physiology of sleep, *Am J Electroneurodiagn Technol* 46(1):18-38, 2006.

Jones KE, Johnson RK, Harvey-Berino JR: Is losing sleep making us obese? *Nutr Bull* 33:272-278, 2008.

Kotagal P, Yardi N: The relationship between sleep and epilepsy, *Semin Pediatr Neurol* 15:42-49, 2008.

McCance KL, Huether SE: *Pathophysiology: The biologic basis for disease in adults and children*, ed. 5, St. Louis, 2006, Mosby.

Mendez JL, Olson EJ: Obstructive sleep apnea syndrome. I: Identifying the problem, *J Respir Dis* 27(5):144, 2006.

Mullington JM, Haack M, Toth M, et al: Cardiovascular, inflammatory, and metabolic consequences of sleep deprivation, *Progr Cardiovasc Dis* 51(4):294-302, 2009.

National Heart, Lung, and Blood Institute: National Institutes of Health Sleep disorder research plan, 2011. Retrieved from *www.nhlbi.nih.gov/health-pro/resources/sleep/nih-sleep-disorders-research-plan-2011.htm.*

National Institute of Child Health and Human Development: About SIDS and safe infant sleep, 2013. Retrieved from *www.nichd.nih.gov/sts/about/Pages/default.aspx.*

National Institute of Neurological Disorders and Stroke: Restless legs syndrome information page, 2013. Retrieved from *www.ninds.nih.gov/disorders/restless_legs/restless_legs.htm.*

National Institute of Neurological Disorders and Stroke: Sleep apnea information page, 2014a. Retrieved from *www.ninds.nih.gov/disorders/sleep_apnea/sleep_apnea.htm.*

National Institute of Neurological Disorders and Stroke: Narcolepsy information page, 2014b. Retrieved from *www.ninds.nih.gov/disorders/narcolepsy/narcolepsy.htm.*

National Institutes of Health: National Heart, Lung and Blood Institute's Your guide to healthy sleep, 2011. Retrieved from *www.nhlbi.nih.gov/health/resources/sleep/healthy-sleep.htm.*

National Institutes of Health: Night terrors, 2014. Retrieved from *www.nlm.nih.gov/medlineplus/ency/article/000809.htm.*

Smyth CA: Evaluating sleep quality in older adults: The Pittsburgh Sleep Quality Index can be used to detect sleep disturbances or deficits, *Am J Nurs* 108(5):42-50, 2008.

U.S. National Library of Medicine: *Bruxism*, 2014. Retrieved from *www.nlm.nih.gov/medlineplus/ency/article/001413.htm.*

Zadra A, Pilon M, Montplaisir J: Polysomnographic diagnosis of sleepwalking: Effects of sleep deprivation, *Ann Neurol* 63(4):513-519, 2008.

CHAPTER 34

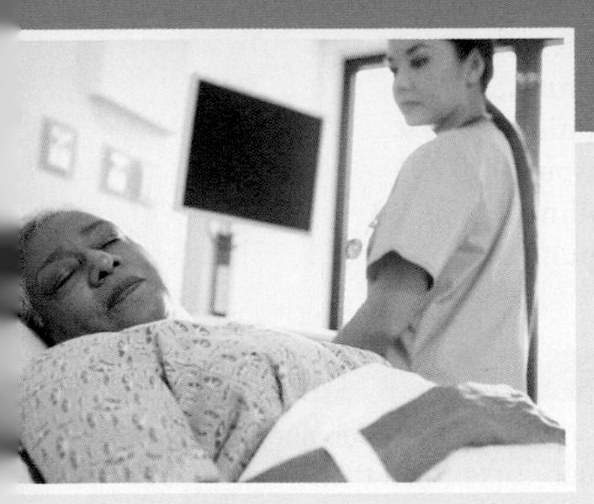

Diagnostic Testing

EVOLVE WEBSITE

http://evolve.elsevier.com/YoostCrawford/fundamentals/

- Additional Evolve-Only Review Questions With Answers
- Answers and Rationales for Text Review Questions
- Answers to Critical-Thinking Questions
- Case Study With Questions
- Glossary
- Video Skills Clips
- Conceptual Care Map Creator
- Skills Checklists
- Animation

LEARNING OUTCOMES

Comprehension of this chapter's content will provide students with the ability to:

LO 34.1 Recall the types of cells found in blood and their functions.
LO 34.2 Identify common blood tests, their purposes, and their normal values.
LO 34.3 Discuss other laboratory tests, such as urine and stool studies, and their purposes and normal values.
LO 34.4 Explain the purpose of common diagnostic tests.
LO 34.5 Describe assessment procedures for patients undergoing diagnostic tests.
LO 34.6 Choose appropriate nursing diagnoses associated with diagnostic testing.
LO 34.7 Select goals to meet individual patient problems.
LO 34.8 Describe the nurse's role before, during, and after diagnostic tests and procedures.

KEY TERMS

activated partial thromboplastin time, p. 772
alanine aminotransferase, p. 776
albumin, p. 772
alkaline phosphatase, p. 776
arterial blood gas, p. 779
aspartate aminotransferase, p. 776
basophils, p. 771
bilirubin, p. 776
biopsy, p. 784
blood urea nitrogen, p. 776
brain natriuretic peptide, p. 779
C-reactive protein, p. 779
cholesterol, p. 776
computed tomography, p. 782
creatine kinase, p. 777
creatinine, p. 776
electrocardiogram, p. 783
endoscopy, p. 783
eosinophils, p. 771
erythrocytes, p. 771
fiberoptics, p. 783
fibrinogen, p. 772
gamma-glutamyl transpeptidase, p. 776
globulins, p. 772
Hemoccult, p. 791
hemoglobin, p. 771
hemolysis, p. 776
high-density lipoproteins, p. 776

KEY TERMS

homocysteine, p. 779
international normalized ratio, p. 772
leukocytes, p. 771
low-density lipoproteins, p. 776
lymphocytes, p. 771
magnetic resonance imaging, p. 782
mammograms, p. 781
monocytes, p. 771
myoglobin, p. 779
neutrophils, p. 771
paracentesis, p. 784
prealbumin, p. 776
prothrombin time, p. 772
radiography, p. 781
steatorrhea, p. 781
thoracentesis, p. 784
thrombocytes, p. 771
triglycerides, p. 776
troponin I, p. 779
troponin T, p. 779
ultrasound, p. 783
urobilinogen, p. 781
venipuncture, p. 789

CASE STUDY

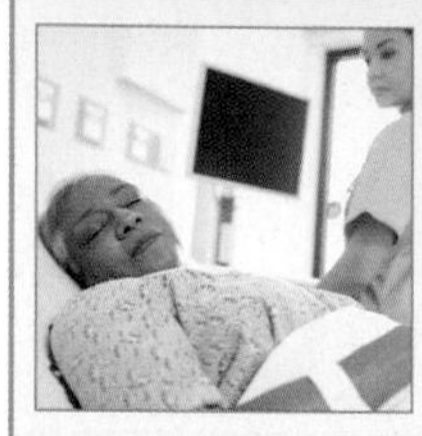

Mrs. Rees, a 68-year-old female, was admitted to the hospital with loss of appetite and fatigue and was evaluated to rule out gastrointestinal bleeding. She says that her "stools have been darker than they normally are." She has a medical history of osteoarthritis, diabetes mellitus, and hypertension. She has no known drug allergies (NKDA) and has full-code status. "I don't have the energy to do anything anymore. I don't know what's wrong with me." Her vital signs on admission are T 36.8° C (98.2° F), P 110 regular and bounding, R 26 and labored, and BP 138/86, with a pulse oximetry reading of 91% on room air. She denies having pain, but says she is very tired. Admitting blood work was normal except for the following: RBC 3.8 cells/mm^3, Hgb 8.6 g/dL, Hct 34%, and glucose 210 mg/dL.

During the assessment, Mrs. Rees says, "I'm worried about that test tomorrow. I just know they're going to find cancer. My father died of stomach cancer, and it was horrible."

The patient states that she takes a regular aspirin every day. She says, "I saw on TV that it's supposed to prevent heart attacks." She is scheduled for an esophagogastroduodenoscopy (EGD) tomorrow.

Medications are as follows:

- Sliding-scale insulin for Humulin R subcut with dose based on fingerstick blood glucose result:

Less than 150 mg/dL	No insulin
150-200 mg/dL	4 units
200-249 mg/dL	6 units
250-299 mg/dL	8 units
300 mg/dL or higher	Call health care provider

- Intravenous (IV) 1000 mL D_5 0.45%NS at 50 mL/hr
- Versed 2.5 mg IV on call for the EGD
- She takes the following medications on a daily basis, which are currently on hold:
  - Humulin N 10 units/Humulin R 5 subcut units q A.M.
  - Humulin N 5 units subcut q P.M. before dinner
  - Celebrex 200 mg po q A.M.
  - Lisinopril 10 mg po q A.M.

Treatment orders are as follows:

- Vital signs, including pulse oximetry, q 4 hr
- 2 to 4 L of O_2 per nasal cannula; titrate to keep SpO_2 > 93%
- Clear liquids; nothing by mouth (NPO) after midnight
- EGD in A.M.
- Fingerstick blood sugar before meals and at bedtime
- Bed rest with bathroom privileges
- Complete blood count (CBC) q A.M.
- Stools × 3 for occult blood

Refer back to this case study to answer the critical-thinking question throughout the chapter.

An essential aspect of patient care is identifying diseases and disorders. Diagnostic test results are examined and combined with patient assessment data to identify, determine the severity of, and evaluate therapy effectiveness for a disease or disorder. Diagnostic tests are used to examine different aspects of the body and assess indicators that the body may not be healthy. Whether it is a fractured ankle seen on an x-ray or low blood glucose level determined from a fingerstick blood sample, diagnostic tests assist health care providers in determining the best possible treatment for the patients in their care. Nurses must be able to perform, understand, and communicate the results of diagnostic tests to their patients.

NORMAL STRUCTURE AND FUNCTION OF BLOOD CELLS LO 34.1

On average, a person has approximately 5 liters of blood circulating throughout the body. Approximately 3 liters are plasma, the fluid portion, and 2 liters are cells.

CELL TYPES

Three types of cells are found in blood: erythrocytes, thrombocytes, and leukocytes (Figure 34-1). The **erythrocytes** (red blood cells [RBCs]) contain **hemoglobin** (Hgb), which is a protein primarily responsible for oxygen transport to and carbon dioxide transport from the erythrocytes. The red blood cells have an important role in maintaining normal acid-base balance. Development of new erythrocytes occurs in the bone marrow.

Thrombocytes, also called *platelets*, are an integral part of blood clotting. When a blood vessel ruptures, platelets clump together to form a plug to seal the vessel. Platelets are formed in the bone marrow.

The **leukocytes** (white blood cells [WBCs]) are primarily responsible for the inflammatory and immune response in the body (Table 34-1). Leukocytes are classified as **lymphocytes** (T and B), **monocytes**, **eosinophils**, **neutrophils**, and **basophils**. Leukocytes are formed primarily in the bone marrow, except for T lymphocytes, which are produced in the thymus.

TABLE 34-1 Normal White Blood Cell Count Differential

TYPE	PROPORTION OF 100 WBCs (%)	FUNCTION
Neutrophils	55-70	Are first defenders against bacterial and fungal infections, foreign antigens, and cell debris
Lymphocytes	20-40	Recognize foreign antigens; produce antibodies; create memory cells
Monocytes	2-8	Involved in phagocytosis; become macrophages
Eosinophils	1-4	Destroy parasites; involved in allergic reactions
Basophils	0.5-1.0	Involved in the inflammatory response to injury; release histamine

Adapted from Pagana KD, Pagana TJ: *Mosby's manual of diagnostic and laboratory tests,* ed. 5, St. Louis, 2014, Mosby.

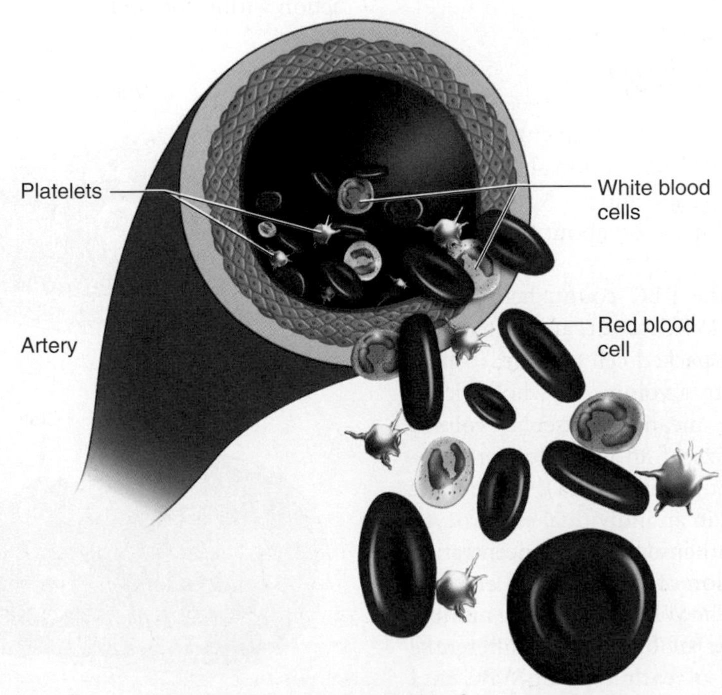

FIGURE 34-1 Formed elements of blood.

PLASMA

Plasma is the fluid portion of the blood. It contains various substances vital to homeostasis, and water is the primary carrier of these substances. Electrolytes, such as sodium, potassium, calcium, magnesium, chloride, and bicarbonate, are transported to and from the cells in the plasma. Chapter 39 provides an in-depth discussion of electrolytes.

Plasma proteins include albumin, fibrinogen, and globulins. **Albumin** is the major plasma protein, primarily responsible for maintaining fluid balance by providing colloidal osmotic pressure in the blood. **Fibrinogen** plays an integral part in blood coagulation by converting into fibrin threads in the presence of ionized calcium. Fibrin is the essential component of blood clots. **Globulins** are classified as alpha, beta, and gamma globulins. Some globulins function as antibodies, and others are responsible for enzymatic functions and the transport of lipids, iron, and copper in the blood.

Plasma contains various nutrients, primarily glucose, amino acids, fatty acids, and vitamins. Hormones are transported throughout the body in blood plasma. The blood also transports waste products such as urea and creatinine to be excreted by the kidney.

LABORATORY TESTS: BLOOD LO 34.2

A venous blood sample can be tested for many different components. Blood tests are common diagnostic tools that are used frequently in inpatient and outpatient settings. Venous blood is the primary source of sampling for these tests. Arterial blood samples are used for determination of arterial blood gases. Capillary blood samples are often used for fingerstick glucose tests.

COMPLETE BLOOD CELL COUNT

A complete blood cell count (CBC) is a frequently ordered diagnostic test designed to provide information about oxygen and carbon dioxide transport capabilities. A differential blood cell count can provide information about the status of the immune response.

CBC components include the RBC count, hemoglobin level, hematocrit, RBC indices, WBC count, and differential WBC count. Hematocrit is the packed cell volume; it measures the proportion of RBCs in a volume of whole blood. The RBC indices include the mean corpuscular volume (MCV), which is the average size of an individual erythrocyte; the mean corpuscular hemoglobin (MCH), which is the average amount of hemoglobin in an individual erythrocyte; and the mean corpuscular hemoglobin concentration (MCHC), which is the proportion of an individual erythrocyte occupied by hemoglobin. The WBC count is the number of WBCs in a cubic millimeter of blood. The differential WBC count is the proportion of each type of WBC in a sample of 100 WBCs (see Table 34-1). Table 34-2 lists the CBC components, normal values, and common explanations for abnormal levels.

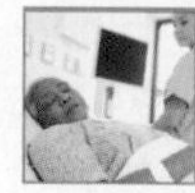

1. Explain the relationship between Mrs. Rees's laboratory results and her vital signs. Provide possible explanations for the abnormal results.

COAGULATION STUDIES

Three mechanisms are activated by injury to a blood vessel: vascular spasm, plug formation, and blood clotting (Figure 34-2). In an attempt to prevent additional blood loss, the injured vessel constricts. This vasoconstriction lasts only a few minutes but provides the needed time and decreased surface area to facilitate platelet aggregation. The platelets clump together and form a temporary plug to seal the injured vessel. The final mechanism to protect against blood loss is coagulation, or clotting, of the blood. This complex process involves the conversion of fibrinogen to fibrin. The fibrin then adheres to the platelets and other blood cells to form a more permanent seal to the injured blood vessel (Figure 34-3).

Five diagnostic tests are used to monitor hemostasis, the blood's ability to stop bleeding. They measure (1) platelets, (2) bleeding time, (3) **prothrombin time** (PT) or **international normalized ratio** (INR), (4) **activated partial thromboplastin time** (APTT), and (5) fibrinogen. These tests, the normal values, and abnormal findings are summarized in Table 34-3.

Newer anticoagulants are being used in some patients. Some of these drugs are monitored by the CBC and others by clotting factors, depending on the medication and its action within the body.

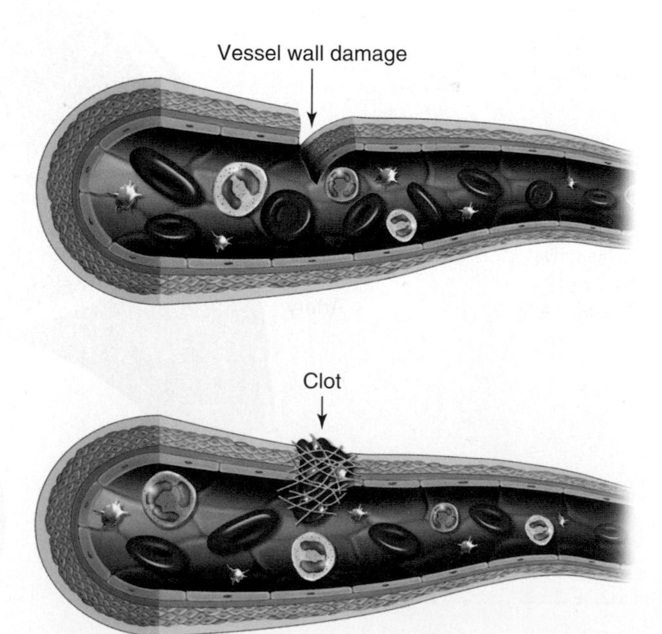

FIGURE 34-2 Blood clotting.

TABLE 34-2 Complete Blood Cell Count

COMPONENT	NORMAL VALUE	CLINICAL SIGNIFICANCE OF ABNORMAL VALUES: DECREASED LEVELS	CLINICAL SIGNIFICANCE OF ABNORMAL VALUES: INCREASED LEVELS
Red blood cells (cells/mm^3)	Adult male: 4.7-6.1 Adult female: 4.2-5.4 Newborn: 4.8-7.1 Child 8-12 yr: 4.0-5.5	Anemia Bone marrow suppression Chronic infection Hemorrhage Renal disease Vitamin B_6, B_{12}, or folic acid deficiency	Major burns Cardiovascular disease Chronic lung disease Congenital heart defect Polycythemia vera
Hemoglobin (g/dL)	Adult male: 14-18 Adult female: 12-16	Anemia Bone marrow suppression Chronic infection Hemorrhage Renal disease Vitamin B_6, B_{12}, or folic acid deficiency	Major burns Cardiovascular disease Chronic lung disease Congenital heart defect Polycythemia vera
Hematocrit (%)	Adult male: 42-52 Adult female: 37-48	Anemia Bone marrow suppression Chronic infection Hemorrhage Renal disease Vitamin B_6, B_{12}, or folic acid deficiency	Major burns Cardiovascular disease Chronic lung disease Congenital heart defect Polycythemia vera
Red Blood Cell Indices			
Mean corpuscular volume (cells/mm^3)	80-95	Iron-deficiency anemia Lead poisoning Thalassemia minor and major	Pernicious anemia Folic acid deficiencies Chronic liver disease
Mean corpuscular hemoglobin (pq/cell)	27-31	Iron-deficiency anemia Lead poisoning Rheumatoid arthritis Sickle cell anemia	Alcohol abuse Chronic liver disease Folic acid deficiency Hypothyroidism
Mean corpuscular hemoglobin concentration (g/dL)	32-36	Iron-deficiency anemia Lead poisoning	Normal finding in infancy
White blood cells (cells/mm^3)	Adult: 5000-10,000 Child >2 yr: 5000-10,000 Newborn: 9000-30,000	Chronic leukemia Aplastic anemia	Acute leukemia Infections Surgery Trauma
Differential White Blood Cell Count*			
Neutrophils (cells/mm^3)	Segmented: 2500-8000	Anaphylactic shock Anorexia nervosa Leukemia Rheumatoid arthritis Septicemia Stress Viral infection (measles, rubella, infectious mononucleosis, hepatitis)	Acidosis Acute hemolysis of red blood cells Acute pyogenic infections Cancer of liver, gastrointestinal tract, or bone marrow Emotional stress Physical stress Hemorrhage Septicemia Tissue necrosis (surgery, major burns, myocardial infarction)

Continued

TABLE 34-2 Complete Blood Cell Count—cont'd

COMPONENT	NORMAL VALUE	CLINICAL SIGNIFICANCE OF ABNORMAL VALUES: DECREASED LEVELS	CLINICAL SIGNIFICANCE OF ABNORMAL VALUES: INCREASED LEVELS
Lymphocytes (cells/mm^3)	1000-4000	Acute tuberculosis Acquired immunodeficiency syndrome (AIDS) Congestive heart failure Hodgkin disease Myasthenia gravis Renal failure Systemic lupus erythematosus	Crohn disease Drug hypersensitivity Infectious mononucleosis Ulcerative colitis Viral disorders (mumps, rubella, rubeola, hepatitis, varicella)
Monocytes (cells/mm^3)	100-700	Acute stress reaction Overwhelming infection	Chronic inflammatory disorders Chronic ulcerative colitis Syphilis Tuberculosis
Eosinophils (cells/mm^3)	50-500	Severe infection Shock Stress Trauma	Allergic disease Cancer of lung, stomach, or ovary Hodgkin disease Parasitic infection Polycythemia Ulcerative colitis
Basophils (cells/mm^3)	25-100	Acute infection Graves disease Pregnancy Shock Stress	Chickenpox Chronic sinusitis Measles Ulcerative colitis

Adapted from Pagana KD, Pagana TJ: *Mosby's manual of diagnostic and laboratory tests,* ed. 5, St. Louis, 2014, Mosby.
*Proportion of each type of white blood cell observed on the blood smear.

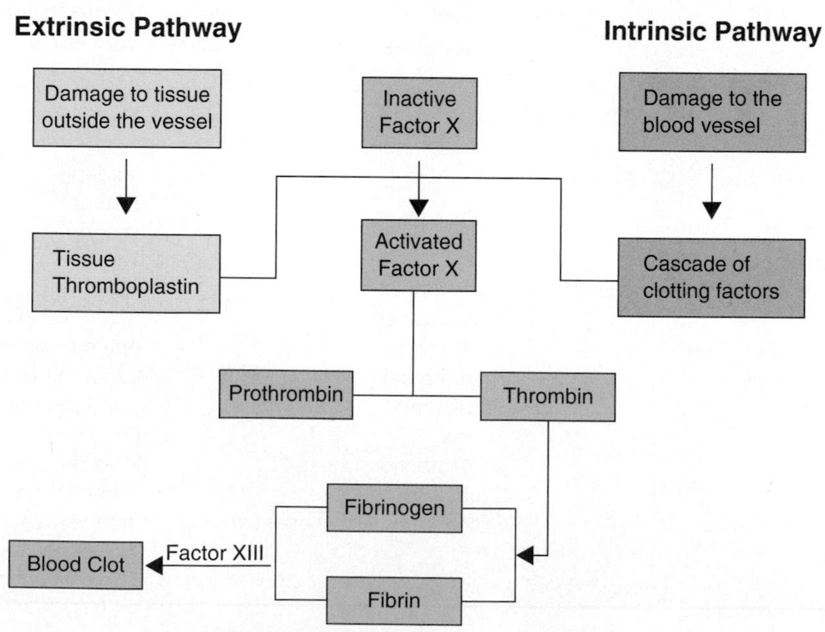

FIGURE 34-3 Pathways of coagulation.

TABLE 34-3 Coagulation Studies

COMPONENT	FUNCTION	NORMAL VALUE	CLINICAL SIGNIFICANCE OF ABNORMAL VALUES	
			DECREASED LEVELS	INCREASED LEVELS
Platelets (cells/mm^3)	Measures number, size, and shape of cells	150,000-400,000	Pernicious, aplastic, and hemolytic anemias Multiple transfusions of packed red blood cells HIV infection Result of chemotherapy and radiation therapy	Leukemias Splenectomy Iron-deficiency anemia Rheumatoid arthritis Acute infection or inflammatory diseases
Prothrombin time	Can detect bleeding disorders caused by abnormalities of the extrinsic clotting system Used to monitor effectiveness of warfarin sodium (Coumadin) therapy	11-12.5 sec Therapeutic level for anticoagulant therapy: 1.5-2.0 times the control value	NA	Acute leukemia Congestive heart failure Chronic pancreatitis Hepatitis Liver disease Oral anticoagulant therapy (Coumadin)
International normalized ratio (INR)	Used to monitor effect of anticoagulant therapy	0.8-1.1 for patient not on anticoagulant 2.0-3.0 for prophylaxis or treatment of venous thrombosis 3-4 for prosthetic cardiac valve replacement	NA	Acute leukemia Congestive heart failure Chronic pancreatitis Hepatitis Liver disease Oral anticoagulant therapy (Coumadin)
Activated partial thromboplastin time	Can detect bleeding disorders caused by abnormalities of the intrinsic clotting system Used to monitor effectiveness of heparin therapy	30-40 sec Therapeutic level for anticoagulant therapy: 1.5-2.5 times the control value	Acute hemorrhage Advanced stages of cancer	Hemophilia Cirrhosis Hemodialysis Liver disease Heparin therapy Vitamin K deficiency
Fibrinogen (mg/dL)	Used to identify suspected bleeding disorders Used to monitor progressive liver disease	200-400	Anemia Cirrhosis Hemophilia Leukemia Liver disease Malnutrition	Acute infection Major burns Heart disease Hepatitis Nephrosis Cancer (breast, kidney, stomach) Myocardial infarction

Adapted from Pagana KD, Pagana TJ: *Mosby's manual of diagnostic and laboratory tests*, ed. 5, St. Louis, 2014, Mosby.
HIV, Human immunodeficiency virus; *NA*, not applicable.

BLOOD CHEMISTRY

When electrolytes are dissolved, they become electrically charged particles known as *cations* (positively charged) or *anions* (negatively charged). The most commonly monitored cations include sodium (Na^+), potassium (K^+), calcium (Ca^{2+}), and magnesium (Mg^{2+}). Anions that are commonly monitored include chloride (Cl^-), bicarbonate (HCO_3^-), and phosphate (HPO_4^-). Chapter 39 discusses the functions of these intracellular and extracellular electrolytes, the normal values, and the common causes of abnormal values.

Glucose, an energy source necessary for cellular metabolism, is an end product of carbohydrate metabolism. Excess glucose is converted to glycogen and is stored in the liver. Normal glucose levels are controlled by the release of two hormones: glucagon and insulin. Glucagon raises blood levels of glucose by facilitating the breakdown of glycogen. Insulin lowers blood glucose levels by acting as a carrier to transport glucose into the cells, where it is available for use.

Monitoring serum levels of glucose is useful in detecting abnormal glucose metabolism. Although there are several causes for abnormal glucose metabolism, the most common is diabetes mellitus. Blood glucose levels can be monitored with a venous sample in conjunction with other laboratory tests. It is frequently monitored using a capillary blood sample.

Hemoglobin A_{1c} (Hgb A_{1c}), or glycosylated hemoglobin, testing evaluates blood sugar levels over a period of 2 to 3 months This blood test is performed to provide the primary care provider (PCP) with information about long-term blood sugar control. The normal value of Hgb A_{1c} in patients without diabetes is 4% to 5.9% of hemoglobin. In patients with their diabetes under control, the value is below 7%. A level higher than 9% indicates that the patient has had poor blood glucose control with hyperglycemia during the past few weeks.

LIPID PROFILE

A lipoprotein profile is used to diagnose hyperlipidemia and monitor treatment effectiveness. It usually consists of four tests: total cholesterol, low-density lipoprotein (LDL) cholesterol, high-density lipoprotein (HDL) cholesterol, and triglycerides. **Cholesterol** is a sterol (i.e., modified steroid) that is mostly synthesized in the liver from dietary fats. It can be found in cell plasma membranes and is a precursor for vitamin D, steroid hormones, and sex hormones.

Low-density lipoproteins transport cholesterol from the liver to various parts of the body. LDL cholesterol is considered "bad cholesterol" because of its role in atherosclerotic disease. **High-density lipoproteins** transport excess cholesterol from the tissues back to the liver, where it is broken down and excreted in bile. HDL cholesterol is considered "good cholesterol" because high levels reduce the risk of heart disease.

Triglycerides are composed of fatty acids, proteins, and glucose. They are synthesized in the liver and stored in adipose tissue and muscle. They can be retrieved when additional energy is needed to meet metabolic demand. Measurement of triglycerides is used to calculate LDL cholesterol levels with the following formula (Pagana and Pagana, 2014):

LDL cholesterol =
Total cholesterol − (HDL cholesterol + [Triglycerides ÷ 5])

Normal values for blood chemistries and lipid levels and the disorders that lead to abnormal values are summarized in Table 34-4.

LIVER FUNCTION TESTS

A liver profile usually consists of serum levels of albumin, bilirubin, and the following four liver enzymes: alanine aminotransferase, alkaline phosphatase, aspartate aminotransferase, and gamma-glutamyl transpeptidase.

Albumin is one of the plasma proteins synthesized by the liver. It is an essential component of fluid balance, responsible for maintaining colloidal oncotic pressure in the vascular and extravascular spaces. Low levels of albumin may indicate malnutrition.

Prealbumin is another plasma protein synthesized by the liver. It has a much shorter half-life than albumin and is therefore considered a more precise measure of current nutritional status.

Bilirubin, one of the components of bile, is synthesized in the liver, spleen, and bone marrow. Bilirubin is also a by-product of **hemolysis**, or RBC destruction. Total bilirubin levels are increased in jaundice. The animation "Hemoglobin Breakdown" illustrates the process of hemolysis.

Alanine aminotransferase (ALT) is an enzyme found primarily in the liver, but it also is found in the kidneys, heart, and skeletal muscle. It is a catalyst for amino acid production. Serum levels are used to monitor liver disease progression and the effect of hepatotoxic drugs.

Alkaline phosphatase (ALP) is an enzyme found primarily in the liver. It also is found in the bone, placenta, intestine, and kidneys. Serum levels are useful indicators of liver and bone disease.

Aspartate aminotransferase (AST) is an enzyme found primarily in the heart, liver, and muscle. It is released after cell death or injury. Serum levels are measured primarily to assess the severity of liver damage and disease.

Gamma-glutamyl transpeptidase (GGTP) is found primarily in the liver and biliary tract. This enzyme assists the transportation of amino acids across cell membranes. Elevated serum levels may indicate liver disease.

Normal values for liver function test results and disorders that lead to abnormal values are summarized in Table 34-5.

KIDNEY FUNCTION TESTS

Two blood tests are used to monitor renal function and assess damage: blood urea nitrogen (BUN) and serum creatinine. Urea is a by-product of protein metabolism. It is excreted by the kidneys and measured as **blood urea nitrogen.** Elevated BUN levels may indicate decreased renal glomerular function. BUN levels also may be elevated as a result of a high-protein diet or with dehydration. The glomerular filtration rate (GFR) is another essential test of renal function. A level less than 60 mL/min/1.73 m^2 may be a sign of renal failure.

Serum **creatinine** is a waste product of skeletal muscle metabolism. It is excreted by the kidneys. Because creatinine is excreted at a more consistent rate than BUN, serum-level values tend to be more sensitive in detecting renal impairment. The normal ratio of BUN to creatinine is between 6 and 25.

TABLE 34-4 Blood Chemistries and Lipid Studies

		CLINICAL SIGNIFICANCE OF ABNORMAL VALUES	
COMPONENT	**NORMAL VALUE**	**DECREASED LEVELS**	**INCREASED LEVELS**
Glucose (mg/dL)	60-110	Anxiety Excessive exercise Malabsorption Excessive insulin	Diabetes mellitus Obesity Liver disease Pancreatitis Trauma Reactive hypoglycemia due to high carbohydrate intake
Total cholesterol (mg/dL)*	<200	Acquired immunodeficiency syndrome (AIDS) Chronic anemia Liver disease Malabsorption Malnutrition Sepsis Stress	Atherosclerosis Cardiovascular disease Hyperlipidemia Nephrotic syndrome Obesity Uncontrolled diabetes mellitus
High-density lipoprotein cholesterol (mg/dL)*	Males: >45 Females: >55	Chronic inactivity Diabetes mellitus End-stage liver disease Obesity Renal failure Smoking Stress	Alcoholism Chronic liver disease Long-term aerobic exercise
Low-density lipoprotein cholesterol (mg/dL)*	<130 Borderline high risk: 130-159 High risk: >159	Cancer Malabsorption Malnutrition	Chronic renal failure Diabetes mellitus High-cholesterol diet Hyperlipidemia Nephrotic syndrome
Triglycerides (mg/dL)*	Males: 40-160 Females: 35-135 Borderline high: 160-199 High: 200-499 Very high: >500	Chronic obstructive pulmonary disease Low-fat diet Malabsorption Malnutrition	Alcohol abuse Cirrhosis Diabetes mellitus Low-protein, high-carbohydrate diet Familial hyperlipoproteinemia Gout Hypertension Nephrotic syndrome Pancreatitis

Adapted from Pagana KD, Pagana TJ: *Mosby's manual of diagnostic and laboratory tests*, ed. 5, St. Louis, 2014, Mosby.
*Test requires fasting.

The creatinine clearance tests renal function and is a 24-hour urine collection test used to measure the glomerular filtration rate. A level below 60 mL/min/1.73 m^2 may indicate renal failure.

CARDIAC MARKERS

Cardiac markers are proteins that leak out of injured heart muscle cells into the bloodstream. A series of tests is used to detect abnormal levels of these markers, which can indicate myocardial damage due to coronary artery occlusion. Tests are conducted for the following markers: creatine kinase (CK) and the CK-MB isoenzyme, myoglobin, and troponin I and troponin T.

Creatine kinase is an enzyme found primarily in skeletal muscle, cardiac muscle, and brain tissue. Elevated CK levels usually indicate damage in one of these three areas. CK occurs is further broken down into three isoenzyme forms. CK1 (CK-BB) is found primarily in brain tissue. CK2 (CK-MB) is found in cardiac tissue. CK3 (CK-MM) is found primarily in skeletal tissue. Normal levels of CK consist primarily of the CK-MM isoenzyme. Elevated levels of isoenzymes can be

TABLE 34-5 Liver and Kidney Function Tests

COMPONENT	NORMAL VALUE	CLINICAL SIGNIFICANCE OF ABNORMAL VALUES	
		DECREASED LEVELS	INCREASED LEVELS
Albumin (g/dL)	3.3-5	Diabetes mellitus Glomerular protein loss Hepatic disease Malnutrition Renal disease Rheumatoid arthritis Stress	Acute pancreatitis Dehydration
Bilirubin (mg/dL)*	0.3-1.0	NA	Biliary obstruction Cirrhosis Hepatitis Hemolytic transfusion reaction Tissue hemorrhage
Alanine aminotransferase (units/L)	4-36	NA	Biliary obstruction Cirrhosis Hepatitis Muscle inflammation Pancreatitis Shock Trauma
Alkaline phosphatase (units/L)	30-120	Chronic nephritis Hypothyroidism Malnutrition Excessive vitamin D intake	Biliary obstruction Cirrhosis Hepatitis High-fat intake Pancreatitis Vitamin D deficiency
Aspartate aminotransferase (units/L)	0-35	Diabetic ketoacidosis Pregnancy Uremia	Acute renal disease Biliary obstruction Cirrhosis Hepatitis Pancreatitis Trauma
Gamma-glutamyl transpeptidase (units/L)	Males and females >45 yr: 8-38 Females <45 yr: 5-27	NA	Acute pancreatitis Alcoholism Biliary obstruction Cirrhosis Congestive heart failure Hepatitis Myocardial infarction
Blood urea nitrogen (mg/dL)	10-20	Alcohol abuse Diet inadequate in protein Hepatitis Liver failure Malnutrition	Acute glomerulonephritis Congestive heart failure Diabetes mellitus High-protein diet Nephrotic syndrome Renal disease Severe dehydration Severe infection Shock
Serum creatinine (mg/dL)	Females: 0.5-1.1 Males: 0.6-1.3	Atrophy of muscle Pregnancy	Congestive heart failure Dehydration Diabetes mellitus Glomerulonephritis Renal failure Rheumatoid arthritis Shock Uremia

Adapted from Pagana KD, Pagana TJ: *Mosby's manual of diagnostic and laboratory tests,* ed. 5, St. Louis, 2014, Mosby.
NA, Not applicable.
*Test requires fasting.

TABLE 34-6 Cardiac Markers

MARKER	NORMAL VALUE	ABNORMAL VALUE	BEGINS TO RISE (hr)	PEAK (hr)	RETURNS TO NORMAL (days)
Total creatine kinase (units/L)	Females: 30-135 Males: 55-170	Females: >150 Males: >174	3-6	18	2-3
CK-MB (%)	<0%	>3%	3-6	12-24	½-2
Myoglobin (ng/mL)	<90	>90	2-6	8-12	Within 1
Troponin I (ng/mL)	<0.03	>0.04	2-3	14-20	7-10
Troponin T (ng/mL)	<0.1	>0.1	2-3	12-24	10-14

Adapted from Pagana KD, Pagana TJ: *Mosby's manual of diagnostic and laboratory tests*, ed. 5, St. Louis, 2014, Mosby.
CK-MB, Creatine kinase MB isoenzyme found primarily in heart muscle.

useful in diagnosing and differentiating between myocardial damage and skeletal and inflammatory disorders. Correct timing of these tests is essential for accurate diagnosis.

Myoglobin is an oxygen-transporting and storage protein found in cardiac and skeletal muscle. When damage to a muscle cell occurs, myoglobin is released, and blood levels of the protein rise. Because myoglobin is found primarily in cardiac and skeletal muscles, elevated levels can be diagnostic of myocardial infarction (MI) or skeletal muscle trauma.

Troponin is a complex of three proteins found in cardiac and skeletal muscle. Two of the proteins, **troponin I** and **troponin T**, are found exclusively in cardiac muscle. These proteins are released during myocardial damage and can be detected within 3 hours of an MI, even with small areas of cardiac muscle injury. Tests for troponins are much more sensitive to the early onset of an MI and are used much more frequently in the clinical setting to detect an MI than CK-MB or myoglobin. Table 34-6 lists the onset, peak, and return-to-normal times for the cardiac markers previously discussed.

Homocysteine is an amino acid formed in the conversion of methionine to cysteine. Folate and vitamins B_6 and B_{12} are necessary for the body to metabolize homocysteine. Normal levels for homocysteine are 4 to 14 μmol/L. High levels of homocysteine are associated with an increased risk of cardiovascular disease, although it is not known whether increased levels are a precursor to or a result of the disease. Smoking and vitamin deficiencies, specifically folate and vitamins B_6 and B_{12}, seem to play a role in elevating levels. Adding these vitamins to the diet can lead to lower serum levels of homocysteine.

Brain natriuretic peptide (BNP) is a hormone produced by myocardial cells. It is released from the ventricle during times of increased pressure or overload. BNP causes vasodilation by opposing the action of angiotensin II and increases sodium excretion and urine output. Elevated levels are often found in patients with heart failure, and plasma concentrations reflect the severity of cardiac failure. Normal levels are below 100 pg/mL.

C-reactive protein (CRP) is produced by the liver in response to inflammation, tissue damage, and infection. Blood levels of CRP have been used as a marker for inflammatory and autoimmune disorders such as rheumatoid arthritis, lupus, and inflammatory bowel syndrome. CRP is a marker for vascular inflammation—an important factor in atherosclerosis. The high-sensitivity CRP (hs-CRP) blood test is used to measure the CRP level. Levels below 1 mg/L indicate a low risk, levels between 1 and 3 mg/L indicate average risk, and levels above 3 mg/L indicate high risk. CRP is now used as a screening for coronary artery disease and as a predictor of future cardiac events.

The **arterial blood gas** (ABG) diagnostic test is used to examine arterial blood and assess a patient's oxygenation status and acid-base balance. Chapter 39 provides more information on this topic.

LABORATORY TESTS: URINE AND STOOL — LO 34.3

Tests are commonly ordered for urine, stool, and other bodily fluid specimens. In many circumstances, it is the nurse's responsibility to collect these specimens or to delegate the collection to unlicensed assistive personnel (UAP).

URINALYSIS

Urinalysis is a common diagnostic test. It is frequently ordered on admission to the hospital and as part of a routine physical examination. It is used to diagnose urinary tract infections and is helpful in detecting diseases and disorders unrelated to the renal system. An overview of the components of the urinalysis, the normal values, and the disorders related to abnormal values can be found in Table 34-7.

STOOL

The excreted waste products of digestion are known as *stool* or *feces*. Stool analysis is useful in identifying disorders of the gastrointestinal (GI) tract, liver, and pancreas. Analysis is commonly ordered to test for occult blood, fecal fat, urobilinogen levels, and ova and parasites.

TABLE 34-7 Urinalysis Findings

COMPONENT	NORMAL VALUE	ABNORMAL VALUES
Color	Light yellow to amber	Dark yellow to amber: • Concentrated urine • Presence of bilirubin Blue/green: • Pseudomonal urinary tract infection Light straw/very pale yellow: • Alcohol • High fluid intake • Dilute urine Orange: • Presence of bile • Fever • Several drugs known to alter the color of urine
Clarity	Clear to slightly hazy	Cloudy: may indicate bacteria and red or white blood cells
Specific gravity	1.005-1.030	Increased: • Acute glomerulonephritis • Congestive heart failure • Dehydration • Diabetes mellitus • Low fluid intake • Liver failure • Vomiting and diarrhea Decreased: • Antidiuretic hormone deficiency • Chronic pyelonephritis • Diuretics • High fluid intake
Potential hydrogen (pH)	4.6-8.0	Increased: • Bacteriuria • Chronic renal failure • Metabolic alkalosis • Urinary tract infection • Starvation Decreased: • Dehydration • Diabetes mellitus • Diarrhea • Fever • Urinary tract infection
Glucose	Negative	Increased: • Diabetes mellitus • Infection • Stress
Ketones	Negative	Increased: • Alcoholism • Anorexia • Diabetes mellitus • Diarrhea • Fasting • Fever • High-protein diet • Postanesthesia • Starvation • Vomiting
Red blood cells	≤2	Increased: • Acute tubular necrosis • Benign prostatic hypertrophy • Renal calculi • Hemophilia • Renal trauma • Urinary tract infection • Menstruation
Protein	0-8 mg/dL	Increased: • Diabetes mellitus • Emotional stress • Exercise • Glomerulonephritis • Pyelonephritis
Bilirubin	Negative	Increased: • Cirrhosis of the liver • Hepatitis • Obstructive jaundice
Bacteria	Negative	Increased: • Urinary tract infection

Adapted from Pagana KD, Pagana TJ: *Mosby's manual of diagnostic and laboratory tests,* ed. 5, St. Louis, 2014, Mosby.

Bleeding anywhere along the GI tract results in blood in the stool. Bleeding that occurs in the upper GI tract produces stools that are black and tarry in appearance. Bleeding from the lower tract results in stools with bright red blood. The testing for occult blood in the stool can detect very small amounts of blood, as little as 5 mL per day. Results that are positive for occult blood may indicate several disorders, including peptic ulcer disease, inflammatory bowel disease, hemorrhoids, and trauma to the GI tract. Positive occult blood findings also can indicate gastric or colon cancer. The American Cancer Society (2013) recommends screening for colorectal cancer using fecal occult blood testing, sigmoidoscopy, or colonoscopy in adults beginning at age 50 years.

Examination of the stool can provide diagnostic information about the effectiveness of the digestive system. Fecal fat, or **steatorrhea**, indicates a failure to digest and absorb dietary fat. Steatorrhea is usually a result of malabsorption syndrome, deficiency of pancreatic enzymes, or deficiency of bile (usually due to biliary obstruction).

Urobilinogen is produced by the breakdown of bilirubin and is responsible for the brown color of stool. Normal levels are 50 to 300 mg per 24 hours. Increases in urobilinogen result from increased RBC destruction, as in hemolytic anemia. Decreased levels are seen in biliary obstruction or in severe liver disease.

Parasites and their eggs (ova) in the stool can lead to GI symptoms such as diarrhea. Common parasites are roundworm, pinworm, hookworm, tapeworm, and *Trichinella spiralis.* With the exception of pinworms, common parasites are ingested by consuming contaminated food or water. Stool collected for ova and parasite examination must be delivered to the laboratory while still warm.

CULTURE AND SENSITIVITY

When an infection is suspected, culture specimens can be obtained from body fluids to identify the pathogen responsible. Common sources of specimens are blood, throat, sputum, stool, urine, and wounds. The collected specimen is sent to the laboratory, where a section is placed on a culture medium. A culture is considered positive when bacteria are found growing on the medium. After the pathogen has been identified, it is exposed to various antibiotics, and the bacterial growth is monitored to determine *sensitivity*, or which antibiotic therapy would be most effective in treating the infection. Bacteria are considered susceptible when the antibiotic kills or inhibits growth, whereas resistant bacteria continue to grow despite the presence of the antibiotic.

DIAGNOSTIC EXAMINATIONS LO 34.4

In addition to having their blood and body fluids tested in the laboratory, patients may have orders for diagnostic tests such as radiography, computed tomography, magnetic resonance imaging, electrocardiography, endoscopy, ultrasound, and needle aspirations and biopsies. Nursing responsibilities for these tests depend on the setting and the particular test.

RADIOGRAPHY

Radiography is the use of x-rays to visualize bones, organs, and soft tissues for abnormalities. X-rays are electromagnetic vibrations that travel in a straight line. When the x-ray passes through matter, some of the intensity is absorbed; the denser the matter, the higher the degree of absorption. This absorption can be captured on film, with the differences in density appearing as various shades of darkness. High-density matter, such as bone, appears to be white, and air-filled areas appear to be black.

Noncontrast Studies

X-rays are routinely ordered as diagnostic examinations for the chest, bones, abdomen, and breasts. These x-rays are considered noncontrast studies because they do not require administration of contrast material before the examination.

Chest x-rays are one of the most frequently ordered radiographs. A chest x-ray can be used to diagnose several pulmonary disorders, such as tuberculosis, cancer, and pneumonia. Chest x-rays are also used to determine the correct placement of treatment devices, such as chest tubes, central line infusion catheters, and pacemakers.

X-rays are also used to diagnose fractures in bones and joints. Other disorders that can be diagnosed with orthopedic x-rays include osteoporosis, osteomyelitis, arthritis, and tumors.

Mammograms are soft tissue x-rays that allow visualization of the underlying breast tissue. Mammography is used primarily as a screening tool for the detection of tumors or cysts that are missed by palpation. The American Cancer Society (2013) recommends yearly mammograms for all women who are 40 years of age or older.

Contrast Studies

In some situations, visualization requires the use of contrast media to highlight the details not seen on a noncontrast x-ray. The ideal contrast material has low toxicity, is nonallergenic, has no effects on normal physical function, and is relatively low in cost. All contrast materials have the potential for causing allergic reactions, ranging from mild responses (e.g., nausea, vomiting, localized rash) to severe anaphylaxis.

Disorders of the GI tract, including gastric ulcers, pyloric stenosis, hiatal hernias, and carcinoma of the stomach, are commonly tested for using contrast x-rays. The upper GI series consists of a series of x-rays of the esophagus, stomach, duodenum, and upper portion of the jejunum. Before the examination, the patient drinks a contrast agent, usually barium sulfate; the upper GI series is sometimes referred to as a *barium swallow.* The contrast medium outlines the organs seen on x-ray, thereby aiding in identification of any abnormality.

The lower GI tract can also be visualized using barium sulfate. The contrast medium is introduced through a rectal tube or an enema. Examination of the ascending, transverse, and descending colons, as well as the sigmoid colon and rectum, is useful in diagnosing colon cancer, obstructions, and chronic disorders such as ulcerative colitis. For the upper and lower GI barium studies, it is the nurse's responsibility to monitor the patient until the barium is expelled. Patients should increase their fluid intake, and some may need a mild laxative to aid in the elimination of the barium.

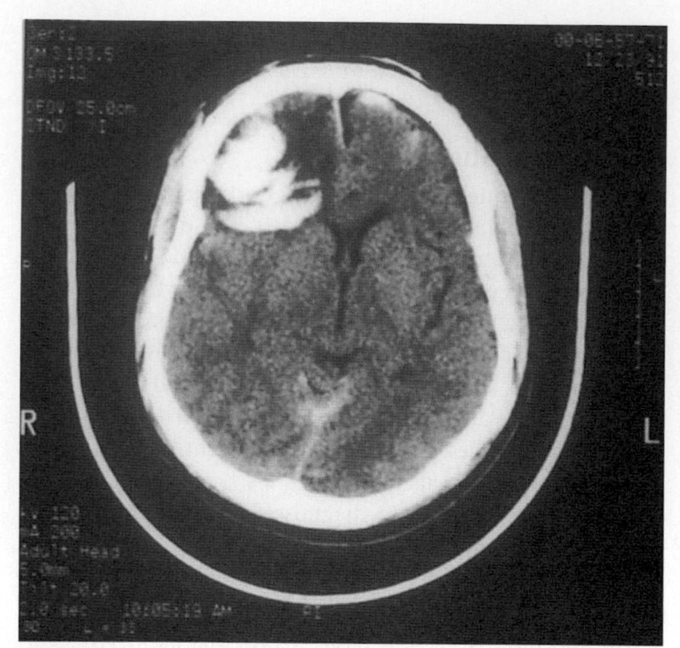

FIGURE 34-4 Computed tomography scan. (From Black JM, Hawks JH: *Medical-surgical nursing: clinical management for positive outcomes*, ed. 8, St. Louis, 2009, Saunders.)

COMPUTED TOMOGRAPHY

Computed tomography (CT) is a radiologic procedure in which the use of a special scanner allows cross-sectional images of an organ to be visualized (Figure 34-4). CT scans can be done with or without the use of a contrast medium. Table 34-8 lists specific examinations and abnormal findings.

MAGNETIC RESONANCE IMAGING

Magnetic resonance imaging (MRI) is the most common diagnostic examination for brain pathology and joint visualization (Figure 34-5). It involves the use of a superconducting magnet and radiofrequency waves that cause hydrogen nuclei to emit signals. A computer translates the signals into a well-defined image of the structure.

MRI produces a cross-sectional image of the body, similar to a CT scan, but without radiation exposure. It allows better visualization of blood vessels and signs of hemorrhage within hours of the event. It can be used with or without contrast media. Table 34-9 lists the most common sites studied with MRI and examples of abnormal findings.

MRI has some disadvantages. It tends to be more expensive than CT. The magnet can affect the functioning of computerized equipment such as IV infusion pumps and mechanical ventilators. Because the magnet can move metal objects implanted in the body, it is contraindicated for patients with pacemakers, inner ear implants, fragments from gunshot wounds, or other metal objects in the body. All jewelry is removed before the test. Some patients experience claustrophobia because the test is sometimes performed with

TABLE 34-8 Computed Tomography Findings

SITE	ABNORMAL FINDINGS
Abdomen	Abdominal aortic aneurysm Appendicitis Bile duct dilation Gallstones Hemorrhage Infection Tumors
Brain	Abscess Cerebral infarction Aneurysms Hemorrhage Hydrocephalus Tumors
Chest	Aortic aneurysm Enlarged lymph nodes Esophageal tumors Hiatal hernia Pleural effusion Pulmonary embolism
Kidneys, ureters	Urinary calculi Tumors

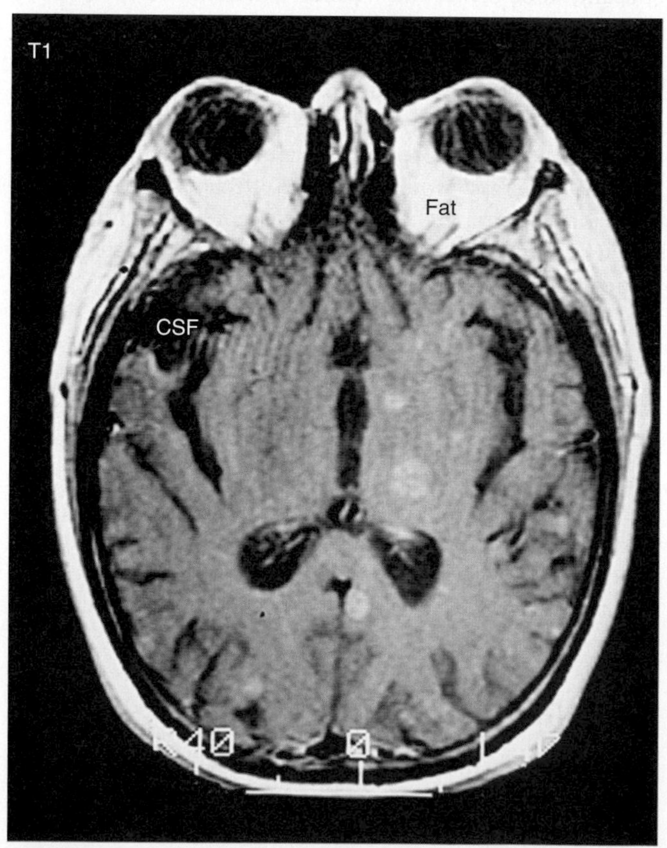

FIGURE 34-5 Magnetic resonance imaging scan. (From Mettler FA: *Essentials of radiology*, ed. 3, St. Louis, 2014, Saunders.)

TABLE 34-9 Magnetic Resonance Imaging Findings

SITE	ABNORMAL FINDINGS
Abdomen, pelvis	Cancers in the peritoneal area Abdominal aortic aneurysm Acute tubular necrosis
Brain	Acute head injury Stroke Subarachnoid hemorrhage Cerebral abscess Hydrocephalus Tumors
Breast	Cancer Benign lesions
Heart	Congenital heart disease Atherosclerotic plaques Myocardial infarction
Spine	Spinal cord lesions Spinal cord compression Disk herniation Spinal stenosis

the patient in a tunnel-like machine for 30 to 90 minutes. Rarely, people with a tattoo have reported burning and swelling in the area of the tattoo after MRI (Food and Drug Administration, 2014).

POSITRON EMISSION TOMOGRAPHY

Positron emission tomography (PET) is a nuclear study performed after injection of a radionuclide into a vein. The PET scan is then performed, and the organ or organs being studied appear as color-coded images that can be analyzed.

ELECTROCARDIOGRAM

An **electrocardiogram** (ECG), also called EKG, is a recording of the electrical current generated by the heart during depolarization and repolarization of the cardiac muscle. The ECG is composed of several waveforms that reflect different aspects of cardiac contraction: P wave (atrial depolarization), QRS wave (ventricular depolarization), and T wave (ventricular repolarization).

The ECG is recorded on special paper that allows measurement of the waveforms in terms of time and shape. Increases in the duration of any waveform can indicate injury to or disorders of the cardiac conduction system. Chapter 38 provides more information on ECGs.

ENDOSCOPY

Endoscopy is a general term used to describe the examination of the interior of an organ or cavity by means of a fiberoptic

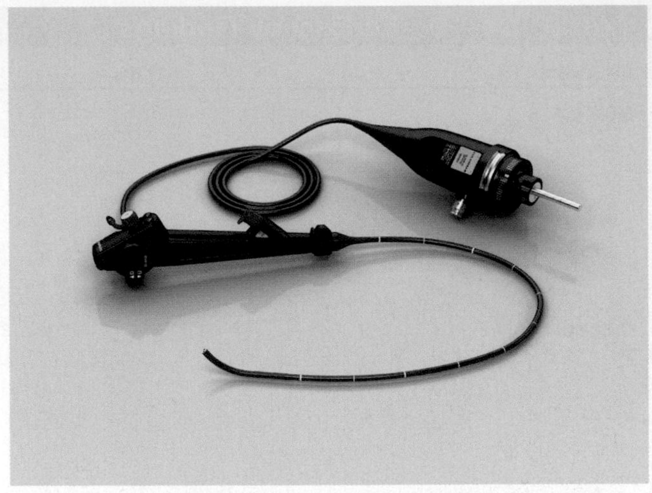

FIGURE 34-6 Fiberoptic scope. (Courtesy Olympus America, Inc, Mehlville, NY.)

scope (Figure 34-6). **Fiberoptics** is a system in which flexible glass or plastic fibers are used to transmit light around curves and corners. This allows direct visualization of the area of interest. Separate ports allow instillation of drugs, suction, and insertion of instruments for tissue or foreign object removal. Endoscopic examination is often used to identify tumors and to remove tissue samples for biopsy (Evidence-Based Practice and Informatics box). Table 34-10 summarizes the most common types of tests and the significance of abnormal findings.

EVIDENCE-BASED PRACTICE AND INFORMATICS

Colorectal Cancer Guidelines

The American Cancer Society has recommended the following examinations for early detection of colorectal cancer for people of average risk who are asymptomatic:

- Fecal occult blood test annually starting at age 50 (if the test is positive, a colonoscopy should be performed)
- Flexible sigmoidoscopy every 5 years starting at age 50 (if the test is positive, a colonoscopy should be performed) *or* colonoscopy every 10 years starting at age 50 *or* double-contrast barium enema every 5 years *or* CT colonography every 5 years

Patients considered at higher risk undergo the examinations at more frequent intervals.

From American Cancer Society: *Guidelines for early detection of cancer*, 2013. Retrieved from *www.cancer.org/healthy/findcancerearly/cancerscreeningguidelines/index.*

ULTRASOUND

Ultrasound is a procedure that provides visualization of soft tissue organs by recording and measuring the reflection of ultrasonic waves. The reflected waves are received by a transducer that converts them into electrical signals. A computer

TABLE 34-10 Endoscopy Findings

EXAMINATION	SITE	ABNORMAL FINDINGS
Arthroscopy	Joint structure	Cysts Degenerative joint changes Fractures Meniscal injury or disease Osteoarthritis Rheumatoid arthritis Synovitis
Bronchoscopy	Larynx, trachea, and bronchi	Cancer Foreign body Hemorrhage Infection Lung abscess Tracheal stenosis
Colonoscopy	Large intestine	Colon cancer Crohn's disease Diverticulosis Hemorrhoids Polyps Ulcerative colitis
Cystoscopy	Bladder and urethra	Calculi Diverticula Prostatic hypertrophy Tumors Urethral stricture
Esophagogastroduodenoscopy	Esophagus, stomach, and upper duodenum	Diverticula Esophageal hiatal hernia Esophageal stenosis Gastritis Pyloric stenosis Tumors Varices Ulcers
Sigmoidoscopy	Distal sigmoid colon, rectum, and anus	Anal fistula Abscesses Crohn's disease Hemorrhoids Irritable bowel syndrome Tumors Ulcerative colitis

translates these signals into a visual image. This allows a direct view of various organ structures and soft tissues, such as muscles and tendons. Fetal ultrasound is commonly used to determine fetal age, growth, and presence of congenital abnormalities. Abnormal organ growth, lesions or tumors, and structural damage can also be seen with ultrasound. Table 34-11 summarizes the most common examinations done with ultrasound and the significance of abnormal findings.

NEEDLE ASPIRATIONS AND BIOPSIES

Needle aspirations are procedures that are used to remove fluid and tissue for testing. Fine-needle aspiration is a method for obtaining samples with minimal trauma to the underlying organ or structure. A **paracentesis** involves removing fluid from the peritoneal cavity; a **thoracentesis** removes fluid from the pleural space. A **biopsy** involves removing a larger collection of cells, as in a tumor or mass, and may be used to

TABLE 34-11 Ultrasound Findings

EXAMINATION	SITE	ABNORMAL FINDINGS AND USES
Abdominal	Hepatobiliary system	Organ enlargement Presence of masses Tumors Calculi Cirrhosis
	Pancreas	Tumor Pseudocysts Inflammation
	Kidneys	Cysts Calculi Masses Hydronephrosis
	Aorta	Aneurysms Clots Tumors
	Spleen and lymph nodes	Organ enlargement Metastatic spread of cancer
Pelvic (gynecologic)	Bladder, uterus, and ovaries	Organ enlargement Follicle development and oocyte retrieval during infertility treatments Tumors
Breast	Breast	Cysts Tumors
Carotid Doppler	Carotid arteries	Aneurysm Occlusive disease
Pelvic (obstetric)	Uterus	Fetal health, age, and size Level of amniotic fluid Placenta abnormalities
Heart (echocardiogram)	Heart	Heart size, shape, position, and thickness Heart valve abnormalities Abnormal blood flow

detect cancer in the skin, breast, or liver. Samples can be obtained from any part of the body that can be accessed by the needle. Bacteriologic examination may be conducted on the samples aspirated. Table 34-12 summarizes four of the more common types of aspirations ordered.

ASSESSMENT LO 34.5

The nurse begins a preprocedure assessment by collecting basic health history information. Some example questions can be found in the Health Assessment Questions box.

Several factors need to be assessed before a patient undergoes a diagnostic test. Table 34-13 summarizes some aspects that are applicable to most diagnostic tests. The nurse should check the facility's procedure manual or a diagnostic handbook for care specific to each test.

It is common for diagnostic procedures to be scheduled on an outpatient basis. This means that the patient is not hospitalized but comes in for the procedure before the

HEALTH ASSESSMENT QUESTIONS

Diagnostic Test Focus

- What medications do you take on a daily basis (include prescription, herbal, and over-the-counter medications)?
- Do you have any allergies to food or medications? What happens if you take them?
- What is your understanding of the test? Do you have any questions?
- What medications did you take before the examination? Prescriptions? Over-the-counter medications?
- Have you smoked or consumed alcohol in the past 24 hours?
- When was the last time you had anything to eat or drink?
- For females: Is there any chance that you may be pregnant? When was your last menstrual period?
- What preparation did you make for this test (e.g., laxatives, NPO)?

scheduled time. As a result, the patient may be required to follow certain instructions at home. The Patient Education and Health Literacy box describes some of these instructions.

TABLE 34-12 Needle Aspiration Findings

EXAMINATION	SITE	ABNORMAL FINDINGS
Bone marrow aspiration	Iliac crest, sternum	Agranulocytosis Cancer Infection Iron-deficiency anemia Leukemia Lymphoma Platelet dysfunction
Lumbar puncture	Lumbar vertebrae	Infection Brain infarction Meningitis Tumor
Paracentesis	Peritoneal cavity	Cirrhosis Congestive heart failure Nephrotic syndrome Malignancy Peritonitis Pancreatitis
Thoracentesis	Pleural cavity	Infection Malignancy Metastasis Chest trauma Hemothorax

PATIENT EDUCATION AND HEALTH LITERACY

Preparation for Procedures

Patients often need to complete preprocedure preparation at home. These preparations may include the following:

- A special diet (e.g., clear liquids, NPO)
- Laxatives, cathartics, or enemas
- Cessation of certain daily medications (e.g., a patient who takes a daily aspirin may need to stop taking it 1 week before the scheduled examination)

It is important that the nurse assess the patient's level of understanding when first discussing the procedure. When the nurse performs the preprocedure assessment, determining compliance with these instructions is a critical nursing responsibility.

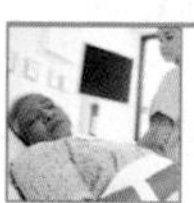

2. List at least three focused assessments for Mrs. Rees before her esophagogastroduodenoscopy (EGD).

◆ NURSING DIAGNOSIS LO 34.6

Nursing diagnoses are statements based on subjective and objective assessment information, and they are used to develop and evaluate the effectiveness of the plan of care. The following are common diagnoses related to diagnostic testing:

TABLE 34-13 Assessment Factors and Interventions Associated With Diagnostic Testing

FOCUS	NURSE'S RESPONSIBILITY
Identification (ID) band	Check for the presence of an ID band. Ensure that the band is on the patient and is correct.
Database, medical history	Review the medical record for a history of medical disorders that may signal a high risk for complications (e.g., bleeding disorders, hypertension).
Allergies	Check for allergies to food or medications. If the patient is undergoing an examination that involves an iodine contrast medium, check for a history of adverse reactions or allergies to iodine-containing food (e.g., shellfish, cabbage, kale, iodized salt).
Consent	Check that the consent form has been signed and witnessed.
Baseline vital signs	Obtain and document a complete set of vital signs. This provides a baseline for comparison during the procedure.
Medications	Consult with the primary care provider about whether regularly scheduled medications should be administered before the diagnostic test.
Nothing by mouth (NPO)	When appropriate, ensure that the patient has maintained NPO status.
Preparations	Determine whether the ordered preparations (e.g., laxatives, cathartics) were taken by the patient. Document the results.
Intravenous (IV) access	If the procedure requires IV access for the administration of medications or contrast media, be sure the IV line is patent and well secured.
Preprocedure medications	If a preprocedure sedative or analgesic has been ordered, ensure that the medication is given at the appropriate time.

- *Readiness for Enhanced Knowledge* regarding the diagnostic test purpose, procedure, and care required as evidenced by patient's statement about wanting to know what is wrong
- *Risk for Injury* with risk factor of preprocedure medications that cause changes in the sensorium
- *Fear* related to loss of control and unpredictable outcome due to invasive procedures as evidenced by patient's statement of being scared about the outcome
- *Anxiety* related to actual or perceived threat to biologic integrity due to invasive procedures as evidenced by fidgeting and insomnia

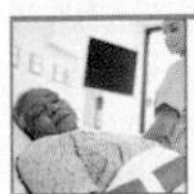

3. Identify two nursing diagnoses appropriate for Mrs. Rees. Include related factors and defining characteristics.

PLANNING LO 34.7

During the planning phase, the assessment data and nursing diagnoses are used to develop individualized goals and interventions (Table 34-14). The following examples of goal statements reflect the desired outcomes of patients undergoing diagnostic testing:

- Patient will state how and why the procedure is performed before the test.
- Patient will remain free from injury in the preprocedure time period.
- Patient will exhibit coping skills by learning about the test and results before the procedure.
- Patient will sleep 6 to 7 hours the night before the diagnostic procedure.

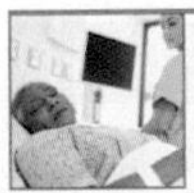

The conceptual care map for Mrs. Rees can be found at *http://evolve.elsevier.com/YoostCrawford/fundamentals/*. It is partially completed to indicate how to use the map as a learning tool. Complete the nursing diagnoses using the example conceptual care maps shown in Chapters 8 and 25 to 33.

IMPLEMENTATION AND EVALUATION LO 34.8

The nurse's responsibility during a diagnostic procedure is to monitor the patient and assist the health care provider. A time out must be called prior to any procedure to properly identify the correct patient with the correct procedure and correct site. It is not uncommon for a mild antianxiety or analgesic medication to be administered before and during the examination. The nurse should monitor the vital signs and oxygenation and provide supportive interventions as needed (e.g., oxygen). Post procedure, the nurse's responsibility is to monitor vital signs and assess for any complications that may arise from a procedure such as hemorrhage, pain, allergic reaction, and infection.

Many diagnostic procedures require that the patient be positioned in a certain way. Often, the nurse needs to assist the patient in maintaining this position throughout the procedure. When positioning the patient, make sure that bony prominences are protected and the patient is as comfortable as possible.

During these procedures, patients are usually conscious, although somewhat drowsy. When needed, the nurse should provide emotional support by explaining the procedure and answering questions. Never underestimate the support provided by simply holding the patient's hand.

Many diagnostic procedures involve the risk of exposure to the patient's blood and body fluids. Universal or standard precautions and medical asepsis should always be maintained. When sterile technique is required, it is the nurse's responsibility to assist in maintaining the sterile field.

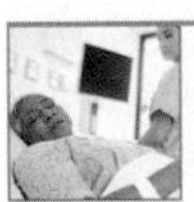

4. List at least five nursing interventions for this diagnosis: *Risk for Injury* with risk factors of the effects of Versed on the sensorium. Include focused assessment data and teaching points.

It is not uncommon for biopsies or specimens to be collected during procedures. The nurse makes sure that each specimen is placed in the appropriate container and labeled

TABLE 34-14 Care Planning

NANDA-I NURSING DIAGNOSIS LABEL WITH NURSING DIAGNOSIS STATEMENT	NURSING OUTCOME CLASSIFICATION (NOC)	NURSING INTERVENTION CLASSIFICATION (NIC)
Readiness for Enhanced Knowledge regarding the diagnostic test purpose, procedure, and care required as evidenced by patient's statement about wanting to know what is wrong	*Knowledge: Health behavior* (1805) Health promotion services (180516)	*Health education* (5510) Determine current health knowledge and lifestyle behaviors of individual, family, or target group.

From Bulechek G, Butcher H, Dochterman J, et al (Eds): *Nursing interventions classification (NIC)*, ed. 6, St. Louis, 2013, Mosby; Moorhead S, Johnson M, Maas M, et al (Eds): *Nursing outcomes classification (NOC)*, ed. 5, St. Louis, 2013, Mosby; NANDA International: *Nursing diagnoses: Definitions and classification, 2012–2014*, West Sussex, England, 2012, Wiley-Blackwell. Reprinted with permission from NANDA International, Inc.

with the patient's identification information. The date and time of the collection should be noted on the label and the laboratory requisition slip.

SPECIMEN COLLECTION

The scheduling and collection of specimens for ordered tests is a primary responsibility of the nurse (Collaboration and Delegation box). Although many of the specimens can be collected by UAP, it remains the nurse's role to ensure that the samples are collected correctly and in a timely manner. Before the start of any procedure, the nurse must ensure that consent forms are signed and the patient has been correctly identified with the correct specimens being collected (Ethical, Legal, and Professional Practice box). Certain types of specimen collection can be performed at home; it is important that the nurse assess the ability of the patient or the caregiver to carry out the collection following the correct technique (Home Care Considerations box).

COLLABORATION AND DELEGATION

Specimen Collection and Diagnostic Tests

- Many specimens are collected by trained unlicensed assistive personnel (UAP). It is important for the nurse to understand which specimen collection can be delegated and to whom (i.e., nursing assistants, laboratory technicians).
- The nurse is responsible for ensuring that the specimen is collected correctly and sent to the laboratory in a timely manner. The nurse documents the appropriate information in the patient record.
- It is important for the nurse to communicate to other members of the health care team when preprocedure medications or treatments may alter the plan of care. For example, if the nurse has administered a preprocedure sedative, the other members of the health care team should be aware of an increased risk for sedation, breathing difficulties, or injury related to falls.
- When multiple tests are ordered, the nurse is responsible for coordinating and scheduling the tests. For example, if a patient is ordered to have a chest x-ray and a colonoscopy, it would be important to wait until after the chest x-ray is completed before administering the preprocedure cathartics.

An essential component of the collection process is obtaining the specimen from the correct patient (Evidence-Based Practice and Informatics box). The National Patient Safety Goals established by The Joint Commission (2014) address patient safety concerns. Goal 1, *identify patients correctly,* directly relates to specimen collection.

Blood Collection

Blood specimens are collected by venipuncture, which accesses a vein; arterial puncture, which accesses an artery; and fingerstick, which collects capillary samples.

ETHICAL, LEGAL, AND PROFESSIONAL PRACTICE

Informed Consent and Communication of Examination Results

- Many diagnostic examinations require informed consent. It is the nurse's responsibility to ensure that the physician has explained the procedure and the consent form is signed before the procedure begins.
- The nurse communicates test and diagnostic examination results to the appropriate health care team members in a timely manner.
- The Health Insurance Portability and Accountability Act (HIPAA) protects the patient by requiring that testing results be shared only with health care professionals who need the information to provide treatment and with individuals designated in writing by the patient. Chapter 11 provides more information on HIPAA.

HOME CARE CONSIDERATIONS

Specimen Collection at Home

It is not uncommon for the patient to be asked to collect a specimen at home and transport it to the health care center. To ensure accurate test results, the nurse should assess the following factors:

- Does the patient understand the collection instructions? They include timing of the collection, cleansing procedures, and contamination precautions.
- Does the patient have the appropriate equipment and containers to collect the specimen?
- How is the specimen to be transported?
- Does it need to be kept warm or cold?
- When does it need to be transported? Immediately or within a few hours?

SAFE PRACTICE ALERT

The nurse must check that the consent form has been signed *before* preprocedure sedatives or narcotics are administered.

EVIDENCE-BASED PRACTICE AND INFORMATICS

National Patient Safety Goals

- Identifying patients correctly continues to be a top National Patient Safety Goal.
- Two patient identifiers are used when collecting blood samples and other specimens for clinical testing.
- The patient's room number or physical location is not used as an identifier.
- Containers used for blood and other specimens are labeled in the presence of the patient.

Modified from The Joint Commission: National Patient Safety Goals, 2014. Retrieved from *www.jointcommission.org/assets/1/6/HAP_NPSG_Chapter_2014.pdf.*

Venipuncture is performed by nurses in some settings but is commonly performed by phlebotomists. This skill is discussed later in this chapter and in Chapter 39, where it is covered in Skill 39-1 in relation to starting a peripheral IV line. Arterial samples are usually collected by a phlebotomist or nurse who has been specially trained in drawing arterial blood. Capillary samples are routinely obtained by the nurse and sometimes by the UAP, according to facility policy.

Venipuncture

Some of the most frequently ordered diagnostic tests require a sample of the patient's blood. This sample is usually obtained by **venipuncture**, insertion of a needle directly into the vein and withdrawal of the needed amount of blood (Diversity Considerations box). When venipuncture is required, the timing of the test may be important. For example, some tests require the patient to fast for a specified time period. If the purpose of the test is to monitor blood levels of a medication, venipuncture must be done at a precise time after the medication is administered.

DIVERSITY CONSIDERATIONS

Life Span

- Obtaining a blood sample from infants and children can be difficult due to the small size of the veins.
- Capillary blood from heelsticks is sometimes used for testing in newborns and infants.
- Elderly people commonly have veins that are fragile, increasing the risk of hemorrhage and bruising after venipuncture.

Morphology

- It is often difficult to visualize and access veins in people who are obese.

! SAFE PRACTICE ALERT

Venipuncture is an invasive procedure that may expose the nurse to blood-borne organisms and contaminated needles. The nurse must wear gloves throughout the procedure and properly dispose of the collection needles in the sharps container immediately after the specimen is obtained.

Other factors that can influence test results include hemoconcentration and hemolysis. Hemoconcentration, which is an increased concentration of red blood cells compared with plasma volume, can result from the tourniquet being applied for too long. The nurse should minimize the time that the tourniquet is on the patient's arm and release it as soon as the specimens are collected.

Hemolysis is the breakdown of red blood cells and the subsequent release of hemoglobin. Hemolysis occurs when the needle used for venipuncture is too small and the red blood cells are damaged as a result of the negative pressure.

Certain blood collection tubes are specific for venipuncture. These tubes are made of glass or plastic and are attached to a needle and a holder. The tubes are sealed with a partial negative vacuum (i.e., the pressure within the tube is less than that outside the tube). The needle is inserted into the vein, with the collection tube attached in the holder; the negative pressure causes blood to flow into the tube to a predetermined point. The rubber stopper seals are different colors based on the additive contained inside. Table 34-15 lists the most common stopper colors, the additive contained in the tube, and the corresponding test. The ordered serum samples must be collected in a specific order to avoid cross-contamination of the additives from one tube to another. The chart lists the tubes in the order of collection. Nurses should be aware of facility policy regarding the collection of blood and containers available.

QSEN FOCUS!

Safety is demonstrated when the nurse values the contributions of standardization.

Although venipuncture is commonly performed by certified phlebotomists, there are situations and times when it is the nurse's responsibility to obtain the blood sample.

QSEN FOCUS!

When collecting blood samples, the nurse uses evidence-based practice and demonstrates knowledge of basic scientific methods and processes.

! SAFE PRACTICE ALERT

It is important to assess the venipuncture site in patients who are on anticoagulant therapy (e.g., Coumadin, heparin, Lovenox) or take aspirin on a daily basis. They are at higher risk for continued bleeding.

Blood Glucose Monitoring Device

Frequent monitoring of blood glucose levels by the nurse or self-monitoring by the patient is easily done with the use of a glucose monitoring device (Home Care Considerations box). A drop of capillary blood is obtained by puncturing the end of a finger with a sterile lancet. A test strip with a specific reagent is placed in the monitoring device and the drop of blood is placed on the test strip. The devices use a light beam or an electric charge to interpret the changes on the test strip (Skill 34-1). The accuracy of the capillary reading can be influenced by hypoxia, markedly abnormal hemoglobin levels, or a glucose level higher than 800 mg/dL (Corbett and Banks, 2013). Most monitors cannot detect glucose levels greater than 600 mg/dL. Test strip factors and contaminants on the patient's hand can also have an impact on the accuracy of capillary readings.

TABLE 34-15 Blood Collection Tubes

STOPPER COLOR	ADDITIVE	SPECIMEN USE
Yellow	Sodium polyanethol sulfonate (SPS)	Blood culture
Light blue	Sodium citrate	Coagulation studies: PT, PTT, and fibrinogen
Red	No additive	Most blood chemistries and serology tests Blood bank testing
Red/black	Silicone	Most blood chemistries and serology tests
Green	Heparin	Stat (immediate) blood chemistries
Lavender	Ethylenediaminetetraacetic acid (EDTA)	Hematology studies
Gray	Potassium oxalate and sodium fluoride *or* Lithium iodoacetate and heparin	Glucose Blood alcohol levels Lactic acid

(From Warekois RS, Robinson R: *Phlebotomy*, ed. 3, St. Louis, 2012, Saunders.)

PT, Prothrombin time; *PTT*, partial thromboplastin time.

HOME CARE CONSIDERATIONS

Blood Glucose Monitoring

Patients with diabetes mellitus are asked to monitor their blood glucose levels on a daily basis at home. It is important to assess their ability to comply with this testing regimen.

- Does the patient understand the procedure and frequency of testing? A return demonstration is helpful in assessing the patient's level of understanding.
- Are there financial concerns regarding testing? Although testing supplies may be expensive, most insurance companies cover the cost. For uninsured patients, there are programs that assist with the costs.
- Is the patient compliant with the testing? Frequent testing can be an essential component of blood glucose control.

Urine Collection

Urinalysis is one of the most frequently ordered diagnostic tests. Urine samples are relatively easy to obtain and are inexpensive. Testing components of urine can provide diagnostic information about renal function, fluid balance, and the existence of infection and other disorders. The nurse is responsible for ensuring that the urine sample is collected accurately. Urine tests can require a one-time voided sample or a timed collection in which all the urine within a specific time period (e.g., 24 hours) is collected and saved.

! SAFE PRACTICE ALERT

It is essential that the nurse maintain standard precautions when collecting urine and stool specimens. These precautions include washing hands before and after collection, wearing gloves during the procedure, and storing the specimen in a biohazardous material container or plastic bag during transport to the laboratory.

A random (clean-voided) specimen is usually adequate for routine urinalysis and random drug testing. Most patients are able to obtain a specimen independently and with minimal direction. The clean specimen can be collected in a new urinal or bedpan or directly into the specimen container.

When a urine sample is needed for culture and sensitivity, a clean-catch (midstream) collection method is used. The clean-catch process requires cleaning of the urethral meatus and surrounding area with antiseptic wipes. The patient begins voiding, allowing the first part of the stream to pass. The container is placed under the stream to collect the urine midstream (Skill 34-2). With a random or clean-catch specimen, it is essential that the specimen be free from fecal matter. If a woman is menstruating, that information should be included on the test requisition slip and communicated to the laboratory. If a patient has an indwelling Foley catheter, a sterile urine specimen can be obtained through the collection port of the catheter tubing.

A timed specimen requires all urine to be collected within a specified time period, which can range from 1 to 24 hours. The patient is instructed to discard the first voiding and then collect all subsequent urine for the time period. Depending on the test ordered, the urine may require refrigeration or a special container with preservatives. If unsure, the nurse should check with the laboratory personnel for specific instructions. Signs should be posted in the bathroom, instructing health care personnel to save all urine for the required time period.

Stool Collection

The amount of stool collected depends on the purpose of the test. A specimen to be tested for occult blood requires only a small amount of stool, which is placed on a **Hemoccult** test strip. A Hemoccult strip contains chemically altered filter paper that changes color when stool containing blood is placed on it. Specimens that are cultured to detect, for example, bacterial or viral infection require only a small amount of stool. Testing for ova and parasites usually requires a larger sample, typically 1 inch of solid stool or 15 to 30 mL of liquid stool (Skill 34-3). Specimens should be obtained from different areas in the stool.

When handling stool, the nurse must always maintain medical asepsis. The nurse wears gloves throughout the specimen collection and makes sure that there is no stool on the outside of the container. After the stool is in the container, the lid is firmly applied, and the container is placed in a biohazard bag. The specimen is transported to the laboratory immediately after collection.

Sputum Collection

Sputum is the mucus that is found in the lungs, bronchial tubes, and trachea in cases of inflammation or infection. A sputum sample is often ordered when an infectious disease, such as pneumonia or tuberculosis, is suspected. Subsequent sputum specimens can be used to evaluate the effectiveness of antibiotic or antiviral therapy. Sputum analysis can identify abnormal cells that may indicate a tumor or malignancy (Nursing Care Guideline: Sputum Specimen Collection box).

The nurse should provide clear instructions to the patient to ensure that the specimen is sputum and not saliva. Normally, the patient is instructed to expectorate the sputum directly into a sterile container. When sputum is being tested for tuberculosis, a special container may be required.

Throat Culture

A throat culture is obtained in a variety of settings. The nurse may collect a culture in a medical office or in the hospital setting. Guidelines for obtaining a throat culture are outlined in the Nursing Care Guideline: Throat Culture box.

Wound Drainage Collection

Wound infections can occur as a complication of surgery, trauma, or underlying disease processes. Infection slows the healing process by prolonging the inflammatory phase of healing, increasing the need for nutrients and energy, and producing enzymes that are damaging to surrounding tissues.

The nurse assesses the wound on a frequent basis, looking for signs of infection. Changes in the appearance and amount of drainage can indicate an underlying wound infection. Obtaining a sample of the drainage for culture is an important step in identifying the presence of an infection and determining appropriate treatment (see Skill 29-3).

INTERVENTIONS AFTER INVASIVE PROCEDURES

Most invasive procedures require ongoing nursing assessment and care. After the procedure, it is important to continue to monitor the patient's vital signs, airway, and oxygenation status. There are specific responsibilities for postprocedure care, depending on the type of procedure. Table 34-16 describes postprocedure care and possible com plications for the various types of endoscopy discussed in Table 34-10.

Needle aspirations require patient positioning and special care during and after the procedure. Table 34-17 summarizes the essential aspects that the nurse should consider. For detailed information on the care during and after specific procedures, the nurse should consult the facility procedure book or a diagnostic testing handbook.

COMMUNICATION OF RESULTS

A primary responsibly of the nurse is communicating the test results to the ordering health care provider in a timely manner. The Joint Commission's (2014) second National Patient Safety Goal is to *improve the effectiveness of communication among caregivers*. Promptly ommunicating test results to the right staff person is part of this goal.

QSEN FOCUS!

Informatics is used when technology and information management tools are applied to support safe processes of care, such as communication of laboratory and diagnostic test results to the appropriate care providers.

NURSING CARE GUIDELINE

Sputum Specimen Collection

Background

- A sputum specimen is a sample of mucus used for diagnostic testing to look for specific microorganisms and to determine optimal treatment options.
- Unless suctioning techniques are used, obtaining a sputum specimen can be delegated to unlicensed assistive personnel (UAP) who have been educated and trained in the procedure, according to the patient's care plan, the nurse's judgment, or the facility policy and procedure.
- UAP education includes appropriate collection and handling of the specimen and reporting of procedural or physiologic difficulties.

Procedural Concerns

- The specimen cup is sterile so that bacteria from the environment are not introduced into the sample. Do *not* touch the inside of the cup. Wear clean gloves when handling the sputum cup.
- Obtain the sample first thing in the morning if possible.
- Provide oral care (see Chapter 27, Skill 27-6).
- Instruct the patient to breathe deeply and cough to expectorate sputum into the cup.
- If a sample cannot be obtained in this manner, alternative procedures may be used, for which an order from the primary care provider may be needed. The following are alternative methods:
  - Expectorants
  - Chest physiotherapy
  - Aerosols or nebulizers
  - Suctioning, using tracheostomy suctioning or nasotracheal suctioning (see Skill 38-1) or a sputum trap
- Obtain 2 to 10 mL of sputum for routine testing to ensure accurate results.
- Provide oral care.
- Label the container, place it in a biohazard bag, and transport the sample to the laboratory.

Documentation Concerns

- Document assessment of the sample for quantity, color, type, odor, and consistency of the sputum.
- Document assistance required by the patient or caregiver in obtaining the sample.
- Describe the patient's reaction to the procedure.
- Note that the order has been completed.

NURSING CARE GUIDELINE

Throat Culture

Background

- A throat culture is used for diagnostic testing to look for specific microorganisms, to determine whether an infection exists and the source of that infection, and to determine optimal treatment options.
- Obtaining a throat culture should *not* be delegated to unlicensed assistive personnel.

Procedural Concerns

- Wear gloves.
- The swab end of the Culturette is sterile. Touch only the potentially infected areas of the oropharynx and tonsils with the swab to avoid cross-contamination.
- Depress the tongue, and use a light to see the interior of the mouth and throat. Run the swab over reddened or draining areas.
- The procedure may cause gagging, which can be alleviated by several measures:
  - Instructing the patient to sit upright and say "ahhh"
  - Placing the swab off center
  - Swabbing quickly
- Place the swab in its tube, and seal it immediately. Specialized chemicals in the tube promote the growth of microorganisms.
- Label the container, place it in the biohazard bag, and transport it to the laboratory.

Documentation Concerns

- Document assessment of the throat, including swelling, redness, presence and color of discharge, and pustules.
- Document that the culture has been completed.
- Note pain, discomfort, or other patient concerns.

Evidence-Based Practice

- Rapid antigen detection testing (RADT) has been developed for use in outpatient and emergency department settings. The test is performed in the manner described in the Procedural Concerns section and does not require a wait time to retrieve results.
- There is slightly conflicting evidence regarding the validity of the results, but most studies have found a high correlation for positive and negative results. A patient with a positive RADT result should begin treatment without having a follow-up culture sent to the laboratory. If the RADT result is negative and clinical symptoms suggest pharyngitis, the primary care provider may consider ordering a follow-up throat culture to be sent to the laboratory and may withhold treatment until the results are received (Al-Najjar and Uduman, 2008; Llor, Calviño, Hernández, et al., 2009; Sarikaya, Aktas, Ay, et al., 2010).

TABLE 34-16 Care After Endoscopy and Possible Complications

EXAMINATION	POSTPROCEDURE CARE	POSSIBLE COMPLICATIONS
Arthroscopy	Assess the neurovascular status of the affected limb, including pain, pallor, paresthesia, paralysis, and pulse. Elevate the extremity and apply ice. Administer analgesics PRN. Instruct the patient to avoid alcohol for 24 hr.	Thrombophlebitis Compartment syndrome
Bronchoscopy	Keep patient NPO until swallow, gag, and cough reflexes have returned. Provide gargles for mild pharyngitis. Monitor respiratory status, including lung sounds and sputum. Maintain oxygen as ordered.	Shock Bleeding from biopsy Hypoxemia Bronchospasm/laryngospasm Infection Pneumothorax
Colonoscopy, sigmoidoscopy	Monitor vital signs until the patient is fully awake. Encourage a liquid diet or light meal for the first 6 hr after the procedure. Observe stools for visible blood. Instruct the patient to report any abdominal pain.	Perforation of bowel Hypotension Hemorrhage
Cystoscopy	Monitor voiding patterns. Inspect urine for blood or clots. Instruct the patient that frequency, dysuria, and pink to light red urine are common after the procedure.	Bladder edema or perforation Infection Hematuria Urinary retention
Esophagogastroduodenoscopy	Maintain NPO until the gag reflex returns. Position the patient on the left side until fully awake to prevent aspiration.	Perforation Bleeding Aspiration Infection

TABLE 34-17 Care During and After Needle Aspirations and Biopsies

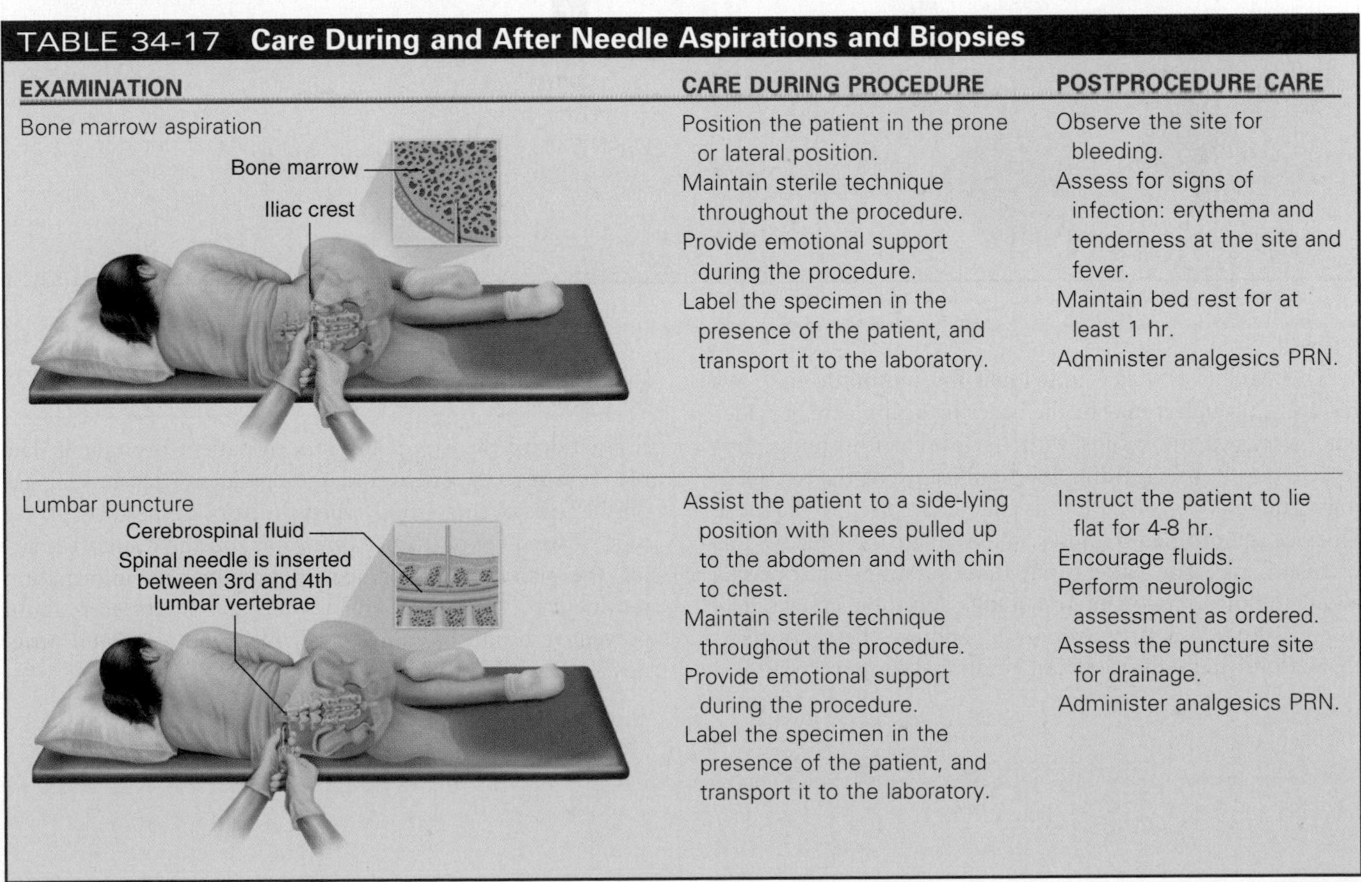

EXAMINATION	CARE DURING PROCEDURE	POSTPROCEDURE CARE
Bone marrow aspiration	Position the patient in the prone or lateral position. Maintain sterile technique throughout the procedure. Provide emotional support during the procedure. Label the specimen in the presence of the patient, and transport it to the laboratory.	Observe the site for bleeding. Assess for signs of infection: erythema and tenderness at the site and fever. Maintain bed rest for at least 1 hr. Administer analgesics PRN.
Lumbar puncture	Assist the patient to a side-lying position with knees pulled up to the abdomen and with chin to chest. Maintain sterile technique throughout the procedure. Provide emotional support during the procedure. Label the specimen in the presence of the patient, and transport it to the laboratory.	Instruct the patient to lie flat for 4-8 hr. Encourage fluids. Perform neurologic assessment as ordered. Assess the puncture site for drainage. Administer analgesics PRN.

Continued

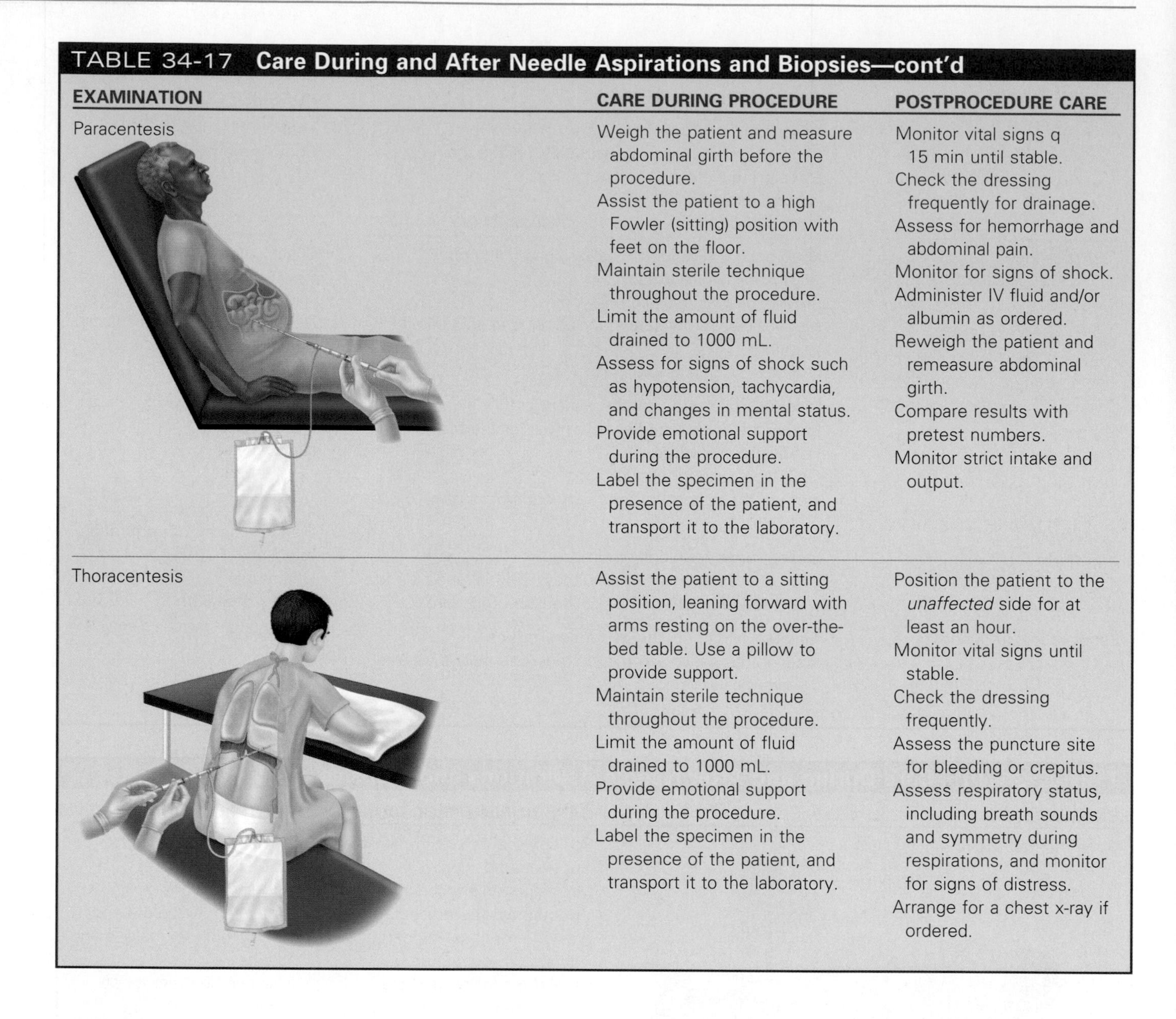

TABLE 34-17 Care During and After Needle Aspirations and Biopsies—cont'd

EXAMINATION	CARE DURING PROCEDURE	POSTPROCEDURE CARE
Paracentesis	Weigh the patient and measure abdominal girth before the procedure. Assist the patient to a high Fowler (sitting) position with feet on the floor. Maintain sterile technique throughout the procedure. Limit the amount of fluid drained to 1000 mL. Assess for signs of shock such as hypotension, tachycardia, and changes in mental status. Provide emotional support during the procedure. Label the specimen in the presence of the patient, and transport it to the laboratory.	Monitor vital signs q 15 min until stable. Check the dressing frequently for drainage. Assess for hemorrhage and abdominal pain. Monitor for signs of shock. Administer IV fluid and/or albumin as ordered. Reweigh the patient and remeasure abdominal girth. Compare results with pretest numbers. Monitor strict intake and output.
Thoracentesis	Assist the patient to a sitting position, leaning forward with arms resting on the over-the-bed table. Use a pillow to provide support. Maintain sterile technique throughout the procedure. Limit the amount of fluid drained to 1000 mL. Provide emotional support during the procedure. Label the specimen in the presence of the patient, and transport it to the laboratory.	Position the patient to the *unaffected* side for at least an hour. Monitor vital signs until stable. Check the dressing frequently. Assess the puncture site for bleeding or crepitus. Assess respiratory status, including breath sounds and symmetry during respirations, and monitor for signs of distress. Arrange for a chest x-ray if ordered.

The patient is a key individual in communicating test results. Although it may be the ordering health care provider who discusses the results with the patient, the nurse may receive questions regarding the significance of the test findings. The tests described in this chapter are used to diagnose illnesses, determine prognoses, and evaluate the effectiveness of treatments. The patient may have questions or concerns about the meaning of the test results and their impact. The nurse is in a unique position to address these concerns through further education and emotional support.

EVALUATION

Evaluation of the care plan for each patient is ongoing. The plan of care for a patient undergoing diagnostic tests changes on the basis of the setting, when the tests are performed, the type of tests, the postprocedure care, and the results. Updating the plan of care to include teaching and information pertinent to the results enables the patient to learn about preventive health measures, available treatments, and prognoses for specific diseases.

SKILL 34-1 Blood Glucose Testing

PURPOSE

- Monitoring glucose levels in blood
- Monitoring the response to insulin therapy
- Gauging the amount of insulin needed for a sliding scale

RESOURCES

- Sterile lancet or automatic lancing device
- Blood glucose testing reagent strips
- Blood glucose meter
- Soap and warm water or alcohol wipes
- 2- × 2-inch gauze sponges
- Adhesive bandage
- Sharps container
- Clean gloves
- Personal protective equipment (PPE) as needed

COLLABORATION AND DELEGATION

- Blood glucose testing may be delegated to unlicensed assistive personnel (UAP) without a nurse's assistance after appropriate training and certification in accordance with state and institutional guidelines.
- UAP should report the following:
  - Completion of the procedure
  - Timely notification of results to professional personnel
  - Difficulties in the procedure or other concerns verbalized by the patient
- UAP should be instructed in the following:
  - Timing of the procedure according to orders (frequently before meals and at bedtime)
  - Avoidance of extremities on which cuts or bruises are observed
  - Preferred sites of fingers or forearms, depending on the testing meter
- Specificities of techniques such as milking, massaging, using alcohol wipes, and not wasting the first drop vary for different glucometers. Check the manufacturer's instructions for further information.

SPECIAL CIRCUMSTANCES

1. **Assess:** Is there difficulty obtaining the specimen?
   Intervention: Warming the extremity increases vasodilation.
2. **Assess:** Is the reagent strip discolored?
   Intervention: Obtain a new bottle and strip.
   - Check the expiration date.
   - Label the date of opening with initials.
   - Calibrate the meter.
   - Always cap the container immediately after taking the strip, because humidity and light can affect strip validity.
3. **Assess:** Is the result out of normal range for the patient?
   Intervention: Assess the patient; troubleshoot the meter.
   - Ensure that hands were washed.
   - Assess for signs and symptoms of hypoglycemia or hyperglycemia.
   - Verify the time of the last meal or insulin dose.
   - Ensure that an adequate sample was obtained.
   - Check that strip codes match the meter.
   - Verify the last calibration. Check the meter with control samples.
   - Make sure that batteries are charged.

PREPROCEDURE

I. Check PCP orders and the patient care plan.
Knowledge of patient-specific orders is critical for safe patient care.

II. Gather supplies and equipment.
Preparing for the patient encounter saves time and promotes patient trust.

III. Perform hand hygiene.
Frequent hand hygiene prevents the spread of microorganisms.

IV. Maintain standard precautions.
Use of the correct personal protective equipment (PPE) is required whenever contact with bodily fluids is possible, to reduce the transfer of pathogens.

V. Introduce yourself.
Initial communication establishes the role of the nurse and begins a professional relationship.

VI. Provide for patient privacy.
It is important to maintain patient dignity.

VII. Identify the patient, using two identifiers.
Identifying a patient involves scanning barcodes or comparing the patient's stated name and birthdate to information on the patient's wristband or health record. The correct person must receive the correct treatment.

VIII. Explain the procedure to the patient.
The nurse has a responsibility to inform a patient before initiating care. Information may ease patient anxiety and facilitate cooperation.

PROCEDURE

Blood Glucose Testing

Follow preprocedure steps I through VIII.

1. Raise the bed (working height) and lower the side rails as appropriate and safe.
Proper positioning of equipment prevents provider discomfort and possible injury.

2. Select the site, which depends on the meter:
- **a.** Use the middle or ring finger, along either side about halfway between the end of the finger and the first joint.
- **b.** Follow the manufacturer's instructions for other sites.
- **c.** Avoid nonintact skin.

Correct site selection promotes patient comfort, provides accurate results, and prevents nerve, skin, or bone injury.

3. Apply clean gloves.
Use of gloves prevents the spread of microorganisms and protects caregivers from injury.

4. Remove the reagent strip from the container and recap:
- **a.** Ensure that the strip is not expired.
- **b.** Ensure that the strip is intact.
- **c.** Check that the code on the container matches the code programmed in the meter.
- **d.** Follow the manufacturer's instructions on when to place the strip in the glucometer.

Performing the procedure properly ensures accurate results.

5. Cleanse the site: Have the patient wash hands with soap and warm water, or wipe the finger with an alcohol wipe. Allow the finger to dry thoroughly before testing. Lower the hand below the heart to facilitate capillary blood flow.
Disinfection prevents microorganisms or other particulates from contaminating the site. Warm water increases vasodilation, and thorough drying prevents contamination of the sample.

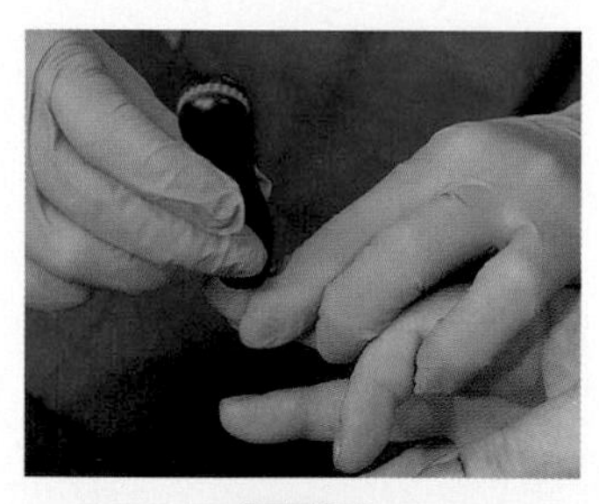
STEP 6

6. Quickly puncture the capillary site. Use a lancing device, following the manufacturer's instructions and facility policy and procedures.
Correct technique reduces pain, promotes patient comfort, and promotes safe, quality patient care.

7. Using a 2 × 2 gauze pad, wipe off the first drop of blood and any remaining alcohol.
This method ensures accurate results because the first drop of blood may contain higher amounts of serous fluids, and alcohol may change the results.

8. Place blood on reagent test strip according to the manufacturer's instructions.
Following instructions ensures accurate results. A full sample is required.

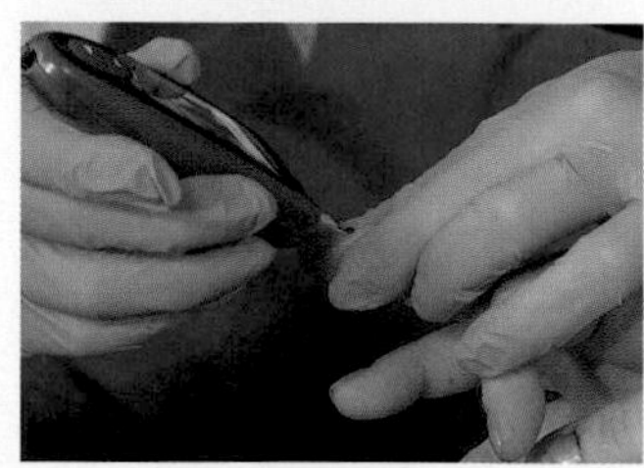
STEP 8

9. The meter calculates results and displays them when complete.
Automatic computation ensures accurate results. The time needed to produce results depends on the manufacturer; most meters are automatically timed.

10. Apply gauze and pressure to the site.
The risk of bleeding and complications is decreased.

11. Discard the lancet into the sharps container.
Proper disposal prevents an accidental needlestick.

12. Check the site; apply an adhesive bandage if needed.
Covering the site decreases the risk of bleeding and complications.

13. Remove gloves.

Follow postprocedure steps I through VI.

POSTPROCEDURE

I. Return the bed to its lowest position, raise the top side rails, and verify that the call light is within reach of the patient.
Precautions are taken to maintain patient safety. Top side rails aid in positioning and turning. Raising four side rails is considered a restraint.

II. Assess for additional patient needs and state the time of your expected return.
Meeting patient needs and offering self promote patient satisfaction and build trust.

III. Properly dispose of PPE.
Gloves, gowns, and masks must be appropriately discarded to prevent the spread of microorganisms.

IV. Clean equipment if it was in contact with the patient; see specific manufacturer instructions.
Disinfection eliminates most microorganisms from inanimate objects.

V. Perform hand hygiene.
Frequent hand hygiene prevents the spread of infection.

VI. Document the date, time, assessment, procedure, and patient's response to the procedure.
Accurate documentation is essential to communicate patient care and to provide legal evidence of care.

SKILL 34-2 Urine Specimen Collection

PURPOSE

- Collecting a urine sample for diagnostic testing
- Testing a urine sample for specific substances
- Determining whether specific microorganisms are growing in the urinary system
- Determining the optimal treatment options for urinary system infections

RESOURCES

- Appropriate collection container:
  - Sterile specimen cup
  - Nonsterile, large, 24-hour collection container (may contain a chemical preservative)
- Diagnostic test reagent strips (specified for substance testing)
- Washbasin with ice (for 24-hour collection)
- Syringe with Luer-Lok tip or blunt, needleless cannula (for catheter collection)
- Antiseptic/disinfectant towelettes
- Toilet paper
- Biohazard bag for laboratory transport
- Patient identification labels
- Clean, nonsterile gloves
- Personal protective equipment (PPE) as needed

COLLABORATION AND DELEGATION

- Voided urine specimen collection (not collection from a catheter) may be delegated to unlicensed assistive personnel (UAP) without a nurse's assistance after appropriate training in accordance with state and facility guidelines.
- UAP should report the following to the nurse:
  - Completion of the procedure
  - Sample color, odor, and consistency
  - Blood, mucus, or foul odors in the specimen, or any breaks in specimen collection technique
  - Difficulties in performing the procedure or other concerns verbalized by the patient
- UAP should be instructed in the following:
  - Timing of the specimen collection
  - Sterile technique
  - Midstream clean-catch process
  - Appropriate documentation

SPECIAL CIRCUMSTANCES

1. **Assess:** Is a random urine sample being obtained by using the nonsterile or clean-catch technique?
   Intervention: Document which technique was used; contamination may have occurred, causing inaccurate or unexpected results.
2. **Assess:** Was there a urine specimen that missed collection or a spilled urine specimen during a 24-hour collection period?
   Intervention: Document the problem, and start the procedure over.
3. **Assess:** Is a 24-hour urine collection being obtained from an indwelling catheter?
   Intervention: Replace the drainage collection bag at the start of the procedure, and keep the bag on ice.
4. **Assess:** Is the test strip for reagent testing discolored or otherwise not intact?
   Intervention: Obtain a new container of test strips:
   - Check the expiration date on the container.
   - Label the container with the date of opening and your initials.
   - Always cap the container immediately after removing a strip; humidity and light can affect strip validity.

PREPROCEDURE

I. Check PCP orders and the patient care plan.
Knowledge of patient-specific orders is critical for safe patient care.

II. Gather supplies and equipment.
Preparing for the patient encounter saves time and promotes patient trust.

III. Perform hand hygiene.
Frequent hand hygiene prevents the spread of microorganisms.

IV. Maintain standard precautions.
Use of the correct personal protective equipment (PPE) is required whenever contact with bodily fluids is possible, to reduce the transfer of pathogens.

V. Introduce yourself.
Initial communication establishes the role of the nurse and begins a professional relationship.

VI. Provide for patient privacy.
It is important to maintain patient dignity.

VII. Identify the patient, using two identifiers.
Identifying a patient involves scanning barcodes or comparing the patient's stated name and birthdate to information on the patient's wristband or health record. The correct person must receive the correct treatment.

VIII. Explain the procedure to the patient.
The nurse has a responsibility to inform a patient before initiating care. Information may ease patient anxiety and facilitate cooperation.

PROCEDURE

Urinalysis (Clean Catch): Female

Follow preprocedure steps I through VIII.

1. Assist the patient to the bathroom, onto a bedside commode, or onto a new bedpan.
Prepare the patient for the procedure in a safe and proper environment. Precautions must be taken to maintain patient safety and prevent provider injury.
2. If the patient will be collecting the sample, have her wash her hands.
Handwashing prevents microorganisms from contaminating the specimen and ensures accurate results.
3. Remove the lid from a sterile specimen cup, and place it on a flat surface with the inside of the lid facing up.
Proper technique avoids contamination of the specimen with microorganisms and ensures accurate results.
4. Instruct the patient to separate the labia with the second and third fingers on the non-dominant hand.
Spreading the labia exposes the urinary meatus and prevents microorganisms from contaminating the specimen; it ensures more accurate results.
5. Have the patient cleanse the perineum using an antiseptic wipe or swab while keeping the labia spread (depending on the facility-provided kit or supplies). Instruct the patient to use the following method:
   - **a.** Wipe from the front to the back (toward the rectum)
   - **b.** Use a new wipe or swab for each wipe
   - **c.** Wipe one side of the labia, then cleanse the other side, and then the center of the perineum

   Proper cleaning should be used to prevent the spread of microorganisms and to prevent microorganisms from contaminating the specimen. Washing should be done from the least contaminated area to the most contaminated area (i.e., from the area of fewer microorganisms to the area of more microorganisms) to ensure accurate results.
6. While keeping the labia spread, instruct the patient to urinate a small amount but not into the specimen cup.
Urinating a small amount before taking the specimen flushes contaminants from the urethra and prevents microorganisms from contaminating the specimen, ensuring more accurate results.
7. Instruct the patient to place the cup into the urine stream; the cup must not touch skin or the perineum.
This method prevents microorganisms from contaminating the specimen and ensures accurate results.
8. Collect 90 to 120 mL of urine if possible. A minimum of 30 mL is needed for some tests.
Routine urine testing requires at least 30 mL to ensure accurate results. Check with the laboratory for amounts necessary for specific tests.
9. Instruct the patient to remove the cup from the urine stream before she has finished urinating.
Avoiding collection of the last quantity of urine eliminates contamination from skin flora.
10. Instruct the patient to finish urinating and immediately cap the container.
Completing urination avoids complications from not emptying the bladder. Immediate capping of the container prevents microorganisms from contaminating the specimen and ensures accurate results.

11. The nurse should handle the container with gloves. Wipe and dry the outside of the container with a paper towel.
    Precautions must be taken to protect caregivers and prevent the spread of microorganisms.
12. Label the container according to facility policy and procedure. A note should be placed on label if patient is menstruating.
    Proper labeling of samples prevents adverse events and medical errors.
13. Place the container in a biohazard bag. Remove gloves and perform hand hygiene.
    Precautions must be taken to protect caregivers and prevent the spread of microorganisms.
14. Transport the specimen to the laboratory. If it is not possible to get the specimen to the laboratory within 15 minutes of collection, place the specimen in the refrigerator.
    Many tests are time or temperature sensitive; urine tests are especially temperature sensitive. Refrigeration slows microorganism growth.
15. Communicate in a report and in the chart or electronic health record that the test is complete.
    Communicate essential information to provide safe, timely, and efficient quality patient care and to prevent adverse events and medical errors.

Follow postprocedure steps I through VI.

Urinalysis (Clean Catch): Male

Follow preprocedure steps I through VIII.

1. Follow procedure steps 1 through 3 in the Urinalysis (Clean Catch): Female section.
2. If the patient has not been circumcised, have him retract the foreskin and *not* release it.
   Retracting the foreskin exposes the urinary meatus and prevents microorganisms from contaminating the specimen, ensuring more accurate results.
3. Have the patient cleanse the top of the penis using an antiseptic wipe or swab (depending on the facility-provided kit or supplies). Instruct the patient to use the following method:
   a. Clean from the meatus to the base of the glans using a circular outward motion
   b. Use a new wipe or swab for each cleansing
   c. Repeat the cleansing a total of three times
   Proper cleaning should be used to prevent the spread of microorganisms and to prevent microorganisms from contaminating the specimen. Washing should be done from the least contaminated area to the most contaminated area (i.e., from the area of fewer microorganisms to the area of more microorganisms) to ensure accurate results.

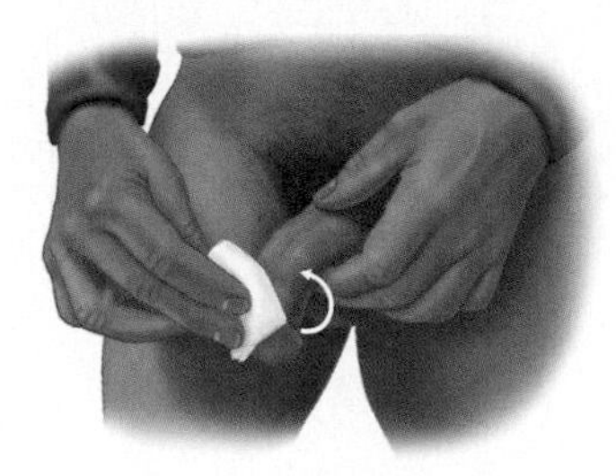

STEP 3a

4. Instruct the patient to urinate a small amount but *not* into the specimen cup.
   Urinating a small amount before obtaining the specimen flushes contaminants from the urethra and prevents microorganisms from contaminating the specimen, ensuring more accurate results.
5. Instruct the patient to place the cup into the urine stream; the cup must *not* touch skin or the penis.
   This prevents microorganisms from contaminating the specimen and ensures accurate results.
6. Collect 90 to 120 mL of urine if possible. A minimum of 30 mL is needed for some tests.
   Routine urine testing requires at least 30 mL to ensure accurate results. Check with the laboratory for amounts necessary for specific tests.
7. Instruct the patient to remove the cup from the urine stream *before* he has finished urinating.
   Avoiding collection of the last quantity of urine eliminates contamination from skin flora.
8. Instruct the patient to finish urinating and then immediately cap the container.
   Completing urination avoids complications from not emptying the bladder. Immediate capping of the container prevents microorganisms from contaminating the specimen and ensures accurate results.
9. Follow procedure steps 11 through 15 in the Urinalysis (Clean Catch): Female section.

Follow postprocedure steps I through VI.

Urinalysis: Quick Reagent Strips and Urine Culture and Sensitivity

Follow preprocedure steps I through VIII.

1. Follow procedure steps 2 through 8 in the Urinalysis (Clean Catch): Female section.
2. Depending on the test, do *not* allow the cup to touch the skin, perineum, or penis. Collect an appropriate quantity of urine. Depending on the test and results, the sample may be sent for a urinalysis and culture and sensitivity. The total amount of urine needed is 13 to 35 mL:
   a. Urinalysis requires 10 to 30 mL.
   b. Urine culture and sensitivity requires 3 to 5 mL.
   Avoid touching the patient with the cup to prevent microorganisms from contaminating the specimen and to ensure accurate results. Accurate testing requires the minimum quantity specified.
3. Follow procedure steps 10 through 11 in the Urinalysis (Clean Catch): Female section. For urinalysis using a quick reagent strip proceed to step 4. For urine culture and sensitivity skip to step 6.

For Urinalysis Using Quick Reagent Strips

4. Obtain a quick reagent test strip for the ordered test, and dip it in the urine sample. Follow the manufacturer's instructions on the test strip container for the amount of time to wait between immersing the strip in urine and reading the result, the minimum quantity of urine that must be used for accuracy, and result interpretation.
   The use of proper equipment for a specific test ensures the accuracy of the reading.
5. Compare the colors on the quick reagent strip with those from the testing bottle after the designated time for results has elapsed. Document the results, and notify the primary care provider (PCP) if needed.
   Obtaining a quick and accurate test result facilitates diagnostic decision making. Proper record keeping is essential because it communicates important information needed for patient care and provides legal evidence of care. Ensure quality patient care by communicating promptly with the PCP if needed.

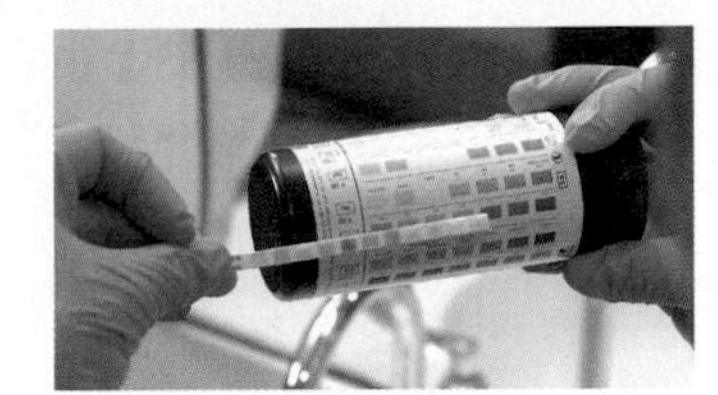

STEP 5

For Urine Culture and Sensitivity

6. Transfer the urine to a special culture collection container. The method used depends on facility policies and procedures. Follow the manufacturer's instructions.
7. Follow procedure steps 12 through 15 in the Urinalysis (Clean Catch): Female section.

Follow postprocedure steps I through VI.

Foley Catheter Urine Specimen Collection

Follow preprocedure steps I through VIII.

1. Ensure that the urine in the tubing is emptied into the drainage bag.
   Emptying the tubing provides an accurate baseline assessment, and it prevents microorganisms from contaminating the specimen, which can interfere with obtaining accurate results.
2. Clamp the catheter tubing below the specimen port.
   Fresh urine will collect but not drain into the bag. Microorganisms grow quickly in urine at room temperature.
3. Wait 10 to 30 minutes to allow urine to accumulate.
   The specimen cannot be obtained from the drainage bag because the urine in the bag is not sterile. Allowing urine to accumulate in the upper part of the tubing ensures a sterile specimen.
4. When the appropriate amount of urine has accumulated, begin collecting the specimen using aseptic technique.
   Proper aseptic technique should be used to prevent the spread of microorganisms and ensure accurate results.

5. If there is a sufficient length of catheter tubing to work with from the anchoring device to the injection port, leave the catheter anchored; otherwise, remove the catheter from the anchoring device, and be careful when working with it to avoid inadvertent dislodgement.
   Avoiding inadvertent dislodgement of the catheter maintains patient safety and comfort.
6. Place a waterproof pad under the catheter at the injection port.
   The pad protects linens and maintains skin integrity.
7. Put on clean gloves. Clean the specimen port or injection port with an antiseptic wipe in accordance with facility policy and procedure.
   Proper antiseptic procedures should be used to prevent the spread of microorganisms and reduce the risk of infections.

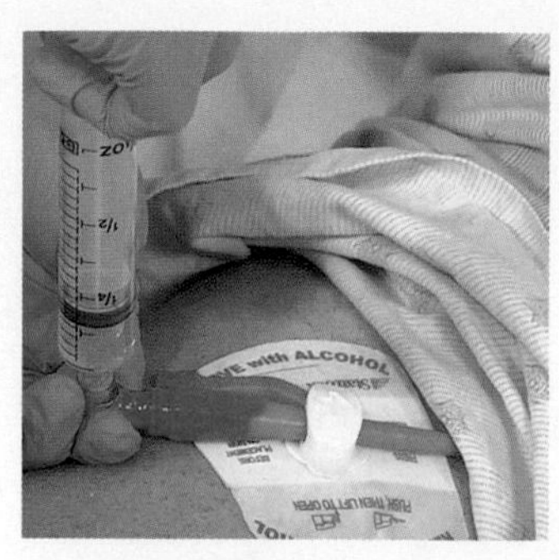

STEP 8

8. Connect a syringe to the specimen port:
   a. If a needleless catheter system (Luer-Lok) is in place, twist a syringe onto the port.
   b. If an access port is in place, insert a blunt, needleless cannula at a 30-degree angle with the bevel in the direction of the bladder.
   c. Pull back on the syringe plunger to obtain a sample.
   The specimen port and needleless syringe are used to prevent possible provider injury. A 30-degree angle allows urine to be withdrawn easily and prevents puncture of the catheter and specimen port.
9. Withdraw the syringe, and transfer the urine directly from the syringe to an appropriate sterile collection container.
   Proper technique avoids contamination of the specimen from microorganisms and ensures accurate results.
10. Remove the clamp, and secure the catheter before leaving the bedside.
    Removing the clamp allows drainage to occur by gravity. Securing the catheter reduces the risk of damage to urinary tissues and inadvertent removal of the catheter.
11. Follow procedure steps 12 through 15 in the Urinalysis (Clean Catch): Female section.

Follow postprocedure steps I through VI.

24-Hour Urine Specimen Collection

Follow preprocedure steps I through VIII.

1. Label a special 24-hour collection container according to facility policy and procedure.
   Proper labeling of samples prevents adverse events and medical errors.
2. Ensure that all samples are collected:
   a. Place a sign in the patient's bathroom and on the patient's chart or a notation in the electronic health record.
   b. Remind the patient of the necessity of collecting all urine samples for the 24-hour period.
   c. Communicate testing in a report at the end of the shift and in the chart or electronic health record.
   Proper communication of instructions enhances patient cooperation, prevents adverse events and medical errors, and ensures accurate results. Proper record keeping is essential because it communicates important information needed for safe, efficient, and timely quality patient care and provides legal evidence of care.
3. Prepare for the procedure by placing a basin filled with ice in the bathroom or ensuring that a designated refrigerator is available for storing the specimens. Collect the urine in a new container (i.e., urinal, graduated hat, or bedpan). Always wear clean gloves when handling urine specimens.
   Urine tests are especially temperature sensitive; refrigeration slows microorganism growth and ensures accurate results.
4. If possible, begin the test in the morning:
   a. Have the patient void. Document the quantity, color, and clarity of urine for the first morning void.
   b. Discard the first morning void.
   c. Note the time of day that the test was started.
   Discard the first morning void to provide an accurate baseline assessment; the urine in the first morning void was produced before the 24-hour test period.

5. Immediately empty each specimen completely into a special collection container:
   a. Do *not* splash the urine.
   b. Depending on the test, separate containers may be required; document the time and quantity on each container.
   c. Document the time, quantity, color, and clarity of the urine for each void in the chart or electronic health record. Record the quantity on the patient's flow sheet if on intake and output.
   d. Ensure that the specimen is labeled and on ice or refrigerated.

   Splashing causes loss of specimen volume, which may result in inaccurate results. Proper labeling of samples prevents adverse events and medical errors. Refrigeration or use of ice decreases the growth of microorganisms.
6. At the end of the 24-hour collection time:
   a. Obtain the last urine sample.
   b. Remove the signs from the patient bathroom and from the patient chart or the notation in the electronic health record.
   c. Communicate that the testing is complete in a report and in the patient's health record.

   Proper communication of instructions prevents adverse events and medical errors and ensures accurate results. Proper record keeping is essential because it communicates important information needed for safe, efficient, and timely quality patient care and provides legal evidence of care.
7. Follow steps 12 through 15 in the Urinalysis (Clean Catch): Female section.

Follow postprocedure steps I through VI.

POSTPROCEDURE

I. Return the bed to its lowest position, raise the top side rails, and verify that the call light is within reach of the patient.
Precautions are taken to maintain patient safety. Top side rails aid in positioning and turning. Raising four side rails is considered a restraint.

II. Assess for additional patient needs and state the time of your expected return.
Meeting patient needs and offering self promote patient satisfaction and build trust.

III. Properly dispose of PPE.
Gloves, gowns, and masks must be appropriately discarded to prevent the spread of microorganisms.

IV. Clean equipment if it was in contact with the patient; see specific manufacturer instructions.
Disinfection eliminates most microorganisms from inanimate objects.

V. Perform hand hygiene.
Frequent hand hygiene prevents the spread of infection.

VI. Document the date, time, assessment, procedure, and patient's response to the procedure.
Accurate documentation is essential to communicate patient care and to provide legal evidence of care.

SKILL 34-3 Stool Specimen Collection

PURPOSE

- Use for diagnostic testing
- Testing for specific agents
- Determining the specific microorganisms growing in the gastrointestinal system
- Determining optimal treatment options for gastrointestinal system infections
- Testing for blood in the gastrointestinal system

RESOURCES

- Stool collection container with a lid (for stool culture)
- Hemoccult cardboard test slide and developing solution per facility policy (for occult blood)
- New bedpan, graduated specimen hat, or bedside commode
- Tongue blades
- Biohazard bag for laboratory transport
- Patient identification labels
- Clean gloves and other personal protective equipment (PPE) as needed.

COLLABORATION AND DELEGATION

- Collecting a stool specimen and testing stool for occult blood may be delegated to unlicensed assistive personnel (UAP) without a nurse's assistance after appropriate training in accordance with state and facility guidelines.
- UAP should report any of the following to the nurse:
  - Positive results of occult blood (immediate report to nurse)
  - Completion of the procedure
  - Sample color, odor, and consistency
  - Difficulties encountered in the procedure or other concerns verbalized by the patient
- UAP should be instructed in the following:
  - Timing of the procedure
  - Necessity of ensuring that the sample is free of other bodily fluids and toilet paper
  - Appropriate documentation

EVIDENCE-BASED PRACTICE

When patients are being tested for occult blood with a guaiac-based fecal occult blood test (gFOBT), it is important that "patients … adhere to a 72-hour diet free of … [foods such as] meat, poultry, fish, and leafy green vegetables before testing to avoid false-positive results. Medications … , such as aspirin and antiinflammatory agents, iron and oxidizing drugs, and potassium preparations, may cause false-positive results, and ascorbic acid use may result in false-negative results" (Jessee, 2010, p. 134).

SPECIAL CIRCUMSTANCES

1. **Assess:** Has measurement of intake and output been ordered?
   Intervention: Two graduated collection hats are needed in the patient's bathroom: one for urinary collection and measurement and the other for collection of stool samples.
2. **Assess:** Is the sample contaminated with bodily fluids, toilet paper, or toilet water?
   Intervention: Obtain a new sample.
3. **Assess:** Are multiple specimens required? The test is often ordered in sets of three.
   Intervention: Communicate and document information:
   - Place a sign in the patient's bathroom and on the patient's health record.
   - Remind the patient that samples are needed, and provide other procedural information.
   - Communicate information in the report and the patient's health record.
   - Ensure that valid samples are not discarded.
   - Remove the signs when the last sample has been obtained.
4. **Assess:** Is the patient on antimicrobial therapy?
   Intervention: Note the medication and dose on the laboratory slip; medication may affect test results.

PREPROCEDURE

I. Check PCP orders and the patient care plan.
Knowledge of patient-specific orders is critical for safe patient care.

II. Gather supplies and equipment.
Preparing for the patient encounter saves time and promotes patient trust.

III. Perform hand hygiene.
Frequent hand hygiene prevents the spread of microorganisms.

IV. Maintain standard precautions.
Use of the correct personal protective equipment (PPE) is required whenever contact with bodily fluids is possible, to reduce the transfer of pathogens.

V. Introduce yourself.
Initial communication establishes the role of the nurse and begins a professional relationship.

VI. Provide for patient privacy.
It is important to maintain patient dignity.

VII. Identify the patient, using two identifiers.
Identifying a patient involves scanning barcodes or comparing the patient's stated name and birthdate to information on the patient's wristband or health record. The correct person must receive the correct treatment.

VIII. Explain the procedure to the patient.
The nurse has a responsibility to inform a patient before initiating care. Information may ease patient anxiety and facilitate cooperation.

PROCEDURE

Stool Culture

Follow preprocedure steps I through VIII.

1. Assist the patient to the bathroom, where a new collection hat has been placed in the toilet, onto the clean bedside commode, or onto a new bedpan. Inform the patient to use the call light when finished defecating.
   Prepare the patient for the procedure in a safe and private environment. Precautions must be taken to maintain patient safety and prevent provider injury.
2. Instruct the patient to perform hand hygiene.
   Hand hygiene prevents the spread of microorganisms.
3. Assist the patient back to bed.
   Assistance promotes comfort and dignity.
4. Apply clean gloves.
   Using gloves prevents the spread of microorganisms and protects caregivers from injury.
5. Remove the lid from the specimen cup and place it on a flat surface with the inside of the lid facing up.
   Proper technique avoids contamination of the specimen from microorganisms and ensures accurate results.
6. Use a wooden tongue blade or applicator stick to collect a 1-inch diameter specimen of solid stool or 15 to 30 mL of liquid stool. Samples should be collected from different areas of the specimen. The nurse should handle the container or specimen only while wearing gloves.
   A minimum quantity of stool is required to ensure accurate test results. Using a wooden tongue blade or applicator stick prevents microorganisms from contaminating the specimen.
7. Cap the container when finished. The nurse should handle the container and/or specimen only while wearing gloves.
   Immediate capping of the container prevents microorganisms from contaminating the specimen and ensures accurate results.
8. Clean the outside of the container with a paper towel. The nurse should handle the container or specimen only while wearing gloves.
   Precautions must be taken to protect caregivers and prevent the spread of microorganisms.
9. Label the container in accordance with facility policy and procedure.
   Proper labeling of the sample prevents adverse events and medical errors.
10. Place the container in a biohazard bag. Remove gloves and perform hand hygiene.
    Precautions must be taken to protect caregivers from infection and to prevent the spread of microorganisms.
11. Transport the specimen to the laboratory. If it is not possible to get the specimen to the laboratory within 15 minutes of collection, check the facility or laboratory policy and procedure for storage recommendations.
    Many tests are time or temperature sensitive; stool samples undergo changes due to normal bacterial flora that affect test results.

12. Communicate in a report, and document, that the test is complete.
 Communicate essential information to provide safe, timely, and efficient quality patient care and to prevent adverse events and medical errors.

Follow postprocedure steps I through VI.

Occult Blood Testing (Guaiac-Based Fecal Occult Blood Test)

Follow pre-procedure steps I through VIII.

1. Follow procedure steps 1 through 3 in the Stool Culture section.
2. Apply clean gloves.
 Using gloves protects the provider, prevents the spread of microorganisms, and prevents microorganisms from contaminating the specimen, ensuring more accurate results.
3. Open a Hemoccult test slide.
 Prepare needed equipment before beginning the test.
4. Use a wooden tongue blade or applicator stick to collect a thin smear from the center of the specimen, and apply a smear of the stool sample to the center of the first test window of the Hemoccult test slide.
 Samples taken from the edge of the stool specimen may be contaminated from straining or hemorrhoids; using a sample from the center of the specimen ensures more accurate results.
5. Use a new tongue blade or applicator stick to collect a thin smear from a different area of the specimen (avoiding the edges of the sample), and apply a smear of the stool sample to the center of the second test window.
 Samples taken from the edge of the stool specimen may be contaminated from straining or hemorrhoids. Sampling different areas of the fecal specimen ensures more accurate test results; blood may not be in every area of the sample.

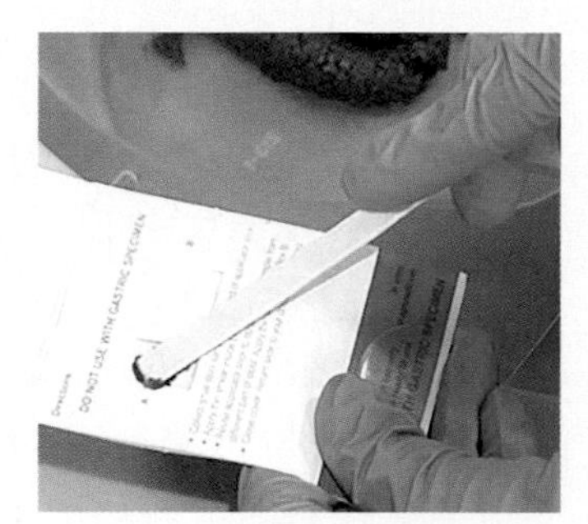

STEP 5

6. Close the Hemoccult test slide. Follow facility policy for development of fecal occult. If your facility permits the testing of fecal occult on the nursing unit, follow steps 7 to 10. If not, skip to step 10.
 Closing the slide protects the provider and prepares the test for processing.
7. Wait 3 to 5 minutes; see the manufacturer's instructions.
 The stool must have sufficient time to adhere to the slide for processing to ensure accurate results.
8. Develop the results:
 a. Open the reverse side of the Hemoccult test slide.
 b. Apply two drops of developing solution to each of the three windows (i.e., first and second test windows and the control window).
 c. Wait 30 to 60 seconds, according to the manufacturer's directions.
 The developing solution chemically reacts with the blood; the solution soaks through the paper to the stool; and proper timing ensures accurate results. The control window ensures valid testing of the solution and the slide.

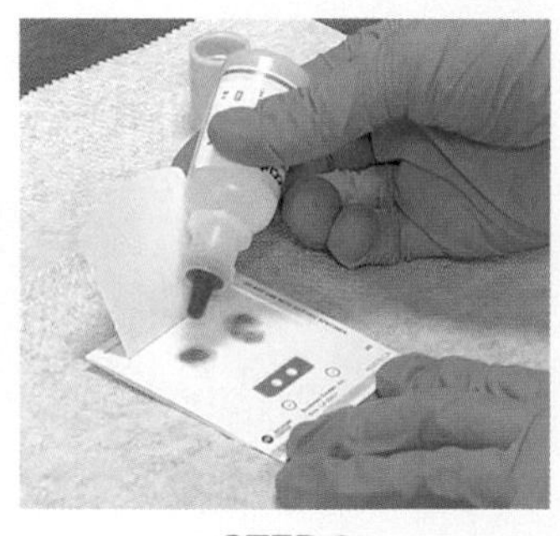

STEP 8

9. A bluish color indicates the presence of blood. Document the test results according to facility policy and procedure, and notify the primary care provider if needed.
 The solution chemically reacts with blood, producing a blue color when blood is present. Proper record keeping is essential because it communicates important information needed for patient care and provides legal evidence of care.
10. Label the test slide, and send it to the laboratory in a biohazard bag in accordance with facility policy and procedure.
 Proper labeling of samples prevents adverse events and medical errors.
11. Remove gloves and perform hand hygiene.
12. Communicate in a report and document that the test is complete.

Communicate essential information to provide safe, timely, and efficient quality patient care and to prevent adverse events and medical errors. Because blood may not be in all areas of the sample, performing multiple tests optimizes the chances of identifying occult blood.

Follow postprocedure steps I through VI.

POSTPROCEDURE

I. Return the bed to its lowest position, raise the top side rails, and verify that the call light is within reach of the patient.
Precautions are taken to maintain patient safety. Top side rails aid in positioning and turning. Raising four side rails is considered a restraint.

II. Assess for additional patient needs and state the time of your expected return.
Meeting patient needs and offering self promote patient satisfaction and build trust.

III. Properly dispose of PPE.
Gloves, gowns, and masks must be appropriately discarded to prevent the spread of microorganisms.

IV. Clean equipment if it was in contact with the patient; see specific manufacturer instructions.
Disinfection eliminates most microorganisms from inanimate objects.

V. Perform hand hygiene.
Frequent hand hygiene prevents the spread of infection.

VI. Document the date, time, assessment, procedure, and patient's response to the procedure.
Accurate documentation is essential to communicate patient care and to provide legal evidence of care.

SUMMARY OF LEARNING OUTCOMES

LO 34.1 *Recall the types of cells found in blood and their functions:* Three types of cells are found in blood: erythrocytes, which contain hemoglobin; thrombocytes, which are necessary for blood clotting; and leukocytes, which are responsible for the inflammatory and immune responses.

LO 34.2 *Identify common blood tests, their purposes, and their normal values:* Complete blood counts, coagulation studies, blood chemistries, liver and kidney function tests, and cardiac markers are the most common blood tests ordered for diagnostic and treatment purposes.

LO 34.3 *Discuss other laboratory tests, such as urine and stool studies, and their purposes and normal values:* Urine and stool studies provide additional diagnostic information that is not always available with blood tests. They include urinalysis and stool analysis for occult blood. Culture and sensitivity analysis can be performed on blood, stool, urine, the throat, sputum, and wounds.

LO 34.4 *Explain the purpose of common diagnostic tests:* Common radiographic studies are useful in visualizing structural abnormalities and disorders in the skeletal system, GI tract, and other body systems. Other studies that visualize structure include computed tomography, magnetic resonance imaging, ultrasound, and endoscopy. Electrocardiograms measure the electrical activity of the heart.

LO 34.5 *Describe assessment procedures for patients undergoing diagnostic tests:* The nurse assesses baseline information before the patient undergoes diagnostic tests, including any preparation the patient has performed at home before the test.

LO 34.6 *Choose appropriate nursing diagnoses associated with diagnostic testing: Anxiety, Fear,* and *Readiness for Enhanced Knowledge* are common nursing diagnoses associated with diagnostic testing.

LO 34.7 *Select goals to meet individual patient problems:* Goals are written to meet individual patient problems, and they depend on the diagnostic tests being performed and the patient's level of knowledge and particular nursing diagnosis.

LO 34.8 *Describe the nurse's role before, during, and after diagnostic tests and procedures:* The nurse's role before, during, and after diagnostic procedures includes conducting the baseline assessment, monitoring patient status, and assessing for potential complications. The nurse may be responsible for collecting some specimens.

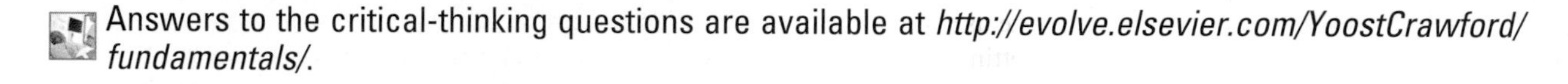
Answers to the critical-thinking questions are available at *http://evolve.elsevier.com/YoostCrawford/fundamentals/.*

REVIEW QUESTIONS

1. Which laboratory result should immediately be reported by the nurse to the primary care provider?
   a. Hemoglobin: 15.6 g/dL
   b. Hematocrit: 32%
   c. Red blood cells: 5.3 cells/mm^3
   d. White blood cells: 6000 cells/mm^3
2. The patient states that he has been taking Coumadin, an anticoagulant, for several years. The nurse notices several bruised areas on his arms. Which of the following laboratory results is clinically significant?
   a. Platelets: 450,000 cells/mm^3
   b. Prothrombin time: 24.2 seconds
   c. Activated partial thromboplastin time: 30 seconds
   d. Fibrinogen: 350 mg/dL
3. The patient tells the nurse that she has been on a high-protein, low-carbohydrate diet for the past 6 months. Which blood test results could be influenced by her diet?
   a. Bilirubin
   b. Creatinine
   c. Blood urea nitrogen
   d. Creatine kinase
4. The nurse is working at a health fair and providing information about reducing the risk of heart disease. A man asks what his ideal numbers should be for cholesterol and triglycerides. Which of the following is correct?
   a. Total cholesterol: >200 mg/dL
   b. HDL: >45 mg/dL
   c. LDL: >100 mg/dL
   d. Triglycerides: >160 mg/dL
5. The nurse is preparing a patient for an esophagogastroduodenoscopy (EGD). Which statements by the patient indicate that the patient has understood the nurse's teaching? *(Select all that apply.)*
   a. "The doctor will be able to view my stomach during the test."
   b. "I will be able to have something to drink immediately after the test."
   c. "There are no risks involved with this test."
   d. "The doctor will be able to see whether there is an ulcer in my stomach."
   e. "I will be NPO for 8 hours before the test."

6. A 24-hour urine specimen for creatinine clearance is ordered for a patient. Which instruction is correct?
   a. "Collect all urine from the time the collection begins until it ends."
   b. "Save only a sample from each voiding."
   c. "Clean the perineal area three times each time before you begin to urinate."
   d. "Discard the first urine specimen, and then collect all urine until the time period expires."
7. Which specimens should be collected using sterile technique in a sterile container? *(Select all that apply.)*
   a. Clean-catch urine
   b. Stool for occult blood
   c. Wound drainage
   d. Sputum
   e. Urine from a Foley catheter
8. Which blood test is used to monitor renal function?
   a. Creatine kinase
   b. Triglycerides
   c. Creatinine
   d. Alkaline phosphatase
9. For which patient is magnetic resonance imaging contraindicated?
   a. A patient with an allergy to latex
   b. A patient with an infection
   c. A patient with a pacemaker
   d. A patient with a head injury
10. The nurse is attempting a fingerstick on a diabetic patient and is having difficulty obtaining a suitable drop of blood. Which interventions may facilitate this process?
   a. Applying a tourniquet above the hand
   b. Asking the patient to close and open her hand several times
   c. Applying warm compresses
   d. Elevating the hand on a pillow

Answers and rationales to the review questions are available at *http://evolve.elsevier.com/YoostCrawford/fundamentals/.*

REFERENCES

Al-Najjar FY, Uduman SA: Clinical utility of a new rapid test for the detection of group A *Streptococcus* and discriminate use of antibiotics for bacterial pharyngitis in an outpatient setting. *Int J Infect Dis*, 12(3):308-311, 2008.

American Cancer Society: Guidelines for early detection of cancer, 2013. Retrieved from *www.cancer.org/healthy/findcancerearly/cancerscreeningguidelines/index.*

Corbett JV, Banks A: *Laboratory tests and diagnostic procedures with nursing diagnoses*, ed. 8, Upper Saddle River, N.J., 2013, Pearson Prentice Hall.

Cronenwett L, Sherwood G, Barnsteiner J, et al: Quality and safety education for nurses. *Nurs Outlook*, 55(3):122-131, 2007.

Food and Drug Administration: Think before you ink: Are tattoos safe? 2014. Retrieved from *www.fda.gov/forconsumers/consumerupdates/ucm048919.htm.*

Jessee MA: Stool studies: Tried, true, and new. *Crit Care Nurs Clin North Am*, 22(1):129-145, 2010.

The Joint Commission: National Patient Safety Goals, 2014. Retrieved from *www.jointcommission.org/assets/1/6/HAP_NPSG_Chapter_2014.pdf.*

Llor C, Calviño O, Hernández S, et al.: Repetition of the rapid antigen test in initially negative supposed streptococcal pharyngitis is not necessary in adults. *Int J Clin Pract*, 63(9):1330-1340, 2009.

Pagana KD, Pagana TJ: *Mosby's manual of diagnostic and laboratory tests*, ed. 5, St. Louis, 2014, Mosby.

Sarikaya S, Aktas C, Ay D, et al.: Sensitivity and specificity of rapid antigen detection testing for diagnosing pharyngitis in the emergency department. *Ear Nose Throat J*, 89(4):180-182, 2010.

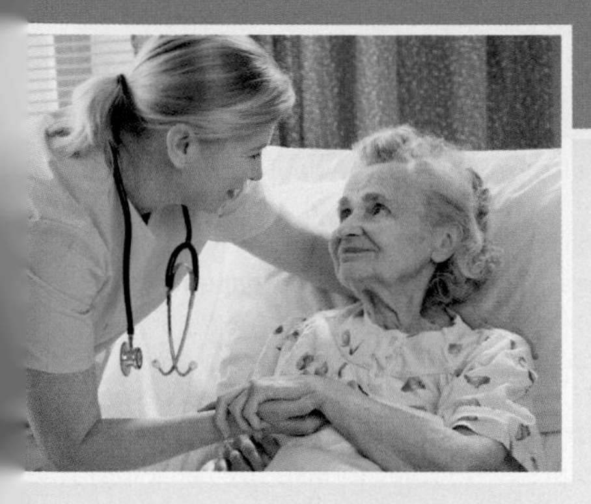

CHAPTER 35

Medication Administration

EVOLVE WEBSITE

http://evolve.elsevier.com/YoostCrawford/fundamentals/

- Additional Evolve-Only Review Questions With Answers
- Answers and Rationales for Text Review Questions
- Answers to Critical-Thinking Questions
- Case Study With Questions
- Video Skills Clips
- Conceptual Care Map
- Animations
- Skills Checklists
- Glossary

LEARNING OUTCOMES

Comprehension of this chapter's content will provide students with the ability to:

LO 35.1 Recall how government, facility, and professional regulations affect medication administration by nurses.

LO 35.2 Explain the physiologic outcomes of medication actions.

LO 35.3 Identify differences between prescription and nonprescription medications.

LO 35.4 Summarize common medication forms and routes.

LO 35.5 Describe measures for administering medications safely.

LO 35.6 Discuss assessments necessary for safe medication administration.

LO 35.7 Choose nursing diagnoses related to safe medication administration.

LO 35.8 Determine individual patient goals.

LO 35.9 Implement guidelines and essential nursing actions for safely administering medications.

KEY TERMS

absorption, p. 815
adverse effects, p. 816
allergic reactions, p. 816
anaphylactic reaction, p. 816
antagonism, p. 817
buccal, p. 821
controlled substances, p. 813
distribution, p. 815
drug, p. 813
drug incompatibility, p. 817
excretion, p. 815
generic name, p. 813
half-life, p. 815
idiosyncratic reaction, p. 816
inhalation, p. 823
intradermal, p. 823
intramuscular, p. 823
intravenous, p. 823
medication, p. 813
medication error, p. 826
medication interactions, p. 817
metabolism, p. 815
NPO, p. 833
onset of action, p. 816
oral, p. 821
parenteral, p. 821
peak plasma level, p. 816
pharmacodynamics, p. 814
pharmacokinetics, p. 814
prescription, p. 818
side effects, p. 816
Six Rights of Medication Administration, p. 828
subcutaneous, p. 823
sublingual, p. 821
synergistic effect, p. 817
therapeutic effect, p. 815
topical, p. 821
toxic effects, p. 816
trade name, p. 813
transdermal patch, p. 823
trough, p. 816

CASE STUDY

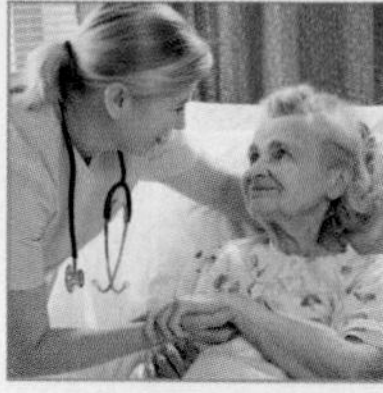

Mrs. Petros is a 82-year-old female admitted to the hospital 4 hours earlier after a fall at home caused by dizziness and weakness. She was initially brought to the emergency department by her daughter, who checked on her after not reaching her by phone. Her medical history includes hypertension, osteoarthritis, and a hysterectomy at age 50. She states that she has an allergy to penicillin, and she has full-code status. The patient has lived alone since the death of her spouse 3 months ago. She brought a small plastic bag with multiple medications in it because, as she said, "I can't open my medication bottles because of my arthritis."

Mrs. Petros's vital signs are T 36.5° C (97.7° F), P 92 and regular, R 20 and unlabored, BP 172/92, with a pulse oximetry reading of 98% on room air. She reports a pain level of 8 of 10 in her left hip. She also reports a pain level of 5 of 10 in her hands from her arthritis. As the nurse completed the admission assessment, Mrs. Petros stated, "I forgot to take my Lasix in the morning, so I took both tablets before bed. I was up and down to the bathroom a lot, and fell because I was dizzy and my legs gave out early this morning. My daughter came to get me. Right now my hip and leg hurt when I move."

She further reported, "I always have some pain in my hands and have to take medicine for that sometimes, but I don't like to because then I get constipated. I take a tablet of the over-the-counter herb, feverfew, every day to help with my arthritis pain." The nurse notes a 4- × 5-cm bruise on the left hip. The patient's Braden score is 20, and her Morse Fall score is 40. Her left hip x-ray on admission showed no acute fracture. Serum potassium level is 3.3 mEq/L.

Treatment orders are as follows:

- Vital signs q 4 hr
- No-added-salt diet
- Activity as tolerated with assistance
- Intake and output
- Electrolyte panel in A.M.

Medication orders are as follows:

- Continue home medications of
  - Furosemide 40 mg PO bid
  - Hydrocodone 5 mg PO q 4 hr PRN for pain
  - K-Lor 8 mEq daily
- Start Colace 50 mg PO daily
- Start intravenous infusion of 5% dextrose in half normal saline (D_5 ½NS) with 20 mEq of KCl to run at 75 mL/hr

Refer back to this case study to answer the critical-thinking exercises throughout the chapter.

Historically, nurses administered prescribed medications at scheduled times by the prescribed route with minimal assessment and documentation. Today, the nurse's role and responsibility in medication administration are much more complex. Safe nursing practice includes knowledge about medication actions; side effects; interactions with foods, herbs, and other medications; associated assessment and evaluation; ethical considerations; and legal aspects of medication therapy. Patients with acute and chronic illnesses seek treatment for their symptoms, with medications often prescribed to help diagnose, treat, or prevent illness; relieve symptoms; or cure illness. The nurse must integrate into the plan of care the self-prescribed medications and herbs that patients use to prevent or treat self-identified illnesses.

Medication management requires the collaborative efforts of many health care providers, such as the prescribing primary care provider, pharmacist, respiratory therapist, and dietician. Nurses, however, have the specialized knowledge, clinical judgment, and skills employed in health care and community settings that are needed for the essential role of educating patients about medications, administering medications according to accepted protocols, and evaluating the patient's response to medications. Patient education by nurses on the correct use of medications is an important responsibility to prevent illness relapse, new medical problems, and patient injury. Often, family members or caregivers are included in medication teaching to meet the patient's needs. Clinical judgment is needed before, during, and after administering medications to patients as assessments are made about the effectiveness of medications in restoring or maintaining patients' health. Continuing education of nurses is needed to ensure that standards of practice are met, new or unfamiliar medications are administered properly, and medication administration technology is used correctly.

MEDICATIONS AND REGULATIONS LO 35.1

Medications are substances that can prevent, improve, or reduce the symptoms of a medical condition, and the objective of drug therapy is to provide maximum benefit with minimum harm to the patient. Ongoing research provides the scientific foundation for the use of medications. The chemical makeup of the medication determines its actions in the human body.

DRUGS AND MEDICATIONS

A **drug** is any substance that positively or negatively alters physiologic function. A **medication** is a drug specifically administered for its therapeutic effect on physiologic function. Medications and preparations may be researched by using drug textbooks or point-of-care software on hand-held devices or computers.

Medications can have up to four designations: chemical name, official name, generic name, and trade (brand) name. The chemical name describes the elements of the medication's molecular structure. The official name is assigned by the U.S. Adopted Names Council, and it is usually the **generic name**, which is simpler than the chemical name. The generic name is not capitalized and often contains a prefix or suffix that helps to identify the drug class. For example, beta blockers are drugs that are prescribed for cardiac conditions; their generic names frequently end in *-olol:* propranolol, metoprolol, labetalol. The **trade name**, or brand name, is a registered name assigned by the drug manufacturer. Because one type of medication can be manufactured by several companies, it can have several different trade names while having a common generic and chemical name:

Chemical Name	Generic Name	Trade Names
2-(4-isobutylphenyl) propionic acid	Ibuprofen	Motrin, Advil, Nuprin

MEDICATION STANDARDS AND REGULATIONS

Medications are synthesized in a laboratory or developed from plant, mineral, or animal sources. Because medications vary in purity, potency, efficacy, safety, and toxicity, the United States and many other governments have developed standards to ensure uniform quality so that the effects are predictable. In the United States, official medication lists have been reported in the *United States Pharmacopeia* (USP) since 1820 and the *National Formulary* (NF) since 1898. These sources help protect public safety by identifying medication properties that show an appropriate range of quality and purity.

Medication administration in the United States is regulated by law. The Pure Food and Drug Act of 1906 designated the USP and NF as the only official authorities to establish drug standards, including the requirement that medications be free of impurities. Subsequent legislation has continued to set standards related to the safety, potency, sales, distribution, and efficacy of medications and the regulation of **controlled substances**, which have regulated manufacturing, prescribing, and dispensing requirements. Table 35-1 summarizes U.S. drug legislation. Enforcement of medication legislation in the United States is the responsibility of the U.S. Food and Drug Administration (FDA), which mandates that all medications undergo safety testing before being released to the public.

TABLE 35-1 U.S. Drug Legislation

YEAR	LEGISLATION
1912	*Sherley Amendment:* prohibits labeling of medicines with false therapeutic claims intended to defraud the purchaser. (Mrs. Winslow's Soothing Syrup for teething and colicky babies, laced with morphine, killed many infants.)
1914	*Harrison Narcotic Act:* classified medications thought to be habit-forming as narcotics; regulates the use of narcotic substances, including increased record keeping for physicians and pharmacists who dispense narcotics.
1938	*Federal Food, Drug, and Cosmetic (FDC) Act:* requires that labels be accurate and that all drugs be tested for harmful effects; added the *Homeopathic Pharmacopeia* as a third medication standard.
1951	*Durham-Humphrey Amendment:* defines the kinds of drugs that cannot be safely used without medical supervision; restricts their sale to prescription by a licensed practitioner (before this amendment, all medications could be purchased over the counter).
1962	*Kefauver-Harris Drug Amendments:* require proof of drug safety and efficacy before marketing and greater controls on investigational medications (passed in response to birth defects associated with thalidomide).
1970	*Patient package insert requirement:* mandates that oral contraceptives contain information for the patient about specific risks and benefits. *Comprehensive Drug Abuse Prevention and Control Act:* replaces previous laws and categorizes drugs on the basis of their abuse and addiction potential compared with their therapeutic value (i.e., controlled substances addiction potential); made it illegal to possess a controlled substance without a prescription.
1997	*Food and Drug Administration Modernization Act:* contains the most wide-ranging reforms in agency practices since 1938. Provisions include measures to accelerate the review of devices, regulate advertising of unapproved uses of approved drugs and devices, and regulate health claims for foods.

From U.S. Food and Drug Administration: *Significant dates in U.S. food and drug law history,* Washington, D.C., 2010, U.S. Department of Health and Human Services.

TABLE 35-2 Controlled Substances

CATEGORY	DESCRIPTION	EXAMPLES
Schedule I	High potential for abuse No currently accepted medical use in treatment in the United States	Heroin, LSD, and methaqualone
Schedule II	High potential for abuse; may lead to severe psychological or physical dependence Has a currently accepted medical use with severe restrictions	Morphine, cocaine, methadone, and methamphetamine
Schedule III	Lower potential for abuse compared to the drugs in schedules I and II in regard to moderate dependence Has a currently accepted medical use	Anabolic steroids, narcotics such as codeine or hydrocodone with aspirin or acetaminophen, and some barbiturates
Schedule IV	Lower potential for abuse relative to the drugs in schedule III; may lead to limited dependence Has a currently accepted medical use	Pentazocine, meprobamate, diazepam, and alprazolam
Schedule V	Low potential for abuse relative to the drugs in schedule IV Has a currently accepted medical use in treatment in the United States.	Over-the-counter cough medicines with codeine

From U.S. Department of Justice, Drug Enforcement Administration: *Mid-level practitioners authorization by state*, Washington, D.C., n.d., U.S. Department of Justice.

CONTROLLED SUBSTANCES

A specific aspect of nursing practice governed by law is the use of controlled substances. In the United States, the Comprehensive Drug Abuse Prevention and Control Act (1970), known informally as the Controlled Substances Act (CSA), established five categories of scheduled drugs, referred to as *controlled substances* (Table 35-2). One objective of the CSA is to reduce opportunities for drugs to be diverted from legitimate sources to drug abusers. In working toward this goal, the CSA mandates regulations for the handling and distributing of controlled substances by manufacturers, distributors, pharmacists, nurses, and care providers. Compliance with these regulations is monitored by the Drug Enforcement Administration (DEA), an office within the U.S. Department of Justice.

A written record is required to track all transactions involving controlled substances that originate from legitimate sources. Every time a controlled substance is purchased or dispensed, an accurate record must be documented. An inventory must be kept of all controlled substances in stock, and this inventory must be reported to the DEA every 2 years. Although not required by the CSA, many hospitals and clinics require that floor stock of controlled substances be accounted for at the beginning and end of each nursing shift.

If a controlled drug needs to be wasted (e.g., only a partial amount is needed for the prescribed dose), two licensed clinical staff members must witness the disposal of the substance and document the wasting of the drug in the appropriate manner.

STATE AND LOCAL MEDICATION REGULATIONS

Health care facilities develop policies and procedures that must be in compliance with federal, state, and local regulations and may be more restrictive than government controls. The goal of these regulations is to prevent adverse patient outcomes. The functions and professional responsibilities of nurses are defined by each state's nurse practice act. Health care facilities cannot modify or expand the nurse practice act. It is the nurse's responsibility to understand and follow the nurse practice act and policies of the facility when administering any medication, particularly controlled substances. Violations of regulations can result in fines, imprisonment, and the loss of nurse licensure.

PRINCIPLES OF DRUG ACTIONS LO 35.2

The nurse should understand how a drug exerts its effects on the body. **Pharmacokinetics** is the study of how a medication enters the body, moves through the body, and ultimately leaves the body. **Pharmacodynamics** is the process in which a medication interacts with the body's cells to produce a biologic response. Understanding these processes helps the nurse evaluate the *therapeutic,* or intended, response and *adverse,* or unintended, effects caused by the administered medication.

PHARMACOKINETICS

The **therapeutic effect**, or intended effect, is the desired result or action of a medication. To achieve a therapeutic effect, the medication must be taken into the body, be absorbed and distributed in cells and tissues, and alter physiologic functioning. Effectiveness is influenced by the medication dose, route of administration, frequency of administration, function of metabolizing organs such as the liver or kidneys, and age of the patient (Diversity Considerations box). Prescribing practitioners and nurses providing care monitor the patient's response to the medication. Laboratory and diagnostic studies measure medication effects. Medication actions depend on absorption, distribution, metabolism, and excretion properties.

DIVERSITY CONSIDERATIONS

Life Span

- *Pregnancy:* Nurses must take extreme care when administering medications during pregnancy, especially in the first trimester, due to the risk of harm to the developing fetus.
  - The U.S. Food and Drug Administration has established categories for pregnant women for each drug.
  - Category A drugs have no demonstrated risk, whereas category D or X drugs have positive evidence of risk or harm to the fetus.
- *Infants:* Infants require small doses because of their body size and immature organs.
- *Infants and children:* Medication doses are often based on weight.
- *Older adults:* Age-related changes, such as increased fat deposits, decreased gastric mobility, decreased renal and liver function, and changes in the blood-brain barrier, can lead to increased side effects of medications.

Gender

- Distribution of body fat and hormone levels are different in men and women, leading to differences in drug actions.

Culture, Ethnicity, and Religion

- Genetic factors affect drug metabolism and influence dosage needs.
- Cultural factors may affect drug action.
  - Herbal medicine used in a culture may affect the action of prescribed medications.
  - Certain cultural and religious groups have beliefs that discourage the use of medications other than natural remedies.

Absorption

Absorption is the passage of a drug from the administration site into the bloodstream. Several factors affect absorption: route of administration, ability of the drug to dissolve or become soluble, blood flow to the administration site, body surface area, and patient age. Administration of a medication intravenously, or directly into a blood vessel, results in the quickest rate of absorption, followed in descending order by intramuscularly, subcutaneously, and orally administered medications.

Distribution

Distribution is the process of delivering the medication to tissues and organs and ultimately to the specific site of action. Distribution is affected by the chemical properties of the drug, the effectiveness of the cardiac system, the ability to pass through tissue and organ membranes, and the extent to which the drug binds to proteins or accumulates in fatty tissue.

Metabolism

Metabolism is the process by which a drug is altered to a less active form to prepare for excretion. The products of this process are called *metabolites.* Most metabolism takes place in the liver, and it may be slowed in elderly individuals or anyone with impaired liver function. Care is taken in administering medications to these populations because toxic levels of a medication can build up if the liver is not able to break the drug down to a less active form.

Excretion

The **excretion** process removes the less active drug or its metabolites. Most metabolites exit the body through the kidneys, but some may be excreted in feces, breath, saliva, sweat, and breast milk. The drug may accumulate to unwanted levels in elderly individuals and people with impaired kidney function, necessitating prescription of smaller doses with longer durations between doses.

PHARMACODYNAMICS

Drug activity results from chemical interactions between a medication and the cells of the body, causing a biologic response. The biochemical response can be systemic, such as the effects seen when an administered pain medication affects the nervous system (sedation), respiratory system (change in respiratory rate), and gastrointestinal system (constipation). The response can be local, as occurs when an antipruritic lotion is applied to an insect bite. The biochemical response is typically evaluated on the basis of changes in the patient's clinical condition. Improvement is seen when a therapeutic effect is achieved with the medication, but unexpected or unwanted effects may occur, and different patients may respond differently to the same medication.

The desired drug action is produced by maintaining a constant drug level in the body and is based on the **half-life** of the drug. A drug's half-life is the expected time it takes for the blood concentration to measure one half of the original drug dose due to drug elimination. For example, if a drug has a half-life of 12 hours, 50% of the drug's original dose remains in the bloodstream 12 hours after administration. Repeated doses are usually required to maintain the desired drug level. Correct spacing of doses to maintain consistent drug levels and obtain therapeutic effects is based on the drug's half-life and is an important consideration when medications are prescribed.

Nurses must account for other drug action factors. **Onset of action** is the time the body takes to respond to a drug after administration. Onset is affected by the administration route, drug formulation, and pharmacokinetic factors. For example, the onset of action for insulin varies greatly, depending on the route (intravenous versus subcutaneous) and on the type of insulin (e.g., Humalog versus Lantus). **Peak plasma level** indicates the highest serum (blood) concentration. After the peak is reached, serum levels decrease until another dose is administered. Conversely, the **trough** is the lowest serum level of the medication. The peak and trough levels of a medication are measured with serum laboratory tests, and results are used to adjust dose amounts and monitor for toxicity. Blood samples for peak serum levels are drawn at specified times after administration on the basis of the drug half-life; samples for trough levels are drawn just before the administration of a scheduled dose.

SIDE EFFECTS, ADVERSE EFFECTS, AND INTERACTIONS

Side effects are predictable but unwanted and sometimes unavoidable reactions to medications. Side effects may be minor and harmless, or they may cause patient injury. Patients may refuse to continue a medication because of side effects. Patient education regarding how to handle expected side effects can offset these reactions. For example, if nausea is a frequent side effect of a medication, the drug can be taken with a light meal to reduce this sensation. Nurses must be particularly alert for side effects when a new medication is started or the dose is increased.

Adverse effects are severe, unintended, unwanted, and often unpredictable drug reactions. An adverse effect may occur after one dose, such as a severe allergic response, or it may develop over time, such as the development of anemia associated with a medication. When an adverse reaction occurs, the medication is immediately stopped. Adverse reactions are reported by health care providers to the FDA by using the MedWatch program (U.S. Food and Drug Administration, 2014).

Toxic effects result from a medication overdose or the buildup of medication in the blood due to impaired metabolism and excretion. Toxic levels of a drug can lead to serious physiologic effects that may be lethal. For example, toxic levels of a pain medication such as morphine sulfate may cause respiratory depression, leading to respiratory arrest. Other organs that can be damaged from drug toxicity include the kidneys (nephrotoxicity), liver (hepatotoxicity), organs of hearing (ototoxicity), and heart (cardiotoxicity). Most drug toxicity is avoidable with careful patient monitoring, especially of kidney and liver function.

Allergic reactions are unpredictable immune responses to medications. When a patient is first exposed to a foreign substance (antigen), the body produces antibodies. The medication, a chemical preservative, or one of the metabolites can initiate the immune response. On exposure, the patient reacts to the antigen with an allergic reaction that ranges from minor to severe. Minor allergic reactions include a rash, itching of the skin, inflammation of the nasal passages causing swelling and a clear discharge, and raised skin eruptions (hives).

A severe allergic reaction is called an **anaphylactic reaction**, and it is a medical emergency. Anaphylaxis can occur immediately after the administration of medication and can be fatal. Treatment includes immediate discontinuation of the drug and administration of epinephrine (an antagonist), intravenous (IV) fluids, steroids, and antihistamines while providing respiratory support. Patients who have experienced a severe allergic reaction to a medication need to wear an identification bracelet or tag identifying the drug or substance (Figure 35-1). The bracelet or tag alerts medical staff to the allergy if the patient is unable to communicate.

! SAFE PRACTICE ALERT

Many community-based health facilities require patients to remain in the facility for 20 to 30 minutes after receiving medications to be monitored for a severe allergic reaction. Treatment can be initiated immediately if a reaction occurs.

! SAFE PRACTICE ALERT

To avoid initiating an allergic response, always check for patient allergies before administering medication.

An **idiosyncratic reaction** is an unpredictable patient response to medication. This response can be an overresponse, underresponse, or abnormal reaction to the medication. For example, a patient receiving an antihistamine may

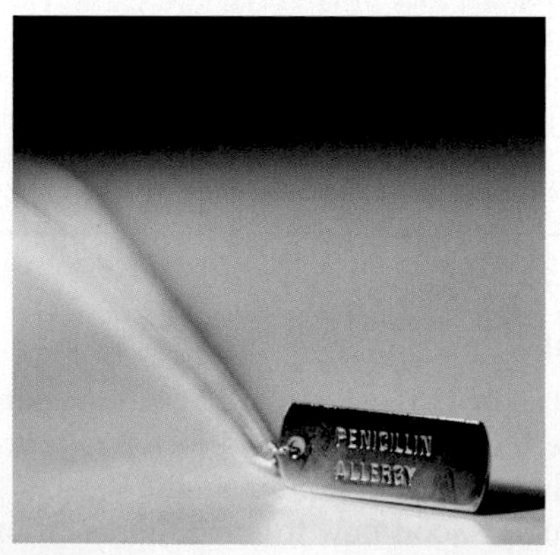

FIGURE 35-1 Patient allergy necklace.

become overly alert and be unable to sleep rather than being drowsy, as expected.

Medication interactions occur when the drug action is modified by the presence of a certain food or herb or another medication. The interaction can alter the way the medication is absorbed, metabolized, or eliminated. A **synergistic effect** occurs when the combined effect is greater than the effect of either substance if taken alone. Alcohol, for example, is a central nervous system depressant that has an increased effect when taken with antihistamines, antidepressants, or barbiturates. A synergistic effect may be specifically sought by the health care provider; for example, a patient with hypertension may receive a diuretic and a vasodilator to achieve a greater antihypertensive response than would be achieved by either drug alone. **Antagonism** occurs when the drug effect is decreased by taking the drug with another substance, including herbs. For example, antibiotics can lessen the effect of birth control medications, and grapefruit juice alters the absorption of statins, a class of lipid-lowering drugs.

Special care is taken when administering parenteral medications. Mixing medications in a solution that causes precipitation or combining a drug with another drug that causes an adverse chemical reaction is called **drug incompatibility**. Compatibility must be assessed before mixing or administering medications with a syringe or through intravenous tubing. If medications that are not compatible are prescribed, they must be administered separately with appropriate safety measures, such as flushing the intravenous tubing between medications.

NONPRESCRIPTION AND PRESCRIPTION MEDICATIONS LO 35.3

Medications are classified as those that require a legal prescription and those that can be obtained without a health care provider's authorization. Nurses need to assess patient use of nonprescription and prescription substances and provide teaching on possible interactions among the substances.

NONPRESCRIPTION MEDICATIONS

Many medications, vitamins, herbs, and supplements can be obtained without a prescription from a heath care provider. They are referred to as *over-the-counter* (OTC) medications. Examples are cold medicines, mild analgesics, diet and nutrition supplements, and sleep aids. The FDA regulates OTC medications relative to safety and recommended dosage, but it does not regulate all supplements. Most people take OTC medications responsibly, but there is potential for misuse, including inappropriate dosing, delay in seeking evaluation by a health care provider, and lack of knowledge about interactions with prescription medications. It is important for the nurse to educate patients about following the package directions and notifying the health care provider that OTC medications are being used.

Factors to consider when selecting an OTC medication include clearly understanding the desired effect and potential side and adverse effects of all ingredients in the medication, possible allergic reactions, potential interactions with other medications and herbs, warnings, directions and dosage, and features such as safety caps. The FDA developed Choosing the Right Over-the-Counter Medicine, a checklist for use when selecting OTC medications *(www.fda.gov/downloads/Drugs/ResourcesForYou/UCM133407.pdf)*.

Vitamins

The vitamins needed by the body are usually acquired from food that is eaten. The body uses vitamins for the biologic processes of growth, digestion, and nerve function. Water-soluble vitamins are excreted by the body through the kidneys. They are the B complex and C vitamins. Fat-soluble vitamins are stored by the body for use as needed; however, excess can build up in the liver, so they must be used with caution. They are the A, D, E, and K vitamins. There are certain conditions in which vitamins should be considered for use. They include pregnancy, breastfeeding, a vegetarian or vegan diet, an illness or condition that prevents oral consumption of foods, and the need for dietary supplements.

Vitamin use should be recorded as part of the patient history. Vitamins can have side effects such as anticoagulation and interfering with the results of medical tests (Table 35-3). Vitamin products are regulated by the FDA as dietary supplements, with testing for purity, strength, and composition.

Alternative Therapies

Many people take herbal supplements to support and maintain their health. Herbal therapy has roots that date back to ancient times. In a 2007 survey conducted by the National Center for Complementary and Alternative Medicine (NCCAM), more than 38 million people in the United States reported using a herb or supplement. Among the top 10 were Echinacea, flaxseed, ginseng, ginkgo, and garlic (NCCAM, 2009)

Herbal medications come from plants or a plant part and are found in many foods. Herbs can be dried and processed to make a more concentrated product that is delivered in a capsule or pill. Many commercial herbal preparations contain more than one herb. Many nonprescription and prescription drug formulations include a plant or plant extract. Common examples are aspirin (willow tree bark), morphine (opium poppy), and digitalis (foxglove).

The FDA regulates herbs and dietary supplements through the Dietary Supplement Health and Education Act (DSHEA). This form of regulation is different from that for prescription medications, despite the fact that herbs and prescription medications can act in the human body in the same way. The effects of herbals and dietary supplements necessitate that health care providers be informed about these products so that they can educate consumers. More detailed information

TABLE 35-3 Vitamins and Adverse Effects

VITAMIN	ADVERSE EFFECTS
Water-Soluble Vitamins	
B_3 (niacin)	Flushing, redness of the skin, upset stomach
B_6 (pyridoxine, pyridoxal, and pyridoxamine)	Nerve damage to the limbs, which may cause numbness, trouble walking, and pain
C (ascorbic acid)	Upset stomach, kidney stones, increased iron absorption
Folic acid (folate)	At high levels, especially in older adults, may hide signs of B_{12} deficiency
Fat-Soluble Vitamins	
A (retinol, retinal, retinoic acid)	Nausea, vomiting, headache, dizziness, blurred vision, clumsiness, birth defects, liver problems, possible risk of osteoporosis
D (calciferol)	Nausea, vomiting, poor appetite, constipation, weakness, weight loss, confusion, heart rhythm problems, deposits of calcium and phosphate in soft tissues

From U.S. Food and Drug Administration: *Fortify your knowledge about vitamins*, Washington, D.C., 2009, U.S. Department of Health and Human Services.

TABLE 35-4 Common Herb Side Effects and Drug Interactions

HERB	USES	SIDE EFFECTS AND DRUG INTERACTIONS
Echinacea	Stimulates the immune system; facilitates wound healing; fights flu and colds	Possible liver inflammation and damage if used with anabolic steroids or methotrexate
Feverfew	Alleviates and helps prevent migraines; relieves pain of arthritis	Increased bleeding; potentiates action of anticoagulants
Garlic	Lowers blood pressure and cholesterol and triglyceride levels	Increased bleeding; potentiates action of anticoagulants
Ginkgo biloba	Improves memory and mental alertness	Increased bleeding; potentiates action of anticoagulants
Ginseng	Increases physical stamina and mental concentration	Can increase heart rate and blood pressure; decreases effectiveness of anticoagulants
Saw palmetto	Helps with enlarged prostate and urinary inflammation	Interacts with other hormones
St. John's wort	Alleviates mild to moderate depression, anxiety, and sleep disorders	Interacts with antidepressants, birth control pills, cyclosporine, digoxin, and human immunodeficiency virus (HIV) and cancer medications

From National Center for Complementary and Alternative Medicine: *Herbs at a glance*, Bethesda, Md., 2009, National Institutes of Health.

on labeling and health claims can be found on the FDA website *(www.fda.gov)*.

Herbs are often taken for specific symptoms and for a limited period of time. Because they act in the body similar to the way that prescription medications act, they should be used with caution, and many need to be discontinued several days before a surgical procedure. Many consumers are reluctant to inform their health care provider about their use of herbal supplements, and this increases the possibility of an adverse reaction among prescribed medications and the supplements (Table 35-4).

Herbs can be grown in many regions with different soil, water, and atmospheric conditions. For this reason, standardization and quality control are difficult. The nurse must be vigilant in obtaining an accurate patient medication history that includes the use of herbs, extracts, teas, tinctures, and dietary supplements. Because many herbs have the same properties as prescription medications, the patient taking a herb and prescription medication for the same effect could experience a toxic reaction. To determine specific side effects and possible drug interactions, each preparation needs to be researched individually.

PRESCRIPTION MEDICATIONS

Medications are usually dispensed by a pharmacist on receipt of written directions, or **prescription** (Figure 35-2). Legally, prescribing medications is limited to physicians, dentists, specially qualified nurse practitioners or other advanced practice nurses, and physician assistants. It is illegal to dispense

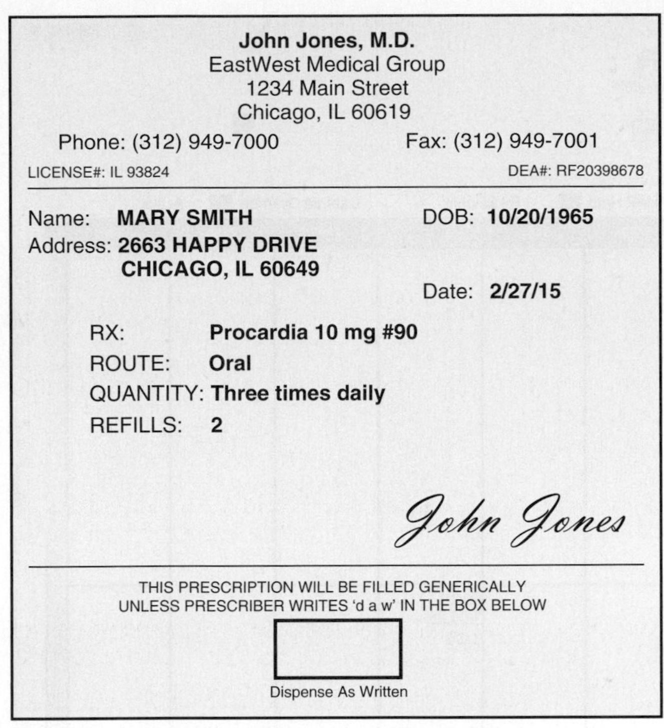
John Jones, M.D.
EastWest Medical Group
1234 Main Street
Chicago, IL 60619
Phone: (312) 949-7000 Fax: (312) 949-7001
LICENSE#: IL 93824 DEA#: RF20398678

Name: **MARY SMITH** DOB: **10/20/1965**
Address: **2663 HAPPY DRIVE**
CHICAGO, IL 60649
Date: **2/27/15**

RX: **Procardia 10 mg #90**
ROUTE: **Oral**
QUANTITY: **Three times daily**
REFILLS: **2**

John Jones

THIS PRESCRIPTION WILL BE FILLED GENERICALLY
UNLESS PRESCRIBER WRITES 'd a w' IN THE BOX BELOW

Dispense As Written

FIGURE 35-2 Sample prescription.

medications without a legal prescription. A medication order from any health care setting must have several components to be a legally valid medication prescription:

- Patient's name
- Date and time the order is written
- Name of drug to be administered
- Dosage of the drug
- Route of drug administration
- Frequency of drug administration
- Signature of the person writing the order

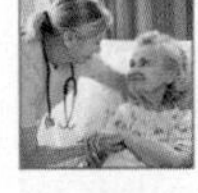

1. Mrs. Petros has requested medication for pain in her bruised hip. When the nurse accesses the locked narcotic cabinet, she finds that the narcotic count for the pain medication prescribed does not match the computer count. What action does the nurse take?

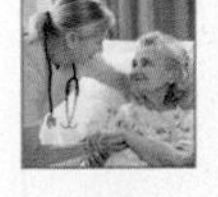

2. The health care provider phones in an order for Mrs. Petros for "Colace daily" and the order needs to be added to her chart. What additional actions are needed for the nurse to safely administer this medication?

Each patient in a health care facility has a medication administration record (MAR). The MAR includes the patient's name, full name of medication, administration time, dose, route, frequency, site of administration for parenteral medications, and the nurses' initials and signatures. The prescribing health care provider may also be identified. The MAR shows when previous doses were administered and by whom, along with any as needed (PRN) or intermittent (one-time) medications. Figure 35-3 shows a legal medication order for inpatient settings. Computerized charting meets all of these requirements. Specific documentation is needed when a medication is not administered as prescribed such as when a patient refuses a medication or the nurse purposefully holds a medication before a procedure.

Technological advances, such as bar codes, electronic medication administration records (eMARs), computerized provider order entry (CPOE), intravenous smart pumps, and clinical decision support systems (CDSSs), have reduced medication errors and prevented adverse events by providing legibility, nurse and physician reminders, and patient condition change alerts (Forni, Chu, and Fanikos, 2010; George, Henneman, and Tasota, 2010; Poon, Keohane, Yoon, et al, 2010).

QSEN FOCUS!

Using informatics, the nurse applies technology and information management tools to support safe processes of care. The nurse values technologies that support error prevention in medication administration.

Nurses need to know why a medication is ordered for certain times and whether the times can be altered. For example, there is a difference between medications ordered every 6 hours (q 6 hr) and those ordered four times per day (qid), even though the four doses of medication are administered in a 24-hour period. A medication ordered q 6 hr is given at regular intervals around the clock (e.g., at 6 A.M., 12 P.M., 6 P.M., and midnight) to maintain a constant blood level. A medication given qid (e.g., at 9 A.M., 1 P.M., 5 P.M., and 9 P.M.) is administered during waking hours.

Medication orders can change on the basis of the status of the patient. For example, a sudden change in condition, an adverse response to a medication, or a patient transfer to a different care unit can necessitate a change in medication orders. Medications may need to be reordered after surgical procedures or on discharge. Insulin is often prescribed to be taken at a specific time before meals; other medications may be ordered to be taken after meals to ensure that food is in the patient's system.

The five common types of medication orders in acute care settings are based on administration frequency or urgency: routine, PRN (as needed), one-time or on-call, stat, and now orders (Table 35-5). Stat medications are given immediately. The nurse is notified of when to give an on-call medication; the time is based on when a treatment or procedure is scheduled to start, such as when the operating room staff is ready to transport a patient to the surgical department for surgery. A PRN medication is administered as needed but still within identified time constraints. Each facility's pharmacy has guidelines for medication administration times. It is not

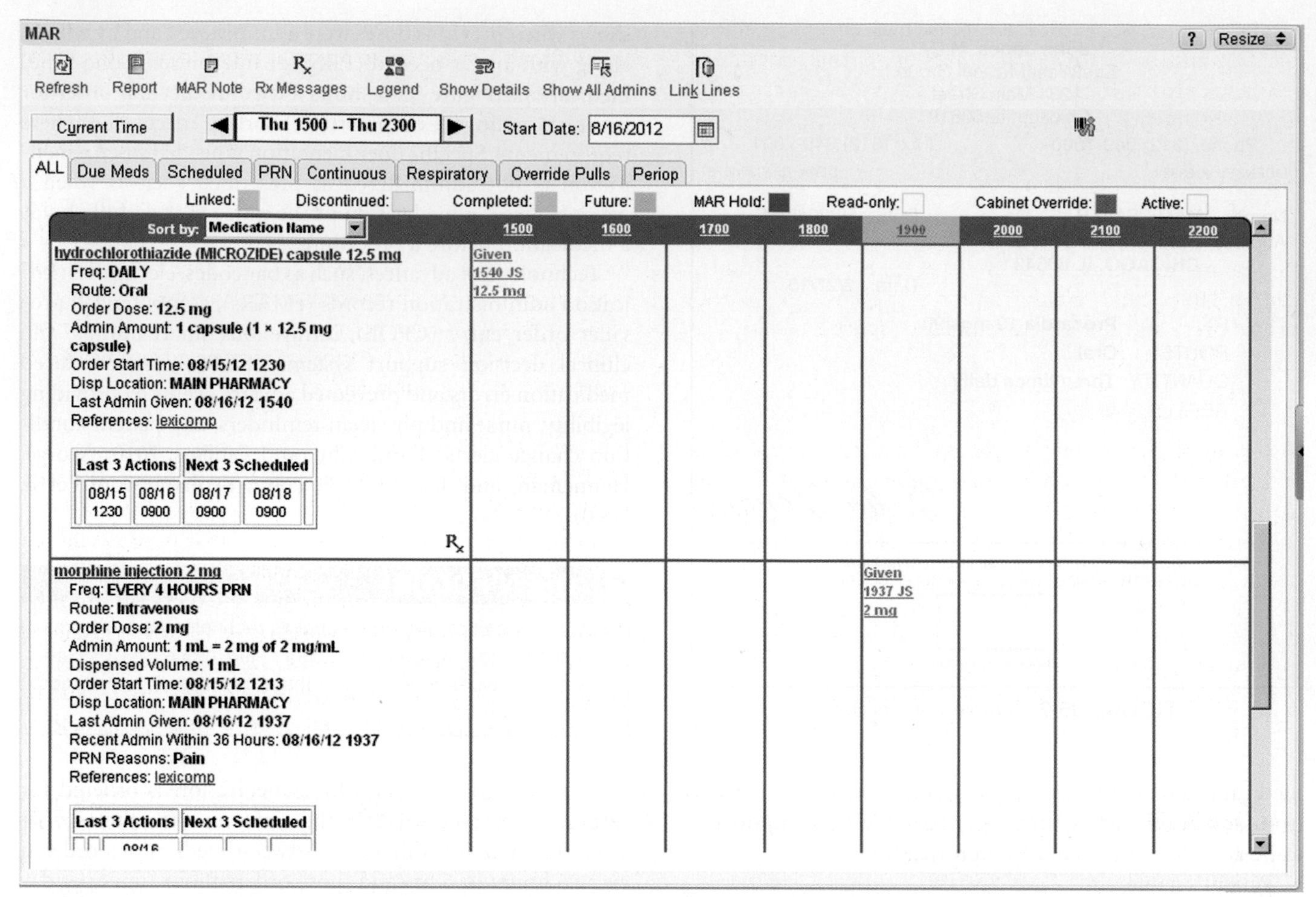

FIGURE 35-3 Medication administration record. (Courtesy Epic Systems Corporation, 2012.)

TABLE 35-5 Types of Medication Orders

TYPE	DESCRIPTION	EXAMPLES
Routine order	Administered until the health care provider discontinues the order or until a prescribed number of doses or days have occurred.	Digoxin 0.125 mg PO daily Amoxicillin 250 mg PO q 8 hr × 10 days
PRN order	Given only when the patient requires it. Use determined by objective and subjective assessment and clinical judgment of the nurse.	Morphine sulfate 4 mg IV q 2 hr PRN pain
One-time or on-call order	Given only once at a specified time, often before a diagnostic or surgical procedure.	Ativan 1 mg IV on call surgery
Stat order	Given immediately and only once in a single dose; frequently given for emergency situations.	Diazepam 10 mg IV stat for seizure
Now order	Used when a medication is needed quickly but not as immediately as a stat medication; given one time.	Vancomycin 1 g IV now, on admit

within the scope of practice for a nurse to determine medication administration times. The hours of administration per pharmacy protocol must be adhered to, unless ordered differently by the healthcare provider.

FORMS OF MEDICATION AND ROUTES OF ADMINISTRATION LO 35.4

Medications are formulated for a specific route of administration. The route of administration is specified on the prescribed order and refers to how the drug is absorbed.

FORMS OF MEDICATION

Nurses must administer the correct form of a medication (Table 35-6) by the correct route for optimal effectiveness and patient safety. Patient education on correct administration by the correct route is an important responsibility for nurses.

ROUTES OF MEDICATION ADMINISTRATION

Although the pharmacy should dispense the correct form, the nurse ensures that the medication is the correct form for the route of administration. Medication preparations are not interchangeable for alternate routes. For example, if a patient has difficulty swallowing a medication tablet, the nurse cannot substitute a liquid form without consulting the health care provider. A liquid form may be a different concentration or have a different absorption rate, which requires a change in dose or time of administration.

Common routes of administration include **oral** (by mouth), **buccal** (against the cheek), **sublingual** (under the tongue), **parenteral** (by injection or infusion), **topical** (on skin or mucous membranes), by inhalation, and through a medical tube (e.g., a nasogastric tube, percutaneous endoscopic gastrostomy [PEG] tube). Each route has advantages and disadvantages (Table 35-7).

Oral Administration

Medication is most commonly administered by the oral route, abbreviated as *PO* (Latin: *per os,* which means "by mouth"). These medications are designed to be swallowed with fluid, which is the safest, most convenient, and least expensive method for administration. Medications given by the oral route have a slower onset of action than parenteral medications. Nurses are responsible for ensuring that all medications taken by the oral route are swallowed. Patients with difficulty swallowing may hold medications in their

TABLE 35-6 Common Forms of Medication

FORM	DESCRIPTION AND USES
Tablets	Medication is compressed with binding substances and disintegrating agents; may have flavoring added to improve taste; used for oral, sublingual, and buccal routes. *Enteric coated tablets* have a special outer covering that delays absorption as it dissolves in the intestines.
Capsules	Medications are enclosed in cylindrical gelatin coatings. *Time-release capsules* have medication particles encased in smaller casings that deliver medication over an extended period.
Powders	Ultrafine drug particles in a dry form; depending on the medication, may be inhaled, mixed with food, or dissolved in liquids immediately before administration.
Troches or lozenges	Medications prepared to dissolve in the mouth.
Solutions	Medications already dissolved in liquid. *Syrups* are mixed with sugar and water. *Suspensions* are finely crushed medications in liquid. *Elixirs* are medications dissolved in alcohol and water with glycerin or other sweeteners. *Drops* are a sterile solution or suspension administered directly into the eye, outer ear canal, or nose or sublingually. *Injectable solutions* are sterile suspensions supplied in ampules, vials, prefilled syringes, bags, or bottles.
Inhalants or sprays	Medications inhaled or sprayed into the mouth or nose; may have local or systemic effects. Some are delivered in fixed doses.
Skin preparations	Ointments (spreadable, greasy preparations), creams (not greasy but used on skin only), and lotions (solutions or suspensions used on skin and not as sticky as creams or ointments). *Transdermal patches* contain medication absorbed through the skin over an extended period.
Suppositories	Bullet-shaped gelatin tablets commonly administered rectally or vaginally, depending on the medication. Urethral preparations are used for erectile dysfunction.

TABLE 35-7 Medication Administration Routes

ROUTE	ADVANTAGES	DISADVANTAGES
Oral	Convenient, cost-effective, and comfortable, with low stress for the patient. Certain oral tablets formulated to dissolve on contact with the tongue	Inappropriate for patients with nausea or vomiting; contraindicated for patients with swallowing difficulty Can irritate gastrointestinal lining, have unpleasant taste, or discolor teeth Patient must be alert and oriented to safely administer Cannot be used with simultaneous gastric suctioning or before various diagnostic or surgical procedures Possible irregular or slow absorption
Sublingual or buccal	As above plus more potent because the drug bypasses the liver and enters the bloodstream directly	May be inactivated by gastric juices if swallowed
Topical	Local effect with few side effects	Absorption may be irregular if skin breaks are present, and it may be slow
Transdermal	Prolonged systemic effects without gastrointestinal absorption problems	May leave residue on clothes
Mucous membranes (eyes, ears, nose, vagina, rectum, ostomy)	Local effects to involved sites with systemic effects possible; readily absorbed; may be used if the oral route is contraindicated	Mucous membranes are highly sensitive to concentrated medications Dose absorption may be unpredictable Procedure may be messy
Inhalation	Rapid localized effect; may be administered to unconscious patients	May cause serious systemic effects; can be used only through the respiratory system
Parenteral (intramuscular, intradermal, subcutaneous, intravenous)	Can be used if the oral route is contraindicated; more rapid response than the oral or topical route; can be used for critically ill patients and long-term therapy Intravenous (IV) route can decrease discomfort and can better control absorption if peripheral perfusion is compromised	Sterile technique must be used as the skin barrier is compromised More costly to formulate and administer; useful for small volumes only, except by IV route; affected by circulatory status; can produce patient anxiety

mouths, or patients with cognitive or mental health issues may pocket medications in the cheeks.

The sublingual and buccal oral routes are used for absorbing small amounts of medications quickly through the oral mucosa; this prevents destruction of the medication by gastric or intestinal secretions. For the **s**ublingual route, medications are placed under the tongue to dissolve (Figure 35-4). Nitroglycerin for chest pain is administered by this route. For the buccal route, medications are placed against the mucous membrane of the cheek until completely dissolved (Figure 35-5). Medications administered by the buccal route include antiemetics and opiate pain medications.

Oral medication can be administered through nasogastric, gastric, intestinal, and jejunal tubes. Tube placement is checked before medication administration. Chapter 30 provides more information about checking tube placement before medication administration. Special safety precautions need to be taken to prevent aspiration or clogging of the

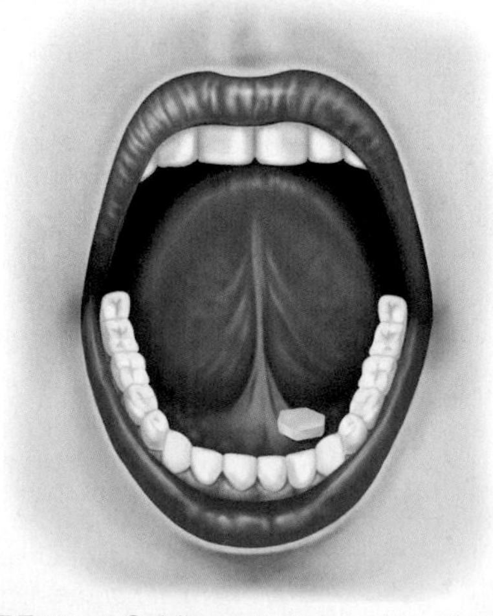

FIGURE 35-4 Sublingual placement of a tablet.

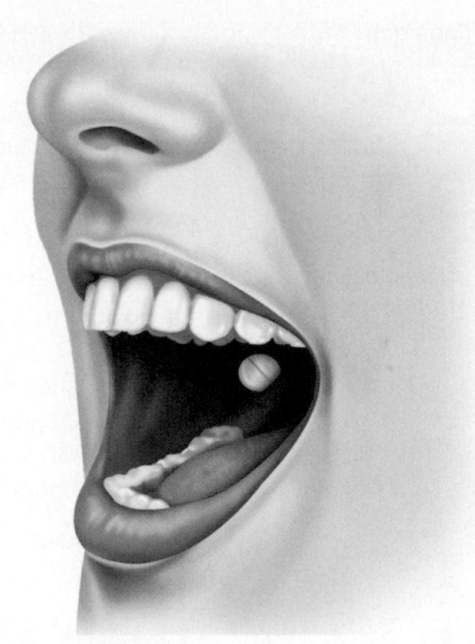

FIGURE 35-5 Buccal placement of medication.

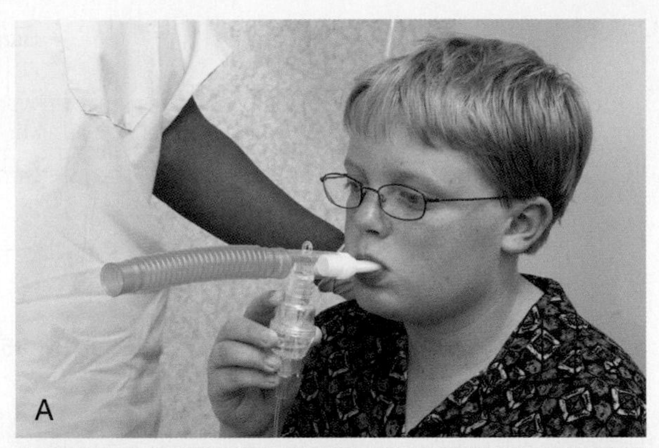

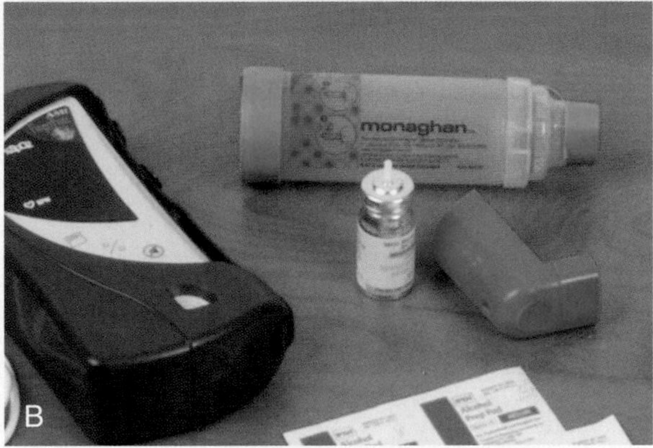

FIGURE 35-6 Inhaled medication delivery systems. **A,** Nebulizer. **B,** Metered-dose inhaler and spacer. (**A,** from Lilley LL, Collins SR, Snyder JS: *Pharmacology and the nursing process*, ed. 7, St. Louis, 2014, Mosby.)

tube when administering medications through small-bore feeding tubes.

> **! SAFE PRACTICE ALERT**
>
> Remember that not all medications can be crushed for administration through a tube. Enteric-coated, time-release, sublingual, buccal, and other medications with special coatings cannot be administered through a tube. Contact the health care provider to safely change the prescribed medication to an alternate administration route or formulation.

Topical Medications

Medications formulated for topical application are applied to a specific skin surface or mucous membrane of a body cavity. Nurses administer medications to the skin and mucous membranes in a variety of ways. Liquids and ointments can be directly applied to the eyes. Suppositories can be inserted into the rectum or vagina. Fluids can be instilled into a body cavity such as the ear, nose, bladder, or rectum. Body cavities such as the eye, ear, vagina, bladder, and rectum can be flushed with a medicated solution. A spray can be applied to the throat. Lotions and ointments can be applied to any skin surface.

Absorption is affected by the vascularity of the application site and typically requires additional applications each 24-hour period. A **transdermal patch** is a topical preparation designed to deliver medication slowly for systemic effects (e.g., nicotine, pain medication such as fentanyl, nitroglycerin for angina).

Inhaled Medications

Inhalation medications are taken into the body through the respiratory tract. The deeper passages of the respiratory tract provide a large surface for medication absorption. Inhaled medications are effectively used to induce anesthesia and to treat respiratory disorders. Nurses administer inhaled medications through nasal passages, oral passages, an endotracheal tube, or a tracheostomy tube (Figure 35-6). Means of delivery include small amounts of fluids, metered-dose inhalers (MDIs), turbo-inhalers, and nebulizers.

Parenteral Medications

Parenteral medications are administered through a needle by a route other than topical or through the gastrointestinal or respiratory tract. Absorption is usually faster and more complete by a parenteral route than the oral route. Aseptic technique is used because the protective skin barrier is bypassed with this route, resulting in infection risk. Safe injection practices maintain basic levels of patient safety and provider protection by combining aseptic technique with standard precautions (Centers for Disease Control and Preventions [CDC], 2014). Tissue damage is another risk when medications are administered into tissue, muscle, or blood vessels. There are four major sites of injection:

1. **Intradermal** (ID): Shallow injection into the dermal layer just under the epidermis
2. **Subcutaneous** (Sub-Q, subQ): Injection into the subcutaneous tissue just below the skin
3. **Intramuscular** (IM): Injection into a muscle of adequate size to accommodate the amount and type of medication
4. **Intravenous** (IV): Injection into a vein

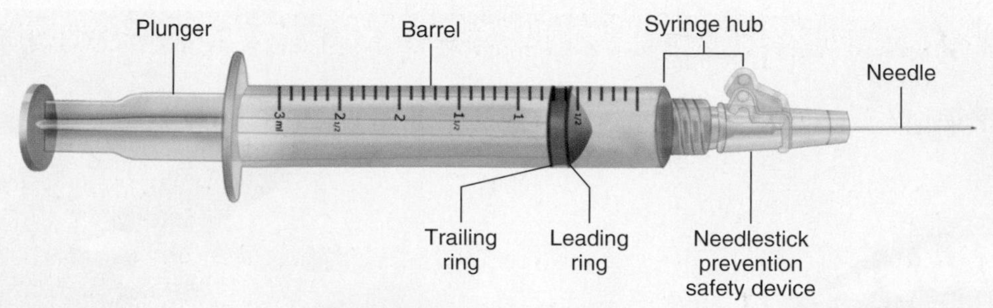

FIGURE 35-7 Parts of a syringe.

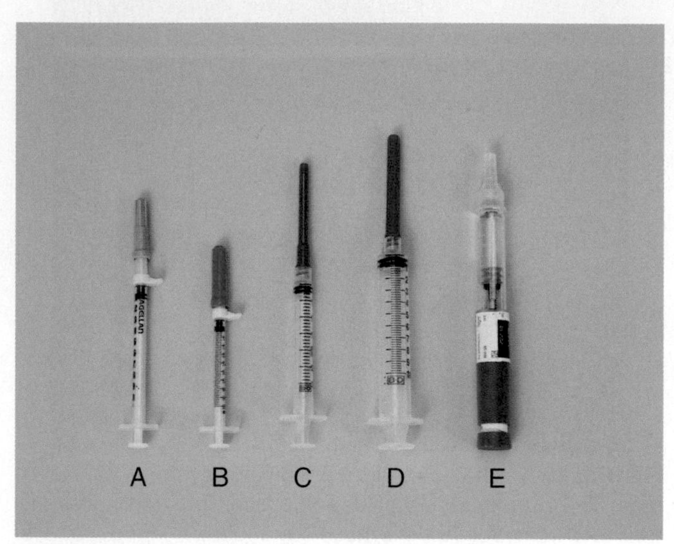

FIGURE 35-8 Types of syringes: tuberculin *(A)*, insulin 50 units *(B)*, standard 3 mL *(C)*, and standard 10 mL *(D)*, insulin pen *(E)*.

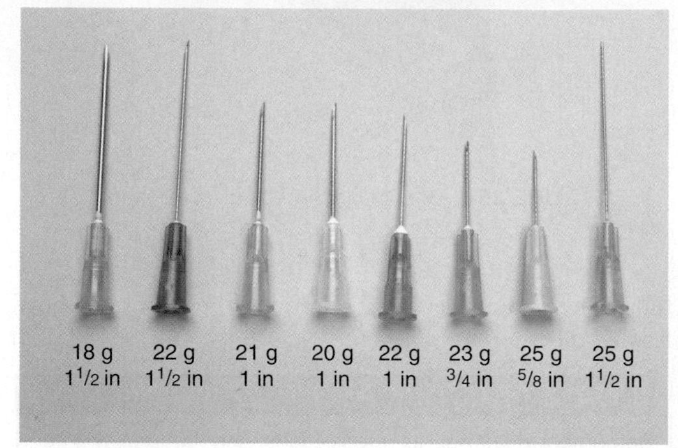

FIGURE 35-9 Needle sizes. (From Lilley LL, Collins SR, Snyder JS: *Pharmacology and the nursing process*, ed. 7, St. Louis, 2014, Mosby.)

Parenteral Medication Preparation

Various supplies are needed to administer parenteral medications. Syringes are usually made of plastic and have a barrel, plunger, and syringe tip (Figure 35-7). The plunger fits within the barrel. Moving the plunger in and out of the barrel allows fluid or air to move in or out of the syringe. With a Luer-Lok syringe, the needle is secured onto the end of the syringe with a twist motion. A Luer-Lok syringe can be directly attached to an access port on the IV tubing or saline lock without the use of a needle. Other syringes have needles that slide onto the end. The nurse may touch the outside of the syringe barrel and the handle of the plunger, but a nonsterile object should not touch the tip of the barrel, inside of the barrel, shaft of the plunger, or needle. Common syringes range from very small, 0.5-mL sizes for intradermal and subcutaneous injections to 60 mL for irrigations and tube feeding. Larger syringes are available for special uses. The three common types of syringes are standard, tuberculin, and insulin (Figure 35-8).

Most needles are made of stainless steel. The hub of the needle fits onto the tip of the syringe, the shaft of the needle is metal, and the bevel is the slanted tip of the needle. The needle diameter, or gauge, is identified by a number. Common gauges range from 18 to 30; the larger gauges, such as 16 or 14, are used in emergency departments or operating rooms (Figure 35-9). As the gauge number decreases, the diameter of the needle increases. For example, an 18-gauge needle has a larger diameter than a 25-gauge needle. The nurse selects a needle gauge based on the viscosity, or thickness, of the medication to be injected and the route of administration. Long-acting medications formulated in an oil base for sustained release require a larger gauge than thinner, water-based medications.

Needle length varies from 0.25 to 3 inches. Proper needle length depends on the age and size of the patient and the route of administration. Shorter needles are used for children and thin adults.

Standard syringes are 1-, 3-, 5-, and 10-mL sizes. Subcutaneous injections are typically administered with a 1-mL syringe and a ⅜- to ⅝-inch, 25- to 31-gauge needle. Intramuscular injections are usually administered with a 3-mL syringe and a 1- to 3-inch, 19- to 25-gauge needle. Intradermal injections require a 1-mL tuberculin syringe with a short, ¼- to ⅝-inch needle. U-100 (meaning there are 100 units per mL) insulin syringes are calibrated in units and millimeters and are supplied in three sizes: 30 units (0.3 mL), 50 units (0.5 mL), and 100 units (1 mL), each with a 26- to 31-gauge needle. Insulin may be administered by a prefilled insulin pen (see Figure 35-8), which combines the insulin container and syringe. Table 35-8 lists route, site selection, and appropriate syringe and needle sizes.

TABLE 35-8 Syringe and Needle Sizes

PARENTERAL ROUTE	SYRINGE SELECTION	NEEDLE SELECTION	SITE SELECTION
Subcutaneous	1-3 mL Insulin syringe: 0.5-1 mL with preattached needle	27-25 gauge, 3/8-5/8 inch Insulin syringe: 26-31 gauge, 5/16-1/2 inch*	Abdomen, lateral aspects of the upper arm and thigh, scapular area of the back, and upper ventrodorsal gluteal area
Intradermal	1-mL tuberculin syringe	Preattached 25-27 gauge, 1/4-5/8 inch	Inner forearm, upper arm, and across the scapula
Intramuscular	Adults: up to 3 mL depending on site Infants, small children: 0.5-1 mL	20-25 gauge, 1-3 inch Oil-based solutions: 18-20 gauge	Ventrogluteal, vastus lateralis, and deltoid Age of patient and corresponding site†: Infant: vastus lateralis Children: vastus lateralis or deltoid Adult: ventrogluteal or deltoid
Intravenous	Depends on amount of medication to be infused	Typically a large-gauge, 1-inch needle; needleless, blunt-tip cannula or Luer-Lok used with associated intravenous ports. (Do not use needles in a needless system to access IV ports.)	Vein

*From American Diabetes Association: Insulin (and other injected drugs). *Diabetes Forecast, 62*(1), 2009.
†From Nicoll LH, Hesby A: Intramuscular injection: An integrative research review and guideline for evidence-based practice. *Appl Nurs Res, 16*(2), 149-162, 2002.

Only advance practice nurses in specialty areas administer medication by epidural, intrathecal, intraosseous, intraperitoneal, or intraarterial parenteral routes. The nurse is responsible for monitoring the integrity of the delivery system, understanding the desired outcome of the medication, and evaluating the patient response to the medication for all routes of delivery.

Filter needles or straws are used when medications are being withdrawn from a glass ampule. The filter traps glass fragments. A filter needle or straw must be replaced with a regular needle before injecting the medication into the patient.

Needleless delivery systems significantly decrease needlestick injuries and exposure to blood-borne pathogens. Needleless systems are available for intravenous medication administration and require special tubing ports and blunt-tip cannulas that attach to the syringe in place of a needle. Some needleless systems allow syringes to connect directly to the intravenous tubing port. Adapters are available for vials that allow access to the contents of the vial by needleless cannulas. Needleless devices are disposed of in the same manner as regular needles.

SAFE MEDICATION ADMINISTRATION LO 35.5

The nurse is accountable for adherence to professional standards that apply to medication administration. Accountability is based on facility policies and procedures and on the American Nurses Association's *Nursing: Scope and Standards of Practice* (2010) for medication protocols and legal expectations. Before administering a medication, the nurse should check the patient's MAR or the health care provider's prescription, review diet and fluid orders, review relevant laboratory values, and perform a brief physical assessment.

To decrease medication errors, safe practice standards dictate that the nurse should follow only written orders. In an emergency situation, a verbal order from a health care provider may be given to the nurse or pharmacist, but the order must be put in writing as soon as possible. In most settings, student nurses are not allowed to transcribe written orders or accept verbal orders.

! SAFE PRACTICE ALERT

Nurses are legally accountable for medications they administer and for recognizing side effects and adverse reactions. Questions regarding the purpose, dose, route, time, abbreviations, relation to laboratory values, potential interactions, allergies, or patient response must be resolved with the health care provider or pharmacist before the nurse administers the medication. The nurse has the right and responsibility to refuse to administer a medication if he or she feels that the prescribed medication endangers the safety of the patient, but the health care provider must be notified of the refusal to administer the medication.

INTERPRETING THE ORDER

Special care is taken by the nurse to correctly read and interpret the initial medication order. The order must be clearly written or entered correctly into an electronic system. Clinical judgment is needed to evaluate whether the medication, amount prescribed, and route are safe for the patient. The nurse must understand the purpose, typical dosage, route, and side effects of the medication before administration. Interpreting the order is a step that should not be overlooked because the nurse assumes legal responsibility for all medications he or she administers. The nurse should clarify orders with the prescriber that are difficult to read, do not contain all of the critical information needed for safe administration, or contain prohibited or unfamiliar abbreviations (Ethical, Legal, and Professional Practice box).

ETHICAL, LEGAL, AND PROFESSIONAL PRACTICE

Calling the Health Care Provider About a Medication Order

The nurse is preparing the prescribed daily dose of warfarin for Mr. Andrews. As part of the nurse's assessment, the nurse reviews the international normalized ratio (INR) in the laboratory results obtained earlier in the morning. The INR level is 4.2, and the nurse recognizes that it would be unsafe to administer the prescribed warfarin. Additional investigation reveals that, unknown to the nursing staff, Mr. Andrews's wife has been administering his prehospitalization prescribed medications while he has been in the hospital. These medications include warfarin. The situation is reported by the nurse to the health care provider using the SBAR format:

S: Situation. Mr. Andrews's warfarin dose was held today because his INR result is 4.2.

B: Background. Mr. Andrews, age 79, was admitted 2 days ago with a third occurrence of deep vein thrombosis. His wife has been giving him his home medication of warfarin without telling the nursing staff. He has a history of gastrointestinal (GI) bleeding requiring transfusions.

A: Assessment. The warfarin was held today based on the INR results and his history of GI bleeding. Mr. Andrews's home medications have been sent to the pharmacy for safekeeping until he is discharged to prevent duplication of medications.

R: Recommendation. Do you want to monitor the INR daily and guaiac stools? What INR parameters should be used for resuming administration of the warfarin and at what dose? We will monitor for bruising, bleeding gums, and bloody urine or stools and have the patient use a soft toothbrush and safety razor.

MEDICATION ERRORS

Prevention of medication errors is the first step in medication safety. According to the Institute of Medicine (IOM), medication errors injure 1.5 million Americans each year and kill an estimated 7000 people. The financial costs are high: Among hospitalized patients alone, treatment of drug-related injuries costs about $3.5 billion in lost productivity, wages, and additional expenses (IOM, 2006).

The National Coordinating Council for Medication Error Reporting and Prevention (NCCMERP, 2011) defines a **medication error** as any preventable event that may cause or lead to inappropriate medication use or patient harm while the medication is in the control of the health care professional, patient, or consumer. These events may be related to professional practice, health care products, procedures, and systems, including prescribing; order communication; product labeling, packaging, and nomenclature; compounding; dispensing; distribution; administration; education; monitoring; and use.

QSEN FOCUS!

An understanding of safety is evident when the nurse delineates general categories of errors and hazards in care. The nurse values his or her own role in preventing errors.

Medication errors can occur anywhere in the medication system, from the manufacturer to patients and their families. Mistakes can occur during any of the many steps in the process of medication administration. Fortunately, mistakes can be caught at any of the preadministration steps. Multidisciplinary collaboration for medication administration helps safeguard against errors (Collaboration and Delegation box). Because the nurse is typically the last person in the sequence of administering medications in a health care facility, the nurse is the patient's last line of defense against mistakes. Many facilities have a No Interruption Zone policy for medication administration, requiring the nurse to prepare medications in a quiet setting without interruptions by other staff, patients, or phone calls. Focusing only on preparing the correct medications helps to decrease errors.

COLLABORATION AND DELEGATION

Medication Administration in the Acute Care Setting

- Collaboration with the patient and family or support person promotes the proper use of medications, ensuring their desired effects occur.
- Family members may be assisting the patient with medication use after discharge and need to understand how to monitor for therapeutic and adverse effects.
- Care providers, pharmacists, and case managers or social workers can ensure that the patient has the resources to obtain needed medications.
- Dieticians are involved with dietary requirements associated with medications, especially for patients with diabetes or cardiac disorders requiring special dietary intake to increase medication effects.
- Medication administration cannot be delegated to unlicensed assistive personnel (UAP) in the acute care setting. UAP usually are informed of any medication effects that are anticipated or being monitored. For example, UAP are told to expect that the patient may be dizzy when getting up after taking an antihypertensive medication that lowers the blood pressure.

There are several types of medication errors. Some can cause harm to the patient directly (e.g., giving an excessive dose of medication). Others fail to treat the patient's illness (e.g., giving too little medication). Other errors include giving the wrong drug, giving a medication to the wrong patient, or using the wrong route. Human factors include knowledge or performance deficits (e.g., administering a drug intravenously rather than intramuscularly), miscalculation of dosage, stress, and lack of sleep. Name confusion arises from medications with names that look or sound alike.

If a medication error occurs, the nurse's priorities are to determine the effect on the patient and intervene to offset any adverse effects of the error. Actions include immediate and ongoing assessment, notification of the prescribing health care provider, initiation of interventions as prescribed to offset any adverse effects, and documentation related to the event. Error reporting is an essential component of patient safety and should be completed as soon as the patient is assessed and stable. The nurse should follow facility guidelines for medication error reporting.

QSEN FOCUS!

Creating a culture of safety, the nurse describes factors such as open communication strategies and organizational error reporting systems. The nurse uses organizational error reporting systems for any medication error.

Measures that can be especially effective in reducing errors include replacing handwritten medication orders with a computerized provider order entry system and using a bar code system when administering medications. Bar codes verify that the patient and drug match and that adverse interactions are unlikely. The Institute for Safe Medication Practices has compiled a list of error-prone abbreviations, symbols, and dose designations that should be avoided to decrease errors.

ABBREVIATIONS

The safe use of abbreviations is important in preventing medication errors. The National Patient Safety Goals developed by The Joint Commission emphasize prevention of medication errors. From this effort came The Joint Commission's Do Not Use list of abbreviations that were identified as contributing to medication errors. This list is included in Chapter 10. Table 35-9 identifies some commonly approved abbreviations used in medication administration.

QSEN FOCUS!

When administering medications, the nurse examines medication administration factors, basic safety design principles, and commonly used unsafe practices such as dangerous abbreviations.

DOSAGE CALCULATION

Three types of measurement systems are used in medication calculations: metric, apothecary, and household. The nurse must understand all three to accurately administer the prescribed medication. A nurse may need to convert the ordered dose to what is dispensed by the pharmacy.

TABLE 35-9 Common Abbreviations Related to Medication Administration

ABBREVIATION	MEANING
ac	Before meals
pc	After meals
h *or* hr	Hour
bid	Two times per day
tid	Three times per day
qid	Four times per day
q	Every
g *or* gm	Gram
mcg	Microgram
mg	Milligram
mL	Milliliter
IM	Intramuscular
IV	Intravenous
PO *or* po	By mouth, orally
NPO *or* npo	Nothing by mouth
PRN *or* prn	As needed
SL	Sublingual
STAT	Immediately

Basic measures of the metric system include gram (weight), liter (volume), and meter (linear). The metric system has a basic unit of 10, and calculations are performed by dividing or multiplying in increments of 10. Because 1 g is equal to 1000 mg, to change milligrams to grams, the number of grams is multiplied by 1000. An example is 0.5 g = 500 mg.

SAFE PRACTICE ALERT

When noting a metric dose, always place a zero in front of the decimal point, and never have a trailing zero. For example, doses are identified as 0.5 mL instead of .5 mL and as 5 mL instead of 5.0 mL.

The apothecary system is older than the metric system. It has a basic measure called the *minim* (volume). The minim is followed in increasing order by the dram, ounce, pint, quart, and gallon. Weight in the apothecary system is based on 1 grain of wheat, which is abbreviated as *gr*. The apothecary system is no longer used on any drug labels. Medications should be prescribed and calculated using the metric system. Occasionally, the nurse may find a prescription written in terms of fluid ounces or grains.

The household system is the one with which most people in the United States are familiar. It is the most inaccurate of the three systems. The base unit of measurement is the drop (gt). The drop is followed in increasing order by the teaspoon (tsp), tablespoon (Tbsp), and cup. The use of the teaspoon as a measurement is familiar and widely practiced by many. If strictly accurate dosing is needed, it is important to convert to a metric equivalent. These conversions are done by memorizing equivalents and then calculating the conversion. For example, a teaspoon is 5 mL and a tablespoon is 15 mL.

Calculation Methods

Several formulas or methods can be used to calculate the dosage of medications. Regardless of the method chosen, it is important to identify the available quantity of medication and the desired (prescribed) quantity.

Although a ratio proportion or formula method of dosage calculation may be used, the dimensional analysis method removes the need for multiple-step calculations and provides a consistent method for calculating medication dosages. This formula can be used in all situations, from doing basic calculations to determining pediatric doses to calculating titration of potent drugs in critical care units.

The nurse begins a dosage calculation by identifying the units of measure (e.g., mg, capsule) needed for the answer to the problem. The unit used in the answer must have the same unit as the numerator, or top of the equation, and the denominator, or bottom of the equation. Start the equation with the dose to be given, then the concentration or supply available. For example, the prescribed medication is "amoxicillin 0.5 g every 8 hours," and the available quantity is amoxicillin 250 mg per 1 capsule. A unit conversion is needed from grams to milligrams. Notice that *capsule* must be in the numerator in the problem because it is the unit needed in the answer; the nurse needs to figure out how many capsules to administer per dose.

$$\frac{0.5\ \text{g}}{1\ \text{dose}} \times \frac{1\ \text{capsule}}{250\ \text{mg}} \times \frac{1000\ \text{mg}}{1\ \text{g}} =$$

In dimensional analysis, the first step is to cross off units that appear in both the numerator and denominator:

$$\frac{0.5\ \cancel{\text{g}}}{1\ \text{dose}} \times \frac{1\ \text{capsule}}{250\ \cancel{\text{mg}}} \times \frac{1000\ \cancel{\text{mg}}}{1\ \cancel{\text{g}}} =$$

After the units occurring in both numerator and denominator are crossed off, the only units left in the equation are the correct ones for the answer to the nurse's question. Next, the numbers on the top of the equation are multiplied, and the numbers on the bottom are multiplied. The final step is to divide the numerator by the denominator and add the correct units to the numeric answer:

$$\frac{500\ \text{capsules}}{250\ \text{doses}} = 2\ \text{capsules/dose}$$

Using a consistent approach in calculating medication dosages can greatly reduce the potential for medication errors resulting from miscalculations.

ADMINISTERING MEDICATIONS BY USING THE SIX RIGHTS

The **Six Rights of Medication Administration** were developed to help the nurse prevent mistakes. Confirming that the medication order is safe and following the Six Rights during each patient interaction can prevent medication errors. The Six Rights of Medication Administration are the right drug, right dose, right time, right route, right patient, and right documentation (Nursing Care Guideline: Six Rights of Medication Administration box).

Before administering a medication, the nurse carefully reads the medication record and does three checks with the labeled medication. The first check consists of verifying that the label of the medication matches the MAR, performing a dosage calculation, and checking the expiration date of the medication. The second check consists of preparing the medication and again checking the medication label against the MAR. The third check is a recheck of the label on the medication before returning the medication to its storage place *or* a recheck of the medication label a final time against the MAR before opening the package at the bedside.

High-Risk Situations for Medication Administration

Many situations can increase the risk of making a medication error and causing patient injury (Table 35-10). Safeguards for preventing medication errors include following facility policies regarding patient identification, giving medications prepared by the person administering them, double-checking doses, verifying high-risk drug doses with a second nurse, addressing patient questions about medication, and understanding why the patient is receiving a specific medication.

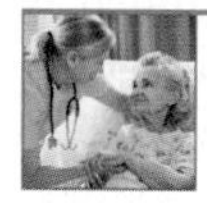

3. The nurse accidentally administers Mrs. Petros's prescribed diuretic, potassium, and stool softener to Mrs. Peters, the patient in the next room. Identify at least four safety measures that can prevent medication errors when properly followed, and list the actions the nurse needs to take now.

Patient Rights

In 2003, the American Hospital Association developed the Patient Care Partnership program to help patients understand their rights while in the hospital. Patient rights related to medication administration include the following:

- The right to be informed of the name, purpose, and potential side effects of medications
- The right to refuse a medication

NURSING CARE GUIDELINE

Six Rights of Medication Administration

Background

- Six Rights of Medication Administration:
  - The right drug
  - The right dose
  - The right time
  - The right route
  - The right patient
  - The right documentation
- Never administer medication that you did not prepare. This task cannot be delegated, even to other professionals.
  - Unlicensed assistive personnel (UAP) may not administer medications unless they are in a state that allows designation of certified medication technicians in certain facilities.
  - These technicians may administer certain medications. Check with the state's nurse practice act and the facility's policies and procedures.
  - The task is not being delegated; the technician is assuming responsibility.
- If there is any question regarding the medication order by the nurse or the patient, do not administer the medication. Contact the primary care provider or pharmacist for clarification.
- Never leave the medication unattended at the bedside.

Procedural Concerns

Verification

- The Six Rights require that verifications be made.

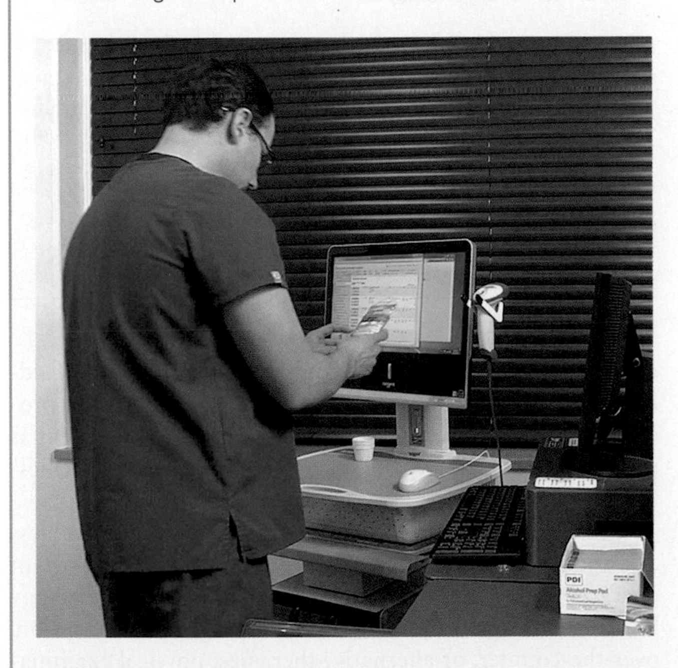

- Verify that the drug is the right drug at each of these three points:
  - When taking the drug out of the drawer or dispensing unit
  - When comparing it with the MAR as the drug is being prepared
  - At the bedside immediately before administration
- Verify that the right dose will be given by confirming the following:
  - The calculation of the dose is correct.
  - Its strength is correct.
  - The dose prescribed is appropriate for the patient.
- Additional verification is provided by the following:
  - Have another nurse check critical dosage calculations.
  - Be aware that unit-dose systems were developed to decrease errors related to dose amounts.
  - Use standard measurement devices such as graduated medication cups, syringes, and calibrated droppers when preparing medications.
- Verify that the medication will be administered at the right time:
  - Administer medications within the appropriate time frame (usually between the half hour before and the half hour after the scheduled time; check facility and state policy) or administer as specified (e.g., before meals).
  - Make sure it will be administered with the correct frequency.
  - Use the correct time system. Many health centers use military time to avoid the confusion that can result when using A.M. and P.M.
- Verify that the medication will be administered by the right route to ensure compatibility:
  - Possible routes of administration are oral (PO), sublingual, buccal, rectal, vaginal, topical, transdermal, subcutaneous, intramuscular (IM), intradermal (ID), intravenous (IV), and inhalation.
  - Before administering parenteral medications, check compatibility, need for dilution, and rate of administration.
  - When medications are mixed in the same syringe, there may be a time limit between when the drugs are mixed and when they are administered. Always verify timing of administration.
  - Some medications may be cut or crushed.
- Verify that the medication will be administered to the right patient by using one of the following:
  - A bar code scanning system or at least two identifiers, such as full name of the patient, date of birth, and current photograph (but *not* the patient's room or physical location)
  - The medical record number on the patient's wristband

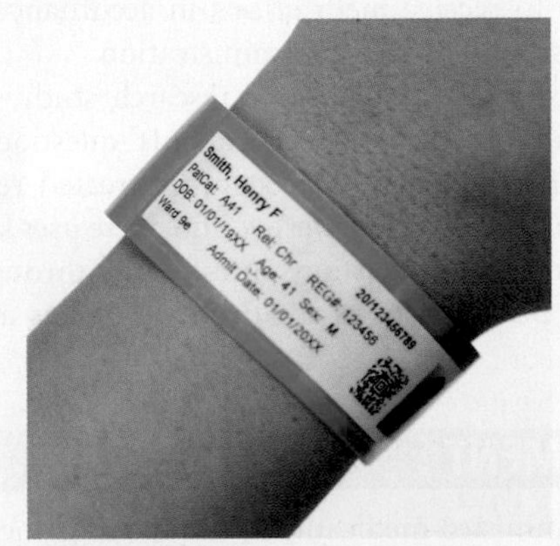

(Courtesy GBS Corp, *www.gbscorp.com*.)

Continued

NURSING CARE GUIDELINE—cont'd

- Complete the right documentation after administration:
  - Verify that it is accurate and complete according to facility policy and procedure.
  - It should account for adverse effects.
  - It should include communication with other health care providers.
  - It must include the patient's response.

Other Considerations

- Verify that the medication is being given for the right reason (i.e., medication is correct for the patient's condition). Know what outcome from the medication is expected for the patient.
- Complete an assessment, and verify the observations:
  - The appropriate vital signs are taken before and after administration.
  - The patient has no allergies to the drug.
  - The appropriate laboratory data are obtained.
  - The appropriate physical assessment data are collected.
  - The patient's pain levels are known.
- When the nurse is administering a medication, patient teaching is essential and should include the name of the drug, what it is for, the dosage, and pertinent side effects.
- Complete an evaluation of medications, and verify that required follow-up assessments are performed.

Patient Concerns

- If the patient questions or refuses the medication, stop the administration, verify the information, and proceed accordingly.
- The patient has the right to refuse medications.

Documentation Concerns

- Do not document administration of the medication until it is given to the patient.
- Documentation using paper charting may be necessary if the situation is an emergency or the computer system is not operational for some reason. The following are special considerations for paper charting.
  - Ensure the legibility of orders and documentation.
  - The appropriate ink color, depending on facility policy, must be used. Some facilities require black ink so that documents can be scanned and stored electronically. Other facilities require that each shift document in a different ink color.
  - Never leave blanks or spaces in documentation.
  - Chapter 10 further discusses paper charting and correction of errors.
- Documentation using computerized charting:
  - Ensure that the entries are in the appropriate location.
  - Ensure that the actual caregiver is logged on and that entries are submitted or saved.
  - If a manual override is used, document the reason for using it.
- Documentation using both computerized and paper charting:
  - Use appropriate abbreviations, avoiding abbreviations as listed in the following references:
    - The Do Not Use list published by The Joint Commission
    - The Error-Prone Abbreviations, Symbols, and Dose Designations list published by the Institute for Safe Medication Practices (ISMP)
  - Use correct grammar and spelling.
  - Record the correct time.
  - Perform charting promptly.
- Document adverse effects reported by the patient or observed during evaluation.

Evidence-Based Practice

- The ISMP (2010) independently collects data and promotes educational tools to prevent medication errors. The institute collaborates with multiple agencies to assist facilities with implementing the best evidence-based practices in regard to medication administration.
- Use of evidence-based practices has reduced medication errors and prevented adverse events.

- The right to have an accurate medication history taken by a qualified person
- The right to receive medications in accordance with the Six Rights of Medication Administration

If the medication is part of a research study, the nurse should be informed of this fact. Patients' questions or concerns regarding medication need to be treated respectfully and questions should be answered. The nurse uses knowledge and caring to answer questions and follows through appropriately if a patient refuses medications or has an adverse effect.

◆ ASSESSMENT LO 35.6

To safely administer medications, the nurse gathers patient assessment data. Information about a patient's allergies to drugs and food and the patient's pregnancy or breastfeeding status is especially critical. The initial assessment produces baseline data, and medication-specific assessment is part of ongoing care by the nurse (Health Assessment Questions box).

Ongoing assessment evaluates medication effectiveness and enables early identification of adverse effects. Important data to be collected are the patient's medical history; allergy information; medication history, including any prescription, over-the-counter, or alternative therapies; physical examination results, with a focus on medication effects on the body; and relevant laboratory results. Assessment questions are adapted to meet the patient's needs and are asked in terms that the patient can understand. Responses to medication assessment questions should be documented in the appropriate sections of the health record.

TABLE 35-10 High-Risk Situations for Medication Administration

MEDICATION ADMINISTRATION RIGHTS	HIGH-RISK SITUATIONS
Right drug	Incorrectly dispensing and giving a medication with a similar name to the one prescribed Administering a medication that the nurse did not prepare Incorrectly identifying a medication Not listening to a patient who reports that the medication looks different from that given previously
Right dose	Needing multiple tablets, capsules, or medication cups to prepare a single dose Having a large change in dosage prescribed Having a unit dose or dose supplied by the pharmacy that does not match the prescribed dose Not listening to a patient who states that the dose being offered is different from that normally taken Using nonstandardized measuring devices, such as a plastic spoon Breaking tablets that are not scored into pieces or not using an accepted cutting device to split a tablet Leaving part of crushed medication behind in the crushing device or the patient's not eating all of the food or liquid in which the crushed medication is mixed
Right time	Giving all medications at convenient times for the nurse instead of at the times they will be most effective or are specifically prescribed Not administering medications according to specific needs, such as with food or on an empty stomach Missing doses and needing to reschedule times
Right route	Not knowing the medication's usual route Not looking up unfamiliar medications Preparing parenteral doses that are not designed for the parenteral route
Right patient	Incorrectly identifying patients with similar names (who often require additional safety measures such as flagging the medication administration record [MAR]) Bypassing the identification process and relying on memory of previous patient interactions Preparing medications for more than one patient at a time Relying on unsafe identification means, such as a room number Using a smudged or illegible name band as an identifier
Right documentation	Using incomplete, inaccurate, or illegible medication information Lacking documentation of the assessment data required for the medication, such as laboratory values or apical heart rate Documenting before medication is administered Failing to document the medications administered, which is especially dangerous for medications scheduled at shift-change times (e.g., morning insulin doses) Failing to document the patient response to medications

! SAFE PRACTICE ALERT

Patient allergies to foods, drugs, and other substances are noted in the medical record in the history and physical section and on the medication administration record. The pharmacy and dietary departments are notified about allergies, and an allergy band is placed on the patient's wrist.

The body's response to some medications is monitored over time to establish therapeutic effects or watch for adverse effects. Common laboratory measures monitored to assess medication responses include electrolytes, serum glucose, complete blood count (CBC), white blood cell (WBC) count, bleeding time, blood urea nitrogen (BUN), creatinine, and serum levels of specific medications.

The nurse completes a physical assessment to identify body systems that may be affected by prescribed medications. For example, a respiratory assessment is performed before the administration of a bronchodilator treatment for a patient having an asthma attack. This assessment includes respiratory rate, auscultation of lung sounds, use of accessory muscles, and oxygen saturation levels. The assessment is repeated after medication administration to determine the effectiveness of the intervention.

Because medications may affect temperature, pulse, respirations, and blood pressure, vital signs that may be affected should be measured before and after administering a medication. For example, the apical pulse for 1 minute is obtained before administering digoxin (i.e., cardiac medication that slows the heart rate) because it is common to withhold administration if the patient's heart rate is less than 60 beats/min; blood pressure is monitored before and after an antihypertensive is administered; the patient's temperature is measured before and after an antipyretic (medication to decrease

HEALTH ASSESSMENT QUESTIONS

Drug History and Current Use
- What food or drug allergies do you have? Describe the reaction.
- What prescribed medications are you currently taking? Do you have them with you?
- Which over-the-counter medications and herbs do you take on a regular basis (e.g., antacids, laxatives, aspirin, creams, or lotions)?
- What is your alcohol intake? Caffeine intake? Use of home remedies?
- What medications have you stopped taking recently?
- Do you use any other methods to relieve your symptoms?
- Do you have any cultural or religious considerations regarding medications?

Medical History
- Do you have any ongoing illnesses?
- What surgeries have you had?
- Are you up to date on your immunizations?
- Are you pregnant or breastfeeding?
- Have you been hospitalized? For what?

Medication Schedule
- What times do you take your medications?
- Do you prepare your medications in a special way (e.g., crushed in applesauce, taken with a meal)?
- How do you remember to take your medications on schedule?

Medication Response
- What response have you had to your medications?
- Have you had any side effects or adverse reactions from medications?

Medication Compliance
- Can you tell me why you take this medication?
- Are there problems that prevent you from taking your medications (e.g., cost, access at work or school, irregular meal schedules)?
- Do you have vision problems? Hearing problems? Difficulty opening medication containers? Mobility difficulties? Trouble remembering to take medications? Trouble swallowing?
- How do you feel about taking medications?

Medication Safety
- Where are your medications kept at home?
- Do others have access to your medications? Any children?
- Do you have medications at home that you no longer take regularly? How long do you keep your medications?
- How do you dispose of medications that you are no longer taking?
- Do you do any special monitoring for these medications (e.g., blood levels, blood glucose monitoring)?

fever) is administered; and respiratory rate and blood pressure are measured before administration of an opiate that can decrease these vital signs.

Assessing the patient's ability to swallow is important before administration of an oral medication. Adequate muscle mass is needed for proper absorption of intramuscular medications, and patent venous access must be available for intravenously administered medications. The skin site for topical medications must be inspected.

The most important steps for the nurse to take when preparing to administer medications are assessment of the patient and adherence to the Six Rights of Medication Administration (see Nursing Care Guideline: Six Rights of Medication Administration box).

NURSING DIAGNOSIS LO 35.7

The nurse analyzes subjective and objective assessment data to identify actual or potential problems to develop a nursing diagnosis. It is important to have thorough data in determining the nursing diagnosis, which leads to developing the appropriate nursing interventions. The following are examples of common nursing diagnoses related to medication administration:

- *Deficient Knowledge* related to lack of exposure to information as evidenced by patient's taking a double dose of Lasix and not being aware of possible side effects
- *Constipation* related to opioid pain medication use as evidenced by reported hard, painful stools
- *Noncompliance* related to deficient knowledge as evidenced by refusal to continue prescribed medications

PLANNING LO 35.8

The nurse develops patient goals and plans care on the basis of the nursing diagnoses, assessment of the patient's ability to perform needed tasks, and realistic expectations for achieving the goals (Table 35-11). The following are patient goals based on the nursing diagnoses:

- The patient will verbalize side effects of medications before discharge.
- During outpatient visit, the patient will demonstrate understanding about the need for adequate fluid and fiber intake to prevent constipation.
- The patient will take medications daily until the next appointment.

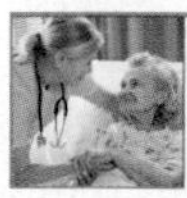

The conceptual care map for Mrs. Petros can be found at *http://evolve.elsevier.com/YoostCrawford/fundamentals/*. It is partially completed to indicate how to use the map as a learning tool. Complete the nursing diagnoses using the example conceptual care maps shown in Chapter 8 and Chapters 25 to 33.

TABLE 35-11 Care Planning

NANDA-I NURSING DIAGNOSIS LABEL WITH NURSING DIAGNOSIS STATEMENT	NURSING OUTCOME CLASSIFICATION (NOC)	NURSING INTERVENTION CLASSIFICATION (NIC)
Deficient Knowledge related to lack of exposure to information, as evidenced by patient's taking a double dose of Lasix and not being aware of possible side effects	*Knowledge: Medication* (1808) Medication adverse effects (180820)	*Teaching: Prescribed medication* (5616) Instruct patient on possible adverse side effects of each medication.

From Bulechek G, Butcher H, Dochterman J, et al (Eds): *Nursing interventions classification (NIC),* ed. 6, St. Louis, 2013, Mosby; Moorhead S, Johnson M, Maas M, et al (Eds): *Nursing outcomes classification (NOC),* ed. 5, St. Louis, 2013, Mosby; NANDA International: *Nursing diagnoses: Definitions and classification, 2012–2014,* West Sussex, England, 2012, Wiley-Blackwell. Reprinted with permission from NANDA International, Inc.

IMPLEMENTATION AND EVALUATION LO 35.9

The nurse implements the plan of care through identified nursing interventions based on the nursing diagnosis, goals, and desired outcomes. Evaluation of the effectiveness of those interventions occurs within the specific time frames that the nurse established in the plan. Using the goals and outcomes provides an objective, measurable way to conduct the evaluation.

MEDICATION ADMINISTRATION

Each medication that a nurse administers must be prescribed by a health care provider and be appropriate for the patient. The order may be handwritten on a patient chart or electronically entered into the medication system, where it is then transcribed onto the electronic health record (EHR) or medication administration record (MAR). The nurse uses the MAR when preparing and administering all medications.

Medications are administered through several different routes, and nurses must follow established protocols for administering medications safely by each route. Clinical judgment acknowledges that special techniques be used for children and elderly individuals to facilitate the administration of medications (Diversity Considerations box).

Oral Medications

The easiest and most convenient administration route is by mouth (PO), which is discussed in Skill 35-1. Drugs administered by this route are intended to be absorbed in the stomach and small intestine. The patient's ability to swallow, level of consciousness, gag reflex, and whether the patient is experiencing nausea and vomiting are assessed to ensure the patient's ability to take medications by the oral route and to prevent aspiration (i.e., inhalation of gastric contents into the respiratory system). If a patient should receive nothing by mouth (**NPO**), an alternate route is used or an order is obtained for the patient to be NPO except for medications. After oral medication has been taken, the nurse verifies that the medication was swallowed and encourages the patient to drink fluids to ensure that medication has not lodged in the esophagus. If the patient feels that medication is stuck in the throat, eating a small amount of soft food, such as oatmeal or a slice of bread, helps the medication move from the esophagus.

Special techniques are used for the patient who has difficulty swallowing large tablets. Some capsules may be opened and the contents added to a small amount of applesauce, pudding, or ice cream. Certain tablets may be crushed and

DIVERSITY CONSIDERATIONS

Life Span

Children

- Liquid forms of oral medications are preferred for children younger than 5 years of age.
- Parents or caregivers may need instruction with pictures and written directions about home medication administration.
- A calibrated dropper is used for infants or very young children. Place the medication between the gum and cheek to prevent aspiration.
- Uncoated tablets or soft capsules may be crushed and sprinkled over a small amount of food. Do not use a favorite food or formula because the child may avoid food associated with medicines in the future.
- Warn the child if the medication has an unpleasant taste; this helps to increase future trust in the nurse.
- Praise the child after the medication is swallowed.

Older Adults

- Do not rush medication administration. Allow time for understanding of treatment and slower swallowing.
- Crushed or liquid forms of medications may be easier to swallow.
- Normal aging processes (e.g., decreased renal and hepatic function) may affect the dosage needed because drugs may be metabolized slower. Adverse effects may be increased in elderly individuals.
- Patients may need instruction on medications to be taken at home. Focus on the name and purpose of the drug, because the color may vary by manufacturer.
- Loss of dexterity and the ability to open pill bottles, visual impairment, and cognitive impairment in the elderly can affect safe medication administration.

added to food in a similar manner. Use a small amount of food so that the entire dose is administered if the patient eats only a small amount.

! SAFE PRACTICE ALERT

Enteric-coated or sustained-release tablets should never be crushed. The enteric coating protects the oral and gastric mucosa from irritating medications. Crushing a sustained-release medication allows absorption to occur all at once rather than the desired absorption over time.

Liquid medications often come in premeasured packages. If not, a calibrated syringe or medication cup is used to accurately measure the prescribed amount. Antifungal liquid medications (e.g., nystatin) may need longer contact with mucous membranes and be prescribed as "swish and swallow." The patient swishes the medication back and forth in the mouth several times and then swallows it. This should be the last oral medication administered so that additional use of fluids to swallow the other medications does not rinse the medication from the mucous membranes.

Medication is never given from a container with a label that is missing or difficult to read. Unused medication is not returned to a multidose container and should not be placed in unlabeled containers. Medication that has changed color or does not stay in solution is discarded. Offer oral hygiene after medication with an unpleasant taste.

! SAFE PRACTICE ALERT

Never return unused medication to a multidose container. Never administer medication that is not labeled.

Medication may be administered by the enteral route (i.e., through a gastrointestinal tube). Liquid medication is preferred, although some tablets may be finely crushed and dissolved in water. Care is taken that the tube is flushed before and after administration with 30 to 45 mL of water (or in accordance with facility policy) to clear the tube of medication and prevent clogging of the tube. Having the patient sit as upright as possible decreases the risk of aspiration. The patient should remain with the head elevated for at least 30 minutes after administration. To allow absorption time, gastric suction should not be used for 20 to 30 minutes after administration. Water intake associated with medication administration is counted as intake on the intake and output record.

Sublingual and Buccal Medications

The sublingual and buccal routes allow rapid absorption of medications such as nitroglycerin for chest pain. A sublingual medication is placed under the tongue and allowed to dissolve. The patient should not eat or drink anything until the medication is completely dissolved. A medication given by the buccal route (e.g., antiemetic, sedative, opiate) is placed in the side of the mouth against the inner cheek. Patients are taught to alternate cheeks to avoid mucosal irritation. Buccal medication should not be chewed, swallowed, or taken with liquids. Standard precautions are used by the nurse administering medications by the sublingual or buccal route because the nurse's hand may come in contact with oral secretions.

Topical Medications

Topical medications are placed on the skin surface, on mucous membranes, or in body cavities (Nursing Care Guideline: Topical Medication Administration box). Placement sites in addition to the skin include eyes, ears, nose, rectum, vagina, and lungs. Drugs applied directly to skin for a local effect include lotions, creams, powders, and aerosol sprays. Cleanse the skin before applying topical medications to remove body oils or dry skin, which can impair medication absorption. Gauze dressing may be applied over the medication to prevent removal of the medication by clothing. Gloves and applicators are used to avoid absorption through the nurse's skin during placement of topical medications.

Transdermal Medications

Medications designed to be absorbed through the skin for systemic effect are administered transdermally, usually in the form of a patch. The skin site must be cleansed because skin oils may interfere with the adhesive on these products. A previously placed patch and remaining medication are removed. Patches are disposed of according to facility policy, especially if the patch contains a controlled substance. Placement sites are rotated to avoid skin irritation. Placement of the new patch and removal of the old patch are recorded in the MAR.

Ophthalmic Instillation

Ophthalmic medications (i.e., eyedrops and ointments), including over-the-counter preparations, are used to treat eye irritation, infections, or disorders such as glaucoma (Nursing Care Guideline Ophthalmic Medication Administration box). Eyedrops can be used for diagnostic procedures or to anesthetize the eye for procedures. Cross-contamination is a potential problem with eye medications. Each patient has an individual bottle of eye medication. Care is taken not to touch the tip of the dropper or tube to the patient's eye because infection can be transferred from one eye to another if the applicator touches the eye.

Otic Instillation

Solutions administered to the ear canal are otic medications (Nursing Care Guideline: Otic Medication Administration box). Eardrops are used to treat ear infections and associated pain, soften earwax to ease removal, apply a local anesthetic, and destroy insects trapped in the ear canal. The internal ear is very sensitive to temperature changes, and it is important to use eardrops at room temperature to prevent nausea, pain, and dizziness. If the tympanic membrane has been damaged,

NURSING CARE GUIDELINE

Topical Medication Administration

Background

- Always follow the Six Rights of Medication Administration.
- Medications are applied to skin for many reasons:
  - Hormone treatment
  - Administration of cardiac medications
  - Application of narcotic analgesics
  - Assistance with overcoming nicotine addiction
  - Treatment of pruritus
  - Provision of a protective coating on the skin
  - Treatment or prevention of infection
- The following are types of topical medications:
  - Creams or oils (for lubrication)
  - Lotions (to protect and soothe)
  - Powders (for drying surface moisture and decreasing friction)
  - Ointments (to provide prolonged contact with the medication and to soften)
  - Transdermal patches or disks (for continuous medication administration for several hours to several days)
- Absorption of medication through the skin is called *inunction.*

Procedural Concerns

All Topicals

- Apply gloves to avoid being exposed to the patient's medication that is absorbed through the skin.

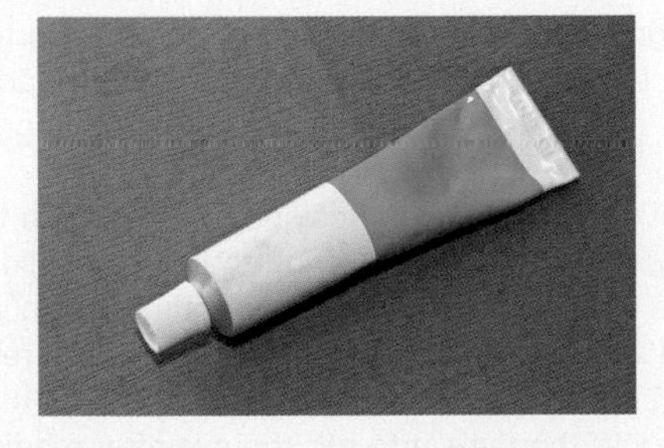

Transdermal Patches

- Remove the old patch from the patient's skin; fold it so that it sticks to itself instead of having exposed adhesive surfaces.

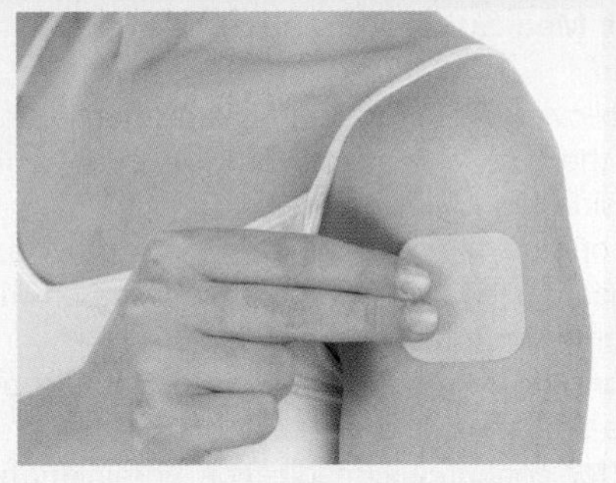

- Assess, clean, and dry new and old sites:
  - Rotate application sites.
  - Ensure that each site is free from hair and is not located over a bony prominence.
  - Note any redness, irritation, or skin breakdown; do not apply a new patch to an area of skin irritation or breakdown.
  - Never apply a patch over a pacemaker or implanted port.
- Remove the new patch from the package; mark the patch with your initials, date, and the time of day it was applied.
- Remove the covering, and apply the patch to the skin:
  - Apply gentle pressure with the palm of your hand for 10 to 15 seconds.
  - Do not massage the patch.
- Each new patch should be applied at the same time of day and on the days ordered.

Documentation Concerns

- Follow all documentation procedures discussed in the Nursing Care Guideline: Six Rights of Medication Administration box.
- Document the body site where the topical medication was applied and skin changes observed at old or current application sites.

Evidence-Based Practice

- If the patient is in a cardiac emergency, remove transdermal patches before defibrillation. Many patches have an aluminum backing that can cause second-degree burns with defibrillation.
- If removal is not possible, it is necessary to check the patient after the event for patches and treat accordingly (Brown, Denman, and Platts, 2009).

all procedures are performed with sterile technique to prevent infection. Medication should not be forced into the ear canal because forcing may rupture the tympanic membrane.

Nasal Medications

Nasal medications are administered by drop or nebulizer formulations into the nose (Nursing Care Guideline: Nasal Medication Administration box). The nose is a clean, not sterile, cavity, but the nurse uses medical asepsis when administering nasal preparations because of the connection of the nose to the sinuses. Decongestant sprays or drops to relieve symptoms of sinus congestion are the most common medications administered through nasal instillation. When these medications are used in excess, they may have systemic effects such as increased heart rate and a rebound effect that increases congestion.

Inhaled Medications

The nose and mouth provide entry to the lower respiratory system. MDIs and dry powder inhalers (DPIs) are small, hand-held devices that a patient activates before inhaling (Skill 35-2). Each time the device is pressed, a specific dose is

NURSING CARE GUIDELINE

Ophthalmic Medication Administration

Background

- Always follow the Six Rights of Medication Administration.
- Because the cornea is sensitive, most eye medications are placed inside the lower eyelid.
- Types of ophthalmic medication:
  - Eyedrops (for treatment of eye diseases or irritations)
  - Ointments (for infections or irritations)
  - Irrigations (to remove secretions or foreign bodies or to cleanse and sooth the eye)
  - Disks (for continuous medication administration up to a week), which are similar to a contact lens, usually placed in the eye at night because they may cause blurriness of vision, and may stay in place for a week

Procedural Concerns

- Always wear gloves.
- Do not let anything touch the applicator (i.e., maintain medical asepsis).
- All types of ophthalmic medications:
  - Hand the patient tissues (to blot eye overflow from the face).
  - Tilt the patient's head back.
  - Have the patient look up.
  - Pull the patient's lower eyelid down to form a pouch.
- Eyedrops
  - Hold the bottle above the eye that is to be treated.
  - Place drops into the pouch formed by the lower eyelid in the lower conjunctival sac.
  - Maintain slight pressure on the inner canthus to prevent loss of medication through the tear duct and reduce systemic effects of the medication.

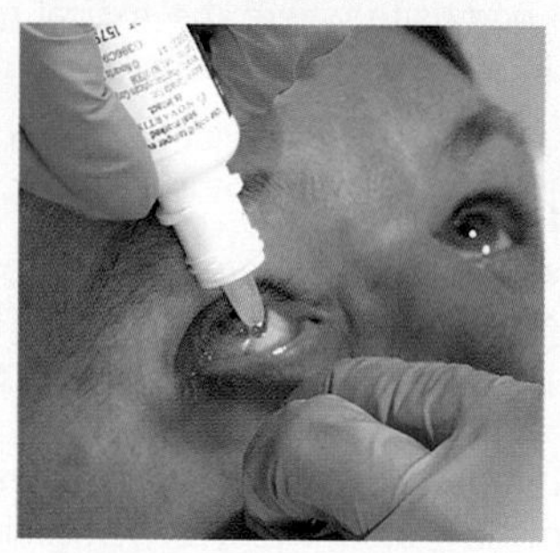

- Ointments:
  - Squeeze a ½-inch strip of ointment from the tube into the lower eyelid, moving from the inner canthus to the outer canthus.
  - Instruct the patient to close and roll the eyes around.
  - Inform the patient that the medication may temporarily blur vision.
- Irrigations:
  - Fill a sterile irrigation syringe with warmed sterile irrigation solution.
  - Place a basin below the patient's face, and offer the patient a towel.
  - Hold the patient's eye open with the nondominant hand.
  - Hold the syringe 1 inch above the eye and at an angle from the inner canthus toward the outer canthus.
  - Flush the eye until the solution exiting the eye is clear or the foreign particle is removed.
- Disks:

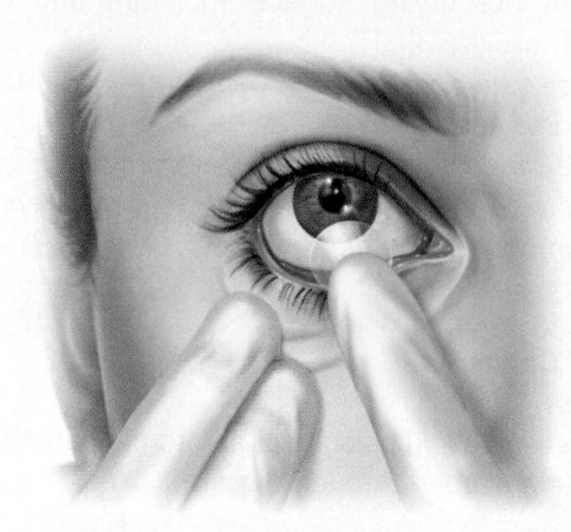

  - Position the medicated disk on a gloved fingertip.
  - Place the disk in the conjunctival sac, and position the lower eyelid over the top of it. The disk should not be visible.
  - Remove the disk at the designated or ordered time:
    - Expose the disk by lowering the lower eyelid.
    - Use a gloved index finger and thumb to pinch the disk and break the suction with the eye, and remove the disk.
- Do not allow the patient to rub the eye after medication has been inserted.

Documentation Concerns

- Follow all documentation procedures discussed in the Nursing Care Guideline: Six Rights of Medication Administration box.
- Document the eye or eyes in which medication was instilled and the patient's response to the medication.

released. Medication absorption is very rapid. Spacers can be used with the MDI to trap the medication and allow inhalation over several breaths. A spacer is especially helpful for children or a patient who cannot inhale slowly.

Nebulizers are used to aerosolize medication into a fine droplet or gas form that is then inhaled for delivery to the lungs, where the particles are absorbed almost immediately. Common uses for inhaled medications are to induce anesthesia during surgery and to treat respiratory disorders such as asthma or chronic lung disease. Bronchodilation is a desired local effect from inhaled medications for respiratory disorders. Some medications, such as inhaled steroids for inflammation, can cause systemic effects.

! SAFE PRACTICE ALERT

Rinsing the mouth and oral care should be performed by the patient receiving steroids by inhalation. This prevents irritation to the oral mucosa and tongue and prevents oral fungal infections.

NURSING CARE GUIDELINE

Otic Medication Administration

Background

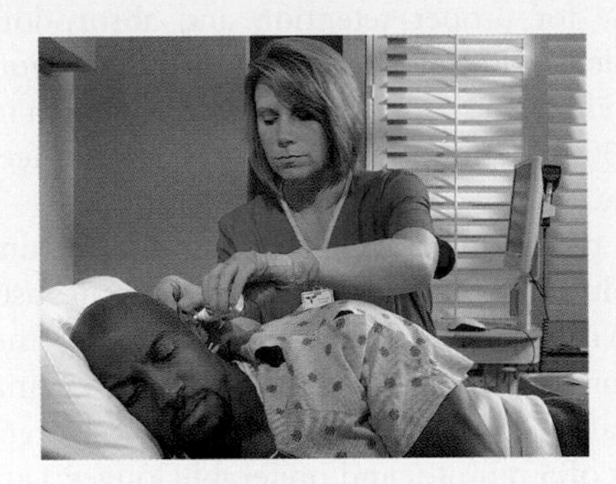

- Always follow the Six Rights of Medication Administration.
- Medications are placed in the ear to soften cerumen (earwax), destroy insects or organisms inside the ear, relieve pain, or act as a local anesthetic.
- Types of otic medications:
  - Eardrops (to treat infections or soften cerumen)
  - Irrigations (to remove secretions or foreign bodies and clean the ear)

Procedural Concerns

- Do not let anything touch the applicator (maintain medical asepsis).
- All types of otic medications:
  - Hand the patient tissues to blot overflow from the ear.
  - Clean the ear if needed.
- Eardrops:
  - Have the patient lie with the ear to be treated in the uppermost position.
  - Hold the medication bottle above the ear.
  - Straighten the auditory canal of an adult patient by gently pulling the pinna up and back.
  - Place the specified number of drops into the ear canal.
  - Release the pinna, and press on the tragus several times to prevent loss of medication and reduce systemic effects from the medication.
  - If ordered, place cotton loosely in the auditory canal.
  - Wait 5 minutes before administering medication in the other ear (if bilateral administration is ordered).
- Irrigations:
  - Fill a sterile irrigation syringe with warmed sterile irrigation solution.
  - Place a basin at face level and under the ear, and offer the patient a towel.
  - Clean the pinna and meatus of the ear canal.
  - Straighten the auditory canal of an adult patient by gently pulling the pinna up and back.
  - Hold the syringe at an upward angle at the entrance to the ear.
  - Flush the ear until the solution exiting the ear is clear or the foreign particle is removed.
  - Place cotton loosely in the ear, and offer the patient a towel.
  - Have the patient lie down on another towel placed under the head; the patient should be in a side-lying position with the affected side down to help drain excess fluid by gravity.
  - Remove the cotton in 10 to 15 minutes to allow fluid to flow freely outward.
- If the patient complains of pain or dizziness during the procedure, stop and assess the complaint.

Documentation Concerns

- Follow all documentation procedures discussed in the Nursing Care Guideline: Six Rights of Medication Administration box.
- Document the ear or ears in which medication was instilled and the patient's response to the procedure.

NURSING CARE GUIDELINE

Nasal Medication Administration

Background

- Always follow the Six Rights of Medication Administration.
- Nasal medications are used to treat allergies, sinus infections, nasal congestion, and inflammation. Chronic use of nasal decongestants may lead to rebound effect (i.e., increased nasal congestion).

Procedural Concerns

- Have the patient blow the nose first.
- Medication administration:
  - Tilt the patient's head slightly back, or have the patient lie in the supine position with the head tilted backward.
  - Have the patient breathe out through the mouth.
  - Insert the end of the delivery device $\frac{1}{3}$ inch into one nostril. Have the patient plug the opposite nostril. Do not touch the insides of the nares with the device because doing so may cause sneezing and contamination.

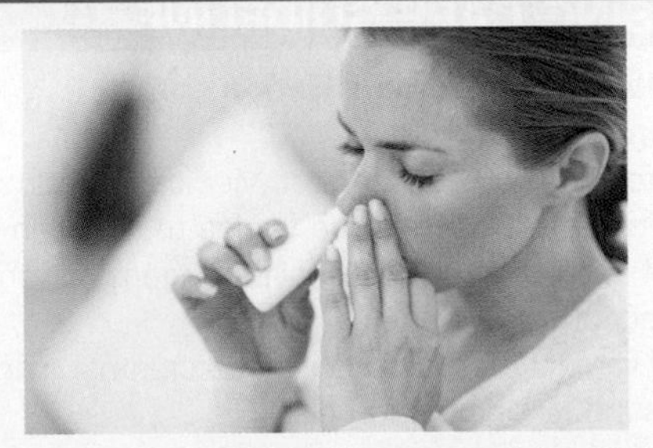

  - Administer the drops or spray as the patient inhales through the nose.
  - Have the patient exhale through the mouth.
- Keep the patient's head tilted back for several minutes while the patient continues to breathe through the mouth.

Documentation Concerns

- Follow all documentation procedures discussed in the Nursing Care Guideline: Six Rights of Medication Administration box.
- Document whether medication was instilled into one or both nares and the patient's response to the procedure.

Assessment before and after administration of inhaled medications includes assessment of breathing status, breath sounds, respiratory rate, and use of accessory muscles. The nurse assesses the patient's use of inhalers because the MDI is often used incorrectly. Important patient education includes determining when the inhaler is empty and needs to be replaced. It is recommended that the number of doses in the container be divided by the number of doses the patient takes in a day. The patient should keep a record of doses to obtain a refill of the medication canister before it runs out (Mayo Foundation for Medical Education and Research, 2014). Proper use of the medication ensures optimal outcomes. The ability to compress the inhaler is affected by hand strength, flexibility, and the hand size of a child or adult.

Vaginal Medications

Creams, foams, tablets, liquids (i.e., douche), suppositories, and gels can be administered vaginally (Nursing Care Guideline: Vaginal Medication Administration box). They are used for infection, itching, antibacterial preparation before surgery, contraception, or induction of labor in women after the fetus dies early in pregnancy. Proper placement often requires a special applicator. Vaginal suppositories are typically refrigerated until use because they melt at body temperature. Patients should be offered an absorbent pad and a comfortable undergarment to collect medication drainage. Tampons should not be used after vaginal medication instillation because the tampon can absorb the medication intended for mucosal absorption.

Rectal Medications

Rectal suppositories are thinner than vaginal suppositories. Medication effects from this route can be local (e.g., laxative or stool softener effect) or systemic (e.g., antiemetic or antipyretic effect). Rectal suppositories are often stored in the refrigerator. Clean, disposable gloves are used when administering suppositories. The unwrapped suppository is placed above the internal anal sphincter and against the mucous membrane for proper retention and absorption (Nursing Care Guideline: Rectal Medication Administration box). For a laxative effect, the suppository needs to remain in the rectal vault for 30 to 45 minutes or until the patient feels the urge to defecate.

Liquid medications are instilled in the rectum using an enema solution. An enema solution can be used to treat patients with high potassium levels or to rid the bowel of stool before a procedure. Small-volume enemas contain approximately 100 mL of fluid and need to be retained for a minimum of 5 minutes and preferably longer. Large-volume enemas contain up to 1000 mL of fluid and need to be retained as long as possible for maximum benefit.

Parenteral Medications

Parenteral medications are administered by injection into tissue, muscle, or a vein. Patients may refer to any parenteral medication as a *shot*. Standard precautions and sterile technique are followed when using the parenteral route because the skin barrier is broken. The effects of parenterally administered medications occur rapidly, depending on the rate of absorption, and the nurse must closely observe the patient for medication responses.

Equipment needed to administer parenteral medications includes syringes, needles, or another injection mechanism and the vial or ampule from the pharmacy that contains the medication. Many types of syringes and needles are available. The nurse must select the correct syringe and needle to administer the type and amount of medication solution into the prescribed site. All syringes and needles have safety devices

NURSING CARE GUIDELINE

Vaginal Medication Administration

Background

- Always follow the Six Rights of Medication Administration.
- Medications are placed in the vagina to maintain the normal acidity of secretions and normal pathogens and to combat or treat infections.
- Types of vaginal medications include creams, foams, tablets, liquids, suppositories, and gels.

Procedural Concerns

- Have the patient empty her bladder.
- Instruct the patient to lie on her back with knees flexed (i.e., dorsal recumbent position), or if unable to tolerate the dorsal recumbent position, have her lie in the Sims position.
- Don gloves.
- Lubricate the applicator or suppository using a water-soluble gel.
- Separate the labia with the nondominant hand to expose the vaginal opening.
- Cleanse the vaginal opening (see Skill 27-2).
- Fully insert the applicator or suppository. Use a rolling motion, inserting downward and backward.
- Remove gloves, turning them inside out to prevent the spread of microorganisms.
- Instruct the patient to remain on her back, in a side-lying position, or with hips elevated on a pillow for 5 to 10 minutes.
- Offer the patient a perineal pad.

Documentation Concerns

- Follow all documentation procedures discussed in the Nursing Care Guideline: Six Rights of Medication Administration box.
- Document the patient's response to the procedure.

NURSING CARE GUIDELINE

Rectal Medication Administration

Background

- Always follow the Six Rights of Medication Administration.
- Medications are placed in the rectum when a patient is unable to take a medication by mouth or when a more rapid effect is required.
- Types of rectal suppositories are antipyretics, antiemetics, and laxatives.

Procedural Concerns

- Position the patient on the left side, with the upper knee flexed (i.e., Sims position) (see Figure 28-21).
- Unwrap the suppository and lubricate it and a gloved index finger, using water-soluble gel.

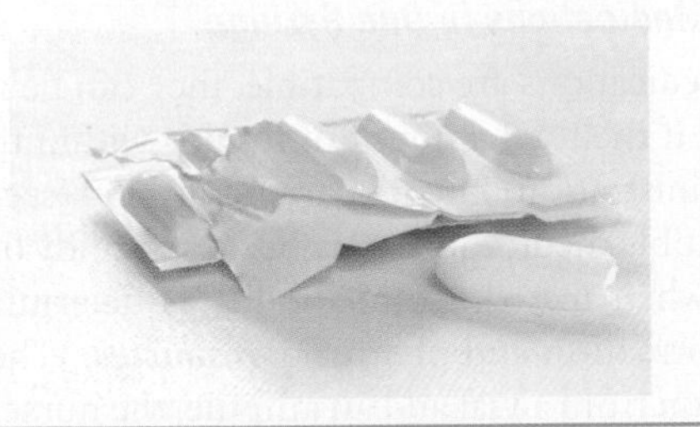

- Separate the buttocks to expose the anus.
- Have the patient breathe slowly and deeply.
    - Insert the suppository with the rounded end inserted first.
    - Gently push the suppository along the rectal wall; avoid embedding it in feces.
    - Continue until the suppository is inserted past the internal sphincter (approximately 3 to 4 inches).
- Cleanse excess lubricant or stool from the patient's perirectal area.
- Instruct the patient to remain in left lateral position with buttocks pressed together for 5 to 10 minutes; if a laxative was inserted, the patient should remain supine for 35 to 45 minutes.
- Remove gloves, turning them inside out to avoid possible contamination with microorganisms.
- Wash hands thoroughly.

Documentation Concerns

- Follow all documentation procedures discussed in the Nursing Care Guideline: Six Rights of Medication Administration box.
- Document the patient's response to the procedure and, in the case of a laxative, how long the patient was able to retain the medication.

or coverings to help prevent needlestick injuries. Syringes may come packaged with a needle attached, but needles also come packaged individually to allow the nurse to select the best needle size for the patient and medication. All needles are safety covered and are disposed of immediately in an approved puncture-resistant container in accordance with facility policy.

QSEN FOCUS!

The nurse demonstrates safety by the effective use of strategies to reduce the risk of harm to self or others by immediately activating the safety mechanism on a syringe after administering an injection.

! SAFE PRACTICE ALERT

After use, a needle should not be recapped (placing the protective cap back over the needle). Most needlestick injuries occur during recapping. Needlesticks expose health care workers to blood-borne pathogens such as human immunodeficiency virus (HIV) and hepatitis B and C viruses.

! SAFE PRACTICE ALERT

The needle safety mechanism is activated immediately after the syringe and needle are used for medication administration. Covering the needle is critical in preventing a needlestick injury.

Preparing Parenteral Medications

Parenteral medications may be premixed and packaged as a unit dose, or they may have to be prepared by the nurse. Medications may be prepared from ampules or vials and may come in a powder form that needs to be reconstituted before it is administered (Skill 35-3).

Ampules and Vials

An ampule is a small glass container that holds a single liquid dose of medication (Figure 35-10). Ampules range in size from 1 mL to 10 mL (or larger), but all have a constricted neck area that is snapped off to allow access to the medication. A colored ring around the narrow neck identifies where

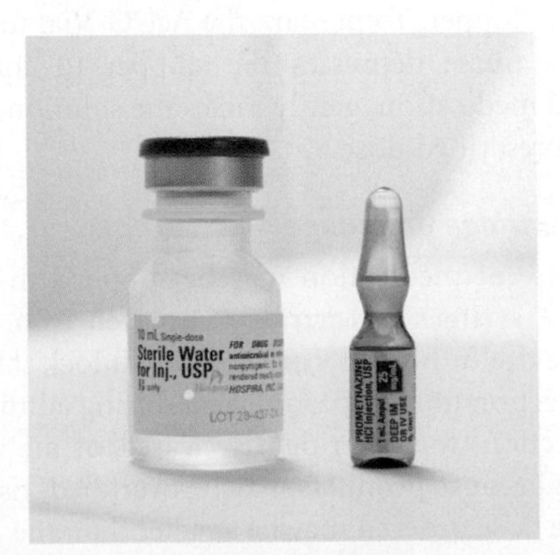

FIGURE 35-10 A vial *(left)* and an ampule *(right)*.

the glass is prescored to be broken. The ampule neck is cleaned with an alcohol swab. A protective sleeve or sterile 2- × 2-inch gauze is used when breaking the ampule top to protect the nurse from being cut by the glass. After the needed dose of medication has been drawn, the ampule is discarded in a sharps container along with any unused medication.

A vial is a glass or plastic container holding one or more doses of a solution or medication (see Figure 35-10). It has a self-sealing rubber seal at the top and a soft metal or plastic cap that is easily removed to access the rubber seal. A needle attached to a syringe is used to pierce the rubber seal, and the proper amount of fluid is drawn into the syringe. Alternatively, an adapter for use with a needleless cannula may be used if multiple doses are to be drawn from the vial. If more than one dose is to be used from the vial, the vial must be labeled with the date and time it is opened and the initials of the nurse opening it. The medication is stored in a locked medication cart or room and used or discarded within a designated time to protect from possible microbial growth in the vial. Multidose vials should be dedicated to one patient whenever possible. The rubber seal is cleaned with alcohol each time the vial is accessed for additional doses. The vial is a closed system, and air equivalent to the amount of liquid to be withdrawn is injected into the vial. Injecting air prevents a vacuum from forming in the vial, which would make withdrawing the medication difficult.

Reconstituting Powdered Medications

Some medications are supplied as a powder in a vial. They are reconstituted by adding a liquid, or diluent, to the powder. Powdered medications are carefully reconstituted by adding only the proper amount and type of diluent identified by the manufacturer. Sterile normal saline and sterile distilled water are common diluents used for reconstituting medications. Specific directions printed on the vial or package insert identify the type and amount of diluent needed for reconstitution and the resulting concentration of medication.

An Act-O-Vial system (i.e., dual-compartment vial) is another approach for administering powdered medication. In this system, the medication powder (e.g., Solu-Medrol) and diluent are in two compartments of a single vial, separated by a rubber stopper. To prepare the Act-O-Vial for administration, the nurse depresses the stopper to combine the diluent and medication, gently mixes the solution, and withdraws the prescribed dose.

Prefilled Cartridge or Syringe

A single dose of medication may be supplied in a prefilled cartridge or syringe. A cartridge is placed into a reusable injection device or holder. Care is taken to lock the cartridge into the injection holder to stabilize it during administration. Before injection, the cartridge is cleared of air and excess medication because products may be overfilled, risking overdose, or the dose ordered may be smaller than the amount of medication contained in the cartridge. After administration, the cartridge is removed from the holder and placed in the appropriate disposal container. Examples of prefilled cartridge holders include Tubex and Carpuject appliances. This method is used if a needleless system is in place or a safety needle can be used. Some medication supplied in cartridges is withdrawn using an appropriate syringe and is then administered with the syringe. Withdrawing medication from a cartridge is similar to using a vial, except that no air is injected into the cartridge before the medication is withdrawn.

Prefilled syringes are similar to prefilled cartridges. A single dose of medication is in a syringe with a needle attached. Excess air or medication may need to be expelled from the syringe; however, some prefilled medication syringes, such as Lovenox, contain air that should not be removed before administration.

Mixing Medications in One Syringe

If two medications are compatible, they can be mixed in one injection if the total amount of fluid is within the guidelines for administration into a parenteral site (see Skill 35-3). Incompatible medications may become cloudy or form a precipitate when mixed. Compatibility is determined through drug information and pharmacy resources. When preparing medication from a vial and an ampule, the nurse prepares the medication from the vial first and then uses the same syringe and a filter needle or straw to withdraw the medication from the ampule. When mixing medications from two vials (Skill 35-4), the nurse takes care to ensure that the final dose is correct. Aseptic technique is used.

Administering Parenteral Medications

The depth of penetration, needle angle, and site selection determine whether the medication is an intradermal, subcutaneous, or intramuscular dose (Skill 35-5). Figure 35-11 illustrates the angle of insertion into tissue levels for parenteral injections.

Intradermal Administration

Intradermal injections are given into the dermis, the layer of tissue just below the skin surface. The intradermal route is often used to administer local anesthetics, to test for allergies, and to test for tuberculosis exposure. Drugs are absorbed slowly through the dermal tissue, and only small amounts of medication (0.01 to 0.1 mL) can be instilled. Common sites for injection are the inner forearm, the upper arm, and the scapular area. A 1-mL tuberculin syringe with a 25- to 27-gauge, ¼- to ⅝-inch needle is used to provide accurate measurement of the small dose and shallow penetration through the epidermis layer of the skin. Pressure should not be applied to the site, and the site should not be massaged after injection. The location of the injection is documented.

Subcutaneous Administration

Subcutaneous tissue is the layer of fat located below the dermis and above muscle tissue (see Skill 35-5). Insulin and

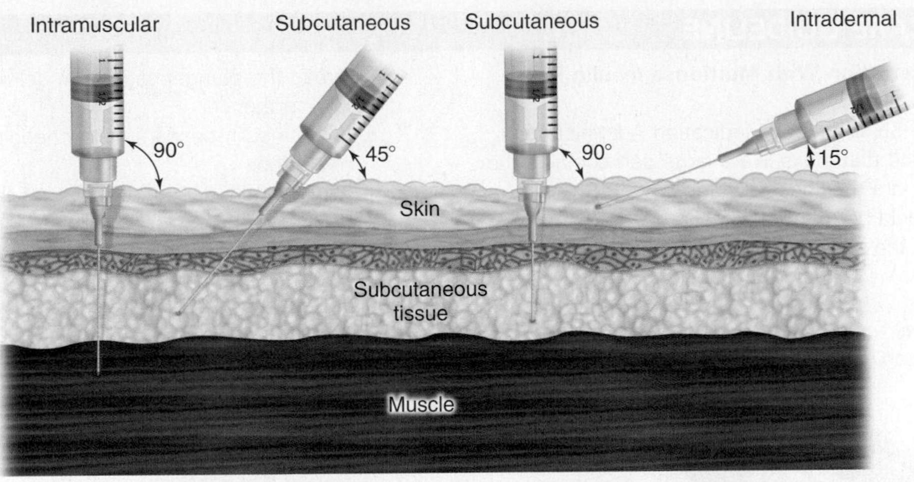

FIGURE 35-11 Insertion angles for parenteral injections.

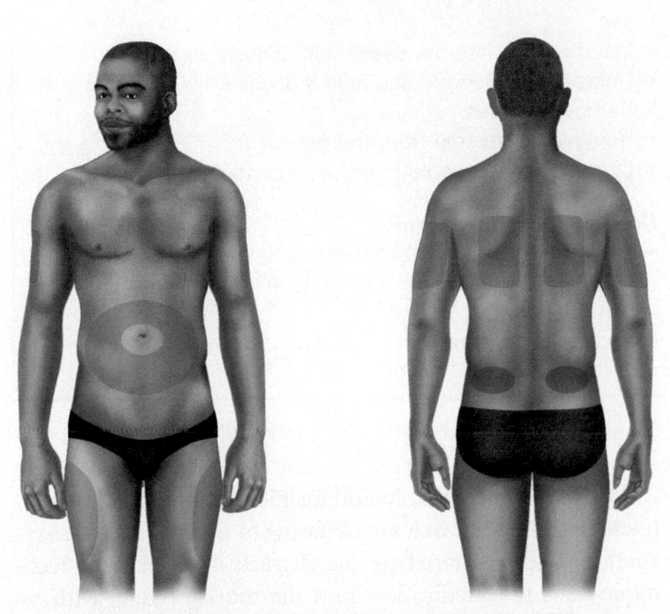

FIGURE 35-12 Subcutaneous injection sites.

heparin are medications commonly administered by the subcutaneous route. Absorption is slow, with a sustained effect. Because the subcutaneous area is less vascular, injection into a blood vessel is rare. Aspiration is therefore not required for subcutaneous injections (American Diabetes Association, 2004). The volume of medication administered should not exceed 1 mL by this route.

Common subcutaneous sites include the abdomen, lateral aspects of the upper arm and thigh, scapular area of the back, and upper ventrodorsal gluteal area (Figure 35-12). The injection site should be rotated to avoid the development of hard, painful areas where injections are given. A 0.5- to 3-mL syringe with a 25- to 31-gauge, ⅜- to ⅝-inch needle is used. Typically, the nurse pinches approximately 2 inches of tissue between two fingers and inserts the needle at a 90-degree angle. If less tissue is available, the nurse pinches 1 inch of tissue and inserts the needle at a 45-degree angle.

Some types of insulin are supplied in special multidose devices called *insulin pens* (Nursing Care Guideline: Medication Administration with Multidose Insulin Pens box). These pens are easier for some patients to use at home because the medication does not have to be drawn up. Instruct the patient to use caution when more than one kind of insulin is supplied in pen form. The pens look very similar, and double-checking that the correct insulin is being administered is recommended. For a description of the use of insulin in diabetes, view the "Type 1 Diabetes" and "Type 2 Diabetes" animations.

A child may require a shorter needle, whereas an obese adult may require a longer one. The angle of insertion for the needle is 45 to 90 degrees, depending on the weight of the patient. A 45-degree angle may be used to give a subcutaneous injection to a very thin patient to ensure that the medication is injected into fatty tissue. A 90-degree angle can be used in a patient with adequate subcutaneous tissue. The length of the needle should be approximately half the depth of the pinched skin fold.

Intramuscular Administration

Because there are more blood vessels in muscles than in subcutaneous tissue, intramuscular (IM) injections are absorbed rapidly if the patient has adequate circulation. When preparing to administer an IM injection, the nurse considers the volume of fluid to be injected, medication being administered, injection technique, site selection, and syringe and needle selection. Other factors include the patient's age, physical build, and underlying medical disorders such as a bleeding disorder (Malkin, 2008).

The three common IM injection sites are ventrogluteal, vastus lateralis, and deltoid (Figure 35-13). Injections into the deltoid are limited to 2 mL or less. Well-developed adults can tolerate up to 3 mL of medication injected into the larger muscles. In 2004, the World Health Organization recommended that a fourth site, the dorsogluteal muscle, *not* be

NURSING CARE GUIDELINE

Medication Administration With Multidose Insulin Pens

Background

- Always follow the Six Rights of Medication Administration.
- A specialized device that looks like a large pen contains the prescribed insulin in a multidose syringe.
- Injection sites should be rotated.
- Patients must dial the correct dose and attach a new needle for each injection.

Procedural Concerns

- Remove the pen cap.

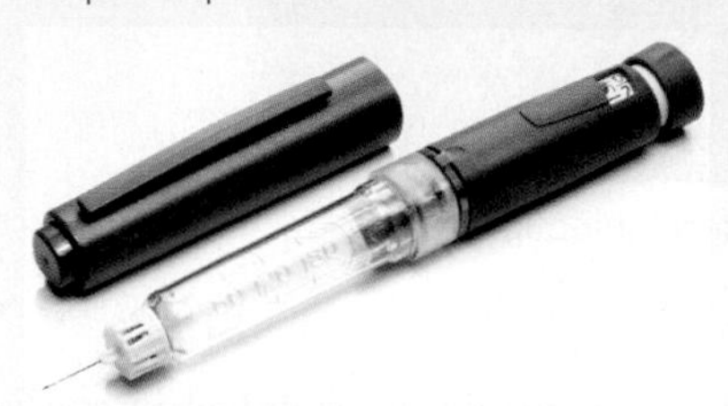

- Clean the pen tip with alcohol.
- If an insulin suspension is prescribed, invert the pen 20 times to mix a suspension.
- Remove the protective tab on a new needle.
- Attach the needle to the pen; needles usually screw onto the pen.
- Remove the cap on the needle.
- Prime the pen:
  - Dial the dose to 2 units.
  - Hold the pen with the needle pointing up, making sure all air rises to the top of the pen.
  - Depress the plunger slightly to deliver the 2-unit dose of insulin to the air.
    - If the insulin appears at the needle tip, proceed to the next step.
    - If the insulin does not appear at the needle tip, repeat the 2-unit dose to the air.
- If a previously used cartridge is to be used, check the insulin reservoir:
  - If there is enough insulin remaining for a complete dose, proceed with the injection.
  - If there is not enough insulin remaining for a complete dose, replace the pen with a new one, or in pens with replaceable cartridges, replace the cartridge.
- Verify that the dial is at 0 units.
- Dial the needed dose.
- Clean the injection site with alcohol, and allow it to air-dry.
- Hold the pen as you would a dart, directed at the chosen site.
- Insert needle into the tissue with a quick motion.
- Depress the plunger, and hold it down while counting to 6.
- Remove the pen.
- Remove the needle from the pen.
- Dispose of the needle in a sharps container.

Documentation Concerns

- Follow all documentation procedures discussed in the Nursing Care Guideline: Six Rights of Medication Administration box.
- Document the site of the injection.

used routinely for IM injections due to the proximity to the sciatic nerve and superior gluteal artery and the increased risk of injecting into the thick layer of fat present. If the dorsogluteal site is used because no other site is available, aspiration for blood before administration of medication should be performed to prevent inadvertent injection into the gluteal artery. Aspiration for blood is no longer recommended for other IM sites. The primary site for administering an IM injection for patients older than 7 months of age is the ventrogluteal site, which is free of major blood vessels, nerves, and fat and is associated with lower rates of injury (Nicoll and Hesby, 2002). The vastus lateralis site has no large blood vessels or nerves and can safely be used for most patients. The deltoid site lies close to the radial nerve and brachial artery; care must be taken to properly locate the muscle for safe injection. Each IM site is located according to specific anatomic landmarks.

SAFE PRACTICE ALERT

Failure to correctly find the correct injection site by using anatomic landmarks before injecting medication can result in tissue, bone, or nerve damage.

Most IM injections, including medications that discolor tissue (e.g., iron) or that are irritating to tissue (e.g., hydroxyzine), are administered by the Z-track method. This technique seals the medication into the muscle tissue, with no tracking of medication into the subcutaneous tissue when the needle is withdrawn. After the medication dose is prepared, a new needle is placed on the syringe so that no medicine is on the outside of the needle. A large muscle site, such as the ventrogluteal area, is selected. The site is prepared with an antiseptic cleanser, and the overlying skin and subcutaneous tissue are then pulled approximately 2.5 cm (1 inch) laterally to the side (Figure 35-14). The skin is held taut in this position with the nondominant hand, the needle is inserted deep into the muscle, and the medication is injected. The needle is held in place approximately 10 seconds to allow medication dispersion. The needle is then withdrawn, and the skin is immediately released. A zigzag path is left that seals the medication into the muscle.

Special medication administration devices include EpiPens, which are used for severe allergic reactions. An EpiPen IM injection is given in the vastus lateralis muscle by means of the special technique described in Nursing Care Guideline: Medication Administration with EpiPens box.

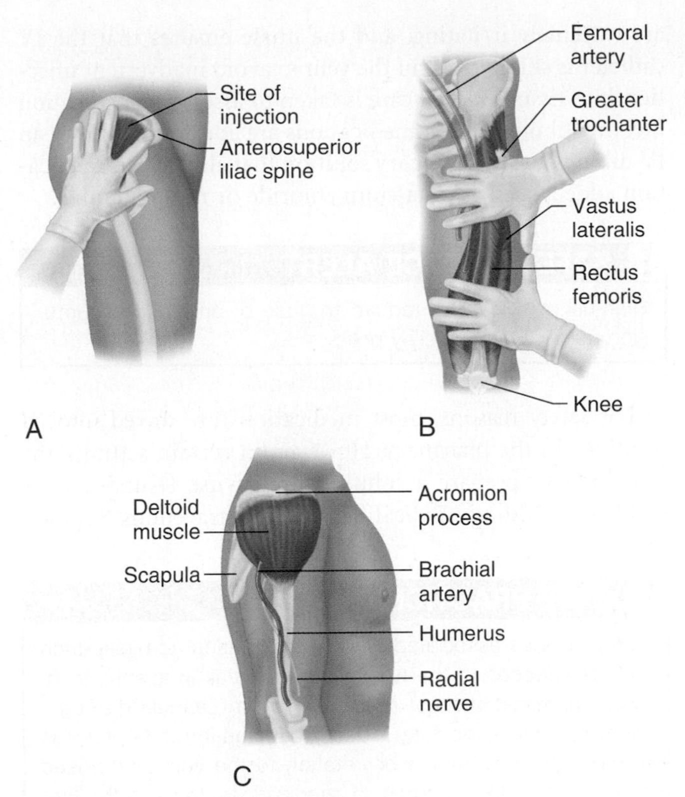

FIGURE 35-13 Intramuscular injection sites. **A,** Ventrogluteal. **B,** Vastus lateralis. **C,** Deltoid.

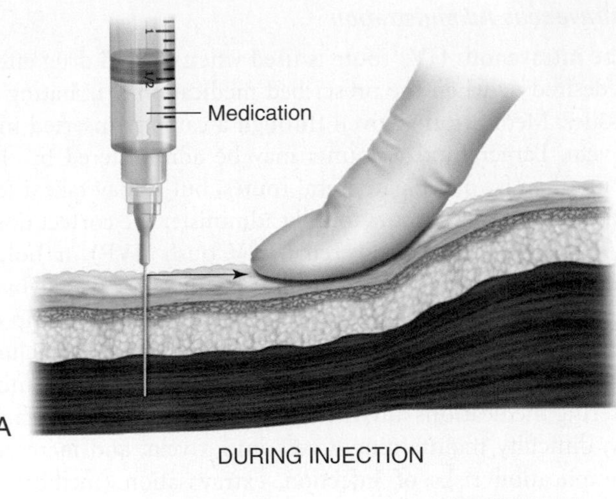

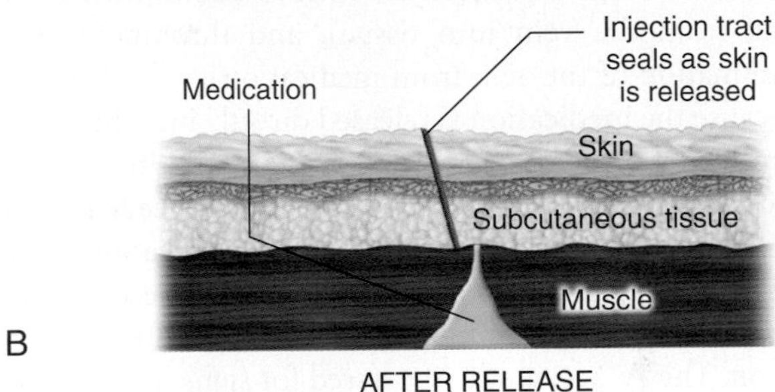

FIGURE 35-14 Z-track injection technique. **A,** During injection. **B,** After release.

NURSING CARE GUIDELINE

Medication Administration With EpiPens

Background

- Always follow the Six Rights of Medication Administration.
- An EpiPen is a specialized device that looks like a large pen and consists of a needle and a syringe; it contains one dose of epinephrine.

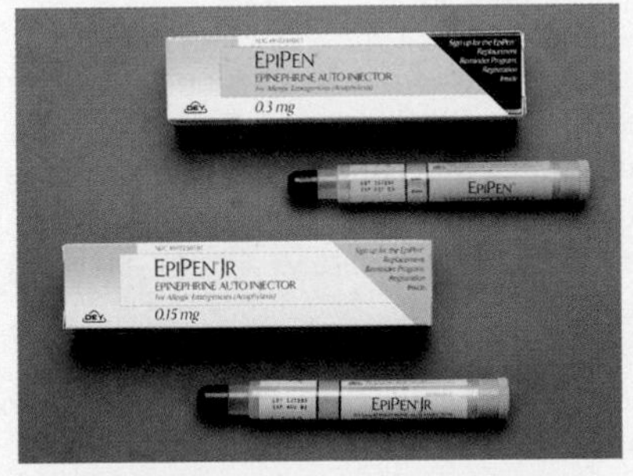

(From Proctor DB, Adams AP: *Kinn's the medical assistant,* ed. 11, St. Louis, 2011, Saunders.)

- It is used for the emergency treatment of severe allergic reactions, or anaphylaxis, caused by allergens, exercise, or unknown triggers and for patients who are at increased risk for these reactions.
- Two doses are available:
  - An adult dose (0.3 mg) for individuals weighing more than 66 lb
  - A junior dose (0.15 mg) for individuals weighing 33 to 66 lb
- The injection site for the patient is the lateral aspect of the thigh, the vastus lateralis (see the Injections: Intramuscular section of Skill 35-5).
- EpiPens are stored at room temperature in their plastic storage tubing.

Procedural Concerns

- Inspect the EpiPen for expiration date and solution color. The solution should be clear.
- Remove the EpiPen from its plastic storage tubing.
- Remove the blue safety top from the EpiPen.
- Wrap your hand around the EpiPen.
- Point the orange pen tip against the patient's thigh. The dose can be administered through the patient's clothes.
- Quickly dart the EpiPen into the thigh.
- Hold the pen in place for 5 to 10 seconds.
- Remove the pen.
- The needle has an automatic safety shield that covers the needle before use and locks in the covered position after the injection.
- Seek medical attention for the patient.

Documentation Concerns

- Follow all documentation procedures discussed in the Nursing Care Guideline: Six Rights of Medication Administration box.
- Document whether the injection was given in the left or right thigh.
- Document the patient's vital signs and response to the injection.

Intravenous Administration

The intravenous (IV) route is used when a rapid drug effect is desired or when the prescribed medication is irritating to tissues. Medication is given through a catheter inserted into a vein. Larger fluid amounts may be administered by this route than by other parenteral routes, but it may take a few minutes to several hours to fully administer the correct dose. IV medications are delivered by IV push (IVP) or bolus, intermittent small-volume administration or IV piggyback (IVPB), or volume control administration set (IV pump or controller) (Skill 35-6). Disadvantages of the IV route include the cost of preparation and administration, difficulty administering medications anywhere other than a health care facility, difficulty maintaining access into a vein, and increased complication risks of infection, extravasation (medication leaking from the vein into tissue), and thrombophlebitis (inflammation of the vein from medication).

Because the medication is released directly into the bloodstream, extra care is taken in preparing and administering medication by the IV route. Assessment data needed before administration include patient allergies, medication or IV solution incompatibilities, the amount and type of diluent needed for the medication, and the rate of medication administration. The IV access site is assessed for signs or symptoms of infiltration (swelling and discomfort at the site) and thrombophlebitis. Medications are prepared in a sterile manner. Some medications have pH or osmolarity levels that are extremely irritating, and the nurse ensures that the IV catheter is still in place in the vein to avoid inadvertent injection into tissue. Special care is taken to assess for medication incompatibilities when medications are administered into an IV tubing port of a primary solution that already has medication added, such as potassium chloride or multivitamins.

> **! SAFE PRACTICE ALERT**
>
> High-risk medications require the use of an electronic infusion pump. Follow facility policy.

For safety reasons, most medications are mixed into IV solutions in the pharmacy. However, in certain settings, the nurse has to prepare a solution for IV use (Nursing Care Guideline: Adding Medications to an Intravenous Solution box).

> **! SAFE PRACTICE ALERT**
>
> Complications associated with IV medication administration include infection of the IV site from a break in aseptic technique; administration of medication from cannula dislodgement into tissue, resulting in tissue damage; thrombophlebitis in the vein from trauma or irritation to the vein; and speed shock from administration of medications too rapidly. Frequent assessment of the IV site for infection and infiltration is essential.

NURSING CARE GUIDELINE

Adding Medications to an Intravenous Solution

Background

- Always follow the Six Rights of Medication Administration.
- Medications may be added to an intravenous solution for diluted delivery.
- Addition of medications should be performed only under sterile, aseptic, specialized conditions by licensed personnel with specialized knowledge.
- The nurse should be uninterrupted, strictly adhere to the Six Rights of Medication Administration (see the Nursing Care Guideline: Six Rights of Medication Administration box) and aseptic technique, and be extremely familiar with the principles of reducing and preventing medication errors.
- Most facilities require that nurses demonstrate competency to perform this skill.

Procedural Concerns

- Inspect the medication and the IV solution for expiration date and solution color.
- Verify compatibility between the medication and the IV solution.
- Clean the port on the IV bag and vial top with an alcohol swab.
- Follow the medication reconstitution and dilution instructions carefully.
- Use the proper equipment and procedure to draw the medication from the ampule or vial (see Skill 35-3).
- After ensuring that the proper technique has been used and the correct dosage has been drawn into the syringe, clean the port on the IV bag again with an alcohol swab, and allow it to dry completely.
- Inject the medication from the syringe into the IV bag. The IV flow clamp should be closed to prevent the medication from infusing into the patient in its concentrated dose and to allow the medication to properly dilute in the IV solution.
- Label the IV bag immediately! Check facility policies and procedures for specifics.
- Verify the medication vial, ampule, or container against the IV bag label and against the primary care provider's order before hanging the medication.
- Regulate the flow rate according to dosage requirements.
- Monitor the patient and the infusion.

Documentation Concerns

- Follow all documentation procedures discussed in the Nursing Care Guideline: Six Rights of Medication Administration box.
- Document the patient's response to the medication.

MEDICATIONS AND HOME CARE

Patient education regarding medications is an important responsibility for the nurse. Education may be directed to the patient, a family member, or a caregiver. When providing medication instruction, it is important to prioritize what the patient, family member, or caregiver needs to know about each medication and supplement being taken.

Oral medications have long been administered in the home. Long-term transdermal, peritoneal dialysis, and IV treatments with infusion pumps are now being administered in the home under supervision of an interdisciplinary team that includes equipment providers, pharmacists, care agencies, care providers, and nurses (Home Care Considerations box).

HOME CARE CONSIDERATIONS

Medication Administration in the Home

- Discharge planning should include teaching patients, family members, and caregivers how to safely administer medications in the home.
- Patients should be encouraged to keep an updated list of medications and bring this list with them anytime they have an encounter in the healthcare system.
- Nurses must follow the state nurse practice act and comply with laws relevant to the storage, use, and disposal of medications in the home, especially in regard to controlled substances.
- A medication regimen for each patient must account for lifestyle, be easy to remember, and be convenient for the patient. Assistive devices, such as a pill organizer or an automated phone reminder system, can help patients remember to take medications (Figure 35-15).
- Linking medication times to normal events in the day, such as meals or bedtime, increases accurate and continued use of medications. These events must be assessed carefully because patients may have schedules that vary from the expected, such as eating only two meals per day.
- Nurses should carefully assess for factors that may affect the safe use of medications, such as poor memory or poor vision.
- Referrals to social services for financial assistance programs and drug company assistance programs can help address financial needs for obtaining medications.
- Medications disposed of in the trash or flushed down the toilet can leak into the water supply and contaminate it. Many pharmacies have designated specific days when patients may safely dispose of expired or unused medications by returning them to the pharmacy.
- Patients are educated about proper disposal of needles. Sharps disposed of in the trash have the potential of injuring sanitation workers.

When providing patient education, the nurse must use language that the patient can understand. The patient, family, or caregiver should be able to repeat to the nurse the following information for each medication being taken: the name

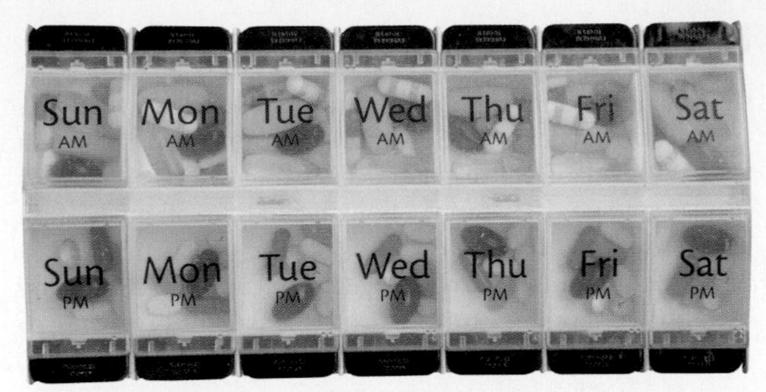

FIGURE 35-15 Weekly medication organizer.

of the medication; the reason for taking it; how and when to take it; food, drinks, over-the-counter medications, and herbs that can affect the action of the drug; safety concerns, such as activities affected by use of the drug (e.g., driving a car); usual side effects; usual adverse reactions; and special instructions about the prescribed route of the medication (Patient Education and Health Literacy box).

The nurse must emphasize that the patient should take medications in the amounts and for the length of time prescribed. It is important to discuss with the patient and family what action should be taken if a dose is missed, the importance of not sharing medications with others, and how to dispose of unused or outdated medications. The patient should demonstrate new skills, such as self-administering insulin, to the nurse after teaching is completed. Documentation of teaching the patient and family and of the planned outcomes is the last step of patient teaching.

PATIENT EDUCATION AND HEALTH LITERACY

Self-Administration of Medications

- Patients who understand medication instructions make fewer mistakes, get well sooner, and better manage chronic health conditions than those who lack understanding.
- It is essential that patients be assessed regarding their ability to understand these materials.
- Large pharmacies can provide patients with translated medication instructions.
- The National Patient Safety Foundation has developed the Ask Me 3 program, which emphasizes questions patients should ask during each health care encounter:
  - What is my main problem?
  - What do I need to do?
  - Why is it important for me to do this?

From National Patient Safety Foundation: Ask me 3, 2007, *www.npsf.org/for-healthcare-professionals/programs/ask-me-3/*.

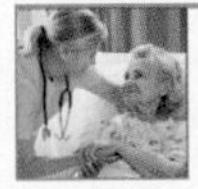

4. Mrs. Petros verbalizes the concern that she will not take her medications correctly when she returns home. What plan can the nurse implement to help the patient safely take her medications?

EVALUATION

Clinical observation is an important way to evaluate the effectiveness of medications. Subjective data (e.g., "My pain is a level 2") and objective data (e.g., patient's apical pulse is regular and 88 beats/min) show evaluation of medication responses. The nurse assesses for adverse effects of medications, such as nausea, rash, change in vital signs, and difficulty breathing. Laboratory tests indicate the patient's response to some medications. Monitoring drug levels in the blood determines whether they are within the therapeutic range desired or dose adjustments are needed. Electronic monitoring can reflect outcomes from medication treatment, such as the oxygen saturation of a patient after respiratory medications are administered or a change in heart rate or rhythm on a cardiac monitor after medication treatment for arrhythmias. Significant deviations from normal response must be reported to the health care provider.

SKILL 35-1 Oral Medication Administration

PURPOSE

- The administration of oral medications must be done appropriately and safely and should follow the Six Rights of Medication Administration:
  - The right medication
  - The right dose
  - The right time
  - The right route
  - The right patient
  - The right documentation

RESOURCES

- Medication cup:
  - Plastic graduated cup for liquid medication
  - Paper soufflé cup for tablets and capsules
- Oral syringe for liquid medication doses less than 10 mL
- Water or another drink, as appropriate, with medication
- Food or a snack, as appropriate, with medication
- A straw, as appropriate, for the medication or for the patient
- Medication administration resource guide or software or a drug handbook
- Pill crusher (i.e., commercial, industrial, or mortar and pestle), as needed
- Pill splitter, as needed

COLLABORATION AND DELEGATION

- Refer to the Nursing Care Guideline: Six Rights of Medication Administration box.
- Medication administration may not be delegated.
- Unlicensed assistive personnel should report the following to the nurse:
  - Changes in vital signs or patient complaints or discomfort
  - Medication found in the patient's room
  - Patient questions regarding medication
- The timing for administering many medications in regard to meals is important. Ensure proper administration and collaboration with the dietary staff.
- Collaborate with the pharmacist on medication questions before administration.

EVIDENCE-BASED PRACTICE

- Medication errors can be prevented by having as much data available as possible when preparing and administering medications.
- Data gathering includes observation and assessment of the patient, the patient's chart, and traditional book resources.
- Implementing new technological innovations can further reduce the risk of medication errors by providing additional resources and prompts to assist the licensed professional in ultimately providing safe, quality patient care (George, Henneman, and Tasota, 2010).

SPECIAL CIRCUMSTANCES

1. **Assess:** Does the patient have an aspiration risk or difficulty swallowing?
   Intervention: Medication may have to be crushed and mixed with fluid or food.
   - Verify that the patient's required medication may be crushed or the capsule opened.
   - When crushing tablets:
     - Clean the compartment of the pill crusher by following the manufacturer's instructions.
     - Place the pill into the container following the manufacturer's instructions.
     - Place the powder in an appropriate food or fluid.
     - Following the manufacturer's instructions, clean the compartment to remove any pill residue.
   - For medication that in capsule form:
     - Gently hold the two ends of the capsule.
     - While holding the capsule above the appropriate food or fluid, twist the ends in opposite directions.
     - Empty the powder from the capsule into the food or fluid.
     - If all powder does not release from the capsule, gently pinch and twist the capsule or tap the edges of the capsule with your finger.
     - Discard the empty capsule in accordance with facility policies and procedures.
2. **Assess:** Is the pill dosage larger than what was ordered?
   Intervention: The medication should be divided appropriately.
   - Capsules cannot be divided for any reason. Call the pharmacist or primary care provider (PCP) to obtain a different dosage or form of the medication.
   - Check with the pharmacist before dividing medication to verify whether the exact dosage is available; dividing medication is not as accurate as obtaining whole tablets or liquids.
   - If a tablet or pill is enteric coated, it *cannot* be split or crushed. Call the pharmacist or PCP for an alternate route or form of medication.
   - If a tablet or pill is extended-release, it *cannot* be split or crushed. Call the pharmacist or PCP for an alternate route or form of medication.
   - If the medication surface is scored to facilitate splitting, it can be split.
   - To use a pill splitter:
     - Clean the pill splitter by following the manufacturer's instructions.
     - Place the tablet on the pill splitter with the scoring aligned with the blade.

- Bring the handle down.
- Remove the two halves. Follow facility policies and procedures for safe disposal of the second half of the pill.
- Clean the pill splitter by following the manufacturer's instructions.

- To break a pill:
  - Apply new nonsterile gloves.
  - Grasp half of the pill on one side of the scored line between the thumb and forefinger of one hand, and grasp the other half of the pill on the other side of the scored line between the thumb and forefinger of the other hand.
  - Bend the pill. The pill should break evenly along the scored line.
  - Follow facility policies and procedures for safe disposal of the other half of the pill.
- If the medication surface is *not* scored:
  - Call the pharmacist or use electronic or printed resources to determine whether the medication may be split.
  - If the pill may be split, use only a commercial pill splitter.

3. **Assess:** Has the medication been dropped on the floor or other unclean surface?
   Intervention: Discard the medication appropriately, and document in accordance with facility policies and procedures. Repeat the preparation with a new pill.
4. **Assess:** Is the patient questioning or refusing the medication?
   Intervention: Stop the administration.
   - The patient has the right to refuse medication.
   - If the patient continues to refuse although the medication is correct, document this in accordance with facility policies and procedures and notify the PCP.
5. **Assess:** Does the medication require special administration?
   Intervention: Use drug resources, or consult with a pharmacist.
   - Some medications require administration with food.
   - Some medications require administration on an empty stomach.
   - Some liquid medications require administration through a straw to avoid staining the teeth.
   - Some medications cannot be crushed. Refer to the Institute of Safe Medication Practice's Do Not Crush list *(www.ismp.org/Tools/DoNotCrush.pdf)*.
   - Some medications cannot be split.
   - Some medications cannot be given with other medications.
   - Some medications cannot be given with certain foods or fluids.
6. **Assess:** Is the liquid medication from the unit-dose container the incorrect dosage for the patient?
   Intervention: Measure the correct dosage of medication, and dispose of the excess as waste in accordance with facility policies and procedures.
   - If the needed dosage is less than 10 mL, use an oral syringe to draw up the medication.
   - If the needed dosage is more than 10 mL, use a plastic graduated medication cup.
   - Measure the dosage in a medication cup at eye level to ensure accuracy.
7. **Assess:** What is the proper method of disposing of excess medication that is a controlled substance?
   Intervention: Follow facility policies and procedures; disposal requires witnessing by a second licensed professional.
8. **Assess:** Has the medication expired?
   Intervention: Do not administer expired medication.
   - Notify the pharmacy of any expired medication.
   - Follow facility policies and procedures for disposal of expired medication.
   - Obtain new medication to administer to the patient, and restart the procedure.

PREPROCEDURE

I. Check PCP orders and the patient care plan.
Knowledge of patient-specific orders is critical for safe patient care.

II. Gather supplies and equipment.
Preparing for the patient encounter saves time and promotes patient trust.

III. Perform hand hygiene.
Frequent hand hygiene prevents the spread of microorganisms.

IV. Maintain standard precautions.
Use of the correct personal protective equipment (PPE) is required whenever contact with bodily fluids is possible, to reduce the transfer of pathogens.

V. Introduce yourself.
Initial communication establishes the role of the nurse and begins a professional relationship.

VI. Provide for patient privacy.
It is important to maintain patient dignity.

VII. Identify the patient by using two identifiers.
Identifying a patient involves scanning barcodes or comparing the patient's stated name and birthdate to information on the patient's wristband or health record. The correct person must receive the correct treatment.

VIII. Explain the procedure to the patient.
The nurse has a responsibility to inform a patient before initiating care. Information may ease patient anxiety and facilitate cooperation.

PROCEDURE

Oral Medication: Tablets and Capsules

Follow preprocedure steps I through VIII.

1. Ask the patient whether a preferred drink or snack is desired, if appropriate, or obtain it before preparing the medication.
Asking about the patient's preferences promotes compliance. Preparing supplies in advance avoids interruption during the procedure and possible medication errors.
2. Prepare medications in a No Interruption Zone according to facility policy. Obtain the medication. Verify that the label of the medication matches the medication administration record (MAR), perform any dosage calculation, and check the expiration date of the medication.
   a. If an automated dispensing system is used, enter the appropriate information, and remove the medication. Verify the correct dose, but do not pour or open.
   b. If bar coding is used, scan the MAR and medication. Verify the correct medication and dosage, but do not prepare or open.
   c. If a medication cart is used, unlock the cart, locate the correct patient drawer, pull the medication, and verify the correct dose. Do not prepare or open.
Avoid possible medication errors by adhering to the Six Rights of Medication Administration and by checking the medication with the MAR three times. Most medication is prepared at the bedside.
3. Prepare the medication and check the medication label against the MAR a second time.
   a. If a multidose bottle is used, pour the medication onto the open lid of the bottle until the appropriate number of tablets or capsules has been counted out, and then pour them into a medication cup.
   b. If a unit dose is used, verify the correct dose. Split whole tablets if needed and appropriate, but otherwise do *not* remove the medication from the wrapping until ready to administer at the patient's bedside.
Verification ensures the accuracy of the dose. Avoid possible medication errors by adhering to the Six Rights of Medication Administration and by checking the medication with the MAR three times. Pouring into the lid avoids touching the medication, preventing the spread of microorganisms. Not removing medication from the wrapping allows another check and patient education at the bedside.
4. Enter the patient's room, perform patient identification, check patient allergies, assess patient knowledge, and educate the patient as needed.
Communication with the patient facilitates cooperation. Avoid possible medication errors by adhering to the Six Rights of Medication Administration.
5. Recheck the label on the medication with the MAR a third time before returning the medication to its storage place *or* before opening the package at the bedside. Prepare or open unit-dose medication.
   a. Perform premedication assessments as needed including the patient's ability to swallow.
   b. If using a bar-coding device, scan the medication and the patient identification, and enter any pertinent information.
   c. Open the medication packages one at a time, and place them in a medication cup. Do *not* touch the tablets or capsules.

Avoid possible medication errors by adhering to the Six Rights of Medication Administration and by checking the medication with the MAR three times. Avoid direct contact with the medication to prevent the spread of microorganisms.

6. Administer medication with water while the patient is sitting or has the head of the bed elevated. Assist as needed (see Chapter 30, Nursing Care Guideline: Assisting an Adult With Feeding box), and ensure that all the tablets or capsules are swallowed.
   Patient position is important to prevent aspiration. Providing assistance to the patient promotes compliance, avoids medication errors, and promotes safety and quality care.
7. If a medication requires a follow-up assessment of the patient, return to obtain information within an appropriate time frame. Educate the patient about the expected effect of the medication and the time of your return.
   Completing the necessary follow-up prevents adverse effects and promotes patient compliance. Communication with the patient eases anxiety and gives the patient control.

Follow postprocedure steps I through VI.

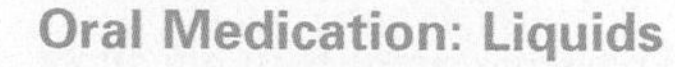

Oral Medication: Liquids

Follow preprocedure steps I through VIII.

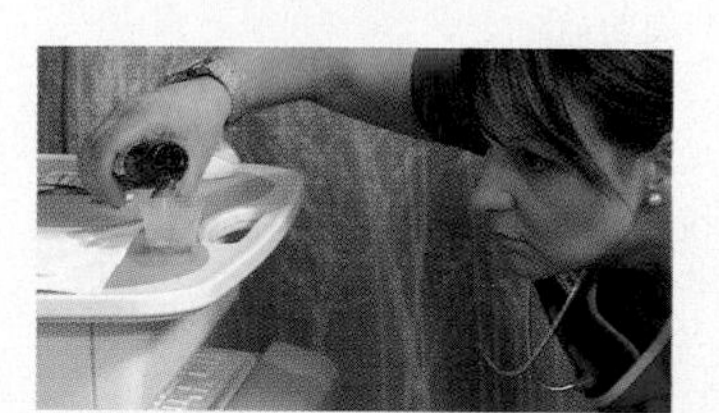

STEP 2a(1)

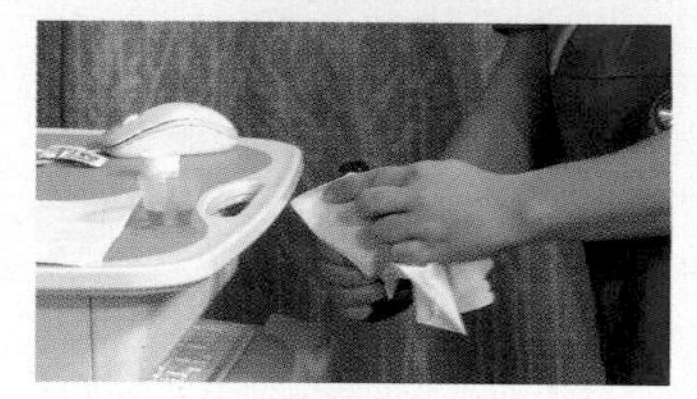

STEP 2a(2)

1. Follow procedure step 2 in the Oral Medication: Tablets and Capsules section.
2. Verify the needed medication dosage. Prepare the medication and check the medication label against the MAR a second time:
   a. If using a multidose bottle and if less than 10 mL is needed, use a syringe to measure the dosage. If more than 10 mL is needed, use a graduated medication cup. Shake the bottle gently if doing so is not contraindicated on the label, and remove the lid, placing it upside down on the counter. Pour or draw the dose at eye level. When pouring, hold the bottle with the label in your palm; wipe the lip of the bottle as needed with a paper towel, and replace the lid.
   b. If using a unit dose, verify the correct dose; gently shake the container but do *not* open it.
   Avoid possible medication errors by adhering to the Six Rights of Medication Administration and by checking the medication with the MAR three times. Shaking mixes the medication and ensures the accuracy of the dose. Lid placement prevents the spread of microorganisms. Measuring at eye level ensures accuracy. Positioning the label in the palm ensures that the medication does not spill onto the label and promotes safety for the person pouring the medication. Not opening the unit-dose container allows another check to be performed, along with patient education, at the bedside, thus further promoting patient safety and cooperation.
3. Enter the patient's room, perform patient identification, check patient allergies, assess patient knowledge, and educate the patient as needed.
   Communication with the patient facilitates cooperation. Avoid possible medication errors by adhering to the Six Rights of Medication Administration.
4. Recheck the label on the medication with the MAR a third time before returning the medication to its storage place *or* before opening the package at the bedside. Prepare the medication for administration:
   a. Perform premedication assessments as needed.
   b. If using a bar-coding device, scan the medication and the patient identification, and enter pertinent information.
   c. If using a unit dose, open the medication, and administer from the original container. Do *not* touch the medication.
   Avoid possible medication errors by adhering to the Six Rights of Medication Administration and by checking the medication with the MAR three times. Avoid direct contact with the medication to prevent the spread of microorganisms.

5. Administer medication while the patient is sitting or has the head of the bed elevated. Assist as needed (see Chapter 30, Nursing Care Guideline: Assisting an Adult With Feeding box), and ensure that all medication is swallowed.
Patient position is important to prevent aspiration. Providing the patient assistance promotes compliance, avoids medication errors, and promotes safety and high-quality care.
6. If a medication requires a follow-up assessment of the patient, return to obtain information within an appropriate time frame. Educate the patient about the expected effect of the medication and the time of your return.
Completing the necessary follow-up prevents adverse effects and promotes patient compliance. Communication with the patient eases patient anxiety and gives the patient control.

Follow postprocedure steps I through VI.

Oral Medication: Sublingual and Buccal

Follow preprocedure steps I through VIII.

1. Follow procedure steps 2 and 3 in the Oral Medication: Tablets and Capsules section.
2. Enter the patient's room, perform patient identification, check patient allergies, assess patient knowledge, and educate the patient as needed.
Communication with the patient facilitates cooperation. Avoid possible medication errors by adhering to the Six Rights of Medication Administration.
3. Recheck the label on the medication with the MAR a third time before returning the medication to its storage place *or* before opening the package at the bedside. Prepare unit-dose medication.
   a. Perform premedication assessments as needed and explain how sublingual or buccal medication is absorbed to the patient.
   b. If using a bar coding device, scan the medication and the patient identification, and enter pertinent information.
   c. Open medication, and place in a medication cup. Do *not* touch the medication.
   d. Don clean gloves.
      - Place sublingual medication under the tongue until dissolved.
      - Place buccal medication between the cheek and gums until dissolved.
      - Do *not* administer either form of medication with food or fluid. Instruct the patient *not* to chew or swallow the medication.

   Avoid possible medication errors by adhering to the Six Rights of Medication Administration and by checking the medication with the MAR three times. Avoid direct contact with the medication to prevent the spread of microorganisms. Gloves should be worn whenever contact with mucous membranes or bodily fluids is possible. Foods, fluids, and stomach acid can diminish the effectiveness of the medication.
4. Administer medication while the patient is sitting or has the head of the bed elevated. Assist as needed (see Chapter 30, Nursing Care Guideline: Assisting an Adult With Feeding box), and ensure that all medication is dissolved.
Patient position is important to prevent aspiration. Providing the patient assistance promotes compliance, avoids medication errors, and promotes safety and quality care.
5. If any medication requires a follow-up assessment of the patient, return to obtain information within an appropriate time frame. Educate the patient about the expected effect of the medication and the time of your return.
Completing the necessary follow-up prevents adverse effects and promotes patient compliance. Communication with the patient eases anxiety and gives the patient control.

Follow postprocedure steps I through VI.

POSTPROCEDURE

I. Return the bed to its lowest position, raise the top side rails, and verify that the call light is within reach for the patient.
Precautions are taken to maintain patient safety. Top side rails aid in positioning and turning. Raising four side rails is considered a restraint.

II. Assess for additional patient needs and state the time of your expected return.
Meeting patient needs and offering self promote patient satisfaction and build trust.

III. Properly dispose of PPE.
Gloves, gowns, and masks must be appropriately discarded to prevent the spread of microorganisms.

IV. Clean equipment if it was in contact with the patient; see specific manufacturer instructions.
Disinfection eliminates most microorganisms from inanimate objects.

V. Perform hand hygiene.
Frequent hand hygiene prevents the spread of infection.

VI. Document immediately after medication administration. Include the medication, dose, route, date, time, assessment, and the patient's response to the medication in the documentation.
Accurate documentation is essential to communicate medications administered and to provide legal evidence of care. Avoid possible medication errors by adhering to the Six Rights of Medication Administration.

SKILL 35-2 Inhaled Medication Administration

PURPOSE

- The administration of inhaled medications must be done appropriately and safely and should follow the Six Rights of Medication Administration:
  - The right medication
  - The right dose
  - The right time
  - The right route
  - The right patient
  - The right documentation
- Inhaled medication is administered to improve or maintain the patient's underlying pathophysiology. Nebulizers allow medication to reach smaller airways by delivering finer particles:
  - They promote bronchodilation and inhibit inflammation by delivering various pharmacologic agents.
  - They promote expectoration of pulmonary secretions by delivering aerosolized mucolytic agents or humidity.
  - They treat and prevent pulmonary-specific infections by delivering antiinfective agents.

RESOURCES

- Spacer, if required, for a metered-dose inhaler (MDI)
- An MDI
- Warm water to rinse the patient's mouth after administration, depending on the pharmacologic agent
- Emesis basin
- Nebulizer setup and tubing for nebulizer administration

COLLABORATION AND DELEGATION

- Refer to the Nursing Care Guideline: Six Rights of Medication Administration box.
- The administration of medication may not be delegated; however, the patient may self-administer medication under the supervision of the nurse. Supervision cannot be delegated.
- Unlicensed assistive personnel should report any of the following to the nurse:
  - Changes in vital signs or any patient complaints or discomforts
  - Medication found in the patient's room
  - Patient questions regarding medication
- The timing of inhaled medication is important:
  - Ensure that the proper administration takes place and is performed in collaboration with a respiratory therapist as appropriate or indicated.
  - Ensure that the order of administration of inhaled medication is appropriate (e.g., use rescue inhalers before maintenance).
- In many facilities, a respiratory therapist is responsible for inhaled medication administration. Collaborate and consult with the respiratory therapist as necessary and in accordance with facility policies and procedures.
- Collaborate with the pharmacist about medication questions before administration.

SPECIAL CIRCUMSTANCES

1. **Assess:** What is the patient's respiratory status?
   Intervention: Document the patient's preadministration and postadministration status, including the following:
   - Auscultation of lung fields
   - Respiratory and heart rates
   - Pulse oximetry
   - Patient report of breathing status
   - Patient complaints and discomfort
2. **Assess:** Is a spacer being used?
   Intervention: Properly insert the spacer:
   - Ensure that the spacer is clean.
   - Fit the mouthpiece of the MDI into the end of the spacer or into the MDI cradle port, depending on the brand of spacer.
   - Have the patient use the mouthpiece of the spacer instead of that of the MDI.
   - Clean the spacer:
     - Once each day with warm running water
     - Once each week with mild soap and water
3. **Assess:** Has the medication expired?
   Intervention: Do not administer expired medication.
   - Notify the pharmacy about expired medication.
   - Follow facility policies and protocols.

PREPROCEDURE

I. Check PCP orders and the patient care plan.
Knowledge of patient-specific orders is critical for safe patient care.

II. Gather supplies and equipment.
Preparing for the patient encounter saves time and promotes patient trust.

III. Perform hand hygiene.
Frequent hand hygiene prevents the spread of microorganisms.

IV. Maintain standard precautions.
Use of the correct personal protective equipment (PPE) is required whenever contact with bodily fluids is possible, to reduce the transfer of pathogens.

V. Introduce yourself.
Initial communication establishes the role of the nurse and begins a professional relationship.

VI. Provide for patient privacy.
It is important to maintain patient dignity.

VII. Identify the patient by using two identifiers.
Identifying a patient involves scanning barcodes or comparing the patient's stated name and birthdate to information on the patient's wristband or health record. The correct person must receive the correct treatment.

VIII. Explain the procedure to the patient.
The nurse has a responsibility to inform a patient before initiating care. Information may ease patient anxiety and facilitate cooperation.

PROCEDURE

Inhaled Medication: Metered-Dose Inhaler (MDI)

Follow preprocedure steps I through VIII.

1. Provide a glass of warm water for the patient to rinse the mouth after inhalation.
   Preparing supplies in advance avoids interruption during the procedure, thereby avoiding possible medication errors.
2. Prepare medications in a No Interruption Zone according to facility policy. Obtain the medication. Verify that the label of the medication matches the medication administration record (MAR), perform any dosage calculation, and check the expiration date of the medication.
   a. If using an automated dispensing system, enter the appropriate information, and remove the medication from the dispenser. Verify that the correct medication and dosage has been dispensed. Store unused medication doses according to facility policy.
   b. If using bar coding, scan the MAR and the medication. Verify that the correct dose has been dispensed.
   c. If using a medication cart, unlock the cart, and find the patient's drawer. Remove the patient's medication from the drawer, and verify that they are the correct dose.
   Avoid possible medication errors by adhering to the Six Rights of Medication Administration and by checking the medication label against the MAR three times.
3. Ensure that a canister of medication is in the holder, and check the expiration date. Check the medication label against the MAR a second time.
   Medication must be in the container so that the patient receives the ordered dose. Avoid possible medication errors by adhering to the Six Rights of Medication Administration and by checking the medication with the MAR three times.
4. Prime the MDI. If there is a priming button on the bottom, push the button.
   Proper preparation of the MDI ensures that the medication is delivered.
5. Perform patient identification, assess the patient's knowledge, and educate the patient as needed. Ask the patient about any allergies.
   The correct individual must receive the correct treatment. Communication with the patient facilitates patient cooperation. Avoid possible medication errors by adhering to the Six Rights of Medication Administration.
6. Perform premedication respiratory assessments including respiratory rate and pulse oximetry.
   Promote safe, quality patient care by providing baseline assessment data to evaluate the patient's response to medication.

7. If using a bar-coding device, scan the medication and the patient identification. Enter any pertinent information. Recheck the label on the medication with the MAR a third time before returning the medication to its storage place *or* before opening the package at the bedside.
Avoid possible medication errors by adhering to the Six Rights of Medication Administration and by checking the medication with the MAR three times.
8. Discuss the purpose of an MDI and how it works.
9. Administer the medication. Assist the patient as needed, or the patient may self-administer the medication.
   a. The patient may sit, stand, or lie in bed with the head of the bed elevated at least 30 degrees.
   b. The patient shakes the MDI.
   c. The patient must take a deep breath in and then blow out completely.
   d. The patient places the mouthpiece of the inhaler into the mouth.
   e. The patient should inhale slowly. With a traditional MDI, pushing the canister releases the medication; with an inhalation-activated MDI, inhaling releases the medication.
   f. The patient should continue the deep inhale over a period of 3 to 5 seconds and then should hold that breath for 5 to 10 seconds. The patient removes the inhaler from the mouth.
   g. The patient exhales through the nose or through pursed lips.
Patient position promotes optimal lung expansion. Shaking the MDI ensures the medication is mixed and improves dose accuracy through the delivery of fine particles. The breathing procedure promotes medication effectiveness and keeps the small airways patent.

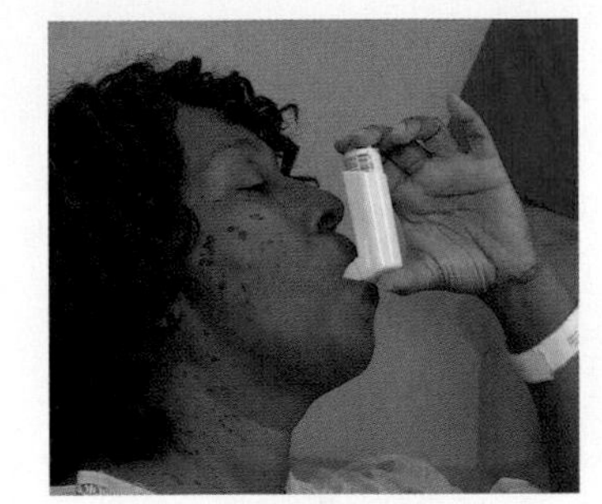
STEP 9d

10. If more than one inhalation of the same medication is ordered, wait at least 20 to 30 seconds (check recommendation for specific medications) between doses. If a different medication is ordered, allow 2 to 5 minutes between the inhalation.
Pausing between doses allows the earlier medication dose to become effective before the next dose is administered.
11. After 2 minutes, have the patient rinse the mouth with warm water and spit it into the emesis basin.
Take steps to prevent infection (such as yeast infections) or soreness in the patient's mouth to reduce the adverse effect of some inhaled medication.
12. Clean the inhaler holder and cap with warm running water after each use. Allow to dry completely.
Cleaning of equipment should be performed to prevent the spread of microorganisms and ensure proper functioning of equipment.
13. Perform a medication follow-up assessment: Return to obtain information within an appropriate time frame. Assess the respiratory status and compare to the pre-administration assessment. Encourage the patient to demonstrate self-administration of medication. Educate the patient on the expected effect of the medication.
Prevent adverse effects by performing the appropriate follow-up. Communication with the patient eases anxiety, facilitates cooperation, and gives the patient control.
14. If the canister is new, mark the date on the canister and calculate the number of doses of medication.

Follow postprocedure steps I through VI.

Inhaled Medication: Dry Powder Inhalation

Follow preprocedure steps I through VIII.

1. Follow procedure steps 1 through 7 in the Inhaled Medications: Metered-Dose Inhaler section. *Exceptions:* Priming, shaking, and using a spacer are not indicated with a dry powder inhaler (DPI).
2. If the patient is receiving a DPI for the first time, explain that a training device will be used prior to the administration of the medication. Administer the medication. Assist the patient as needed, or the patient may self-administer the medication.
   a. Have the patient sit, stand, or lie in bed with the head of the bed elevated.
   b. Assess the patient's ability to hold, manipulate, and activate the DPI.
   c. Point out the dose indicator on the DPI.
   d. Follow the manufacturer's instructions to prepare for administration.
   e. Follow the manufacturer's instructions for correct positioning of the DPI during administration.
   f. Have the patient take a deep breath in and then blow out completely.
   g. Place the mouthpiece of the inhaler into the patient's mouth.
   h. For dosing, puncture a capsule or trigger a spring-loaded mechanism while having the patient begin inhaling slowly.
   i. Ask the patient to hold that breath for 5 to 10 seconds. Remove the inhaler from the patient's mouth.
   j. Have the patient exhale through pursed lips.
   k. Instruct the patient to clean the device after each use.

   Positioning promotes optimal lung expansion. Manufacturer's instructions delineate priming and appropriate medication delivery for accurate dosing.
3. If more than one inhalation of the same medication is ordered, wait at least 1 minute between doses.
   Pausing between doses allows the earlier medication dose to become effective before the next dose is administered.
4. After 2 minutes, have the patient rinse the mouth with warm water and spit the solution into an emesis basin.
   Take steps to prevent infection (specifically thrush) or soreness in the patient's mouth to reduce the adverse effect of some inhaled medications.
5. Perform a medication follow-up assessment: Return to obtain information within an appropriate time frame. Assess the respiratory status and compare to the pre-administration assessment. Encourage the patient to demonstrate self-administration of medication. Educate the patient on the expected effects of the medication.
   Prevent adverse effects by performing the appropriate follow-up. Communication with the patient eases anxiety, facilitates cooperation, and gives the patient control.

Follow postprocedure steps I through VI.

Inhaled Medication: Nebulizer

Follow preprocedure steps I through VIII.

1. Follow procedure steps 1 through 7 in the Inhaled Medications: Metered-Dose Inhaler section. *Exceptions:* Priming, shaking, and using a spacer are not indicated with nebulizers.
2. If other inhaled medication has been ordered, administer those delivered through the nebulizers first, unless contraindicated; then wait 5 minutes before administering the other medication.
   The sequence and timing of administration of inhaled medications allows the first medication to become effective before the next one is administered.
3. In addition to respiratory assessment, monitor the pulse during the procedure especially if beta-adrenergic bronchodilators are used.
   Promote safe, quality patient care by providing baseline assessment data to evaluate the patient's response to medication.

4. Assemble the nebulizer (model with mouthpiece):
   a. Connect the tubing to the air compressor source (i.e., nebulizer machine, compressed air source, or compressed oxygen source) following manufacturer's instructions.
   b. Connect the other end of the tubing to the bottom of the nebulizer chamber.
   c. Place the medication in the nebulizer chamber in accordance with the PCP order; ensure that saline for inhalation has been added if it is needed.
   d. Close the nebulizer chamber (the top screws onto the bottom).
   e. Connect the T-piece connector to the top of the chamber.
   f. Place the mouthpiece in one end of the T-piece.

   Proper assembly ensures correct and accurate medication administration. Avoid wasting medication by using reservoir tubing.
5. Assemble the nebulizer (face mask model):
   a. Follow procedure step 4 A through D.
   b. Place the nebulizer face mask on top of the chamber.

   Patients may be unable to hold the delivery device for the entire treatment; the face mask allows medication delivery with minimal patient effort.
6. Administer treatment:
   a. Have the patient sit or lie in bed with the head of the bed elevated at least 30 degrees.
   b. Turn on the nebulizer machine, or turn on the compressed air or oxygen to 6 to 8 L/min.
   c. Check that the mode for administration of medication is set to *misting.*
   d. If a mouthpiece will be used, hand the patient the setup or secure the face mask on the patient.
   e. Encourage the patient to take slow, deep breaths throughout the treatment.

   Proper patient positioning promotes optimal lung expansion. Placing the face mask or delivery device with the patient as the last step ensures equipment functioning and prevents oxygen deprivation.

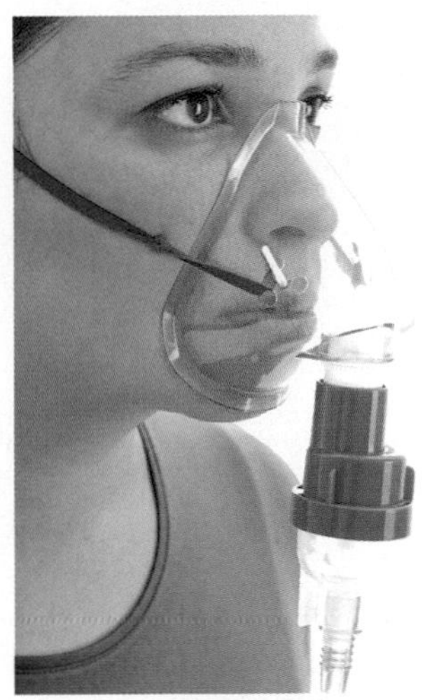

STEP 6

7. When the nebulizing is complete, discontinue the treatment:
   a. If medication drops are adhering to the side of the chamber, tap the chamber until the misting is complete.
   b. Remove the mask or mouthpiece setup from the patient.
   c. Turn off the compressed air source.
   d. Disconnect the tubing from the nebulizer chamber and air source.

   Nebulizing occurs by airflow from the bottom of the chamber. Ensuring that all droplets are at the bottom of the chamber promotes full-dose administration.
8. Have the patient rinse the mouth with warm water and spit the solution into an emesis basin.

   Take steps to prevent infection or soreness in the patient's mouth to reduce the adverse effect of some inhaled medications.
9. Clean the nebulizer administration setup.
   a. After each use with warm running water.
   b. Once each week with mild soap and warm water.
   c. Once each month, soaking it for 30 minutes in a solution of three parts water to one part vinegar. Allow it to air-dry while covered by a paper towel.
   d. Certain medications cannot share nebulizers; follow the policy and procedure of the facility. Change nebulizers according to facility policy and procedure.

   Store the setup in a clean plastic bag. Proper cleaning should be done to prevent the spread of microorganisms. Air-drying and bag storage prevents lint and other particles from getting into the delivery device and possibly entering the respiratory system in a future administration.

10. Perform a medication follow-up assessment. Return to obtain information within an appropriate time frame. Educate the patient on the expected effect and the time of your return. Assess the respiratory status and pulse, and compare to the pre-administration assessment. Encourage the patient to demonstrate self-administration of medication. Educate the patient on the expected effect of the medication.
Assess the patient to evaluate the effectiveness of the medication and treatment and prevent adverse effects. Communication with the patient eases anxiety, promotes compliance, and gives the patient control.

Follow postprocedure steps I through VI.

POSTPROCEDURE

I. Return the bed to its lowest position, raise the top side rails, and verify that the call light is within reach for the patient.
Precautions are taken to maintain patient safety. Top side rails aid in positioning and turning. Raising four side rails is considered a restraint.

II. Assess for additional patient needs and state the time of your expected return.
Meeting patient needs and offering self promote patient satisfaction and build trust.

III. Properly dispose of PPE.
Gloves, gowns, and masks must be appropriately discarded to prevent the spread of microorganisms.

IV. Clean equipment if it was in contact with the patient; see specific manufacturer instructions.
Disinfection eliminates most microorganisms from inanimate objects.

V. Perform hand hygiene.
Frequent hand hygiene prevents the spread of infection.

VI. Document immediately after medication administration. Include the medication, dose, route, date, time, assessment, and the patient's response to the medication in the documentation.
Accurate documentation is essential to communicate medications administered and to provide legal evidence of care. Avoid possible medication errors by adhering to the Six Rights of Medication Administration.

SKILL 35-3 Preparing Injections: Ampules, Multidose Vials, and Reconstituting Medications

PURPOSE

- Preparing medications from ampules and multidose vials and reconstituting medications must be done appropriately and safely and should follow the Six Rights of Medication Administration:
  - The right medication
  - The right dose
  - The right time
  - The right route
  - The right patient
  - The right documentation
- Medications from ampules and multidose vials and reconstituted medications are administered to improve or maintain the patient's underlying pathophysiology.
- When compatible, medications given by the same route should be prepared in one syringe for one injection to minimize discomfort and inconvenience to the patient.

RESOURCES

- Filter needle or straw for withdrawing medication from ampules
- Needle or blunt-tip cannula for withdrawing medication from vials
- Appropriate syringe and needle (see Skill 35-5 and Skill 35-6)
- Alcohol swabs
- 2 × 2 gauze pad
- Reconstitution solution for powdered medication vials according to the medication manufacturer's instructions

Collaboration and Delegation

- Refer to the Nursing Care Guideline: Six Rights of Medication Administration box.
- Medication administration may not be delegated.
- Unlicensed assistive personnel should report any of the following to the nurse:
  - Changes in vital signs and any patient complaints or discomforts
  - Medication found in the patient's room
  - Patient questions regarding medication
- Collaborate with the pharmacist on any medication questions before or during preparation.

EVIDENCE-BASED PRACTICE

- Many of the techniques in this skill apply to medications produced by mixing two or more substances together (i.e., admixtures) rather than the traditional procedure of drawing up medications for administration in an injection.
- Many medication errors and adverse events occur during these processes. George, Henneman, and Tasota (2010) explain the concerns: "IV admixture is known to be an error-prone procedure. Limiting the number of people who mix medications can minimize this, and assigning this responsibility to pharmacists is a common safety measure. However, because of the timing of pharmacy delivery of premixed agents and the need to start medications emergently, nurses may need to mix infusions. Nurses mixing medications must be knowledgeable about standard concentrations and procedures. They must alert the pharmacy if they have deviated from the standard concentration so that subsequent bags are mixed appropriately to avoid alteration in subsequent dose concentrations" (p. S141).
- Single-dose vials are preferred for any medication preparation; whenever possible, multidose vials and ampules should be avoided to prevent contamination, spread of microorganisms, and infections (World Health Organization, 2010).
- If possible, multidose vials should be used only for a single patient. Assign the medication to that patient for reuse, rather than using the vial for multiple patients (Centers for Disease Control and Prevention, 2012; World Health Organization, 2010).

SPECIAL CIRCUMSTANCES

1. **Assess:** How should an ampule be broken?
   Intervention:
   - Hold the ampule in the nondominant hand.
   - Use the dominant hand to grasp the top of the ampule with 2 × 2 gauze pad or an ampule sleeve.
   - Push the middle of the ampule (neck) away from the hands.
   - Dispose of the ampule tip in a sharps container.
2. **Assess:** Did the ampule break in a jagged manner so that it obviously does not have an even break around the neck?
   Intervention: Discard the ampule and its solution, and restart the procedure.
3. **Assess:** How should a needle be covered to safely transport the injection to the bedside?
   Intervention:
   - Place the syringe cap on a counter surface.
   - Hold the syringe with one hand; do *not* stabilize the cap with your hand.
   - Use a scooping motion to pick up the cap with the needle. Do *not* let the needle touch any other surface.
   - After the cap is on the needle, hold the syringe vertically.
   - Snap the cap tightly onto the syringe by holding the sides of the cap. Do *not* push the cap on while holding the top of the cap.

4. **Assess:** What additional steps should be taken when opening a new multidose vial?
Intervention: Appropriately open and label the vial:
- Check the expiration date, and examine the solution.
- Add the date, time of day, and your initials to the label (in ink).
- Remove the plastic top of the vial.

5. **Assess:** Is there a reconstitution solution attached to the powdered medication vial?
Intervention: Follow the manufacturer's instructions to reconstitute the solution:
- Typically, the vial with the reconstitution solution is on top of the vial with the powder.
- Usually, the two vials are pushed into each other to mix the solution and powder.
- Roll the vial between your palms to ensure that the solution and powder are mixed evenly.

PREPROCEDURE

I. Check PCP orders and the patient care plan.
Knowledge of patient-specific orders is critical for safe patient care.

II. Gather supplies and equipment.
Preparing for the patient encounter saves time and promotes patient trust.

III. Perform hand hygiene.
Frequent hand hygiene prevents the spread of microorganisms.

IV. Maintain standard precautions.
Use of the correct personal protective equipment (PPE) is required whenever contact with bodily fluids is possible, to reduce the transfer of pathogens.

V. Introduce yourself.
Initial communication establishes the role of the nurse and begins a professional relationship.

VI. Provide for patient privacy.
It is important to maintain patient dignity.

VII. Identify the patient by using two identifiers.
Identifying a patient involves scanning barcodes or comparing the patient's stated name and birthdate to information on the patient's wristband or health record. The correct person must receive the correct treatment.

VIII. Explain the procedure to the patient.
The nurse has a responsibility to inform a patient before initiating care. Information may ease patient anxiety and facilitate cooperation.

PROCEDURE

Ampules

Follow preprocedure steps I through VIII.

1. Prepare medications in a No Interruption Zone according to facility policy. Obtain the medication. Verify that the label of the medication matches the medication administration record (MAR), perform any dosage calculation, and check the expiration date of the medication and make sure the solution has no sediment. Check the expiration date of the syringe and filter needle or straw packaging.
   a. If an automated dispensing system is used, enter the appropriate information, and remove the medication. Verify the correct medication, dose, and form.
   b. If bar coding is used, scan the MAR and medication. Verify the correct medication, dose, and form.
   c. If using a medication cart, unlock the cart, and locate the correct patient drawer. Remove the medication from the drawer, and verify the correct medication, dose, and form.
   d. If the medication is in a refrigerator: Unlock the refrigerator, find the vial or ampule, and verify that it is the correct medication, dose, and form.

   Avoid possible medication errors by adhering to the Six Rights of Medication Administration and by checking the medication with the MAR three times.

2. Perform hand hygiene.
Frequent hand hygiene prevents the spread of microorganisms.
3. Tap the top of the ampule, and verify that the solution is entirely below the neck of the ampule.
The entire dose should be below the ampule neck to ensure that the entire dose can be withdrawn.
4. Unwrap the syringe, and place the filter needle or straw on the syringe.
The filter needle or straw prevents fragments of glass from entering the medication solution as it is drawn up into the syringe.
5. Open the ampule.
   a. Clean the ampule head with an alcohol swab.
   b. Hold the ampule in the nondominant hand.
   c. Use the dominant hand to grasp the top of the ampule with 2 × 2-inch gauze.
   d. Snap off the top of the ampule. Use a quick and smooth motion towards you.
   e. Dispose of the ampule top in a sharps container.
Using the proper technique to open an ampule prevents the spread of microorganisms and prevents cross-contamination. The top should be snapped towards the nurse to avoid fragments of glass from hitting the nurse. Proper disposal of waste protects caregivers from injury and reduces the spread of microorganisms.

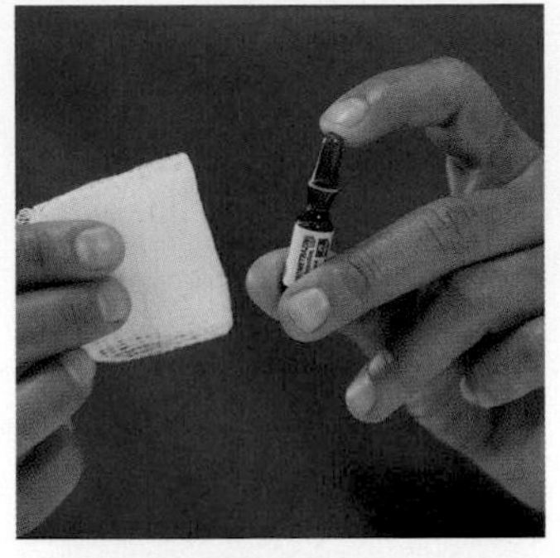
STEP 5b

6. Remove the cap of the filter needle or straw. Place the cap on the medication cart.
Protects the caregiver from injury and prevents the spread of microorganisms.
7. Draw the solution into the syringe:
   a. Place the ampule on the counter, and hold it with the nondominant hand.
   b. Fully insert a filter needle or straw into the center of the ampule.
   c. Withdraw the entire solution from the ampule into the syringe with the ampule upright or inverted while keeping the needle in the solution.
   d. Remove the syringe from the ampule.
By avoiding exposure of the solution to open air, contamination of the solution and the spread of microorganisms diminish.

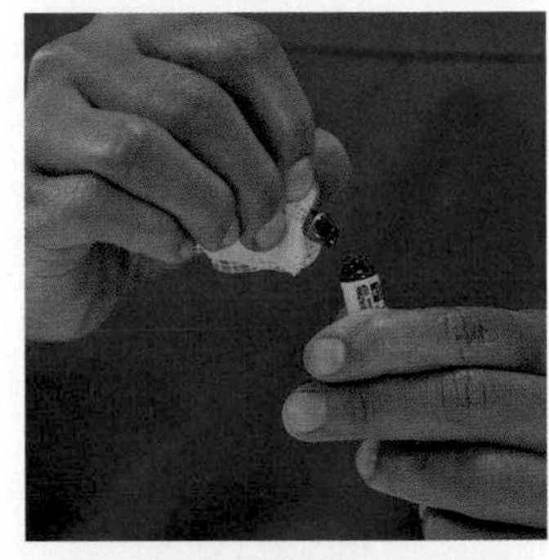
STEP 5d

8. Engage the safety device or re-cover the filter needle or straw by scooping the cap from the medication cart.
Proper procedure protects the caregiver from injury.
9. If there is excess air in the syringe, invert the syringe and expel the air.
Air rises to the top of the syringe, making it easier to expel.
10. Verify that the appropriate dose has been drawn into the syringe; work over a sink, and adjust to the ordered dose while holding the syringe at eye level with the needle pointing upward.
Holding the syringe at eye level ensures accuracy of the measurement.
11. Remove the filter needle or straw from the syringe, and dispose of it in a sharps container.
Proper disposal protects the caregiver from injury.

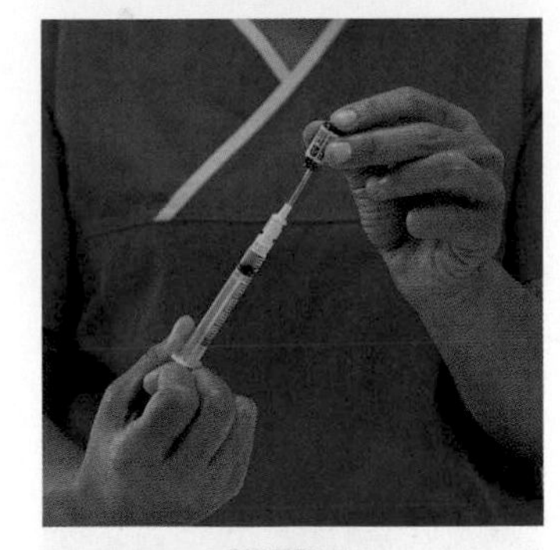
STEP 7c

12. Attach the appropriate needle for medication administration using aseptic technique.
Aseptic technique is used for preparation and administration of all parenteral medications.
13. Double-check the dose and check the medication label against the MAR a second time before disposing of the ampule in the sharps container.
Verification of the dose promotes ultimate safe, quality care and avoids possible medication errors by adhering to the Six Rights of Medication Administration and by checking the medication with the MAR three times. Proper disposal of the ampule prevents possible injury.
14. Administer the medication immediately after completing its preparation. If unable to administer immediately, label the syringe with name of medication and the amount in the syringe.

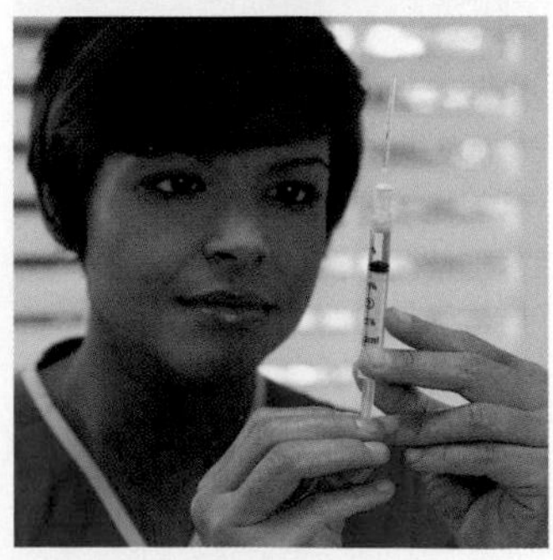
STEP 10

Follow postprocedure steps I through VI.

Multidose Vials

Follow preprocedure steps I through VIII.

1. Prepare medications in a No Interruption Zone according to facility policy. Obtain the medication. Verify that the label of the medication matches the medication administration record (MAR). Perform any dosage calculation including concentration of drug, volume of drug to be drawn, and which medication require verification by a second RN. Check the expiration date of the medication vial and make sure the solution has no sediment. Check the expiration date of the syringe and blunt cannula or needle packaging:
   - **a.** If an automated dispensing system is used, enter the appropriate information, and remove the medication. Verify the correct medication, dose, and form.
   - **b.** If bar coding is used, scan the MAR and medication. Verify the correct medication, dose, and form.
   - **c.** If using a medication cart, unlock the cart, and locate the correct patient drawer. Remove the medication from the drawer, and verify the correct medication, dose, and form.
   - **d.** If the medication is in a refrigerator: Unlock the refrigerator, find the vial or ampule, and verify that it is the correct medication, dose, and form.

   Avoid possible medication errors by adhering to the Six Rights of Medication Administration and by checking the medication with the MAR three times.
2. Perform hand hygiene.
   Frequent hand hygiene prevents the spread of microorganisms.
3. Clean the top of the vial with an alcohol swab.
   Proper antiseptic procedures should be used to prevent the spread of microorganisms.
4. Unwrap the syringe, and place the needle or blunt cannula on the syringe. Check medication administration instructions to see if a filter needle is required.
   Some medications may require the use of a filter needle
5. Remove the cap of the needle or blunt cannula, and place it on the medication cart.
   Protects the caregiver from injury and prevents the spread of microorganisms.
6. Draw sufficient air into the syringe to equal the ordered dose.
   Air injection creates pressure in the vial to facilitate withdrawal of the solution in a later procedural step.
7. Keep the multidose vial on the counter.
   - **a.** Insert the needle or blunt cannula straight into the vial.
   - **b.** Inject the air from the syringe into the vial; keep the plunger depressed.
   - **c.** Invert the bottle with the syringe.
   - **d.** Withdraw the ordered dose keeping the end of the needle in the fluid.
   - **e.** Remove the syringe from the vial.
   - **f.** Check the dose and remove any air or excess medication from the syringe. Work over a sink, and adjust to the ordered dose while holding the syringe at eye level with the needle pointing upward.

   Keeping the vial on the counter while inserting the needle establishes stability and promotes safety. Air injection creates pressure in the vial to facilitate withdrawal of solution. Holding the syringe at eye level ensures accuracy of the measurement.

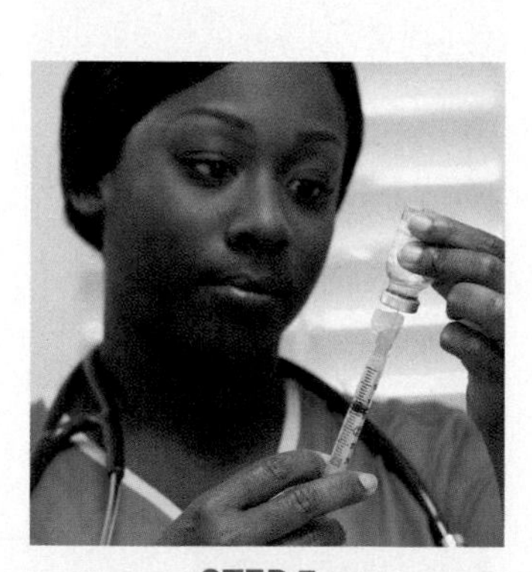

STEP 7c

8. Re-cover the needle or cannula by scooping the cap from the medication cart.
   Proper procedure protects the caregiver from injury.
9. Remove the needle or cannula from the syringe, and dispose of it in a sharps container.
   Proper procedure protects the caregiver from injury.
10. Attach the appropriate needle for medication administration using sterile technique.
11. Double-check the dose against the MAR one more time.
    Verification of the dose promotes ultimate safe, quality care and avoids possible medication errors by adhering to the Six Rights of Medication Administration.

12. Administer the medication immediately after completing its preparation. If unable to administer immediately, label the syringe with name of medication and the amount in the syringe.
13. If using a multidose vial, mark it with the date and your initials.
Once opened medications have to be used within a certain time frame according to manufacturer's recommendations.

Follow postprocedure steps I through VI.

Reconstituting Medications

Follow preprocedure steps I through VIII.

1. Prepare medications in a No Interruption Zone according to facility policy. Obtain the medication. Verify that the label of the medication matches the MAR, perform any dosage calculation, and check the expiration date of the medication.
   a. If an automated dispensing system is used, enter the appropriate information, and remove the medication. Verify the correct medication, dose, and form.
   b. If bar coding is used, scan the MAR and medication. Verify the correct medication, dose, and form.
   c. If a medication cart is used, unlock the cart, and locate the correct patient drawer. Remove the medication, and verify the correct medication, dose, and form.
Avoid possible medication errors by adhering to the Six Rights of Medication Administration and by checking the medication with the MAR three times.
2. Obtain the correct reconstitution or diluent solution according to the manufacturer's instructions.
The correct reconstitution solution or diluent must be used to ensure compatibility and the correct concentration after reconstitution. Avoid possible medication errors by adhering to the Six Rights of Medication Administration.
3. Perform hand hygiene.
Hand hygiene prevents the spread of microorganisms.
4. Clean the top of the vial with an alcohol swab.
Proper antiseptic procedures should be used to prevent the spread of microorganisms.
5. Unwrap the syringe, and place the needle or blunt cannula on the syringe. Check medication administration instructions to see if a filter needle is required.
Some medications may require the use of a filter needle.
6. Remove the cap of the needle or blunt cannula, and place it on the medication cart.
Protects the caregiver from injury and prevents the spread of microorganisms.
7. Draw sufficient air into the syringe to equal the ordered dose of the reconstitution or diluent solution.
Air injection creates pressure in the vial to facilitate withdrawal of the solution in a later procedural step.
8. Keep the multidose vial on the counter:
   a. Insert the needle or blunt cannula straight into the vial.
   b. Inject the air from the syringe into the vial; keep the plunger depressed.
   c. Invert the bottle with the syringe.
   d. Withdraw the ordered dose of solution keeping the end of the needle in the fluid.
   e. Remove the syringe from the vial.
   f. Check the dose and remove any air or excess solution from the syringe. Work over a sink, and adjust to the ordered dose while holding the syringe at eye level with the needle pointing upward.
Keeping the vial on the counter when inserting the needle establishes stability and promotes safety. Air injection creates pressure in the vial to facilitate withdrawal of solution. Holding the syringe at eye level ensures accuracy of the measurement.

9. Re-cover the needle or blunt cannula by scooping the cap from the medication cart.
Proper procedure protects the caregiver from injury.
10. Remove the cap from the powdered medication vial.
11. Clean the top of the vial with an alcohol swab.
Proper antiseptic procedures should be used to prevent the spread of microorganisms.
12. Remove the cap of the needle or blunt cannula, and place the cap on the medication cart.
Proper procedure protects the caregiver from injury and prevents the spread of microorganisms.
13. Keep the powdered medication vial on the counter:
a. Insert the needle straight into the vial.
b. Inject the reconstitution or diluent solution.
c. Remove the syringe from the vial.
Keeping the vial on the counter establishes stability and safety.
14. Re-cover the needle or cannula by scooping the cap from the medication cart.
Proper procedure protects the caregiver from injury.
15. Roll the vial between your palms. Make sure that all the powder dissolves and the solution contains no sediment.
Proper procedure ensures that the medication is evenly mixed.
16. Draw sufficient air into the syringe to equal the ordered dose.
Air injection creates pressure in the vial to facilitate withdrawal of the solution in a later procedural step.
17. Place the medication vial on the counter.
a. Insert the needle straight into the vial.
b. Inject the air from the syringe into the vial; keep the plunger depressed.
c. Invert the vial with the syringe.
d. Make sure the needle stays within the fluid.
e. Withdraw the ordered dose.
f. Remove the syringe from the vial.
Keeping the vial on the counter establishes stability while inserting the needle and promotes safety. Air injection creates pressure in the vial to facilitate withdrawal of the solution. Inverting the vial ensure that the needle is in the fluid for withdrawal into the syringe.
18. Re-cover the needle or blunt cannula by scooping the cap from the medication cart.
Proper procedure protects the caregiver from injury.
19. Remove the blunt cannula if used, and dispose of it in a sharps container.
Proper procedure protects the caregiver from injury.
20. Attach the appropriate needle for medication administration using sterile technique, or use the needle that was used to draw up the medication if appropriate.
Proper procedure protects the patient from microorganisms.
21. Double-check the dose against the MAR. Check the medication label against the MAR a second time. Check the medication label against the MAR a third time before administration.
Verification of the dose promotes ultimate safe, quality care and avoids possible medication errors by adhering to the Six Rights of Medication Administration and by checking the medication with the MAR three times.
22. Administer the medication immediately after completing its preparation.

Follow postprocedure steps I through VI.

POSTPROCEDURE

I. Return the bed to its lowest position, raise the top side rails, and verify that the call light is within reach for the patient.
Precautions are taken to maintain patient safety. Top side rails aid in positioning and turning. Raising four side rails is considered a restraint.

II. Assess for additional patient needs and state the time of your expected return.
Meeting patient needs and offering self promote patient satisfaction and build trust.

III. Properly dispose of PPE.
Gloves, gowns, and masks must be appropriately discarded to prevent the spread of microorganisms.

IV. Clean equipment if it was in contact with the patient; see specific manufacturer instructions.
Disinfection eliminates most microorganisms from inanimate objects.

V. Perform hand hygiene.
Frequent hand hygiene prevents the spread of infection.

VI. Document immediately after medication administration. Include the medication, dose, route, date, time, assessment, and the patient's response to the medication in the documentation.
Accurate documentation is essential to communicate medications administered and to provide legal evidence of care. Avoid possible medication errors by adhering to the Six Rights of Medication Administration.

SKILL 35-4 Medication Administration: Mixing Insulin

PURPOSE

- The mixing and administration of insulin must be done appropriately and safely and should follow the Six Rights of Medication Administration:
  - The right medication
  - The right dose
  - The right time
  - The right route
  - The right patient
  - The right documentation
- Insulin is administered to improve or maintain the patient's underlying pathophysiology and prevent complications by regulating blood glucose levels.
- The ordered insulin should be prepared in one syringe for one injection, if not contraindicated, to minimize discomfort and inconvenience to the patient.

RESOURCES

- Insulin syringe (50 or 100 units)
- Multidose insulin vials
- Alcohol swabs

COLLABORATION AND DELEGATION

- Refer to the Nursing Care Guideline: Six Rights of Medication Administration box.
- Medication administration (including the mixing of insulin) may not be delegated.
- Unlicensed assistive personnel should report any of the following to the nurse.
  - Changes in vital signs and any patient complaints or discomforts
  - Medication found in the patient's room
  - Patient questions regarding medication
- The timing of insulin administration is important.
  - Ensure proper administration and collaboration with dietary administration in the facility; insulin must be administered with regard to meals.
  - Administer insulin immediately after its preparation.
  - Immediate administration ensures that the medication remains mixed appropriately within the syringe.
  - Rapid-acting insulin can reduce the effectiveness of long-acting insulin after the two are mixed.
- Collaborate with the pharmacist about medication questions before or during preparation.

SPECIAL CIRCUMSTANCES

- Intermediate-acting insulin is cloudy. Rapid-acting and short-acting insulin are clear.
- Key mnemonic: *clear before cloudy.*

1. **Assess:** While injecting air into intermediate-acting (cloudy) insulin, did you let the needle touch the solution?
   Intervention: Obtain a new syringe for the next step.
2. **Assess:** While withdrawing intermediate-acting (cloudy) insulin, did you accidentally inject clear insulin?
   Intervention: Start the procedure over.
   - Dispose of the intermediate-acting (cloudy) vial according to facility policies and procedures.
   - Obtain a new intermediate-acting (cloudy) vial.
3. **Assess:** While withdrawing intermediate-acting (cloudy) insulin, did you overdraw the total amount calculated?
   Intervention: Discard the syringe, and start the procedure over.

PREPROCEDURE

I. Check PCP orders and the patient care plan.
Knowledge of patient-specific orders is critical for safe patient care.

II. Gather supplies and equipment.
Preparing for the patient encounter saves time and promotes patient trust.

III. Perform hand hygiene.
Frequent hand hygiene prevents the spread of microorganisms.

IV. Maintain standard precautions.
Use of the correct personal protective equipment (PPE) is required whenever contact with bodily fluids is possible, to reduce the transfer of pathogens.

V. Introduce yourself.
Initial communication establishes the role of the nurse and begins a professional relationship.

VI. Provide for patient privacy.
It is important to maintain patient dignity.

VII. Identify the patient by using two identifiers.
Identifying a patient involves scanning barcodes or comparing the patient's stated name and birthdate to information on the patient's wristband or health record. The correct person must receive the correct treatment.

VIII. Explain the procedure to the patient.
The nurse has a responsibility to inform a patient before initiating care. Information may ease patient anxiety and facilitate cooperation.

PROCEDURE

Mixing Insulin

Follow preprocedure steps I through VIII.

1. Prepare medications in a No Interruption Zone according to facility policy. Obtain the medication. Verify that the label of the medication matches the medication administration record (MAR). Perform any dosage calculation and determine the total volume of insulin to be administered. Check the expiration date of the medication:
   a. If an automated dispensing system is used, enter the appropriate information, and remove the medication. Verify that the device contains the correct type of insulin.
   b. If bar coding is used, scan the MAR and medication. Verify the correct insulin type.
   c. If a medication cart is used, unlock the cart, locate the correct patient drawer, remove the medication, and verify the correct insulin type.
   d. If the medication is in a refrigerator, unlock the refrigerator, find the multidose vials, and verify that you have the correct insulin type. Allow the insulin to come to room temperature before administration.

   Avoid possible medication errors by adhering to the Six Rights of Medication Administration and by checking the medication with the MAR three times.
2. Perform hand hygiene.
   Frequent hand hygiene prevents the spread of microorganisms.
3. If the insulin is cloudy, roll the vial between your hands. Do *not* shake it.
   Rolling the vial mixes the insulin to ensure an even suspension of the dose.
4. Place both vials on the counter, and clean their tops with alcohol swabs.
   Proper cleaning should be used to prevent the spread of microorganisms.
5. Use an insulin syringe of the appropriate size (50 or 100 units) based on the calculation of total insulin units ordered.
6. Check the expiration date on the syringe packaging.
   Avoid possible medication errors by adhering to the Six Rights of Medication Administration; they apply to the equipment and the medication.
7. Unwrap the syringe; remove the cap, and place it on the medication cart.
   Careful handling of the syringe protects caregivers from injury and reduces the spread of microorganisms.
8. Draw sufficient air into the syringe to equal the number of ordered units of cloudy, intermediate-acting insulin.
   Air injection creates pressure in the vial to facilitate withdrawal of the solution in a later procedural step.
9. Keep the vial of cloudy, intermediate insulin on the counter:
   a. Insert the needle straight into the vial; do *not* let the needle touch the solution.
   b. Inject the air from the syringe into the vial; keep the plunger depressed.
   c. Remove the syringe from the vial.

   Keeping the vial on the counter establishes stability and promotes safety. Not letting the needle touch the solution avoids contamination of the next insulin solution. Air injection creates pressure in the vial, which facilitates withdrawal of the solution in a later procedural step. Keeping the plunger depressed while removing the needle from the vial prevents the accidental withdrawal of insulin.

10. Draw sufficient air into the syringe to equal the number of ordered units of clear, rapid- or short-acting insulin.
Air injection creates pressure in the vial to facilitate withdrawal of the solution.
11. Keep the vial of clear, rapid- or short-acting insulin on the counter:
  a. Insert the needle straight into the vial.
  b. Inject the air from the syringe into the vial; keep the plunger depressed.
  c. Invert the vial with the syringe.
  d. Withdraw the ordered number of units of rapid- or short-acting insulin.
  e. Remove the syringe from the vial.
Keeping the vial on the counter while inserting the needle establishes stability and promotes safety. Air injection creates pressure in the vial to facilitate withdrawal of the solution. Inverting the vial ensures that the needle reaches the solution in order to withdraw the ordered amount of medication.
12. Check the medication label against the MAR a second time. Verify the dose with a second licensed nurse according to facility policy.
Verification of the dose promotes ultimate safe, quality care and avoids possible medication errors by adhering to the Six Rights of Medication Administration and by checking the medication with the MAR three times.
13. Verify the calculation; final units in syringe = first-ordered insulin units + second-ordered insulin units.
Having the correct calculation is important for the next procedural step; it promotes ultimate safe, quality care and avoids possible medication errors by adhering to the Six Rights of Medication Administration.
14. Keep the vial of cloudy, intermediate insulin on the counter:
  a. Insert the needle straight into the vial, but do *not* push on the plunger.
  b. Invert the vial with the syringe.
  c. Withdraw insulin to obtain the total number of units calculated.
  d. Remove the syringe from the vial.
Keeping the vial on the counter while inserting the needle establishes stability and promotes safety. Not pushing on the plunger keeps the correct dose of the first insulin in the syringe.
15. Verify the dose with a second licensed nurse according to facility policy.
Verification of the dose promotes ultimate safe, quality care and avoids possible medication errors by adhering to the Six Rights of Medication Administration.
16. Re-cover the syringe by scooping the cap from the medication cart.
Careful handling of the syringe protects caregivers from injury and reduces the spread of microorganisms.
17. Verify the dose against the MAR one more time.
Rechecking the dosage promotes ultimate safe, quality care and avoids possible medication errors by adhering to the Six Rights of Medication Administration.
18. Administer the medication within 5 minutes of completing procedure step 17; use the subcutaneous injection technique.
Prompt administration of the medication ensures that it remains mixed appropriately within the syringe.
19. Dispose of the needle and syringe in a sharps container according to facility policies or procedures.
Proper disposal of waste reduces the spread of microorganisms and protects caregivers from injury.

Follow postprocedure steps I through VI.

POSTPROCEDURE

I. Return the bed to its lowest position, raise the top side rails, and verify that the call light is within reach for the patient.
Precautions are taken to maintain patient safety. Top side rails aid in positioning and turning. Raising four side rails is considered a restraint.

II. Assess for additional patient needs and state the time of your expected return.
Meeting patient needs and offering self promote patient satisfaction and build trust.

III. Properly dispose of PPE.
Gloves, gowns, and masks must be appropriately discarded to prevent the spread of microorganisms.

IV. Clean equipment if it was in contact with the patient; see specific manufacturer instructions.
Disinfection eliminates most microorganisms from inanimate objects.

V. Perform hand hygiene.
Frequent hand hygiene prevents the spread of infection.

VI. Document immediately after medication administration. Include the medication, dose, route, date, time, assessment, and the patient's response to the medication in the documentation.
Accurate documentation is essential to communicate medications administered and to provide legal evidence of care. Avoid possible medication errors by adhering to the Six Rights of Medication Administration.

SKILL 35-5 Subcutaneous, Intramuscular, and Intradermal Injections

PURPOSE

- The administration of injected medication must be done appropriately and safely and should follow the Six Rights of Medication Administration:
  - The right medication
  - The right dose
  - The right time
  - The right route
  - The right patient
  - The right documentation
- Injected medication is administered to improve or maintain the patient's underlying pathophysiology.

RESOURCES

- Alcohol swab (or approved cleansing agent in accordance with facility policies and procedures)
- 2 × 2 gauze pad
- Adhesive bandage
- Nonsterile gloves
- For subcutaneous injections:
  - Syringe: 0.5- to 3-mL or U-100 insulin syringe
  - Needle: 25 to 31 gauge, ⅜ to ⅝ inch (up to 1 inch for an obese patient)
- For intramuscular injections:
  - Syringe: 2 to 3 mL (adult); 0.5 to 1 mL (pediatric)
  - Needle: 19 to 25 gauge, 1 to 3 inches (adult); 22 to 25 gauge, ⅝ to 1 inch (pediatric)
- For intradermal injections:
  - Syringe: up to 1-mL tuberculin syringe
  - Needle: 25 to 27 gauge, ¼ to ⅝ inch

COLLABORATION AND DELEGATION

- Refer to the Nursing Care Guideline: Six Rights of Medication Administration box.
- Medication administration may not be delegated.
- Unlicensed assistive personnel (UAP) should report the following to the nurse:
  - Changes in vital signs or any patient complaints or discomforts
  - Medications found in the patient's room
  - Patient questions regarding medications
- Collaborate with the pharmacist about medication questions before administration.

EVIDENCE-BASED PRACTICE

- Aspiration of blood for any injection is no longer recommended. The rationale for this technique had been to verify correct placement and to ensure that the injection was not entering a large blood vessel. Aspiration most commonly occurred at the dorsogluteal site.
- Because the dorsogluteal site has the highest risk of incorrect placement and entry into a large blood vessel, it is no longer used, and aspiration is no longer necessary for injections into muscle tissue. This approach is endorsed by many major health organizations, including World Health Organization (WHO), Centers for Disease Control and Prevention (CDC), Advisory Committee on Immunization Practices (ACIP), American Academy of Family Physicians (AAFP), and the U.K. Department of Health (DoH) (Crawford and Johnson, 2009; Malkin, 2008).
- In regard to "eliminating unnecessary injections," the World Health Organization (2010) states that "when effective treatment can be given by other routes (oral or rectal), this is preferred, because it reduces potential exposure to blood and infectious agents and reduces infection risks" (p. 4).

PREPROCEDURE

I. Check PCP orders and the patient care plan.
Knowledge of patient-specific orders is critical for safe patient care.

II. Gather supplies and equipment.
Preparing for the patient encounter saves time and promotes patient trust.

III. Perform hand hygiene.
Frequent hand hygiene prevents the spread of microorganisms.

IV. Maintain standard precautions.
Use of the correct personal protective equipment (PPE) is required whenever contact with bodily fluids is possible, to reduce the transfer of pathogens.

V. Introduce yourself.
Initial communication establishes the role of the nurse and begins a professional relationship.

VI. Provide for patient privacy.
It is important to maintain patient dignity.

VII. Identify the patient by using two identifiers.
Identifying a patient involves scanning barcodes or comparing the patient's stated name and birthdate to information on the patient's wristband or health record. The correct person must receive the correct treatment.

VIII. Explain the procedure to the patient.
The nurse has a responsibility to inform a patient before initiating care. Information may ease patient anxiety and facilitate cooperation.

PROCEDURE

Injections: Subcutaneous

Follow preprocedure steps I through VIII.

1. Prepare medications in a No Interruption Zone according to facility policy. Obtain the medication. Verify that the label of the medication matches the medication administration record (MAR), perform any dosage calculation, and check the expiration date of the medication:
   a. If using an automated dispensing system, enter the appropriate information, and remove the medication. Verify the correct dose.
   b. If using bar coding, scan the MAR and medication. Verify the correct dose.
   c. If using a medication cart, unlock the cart, locate the correct patient drawer, remove the medication, and verify the correct dose.

   Avoid possible medication errors by adhering to the Six Rights of Medication Administration and by checking the medication with the MAR three times.
2. Perform hand hygiene.
   Frequent hand hygiene prevents the spread of microorganisms.
3. Check the medication label against the MAR a second time. Verify that the correct medication and dosage have been obtained, and draw up the medication in an appropriate syringe with an appropriate needle (see Skill 35-3).
   a. An appropriate fluid amount is 0.5 to 1 mL.
   b. Some syringes are prefilled (multidose-unit pens) (see the Nursing Care Guideline: Medication Administration With Multidose Insulin Pens box).

   Avoids possible medication errors by adhering to the Six Rights of Medication Administration and by checking the medication with the MAR three times.
4. Assess the patient's knowledge, and educate the patient about the procedure as needed.
   Communication with the patient eases anxiety and facilitates cooperation.
5. Perform premedication assessments as indicated.
   Evaluation of the patient before administering medication promotes safe, quality patient care and provides baseline assessment data to evaluate the effectiveness of the medication and interventions.

6. If using bar coding, scan the medication and the patient identification. Enter pertinent information. Recheck the label on the medication with the MAR a third time before returning the medication to its storage place *or* before opening the package at the bedside.
   Avoid possible medication errors by adhering to the Six Rights of Medication Administration and by checking the medication with the MAR three times.
7. Determine an appropriate injection site:
   a. Does the medication require that a specific injection site be used?
   b. Should the injection site be rotated on a schedule?
   c. Assess the skin and tissue of the selected site to be sure the site is acceptable.
   d. Allow patient choice or input if possible.
   Some medications absorb better in certain sites. The injection sites for routine medications are rotated to prevent tissue damage. Obvious skin or tissue integrity issues such as scars, moles, or rashes require avoidance of the site. Permitting patient input promotes compliance and gives the patient control.
8. Site locations, beginning with the most common (see Figure 35-13).
   a. Lateral aspect of the upper arm
   b. Abdomen, below the costal margin to the iliac crests (avoid injections within 2 inches of the umbilicus)
   c. Lateral anterior thigh
   d. Upper ventrodorsal gluteal area
   e. Upper back or scapular areas
   Subcutaneous injection areas are not bony, muscular, or dense with nerves or blood vessels. Correct anatomic placement of the injection prevents injury.
9. Position the patient for optimal access to the chosen site.
   Proper patient position promotes optimal administration and technique for ultimate safe, quality care and promotes patient comfort during administration.
10. Perform hand hygiene, and apply clean gloves.
    Frequent hand hygiene and proper glove use prevent the spread of microorganisms.
11. Clean the site with an alcohol swab, using a circular motion that moves from the center outward 2 inches, *or* follow facility policies and procedures. Allow the site to air-dry.
    Proper antiseptic procedures should be used to prevent the spread of microorganisms.
12. Administer the injection:
    a. Have the patient relax.
    b. Hold a piece of gauze in the third and fourth fingers of the nondominant hand.
    c. Pull the needle cap straight off, and set the cap aside.
    d. Hold the syringe as you would a pen or dart, with the thumb and tips of one or two (forefinger and middle) fingers of the dominant hand and with the palm of the hand directed downward.
    e. Pinch or stretch the tissue at the site with the nondominant hand.
    f. Insert the needle quickly, with the bevel up at a 45- to 90-degree angle. The nondominant hand releases the pinched tissue and stabilizes the syringe.
    g. Use the dominant hand to slowly depress the plunger and inject the medication.
    Relaxing the muscles facilitates injection into the subcutaneous tissue rather than inadvertent injection into muscle. Proper technique promotes minimal discomfort and easy manipulation of supplies. Taking proper precaution to remove the needle cap prevents the spread of microorganisms. Pinching the skin allows smooth injection. Keeping the bevel up and using the appropriate needle angle promote proper medication administration into subcutaneous tissue rather than into muscle (avoiding possible errors) and promote safe, quality patient care.

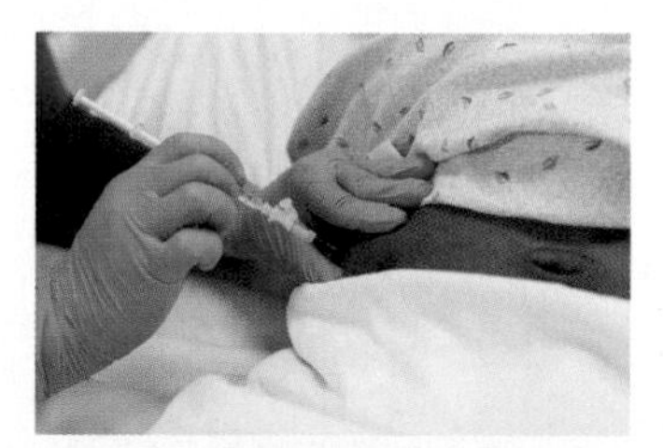

STEP 12d

13. Perform the following steps in quick succession:
    a. With the dominant hand, withdraw the syringe.
    b. With the dominant hand, activate the needle safety protection device.
    c. With the nondominant hand, apply the gauze and slight pressure to the site; do *not* massage the site.
    d. Apply an adhesive bandage as needed.
    Following this procedure minimizes discomfort and tissue damage. Massage can damage tissue by pushing the medication into surrounding tissues and may cause the medication to be absorbed faster than intended. The needle safety device protects caregivers from injury.
14. Dispose of the needle and syringe in a sharps container according to facility policy.
    Proper disposal of waste reduces the spread of microorganisms and protects caregivers from injury.
15. If the medication requires follow-up assessment, return to obtain information within an appropriate time frame. Educate the patient on the expected effect of the medication.
    Performing a follow-up assessment can prevent adverse effects and provides information regarding the effectiveness of the medication administered. Communication with the patient eases anxiety and facilitates cooperation.

Follow postprocedure steps I through VI.

Injections: Intramuscular

Follow preprocedure steps I through VIII.

1. Prepare medications in a No Interruption Zone according to facility policy. Obtain the medication. Verify that the label of the medication matches the MAR, perform any dosage calculation, and check the expiration date of the medication.
    a. If using an automated dispensing system, enter the appropriate information, and remove the medication. Verify the correct dose.
    b. If using bar coding, scan the MAR and medication. Verify the correct dose.
    c. If using a medication cart, unlock the cart, locate the correct patient drawer, remove the medication, and verify the correct dose.
    Avoid possible medication errors by adhering to the Six Rights of Medication Administration and by checking the medication with the MAR three times.
2. Perform hand hygiene.
    Frequent hand hygiene prevents the spread of microorganisms.
3. Check the medication label against the MAR a second time. Verify that the correct medication and dosage have been obtained, and draw up the medication in an appropriate syringe with an appropriate needle (see Skill 35-3).
    a. The fluid amount for IM injections is up to 3 mL, depending on the site.
    b. Some syringes are prefilled (e.g., EpiPens, multidose-unit pens) (the Nursing Care Guideline: Medication Administration With EpiPens box).
    This approach avoids possible medication errors by adhering to the Six Rights of Medication Administration and by checking the medication with the MAR three times.
4. Follow procedure steps 4 through 7 in the Injections: Subcutaneous section.
5. Locate the intramuscular (IM) injection site.
    a. For ventrogluteal injection, place the heel of the hand over the greater trochanter of the patient's femur; the thumb should point toward the pelvic area. If the patient's right ventrogluteal area is the injection site, the left hand is used; if the patient's left ventrogluteal area is the injection site, the right hand is used. The index finger should be over the anterior superior iliac spine, and the index and middle fingers spread to form a V shape as far apart over the iliac crest as possible. The point of injection is between the index and middle fingers in the middle of the V shape.

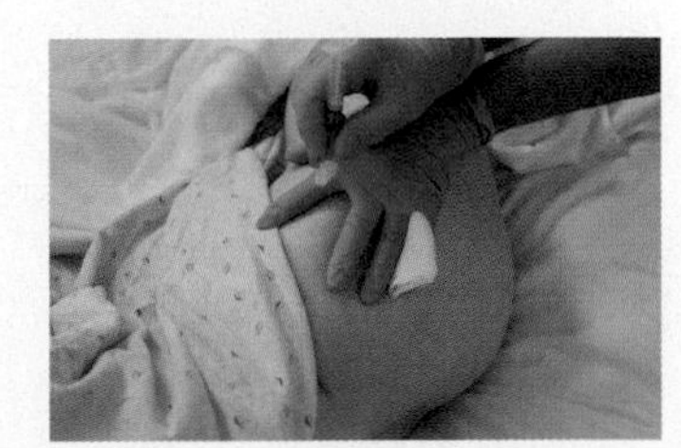

STEP 5a

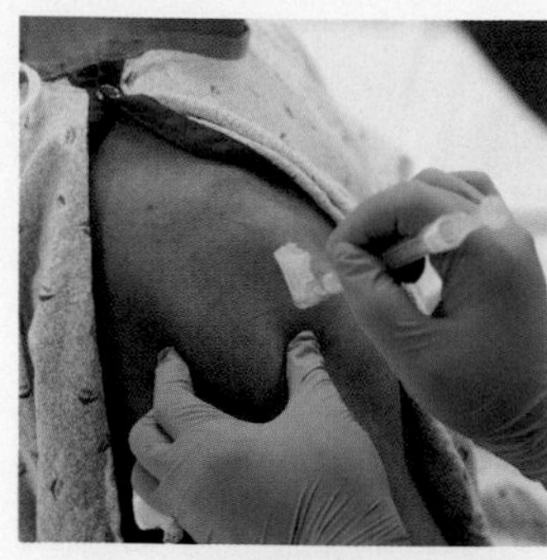
STEP 5b

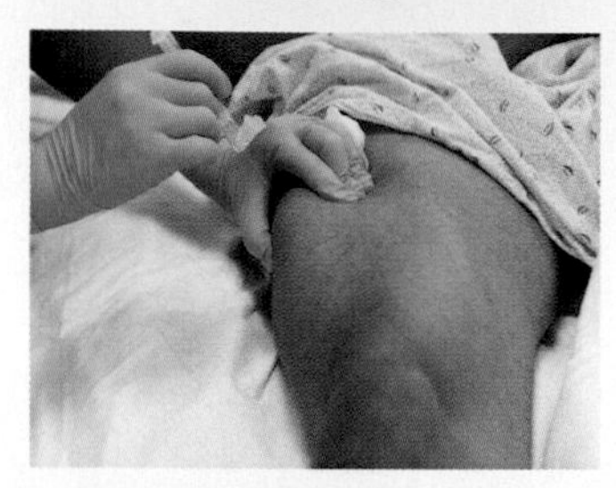
STEP 5c

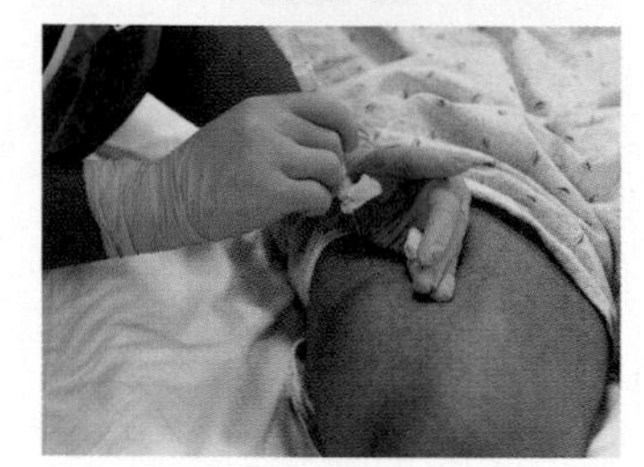
STEP 7

b. For deltoid muscle injection, place the ring finger along the lower edge of the acromial process, with the middle finger (and possibly index finger) joined with the ring finger. The point of injection is just posterior to midline immediately below the middle or index finger, in line with the axilla.
c. For vastus lateralis injection, place one hand below the greater trochanter of the femur, with the thumb pointing toward the knee to form an L or backward-L shape. Place the other hand above the knee, with the thumb pointing toward the hip to form an L or backward-L shape. The point of injection is in the center third of the lateral thigh between the hands and at the center of the side of the leg.

A ventrogluteal site is preferred due to muscle size. Intramuscular injection areas are not bony, are highly muscular, and have low density of pertinent nerve areas or major blood vessels. The correct anatomic placement of an injection prevents injury to the patient.

6. Follow procedure steps 9 through 11 in the Injections: Subcutaneous section.
7. Use the Z-track method to insert the needle.
   a. Remember the injection site.
   b. Use the third and fourth fingers of the nondominant hand to hold the gauze.
   c. Pull the needle cap straight off.
   d. Use the thumb and tips of the one or two (forefinger and middle)fingers to hold the syringe, palm down, as you would a pen or dart.
   e. Use the side of the nondominant hand to pull the skin tight below the injection site or to the side (Z-track).
   f. Insert the needle quickly at a 90-degree angle.
   g. Continue to pull on the skin with the side of the nondominant hand; use the thumb and index finger to stabilize the barrel of the syringe.
   h. Move the dominant hand up on the barrel to the end of the plunger.

   The Z-track technique ensures that medication is "locked" into the muscle. The procedure promotes injection into the muscle, provides minimal patient discomfort, and allows accessibility of supplies. Uncapping the needle by pulling the cap straight off prevents the spread of microorganisms. The angle of needle entry promotes medication administration into the muscle rather than inadvertent administration into other tissue, and it avoids possible medication errors and promotes patient safety and quality care.
8. Administer the medication by slowly depressing the plunger, delivering 1 mL of medication over 10 seconds. Hold the needle in place for 10 seconds after the medication is administered.

   Injecting the medication slowly minimizes patient discomfort and tissue damage. Holding the needle in place allows the medication to disperse into the tissue.
9. Perform the following steps in quick succession:
   a. Withdraw the needle and syringe with the dominant hand.
   b. Activate the needle safety protection device with the dominant hand.
   c. Release the Z-tracked tissue from the nondominant hand.
   d. Apply gentle pressure with the gauze with the nondominant hand. Do *not* massage the site.
   e. Apply an adhesive bandage if needed.

   Following this procedure minimizes discomfort and tissue damage. Massage can damage tissue by pushing the medication into surrounding tissues and may cause the medication to be absorbed faster than intended. The needle safety device protects caregivers from injury.
10. Follow procedure steps 14 and 15 in the Injections: Subcutaneous section.

Follow postprocedure steps I through VI.

Injections: Intradermal

Follow preprocedure steps I through VIII.

1. Prepare medications in a No Interruption Zone according to facility policy. Obtain the medication. Verify that the label of the medication matches the MAR, perform any dosage calculation, and check the expiration date of the medication.
   a. If using an automated dispensing system, enter the appropriate information, and remove the medication. Verify the correct dose.
   b. If using bar coding, scan the MAR and medication. Verify the correct dose.
   c. If using a medication cart, unlock the cart, locate the correct patient drawer, remove the medication, and verify the correct dose.

   Proper procedure to avoid possible medication errors by adhering to the Six Rights of Medication Administration and by checking the medication with the MAR three times.
2. Perform hand hygiene.

   Frequent hand hygiene prevents the spread of microorganisms.
3. Verify the correct medication and dosage. Check the medication label against the MAR a second time.
   a. Draw up the medication in an appropriate syringe with an appropriate needle (see Skill 35-3).
   b. The usual amount for an intradermal (ID) injection is 0.1 mL.

   Proper procedure avoids possible medication errors by adhering to the Six Rights of Medication Administration and by checking the medication with the MAR three times.
4. Follow procedure steps 4 through 7 in the Injections: Subcutaneous section.
5. Locate the injection site.
   a. For the anterior forearm, locate a site that is three to four finger widths below the antecubital area and one hand width above the wrist. If the skin at the injection point is intact, proceed with the injection.
   b. For the upper back, use the scapular area.
   c. If the upper back is not acceptable, use another subcutaneous site (see procedure step 9 in the Injections: Subcutaneous section).

   The anterior forearm is the preferred site for ID injections. The skin must be intact and without blemishes, marks, or scars for proper interpretation of results.
6. Follow procedure steps 9 through 11 in the Injections: Subcutaneous section
7. Administer the injection.
   a. Use the third and fourth fingers of the nondominant hand to hold the gauze.
   b. Pull the needle cap straight off.
   c. Use the thumb and tip of the forefingers of the dominant hand to hold the syringe.
   d. Use the thumb and forefinger of the nondominant hand to apply outward traction to the skin around the injection site.
   e. Insert the needle against the skin, with the bevel up and at a 5- to 15-degree angle; the needle should be visible under the skin.
   f. Release the skin, and use the thumb and forefinger of the nondominant hand to stabilize the barrel of the syringe.
   g. Move the dominant hand up on the barrel to the plunger.

   Stretching the skin facilitates the needle entering the dermis rather than underlying tissue. Following this procedure promotes accessibility of supplies, prevents the spread of microorganisms, and promotes patient safety and quality care. The needle and syringe angle promotes medication administration into the dermis rather than inadvertent administration into other tissue and avoids possible medication errors. Stabilization of the syringe minimizes patient discomfort.

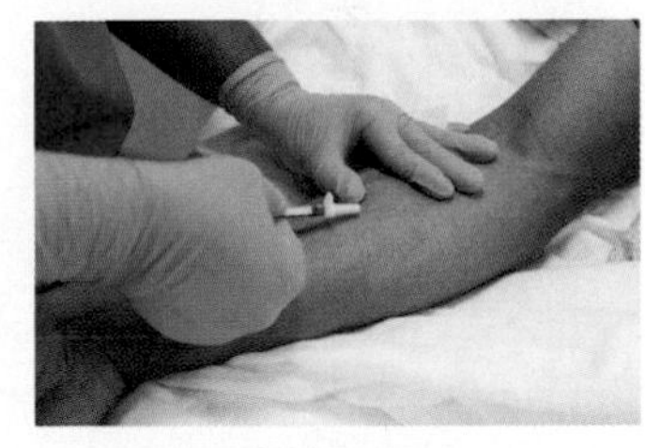

STEP 7e

8. Administer the medication by slowly depressing the plunger. Observe the resulting bubble formation; a wheal should appear at the injection site when the medication has been properly injected into the dermis.
   Using this technique ensures intradermal placement; resistance indicates dermal administration. Injecting the medication slowly minimizes patient discomfort and tissue damage. A bubble or wheal indicates dermal administration has occurred.
9. Perform the following steps in quick succession.
   a. Withdraw the needle and syringe at the same angle as that of insertion, using the dominant hand.
   b. Activate the needle safety protection device with the dominant hand.
   c. Use the nondominant hand, apply gauze gently to the site. Do *not* massage it.
   Following this procedure minimizes discomfort and tissue damage. Massage can damage tissue by pushing the medication into surrounding tissues and may cause the medication to be absorbed faster than intended. The needle safety device protects caregivers from injury.
10. Follow procedure steps 14 and 15 in the Injections: Subcutaneous section.

Follow postprocedure steps I through VI.

POSTPROCEDURE

I. Return the bed to its lowest position, raise the top side rails, and verify that the call light is within reach for the patient.
Precautions are taken to maintain patient safety. Top side rails aid in positioning and turning. Raising four side rails is considered a restraint.

II. Assess for additional patient needs and state the time of your expected return.
Meeting patient needs and offering self promote patient satisfaction and build trust.

III. Properly dispose of PPE.
Gloves, gowns, and masks must be appropriately discarded to prevent the spread of microorganisms.

IV. Clean equipment if it was in contact with the patient; see specific manufacturer instructions.
Disinfection eliminates most microorganisms from inanimate objects.

V. Perform hand hygiene.
Frequent hand hygiene prevents the spread of infection.

VI. Document immediately after medication administration. Include the medication, dose, route, date, time, assessment, and the patient's response to the medication in the documentation.
Accurate documentation is essential to communicate medications administered and to provide legal evidence of care. Avoid possible medication errors by adhering to the Six Rights of Medication Administration.

SKILL 35-6 Administering Intravenous Medications and Solutions

PURPOSE

- The administration of intravenous medications (IV) and solutions must be done appropriately and safely and should follow the Six Rights of Medication Administration:
  - The right medication
  - The right dose
  - The right time
  - The right route
  - The right patient
  - The right documentation
- Peripheral intravenous (IV) lines are used to:
  - Prevent infections.
  - Provide fluids.
  - Administer medications.
  - Replace electrolytes.
  - Promote comfort.
  - Provide nutrition.
  - Maintain emergency access for medications.

RESOURCES

- 3- to10-mL prefilled saline flush
- Antiseptic or alcohol swabs
- IV solution in accordance with the primary care provider (PCP) order
- Infusion-set tubing, primary or secondary, appropriate for the pump; needle or blunt cannula if applicable
- Clean gloves
- IV pole and pump
- Personal protective equipment (PPE), as required

COLLABORATION AND DELEGATION

- Maintaining a peripheral IV line, including changing tubing or solutions, may not be delegated to unlicensed assistive personnel (UAP).
- UAP may observe a peripheral IV site and running infusions during other procedures and should report the following to the nurse:
  - Burning, redness, pain, coolness, leaking, or swelling at the peripheral IV site
  - Patient concerns or complaints
  - Low volume in any IV bag
  - Alarms being produced by IV equipment
  - Changes in vital signs
- Many facilities have an IV therapy team that maintains IV sites. For the comfort and safety of the patient, nurses should coordinate with this team in accordance with facility policy and procedure and their own skill level.

SPECIAL CIRCUMSTANCES

1. **Assess:** Is the IV solution discolored, leaking, or expired?
   Intervention: Discard the IV solution, and obtain a new solution; document according to facility policy and procedure.
2. **Assess:** Is the IV solution in a bottle instead of a bag?
   Intervention: Clean the port on the bottle with an antiseptic swab, and insert a spike into the port on the bottle.
3. **Assess:** Was the tubing spike touched by anything other than the clean port of an IV bottle?
   Intervention: Discard the spike, and restart with a new one.
4. **Assess:** What should be done if an IV solution will not infuse?
   Intervention: Check the tubing, and assess the IV site.

PREPROCEDURE

I. Check PCP orders and the patient care plan.
Knowledge of patient-specific orders is critical for safe patient care.

II. Gather supplies and equipment.
Preparing for the patient encounter saves time and promotes patient trust.

III. Perform hand hygiene.
Frequent hand hygiene prevents the spread of microorganisms.

IV. Maintain standard precautions.
Use of the correct personal protective equipment (PPE) is required whenever contact with bodily fluids is possible, to reduce the transfer of pathogens.

V. Introduce yourself.
Initial communication establishes the role of the nurse and begins a professional relationship.

VI. Provide for patient privacy.
It is important to maintain patient dignity.

VII. Identify the patient by using two identifiers.
Identifying a patient involves scanning barcodes or comparing the patient's stated name and birthdate to information on the patient's wristband or health record. The correct person must receive the correct treatment.

VIII. Explain the procedure to the patient.
The nurse has a responsibility to inform a patient before initiating care. Information may ease patient anxiety and facilitate cooperation.

PROCEDURE

IV Piggyback Medication, or Intermittent Infusion

Follow preprocedure steps I through VIII.

1. Follow instructions in the Nursing Care Guideline: Six Rights of Medication Administration box. Prepare medications in a No Interruption Zone according to facility policy.
Avoid possible medication errors by adhering to the Six Rights of Medication Administration and by checking the medication with the MAR three times.
2. Obtain all medication for the assigned time before entering the patient's room.
Promote patient rest through minimal interruptions.
3. Perform hand hygiene.
Frequent hand hygiene prevents the spread of microorganisms.
4. Verify medication, dosage, and solution compatibility with any IVs already infusing.
Verification of compatibility is critical to reduce medication errors and promote patient safety.
5. Obtain the prescribed IV medication or solution bag. Medication should be prepared by the pharmacy.
The Joint Commission's Standard MM.4.20, EP 1, states: "When an on-site, licensed pharmacy is available, only the pharmacy compounds or admixes all sterile medications, IV admixtures, or other drugs except in emergencies or when not feasible."
6. Check the IV medication or solution bag against the MAR a second time. Verify that the correct medication and dosage have been obtained.
This approach avoids possible medication errors by adhering to the Six Rights of Medication Administration and by checking the medication with the MAR three times.
7. Connect the tubing to the IV solution.
   a. Open the tubing package, slide a roller clamp 2 inches below the drip chamber, and roll the clamp closed.
   b. Remove the sterile protections. Pull or snap off the cover from the port on the bag, and slide off the cover from the spike on the tubing.
   c. Use sterile technique to insert the spike into the port with a twisting motion. Ensure that it is fully inserted.

   Using a roller clamp ensures the accuracy of drip regulation and prevents wasting of solution during preparation. Maintain sterility while preparing the port and spike to prevent the spread of microorganisms.

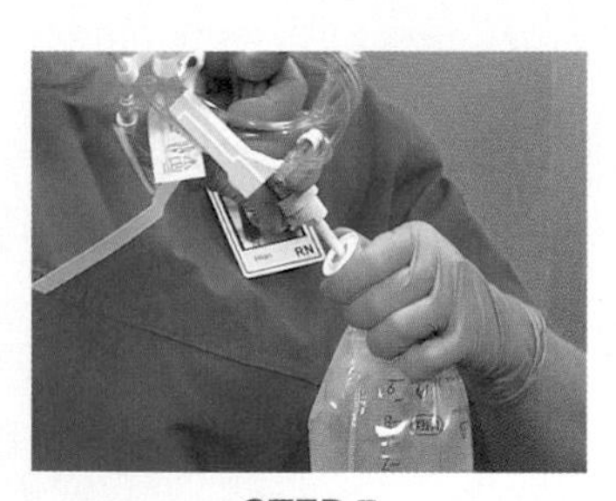

STEP 7

8. Squeeze the drip chamber, and then fill it one-third to half-full with the IV solution.
Squeezing removes air from the tubing and creates suction.
9. Prime or fill the tubing with solution.
   a. Remove the cap on the end of the tubing if necessary; do *not* discard the cap, and keep it sterile. Place the end of the tubing over the sink; do *not* touch the sink.
   b. Slowly open the clamp.
   c. Allow the solution to run through the tubing. Hold the tubing upside down, and tap the ports to release the air and fill the ports.
   d. Close the clamp when the tubing is full.
   e. Replace the cap on the tubing.

   Maintain sterility and prevent contamination. Proper preparation of the tubing and ports prevents air from entering the tubing and prevents loss of solution.

10. Inspect the tubing for air. If air is present, tap the tubing to move the air up.
    Remove air from the tubing to prevent adverse events and complications.
11. If a saline lock is being used, clean the injection port with an alcohol swab and connect the tubing to the port by screwing the tubing into the port or using a needleless cannula, depending on the type of equipment (see Chapter 39, Nursing Care Guideline: Converting an Intravenous Line: Continuous to Intermittent to Continuous box).
12. Program the IV pump with the correct mL/hr for the infusion, following the manufacturer's instructions.
    Use the correct infusion volume and time to prevent adverse events and medical errors.
13. Ensure that the tubing and solution is labeled in accordance with facility policies and procedures.
    Proper labeling of solutions prevents adverse events and medical errors.
14. If using bar coding, scan the IV medication or solution bag and the patient identification. Enter pertinent information. Recheck the label on the IV medication or solution bag with the MAR a third time.
    Avoid possible medication errors by adhering to the Six Rights of Medication Administration and by checking the medication with the MAR three times.
15. If a continuous infusion is already in place, connect the tubing to a port above the pump. Ensure that the secondary medication and its IV solution are compatible with the primary IV solution.
    a. Wipe the port with an alcohol swab.
    b. Connect the tubing by screwing it into the port or using a needleless cannula, depending on the equipment type.
    c. Program the pump following the manufacturer's instructions.
    d. Verify that the tubing and solution are labeled according to facility policy and procedure.

    Knowledge of medication interactions is critical for safe patient care. Proper antiseptic procedures should be used to prevent the spread of microorganisms and prevent infection. Proper labeling of samples prevents adverse events and medical errors.
16. When the infusion is complete, disconnect the tubing in accordance with the type of infusion.
    a. If using a saline lock, see Chapter 39, Nursing Care Guideline: Flushing an IV box.
    b. If using a continuous infusion, ensure that the solution containing medication is empty, stop the pump (follow the manufacturer's instructions), and clamp the tubing. The tubing may be left in place. Reset the pump for the maintenance IV infusion solution. Some pumps will automatically revert to the primary IV solutions when the piggybacked solution is completed.

    Discontinuing the infusion at the appropriate time prevents adverse events and medication errors. Leaving the tubing in place reduces the spread of microorganisms by keeping the system closed.

Follow postprocedure steps I through VI.

IV Push or IV Bolus

Follow preprocedure steps I through VIII.

1. Follow procedure steps 1 through 6 in the IV Piggyback Medication or Intermittent IV section.
2. If using bar coding, scan the medication and the patient identification. Enter pertinent information. Recheck the label on the medication with the MAR a third time before returning the medication to its storage place *or* before opening the package at the bedside.
   Avoid possible medication errors by adhering to the Six Rights of Medication Administration and by checking the medication with the MAR three times.

3. If using a saline lock:
   a. Use an alcohol swab to clean the injection port of the saline lock.
   b. Flush the IV line (see Chapter 39, Nursing Care Guideline: Flushing an IV box).
   c. Attach the syringe by screwing it into the port or using a needleless cannula depending on the equipment available.
   d. Inject the medication, adhering to safe medication guidelines (see the Nursing Care Guideline: Six Rights of Medication Administration box).
   e. Flush the IV line (see Chapter 39, Nursing Care Guideline: Flushing an IV box).

   Injection rates for IV medication given via IV push vary; knowledge of safe guidelines is essential for patient safety.
4. If using a continuous infusion:
   a. Place the pump on hold.
   b. Use an alcohol wipe to clean the injection port that is closest to the saline lock.
   c. Flush the IV line (see Chapter 39, Nursing Care Guideline: Flushing an Intravenous Line).
   d. Attach the medication syringe by screwing it into the port or using a needleless cannula depending on the equipment available.
   e. Inject the medication, adhering to safe medication guidelines (see the Nursing Care Guideline: Six Rights of Medication Administration box).
   f. Flush the IV line (see Chapter 39, Nursing Care Guideline: Flushing an Intravenous Line box).
   g. Restart the infusion pump.

   Stopping the pump and flushing with saline prevents adverse events and medication errors. Because saline is compatible with all medications, it is used to flush the line to prevent incompatible medications from mixing. Keeping the system closed reduces the risk of spreading microorganisms. Injections rates for IV medication given by IV push vary; knowledge of safe guidelines is essential for patient safety.

Follow postprocedure steps I through VI.

POSTPROCEDURE

I. Return the bed to its lowest position, raise the top side rails, and verify that the call light is within reach for the patient.
Precautions are taken to maintain patient safety. Top side rails aid in positioning and turning. Raising four side rails is considered a restraint.

II. Assess for additional patient needs and state the time of your expected return.
Meeting patient needs and offering self promote patient satisfaction and build trust.

III. Properly dispose of PPE.
Gloves, gowns, and masks must be appropriately discarded to prevent the spread of microorganisms.

IV. Clean equipment if it was in contact with the patient; see specific manufacturer instructions.
Disinfection eliminates most microorganisms from inanimate objects.

V. Perform hand hygiene.
Frequent hand hygiene prevents the spread of infection.

VI. Document immediately after medication administration. Include the medication, dose, route, date, time, assessment, and the patient's response to the medication in the documentation.
Accurate documentation is essential to communicate medications administered and to provide legal evidence of care. Avoid possible medication errors by adhering to the Six Rights of Medication Administration.

SUMMARY OF LEARNING OUTCOMES

LO 35.1 *Recall how government, facility, and professional regulations affect medication administration by nurses:* Medication production, distribution, prescription, and administration are regulated by law. Controlled substances have additional regulations governing their use.

LO 35.2 *Explain the physiologic outcomes of medication actions:* A medication's action results from chemical interactions between the medication and the cells of the body, producing a physiologic response. Medication response can be altered by absorption, distribution, metabolism, or excretion of the drug.

LO 35.3 *Identify differences between prescription and nonprescription medications:* Medications that are obtained with a prescription are used to treat many illnesses and symptoms. Many patients use alternative and over-the-counter therapies to self-treat health conditions. To prevent potential interactions with prescribed medications, nurses need to assess for and identify all therapies used by the patient.

LO 35.4 *Summarize common medication forms and routes:* Medications come in many forms, including tablets, capsules, powders, solutions, inhalants, ointments, lotions, and suppositories. Routes of medication administration include oral, topical, transdermal, inhalation, and parenteral, which includes intramuscular, subcutaneous, intradermal, and intravenous routes.

LO 35.5 *Describe measures for administering medications safely:* To ensure patient safety, the nurse must follow the Six Rights (i.e., the right drug in the right dose at the right time by the right route to the right patient with the right documentation). To follow the Six Rights, the nurse needs to be able to interpret medication orders and calculate safe medication dosages.

LO 35.6 *Discuss assessments necessary for safe medication administration:* The nurse is responsible for assessing subjective and objective data and following established administration guidelines before administering medications.

LO 35.7 *Choose nursing diagnoses related to safe medication administration*: The nurse bases nursing diagnoses for each patient on individual data collected during assessment.

LO 35.8 *Determine individual patient goals:* Patient goals are based on the problem as stated in the nursing diagnosis. Patient goals are measurable.

LO 35.9 *Implement guidelines and essential nursing actions for safely administering medications:* Nursing knowledge of safe medication administration includes applying the Six Rights of Medication Administration using proper administration techniques and conducting ongoing evaluation of the nursing care plan.

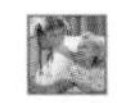
Answers to critical-thinking questions are available at *http://evolve.elsevier.com/YoostCrawford/fundamentals/.*

REVIEW QUESTIONS

1. The nurse is teaching a patient about how to take a sublingual nitroglycerin tablet. Which statement by the patient best demonstrates understanding of the teaching?
   a. "I will hold the tablet next to my skin."
   b. "I will put the tablet inside my cheek."
   c. "I will put the tablet under my tongue."
   d. "I will place the tablet in the lower lid of my eye."
2. The nurse is caring for a critically ill patient. What are the contraindications for administering medications by the oral route for this patient? *(Select all that apply.)*
   a. Vomiting
   b. Unconsciousness
   c. Fractured leg
   d. Penicillin allergy
   e. Family visitor
   f. Diarrhea
3. The nurse is about to administer a new medication to a patient. Which action best demonstrates awareness of safe, proficient nursing practice?
   a. Identify the patient by comparing her name and birth date to the medical administraton record (MAR).
   b. Determine whether the medication and dose are appropriate for the patient.
   c. Make sure the medication is in the medication cart.
   d. Check the accuracy of the dose with another nurse.

4. A patient has been using herbal medication as part of her daily routine. Which actions should the nurse take? *(Select all that apply.)*
   a. Document the herbs as part of the medication history.
   b. Recommend a reputable company from which to buy herbs.
   c. Allow the patient to self-administer the herbs with her morning medications.
   d. Inform the health care provider of the findings.
   e. Identify possible adverse effects of the herbal medications.
5. A nurse must give 1 g of Keflex, PO, q 6 hr × 3 days. The supply on hand is 500 mg/capsule. How many capsules should the nurse administer at each dose?
6. The health care provider prescribes a medication that is administered transdermally. The nurse understands what feature of the transdermal route?
   a. It is inhaled into the respiratory tract.
   b. It is dissolved inside the cheek.
   c. It is absorbed through the skin.
   d. It is inserted into the vaginal cavity.
7. The nurse is caring for a patient who is unable to hold a cup or spoon. How should the nurse administer oral medications to the patient?
   a. Crush the pills and mix them in pudding before administering.
   b. Ask the pharmacist to change all of the medications to a liquid form.
   c. Use a small paper cup to put the pills into the patient's mouth.
   d. Place the pills on the table and have the patient take the pills by hand.
8. What should the nurse do first when preparing to administer medications to a patient?
   a. Check the medication expiration date.
   b. Check the MAR.
   c. Call the pharmacy for administration instructions.
   d. Check the patient's name band.
9. The nurse is preparing a plan of care for a patient. What is the most appropriate goal for a patient related to medications?
   a. The patient will administer all medications correctly by discharge.
   b. The patient will be taught common side effects of prescribed medications.
   c. The patient will have a good understanding of prescribed medications.
   d. The patient will have all medications administered by staff as prescribed.
10. The nurse reviews a physician's order and finds that the medication amount is greater than the standard dose. What should the nurse do?
   a. Give the standard dose rather than the one that is ordered.
   b. Inform the nursing supervisor.
   c. Call the physician to discuss the order.
   d. Give the drug as ordered by the physician.

ⓔ Answers and rationales to review questions are available at *http://evolve.elsevier.com/YoostCrawford/fundamentals/*.

REFERENCES

American Diabetes Association: Insulin administration position statement. *Diabetes Care,* 27(S1):S106-S109, 2004.

American Nurses Association: *Nursing: Scope and standards of practice,* ed 2, Silver Spring, Md., 2010, Author.

Brown MR, Denman R, Platts D: Analgesic patches and defibrillators: A cautionary tale. *Europace,* 11(11):1552-1553, 2009.

Centers for Disease Control and Prevention (CDC): Injection safety 2014. Retrieved from *www.cdc.gov/injectionsafety/.*

Centers for Disease Control and Prevention (CDC): The one and only campaign, 2012. Retrieved from *http://oneandonlycampaign.org/.*

Crawford CL, Johnson JA: To aspirate or not to aspirate, that is the question: An integrative review of the evidence [PowerPoint]. Sigma Theta Tau International Nursing Research Congress, Vancouver, Canada, 2009.

Cronenwett L, Sherwood G, Barnsteiner J, et al: Quality and safety education for nurses. *Nurs Outlook,* 55(3):122-131, 2007.

Forni A, Chu HT, Fanikos J: Technology utilization to prevent medication errors. *Curr Drug Safety,* 5(1):13-18, 2010.

George EL, Henneman EA, Tasota FJ: Nursing implications for prevention of adverse drug events in the intensive care unit. *Crit Care Med,* 38(6):S136-S144, 2010.

Institute for Safe Medication Practices (ISMP): *List of error-prone abbreviations, symbols, and dose designations,* Horsham, Pa., 2010, Author.

Institute of Medicine (IOM): *Preventing medication errors: Quality chasm series,* Washington, D.C., 2006, Author.

Malkin B: Are techniques used for intramuscular injection based on research evidence? *Nurs Times,* 104(50/51):48-51, 2008.

Mayo Foundation for Medical Education and Research: Ipratropium (inhalation route), 2014. Retrieved from *www.mayoclinic.org/drugs-supplements/ipratropium-inhalation-route/description/drg-20067557.*

National Center for Complementary and Alternative Medicine (NCCAM): *Herbs at a glance*. Bethesda, Md., National Institutes of Health, 2009.

National Coordinating Council for Medication Error Reporting and Prevention (NCCMERP): *About medication errors*, Rockville, Md., U.S. Pharmacopeia, 2011.

Nicoll LH, Hesby A: Intramuscular injection: An integrative research review and guideline for evidence-based practice. *Appl Nurs Res*, 16(2):149-162, 2002.

Poon EG, Keohane CA, Yoon CS, et al: Effect of bar-code technology on the safety of medication administration. *N Engl J Med*, 362:1698-1707, 2010.

U.S. Food and Drug Administration: *MedWatch*, 2014. Retrieved from *www.fda.gov/safety/medwatch/default.htm.*

World Health Organization: WHO best practices for injection and related procedures toolkit, Geneva, Switzerland, 2010, WHO Document Production Services.

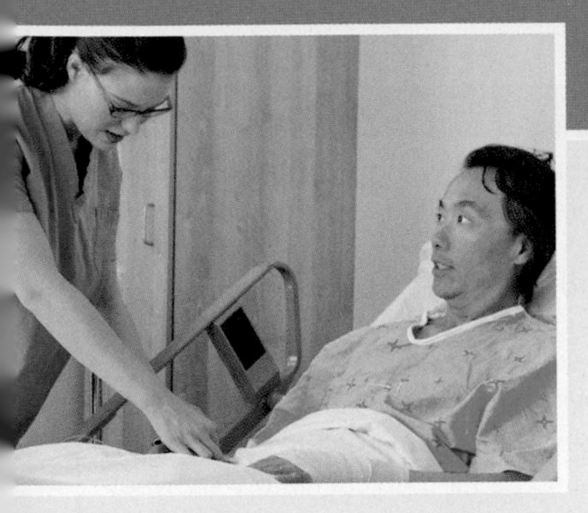

CHAPTER 36

Pain Management

EVOLVE WEBSITE

http://evolve.elsevier.com/YoostCrawford/fundamentals/

- Additional Evolve-Only Review Questions With Answers
- Answers and Rationales for Text Review Questions
- Answers to Critical-Thinking Questions
- Case Study With Questions
- Conceptual Care Map Creator
- Glossary

LEARNING OUTCOMES

Comprehension of this chapter's content will provide students with the ability to:

LO 36.1 Define pain.
LO 36.2 Describe the role of the nurse in pain management.
LO 36.3 Explain the physiology of pain and its perception.
LO 36.4 Articulate factors that influence pain perception and response.
LO 36.5 Determine individual physiologic, behavioral, and psychosocial responses to pain during patient assessment.
LO 36.6 Identify nursing diagnoses for patients experiencing pain.
LO 36.7 Generate nursing care goals and outcome criteria for patients experiencing pain.
LO 36.8 Plan pain management care that includes implementation and evaluation of pharmacologic and nonpharmacologic interventions for pain.

KEY TERMS

A-delta fibers, p. 887
acute pain, p. 890
analgesic, p. 887
C fibers, p. 887
chronic pain, p. 890
coanalgesic medications, p. 903
drug tolerance, p. 903
multimodal analgesia, p. 899
nerve block, p. 903
neuropathic pain, p. 890
neurotransmitters, p. 887
nociceptive pain, p. 890
nociceptors, p. 887
nonopioid analgesics, p. 901
nonsteroidal anti-inflammatory drugs, p. 901
opioid analgesics, p. 901
pain threshold, p. 889
pain tolerance, p. 889
patient-controlled analgesia, p. 901
phantom pain, p. 890
preemptive analgesia, p. 901
psychogenic pain, p. 891
radiating pain, p. 890
referred pain, p. 890
somatic pain, p. 890
visceral pain, p. 890

CASE STUDY

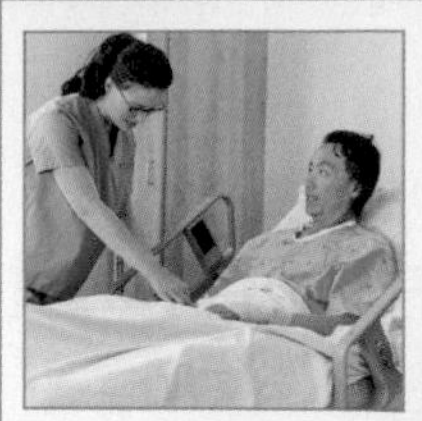

Mr. Charles is a 45-year-old man who was admitted to the emergency department with a fracture of his left femur. He was riding a four-wheeler downhill when it overturned and pinned his left leg, causing edema and pain with movement.

On admission, Mr. Charles's vital signs are T 37.5°C (99.6°F), P 100 and regular, R 24 and unlabored, BP 150/88, with a pulse oximetry reading of 94% on 4 L of oxygen by nasal cannula. His left leg skin color is pale and cool to touch, with a large ecchymotic area of the mid-thigh and decreased sensation in the left foot. Pulses distal to the fracture are weak. Capillary refill is 4 seconds in the left foot. Mr. Charles complains of sharp, stabbing pain on movement of the left leg, with a pain rating of 10 of 10. He is grimacing and visibly restless. He states, "My leg is killing me. Please give me something for pain." His code status is full. He is allergic to aspirin and has a medical history of hypertension. A left leg x-ray shows a closed, displaced fracture of the mid-femur. Mr. Charles is taken to surgery for internal fixation to reduce and immobilize the fracture.

Postoperative treatments are as follows:

- Vital signs with neurovascular checks of the left leg every 15 minutes for the first hour, then hourly for 4 hours, and then q 4 hr
- Keep left leg elevated
- Ice packs to left leg as needed for relief of pain or swelling PRN
- Up in chair and bathroom privileges with assistance

Medication orders are as follows:

- Morphine patient-controlled analgesia (PCA) per anesthesia dose for 24 hours
- Lactated Ringer intravenous (IV) solution at 125 mL/hr
- Oxycodone/acetaminophen (Percocet) 10/325 mg, one or two tablets q 4 hr PRN for pain
- Atenolol (Tenormin) 50 mg PO every morning
- Diphenhydramine (Benadryl) 10 mg intravenously q 4 hr PRN
- Senna (Senokot) two tablets PO every morning

Refer back to this case study to answer the critical-thinking questions throughout the chapter.

Pain is the most common reason people seek health care. Acute or chronic pain from any cause affects more individuals than do diabetes mellitus, cancer, and cardiac disease combined, and it remains undertreated. The Institute of Medicine (2011), in its report *Relieving Pain in America*, estimates that approximately 100 million adults in the United States suffer from chronic pain. The World Health Organization (WHO, 2009) estimates that 5 billion people worldwide suffer from pain due to insufficient treatment or no treatment.

THE CONCEPT OF PAIN LO 36.1

Pain has physical and emotional aspects. It is what the person feels and how the person perceives how it feels. Margo McCaffery, a pain management nurse expert, developed a definition of pain in 1968 that has served as a practical guide for health care providers for many years. McCaffery maintains that pain is whatever the person with the pain says it is and that it exists whenever the person says it does, leaving pain *open to interpretation* (Pasero and McCaffery, 2011).

In 1979, the International Association for the Study of Pain (2014) defined pain as an "unpleasant sensory and emotional experience associated with actual or potential tissue damage or described in terms of such damage." This is the most widely used definition today. Pain prevents injury in some cases (such as when a person instantly withdraws a hand after touching a hot surface) and results from injury in other cases (such as the pain of a fractured hip from a fall). Long-term disability is most commonly the result of chronic pain (Nicholson and Passik, 2007). As the population ages, the number of people who need pain management for back disorders, degenerative joint diseases, rheumatologic conditions, visceral diseases, and cancer is expected to rise.

Pain is the most subjective of all symptoms that patients experience, and it is felt differently by each individual. Cognitive, affective, behavioral, and sensory factors can influence pain. An alert, oriented patient knows what pain is, can verbalize what it is, knows what it feels like, and can perform behaviors to prevent or alleviate it. Unrelieved pain can result from the health care professional's failure to assess pain, failure to accept a patient's reported pain, and failure to initiate pain relief (Pasero and McCaffery, 2011). Nurses must be aware of their own attitudes and expectations regarding pain. Awareness allows the nurse to focus on the patient's experience of reported pain. All patients have a right to effective management of pain.

NURSING AND PAIN MANAGEMENT LO 36.2

The importance of assessing pain has resulted in pain becoming known as the *fifth vital sign*. Connecting pain assessment to routine vital sign assessment and documentation makes it a routine standard of care for every patient. In 1999, The Joint Commission developed a standard of pain management for the care of hospitalized patients (Berry and Dahl, 2000). This standard resulted from the undertreatment of pain. Since 2001, The Joint Commission has required every patient to be assessed and treated for pain. Pain must be assessed on a regular basis, along with temperature, pulse, respiration, and blood pressure. Nurses assess pain using various pain assessment tools or strategies, and they document the patient's response when vital signs are taken and before and after pain control interventions are performed or **analgesic** (pain-reducing) medication is administered.

Pain management and pain relief are essential elements of nursing practice. In addition to assessing pain, the nurse monitors pain management, evaluates the level of pain relief, advocates for the patient, and educates the patient about treatment options for pain management. In most health care settings, only advanced practice nurses and physicians can prescribe medications for pain relief. To understand how patients perceive pain, the nurse must understand its physiology.

NORMAL STRUCTURE AND FUNCTION LO 36.3

The nature of pain is complex and poorly understood. It may be a protective mechanism, a warning signal, an unmet need, or a malfunction of the nervous system secondary to a disease process. It is a motor, sensory, and emotional response to a subjective feeling. It may be a symptom of a problem or disease, but it is also a disease entity that can be treated. Pain may arise from many factors: thermal or heat injury, mechanical injury (such as a fracture), chemical injury (as the result of inhalation), or ischemic pain from lack of oxygen in tissues.

The peripheral and central nervous systems are involved in processing painful stimuli. Various structures and mechanisms in the nervous system are part of pain transmission, including nociceptors. **Nociceptors** are the free endings of afferent nerve fibers, which are sensory neurons that are sensitive to noxious thermal, mechanical, or chemical stimuli. These pain receptors are distributed throughout the body, although the highest density is found in the skin, making the skin extremely sensitive to pain. The joints, tissues, and organs have nociceptors, although the internal organs have the lowest density of receptors that respond only to painful stimuli.

NOCICEPTION

Nociception is the process by which the sensation of tissue injury is conducted from the peripheral to the central nervous system (Figure 36-1). The four steps in this process: are transduction, transmission, modulation, and perception.

Transduction

At the site of tissue injury, nociceptors detect pain stimuli and convert (transduce) this electrochemical response into an electrical impulse (signal). This process is called *transduction.* Tissue injury initiates the release of **neurotransmitters**, chemicals that transmit signals across synapses from one neuron to another. This release of neurotransmitters is part of the inflammatory response. Release of bradykinin, substance P, histamine, serotonin, cytokines, calcium ions, potassium ions, sodium ions, and prostaglandins further activates pain receptors and amplifies the inflammatory response (Table 36-1). The inflammatory process may be the most significant cause of generalized pain.

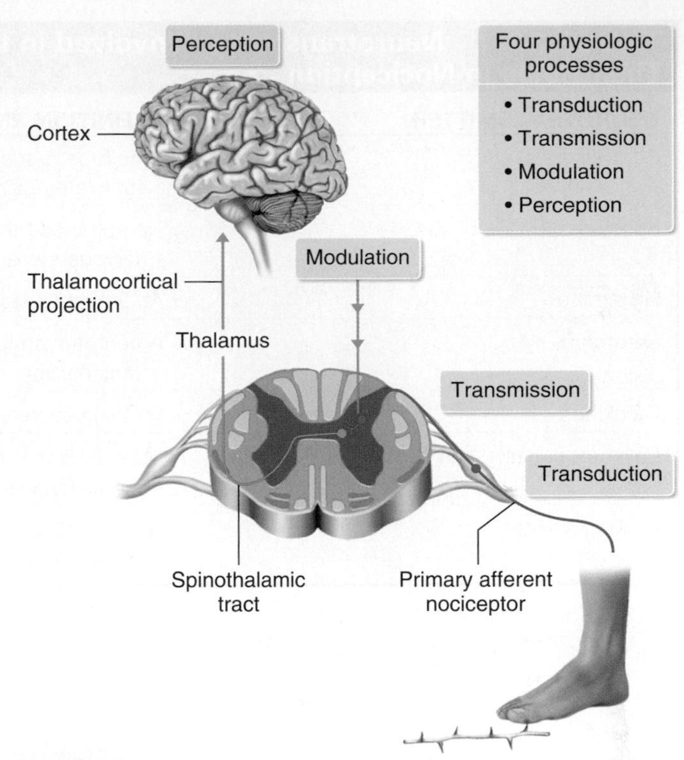

FIGURE 36-1 Four physiologic processes conduct pain from injured tissue to the peripheral and central nervous systems.

Transmission

After transduction takes place, the action potential, or electrical signal, is transmitted through an afferent nerve to the spinal cord and brain. This process is called *transmission.* Substance P, which transmits the pain impulses in nerve fibers, is one of the most important neurotransmitters in the transmission process.

Signals from the nociceptors travel along two types of afferent (sensory) nerve fibers: **A-delta fibers,** which are large-diameter, myelinated fibers with rapid conduction of signals that are translated as sharp, acute pain, and **C fibers,** which are smaller, unmyelinated fibers with slow conduction of signals that are translated as diffuse, dull, and longer-lasting pain. The signals are transmitted by the spinothalamic pain transmission route (Figure 36-2). A-delta and C fibers in the peripheral tissues carry impulses to the dorsal root ganglia and then on to the spinal dorsal horn, the spinothalamic tract, the brainstem, the thalamus, and the cerebral cortex.

TABLE 36-1 Neurotransmitters Involved in the Inflammatory Response: Their Roles in Nociception

NEUROTRANSMITTER	DEFINITION AND FUNCTION
Bradykinin	A peptide produced in the blood that mediates the inflammatory response and stimulates pain receptors
Substance P	Neuropeptide that transports pain impulses from the periphery to the central nervous system
Histamine	An amine released by immune cells in response to inflammation
Serotonin	A neurotransmitter released from the brainstem and dorsal horn that inhibits pain transmission
Cytokines	Proteins secreted by immune system cells that control inflammation
Calcium, sodium, and potassium ions	Molecules that activate nerve endings (synapses), which respond to painful stimuli by changing ionic movement into and out of nerve cells
Prostaglandins	Hormone-like compounds derived from fatty acids that are thought to increase sensitivity to pain by stimulating pain receptors on neurons

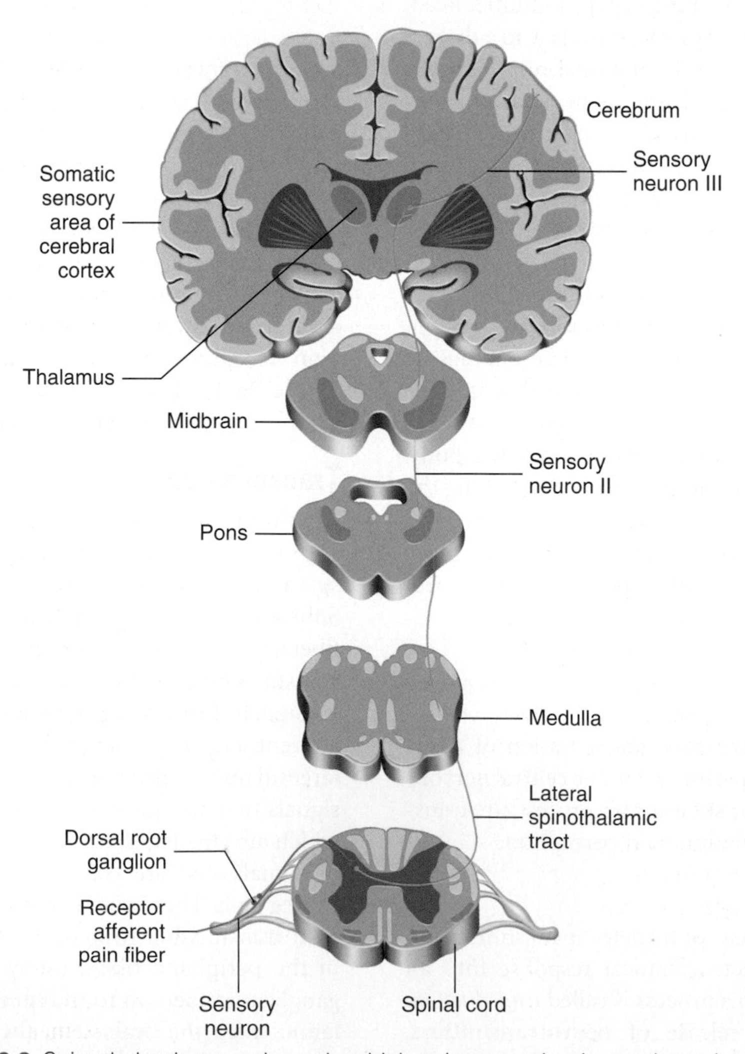

FIGURE 36-2 Spinothalamic tract through which pain sensation is conducted to the brain.

In addition to the signals traveling along the sensory transmission pathways, motor reflexes, when intact, are initiated as a protective mechanism that causes withdrawal from a pain source, as occurs when a person touches a hot item. The action potential, or electrical impulse, is propagated along nerve fibers, causing contraction of the muscle and withdrawal from the heat source (Pasero and McCaffery, 2011).

Perception

Perception (recognition) of pain occurs when the brain translates the afferent nerve signals as pain. The thalamus sends the impulse to the somatosensory cortex, which perceives physical sensations about the location, intensity, and quality of pain; to the limbic system, which controls emotional reactions to stimuli; and to the frontal cortex of the brain, which is involved in thought and reason. The stimulation of these areas allows a person to perceive pain.

The **pain threshold** is the lowest intensity at which the brain recognizes the stimulus as pain. This threshold varies from person to person. For instance, one person may report pain from a fracture injury as being severe, whereas another person may report pain from the same type of fracture injury as being moderate. **Pain tolerance** is the intensity or duration of pain that a patient is able or willing to endure. Tolerance varies from person to person and from one injury to another. For example, one patient in early labor may request pain medication as soon as possible because she has a low tolerance for pain. Another patient may not request pain medication until she is in active labor because she has a high tolerance for pain. People who have a decreased or lack the ability to sense pain, such as the elderly or diabetics with neuropathy, are at risk for tissue injury because tissue damage may occur before the individual is aware of any problems.

Modulation

Once pain is recognized, the brain can change the perception of it by sending inhibitory input to the spinal cord to impede the transmission through a process called *modulation.* The brainstem activates descending nerve fibers to send the signal back to the spinal cord. This triggers the release of natural analgesic neurotransmitters called *endogenous opioids* (i.e., enkephalins, beta-endorphins, dynorphins). Enkephalins influence the perception of pain and the associated emotional aspects. Beta-endorphins act on the central and peripheral nervous systems to reduce pain. Dynorphins are modulators of pain that may stimulate pain or reduce it, depending on which receptors are activated. These three types of neurotransmitters inhibit the transmission of pain impulses and the release of substance P by binding to opiate receptor sites in the central and peripheral nervous systems.

PAIN THEORIES

Although the physiology of pain is not totally understood, many researchers have worked to gain a clearer idea of how pain affects the human body. Three key theories have significantly influenced current nonpharmacologic and pharmacologic interventions in pain management.

Pattern Theory

As early as 1953, Willem Noordenbos proposed that when an injury occurs, a signal is carried along large-diameter nerve fibers (touch fibers) that may inhibit a signal carried by thin fibers (pain fibers). He thought that the difference between a large-diameter signal and a small-diameter signal determined whether a person felt pain. Patterns of stimulation of the nerve endings determined whether the brain interpreted the stimuli as pain (Todd and Kucharski, 2004). Noordenbos's pattern theory hinted at the physiology of pain that is now accepted science and provided a foundation for the gate control theory.

Gate Control Theory

Melzack and Wall (1965) proposed the gate control theory of pain to explain why thoughts and emotions influence pain perception. Tissue injury causes the release of bradykinin, histamine, potassium ions, sodium ions, calcium ions, prostaglandins, and serotonin. Movement of these substances in and out of the cell creates an action potential (electrical impulse). This action potential can travel along sensory nerve A-delta fibers and be translated by the brain as sharp pain, or it can travel along sensory nerve C fibers and be interpreted as chronic or persistent pain.

According to the theory, a gating mechanism exists in the dorsal horn of the spinal cord. The interplay of signals from different nerve fibers at this *gate* determines whether painful stimuli are stopped or go on to the brain. If unimpeded, impulses transmitted by activated A-delta fibers or C fibers enter the spinal cord through the gate and travel to the brain, where they are perceived as pain. If the impulses are stopped at the spinal cord gate by competing signals, they are not transmitted to the brain, and there is no perception of pain.

Endorphins and enkephalins produced in the body fight pain by binding to opioid receptors at synaptic nerve terminals. Receptor binding closes the gate, inhibiting signal transmission to the brain and decreasing or eliminating pain. Opioid medications, massage, non-painful stimuli, and topical analgesics stimulate various nerve fibers, which close the gate, inhibit impulse transmission to the brain, and reduce the recognition of C fiber signals, resulting in analgesia (Helms and Barone, 2008).

Neuromatrix Theory

More recently, Melzack (2001) introduced a pain theory suggesting that pain is a multidimensional experience controlled by a body-self neuromatrix. This contemporary pain theory seeks to address the distinctive experience of pain as it is perceived and regulated by each person. The neurometrix theory proposes that each person has a genetically controlled network of neurons that is unique and affected by

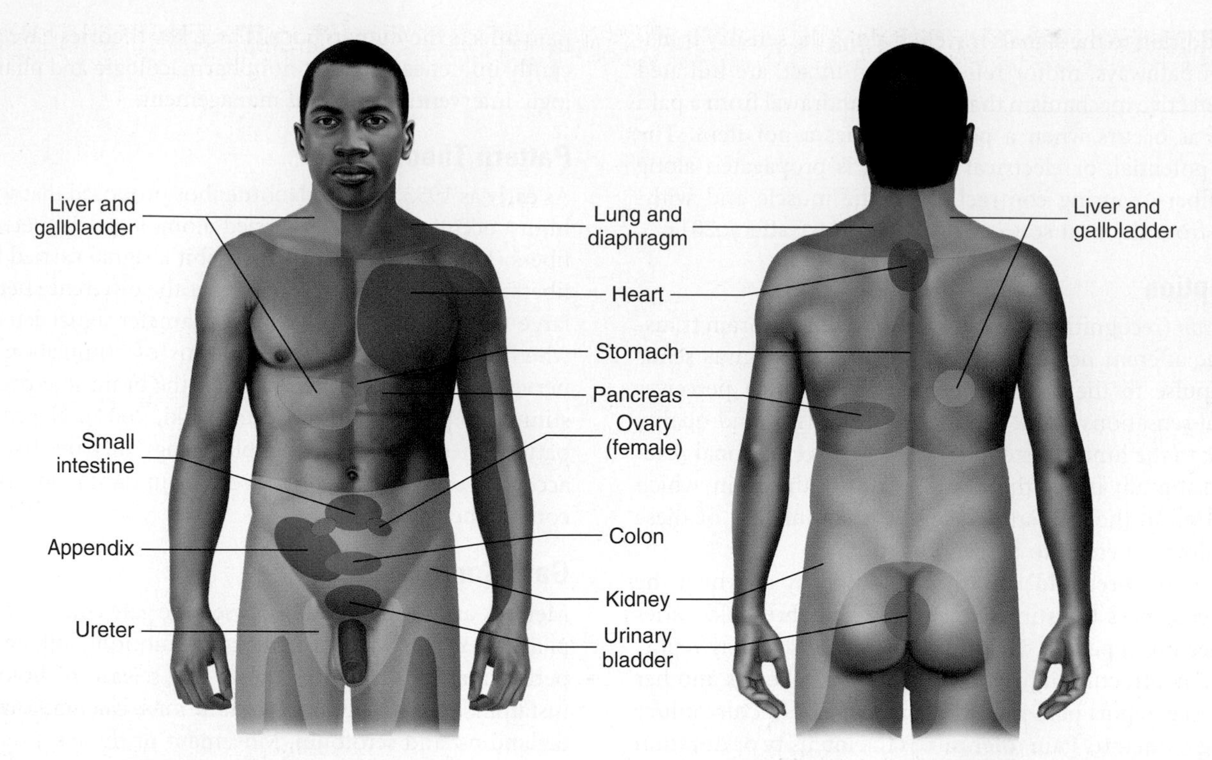

FIGURE 36-3 Pain may be referred from its site of origin to different areas of the body.

that person's physical, psychological, cognitive, and life experiences. This theory seeks to take into consideration additional factors in the pain experience other than the direct relationship between tissue injury and pain (Helms and Barone, 2008).

TYPES OF PAIN

Pain can be classified in many different ways. It can be classified by its cause: cancer pain or noncancer pain. It can be categorized by the underlying pathophysiology: nociceptive or physiologic pain, and neuropathic or nervous system pain (Pasero and McCaffery, 2011). Pain also can be classified by its duration. **Acute pain** is pain that lasts less than 6 months, and **chronic pain** persists longer than 6 months. Treatment for each type of pain is different, as is each patient's response to the various types of pain.

Nociceptive Pain

Nociceptive pain is the most common type of pain. This type of physiologic (physical) pain occurs when nociceptors are stimulated in response to trauma, inflammation, or tissue damage from surgery. Characteristically, nociceptive pain may be sharp, burning, aching, cramping, or stabbing. Nociceptive pain originates in visceral and somatic locations. **Visceral pain** arises from the organs of the body and occurs in conditions such as appendicitis, pancreatitis, inflammatory bowel disease, bladder distention, and cancer. **Somatic pain** results from injury to skin, muscles, bones, and joints. Somatic pain occurs in conditions such as sunburn, lacerations, fractures, sprains, arthritis, and bone cancer.

Two types of symptoms are related to pain: referred pain and radiating pain. **Referred pain** originates in one area but hurts in another area, such as pain from a myocardial infarction (i.e., heart attack) (Figure 36-3). The pain is caused by lack of oxygen to the heart muscle, but the pain may be felt in the jaw or down the left arm. **Radiating pain** extends from the source to an adjacent area of the body. For example, in gastroesophageal reflux, pain in the stomach radiates up the esophagus.

Neuropathic Pain

Neuropathic pain results from nerve injury, and the pain continues even after the painful stimuli are gone. Sometimes referred to as *pathologic pain,* neuropathic pain may stem from injury to nerves in the central or peripheral nervous system (Mitchell, 2010). It is usually chronic pain that may be continuous or episodic. Characteristically, neuropathic pain may be burning, aching, crushing, stabbing, shooting, tingling, or numbing.

Patients may have dysesthesia (unpleasant, abnormal sensation), allodynia (pain from noninjury stimuli), hyperalgesia (excessive sensitivity), or hyperpathia (greatly exaggerated pain reaction to stimuli). Sources of neuropathic pain include neuropathies, tumors, infection, and chemotherapy. Examples of disease processes that may invoke or involve secondary neuropathic pain are diabetes mellitus, cerebrovascular accident (such as brain attack or stroke), viral infections, carpal tunnel syndrome, and phantom limb pain. **Phantom pain** occurs when the brain continues to receive messages from the area of an amputation. Over time, the brain adapts to the loss

TABLE 36-2 Types of Pain

PAIN TYPE	DEFINITION	SOURCES OF PAIN
Acute	Pain that results from an acute injury, has a rapid onset and short duration, and subsides when the injury is healed	Trauma, surgery, labor, acute disease
Cancer (malignant)	Pain that stems from cancer or cancer treatment	Tumor pressing on a bone or nerve, organ obstruction, toxicity from chemotherapy
Noncancer	Acute pain that becomes chronic pain and may be prolonged and potentially life-threatening	Whiplash injury, low back pain, osteoarthritis, sickle cell disease, neuralgia
Chronic	Persistent pain that lasts longer than 6 months, may be episodic or continuous, and may lead to disability	Arthritis, fibromyalgia, neuropathy
Neuropathic	Episodic or continuous pain that results from a nerve injury and persists even without painful stimuli	Tumor, infection, toxicity from chemotherapy, neuropathy
Nociceptive	Physiologic pain that results from nociceptor stimulation in response to an injury or tissue damage	Surgery, inflammation, trauma
Visceral	Nociceptive or physiologic pain	Organs, such as heart, lungs, kidneys, gallbladder
Referred	Pain in an area other than the area causing the pain	Jaw and left arm pain with a myocardial infarction
Radiating	Pain that extends to other areas	Gastroesophageal reflux, extending to the thorax
Somatic	Nociceptive or physiologic pain	Bone, skin, joint, muscle
Phantom	Neuropathic or pathologic pain from loss of a body part	Amputated extremity
Psychogenic	Perceived pain without a physical cause	Headache, backache, stomachache
Breakthrough	Spike in pain when chronic pain already exists	Surgery, injury, fluctuation in pain associated with existing condition such as cancer

of the limb, and the pain stops. This adaption is called *plasticity* (Mitchell, 2010).

Psychogenic Pain

Pain that is perceived by an individual but has no physical cause is called **psychogenic pain**. It may be caused, increased, or prolonged by mental, emotional, or behavioral factors. Some patients may report headaches, back pain, or stomach pain that is psychogenic pain. Even though there is not a physical cause, the pain is treated through a variety of interventions to alleviate the patient's distress (WHO, 2007). Table 36-2 outlines the various types of pain.

ALTERED STRUCTURE AND FUNCTION LO 36.4

Pain is a complex collection of physical sensations and emotional responses that can be altered by many variables. Physiologic changes, age, gender, emotions, cognitive function, sociocultural factors, and the ability to communicate may influence the sensation of pain.

ALTERATIONS IN PAIN PATHWAYS

Damage and hypersensitivity anywhere along the pain pathway—in pain receptors, the spinal cord, or cerebral cortex—can alter a patient's perception of pain. Neurologic injuries that result in permanent damage to the spinal cord, such as paraplegia or quadriplegia, prevent a person from feeling pain in areas below the level at which the spinal cord was injured or severed. Neurologic damage resulting from disease processes such as peripheral neuropathy due to diabetes mellitus alters pain perception. Psychological dysfunction may result from or lead to altered pain perception.

PHYSIOLOGIC ALTERATIONS CAUSED BY PAIN

Acute injury or tissue damage triggers physiologic stress responses, which are attempts by the body to protect itself. These responses may have adverse effects for the patient if pain is left untreated. The sympathetic nervous system is stimulated first, and if the pain is not relieved, the parasympathetic nervous system is stimulated. Each body system has its specific response to pain (Pasero and McCaffery, 2011):

- *Endocrine system:* Pain triggers the release of excessive amounts of hormones, including cortisol, adrenocorticotropic hormone (ACTH), antidiuretic hormone (ADH), growth hormone, catecholamines, glucagon, insulin, and testosterone. The release of these hormones results in carbohydrate, protein, and fat catabolism (breakdown), and poor use of glucose, leading to hyperglycemia (high blood glucose levels).
- *Cardiovascular system:* Pain increases cardiac workload and oxygen demand. Decreased oxygen delivery to the cells leads to increases in the heart rate and force of contraction. Blood pressure increases, and increased workload may cause plaque formation, narrowing of the arteries, possible blood clot formation, and increased risk for myocardial infarction (heart attack). In situations of prolonged or unrelieved pain, blood pressure and pulse may decrease due to parasympathetic stimulation.
- *Respiratory system:* Pain reduces tidal volume (air exchange) and increases inspiratory and expiratory pressures. The respiratory rate increases and becomes irregular in an attempt to distribute more oxygen to the cells. Prolonged pain may cause a reluctance to breathe deeply, which limits thoracic expansion. If this continues, pneumonia and atelectasis may occur.
- *Musculoskeletal system:* Pain impairs muscle function and the capacity to perform activities of daily living (ADLs). The patient experiences muscle spasms, muscle tension, and fatigue. A withdrawal response is initiated by the patient's prolonged pain.
- *Genitourinary system:* Pain causes the release of ACTH, catecholamines, aldosterone, angiotensin II, cortisol, and prostaglandins. Blood pressure increases through activation of the renin-angiotensin system. Urine output decreases, and urinary retention increases. Fluid overload and hypokalemia may result.
- *Gastrointestinal system:* Pain decreases gastric emptying and motility, increases gastrointestinal secretions, and increases smooth muscle tone. Metabolism is slowed, resulting in indigestion from the slow movement of food in the gastrointestinal tract. Constipation may develop from decreased intestinal motility.
- *Immune system:* The inflammatory response is initiated by painful stimuli. Inflammatory mediators are released in an attempt to prevent further tissue injury, fight infection, and reduce pain. Some of the inflammatory mediators that are released may contribute to persistent pain.

FACTORS INFLUENCING PAIN

Differences in individual characteristics—age, gender, morphology, disabilities, culture, ethnicity, and religion—play a role in the behavioral reaction to pain and in the perception of pain. Reactions to pain and perceptions of pain vary among individuals, even within the same culture. The nurse must understand differences in cultures and attend to the particular needs of each patient. When providing culturally sensitive nursing care, the nurse adjusts the plan of care to incorporate the patient's needs.

The meaning of pain varies among individuals. Pain is physical, part of a disease entity or a symptom of an injury, but it can also result from emotional or psychological distress. For example, unresolved psychological pain may result in posttraumatic stress disorder, anxiety, or depression. In cases of acute pain, anxiety increases the severity of the pain experienced, reduces the individual's tolerance to pain, and decreases the ability to cope with pain. Individuals with chronic pain are more likely to suffer from depression and fatigue and are more likely to attempt suicide (Schneider, 2004). Current pain is influenced by an individual's previous experiences with pain. Having had an injury or surgery previously, a patient has a preconceived idea about what the pain will feel like and what methods are effective for pain relief.

Just as the meaning of pain and the perception of pain are individualized responses, the response to drugs is influenced by each person's genetic makeup (Box 36-1). Differences in pain perception and management are described in the Diversity Considerations box.

BOX 36-1 Genetics and Medication Metabolism

Research is being conducted to determine the degree to which genetic makeup influences how individuals respond to medications:

- Pharmacogenetics looks at a person's genotype to determine how the individual metabolizes medications.
- Genetic testing can predict how individuals are likely to respond to certain drugs (National Center for Biotechnology Information, 2004).
- Pharmacogenomics is the study of how genetic expression influences drug behavior in the body (Kudzma and Carey, 2009).
- In the future, dosages will be based on the patient's ability to metabolize medications (Eichelbaum, Ingelman-Sandberg, and Evans, 2006).

! SAFE PRACTICE ALERT

When treating an elderly patient for pain, start with a low dose within the prescribed range and slowly increase the dosage to relieve pain. Opioid doses should start 50% to 75% lower than the normal adult dose to avoid oversedation (D'Arcy, 2009).

DIVERSITY CONSIDERATIONS

Life Span

Infants and Children

- Preterm infants may display behaviors different from those of term infants due to neurologic immaturity (Holsti and Grunau, 2007).
- Infants and young children often demonstrate physical and emotional pain by crying.
- Parents or caregivers may hold infants or children during painful procedures to promote comfort.
- Toys, video games, or other forms of entertainment may be used to distract children undergoing painful procedures.
- Age-appropriate language should be used with children to prevent unnecessarily frightening them before a potentially painful treatment.
- Undertreatment is more prevalent in the pediatric population than among adults (Mitchell, 2010).

Older Adults

- Pain is not a consequence of natural aging (D'Arcy, 2009). All pain needs to be investigated by the health care provider.
- The sensation of pain is just as acute in elderly patients as it is in young-adult patients, but among elderly patients, the transmission of pain impulses may be altered by chronic diseases or disorders causing a decreased or increased sensation of pain with diabetes mellitus and peripheral neuropathies, or an increased sensation of pain with arthritis (D'Arcy, 2009).
- The ability of elderly individuals to recognize pain may be blunted or masked by illness and medications.
- Elderly people who are depressed or cognitively impaired may be unable to tell others that they are in pain. Elderly patients, like all adults, may be reluctant to take pain medications for fear of addiction (Hutt, Buffum, Fink, et al, 2007).
- Decreased metabolism and clearance of drugs may lead to toxic levels in older adults; therefore, many medications need to be administered in lower doses (Bruckenthal and D'Arcy, 2007).
- Polypharmacy is a common concern with elderly or chronically ill patients who take multiple medications simultaneously, including prescription drugs, over-the-counter medications, and herbal supplements (D'Arcy, 2009).
- Patients should be encouraged to keep all medications in their original containers to prevent confusion and to facilitate medication reconciliation by health care personnel in the event of an individual's hospitalization.

Gender

- Compared with men, women have reported being in more pain, which may be due to differences in estrogen and testosterone levels (Mitchell, 2010).
- Women seek help for pain more often than men do, but women are less likely to receive treatment (Partners Against Pain, 2014).
- Women are more likely to be given sedatives for pain, and men are more likely to be given analgesics for pain (Partners Against Pain, 2014).

Culture, Ethnicity, and Religion

- Not all individuals of the same culture or ethnicity express pain in the same manner.
- Acceptable treatment for pain may vary depending on an individual's religious beliefs.
- Non-Hispanic white adults report more pain than other races (Mitchell, 2010).
- African Americans and Hispanics are undertreated and wait until their pain is severe before calling for pain medication (Mitchell, 2010).
- Patients of Asian descent may try to hide cancer pain because it is believed by some to be a punishment for sins of the past (Im, Lee, Lim, et al, 2009).
- Education regarding pain management strategies and medication administration information should be provided in the patient's native language to enhance comprehension and effectiveness.

Disability

- A patient with impaired cognition may not be able to communicate pain. Facial expressions, vocalization of noises, or changes in physical activity or routines may be signs of pain.
- Noncognitive pain assessment tools such as the Wong-Baker Facial Grimace Scale may be used to assess pain levels (Mann, 2010).
- Patients who are intubated may be able to write or point to a pain assessment tool to indicate their level of pain.
- Restlessness and elevated blood pressure and/or pulse rate may signal increased pain levels in patients who are intubated and sedated and unable to communicate verbally or in writing.

Morphology

- Research indicates that obese people tend to experience more pain in more locations than individuals of average weight (Janke, Collins, and Kozak, 2007).
- Pain medication dosages need to be adjusted on the basis of the height and weight of patients of all ages due to body surface area and metabolic differences.

◆ ASSESSMENT LO 36.5

Completing a thorough pain assessment helps the nurse to develop a profile of the patient, facilitating the identification of patient needs or problems in relation to pain. The Health Assessment Questions box contains sample questions to ask patients about their pain. Except in emergent situations, the nurse begins a thorough, focused assessment by obtaining a health history specifically related to the patient's complaint of pain.

HEALTH ASSESSMENT QUESTIONS

- What is the intensity of your pain? Would you describe your pain as mild, moderate, or severe? On a pain scale with 0 being no pain and 10 being excruciating pain, how do you rate your pain?
- How long have you been experiencing this pain? Has the pain begun recently, or have you been in pain longer than 6 months?
- Where is the pain you are experiencing? Does it radiate anywhere? Point to exactly where the pain is and where it radiates to, if it does.
- Have you noticed any pattern with the pain you are experiencing? Does the pain occur in the morning, occur when you are ambulating, or awaken you during the night?
- Is the pain sharp or dull, aching or throbbing, or burning? Is the pain constant or intermittent (comes and goes)?
- Are there precipitating factors that occur before the pain is felt? What have you tried for pain relief? Have you tried applying heat or massaging or rubbing the area? Has what you have tried helped?
- What medications are you currently using or have you taken in the past to relieve pain?

If a patient is in excruciating pain due to trauma or an ischemic attack, a rapid, narrowly focused assessment to determine the location, onset, quality, and severity of the pain must be completed before appropriate emergency treatment can be initiated. In these emergent situations, the more complete pain assessment may be deferred until some degree of pain relief is achieved. Patients who are in severe pain are unable to focus on answering open-ended questions designed to gather extensive information. When patients are exhibiting signs of severe pain, nurses must use short, closed-ended questions to gather specific information in the most expedient manner possible.

PAIN HISTORY AND ASSESSMENT

Because pain is a very individual, subjective experience, nurses cannot objectively assess pain in patients. Completing a thorough pain assessment requires nurses to ask patients about several critical areas of concern: pain location, onset, quality, intensity, and pattern; precipitating and alleviating factors; and associated symptoms. The acronym SOCRATES is used by many health care personnel to help them remember each area of pain assessment (Value MD, 2010). The letters in SOCRATES have the following meanings:

S: Site (Where is the pain located?)
O: Onset (When did the pain start? Was it gradual or sudden?)
C: Character (What is the quality of the pain? Is it stabbing, burning, or aching?)
R: Radiation (Does the pain radiate anywhere?)
A: Associations (What signs and symptoms are associated with the pain?)
T: Time course (Is there a pattern to when the pain occurs?)
E: Exacerbating or relieving factors (Does anything make the pain worse or lessen it?)
S: Severity (On a scale of 0 to 10, what is the intensity of the pain?)

In addition to asking about the previous factors, nurses should ask patients who are experiencing pain about past pain experiences, the effect their pain is having on ADLs, the meaning patients associate with their pain, and coping strategies that they are using to deal with the discomfort. Nurses should observe carefully the emotional response of patients who are in pain. When patients are unable to communicate verbally, nurses must observe for signs or symptoms of pain and evaluate precipitating factors that could result in pain. Although there are no laboratory or diagnostic studies that assess for pain level, many types of pain assessment tools have been developed to assist patients of all ages.

Pain Assessment Tools

Pain can be assessed with the use of tools specifically designed to help patients evaluate the intensity and location of their pain and to aid health care team members in evaluating the effectiveness of pain management. Many types of pain assessment tools are available, including cognitive and noncognitive scales. The basic pain assessment tool is the 0-10 numeric pain scale, which allows patients to verbally report their pain level. The most reliable indicator of the existence and intensity of pain is the patient's self-report. A reported pain level of 1 to 3 is considered mild pain. Pain reported in the range of 4 to 7 is moderate pain. Pain of 8 to 10 is interpreted as severe pain (Glassford, 2008). A numeric scale quantifies pain.

Descriptors of pain are denoted verbally in the Verbal Descriptor Scale and the Wong-Baker Facial Grimace Scale. The Universal Pain Assessment Tool (Figure 36-4) is a combination of the Verbal Descriptor Scale, Wong-Baker Facial Grimace Scale, and Activity Tolerance Scale, which is available with foreign-language phrases explaining the pain levels. This tool can be used worldwide for assessing pain (Mitchell, 2010).

Table 36-3 shows the Neonatal Infant Pain Scale that is recommended for use with children younger than 1 year of age. A score higher than 3 indicates that the child is in pain. It is used as a noncognitive pain assessment scale in the neonatal intensive care unit (NICU), newborn nursery, and

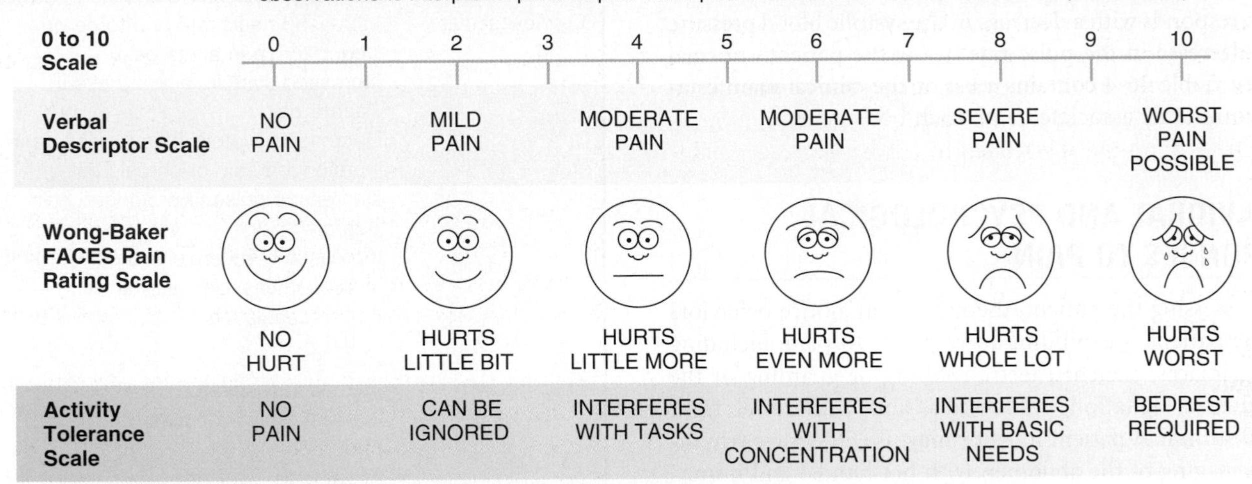

FIGURE 36-4 Visual cues, descriptive terms, and activity levels can be useful in helping patients identify their level of pain if they are unable to relate to the numeric scale. (From Hockenberry MJ, Wilson D: Wong's nursing care of infants and children, ed 10, St. Louis, 2015, Mosby.)

TABLE 36-3 Neonatal Infant Pain Scale

PAIN ASSESSMENT	EXAMPLE	SCORE
Facial expression	Restful face, neutral expression	0 (relaxed muscles)
	Tight facial muscles; furrowed brow, chin, and jaw (negative facial expression, including nose, mouth, and brow)	1 (grimace)
Cry	Quiet, not crying	0 (no cry)
	Mild moaning, intermittent	1 (whimper)
	Loud scream; rising, shrill, continuous (If baby is intubated, silent cry as evidenced by obvious mouth and facial movement may be scored.)	2 (vigorous cry)
Breathing patterns	Usual pattern for this infant	0 (relaxed)
	Indrawing, irregular, faster than usual; gagging; breath-holding	1 (change in breathing)
Arms	No muscular rigidity; occasional random movements of the arms	0 (relaxed/restrained)
	Tense, straight legs; rigid and/or rapid extension, flexion	1 (flexed/extended)
Legs	No muscular rigidity; occasional random leg movement	0 (relaxed/restrained)
	Tense, straight legs; rigid and/or rapid extension, flexion	1 (flexed/extended)
State of arousal	Quiet, peaceful sleeping or alert random leg movement	0 (sleeping/awake)
	Alert, restless, and thrashing	1 (fussy)

From Hudson-Barr D, Capper-Michel B, Lambert S, et al: Validation of the pain assessment in neonates (PAIN) scale with the neonatal infant pain scale (NIPS), *Neonatal Netw* 21(6):15-21, 2002.

pediatrics department to determine pain levels of newborns and infants. On the basis of the score, the nurse can determine the need for pain medication.

Vital Signs

Physical assessment of the patient with pain begins with vital sign assessment. Vital signs may vary according to how the patient perceives pain. Elevated pulse and blood pressure values may indicate acute pain and a need for pain medication. A decrease in blood pressure and pulse rate may indicate chronic pain. While taking vital signs, the nurse asks the patient what his or her pain level is or, for the nonverbal patient, determines the pain level on a noncognitive pain scale. The nurse can perform measures such as repositioning the patient or therapeutically touching the patient in an effort to decrease the pain level before administering pain medication.

PHYSIOLOGIC RESPONSES TO PAIN

Multiple systems of the body may be affected by pain, depending on its severity and duration. For instance, if a patient is in acute pain, the patient's heart rate, respiratory rate, and blood pressure increase above the patient's normal baseline due to a response by the sympathetic nervous system. With chronic or prolonged pain, the parasympathetic nervous system responds with a decrease in the systolic blood pressure and a decrease in the pulse rate below the patient's normal baseline. Table 36-4 contains a list of the clinical manifestations commonly associated with each body system.

TABLE 36-4 Clinical Manifestations of Pain

BODY SYSTEM	CLINICAL MANIFESTATIONS
Cardiovascular	Increased heart rate and force of contraction in acute pain Increased systolic blood pressure in acute pain Decreased systolic blood pressure in prolonged pain or chronic pain Decreased pulse in prolonged pain or chronic pain Increased myocardial oxygen demand Increased vascular resistance Hypercoagulation Chest pain
Respiratory	Increased respiratory rate Increased bronchospasms Pneumonia Atelectasis
Gastrointestinal	Delayed gastric emptying Decreased intestinal motility Constipation Anorexia Weight loss
Musculoskeletal	Muscle spasms Increased muscle tension Impaired mobility Weakness Fatigue
Endocrine	Fever Shock
Genitourinary	Decreased urine output Urinary retention Fluid overload Hypokalemia
Sensory	Pallor Diaphoresis Dilated pupils in acute pain Constricted pupils in deep or prolonged pain Rapid speech in acute pain Slow speech in deep or prolonged pain
Immune	Impaired immune function Infection

BEHAVIORAL AND PSYCHOLOGICAL RESPONSES TO PAIN

While assessing the patient, the nurse may notice behaviors that the patient is exhibiting in response to pain, including facial grimaces, clenched teeth, rubbing or guarding of the painful area, agitation, restlessness, and withdrawal from painful stimuli. A patient in labor may use effleurage (rhythmic massaging of the abdomen with her hands) and immobilization to help deal with uterine contraction pain. Vocalizations of pain may be expressed as crying, moaning, or screaming.

Patients may exhibit psychological responses to pain, including anxiety, fear, depression, anger, irritability, helplessness, and hopelessness. When a patient is anxious, fearful, or angry, the nurse addresses the patient's physical needs first. The nurse provides a comfortable environment and privacy for the patient. Then the nurse communicates with clear, simple validating statements to relieve the stress of the situation and to develop a trusting relationship with the patient. The nurse needs to allow time for the patient to verbalize feelings and concerns regarding pain relief to assess the patient's coping abilities. The nurse acknowledges the patient's pain experience and expresses acceptance of the patient's response to pain. After pain has been assessed, the nurse uses nursing diagnoses to develop a plan of care for the patient.

◆ NURSING DIAGNOSIS LO 36.6

Nurses should carefully document all physiologic, behavioral, and psychological responses observed during assessment so that appropriate nursing diagnoses and goals can be formulated, making holistic pain management possible. After a thorough pain assessment, the type and meaning of a patient's pain are established, allowing appropriate nursing diagnoses to be identified, goals and outcomes to be set, and adequate pain management to take place.

Nursing diagnoses for pain are developed on the basis of objective and subjective patient data collected by the nurse during the patient's assessment. Common nursing diagnoses directly associated with pain are *Acute Pain, Chronic Pain, Ineffective Coping, Anxiety, Disturbed Sleep Pattern,* and *Readiness for Enhanced Comfort.* The following are examples of nursing diagnostic statements.

- *Acute Pain* related to long-bone fracture as evidenced by reported pain of 10 of 10, pain with movement, and request for pain medication
- *Chronic Pain* related to deformity of joints as evidenced by limited mobility, inability to manage activities of daily living, and feelings of helplessness
- *Ineffective Coping* related to severe pain as evidenced by inability to ask for help, lack of appetite, and poor concentration

- *Anxiety* related to fear of increasing pain levels as evidenced by restlessness, quivering voice, and increased blood pressure
- *Disturbed Sleep Pattern* related to pain from chronic illness as evidenced by verbal complaints of inability to sleep, dark circles under the eyes, and frequent yawning
- *Readiness for Enhanced Comfort* as evidenced by inquiry regarding use of decreasing dosage of pain medication for comfort and by pain rating of 2 of 10

After nursing diagnoses are identified from the assessment information, the nursing care plan is developed, starting with goal development.

◆ PLANNING LO 36.7

Reviewing data collected during the assessment phase of the nursing process helps the nurse to identify and prioritize nursing diagnoses and set realistic outcome criteria based on a patient's condition and capabilities. Goals and expected outcomes must take into consideration the economic, psychosocial, physical, and other resources available in individual situations.

GOALS AND OUTCOME STATEMENTS

The following are examples of goals or outcome statements:

- Patient will report a pain level of less than 3 of 10 within 5 postoperative days.
- Patient will perform activities of daily living on a daily basis, reporting chronic pain at a level of 3 or less within 1 week of starting on newly prescribed pain medication.
- Patient will report increased ability to concentrate on routine activities within 2 hours of receiving the prescribed dose of analgesia.
- Patient will report decreased anxiety, with no signs of restlessness, within 3 days of hospitalization.
- Patient will state being able to sleep for 6 to 8 hours each night within 3 days of hospitalization.
- Patient will meet with a pain specialist to outline a plan for decreasing analgesia dosage within the next 2 weeks.

Because various members of the health care team specialize in different ways of accomplishing pain relief, a multidisciplinary approach is often needed to achieve pain relief goals. The multidisciplinary team collaborates to develop a plan of care for the patient's pain management. While maintaining ultimate responsibility for overseeing the implementation and proper completion of duties, the nurse may delegate appropriate duties to unlicensed assistive personnel (UAP) (Collaboration and Delegation box).

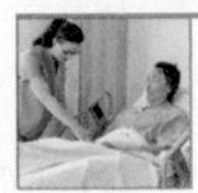

1. Write a short-term and long-term goal or outcome for Mr. Charles's postoperative nursing diagnosis: *Acute Pain* related to surgical repair as evidenced by increased heart rate, reluctance to move, and reported pain level of 8 of 10 (8/10).

COLLABORATION AND DELEGATION

Complementary Pain Therapy

- The patient with pain needs a multidisciplinary treatment plan to ensure pain management and relief.
- Music therapy, massage therapy, physical therapy, and the services of health care providers specializing in pain management provide exercise, muscle manipulation, and other complementary therapies to manage pain in addition to medication.
- The nurse can delegate unlicensed assistive personnel to perform nonpharmacologic pain management techniques, such as administering back rubs, repositioning the patient, performing oral hygiene, changing the linens, talking to the patient, and darkening the room, to help make the patient more comfortable and assist in decreasing pain.

While planning care, the nurse must consider ethical and legal aspects of managing pain to comply with the American Nurses Association (ANA) standards of practice and Code of Ethics for Nurses and with the regulatory standards of The Joint Commission. The most commonly encountered ethical dilemmas are undertreatment of pain, especially among elderly patients, and thorough management of pain. The nurse has a legal obligation to act on behalf of patients to ensure pain relief (Zalon, Constantino, and Andrews, 2008) (Ethical, Legal, and Professional Practice box).

When the pain assessment has been completed and the plan of care has been formulated with nursing diagnoses and goals appropriate for the patient, implementation of the plan of care begins (Table 36-5).

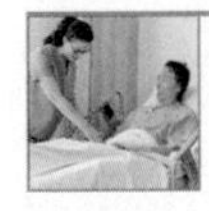

The conceptual care map for Mr. Charles can be found at *http://evolve.elsevier.com/YoostCrawford/fundamentals/*. It is partially completed to indicate how to use the map as a learning tool. Complete the nursing diagnoses using the example conceptual care maps shown in Chapters 8 and 25-33.

◆ IMPLEMENTATION AND EVALUATION LO 36.8

Implementation of the plan of care is performed in response to the patient's needs. The plan of care is modified as the patient's status changes. The goal of implementation is to progress toward the desired outcomes of care. The Joint Commission developed standards for pain assessment and management in an attempt to improve the management of pain relief (Box 36-2).

A variety of treatments may be used to provide holistic pain management, including nonpharmacologic interventions, nonopioid analgesics, opioid analgesics, and adjuvant analgesics (coanalgesics).

TABLE 36-5 Care Planning

NANDA-I NURSING DIAGNOSIS LABEL WITH NURSING DIAGNOSIS STATEMENT	NURSING OUTCOME CLASSIFICATION (NOC)	NURSING INTERVENTION CLASSIFICATION (NIC)
Acute Pain related to long-bone fracture as evidenced by reported pain of 10 of 10, pain with movement, and request for pain medication	*Pain control* (1605) Reports pain controlled (160511)	*Pain management* (1400) Select and implement a variety of measures (e.g., pharmacological, nonpharmacological, interpersonal) to facilitate pain relief as appropriate.

From Bulechek G, Butcher H, Dochterman J, et al (Eds): *Nursing interventions classification (NIC),* ed. 6, St. Louis, 2013, Mosby; Moorhead S, Johnson M, Maas M, et al (Eds): *Nursing outcomes classification (NOC),* ed. 5, St. Louis, 2013, Mosby; NANDA International: *Nursing diagnoses: Definitions and classification, 2012–2014,* West Sussex, England, 2012, Wiley-Blackwell. Reprinted with permission from NANDA International, Inc.

ETHICAL, LEGAL, AND PROFESSIONAL PRACTICE

Meeting Pain Management Standards

When patients are satisfied with nursing care and obtain pain relief and no adverse effects from medication or errors in administration occur, patients are more likely to report satisfaction with their care. Several strategies can be implemented by nurses to ensure ethical compliance with pain management standards and to reduce legal risks of medication administration:

- Check patient allergies and sensitivities before administering any medication.
- Use the Six Rights of Medication Administration when administering medications.
- Follow the steps of the nursing process.
- Monitor for side effects or adverse effects of medication.
- Report uncommon patient responses to analgesia to the patient's primary care provider (PCP).
- Communicate effectively with the patient.
- Teach the patient about the use of medications and potential side effects.
- Evaluate the effect of medication on the patient, and document the patient's response. Use equipment such as patient-controlled anesthesia pumps properly.
- Document accurately and in a timely manner.
- Follow the facility's policies and procedures.
- Arrange for appropriate referrals to meet the needs of the patient.

BOX 36-2 The Joint Commission's Pain Assessment Standards

The Joint Commission requires all organizations to meet certain pain assessment standards:

- Recognize the right of patients to have appropriate assessment and management of their pain.
- Identify patients with pain in an initial screening assessment.
- Perform a more comprehensive pain assessment when pain is identified.
- Record the results of the assessment in a way that facilitates regular reassessment and follow-up.
- Educate relevant providers in pain assessment and management.
- Determine and ensure staff competency in pain assessment and management.
- Address pain assessment and management in the orientation of all new staff.
- Establish policies and procedures that support appropriate prescribing and ordering of effective pain medications.
- Ensure that pain does not interfere with participation in rehabilitation.
- Educate patients and their families about the importance of effective pain management.
- Address patient needs for symptom management in the discharge planning process.
- Collect data to monitor the appropriateness and effectiveness of pain management.

From Berry P, Dahl J: The new JCAHO pain standards: Implications for pain management nurses, *Pain Manage Nurses* 1(1): 3-12, 2000.

NONPHARMACOLOGIC PAIN MANAGEMENT AND ALTERNATIVE AND COMPLEMENTARY THERAPIES

Nonpharmacologic pain management, alternative and complementary therapies are recommended for patients with mild pain who do not want to use medication to control pain. These therapies are often used concurrently with medication administration and counseling to support patients with intractable or chronic pain. Alternative therapies take the place of pharmacologic interventions, and complementary therapies are implemented to enhance the effect of pharmacologic treatment. During the assessment process, nurses should inquire about the patient's use of herbal remedies to avoid potential medication interactions if analgesics are included in the plan of care.

There are many types of social interaction and therapies that target the mind, body, and spirit and help alleviate pain. Many are independent nursing interventions that do not require a practitioner order. They may include the positioning of patients for comfort and for proper body alignment (see Chapter 28); postoperative splinting (see Chapter 37); massage to promote relaxation and decrease muscle tension and pain perception (see Chapter 27); and progressive relaxation techniques, guided imagery, and meditation (see Chapter 32).

Distracting patients by encouraging them to watch television or listen to music may lessen their focus on and awareness of pain. Engaging patients in conversation and singing are other forms of distraction. Spiritual support, such as prayer or meditation, can be encouraged in individual circumstances to draw on the patient's beliefs and faith as a means of diminishing pain. Additional alternative and complementary pain therapies are listed in Box 36-3.

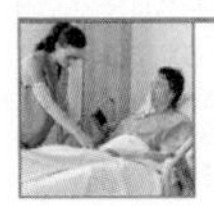

2. Identify a minimum of five nursing interventions to decrease Mr. Charles's pain using nonpharmacologic methods.

Neurologic and neurosurgical pain therapies using electrical stimulation of the area of pain and brain stimulation are options for dealing with chronic pain, as are types of neurosurgery (Box 36-4). Although many of these therapies are not independent nursing actions, the nurse should understand these interventions to better support patients in need of such treatment. When patients experiencing chronic pain have decided to try alternative or complementary therapies for pain relief, it is important that nurses listen and support their requests. Increasing numbers of patients are embracing nonpharmacologic pain interventions on the basis of research they have done and fear of addiction or side effects from narcotic analgesics (Shumay, Maskarinec, Kakai, et al, 2001).

BOX 36-3 Alternative and Complementary Pain Therapies

- *Herbal remedies:* The use of certain herbal mixes relieves pain; examples are ginger, rosehips, feverfew, and black cohosh.
- *Yoga:* Slow stretches and deep breathing build strength, release muscle tension, and improve flexibility to bring the body into balance and the mind into a focus on something other than pain.
- *Biofeedback:* Taking control of body responses to pain is achieved through voluntary control over physiologic body activities, such as relieving muscle tension.
- *Meditation:* Meditating restores the body to a calm state through controlled breathing and relaxation to decrease stress and pain.
- *Hypnosis:* Used for all types of pain, hypnosis alters the state of consciousness to modify memory and perception of pain and reduces cortical activation associated with painful stimuli.
- *Reiki and therapeutic touch:* Hand placement to correct or balance energy fields restores health by restoring communication between cells, thereby diminishing pain.
- *Traditional Chinese medicine:*
  - *Acupuncture:* The insertion of fine needles into the skin at various depths causes secretion of endorphins and interferes with transmission of pain impulses.
  - *Acupressure:* The application of pressure at acupuncture sites interferes with transmission of pain impulses.

PHARMACOLOGIC PAIN MANAGEMENT

The nurse's role in pharmacologic pain management is to assess for pain, to administer pain medication accurately and safely, and to teach the patient about medication self-administration (Patient Education and Health Literacy box). To safely administer medications, the nurse needs to understand many routes of administration (Evidence-Based Practice and Informatics box). Administration is achieved by oral, transmucosal, sublingual, rectal, intradermal, subcutaneous, intramuscular, transdermal, and intravenous routes, as well as by gastric tube and inhaler.

QSEN FOCUS!

Nurses must read about current research to be familiar with pain relief options and provide evidence-based care that is acceptable to each patient.

Two therapeutic strategies used to manage pain are multimodal analgesia and preemptive analgesia. **Multimodal analgesia** is the use of more than one means for controlling pain. When more than one type of agent is used, analgesia is more effective, requires lower doses of each agent, and produces fewer side effects. Multimodal analgesia may be two medications (e.g., acetaminophen with codeine, morphine sulfate with gabapentin) or a medication used in combination with a complementary therapy (e.g., topical ointment

BOX 36-4 Neurologic and Neurosurgical Pain Therapies

- *Spinal cord stimulation* (SCS): Implantation of a device into the epidural space treats chronic neurologic pain by producing a tingling sensation that alters pain perception. Leads are connected to a generator in the abdomen or buttocks.
- *Transcutaneous electrical nerve stimulation* (TENS): Stimulation of selective receptors by applying low-intensity current through skin electrodes interferes with transmission of pain impulses in nerve fibers, reducing pain and analgesia use and improving mobility. A TENS unit is a portable, battery-operated stimulator with a lead wire and electrode pads that are applied to the skin in the area of pain. It is contraindicated for patients with pacemakers or cardiac arrhythmias.
- Application of heat and cold:
  - *Cryotherapy*: Application of cold decreases swelling and pain, produces local analgesia, and slows nerve conduction, which improves functioning. Examples of cold therapy are ice bags and cold compresses.
  - *Thermotherapy:* Application of heat decreases pain by producing local analgesia, dilating blood vessels, and improving functioning. Examples of heat therapy are hot compresses, heating pads, and sitz baths.
  - Apply heat or cold for 15 minutes to avoid tissue injury.
- *Cordotomy:* Surgical procedure in which pain-conducting tracts in the spinal cord are disabled to diminish severe pain and cancer pain.
- *Neurectomy:* Surgical removal of a nerve or a section of nerves to treat chronic pain when other treatments fail.
- *Rhizotomy:* Surgery to sever nerve roots in the spinal cord for neuromuscular conditions such as spastic cerebral palsy and back pain.
- *Sympathectomy:* Surgical dissection of nerve tissue of the sympathetic nervous system in the cervical, thoracic, or lumbar spine to disrupt signals to the brain.

PATIENT EDUCATION AND HEALTH LITERACY

Empowering Patients Experiencing Pain

- Teach patients to keep a journal of the type of pain, onset of pain, activity related to the pain, intensity of the pain, and nonpharmacologic and pharmacologic measures used to relieve pain.
- Teach patients methods of nonpharmacologic treatment to relieve pain, such as massage, guided imagery, muscle relaxation, and distraction.
- Instruct patients to consult with their primary care provider (PCP) before using herbal remedies because this helps avoid interactions with pharmacologic agents.
- Teach patients to take pain medication before the pain becomes severe or occurs around the clock. This helps to maintain a consistent blood level of medication, producing sustained analgesia.
- Instruct patients about when to contact their PCP or pain specialist, and stress the importance of doing so in the event that the pain control measures used are ineffective.
- Offer information on community agencies or resources and support groups that provide information and educational materials.

EVIDENCE-BASED PRACTICE AND INFORMATICS

Postoperative Pain Management

Research on pain management is ongoing. Development of devices that promote patient mobility should improve postoperative recovery and reduce the resources required by nurses to help patients complete tasks such as ambulation and personal care. An evidence-based research study compared traditional morphine patient-controlled analgesia (PCA) with a needleless, self-contained fentanyl HCl transdermal pain relief system. The fentanyl HCl transdermal system is a very small, self-contained, adhesive, on-demand device applied directly to the patient's skin. Patients received the patient-controlled fentanyl transdermal system or intravenous morphine PCA for up to 72 hours after major surgery. The study found that the fentanyl HCl transdermal system was preferred:

- It eliminated having to program an intravenous pump.
- It minimized preparation time, making it less time-consuming for nurses.
- It eliminated medication errors.
- It provided greater pain control for patients.
- It enabled patients to perform daily activities more easily due to the lack of an intravenous line.
- It enabled patients to move and ambulate earlier due to improved pain control.

Adapted from Pennington P, Caminiti S, Schein J, et al: Patients' assessment of the convenience of fentanyl HCl Iontophoretic transdermal system (ITS) versus morphine intravenous patient-controlled analgesia (IV PCA) in the management of postoperative pain after major surgery, *Pain Manage Nurs* 10(3): 124-133, 2009.

with massage therapy). **Preemptive analgesia** is the administration of medications before a painful event to minimize pain. Medications administered before surgery or before dressing changes are examples of preemptive analgesia.

> **! SAFE PRACTICE ALERT**
>
> Check for allergies before administering medications. Watch the patient for at least 30 minutes after administering a medication to assess for an anaphylactic reaction. Allergic responses may occur with initiation of an agent or after sensitization to the medication on the first, second, or later exposure to the drug. Spending a short time on monitoring the patient may save the patient's life.

Nonopioid Analgesics

Nonopioid analgesics include acetaminophen and **nonsteroidal anti-inflammatory drugs** (NSAIDs) such as ibuprofen and aspirin. These drugs are used in the treatment of many types of mild to moderate pain. Mild pain is rated as 1 to 3 on a numeric pain scale; it may be an achy feeling to the patient. Moderate pain is classified as 4 to 7 on a numeric pain scale; it may be the type of pain a patient experiences on day 3 after surgery. Nonopioids are not addictive and are safer for the patient to use than narcotic analgesics, although patients may become dependent on nonopioids for pain relief.

Acetaminophen has analgesic and antipyretic capabilities and is a safe pain relief agent for most patients, including those with liver disease, if monitored closely and administered within the safe dosage range. Special caution should be taken when giving acetaminophen to infants, children and the elderly. Long-term use may result in hepatotoxicity, renal damage, or leukopenia. The total daily dose should not exceed 3 to 4 g. An overdose may cause liver damage and can be fatal. Acetaminophen is used for fever reduction and for mild to moderate pain from conditions such as a mild headache or general achiness.

NSAIDs are more useful than acetaminophen in treating inflammatory pain and bone pain. NSAIDs have anti-inflammatory effects in addition to analgesic and antipyretic qualities. Aspirin is also an effective agent for decreasing platelet aggregation in patients who are prone to blood clots or at risk for myocardial infarction.

Unfortunately, NSAIDs have significant side effects, including possible gastrointestinal upset and bleeding and cardiac and renal complications. These side effects may be avoided by taking the drugs with food and taking the prescribed dose. Proton pump inhibitors (PPIs) or histamine H_2-receptor blockers are often prescribed for patients who are on long-term NSAID therapy to help reduce the incidence of stomach ulcers.

Opioid Analgesics

Opioid analgesics are the most effective agents for relief of moderate to severe pain. These narcotic drugs work by binding to the opioid receptors in the nervous system, which are sites of endorphin action. There are many types of opioid analgesics, including agonist analgesics and agonist-antagonist analgesics.

Agonist analgesics, such as morphine, hydromorphone, oxycodone, fentanyl, and meperidine, are the most effective agents for relief of severe pain, which is rated 7 to 10 on a numeric pain scale. They may change the patient's perception of pain while relieving the pain. The normal route of administration is oral, intramuscular, or intravenous. When it is administered intramuscularly or intravenously, it may be given every 1 to 3 hours, depending on the dose administered. The nurse needs to be aware of adverse effects such as respiratory depression, seizures, nausea, vomiting, constipation, itching, and urinary retention. The nurse may administer an antagonist analgesic for the respiratory depression, antiemetics for the nausea and vomiting, and an antihistamine for itching. Dizziness, blurred vision, confusion, and orthostatic hypotension may occur.

Agonist-antagonist analgesics include pentazocine, butorphanol, dezocine, and nalbuphine. These medications are used for moderate to severe pain. They depress the pain-impulse transmission at the spinal cord by acting with opioid receptors. They are normally administered by the intramuscular or intravenous route. Dosing is every 1 to 4 hours, depending on the drug. The nurse needs to be aware of patient drowsiness, dizziness, nausea, vomiting, itching, and respiratory depression. Treatment for these adverse effects is the same as that for the adverse effects associated with agonist analgesics.

Antagonist analgesics such as naloxone (Narcan) are used for the treatment of opioid analgesic overdose. They compete with opioids at the opioid receptor sites, decreasing the side effects of opioids. They are administered intravenously, intramuscularly, or subcutaneously every 2 to 3 minutes until symptoms of opioid overdose subside. Signs of opioid withdrawal, such as vomiting, hypertension, and anxiety, may occur up to 2 hours after administration.

> **! SAFE PRACTICE ALERT**
>
> Check vital signs before administering opioid analgesics. Overdose of opioids may cause respiratory depression. Respiratory depression is defined as fewer than 10 respirations per minute. Administer 0.4 to 2 mg of naloxone every 2 to 3 minutes to a maximum dose of 10 mg to increase the respiratory rate to more than 10 respirations per minute. Administering opioids when a patient is hypotensive (systolic blood pressure of 90 or less) also may cause hypoperfusion.

Patient-controlled analgesia (PCA) is a system in which an electronically controlled infusion pump immediately delivers a prescribed amount of analgesic to the patient when he or she activates a button, without the need for a nurse to administer it (Nursing Care Guideline box). The purpose of

NURSING CARE GUIDELINE

Patient-Controlled Analgesia

Background

- Patient-controlled analgesia involves the intravenous administration of a controlled substance as a pain medication.
- Patient control of the infusion pump is restricted to certain parameters, as prescribed by the primary care provider (PCP):
  - The PCP may prescribe continuous doses of pain medication with additional boluses administered by the patient as needed.
  - The PCP orders a specific lockout time between patient doses to avoid overdosing.
  - PCA by proxy is unauthorized activation of the PCA pump by someone other than the patient. The PCP may order authorized nurse-controlled or caregiver-controlled anesthesia by PCA pump when a patient is unable to activate the dosing button. This type of order is indicated for young children and unconscious or incompetent adults.
- Nurses should refer to the manufacturer's instructions for pump operation.
- Nurses should follow facility policies and procedures for frequency of assessment and documentation of PCA use.

Procedural Concerns

- Perform assessments:
  - Assess the patient at the beginning of PCA use and again one-half hour later.
  - Check the patient every hour for the first 8 hours of PCA use after the initial assessments.
  - After the first 8 hours, assess the patient as specified in the PCP order or every 4 hours at a minimum. Assessment may be done more frequently in accordance with nursing judgment, depending on patient status.
- Take precautions:
  - Ensure that only the patient operates the PCA pump. Family members should never activate the pump for the patient.
  - Keep naloxone or another specifically indicated antagonist analgesic immediately accessible in case of an overdose or emergency.
  - Follow the PCP order for medications, dosage, and pump settings.
- Two nurses must verify or witness medication changes and check orders against pump settings at the change of shift and with any changes in pump settings. Conscientiously monitor the following:
  - Proper PCA pump function
  - Fluid levels
  - IV line patency
  - Respiratory rate, level of consciousness, and blood pressure
  - Pain level and itching, nausea, and vomiting (common side effects of opiates)

Documentation Concerns

- Note the patient and family education that was provided.
- Education may initially occur preoperatively.
- Education must be reinforced postoperatively.
- Record assessment and monitoring results.
- Document the medications administered, medications remaining, and pump settings on each shift.

Evidence-Based Practice

- Benefits for a patient using a PCA pump include satisfaction related to control of pain and self-management rather than having to ask for or wait for the nurse to administer medication.
- Benefits for a nurse with a patient on PCA include increased time available for patients due to decreased requests for what could be hourly pain medication administration.
- With proper education, policies, and procedures in place, PCA can be a safe method of pain management for the patient and the provider (Taylor, 2010).

PCA is improved pain control. PCA uses more frequent but smaller doses of medication, usually opioids (i.e., morphine sulfate, fentanyl, or hydromorphone), and provides more even levels of medication in the patient's body. The PCA pump can deliver medicine into a vein (intravenously, the most common method), under the skin (subcutaneously), or between the dura mater and the spinal cord (epidurally). When the medication is delivered intravenously, the site must be monitored for infiltration and phlebitis.

! SAFE PRACTICE ALERT

Administer the prescribed medication dose that best manages pain and has the fewest side effects.

The following are additional methods by which opioids are delivered:

- On-Q infusion pump provides continuous infusion of local anesthesia through an antimicrobial catheter, which destroys or inhibits microorganism growth on the catheter. It is most often used for postoperative pain control following abdominal surgery.
- Transdermal administration consists of a medicated adhesive patch (e.g., fentanyl patch) that is placed on the skin to deliver a specific dose of medication through the skin, allowing absorption into the bloodstream.
- Intrathecal injection or infusion of a narcotic or local anesthetic into the subarachnoid space through a needle or catheter provides pain relief to a large area of the body. It may be used as spinal anesthesia for surgery, cancer pain, or relief from spasms that occur with spastic cerebral palsy.
- Epidural analgesia is continuous infusion of a narcotic or local anesthetic into the epidural space by insertion of a needle or catheter for relief of acute or chronic pain. It is used for labor pain, surgery, and cancer pain because it numbs the nerve endings in a local area of the body.

- **Nerve block** is an injection of a local anesthetic into or near spinal nerves for temporary pain control. The anesthetic can be injected into the cervical, thoracic, lumbar, and sacral areas of the spinal column. Nerve blocks can be used for migraine headaches, dental work, back pain, herniated disks, and cancer pain.

Opioid analgesics are essential in adequate pain management, although risks of tolerance, physical dependence, and addiction are associated with their use. The nurse needs to understand these risks and be able to differentiate them. **Drug tolerance** is an adaptation to the medication, which eventually leads to less effective pain relief. It is better to change to another medication than to continue increasing the dose of the same medication. Physical dependence builds as the body becomes unable to function normally without the medication, reaching the point of withdrawal symptoms on abrupt cessation of the medication. Addiction is a psychological or emotional dependence on a medication. The addicted individual craves the medication and engages in compulsive use, or abuse, regardless of the consequences (D'Arcy, 2010). Estimates of addiction among people with chronic pain vary between 3% and 40% (National Institute on Drug Abuse, 2011).

Adjuvant or Coanalgesic Medications

Adjuvant medications, or **coanalgesic medications**, work synergistically with standard pain medications to enhance pain relief and to treat side effects of the medication. For example, tricyclic antidepressants and anticonvulsants may be used together to treat neuropathic pain. Antiemetics are often administered with opioid analgesics to counteract the nausea and vomiting. Laxatives or stool softeners (e.g., senna, docusate) are prescribed to prevent constipation, and antihistamines (e.g., diphenhydramine) are given to decrease the itching side effect of morphine. Ketorolac (Toradol) is an NSAID used along with opioid analgesics to enhance pain relief. Caffeine is used with analgesics to treat migraine headaches.

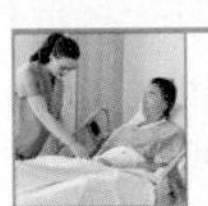

3. Explain why Mr. Charles's medication orders include the stool softener Senokot and the antihistamine Benadryl.

PALLIATIVE CARE

Another option for pain relief is palliative nursing care. The goal of palliative care is to help relieve pain caused by serious illness, regardless of the patient's prognosis. Palliative care is appropriate for patients of any age and for any stage of serious illness. Typically, a group of physicians, nurses, and social workers work as a team to provide the appropriate treatment for the patient. Palliative care improves the quality of life of patients and families who face a life-threatening illness by providing pain and symptom relief and supplying spiritual and psychosocial support from diagnosis to the end of life and bereavement (WHO, 2012a).

THERAPEUTIC DECISION MAKING

The nurse evaluating and administering care to the patient makes the therapeutic decision about the best treatment for that individual on the basis of knowledge of pain relief techniques and the primary care provider (PCP) orders. After vital sign and pain scale assessments are completed, the nurse determines what level of intervention the patient needs. When the PCP has ordered a range of pain medication for a patient, the nurse can titrate the dose on the basis of the patient's pain assessment. If the pain is severe, the nurse may begin with a higher dose or stronger opioid to obtain pain relief. If the patient complains of moderate pain, the nurse may try giving a nonopioid pain medication, such as acetaminophen or ibuprofen. For mild pain, the nurse may try nonpharmacologic interventions before administering a nonopioid pain medication if ordered.

The timing of pain medication administration can be critical in providing adequate pain relief. There is strong support for providing around-the-clock (ATC) dosing of analgesia to prevent pain levels from getting too high. Consistent analgesia helps to maintain medication blood levels and prevent pain recurrence (Vallerand, 2003). If a patient delays asking for pain medication until the pain is severe, the nurse may need to administer higher doses of analgesia or stronger medications to initially get the patient's pain under control. Relief from pain may take longer. In light of this, nurses should administer or encourage patients to take (or request) pain medicine on a scheduled basis, especially when patients are recovering from surgical or diagnostic procedures known to cause moderate to severe pain or when they are experiencing chronic pain.

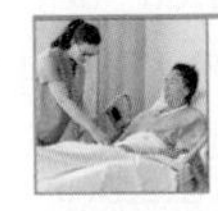

4. Provide the rationale for administering postoperative pain medications intravenously to Mr. Charles instead of orally or intramuscularly.

To determine whether pain relief methods are effective, the nurse evaluates the patient's level of pain relief and documents the results in the patient's chart. The World Health Organization's (2012b) pain relief ladder is a tool that helps health care providers determine which pain medication and adjuvant therapy may be most effective on the basis of the intensity of the reported pain.

BARRIERS TO ADEQUATE MANAGEMENT

There are many barriers to adequate pain management, including a patient's personal barriers (Duigan and Dunn, 2009). Fear of addiction or tolerance to the drug may cause an individual to refuse medication for pain. The cost of medication and no access to health care may be factors. Some people think that pain is inevitable and should be tolerated, believing that "good" patients do not complain about pain.

Health care providers may have barriers as well. Adequate pain relief for patients may be compromised by poor pain assessment skills, inaccurate beliefs, or prejudicial attitudes on the part of health care team members about the experience of pain. Forgetting to consider the culture and personal experiences of patients related to pain may thwart nurses from providing patients with acceptable pain relief. A lack of education regarding physical dependence and addiction may also be a hindrance. The PCP may be overly concerned about the side effects associated with the drugs or about tolerance developing. Sometimes pain relief medication cannot be prescribed until after the patient has been diagnosed, which can cause pain levels to increase so significantly that they become very difficult to get under control.

Pain Management for Addicted Patients

Although addicted patients are entitled to receive pain relief, many PCPs and nurses are reluctant to address their needs or are unsure about how best to do so. The American Society for Pain Management Nursing (ASPMN) provides guidelines for pain management in patients with substance use disorders (Oliver, Coggins, Comptom, et al, 2012). Addicted patients are different from opioid-dependent patients who rely on analgesia for treatment of chronic conditions. Whereas addicted patients exhibit a lack of control and a compulsive need for medication, dependent patients experience an improved quality of life and increased level of function with treatment. Nurses who work with addicted individuals collaborate with PCPs to closely monitor prescription control, document the patient's complaints of pain, and report the effectiveness of prescribed medication (D'Arcy, 2012).

Barriers Within the Health Care System

The barriers to adequate pain management are especially high within the health care system. Pain is often not a high priority for treatment. Systematic pain management approaches and pain management teams may not be in place. There may be inadequate reimbursement for pain medications, and regulations may restrict access to medications.

Patients have a right to pain relief. Inadequate pain management may lead to detrimental outcomes such as:

- Impaired recovery and progression to chronic pain
- Compromised ability to carry out ADLs
- Inability to get adequate rest and sleep, leading to a diminished quality of life
- Significant suffering, with increasing anxiety, depression, fear, and anger
- Work absenteeism and potential underemployment or loss of employment
- Increased health care costs
- Difficulty accessing disability compensation

Patients are not the only ones affected. Relationships with family and friends may be stressed and strained. It is the nurse's responsibility to provide every patient with adequate pain management to ensure maximum relief with the fewest side effects that leads to the highest quality of life possible.

EVALUATION

Evaluation of treatment interventions for patients with pain is based on the attainment of goals and is an ongoing process. If medication intervention is required for pain management, the pain is reassessed and documented. Time intervals for reassessment are patient specific and depend on the route of administration:

Nonpharmacologic techniques	30 to 60 min after intervention
IM, subQ, or PO administration	30 to 60 min after intervention
Transdermal administration	12 to 16 hr after intervention
IV or sublingual administration	15 to 30 min after intervention

The nurse documents the time the medication is given and the time of postintervention reassessment. The nurse is required to document the pain scale on every shift, whether the patient is having pain or is pain free.

When discharging a patient, the nurse is responsible for educating the patient, family, and support persons about the proper administration of medications. Patient education must be documented in the nurse's notes and on the patient education sheet. The patient is given a copy of the education sheet, which explains the medication, its intended purpose, how to take it, and side effects (Patient Education and Health Literacy box).

PATIENT EDUCATION AND HEALTH LITERACY

Providing Medication Education

- When educating the patient about medication administration, turn off the television and hand-held devices to minimize interruptions.
- Make sure the patient has assistive devices in place, such as glasses and hearing aids.
- Teach the patient about the medication currently prescribed, including the name of the medication, the dose, why it is prescribed, when to take it, side effects or adverse effects, and special considerations for taking the medication.
- Provide written instructions for reference after discharge. Include family members and significant others in the teaching, as appropriate.
- Instruct the patient on when to call the health care provider with questions or concerns about the medication.

To provide appropriate nursing care for a patient in pain, the nurse must have an understanding of the pathophysiology of pain, types of pain, physiologic alterations caused by pain, and factors influencing pain. With this knowledge, the nurse can apply the nursing process to develop a patient-centered plan of care, incorporating nonpharmacologic and pharmacologic treatments, and educating the patient and caregivers about the treatment methods. If pain relief goals are unmet, the nurse needs to collaborate with other health care team members and the patient to determine other options for treatment. Nurses must advocate for the most effective pain management regimen possible for every patient.

SUMMARY OF LEARNING OUTCOMES

LO 36.1 *Define pain:* Pain is a subjective sensation that involves the total person, including psychological and physiologic responses. Any definition of pain must include the perceptions of pain and its associated sensations.

LO 36.2 *Describe the role of the nurse in pain management:* The nurse assesses pain using a pain assessment tool and documents the patient's response when vital signs are taken and before and after pain control interventions are performed or analgesics are administered. Pain management and pain relief are essential elements of nursing practice.

LO 36.3 *Explain the physiology of pain and its perception:* Acute injury or tissue damage to the body leads to physiologic stress responses, which are an attempt by the body to protect itself. First, the sympathetic nervous system is stimulated; if pain is not relieved, the parasympathetic nervous system is stimulated. Each body system has its specific response to pain.

LO 36.4 *Articulate factors that influence pain perception and response:* Individual characteristics, such as age, gender, morphology, disabilities, culture, ethnicity, and religion, affect each person's behavioral reaction to pain and its perception. Past experiences with pain and emotional issues may also have an impact on patient response.

LO 36.5 *Determine individual physiologic, behavioral, and psychosocial responses to pain during patient assessment:* The nurse uses cognitive and noncognitive tools to assess physical changes in the patient that are caused by pain, such as increased blood pressure and pulse rate, and behavioral and psychological changes, such as anxiety, fear, and impatience.

LO 36.6 *Identify nursing diagnoses for patients experiencing pain:* Typically, the highest-priority nursing diagnoses for pain are *Acute Pain* and *Chronic Pain.* Other concerns that may need to be addressed when pharmacologic pain interventions are implemented are gastric distress and respiratory depression. Other nursing diagnoses related to emotional distress, such as *Anxiety* or *Fear,* may be associated with pain.

LO 36.7 *Generate nursing care goals and outcome criteria for patients experiencing pain:* The pain level is the primary outcome criterion used in developing pain management goals. The patient's vital signs and changes in behavior may be incorporated into pain-related goals.

LO 36.8 *Plan pain management care that includes implementation and evaluation of pharmacologic and nonpharmacologic interventions for pain:* The nurse talks with the patient, reviews the latest research, and consults other members of the health care team to determine the best course of pain management. Medication, alternative, and complementary therapies may be implemented to provide holistic pain relief.

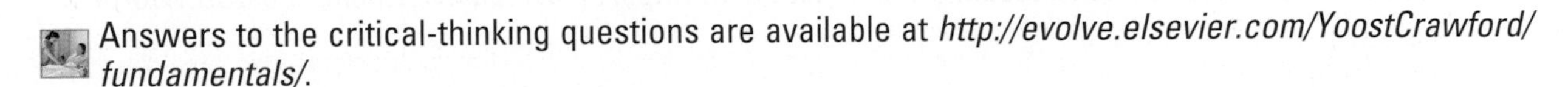

Answers to the critical-thinking questions are available at *http://evolve.elsevier.com/YoostCrawford/fundamentals/.*

REVIEW QUESTIONS

1. When assessing the patient for pain, which factors should the nurse consider? *(Select all that apply.)*
   - **a.** Previous medical history
   - **b.** Physical appearance
   - **c.** Age, gender, and culture
   - **d.** Lifestyle and loss of appetite
   - **e.** Hair color and style

2. Which statement best describes the dosage of pain medication that a nurse should administer given pharmacologic treatment considerations?
   - **a.** The smallest dose possible to avoid opioid addiction
   - **b.** The smallest dose possible to decrease adverse effects
   - **c.** A dose that best manages pain with fewest side effects
   - **d.** A large dose initially to decrease the initial level of pain

3. Which method is the most accurate way to determine the pain level of a patient who is alert and oriented?
   a. Evaluate whether the patient is crying or grimacing.
   b. Assess the patient's heart rate and blood pressure.
   c. Consider the seriousness of the patient's condition.
   d. Use a pain assessment tool and ask the patient to rate the pain level.
4. A patient who has a serious back injury received intravenous medication for pain approximately 1 hour earlier. The patient practices relaxation techniques but still is reporting pain at a level of 9 of 10. What intervention should the nurse implement next?
   a. Report the lack of pain relief to the primary care provider.
   b. Tell the patient to give the medication more time.
   c. Reposition the patient, and try diversion activities.
   d. Document in the nurse's notes that the patient has a low pain tolerance.
5. Which symptom does the nurse recognize as a physiologic response to acute pain?
   a. Increased blood pressure
   b. Decreased pulse
   c. Increased temperature
   d. Restlessness
6. When administering medications to elderly patients, what information does the nurse need to understand?
   a. Start with a low dosage, and increase the dosage as needed for pain relief.
   b. Start with a high dosage, and decrease the dosage as pain is relieved.
   c. Start with a mid-range dosage, and increase or decrease the dosage as needed for pain.
   d. Start with a low dosage, and decrease the dosage as indicated for pain.
7. The nurse administered intravenous morphine at 0830. At what time will the nurse ask the patient if pain relief was obtained?
   a. 1000
   b. 1030
   c. 0900
   d. 0930
8. The patient who had a below the knee amputation 3 days ago complains of pain from the amputated extremity. Which statement by the nurse best explains what the patient is experiencing?
   a. "The phantom pain will subside when the brain realizes the lower extremity is no longer there."
   b. "The radiating pain will continue for months because the lower extremity is no longer there."
   c. "You are suffering from referred pain, which you will always have, but it will lessen with time."
   d. "You are experiencing psychogenic pain because loss of an extremity is an emotional loss."
9. The endocrine system releases excessive hormones during episodes of acute pain. The nurse should monitor patients experiencing acute pain for which potential problem?
   a. Hyperglycemia
   b. Migraine headache
   c. Hyperkalemia
   d. Diarrhea
10. A patient with a fractured femur thinks about vacationing on the beach to relieve pain. What nonpharmacologic pain relief technique should the nurse document the patient is using?
    a. Distraction
    b. Imagery
    c. Relaxation
    d. Biofeedback

ⓔ Answers and rationales for the review questions are available at *http://evolve.elsevier.com/YoostCrawford/fundamentals/*.

REFERENCES

Berry P, Dahl J: The new JCAHO pain standards: Implications for pain management nurses. *Pain Manag Nurses*, 1(1):3-12, 2000.

Bruckenthal P, D'Arcy Y: Assessment and management of pain in older adults: A review of the basics. *Topics Adv Pract Nurs eJ*, (1):1-8, 2007

Cronenwett L, Sherwood G, Barnsteiner J, et al: Quality and safety education for nurses. *Nurs Outlook*, 55(3):122-131, 2007.

D'Arcy Y: Overturning barriers to pain relief in older adults. *Nursing*, 39(10), 32-39, 2009.

D'Arcy Y: Managing chronic pain in acute care. *Nurse Pract*, 35(12):14-16, 2010.

D'Arcy Y: Treating pain in addicted patients, 2012. Retrieved from *http://nurse-practitioners-and-physician-assistants.advanceweb.com/continuing-education/ce-articles/treating-pain-in-addicted-patients.aspx*.

Duigan M, Dunn V: Perceived barriers to pain management. *Emerg Nurse*, 16(9):31-35, 2009.

Eichelbaum M, Ingelman-Sandberg M, Evans W: Pharmacogenomics and individualized drug therapy. *Annu Rev Med*, 57:119-137, 2006.

Glassford B: Range orders for pain medication. *Crit Care Nurse*, 28(4):66-67, 2008.

Helms J, Barone C: Physiology and treatment of pain. *Crit Care Nurse*, 28(6):38-50, 2008.

Holsti L, Grunau R: Initial validation of the behavioral indicators of infant pain. *Pain*, 132(3):264-272, 2007.

Hutt E, Buffum M, Fink R, et al.: Optimizing pain management in long-term care residents. *Geriatrics Aging*, 10(8):523-527, 2007.

Im E, Lee SH, Lim H, et al: A national online forum on ethnic differences in cancer pain experience. *Nurs Res*, 58(2):86-94, 2009.

Institute of Medicine: Relieving pain in America: A blueprint for transforming prevention, care, education and research, 2011. Retrieved from *www.iom.edu/Reports/2011/Relieving-Pain-in-America-A-Blueprint-for-Transforming-Prevention-Care-Education-Research.aspx.*

International Association for the Study of Pain: IASP taxonomy, 2014. Retrieved from *www.iasp-pain.org/Education/Content.aspx?ItemNumber=1698#Pain.*

Janke E, Collins A, Kozak A: Overview of the relationship between pain & obesity: What do we know? Where do we go next? *J Rehabil Res Dev*, 44(2):245-262, 2007.

Kudzma E, Carey E: Pharmacogenomics: Personalizing drug therapy. *Am J Nurs*, 109(10):50-57, 2009.

Mann A: Pharmaceutical pain management, 2010. Retrieved from *http://nursing.advanceweb.com/Article/Pharmaceutical-Pain-Management.aspx.*

Melzack, R: Pain and the neuromatrix in the brain. *J Dent Educ*, 65(12):1378-1382, 2001.

Melzack R, Wall P: Pain mechanisms: A new theory. *Science*, 150:971, 1965.

Mitchell E: Pain control. In F Smith (Ed), *Topics in critical care medicine*, New York, 2010, Cambridge University Press.

National Center for Biotechnology Information: One size does not fit all: The promise of pharmacogenomics, 2004. Retrieved from *www.ncbi.nlm.nih.gov/About/primer/pharm.html.*

National Institute on Drug Abuse (2011). Chronic pain treatment and addiction, 2011. In Prescription Drug Abuse. Retrieved from *www.drugabuse.gov/publications/research-reports/prescription-drugs/chronic-pain-treatment-addiction.*

Nicholson B, Passik S: Management of chronic noncancer pain in the primary care setting. *Southr Med J*, 100(10):1028-1036, 2007.

Oliver J, Coggins, C, Compton, P, et al: American Society for Pain Management Nursing position statement: Pain management in patients with substance use disorders, *Pain Manag Nurs*, 13(3): 169-183, 2012.

Partners Against Pain: Gender and pain management, 2014. Retrieved from *www.partnersagainstpain.com/hcp/pain-management-resources/gender-pain.aspx*

Pasero C, McCaffery M: *Pain assessment and pharmacologic management*, St. Louis, 2011, Mosby.

Schneider JP: *Living with chronic pain*, New York, 2004, Harleigh Press.

Shumay D, Maskarinec G, Kakai H, Gotay C: Why some cancer patients choose complementary and alternative medicine instead of conventional treatment. *J Fam Pract*, 50(12):1067, 2001.

Taylor S: Safety and satisfaction provided by patient-controlled analgesia. *Dimens Crit Care Nurs*, 29(4):163-166, 2010.

Todd E, Kucharski A: Pain: Historical perspectives. In CA Warfield, ZH Bajwa (eds), *Principles and practice of pain medicine*, ed. 2, New York, 2004, McGraw-Hill.

Vallerand A: The use of long-acting opioids in chronic pain management. *Nurs Clin North Am*, 38(3):435-445, 2003.

Value MD: Clinical mnemonics, 2010. Retrieved from *www.valuemd.com.*

World Health Organization (WHO): Access to medications. *WHO Drug Inform*, 21(1):16-17, 2007.

World Health Organization: Access to controlled medications programme: Improving access to medications controlled under international drug conventions [World Health Organization briefing note], 2009. Retrieved from *www.who.int/medicines/areas/quality_safety/ACMP_BrNoteGenrl_EN_Feb09.pdf.*

World Health Organization: WHO definition of palliative care, 2012a. Retrieved from *www.who.int/cancer/palliative/definition/en/.*

World Health Organization: WHO's pain ladder, 2012b. Retrieved from *www.who.int/cancer/palliative/painladder/en/index.html.*

Zalon M, Constantino R, Andrews K: The right to pain treatment: A reminder for nurses. *Dimens Crit Care Nurs*, 27(3):93-101, 2008.

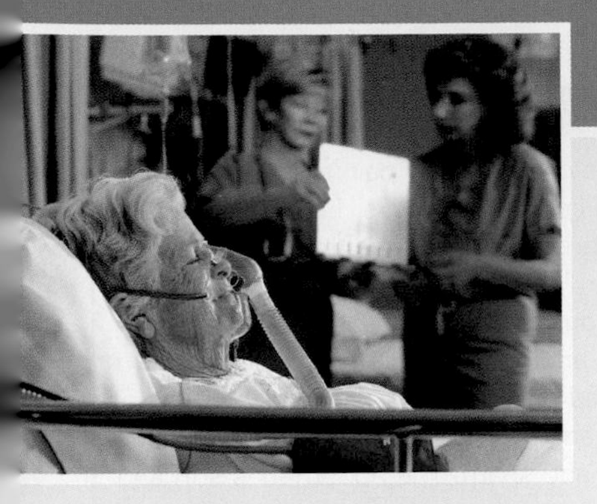

CHAPTER 37

Perioperative Nursing Care

EVOLVE WEBSITE

http://evolve.elsevier.com/YoostCrawford/fundamentals/

- Additional Evolve-Only Review Questions With Answers
- Answers and Rationales for Text Review Questions
- Answers to Critical-Thinking Questions
- Case Study With Questions
- Conceptual Care Map
- Video Skills Clips
- Skill Checklist
- Glossary

LEARNING OUTCOMES

Comprehension of this chapter's content will provide students with the ability to:

LO 37.1 Differentiate between the phases of the perioperative period.
LO 37.2 Classify different types of surgery.
LO 37.3 Discuss safety during the perioperative period.
LO 37.4 Describe alterations that can occur during the perioperative period.
LO 37.5 Identify vital perioperative assessment data.
LO 37.6 Select nursing diagnoses for each perioperative stage.
LO 37.7 Establish nursing care goals and outcome criteria for surgical patients.
LO 37.8 Evaluate the effectiveness of the perioperative nursing interventions.

KEY TERMS

airway obstruction, p. 933
anesthesia, p. 911
atelectasis, p. 935
bier block, p. 920
circulating nurse, p. 912
elective surgery, p. 914
emergency surgery, p. 914
epidural anesthesia, p. 920
general anesthesia, p. 919
hemorrhage, p. 933
informed consent, p. 926
intraoperative phase, p. 911
laryngospasm, p. 917
local anesthesia, p. 920
major surgery, p. 914
malignant hyperthermia, p. 917
minor surgery, p. 914
moderate sedation, p. 918
nerve block, p. 920
perioperative nursing, p. 910
perioperative period, p. 910
pneumonia, p. 934
postoperative phase, p. 912
preoperative phase, p. 910
pulmonary embolism, p. 934
regional anesthesia, p. 919
scrub nurse, p. 922
sedation, p. 918
shock, p. 934
spinal anesthesia, p. 920
thrombophlebitis, p. 934
topical anesthesia, p. 920
urgent surgery, p. 914

CASE STUDY

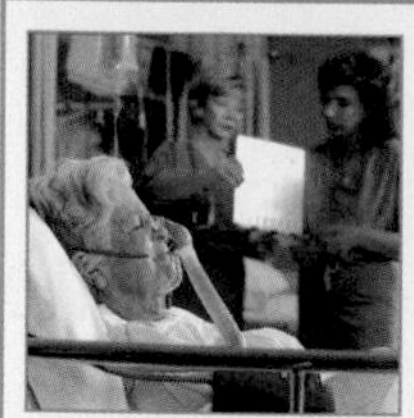

Mrs. Logan is a 72-year-old female admitted to the hospital with a diagnosis of abdominal pain and cholecystitis that requires surgery. She has no known drug allergies (NKDA) and has full code status. Mrs. Logan states that she is "afraid of surgery and nervous about being under anesthesia." She has never had surgery before and states she "doesn't know what to expect." Her preoperative vital signs are T 37° C (98.6° F), P 104 and regular, R 24 and shallow, BP 150/88, with a pulse oximetry reading of 94% on room air and pain level of 4 of 10.

A laparoscopic cholecystectomy is performed under general anesthesia, and Mrs. Logan is transferred from the postanesthesia care unit (PACU) to a surgical unit. Her vital signs on admission to the surgical floor are T 36.8° C (98.2° F), P 74 and regular, R 18 and unlabored, BP 138/82, with a pulse oximetry reading of 98% on 2 L of O_2 via face mask and pain level of 6 of 10. The pain is located in her abdomen and described as throbbing and sharp. The abdomen is soft and tender with three adhesive bandages over the puncture wounds where the laparoscopic instruments were inserted during surgery, and one 2 × 2 gauze pad applied over the small incisions near the umbilicus where the laparoscope was inserted. All dressings are dry and intact. She has a history of hypertension.

Treatment orders are as follows:

- Vital signs with O_2 saturation q 4 hr
- Incentive spirometry q 1 hr while awake
- Bed rest with bathroom privileges (BRP) with assistance
- Sequential compression devices (SCDs) while in bed
- Intake and output (I&O) every shift
- Assess voiding, bladder scan if unable to void in 6 hours
- Abdominal dressing change every shift
- Advance to clear liquid diet when bowel sounds return

Medication orders are as follows:

- Intravenous (IV) 5% dextrose and 0.9% sodium chloride at 100 mL/hr
- Ancef 2 g intravenous piggyback (IVPB) q 8 hr
- Hydrochlorothiazide 25 mg PO daily
- Potassium 20 PO mEq daily
- Lovenox 40 mg subcut daily
- Tylenol #3, 2 tablets PO q 4 hr PRN for moderate pain
- Morphine 10 mg IV q 4 hr PRN for severe pain
- Zofran 4 mg IV q 8 hr PRN for nausea

Refer back to this case study to answer the critical-thinking exercises throughout the chapter.

Surgery is a significant event in an individual's life. It is a major decision involving the patient's body and health. Surgery may be performed to diagnose a medical disease, reconstruct or remove diseased tissue or organs, improve appearance, or relieve symptoms or pain.

The patient undergoing planned or unplanned surgery experiences unique physical adaptations. The operation becomes the central focus for these patients, and the thought of having surgery can cause stress and anxiety. The patient and family may have to adapt physically, socially, and psychologically before and after the surgical procedure.

Perioperative nursing is the care nurses provide for patients before, during, and after surgery. Perioperative nurses plan, direct, and coordinate the care of every patient undergoing operative and other invasive procedures. They are responsible for patient outcomes resulting from the nursing care provided during the perioperative experience.

PHASES OF SURGERY LO 37.1

The patient having a procedure goes through three phases: preoperative, intraoperative, and postoperative. Each patient receives individualized care with safety as a priority to minimize risks and complications. The three phases together are known as the **perioperative period.**

PREOPERATIVE PHASE

The first phase of surgery is known as the **preoperative phase**. Depending on the patient's health status, this phase may last for several months. In an emergency situation, the preoperative period may be a few hours or less. It begins when the patient decides to have surgery. Typically, patients, or their families when the patient is not cognitively or emotionally competent, make this decision in collaboration with a surgeon. The agreement to have surgery validates the patient's want or need for surgery and confirms that the procedure will take place.

After the agreement, the patient undergoes diagnostic testing and other procedures. Nursing activities focus on preparing the patient for surgery. The ultimate goal of nursing care is to promote positive surgical outcomes. The nurse assesses the patient and identifies actual or potential health problems. All preoperative forms are completed. Physician's orders are implemented. Preoperative teaching begins, and supportive care is provided. This includes explaining the necessity for preoperative tests. Risk assessment by a member of the anesthesia team is performed during this period.

In an emergency situation, there is not always time for all of the preoperative activities to occur. The surgeon decides how soon surgery needs to be performed and which diagnostic tests and assessments are required. The preoperative phase ends when the patient is transferred to the operating room.

INTRAOPERATIVE PHASE

The second phase is known as the **intraoperative phase**. It begins when the patient enters the operating room. During this phase, the patient is anesthetized, monitored, prepped, and draped, and the surgical procedure is performed. The Agency for Healthcare Research and Quality (AHRQ, 2009b) and The Joint Commission (2014) recommend implementing a time out before the procedure begins to help eliminate risk. During the time out, all personnel in the operating room stop what they are doing and use active communication. This allows a final assessment to verify the correct patient, procedure, and surgical site. The time out is documented. Throughout the intraoperative phase, nursing activities focus on safety, infection prevention, and physiologic response to **anesthesia**, which is provided by an agent (anesthetic) that makes the patient insensitive to pain and sensation.

Positioning

An important task of the surgical team is properly positioning the patient. Intraoperative injuries can occur and have devastating effects on the patient. Injuries resulting from improper positioning can be short term, such as minor discomfort, or long term, such as pressure ulcers or nerve damage. The patient is commonly positioned for the surgical procedure after having anesthetized. Proper positioning allows safety to be maintained. The patient is placed in a functional position with good body alignment. Pressure points are padded, and an electrical grounding pad is placed under the patient. Special precautions are taken when a patient is very thin, obese, or elderly or has a physical deformity.

The entire surgical team is responsible for properly positioning the patient. Attachments to the operating table, straps, pillows, and wedges are used to ensure proper positioning. Proper positioning allows access to the patient's airway and the surgical site, and it permits the nurse to monitor vital signs, IV lines, and comfort level. Common positions used in the operating room include supine or dorsal recumbent, prone, lithotomy, sitting, lateral, Trendelenburg, and jackknife (Litwack, 2009). Figure 37-1 shows these surgical positions, and Table 37-1 describes their use.

> **! SAFE PRACTICE ALERT**
>
> The supine position ensures a significant degree of patient immobility and access to many surgical sites.

> **! SAFE PRACTICE ALERT**
>
> Obese patients with respiratory and cardiovascular disease may have difficulty lying supine, which may result in hypotension and spinal occlusion of the inferior vena cava. A towel can be positioned under the right lower back and hip to correct the inferior vena cava occlusion by causing the patient to shift to the left side.

Preparing the Surgical Site

After positioning, the skin is prepared for the surgical procedure to minimize the risk of postoperative infection. Skin preparation consists of removing the hair, cleansing the skin, and using an antimicrobial agent (Evidence-Based Practice and Informatics box). Hair is left in place on the surgical site when possible. Some procedures may require the hair to be removed preoperatively. Hair removal depends on the location of the surgical incision, the type of surgery, and the amount of hair at the incision site. If hair is removed, precautions must be taken to prevent injury to the skin. Clippers can be used for hair removal. If hair is removed from the head, the patient is asked preoperatively how he or she would like the hair to be cared for. Some patients may want to save the hair for cultural or religious reasons.

> **EVIDENCE-BASED PRACTICE AND INFORMATICS**
>
> **Preoperative Preparations**
>
> - *Shower:* The patient is instructed to shower or bathe with an antimicrobial soap the day of surgery or the day before the surgical procedure if outpatient surgery is planned. A shower or bath is given preoperatively if the patient is hospitalized. Assistance is provided if the patient is unable to bathe independently.
> - *Hair removal:* To decrease the risk of infection, hair is not routinely removed from the surgical site. The surgeon decides whether hair removal is indicated. Electric clippers are used. The clippers should have a head that can be sterilized before it is used again or a disposable head. Razors are not recommended because they can increase the risk of infection.
> - *Documentation:* Skin preparation is documented on the intraoperative record. More information is available from *www.ncbi.nlm.nih.gov/pubmed/18616201* and the Agency for Healthcare Research and Quality (AHRQ, 2008).

The skin is cleansed and dried with a sterile towel. After the skin has been prepped, surgical draping begins. Drapes are applied to create a sterile field, maintain the patient's privacy, and only expose the surgical site.

Safety is a priority of all surgical team members during the intraoperative period because the patient is totally dependent on the team while under anesthesia. The intraoperative period ends when the patient is transferred to the postanesthesia care unit (PACU), also called the recovery room.

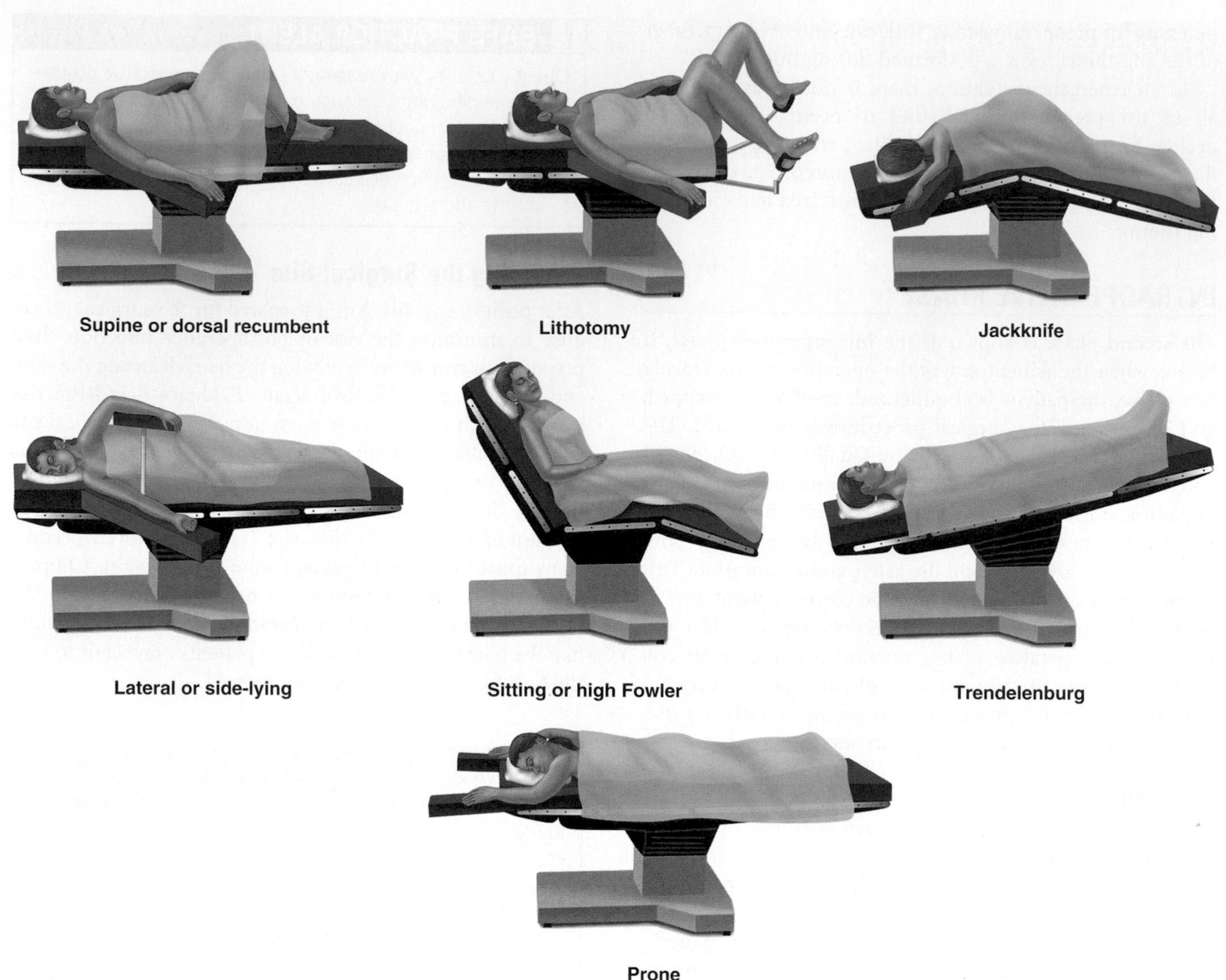

FIGURE 37-1 Surgical positions.

POSTOPERATIVE PHASE

The **postoperative phase** is the third phase of surgery. It begins when the patient is admitted to the PACU and ends when the patient has completely recovered from the surgical procedure, which may be several months. To ensure a smooth transition to the PACU, the anesthesiologist and **circulating nurse**, who is the patient's advocate and a liaison between scrubbed personnel and the surgical team, often accompany the patient to the PACU. The Joint Commission recommends using hand-off communication, which takes place between the intraoperative nurse and the postoperative nurse. The anesthesiologist also may provide hand-off communication to the postoperative nurse. The communication should include an update on the status of the patient and medications given during the procedure.

During the postoperative phase, the patient begins to recover from surgery and anesthesia. The postoperative nurse assesses the patient's response to the surgical procedure, carries out nursing interventions to prevent complications, and promotes healing (Woodruff, 2008). Priority nursing assessments include assessing the respiratory, circulatory, and neurologic status of the patient. The pain level is monitored. Blood pressure, pulse oximetry, and cardiac monitoring are initiated.

TYPES OF SURGERY LO 37.2

Surgical procedures can be classified according to the purpose, degree of urgency, and degree of risk. The classifications assist the nurse in recognizing the level of care that is required for a patient. Keep in mind that these classifications can overlap.

CLASSIFICATION BY PURPOSE

Surgical procedures can be grouped based on their purpose. Terms used to classify surgical procedures are diagnostic,

TABLE 37-1 Positions for Surgical Procedures

POSITION	DESCRIPTION AND TYPE OF SURGERY	POTENTIAL POSITIONING INJURIES
Supine (horizontal recumbent)	Flat on back (thoracic, heart, abdominal)	Backache Nerve injury Postural hypotension Pressure alopecia Pressure point compression
Dorsal recumbent	Flat on back with knees flexed and hips externally rotated (thoracic, heart, vaginal)	Backache Nerve injury Postural hypotension Pressure alopecia Pressure point compression Hip and leg discomfort
Prone	Flat on abdomen (posterior thorax, spine, back of legs)	Neck pain Nerve injury Joint damage Eye abrasion Ear abrasion Reduced respiratory circulation Injury to breasts and male genitalia
Lithotomy	Flat on back and legs up in stirrups (gynecologic, perineal, rectal, genitourinary)	Lower back pain Perineal nerve injury related to stirrups Hypotension
Sitting	Upright or semi-reclining with legs elevated to the level of the heart (breast, thoracic, head, neck)	Airway edema Cerebral air embolism Facial edema Hypotension Tachycardia
Lateral	Side-lying (thoracic, kidney, hip)	Neck pain Nerve injury Ventilation-perfusion mismatch Eye abrasion Ear abrasion Venous pooling in dependent extremities
Trendelenburg	Flat on back, head down, feet elevated	Airway problems Difficulty breathing Backache Nerve injury
Jackknife	Placed on abdomen, head lowered, feet lowered, buttocks up (rectal)	Neck pain Nerve injury Joint damage Eye abrasion Ear abrasion Reduced respiratory circulation

BOX 37-1 Purposes of Surgical Procedures

- *Diagnostic:* Establishes or confirms a diagnosis (e.g., laparoscopy of the abdomen)
- *Ablative:* Removes a part of the body that is diseased (e.g., removal of a gangrenous toe)
- *Constructive:* Restores functioning that has been lost or reduced (e.g., cleft lip or palate)
- *Reconstructive or restorative:* Restores function or appearance of traumatized or malnourished tissues (e.g., skin graft for a burn victim, reconstruction after cancer surgery)
- *Transplantation:* Replaces dysfunctional body part (e.g., heart, kidney)
- *Palliative:* Improves comfort and decreases pain or symptoms but does not cure (e.g., back surgery to decrease pressure).
- *Cosmetic:* Improves personal appearance (e.g., liposuction)

ablative, constructive, reconstructive or restorative, transplantation, palliative, and cosmetic (Box 37-1).

CLASSIFICATION BY DEGREE OF URGENCY

The degree of urgency is determined by the surgeon. All presurgical screening examinations and diagnostic testing results are reviewed. After the degree of urgency has been determined, the operating room can be scheduled for the appropriate time.

Elective Surgery

Elective surgery is a procedure that is performed to improve the patient's quality of life. The patient's health may improve physically and psychologically. Elective procedures are planned in advance, and the patient chooses when to undergo surgery. The date selected to perform the procedure is based on the convenience of the patient and surgeon. Other factors to be considered are adequate time for preparation, planning, and evaluation of the patient.

Elective surgery is not considered an urgent procedure. Examples of elective surgery include hysterectomy for uterine fibroids and cholecystectomy for chronic gallbladder disease.

Urgent Surgery

Some patients have a medical problem that has the potential for complications to develop if a surgical procedure is not performed. **Urgent surgery** is performed when the patient's health condition is not immediately life-threatening. Failure to have the surgical procedure performed may result in complications or death. Surgery is required within 24 hours of the diagnosis to avoid preventable complications.

Because urgent surgery does not need to be performed immediately, the patient can continue to be evaluated over the next 24 hours. Examples of urgent surgery include hip pinning for a hip fracture and bowel resection to remedy a bowel obstruction.

Emergency Surgery

When a patient has a critical medical problem, emergency surgery may be needed. **Emergency surgery** is a procedure that is unanticipated and is performed immediately to preserve the life of the patient, a body part, or body function. Delay of this surgery can have a detrimental effect on the patient. Morbidity and mortality rates increase with emergency surgery because of risks associated with the underlying medical problem, surgical procedure, and medications administered during and after surgery. Examples of emergency surgery include control of internal bleeding caused by a gunshot wound and appendectomy to treat a perforated appendix.

CLASSIFICATION BY DEGREE OF RISK

The degree of risk of a surgical procedure depends on the surgical procedure, health status, coexisting illnesses, and physical fitness. A healthy person with no preexisting health conditions has a better chance of surviving surgery without complications. Some health conditions increase risk and may cause surgery to be cancelled until the patient's health has improved. Based on the degree of risk, surgery can be classified as major or minor.

Minor Surgery

When surgical alteration of the body is minimal and there is low risk to the life of the patient, the operation is classified as **minor surgery**. Many minor surgical procedures require little or no anesthesia and respiratory assistance. Most minor procedures are associated with few postoperative complications. Cataract surgery and a breast biopsy are examples of minor surgical procedures.

Major Surgery

When there is a higher risk to the life of the patient and surgery involves reconstruction or alteration of a body part, it is classified as **major surgery**. Anesthesia and respiratory assistance are usually required. Major surgery may be a complicated or prolonged procedure with a large amount of blood loss involving vital organs, and it may have a higher risk of postoperative complications. Mastectomy and a bowel resection are examples of major surgery.

Factors Affecting the Degree of Risk

All surgical procedures have some degree of risk. People in good health have lower risks. Certain health conditions increase the surgical risk for complications such as infection, delayed wound healing, and anesthesia reactions (Diversity Considerations box).

DIVERSITY CONSIDERATIONS

Life Span

- Older adults and children have greater risks associated with surgery.
- Infants have an immature sympathetic nervous system, which can increase the risk of bradycardia during surgery.
- Infants have lower blood volumes, and blood loss can contribute to dehydration and the inability to respond to an increased oxygen demand.
- The infant's renal system metabolizes drugs slower, and the immature liver can lead to lengthened effects of narcotic medications.
- Shivering reflexes are not well developed in infants, and they have a relatively large body surface area that contributes to difficultly maintaining a stable body temperature, resulting in hyperthermia or hypothermia.
- The immune system is immature in infants, which compromises the ability to resist infection.
- Older adults may have unique physical, physiologic, and pharmacologic changes that can influence how the body responds to anesthesia, which affects preoperative and postoperative care.
- Many older adults have a decreased physiologic reserve that can reduce the ability to compensate for changes that take place during the surgical procedure.
- Certain disorders combined with anesthesia and surgery amplify the surgical risk for older adults. Complications may include infection, anemia, and hemorrhage.
- There is the potential for a fluid and electrolyte imbalance because older adults have a smaller percentage of body water, a decreased thirst response, and decreased kidney function.

Culture, Ethnicity, and Religion

- Cultural influences, beliefs, and practices can influence how a patient responds to surgery and pain, which can have a positive or negative impact on the patient. Cultural beliefs may contribute to stress, anxiety, and fear related to surgery.
- Patients who do not speak English may have difficulty understanding, which can increase stress, anxiety, and fear related to the surgical procedure.
- Certain groups do not believe in blood transfusions, which can present a risk in operations in which a large volume of blood is lost. Some of these patients may be able to donate and store their own blood before surgery.

Disability

- Any disorder that causes extreme anxiety, hinders the ability to understand, interferes with coping with the stress of surgery, or impedes the patient's ability to respond appropriately can increase the risks of surgery and postoperative complications.

Morphology

- Malnutrition can lead to a delay in wound healing, infection, fluid and electrolyte imbalances, and fatigue.
- Obesity can cause significant mechanical difficulty for the surgeon. It can lead to excessive blood loss and problems exposing, accessing, and retracting tissue of the surgical site.
- During the postoperative phase, the obese patient may have difficulty with lung expansion, which can contribute to the development of pneumonia and wound infections. The increased depth and size of the surgical wound may cause wound infections and poor wound healing.
- People who are obese have higher risks of delays in metabolizing medications, hypertension, and cardiovascular, respiratory, and gastrointestinal complications.
- Hypoxemia is often associated with obesity due to increased respiratory effort, ventilation-perfusion mismatch, closure of small airways, and reduced total lung capacity.

General Health

All patients who are scheduled to have surgery have a careful review of their current health status. When a person is in a poor state of health, surgery may be delayed or cancelled. When a patient's risk for infection is high, antibiotics are given prophylactically to allow the medication to reach therapeutic levels in tissues before surgery.

Medications

Over-the-counter, prescribed, or herbal medications can increase surgical risk and affect how the patient responds to the stress of undergoing surgery or anesthesia. During assessment, the nurse questions the patient about all medications taken at home. The following adverse interactions occur when medications are combined with surgery or anesthetic agents:

- Diuretics contribute to fluid and electrolyte imbalances.
- Anticoagulants increase the risk for bleeding and are discontinued before surgery.
- Tranquilizers increase the risk of respiratory depression.
- Corticosteroids increase the risk of bleeding, increase the risk of infection, and delay wound healing and immune response.
- Medications that affect the central nervous system can interfere with anesthesia.
- Herbal medications can affect the patient's reaction to the stress of surgery. Some herbal medications may potentiate the action of some anesthetic agents, and others may increase the risk of bleeding.

! SAFE PRACTICE ALERT

When conducting a health assessment, ask about herbal and over-the-counter medications.

Mental and Cognitive Status

Disorders that affect cognitive functioning, such as schizophrenia, dementia, developmental delay, and mental retardation, compromise a person's ability to interpret and understand medical information. These disorders can increase the surgical risk and interfere with the patient's ability to follow instructions and care for the surgical wound. Some individuals may be prescribed antipsychotic or anticonvulsant medications, which can interact with anesthetic agents.

Surgery is a major psychological stressor. Extreme anxiety and fear increase the surgical risk and cause the patient to have difficulty understanding information. Anxiety may be expressed as frustration, anger, withdrawal, crying, or questioning. Patients commonly fear that they will experience severe pain after surgery, the anesthesia will not put them to sleep, they will not be able to tell anyone that they feel intense pain, or they will not wake up from the anesthesia. Patients fear the unknown, and education about what to expect in each phase of the perioperative period helps to allay some fears and to decrease stress and anxiety. Nurses encourage patients to verbalize concerns and fears. In some cases, patients may need counseling before the surgical procedure. Nurses determine the support systems and coping skills of the patient before the surgical procedure.

Nutrition

Malnutrition and obesity increase surgical risks. Nutrients are necessary to promote wound healing and resist infection. Protein and vitamin K deficiencies contribute to poor wound healing, respiratory depression, sedation, and clotting disorders. A protein deficiency interferes with a drug's ability to bind with proteins. As a result, plasma concentrations of drugs can remain elevated, increasing the risk for side effects and adverse effects of medications given. Vitamin K deficiency can lead to increased bleeding.

Cardiac Disorders

Cardiovascular diseases increase the risk of surgery. Disorders such as myocardial infarction (MI), dysrhythmias, chest pain, hypertension, and heart failure (HF) need to be managed or controlled before surgery. Recent MI, chest pain, and dysrhythmias increase the risk of a second MI and life-threatening dysrhythmias. When a patient has hypertension, the scheduled dose of antihypertensive medication may be given before surgery. If hypertension is not controlled, the risk of anesthesia and surgical complications significantly increases. In some cases, diuretics are withheld if the patient does not have a Foley catheter inserted or fluid loss is expected during surgery. HF may cause surgery to be delayed due to the risk of additional fluid and electrolyte imbalances.

Blood Coagulation Disorders

Bleeding, hemorrhage, blood clots, and shock can be caused by coagulation disorders, which can significantly increase surgical risk. Laboratory results for prothrombin, thrombin, platelets, red blood cells, hemoglobin, and hematocrit are monitored to help identify potential risks.

Respiratory Disorders

A thorough assessment of the respiratory system is completed before surgery. Some anesthetics cause respiratory depression, predisposing the patient to greater surgical risk. Respiratory disorders such as chronic obstructive pulmonary disease (COPD) and pneumonia can increase the risk of respiratory depression during surgery.

Renal Disorders

Renal disorders contribute to fluid and electrolyte imbalances, which can increase the risk of surgery. People with acute or chronic renal failure may not be good surgical candidates. They have the additional risks of blood pressure abnormalities, acid-base imbalances, fluid instability, and a metabolism that is not able to excrete drugs properly.

Liver Disease

Liver disease interferes with metabolism, protein synthesis, coagulation, and glucose homeostasis. These manifestations of liver disease can contribute to fluid and electrolyte imbalances, acid-base imbalances, and altered excretion and metabolism of drugs, each of which can increase surgical risk.

Diabetes Mellitus

Diabetes can increase the risk of delayed wound healing. On the day of surgery, patients may not be able to have anything by mouth (NPO). Glucose levels are monitored closely, and insulin doses are adjusted accordingly. Oral hypoglycemic agents may be withheld. Glucose levels may fluctuate in people with diabetes because of the stress of surgery resulting in hypoglycemia or hyperglycemia. The stress of surgery often causes elevated glucose levels. This may result in patients temporarily receiving insulin even when this is not part of their preoperative medication regimen. IV insulin is often used during surgical procedures.

! SAFE PRACTICE ALERT

It is important to monitor glucose levels closely because they may elevate due to the stress of surgery.

Use of Illicit Drugs and Nicotine

People who use illicit drugs and nicotine have a higher risk of adverse drug interactions. Certain drugs change the way anesthetics work during surgery. Drugs that are commonly abused include cocaine, marijuana, alcohol, and opiates. When these drugs are taken, a potentially dangerous situation can develop for the patient.

Wound healing is compromised if a patient smokes because smoking causes vasoconstriction, resulting in decreased blood flow. Smoking contributes to decreased ciliary action in the tracheobronchial tree, and mucous secretions may increase. The tracheobronchial tree may become chronically irritated, and anesthesia can increase this irritation.

Before surgery is an excellent time to teach a smoker about the effects and risks of smoking. Smoking puts a person at risk for reactive airway disease, which can contribute to complications such as laryngospasm. A **laryngospasm** causes the laryngeal muscle to suddenly contract (spasm), blocking air inflow. A laryngospasm typically lasts for less than 1 minute, during which the patient has trouble speaking and breathing. If intubation is required, it may be very difficult. When possible, patients are encouraged to stop smoking 6 weeks before having surgery. If patients are unable to cease smoking weeks ahead of surgery, abstaining for 24 to 48 hours before surgery can have a positive impact.

Family History

Understanding family history is important. It should be determined whether family members had surgery in the past and whether there were complications associated with surgery or anesthesia. Obtaining a thorough history of anesthesia problems of family members or the patient can help to determine the likelihood of complications developing in the current situation. If a patient reveals there were complications related to anesthesia in the past, their causes are discussed.

Malignant hyperthermia (MH) is a rare, hereditary, and life-threatening condition that usually occurs when inhaled general anesthetics or a neuromuscular blocking agent is administered. Susceptibility to MH is inherited as an autosomal dominant disorder, which occurs when one parent carries the trait (mutated gene) for the disease. It usually occurs during the intraoperative or early postoperative phases, but it has occurred during exercise and on exposure to hot environments.

MH causes severe muscle contractions and a rapid elevation of the body temperature. During an acute episode, the patient can develop a very high fever, cyanosis, muscle rigidity, hypertension, tachycardia, tachypnea, hyperkalemia, dysrhythmias, and acidosis. This change in body chemistry can be life-threatening, and result in death without proper treatment. Even with treatment, the patient may die of MH. The signs of this disorder must be recognized early so that treatment can begin promptly. When MH occurs, surgery is stopped, and anesthesia is discontinued. Treatment consists of oxygen, IV fluids, and cooling the patient. Dantrolene sodium (Dantrium) is used to alleviate muscle spasms.

Previous Surgery

Previous operations and the patient's response to anesthesia are assessed. If there were complications from surgery or anesthesia, the surgical risk is increased because of the potential for these problems to occur again. It is possible for previous operations to influence a patient's psychological and physiologic response to subsequent surgery. A past negative surgical experience may contribute to the patient experiencing stress, anxiety, and fear.

SURGICAL SETTINGS

Surgical procedures traditionally occur in the hospital setting (Figure 37-2). Most hospitals are able to accommodate a wide variety of surgical procedures, including complex procedures with a high degree of risk. Patients may be hospitalized and transferred to the operating room or admitted the day of surgery to decrease costs. For patients admitted the day of surgery, all laboratory and diagnostic tests are performed

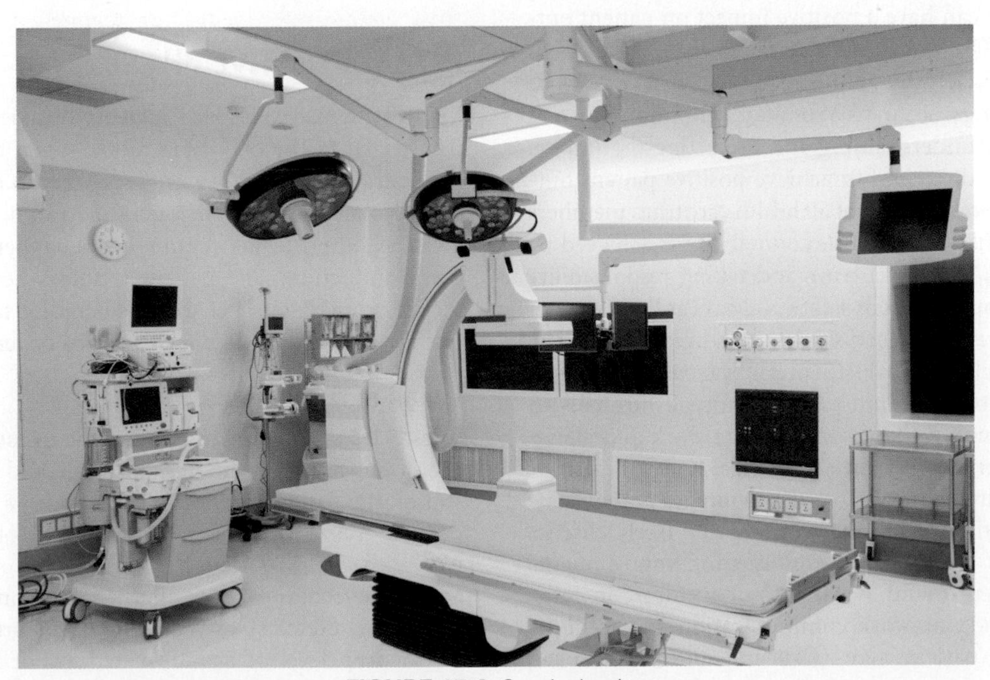

FIGURE 37-2 Surgical suite.

before the day of surgery. The patient's response to surgery and anesthesia is evaluated. The physician determines whether the patient is admitted to the hospital after surgery or discharged to home.

Many operations that used to require a hospital stay are now much less invasive and commonly performed on an outpatient basis. This decreases costs associated with hospitalization. Operations can be performed in ambulatory care centers, same-day surgery centers, and outpatient centers. These facilities are designed for the patient to be admitted the morning of surgery and go home the same day. The centers can be freestanding or affiliated with a hospital. Some centers perform a variety of procedures, and some specialize in a particular area. Examples of specialized ambulatory centers are eye surgery centers and plastic surgery centers.

SAFETY CONCERNS DURING SURGERY LO 37.3

The Association of periOperative Registered Nurses (AORN) has identified patient safety as a major goal. Perioperative nurses should be knowledgeable about AORN's Perioperative Standards and Recommended Practices (AORN, 2012). These standards should be integrated into clinical practice, such as during surgery.

Nurses participate in patient safety programs and hold peers accountable for all safety standards (Banschbach, 2008). Communication is important in the operating room to ensure patient safety. If the sterile field or technique is broken, the behavior that does not follow patient safety guidelines is addressed immediately, such as with the following examples: "You contaminated your glove," and "The patient's arm is not straight; it needs to be repositioned." The communication style of the nurse can have a positive impact on patient outcomes (Beyea, 2008). Being assertive rather than aggressive is viewed more positively.

Successful surgery occurs as a result of a common goal and the surgical team understanding and respecting the importance of each person's role. To achieve positive patient outcomes, mutual accountability of all health care team members is needed (Banschbach, 2008). Accountability is achieved by preventing errors from occurring and taking responsibility when they do happen. Patient safety is always at the forefront of the health care team's actions in the surgical suite. The Joint Commission's National Patient Safety Goals (2014) state that a universal protocol must be used by all hospitals to create an environment that promotes teamwork and allows employees to promote patient safety. Health care organizations create a culture of safety that encourages an environment in which the perioperative team can freely discuss concerns such as errors and suggestions for improvements without fear of reprimand. A patient safety culture in combination with good teamwork, communication, and accountability improves patient care (Catalano and Fickenscher, 2008).

> **! SAFE PRACTICE ALERT**
>
> Patient safety is always at the forefront of the health care team's actions. The nurse uses at least two patient identifiers before administering nursing care, treatments, or procedures.

ALTERED STRUCTURE AND FUNCTION DURING PHASES OF SURGERY LO 37.4

Physiologic and psychological alterations may occur in each phase of surgery. The extent of the alteration depends on the individual patient's physical and emotional state, the type of surgery and anesthesia used, and the patient's individual risk factors.

PREOPERATIVE PHASE

The thought of having surgery can cause emotional responses by the patient and their family members. The patient scheduled for surgery often experiences stress, anxiety, and fear. The patient is encouraged to ask questions before the surgical procedure (American College of Surgeons, 2014). The nurse can use therapeutic communication to establish a positive and trusting nurse-patient relationship. When attempting to decrease stress, anxiety, and fear, it is important for the nurse to avoid providing the patient false reassurance. Providing information and preoperative teaching on the surgery, pain management, and how to perform activities to reduce the risk for postoperative complications can help patients and allay some of their concerns (Litwack, 2009).

INTRAOPERATIVE PHASE

Many patients experience increased anxiety after they are transferred to the operating room. When the patient enters the operating room, they are told what to expect and introduced to all people in the operating room. Explanations are given in simple terms about what is happening before anesthesia induction. The patient is told when they are being moved from a stretcher to the operating table, when an IV line is started, and when anesthesia is begun.

Types of Anesthesia

Anesthetic agents are chosen by the anesthesia team. This decision is based on the type, location, and length of surgery and on the patient's condition.

Sedation

Moderate sedation, also known as conscious sedation, induces an altered state of consciousness providing a moderate to deep level of **sedation** (a state of calm or reduced anxiety), amnesia, and analgesia that minimizes pain and discomfort. This is achieved by using pain medications and sedatives. Patients receiving conscious sedation may be asked to speak or respond to verbal cues during the surgical procedure. They are able to communicate discomfort experienced and are able to maintain an open airway. For some patients, a short period of amnesia obliterates their memory of the procedure.

When the patient is not being monitored by the anesthesia team, the registered nurse monitors the patient. Nurses who provide sedation conduct an airway and presedation assessment (Ogg and Burlingame, 2008). The nurse monitoring the patient who is receiving sedation does not leave the patient unattended and must be able to identify adverse reactions. The nurse is prepared to respond appropriately if the patient becomes heavily sedated or other complications develop.

General Anesthesia

Major operations are performed under **general anesthesia**, which causes central nervous system depression and puts the patient in a drug-induced coma. This type of anesthesia causes a loss of consciousness, loss of sensation, amnesia, analgesia, and skeletal muscle relaxation. It is considered very safe and has few side effects. The term *balanced anesthesia* is often used to describe general anesthesia because the goal is to attain a balance among analgesia, hypnosis, and immobility.

Risks associated with general anesthesia are circulatory and respiratory depression. General anesthesia is commonly administered by gases, volatile liquids that are vaporized and inhaled with oxygen, or intravenous drugs. A blend of inhaled gases and intravenous drugs is commonly used. Patients who receive general anesthesia cannot be aroused, even in response to painful stimulation. Individuals undergoing general anesthesia may not be able to maintain their airway or breathe on their own. Most inhaled anesthetic agents can be rapidly modified if necessary. Anesthetics given intravenously are more difficult to change or modify after they have been administered.

The four stages of general anesthesia were developed to help health care providers evaluate induction of and emergence from anesthesia. When general anesthesia is given, the patient moves through stages I and II to stage III. Surgery is performed during stage III. After anesthetic agents have been discontinued, patients can emerge from anesthesia into consciousness backward through all three stages. During induction, a patient can move to stage IV (anesthetic overdose); this stage represents a great danger and can result in death. Table 37-2 describes the stages of general anesthesia.

The nurse should have an understanding of the anesthetic agents used, including the actions, indications for use, and potential side effects. Monitoring for malignant hyperthermia (discussed earlier) is a concern for the entire surgical team. A combination of medications can be administered when a patient receives general anesthesia. Some medications decrease anxiety, promote sedation, and cause rapid induction, maintenance of anesthesia, loss of consciousness, skeletal muscle relaxation, and temporary paralysis.

TABLE 37-2 Stages of General Anesthesia

STAGE	DESCRIPTION
I: Analgesia	Patient is awake, becomes drowsy, and loses consciousness Experiences analgesia or a loss of pain sensation
II: Excitement	Begins with loss of consciousness Excitement of muscles Involuntary movement Muscles become tense Breathing may be irregular Ends with regular breathing and loss of eyelid reflexes
III: Surgical anesthesia	Vital signs and reflexes are depressed Skeletal muscles relax Breathing is regular Operation begins
IV: Medullary paralysis	Respiratory centers in the medulla oblongata of the brain, which control breathing and other vital functions, cease to function Complete respiratory depression Cardiopulmonary resuscitation (CPR) needed Death can occur

! SAFE PRACTICE ALERT

Some medications administered during surgery and postoperatively to decrease pain can cause respiratory depression. All patients receiving medications that can cause respiratory depression monitoring of vital signs, including pulse oximetry, and oxygen therapy as indicated.

! SAFE PRACTICE ALERT

When reversal agents are used, they reverse the effects of anesthesia, pain medication, and sedation. The nurse conducts an assessment, including a pain assessment, when these agents are used.

Regional Anesthesia

Regional anesthesia disrupts the transmission of nerve impulses to a specific area of the body. It is achieved by performing spinal, epidural, or peripheral nerve blocks. The application of regional anesthetics blocks pain impulses. With this type of anesthesia, there is no loss of consciousness, the patient is not intubated, and the need for additional pain medication may decrease. The patient remains awake. The area of the body that is anesthetized becomes numb and loses sensation. Some medications may cause reflexes in the area to be temporarily lost. Regional anesthesia is preferred for patients who are hemodynamically compromised.

Regional anesthetic that is injected into a particular nerve, group of nerves, or surrounding tissue is called a **nerve block**. When a nerve block is used, intraoperative anesthesia and postoperative analgesia are provided. Injections are given in the head, neck, extremities, or trunk.

A **bier block** involves injection of anesthetic agents into the venous circulation of an extremity. This type of regional anesthesia is commonly used when the surgical procedure involves an extremity, or it can be used to help manage chronic pain. A tourniquet is used to keep venous blood from entering the surgical site and entrapping the anesthetic in the extremity. Major concerns for this type of anesthesia consist of failure of the tourniquet and premature releasing of the tourniquet. It is important to document the time the tourniquet is inflated. Surgery is completed within the specified time to prevent complications developing in the extremity.

When an anesthetic agent is injected into the epidural space in the lumbar or thoracic region, **epidural anesthesia** is achieved. Narcotics may be combined with the local anesthesia to produce a better analgesic effect. Low concentrations of local anesthetics allow sensory pathways to be blocked. Higher concentrations of local anesthetics also cause motor pathways to be blocked. The epidural catheter may remain in place to assist with postoperative pain control. It is possible for the epidural catheter to be advanced too far. When this happens, the catheter punctures the dural membrane, causing cerebrospinal fluid to leak into the epidural space.

With **spinal anesthesia,** an anesthetic agent is injected into the subarachnoid space. This blocks sensations in the lower body. Sensory and motor sensations are inhibited by the anesthetic. Figure 37-3 illustrates placement of the needle for epidural and spinal anesthesia.

Many people experience severe headaches known as spinal or postspinal headaches. If the headache does not resolve, a blood patch may be placed over the dura hole. Blood is removed from the patient's arm and injected into the epidural space at the level of the dura hole. Many patients receive immediate relief. The patient must remain flat for approximately 2 hours after this procedure.

When minor surgical procedures require anesthesia to numb a certain area of the body requiring surgery, this type of anesthesia is administered by injecting an anesthetic into that specific site to block pain and other sensation in either a small or large region of the body. The application or injection of anesthetic drugs subcutaneously to a specific area of the body is called **local anesthesia**. The medication is often injected into the tissue surrounding the affected area and is designed to block nerve stimuli at their origin. It can be applied as drops to numb the eye or topically to relieve pain and itching. Consciousness is not altered. **Topical anesthesia** is a type of local anesthesia often used to decrease discomfort.

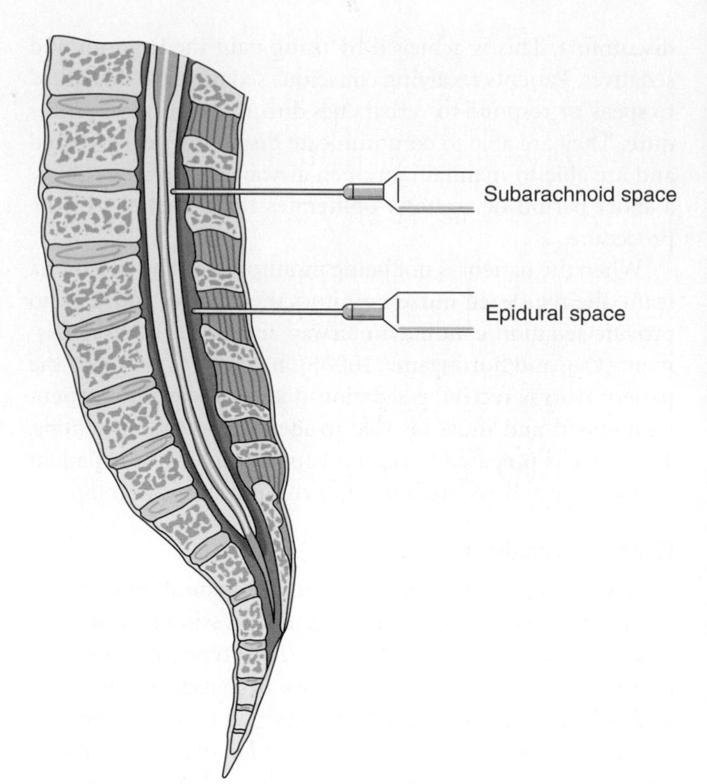

FIGURE 37-3 Placement of the needle for epidural and spinal anesthesia. (From Monahan FD, Sands JK, Neighbors M, et al: *Phipps' medical-surgical nursing: health and illness perspectives*, ed. 8, St. Louis, 2007, Mosby.)

It can be used to numb the surface of a specific area of the body, such as the mucous membranes, ear, or skin.

POSTOPERATIVE PHASE

Many patients are not alert and oriented when they are transported to the PACU. The gag reflex may be suppressed, and the patient may still be intubated. Depending on the operation and anesthetic agent, the patient may have decreased or absent peristalsis, decreased urine production, and a decreased level of consciousness. Patients may have surgical dressings, which are monitored for drainage. Vital sign changes can signify hemorrhage or shock. As the effects of anesthesia wear off, the patient may experience pain.

◆ ASSESSMENT LO 37.5

The nurse assesses the patient during each phase of the perioperative period: preoperative, intraoperative, and postoperative. Assessment data assist the nurse in planning care of the patient. The nurse gathers patient health data by collaborating with the patient and family if appropriate. Information is obtained from the medical record and the patient (Health Assessment Questions box). It is important for the nurse to validate all information obtained. The data are evaluated, interpreted correctly, and prioritized.

HEALTH ASSESSMENT QUESTIONS

Preoperative Phase
- Do you have medication, food, or contact allergies?
- What operations have you had in the past, and when were they performed?
- Have you or family members had problems with anesthesia?
- What prescription medications are you currently taking?
- Do you take over-the-counter medications?
- Do you take herbal medications or vitamin supplements?
- Is there a possibility you may be pregnant?
- Do you smoke?
  - How often you do smoke, and how long have you smoked?
- How much alcohol do you drink in a typical day or week?
- Do you use recreational marijuana or drugs?

Intraoperative Phase
- Are you comfortable? What is your pain rating?
- Do you have questions or concerns?

Postoperative Phase
- How is your breathing?
- Can you take several slow, deep breaths?
- What is your name?
- Do you know where you are?
- How do you feel?
- Are you having pain?
- Would you like a warm blanket?

PREOPERATIVE HEALTH HISTORY AND PHYSICAL ASSESSMENT

During the preoperative phase, the nurse conducts a health history and physical assessment to identify physical and psychosocial risk factors and strengths. Additional information gathered consists of sociocultural needs, coping patterns, support systems, and the patient's knowledge, understanding, and perception of the surgical procedure. Obtaining this information assists the nurse in individualizing the preoperative assessment and developing interventions to decrease surgical risk and complications such as infections, atelectasis, deep vein thrombosis, and constipation.

The preoperative assessment serves as a screening process to determine whether patients are in the best possible state of health before surgery and to establish baseline data to be compared with postoperative assessments. Preoperative assessments and interventions have an influence on quality improvement and patient outcomes because potential problems are identified (Putnis, Nanuck, and Heath, 2008). During the preoperative phase, the patient communicates their concerns and fears about the procedure. This allows discussions to occur and helps to alleviate some of the stress, anxiety, and fear related to the surgical procedure. The nurse provides information that improves the outcome of surgery, such as facts about smoking cessation and weight loss.

Discharge planning begins in the preoperative phase. A successful discharge plan is achieved by identifying potential problems preoperatively. During the preoperative assessment, the nurse evaluates the home environment and familial support. This can assist the nurse in identifying special needs or arrangements required to prepare the patient for discharge and the need for assistance from other health care team members, such as a case worker or social worker.

In addition to a complete head-to-toe assessment by the nurse, the surgeon and anesthesia team evaluate the patient. Careful assessment of the cardiovascular and respiratory systems, including the airway, is completed before surgery. Preexisting conditions are evaluated to determine their relevance to the procedure and consider the problems or complications that could occur. A member of the anesthesia team assesses the patient's physical and emotional health preoperatively. The patient's past experiences and adverse effects from anesthesia are reviewed to determine anesthesia risks. The surgeon or anesthesiologist orders preoperative testing.

After performing the history and physical assessment, the nurse prepares the patient for surgery, reviews preoperative testing results, and verifies that consent has been obtained. Abnormal preoperative testing results are reported to the physician. Based on the results of testing, additional tests may be ordered to provide more detailed information regarding the health status of the patient.

! SAFE PRACTICE ALERT

Preoperative assessments can improve patient safety and patient outcomes by identifying potential risk factors that can increase the patient's surgical risk.

Activity Level and Level of Consciousness

A baseline assessment of the patient's level of consciousness, orientation, the ability to maintain thought patterns, follow commands, and respond to questions and tactile simulation is obtained. During the postoperative phase, a comparison with the preoperative neurologic assessment can be used to determine changes. This information assists the nurse in planning and implementing safe care.

Vital Signs

Preoperative vital signs are taken to establish baseline data. The patient's blood pressure, pulse, respiratory rate, temperature, and pain level can alert the nurse and health care team to current problems. During the intraoperative and postoperative phases of surgery, vital signs are compared with the preoperative vital signs to detect changes that may herald complications.

Laboratory and Diagnostic Examinations

When a patient is scheduled for surgery, diagnostic preoperative tests may be ordered to provide baseline data and identify problems that may contribute to postoperative complications. The type of testing is based on the patient's current medical problem, preexisting illness, overall health status, and age and on the surgical procedure to be performed. Table 37-3 lists common preoperative diagnostic tests and detailed nursing assessment information.

INTRAOPERATIVE PHASE

During the intraoperative phase, the nurse assesses the patient's response to surgery. An important role for the circulating nurse is to be the patient advocate because anesthetized patients cannot speak for themselves. Safety is evaluated in the operating room throughout the intraoperative phase.

Continuous Monitoring of Vital Signs

During the intraoperative phase, the nurse and the anesthetist continuously monitor the patient's vital signs, including temperature, heart rate, blood pressure, respiration, oxygen saturation, intake and output, and the electrocardiogram. The amount of blood loss is always assessed. Continuous monitoring is essential to quickly distinguish adverse effects from the effects of anesthesia or the surgical procedure. Prompt interventions can help control the adverse effects and prevent further complications from developing.

Assessment of Positioning and Other Safety Concerns

An important task for the circulating nurse is assessment of safe and proper positioning. The surgical team places the patient in a position that allows access to the patient's airway and surgical site. Safety, comfort, and monitoring vital signs are considered when the patient is being positioned.

The circulating nurse assists in managing other safety concerns. The **scrub nurse** prepares and maintains the sterile field. The circulating nurse can provide assistance to the scrub nurse by transferring equipment and supplies to the sterile field. Sharps, sponges, and instruments are counted as they are added to the sterile field. Additional counts are performed before the surgery is completed to ensure that supplies are not left inside the patient. Specimens obtained during surgery are labeled and handled appropriately to ensure proper evaluation. All specimens, sharps, sponges, and instrument counts are documented on the intraoperative record (Goldberg and Feldman, 2012).

POSTOPERATIVE PHASE

After surgery has been completed, the patient is transferred to the PACU. Often, two or more individuals from the surgical team, including the anesthesia provider, accompany the patient to the PACU. The patient may be awake, alert, drowsy, sedated, or intubated. This is a critical time for the patient. Sudden or rough handling can cause injury, hypotension, or cardiac arrest.

The PACU nurse receives a report on the patient that includes the following:

- Patient identification
- Type of anesthesia received
- Name of the procedure performed
- Location and number of drains and dressings
- Estimated blood loss
- Name and amount of fluid received
- Vital signs
- Oxygenation saturation
- Urinary output

In the postoperative phase, the nurse assesses the patient's physical response to surgery and monitors for postoperative complications. The PACU nurse immediately assesses the patient, including airway, breathing quality, vital signs, level of consciousness, orientation, speech pattern, motor and sensory ability, and dressings. Ongoing detailed assessments include the following data:

- General health and appearance
- Level of consciousness and neurologic status
- Vital signs and pain level
- Respiratory system: breath sounds, rate rhythm, depth, use of accessory muscles, gag reflex
- Oxygenation saturation and capillary refill
- Skin color and temperature
- Patency of IV lines, IV fluids, and infusion rate
- Patency of drains
- Urinary output
- Surgical site
- Dressing drainage (type, amount, and color)
- Drainage under the patient
- Ability to move all extremities
- Nausea
- Emesis
- Laboratory results

Based on the patient's health status and the surgical procedure, additional assessments may be needed. The frequency of postoperative assessments is based on the physician's orders, the patient's condition, identified risk factors, and hospital policies. Commonly, assessments are made every 15 minutes during the first hour and then every 30 minutes for the next 2 hours. If the patient is unstable, assessments are performed more frequently.

Vital Signs

The nurse assesses patient vital signs throughout the postoperative period. The temperature, heart rate, blood pressure, respiration, and oxygen saturation are monitored every 15 minutes until the patient stabilizes. Some facilities may have different protocols. It is important for the nurse to follow the facility's protocol and policy. The postoperative vital signs are compared with the preoperative vital signs. The nurse assesses postoperative problems such as pain, hypovolemia, hemorrhage, and shock that can affect vital signs.

TABLE 37-3 Common Preoperative Diagnostic Tests

Before all blood tests and procedures, explain the procedure and purpose to the patient.
After blood tests, apply pressure to the venipuncture site.

TEST	RATIONALE	NURSING ASSESSMENT
Complete blood count (CBC)	To detect hemorrhage, dietary deficiencies, anemia, hydration status, coagulation ability, and infection	Assess overall appearance for nutritional and hydration status. Assess vital signs to detect anemia, infection. Assess for signs of blood loss to detect hemorrhage or anemia.
Electrolytes	To monitor fluid and electrolyte balance and therapy	Assess preoperative medications for diuretics, potassium supplements, or other medications that affect electrolyte levels. Assess cardiac and neurologic function.
Blood type and crossmatch	To determine blood type before donating or receiving blood	Assess the patient's views on blood transfusions.
BUN and creatinine	To measure renal function	Assess intake and output.
Pulmonary function test	To assess lungs and pulmonary reserve before anesthesia, to assess response to bronchodilator therapy, and to detect pulmonary deficiencies.	Assess patient medications and respiratory status.
Chest x-ray	To obtain information about the heart, lungs, bone structure and large blood vessels in the chest.	Ask female patient if she is pregnant or suspects being pregnant. Have the patient remove clothing and metal objects (e.g. necklaces, pins) from the neck to the waist.
Blood glucose	To directly measure blood glucose used to evaluate diabetic patients	Assess for preoperative diabetic medications, hyperglycemia and hypoglycemia.
ALT (formerly SGPT), AST	To identify disease of the liver	Assess for signs of jaundice.
Coagulation studies	To evaluate clotting mechanisms	Assess preoperative anticoagulant medications. Check skin color and monitor for bleeding.
Electrocardiogram	To evaluate arrhythmias, conduction defects, myocardial injury and damage, and pericardial disease	Assess preoperative cardiac and antihypertensive medications. Assess cardiac status.
Urinalysis	To detect urinary tract disease, and to gain basic information about kidneys and other metabolic processes	Assist with collection as needed. Assess the patient's intake and output.
Human chorionic gonadotropin	To diagnose pregnancy	Assess the patient's pregnancy history, last menstrual period, and prenatal care if results are positive.

Adapted from Pagana KD, Pagana TJ: *Mosby's manual of diagnostic and laboratory tests,* ed. 5, St. Louis, 2014, Mosby.
ALT, Alanine aminotransferase; *AST, Aspartate Aminotransferase*; *BUN,* blood urea nitrogen; *SGPT,* serum glutamic pyruvic transaminase.

Monitoring Dressings, Drains, and Tubes

Dressings are monitored for drainage. The amount and type of drainage is documented by measuring the diameter of the drainage on each dressing. The surgeon often prefers to be the first person to change the surgical dressing. As a result, the nurse may need to reinforce the dressing. The amount of reinforcement dressing applied is documented.

Drainage that accumulates on a dressing, on clothing, and underneath the patient is monitored for odor, amount, color, and consistency. Drains and tubes are positioned to facilitate proper functioning and patency. Excessive drainage from dressings, drains, and tubes may indicate hemorrhage and the need to notify the surgeon.

Neurologic Assessment

A neurologic assessment is conducted as soon as the patient enters the postoperative phase. This allows the nurse to establish the current functioning of the patient's neurologic system and to determine changes from assessments that were previously conducted. The neurologic assessment includes level of consciousness, orientation, pupillary responses, muscle strength, and movement of the extremities. The patient's response to verbal or tactile stimulation and the ability to sense touch and pain are assessed.

Elimination

Urinary and bowel elimination are monitored during the postoperative phase. Anesthesia and anticholinergic medication can decrease muscle tone, contributing to an accumulation of urine in the bladder and resulting in urinary retention. The nurse monitors the patient for restlessness, diminished urinary output, bladder distention, difficulty or inability to void, and hypertension.

Opioid medications, anesthesia, and immobility can decrease peristalsis. Decreased peristalsis can contribute to the development of hard stool and constipation. Some patients may develop ileus due to a decreased peristalsis from anesthesia or manipulation of intestinal contents during the surgical procedure. The nurse assesses the patient for abdominal distention, flatus, and a change in bowel habits.

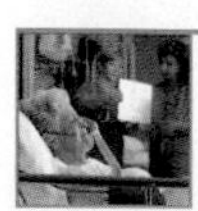

1. List focused assessments and rationales for each assessment to be completed on Mrs. Logan the first postoperative day.

◆ NURSING DIAGNOSIS LO 37.6

The perioperative nurse analyzes the assessment data and makes judgments regarding the information collected. Actual or potential nursing diagnoses are developed based on the interpretation of data about the patient's health problems, needs, or health status. Nursing diagnoses are developed for each perioperative period:

- Preoperative phase
  - *Anxiety* related to a change in health status and fear of the unknown as evidenced by increased blood pressure, heart rate, respiratory rate and verbal reports of feeling nervous
  - *Insomnia* related to anxiety about surgical procedure as evidenced by inability to sleep and restlessness
  - *Deficient Knowledge* related to preoperative procedures as evidenced by asking questions and the need for explanations
- Intraoperative phase
  - *Ineffective Breathing Pattern* related to the effects of anesthesia and narcotic medications as evidenced by shallow breathing, tachypnea (or bradypnea), and abnormal blood gas results
  - *Ineffective Tissue Perfusion* related to decreased peripheral circulation and immobility as evidenced by altered skin color and temperature, and diminished pulses.
  - *Risk for Perioperative Positioning Injury* with risk factors of improper positioning during the surgical procedure
- Postoperative phase
  - *Acute Pain* related to tissue injury at the surgical site as evidenced by verbal reports of pain; rubbing and guarding the surgical site; increase in blood pressure, heart rate, and respiratory rate; and loss of the ability to sleep, ambulate, and perform activities of daily living
  - *Nausea* related to manipulation of the gastrointestinal tract and anesthesia as evidenced by nausea and vomiting
  - *Risk for Infection* with a risk factor of invasive surgical procedure

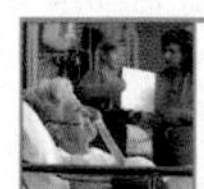

2. Write two nursing diagnoses for Mrs. Logan in the postoperative period.

◆ PLANNING LO 37.7

During the preoperative phase, the nurse plans for the entire perioperative period (Table 37-4). This includes the expected outcomes and the nursing interventions to achieve the identified outcomes. The nurse reviews these expected outcomes with the patient and family before surgery. Collaboration with other members of the health care team is necessary during the perioperative period (Collaboration and Delegation box).

The perioperative nurse determines goals for patients having surgery. In the perioperative period, goals are developed from nursing diagnoses and interventions to correct, modify, or maintain the nursing diagnoses. It is important to individualize the goals based on the priority needs of the patient. All goals must be realistic, specific, and measurable. This helps guide the nurse when providing nursing care. The

TABLE 37-4 Care Planning

NANDA-I NURSING DIAGNOSIS LABEL WITH NURSING DIAGNOSIS STATEMENT	NURSING OUTCOME CLASSIFICATION (NOC)	NURSING INTERVENTION CLASSIFICATION (NIC)
Anxiety related to a change in health status and fear of the unknown as evidenced by increased blood pressure, heart rate, respiratory rate, and verbal reports of feeling nervous	*Coping* (1302) Reports decrease in physical symptoms of stress (130216)	*Anxiety reduction* (5820) Explain all procedures, including sensations likely to be experienced during the procedure.

From Bulechek G, Butcher H, Dochterman J, et al (Eds): *Nursing interventions classification (NIC)*, ed. 6, St. Louis, 2013, Mosby; Moorhead S, Johnson M, Maas M, et al (Eds): *Nursing outcomes classification (NOC)*, ed. 5, St. Louis, 2013, Mosby; NANDA International: *Nursing diagnoses: Definitions and classification, 2012–2014*, West Sussex, England, 2012, Wiley-Blackwell. Reprinted with permission from NANDA International, Inc.

COLLABORATION AND DELEGATION

Multidisciplinary Care of the Perioperative Patient

- Physical therapy and occupational therapy provide assistance with ambulatory support and the use of assistive devices.
- Unlicensed assistive personnel (UAP) help with turning immobilized patients at least every 2 hours.
- UAP encourage and assist the patient to move in bed, ambulate, eat, and increase fluid intake.
- Dietitians provide support for nutritional problems and concerns.
- The application of sequential compression devices can be delegated to UAP who have had training in this task.
- Leg exercises are taught initially by a registered nurse. Reinforcement of performing leg exercises can be delegated to UAP.

following are examples of goals for the nursing diagnoses listed earlier:

- Patient will exhibit vital signs within normal limits in the preoperative period.
- Patient will sleep at least 6 hours the night before surgery.
- Patient will verbalize understanding of the surgical procedure before the operation.
- Patient's airway will remain patent during surgery.
- Patient will remain hemodynamically stable during the intraoperative period.
- Patient will be positioned appropriately during surgery.
- Patient will report a pain level of 3 or less in the postoperative period.
- Patient will be free from nausea and vomiting after surgery.
- Patient will remain free from infection in the postoperative period.

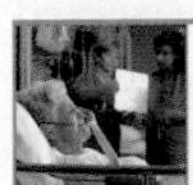

The conceptual care map for Mrs. Logan can be found at *http://evolve.elsevier.com/YoostCrawford/fundamentals/*. It is partially completed to indicate how to use the map as a learning tool. Complete the nursing diagnoses using the example conceptual care maps shown in Chapters 8 and 25 to 33.

IMPLEMENTATION AND EVALUATION LO 37.8

Nursing interventions and evaluations provide the patient with an understanding of the surgical procedure and expectation after surgery and with care during all phases of the perioperative period. The patient is prepared psychologically and physically. The nurse is alert for potential problems and complications as the patient moves through each phase.

INTERVENTIONS

The perioperative nurse implements nursing interventions to help the patient achieve goals that have been identified. This includes physiologic and psychological preparation for surgery, the immediate postoperative phase, and the patient's discharge to home. Many nursing interventions are carried out in the perioperative period, and they all are focused on achieving positive outcomes.

Preoperative Phase

During the preoperative phase, nurses are focused on assessment and teaching in preparation of the patient for surgery. Patient teaching before surgery enhances postoperative care because the patient knows what to expect and how to respond ahead of time.

Preoperative Teaching

Many surgical patients experience stress, anxiety, and fear, which may result from the recognition of a lack of control. Preoperative teaching can help decrease fear, anxiety, and stress and reduce postoperative complications by preparing the patient for the surgical procedure and the postoperative period.

Some people fear the unknown, including surgery, anesthesia, and death. It is important for nurses to acknowledge these concerns and fears and address them with the preoperative patient. Educating the patient and family can help to alleviate some of their concerns. When a patient is scheduled for surgery, teaching starts as early as possible to allow the patient to seek clarity and make appropriate decisions. Teaching may begin in the physician's office and includes the family when appropriate. The purpose is to prepare the patient for surgery and discharge. Information can be given when the patient comes for diagnostic testing and when they have been admitted for surgery. Nurses should give information in several sessions so that the patient has time to assimilate the information provided.

Preoperative teaching helps the patient and family understand what is required before, during, and after the procedure (Litwack, 2009). For teaching to be effective, the nurse provides information at a level that the patient and family understand. The patient's cultural background is considered. If there is a language barrier between a patient and a nurse, it may be necessary to arrange for a hospital-provided translator to explain information to the patient.

If the patient needs to perform certain activities in the initial postoperative phase, explaining these activities preoperatively gives the patient the opportunity to learn and practice. Teaching includes information about postoperative bandages, tubes, drains, medications, exercises, pain control, turning, antiembolism measures, assistive devices, and dietary guidelines. The Patient Education and Health Literacy box details areas to include in preoperative teaching. The nurse develops an understanding of what the preoperative patient knows and what they need to know.

Pain Management Plan

The patient having surgery often has anxiety and fear related to pain. The surgical patient can expect to experience some type of pain from surgery. The patient is informed of the treatment plan to help manage pain. It is important for the patient to understand that the pain must be controlled to allow maximized participation in postoperative therapy (AHRQ, 2009a).

Pain levels should be monitored frequently by using a pain scale. An assessment is conducted to determine aggravating and alleviating factors related to pain. If patient-controlled analgesia (PCA) is ordered for pain control, the patient is taught how to push the button for pain moderation. Cultural beliefs and expectations regarding pain management are considered. Effective pain management strategies and therapies used in the past are explored. Alternative methods of pain management such as distraction, guided imagery, and relaxation can be used in the postoperative period. Chapter 36 provides more information on pharmacologic and nonpharmacologic control of pain.

Informed Consent

When surgery is recommended for treatment, patients must be given information that allows them to make informed decisions. Having a good understanding of proposed procedures allows a patient to select or reject treatment options.

PATIENT EDUCATION AND HEALTH LITERACY

Preoperative Teaching

Before admission to the hospital, the patient receives information that explains perioperative care and routines. Preadmission education can increase compliance, decrease anxiety, and contribute to better performance of exercises.

- Explain preoperative testing (e.g., laboratory tests, x-rays, electrocardiogram). This helps the patient understand how to prepare for surgery.
- Teach the patient about preoperative washing and antibacterial products that may be used to prepare the skin before surgery. Education can decrease postoperative anxiety.
- Exercises and activities that need to be performed are reviewed with the patient. This includes leg exercises, coughing, deep breathing, and incentive spirometry. Preoperative instruction can help the patient to successfully perform postoperative exercises.
- Explain the importance of deep breathing, coughing, splinting, and leg exercises. Coughing and deep breathing helps to expand the lungs and improve ventilation (Nursing Care Guideline: Cough and Deep-Breathing Techniques box). Splinting helps to support the incision and promote comfort (Nursing Care Guideline: Postoperative Splinting box). Leg exercises help stimulate circulation and minimize the risk of thrombus formation.
- The patient performs a return demonstration of exercises before surgery. Return demonstration is an effective method to evaluate learning and reinforce instruction.
- Teach the patient how to move in bed and out of bed after surgery. This enables the patient to assist with turning and changing positions in bed.
- Explain that pain medication will be given to help manage pain. Providing information can promote comfort, help the patient understand what to expect after surgery, and decrease fear and anxiety.
- Describe the type of assessments that will be conducted. This enables the patient to become knowledgeable about dressings, drains, and equipment.
- Explain that the patient will be cared for in the PACU immediately after surgery. After a period of observation, the patient will be discharged home or sent to a surgical unit.
- If the patient is going to be discharged after surgery, provide instructions on what to wear the day of surgery, and inform the patient that another adult will need to drive home. This will help familiarize the patient with how they will be cared for.

The physician is responsible for obtaining the informed consent for surgery (Ellis and Hartley, 2012). The signed **informed consent** document gives legal authorization for the surgical procedure, and it helps to protect the patient from having unauthorized procedures performed. It can protect the health care team and hospital from claims by the patient that an unauthorized procedure was performed.

NURSING CARE GUIDELINE

Cough and Deep-Breathing Techniques

Background

- The following breathing techniques are used by postoperative patients:
  - Controlled cough
  - Deep breaths in through the nose and exhaled through the mouth
  - Diaphragmatic breathing
  - Pursed-lip exhalation
- The techniques have the following benefits:
  - Maintenance of lung expansion
  - Prevention of atelectasis and pneumonia
- If surgery is planned, the patient can benefit from being taught one or more of these techniques *before* surgery to allow time to practice them before they are needed.

Procedural Concerns

- The patient should be in an upright position (semi-Fowler or Fowler if possible).
- Instruct the patient in deep breathing:
  - Rest the palms of the hands below the rib cage, with the middle fingers touching.
  - Take slow, deep breaths:
    - Inhale through the nose.
    - Feel the abdomen push against the hands.
    - Keep the chest and shoulders still.
  - Inhale as deeply as possible.
  - Hold that breath for 3 to 5 seconds.
  - Exhale slowly through pursed lips (see the pursed-lip breathing instruction), and stop exhaling when the middle fingers touch again.
  - Perform each inhalation and exhalation three to five times before resting.
  - Perform all of these steps 10 times every hour if possible.
- Controlled coughs:
  - If the patient has an abdominal or thoracic incision, provide a splint (see the Nursing Care Guideline: Postoperative Splinting box).
  - Have the patient take two deep breaths in and out.
  - The patient then inhales as deeply as possible and holds it for 3 to 5 seconds.
  - Release the breath as a full cough; cough two or three times, but do not inhale between coughs if possible.
  - Perform these steps two or three times every 2 hours if possible.
- Pursed-lip breathing:
  - Have the patient purse the lips as if to make a whistling sound (into an O shape) and then release a slow, controlled exhalation.

Documentation Concerns

- Document the patient education concerning correct procedure and performance times.
- Note patient concerns or discomfort, and document noncompliance issues.
- Include the respiratory assessment before and after the procedure.
- Document the number of times the patient performed each step and the patient's tolerance of the procedure.

Evidence-Based Practice

- Deep-breathing exercises are included as part of the routine guidelines and taught preoperatively to maximize understanding on the part of the patient when not impaired by the effects of medications.
- There is a definitive fall in lung volume postoperatively, and these exercises are as effective as continuous positive airway pressure in increasing lung volume (Eagle and Smetana, 2006).

QSEN FOCUS!

Patient-centered care is facilitated through informed consent and by informing the patient of care that will be provided throughout the peroperative period. The preoperative nurse witnesses the informed consent for surgery and explains the care that will be provided.

The written signature enables the consent form to become a legal document. After the patient signs the document, the consent form becomes a permanent part of the medical record. The consent form is signed before the patient is given analgesics or sedative medications.

Before consent is obtained, the patient is given a description of the surgical procedure, benefits, risk factors, potential complications, expected outcome, and postoperative recovery by the surgeon. Additional information regarding the procedure or the health status of the patient is provided. The consent form (Figure 37-4) discloses enough information to allow the person to make an informed decision. The informed consent includes documentation of the patient's mutual understanding of and agreement to treatment and care. A patient needs to voluntarily give consent without persuasion or threats to influence the patient to agree to the procedure.

Failure to obtain an informed consent can have legal consequences. If a surgical procedure is performed without consent, it can be viewed as assault, battery, or malpractice. The Ethical, Legal, and Professional Practice box provides information that is included in a consent form. Barriers to understanding the informed consent are cultural issues, font size, forms that are too long, and a patient's lack of medical knowledge and education (Lorenzen, Melby, and Earles, 2008).

Informed consent is not needed in emergency circumstances. When the patient is not able to give consent, the physician attempts to obtain the consent from the next of kin or legal guardian. The consent may be obtained by telephone

Date of procedure: ____/____/____

CONSENT FOR PROCEDURE

I,________________________________, request and give consent to ________________________________
(Type or print patient name) (Type or print doctor or practitioner name(s))

to perform the following procedure(s) ________________________________
(Please list site and side if appropriate)

____

____

The benefits, risks, complications, and alternatives to the above procedure(s) have been explained to me.

I understand that the procedure(s) will be performed at the facility by and under supervision of my doctor or practitioner. My doctor or practitioner may use the services of other doctors or practitioners, or members of the resident staff as he or she deems necessary or advisable.

I authorize my doctor or practitioner and his or her associates and assistants to perform such additional procedures, which in their judgment are necessary and appropriate to carry out my diagnosis or treatment.

I authorize the hospital to retain, photograph, preserve and use for scientific, teaching purposes, or to make other dispositions of, at their convenience, any specimens, tissues, or parts taken from my body during the course of this operation.

I consent to observers in the procedure area in accordance with hospital policy. I consent to a healthcare industry representative being present during the procedure, if necessary, to provide technical assistance or to perform calibration of equipment. I consent to photography or video taping of my surgical procedure for educational purposes, provided my identity remains anonymous and confidential.

I consent to the administration of sedation or analgesia during my procedure. The risks, benefits, and alternatives to receiving sedation or analgesia have been explained to me.

If anesthesia is required, I consent to the administration of anesthesia by members of the Department of Anesthesiology. I also consent to the use of non-invasive and invasive monitoring techniques as deemed necessary. I understand that anesthesia involves risks that are in addition to those resulting from the operation itself including, but not limited to, dental injury, hoarseness, vocal cord injury, infection, nerve injury, corneal abrasion, seizures, heart attack, stroke and even death.

If applicable, I consent to the use of fluoroscopy. I understand that prolonged exposure to fluoroscopy may result in skin reactions, such as redness, irritation or a burn.

Please initial one of the following statements (females 55 years and under):

______To the best of my knowledge I am not pregnant. ______I believe I am pregnant.

I certify that I have read and understand the above consent statements. In addition, I have been offered the opportunity to ask my doctor or practitioner any questions I have regarding the procedure(s) to be performed and they have been answered to my satisfaction. I acknowledge that I have been given no guarantee or assurance as to the results that may be obtained from the procedure(s).

________________ ____/____/____ ________
Signature of Patient or Decision Maker Date Time

____
Relationship to Patient

________________ ____/____/____ ________
Witness Signature Date Time

____
Witness Print Name

________________ ____/____/____ ________
Doctor or Practitioner Signature/Title Date Time

____
Doctor or Practitioner Print Name or ID#

Telephone Consent:

____
Name of person providing consent

________________ ____/____/____ ________
Witness Signature Date Time

____
Witness Print Name

____
Relationship to Patient if Decision Maker

________________ ____/____/____ ________
Witness Signature Date Time

____
Witness Print Name

Interpretation: The information presented orally to the O patient O representative O decision maker was interpreted into (language): ____________. The person for whom the information was interpreted stated s/he understood the interpretation.

____
Interpreter Name

____
Agency and ID# (if applicable)

________________ ________________ ____/____/____ ________
Staff Signature/Title Print Name or ID# Date Time

FIGURE 37-4 Sample informed consent document. (Courtesy Christiana Care Health Services, Newark, Del.)

NURSING CARE GUIDELINE

Postoperative Splinting

Background

- Postoperative splinting is used to support an incision and to promote comfort by decreasing pressure, discomfort, and pain related to an incision.
- It is used during coughing, deep breathing, or movement that may cause sutures to tear.
- Postoperative splinting is used primarily for incision sites on the abdomen and the thorax.

Procedural Concerns

- One of the patient's hands is placed on top of the incision; the other hand is placed on top of the first.
- For comfort, the patient may use a pillow, holding it under the hands and over the incision.

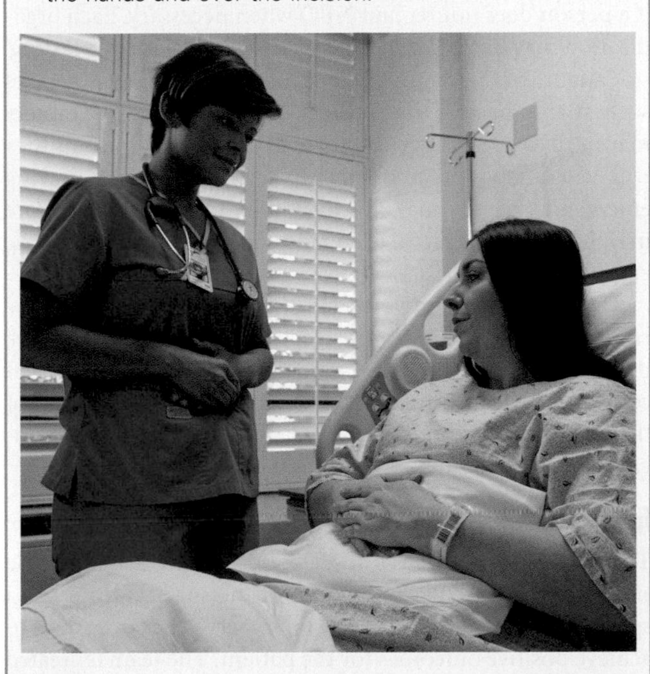

- After placement, the patient may continue with controlled coughing or deep-breathing procedures (see Nursing Care Guideline: Cough and Deep-Breathing Techniques box) or with repositioning and getting out of bed.

Documentation Concerns

- Document that the patient has been educated about how to correctly perform the procedure.
- Note the patient's concerns and discomfort, and document incidences of noncompliance.
- Include assessments of the incision.

! SAFE PRACTICE ALERT

The physician or surgeon is responsible for obtaining informed consent. The preoperative nurse is responsible for making sure the consent is signed by the patient and placed in the patient's chart.

ETHICAL, LEGAL, AND PROFESSIONAL PRACTICE

Informed Consent

Informed consent discloses the following:

- Medical diagnosis and reason for treatment
- Procedure to be performed
- The name of the person performing the procedure
- Qualifications of the person performing the procedure
- Names of individuals assisting with the procedure
- Risks and benefits of the procedure
- Alternative treatments
- The right to refuse or withdraw consent at a later date

Ethical and Legal Concerns

- Every person has the right to agree to or refuse health care treatment.
- When informed consent is given, the person understands the treatment options.
- Consent is given voluntarily.
- The law requires the medical provider to obtain consent for medical treatment.
- The nurse may sign a consent form as a witness to the patient's signature.
- A legal guardian may give consent for a minor child, an unconscious patient, or someone with dementia (Ellis and Hartley, 2012).
- If there is a question about an individual's competency, a court will make a determination. A legal guardian is appointed by the court if a person is determined incompetent.

or court order. If time does not allow for this, the physician has the responsibility of documenting the need for treatment to save the patient's life in the medical record. The physician also considers the organizational policy and state laws when emergency surgery is needed and the consent has not been obtained.

During the consent process the nurse provides information about nursing care, facilitates preoperative teaching, and reinforces information about the procedure. The nurse is a witness to the patient's signature and to the patient being competent and signing voluntarily. If the nurse finds that the patient does not understand the procedure or that the patient is unsure about signing the consent form, the nurse informs the physician of the situation and asks the physician to talk to the patient (Nursing Care Guideline: Obtaining and Completing Informed Consent box).

! SAFE PRACTICE ALERT

A nurse acts as a patient advocate before the consent form is signed, ensuring that the patient has been informed about the surgical procedure and has no further questions for the physician. If the patient does not have additional questions, the nurse has the responsibility to act as a witness to the patient signing the consent form.

NURSING CARE GUIDELINE

Obtaining and Completing Informed Consent

Background

- Obtaining and completing the informed consent document is the responsibility of the surgeon.
- Witnessing a consent form means
  - The nurse has watched the correct patient signing the form.
  - The nurse has verified the correct identity of the patient who is signing the form.
  - The nurse signs the form as a witness to the preceding two events.
- Be aware of individual facility policy and procedures.

Procedural Concerns

- Never witness a blank or incomplete informed consent form. Ensure all the information is complete.
- Do *not* administer analgesic or sedative medications before the informed consent form is signed by the patient.
- If the patient does not understand any aspect of informed consent, contact the surgeon to speak with the patient again and to answer questions before sedation.
- To sign the informed consent, the patient must
  - Be mentally sound
  - Have all information in the patient's primary language
  - Be of legal age
  - Not be under sedation
- The patient has the right to withdraw consent at any time and refuse treatment.

Documentation Concerns

- Document that consent was obtained.
- Indicate that all information is complete.
- Include the preoperative checklist.

Evidence-Based Practice

- Health literacy is often overlooked on an informed consent form, but it should be considered to ensure that the consent is valid.
- Lorenzen, Melby, and Earles (2008) purport that incorporating language that is in terms an average person can read, shortening the form, increasing the font size, bulleting information, and using a teach-back technique (i.e., the patient restates information) can enhance the intended meaning and value of informed consent.

After consent has been obtained, the signed and witnessed form is a legal document that becomes a part of the patient's chart. Consent forms are not legal if the patient is sedated, confused, or incompetent. When a patient refuses to sign the consent form, the nurse documents in the patient's medical record that the patient refused to consent to surgery. Some organizations request that the patient sign a release form that identifies the refusal to consent.

Patient Preparation

The type of surgery dictates the preparation necessary to get a patient ready for surgery. When scheduled for an elective or urgent procedure, some patients are required to fast before surgery. Some anesthetics delay normal reflexes so that the body's usual defenses may not be working properly. An empty stomach helps to decrease the chances of regurgitating undigested food or liquids. Aspiration of gastric contents during the intraoperative or postoperative period may lead to aspiration pneumonia. If a patient is ordered to be NPO but has scheduled oral medications, the nurse needs to clarify with the physician which medications are to be given. The physician may order some medications to be given with sips of water the day of surgery. Surgery may be cancelled or delayed if a person does not remain NPO when necessary. Each organization may have policies that provide guidelines for fasting.

Patients who are admitted because of medical emergencies such as trauma and those whose health deteriorates rapidly may need to have surgery performed quickly. This means they will have a shortened preoperative phase. Patients having emergency surgery may not have time to fast and therefore may have a nasogastric tube inserted to assist with gastric emptying.

Usually a preoperative checklist (Figure 37-5) needs to be completed on paper or in the electronic health record before the surgical procedure. The nurse has the responsibility of completing the information on the checklist. If some areas of the checklist have not been completed, the nurse communicates this information to the health care team.

Intraoperative Phase

The operating room has a specialized team to assist with the surgical procedure. Each member of the surgical team has a specific job and function. All members work together to achieve positive outcomes for the patient. The team is created with the primary goal of maintaining patient safety.

Nursing Roles During Surgery

Table 37-5 lists the surgical team members and their functions. The members of the team vary slightly based on the procedure being performed, the type of anesthesia being administered, and the hospital policy. Each sterile (scrubbed) member of the team performs surgical scrub, gowning, and gloving before the operation or procedure (Skill 37-1).

Anesthesia

Shortly before the intraoperative phase begins, some patients may be given medications to help them relax and to dry secretions. The patient's transfer by cart, bed, or wheelchair to the operating room begins the intraoperative phase. Assistance is provided to transfer the patient to the operating room table. For safety, the patient is strapped to the table. Members of the surgical team are introduced to the patient. At this time,

PREOPERATIVE CHECKLIST

Preoperative Requirements	Initials	Day of Surgery	Initials
Height _____ Weight _____		Surgical site marked Y or NA	
Isolation Y or N Type _____		ID band on patient Y or N	
Allergies noted on chart Y or N		Allergy band on patient Y or NA	
Vital signs (baseline) T _____ P _____ R _____ BP _____ Pulse Ox _____		Vital signs Time _________ T _____ P _____ R _____ BP _____ Pulse Ox _____	
Chart Review		**Procedures**	
H&P on chart		NPO since _____	
H&P within 30 days? Y or N		Capillary blood glucose Result: _____ NA	
Signed and witnessed informed consent form on chart Y or N		Voided/catheter Time _____	
Signed consent for blood administration Y or NA		Preoperative medications given Time _____ NA	
Blood type and crossmatch Y or NA		Preoperative antibiotics given Time _____ NA	
Name plate on chart Y or N		Preoperative skin prep Y or NA Shower_____ Scrub_____ Clip_____	
Diagnostic Results		Makeup, nail polish, false fingernails, and false eyelashes removed Y or NA	
Hgb/Hct _____ /_____ NA		Hospital gown applied Y or NA	
PT/INR/PTT _____ /_____ /_____ NA			
CXR _____ NA		**Valuables**	
ECG _____ NA hCG _____ Negative _____ Positive _____NA		Dentures Y or N	
Other labs		Wig or hairpiece Y or N	
Final Chart Review		Eyeglasses Y or N	
Additional forms attached		Contact lenses Y or N	
		Hearing aid Y or N	
		Prosthesis Y or N	
		Jewelry Y or N Piercings with jewelry Y or N	
		Clothing Y or N	
		Disposition of valuables: Hearing aid in place Y or NA	

Time to OR _______________ Date _______________
Transported to OR by _______________
Final check by _______________ RN _______________

FIGURE 37-5 Sample preoperative checklist. (From Lewis SL, Dirksen SR, Heitkemper MM, et al: *Medical-surgical nursing: assessment and management of clinical problems*, ed. 9, St. Louis, 2014, Mosby.)

the administration of anesthesia begins. Until anesthesia induction, the patient is kept informed about what is happening to help decrease anxiety.

! SAFE PRACTICE ALERT

Patient safety is the nurse's first priority. The circulating nurse maintains patient safety during the surgical procedure by monitoring the patient's condition and surgical asepsis.

Surgical procedures can be very uncomfortable. Anesthesia allows surgery to be performed, making the patient insensitive to pain and sensation. The type of anesthetic agent to be administered is largely determined by the anesthesia provider, the type of surgery, and the patient's health. When there are preexisting illnesses, certain types of anesthesia may be used to help manage the underlying health condition of the patient. The surgeon collaborates with the anesthesia provider to determine the type of anesthesia used, but the anesthesia provider makes the final decision. The anesthesia provider is in charge of the medical management and anesthetic care of the patient during surgery.

Support is given to the patient on induction of anesthesia, during the procedure, and as he or she emerges from anesthesia. The patient's responses to anesthesia are monitored during surgery. Continuous medical assessment of the patient

TABLE 37-5 Intraoperative Surgical Team

TEAM MEMBER	FUNCTION
Surgeon (physician)	Treats malformations, injuries, and diseases by manipulation or operation
Scrub nurse/assistant (registered nurse or surgical technologist)	Prepares the surgical setup, handling instruments Maintains surgical asepsis while draping Assists the surgeon by passing instruments, sutures, and supplies
Circulating nurse (registered nurse)	Acts as the patient's advocate and a liaison between scrubbed personnel and the surgical team Coordinates the needs of the surgical team by obtaining supplies and carrying out the nursing care plan Assesses patient safety and aseptic practice Documents in the EHR
Anesthesiologist (physician)	Administers anesthesia Monitors the patient during surgery
Certified registered nurse anesthetist (CRNA)	Administers anesthesia and collaborates with the anesthesiologist Monitors the patient during surgery
Registered nurse first assistant (RNFA)	Collaborates with the surgeon and health care team members during the procedure

includes monitoring and controlling the heart rate, heart rhythm, blood pressure, temperature, fluid balance, pain, breathing, and level of consciousness. Care is taken to match the anesthetic needs and the medical condition of the patient.

General anesthesia causes a drug-induced coma, not a sleeplike state. When the medications begin to be metabolized and excreted, the patient gradually begins to recover consciousness. It takes time for this to happen. Patients are at risk for a variety of medical problems as they emerge from the anesthesia. Complications that can occur include injury to the throat or vocal cords, laryngeal edema, and laryngospasms. The nurse monitors the patient closely and is must be prepared to provide assistance to support the respiratory system.

! SAFE PRACTICE ALERT

Airway and ventilation status is assessed for all patients receiving anesthesia.

During the intraoperative phase, perioperative nurses document appropriately. This includes documenting how the patient is positioned, the start of surgery, medications, drains, specimens, instrumentation, sponges, needles, dressings, and the end of surgery.

Postoperative Phase

The postoperative period begins with transfer to the PACU. The postanesthesia nurse provides care to the patient after the surgical procedure in the PACU. Postoperative care consists of caring for the patient and providing intensive support in the immediate postoperative phase. The nurse focuses on quickly recognizing the best way to reestablish a normal homeostatic balance for the patient. The nurse orients the patient and informs the patient that surgery is over. To promote comfort and decrease anxiety, the nurse pays special attention to the patient's pain level, position, and need to urinate. Bright overhead lights and a noisy environment are avoided, and room temperature is kept at a level comfortable for the patient (Litwack, 2009).

Airway Management

Maintaining the patient's airway is the nurse's first priority. The patient is positioned in a manner that facilitates breathing. The surgical procedure and preexisting health problems are considered when positioning the patient. The patient is positioned to prevent aspiration, facilitate respiration, promote comfort, and accommodate tubes, casts, and incisions.

Monitoring Vital Signs

Vital signs are monitored during the postoperative phase. Nursing assessments and interventions focus on temperature, blood pressure, pulse, respiration, and oxygen saturation. All vital signs are compared with the baseline data, and deviations from the preoperative vital signs are documented and reported. Changes in vital signs can be symptomatic of many complications. Diligent assessment of the patient is conducted to quickly identify problems or complications.

Monitoring Neurologic Status

Assessing the patient's neurologic system provides data for nursing interventions to reduce surgical risk factors and postoperative complications. The nurse compares the postoperative data with preoperative baseline data to plan interventions. The PACU nurse orients the patient to the environment, monitors mental status, and provides a calm environment in the immediate postoperative setting.

Pain Management

Surgery is an invasive procedure, and pain is an expected outcome. It is difficult to eliminate pain completely after a major surgical procedure. Pain stimulates the sympathetic nervous system, resulting in tachycardia, immobility, shallow breathing, and impaired gas exchange. Each of these effects is potentially harmful. The nurse thoroughly assesses a patient and the response to pain in the postoperative period at least every 2 hours and treats accordingly. If the patient's pain is poorly controlled, assessment is performed more frequently. If a patient does not experience a significant decrease in pain, the nurse should consider revising the plan of care and notify the surgeon. Education is necessary if a patient is being sent home on pain medications.

> **! SAFE PRACTICE ALERT**
>
> The patient's report of pain, the type of pain medication, the medication order, and vital signs determine pain management strategies. The only exception to this is when the patient is not able to communicate.

It is difficult to manage acute pain in patients who use opioids for chronic pain. These patients use opioids to achieve pain control on a daily basis. Surgery causes acute pain, and additional doses of pain medication may be necessary. A pain management plan can determine how to better manage a patient's pain.

After the immediate postoperative period, a patient whose pain is controlled is more likely to perform leg exercises, ambulate, cough and deep-breathe, turn, and use the incentive spirometer, decreasing the likelihood of postoperative complications. Administering pain medications and using nonpharmacologic pain management techniques enable the patient to feel more comfortable. Pain is managed by a variety of medications, including narcotics, nonopioid medications, and analgesics. Activities such as distraction, relaxation, music, and imagery techniques create comfort and decrease anxiety (see Chapter 36). Heat and cold applications are used as therapies in pain management (see Chapter 29). It is important for the nurse to follow the primary care provider's orders and understand hospital policy to determine which applications are appropriate for the patient.

Postoperative Safety

Safety measures are carefully implemented for postoperative patients. In the postoperative phase, the top side rails are kept up and the call light in reach. Pillows are not used with unconscious patients to decrease the risk of airway complications, such as accidental suffocation. When unconscious patients begin to wake up, the nurse orients them to where they are, informs them that the surgical procedure has been completed, and gives additional instructions or information they may need.

Nursing Care of Common Postoperative Complications

Postoperative complications are a major concern. Many postoperative complications and problems rapidly become critical situations. A patient can be at risk for postoperative complications for numerous reasons.

Many postoperative complications can be prevented by preoperative assessments, vigilance during the immediate postoperative period, and nursing interventions. Understanding how adverse events and errors occurred can prevent future errors and improve morbidity and mortality rates (Beyea, 2009). If a postoperative complication does occur, the nurse performs an assessment, provides nursing care, and carries out the interventions designed to minimize the effects of the complication. During this time, the nurse may need to provide the patient and family emotional support.

Airway Obstruction

An **airway obstruction** is a life-threatening emergency that produces reduced airflow. It is a common postoperative complication. Airway obstruction can occur when the tongue falls back into the pharynx, or it can result from laryngospasm, bronchospasm, or aspiration of gastric contents. It often occurs when the patient is lying in a supine position and is very relaxed.

Airway obstruction is a high priority because it interferes with the delivery of oxygen to vital organs. Nursing care of a patient with an airway obstruction includes manual opening of the airway with a jaw-thrust or chin-lift maneuver. Close assessment determines whether there is an obvious obstruction such as the tongue, vomit, blood, secretions, loose teeth, or a foreign body that needs to be removed. Suctioning can be performed to remove vomit, blood, and secretions. Interventions performed are evaluated to determine their effectiveness. The patient with an advanced airway problem sometimes needs the assistance of an anesthesiologist. Manual resuscitation with an Ambu bag or bag-valve-mask device or re-intubation may be necessary to force oxygen into the lungs and facilitate obtaining a patent airway.

Hemorrhage

A large amount of bleeding, or **hemorrhage**, can occur in the immediate postoperative period from internal or external blood loss. During the postoperative phase, hemorrhage can occur from a weak suture, stress on the surgical site, medications, or a clot that has become dislodged.

Nursing care focuses on controlling the bleeding and replacing blood volume if needed. Careful assessment is performed to look for clinical indications of hemorrhage, such as anxiety; restlessness; cold, clammy skin; a weak, thready, rapid pulse; hypotension; respirations that are rapid and deep; increased thirst; and decreased urine output. The nurse pays close attention to the surgical dressing.

When assessing for bleeding, the nurse observes the color of the blood. Bright red blood suggests recent bleeding; dark, brownish blood indicates that the bleeding is not fresh. The perimeter of the blood stain on the original dressing is outlined. Reinforcement of the original dressing may be needed. The date and time the outline was made is noted on the dressing. When external bleeding occurs, pressure is applied to the site manually with gloved hands or with a pressure dressing. Manual pressure is performed with caution to prevent further injury to the affected area. If bleeding is severe, the patient may need to return to the operating room.

! SAFE PRACTICE ALERT

Always wear gloves when changing or reinforcing dressings or when applying manual pressure over a wound that is bleeding.

Shock

When the circulatory system fails to maintain adequate perfusion to the vital organs, **shock** occurs. As a result, the heart is unable to pump enough blood to the body. This is a life-threatening postoperative complication, and cell and organ death will occur if it is untreated. Hypovolemic shock is the most common type of shock seen in postoperative patients. It occurs when there is a decrease in circulating blood volume due to hemorrhage or dehydration.

Common assessment findings are similar to those identified for hemorrhage. Hypovolemic shock is considered a medical emergency. The symptoms and prognosis can vary according to the amount of blood volume lost, the rate of blood loss, and the underlying cause of shock.

The goals of treatment for shock consist of improving and maintaining tissue perfusion by correcting the cause of shock. Nursing care is focused on establishing a patent airway, monitoring vital signs, administering oxygen as ordered, maintaining a flat position with the legs elevated to increase venous return, and monitoring laboratory test results (e.g., arterial blood gases, complete blood count). Additional interventions include maintaining body temperature and administering blood, IV fluids, and prescribed medications.

Thrombophlebitis

Thrombophlebitis is inflammation of a vein with the formation of a thrombus (i.e., blood clot). For postoperative patients, a blood clot commonly originates in the deep veins of the legs, known as *deep vein thrombosis.* It can result from trauma during surgery, decreased blood flow, immobility, and varicose veins. Patients have cramping, pain, redness, and swelling in the extremity with the thrombus. A venous Doppler ultrasound can be used as a diagnostic test and to guide treatment.

Nursing care focuses on preventing clots from developing and preventing a thrombus from becoming detached. Antiembolism stockings (see Chapter 28, Skill 28-4), sequential compression devices (see Chapter 28, Skill 28-5), leg exercises, and ambulation can be used to promote circulation and help prevent a thrombus from forming. If thrombophlebitis occurs, treatment consists of the administration of anticoagulants and analgesics, bed rest, elevation of the affected extremity, and measuring the circumference of the affected extremity every shift. Laboratory values for clotting times are monitored, and the patient is instructed not to rub or massage the affected extremity.

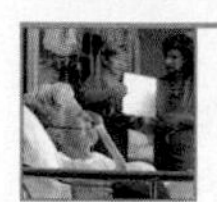

3. Identify at least three nursing interventions to prevent the postoperative complication of deep vein thrombosis for Mrs. Logan.

Pulmonary Embolism

A blood clot that detaches and lodges in the pulmonary artery is called a **pulmonary embolism**. Fat droplets, air bubbles, venous stasis, amniotic fluid, tumor cells, and clotting disorders contribute to the development of a pulmonary embolism. Venous stasis, which is commonly seen in postoperative patients, is a risk factor for development and dislodgment of a thrombus, a portion of which may break away from the wall of the vein and travel to the heart, lungs, or brain. Pulmonary embolism is a life-threatening complication, and immediate intervention is needed to sustain life. Patients have the following signs and symptoms at clinical presentation:

- Anxiety
- Restlessness
- Chest pain
- Dyspnea
- Cough
- Cyanosis
- Leg pain and swelling (in one or both legs)
- Dysrhythmias
- Tachypnea
- Tachycardia
- Hypotension

Nursing care includes stabilizing the respiratory and cardiovascular systems. A concern for these patients is the potential development of other emboli. Treatment consists of administering anticoagulants, analgesics, and sedatives. The patient is administered oxygen and placed on bed rest. The head of the bed is elevated to facilitate breathing. The nurse provides instructions to the patient to avoid activities that increase intrathoracic pressure (Valsalva maneuver), which can increase the risk of more emboli traveling to the pulmonary artery. The nurse monitors vital signs, pulse oximetry, laboratory tests for clotting times, and the cardiovascular and respiratory systems.

Pneumonia

Pneumonia is inflammation of the lungs. It is usually caused by an infection or foreign material. In postoperative patients, pneumonia may occur (usually 48 to 72 hours postoperatively) as a result of aspiration, excessive pulmonary secretions, immobility, failure to cough deeply, and a depressed cough reflex. Assessment of the patient reveals dyspnea, adventitious breath sounds, chest pain, chills, fever, and cough. The cough may be productive with purulent or rust-colored secretions.

Treatment includes promotion of lung expansion and preventing the spread of infection. Nursing care includes interventions to improve lung function, such as encouraging the use of the incentive spirometer (Nursing Care Guideline: Incentive Spirometry box), nebulizer treatments, and intermittent positive-pressure breathing (IPPB). Antibiotics are given to treat the infection. Other treatments are expectorants, antipyretics, and analgesics. The patient is positioned in a semi-Fowler or Fowler position to facilitate expansion of the lungs. Hydration orally and with IV fluids helps to liquefy secretions. Oxygen is administered as ordered to maintain adequate oxygen saturation levels for the patient.

Atelectasis

Atelectasis is the collapse of all or part of the lung. It is caused by pressure on the outside of the lung or a blockage of the air passages (bronchus or bronchioles). As a result,

NURSING CARE GUIDELINE

Incentive Spirometry

Background

- An incentive spirometer is used by the patient to practice inhalation.
- The patient attempts to reach a set inhalation volume.
- The volume may be set by the primary care provider (PCP) or respiratory therapy specialist or calculated from standardized charts.
- The technique encourages deep breathing, maintains lung expansion, and helps to prevent atelectasis and pneumonia.
- If surgery is planned, the technique is taught to the patient before surgery to allow time for practice.

Procedural Concerns

- The patient should be in an upright position (semi-Fowler or Fowler) if possible.
- The patient's goal is to have a steady rise of a marker in the device to achieve a specific inhalation volume, which is marked on the device.

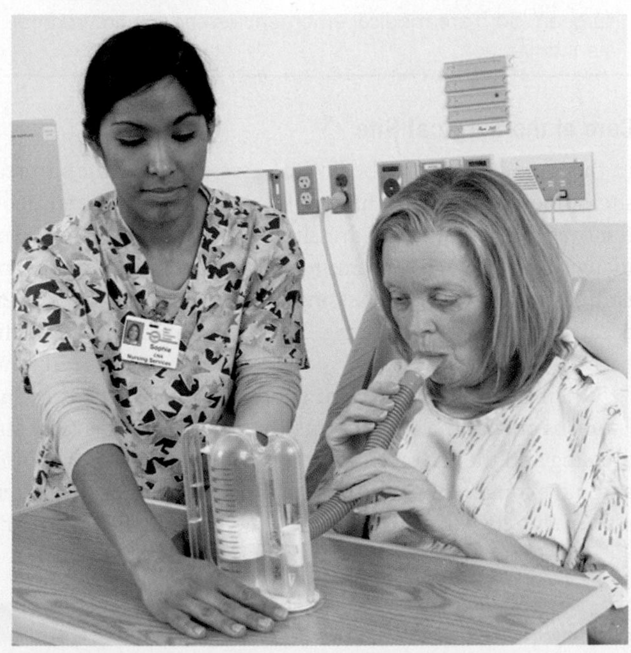

(From Sorrentino SA, Remmert L: *Mosby's textbook for nursing assistants*, ed. 8, St. Louis, 2012, Mosby.)

- Instruct the patient to inhale slowly with the mouth on the mouthpiece.
  - Inhale as much as possible, and hold that breath for 3 to 5 seconds.
  - Slowly exhale.
  - Repeat each inhalation and exhalation 5 to 12 times.
  - End with two controlled coughs (see Nursing Care Guideline: Cough and Deep-Breathing Techniques box).
- Perform this exercise every 1 to 2 hours per orders.

Documentation Concerns

- Document the patient education concerning correct procedure and performance times.
- Note the patient's concerns and discomfort, and document noncompliance issues.
- Include a respiratory assessment before and after the procedure.
- Document the patient's use of the incentive spirometer and tolerance of the procedure.

Evidence-Based Practice

- Pulmonary therapy, including incentive spirometry breathing (ISB), was found to decrease recovery time and improve lung functioning of obese patients if begun immediately after surgery in recovery and the PACU.
- Lung function was significantly improved for 24 hours postoperatively (Zoremba, Dette, Gerlach, et al, 2009).

pulmonary secretions are retained, and the patient has poor gas exchange. Common assessment findings are cough, dyspnea, anxiety, chest pain, cyanosis, diminished breath sounds over the affected area, and crackles.

Treatment focuses on promoting expansion of the lung and improving oxygenation. Nursing care includes administering oxygen and analgesics as ordered, positioning in a Fowler or semi-Fowler position, ambulation, hydration, coughing, deep breathing, incentive spirometry, and turning every 2 hours.

Wound Complications

Surgery may cause a disruption in skin integrity. This endangers the skin's ability to protect against infection. A wound infection is a common postoperative complication (Allen, 2009), and it usually occurs 48 to 72 hours postoperatively.

The edges of a healing surgical wound should be pink with healthy granulation tissue. They should be well approximated. This means the edges precisely meet together. Incisions may be held together by staples, sutures, surgical super glue, or Steri-Strips. A delay in wound healing can be caused by infection, blood clots, tissue hypoxia, trauma, advanced age, abnormal laboratory values, obesity, undernourishment, immunosuppression, and systemic diseases such as diabetes. Chapter 29 provides more information on wound healing.

When wound dehiscence occurs, the surgical incision fails to remain closed. The edges of the incision separate without organs protruding (Figure 37-6). This can occur in any wound but is commonly seen after abdominal surgery. With dehiscence, the surgical dressing reveals a large amount of serosanguineous fluid. If dehiscence occurs or is suspected, the nurse assists the patient into a position that allows minimal strain to be placed on the incision. The wound is covered with a sterile saline dressing, and the surgeon is notified immediately. Dehiscence usually is a later postoperative wound complication, occurring 48 to 72 hours after surgery.

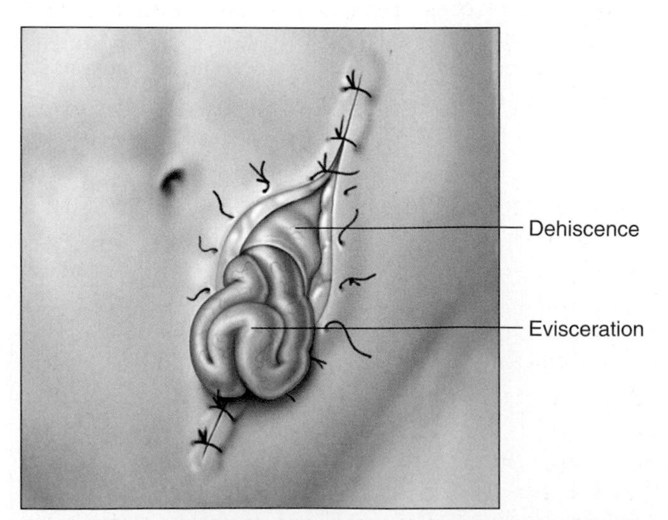

FIGURE 37-6 Dehiscence and evisceration. (From Harkreader H et al: *Fundamentals of nursing: caring and clinical judgment*, ed. 3, St. Louis, 2007, Saunders.)

Evisceration occurs when the surgical incision fails to remain closed and organs protrude. The patient may report feeling the wound "coming loose." When this occurs, the patient is placed in a position that puts the least amount of strain on the incision. The semi-Fowler position is often used. Sterile gauze soaked in sterile saline is placed on the incision, and the surgeon is notified immediately. The patient is encouraged to remain calm.

Dehiscence and evisceration are medical emergencies. Surgical repair is often needed. Both wound complications can be caused by delayed wound healing or sutures that have been removed too soon. When the sutures have been removed too early, deep muscle support to maintain the closure of the wound may be decreased. The length of time sutures remain in the patient depends on the type of sutures used, the procedure, the length of the incision, and the size of the patient. Sutures are commonly removed when the edges of a healing wound appear pink and slightly raised.

Smoking, medications, and preexisting medical problems contribute to poor wound healing. Additional causes for dehiscence and evisceration are wound infection, defective sutures, allergic reaction to sutures, obesity, sneezing, coughing, and vomiting.

> **! SAFE PRACTICE ALERT**
>
> When dehiscence or evisceration occurs, the patient is placed in a position that produces minimal strain on the surgical wound. Apply a sterile saline dressing, and call the surgeon. Both are medical emergencies and require immediate intervention.

Care of the Surgical Site

In the PACU, there may be limited assessment of the surgical site. Some hospitals may have policies stating that the surgeon removes the first surgical dressing, which is the preference of many surgeons. Every attempt is made to reinforce a postoperative dressing, but the dressing sometimes must be removed because of excessive bleeding. The surgeon is notified if this occurs.

When a wound assessment is performed and the dressing is not removed, the nurse notes the location and size of the dressing and the characteristics of the drainage, such as color, amount, consistency, and odor. Box 37-2 shows a wound assessment checklist for use when the dressing is removed.

> **! SAFE PRACTICE ALERT**
>
> Until orders have been given to remove the dressing, the initial surgical dressing is not removed.

BOX 37-2 Wound Assessment Checklist

When dressings are being removed, the nurse assesses the following wound characteristics:

- Size (current size; size may decrease with healing)
- Type of closure (transverse, midline, horizontal)
- Edges (well approximated with staples, sutures, Steri-Strips, or surgical glue)
- Drains (type of drain; amount and type of fluid in drains)
- Drainage (type, consistency, color, amount, and odor for the type)
- Signs of infection (redness in the surrounding skin, yellow wound bed, purulent drainage, and foul-smelling drainage)

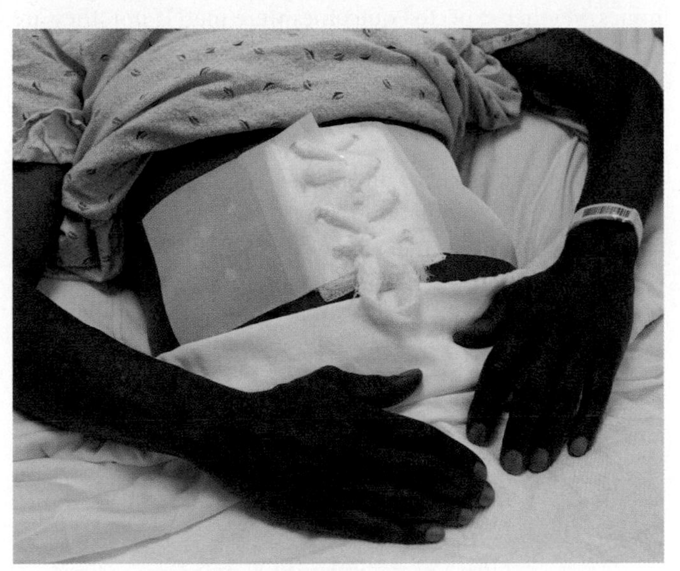

FIGURE 37-7 Montgomery straps.

When a patient has a wound with excess drainage, dressings may need to be changed frequently. Tape can be very irritating to the skin. In some cases, Montgomery straps (ties) are used when surgical dressings are in place for extended periods, and the dressing is changed frequently (Figure 37-7). The straps are designed to decrease the skin irritation and discomfort that are caused by repeated removal of tape.

Postoperative Care After the Postanesthesia Care Unit

Specific discharge criteria must be met for the patient to be discharged from the PACU. Criteria include the patient's vital signs, respiratory status, level of consciousness, and activity level. The Aldrete score was developed in 1970 (Aldrete and Kroulik) to provide concrete criteria for PACU discharge. This score has since been modified for use with ambulatory and outpatient surgery patients.

For patients being admitted to a nursing unit, the PACU nurse gives a report on the patient's postoperative status to the unit nurse when the patient is transferred. After arrival in the nursing unit, the patient is moved to a bed. The unit nurse assesses the patient's vital signs and respiratory status, dressings and drains, and level of consciousness and provides care according to the patient's needs. Before the nurse leaves the patient, the top side rails on the bed are raised, the bed is returned to the lowest position, and the call light is placed within reach.

Early Ambulation

The nurse instructs the patient to call for assistance when he or she wants to get out of bed. Many patients feel weak and dizzy the first time they ambulate after surgery. Dangling before attempting to stand up for ambulation helps to prevent injury to patients who have been immobile for some time. Having one or two caregivers to assist the first time the patient gets out of bed is recommended. Early ambulation helps to prevent many complications postoperatively, including constipation, deep vein thrombosis, atelectasis, pneumonia, and urinary stasis. Many patients who experience abdominal distention and gas pain obtain some relief from ambulating.

Fluids and Hydration

To maintain fluid volume, IV fluids are infused at the ordered rate. The intake and output values are monitored to determine fluid imbalances. The IV site, IV solution, infusion rate, and patency are assessed. Adequate fluid intake helps to keep stools soft, ease the passage of stool, keep lung secretions thin, and prevent urinary complications.

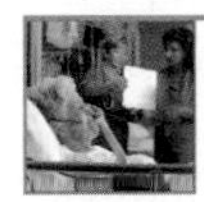

4. Name at least three nursing actions to prevent postoperative respiratory complications for Mrs. Logan.

Diet Advancement

Patients remain NPO until the gag reflex returns. Ice chips and oral fluids can be administered as prescribed. Oral feedings may be delayed until peristalsis returns. The abdomen is assessed for bowel sounds, flatus, and distention. Many patients move from a clear diet to a regular diet very quickly.

Discharge

During the postoperative phase, the nurse, patient, and family collaborate to prepare the patient for discharge. Discharge instructions are given to the patient. Additional information is provided to the patient about medications, wound care, activity level, and diet (Home Care Considerations box). Specific information related to the disease process and the surgical procedure is given. Some patients may be required to urinate before they can be discharged. The physician determines the readiness for discharge and writes an order for the patient to be discharged from the hospital. When anesthesia has been administered, patients are not allowed to drive themselves home because of the effects of anesthetic medications.

HOME CARE CONSIDERATIONS

Postoperative Care in the Home

The patient and family are evaluated to determine their ability to manage required care after the patient is discharged. Some patients may require medications, dressing changes, activity limitations, and physical therapy. Patients may be at risk for complications.

- Do the patient and family understand the signs and symptoms that may require follow-up with a physician?
- Do the patient and family have a plan to meet the needs of the patient?
- How often will caregivers or support people be able to provide assistance?
- Is a referral for home care needed to assist with self-care activities?
- Can the home be modified to allow necessary medical equipment to be moved into the home?

If a patient is admitted to a nursing unit after surgery, the length of stay depends on the disease process and the surgical procedure. Inpatients must meet clinical discharge criteria that are determined by the physician and receive discharge instructions before leaving the hospital.

Many patients want to be discharged from the hospital as soon as possible. After the physician has indicated the patient can leave the hospital, the discharged process is completed as quickly as possible. Often, nurses make follow-up calls to patients within 24 hours after discharge to determine whether the patient has questions or concerns. This promotes comfort and reassures the patient as he or she heals and returns to a preoperative state of health.

EVALUATION

In each phase of the perioperative period, the nurse evaluates the effectiveness of all nursing interventions. The nurse determines whether expected outcomes were met. If not, they are reevaluated. If outcomes are met, the nurse evaluates whether continuing the interventions is appropriate. Throughout the perioperative period, ongoing assessments are consistently made.

The nurse documents during each phase of the perioperative period. Documentation reflects the plan of care, nursing assessments, diagnosis, outcome identification, planning, interventions, and evaluations. The perioperative record reflects continuous evaluation of nursing care and the patient's response to all treatments and nursing interventions.

SKILL 37-1 Surgical Scrub, Gowning, and Gloving

PURPOSE

- Surgical handwashing prevents the spread of microorganisms.
- Wearing a surgical gown prevents the spread of microorganisms and allows the wearer to perform activities in the operating room in comfort while maintaining sterility.
- Surgical gloving is used to prevent the spread of microorganisms, protect the provider and patient from infection, and perform activities in the operating room in comfort while maintaining sterility.

RESOURCES

- Sink with knee or foot controls
- Antimicrobial soap per facility policy and procedures
- Surgical scrub sponge
- Plastic nail pick
- Sterile towels
- Sterile surgical gown
- Adjunct surgical clothing: face mask, cap, shoe covers
- Work area above waist height, located near the procedure
- Sterile surgical gloves of the correct size

COLLABORATION AND DELEGATION

- Surgical handwashing is required for all health care workers who will be sterile or scrubbed in the surgical environment.
- Surgical handwashing is essential to prevent infections. Team members should speak up when they see anyone breaking surgical technique. Handwashing should start over if sterile technique is broken.
- The scrub nurse/assistant may assist with certain aspects of the procedure.
- Surgical gowning is performed by any health care provider who may be participating in a procedure that requires sterile surgical technique.
- Unlicensed assistive personnel (UAP) who are assisting in a procedure and have been trained in the proper application may perform surgical gowning and gloving. Check with the state board of nursing for specific policies.
- Surgical gloving is completed by all health care providers who participate in a procedure that requires sterile surgical technique.

EVIDENCE-BASED PRACTICE

- Natural fingernails should be kept less than ¼ inch long. Clear nail polish that has been applied within the past 4 days and is not chipped is acceptable. Rings are removed because the evidence has associated even a plain band with a higher bacterial count. Artificial nails may not be worn (AORN, 2005).
- The Association for Perioperative Practice (AfPP) (2007) and the Operating Room Nurses Association of Canada (ORNAC) (2005) point out that "it is important to be aware that the gown is considered sterile only in the area between the chest and the level of the sterile field and that, in relation to the sleeves, this is from 2 inches above the gown cuff or from the glove cuff to the elbow. All other areas are considered unsterile, even though they have not been contaminated" (Pirie, 2010).
- Due to the risk of tearing a hole in the gloves and therefore increasing the risk of contamination, many organizations such as the Association of periOperative Registered Nurses (AORN), the ORNAC, the AfPP, and the Australian College of Operating Room Nurses (ACORN) recommend double-gloving in certain situations to protect the provider (Pirie, 2010).

SPECIAL CIRCUMSTANCES: SURGICAL SCRUB

1. **Assess:** Are there cuts, open sores, hangnails, or breaks in the skin or around cuticles?
   Intervention: Cover them with an appropriate dressing after cleaning.
2. **Assess:** Are there long nails, artificial nails, or nail polish?
   Intervention: File long nails, remove artificial nails, and remove nail polish. Check facility policy; only clear nail polish usually is allowed, and if it has been on the fingernails longer than 4 days, it should be removed because it is a place for microorganisms to grow.
3. **Assess:** Is the surgical team member wearing jewelry, a watch, or long sleeves?
   Intervention: Remove the jewelry, watch, and long sleeves.
4. **Assess:** Are there visible marks, spots, or dirt to be removed?
   Intervention: Use the soap and water method to remove them.
5. **Assess:** Have hands (skin) directly touched the sink, body, or another surface?
   Intervention: Start handwashing again.
6. **Assess:** Did hands (skin) touch another surface when retrieving the sterile towels?
   Intervention: Start handwashing again.

SPECIAL CIRCUMSTANCES: GOWNING

1. **Assess:** Has there been inadvertent contamination of the gown against the wearer's body or an object?
   Intervention: Obtain a new gown and start the procedure over.

2. **Assess:** Has the skin touched a sterile part of the gown or sterile field, or has the gown touched the skin or anything outside of the sterile field?
   Intervention: Obtain a new gown and start the procedure over.
3. **Assess:** Have the surgical team members turned their backs on the opened sterile gown or sterile area?
   Intervention: Obtain new gowns and start the procedure over.
4. **Assess:** Did the gown tear during the procedure?
   Intervention: Obtain a new gown and start the procedure over.

SPECIAL CIRCUMSTANCES: GLOVING

1. **Assess:** Is the surgical team member wearing jewelry?
   Intervention: Remove *all* jewelry before surgical gloving to avoid the possibility of tearing the gloves.
2. **Assess:** Is the glove package damaged, or has it expired?
   Intervention: Obtain a new pair of gloves.
3. **Assess:** Is any part of the work area below waist level?
   Intervention: Raise the work area, and find a new area to place surgical gloves.
4. **Assess:** Has skin directly touched a sterile part of the glove or sterile field, or has the glove touched skin or anything outside of the sterile field?
   Intervention: Obtain a new pair of gloves and start over.
5. **Assess:** Have scrubbed members of the surgical team turned their backs on the opened package of gloves or sterile area?
   Intervention: Obtain a new pair of gloves and start over.
6. **Assess:** Did the gloves tear during the procedure?
   Intervention: Obtain a new pair of gloves and start over.

PROCEDURES

Surgical Scrub

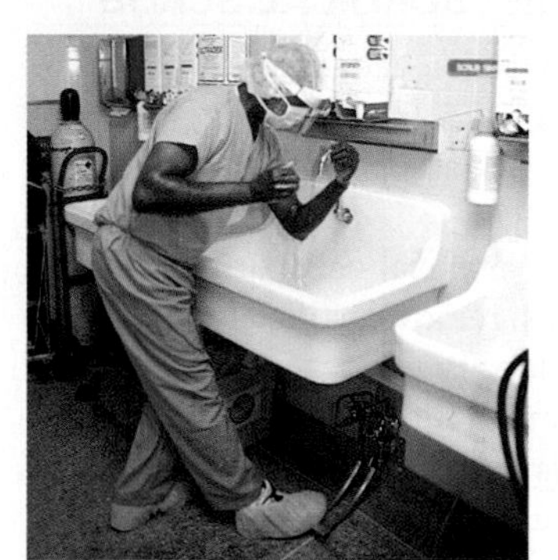

STEP 2
(From Ignatavicius and Workman, 2013.)

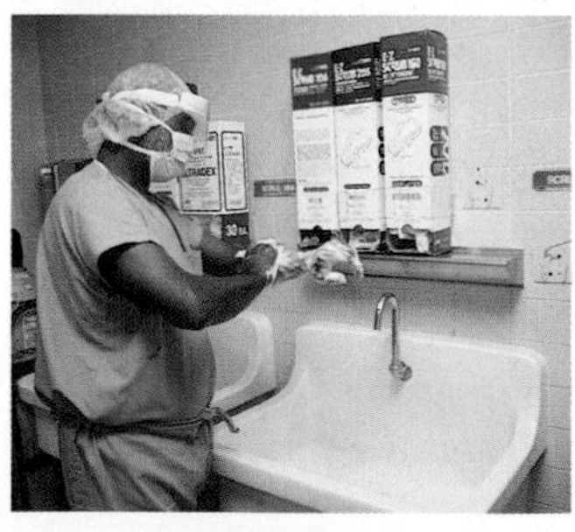

STEP 4
(From Ignatavicius and Workman, 2013.)

1. Apply the adjunct surgical clothing (i.e., surgical cap, face mask, and shoe covering) before entering the surgical area. Use the knee or foot controls to turn on warm water at a medium flow.
   Adjunct surgical clothing is applied before entering the surgical area and before the surgical scrub and the donning of sterile gown and gloves. Warm water helps remove dirt and microorganisms but not protective skin oils. Use medium flow to avoid splashing.
2. Wet the skin from 2 inches above the elbows to the hands; hands remain above the elbows.
   Hands should be the least contaminated when finished washing if this procedure has been followed.
3. Apply soap.
   Using soap reduces microorganisms.
4. Prescrub: Lather, rub using a circular movement, and wash for 20 seconds in the following order:
   a. Fingertips (clean under the nails with a pick)
   b. Fingers
   c. Between fingers (interlaced, including the thumbs)
   d. Palm of hands with fingertips
   e. Back of hands
   f. Wrists
   g. Forearms
   h. Elbows
   Friction helps remove microorganisms; the presence of lather indicates friction has occurred.
5. Rinse from fingertips to elbows. Keep the hands above the elbows.
   Proper technique and hand position prevent the spread of microorganisms.
6. Scrub with a surgical brush in the order specified:
   a. Fingers, hands, arms (four strokes each)
   b. Nails (15 strokes each with the brush)
   c. Palm, back of hand, thumb, fingers (all sides receive10 strokes each with the brush)
   d. Arm (divide the arm into thirds; scrub each third with 10 strokes with the brush)
   e. Rinse the brush; repeat on the other arm.
   f. Throw away the brush.
   Scrubbing removes microorganisms.

7. Rinse from fingertips to elbows. Keep the hands above the elbows.
   Proper technique and hand position prevents the spread of microorganisms.
8. Turn off the water using the knee or foot controls; hold arms in the air in front with hands raised, if indicated.
   This maintains sterility of the hands by using the knee or foot controls to turn off the water. Keeping the hands raised and avoiding touching anything with them prevents contamination.
9. Obtain one sterile towel. Dry one arm from the fingertips to the elbows, using a patting motion.
   Use a dry, sterile towel to prevent the spread of microorganisms; microorganisms like dampness. Avoid injury to the skin from rubbing.
10. Drop the towel into the linen hamper, or the circulating nurse collects it in outstretched hands.
    Proper disposal of the towel maintains sterility and prevents contamination.
11. Repeat procedure steps 9 and 10 for the other arm.

Applying a Gown

1. Perform the surgical scrub procedure as described earlier.
2. Obtain a sterile gown:
   a. Reach for the gown from the circulating nurse by grasping the gown inside just below the neckband.
   b. Alternatively, lift the gown from the sterile table by grasping the inside of the gown and stepping away from the table.
   The circulating nurse assists with sterile technique and proceeds in such a way as to avoid inadvertent contamination of the gown.
3. Open the gown by grabbing the inside of the gown below the neckline and allowing it to unfold in front and away from the body.
   Maintain sterility by avoiding inadvertent contamination of the gown.

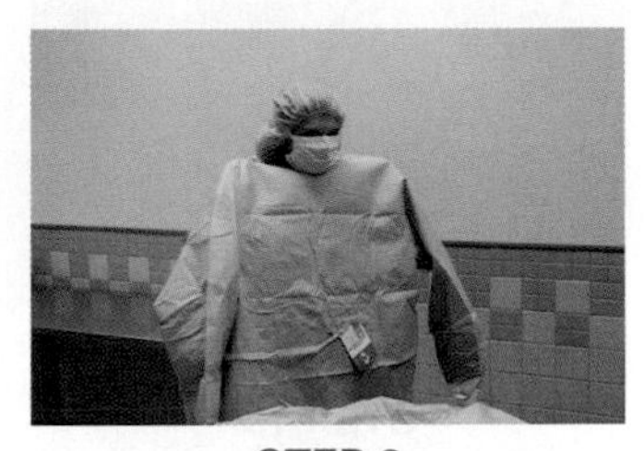

STEP 3
(From Ehrlich, 2013.)

4. Put the gown on:
   a. Place both arms inside the sleeves. Do *not* touch the outside of the gown.
   b. Have the circulating nurse pull the gown on and tie it in the back.
   c. Do *not* put hands through the sleeve openings.
   Avoid inadvertent contamination of the gown by allowing the circulating nurse to assist with sterile technique and by keeping the hands inside the gown for a closed gloving procedure. The back of the gown is not considered sterile.

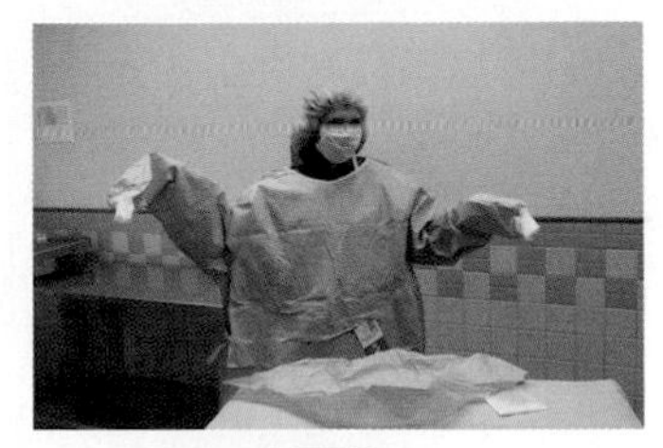

STEP 4
(From Ehrlich, 2013.)

5. Apply sterile gloves (see the Applying Surgical Gloves section).
6. If needed, complete the remainder of the gown preparation and securing according to the manufacturer's instructions.

Applying Surgical Gloves

1. Perform the surgical scrub procedure (see the Surgical Scrub section).
2. Perform the surgical gowning procedure, if needed (see the Applying a Gown section).
3. Keep hands inside the surgical gown sleeves. The circulating nurse opens the outer sterile glove package and places the inner sterile glove package on a sterile field.
   The circulating nurse assists with sterile technique; the provider who will wear the gloves keeps hands inside the gown for the closed gloving procedure.
4. Open the inner sterile glove package while keeping the hands inside the gown.
   This maintains sterility and prevents the spread of microorganisms.
5. If right handed, use the right hand as the working hand to grab the cuff of the glove for the left hand; if left handed, use the left hand to grab the cuff of the glove for the right hand.
   Grabbing the cuffs of the gloves prevents contamination.
6. Prepare to put on the glove. Extend the forearm straight out from the body, with the elbow held at a 90-degree angle and the palm facing upward.
   Arm and hand positions are intended to maintain sterility.

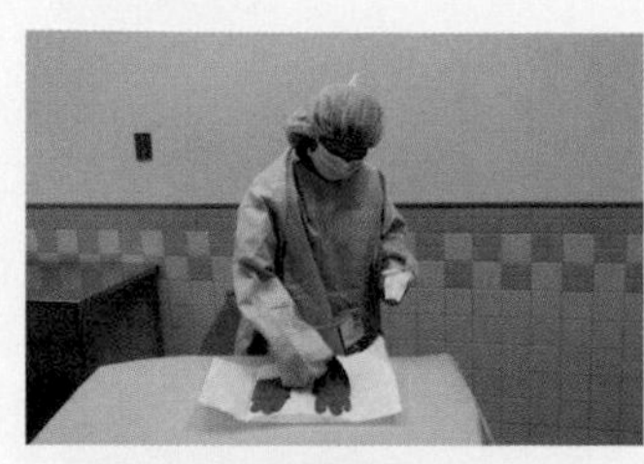

STEP 7
(From Ehrlich, 2013.)

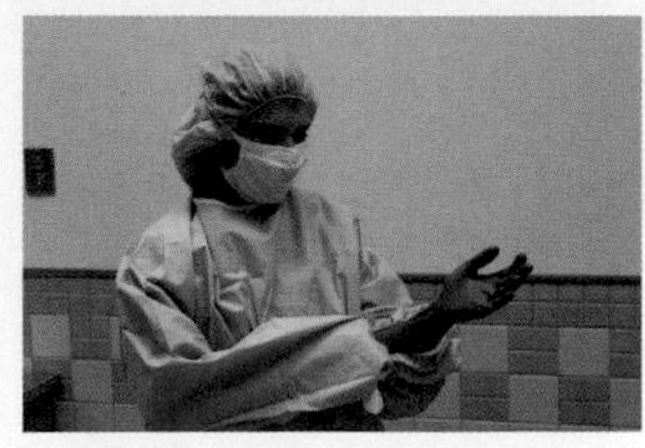

STEP 8
(From Ehrlich, 2013.)

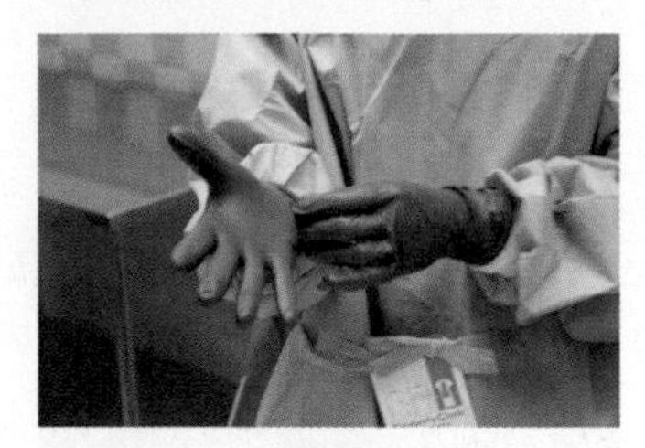

STEP 10
(From Ehrlich, 2013.)

7. Put the glove over the gowned hand:
   a. The working hand is used to pull the glove cuff over the gowned (sleeve-covered) hand.
   b. Unfold the glove while pulling it over the gowned hand.
   c. The fingers of the glove need to fall or point toward the elbow, *not* toward the floor.

   This creates a glove-gown seal and prevents the spread of microorganisms.
8. Insert fingers into the glove:
   a. With the ungloved, gown-covered hand, hold the glove with the glove fingers up.
   b. Push the partially gloved hand out of the gown and into the glove, extending the fingers into the fingers of the glove.
9. Repeat procedure steps 5 through 8 for applying the opposite glove.
10. Ensure both gloves are fitted properly. Avoid snapping the cuffs and ensure the cuffs are completely unrolled and covering the cuff of the gown.
    This creates a sealed sterile gown and glove combination.
11. Maintain sterility:
    a. Hold both hands together, and interlock the fingers.
    b. Keep the hands above the waist and away from the body at all times.

    Interlocking the fingers helps to ensure the gloves are correctly fitted. Keeping the hands up and away from the body reduces the risk of contamination until ready to begin the procedure.

Removing Surgical Gloves

1. Use the dominant hand to pull off one glove by grasping the outside of the cuff; do *not* touch the skin (see illustrations in the Applying Sterile Gloves and Removing Sterile Gloves sections in Chapter 26, Skill 26-2).
   Grasping the cuff prevents the spread of microorganisms from the contaminated surfaces of the gloves.
2. Hold the glove that was just removed crumpled in the hand that is still wearing a glove.
   Keeping the contaminated gloves together prevents the spread of microorganisms.
3. Using the gloveless hand, slide the thumb under the cuff of the remaining glove (skin to skin) while keeping the ungloved fingers curled.
   Keeping the skin surfaces together and avoiding touching the outer glove surface with bare fingers prevents the spread of microorganisms.
4. Peel off the glove, turning it inside out so that the first glove that was removed is contained inside the last glove that was removed.
   The most contaminated glove surfaces are inside the crumpled gloves to prevent the spread of microorganisms.
5. Throw away the gloves.
   Proper disposal of waste reduces the spread of microorganisms.

Removing the Gown

1. Remove the gloves first as described in the previous section.
   Gloves are contaminated. Removing them first allows the hands to touch the least contaminated portions of other personal protective equipment for removal and prevents the spread of microorganisms.
2. If separate from the mask, remove eyewear, handling it by the ear pieces.
   Eyewear is removed so that the mask can be removed without contamination; holding eyewear by the ear pieces lessens the chance of contaminating the hands.
3. Throw the eyewear into the trash, or place it in an appropriate container for cleaning.
   Proper disposal of the used equipment reduces the spread of microorganisms.

4. Remove the gown:
   a. Untie the waist.
   b. Untie the neck.
   c. Pull the gown off from the back of a shoulder, touching *only* the inside of the gown.
   d. While pulling off the gown, turn it inside out and roll it into a ball.
   The front of the gown and sleeves are contaminated; touching only the inside of the gown prevents the spread of microorganisms.
5. Throw the gown into the trash, or place it in the laundry bin for cleaning.
   Proper disposal of the contaminated gown reduces the spread of microorganisms.
6. Remove the mask:
   a. Untie the bottom of the mask.
   b. Untie the top of the mask and hold onto the ties.
   c. Pull the mask away from the face using the ties. Do *not* touch the outside of the mask.
   Holding the mask by the ties prevents contamination. Removing the mask last prevents the spread of microorganisms.
7. Throw the mask into the trash.
   Proper disposal of waste reduces the spread of microorganisms.
8. Remove the cap and shoe covers, and throw them into the trash.
   Proper disposal of waste reduces the spread of microorganisms.
9. Perform hand hygiene (see Chapter 26, Skill 26-1).
   Frequent hand hygiene prevents the spread of microorganisms.

Photos under "Surgical Scrub" are from Ignatavicius DD, Workman ML: *Medical-surgical nursing: Patient-centered collaborative care,* ed. 7, St. Louis, 2013, Saunders.
Photos under "Applying a Gown" and "Applying Surgical Gloves" are from Ehrlich RA: *Patient care in radiography,* ed. 8, St. Louis, 2013, Mosby.

SUMMARY OF LEARNING OUTCOMES

LO 37.1 *Differentiate between the phases of the perioperative period:* Perioperative nursing includes the care of the patient during three phases: preoperative, intraoperative, and postoperative.

LO 37.2 *Classify different types of surgery:* Surgical procedures are classified by the purpose (e.g., diagnostic, ablative, constructive, reconstructive, transplant, palliative, cosmetic); degree of urgency (e.g., elective, urgent, emergent); and degree of risk (e.g., major, minor). Factors affecting the degree of risk are general health, age, medications, mental status, and nutrition. Disorders of the cardiac, blood coagulation, respiratory, renal, liver, and endocrine systems can increase surgical risks.

LO 37.3 *Discuss safety during the perioperative period:* Safety is the major goal of perioperative care. The nurse is responsible for upholding all operating room safety standards and acting as a patient advocate in the preoperative, intraoperative, and postoperative phases.

LO 37.4 *Describe alterations that can occur during the perioperative period:* Alterations depend on patient factors and the type of surgery. Preoperatively, anxiety can occur. Intraoperative alterations depend on the type of surgery, positioning, and anesthesia. Postoperative alterations may include changes in consciousness, abnormal vital signs, and pain.

LO 37.5 *Identify vital perioperative assessment data:* Preoperative vital signs and physical assessment provide baseline data for comparing with postoperative assessment findings. Intraoperative assessment includes vital signs and safety concerns. The postoperative nurse assesses vital signs,; respiratory status, level of consciousness, dressings and drains, intake and output, and elimination.

LO 37.6 *Select nursing diagnoses for each perioperative stage:* Nursing diagnoses are developed based on interpretation of the data regarding the patient's particular surgery and stage within the perioperative period.

LO 37.7 *Establish nursing care goals and outcome criteria for surgical patients:* Nursing care goals and outcome criteria are based on the specific nursing diagnoses in each phase of the perioperative period.

LO 37.8 *Evaluate the effectiveness of the perioperative nursing interventions:* During the preoperative phase interventions are focused on patient education. Safety interventions are a priority in the operating room. Interventions during the postoperative phase are aimed at promoting healing and comfort, restoring the highest level of wellness, and decreasing the risk for potential complications. All nursing care and patient responses are evaluated during the perioperative period.

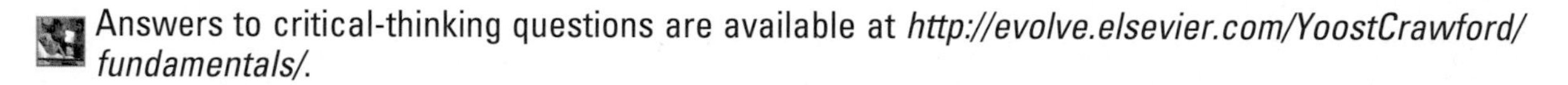
Answers to critical-thinking questions are available at *http://evolve.elsevier.com/YoostCrawford/fundamentals/.*

REVIEW QUESTIONS

1. The nurse is caring for a patient scheduled for a breast reduction to decrease pain in her back. How is this operation classified according to the degree of urgency?
   a. Urgent
   b. Emergency
   c. Emergent
   d. Elective
2. The postanesthesia care recovery unit (PACU) nurse is concerned about postoperative hemorrhage. Which clinical manifestation alerts the nurse to this problem?
   a. Incisional pain
   b. Elevated blood pressure
   c. Increased heart rate
   d. Bradypnea
3. What is the role of the nurse in securing an informed consent for a surgical procedure?
   a. Ensuring that the patient signs the informed consent document
   b. Signing the consent form as a witness
   c. Ensuring that the patient does not refuse treatment
   d. Refusing to participate based on legal guidelines
4. The nurse provided preoperative teaching about pain management to a patient scheduled for surgery. Which postoperative activity by the patient indicates the effectiveness of teaching?
   a. Doing something enjoyable such as relaxing and reading a book
   b. Requesting pain medication when no longer able to tolerate the pain.
   c. Removing the postoperative dressing to see the surgical incision
   d. Refusing to wear anti-embolism stockings while still on bed rest

5. A 55-year-old male is scheduled to have a bowel resection for a diagnosis of colon cancer. He is very nervous about surgery. How can the nurse help to decrease his anxiety?
   a. Ask him if he is concerned the cancer has spread to other areas of his body.
   b. Talk to him to find out what is causing his anxiety.
   c. Question him to find out what the surgeon has told him about the surgery.
   d. Give him a preoperative medication to help him relax.
6. A nurse is providing care to a patient scheduled to have surgery. Which patient data alert the nurse to an increased risk of surgical complications? *(Select all that apply.)*
   a. Daily use of multivitamins
   b. Five pounds overweight
   c. Anticoagulation medication
   d. Uncomplicated family history of previous operations
   e. Blood pressure of 170/98
7. How does malnutrition compromise wound healing?
   a. There is increased stress on the wound.
   b. Blood supply to the wound is increased.
   c. It causes patients to be energized and overexert.
   d. It can increase the risk of infection.
8. Which set of patient information assists the nurse in determining whether the nursing actions taken to prevent airway obstruction have been effective?
   a. Temperature 97.8° F, breathing regular and unlabored, no cough
   b. Intake equals output, denies pain or chest discomfort
   c. O_2 sat 91%, shortness of breath (SOB), R 26
   d. O_2 sat 89%, breathing shallow and regular, R 24
9. A PACU nurse received a patient from the operating room. During surgery, the patient had a loss of consciousness and skeletal muscle relaxation, and the patient does not remember the procedure. When assessing this patient, the nurse should conclude the patient received which type of anesthesia?
   a. General anesthesia
   b. Regional anesthesia
   c. Local anesthesia
   d. Nerve block
10. While conducting a preoperative health assessment, the nurse is informed about a preexisting heart problem. What postoperative interventions should be included in the plan of care for this patient?
   a. Perform a systematic head-to-toe assessment every 4 hours.
   b. Monitor breath sounds and oxygen saturation.
   c. Administer pain medications as needed.
   d. Monitor the electrocardiogram (ECG), apical pulse, and capillary refill.

Answers and rationales to review questions are available at *http://evolve.elsevier.com/YoostCrawford/fundamentals/*.

REFERENCES

Agency for Healthcare Research and Quality (AHRQ): *Surgical site infection: Prevention and treatment of surgical site infection,* Rockville, Md., 2008, U.S. Department of Health and Human Services.

Agency for Healthcare Research and Quality (AHRQ): Post-operative pain management. In *Guidelines on pain management,* Rockville, Md., 2009a, U.S. Department of Health and Human Services.

Agency for Healthcare Research and Quality (AHRQ): *Perioperative protocol. Health care protocol,* Rockville, Md., 2009b, U.S. Department of Health and Human Services.

Aldrete JA, Kroulik D: A post-anesthesia recovery score. *Anesth Analg,* 49:924, 1970.

Allen G: Evidence for practice: Predictive factors for surgical site infection. *AORN J,* 89(2):417-418, 2009.

American College of Surgeons: *Surgical patient education for a better recovery,* 2014. Retrieved from *www.facs.org/patienteducation/surgery.html.*

Association of periOperative Registered Nurses (AORN): *Perioperative standards and recommended practices,* Denver, 2012, AORN.

Association of periOperative Registered Nurses (AORN) Recommended Practices Committee: Recommended practices for surgical attire. *AORN J,* 81(2):413-420, 2005.

Banschbach S: Recommitting your practice to patient safety. *AORN J,* 88(6):887-888, 2008.

Beyea SC: Nursing morbidity and mortality conferences. *AORN J,* 89(2):413-415, 2009.

Beyea SC: Speaking up for quality and safety. *AORN J,* 88(1): 115-116, 2008.

Catalano K, Fickenscher K: Complying with the 2008 National Patient Safety Goals. *AORN J*, 87(3):547-556, 2008.

Cronenwett L, Sherwood G, Barnsteiner J, et al: Quality and safety education for nurses. *Nurs Outlook*, 55(3):122-131, 2007.

Eagle KA, Smetana GW: What the new guidelines offer for preoperative risk reduction. *Patient Care*, 40(10):18-25, 2006.

Ellis JR, Hartley CL: *Nursing in today's world; Trends, issues, and management*, ed. 10, Philadelphia, 2012, Lippincott.

Goldberg JL, Feldman DL: Implementing AORN recommended practices for prevention of retained surgical items. *AORN J*, 95(2):205-216, 2012.

Litwack K: *Clinical coach for effective perioperative nursing care*. Philadelphia, 2009, FA Davis.

Lorenzen B, Melby C, Earles B: Using principles of health literacy to enhance the informed consent process. *AORN J*, 88(1): 23-29, 2008.

Ogg M, Burlingame B: Recommended practices for moderate sedation/analgesia. *AORN J*, 88(2):275-281, 2008.

Pirie S: Surgical gown and gloving. *J Perioper Pract*, 20(6):207-209, 2010.

Putnis S, Nanuck J, Heath D: An audit of preoperative blood tests. *J Perioper Pract*, 18(2):56-59, 2008.

The Joint Commission: National patient safety goals, 2014. Retrieved from *http://www.jointcommission.org/assets/1/6/HAP_NPSG_Chapter_2014.pdf*

Woodruff DW: Pre-op care makes a difference. *RN formation*, 18(1), 2008.

Zoremba M, Dette F, Gerlach L, et al.: Short-term respiratory physical therapy treatment in the PACU and influence on postoperative lung function in obese adults. *Obes Surg*, 19(10):1346-1354, 2009.

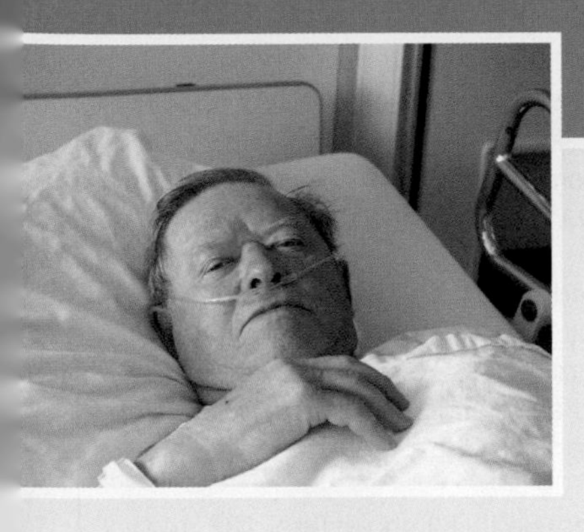

CHAPTER 38

Oxygenation and Tissue Perfusion

EVOLVE WEBSITE

http://evolve.elsevier.com/YoostCrawford/fundamentals/

- Additional Evolve-Only Review Questions With Answers
- Answers and Rationales for Text Review Questions
- Answers to Critical-Thinking Questions
- Case Study With Questions
- Video Skills Clips
- Heart and Lung Sounds
- Conceptual Care Map Creator
- Animations
- Skills Checklists
- Glossary

LEARNING OUTCOMES

Comprehension of this chapter's content will provide students with the ability to:

LO 38.1 Describe the basic anatomy and physiology of the cardiovascular and respiratory systems in relation to ventilation and perfusion.

LO 38.2 Summarize alterations in structure and function of the cardiovascular and respiratory systems.

LO 38.3 Demonstrate assessment of the cardiac and respiratory systems.

LO 38.4 Choose nursing diagnoses for patients with decreased oxygenation.

LO 38.5 Identify goals for patients with complications from decreased oxygenation.

LO 38.6 Evaluate interventions to enhance patient oxygenation, promote safety, and reverse the negative effects of decreased oxygenation.

KEY TERMS

antiembolism hose, p. 968
arrhythmias, p. 956
asthma, p. 952
atelectasis, p. 953
bronchodilators, p. 966
chronic bronchitis, p. 951
chronic obstructive pulmonary disease, p. 951
cyanosis, p. 960
electrocardiogram, p. 956
emphysema, p. 951
endotracheal tubes, p. 964
fraction of inspired oxygen, p. 960
forced expiratory flow, p. 955
forced expiratory volume in 1 second, p. 955
forced vital capacity, p. 955
functional residual capacity, p. 955
hemoptysis, p. 954
hypercapnia, p. 960
hypoxemia, p. 959
nasopharyngeal airway, p. 964
necrosis, p. 955
pleural effusion, p. 956
pneumonia, p. 953
postural drainage, p. 966
reservoir masks, p. 960
residual volume, p. 955
sequential compression devices, p. 968
tracheostomy tube, p. 965
vibration, p. 966

CASE STUDY

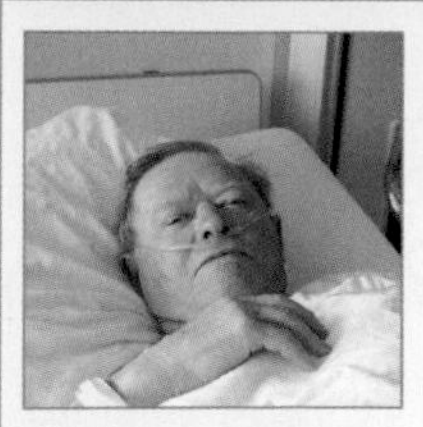

Mr. Ross is a 72-year-old male admitted to the hospital with severe chronic obstructive pulmonary disease (COPD). He has a 40-year history of smoking 2 packs per day and quit 10 years ago, and he has a history of hyperlipidemia.

Mr. Ross's vital signs are T 36.7° C (98° F), P 98 and regular, R 26 and labored, BP 144/73, with a pulse oximetry reading of 90% at rest on 2 liters of oxygen per nasal cannula. He denies pain but complains of difficulty breathing. The patient has a productive cough with thick secretions but has no hemoptysis. Heart sounds are distant. Breath sounds are diminished with inspiratory and expiratory wheezes and a prolonged expiratory phase. The abdomen is protruding without acute changes. Mr. Ross is on an adult regular diet but only ate 25% of his breakfast.

Laboratory and diagnostic test results are as follows:

- Lipids: total cholesterol 242, high-density lipoprotein (HDL) cholesterol 89, low-density lipoprotein (LDL) cholesterol 107, triglycerides 107
- Complete blood count (CBC): white blood cells (WBC) 12.7
- Glucose 122, electrolytes and kidney function values within normal limits
- Arterial blood gases: pH 7.37, PCO_2 57, PO_2 65, HCO_3^- 32
- Chest x-ray indicated increased density in the right lower lobe.

Treatment orders are as follows:

- Physical therapy to help with conservation of energy with activity
- Respiratory therapy for breathing treatments
- Blood glucose level before meals and at bedtime
- Titrate oxygen up to 3 L/min to keep SpO_2 greater than or equal to 92%

Medications are as follows:

- Albuterol (Proventil) nebulizer six times daily
- Simvastatin (Zocor) 5 mg PO daily
- Methylprednisolone (Solu-Medrol) 125 mg IV q 6 hr

Refer back to this case study to answer the critical-thinking questions throughout the chapter.

Human tissues require oxygen to meet metabolic requirements. The purpose of respiration is to deliver oxygen to the cells and remove carbon dioxide. The cardiovascular system moves oxygen from the lungs to the tissues and carbon dioxide from the tissues back to the lungs, where it can be expired (Shier, Butler, and Lewis, 2012). Respiration is controlled by neural and chemical changes that direct the depth and rate of respirations.

Respiratory disorders range from upper respiratory illnesses caused by viruses to life-threatening disorders of the lower respiratory system. Cardiovascular disorders include coronary artery disease, congestive heart failure, arrhythmias, and peripheral vascular disease. This chapter discusses the anatomy and physiology of the cardiovascular and pulmonary systems and provides an overview of disorders that can interfere with respiratory function and tissue perfusion.

NORMAL STRUCTURE AND FUNCTION OF OXYGENATION LO 38.1

Adequate oxygenation of tissues depends on the cardiovascular and respiratory systems working together to oxygenate tissues. Taking in oxygen and delivering it to the bloodstream requires a healthy respiratory system. The ability to circulate oxygen in the body depends on an intact cardiovascular system.

CARDIOVASCULAR SYSTEM

The heart is a hollow, cone-shaped organ. It is normally in the center area of the chest known as the mediastinum and rests on the diaphragm. The size of the heart varies but usually is about 9 cm wide and 14 cm long (Shier, Butler, and Lewis, 2012).

The heart is composed of four chambers divided into the right and left sides (Figure 38-1). The chambers on the top are atria. The lower chambers are ventricles. The wall of the heart is composed of three layers. The epicardium also is known as the visceral pericardium. This outer layer protects the heart and secretes serous fluid. The second layer is the myocardium, which is the cardiac muscle that contracts to push the blood out of the heart chambers. The third layer is the endocardium, which is the innermost layer that provides a protective lining in the chambers and valves of the heart (Shier, Butler, and Lewis, 2012).

Blood returns from the body in the venous system to the heart, where it enters the right atrium (Figure 38-2). It passes through the tricuspid valve to enter the right ventricle during diastole. During systole, the pressure in the right ventricle exceeds the pressure in the pulmonary artery, and the blood passes through the pulmonic valve into the pulmonary artery. From there it flows into the capillary system, where oxygen is picked up by the red blood cells and carbon dioxide is released

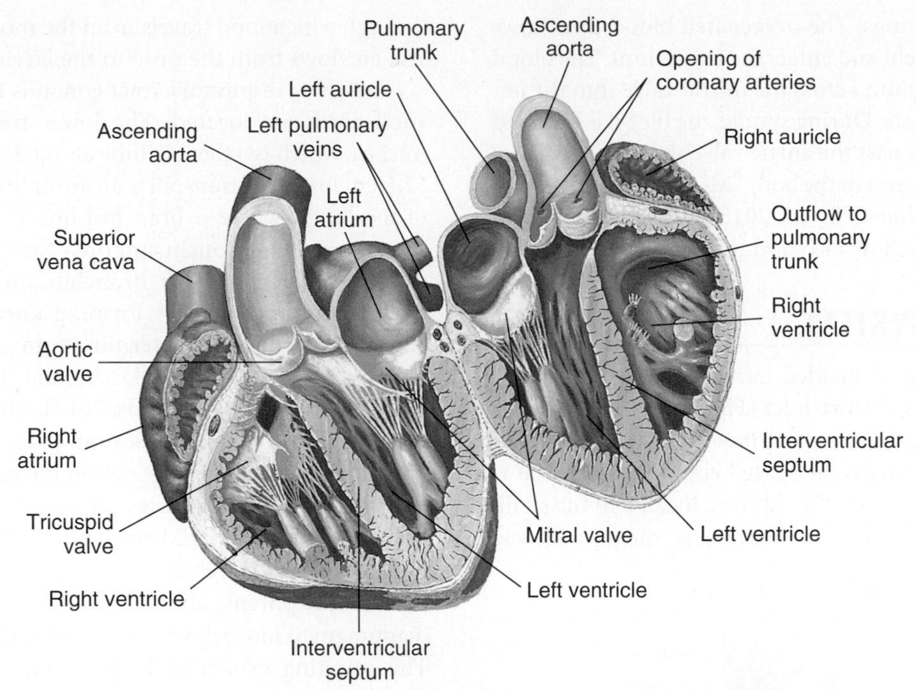

FIGURE 38-1 Cardiac anatomy. (From Ball JW, Dains JE, Flynn JA, et al: *Seidel's guide to physical examination,* ed. 8, St. Louis, 2015, Mosby.)

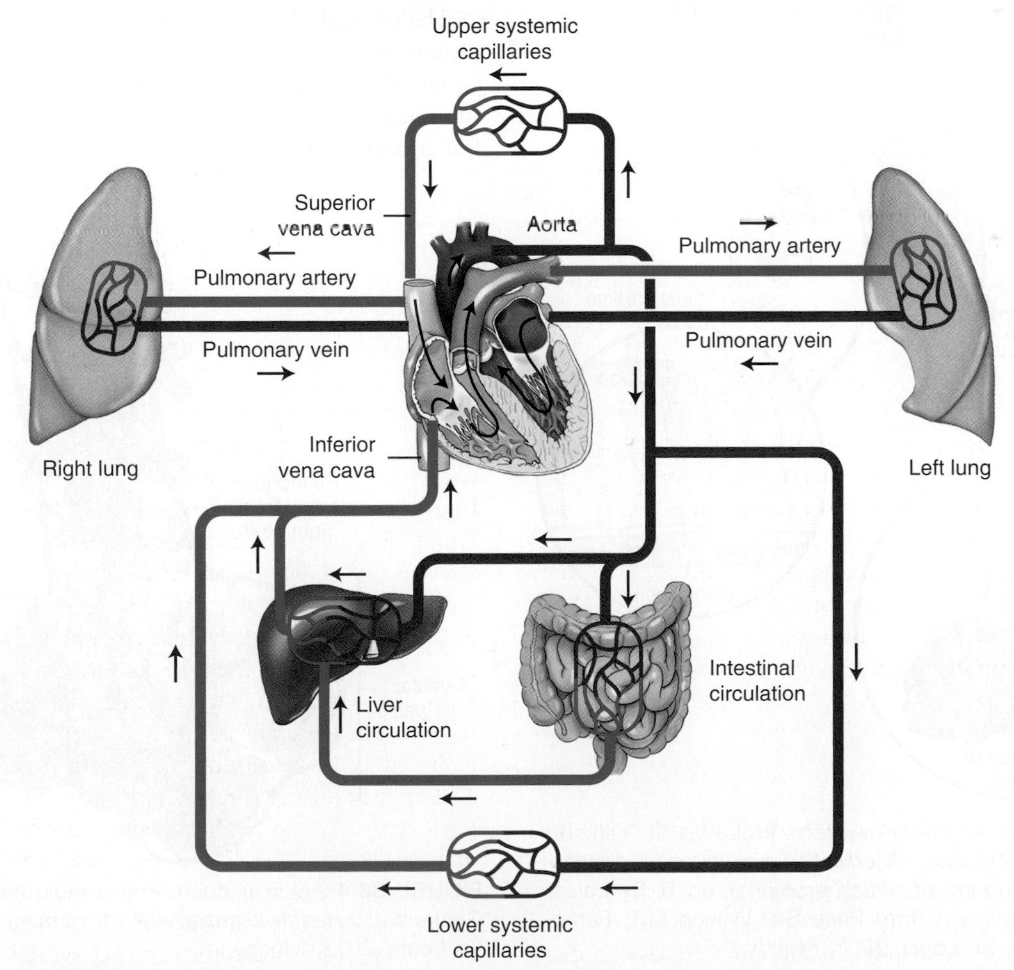

FIGURE 38-2 Circulation of blood in the body. (From Ball JW, Dains JE, Flynn JA, et al: *Seidel's guide to physical examination,* ed. 8, St. Louis, 2015, Mosby.)

to the alveoli of the lungs. The oxygenated blood then flows into the pulmonary vein and enters the left atrium. The blood flows from the left atrium across the mitral valve into the left ventricle during diastole. During systole, the blood is pumped from the left ventricle past the aortic valve into the aorta and then distributed to the rest of the body (McKinley, O'Loughlin, Harris, and Pennefather-O'Brien, 2015). The Cardiac Cycle animation depicts the flow of blood through the heart.

RESPIRATORY SYSTEM

The respiratory system is divided into the upper respiratory tract and the lower respiratory tract (Figure 38-3). The upper respiratory tract includes the nose, nasal cavity, sinuses, and pharynx. The nasal cavity is the space behind the nose that is divided by the nasal septum. The sinuses, located in the skull, are air filled. The pharynx, or throat, is the passageway through which food travels from the mouth to the esophagus and air flows from the nose to the larynx.

The lower respiratory tract contains the larynx, where the vocal cords are located. The lower tract also includes the trachea, which is a flexible tube about 2.5 cm in diameter and 12.5 cm long that transports air from the pharynx and larynx to the lungs, where it branches into right and left bronchi. These mainstem bronchi and their further subdivisions form the bronchial tree. Each bronchus divides repeatedly into increasingly smaller tubes, forming a network of bronchioles and alveolar ducts that terminate in alveoli (Figure 38-4) (McKinley, O'Loughlin, Harris, and Pennefather-O'Brien, 2015; Shier, Butler, and Lewis, 2012). The "Oxygen Transport and Gas Exchange" animation provides more information.

The physiology of oxygenation includes the movement of air into and out of the lungs. Movement of air into the lungs is known as *inspiration.* Inspiration (inhalation) begins with impulses from the respiratory center in the brain that travel through the phrenic and intercostal nerves and stimulate the diaphragm to move downward and the chest cavity to expand. The resulting expanded lung volume decreases the intraalveolar pressure. Atmospheric pressure is then higher than the intraalveolar pressure, causing air to move into the respiratory tract and the lungs to fill with air.

The reversal of air movement is called *expiration.* During expiration (exhalation), the diaphragm relaxes, the elastic tissues of the chest and lungs recoil, and intraalveolar pressures increase, causing air to be forced out of the lungs (Shier, Butler, and Lewis, 2012).

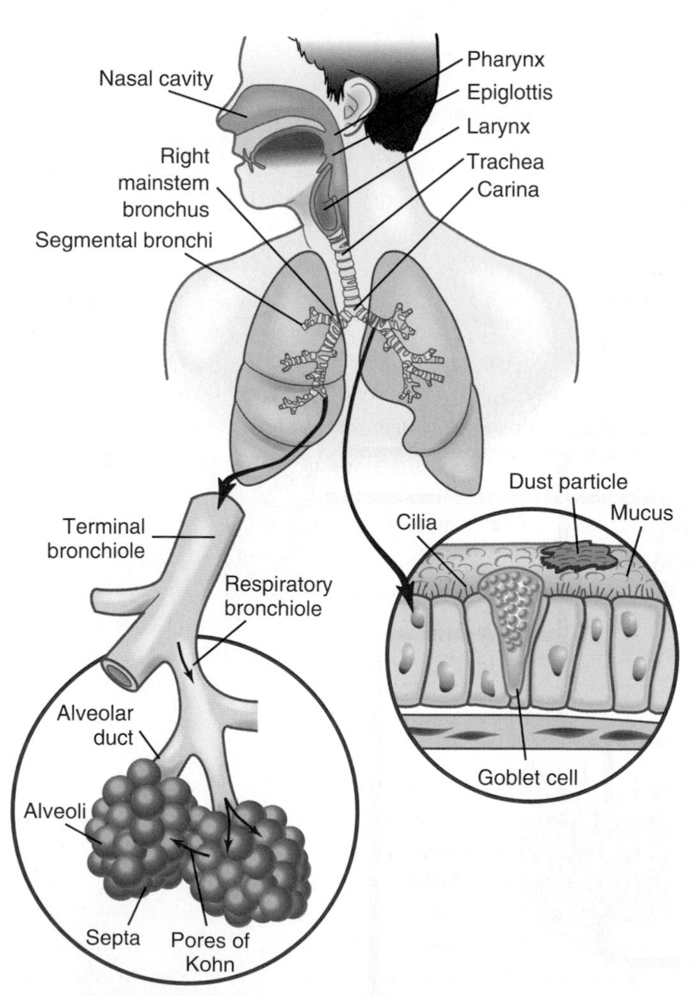

FIGURE 38-3 The respiratory system. (In Lewis SL, Dirksen SR, Heitkemper MM, et al: *Medical-surgical nursing: Assessment and management of clinical problems,* ed. 9, St. Louis, 2014, Mosby. Redrawn from Price SA, Wilson LM: *Pathophysiology,* ed. 6, St. Louis, 2003, Mosby.)

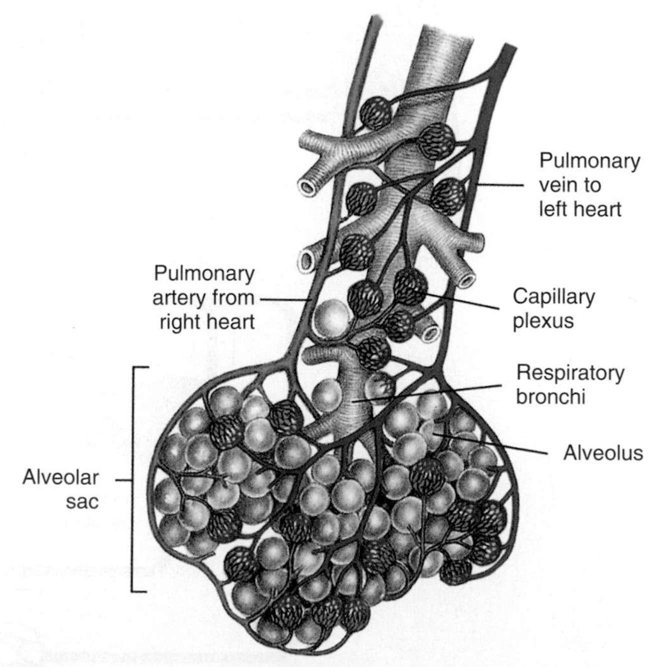

FIGURE 38-4 Alveolar ducts and alveoli. (From Wilson SF, Giddens JF: *Health assessment for nursing practice,* ed. 4, St. Louis, 2013, Mosby.)

ALTERED STRUCTURE AND FUNCTION OF OXYGENATION LO 38.2

The ability to inspire oxygen from the atmosphere depends on intact lung structure. Alteration of lung tissue may decrease delivery of oxygen to the alveoli, impede transfer of oxygen from alveoli to the bloodstream, and hinder expulsion of carbon dioxide.

CARDIOVASCULAR ALTERATIONS

The heart functions as a pump. The heart pumps the oxygenated blood from the lungs to tissues throughout the body, where oxygen is used by the cells. A weakened or diseased heart cannot pump correctly, decreasing the supply of oxygen to tissues and compromising their function.

The coordinated beating of the heart begins with organized impulse generation. The pacemaker of the heart is located in the right atrium and normally generates an impulse that produces a pulse that is 60 to100 beats/min and regular. When the heart beats too slowly, too fast, or irregularly, the ability to pump oxygen to cells can be interrupted.

The heart requires blood flow to the myocardium to continue to beat adequately. Blood is supplied to the heart through the coronary arteries: right coronary artery, left main, left anterior descending, and circumflex arteries (Figure 38-5). Interruption of blood flow to the myocardium (heart muscle) can result from narrowing of the arteries by atherosclerosis, spasms, or congenital malformations. Decreased blood flow to the myocardium decreases the ability of the heart to pump adequately.

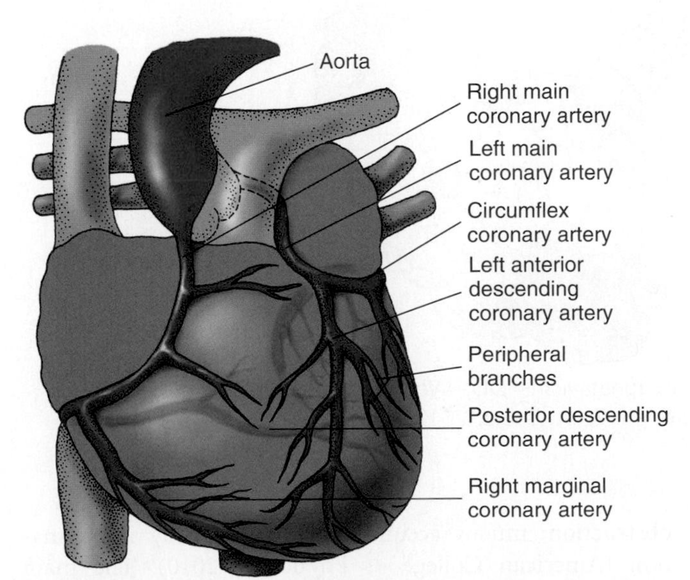

FIGURE 38-5 Coronary arteries. (From Ignatavicius DD, Workman ML: *Medical-surgical nursing: Patient-centered collaborative care,* ed. 7, St. Louis, 2013, Saunders.)

Blood clot formation in the coronary arteries may totally block blood flow to a portion of the myocardium and cause a myocardial infarction. The clinical manifestations of a myocardial infarction include pain or discomfort between the neck and navel. The patient may have associated dyspnea, nausea, and vomiting. The "Coronary Artery Disease" animation shows the progression of this disease.

Other cardiac irregularities may be associated with decreased blood flow, interrupted electrical impulses, or electrolyte disturbances. Assessment may include an irregular heartbeat, difficulty breathing, or dizziness with possible loss of consciousness.

The heart may develop cardiac failure, which decreases contractility and reduces the ability of the heart to meet the needs of the body tissues (Fox, 2013). Causes of heart failure include damage to a heart valve, pressure around the heart, vitamin B deficiency, and damage to blood vessels. The "Heart Failure" animations show the pathophysiology of left- and right-sided heart failure.

RESPIRATORY ALTERATIONS

Chronic obstructive pulmonary disease (COPD) is a general term used for a group of disorders characterized by impaired airflow in the lungs. **Emphysema** is one of the disorders and is characterized by inflamed and damaged alveolar walls in the lungs (Fox, 2013) (Figure 38-6). The clinical manifestation of emphysema is enlargement of small air sacs on the distal end of terminal bronchioles (Sommers and Fannin, 2015). The disorder is characterized by thick mucus and decreased elasticity of the lung tissue. Enzymes damage the walls of the alveoli, and gas exchange is decreased because of decreased surface area due to damage of the alveolar structure (Sommers and Fannin, 2015).

Emphysema may be caused by cigarette smoking or exposure to pollution, and a family history of the disease is a risk factor. Smoking cigarettes is the main risk factor for COPD because it causes oxidative stress, destroys lung tissue, triggers a chronic inflammatory response, and interferes with the lung's ability to repair itself (Sommers and Fannin, 2015).

Chronic bronchitis is another disorder associated with COPD. It is characterized by inflammation of the larger airways, increased production of mucus, and chronic cough (see Figure 38-6). Eventually, the lining of the airways is damaged, increasing the difficulty of clearing mucus. Environmental exposures, including smoking, pollutants in many settings, and second-hand smoke, increase the risk of chronic bronchitis. The "Chronic Obstructive Pulmonary Disease" animation outlines the changes that occur due to this disease.

Frequent bronchopulmonary infections may contribute to COPD (American College of Physicians, 2010). Pulmonary insufficiency, chronic pulmonary emphysema, pneumonia, atelectasis, asthma, and tuberculosis are other disorders that cause respiratory disease.

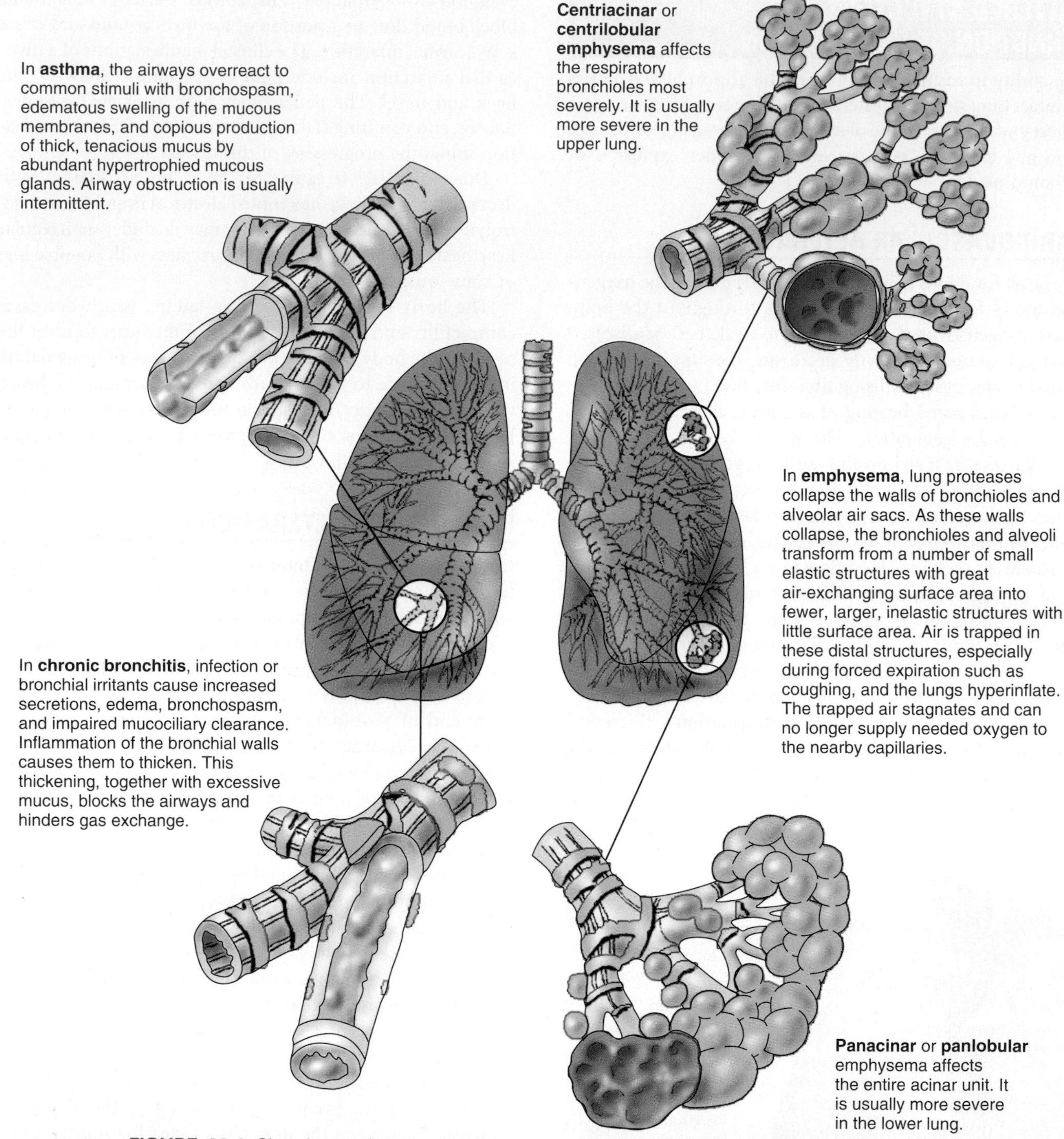

Centriacinar or **centrilobular emphysema** affects the respiratory bronchioles most severely. It is usually more severe in the upper lung.
In **asthma**, the airways overreact to common stimuli with bronchospasm, edematous swelling of the mucous membranes, and copious production of thick, tenacious mucus by abundant hypertrophied mucous glands. Airway obstruction is usually intermittent.
In **emphysema**, lung proteases collapse the walls of bronchioles and alveolar air sacs. As these walls collapse, the bronchioles and alveoli transform from a number of small elastic structures with great air-exchanging surface area into fewer, larger, inelastic structures with little surface area. Air is trapped in these distal structures, especially during forced expiration such as coughing, and the lungs hyperinflate. The trapped air stagnates and can no longer supply needed oxygen to the nearby capillaries.
In **chronic bronchitis**, infection or bronchial irritants cause increased secretions, edema, bronchospasm, and impaired mucociliary clearance. Inflammation of the bronchial walls causes them to thicken. This thickening, together with excessive mucus, blocks the airways and hinders gas exchange.
Panacinar or **panlobular** emphysema affects the entire acinar unit. It is usually more severe in the lower lung.

FIGURE 38-6 Chronic respiratory disorders. (From Ignatavicius DD, Workman ML: *Medical-surgical nursing: Patient-centered collaborative care,* ed. 7, St. Louis, 2013, Saunders.)

Asthma produces symptoms of shortness of breath, intermittent cough, chest tightness, and wheezing heard on auscultation (see Figure 38-6). The disorder may be inherited, begin in childhood and continue into adulthood, and be linked to allergies. The symptoms of asthma are caused by airway spasms, bronchial narrowing or obstruction, mucus accumulation, and airway inflammation (American College of Physicians, 2010). The main feature of asthma is constriction and spasms of airways in response to irritants, allergens, pollutants, or cold air. The Asthma animation depicts the lung changes associated with this disease.

ⓔ

Pneumonia is an infection in the lungs. The clinical manifestations of pneumonia include fever, cough, increased secretions, and difficulty breathing. Key points for nursing management of pneumonia are monitoring gas exchange and maintaining a patent airway. If aspiration is determined to be a contributing cause, swallow precautions are implemented, including thickened liquids and having the patient in an upright position for feeding and drinking.

Atelectasis results from blockage or collapse of air passages in at least one lobe of the lungs. Anesthesia, prolonged bed rest, and shallow breathing can decrease movement of the diaphragm and chest wall, which results in hypoventilation. The process may lead to small airway obstructions from retained secretions. Patients who have had abdominal or chest surgery are at risk for hypoventilation due to the pain caused by deep breathing. Nurses need to encourage patients to maintain adequate ventilation with deep-breathing exercises to prevent atelectasis.

Untreated chronic lung disease may result in respiratory failure (see the "Respiratory Failure" animation). Respiratory failure occurs when the body is unable to maintain sufficient oxygenation to tissues because of disease or injury to the lungs. Early intervention for disease or injury helps prevent respiratory failure. The Diversity Considerations box addresses concerns about the cardiopulmonary system.

ASSESSMENT LO 38.3

A detailed account of the patient's chief complaint and history of current illness can be obtained by asking focused questions (Health Assessment Questions box). Some questions seek specific information, whereas others are open ended to allow the patient more freedom to respond.

HEALTH HISTORY

Assessment of the cardiovascular and pulmonary systems involves gathering subjective and objective data. The subjective information is gathered from the health history and includes information the patient verbalizes throughout the examination. Objective data is gathered from an examination of the patient.

ALTERATIONS OF THE CARDIOPULMONARY SYSTEM

A focused cardiopulmonary assessment is performed for any patient with symptoms of decreased oxygenation, shortness of breath, activity intolerance, or a history of cardiac or respiratory problems. The nurse begins this physical assessment by obtaining a set of vital signs and then performs a cardiac, respiratory, and peripheral vascular assessment, looking for alterations.

Vital Signs

Obtaining objective data begins with taking vital signs that include the blood pressure taken in three positions (lying, sitting, and standing), the respiratory rate, and an apical and peripheral pulse. The apical and peripheral pulses are compared to determine whether a pulse deficit exists. A pulse deficit occurs when the apical pulse rate is higher than the peripheral pulse rate due to some cardiac contractions not

DIVERSITY CONSIDERATIONS

Life Span
- Changes in cardiopulmonary function occur throughout the life span. Maximum predicted heart rate (MPHR = 220 − Age) decreases each year. The maximum oxygen uptake declines for adults after the age of 25.
- Cardiovascular performance declines in the 40s and 50s, even in well-trained athletes.
- Emphysema usually begins in the 30s and 40s, but it becomes severe in the 50s and later (Sommers and Fannin, 2015).
- In pregnancy, cardiac output and blood volume increase, and the growing uterus exerts pressure on the diaphragm, making breathing more difficult.

Gender
- Children's hearts show no significant gender differences. The heart mass of males increases by about 15% to 30% more than that of females after puberty.
- Emphysema occurs more often in men than women.

Culture, Ethnicity, and Religion
- Emphysema does not occur more often in any racial or ethnic groups (Sommers and Fannin, 2015).

Disability
- Scoliosis, a disorder that may begin in childhood, causes the spine to develop a lateral curvature. Kyphosis is an outward deformity of the upper spine. Over time, kyphoscoliosis (combined kyphosis and scoliosis) compromises the respiratory system, resulting in hypoventilation, retention of carbon dioxide, and shortness of breath for the patient.
- Other conditions that limit the ability of the lungs to fully expand, such as being confined to a wheelchair, may contribute to respiratory compromise.

Morphology
- Obesity contributes to diabetes and high cholesterol levels, which are risk factors for coronary artery disease.

HEALTH ASSESSMENT QUESTIONS

Cardiovascular Focus

- Are you having chest pain? If so, rate it on a scale of 0 to 10.
- How long have you had the pain?
- Is the pain located in one area, or does it radiate to other areas?
- Do activities or medications make it worse or better?
- Are symptoms such as shortness of breath or sweating associated with the pain?
- Do you have increased fatigue?
- Have you had recent weight gain?
- Have you had changes in skin texture, color, or temperature?
- Do you take medications that prevent blood clots?
- Have you had sores on your lower extremities that have not healed?
- Have you had episodes of dizziness or loss of consciousness?
- Do you have other chronic diseases?

Pulmonary Focus

- Have you had breathing difficulties when you are exercising or at rest?
- Have you had a loss of appetite, weight loss, or weakness?
- Have you ever smoked?
- If so, are you still smoking, or did you quit smoking?
- Do you sleep on one or more pillows?
- How much do you exercise?
- Do you have wheezing, pain with breathing, or difficulty clearing your secretions?
- Have you had asthma, bronchitis, or other lung diseases in the past?
- Do you use oxygen at home?
- What type of work have you done, and were you exposed to hazardous materials?
- Do you have anxiety related to your breathing condition?
- Do you have a cough? For how long?
- Are you coughing anything up? Color of sputum?
- Is it worse when you lie down?

resulting in peripheral perfusion. Chapter 19 provides more information about pulse and respiration assessment.

Inspection, Palpation, and Auscultation of the Heart and Lungs

The precordium of the chest is visually inspected, noting any musculoskeletal abnormalities. Use of muscles for breathing is evaluated. The use of accessory muscles may indicate respiratory distress. The nurse looks at the precordium to detect movement of the chest wall when the heart contracts. Left ventricular hypertrophy may cause the chest wall to move with each heartbeat. Evaluate the shape of the chest; a barrel-shaped chest may indicate air trapping, which accompanies COPD.

Palpation over the precordium for cardiac function assesses for cardiac enlargement or abnormal vibrations from turbulent blood flow due to hyperactivity or valve disease. Abnormal vibration over the heart is documented as a *thrill*. During auscultation, the vibration may be heard and is referred to as a *murmur*. Auscultation of the heart includes listening for the heart sounds that correlate with closure of the valves of the heart. Chapter 20 provides detailed information about cardiac assessment.

Auscultation of the lungs is completed on the front and back of the chest. Auscultation of the lungs begins at the top of the chest and moves down to below the rib cage. The nurse compares lung sounds side to side. The nurse listens for normal breath sounds and abnormal or adventitious breath sounds that are made when air enters and leaves the lungs through the constricted or diseased airways. A complete discussion of lung assessment can be found in Chapter 20.

Cough Assessment

A patient with a cough needs to be evaluated. Cough may be caused by inflammation or by mechanical or chemical stimulation of the cough receptors in the lung. When taking the history, the nurse determines how long the patient has had the cough and whether the patient has a fever or wheezing. The amount and characteristics of sputum are documented. **Hemoptysis** is the presence of blood in the sputum. The characteristics of the blood—whether it occurs as flecks, streaks, or frank bleeding—are noted. The nurse asks the patient whether the cough is seasonal, which may indicate allergies (Longo, Fauci, Kasper, et al, 2013).

Peripheral Vascular Assessment

An important part of the vascular system assessment is the finding of edema in the extremities. Edema may result from excessive fluid in the vascular system that increases pressure in the capillaries and forces fluid out of the vessels and into the surrounding tissues. Poor venous return may contribute to peripheral edema, particularly in the lower extremities. Another contributing factor is damage to the lymphatic system, which decreases the system's ability to remove excessive fluid from the interstitial spaces. Chapter 20 provides more information on edema.

Peripheral vascular assessment includes evaluation of peripheral pulses, skin color and texture, and capillary refill in the fingers and toes. Patients with cardiopulmonary problems may have thready or absent peripheral pulses, changes in skin color and texture, and slow capillary refill.

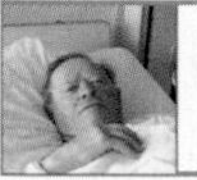

1. List focused assessments that need to be completed for Mr. Ross.

LABORATORY AND DIAGNOSTIC TESTS

Laboratory assessments determine whether the patient has chemical imbalances or abnormal substances in the blood. For example, when cardiac cells die, cardiac enzymes (e.g., troponins) are released into the bloodstream. Measured levels of these enzymes correlate with heart muscle injury. These and other diagnostic tests are performed to determine the function and structure of heart and lung tissues.

Pulmonary Function Tests

Forced vital capacity (FVC) is the amount of air that can be forcefully expelled or exhaled after the lungs are maximally inflated. The normal amount varies by age and size of the patient but is approximately 4 liters in an adult. The amount of air expelled is lower in patients with obstructive pulmonary disease because airways are narrowed (Pagana and Pagana, 2014).

Forced expiratory volume in 1 second (FEV_1) is the volume of air expelled in 1 second from the beginning of the FVC. The expected finding is 75% to 85% of FVC. Patients with obstructive lung disease will have less air expelled than the predicted value (Pagana and Pagana, 2014).

Forced expiratory flow (FEF) is the maximal flow rate that is attained during the middle of the FVC maneuver. The expected findings vary by body size. In cases of emphysema, the result is 25% of the predicted normal value for the patient's size. A low value predicts airway trapping in the patient's small bronchioles (Sommers and Fannin, 2015).

Residual volume (RV) is the amount of air remaining in the lungs after forced expiration. The expected finding is approximately 1 liter. In emphysema, the result may be up to four times the expected normal value (Pagana and Pagana, 2014).

Functional residual capacity (FRC) is the volume of air that is left in the patient's lung after normal expiration. The predicted normal volume is 2.3 liters. In emphysema, it may be increased up to 200% over the expected amount due to air trapping (Pagana and Pagana, 2014).

Complete Blood Count

The complete blood count (CBC) and differential provide information regarding oxygen and carbon dioxide transport capabilities and the status of the immune response. Red blood cell (RBC), hemoglobin, and hematocrit levels indicate oxygen carrying capacity. The hemoglobin level may be decreased in patients with heart failure due to excess fluid in the system that causes hemodilution. It may be increased in COPD patients due to overproduction of RBCs stimulated by low oxygen levels and a resultant increase in the hematocrit. Elevation of the white blood cell (WBC) level indicates an infection, and the WBC differential count shifts to the left, with levels of neutrophils increasing and basophils decreasing. Chapter 34 provides detailed information on the CBC.

Basic Metabolic Panel

The basic metabolic panel is a series of blood tests used to assess a patient's renal function, glucose level, and electrolyte status. A patient with heart failure or hypertension may be on diuretics, some of which can cause hypokalemia and hypomagnesemia. Many electrolyte imbalances can cause cardiac arrhythmias. Chapter 39 provides a detailed discussion of the functions of intracellular and extracellular electrolytes, normal values, and the common causes of abnormal values.

Arterial Blood Gases

Blood samples for arterial blood gas determinations are drawn from patients with decreased oxygenation and a suspected acid-base imbalance. COPD causes impaired gas exchange, leading to decreased oxygen levels and higher circulating levels of carbon dioxide (i.e., respiratory acidosis). Chapter 39 discusses acid-base balance.

EVALUATION OF THE CARDIOPULMONARY SYSTEM

Evaluation of the cardiovascular and pulmonary system includes assessment of blood components, including blood counts, lipids, and cardiac enzymes. Noninvasive assessment includes a 12-lead electrocardiogram (ECG), chest x-ray, echocardiogram, and physical assessment. Invasive assessment may include a cardiac catheterization to evaluate coronary arteries and cardiac structures.

Lipids

A lipoprotein profile is used to diagnose hyperlipidemia, which is a risk factor for coronary heart disease. The profile usually measures four levels: total cholesterol, low-density lipoprotein (LDL) cholesterol, high-density lipoprotein (HDL) cholesterol, and triglycerides. Cholesterol is the primary lipid associated with the development of atherosclerosis if the levels are too high. Cholesterol is evaluated further by measuring HDL and LDL components. A total cholesterol level higher than 200 mg/dL is considered a risk factor for atherosclerosis. The target value for HDL is greater than 45 mg/dL for males and greater than 55 mg/dL for females. The desired value for LDL is less than 130 mg/dL. The desired value for triglycerides is less than 160 mg/dL for males and less than 135 mg/dL for females (Pagana & Pagana, 2014).

Cardiac Enzymes

Cardiac enzymes and other proteins are released when myocardial **necrosis** (death of heart muscle cells) occurs. When a patient has chest pain or related signs and symptoms, enzyme levels are evaluated to determine whether damage to the heart has occurred. Tests assess levels of creatine phosphokinase-MB,

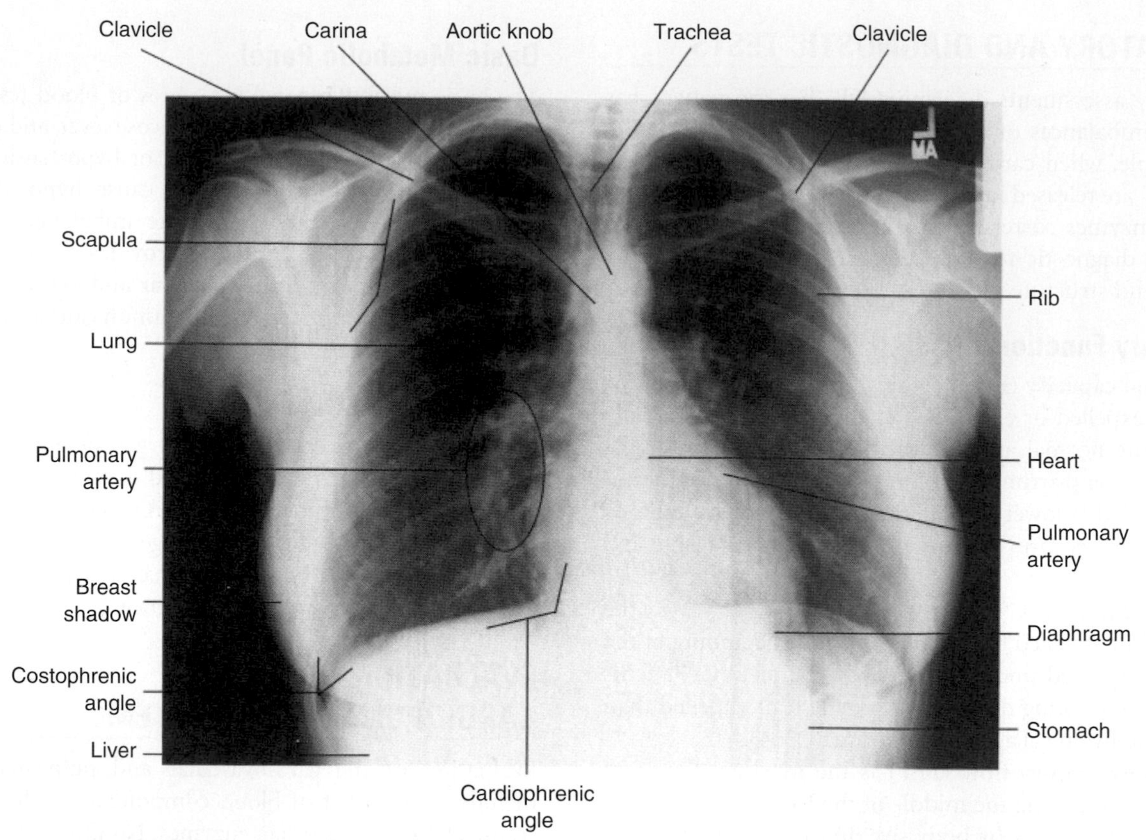

FIGURE 38-7 Chest x-ray. (In Urden LD, Stacy KM, Lough ME: *Critical care nursing,* ed. 7, St. Louis, 2014, Mosby. From Dettenmeier PA: *Radiographic assessment for nurses,* St. Louis, 1995, Mosby.)

troponin T, troponin I, and myoglobin. The cardiac troponin T and I proteins are the most helpful biomarkers for determining whether a myocardial infarction has occurred (Fuster, O'Rourke, Walsh, et al, 2013).

Chest X-ray

A chest x-ray is performed to examine the lungs, heart, and bones of the chest (Figure 38-7). A chest x-ray shows areas of increased density in the lungs, the proximity of organs to each other, and the size of the heart. Abnormal findings include rib fractures, tumors, pneumothorax (air in the pleural cavity), pneumonia (inflammation of the lungs due to infection), **pleural effusion** (excess fluid accumulation in the pleural cavity), pericardial effusion (fluid around the heart), an enlarged heart, and atelectasis. Location and position of the diaphragm may be visualized.

Electrocardiogram

An **electrocardiogram** (ECG; also called EKG) is a graphic representation of the electrical activity that occurs in the heart. The heart's electrical system is an organized series of impulses that transmit a signal from the sinoatrial (SA) node in the right atrium, that travels through the atria and atrioventricular (AV) node to the bundle branches in the ventricles, from which it travels to all parts of the ventricle. The electrical impulses precede the mechanical contraction of the heart. For normal contraction to occur, the impulses travel through the heart in an organized way. The ECG is performed using a 12-lead approach that gathers impulses from 12 areas. The ECG is recorded on special standardized paper (Figure 38-8). Test results are interpreted for rate and rhythm of the heart, lack of blood supply, abnormalities of the conduction system, and **arrhythmias**, which are abnormal rhythms of the heart.

Echocardiogram

An echocardiogram is a noninvasive ultrasound of the heart (Figure 38-9). The examination uses sound waves to visualize the heart structure and evaluate the function of the heart. An echocardiogram shows movement of blood through the heart, and it is used to measure cardiac output. This test can be used to evaluate congenital heart defects, pericardial effusion, disorders of the heart valves, heart size, and effectiveness of cardiac output. Echocardiograms may be obtained alone or in conjunction with a stress test to evaluate the heart when the blood flow to the heart is decreased.

Cardiac Catheterization

Cardiac catheterization uses contrast and a long, flexible catheter to visualize the heart chambers, coronary arteries,

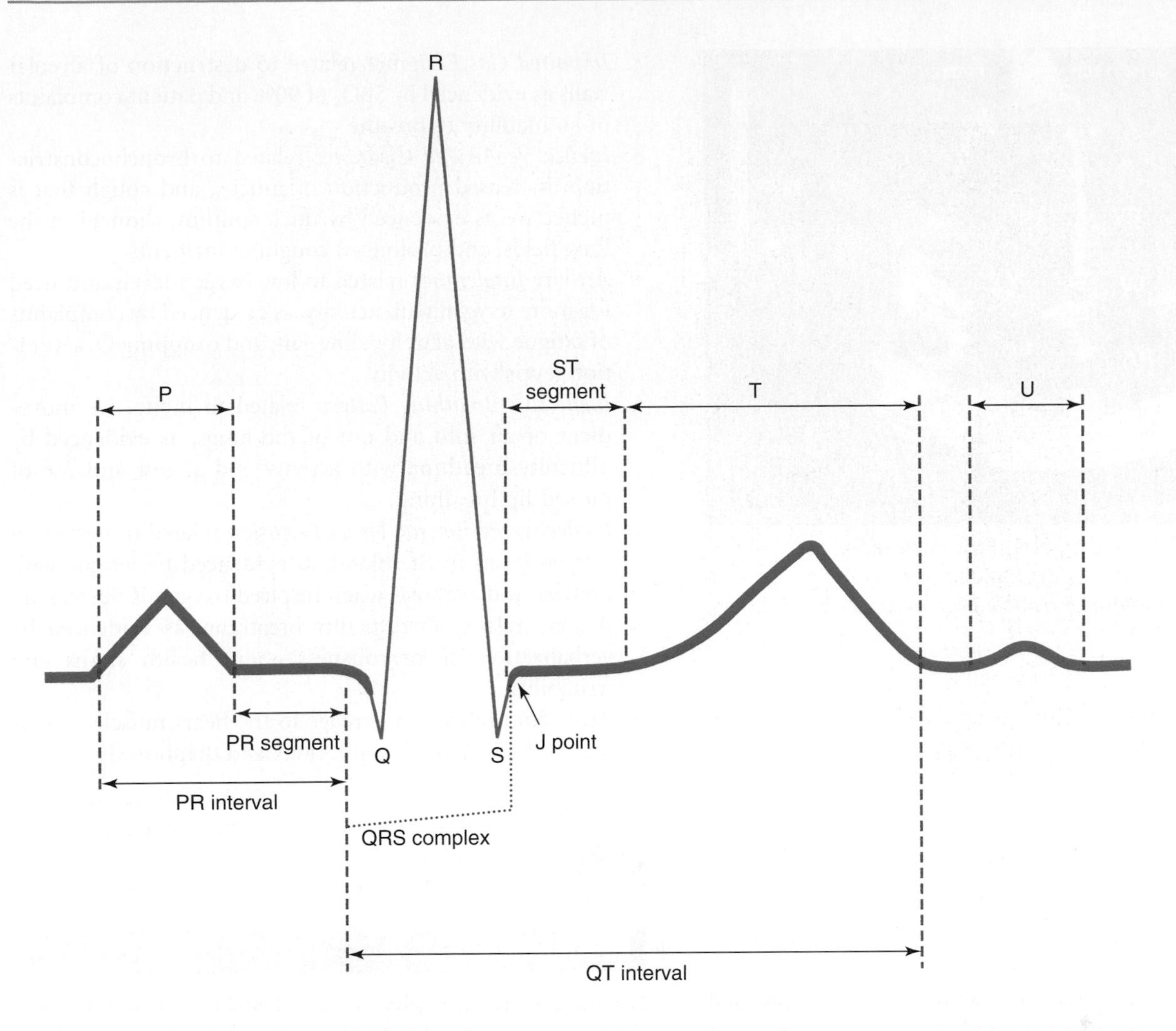

P wave: Represents atrial depolarization.

PR segment: Represents the time required for the impulse to travel through the AV node, where it is delayed, and through the bundle of His, bundle branches, and Purkinje fiber network, just before ventricular depolarization.

PR interval: Represents the time required for atrial depolarization as well as impulse travel through the conduction system and Purkinje fiber network, inclusive of the P wave and PR segment. It is measured from the beginning of the P wave to the end of the PR segment.

QRS complex: Represents ventricular depolarization and is measured from the beginning of the Q (or R) wave to the end of the S wave.

J point: Represents the junction where the QRS complex ends and the ST segment begins.

ST segment: Represents early ventricular repolarization.

T wave: Represents ventricular repolarization.

U wave: Represents late ventricular repolarization.

QT interval: Represents the total time required for ventricular depolarization and repolarization and is measured from the beginning of the QRS complex to the end of the T wave.

FIGURE 38-8 Normal electrocardiogram. (From Ignatavicius DD, Workman ML: *Medical-surgical nursing: Patient-centered collaborative care,* ed. 7, St. Louis, 2013, Saunders.)

and great vessels. It is used to evaluate chest pain, locate the region of coronary artery occlusion, and determine the effects of valvular heart disease. In this invasive procedure, a catheter is inserted into the right femoral or brachial artery to view the left side of the heart and inserted into the antecubital or femoral vein to view structures on the right side of the heart. Cardiac valves, chamber pressures, cardiac output, and the ejection fraction may be assessed using cardiac catheterization. Congenital or acquired structural cardiac abnormalities can be visualized. If a coronary artery is narrowed, a balloon

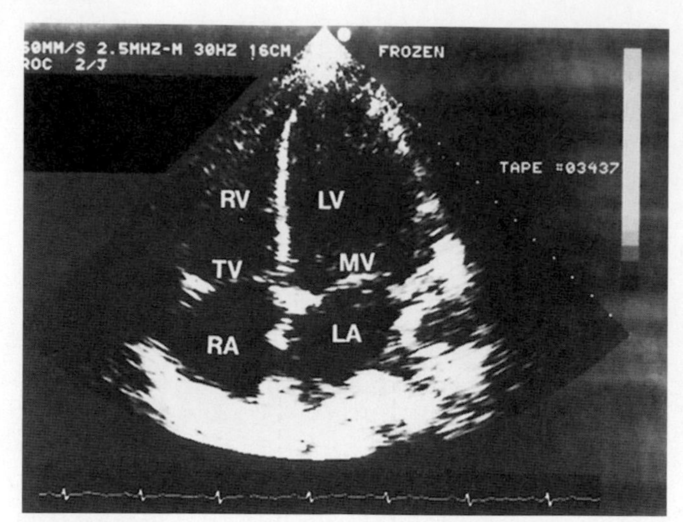

FIGURE 38-9 Echocardiogram. (From Lewis SL, Dirksen SR, Heitkemper MM, et al: *Medical-surgical nursing: Assessment and management of clinical problems,* ed. 8, St. Louis, 2011, Mosby.)

can be used to widen its lumen, or a stent can be placed to permanently keep the vessel open (Pagana and Pagana, 2014).

Cardiac catheterization is performed in a specialized setting by cardiologists using sterile procedures. The patient is given medication to help with relaxation but may be able to follow commands. This is an invasive procedure, and there can be complications such as allergy to the contrast medium, arrhythmias, blood clots, and bleeding at the catheter insertion site. After the procedure, the nurse monitors the patient for signs of an allergic reaction and obtains frequent vital signs according to facility policy. The insertion site is assessed for bleeding and the affected extremity for peripheral pulses, temperature, color, and pain.

◆ NURSING DIAGNOSIS LO 38.4

Selection of the correct nursing diagnosis is important to plan care based on patient needs. Recognition of the potential for decreased oxygen to the tissues directs a focused assessment and the plan for care. The following are common diagnoses related to decreased oxygenation:

- *Impaired Gas Exchange* related to destruction of alveolar walls as evidenced by SpO_2 of 90% and patient complaints of an inability to breathe
- *Ineffective Airway Clearance* related to bronchoconstriction, increased production of mucus, and cough that is ineffective as evidenced by thick sputum, rhonchi in the lung fields, and prolonged coughing incidents
- *Activity Intolerance* related to low oxygen levels and need for more oxygen with activity, as evidenced by complaints of fatigue with activity, slow gait, and dropping O_2 saturation levels with activity
- *Ineffective Breathing Pattern* related to ineffective movement of air into and out of the lungs, as evidenced by difficulty breathing with activity and at rest and use of pursed-lip breathing
- *Ineffective Peripheral Tissue Perfusion* related to decreased oxygen levels in the blood, as evidenced by fatigue with exercise and cyanosis when inspired oxygen is decreased
- *Anxiety* related to difficulty breathing, as evidenced by verbalization of nervousness about health status and irritability
- *Acute pain* related to damage to the heart muscle, as evidenced by increased respirations and diaphoresis

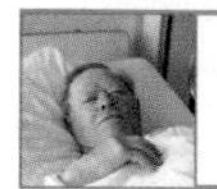

2. List at least two nursing diagnoses that are appropriate for Mr. Ross.

◆ PLANNING LO 38.5

During the planning phase, the assessment data and nursing diagnoses are used to develop individualized goals (Table 38-1). The following examples of goal statements reflect the desired outcomes for patients with decreased oxygenation:

- Patient will maintain SpO_2 at 92% or greater by the end of the shift.
- Patient's lungs will be clear to auscultation within 24 hours.
- Patient will maintain SpO_2 at 92% or greater with activity within 48 hours.
- Patient will report decreased fatigue during hospitalization.

TABLE 38-1 Care Planning

NANDA-I NURSING DIAGNOSIS LABEL WITH NURSING DIAGNOSIS STATEMENT	NURSING OUTCOME CLASSIFICATION (NOC)	NURSING INTERVENTION CLASSIFICATION (NIC)
Impaired Gas Exchange related to destruction of alveolar walls as evidenced by SpO_2 of 90% and patient complaints of inability to breathe	*Respiratory status* (0415) Oxygen saturation (041508)	*Oxygen therapy* (3320) Administer supplemental oxygen as ordered

From Bulechek G, Butcher H, Dochterman J, et al (Eds): *Nursing interventions classification (NIC),* ed. 6, St. Louis, 2013, Mosby; Moorhead S, Johnson M, Maas M, et al (Eds): *Nursing outcomes classification (NOC),* ed. 5, St. Louis, 2013, Mosby; NANDA International: *Nursing diagnoses: Definitions and classification, 2012–2014,* West Sussex, England, 2012, Wiley-Blackwell. Reprinted with permission from NANDA International, Inc.

- Patient will demonstrate a breathing cycle that returns to a normal pattern after aerosol treatments.
- Patient's extremities will be pink and warm to touch after supplemental oxygen is applied.
- Patient will verbalize an increase in psychological and physical comfort within 8 hours.
- Patient's respirations will return to 16 to 20 breaths/min after pain medication is administered before cardiac catheterization.

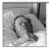

The conceptual care map for Mr. Ross can be found at *http://evolve.elsevier.com/YoostCrawford/fundamentals/*. It is partially completed to indicate how to use the map as a learning tool. Complete the nursing diagnoses using the example conceptual care maps shown in Chapters 8 and 25 to 33.

IMPLEMENTATION AND EVALUATION LO 38.6

The care plan is implemented using safe practices. To determine whether nursing care has been effective, the nurse carefully evaluates the steps that have been taken. Based on the evaluation, the plan of care is revised to provide effective care to the patient.

PROMOTING OPTIMAL CARDIOPULMONARY FUNCTION

Many nursing interventions promote optimal cardiopulmonary function. Placing a dyspneic patient in the semi-Fowler position; aiding airway clearance by teaching the patient to cough, deep-breathe, and use an incentive spirometer; and providing adequate hydration to help thin secretions are examples of nursing measures to promote optimal oxygenation. Nurses are responsible for administering ordered oxygen and medication therapies and for monitoring the effectiveness of treatments (Ethical, Legal, and Professional Practice box).

Oxygen Therapy

Supplemental oxygen can be used on a temporary or permanent basis, depending on the patient's diagnosis and oxygenation status. Oxygen therapy for more than 15 hours per day for patients with COPD improves survival, functioning level, exercise capacity, and mental status (Home Care Considerations box). The goal of long-term therapy is usually to have a baseline PaO_2 of 60 mm Hg at rest and an oxygen saturation level of more than 90%, which represents adequate delivery of oxygen to the tissues (American College of Physicians, 2010). Oxygen saturation may decrease during exercise, sleep, or deterioration of the respiratory status.

ETHICAL, LEGAL, AND PROFESSIONAL PRACTICE

Life and Death Decisions

- When a patient is hospitalized, protocols are in place to begin the lifesaving procedure of cardiopulmonary resuscitation when breathing and heart contractions stop.
- These protocols are not begun if a patient has a do-not-resuscitate (DNR) order.
- The advance directives of a person may determine whether artificial airways and ventilations are given to the patient. An ethical dilemma may occur when a patient is no longer able to make this decision. The family or health care power of attorney decides about advanced procedures for oxygenation.
- Eliott and Olver (2009) examined the decision-making process involved in making a moral judgment about sustaining the patient's life. Hospitals need to develop ethical policies regarding autonomy and surrogacy for patients at the end of life.

HOME CARE CONSIDERATIONS

Oxygen Therapy in the Home

- The order to place oxygen in a home is obtained from a primary care provider and is based on the diagnosis of a medical condition that confirms the need for home oxygen.
- A patient who is using oxygen at home is educated on the proper use and storage of oxygen.
- Signs stating "No Smoking" need to be in place in the home.
- The size and configuration of the home is used to determine the placement of oxygen and length of tubing to allow the patient to go from one room to another.

Oxygen Administration

Oxygen concentration of room air is 21%. When a patient has documented or suspected low oxygen levels, oxygen therapy may be indicated. The goal of oxygen therapy is to decrease the symptoms related to low oxygen levels and decrease the workload on the cardiovascular system. Collaboration with other members of the health care team is essential for patients receiving oxygen therapy (Collaboration and Delegation box).

Clinical practice guidelines for safe and effective patient care include evaluating the indications for oxygen therapy, taking necessary safety precautions, determining the need for oxygen, assessing the outcome of therapy, and monitoring the patient on supplemental oxygen. Assessing the need for oxygen is an important nursing function. Assessment includes using laboratory results to document **hypoxemia**, which is a low level of oxygen in the blood. The low levels can be determined by use of arterial blood gas analysis or measurement of hemoglobin oxygen saturation. Monitoring the patient's condition is another way to evaluate the need for continued oxygen therapy. Hypoxemia may manifest as a

COLLABORATION AND DELEGATION

Multidisciplinary Care of Patients With Oxygenation Problems

- Coordination of care for a patient with oxygenation problems involves collaboration among nurses, physicians, respiratory therapists, speech therapists, and physical therapists.
- The plan of care is based on the physical examination by the primary care provider and is modified based on nursing assessments, including vital signs and ongoing cardiac and pulmonary assessments.
- The medication orders by the primary care provider follow the national hospital inpatient quality measures and the individual needs of the patient. These orders include oxygen therapy, respiratory medications and treatments, and other medications.
- Respiratory therapists initiate the administration of inhaled respiratory medications and assess the patient's status.
- Speech therapists become involved if aspiration is suspected as a contributing factor in the development of the abnormal respiratory status. The speech therapist evaluates swallowing and provides a plan of care using thickened liquids if appropriate.
- Physical therapists evaluate the patient who has the nursing diagnosis of *Activity Intolerance* to assist with a plan of care for mobilization of the patient.

QSEN FOCUS!

Safety requires the nurse to demonstrate effective use of strategies, such as monitoring oxygen therapy and keeping oxygen away from open flames. These measures reduce the risk of harm to patients and health care workers.

! SAFE PRACTICE ALERT

Safe administration of oxygen includes careful assessment and monitoring of the patient. Oxygen is a medication and is used with the same precautions and safety checks as all other medication administration.

high respiratory or heart rate. Other indications may be **cyanosis**, a bluish discoloration of the skin related to deoxygenation of hemoglobin, a decreasing oxygen saturation level, and a feeling of distress.

It is important to use precautions and monitor for complications when administering oxygen. A patient with chronic **hypercapnia**, an abnormally high level of carbon dioxide in the blood (>45 mm Hg in arterial blood), may have respiratory depression when supplemental oxygen levels are too high. A person with chronic hypercapnia may use low oxygen levels as the drive to breathe, and when the levels increase, the person's respiratory rate drops. Respiratory depression increases the risk of $PaCO_2$ levels becoming dangerously high. Another concern about oxygen administration is that when the **fraction of inspired oxygen** (FIO_2, or percentage of oxygen in inspired air) exceeds 50%, atelectasis or oxygen toxicity may occur. High levels of oxygen pose a fire hazard. Nebulizers and humidifiers may have bacterial contamination, promoting infections.

Oxygen Delivery Systems

Devices used to deliver oxygen are categorized as low-flow systems, reservoir systems, and high-flow systems. A commonly used low-flow system is the nasal cannula. Cannulas are contraindicated for newborns and infants with obstructed nasal passages.

Mask delivery systems gather and store oxygen between patient breaths. The mask has holes in the side that allow carbon dioxide to be exhaled. If the unit becomes disconnected from oxygen, the patient can breathe in room air through the holes when inhaling.

! SAFE PRACTICE ALERT

The mask may be uncomfortable for the patient, and the patient may remove the mask when unattended. An alternative oxygen delivery system is required when the patient is eating.

The two other types of masks described in the Nursing Care Guideline: Oxygen Administration Techniques box have similar designs. The partial rebreather mask and nonrebreather mask have a 1-liter reservoir bag that is flexible and has an oxygen inlet. The reservoir allows higher inspired oxygen levels, and these masks can deliver higher levels of oxygen to a patient. The main difference in the types of **reservoir masks** is the valve system. With use of the partial rebreather mask, some exhaled air enters the reservoir bag. As long as the bag remains full, the amount of carbon dioxide that the patient breathes back in is small. The amount of oxygen delivered to the bag typically needs to be greater than 10 liters to prevent the bag from collapsing (White, 2013).

The Nursing Care Guideline: Oxygen Administration Techniques box and Nursing Care Guideline: Continuous Positive Airway Pressure and Bilevel Positive Airway Pressure Applications box provide information about the use of supplemental oxygen and assisted breathing techniques.

Bag-Valve-Mask Device

The bag-valve-mask (BVM) device, also known as an Ambu bag, uses a one-way valve to support, ventilate, and oxygenate a patient who needs ventilatory support (Figure 38-10). All emergency crash carts are supplied with a BVM unit for emergency use. Only personnel who have been properly trained and certified in the use of the devices should administer ventilation using the BVM units.

When it is necessary to use the BVM device, health care personnel should be positioned at the head of the bed. An oral airway is inserted when possible, and the BVM unit is connected to high-flow oxygen. An adequate amount of

NURSING CARE GUIDELINE

Oxygen Administration Techniques

Background

- Oxygen administration provides supplemental oxygen when lungs are not functioning optimally.
- It can provide humidity to increase expectoration and improve lung function.
- Room air is 21% oxygen. Administering higher concentrations of oxygen is considered medication administration.
- All rights of medication administration should be followed (see the Nursing Care Guideline: Six Rights of Medication Administration box in Chapter 35).
- High oxygen levels can be toxic and damage the lungs. High concentrations can damage the retinas of neonates. Careful monitoring and adherence to orders is imperative.

Procedural Concerns

- Thoroughly assess respiratory status:
  - Vital signs
  - Indications of anxiousness, confusion, and restlessness
  - Color, cyanosis
  - Respiratory rate and quality
  - Lung sounds
  - Chest movement and retractions
  - Finger clubbing
- Ensure that orders are obtained for the following:
  - The device
  - Correct flow rate and percent oxygenation
  - Optimal pulse oximetry
- Always ensure oxygen is flowing before placing the oxygen apparatus on the patient.
- If the patient has COPD, use low-flow oxygen delivery *only* (2 L/min or less).
- Monitor the patient for 15 to 30 minutes after starting the oxygen, and repeat assessments as needed, depending on the patient's status.
- Oxygen signage indicates that oxygen is in use.
- The four modes of oxygen delivery are nasal cannula, mask (various types), tracheostomy (trach) mask with collar, and face tent.

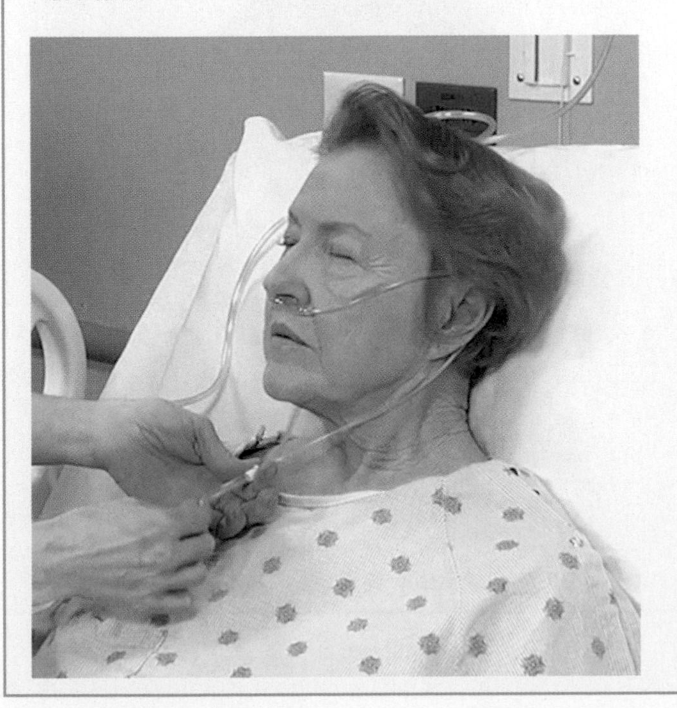

- Oxygen delivery by nasal cannula
  - Correct application:
    - Place the prongs in the patient's nares with the curved side at the top and the prongs pointing toward the back of the head;
    - Loop the tubing around the patient's ears. Gauze or special tubing covers may be used as a cushion where the tubing rests on the ears to prevent sores and protect the skin.
    - Tuck the tubing under the patient's chin and secure it with the sliding adjustment piece.
  - Encourage the patient to breathe through the nose.
  - Flow rates and percent oxygenation values are as follows:
    - 1 L/min = 24%
    - 2 L/min = 28%
    - 3 L/min = 32%
    - 4 L/min = 36%
    - 5 L/min = 40%
    - 6 L/min = 44%
  - Do not administer oxygen through a nasal cannula at greater than 6 L/min.
  - Consider humidification at all levels, especially at flow rates of 4 L/min and higher.
- Oxygen delivery by mask
  - If there is a bag reservoir, ensure it is filled before placing the mask on the patient.
  - Always humidify oxygen delivered by mask.
  - If the patient is able to eat, obtain an order for a nasal cannula during meals.
  - Correct application:
    - Place the mask over the patient's nose and mouth.
    - Secure the mask around the back of the head with the adjustable strap, pulling evenly from both ends of the strap to secure it in place. If the straps are around the ears where they may chafe, cushion the ears with gauze.
    - Adjust the nosepiece by pinching it to provide comfort and ensure fit.
- Oxygen masks include simple face masks, partial rebreather masks, non-rebreather masks, and Venturi masks.
  - Simple face mask

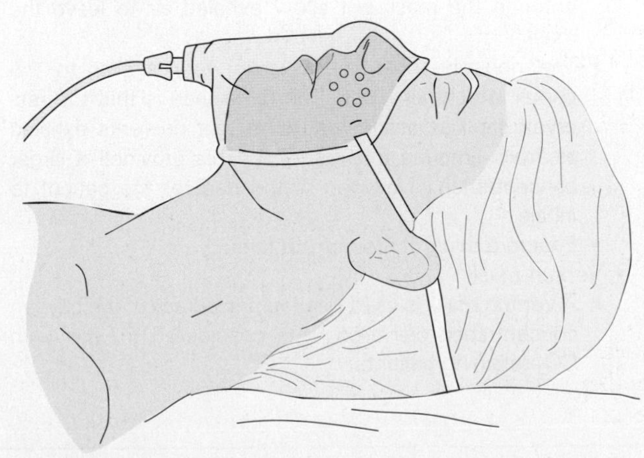

(From Sorrentino SA, Remmert L: *Mosby's textbook for nursing assistants*, ed. 8, St. Louis, 2012, Mosby.)

Continued

NURSING CARE GUIDELINE—cont'd

- There is no reservoir bag.
- Flow rates and percent oxygenation values are as follows:
  - 5 L/min = 40%
  - 6 L/min = 45%
  - 7 L/min = 50%
  - 8 L/min = 55%
  - >8 L/min = 60%

- Partial rebreather mask
  - Flow rates and percent oxygenation values are 6 to 15 L/min and 70% to 90%, respectively.
  - The partial rebreather mask looks very similar to the non-rebreather mask. The partial rebreather masks allows some of the exhaled air to enter the reservoir. The patient rebreathes part of the exhaled air, which contains carbon dioxide and acts as a stimulus to breathe for some patients.
- Non-rebreather mask

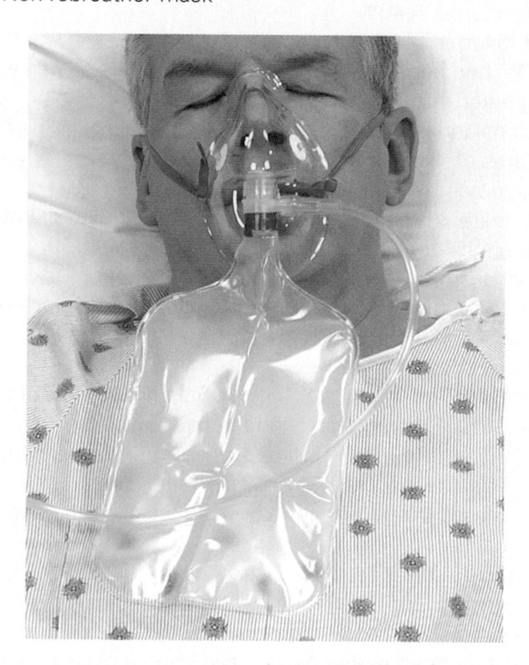

  - Flow rates and percent oxygenation values are 10 to 15 L/min and 60% to 100%, respectively.
  - Special valves on the mask prevent room air from entering the mask but allow exhaled air to leave the mask.
  - The non-rebreather mask looks very similar to the partial rebreather mask. The difference is that the reservoir bag has a one-way valve that prevents exhaled air from entering the reservoir. This provides a larger concentration of oxygen in the bag for the patient to inhale.
  - Ensure a snug fit around the face.
- Venturi mask
  - A Venturi mask is used to ensure accuracy of the oxygen concentration delivered; it is considered for use with CO_2-retaining patients.

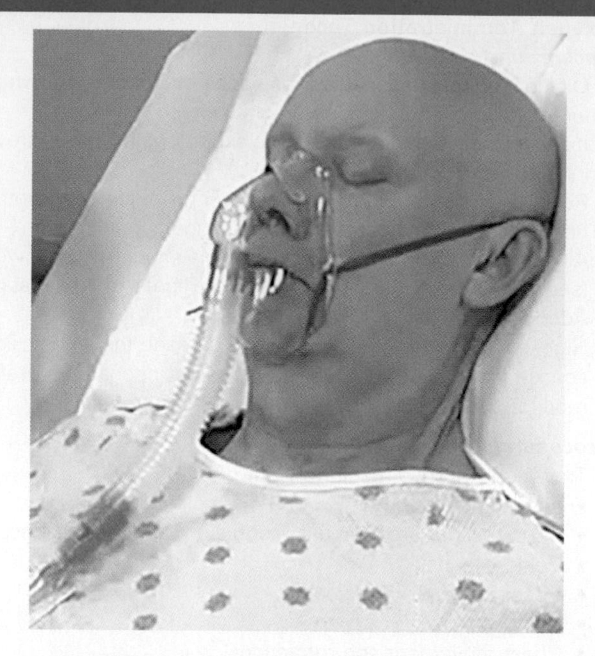

  - Flow rates and percent oxygenation values vary by manufacturer but are in the range of 4 to 12 L/min and 24% to 60%, respectively.
  - Although the manufacturer's instructions need to be consulted for specific details, the Venturi apparatus includes a set of color-coded adaptors (i.e., jets) or a dial.
    - Each color-coded adaptor has a corresponding liters-per-minute setting listed on it for the allowed percent oxygenation. To change the percentage of oxygen being delivered, the adaptor must be changed inside the tubing.
    - If the apparatus has a dial, turn it to set the correct percent oxygenation.
- Trach mask and collar

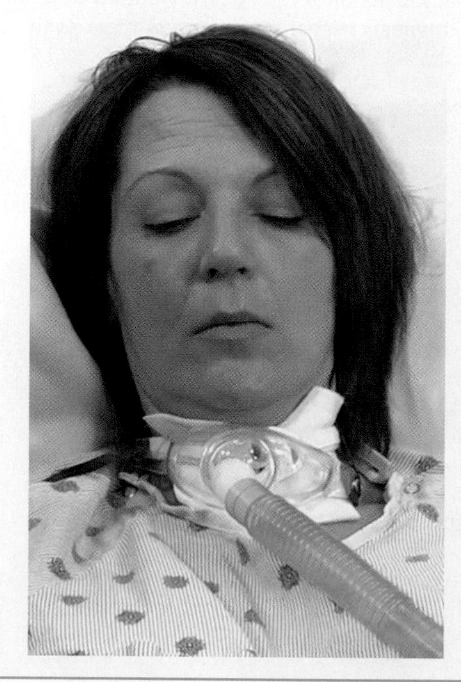

NURSING CARE GUIDELINE—cont'd

- Patients with tracheostomies require a special adaptation for oxygen administration.
- Oxygen is always humidified for tracheostomies.
- Correct application:
  - Center the mask and collar over the tracheostomy.
  - Secure the mask and collar around the back of the patient's neck with the strap, pulling evenly on both ends of the strap to secure it in place.
- Flow rates and percent oxygenation values are similar to those for simple face masks.

- Face tent
  - When a face tent is used, the oxygen is always humidified.

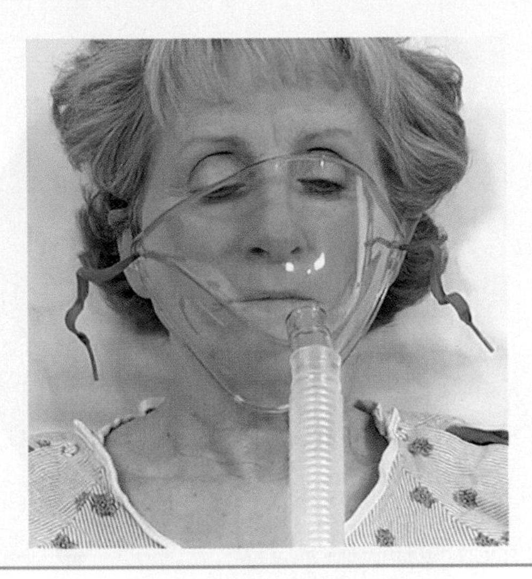

- Correct application:
  - Center the face tent over the face, covering from the jaw upward.
  - Secure it around the top of the patient's head with the strap, pulling evenly on both ends of the strap to secure it in place.
- Flow rates and percent oxygenation values vary.

Documentation Concerns

- Record patient tolerance of the oxygen delivery device.
- Document the respiratory assessment, including information obtained
  - Before initiation of oxygen
  - At initiation of oxygen and 15 to 30 minutes after initiation of oxygen
  - At subsequent times determined by patient status and nursing judgment
- Include the flow rates and percent oxygenation values.

Evidence-Based Practice

- Patients receiving oxygen therapy have up to one-third higher mortality rates than other patients in the hospital. Eastwood and colleagues (2011) found that these patients were missing up to 10% of routine documentations, such as respiratory rates and pulse oximetry readings.
- The lack of documentation indicates a lack of vigilance in monitoring, which can increase the mortality rate.
- Patients on oxygen are high-risk patients, and nurses need to be vigilant in monitoring and documentation to prevent further complications.

NURSING CARE GUIDELINE

Continuous Positive Airway Pressure and Bilevel Positive Airway Pressure Applications

Background

- Positive airway pressure is primarily used in patients with obstructive sleep apnea, pneumonia, and COPD, and to prevent atelectasis.
- Forced air is administered through a mask over the nose or through nasal pillows at the nares, which keeps the airway open at all times.
- There are two types of positive airway pressure applications:
  - Continuous positive airway pressure (CPAP) provides continuous positive airway pressure; that is, it provides the same pressure during both inhalation and exhalation.
  - Bilevel positive airway pressure (BiPAP) provides continuous bilevel positive airway pressure. It uses two pressures: a higher pressure during inhalation and a lower pressure during exhalation.
  - Both types of applications usually deliver room air but can deliver supplemental oxygen if ordered.

Procedural Concerns

- Collaboration is required when either device is used for long periods.
  - A respiratory therapist usually sets up the device and administers therapy to the patient in acute care.
  - The respiratory therapist or nurse may set up the device in long-term care.
  - The patient sets up the apparatus in the home.
- Assessments
  - The patient's tolerance and compliance are evaluated.
  - Necessary assessments are made of the potential barriers to compliance:
    - Dry nares
    - Skin irritation
    - Claustrophobia
    - Perceived inability to breathe against air
    - Noise of the apparatus
- Consultation
  - Follow the primary care provider (PCP) orders for the settings.

Continued

NURSING CARE GUIDELINE—cont'd

- Refer to the manufacturer's instructions for operation of the device.
- Do not initiate the use of or operate the device without proper education.

Documentation Concerns
- Document the patient's tolerance of the device.
- Include the respiratory assessment.
- Note patient compliance issues.
- Include the patient and family education provided.

Evidence-Based Practice
- Nurses must teach patients and families about the effectiveness of CPAP in treating and reducing the negative consequences of obstructive sleep apnea. Education can increase the patient's compliance and ultimately improve quality of life.
- "Despite the effectiveness of CPAP, patient adherence to using CPAP devices varies between 50% and 80%. Patients complain about the rush of air pressure and tend to remove the mask during the night or not wear it at all" (Donohue, 2010, p. 50).
- For patients who are noncompliant, high-flow nasal cannulas are used in some settings to mimic positive airway pressure while promoting patient comfort and compliance (Kernick and Margarey, 2010).

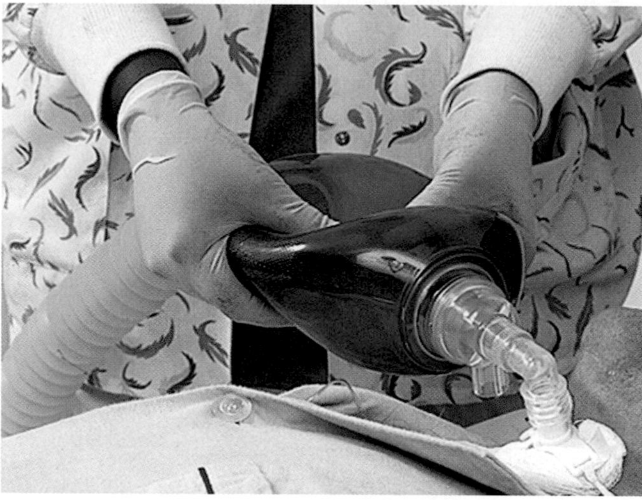

FIGURE 38-10 Bag-valve-mask device. (From Sorrentino SA, Remmert L: *Mosby's textbook for nursing assistants,* ed. 8, St. Louis, 2012, Mosby.)

oxygen and appropriate tidal volume is delivered based on the patient's size. Bags are available in sizes ranging from infant to adult. An adequate seal between the mask and the patient's face, if the patient is not intubated, is necessary to maximize the amount of air that is moved in each ventilation cycle.

Artificial Airways

Pharyngeal Airways

Pharyngeal airways keep obstruction from occurring by pulling the tongue forward and away from the back of the throat (Figure 38-11). Pharyngeal airways are needed most often when a patient has a decreased level of consciousness and loss of muscle tone. The **nasopharyngeal airway** is placed nasally. It is used most often for patients who require frequent nasotracheal suctioning. Oropharyngeal airways are inserted through the mouth. The airway goes over the tongue and is used in unconscious patients. The Nursing Care Guideline: Oropharyngeal and Nasopharyngeal Airway Insertion box provides information about applying these airways.

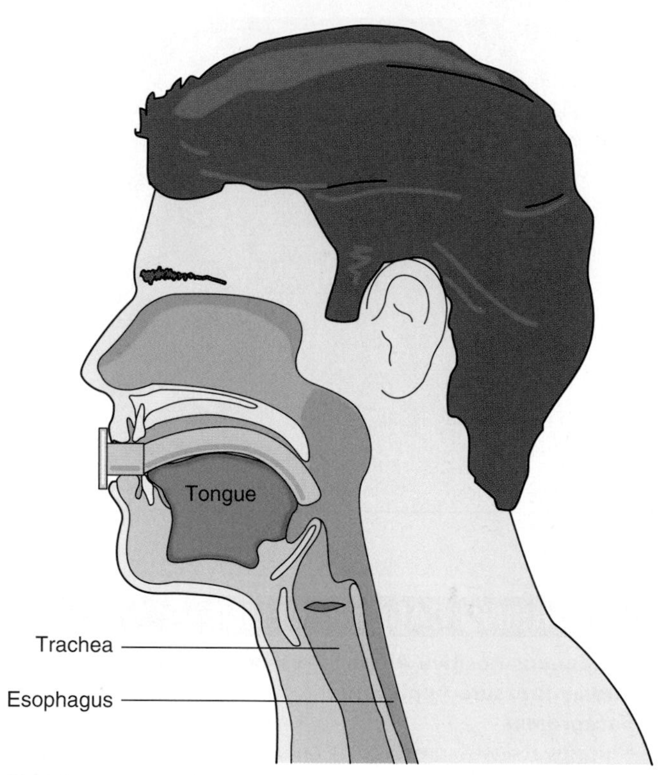

FIGURE 38-11 Pharyngeal airways. (From Monahan FD, Sands JK, Neighbors M, et al: *Phipps' medical-surgical nursing: Health and illness perspectives,* ed. 8, St. Louis, 2007, Mosby.)

! SAFE PRACTICE ALERT

Visually check placement of the airway. Improper placement may result in inadequate ventilation.

Tracheal Airways

Airways that go beyond the pharynx and into the trachea are called *tracheal airways.* **Endotracheal tubes** are semirigid, curved tubes with a cuff at the distal end that seals to prevent aspiration of gastric contents into the lung, allow positive

NURSING CARE GUIDELINE

Oropharyngeal and Nasopharyngeal Airway Insertion

Background

- An artificial airway can be used in an emergency situation to maintain a patent airway in a patient who is otherwise breathing on his or her own.
- Oropharyngeal airway:
  - Keeps the patient's tongue from blocking his or her airway
  - Keeps excessive secretions out of the airway in an unconscious patient
  - Is used primarily for unconscious patients
- Nasopharyngeal airway (i.e., nasal trumpet):
  - Primarily used with patients who require frequent suctioning
  - Acts as a guide for the suction catheter

Procedural Concerns

- Refer to agency policies and procedures and primary care provider (PCP) orders.
- Secure the airway in place with a holder or tape.
- Oropharyngeal airway:
  - The average adult size is 90 mm; it is measured from the mouth opening to the back of the jaw.
  - Insert the airway while directing the curve of the airway at the roof of the mouth, and then rotate the airway 180 degrees after it reaches the back of the throat.
  - Remove the airway every 4 to 8 hours.
- Nasopharyngeal airway:
  - The average adult size is a 28 French, it is measured from the ear tragus to the nostril plus 1 inch.
  - Lubricate the airway before attempting insertion.
  - The airway is inserted gently; if resistance is encountered, try the other nostril.
  - Remove the airway every 8 to 24 hours, and alternate nares.

Documentation Concerns

- Document the reason for insertion of the airway.
- Note patient tolerance of the airway.
- Include mucous membrane assessments and respiratory assessments.
- Document the oral care given.

pressure for ventilation, and keep air from leaking out of the airway.

The **tracheostomy tube** is placed directly in the trachea to control the airway. It is usually made of plastic polymers, but some are made of metal (Figure 38-12). Most plastic tracheostomy tubes have an outer cannula that has a flange and a cuff attached. A removable inner cannula has a standard 15-mm adapter. The inner cannula is removed for cleaning. The tracheostomy tube fits through a stoma in the neck. Suctioning procedures for airways and tracheostomy care are outlined in Skills 38-1 and 38-2.

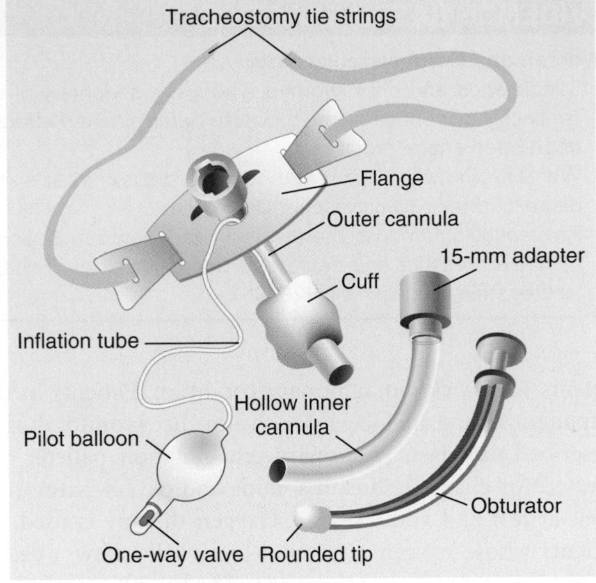

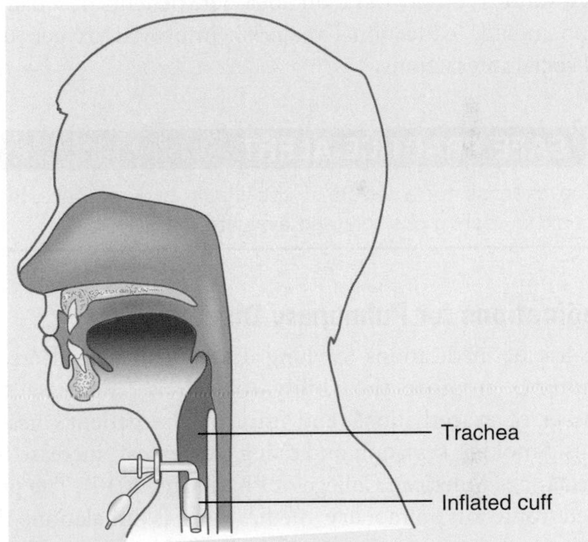

FIGURE 38-12 Tracheostomy components. (From Lewis SL, Dirksen SR, Heitkemper MM, et al: *Medical-surgical nursing: Assessment and management of clinical problems,* ed. 8, St. Louis, 2011, Mosby.)

Diet Therapy

A high-fiber and low-fat diet is recommended for patients at risk for cardiopulmonary disease. The patient is advised to avoid meats that are high in fat and eat lean cuts of meat, such as chicken or turkey breasts. Eating fruits and vegetables is encouraged. Weight management and a high-fiber diet may help to lower LDL cholesterol levels (Evidence-Based Practice box).

Exercise Programs

Regular exercise is recommended for cardiac and pulmonary patients to optimize functioning. Cardiac and pulmonary rehabilitation is an individualized exercise program for

EVIDENCE-BASED PRACTICE

Women and Cardiovascular Risk

- Middle-aged and older women who were sedentary and overweight or obese were studied to determine the effect of an intervention program.
- Women who lost weight and decreased their waist size decreased their cardiovascular disease risk.
- For each kilogram lost, there was an associated reduction of blood pressure and decreased risk of diabetes (Folta, Lichtenstein, Sequin, et al, 2009).

patients with a cardiopulmonary condition. Patients in the outpatient setting are followed with a cardiac monitor during prescribed exercises. Pulmonary rehabilitation patients are assessed for changing breath sounds and oxygen saturation levels at rest and with exercise. Oxygen therapy is used for patients whose oxygen saturation levels fall below a designated value, typically less than 90%. The benefits of rehabilitation include educational material, improved oxygen use, and social interactions.

! SAFE PRACTICE ALERT

Stop exercise for a patient if chest pain occurs. Place the patient in resting position, and evaluate the pain.

Medications for Pulmonary Diseases

The use of medications for lung disease can help decrease symptoms, improve the ability to exercise, decrease the number of exacerbations, and improve the patient's health status. Smoking cessation and using oxygen can increase life expectancy (American College of Physicians, 2010). The preferred route of pulmonary medications is inhalation; the medications can be administered orally and intravenously for serious conditions. Several medications are used for treating pulmonary diseases:

- Oral **bronchodilators** increase the diameter of the bronchi and bronchioles, which decreases wheezing and improves oxygenation.
- Inhalation therapy bronchodilators increase the diameter of the bronchi, which decreases wheezing and improves oxygenation.
- Anticholinergic agents decrease secretions, which improves airway clearance and decreases bronchospasms.
- Corticosteroids decrease inflammation, which improves respiratory function.
- Vaccines provide protection against communicable diseases, including influenza and pneumonia.
- Antibiotics treat infections when they occur.
- Mucolytic therapy decreases the thickness of secretions, which improves airway clearance.
- Leukotriene modifiers decrease inflammation in the airways.

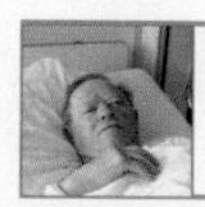

3. Which of Mr. Ross's medications may elevate blood glucose levels?

Medications for Cardiovascular Diseases

Many medications are available to treat cardiovascular diseases. Hypertension is treated with angiotensin-converting enzyme (ACE) inhibitors, angiotensin II receptor antagonists, beta-blockers, calcium channel blockers, and vasodilators. It is important for the nurse to monitor the patient's blood pressure and be alert for adverse reactions to these medications such as dizziness and hypotension. Diuretics may be given to patients with heart failure or edema. Monitoring daily weights and intake and output are appropriate nursing measures for these patients. Antiarrhythmics may be given to patients with arrhythmias or heart failure to slow the heart rate and increase cardiac output.

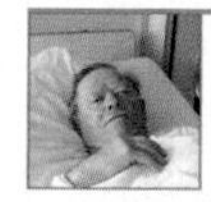

4. Provide at least four nursing interventions with rationales that can help relieve some of Mr. Ross's respiratory distress.

Chest Physiotherapy

Chest physiotherapy includes postural drainage, coughing, deep breathing, and incentive spirometry. **Postural drainage** is a therapeutic way to position a patient to use gravity to help mobilize respiratory tract secretions. Positioning of the patient improves ventilation and perfusion and normalizes the functional residual capacity of the lungs. Postural drainage therapy includes turning, postural drainage, and external manipulation of the thorax using percussion and **vibration** (gently shaking a flat hand against the chest).

Patients who benefit from postural drainage therapy include those who are unable or reluctant to change body positions and patients with unilateral lung diseases that are related to poor oxygenation due to position. Patients who have diseases such as cystic fibrosis or bronchiectasis, or who have difficulty removing secretions may benefit from postural drainage therapy (Flume and Lester, 2009).

The risks of postural drainage therapy should be considered for some patients. Empyema, pulmonary edema, and pulmonary embolism are a few of the conditions for which the therapy is contraindicated. External manipulation of the thorax is contraindicated for patients with a new pacemaker.

Complications of postural drainage therapy include hypoxemia, increased intracranial pressure (ICP), drop in blood pressure during the procedure, vomiting, and bronchospasm. Cardiac dysrhythmias, pain, and injury to the musculoskeletal system may occur. It is important to monitor the patient carefully during the procedure. The cardiac rhythm, breathing patterns, and skin color are assessed to determine oxygenation. Breath sounds, blood pressure, and oxygen saturation levels indicate the movement of air.

Chest Tubes

The physician determines the size of the catheter used for chest drainage tubes; larger chest tubes are more likely to stay patent than smaller tubes. Chest tubes help drain fluid or blood (hemothorax) and excessive air (pneumothorax) from the pleural space. The chest tube is attached to a water-sealed chamber system that helps to regulate the pleural pressure (Figure 38-13). Most chest drainage systems are based on older three-bottle systems but are self-contained plastic units. The three chambers are a collection chamber, a water-seal chamber, and a suction-control chamber. There are also waterless suction chest drainage systems. Skill 38-3 details the care of chest tubes and disposable drainage systems.

Anticoagulant Therapy

Anticoagulation may be used in patients with cardiac arrhythmias such as atrial fibrillation to prevent the formation of blood clots in the atrium. If a clot forms in the left atrium, the patient is at risk for the clot dislodging, entering the cerebral circulation, and causing a cerebral vascular accident.

Anticoagulation is used to prevent venous thromboembolism (VTE) in acutely ill patients. Risk factors for development of VTE include trauma, major surgery, and age older than 40 years. Other risk factors include obesity, varicose veins, and central venous catheter use. A history of smoking during pregnancy, estrogen use, hypercoagulability conditions, and previous deep vein thrombosis increase the risk of VTE. Cancer and cancer therapy may contribute to increased coagulation in patients. Stroke, severe respiratory disease, inflammatory bowel disease, and nephrotic syndrome may increase the risk of VTE (Dobesh, Phillips, and Haines, 2008).

National health policy organizations have described evidence-based practice to prevent deep vein thrombosis. The danger of deep vein thrombosis is the possibility of the blood clot traveling from the deep vein to the pulmonary artery and causing a pulmonary embolus. The development of pulmonary embolism is the most frequent cause of preventable hospital deaths (The Joint Commission, 2014).

To prevent development of VTE, low-dose unfractionated heparin may be injected subcutaneously (Dobesh, Phillips, and Haines, 2008). For patients who have confirmed acute VTE, parenteral drugs for anticoagulation are administered first. Oral anticoagulation with warfarin has a slower onset.

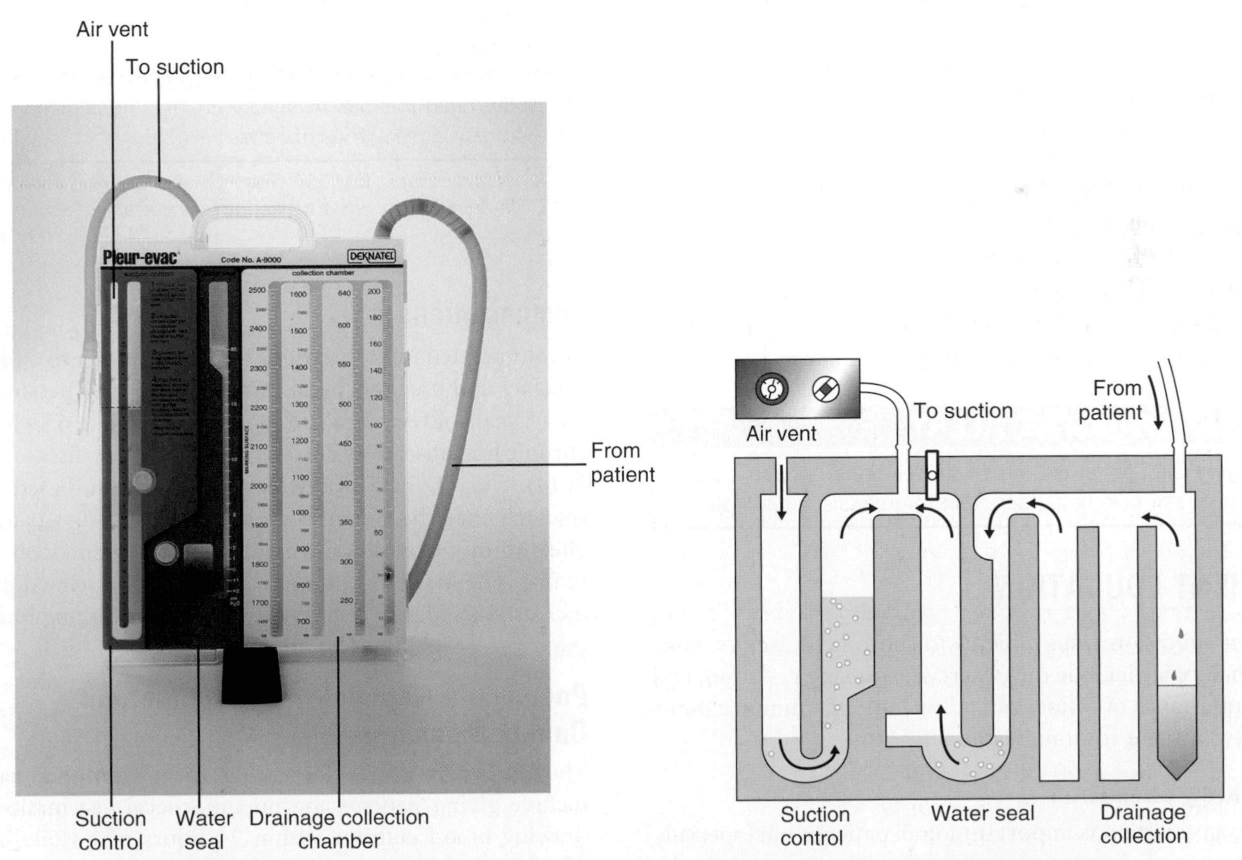

FIGURE 38-13 *Left,* The Pleur-Evac drainage system, a commercial three-bottle chest drainage device. *Right,* Schematic of the drainage device. (From Ignatavicius DD, Workman ML: *Medical-surgical nursing: patient-centered collaborative care,* ed 7, St. Louis, 2013, Saunders.)

Warfarin can be started on the first day of treatment after the parenteral anticoagulation has been started (The Joint Commission, 2014).

Warfarin works by interfering with the synthesis of vitamin K–dependent clotting factors. It takes days to get the anticoagulation levels in the therapeutic range. The adequacy of anticoagulation is monitored using the international normalized ratio (INR). The recommended INR is between 2.0 and 3.0 unless otherwise directed by the health care provider (The Joint Commission, 2014). Discharge teaching for a patient on anticoagulation therapy is crucial. The topics include the importance of compliance with the prescribed regimen, dietary advice regarding controlling foods high in vitamin K, signs of adverse reactions to anticoagulants such as bleeding, and interactions with other medications (The Joint Commission, 2014).

! SAFE PRACTICE ALERT

Patients on anticoagulation need to be monitored carefully for signs and symptoms of bleeding. An INR that exceeds the upper range increases the risk of bleeding.

Antiembolism Hose

Antiembolism hose are tightly fitting, elastic stockings that are used to promote venous blood return and to prevent edema in the lower extremities, deep vein thrombosis, venous stasis, and pulmonary emboli. Refer to Chapter 28, Skill 28-4 for detailed information about antiembolism hose.

Sequential Compression Devices

Sequential compression devices (SCDs) are inflatable sleeves that wrap around the legs of patients. SCDs are used for immobile patients who are at risk for lower extremity venous stasis. Refer to Chapter 28, Skill 28-5 for information about SCDs.

SAFE PRACTICE ALERT

Remove sequential compression devices if a patient complains of calf pain until deep vein thrombosis is ruled out.

PATIENT EDUCATION

Patient education helps patients to control risk factors. Educational topics include diet, exercise, smoking cessation, and the importance of influenza and pneumonia immunizations to prevent these communicable diseases.

Smoking Cessation

Smoking cessation is important for all patients, but especially for those with heart or lung disease. The first step is the patient's desire to stop using tobacco products. An intellectual understanding of the need to stop smoking does not translate into cessation due to the addictive nature of nicotine. Helpful recommendations from the American Lung Association include the use of pharmacologic treatment with medications such as Chantix and Wellbutrin, nicotine replacement, behavioral therapies, and community education programs. Approximately 21% of smokers relapse (Allen, Bade, Hatsukami, et al, 2008).

The Joint Commission's *Specifications Manual for National Hospital Inpatient Quality Measures* (2012) states, "Smoking cessation reduces mortality and morbidity in all populations" (p. HF-4-1). Patients who are given smoking cessation information and counseling from health care providers are more likely to quit smoking permanently (Patient Education and Health Literacy box).

PATIENT EDUCATION AND HEALTH LITERACY

Components of a Smoking Cessation Program

- Education about the dangers of smoking and health benefits of smoking cessation
- Self-help materials
- Being aware of smoking triggers and planning ways to cope with them
- Counseling and support in person or by telephone
- Use of problem-solving approach such as planning a day without smoking
- Nicotine replacements
- Non-nicotine medications (e.g., bupropion works on parts of the brain that are involved with nicotine addiction)
- Alternative therapy approaches

From National Cancer Institute: Tobacco and smoking cessation, 2012. Retrieved from *www.cancer.gov/cancertopics/factsheet/Tobacco.*

Immunizations

Recommended immunizations for adults are yearly influenza vaccines and pneumococcal vaccinations for all persons who are 65 years old or older and those younger than 65 who have chronic lung disease or chronic cardiovascular disease (CDC, 2014). The rationale for the recommendation is based on the research that the pneumococcal vaccination is up to 75% effective in preventing meningitis and pneumococcal bacteremia. The need to immunize patients is related to the increased incidence of antibiotic resistance to pneumococci infections (The Joint Commission, 2014).

Pneumonia National Hospital Inpatient Quality Measures

The quality measures for caring for pneumonia patients include giving patients the pneumococcal vaccination and drawing blood cultures within 24 hours of hospitalization when indicated. If appropriate, the patient should given advice and counseling for smoking cessation. Antibiotic therapy should begin within 6 hours of arrival at the hospital, and influenza vaccination should be administered before the patient is discharged if the immunization was not administered within the recommended time frame (The Joint Commission, 2014).

EVALUATION

The evaluation of the patient's treatment regimen is an ongoing part of the nursing process. Evaluation of goal statements and desired outcomes helps the nurse modify the plan of care according to goal attainment. Not achieving the desired outcomes prompts the nurse to modify the care plan according to current assessment data. Patients with cardiopulmonary disorders often need frequent reevaluation and modification of interventions to meet basic oxygen needs.

SKILL 38-1 Tracheostomy, Nasotracheal, Nasopharyngeal, Oropharyngeal, and Oral Suctioning

PURPOSE

- To remove mucus from the respiratory tract
- To assist the patient in clearing the airway
- To obtain specimens for ordered tests
- To prevent infections

RESOURCES

- Suction kit
- Sterile normal saline solution (NSS)
- Wall suction or portable suction unit
- Suction canister
- Suction tubing
- Yankauer suction catheter
- Oral suction catheter (for oropharyngeal suctioning)
- Bag-valve-mask (BVM) device with 100% oxygenation capability
- Face mask or shield
- Sterile gloves
- Clean gloves
- Personal protective equipment (PPE) as needed

COLLABORATION AND DELEGATION

- Oral and oropharyngeal suctioning may be delegated to unlicensed assistive personnel (UAP) after assessment by a registered nurse according to facility policy and procedures and after completing the appropriate training.
- Tracheostomy and nasotracheal or nasopharyngeal suctioning of a patient may not be delegated to UAP.
- UAP should report any of the following to the nurse:
  - Changes in vital signs, respiratory status, or level of consciousness
  - Pain or discomfort noticed by the patient
  - Skin breakdown or open areas on the oral mucosa
  - Excessive secretions
  - Difficulties encountered during the procedure or other concerns verbalized by the patient
- UAP should be instructed in the following:
  - Appropriate emergency procedures
  - Appropriate equipment use
  - Appropriate documentation
- The respiratory therapist may administer medications that assist with expectoration of secretions. The nurse should time these interventions and coordinate procedures appropriately.
- Depending on the status of the patient, the respiratory therapist may wish to perform the respiratory assessment and suctioning. It is important for the nurse to coordinate procedures with interdisciplinary personnel.

EVIDENCE-BASED PRACTICE

- Many nurses have been taught to instill sterile normal saline into the trachea to facilitate removal of secretions, believing that it would thin secretions and aid in mobilization. However, current evidence shows that this technique has no benefit, because saline does not mix with secretions.
- Introducing a liquid into the respiratory tract can be an emotionally disturbing experience and produce harmful physiologic effects, such as decreasing oxygenation and inducing lower respiratory tract infections. To aid in thinning and mobilization of secretions, airway humidification and adequate hydration should be initiated (Halm and Krisko-Hagel, 2008).

SPECIAL CIRCUMSTANCES

1. **Assess:** Has the patient experienced pain during or after the suctioning procedure?
   Intervention: Consider administering pain medication before suctioning.
   - Ensure there is an appropriate primary care provider (PCP) order. If not, advise the PCP of the patient's pain.
   - Document appropriately.
2. **Assess:** Does the tracheostomy patient have copious amounts of secretions before suctioning?
   Intervention: Ventilate the patient with an appropriate system to avoid worsening the condition.
   - Do *not* use a BVM device to ventilate the patient before suctioning; using the bag pushes the secretions deeper into the lungs.
   - Use a tracheostomy oxygenation mask set for 100% FiO_2 for several respiratory cycles.
3. **Assess:** Are you unable to maintain a sterile hand while ventilating the patient during tracheostomy suctioning?
   Intervention: Obtain a second person to ventilate the patient with a BVM device during the procedure.
4. **Assess:** If nasotracheal or nasopharyngeal suctioning is ordered, have you checked the patient for epistaxis, injuries from the base of the neck up, reactive airway disease, and coagulation problems?
   Intervention: Do *not* suction through the nares (i.e., procedure is contraindicated for all listed conditions). Notify the PCP, and document.
5. **Assess:** Is there difficulty inserting a catheter in a naris during nasotracheal or nasopharyngeal suctioning?
   Intervention: Withdraw the catheter, and attempt the procedure with the other naris.
   - If there is a possible nasal obstruction, do *not* force the catheter into the naris.

- Ensure the catheter is lubricated. If the patient should have NSS only, try a water-soluble lubricant.
- Try inserting a nasal trumpet.
- Ensure the catheter enters along the floor of the nasal passage.

6. **Assess:** Is there difficulty inserting the catheter past the pharyngeal area during nasotracheal suctioning?
   Intervention: Turn the patient's head to one side or the other to elevate the bronchial passages:
   - Turning the patient's head to the left allows right mainstem bronchus entry.
   - Turning the patient's head to the right allows left mainstem bronchus entry.
7. **Assess:** Is the tongue in the way during oral or oropharyngeal suctioning?
   Intervention: Use gauze to physically move the tongue if necessary. Using gauze reduces the risk of trauma.
8. **Assess:** Is the patient unconscious or unable to assist in positioning when nasotracheal, nasopharyngeal, oral, or oropharyngeal suctioning is required?
   Intervention: Position the patient to the side.
   - The tongue falls out of the way of the catheter insertion.
   - The side position prevents aspiration.
   - The side position provides comfort by facilitating procedural technique.

PREPROCEDURE

I. Check PCP orders and the patient care plan.
Knowledge of patient-specific orders is critical for safe patient care.

II. Gather supplies and equipment.
Preparing for the patient encounter saves time and promotes patient trust.

III. Perform hand hygiene.
Frequent hand hygiene prevents the spread of microorganisms.

IV. Maintain standard precautions.
Use of the correct personal protective equipment (PPE) is required whenever contact with bodily fluids is possible, to reduce the transfer of pathogens.

V. Introduce yourself.
Initial communication establishes the role of the nurse and begins a professional relationship.

VI. Provide for patient privacy.
It is important to maintain patient dignity.

VII. Identify the patient, using two identifiers.
Identifying a patient involves scanning barcodes or comparing the patient's stated name and birthdate to information on the patient's wristband or health record. The correct person must receive the correct treatment.

VIII. Explain the procedure to the patient.
The nurse has a responsibility to inform a patient before initiating care. Information may ease patient anxiety and facilitate cooperation.

PROCEDURE

Tracheostomy Suctioning

Follow preprocedure steps I through VIII.

1. Put on specific PPE (e.g., face mask or shield, clean gloves).
   Using gloves and masks controls the spread of microorganisms among patients and providers and protects providers from infection.
2. Ensure the patient is in the Fowler or semi-Fowler position by elevating the head of the bed.
   Elevation of the patient's head and upper body facilitates comfortable respiration, prevents aspiration, and provides comfort to the patient by facilitating procedural technique.
3. Assess the patient's respiratory status.
   Establish baseline status, and assess the need for an appropriate procedure.

4. Place the BVM device at the head of the bed, and ensure it is operational and has 100% oxygen airflow.
   Proper placement of the BVM device prevents disruption of the sterile procedure and ensures quick access during the procedure.
5. Determine the best placement to set up the suction device and tubing:
   a. If right handed, work on the patient's right side; the nurse's right hand is the sterile hand, and left hand is the clean hand.
   b. If left handed, work on the patient's left side; the nurse's left hand is the sterile hand, and right hand is the clean hand.
   Optimal placement promotes sterile technique, prevents contamination by microorganisms in the sterile field, prevents infection, and provides organization to facilitate performing the procedure.
6. Set the pressure of the suction device to 80 to 120 mm Hg continuous, and place the end of the tubing close to the working field.
   This is the optimal pressure setting for the procedure. The tubing needs to be connected quickly to the catheter within the sterile field.
7. Prepare items from the suction kit on the sterile field (see the Sterile Fields section in Chapter 26, Skill 26-4). Use a sterile drape. If doing tracheostomy care, the kit may have a drape.
   a. Open the kit. Create the sterile field.
   b. Before gloving, pour 100 mL sterile NSS into the sterile solution container. To pour liquids into a container within the sterile field, hold the lid of the container in the nondominant hand with the inside facing up. Pour slowly, holding the bottle 2 to 4 inches above the container. (Some kits have rigid plastic containers and some have collapsible cardboard containers lined in plastic.)
   c. Put on sterile gloves (see the Sterile Gloving section in Chapter 26, Skill 26-2).
   d. Place the sterile suction catheter on the sterile field.
   Maintain sterile procedure. Preparation of the work field in this manner reduces microorganisms on the equipment, prevents microorganisms from entering respiratory system and causing infection, and provides organization to facilitate the procedure.
8. Prepare the remainder of the needed items:
   a. Grasp suction catheter with your sterile hand, and wrap the tubing around your fingers.
   b. Grasp the connection tubing with your clean hand.
   c. Connect the catheter to the connection tubing. Be careful not to touch your hands together or to touch the connection tubing with the sterile hand.
   d. Test the functioning of the suction by using your thumb to occlude the suction-control port on the catheter and dipping the catheter tip into the center of the NSS, avoiding the edges of the container. The solution collects in the suction canister. Release the suction-control port on the catheter.
   Maintain sterile procedure to reduce the number of microorganisms on the equipment and prevent microorganisms from entering the respiratory system, where they may cause infection. Avoiding the edges of the solution container prevents microorganisms from entering the respiratory system. Using normal saline solution decreases risk of trauma to respiratory tissues. Testing ensures equipment functioning and prevents adverse events.
9. Use your clean hand to remove the tracheostomy oxygen mask from the patient (if it was needed.)
   Provide access to the tracheostomy to perform the procedure.
10. If the BVM device is not contraindicated (e.g., patient with a tracheostomy who has copious secretions), use your clean hand to give 3 to 5 slow, deep breaths with the BVM device; time the breaths with the patient's inhalations.
    Provide for extra oxygen during the procedure to promote coughing and deep breathing and facilitate secretion removal.

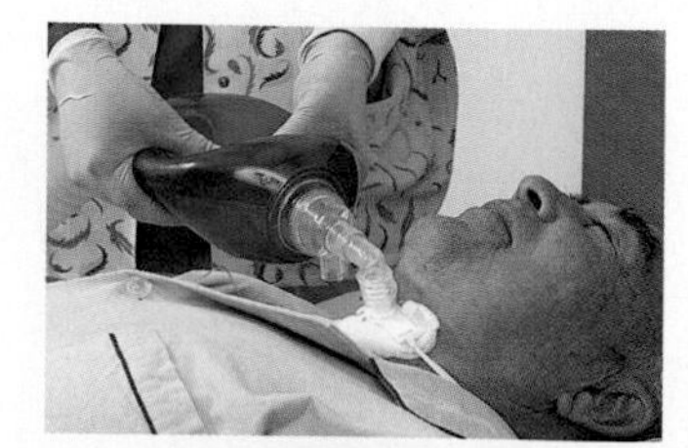

STEP 10
(From Sorrentino and Remmert, 2012.)

11. Suction the patient:
    a. Ensure the suction-control port is open.
    b. With the patient inhaling, gently and quickly insert the catheter approximately 12 to 13 cm into the tracheostomy. If resistance is encountered, pull the catheter back 1 cm.
    c. Withdraw the catheter slowly while rotating it and moving your thumb on and off the suction-control port to promote intermittent suctioning.
    d. The maximum time for each suctioning is 10 to 15 seconds.

    Resistance indicates that the catheter is at the bottom of the trachea, where the bronchi divide. Rotating the catheter allows all areas to be suctioned. Follow the insertion technique to reduce the risk of trauma. Use intermittent suctioning to reduce the risk of trauma to tissues. Restricting the time allotted for each suctioning procedure ensures adequate oxygen levels are maintained for the patient.

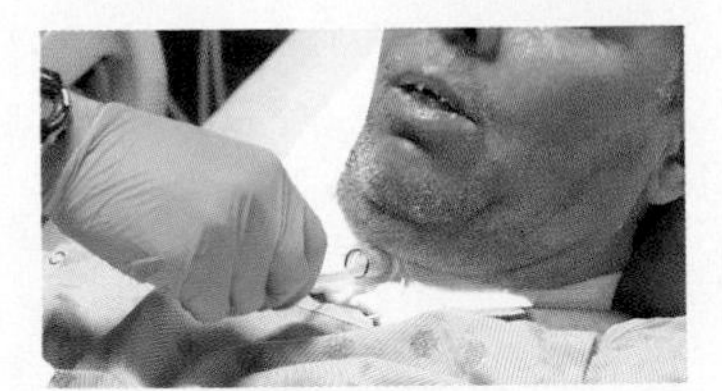
STEP 11c

12. Replace the tracheostomy oxygen mask with your clean hand if it was removed in procedure step 10. Wait 1 to 3 minutes between suctioning.
    Replacing the oxygen source allows oxygen levels to return to normal, promotes comfort, and increases respiratory functioning.
13. Repeat procedure step 8d to clear the suction catheter.
14. Repeat procedure steps 9 through 12 as needed and tolerated.
15. Assess the patient's cardiac and respiratory status after the procedure.
    Observing the patient's cardiac and respiratory status allows the nurse to evaluate the effectiveness of the procedure.

Follow postprocedure steps I through VI.

Nasotracheal or Nasopharyngeal Suctioning

Follow preprocedure steps I through VIII.

1. Follow procedure steps 1 through 8 in the Tracheostomy Suctioning section. Assess the nasal cavity.
   Ensuring that the nasal passages are intact prevents further damage to any areas that are not intact.
2. Hyperextend the patient's head if able and tolerated.
   Hyperextension provides the optimal positioning for the procedure, reduces strain on the caregiver, promotes patient comfort, prevents aspiration, and reduces gagging.
3. Apply water-soluble lubricant to the first 15 cm of the suction catheter tip using sterile technique.
   Water-soluble lubricant may be used in addition to sterile NSS. Lubricant facilitates catheter entry into the naris and reduces the risk of trauma to the nasal tissues.
4. Remove the nasal cannula or oxygen mask from the patient with the clean hand, if applicable.
   Provide access to the nares to perform the procedure.
5. Suction the patient:
   a. Ensure the suction-control port is open.
   b. With the patient inhaling, gently and quickly insert the catheter into a naris, slanting it downward and inserting it to the appropriate depth (15 to 20 cm for nasotracheal; 15 to 18 cm for nasopharyngeal). If resistance is encountered, pull the catheter back 1 cm.
   c. Withdraw the catheter slowly while rotating the catheter and moving the thumb on and off the suction-control port to promote intermittent suctioning. If the patient experiences gagging or nausea, pull the catheter out.
   d. The maximum time for each suctioning pass is 10 to 15 seconds.

   Using a downward slanted entry ensures avoidance of and possible injury to the scroll-shaped bones (i.e., turbinates) in the nose. Resistance indicates that the catheter is at the bottom of the trachea, where the bronchi divide. Gagging or nausea indicates placement is in the esophagus. Rotating the catheter allows all areas to be suctioned and reduces the risk of trauma. Intermittent suctioning reduces the risk of trauma to tissues. Restricting the time allotted for each suctioning procedure ensures adequate oxygen levels are maintained for the patient.

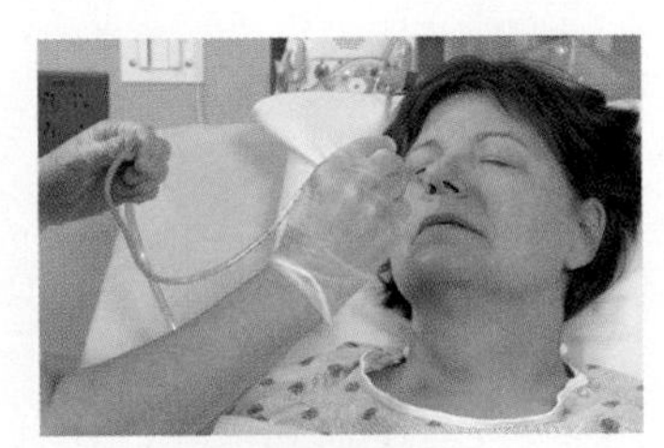
STEP 5b

6. Using your clean hand, replace the nasal cannula or oxygen mask if it was removed in procedure step 4.
   Replacing the oxygen source allows oxygen levels to return to normal, promotes comfort, and increases respiratory functioning.
7. Follow procedure step 8d in the Tracheostomy Suctioning section to clear the suction catheter if needed.
   Greater time causes secretions to accumulate (i.e., body's natural response).
8. Repeat procedure steps 4 through 7 as needed and tolerated.
9. Assess the patient's cardiac and respiratory status following the procedure.
   Noting the patient's cardiac and respiratory status allows the nurse to evaluate the effectiveness of the procedure.

Follow postprocedure steps I through VI.

Oral or Oropharyngeal Suctioning

Follow preprocedure steps I through VIII.

1. Put on specific PPE (e.g., face mask or shield, clean gloves). Assess the oral cavity.
   Using gloves and masks prevents and controls the spread of microorganisms among patients and providers and protects providers from infection. Assessing the oral cavity prevents further damage to areas that are not intact.
2. Place the BVM device at the head of the bed, and ensure it is operational and has 100% oxygen airflow.
   Proper placement of the BVM device ensures quick access during the procedure.
3. Set the pressure of the suction device to 120 mm Hg continuous, and place the end of the tubing close to the working field.
   This is the optimal pressure setting for the procedure. Correct placement of the tubing facilitates timely performance of the procedure.
4. Prepare and test the following items:
   a. Open the suction catheter kit or disposable suction catheter packaging. A Yankauer catheter may be attached in the room.
   b. Obtain the sterile solution container, and place it on the clean work field. Do *not* touch the inside of the container.
   c. Before gloving, pour 100 mL sterile NSS into the sterile solution container.

   Proper preparation of supplies reduces the number of microorganisms, provides organization to facilitate performance of the procedure, and reduces the risk of microorganisms entering the respiratory system. The sterile NSS provides a mechanism to clear the tubing of excessive secretions.
5. Prepare the remainder of the items.
   a. Connect a catheter to the tubing (Yankauer catheter is preferred).
   b. Test the functioning of the suction for the Yankauer catheter by dipping the catheter in NSS; the solution collects in the suction canister.
   c. Alternatively, test the functioning of the disposable suction catheter by using your thumb to occlude the suction-control port on the catheter and then dipping the catheter tip into the center of the NSS, avoiding the edges of the container; the solution collects in the suction canister.

   The Yankauer catheter is larger, is safe for patient use, and has less risk of inducing gagging than the disposable suction catheter. Dipping the catheter tip into the center of the solution prevents microorganisms from being transferred from the edges of the container into the patient's respiratory system. Testing ensures proper functioning of the equipment and prevents adverse events. Using the NSS decreases the risk of trauma to the oral mucosa.
6. Place the patient in a semi-Fowler position. Hyperextend the patient's neck if able and tolerated.
   Use the optimal positioning for the procedure; it reduces strain on the caregiver, promotes comfort, prevents aspiration, and reduces gagging.

7. If used by the patient, remove the oxygen mask; a nasal cannula may remain in place.
   Remove the oxygen mask in use to provide access to the oropharyngeal area for performing the procedure. A nasal cannula may remain in place to allow oxygen levels to remain normal, promote patient comfort, and increase respiratory functioning.
8. Using a disposable suction catheter or Yankauer catheter to suction the patient:
   a. Place the catheter in the patient's mouth.
   b. Slide the catheter down the inner surface of the cheek toward the back of the throat; do *not* apply suction until the catheter reaches the back of the throat. If the patient has gagging or nausea, pull the catheter out without suction. If able, the patient may assist with suctioning.
   c. Apply continuous suction by keeping your thumb on the suction-control port if using a disposable suction catheter.
   d. Encourage the patient to cough, deep breathe, and expectorate.
   e. Or if using a Yankauer catheter, suction only the oral area, and use continuous suction.

   Sliding the catheter down the side of the cheek without suction prevents trauma to the oral mucosa, allows suctioning of secretions deeper in the pharyngeal area, and prevents gagging.

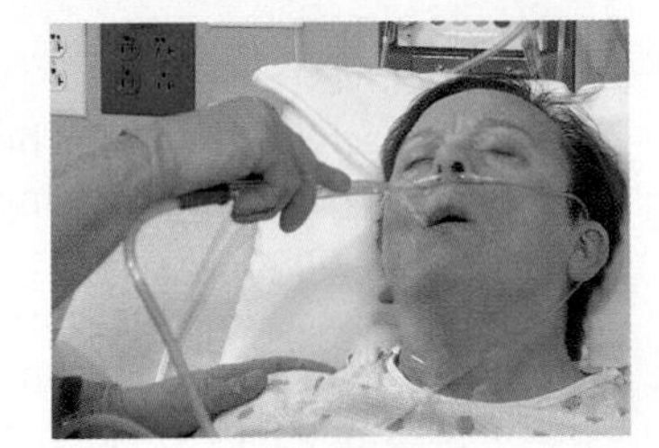
STEP 8

9. Replace the oxygen mask if it was removed in procedure step 7.
   Replacing the oxygen source allows oxygen levels to return to normal, promotes comfort, and increases respiratory functioning.
10. Repeat procedure steps 7 though 9 as needed and tolerated.
11. Clean the equipment.
    a. If using a disposable suction catheter, use a new catheter for each procedure.
    b. If using a Yankauer catheter, rinse it thoroughly with NSS through the suction equipment. Suction air through the catheter to dry the inside, and clean the outside with alcohol wipes or a hydrogen peroxide (H_2O_2) solution.

    Proper cleaning is used to reduce the number of microorganisms on the equipment and to prevent the spread of microorganisms to the respiratory tract.
12. Assess the patient's cardiac and respiratory status after the procedure.
    Observing the patient's cardiac and respiratory status allows the nurse to evaluate the effectiveness of the procedure.

Follow postprocedure steps I through VI.

POSTPROCEDURE

I. Return the bed to its lowest position, raise the top side rails, and verify that the call light is within reach of the patient.
   Precautions are taken to maintain patient safety. Top side rails aid in positioning and turning. Raising four side rails is considered a restraint.
II. Assess for additional patient needs and state the time of your expected return.
   Meeting patient needs and offering self promote patient satisfaction and build trust.
III. Properly dispose of PPE.
   Gloves, gowns, and masks must be appropriately discarded to prevent the spread of microorganisms.
IV. Clean equipment if it was in contact with the patient; see specific manufacturer instructions.
   Disinfection eliminates most microorganisms from inanimate objects.
V. Perform hand hygiene.
   Frequent hand hygiene prevents the spread of infection.
VI. Document the date, time, assessment, procedure, and patient's response to the procedure.
   Accurate documentation is essential to communicate patient care and to provide legal evidence of care.

Step 10 figure from Sorrentino SA, Remmert L: *Mosby's textbook for nursing assistants,* ed. 8, St. Louis, 2012, Mosby.

SKILL 38-2 Tracheostomy Care

PURPOSE

- To prevent skin breakdown at the tracheostomy site
- To prevent infection
- To maintain a patent airway

RESOURCES

- Tracheostomy care kit
  - Three sterile solution containers
  - Sterile brush
  - Sterile field
  - Sterile gloves
  - Clean gloves
  - Velcro tracheostomy tube holder or tracheostomy ties
  - Foam tracheostomy dressing or sterile 2 × 2 gauze pad
  - Sterile cotton swabs
  - Bifurcated 2 × 2 sterile gauze pad tracheostomy dressing
- Sterile normal saline solution (NSS)
- Sterile cotton swabs
- Bag-valve-mask (BVM) device
- Suction canister
- Suction tubing
- Wall suction or portable suction unit
- Oxygenation source with 100% oxygen availability
- Two extra inner cannulas (one the same size as worn by the patient and one a size smaller)
- Two extra outer cannulas (one the same size as worn by the patient and one a size smaller)
- Scissors
- Stethoscope
- Face mask or shield
- Personal protective equipment (PPE) as needed

COLLABORATION AND DELEGATION

- Care of an established tracheostomy may be delegated to unlicensed assistive personnel (UAP) after assessment by a registered nurse according to facility policy and procedures and after appropriate training.
- Care of a new tracheostomy may not be delegated to UAP.
- UAP should report the following to the nurse:
  - Changes in vital signs, respiratory status, or levels of consciousness
  - Problems or tube positioning difficulties
  - Pain or discomfort noted by the patient
  - Skin breakdown or open areas noted at the site of the tracheostomy
  - Excessive secretions
  - Difficulties in performing the procedure or other concerns verbalized by the patient
- UAP should be instructed in the following:
  - Emergency procedures
  - Appropriate equipment use
  - Appropriate documentation
- The respiratory therapist may wish to care for or assist with care of a new tracheostomy, and the nurse should coordinate these procedures appropriately.
- The PCP determines the need for a long-term tracheostomy.

EVIDENCE-BASED PRACTICE

- Tracheostomy twill ties cut into a patient's skin, causing trauma and providing a site for infection. A Velcro tracheostomy tube holder is recommended, because it is easier to use by the patient and provider; it provides soft, cushioned support that prevents injury; and it is preferred by patients. Only a commercially prepared bifurcated tracheostomy dressing should be used to prevent foreign objects from entering the airway.
- If possible, a dressing should be avoided altogether. If it is not possible due to secretions, the current recommendation is to use a 2 × 2 gauze dressing, rather than a 4 × 4 gauze dressing, for minimal to moderate secretions. The larger dressing has a higher rate of inadvertent tracheostomy dislodgment while attempting to fit the dressing under the faceplate. For excessive secretions, a special foam dressing is recommended to prevent the most adverse events (Dennis-Rouse and Davidson, 2008).
- An endotracheal tube may be replaced with a tracheostomy tube when the health professionals determine that long-term airway management is required. Sofi and Wani (2010) studied the effect on pulmonary mechanics with tracheostomies. The researchers determined that tracheostomy tubes were frequently placed when failure of weaning a patient from mechanical ventilation occurred. They determined that the work of breathing was less with the tracheostomy tube than with the endotracheal tube. Some patients therefore benefit from the placement of a tracheostomy tube.

SPECIAL CIRCUMSTANCES

1. **Assess:** Is appropriate equipment within reach to ensure emergency preparedness?
   Intervention: The following items are always kept at the bedside of a tracheostomy patient:
   - BVM device
   - Endotracheal and oropharyngeal suction equipment
   - Waterproof adhesive tape
   - An extra tracheostomy care kit
   - Two extra inner cannulas (one the same size as worn by the patient and one a size smaller)
   - Two extra outer cannulas (one the same size as worn by the patient and one a size smaller) with obturators
   - Scissors
   - Extra tracheostomy ties
   - Oxygenation equipment

2. **Assess:** Has the tracheostomy been dislodged?
   Intervention: Replace the tracheostomy from the emergency supplies at the bedside:
   - Place the obturator in the outer cannula.
   - Insert the outer cannula into the stoma.
   - Remove the obturator.
   - Secure with a tracheostomy tube holder.
   - Assess the tracheostomy for placement and the patient for respiratory status.
   - Insert the inner cannula.
   - Notify the primary care provider (PCP).
3. **Assess:** Is subcutaneous emphysema observed around the stoma?
   Intervention: Assess placement of the tracheostomy and the patient's respiratory status. Notify the PCP.

PREPROCEDURE

I. Check PCP orders and the patient care plan.
Knowledge of patient-specific orders is critical for safe patient care.

II. Gather supplies and equipment.
Preparing for the patient encounter saves time and promotes patient trust.

III. Perform hand hygiene.
Frequent hand hygiene prevents the spread of microorganisms.

IV. Maintain standard precautions.
Use of the correct personal protective equipment (PPE) is required whenever contact with bodily fluids is possible, to reduce the transfer of pathogens.

V. Introduce yourself.
Initial communication establishes the role of the nurse and begins a professional relationship.

VI. Provide for patient privacy.
It is important to maintain patient dignity.

VII. Identify the patient, using two identifiers.
Identifying a patient involves scanning barcodes or comparing the patient's stated name and birthdate to information on the patient's wristband or health record. The correct person must receive the correct treatment.

VIII. Explain the procedure to the patient.
The nurse has a responsibility to inform a patient before initiating care. Information may ease patient anxiety and facilitate cooperation.

PROCEDURE

Tracheostomy Cleaning and Changing the Inner Cannula

Follow preprocedure steps I through VIII.

1. Follow procedure steps 1 through 4 in the Tracheostomy Suctioning section of Skill 38-1.
2. Remove the tracheostomy dressing, and discard according to facility policy and procedures.
   Proper disposal of waste reduces the spread of microorganisms.
3. Assess the tracheostomy site.
   Obtaining an assessment before performing a procedure provides a baseline measurement for subsequent comparisons and determines the need for further intervention.
4. Remove and dispose of gloves, perform hand hygiene.
   Handwashing reduces the spread of microorganisms.

5. Prepare items for the procedure:
   a. Open the sterile tracheostomy kit.
   b. Remove the sterile solution containers (some contain dividers), and place them on the clean work field.
   c. Before sterile gloving, fill each sterile solution container half full with sterile saline. To pour liquids into a container within the sterile field, hold the lid of the container in the nondominant hand with the inside facing up.
   d. Apply sterile gloves (see the Sterile Gloving section in Chapter 26, Skill 26-2.)

   Follow proper procedure to reduce the number of microorganisms and reduce the risk of infection. Preparing items in advance provides organization to facilitate the performance of the procedure.

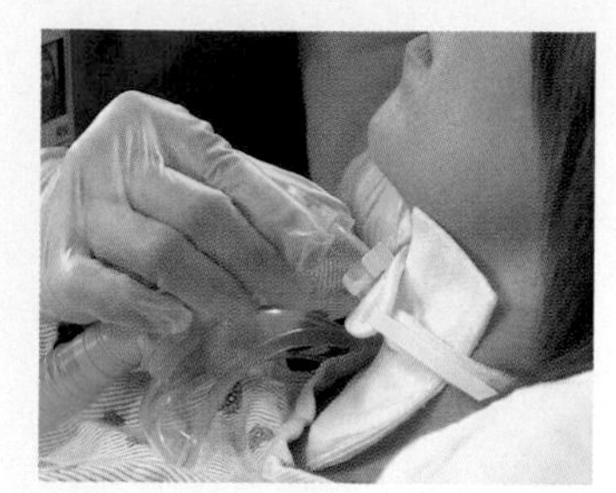

STEP 6

6. Remove the inner cannula, if needed.
   a. Stabilize the faceplate with one hand.
   b. With the nondominant or clean hand, twist the inner cannula to unlock it.
   c. Pull the inner cannula up and out.
   d. If the inner cannula is disposable, replace it with a new cannula (see procedure step 8). If it is not disposable or is to be reused, place the inner cannula in NSS.
7. If using a nondisposable inner cannula, clean it:
   a. Use your clean hand to retrieve the inner cannula from the NSS container; hold the cannula by its edges.
   b. Use your dominant or sterile hand to pick up the sterile brush.
   c. Working above the NSS container, clean the inner cannula with the brush.
   d. Do *not* allow your clean and sterile hands to touch each other.
   e. Rinse the inner cannula in the NSS solution container.
   f. Remove excess NSS from the inner cannula by tapping it on the inside of the NSS container.
   g. Repeat procedure steps c through f as needed.
   h. Allow the inner cannula to air-dry.

   Using a new inner cannula prevents microorganisms from entering the respiratory system and prevents infection. Using the appropriately designated hand and not allowing the two hands to touch maintains sterile procedure, reduces the number of microorganisms, and reduces the risk of infection. Air-drying prevents unintentional contamination.

   Not all tracheostomies have inner cannulas. Stabilize the faceplate to reduce the risk of inadvertent dislodgment. The NSS loosens secretions.
8. Insert a new or cleansed inner cannula:
   a. Use your clean hand to position the inner cannula over the tracheostomy, with the cannula pointing down and inward.
   b. Twist the inner cannula to lock it into place.

   Using the appropriately designated hand reduces the spread of microorganisms and prevents infection. Proper positioning of the cannula prevents microorganisms from entering the respiratory system, where they may cause infection. Locking the cannula secures it in place.

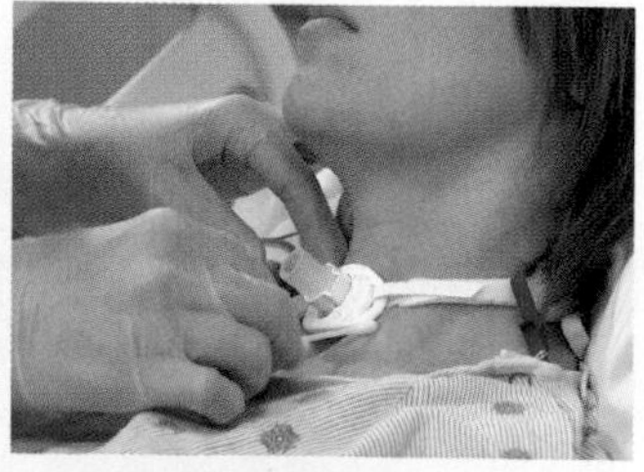

STEP 9

9. Clean the tracheostomy site, including the faceplate, outer cannula, and surrounding areas, one to three times per day:
   a. Use your sterile hand to cleanse the site with sterile cotton swabs; use your clean hand to manipulate the tracheostomy.
   b. Dip a sterile cotton swab into the center of the NSS solution.
   c. Gently cleanse the outer area of the tracheostomy, moving from the stoma outward.
   d. Pat the outer area of the tracheostomy dry with sterile gauze.
   e. Repeat procedure steps b and c as needed.

   Using the appropriately designated hand maintains sterile procedure and reduces the number of microorganisms. Avoiding the more contaminated edges of the NSS solution container reduces the risk of transferring microorganisms to the patient's respiratory system, reducing the risk of infection. Cleaning the skin around the tracheostomy prevents skin breakdown and unintentional contamination. Cleaning from the least-contaminated to the most-contaminated areas prevents infection.

10. Change the Velcro tracheostomy tube holder:
   a. Secure the new holder; do *not* remove the old holder.
   b. Place the holder around the back of the patient's neck.
   c. Insert the ends of the holder in the faceplate, wrap the ends around the back of the neck, and secure them to the Velcro.
   d. Secure the new holder *before* removing the old holder.
   Precautions are taken to maintain patient safety, prevent dislodging the tracheostomy, and prevent necrosis.

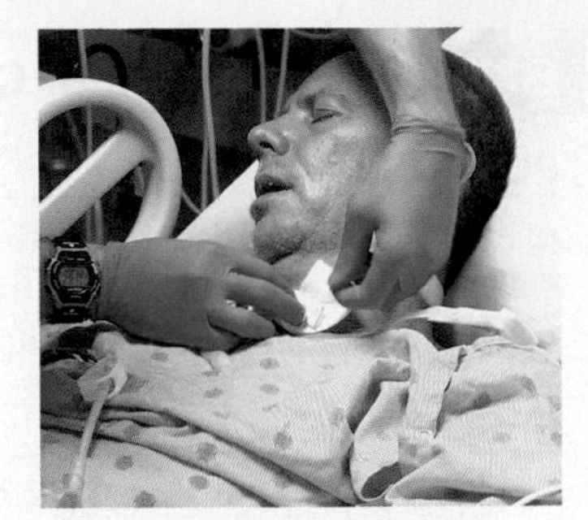

STEP 10

11. If a dressing is required due to secretions, ensure the tube holder is secure:
   a. Use a commercially prepared 2 × 2 bifurcated gauze pad for minimal to moderate secretions.
   b. Use a commercially prepared foam tracheostomy dressing for excessive secretions. Carefully lift one side of the faceplate slightly, and insert the dressing under it; repeat on the other side.
   Smaller dressings prevent accidental dislodgement. Foam dressings absorb excessive secretions and keep moisture away from the skin, preventing skin breakdown.

12. Assess the patient's cardiac and respiratory status following the procedure.
   Observing the patient's cardiac and respiratory status allows the nurse to evaluate the effectiveness of the procedure.

Follow postprocedure steps I through VI.

POSTPROCEDURE

I. Return the bed to its lowest position, raise the top side rails, and verify that the call light is within reach of the patient.
Precautions are taken to maintain patient safety. Top side rails aid in positioning and turning. Raising four side rails is considered a restraint.

II. Assess for additional patient needs and state the time of your expected return.
Meeting patient needs and offering self promote patient satisfaction and build trust.

III. Properly dispose of PPE.
Gloves, gowns, and masks must be appropriately discarded to prevent the spread of microorganisms.

IV. Clean equipment if it was in contact with the patient; see specific manufacturer instructions.
Disinfection eliminates most microorganisms from inanimate objects.

V. Perform hand hygiene.
Frequent hand hygiene prevents the spread of infection.

VI. Document the date, time, assessment, procedure, and patient's response to the procedure.
Accurate documentation is essential to communicate patient care and to provide legal evidence of care.

SKILL 38-3 Care of Chest Tubes and Disposable Drainage Systems

PURPOSE

- To promote optimal respiratory functioning
- To monitor drainage to ensure ultimate lung expansion
- To monitor and prevent complications

RESOURCES

- Emergency equipment at the bedside (see the Special Circumstances section)
- Clean gloves
- Stethoscope
- Hemostats
- Pulse oximeter
- Pen

COLLABORATION AND DELEGATION

- Care of a chest tube may not be delegated to unlicensed assistive personnel (UAP).
- UAP should report the following to the nurse:
  - Changes in vital signs, respiratory status, or levels of consciousness
  - Problems encountered with the procedure or tube positioning difficulties
  - Pain or discomfort expressed by the patient
  - Skin breakdown or open areas observed at the site of the chest tube
  - Other concerns verbalized by the patient
- UAP should be instructed in the following:
  - Appropriate emergency procedures
  - Appropriate equipment use with ambulation or positioning
  - Appropriate documentation
- A respiratory therapist may care for or assist with care of a patient with a chest tube according to facility policy and procedures, and the nurse coordinates procedures appropriately.
- The surgeon assesses chest tube drainage and the insertion site, and the nurse coordinates and documents monitoring and care appropriately.

EVIDENCE-BASED PRACTICE

- Many nurses were taught to "strip" or "milk" the tubing of a chest tube when there was a lack of drainage or an occlusion. However, this practice is outdated and can be dangerous. Evidence shows that it can result in pleural damage, increased bleeding, trauma, and impairment of left ventricular function due to increased intrathoracic pressure (Halm, 2007; Rushing, 2007).

SPECIAL CIRCUMSTANCES

1. **Assess:** Is appropriate equipment within reach to assure emergency preparedness?
   Intervention: The following items are always kept at the bedside of a chest tube patient:
   - Two hemostats with tips covered in soft material (e.g., gauze dressings)
   - Waterproof adhesive tape
   - Occlusive dressing
   - BVM device
   - Oxygenation equipment
2. **Assess:** Has the chest tube become disconnected from the drainage collection device?
   Intervention: Immediately clamp the tube at two places with the covered hemostats.
3. **Assess:** Has the chest tube pulled out from the pleural space?
   Intervention: Immediately cover the insertion site with occlusive dressing. Notify the primary care provider (PCP) immediately.
4. **Assess:** Does the patient require another procedure (e.g., transport) that requires the drainage collection device be lifted above the level of the chest?
   Intervention: Temporarily clamp the tubing at two places with hemostats; release the clamps as soon as possible after the drainage collection device has been restored to the correct position. Tubing is clamped only when the collection device is lifted above the level of the chest, the drainage collection device needs to be changed, or the device breaks.
5. **Assess:** Does the inspiration/expiration water chamber level rise and fall?
   Intervention: Ensure proper functioning of the drainage system and collection device.
   - For a patient who is not being ventilated mechanically, inspiration causes the level to rise, and expiration causes it to fall.
   - For a patient being mechanically ventilated, the opposite occurs. Inspiration causes the level to fall, and expiration causes it to rise.
6. **Assess:** Has the drainage suddenly ceased?
   Intervention: Notify the PCP. Do *not* milk the tubing; trauma or pleural damage may result.
7. **Assess:** Has a large amount of drainage suddenly appeared?
   Intervention: The drainage usually results from positional changes or coughing; assess the patient for a recent position change or coughing. If none is noted, follow the appropriate protocol.
8. **Assess:** Is the tubing free of dependent loops and kinks?
   Intervention: While ensuring that the insertion point of the chest tube into the patient is not moved, straighten the loops or kinks so that drainage is unobstructed.
9. **Assess:** Is the drainage system set to the ordered amount of suction?
   Intervention: Adjust the level of suction as needed to maintain the ordered suction pressure; there should be gentle bubbling in the suction chamber.

10. **Assess:** Is the water level in the water-seal chamber at the marked level?
Intervention: Fill the water-seal chamber to the mark as needed.

11. **Assess:** Is there bubbling in the water-seal chamber?
Intervention: Bubbling indicates an air leak, which may be a sign of a new or persistent pneumothorax. Notify the PCP immediately.

PREPROCEDURE

I. Check PCP orders and the patient care plan.
Knowledge of patient-specific orders is critical for safe patient care.
II. Gather supplies and equipment.
Preparing for the patient encounter saves time and promotes patient trust.
III. Perform hand hygiene.
Frequent hand hygiene prevents the spread of microorganisms.
IV. Maintain standard precautions.
Use of the correct personal protective equipment (PPE) is required whenever contact with bodily fluids is possible, to reduce the transfer of pathogens.
V. Introduce yourself.
Initial communication establishes the role of the nurse and begins a professional relationship.
VI. Provide for patient privacy.
It is important to maintain patient dignity.
VII. Identify the patient, using two identifiers.
Identifying a patient involves scanning barcodes or comparing the patient's stated name and birthdate to information on the patient's wristband or health record. The correct person must receive the correct treatment.
VIII. Explain the procedure to the patient.
The nurse has a responsibility to inform a patient before initiating care. Information may ease patient anxiety and facilitate cooperation.

PROCEDURE

Chest Tube Monitoring and Care

Follow preprocedure steps I through VIII.

1. Adjust patient and bed position to accommodate the patient's diagnosis:
   a. Use the Fowler position for a hemothorax.
   b. Use the semi-Fowler position for a pneumothorax.
   Use the position that promotes optimal drainage of fluid or air.
2. Ensure the tubes are secure and patent:
   a. Check the water-seal vent and the suction-control vent (if suction is used).
   b. Verify that the tubing is resting as close to horizontal as possible on the bed (across a chair if needed) and is directly vertical to the drainage collection device. If coils are made in the tube (not ideal), drain the tube every 15 minutes by moving it. Do *not* lift it above the level of the chest.
   The tubes must be patent for optimal functioning and lung expansion. Coiling may cause resistance and inability to drain.
3. Ensure the drainage collection device placement is upright and *below* the level of the chest tube. *Never* raise the drainage collection device above chest level unless it has been appropriately clamped and then only for as short a period as possible.
   Raising the drainage collection device above the level of the chest causes fluid to reenter the lungs.

4. Check the water-seal chamber; the water level should always rise and fall with the patient's breathing.
   a. For a water-seal system, bubbling is normal for a newly placed chest tube; however, the bubbling should stop when the lung is healing.
   b. For a suction-control chamber, bubbles are normal. Ensure the water is at the prescribed level.
   c. For a waterless system, ensure that the ball in the suction-control chamber is at the prescribed level.

   Following guidelines ensures the system is functioning properly to promote optimal respiratory support. Suction pressure is controlled by the suction-control chamber, not by its connection to wall suction.
5. Drainage assessment:
   a. Assess the type, amount, color, and consistency of the drainage. Notify the PCP of changes.
   b. Mark the quantity, time the assessment was made, and your initials on the drainage collection device at least every 4 hours (more frequently per PCP or facility policy and procedures).
   c. Document assessment findings.

   Increased drainage or a change in the type of drainage can indicate a physiologic change that requires immediate intervention.
6. Dressing assessment:
   a. Verify that the dressing is secure, and reinforce it as needed.
   b. Drainage on the dressing should be minimal (or none).
   c. Document dressing assessment findings.
   d. Reinforce the dressing, but do not change it.

   The dressing must remain secured with occlusive dressing to prevent air from entering the lungs and decreasing respiratory status.

Follow postprocedure steps I through VI.

POSTPROCEDURE

I. Return the bed to its lowest position, raise the top side rails, and verify that the call light is within reach of the patient.
Precautions are taken to maintain patient safety. Top side rails aid in positioning and turning. Raising four side rails is considered a restraint.

II. Assess for additional patient needs and state the time of your expected return.
Meeting patient needs and offering self promote patient satisfaction and build trust.

III. Properly dispose of PPE.
Gloves, gowns, and masks must be appropriately discarded to prevent the spread of microorganisms.

IV. Clean equipment if it was in contact with the patient; see specific manufacturer instructions.
Disinfection eliminates most microorganisms from inanimate objects.

V. Perform hand hygiene.
Frequent hand hygiene prevents the spread of infection.

VI. Document the date, time, assessment, procedure, and patient's response to the procedure.
Accurate documentation is essential to communicate patient care and to provide legal evidence of care.

SUMMARY OF LEARNING OUTCOMES

LO 38.1 *Describe the basic anatomy and physiology of the cardiovascular and respiratory systems in relation to ventilation and perfusion:* The heart is a hollow, cone-shaped organ composed of four chambers divided into right and left sides. The chambers on the top are atria; the lower chambers are ventricles. The respiratory system is divided into the upper (nose, nasal cavity, sinuses, and pharynx) and lower (larynx, trachea, right and left bronchi, bronchioles, alveoli) respiratory tract. The cardiac and pulmonary systems work together to deliver oxygen to tissues. An intact respiratory system is necessary to inspire oxygen and deliver it to the circulatory system. A healthy heart pumps oxygenated blood to tissues through the vascular system.

LO 38.2 *Summarize alterations in structure and function of the cardiovascular and respiratory systems:* Alterations in the cardiovascular and respiratory system may decrease the ability to deliver oxygen to alveoli, absorb oxygen, and expel CO_2.

LO 38.3 *Demonstrate assessment of the cardiac and respiratory systems:* Cardiac and respiratory assessments begin with an assessment of subjective data. Objective data are obtained through vital signs and through inspection, palpation, and auscultation of the heart, lungs, and peripheral vascular system, noting any alterations. Diagnostic tests, including blood work, pulmonary function tests, x-rays, echocardiogram, electrocardiogram, and cardiac catheterization, may be ordered.

LO 38.4 *Choose nursing diagnoses for patients with decreased oxygenation:* Nursing diagnoses for the patient with decreased oxygenation are based on the patient's specific problem. Major diagnoses include *Impaired Gas Exchange, Ineffective Airway Clearance, Activity Intolerance, Ineffective Breathing Pattern, Ineffective Tissue Perfusion,* and *Anxiety.*

LO 38.5 *Identify goals for patients with complications from decreased oxygenation:* Nursing care goals are specific to each patient and reflect the desired measurable outcome for each nursing diagnosis. Goals for patients with decreased oxygenation are designed to meet basic oxygen needs.

LO 38.6 *Evaluate interventions to enhance patient oxygenation, promote safety, and reverse the negative effects of decreased oxygenation:* Interventions for patients with decreased oxygenation include oxygen therapy; artificial airways, including pharyngeal airways, endotracheal airways, and tracheostomies; postural drainage; and pharmacologic therapy.

Answers to the critical-thinking questions are available at *http://evolve.elsevier.com/YoostCrawford/fundamentals/.*

REVIEW QUESTIONS

1. The nurse assesses a patient with chronic obstructive pulmonary disease (COPD). Which finding does the nurse anticipate when inspecting the chest?
   a. A ratio of 1:2 when comparing the side and front views of the chest
   b. A barrel chest
   c. A concave shape to the sternum
   d. A severe lateral curvature of the spine
2. Which is a goal for a patient with the nursing diagnosis of *Ineffective Airway Clearance*?
   a. Patient's respiratory secretions will become thicker so they are not moved when coughing.
   b. Patient's respiratory secretions will have a thinner consistency after being given a mucolytic agent.
   c. Patient will have improved range of motion while in bed.
   d. Patient's respiratory rate will increase to 28 breaths/min during hospitalization.
3. Which position is the priority for a patient experiencing acute shortness of breath?
   a. Supine position
   b. Reverse Trendelenburg position
   c. Face-down position
   d. Upright position
4. Which oxygen delivery setting places a patient in danger of not receiving adequate oxygen?
   a. Nasal cannula at a flow rate of 2 L/min
   b. Nasal cannula at a rate of 5 L/min
   c. Simple mask at a flow rate of 5 L/min
   d. Non-rebreather mask at a flow rate of 5 L/min

5. Which action does a nurse anticipate when suctioning a patient with excessive secretions?
   a. Decrease the patient's oxygen flow rate before beginning the deep suctioning.
   b. Avoid lubricating the catheter tip to prevent getting the substance in the lung tissues.
   c. Limit the time that the catheter is suctioning to prevent excessive loss of oxygen during the process.
   d. Flush the artificial airway with 3 mL of tap water to loosen secretions before suctioning.
6. Which of the chambers of the heart becomes enlarged when mitral valve stenosis occurs?
   a. Right atrium
   b. Right ventricle
   c. Left atrium
   d. Left ventricle
7. Which situation contributes to cyanosis in the pulmonary patient?
   a. Increased $PaCO_2$ levels
   b. Hemoglobin that is not saturated with oxygen
   c. Elevated white blood cell count
   d. Decreased $PaCO_2$ levels
8. A patient with chronic pneumonia may be evaluated by a speech therapist for which cause?
   a. Chronic aspiration of liquids
   b. Hypoventilation due to smoking
   c. Hyperventilation due to anxiety
   d. Decreased respiratory effort due to scolioses
9. A patient with chronic obstructive pulmonary disease (COPD) uses which drive to breathe?
   a. Increased $PaCO_2$
   b. Decreased hemoglobin
   c. Decreased PaO_2 levels
   d. Increased PaO_2 levels
10. Which of the following questions are included in a focused history for a cardiac patient? *(Select all that apply.)*
    a. Are you having pain?
    b. Where is the pain located?
    c. Do you attend religious services regularly?
    d. Do you have increased fatigue?
    e. Do you have any episodes of dizziness?

ⓔ Answers and rationales to the review questions are available at *http://evolve.elsevier.com/YoostCrawford/fundamentals/*.

REFERENCES

Allen S, Bade T, Hatsukami D, Center B: Craving, withdrawal, and smoking urges on days immediately prior to smoking relapse. *Nicotine Tob Res,* 10(1):35-45, 2008.

American College of Physicians: *Pulmonary and critical care medicine,* Philadelphia, 2010, Author.

Centers for Disease Control and Prevention (CDC): Recommended adult immunization schedule, United States, 2014. Retrieved from *www.cdc.gov/vaccines/schedules/hcp/adult.html.*

Cronenwett L, Sherwood G, Barnsteiner J, et al: Quality and safety education for nurses. *Nurs Outlook,* 55(3):122-131, 2007.

Dennis-Rouse MD, Davidson JE: An evidence-based evaluation of tracheostomy care practices. *Crit Care Nurs Q,* 31(2):150-160, 2008.

Dobesh P, Phillips K, Haines S: Optimizing antithrombotic therapy in patients with non-ST segment elevation acute coronary syndrome. *Am J Health Syst Pharm,* 7:22-28, 2008.

Donohue D: Treating obstructive sleep apnea with CPAP. *Nurs Manage,* 41(7):49-50, 2010.

Eastwood GM, Peck L, Young H, et al: Oxygen administration and monitoring for ward adult patients in a teaching hospital. *Intern Med J,* 41(11):784-788, 2011.

Eliott J, Olver I: Choosing between life and death: Patient and family perceptions of the decision not to resuscitate the terminally ill cancer patient. *Bioethics,* 22(3):179-189, 2009.

Flume PA, Lester MK: Airway-clearance therapy guidelines and implementation. *Respir Care,* 54(6):733-753, 2009.

Folta SC, Lichtenstein AH, Sequin RA, et al: The Strong Women-Healthy Hearts program: Reducing cardiovascular disease risk factors in rural, sedentary, overweight, and obese midlife and older women. *Am J Public Health,* 99(7):1271-1277, 2009.

Fox SL: *Human physiology,* ed. 13, New York, 2013, McGraw-Hill.

Fuster V, O'Rourke RA, Walsh J, Fang J (Eds): *Hurst's the heart,* ed. 13, New York, 2013, McGraw-Hill.

Halm MA: To strip or not to strip? Physiological effects of chest tube manipulation. *Am J Crit Care,* 16(6):609-612, 2007.

Halm MA, Krisko-Hagel K: Instilling normal saline with suctioning: Beneficial technique or potentially harmful sacred cow? *Am J Crit Care,* 17(5):469-472, 2008.

Kernick J, Margarey J: What is the evidence for the use of high flow nasal cannula oxygen in adult patients admitted to critical care units? A systematic review. *Aust Crit Care,* 23(2):53-70, 2010.

Longo D, Fauci A, Kasper D, Jameson J, et al: *Harrison's manual of medicine,* ed. 18, New York, 2013, McGraw-Hill.

McKinley M, O'Loughlin VD, Harris R, Pennefather-O'Brien E: *Human anatomy,* ed. 4, Boston, 2015, McGraw-Hill.

National Cancer Institute: Tobacco and smoking cessation, 2012. Retrieved from *www.cancer.gov/cancertopics/factsheet/Tobacco.*

Pagana KD, Pagana TJ: *Mosby's manual of diagnostic and laboratory tests,* ed. 5, St. Louis, 2014, Mosby.

Rushing J: Managing a water-seal chest drainage unit. *Nursing,* 37(12):12, 2007.

Shier D, Butler J, Lewis R: *Hole's human anatomy & physiology,* ed. 13, Boston, 2012, McGraw-Hill.

Sofi K, Wani T: Effect of tracheostomy on pulmonary mechanics: An observational study. *Saudi J Anaesth,* 4(1):2-5, 2010.

Sommers MS, Fannin, E: *Diseases and disorders: A nursing therapeutics manual,* ed. 5, Philadelphia, 2015, FA Davis.

The Joint Commission: Specifications manual for national hospital inpatient quality measures, version 4.0, 2012. Retrieved from *www.jointcommission.org/specifications_manual_for_national_hospital_inpatient_quality_measures/.*

The Joint Commission: Specifications manual for national hospital inpatient quality measures, version 4.3b, 2014. Retrieved from *www.jointcommission.org/specifications_manual_for_national_hospital_inpatient_quality_measures/.*

White G: *Respiratory notes: Respiratory therapist's pocket guide,* ed. 2, Philadelphia, 2013, FA Davis.

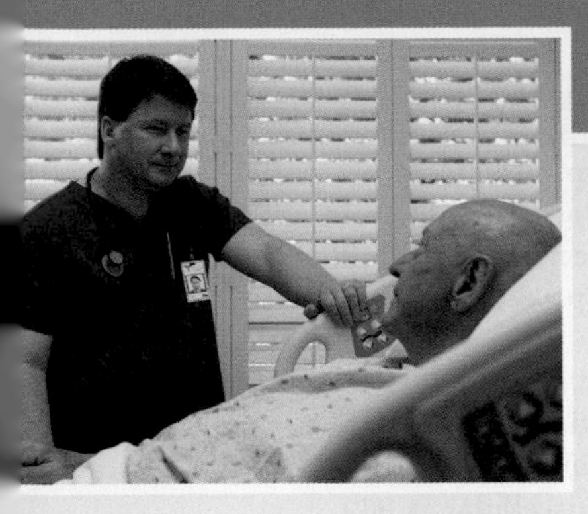

CHAPTER 39

Fluid, Electrolyte, and Acid-Base Balance

EVOLVE WEBSITE

http://evolve.elsevier.com/YoostCrawford/fundamentals/

- Additional Evolve-Only Review Questions With Answers
- Answers and Rationales for Text Review Questions
- Answers to Critical-Thinking Questions
- Case Study With Questions
- Video Skills Clips
- Conceptual Care Map
- Fluids and Electrolytes Tutorial
- Animations
- Skills Checklists
- Glossary

LEARNING OUTCOMES

Comprehension of this chapter's content will provide students with the ability to:

LO 39.1 Discuss the normal structure and function of fluids, electrolytes, acids, and bases in the body.
LO 39.2 Differentiate among common fluid, electrolyte, and acid-base imbalances and their underlying causes.
LO 39.3 Outline assessment priorities for patients with fluid, electrolyte, and acid-base imbalances.
LO 39.4 Identify the most common nursing diagnoses related to fluid, electrolyte, and acid-base imbalances.
LO 39.5 Integrate nursing goals and outcomes into the plan of care for patients with fluid, electrolyte, and acid-base imbalances.
LO 39.6 Carry out nursing interventions to maintain normal fluid, electrolyte, and acid-base balance or to correct imbalances.

KEY TERMS

acid, p. 993
active transport, p. 993
albumin, p. 990
aldosterone, p. 991
antidiuretic hormone, p. 990
arterial blood gases, p. 1007
ascites, p. 1009
atrial natriuretic peptide, p. 991
bases, p. 993
central venous catheter, p. 1015
colloids, p. 989
crystalloids, p. 989
dehydration, p. 996
diffusion, p. 992
edema, p. 997
electrolytes, p. 989
electronic infusion device, p. 1017
extracellular fluid, p. 989
filtration, p. 990
fluid volume deficit, p. 996
fluid volume excess, p. 997
hemolytic reactions, p. 995
homeostasis, p. 990
hydrostatic pressure, p. 990
hypercalcemia, p. 1002
hyperglycemia, p. 1002
hyperkalemia, p. 1001
hypermagnesemia, p. 1002
hypernatremia, p. 998
hyperphosphatemia, p. 1002
hypertonic solution, p. 990
hypocalcemia, p. 1002
hypokalemia, p. 1001
hypomagnesemia, p. 1002
hyponatremia, p. 998
hypophosphatemia, p. 1002

KEY TERMS—cont'd

hypotonic solutions, p. 990
hypovolemia, p. 990
hypoxemia, p. 1008
intermittent infusion device, p. 1014
interstitial fluid, p. 989
intracellular fluid, p. 989
intravascular fluid, p. 989
isotonic solution, p. 989
metabolic acidosis, p. 1004
metabolic alkalosis, p. 1004
milliequivalent, p. 989
oncotic pressure, p. 990
orthostatic hypotension, p. 1005
osmolality, p. 989
osmolarity, p. 989
osmoreceptors, p. 991
osmosis, p. 989
osmotic pressure, p. 989
peripherally inserted central catheter, p. 1016
phlebitis, p. 1014
renin-angiotensin system, p. 990
respiratory acidosis, p. 1002
respiratory alkalosis, p. 1002
selectively permeable membrane, p. 989
solutes, p. 989
solvent, p. 989
tonicity, p. 989
total parenteral nutrition, p. 1028
transcellular, p. 989
vasoconstriction, p. 990

CASE STUDY

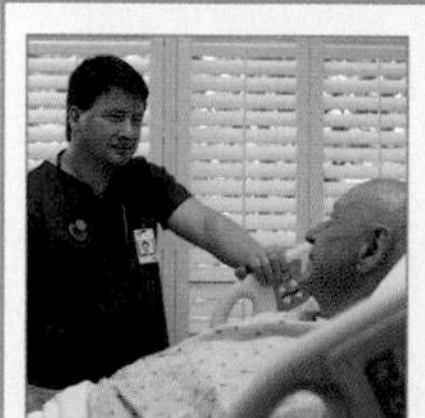

Mr. Abdul is a 76-year-old male who has been admitted to the hospital with a diagnosis of congestive heart failure (CHF). He complains of being tired all the time and barely having enough energy to sit up sometimes. "I think I've put on some weight. My waistband and shoes seem to be tighter and more uncomfortable to wear." He has a history of coronary artery disease. He has smoked one pack of cigarettes per day for 56 years. He has no known drug allergies (NKDA) and has full code status.

Mr. Abdul's vital signs on admission are T 36.5° C (97.7° F), P 118 regular and bounding, R 32 and labored, BP 160/100, with a pulse oximetry reading of 90% on room air. He denies pain and is alert and oriented to person, place, time, and event. He can move all extremities easily but requires assistance with activities of daily living (ADLs) such as bathing and dressing, He becomes short of breath on exertion. He has fine crackles throughout all lung fields and has a moist, nonproductive cough. Bowel sounds are active in all four quadrants. The last bowel movement, a formed brown stool, was yesterday. His skin is warm, dry, and slightly pale. He has +3 pitting edema in both ankles and +1 bilateral dorsalis pedis and posterior tibial pulses.

Admission laboratory test results are as follows:
- Electrolytes: sodium 142 mEq/L; potassium 3.3 mEq/L; chloride 100 mEq/L; bicarbonate 29 mEq/L; blood urea nitrogen 18 mg/dL; creatinine 0.8 mg/dL; glucose 140 mg/dL
- Complete blood count: hemoglobin 15 g/dL; hematocrit 45%; white blood cells 8000 mm^3; platelets 300,000 mm^3
- Arterial blood gases: pH 7.34; PCO_2 56 mm Hg; bicarbonate 32 mEq/L; PO_2 80 mm Hg; O_2 saturation 90%.

Medications are as follows:
- Digoxin 0.125 mg PO q A.M.
- Furosemide 80 mg IV now, then Lasix 40 mg PO q A.M. beginning tomorrow

Treatment orders are as follows:
- O_2 2 L/min per nasal cannula
- Vital signs q 4 hr with pulse oximetry
- Daily weight
- Strict intake and output
- Diet: no added salt
- Activity: bed rest
- Saline lock

Refer back to this case study to answer the critical-thinking exercises throughout the chapter.

The human body is composed primarily of water and chemicals that keep it functioning at optimal levels. Through a series of complex processes, the body is able to maintain normal fluid and chemical balances under various circumstances. However, trauma, disease, and aging can alter the ability to maintain homeostasis and impair normal functioning. The nurse must have an understanding of the homeostatic processes to identify patients at risk for imbalances, recognize when an imbalance has occurred, and intervene appropriately to reestablish equilibrium.

NORMAL STRUCTURE AND FUNCTION OF FLUIDS, ELECTROLYTES, ACIDS, AND BASES LO 39.1

Balanced levels of fluids and various chemicals in the body are essential to maintain health and high-level functioning. Fluctuations in fluid intake and output and alterations brought about by illness can destabilize the balance between fluids and electrolytes. The equilibrium between the acidity and alkalinity of body fluids is acid-base balance, which is regulated by the pulmonary and renal compensatory systems and by chemical (buffering) systems.

COMPOSITION OF BODY FLUIDS

The human body requires sufficient water to survive. Water regulates body temperature, lubricates joints, serves as a shock absorber for internal organs, and transports nutrients and waste products throughout the body. Water is the medium for metabolic reactions within cells.

Total body water (TBW) is the percentage of body weight that consists of water. Almost 60% of a healthy adult's weight is water. However, TBW varies according to age and gender. For example, an infant has a much higher percentage (75%) of TBW than an elderly or obese person (45%). Men tend to have a higher percentage than women (approximately 60% and 50%, respectively).

Body fluid is intracellular or extracellular. Most body fluid is **intracellular fluid** (within the cell). **Extracellular fluid** (fluid outside the cell) is interstitial, intravascular, or **transcellular**, which includes cerebrospinal, synovial, peritoneal, pleural, and pericardial fluids. Vitreous and aqueous fluid in the eye and bile and other digestive fluids are included in this category. **Interstitial fluid** is fluid between the cells of an organ or tissue; it accounts for approximately 25% of total body fluid. **Intravascular fluid**, which is blood plasma, accounts for approximately 8% of body fluid. The remaining includes cerebrospinal, synovial, peritoneal, pericardial, and pleural fluids.

Body fluids are composed of water and solutes. Water moves in and out of the cell, transporting these molecules throughout the body. **Solutes** are chemical substances that dissolve in a liquid (the **solvent**). Solutes that dissolve easily are called **crystalloids**. Substances such as proteins that do not dissolve easily are called **colloids**. Solutes consist of electrolytes and nonelectrolytes, such as, oxygen, carbon dioxide, and glucose.

Electrolytes are charged atoms or molecules (ions) that conduct electrical impulses across cells. They carry a positive charge (cation) or a negative charge (anion). The number of electrolytes that carry a positive charge (cations) and the number that carry a negative charge (anions) should be equivalent. The term **milliequivalent** denotes the ability of cations to bond with anions to form molecules. Electrolytes are measured in milliequivalents per liter of water (mEq/L).

The concentrations of particular electrolytes are measurably different in intracellular fluid and extracellular fluid. The extracellular fluid has essentially the same components in the intravascular and interstitial compartments, with the exception of protein. The intravascular fluid, which is blood plasma, is unique in that it also contains a large amount of proteins, predominantly albumin.

MOVEMENT OF BODY FLUIDS

Water is always moving in and out of cells and throughout the interstitial and intravascular spaces. Movement occurs primarily by two processes: osmosis and filtration.

Osmosis

Osmosis is the movement of water across cell membranes. **Osmotic pressure** is the force created when two solutions of different concentrations are separated by a **selectively permeable membrane**. The cell membrane allows water to move across but not the solutes. Water moves by osmosis from an area of lower concentration of solutes to an area of higher concentration of solutes in an attempt to equalize the concentration across the membrane. The higher the difference in concentration of solutes, the greater the osmotic pressure. The Osmosis animation depicts this process.

Two terms, *osmolality* and *osmolarity*, are often used interchangeably. **Osmolality** refers to the number of osmols (unit of osmotic pressure) per kilogram of solvent, which in this case is water. **Osmolarity** is the number of osmols per liter of solvent. In discussions of body fluids, the differences between the two values are very small. For the purposes of this chapter, osmolarity is used to denote solute concentration.

Another term used to describe osmolarity is **tonicity** of the fluid (Figure 39-1). Tonicity refers to the level of osmotic pressure of a solution. An administered solution that has the same osmolarity as blood plasma is an **isotonic solution**. Normal saline, which is 0.9% sodium chloride, is isotonic.

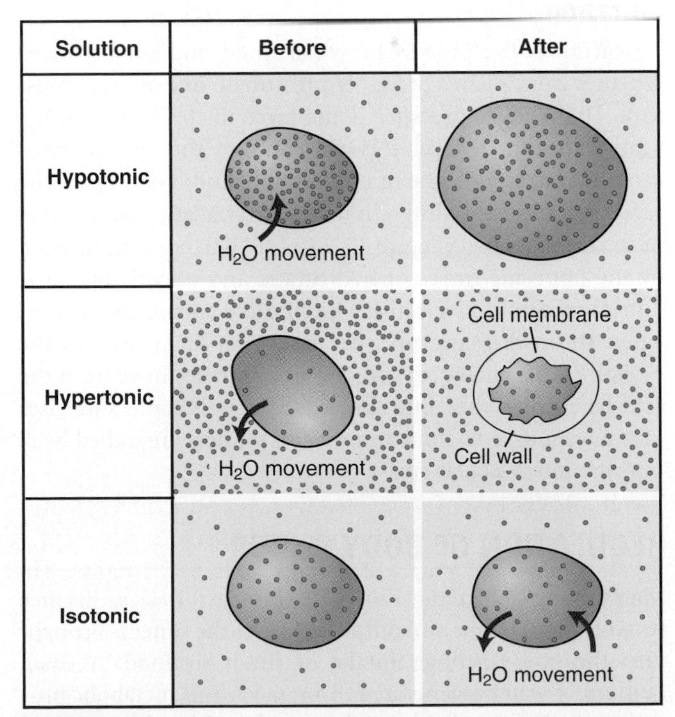

FIGURE 39-1 Effect of tonicity on cells. (From Van Meter KC, Hubert RJ, VanMeter WG: *Microbiology for the healthcare professional*, Philadelphia, 2010, Mosby.)

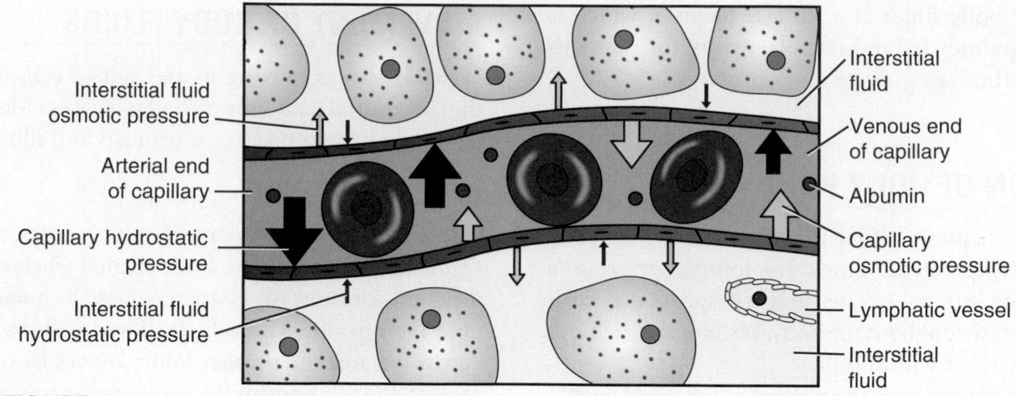

FIGURE 39-2 Filtration pressure changes in a capillary bed. (From Copstead LE, Banasik J: *Pathophysiology*, ed. 5, St. Louis, 2013, Saunders.)

Fluids with a higher osmolarity than body fluids are considered hypertonic. A **hypertonic solution** pulls water from the cell to the extracellular fluid compartment, causing cellular shrinkage. Solutions with a lower osmolarity than body fluids are considered **hypotonic solutions**. Excess water moves into the cells, producing cellular swelling.

Osmotic pressure in the intravascular space is controlled by the concentration of plasma proteins, specifically **albumin**. This is known as colloid osmotic pressure, or **oncotic pressure**. Because these plasma proteins are too large to pass through the capillary membrane, they hold the fluid in the intravascular space.

Filtration

Filtration is the process by which fluid and solutes move together from an area of higher pressure to one of lower pressure. **Hydrostatic pressure** is the force of the fluid pressing against the blood vessel; it is controlled by the force of myocardial contraction, rate of contraction, and blood flow. The force, or pressure, is different on the arterial and venous sides of the capillary bed (Figure 39-2). Fluid balance is influenced by the opposing forces of hydrostatic and oncotic pressure. Filtration across a selectively permeable membrane occurs when the hydrostatic pressure is greater than the oncotic pressure. This allows oxygen and nutrients to move from the arterial capillary bed into the cells. As oncotic pressure rises on the venous side, fluid and waste products are pulled back into the intravascular space.

REGULATION OF BODY FLUIDS

Maintaining adequate fluid volume requires a balance between fluid intake and output. Most of the water is brought into the body through intake of fluids or food. A small amount of water is generated through various metabolic processes, including the breakdown of carbohydrates. Fluid volume and composition are regulated by several body systems, hormones, and other homeostatic mechanisms.

TABLE 39-1 Average Daily Fluid Intake and Output

INTAKE (mL)		OUTPUT (mL)	
Fluids	1600	Urine	1500
Food	700	Feces	200
Metabolism	200	Skin, including perspiration	500
		Lungs	300
Total intake	2500	Total output	2500

Water is lost from the body primarily through the kidneys and excreted as urine. Water loss also occurs through insensible loss, which is moisture lost through respiration and perspiration; a very small amount is lost through feces (Table 39-1).

Homeostasis, the maintenance of fluid balance, is controlled by several physiologic mechanisms, including the renin-angiotensin system (Figure 39-3), the secretion of antidiuretic hormone (Figure 39-4), and the thirst mechanism (Figure 39-5). The **renin-angiotensin system** regulates blood pressure and fluid balance through vasoconstriction and excretion or reabsorption of sodium. **Antidiuretic hormone** (ADH), which is secreted by the pituitary gland, maintains serum osmolality by controlling the amount of water excreted in the urine. Homeostasis is monitored by the kidneys through changes in blood pressure.

A decrease in fluid volume (**hypovolemia**) and a corresponding decrease in blood pressure stimulate the release of the enzyme renin by the kidneys. Renin converts angiotensinogen into angiotensin I. Angiotensin-converting enzyme (ACE), found in the lungs and kidneys, then changes angiotensin I to angiotensin II. Angiotensin II is a hormone that causes several things to occur:

- **Vasoconstriction** (narrowing of blood vessels) throughout the body increases arterial blood pressure.

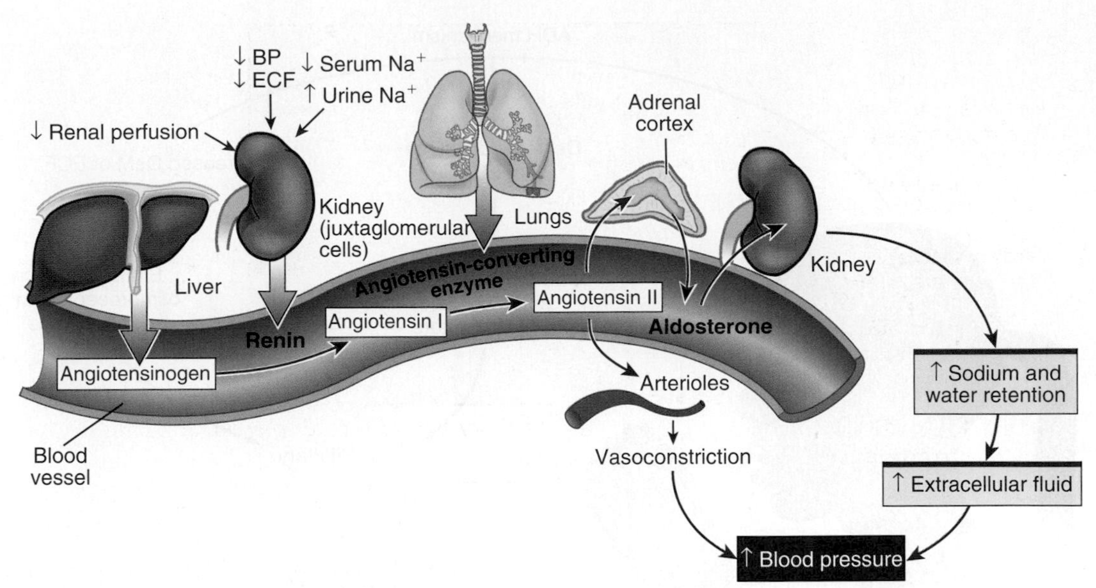

FIGURE 39-3 The renin-angiotensin-aldosterone mechanism. (From Lewis SL, Dirksen SR, Heitkemper MM, et al: *Medical-surgical nursing: Assessment and management of clinical problems,* ed. 9, St. Louis, 2014, Mosby.)

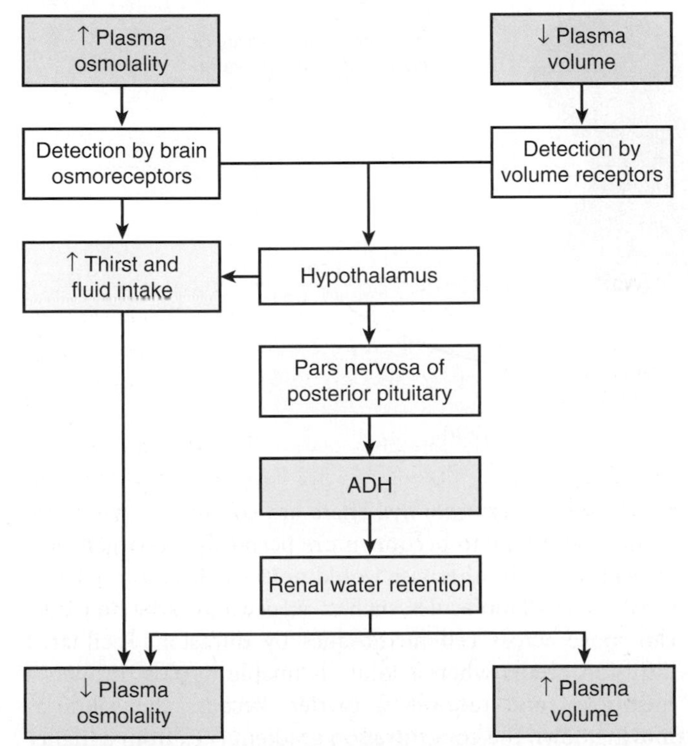

FIGURE 39-4 Action of antidiuretic hormone (ADH). (From McCance KL, Huether SE: *Pathophysiology,* ed. 7, St. Louis, 2014, Mosby.)

- Water from the nephron is reabsorbed back into the intravascular space due to changes in hydrostatic pressure in the nephron.
- Stimulation of the adrenal cortex releases the hormone **aldosterone**. Aldosterone acts on the distal convoluted tubule of the kidney to increase the amount of water and sodium reabsorbed back into the bloodstream.
- ADH is secreted.
- The thirst mechanism is stimulated.

Osmoreceptors, located in the hypothalamus, monitor the osmolarity of blood plasma. When osmolarity increases (becomes more concentrated, as in dehydration), the osmoreceptors stimulate the posterior pituitary to secrete ADH. ADH works on the collecting ducts of the kidneys to reabsorb more water, and less urine is produced as a result (Figure 39-4). As more water moves back into the bloodstream, the plasma osmolarity decreases and returns to normal, and the pituitary stops releasing ADH through a negative feedback loop.

There is an important distinction between aldosterone and ADH. In response to a decrease in circulating blood volume, aldosterone stimulates the reabsorption of water and sodium, thereby increasing volume but not affecting osmolarity. The release of ADH leads to reabsorption of water only. ADH secretion increases fluid volume and decreases plasma osmolarity.

The osmoreceptors, in response to increased osmolarity, stimulate the cerebral cortex to produce a conscious awareness of thirst. As osmolarity returns to normal levels, the thirst sensation subsides (Figure 39-5).

Atrial natriuretic peptide (ANP) is secreted by cells in the atrium of the heart in response to an increase in blood pressure. When released, ANP causes an increase in the glomerular filtration rate (GFR), which leads to increased excretion of water in urine. It inhibits secretion of renin by blocking the renin-angiotensin system, inhibits secretion of ADH, and inhibits reabsorption of sodium chloride and water into the bloodstream (Saladin, 2012).

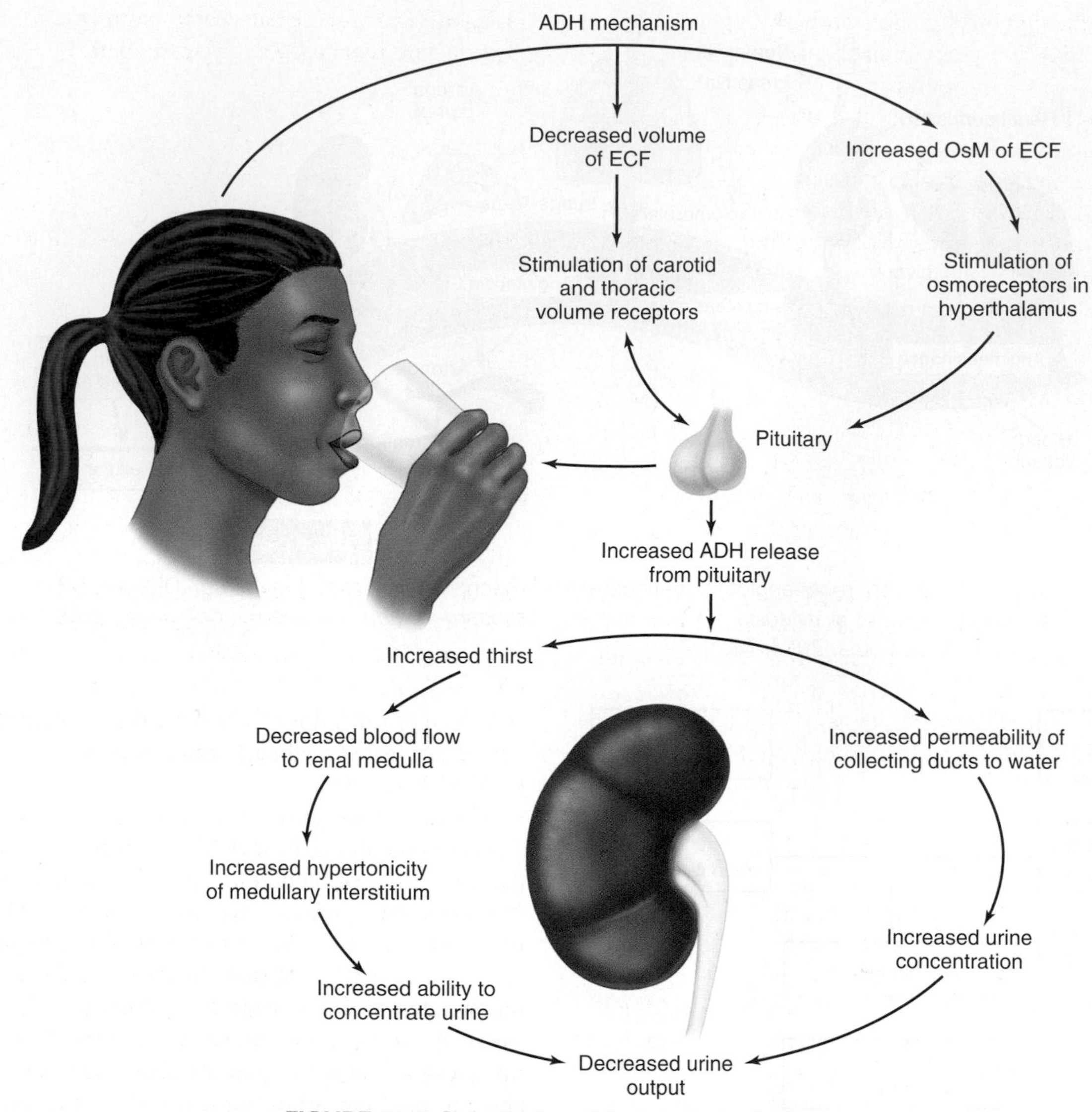

FIGURE 39-5 Dehydration, thirst, and rehydration.

MOVEMENT OF ELECTROLYTES

Electrolytes move in and out of the intracellular and extracellular spaces through three mechanisms: diffusion, filtration, and active transport. **Diffusion** is the movement of solutes across a selectively permeable membrane from areas of higher concentration to areas of lower concentration until equilibrium is reached. The Diffusion animation illustrates this process. The rate of diffusion is influenced by the following factors:

- *Temperature:* The higher the temperature, the faster the particles diffuse.
- *Molecular weight:* Lighter weight molecules (i.e., gases and electrolytes) diffuse more quickly than heavier molecules.
- *Steepness of the concentration gradient:* The more uneven the concentrations on either side of the membrane, the faster solutes move across.
- *Membrane permeability:* There are conditions that cause the membrane to become more permeable to larger molecules, which otherwise would not be able cross.

Many small molecules, such as oxygen and carbon dioxide, can move across cell membranes by diffusion. Facilitated diffusion occurs when a solute is unable to pass through a membrane and requires a carrier. Because the solute is moving down the concentration gradient (i.e., from a higher to a lower concentration), it does not require the use of energy; this is considered a passive process. For example, glucose is unable to move into the cell without insulin as its carrier.

The filtration process described earlier for solvents also applies to the movement of solutes. When water moves as a result of increased pressure, the solutes dissolved in the water also move across the membrane.

The processes of osmosis and diffusion strive to maintain equilibrium of fluids and electrolytes across a membrane.

However, for the body to function properly, higher concentrations of specific substances must be inside or outside the cell. **Active transport** is the transport of a solute from areas of lower to higher concentration; it is the opposite of diffusion. The process is considered active because it requires energy. For example, the exchange of sodium and potassium across the cell membrane is facilitated by the sodium-potassium pump, which is depicted in the Sodium Potassium Pump animation.

REGULATION OF ELECTROLYTES

The major cations are sodium (Na^+), magnesium (Mg^+), potassium (K^+), calcium (Ca^{2+}), and hydrogen (H^+). The major anions are chloride (Cl^-), bicarbonate (HCO_3^-), and phosphate (PO_4^{3-}). Hydrogen and bicarbonate are covered more in depth in the discussion of acid-base balance.

The cellular concentration of these electrolytes is different from their concentration in the extracellular fluid. Potassium and phosphate are found primarily inside the cell, and sodium and chloride are found in highest concentrations in intravascular fluid (i.e., blood plasma). Table 39-2 summarizes the normal serum values, functions, sources, and regulation of these electrolytes.

ACID-BASE BALANCE

For normal cellular functioning to occur, the pH of body fluids must remain balanced. Any disruption of normal acid-base balance can adversely affect cellular functions and metabolic processes. The pH is a measure of the level of acids and bases in a solution and is determined by the concentration of hydrogen ions in the solution. On the pH scale of 0 to 14, 7 is neutral. A pH less than 7 is acidic, and a pH greater than 7 is basic.

An **acid** is a chemical that can release hydrogen ions in solution. Sources of hydrogen include the by-products of the metabolic process, such as ketone bodies, phosphoric acid, carbonic acid, and lactic acid. There is an inverse relationship between pH and the hydrogen ion. The greater the number of hydrogen ions, the lower the pH value. The lower the pH number, the stronger the acid.

Bases are substances that can accept hydrogen ions. Most bases are chemicals that break down into hydroxide ions (OH^-). Hydroxide ions can combine with hydrogen ions to form water, thereby neutralizing the acidic solution. Bicarbonate is a weak base that is found primarily in the plasma; it plays a crucial role in acid-base balance.

Optimal metabolic function can occur only in a constant balance between acids and bases. Blood and body tissues require a pH between 7.35 and 7.45, which is slightly alkaline. There is a complex system in place to maintain normal acid-base balance consisting of three components: chemical buffering systems, which are the primary mechanisms for maintaining acid-base balance; respiratory control of carbon dioxide; and renal control of bicarbonate.

Buffering Systems

A buffering system consists of a weak acid and weak base. It is designed to adjust to small changes in pH. The carbonic acid–bicarbonate system is the primary buffering system in extracellular fluid and is based on the following chemical reaction:

$$CO_2 \text{ (carbon dioxide)} + H_2O \text{ (water)} \rightleftharpoons H_2CO_3 \text{ (carbonic acid)} \rightleftharpoons HCO_3^- \text{ (bicarbonate)} + H^+ \text{ (hydrogen)}$$

This is a reversible chemical reaction. When the reaction moves to the right, carbonic acid breaks down into bicarbonate and hydrogen ions, lowering the pH. When the reaction moves to the left, bicarbonate binds with hydrogen ions and ultimately forms carbon dioxide and water. This buffering system works well because the lungs control the level of hydrogen ions by removing carbon dioxide while the kidneys excrete or reabsorb bicarbonate ions. The normal ratio of bicarbonate to carbonic acid is 20:1 (Figure 39-6). As long as this ratio remains stable, the pH is within a normal range. Any change to this ratio leads to increases or decreases in plasma pH.

The phosphate buffering system is the primary buffering system in the cell. This buffering system is used to a greater degree in the renal tubules than in the cells. It converts alkaline sodium phosphate ($NaHPO_4$) to an acid solution phosphate ($Na_2H_2PO_4$) with the addition of a hydrogen ion.

Potassium and hydrogen ions can be interchanged inside the cell as needed. When there are excess hydrogen ions in the extravascular space, potassium moves out of the cell as the hydrogen ions move into the cell. As a result, acid-base imbalances can affect serum potassium levels, and potassium imbalances can influence acid-base balance.

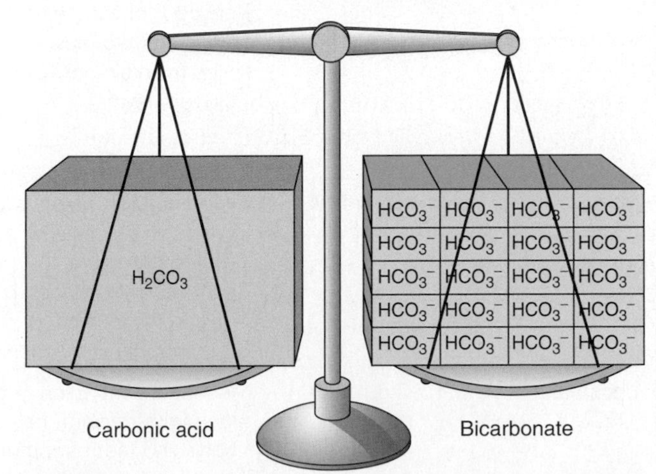

FIGURE 39-6 The bicarbonate–carbonic acid ratio. (From Ignatavicius DD, Workman ML: *Medical-surgical nursing: Patient-centered collaborative care,* ed. 7, St. Louis, 2013, Saunders.)

TABLE 39-2 Electrolyte Function and Homeostasis

ELECTROLYTE	NORMAL LEVELS	FUNCTION	HOMEOSTASIS	SOURCES
Sodium (Na^+)	135-145 mEq/L	Principal ion responsible for resting membrane potential of cells Essential in depolarization needed for nerve and muscle function Principal cation of the ECF; accounts for 90% to 95% of osmolarity Na-K pump important mechanism for producing body heat; essential element for acid-base buffering	Moves out of cell by Na-K pump Regulated by secretion of aldosterone and ANP	Breads, cereals, chips, cheese, processed meats such as lunch meats, hot dogs, bacon, ham Commercially canned foods Table salt
Potassium (K^+)	3.5-5 mEq/L	Along with sodium, produces resting membrane potentials and action potentials of nerve and muscle cells Principal cation of the ICF and responsible for intracellular osmolarity Essential component of Na-K pump and involved in protein synthesis	Moves into the cell by Na-K pump Serum levels regulated by the kidneys through reabsorption or excretion	Fish, excluding shellfish; whole grains, nuts, broccoli, cabbage, carrots celery, cucumbers, potatoes with skins, spinach, tomatoes, apricots, bananas, cantaloupe, nectarines, oranges, tangerines
Calcium (Ca^{2+})	8.5-10.5 mg/dL	Along with phosphate, the primary component of bones and teeth; up to 99% of calcium is found in teeth and bones Role in blood clotting, nerve impulse transmission, cardiac conduction, and muscle contraction	As serum calcium levels drop, parathyroid hormone and calcitriol pull calcium from the bone to maintain normal levels Calcitonin moves excess calcium into the bone	Cheese, ice cream, milk, yogurt, rhubarb, spinach, tofu
Magnesium (Mg^{2+})	1.3-2.1 mEq/L	Found primarily inside cells Key role in production and use of ATP, helps regulate intracellular metabolism by activation of enzymes, part of Na-K pump Required for synthesis of nucleic acids and proteins Helps maintain normal serum calcium levels	Normal levels maintained by increased reabsorption or excretion by the kidneys Additional amount is absorbed through the intestine in the presence of vitamin D and parathyroid hormone	Cashews, halibut, Swiss chard and other green leafy vegetables, tofu, wheat germ, dried fruit
Chloride (Cl^-)	95-105 mEq/L	Most abundant anion in the ECF Key role in maintaining serum osmolarity Required for formation of stomach (hydrochloric) acid Buffering role in acid-base balance	Homeostasis maintained in similar way as sodium; where sodium goes, chloride also goes	Seaweed, rye, tomatoes, lettuce, celery, and olives Table salt, salt substitutes
Phosphate (PO_4^{3-})	1.7-2.6 mEq/L	Most abundant anion in the ICF Along with calcium, helps maintain bone and teeth structure Role in cellular metabolism and ATP production Essential for carbohydrate metabolism	Phosphate has inverse relationship with calcium; as serum calcium levels increase, phosphate levels fall Parathyroid hormone increases excretion by the kidneys	Milk, meat, nuts, legumes, and grains

ANP, Atrial natriuretic peptide; *ATP*, adenosine triphosphate; *ECF*, extracellular fluid; *ICF*, intracellular fluid; *Na-K pump*, Na^+/K^+-ATPase enzyme that pumps sodium out of and potassium into cells.

Several plasma proteins and the hemoglobin in red blood cells have the ability to bind or release hydrogen ions. This helps maintain balance in the intracellular fluid and blood plasma.

Respiratory Regulation

The lungs control the amount of carbonic acid available by retaining or exhaling carbon dioxide. When the pH falls below normal, the lungs exhale more carbon dioxide by increasing the rate and depth of respirations. When the pH is too alkaline (>7.45), respirations slow and become shallower in an effort to conserve carbon dioxide. This compensation occurs very quickly, allowing the return to normal levels.

Renal Regulation

The kidneys neutralize more acid or base than the chemical buffers or the lungs. They do so by excreting or retaining hydrogen ions and excreting or forming bicarbonate ions. It is the only system that removes excess hydrogen ions from the body. When the body is in an acidotic state (<7.35), the kidneys excrete more hydrogen ions and retain bicarbonate. When the pH is abnormally high (i.e., alkalotic, >7.45), the kidneys retain hydrogen ions and excrete bicarbonate ions. Although effective, this mechanism is rather slow. It can take up to 3 days for normal pH levels to be achieved by the renal mechanism.

BLOOD GROUPS

Human blood contains antigens, which are proteins located on the surfaces of red blood cells. Compatibility between the blood donor and recipient antigens is essential in blood transfusion. Many antigens have been identified on human blood cells, but the two types most likely to cause a transfusion reaction are the ABO and Rh groups of antigens.

The ABO system was discovered in 1901 and is still considered the most important antigen group for transfusions. There are four combinations of antigens or blood types, which are based on genes. If a person produces the A antigen, the blood type is classified as A; if a person produces the B antigen, the blood type is classified as B. If the person produces both A and B, the blood type is AB. Type O blood means no antigens are present. Table 39-3 lists the frequency of occurrence of each type.

Individuals with type O blood are classified as universal donors because their blood cells contain no antigens. People with AB blood type are considered universal recipients because their blood cells contain both A and B antigens, and they can receive type A, B, or O blood.

The Rhesus (Rh) factor was discovered in 1940 and is the second most important antigen to test for before blood transfusions. The Rh antigens are responsible for many of the transfusion reactions that occur, especially in newborns.

TABLE 39-3 Blood Types

BLOOD TYPE: ABO, RH	ANTIGENS PRESENT	% OF POPULATION
O+	Rh	35
O–	none	7
A+	A, Rh	35
A–	A	7
B+	B, Rh	8
B–	B	2
AB+	A, B, Rh	4
AB–	A, B	2

From Pagana KD, Pagana TJ: *Mosby's manual of diagnostic and laboratory tests,* ed. 5, St. Louis, 2014, Mosby.

Approximately 85% of white and 95% of African Americans are Rh positive (Rh^+), which means they have the Rh factor on the surface of their red blood cells. Those who do not have the Rh factor are considered Rh negative (Rh^-). When an Rh^- person is exposed to Rh^+ blood for the first time, Rh antibodies develop. This can occur when a pregnant woman who is Rh^- is carrying a fetus who is Rh^+ or an Rh^- person receives Rh^+ blood. After the person has been exposed, subsequent contact with Rh^+ blood can lead to life-threatening destruction of red blood cells, known as **hemolytic reactions.**

Blood Testing

There is a continuing need for donated blood. To be eligible to donate blood, a person must be at least 17 years of age, weigh at least 110 pounds, and have not donated blood within the past 8 weeks. The blood is then tested for ABO and Rh type and antibodies to several viruses, including hepatitis B and C, human immunodeficiency virus (HIV), syphilis, human T-cell lymphotropic virus (HTLV), and in some cases, cytomegalovirus (CMV).

Before administration, the patient's blood is typed for ABO antigens and Rh factor. A crossmatch or mixing of the patient's and donor's blood is performed to detect any incompatibilities. This is carried out in the laboratory before the unit of blood or blood product is released to the nurse.

Blood Components

Whole blood is composed of red blood cells, white blood cells, platelets, and plasma, which contains plasma proteins, antibodies, and electrolytes. Because of the ability to separate the various components, whole blood is used only in situations when the blood components and blood volume are needed, such as massive hemorrhage. Table 39-4 describes the various blood components and their uses.

TABLE 39-4 Blood Components

BLOOD COMPONENT	NURSING CONSIDERATIONS
Whole blood	*Use:* Only used in situations with a major loss of blood (>25% of circulating volume). Available in bags of 500 mL. Must be infused within 4 hr after leaving the laboratory. *Concerns:* Should not be used in patients with a history of congestive heart failure or renal impairment. Cautious use in the elderly, because it can lead to fluid overload. Requires ABO and Rh matching before administering. Patient is monitored for transfusion reactions.
Packed red blood cells (PRBCs)	*Use:* Plasma removal leaves only the red blood cells. Replaces the oxygen-carrying blood cells in patients with anemia or hemorrhage. Can correct blood losses during and after surgery. Must be infused within 4 hr after leaving the laboratory. *Concerns:* Requires ABO and Rh matching before administering. Patient is monitored for transfusion reactions.
Fresh frozen plasma (FFP)	*Use:* FFP contains plasma proteins, fibrinogen, clotting factors, sugar, vitamins, minerals, hormones, and antibodies. Used to treat hemorrhage, as a volume expander, and to correct clotting disorders. Must be infused within 6 hr after leaving the laboratory. *Concerns:* Rh matching before administration. Need to monitor for allergic reactions.
Cryoprecipitate	*Use:* Also known as factor VIII. Used to treat various bleeding disorders *Concerns:* Need to monitor for allergic reactions.
Albumin	*Use:* Available in 5% and 25% concentrations. Contains globulins and other plasma proteins. Used to treat acute renal failure, burns, or trauma. Increases plasma oncotic pressure, causing excess fluid to move from the interstitial space and into the vascular system. *Concerns:* Fluid shifts can lead to fluid overload and congestive heart failure or pulmonary edema. Use cautiously in the elderly and patients with impaired cardiac and/or renal function.
Platelets	*Use:* Indicated for patients with thrombocytopenia or platelet dysfunction and in patients who have had multiple transfusions of PRBCs. Should be infused as quickly as possible, usually within 10 min after leaving the laboratory. *Concerns:* Should be Rh compatible. Monitor patients for allergic reactions.
Autologous blood	*Use:* Also known as autotransfusion, refers to using the patient's own blood or blood components. Blood can be donated before surgery or collected in special containers and infused during and after surgery. *Concerns:* Patients with history of cancer or current infections are not candidates for autotransfusion.

Adapted from Weinstein SM, Hagle, ME: *Plumer's principles & practice of infusion therapy*, ed. 9, Philadelphia, 2014, Lippincott Williams & Wilkins.

ALTERED STRUCTURE AND FUNCTION OF FLUIDS AND ELECTROLYTES LO 39.2

Adequate fluid balance is essential for maintenance of homeostasis. Physical and environmental alterations can affect the stability of fluids, electrolytes and acid-base balance and disrupt essential physiologic processes. The Fluid and Electrolyte Imbalances animation discusses some common imbalances.

FLUID IMBALANCES

Excessive fluid loss or retention can interfere with metabolism and transport of oxygen, nutrients, and waste products (Table 39-5). Excessive fluid loss can lead to decreased circulating volume, which directly affects cardiac output. Fluid volume excess leads to an increase in circulating fluid, thereby increasing the workload of the heart.

Fluid Volume Deficit

Fluid volume deficit (FVD) occurs with excessive loss or inadequate intake of fluid. Two types of fluid deficits can occur: isotonic and hypertonic.

Isotonic fluid deficit, or hypovolemia, occurs when water and sodium are lost at the same rate. In this situation, circulating volume decreases, but serum osmolarity remains unchanged. The other type of fluid volume deficit occurs when water is lost in excess of sodium. Hypertonic fluid volume deficit, or **dehydration**, can be serious if not recognized and treated. As fluid loss continues, the circulating fluid volume decreases, and serum osmolarity increases. When monitoring fluid loss, it is important to remember that even small losses can lead to undesirable consequences. Severity of dehydration is classified by percentage of total body weight:

- A 2% loss is mild dehydration.
- A 5% loss is moderate dehydration.
- An 8% loss is severe dehydration.
- A 15% loss is life-threatening, usually fatal.

TABLE 39-5 Fluid Imbalances

DISORDER	UNDERLYING CAUSES	CLINICAL MANIFESTATIONS	LABORATORY FINDINGS	INTERVENTIONS
Isotonic fluid volume deficit (hypovolemia)	Hemorrhage, burns, vomiting, diarrhea, Addison disease, fever, excessive perspiration	Confusion, thirst, dry mucous membranes, orthostatic hypotension, tachycardia, weak and thready pulse, decreased skin turgor, prolonged capillary refill, and decreased urinary output	Urine specific gravity >1.030 Increased hematocrit Adult males >52 Adult females >48 BUN >20	Administer fluids Monitor vital signs Monitor intake and output Monitor laboratory results, especially hematocrit, BUN, and urine specific gravity
Hypertonic fluid volume deficit (dehydration)	Diabetes insipidus, diabetic ketoacidosis; administration of osmotic diuretics, hypertonic enteral tube feedings, or hypertonic intravenous fluids; prolonged vomiting and diarrhea	Similar to hypovolemia, dry sticky mucous membranes, flushed dry skin, increased body temperature, irritability, convulsions, and coma	Urine specific gravity >1.030 Increased hematocrit Adult males >52 Adult females >48 BUN >20 Serum sodium >145	Administer fluids Monitor vital signs Monitor intake and output Assess for neurologic changes Monitor laboratory results, especially hematocrit, BUN, and urine specific gravity
Isotonic fluid volume excess	Congestive heart failure, renal failure, and cirrhosis	Weight gain, edema in dependent areas, bounding peripheral pulses, hypertension, JVD, dyspnea, cough, abnormal lung sounds	Urine specific gravity <1.005 Decreased hematocrit Adult males <42 Adult females <37 BUN <7	Monitor vital signs Monitor intake and output Assess for edema and JVD Auscultate lung fields Monitor laboratory results, especially hematocrit, BUN, and urine specific gravity
Hypotonic fluid volume excess	Excessive water intake, prolonged use of hypotonic IV solutions, SIADH	Symptoms similar to isotonic fluid volume excess plus neurologic changes that indicate cerebral edema, including decreased level of consciousness, coma, and convulsions	Urine specific gravity <1.005 Decreased hematocrit Adult males <42 Adult females <37 BUN <7 Serum sodium <135	Monitor vital signs Monitor intake and output Assess for neurologic changes Monitor laboratory results, especially hematocrit, BUN, and urine specific gravity

BUN, Blood urea nitrogen; *JVD,* jugular vein distention; *SIADH,* syndrome of inappropriate antidiuretic hormone secretion.

Fluid Volume Excess

Fluid volume excess (FVE) occurs when fluid intake exceeds output. Fluid volume excess is isotonic or hypotonic, depending on corresponding changes in serum osmolarity. Severity of the fluid volume excess is assessed by the corresponding increase in total body weight:

- A 2% gain is mild excess.
- A 5% gain is moderate excess.
- An 8% gain is severe excess.

Edema is the abnormal accumulation of fluid in the interstitial spaces, typically in the face, fingers, abdomen, ankles, and feet. Edema, also known as third spacing, develops when fluid moves into a tissue at a faster rate than it can be reabsorbed into the intravascular space. There are four primary causes of edema formation: increase in hydrostatic pressure due to fluid overload, decreased production of circulating plasma proteins, obstruction of lymphatic drainage, and increased capillary permeability due to tissue damage (Figure 39-7). When fluid is trapped in the interstitial spaces, it is not available for use inside the cell or in the intravascular space.

In isotonic fluid volume excess, there is an equal increase in fluid and sodium retention. The result is an increase in circulating blood volume while serum osmolarity remains

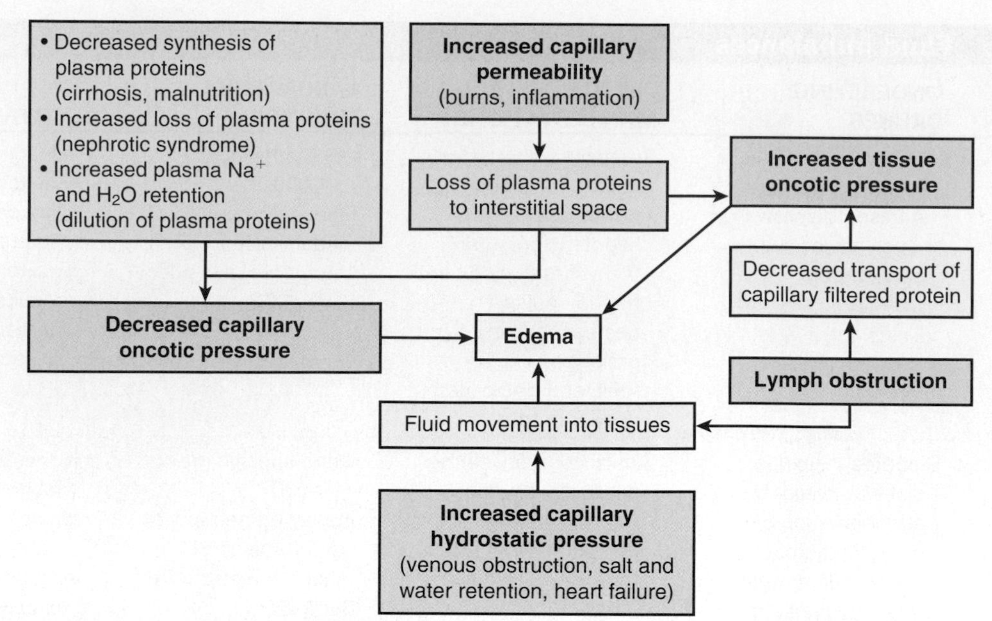

FIGURE 39-7 Mechanisms of edema formation. (From McCance KL, Huether SE: *Pathophysiology*, ed. 7, St. Louis, 2015, Mosby.)

unchanged. Hypotonic fluid volume excess occurs when water is ingested at a rate greater than sodium. Although there is an increase in circulating blood volume, the serum osmolarity decreases as a result of hemodilution. This decrease in serum osmolarity leads to fluid moving into the cells, causing cellular swelling. Swelling leads to pulmonary congestion and cerebral edema. There are situations in which inappropriate secretion of ADH (i.e., syndrome of inappropriate antidiuretic hormone secretion [SIADH]) occurs. Remember that ADH leads to increased retention of fluid and not necessarily sodium. As a result, serum osmolarity decreases. There are several causes of SIADH, including head injury, brain tumors, and postoperative effects of surgery and anesthesia.

Simultaneous Fluid Volume Excess and Deficit

There are situations in which fluid volume excess and fluid volume deficit can occur simultaneously. When the serum albumin level is very low, the hydrostatic pressure is greater than the oncotic pressure, and fluid seeps into the interstitial spaces. As a result, many of the signs of fluid volume excess are present, such as weight gain, pulmonary congestion, and edema. Because this fluid has been lost from the intravascular space, signs of fluid volume deficit are also present, such as hypotension, weak and thready pulse, and tachycardia. In this situation, treatment focuses on replacing the plasma proteins and allowing the fluids to shift back to the intravascular space. Fluid replacement, whether administered orally or intravenously, should begin after this fluid shift has occurred.

ELECTROLYTE IMBALANCES

Although the body has many complex mechanisms to maintain homeostasis, in the presence of disease or trauma, it is not uncommon to have electrolyte imbalances. Understanding the cause and common symptoms of these imbalances helps the nurse identify the patients at risk and recognize electrolyte imbalance in the early stage. Table 39-6 describes the common electrolyte imbalances, causes, symptoms, and interventions.

Hyponatremia and Hypernatremia

Hyponatremia occurs when the sodium level is decreased in relation to body water. It is defined as a serum level less than 135 mEq/L. As a result of the decreased concentration in the extracellular fluid, water moves into the cell, causing cellular swelling.

There are two types of hyponatremia: hypovolemic hyponatremia and hypervolemic hyponatremia. Hypovolemic hyponatremia occurs when there is loss of water and sodium, but the sodium loss is greater. Hypervolemic hyponatremia is also known as dilutional hyponatremia. In this situation, water intake exceeds sodium intake, which leads to an overall decrease in serum sodium levels.

Hypernatremia occurs when the serum sodium level is greater than 145 mEq/L. This imbalance results from a greater loss of water compared with sodium or a greater intake of sodium. As sodium levels increase, water moves from the cells into the intravascular space, which can lead to cellular dehydration. Movement of the fluid into the vascular space can lead to fluid overload, or hypervolemia. Hypernatremia can occur rather quickly or have a slower onset (Box 39-1).

Hypokalemia and Hyperkalemia

Because of the critical role that potassium plays in cellular metabolism, even slight imbalances can affect cardiac and neuromuscular functions. Because the body is unable to conserve potassium, serum levels are easily influenced by

TABLE 39-6 **Electrolyte Imbalances**

DISORDER	UNDERLYING CAUSES	CLINICAL MANIFESTATIONS	INTERVENTIONS
Sodium			
Hyponatremia Na^+ <135 mEq/L	Hypovolemic hyponatremia Diuretics GI fluid loss (vomiting, diarrhea) Profuse diaphoresis Hypervolemic hyponatremia Water intoxication Prolonged use of hypotonic IV solutions SIADH	Lethargy, confusion, weakness Muscle cramping Seizures Anorexia, nausea, vomiting Serum osmolarity <280 mOsm/kg	Monitor vital signs. Monitor intake and output. Monitor laboratory results, especially serum sodium and serum osmolality. Encourage foods high in sodium. Restrict water intake. Administer hypertonic IV saline solutions as ordered.
Hypernatremia Na^+ >145 mEq/L	Excess sodium due to • Excessive sodium intake • Hypertonic IV solutions • Hypertonic enteral feedings without adequate water Excessive loss of water due to • Diarrhea • Inadequate intake of water • Insensible loss due to fever	Thirst, dry sticky mucous membranes, weakness, elevated temperature Severe hypernatremia causing confusion and irritability, decreased levels of consciousness, hallucinations, and convulsions Serum osmolarity >300 mOsm/kg	Monitor vital signs. Monitor level of consciousness. Monitor intake and output. Monitor laboratory results, especially serum sodium and serum osmolarity. Limit salt intake and foods high in sodium. Increase water intake. Administer hypotonic IV solutions as ordered.
Potassium			
Hypokalemia K^+ <3.5 mEq/L	Loss of potassium due to • Vomiting, gastric suction, diarrhea • Laxative abuse, frequent enemas • Use of potassium-wasting diuretics • Inadequate intake seen in anorexia, alcoholism, debilitated patients • Hyperaldosteronism	Weak, irregular pulse Fatigue, lethargy Anorexia, nausea, vomiting Muscle weakness and cramping Decreased peristalsis, hypoactive bowel sounds Paresthesia Cardiac dysrhythmias Increased risk of digitalis toxicity	Monitor vital signs, especially heart rate and rhythm. Monitor cardiac rhythm with ECG. Monitor laboratory results for serum potassium levels. Assess for signs of digitalis toxicity. Encourage foods high in potassium. Administer potassium supplements as ordered; IV potassium is diluted properly and administered slowly, usually by infusion. ***Never*** *administer potassium as an IV bolus or IV push.*
Hyperkalemia K^+ >5.0 mEq/L	Renal failure Massive trauma, crushing injuries, burns Hemolysis IV potassium Potassium-sparing diuretics Acidosis, especially diabetic ketoacidosis	Anxiety, irritability, confusion Dysrhythmias, including bradycardia and heart block Muscle weakness, flaccid paralysis Paresthesia Abdominal cramping	Monitor vital signs, especially heart rate and rhythm. Monitor cardiac rhythm with ECG. Monitor laboratory results for serum potassium levels. Limit potassium-rich foods. Administer cation-exchange resins (Kayexalate) as ordered Administer glucose and insulin as ordered (potassium moves back into cell)

ECG, Electrocardiogram; *GI,* gastrointestinal; *IV,* intravenous; *SIADH,* syndrome of inappropriate antidiuretic hormone secretion.

Continued

TABLE 39-6 Electrolyte Imbalances—cont'd

DISORDER	UNDERLYING CAUSES	CLINICAL MANIFESTATIONS	INTERVENTIONS
Calcium			
Hypocalcemia Ca^{2+} <8.5 mg/dL	Hypoparathyroidism Pancreatitis Vitamin D deficiency Inadequate intake of calcium-rich foods Hyperphosphatemia Chronic alcoholism	Confusion, anxiety Numbness and tingling of extremities Muscle cramps that progress to tetany and convulsions Hyperactive reflexes Cardiac dysrhythmias Positive Chvostek and Trousseau signs	Monitor heart rate and rhythm. Monitor cardiac rhythm with ECG. Institute fall and seizure precautions. Administer oral and/or IV calcium supplements as ordered. Encourage calcium-rich foods.
Hypercalcemia Ca^{2+} >10.5 mg/dL	Prolonged bed rest Hyperparathyroidism Bone malignancy Paget disease Osteoporosis	Lethargy, stupor, coma Decreased muscle strength and tone Anorexia, nausea, and vomiting Constipation Pathologic fractures Dysrhythmias Renal calculi	Monitor heart rate and rhythm. Monitor cardiac rhythm with ECG. Encourage increased fluid intake. Increase patient activity, including active ROM.
Magnesium			
Hypomagnesemia Mg^{2+} <1.3 mEq/L	Decreased intake TPN without magnesium Decreased absorption Nasogastric suction Draining fistulas Prolonged diarrhea Laxative abuse Malabsorption syndrome Ulcerative colitis Crohn's disease Increased renal excretion Diuresis Loop and thiazide diuretics	Irritable nerves and muscles Hyperactive deep tendon reflexes Seizures Dysrhythmias, especially tachyarrhythmias ECG changes Altered level of consciousness Mood swings Delusions, hallucinations Dysphagia, nausea, and vomiting	Assess vital signs, especially heart rate and rhythm. Monitor cardiac rhythm with ECG. Assess mental status, changes in level of consciousness. Monitor laboratory results, including potassium and calcium levels. Assess swallowing before administering medications, food, or fluid. Institute seizure precautions. Administer oral or IV supplements as ordered.
Hypermagnesemia Mg^{2+} >2.1 mEq/L	Excessive intake of magnesium-containing antacids or cathartics TPN with too much magnesium Prolonged use of intravenous magnesium sulfate Renal failure Severe dehydration Adrenal insufficiency Leukemia	Warm, flushed appearance Nausea, vomiting Drowsiness, lethargy Decreased muscle strength Generalized weakness Decreased deep tendon reflexes Hypotension Dysrhythmias, especially bradycardia and heart block Slow, shallow respirations; respiratory arrest	Assess vital signs, especially heart rate and rhythm. Monitor cardiac rhythm with ECG. Assess mental status, changes in level of consciousness. Assess neuromuscular strength and activity. Encourage increased oral intake, increased IV fluids. Administer loop diuretics as ordered. Provide respiratory support (supplemental oxygen or mechanical ventilation) as needed.

TABLE 39-6 Electrolyte Imbalances—cont'd

DISORDER	UNDERLYING CAUSES	CLINICAL MANIFESTATIONS	INTERVENTIONS
Phosphate			
Hypophosphatemia PO_4^{3-} <1.7 mEq/L	Abnormal shift into the cell Hyperventilation Respiratory alkalosis Hyperglycemia Absorption from the GI tract Phosphorus-binding antacids Starvation Malabsorption syndrome Inadequate vitamin D Chronic diarrhea, laxative abuse Increased excretion by kidneys Thiazides and loop diuretics Diabetic ketoacidosis Hyperparathyroidism Hypocalcemia	Weak pulse Shallow respirations Hypotension Decreased cardiac output Hemolytic anemia Bleeding, increased bruising Muscle weakness Decreased deep tendon reflexes Tremors Bone pain Anorexia Increased risk of infection	Assess vital signs, especially respirations, pulse oximetry, and blood pressure. Assess muscle strength and neuromuscular function. Assess for signs of congestive heart failure. Encourage phosphate-rich foods. Instruct patient to avoid phosphorus-binding antacids. Administer oral and IV phosphorus as ordered. Administer pain medications as ordered. Monitor for signs of infection.
Hyperphosphatemia PO_4^{3-} >2.6 mEq/L	Impaired renal function Hypoparathyroidism Acid-base imbalances Cellular injury	Signs of hypocalcemia Tetany Hyperreflexia Muscle spasms, weakness Tachycardia Nausea Diarrhea, cramping	Monitor vital signs. Monitor serum phosphorus and calcium levels. Monitor BUN, creatinine. Assess signs of hypocalcemia. Monitor intake and output. Teach patient to avoid phosphorus-rich foods.

BUN, Blood urea nitrogen; *ECG,* electrocardiogram; *GI,* gastrointestinal; *IV,* intravenous; *ROM,* range of motion; *SIADH,* syndrome of inappropriate antidiuretic hormone secretion; *TPN,* total parenteral nutrition.

BOX 39-1 Onset of Hypernatremia

Rapid Onset
- Severe vomiting
- Hypertonic intravenous fluids
- Excessive sweating

Slow Onset
- Congestive heart failure
- Renal failure
- Increased sodium intake

potassium intake and excretion. These imbalances need to be prevented when possible and identified and treated quickly.

Hypokalemia occurs when the serum potassium level falls below 3.5 mEq/L. Inadequate intake occurs as a result of decreased oral intake or insufficient potassium in intravenous (IV) fluids. The Diversity Considerations box outlines some concerns regarding fluids and electrolytes.

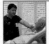

1. On day 2 of his hospital stay, Mr. Abdul begins to complain of increased muscle weakness and cramping. Assessment findings include an irregular apical pulse and hypoactive bowel sounds. Provide a possible explanation for these findings, and identify appropriate nursing action.

DIVERSITY CONSIDERATIONS

Life Span
- Infants are more susceptible to fluid volume deficits or dehydration because of their high percentage of total body water.
- The elderly are more prone to hypokalemia because of increased use of potassium-wasting diuretics.
- Hypokalemia can enhance the effect of digitalis and lead to digitalis toxicity and subsequent cardiac arrest. The elderly are often prescribed both digitalis and potassium-wasting diuretics. They are encouraged to eat foods high in potassium, take prescribed potassium supplements, and learn the signs of hypokalemia.

Gender
- Hormonal fluctuations in females can cause fluid retention.
- Men have a higher total body water percentage than women.

There are primarily four sources of **hyperkalemia** (serum potassium >5.0 mEq/L): excessive intake of potassium, transfusions and medications, impaired renal excretion, and cellular movement. Because potassium levels can be lowered only by renal excretion, homeostasis requires normal renal functioning. In acute and chronic renal failure, the kidneys lose the ability to maintain this homeostatic function. Cells that are damaged due to trauma release intracellular potassium into the extracellular space, raising serum levels.

Hypocalcemia and Hypercalcemia

Hypocalcemia occurs when serum calcium levels fall below 8.5 mg/dL. It occurs as a result of inadequate intake of calcium, lack of absorption, or excessive losses. Decreased serum calcium levels occur when calcium cannot be absorbed from the small intestine. A large portion (40%) of serum calcium is bound to plasma proteins. When the protein stores are decreased, as in malnutrition and cirrhosis, the level of unbound calcium increases, making it available to be excreted by the kidneys. Administration of loop diuretics can lead to increased calcium excretion.

Hypercalcemia occurs when serum calcium levels exceed 10.5 mg/dL. High intake of calcium and increased release of calcium from the bone are the most common reasons for increased serum calcium. An increase in secretion of the parathyroid hormone, as occurs in hyperparathyroidism, leads to increased calcium released from the bones.

Hypomagnesemia and Hypermagnesemia

A decreased serum magnesium level, or hypomagnesemia, is a serum level of less than 1.3 mEq/L. However, most people are not symptomatic until levels fall below 1 mEq/L. Decreased serum levels result from decreased intake, decreased absorption, or increased loss through the kidneys. Hypomagnesemia often occurs in conjunction with hypokalemia and hypocalcemia.

Hypermagnesemia, defined by serum levels greater than 2.1 mEq/L, does not commonly occur. When it does, it is usually due to an excessive intake of magnesium-containing antacids or cathartics. It occurs in patients on total parenteral nutrition (TPN) containing too much magnesium or with the prolonged use of IV magnesium such as magnesium sulfate. Renal failure can lead to decreased excretion of magnesium. Severe dehydration can lead to hemoconcentration of magnesium. Adrenal insufficiency and leukemia also have caused increased serum levels of magnesium.

Hypophosphatemia and Hyperphosphatemia

Hypophosphatemia occurs when serum phosphorus levels fall below 1.7 mEq/L. It normally results from an abnormal shift of phosphate into the cell, decreased absorption of phosphorus from the gastrointestinal tract, or increased excretion of phosphorus by the kidneys. Hyperventilation, which leads to respiratory alkalosis (discussed later), facilitates movement of phosphorus into the cell. Hyperglycemia (increased blood glucose levels) stimulates the pancreas to release insulin, which transports phosphate along with glucose into the cell. Absorption of phosphorus from the gastrointestinal tract can be decreased as a result of phosphorus-binding antacids, starvation, and malabsorption syndrome. Inadequate intake of vitamin D, chronic diarrhea, and laxative abuse can limit absorption. The use of thiazides and loop diuretics increases phosphate loss in the urine. Osmotic diuresis from diabetic ketoacidosis or an increase of parathyroid hormone secretion (as occurs in hyperparathyroidism or hypocalcemia) can lead to increased excretion of phosphate.

Hyperphosphatemia, or serum phosphorus levels greater than 2.6 mEq/L, most often occurs as a result of impaired renal function. As the glomerular filtration rate decreases, the ability of the kidneys to excrete excess phosphate ions diminishes. Increased levels of phosphate ions occur as a result of decreased parathyroid hormone secretion seen in hypoparathyroidism. Acid-base imbalances and cellular injury can cause phosphate ions to shift into the extracellular fluid, increasing serum levels.

ACID-BASE IMBALANCES

For normal cellular functioning to occur, the pH of body fluids must remain in the narrow range between 7.35 and 7.45. Death can occur if the pH falls below 6.9 or rises higher than 7.80. Various chemical buffering systems are designed to maintain normal pH balance. Two compensatory mechanisms, respiratory (carbon dioxide) and renal (metabolic), are designed to help maintain homeostasis.

Four acid-base imbalances can occur: respiratory acidosis and alkalosis and metabolic acidosis and alkalosis (Table 39-7). The animation Acid-Base Imbalances depicts each type.

Respiratory Acidosis

Respiratory acidosis occurs when gas exchange is decreased due to abnormal ventilation, perfusion, or diffusion. This leads to hypercapnia—increased carbon dioxide levels—in the blood. Respiratory acidosis can be acute or chronic. In acute situations, the hydrogen ion concentration is increased, with a pH less than 7.35, and the partial arterial pressure of carbon dioxide ($PaCO_2$) is increased to greater than 45 mm Hg. There is an inverse relationship between the pH and $PaCO_2$. As one increases, the other decreases. Acute respiratory imbalances are not quickly adjusted due to the delay in the renal (metabolic) compensatory mechanism. In chronic respiratory imbalances, such as chronic obstructive pulmonary disease (COPD), the $PaCO_2$ is increased, but the pH is within a normal range. The renal compensation mechanism has time to adjust to the chronic hypercapnia.

Renal compensation of respiratory acidosis focuses on excreting excess metabolic acids and conserving bicarbonate. However, renal compensation is fairly slow, taking 12 to 24 hours to adjust to the abnormal pH levels. As a result of compensation, pH levels move toward the normal range, and bicarbonate levels are abnormally high.

Respiratory Alkalosis

Respiratory alkalosis is a result of hyperventilation and excess exhalation of carbon dioxide. The pH is increased to greater than 7.45, and the $PaCO_2$ is decreased to less than

TABLE 39-7 Acid-Base Imbalances

ACID-BASE IMBALANCE	UNDERLYING CAUSES	CLINICAL MANIFESTATIONS	INTERVENTIONS
Respiratory acidosis	Hypoventilation due to • Chest injury • Asthma attack • Pulmonary edema • Brainstem injury • Medications: anesthetics, opioids, sedatives	Headache Altered level of consciousness, irritability, confusion Dyspnea Tachycardia Muscle twitching Uncompensated ABG results: • pH <7.35 • $PaCO_2$ >45 mm Hg • HCO_3^- normal Partially compensated ABG results: • pH <7.35 • $PaCO_2$ >45 mm Hg • HCO_3^- >26 mEq As compensation continues, the pH increases.	Assess vital signs, especially rate and depth of respirations, pulse oximetry. Assess breath sounds. Assess cardiac rhythm. Administer oxygen as ordered. Monitor ABG results. Have mechanical ventilation available. Encourage deep breathing and coughing. Encourage fluid intake.
Respiratory alkalosis	Pain Hyperventilation Salicylate overdose Nicotine overdose Increased metabolic states	Tachypnea (rapid, shallow breathing) Numbness, tingling of fingers Muscle cramping Palpitations Anxiety, restlessness ECG changes ABG results: • pH >7.45 • $PaCO_2$ <35 mm Hg • HCO_3^- normal Partially compensated ABG results: • pH >7.45 • $PaCO_2$ <35 mm Hg • HCO_3^- <22 mEq As compensation continues, the pH decreases.	Assess vital signs. Encourage patient who is tachypneic to take slow, deep breaths. Have patient breathe into a paper bag. Monitor ABGs. Provide reassurance and emotional support to anxious patient.
Metabolic acidosis	Shock Trauma Cardiac arrest Diabetic ketoacidosis Chronic renal failure Salicylate overdose Sepsis Chronic diarrhea	Kussmaul respirations Hypotension Headache Decreased level of consciousness Weakness Nausea, vomiting, anorexia ABG results: • pH <7.35 • $PaCO_2$ normal • HCO_3^- <22 mEq Partially compensated ABG results: • pH <7.35 • $PaCO_2$ <35 mm Hg • HCO_3^- <22 mEq As compensation continues, the pH increases.	Assess vital signs, especially respiratory rate and rhythm, blood pressure, and pulse oximetry. Monitor cardiac rhythm. Monitor ABGs and serum electrolytes, glucose, and BUN or creatinine. Monitor level of consciousness. Have mechanical ventilation available as needed. Administer sodium bicarbonate as ordered.

ABG, Arterial blood gases; *BUN*, blood urea nitrogen; *ECG*, electrocardiogram.

Continued

TABLE 39-7 Acid-Base Imbalances—cont'd

ACID-BASE IMBALANCE	UNDERLYING CAUSES	CLINICAL MANIFESTATIONS	INTERVENTIONS
Metabolic alkalosis	Vomiting Nasogastric suctioning Overuse of bicarbonate antacids Hypokalemia Loop and thiazide diuretics	Hypotension Mental confusion Muscle twitching, tetany Increased deep tendon reflexes Numbness, tingling of fingers and toes Seizures Anorexia, nausea, vomiting Polyuria ABG results: • pH >7.45 • $PaCO_2$ normal • HCO_3^- >26 mEq Partially compensated ABG results: • pH >7.45 • $PaCO_2$ >45 mm Hg • HCO_3^- >26 mEq As compensation continues, the pH decreases.	Assess vital signs, especially cardiac rate and rhythm, respiration rate and depth, pulse oximetry, blood pressure. Monitor ABGs and serum electrolytes, especially potassium. Assess level of consciousness. Administer oxygen as ordered. Initiate seizure precautions. Treat hypokalemia if appropriate.

ABG, Arterial blood gases; *BUN,* blood urea nitrogen; *ECG,* electrocardiogram.

35 mm Hg. Acute hypoxia leads to an increased respiratory rate by overstimulating the respiratory center of the brain, which leads to hypocapnia (i.e., decreased carbon dioxide levels in the blood). Renal compensation of this imbalance focuses on preserving metabolic acids, thereby decreasing the amount of available bicarbonate. Renal compensation is slow. As compensation occurs, the pH decreases to normal, and the bicarbonate level is below normal levels.

Metabolic Acidosis

Metabolic acidosis, defined as high acid content in the blood, with a pH less than 7.35 and a bicarbonate level less than 22 mEq/L. It occurs when there is a loss of bicarbonate ions or an increase in acids produced as by-products of a metabolic process (i.e., ketones). Lactic acidosis, a result of anaerobic respiration, can quickly lead to a metabolic acidotic state. This occurs in shock, sepsis, or cardiac arrest. Decreased renal function can lead to metabolic acidosis as kidneys lose the ability to secrete hydrogen ions or conserve bicarbonate ions. Loss of intestinal fluids from diarrhea, draining intestinal fistulas, and malabsorption syndrome leads to decreased levels of bicarbonate ions. In metabolic acidosis, the lungs compensate by increasing the rate and depth of respirations in an attempt to remove excess carbon dioxide, thereby lowering the amount of carbonic acid in the blood. This type of deep, rapid breathing is known as *Kussmaul respirations.*

Metabolic Alkalosis

In **metabolic alkalosis**, there is an excess of bicarbonate ions, which raises the pH above 7.45 and produces bicarbonate levels greater than 26 mEq/L. This occurs as a result of excessive intake of bicarbonate-containing medications (i.e., antacids), loss of gastric acids through vomiting or nasogastric suctioning, and frequent blood transfusions (due to the citrate preservative used in the storage of the red blood cells). Loop and thiazide diuretics facilitate increased excretion of hydrogen ions. Hypokalemia can lead to hydrogen ions shifting into the cell in exchange for potassium ions, decreasing circulating blood levels of hydrogen ions. The lungs attempt to compensate by decreasing the rate and depth of respirations. This hypoventilation leads to carbon dioxide retention, increasing carbonic acid levels. Although respiratory compensation can be very effective, it cannot continue indefinitely. It is essential to identify and treat the underlying metabolic disorder.

◆ ASSESSMENT LO 39.3

To provide appropriate nursing care, it is essential for the nurse to understand how trauma, disease, and other disorders lead to fluid, electrolyte, and acid-base imbalances. By conducting a thorough assessment, the nurse identifies patients at risk for these imbalances, recognizes specific imbalances, and develops an individualized plan of care. The nursing assessment includes a thorough health history (Health Assessment Questions box), a focused assessment, and review of diagnostic testing.

HEALTH HISTORY

The health history includes questions designed to highlight recent changes in fluid intake, diet, and other lifestyle habits. It is important to ascertain recent changes in weight (i.e., loss

HEALTH ASSESSMENT QUESTIONS

Fluid and Electrolyte Focus

- What is your normal intake of fluids each day? What type of fluids do you normally drink? Has that changed?
- What do you normally eat in a 24-hour period? (Look for use of processed meats, canned foods, and other high-sodium sources.)
- Do you use salt or salt substitutes?
- How much protein do you typically have in a 24-hour period? What types of protein?
- Do you often feel thirsty?
- Are you on a special diet or have restrictions? Do you have food allergies?
- Have you lost or gained weight recently? If so, how much, and was it intentional?
- What prescription and over-the-counter medications do you take on a routine basis? (Look for diuretics, steroids, nonsteroidal antiinflammatory drugs [NSAIDs], aminoglycosides, sodium-based antacids, lithium, or narcotics.)
- What herbals, vitamins, or mineral supplements do you take on a routine basis and for what reason?
- Do you use laxatives?
- Do you have a history of renal disease, diabetes mellitus, diabetes insipidus, congestive heart failure, thyroid or parathyroid disorders, or pulmonary disease?
- Do you have a recent history of surgery, trauma (including burns), gastroenteritis, head injury, infection, vomiting, diarrhea, or fever?
- Have you noticed swelling of your hands and feet?

or gain). A complete list of over-the-counter and prescription medications helps the nurse identify drug-related influences on homeostasis. Questions regarding the recent medical history, including chronic diseases, surgery or trauma, draining wounds, and changes in elimination patterns, assist the nurse in recognizing patients who are at high risk for or have imbalances.

The health history includes questions about the use of herbal medicines. Certain herbals affect the patient's risk of fluid and electrolyte imbalances (Patient Education and Health Literacy box).

PATIENT EDUCATION AND HEALTH LITERACY

Fluid and Electrolytes Imbalances With Herbals

- Patient education about the effects of herbal supplements can avert side effects that affect fluid and electrolyte balance.
- Teach the patient about the effects of the following herbals:
  - Aloe: acts as a cathartic
  - Artichoke: acts as a diuretic
  - Celery: acts as a diuretic
  - Dandelion: acts as a diuretic
  - Ginseng: contraindicated in renal failure
  - Licorice: pseudoaldosteronism

VITAL SIGNS

A prolonged fever can lead to an increased loss of body fluids. In severe dehydration (i.e., hyperosmolar fluid volume deficit), the body temperature increases, whereas in isotonic fluid volume deficit, the body temperature decreases.

Tachycardia, or increased heart rate, may be the first indication of a fluid volume deficit. When there is a decrease in circulating blood volume, the stroke volume decreases. To ensure adequate oxygenation of the tissues, the heart rate accelerates to maintain normal cardiac output. Alterations in potassium, calcium, and magnesium levels can lead to dysrhythmias, or abnormal heart rhythms. The strength or quality of the pulse is assessed. Fluid volume deficit leads to a weak pulse on palpation, and fluid volume excess causes a strong, bounding pulse.

Changes in respirations are closely linked to acid-base balance. Alterations in respiratory rate, depth, and rhythm can lead to respiratory acid-base imbalance or be a compensatory mechanism for metabolic imbalances. The nurse should be able to differentiate between the underlying disorder and the compensatory mechanism.

Changes in blood pressure can indicate fluid and electrolyte imbalances. With a fluid volume excess, the circulating volume and blood pressure increase. With fluid volume deficit, the blood pressure decreases. It is important to assess for **orthostatic hypotension**, a decrease of more than 20 mm Hg in systolic pressure or 10 mm Hg in diastolic pressure when moving from one position to another, such as sitting to standing. The pulse pressure, which is the difference between the systolic and diastolic blood pressures, is approximately 40 mm Hg. A pulse pressure less than 24 mm Hg can indicate severe fluid volume deficit.

Electrolyte imbalances can affect blood pressure values. Hypernatremia can increase circulating fluid volume, leading to hypertension. Hyperkalemia can cause the blood pressure to decrease.

INTAKE AND OUTPUT

Measurement of intake and output is routinely ordered for patients who are at risk for or who have fluid and electrolyte imbalances. It is important that patients, family members, and health care workers are aware of this intervention.

Oral intake comprises all fluids and foods that become liquid at room temperature, including gelatin, Popsicles, ice cream, and ice chips. Ice chips, when melted, are approximately one half of the frozen amount. For example, one cup of ice chips (240 mL) is equal to 120 mL of water. All IV fluids, including medications and blood products, are recorded as intake. Other sources of fluid intake include enteral tube feedings, nasogastric or bladder irrigations, and large-volume enemas.

Output consists of body fluids and drainage that can be measured. This includes urine, emesis, liquid stool, wound drainage, and drainage from suction devices. Containers with calibrations, such as urinals and urine hats, can be used to collect and measure the fluids.

To measure output in infants and incontinent adults, the diapers or disposable briefs are weighed to determine the amount of fluid. Normally, output is totaled for an 8-hour shift and a 24-hour period. For critically ill patients, insertion of a Foley catheter allows hourly intake and output measurements.

When assessing intake and output, the nurse documents intake and output balance in a 24-hour period (Evidence-Based Practice box). The fluid balance is positive when intake exceeds output, and it is negative when output surpasses intake. Trends over subsequent days should be noted. For example, a 200-mL positive fluid balance for 1 day is not a substantial amount. However, when there is a positive fluid balance for each of the next few days, the excess fluid has a cumulative effect (Figure 39-8).

EVIDENCE-BASED PRACTICE

Alterations in Fluids and Electrolytes With Enteral Tube Feeding

- People who are unable to eat as a result of aging, disease, or injury (e.g., cerebral vascular accident) are often given isotonic nutritional supplements to maintain normal nutritional balance.
- Oh and Seo (2007) examined the fluid intake and output and selected serum electrolyte values for patients who had suffered brain infarctions and were receiving enteral tube feedings.
  - There were no significant imbalances in electrolytes as a result of the enteral feedings.
  - There were significant increases in intake compared with output, leading to fluid excesses.
- Recommendations are to pay close attention to intake and output, daily weights, and assessment findings to detect fluid volume excesses early.

WEIGHT

Despite best intentions, the intake and output record is not always an accurate reflection of changes in fluid balance for various reasons. Patients may forget to save their urine or lose track of the amount of fluids ingested. Daily weights are a more precise method of monitoring changes in fluid balance. A change of 1 kg (2.2 lb) is equivalent to 1 liter (1000 mL) of fluid. Patients are weighed at the same time each day with the same scale and in the same clothes. Daily weights can be initiated by the nurse for any patient considered at high risk for fluid imbalances.

EDEMA

Edema is a significant and visible indication of fluid volume excess. Edema is usually found in the dependent areas of the

Intake/Output

Table | 3-Day | 7-Day | Refresh | I/O Flowsheet

Interval: Shift | Aug 28-Aug 30

Date		08/28/12 0701 - 08/29/12 0700			
Time		0701 - 1500	1501 - 2300	2301 - 0700	Daily Total
IN	**P.O. (mL/kg/hr)**	**575** (0.7)	**300** (0.4)	**625** (0.8)	**1,500** (0.6)
	I.V. (mL/kg)	**260** (2.6)	**260** (2.6)		**520** (5.2)
	Total Intake (mL/kg)	**835** (8.4)	**560** (5.6)	**625** (6.3)	**2,020** (20.2)
OUT	**Urine (mL/kg/hr)**	**825** (1)	**550** (0.7)		**1,375** (0.6)
	Stool (mL/kg)		**1** (0)		**1** (0)
	Total Output (mL/kg)	**825** (8.3)	**551** (5.5)		**1,376** (13.8)
Net I/O		**+10**	**+9**	**+625**	**+644**
Net Since Admission (08/28/12)		**+10**	**+19**	**+644**	**+644**

FIGURE 39-8 The 24-hour intake and output record. (Courtesy Epic Systems Corporation, 2012.)

body. For ambulatory patients or those who spend time sitting in a chair, edema is most prominent in the ankles and feet. For patients who are bedridden, the edema is localized in the sacral area.

Pitting edema is characterized by a lasting indentation in the skin when pressure is applied. To assess edema in the lower extremities, press a finger to the lower tibia and behind the medial malleolus. The edema is graded on a 4+ scale and is based on the depth of the indentation:

- 1+ Slight indentation (2 mm); mild indentation returns to normal fairly quickly
- 2+ Deeper indentation (4 mm); indentation lasts longer
- 3+ Obvious indentation (6 mm); indentation lasts several seconds
- 4+ Deep indentation (8 mm); indentation remains several minutes

Brawny edema occurs when there is obvious swelling, but the tissue is too firm and hard to be indented. Although edema is a definitive indicator of fluid volume excess, it is also considered a fairly late indicator. The circulating volume increases as much as 30% before even 1+ edema is apparent.

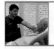

2. List key assessment findings for Mr. Abdul, and explain the underlying physiology.

SKIN TURGOR AND MUCOUS MEMBRANES

Skin turgor can provide an indicator of fluid volume imbalance. With normal fluid balance, pinched skin quickly returns to normal on release. In fluid volume deficit, the skin remains pinched, or tented, after release. Skin turgor is usually assessed at the forehead, anterior chest, and medial forearm.

Visual inspection of the tongue and mucous membranes may reveal hydration. The tongue and mucous membranes are normally moist and pink. In severe fluid volume deficit, they are dry and sticky, with furrows in the tongue. It is common to see dry, cracked lips. Table 39-8 lists assessments of hydration in other body systems.

DIAGNOSTIC TESTS

Several laboratory tests are useful in identifying fluid, electrolyte, and acid-base imbalances. It is the nurse's responsibility to be knowledgeable about these tests and communicate the results to the primary care provider. Tests include serum electrolyte levels, renal function tests, and measurement of oxygen carrying capacity. Urinalysis provides diagnostic information regarding fluid balance. Chapter 34 discusses the specific tests and their diagnostic function.

TABLE 39-8 Assessment of Hydration

BODY SYSTEM	ASSESSMENT
Neurologic	Chvostek sign (spasm of the facial muscle after tapping on the facial nerve) Trousseau sign (spasm of the muscles in the hand and wrist from pressure on the nerves of the upper arm) Deep tendon reflexes Tremors Confusion, agitation, coma
Cardiovascular	Jugular vein distention Electrocardiographic (ECG) waveforms Pulses Blood pressure
Respiratory	Abnormal lung sounds (crackles) Diminished lung sounds Respiratory rate
Musculoskeletal	Muscle strength
Elimination	Frequency and characteristics of stool (constipation or diarrhea) Nausea and vomiting Amount of urine output

Diagnostic Testing for Fluid and Electrolyte Imbalance

Several laboratory tests are available to determine fluid and electrolyte imbalances. Table 39-9 lists the diagnostic tests used for evaluating fluid and electrolyte balance.

Arterial Blood Gases

Measurement of **arterial blood gases** provides essential information on a patient's acid-base balance and oxygenation status (Table 39-10). These test results help to evaluate respiratory function and determine acid-base balance. Interpretation of arterial blood gas requires a systematic approach, keeping in mind the following normal values:

pH	7.35 to 7.45
$PaCO_2$	35 to 45 mm Hg
HCO_3^-	22 to 26 mEq/L
PaO_2	80 to 100 mm Hg
O_2 saturation	95% to 100%

The first step in interpreting arterial blood gasses is to examine the oxygenation status by examining the PaO_2 and O_2 saturation values. Oxygen saturation is the amount of O_2 that is bound to hemoglobin. It accounts for 97% of the oxygen molecules. As oxygen enters the bloodstream from the alveoli in the lungs, it is bound until all the hemoglobin is fully saturated. The PaO_2 represents the free-floating oxygen

TABLE 39-9 Diagnostic Tests for Fluid and Electrolyte Balance

LABORATORY TEST	INFORMATION PROVIDED
Levels of serum electrolytes, including sodium, potassium, magnesium, calcium, chloride, and phosphate	Direct information on extracellular levels and indirect information on intracellular levels of the electrolytes.
Blood urea nitrogen (BUN), creatinine	Indicates renal function.
Serum osmolarity	Information on hydration status; useful in managing fluid requirements.
Red blood cells, hemoglobin, hematocrit	Indicates oxygen-carrying capacity. Hematocrit levels can be influenced by fluid volume, can be diagnostic of fluid volume deficit or fluid volume excess.
Levels of serum albumin	Indicates colloid oncotic pressure capability.
Urinalysis	
• pH	Information about the hydrogen ion concentration in the urine. The pH increases or decreases based on the body's acid-base balance.
• Specific gravity	Increases when fluid volume is concentrated and is low with fluid volume excess.
• Urine osmolarity	Reflects solute concentration of the urine. Urine osmolarity is increased in fluid volume deficit and decreased in fluid volume excess.

TABLE 39-10 Arterial Blood Gas Results for Acid-Base Imbalances

ACID-BASE IMBALANCE	pH	$PaCO_2$	HCO_3^-
Respiratory acidosis	↓	↑	Normal
Respiratory alkalosis	↑	↓	Normal
Metabolic acidosis	↓	Normal	↓
Metabolic alkalosis	↑	Normal	↑

↓, Decreased value; ↑, increased value.

TABLE 39-11 Compensated Acid-Base Imbalances

ACID-BASE IMBALANCE	pH	$PaCO_2$	HCO_3^-
Compensated respiratory acidosis	On the ↓ side of normal	↑	↑
Compensated respiratory alkalosis	On the ↑ side of normal	↓	↓
Compensated metabolic acidosis	On the ↓ side of normal	↓	↓
Compensated metabolic alkalosis	On the ↑ side of normal	↑	↑

↓, Decreased value; ↑, increased value.

molecules. In situations of **hypoxemia** (decreased oxygen concentration in arterial blood), the PaO_2 decreases:

- PaO_2 of 60 to 80 mm Hg: mild hypoxemia
- PaO_2 of 40 to 60 mm Hg: moderate hypoxemia
- PaO_2 less than 40 mm Hg: severe hypoxemia

The second step is to examine the pH and determine whether the value falls within the normal range. If the pH is less than 7.35, there is an underlying acidosis. If the pH is greater than 7.45, the imbalance is alkalotic in nature. The imbalances are caused by a respiratory or metabolic disorder. An underlying compensatory mechanism may be the reason that the pH is normal.

The third step is to examine the $PaCO_2$ and HCO_3^- values to determine whether the underlying disorder is metabolic or respiratory. If the $PaCO_2$ is abnormal and the HCO_3^- is normal, the imbalance results from a respiratory problem. If the $PaCO_2$ is normal and the HCO_3^- is abnormal, there is a metabolic disorder. In respiratory disorders, there is an inverse relationship between the pH and the $PaCO_2$ values.

The fourth step in interpreting arterial blood gasses is to determine whether compensation is occurring. When acid-base imbalances occur, the body attempts to compensate to keep the pH within the normal range (Table 39-11). Compensation can make it more difficult to interpret the arterial blood gas results. The $PaCO_2$ and HCO_3^- may be abnormal, and the pH may be normal. If the pH value is in the normal range, it tends to be near the upper or lower end of the range and provides a clue to the underlying problem. For example, a pH of 7.36 is considered normal but is on the acidotic end. Examine the $PaCO_2$ and HCO_3^- values for an explanation of the imbalance.

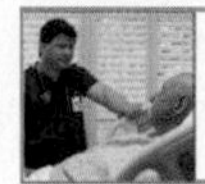

3. Analyze the Mr. Abdul's arterial blood gas results, and identify factors contributing to the results.

FACTORS AFFECTING FLUID, ELECTROLYTE, AND ACID-BASE BALANCES

In assessing an individual for potential fluid, electrolyte, and acid-base imbalances, several factors should be considered, including age, stress, surgery, weight, and medical disorders. Infants are more susceptible to fluid imbalances because their higher metabolic rate creates more toxins, which require additional water to excrete. Their kidneys are not mature, and the ability to concentrate urine is not fully developed. Infants have a greater ratio of body surface area to volume, and more water is lost through evaporation. As a person ages, the thirst sensation tends to decrease. Older adults often drink less fluid than desirable.

Aldosterone production with associated extracellular fluid retention is increased in stress. It leads to increased ADH secretion, which decreases renal excretion of water. Total body fluid is disproportionate to body weight in people who are obese.

Surgery can alter fluid balance in several ways. Preoperatively, patients usually are ordered to have nothing by mouth (NPO). It is common to use cathartics or enemas in preparation for surgery. Intraoperatively, there is an increase in blood loss due to surgery and an increase in insensible fluid loss because the internal structures are exposed to air. Postoperatively, the stress of surgery increases ADH production; there is drainage of body fluids from nasogastric tubes or wounds and postoperative vomiting.

Medical conditions that can affect homeostasis include cardiac, hepatic, renal, and respiratory disorders. When cardiac output decreases (i.e., congestive heart failure), blood pressure decreases. This leads to an increased secretion of aldosterone and ADH, causing retention of excess fluid. Patients with liver failure have decreased plasma levels of albumin, which leads to fluid moving out of the intravascular space and into the interstitial space. **Ascites** is an abnormal collection of fluid in the peritoneal cavity. People with impaired renal function are at a higher risk for fluid and electrolyte imbalances because of the decreased ability to regulate excretion and reabsorption. They are more likely to retain metabolic waste products, which are normally acidic, making these patients more prone to metabolic acidosis. In COPD, the damage to the alveoli limits gas exchange, which leads to decreased oxygen levels and higher circulating levels of carbon dioxide. Chronic respiratory acidosis results.

◆ NURSING DIAGNOSIS LO 39.4

The information that the nurse gathers from the assessment determines the appropriate nursing diagnoses for the patient. Selection of nursing diagnoses related to fluid, electrolyte, and acid-base balance is based on the following considerations:

- Health promotion or identification of high risk
- Actual fluid imbalances
- Possible complications of fluid and electrolyte imbalances
- Conditions that lead to fluid, electrolyte, and acid-base imbalances

The goal for nursing is to prevent imbalances whenever possible. This includes ongoing assessment and instruction to patients, families, and other health care providers on adequate fluid intake and dietary requirements of electrolytes. The following are examples of health-promotion and risk nursing diagnoses:

- *Excess Fluid Volume* related to decreased ability of the heart to pump blood as evidenced by edema in the feet, crackles in lungs, and weight gain
- *Readiness for Enhanced Fluid Balance* with defining characteristics of stable weight, moist mucous membranes, intake equals output, no evidence of edema or dehydration
- *Risk for Imbalanced Fluid Volume* with risk factor of major surgery
- *Deficient Fluid Volume* related to nausea and vomiting as evidenced by output greater than intake, dry mucous membranes, weight loss, excessive thirst
- *Decreased Cardiac Output* related to decreased circulating blood volume as evidenced by low blood pressure, tachycardia, dyspnea, fatigue, and angina

The nurse should remember that fluid and electrolyte imbalances affect function in other areas. Some nursing diagnoses pertaining to a few of the complications that can occur with fluid and electrolyte imbalances are *Acute Confusion, Risk for Injury,* and *Impaired Skin Integrity.*

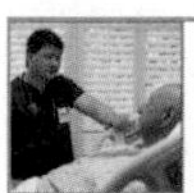

4. Identify two nursing diagnoses appropriate for Mr. Abdul. Include related factors and defining characteristics.

◆ PLANNING LO 39.5

Patient goals are the measures a nurse uses to determine effectiveness of the plan of care (Table 39-12). The goals provide a description of desired outcomes based on the identified nursing diagnoses. For patients who are at risk for or have imbalances, the goals are based on returning to or maintaining normal balance:

- Patient will exhibit no edema within 48 hours.
- Patient's intake and output will be balanced by the end of the next shift.
- Urine specific gravity will be within normal limits on next urinalysis.
- Patient's mucous membranes will be moist by the end of the shift.
- Vital signs will be within patient's normal limits within 24 hours.

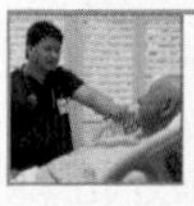

The conceptual care map for Mr. Abdul can be found at *http://evolve.elsevier.com/YoostCrawford/fundamentals/*. It is partially completed to indicate how to use the map as a learning tool. Complete the nursing diagnoses using the example conceptual care maps shown in Chapters 8 and 25 to 33.

TABLE 39-12 Care Planning

NANDA-I NURSING DIAGNOSIS LABEL WITH NURSING DIAGNOSIS STATEMENT	NURSING OUTCOME CLASSIFICATION (NOC)	NURSING INTERVENTION CLASSIFICATION (NIC)
Excess Fluid Volume related to decreased ability of the heart to pump blood as evidenced by edema in the feet, crackles in lungs, and weight gain	*Fluid balance* (0601) Stable body weight (060109)	*Fluid monitoring* (4130) Monitor weight.

From Bulechek G, Butcher H, Dochterman J, et al (Eds): *Nursing interventions classification (NIC)*, ed. 6, St. Louis, 2013, Mosby; Moorhead S, Johnson M, Maas M, et al (Eds): *Nursing outcomes classification (NOC)*, ed. 5, St. Louis, 2013, Mosby; NANDA International: *Nursing diagnoses: Definitions and classification, 2012–2014*, West Sussex, England, 2012, Wiley-Blackwell. Reprinted with permission from NANDA International, Inc.

◆ IMPLEMENTATION AND EVALUATION LO 39.6

Caring for patients with fluid, electrolyte, and acid-base imbalances involves monitoring fluid balance and implementing interventions designed to maintain fluid and electrolyte balance. Replacement of fluids and electrolytes through the use of IV solutions is commonly used to improve fluid and electrolyte balance.

MONITORING FLUID BALANCE

The nurse's role in monitoring fluid balance is to evaluate the impact of disease or effect of treatment on an ongoing basis. Vital signs, intake and output measurement, and daily weights provide valuable information about fluid and electrolyte status. Vital signs are assessed on a regular basis, which is at least every 4 hours for patients with fluid and electrolyte imbalances. When the imbalances are severe and aggressive treatment is required, vital signs are monitored on a more frequent basis.

Daily weights are compared with previous findings to determine changes in fluid status. Depending on the situation, a change in weight is a desired outcome or a significant concern.

Intake and output measurements are usually reviewed at the end of 8 hours and 24 hours. For patients with normal fluid balance, the intake should equal the output at the 24-hour mark. Positive fluid balance (i.e., intake greater than output) can be a desired outcome in patients with fluid volume deficits or can indicate fluid volume excess. It is the nurse's responsibility to evaluate the significance of the daily measurement of intake and output.

It is common for measurement of vital signs, intake and output, and daily weights to be delegated to unlicensed assistive personnel. However, it is important for the nurse to be aware of these assessment findings to evaluate effectiveness of prescribed interventions and nursing care.

Blood tests are often ordered to monitor fluid, electrolyte, and acid-base balance and to assess the effectiveness of prescribed treatments. These tests are commonly ordered to be drawn on a daily or more frequent basis. The nurse is responsible for confirming that the ordered tests have been completed and the results are communicated to the appropriate health care providers.

MAINTAINING FLUID AND ELECTROLYTE BALANCE

Depending on the situation, maintaining fluid and electrolyte balance may require increased intake or restriction of fluids and certain electrolytes. The nurse is essential in determining the appropriate interventions on the basis of the underlying disorder and assessment findings.

Restricting Fluid Intake

When a patient is experiencing severe fluid volume excess, the primary care provider may decide to restrict the amount of fluid the patient takes in. This situation is commonly seen in patients with congestive heart failure and chronic renal failure. Normally, the order indicates the amount of fluid to be consumed in a 24-hour period (e.g., 1000 mL). It is up to the nurse to divide that total into smaller amounts throughout the day. The normal recommendation is to use 50% of the amount during the day, when the patient is most active and consumes two meals. The amount is then further divided into fluid with meals and fluid available between meals and with medication administration. For example, a 1000-mL fluid restriction may be divided as follows:

Breakfast	200 mL
Lunch	200 mL
Dinner	200 mL
Between meals and medications	300 mL
Night shift medications	100 mL

If the patient has IV fluids running, the fluids need to be subtracted from the ordered fluid restriction; the remaining fluid is then divided throughout the 24-hour period. When developing the fluid breakdown, it is essential to involve the patient and incorporate fluid preferences when possible. Several strategies can assist in patient compliance with the restriction:

- Explain the purpose of the restriction. Make sure the patient understands that ice chips, Jello, and ice cream are considered fluids and are included.

- Offer fluids frequently in small amounts. Using a smaller 4- or 6-oz glass offers the impression of more fluid. Give the patient a choice in fluid preferences.
- Instruct the patient to avoid overly sweet or salty foods. Both stimulate the thirst sensation.
- Offer small amounts of ice chips. Remember that 100 mL of ice chips is approximately 50 mL of water.
- Encourage the patient to assist in maintaining the intake and output record. This helps the patient feel more in control of the situation and facilitates compliance with the restriction.

Restricting Electrolyte Intake

Patients with fluid volume excess may need to restrict sodium intake to prevent worsening of the fluid excess. Sodium restrictions are classified as mild, moderate, or severe:

- Mild restriction is 3000 to 4000 mg/day; it is indicated as "no added salt."
- Moderate restriction is 2000 mg/day; it is indicated as the need to consume foods with a low-sodium content.
- Severe restriction is 500 mg/day.

It is important to instruct the patient to avoid the salt shaker. Salt substitutes or herbal seasonings are used to enhance the flavor of food. Canned foods and processed or cured meats are avoided. Encourage the patient to buy fresh or frozen foods whenever possible. Make sure the patient knows how to read and interpret nutrition labels for the amount of sodium per serving. Several over-the-counter medications contain high amounts of sodium. It is important to read the label to determine the amount of sodium contained in the medicine.

Other electrolytes may need to be restricted based on the patient's medical condition. As part of the plan of care, the nurse instructs the patient about the dietary restrictions and common foods to avoid.

ORAL REPLACEMENT OF FLUIDS AND ELECTROLYTES

In situations of fluid volume deficit, the patient may need to increase the amount of fluids taken orally. It is the nurse's responsibility to encourage fluid intake and monitor the patient's response to the increased fluids.

Fluid Replacement

A patient may need to increase fluid intake to offset losses (e.g., mild to moderate diarrhea). This is especially important when the goal is to decrease or eliminate the need for IV fluids.

The same process is used to encourage fluids as when restricting intake. At least 50% of the fluid is taken during the day. The patient avoids drinking large amounts in the evening; it may interrupt sleep with frequent urination. Offer a variety of fluids, and ask the patient's preference. Beverages with caffeine have a diuretic effect and are avoided. Keeping a pitcher of water on hand and within easy reach encourages the patient to drink. For patients who are unable to pour the water, a glass of water is offered every time the nurse enters the room. Encouraging the patient to participate in the planning and involving the patient and family in keeping track of fluid intake helps to meet the desired outcome.

Electrolyte Replacement

In normal situations, the body is able to extract the needed electrolytes from the food consumed. Under certain conditions, it is necessary to supplement dietary intake. The two most commonly prescribed supplements are potassium and calcium.

When a patient is prescribed a potassium-wasting diuretic, such as loop diuretics, it is common for the primary care provider to prescribe a potassium supplement. Several points should be included in the teaching plan:

- Explain the importance of taking the supplement daily as prescribed.
- Taking a supplement with juice can mask an unpleasant taste.
- A change in diuretic therapy may require a change in the potassium dose.
- Many patients use salt substitutes as part of a sodium-restricted diet. It is important to teach that these salt substitutes often use potassium instead of sodium and must be used with caution.

Calcium is essential for bone strength, neuromuscular functioning, and blood clotting. Inadequate intake of milk, milk products, and vitamin D prompts the need for calcium supplements. According to the National Institutes of Health (2011), the adequate intake for adults between the ages of 19 and 70 is 600 IU/day. For adults older than 70 years, the adequate intake increases to 800 mg/day. Those taking calcium supplements should increase fluid intake to at least 2500 mL/day to prevent constipation and reduce the risk of kidney stones.

Excessive loss of fluids and sodium can occur with strenuous exercise or severe diarrhea. It is important to replace the sodium in conjunction with the fluid early and often to prevent severe dehydration (Evidence-Based Practice and Informatics box). Sports drinks contain fluid and electrolytes and are used during and after strenuous exercise. Pedialyte is an electrolyte solution designed specifically for children and is used to replace losses from diarrhea and prevent dehydration.

INTRAVENOUS THERAPY

Patients are often unable to maintain normal fluid balance because of disease, surgery, or trauma. As a result, it is common to replace needed fluids directly into the bloodstream through IV administration. IV fluids are considered medications and are given with the same caution and rights

EVIDENCE-BASED PRACTICE AND INFORMATICS

Hydration During Exercise

- Strenuous and extended physical activity can lead to a significant loss of fluid and electrolytes, especially sodium and potassium. It is recommended that athletes consume fluid before, during, and after strenuous exercise.
- Sports beverages, such as Gatorade and Propel, contain carbohydrates and electrolytes that can help sustain fluid and serum electrolytes during exercise.
- Salty foods and snacks can help replace lost sodium levels and trigger the thirst sensation, leading to increased water consumption.
- Lim (2009) recommends using urine color as an indicator of hydration status. Clear colored urine indicates euhydration (i.e., normal fluid levels), and unclear, yellowish urine indicates dehydration. It is suggested that athletes drink sufficient water or beverage to maintain clear colored urine.
- The Joint Position Statement on Nutrition and Athletic Performance by the American College of Sports Medicine, American Dietetic Association, and Dietitians of Canada (2009) provides more recommendations *(http://journals.lww.com/acsm-msse/Fulltext/2009/03000/Nutrition_and_Athletic_Performance.27.aspx).*

used for medication administration (Ethical, Legal, and Professional Practice box). There are several advantages to using the IV route. It provides immediate access for fluid and electrolyte maintenance or replacement; medications given intravenously have a much faster onset and more predictable effect; and it provides access for supplemental or total nutrition replacement and allows transfusion of blood and blood products to increase oxygen-carrying capacity and reestablish normal oncotic pressure. Concerns related to IV therapy administration are outlined in the Collaboration and Delegation box.

Intravenous Solutions

The type of fluid used and the rate at which it is infused depend on the purpose and desired outcomes. IV fluids are classified broadly as crystalloids or colloids. Crystalloids are solutions with small molecules, usually electrolytes, that are able to pass through cell membranes. These fluids are used primarily for fluid and electrolyte maintenance and replacement.

Crystalloids are further categorized based on the tonicity of the fluid compared with normal blood plasma: hypotonic, isotonic, or hypertonic. Tonicity of blood plasma is 290 mOsm/L. IV solutions with a tonicity significantly less than 290 mOsm/L are hypotonic. Hypotonic fluids lower the osmolarity of blood plasma and cause fluid to shift into the cell. These fluids are used to treat hypernatremia or severe dehydration. Continued use of hypotonic fluids can lead to intracellular swelling or water intoxication. Swelling of brain cells causes increased intracranial pressure.

ETHICAL, LEGAL, AND PROFESSIONAL PRACTICE

Administration of Intravenous Fluids

Intravenous (IV) fluids are considered medications. Before and during IV therapy, check the six Rights of medication administration:

- *Right patient:* Use two unique identifiers, such as patient hospital ID number, patient name, date of birth, picture, or verification from family member. Room and bed number should not be used.
- *Right solution (medication):* Several IV solutions have similar names (e.g., 0.33% NS and 0.9% NS). Make sure the correct solution is infusing.
- *Right rate (dose):* Verify that the IV is infusing at the ordered rate.
- *Right route:* Certain IV fluids, such as total parenteral nutrition (TPN), are too hypertonic to be administered through a peripheral site.
- *Right time:* If infusing correctly, the IV infusion should finish at a designated time. IV bags that need to be replaced early (i.e., infused too quickly) can lead to hypervolemia, whereas IV fluids that are still infusing when a new bag is due to be hung (i.e., infusing too slowly) means the patient is not receiving the prescribed amount of fluid.
- *Right documentation:* IV therapy documentation is ongoing as long as the IV solution is infusing, and it includes the IV site, solution, rate, and patient tolerance.

COLLABORATION AND DELEGATION

Nursing Responsibilities for IV Therapy

- In many states, licensed practical (vocational) nurses (LPN/LVNs) with IV training have the authority to perform many of the functions in IV therapy, including adjusting flow rates, changing IV solutions, administering IV medications, and changing IV tubing and dressings. These functions vary from state to state. Specifics can be found in the state nurse practice act.
- The registered nurse is responsible for delegating these functions only to LPN/LVNs who have received this specialized training.
- The registered nurse is ultimately responsible for assessing the patient and evaluating the effects of IV therapy.

Isotonic solutions have a tonicity essentially the same as blood plasma. These types of fluids increase intravascular volume but do not cause fluid shifts in or out of the cell. When not monitored closely, isotonic fluids can lead to circulatory overload.

Hypertonic fluids have a tonicity that is markedly higher than 290 mOsm/L. These solutions increase the osmotic pressure of plasma and force fluids to move out of the cell and into the bloodstream. This can lead to cellular dehydration and circulatory overload.

The choice of IV fluid is based on the purpose of the therapy. It can contain any or all of the following substances: glucose (in the form of dextrose), sodium, bicarbonate, and chloride. Dextrose is a common element of IV solutions and can provide additional calories for energy. It is usually ordered in 5% or 10% concentrations. An IV solution of 5% dextrose in water (D_5W) is an isotonic solution before it enters the body. The dextrose is quickly broken down, leaving a hypotonic solution circulating.

! SAFE PRACTICE ALERT

Continued use of 5% dextrose in water (D_5W) as a primary infusion can lead to water intoxication or intracellular fluid excess. After the dextrose enters the bloodstream, it is quickly metabolized, leaving only free water, a hypotonic solution.

Saline solutions contain sodium and chloride in various amounts. Normal saline consists of 0.9% NaCl and is considered isotonic. Normal saline is used for replacement of fluid, sodium, and chloride. It is the only fluid used to begin or finish blood transfusions.

! SAFE PRACTICE ALERT

Prolonged use of normal saline can lead to hypernatremia and circulatory overload.

Normal saline solutions have various amounts of NaCl, ranging from 0.33% to 3%. Saline solutions that have greater than 0.9% NaCl are hypertonic, and those that have less than 0.9% are hypotonic. Saline is often combined with dextrose to provide calories along with fluid and electrolyte replacement. This combination solution is considered hypertonic.

Lactated Ringer solution contains sodium, potassium, calcium chloride, and lactate (which metabolizes to bicarbonate) and most closely resembles blood plasma. It is considered a balanced electrolyte solution and is often used after surgery or trauma. Table 39-13 lists common IV solutions, tonicity, and nursing considerations.

! SAFE PRACTICE ALERT

To avoid or treat hypokalemia, IV potassium is often ordered to be added to a continuous IV infusion. IV potassium is always diluted; usually it is added to an IV bag in the pharmacy. The nurse must *never* administer IV potassium as a push or bolus medication.

Colloids, also known as plasma expanders, are solutions that contain protein or starch. The particles remain intact in the solution and are unable to pass through the capillary membrane. They are used to reestablish circulating volume

TABLE 39-13 Common Intravenous Solutions

IV SOLUTION	NURSING CONSIDERATIONS
Hypotonic	
0.33% NS	Provides sodium, chloride, and free water. Allows kidneys to select amount of electrolyte to retain or excrete.
0.45% NS	Useful for determining renal function. Not used as replacement therapy.
Isotonic	
D_5W	Considered isotonic but becomes free water after dextrose is metabolized; then acts as a hypotonic solution. Because it does not contain sodium, continued use can lead to hyponatremia. Useful in IV medication administration.
0.9% NS	Commonly used to reestablish normal extracellular fluid levels in patients with hypovolemia. Not used as a maintenance fluid; continued use can lead to hypernatremia.
D_5 0.2% NS	Useful for maintenance of fluids when less sodium is required. The dextrose provides approximately 170 cal/L.
Lactated Ringer	Most closely resembles blood plasma. Contains sodium, potassium, calcium, chloride, and lactate. Used when there is loss of fluid and electrolytes, as in burns or severe diarrhea.
Hypertonic	
D_5 0.45% NS	Commonly used to treat hypovolemia and maintain normal fluid balance.
D_5 0.9% NS	Used as replacement fluid. Provides calories, sodium, and chloride. Prolonged use can lead to hypernatremia.
D_5 LR	Same content as lactated Ringer solution but adds calories with the dextrose. Useful when patient's caloric intake is reduced.
3% NS	Used to treat severe hyponatremia. Administered in an intensive care setting where the patient can be closely monitored.

D_5, 5% dextrose; *NS*, normal saline; *W*, water.

and oncotic pressure. Examples of colloids include albumin, dextran, Plasmanate, and hetastarch. Blood and blood components are also considered colloids (discussed later).

Intravenous Sites

When a patient requires IV therapy, there are several aspects to consider. What are the purpose (i.e., replacement or maintenance) and expected duration of therapy? Key considerations include the patient's age, diagnosis, health history, and condition of the veins. All of these factors determine whether IV therapy is administered through a peripheral vein or a larger, central vein. Peripheral sites are used when IV therapy will be short term or intermittent or to maintain vascular access with the use of an intermittent infusion device. An **intermittent infusion device** is a saline lock or PRN adapter that allows periodic or emergency venous access. This provides IV access for intermittent infusions or emergency medications. These devices are sometimes capped or have a port that is cleansed before use.

When selecting an appropriate vein for venipuncture, the nurse considers the location and condition of the vein and the purpose and duration of the therapy. The sites most commonly used with peripheral IV therapy are located in the hands and arms and include the cephalic, basilic, accessory and upper cephalic, median basilic, median cubital, and the metacarpal veins of the hands (Figure 39-9). Foot veins are not used in adults because of the risk of thrombophlebitis. In older adults, venous return from the feet and legs may be compromised, causing inconsistent administration of fluids and medications. However, the veins of the feet are often used for infants and children. Scalp veins are a common site for newborns and infants.

It is important to select the most distal site for venipuncture. This preserves the more proximal sites for future insertions. Avoid areas at the wrist and elbow. Flexion of these joints may obstruct IV flow. Venipuncture is contraindicated on an extremity that has been compromised due to surgery (e.g., mastectomy) or injury or if there is a dialysis graft in place.

The condition of the vein is considered. Avoid areas of bruising or **phlebitis** (inflammation of the vein). The vein of choice should feel soft and full, be splinted by bone, and be easily palpated when a tourniquet is applied.

The purpose of IV therapy influences vein selection. Large veins are used when large amounts of fluid need to be infused rapidly or if the fluids are highly viscous, such as packed red

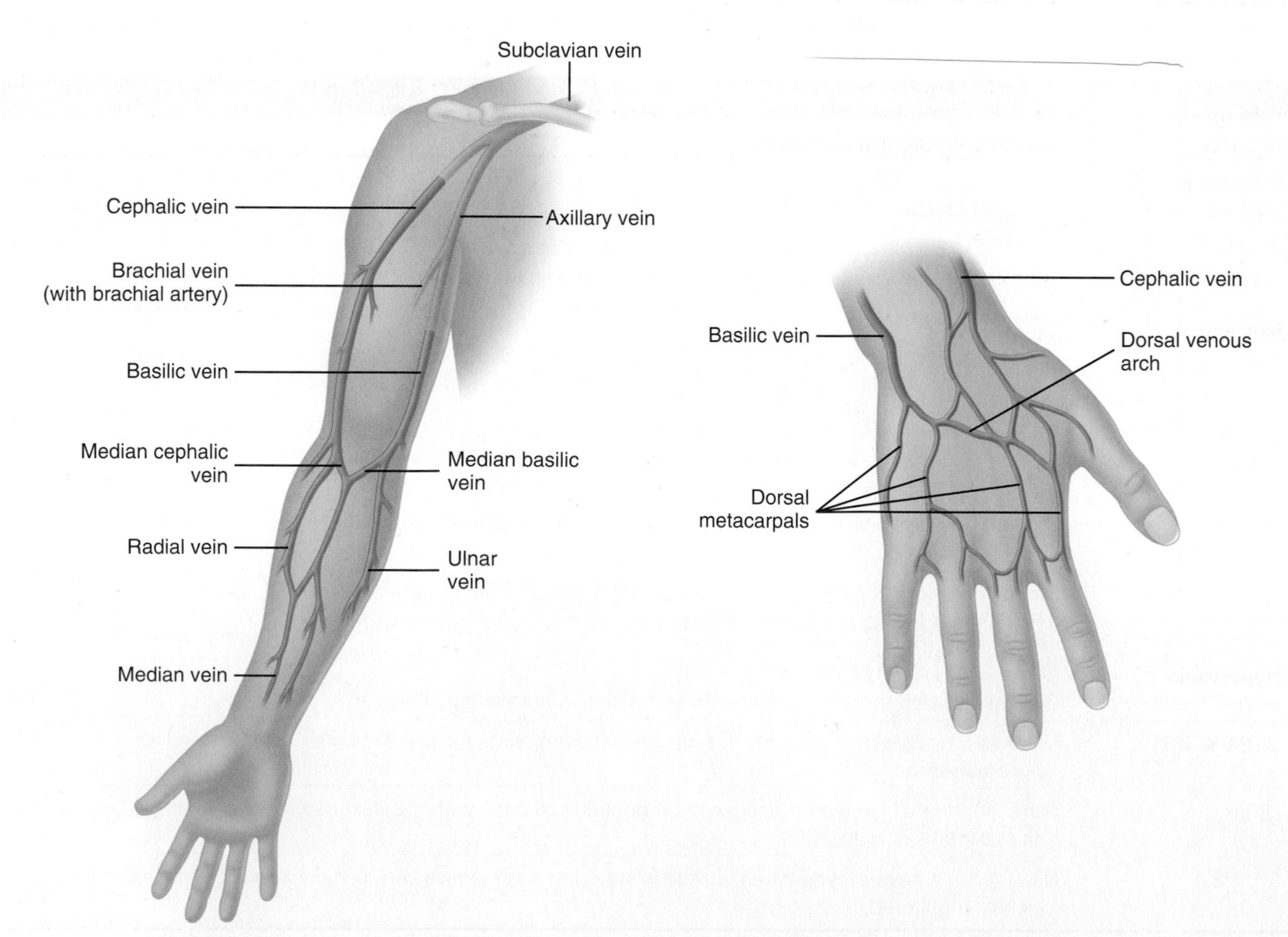

FIGURE 39-9 Veins of the hand and arm. (From Ignatavicius DD, Workman ML: *Medical-surgical nursing: Patient-centered collaborative care,* ed. 7, St. Louis, 2013, Saunders.)

blood cells. When administered through a larger vein, hypertonic fluids and caustic or irritating medications are less likely to cause phlebitis.

Intravenous Catheters

When venous access is necessary to administer fluids or medications, the IV catheter provides that access. The type of catheter chosen depends on the length of time the access is needed, the type of medication or fluid to be administered, and the age and overall health of the patient. The nurse selects the site and catheter that can provide the least risk of complications.

Peripheral Catheters

IV catheters come in several types and sizes. IV catheters are sized by the diameter of the needles, which is known as gauge. The smaller the diameter, the larger the gauge. For example, a 16-gauge needle has a larger diameter than a 24-gauge needle. Selection of the appropriate gauge is important for effective therapy (Table 39-14).

The nurse selects the smallest size needed for IV therapy. The three basic types of peripheral access catheters are as follows:

- Over-the-needle (ONC) catheter, also known as an Angiocath, is a polyurethane or Teflon catheter with a needle stylet inside. After needle insertion, the catheter is threaded into the vein, and the stylet is removed
- Winged infusion needle, also known as a butterfly needle, is a smaller needle commonly used with children and elderly patients for short-term use. The short, steel needle has two flexible wings instead of a catheter hub. The needle is attached to short, flexible extension tubing. The wings are pinched together during insertion and then taped flat to secure the needle.
- Midline catheters are used for longer-term IV therapy and are inserted through a peripheral vein. The catheters are 7 to 8 inches long and are inserted in the antecubital area, with the tip resting in the cephalic or basilic vein, right below the axilla. They are considered inside-the-needle catheters because the catheter remains inside the needle or introducer during insertion. After the catheter is threaded through the vein, the needle is removed. These catheters are inserted by specially trained nurses, and they can remain in place for longer periods, usually 1 to 2 weeks.

TABLE 39-14 Peripheral Intravenous Catheters

NEEDLE GAUGE	COMMON USES
16-18 gauge	Trauma Surgery Rapid infusion of fluids Blood transfusions
20-22 gauge	General and intermittent infusions Blood transfusions
24 gauge	General and intermittent infusions Children and the elderly

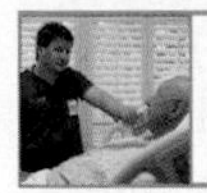

5. Identify five priority interventions for Mr. Abdul and provide the rationales.

Central Venous Catheters

Another type of IV access frequently used is the **central venous catheter** (CVC) or central venous access device (CVAD). The CVC (Figure 39-10) is inserted into a major vein in the arm or chest, and the tip lies in the superior vena cava, outside the right atrium. The CVC has several advantages. It allows rapid infusion of large amounts of fluid; irritating medications and hypertonic solutions (e.g., TPN) are rapidly diluted, reducing the risk of phlebitis; and it allows monitoring of central venous pressure. These are the most common types of CVCs:

- Nontunneled CVC
- Peripherally inserted central catheter (PICC)
- Tunneled CVC
- Implanted port

The nontunneled CVC is commonly used in patients who require short-term but extensive IV therapy (e.g., multiple IV medications), TPN, or recurring blood transfusions. The CVC is inserted by the physician, usually at the bedside, using the subclavian vein. The Centers for Disease Control and Prevention (CDC, 2011) advises avoiding use of the jugular and femoral veins because of the higher incidence of catheter-related infections. These catheters often have double or triple lumens, allowing for simultaneous administration of incompatible medications, fluids, and TPN. They are designed for short-term therapy (days to weeks) and are associated with a

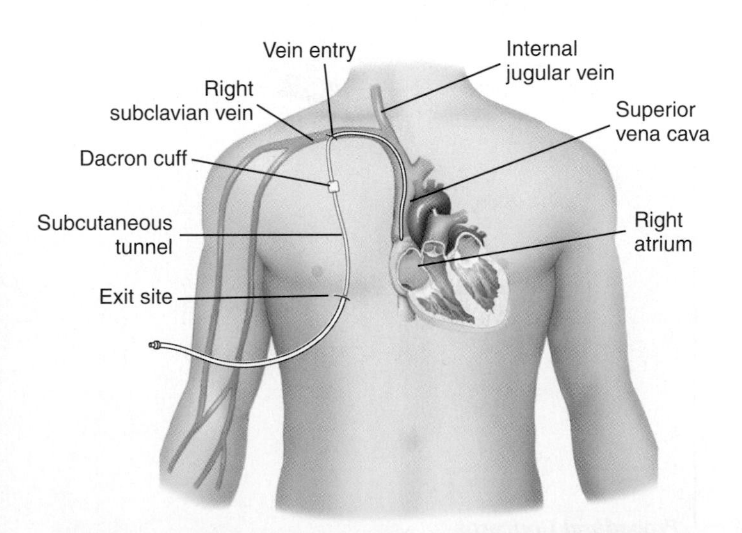

FIGURE 39-10 Tunneled central venous catheter. (From Lewis SL, Dirksen SR, Heitkemper MM: *Medical-surgical nursing: Assessment and management of clinical problems,* ed. 9, St. Louis, 2014, Mosby.)

high risk of complications, including catheter-related infections, pneumothorax, and pulmonary embolism.

The **peripherally inserted central catheter** (PICC) is becoming more common in long-term IV therapy. The PICC has several advantages over the nontunneled CVC: It can be inserted by a specially trained nurse, it can remain in for weeks to months, it does not have the risk of pneumothorax associated with its use, and it is associated with fewer catheter-related infections. The catheter is inserted in the cephalic or basilic veins or antecubital space and threaded up until it rests in the superior vena cava outside the right atrium. Strict aseptic technique is used during insertion and care of PICC lines. PICC lines are inserted by physicians and specially trained registered nurses.

Tunneled CVCs are used for long-term IV therapy. These catheters are inserted into the subclavian or jugular vein and then pulled through (i.e., tunneled) the subcutaneous tissue in the chest wall before exiting the skin. They are initially sutured into place, but they also have a cuff that the subcutaneous tissue eventually adheres to, holding the catheter in proper position.

After an implanted port, or MediPort, is inserted, it can be used for long-term IV therapy that is continuous or intermittent. A tunneled CVC is attached to a port or access device that has been implanted into the subcutaneous tissue in the chest wall, leaving no visible signs of the device. To access the site for IV infusions, the nurse inserts an angled or Huber needle through the skin and into the port. After the infusion is complete, the needle is removed, leaving a closed system (Nursing Care Guideline: Mediport: Access, Dressing Changes, and Care box). According to the CDC (2011), implanted ports have the lowest incidence of catheter-related infections.

! SAFE PRACTICE ALERT

After the central venous catheter is inserted, correct placement is confirmed by radiographic (x-ray) examination before the first use.

Equipment

Before beginning an IV infusion, the nurse gathers and assembles the appropriate equipment. Because of the risk of catheter-related infections, the nurse uses sterile technique when assembling and initiating IV therapy. The equipment needed includes the IV solution bag or container, IV tubing,

NURSING CARE GUIDELINE

Mediport: Access, Dressing Changes, and Care

Background

- A MediPort is a central venous access device with a subcutaneous injection port that is surgically implanted in the upper chest.
- Its primary use is for long-term intravenous access.
- Fewer complications occur with MediPorts.
- They have the lowest risk of catheter-related bloodstream infections (CRBSIs) among vascular access devices (VADs) because the tip of the catheter ends in a large vein and the port is not always accessed (i.e., not open to air).

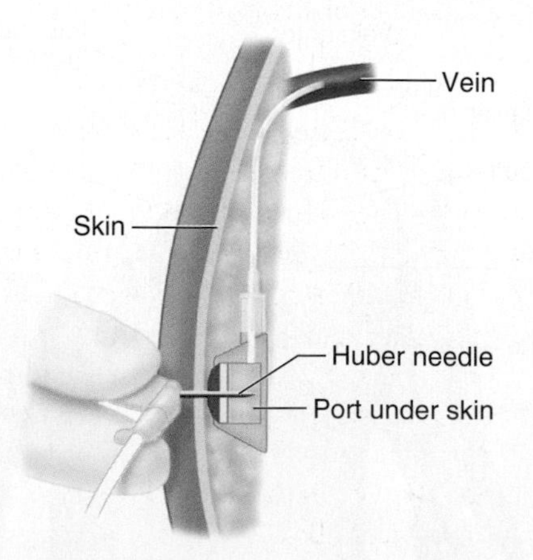

Procedural Concerns

- Follow strict sterile technique to prevent CRBSIs.
- If a dressing change is needed, follow Skill 39-3.
- Accessing a MediPort involves the following steps:
  - Cleanse the site 2 inches around the port with a chlorhexidine preparation.
  - Hold a Huber (noncoring) needle at a 90-degree angle (perpendicular) to the port.
  - For insertion:
    - Hold the port between the thumb and index finger.
    - Fully insert the needle until it meets with resistance and is at the back of the port before inserting fluids.
  - Cover the Huber needle with nontransparent dressing, and reinforce it with tape at its edges.
  - Flush all lumens (see Nursing Care Guideline: Flushing an Intravenous Line):
    - Assess the port for patency.
    - Use a 10-mL sterile syringe to flush it with 10 mL of the prescribed sterile fluid per facility policy or procedure.

Documentation Concerns

- Document the site and catheter assessments.
- Include the type and size of needle used to access the port.
- Report the patency of the port and the type and quantity of solution used.
- Note any problems or patient discomfort with the procedure.

Evidence-Based Practice

- "After the dressing has been applied, reinforce tape around the catheter to secure the dressing-catheter-skin area as this helps to extend adhesion longevity. Label the dressing with the date, initials, and any other data specified by the institution. Maintaining a dressing on an implanted port can be challenging" (Macklin, 2010, p. 115).

peripheral access needle or catheter, and flow monitoring device. All packages are examined for expiration dates and for damage to or breaks in sterile packaging.

IV solutions come in sterile, prefilled plastic bags or, less commonly, glass containers with 50 to 1000 mL of solution. The smaller bags (50 to 250 mL) are used to administer medications, whereas the larger bags are used for continuous infusions of fluids (Figure 39-11). The solution container is checked for the following:

- The correct fluid as ordered by the primary care provider
- Fluid that is clear without evidence of contamination or leaks in the container
- An expiration date that has not passed (questionable IV solution is returned to the pharmacy)

The IV tubing, or administration set, connects the IV solution to the catheter. The tubing consists of an insertion spike, a drip chamber, tubing with at least one secondary port, a roller clamp and slide clamp, and a connection port or hub. The insertion spike and hub are covered with protective caps to maintain sterility. The caps remain in place until the equipment is ready to insert and use.

The drip chamber provides a prespecified amount of fluid per drop (i.e., drop factor). Common drop factors are 10, 15, and 20, known as *macrodrip,* or 60, known as *microdrip.* For IV tubing with a drop factor of 10, 10 drops equals 1 mL of fluid. The drop factor is found on the outside of the package and is used to regulate IV flow rate. Macrodrip tubing is used for most IV infusions. Microdrip tubing is used for very slow infusions and in children and the elderly for whom potential fluid overload is a concern. The roller clamp compresses the tubing to various degrees, allowing regulation of the IV flow rate. The slide clamp is used to completely occlude the IV tubing; it is not used to regulate IV infusion rates. Secondary ports are used to administer medications mixed in IV solutions, IV piggybacks, or IV push medications (see Chapter 35). When a glass container is used, vented IV tubing is needed for the infusion to flow smoothly. This type of tubing allows air to replace the fluid moving out of the container. Plastic bags collapse as the fluid moves through the IV tubing and do not require vented tubing.

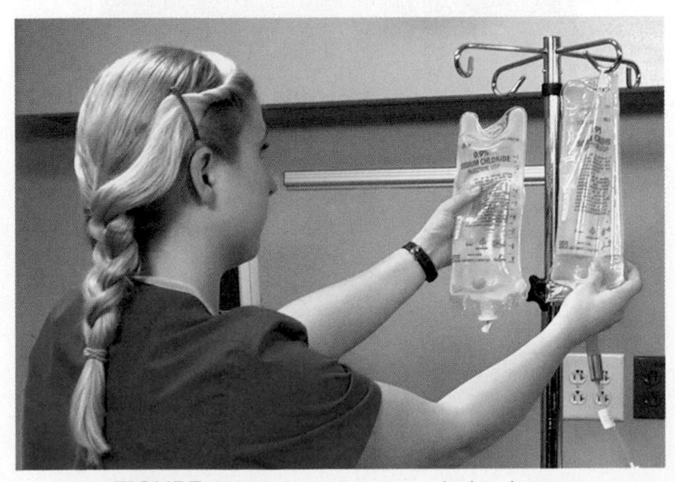

FIGURE 39-11 Intravenous solution bags.

After the supplies have been gathered, the IV tubing is flushed with solution before attaching it to the IV catheter. At this point, the IV catheter is inserted, and the tubing is attached. The tubing is placed in the infusion pump, roller clamp is opened, and the IV begins to flow. Skill 39-1 reviews the procedure for starting a peripheral IV infusion.

When a continuous infusion is no longer needed but IV access is, an intermittent infusion device is attached (Nursing Care Guideline: Converting an Intravenous Line box). These devices are known as saline locks or PRN adapters. When converting a continuous IV to a saline lock, the IV tubing is removed, and the adapter is attached. Some adapters come with extension tubing. It is important to flush the adapter with normal saline before attaching it to prevent an air embolism. The lock is flushed before and after each use, normally with sterile saline (Nursing Care Guideline: Flushing an Intravenous Line box).

! SAFE PRACTICE ALERT

Never use force when flushing an IV catheter with normal saline. Attempting to force the flush may dislodge a clot that can become an embolism.

Flow Rate

Several factors can influence the flow rate: distance, patient position, catheter size, and tubing obstruction. The shorter the distance between the IV bag and IV catheter, the slower the IV infusion flows. To increase the flow, raise the bag to a higher level. Smaller-gauge catheters (e.g., 24 gauge) cannot infuse fluids quickly. For example, if the IV rate needs to be increased to 150 mL/hr, the nurse may need to insert a large-gauge needle to accommodate the new rate. Make sure the tubing is not kinked or obstructed in any way. It is the nurse's responsibility to ensure that the IV solution infuses at the ordered rate.

A volume control device (i.e., Buretrol, Soluset) is often used for infants or children (Figure 39-12). These devices prevent accidental fluid overload due to an improperly regulated IV infusion. The devices usually have a microdrip, or a drop factor of 60 gtt/mL. Another way of manually regulating flow rates is through the use of an inline controller such as a Dial-A-Flo. This is a more precisely calibrated roller clamp and is used when possible fluid overload is a concern.

In most hospitals, an **electronic infusion device** or IV infusion pump (Figure 39-13), is used for even more precise delivery. These devices allow the nurse to program the rate and volume of the fluid to be infused. There are two general types: controllers and pumps. An alarm sounds when the infusion is complete and when there are complications with the flow, such as air in the tubing or obstruction. Controllers operate by gravitational force and regulate the flow using an

NURSING CARE GUIDELINE

Converting an Intravenous Line: Continuous to Intermittent Infusions

Background

- Conversion between continuous and intermittent IV infusions permits administration of intermittent medications and intermittent rehydration.
- This flexibility allows therapeutic interventions to be performed without limiting the patient's mobility, as with a continuous IV infusion.

Procedural Concerns

- Follow strict sterile technique to prevent catheter-related bloodstream infections (CRBSIs).
- Place sterile gauze under the connection hub:
  - This avoids contamination (i.e., maintains sterile technique).
  - It keeps excess fluid away from the skin.
- Ensure all connection hubs and ports are sterile before the connection.
  - Wipe the port and ridges with antiseptic or an alcohol wipe.
  - If there is any question about sterility of the IV tubing, discard the tubing, and obtain a sterile replacement.
- To convert from an intermittent to a continuous infusion:
  - Flush the saline lock (see the Nursing Care Guideline: Flushing an Intravenous Line box).
  - Connect the prepared IV tubing to the port while maintaining sterile technique.
  - Unclamp the IV tubing and extension tubing.
  - Start the infusion.
- To convert from a continuous to an intermittent:
  - Clamp the IV tubing and extension tubing.
  - Disconnect the IV tubing from the extension tubing.
  - Cap the IV tubing with a sterile cap.
  - Flush the saline lock (see the Nursing Care Guideline: Flushing an Intravenous Line box).

Documentation Concerns

- Document the patency of the line, date, and the type and amount of flush.
- Include the site assessment.
- Indicate whether fluids are being started or discontinued.
- Note any problems or patient discomfort with the procedure.

Evidence-Based Practice

- To prevent CRBSIs, all hospitals should have standardized, formal practices in place that address disinfection of the catheter hubs and maintenance of sterility when accessing injection ports according to the National Safety Patient Guidelines (Macklin, 2010; The Joint Commission, 2014).
- Macklin (2010) reports, "Another poor nonaseptic practice that is often overlooked is using clean gloved hands that have been used in non-IV–related patient care before the initiation of nonsterile IV care, such as blood sampling. These gloves are removed, hands rewashed, and new gloves applied before the IV care is initiated" (p. 118).

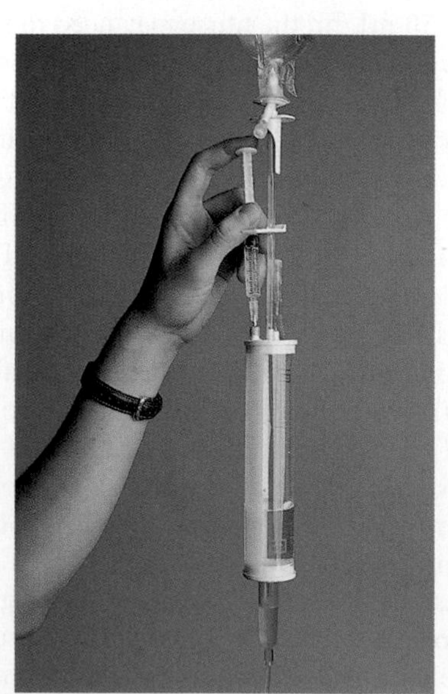

FIGURE 39-12 Volume control device. (From Lilley LL: *Pharmacology for Canadian health care practice,* ed. 2, Toronto, 2010, Mosby.)

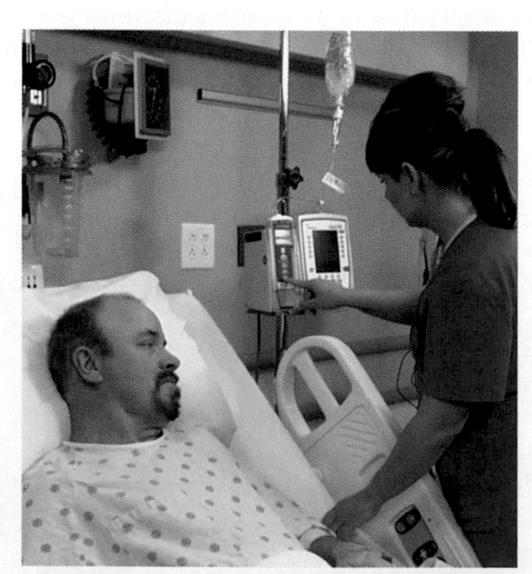

FIGURE 39-13 Electronic infusion pump.

NURSING CARE GUIDELINE

Flushing an Intravenous Line

Background

- Flushing an intravenous (IV) line maintains the saline lock patency.
- Flushing keeps incompatible solutions separate and allows assessment of the IV line.

Procedural Concerns

- Use a prefilled, sterile saline syringe, or fill a syringe with the appropriate quantity of sterile saline solution for injection.
- Wipe the port with antiseptic or an alcohol wipe.
- Wear clean gloves.
- Insert the blunt cannula or needle of the saline syringe into the port on the extension tubing, or screw it into the port, depending on the equipment.
- Unclamp the extension tubing (a saline lock is clamped when not in use).
- Slowly inject the solution over 1 minute into the IV access port.
    - Leave 0.5 mL of solution in the syringe so that air is not injected.
    - Observe for leaking and swelling at the IV site and for resistance when pushing saline. If they are observed, stop the procedure, and discontinue the IV infusion.
- Reclamp the extension tubing.
- Remove the syringe, and discard per institutional policy and procedures.

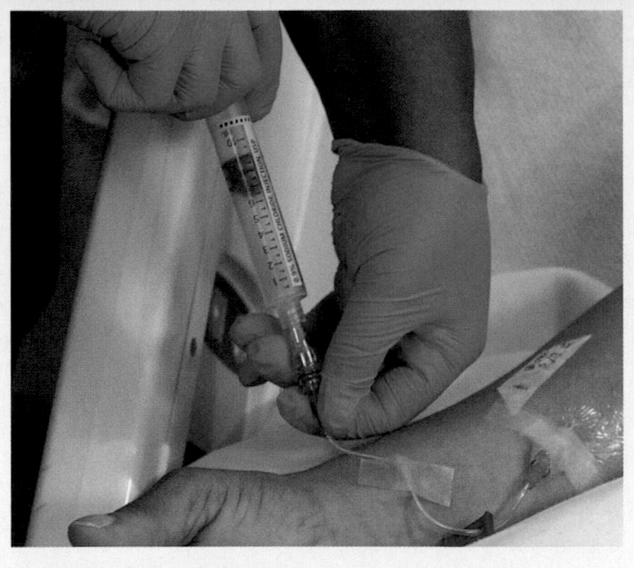

Documentation Concerns

- Document the patency of the line, the date, and the type and quantity of flush used.
- Include all site assessment information.
- Note problems or patient discomfort with the procedure.

Evidence-Based Practice

- Some nurses have been taught to push the saline flush, pause, and then repeat if resistance is felt in the vascular access device, whether it is a central or peripheral line.
- Smooth, steady flushing is recommended, and no evidence exists to support the push-pause-push method. No additional pressure is applied during the flush to overcome resistance (Macklin, 2010).

electronic dispenser. When the rate falls below the programmed rate, an alarm sounds. An infusion pump uses positive pressure to overcome vascular pressure at the insertion site. When the pressure required to infuse the fluid reaches a preset level, an alarm sounds, signaling the nurse to assess for IV patency and tubing obstruction. With controllers and pumps, rates are programmed in milliliters per hour. The nurse programs the ordered rate during the set-up process. Electronic infusion devices are used for patients who have additives such as potassium in their IV solutions, those receiving IV medications, children, the elderly, and any person for whom fluid overload is a concern. Electronic infusion devices are used with all CVCs.

The IV flow rate is the amount of milliliters infused over 1 hour (mL/hr). When the primary care provider orders an IV infusion, the rate usually is written in mL/hr. Sometimes, the order specifies the amount of fluid to be infused in a 24-hour period, and the nurse needs to determine the hourly flow rate.

Complications of Intravenous Therapy

IV therapy is considered an invasive procedure; a needle is entering and resting in a blood vessel. As with any invasive procedure, the risk of infection is increased. Careful sterile technique is essential in preventing catheter-related infections. Other complications associated with IV therapy include occlusion, phlebitis, infiltration, and extravasation. Systemic complications include fluid overload, speed shock, and embolism. Table 39-15 summarizes complications, symptoms, and nursing considerations.

SAFE PRACTICE ALERT

Notify the primary care provider when problems exist with a central venous catheter. Never discontinue a central venous catheter without an order.

Care of the Patient With a Peripheral Intravenous Catheter

When caring for a patient receiving IV fluids or medications, or both, several key nursing assessments and interventions can ensure effective care. When initially assessing patient information, the nurse reviews the IV therapy currently ordered, including the type of catheter, date of insertion, and solution type and rate. The time that the current solution bag was started indicates when the next IV solution should be

TABLE 39-15 Complications of Intravenous Therapy

COMPLICATIONS	SYMPTOMS	NURSING CONSIDERATIONS
Local Complications		
Catheter occlusion: partial or complete obstruction of a vascular access device, caused by clot formation within the catheter or a mechanical obstruction	IV flow is sluggish or stopped. Attempts to flush catheter are met with resistance.	Assess tubing and site for obstructions such as kinked tubing or arm position. Attempt to flush catheter with normal saline. *Do not force.* Forcing the flush can dislodge the clot, which becomes an embolism. If peripheral IV, discontinue the site and restart a new site. If a CVC, notify PCP or IV team.
Catheter-related infection: local infection that occurs at insertion site, if not recognized, can become systemic (septicemia) and possibly life-threatening; usually caused by poor aseptic technique during inserting or dressing or tubing changes; can occur when peripheral site is used for more than 72-96 hr	Local symptoms: pain at site, tenderness, erythema (redness), swelling, increased temperature, purulent drainage Systemic symptoms: fever, chills, tachycardia, hypotension, complaints of headache, backache	Prevention is key. Use aseptic technique during insertion and site care. Rotate sites per agency protocol. Assess site frequently for signs of infection. If symptoms evident, discontinue peripheral IV, and restart in another location. Place used catheter in sterile container and send to laboratory for culture and sensitivity testing. Notify PCP of findings. Replace old IV tubing and solution with new. Do not discontinue a CVC without a physician's order.
Phlebitis: inflammation of the vein caused by poor insertion and care technique, frequent manipulation of IV catheter, size and length of the catheter, use of irritating medications or fluids, and infection	Tenderness, redness, swelling at site Pain, burning, heat along the vein, especially during infusion Palpable venous cord Scale to grade severity: 0: No symptoms 1: Redness at site with or without pain 2: Pain with erythema 3: All the above plus red streak along vein and palpable venous cord 4: All the above plus purulent drainage	Discontinue catheter immediately if infection suspected; send catheter tip for culture and sensitivity testing. Clean insertion site with disinfectant. Apply warm moist compresses for 20 min three or four times per day. When inserting new IV catheter, use opposite extremity if possible. To avoid phlebitis, use smallest gauge possible (22 or 24 gauge), stabilize catheter securely to minimize movement, and rotate sites according to agency policy, usually q 72-96 hr.
Infiltration: infusion of IV solution and/or medications into surrounding tissues, caused by puncturing of the blood vessel through improper insertion or frequent manipulation of IV catheter	Swelling, tenderness, coolness, and firmness of extremity; blanching of skin. Scale to grade severity: 0: No symptoms 1: Skin blanched, edema <1 inch, cool to touch, with or without pain 2: All the above plus edema of 1 to 6 inches 3: All the above plus extremity translucent, edema >6 inches, mild to moderate pain, possible numbness 4: All the above plus tight, leaking skin, deep pitting edema, circulatory impairment, moderate to severe pain	Assess for signs of infiltration. Discontinue infusion, and remove catheter. Apply pressure at site to stop bleeding. Apply warm compresses to increase circulation. If leaking of tissues occurs, cover area with sterile dressing until leaking subsides. Report grade 3 or 4 infiltrations to PCP. Use opposite extremity when inserting new IV catheter.

TABLE 39-15 Complications of Intravenous Therapy—cont'd

COMPLICATIONS	SYMPTOMS	NURSING CONSIDERATIONS
Extravasation: inadvertent infusion of vesicant (causing blisters, tissue sloughing) or irritating solution or medication into surrounding tissues	Similar to infiltration Burning and discomfort Blistering is a late sign.	Know which medications are considered vesicants, including dopamine, norepinephrine, high concentrations of electrolytes, and several antibiotics. Vesicant and irritating solutions or medications are infused slowly and through a larger vein or CVC. If extravasation is suspected, infusion is discontinued immediately. Notify PCP and obtain orders for extravasation treatment and/or antidote. Apply ice to extremity for 24-48 hr and elevate extremity. Use opposite extremity when inserting new IV.
Systemic Complications		
Fluid overload and pulmonary edema: occurs when the volume infused is greater than the cardiovascular system can tolerate; can lead to congestive heart failure, shock, and cardiac arrest	Early signs: restlessness, gradual increase in heart rate, headache, dyspnea, nonproductive cough Late signs: hypertension, severe dyspnea, gurgling respirations, productive cough of frothy sputum, crackles in lung bases, increased jugular vein distention	Prevention is key. Monitor for early signs and symptoms of fluid excess. Use an electronic infusion device for patients at risk, such as those with cardiac disease history or the elderly. Measure daily weights, intake, and output. Frequently assess IV infusion and ensure it is not infusing too rapidly. If fluid overload suspected, provide bed rest in high Fowler position, slow infusion rate to keep vein open, notify PCP immediately, provide oxygen as needed, and administer diuretics and pain medications as ordered.
Speed shock: systemic reaction when medication is administered too quickly	Sudden onset of dizziness, facial flushing, headache, and irregular heart rate during medication administration	Prevention is key. Follow recommended infusion rate for medication. Monitor gravity-flow sets closely during medication administration. Use electronic infusion devices whenever possible for medication administration. If suspected, stop infusion immediately, maintain IV access with IV solution that does not contain medication, notify PCP immediately, and monitor vital signs.
Air embolism: accidental entry of air into bloodstream due to improper preparation of IV tubing or loose connections	Chest pain, shoulder or low back pain, dyspnea, cyanosis, hypotension, tachycardia, syncope, or decreased level of consciousness	Prevention is key. Ensure that catheter and tubing are clamped closed when changing tubing. Use Luer-Lok connections on all tubing. Prime all tubing with IV solution before attaching to catheter. Follow agency protocol when removing a CVC. If IV bag has run dry, inspect tubing closely for air. If air embolism suspected, place patient in Trendelenburg position on left side. Locate the source of air and close off. Notify PCP immediately. Administer oxygen as needed. Have emergency resuscitation equipment available.

Continued

TABLE 39-15 Complications of Intravenous Therapy—cont'd

COMPLICATIONS	SYMPTOMS	NURSING CONSIDERATIONS
Catheter embolism: occurs when a catheter piece breaks off and enters bloodstream, leading to blockage of blood vessel; can occur during insertion when an over-the-needle catheter stylet is partially removed and then reinserted or when a through-the-needle catheter is pulled back and then reinserted through the needle; can occur when the catheter rests over a joint such as wrist or elbow, and the continued flexion weakens the catheter	Depends on where embolism is lodged General signs include cyanosis, hypotension, tachycardia, syncope, and decreased level of consciousness	Prevention is key. Use correct technique when inserting IV catheter. Avoid joints as insertion sites. Apply pressure when removing an IV. If suspected, place tourniquet above insertion site, make sure arterial flow is still intact. Initiate strict bed rest. Notify PCP immediately. Monitor patient for signs of distress. Have emergency equipment available.

Adapted from Infusion Nurses Society: *Policies and procedures for infusion nursing,* ed. 4, Norwood, Mass., 2011, Infusion Nurses Society.
CC, Central venous catheter; *IV,* intravenous; *PCP,* primary care provider.

TABLE 39-16 Intravenous Tubing Change

TYPE OF INFUSION	FREQUENCY OF TUBING CHANGE
Primary IV solution	Continuous: Change primary and secondary (piggyback) tubing q 72-96 hr; check agency policy. Intermittent: Change primary and secondary tubing q 24 hr.
Blood and blood components	Continuous: If multiple units are to be administered continuously, tubing is changed q 4 hr. Intermittent: If only one unit is to be administered, dispose of tubing after infusion is completed and tubing is flushed with saline.
Intravenous fat emulsion (IVFE)	Continuous: If the fat emulsion is to be infused on a continuous basis, the tubing is changed q 24 hr. Intermittent: Dispose of the tubing after the fat emulsion has completely infused; use new tubing with the next dose.
Total parenteral nutrition	Continuous with IVFE: Tubing is changed q 24 hr. Continuous without IVFE: Tubing is changed q 72 hr. Intermittent: Tubing is changed q 24 hr.

From Infusion Nurses Society: *Policies and procedures for infusion nursing,* ed. 4, Norwood, Mass., 2011, Infusion Nurses Society.

ready. A good rule of thumb is to have the new bag ready to hang when there is an hour's worth of fluid left in the bag currently infusing.

On entering a patient's room, there are key areas to assess. Begin at the bag and verify that the correct solution is infusing at the correct rate and the appropriate amount of fluid is in the bag. Examine the drip chamber, make sure it is half full and the IV is dripping. Examine the tubing for kinks or loose connections. Check the date on the tubing. Tubing is changed every 24 to 72 hours, depending on the type of IV therapy (Table 39-16).

Move down to the insertion site, checking for signs of complications. Observe the dressing; it should be clean, dry, and intact. If the dressing is soiled, wet, or loose, it is changed immediately (Skill 39-2). Notice the date of insertion. For peripheral IV lines, the site is rotated every 72 to 96 hours to prevent catheter-related complications. Check the agency policies for specific protocols.

The IV solution, rate, tubing, and insertion site are assessed every hour. Certain catheter-related complications require the IV infusion to be discontinued immediately (Nursing Care Guideline: Discontinuing a Peripheral Intravenous Line box). Assess the patient for systemic complications.

Care of the Patient With Central Venous Access

The assessment and care of a patient with a CVC, including PICCs, is similar to that of a patient with a peripheral IV line (Ethical, Legal, and Professional Practice box and Evidence-Based Practice box). There are some key differences, however.

NURSING CARE GUIDELINE

Discontinuing a Peripheral Intravenous Line

Background

- To avoid catheter-related bloodstream infections (CRBSIs), remove vascular access devices (VADs) if the following occur:
  - The device is no longer needed.
  - It is no longer patent.
  - As soon as one lumen is no longer patent (if the VAD is a central line with more than one lumen).
  - Break in the integrity of the device occurs (notify the primary care provider of the need for removal).
- Remove all IV lines before discharge, unless the VAD is a central line and the patient will be receiving home intravenous therapy.

Procedural Concerns

- Clamp all tubing.
- Wear clean gloves.
- Loosen all dressings and tape.
  - Apply opposing pressure to skin while removing adhesives.
  - Secure the catheter with slight pressure to avoid dislodgement while removing the dressing.
- Holding the gauze over the site with one hand, use the other hand to slide the catheter out.
- Apply pressure over the site using the gauze.
- Dispose of the catheter and dressing per facility policy and procedures.
- Apply a slight pressure dressing to the site.

Documentation Concerns

- Document removal and discontinuation information, including the following:
  - Fluids infused
  - Date
  - Time of day
  - Site
- Record the site and catheter assessment. For example, is the site intact?
- Note any problems or patient discomfort with the procedure.

Evidence-Based Practice

- Webster and colleagues (2010) performed a review of randomized clinical trials to determine whether a peripheral VAD should be routinely changed every 72 hours, as has been a standard in many facilities.
- The results revealed no benefit to this standard and found that a peripheral IV catheter should be changed only if there are patency issues or an indication such as signs of infection.

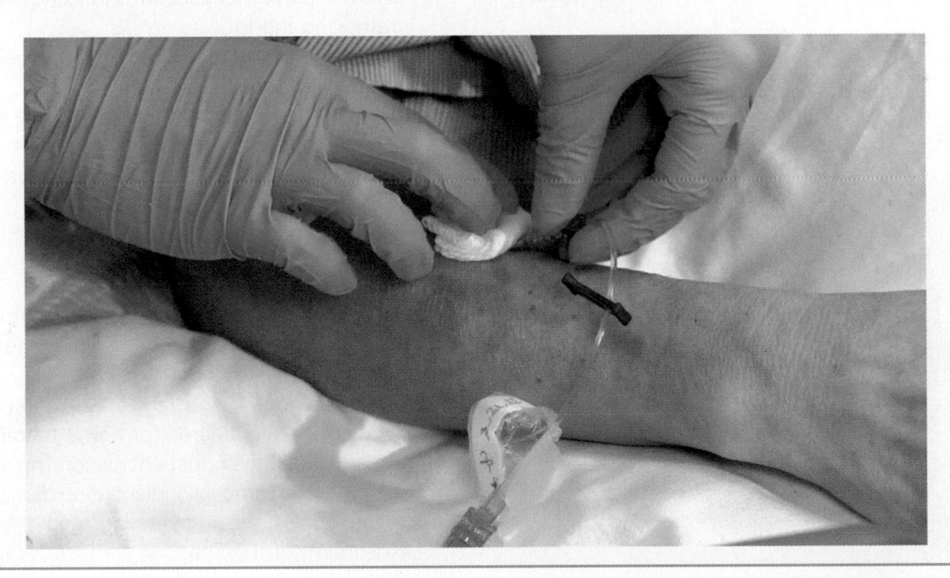

The tubing is changed more frequently, usually every 24 hours. Check the agency policy for specifics. According to the Infusion Nurses Society (INS, 2011), gauze dressings for a CVC should be changed every 48 hours. With transparent dressings, the interval increases to every 3 to 7 days, depending on agency policy. Dressings are changed immediately if wet, soiled, or loose. CVC dressings are changed using strict aseptic, or sterile, technique (Nursing Care Guideline: Peripherally Inserted Central Catheter: Dressing Change and Care box and see Skill 39-3).

ETHICAL, LEGAL, AND PROFESSIONAL PRACTICE

Informed Consent

- Insertion of a central venous catheter (CVC) is considered an invasive procedure and requires a signed consent form.
- It is the responsibility of the primary care provider to obtain written consent from the patient.
- It is the nurse's responsibility to ensure the consent form has been signed and that the patient has no questions or concerns.

EVIDENCE-BASED PRACTICE

Guidelines for Central Venous Catheter Use in Adults

A systematic review of medical and nursing research led to recommendations when caring for a patient with a central venous catheter (CVC):

- Patients should receive clear verbal and written information about CVCs, including the risks and benefits, before providing consent for CVC insertion. Signed consent is obtained by the primary care provider before insertion.
- Ultrasound is recommended for guiding insertion of a peripherally inserted central catheter (PICC) when peripheral veins are not visible or palpable.
- Vigorous cleansing of the skin with chlorhexidine is recommended before insertion.
- Dressings are changed 24 hours after insertion and weekly thereafter when transparent dressings are used.
- Stabilization devices are used in place of sutures. CVCs are not sutured in or around the vein.
- Needle-free connectors are used to reduce risk of infection to patients and needlestick injury to nurses.
- Other recommendations can be found in a systematic review (Bishop, Dougherty, Bodenham, et al, 2007).

NURSING CARE GUIDELINE

Peripherally Inserted Central Catheter: Dressing Change and Care

Background

- Primary use of a peripherally inserted central catheter (PICC) is to permit intermediate-term to long-term intravenous access.
- Fewer complications occur with a PICC than with other IV forms because the tip of the line ends in a large vein.
- The PICC use is beneficial in that it allows therapeutic interventions without hospitalization.

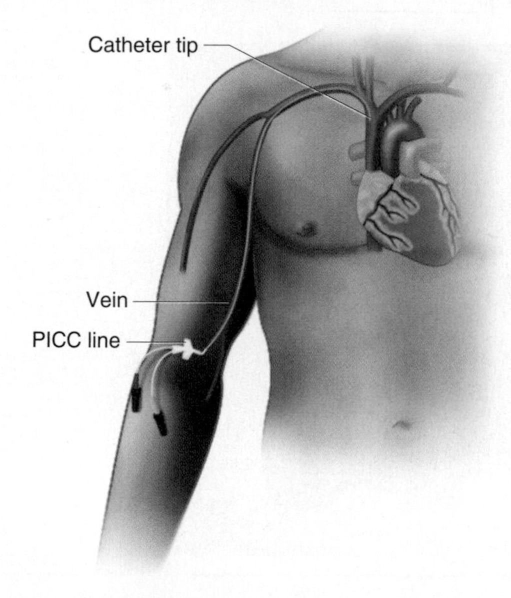

Procedural Concerns

- Follow strict sterile technique to prevent catheter-related bloodstream infections (CRBSIs).
  - Be familiar with individual facility policy and procedures for use of PICCs.
  - Never take a blood pressure on an arm with a PICC.
  - Avoid strenuous exercise of an arm with a PICC.
  - Do not get the site wet.
  - Assess the site.
  - Flush all lumens with 10 mL of preservative-free saline (see the Nursing Care Guideline: Flushing an Intravenous Line box).
- Follow Skill 39-3.
- Some PICCs have an extra catheter from the site to the hub.
  - Ensure the catheter is not moved during the dressing change. Measure the length of the catheter from the site to the hub outside the body to be sure that it has not changed from the previous assessment.
  - Maintain the sterility of the catheter: clean it, and coil it under the dressing.
- Per facility policy and procedures, nurses may be responsible for removing PICCs:
  - Ensure proper education and competency of the nurse removing the PICC.
  - Have the patient bear down (i.e., perform the Valsalva maneuver) when removing the PICC.
  - Gently pull the catheter parallel to the skin to remove it; it should slide out without resistance or discomfort.
  - Apply pressure to the site with a sterile 2 × 2 gauze pad for at least 5 minutes.
  - Apply an occlusive dressing for 24 hours.

Documentation Concerns

- Document the site and catheter assessments.
- Include the measured length of the catheter from the site to the hub outside the body.
- Record the patient and family education that was provided regarding the procedures for home therapy.
- Note any problems or patient discomfort with the procedure.
- Document the removal or discontinuation information, including the fluids infused, the date and time of day, and the assessment of the site.

Evidence-Based Practice

- When assessing patency of a PICC, resistance during a flush does not necessarily indicate occlusion. Do not force the flush or apply more pressure. Instead, reposition the patient or have the patient cough. The tip of the catheter may lie against a structure, which this technique will solve (Macklin, 2010).
- Ensure patency of PICCs with several lumens, because thrombosis may support infection. If a lumen becomes occluded, notify the primary care provider for treatment. If the lumen is unable to become patent, the PICC should be replaced (Macklin, 2010).

Routine site rotation is not needed for CVCs or PICCs. CVCs are discontinued only with a written order from the PCP. A specially trained nurse can remove a nontunneled CVC. To do so, place the patient in a supine position, clamp the infusion, and remove the dressing. Apply clean gloves. If the CVC is sutured in place, remove all sutures. Instruct the patient to take a deep breath and hold it. Grasp the catheter, and remove it in a continuous motion with the dominant hand. Have a sterile dressing ready in the nondominant hand, and place it over the site after the catheter is removed. Instruct the patient to breathe normally while providing direct pressure to the site until bleeding has stopped (at least 1 minute). Cover the site with an occlusive dressing. Inspect the catheter to ensure that it is intact.

Dispose of the catheter, tubing, and dressing in the hazardous waste container. Document the process, significant findings, and patient response. Removal of a PICC is performed by nurses trained in insertion and maintenance of these catheters.

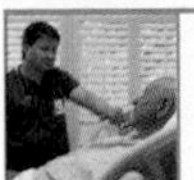

6. List focused assessments leading to a diagnosis of *Fluid Volume Excess* related to sodium and water retention. Include interventions and teaching points.

BLOOD ADMINISTRATION

For patients with fluid volume deficit, IV therapy is effective in restoring fluids and electrolytes to normal levels. However, crystalloids cannot replace the other essential components of blood loss resulting from trauma, anemia, hemorrhage, or surgery. Blood components are necessary to maintain the patient's oxygen and carbon dioxide transport capacity, for

NURSING CARE GUIDELINE

Administering Blood Products

Background

- Blood products are administered to replace lost blood or blood components.
- Ensure the blood that will be administered is the appropriate type for the recipient and that crossmatching was done.
- Informed consent (see Chapter 37, Nursing Care Guideline: Obtaining and Completing Informed Consent box) must be obtained before administration.
- Rapid transfusions may occur through a central line, but blood is warmed before being administered.

Procedural Concerns

- Assessments of the following are performed:
  - Verify patient allergy information.
  - Verify whether the patient has had previous transfusion reactions.
  - If a patient does not already have an 18- to 20-gauge (or larger) IV line in place, start one (see Skill 39-1).
  - The Food and Drug Administration (2011) requires blood products to have bar codes to enable scanning to reduce the incidence of administration errors.
  - Check the blood product that is to be administered to verify that it is not clotted. If it is clotted, do not use it; obtain a replacement bag.
  - Obtain the patient's vital signs.
- Working with another nurse, identify the following:
  - The patient
  - Blood group and type (of the patient and the blood product to be administered)
  - Identification number of the blood product
  - Expiration date of the blood product
- Maintain sterile technique.
- Disconnect running infusions, leaving a saline lock (see the Nursing Care Guideline: Converting an Intravenous Line box).
- Prime a Y-type blood infusion set.
  - It must have an in-line filter.

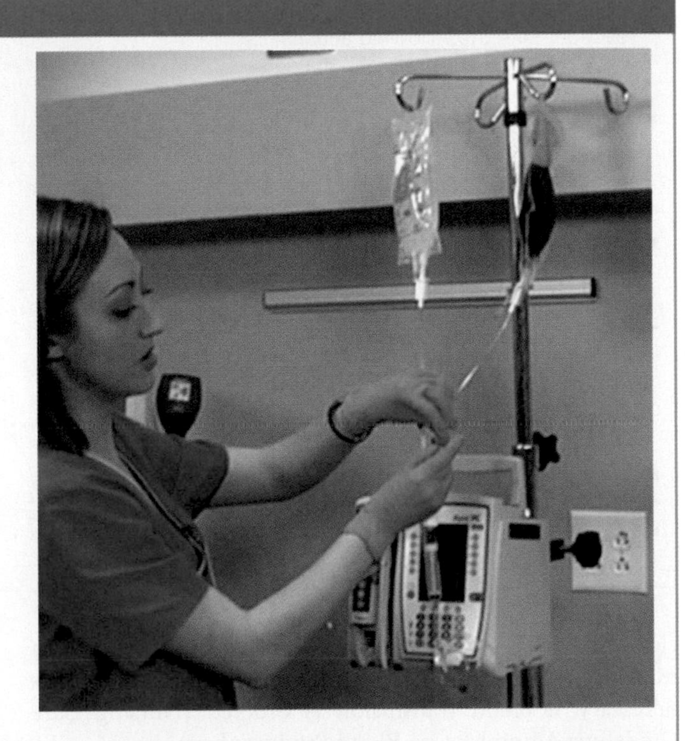

  - Hang it with sterile 0.9% normal saline solution (NSS) on a Y line. Never infuse any other solution or medications with blood products except 0.9% NSS.
  - Use the NSS to prime the infusion set.
- Infuse the blood product slowly over the first 15 minutes.
  - Infusion rate should be 5 to 50 mL/hr.
  - Do not leave the patient.
- Monitor the patient for adverse reactions:
  - Flushing
  - Fever
  - Dyspnea
  - Hypotension
  - Itching
  - Pain

Continued

NURSING CARE GUIDELINE—cont'd

Administering Blood Products—cont'd

Procedural Concerns—cont'd

- Chills
- Shortness of breath
- Nausea
- Unexplained emotions

- Increase the infusion rate if the patient does not demonstrate adverse reactions.
  - Blood products must be infused within 4 hours (maximum) after leaving the laboratory.
  - Minimum infusion rate is determined per facility policy and procedures or per PCP order.
- Continue to monitor the patient frequently. The minimum frequency is as per facility policy and procedures or PCP order.
- Monitoring may be performed more frequently according to nursing judgment and depending on the patient's status. If the patient shows any signs or symptoms of transfusion reaction, take the following actions:
  - Stop the transfusion immediately.
  - Change all tubing and the infusion set.
  - Hang a new IV solution of 0.9% NSS.
  - Notify the PCP.
  - Send the blood product and tubing to the laboratory or blood bank per facility policy and procedures.
- After the transfusion is complete, take the following steps:
  - Disconnect the tubing from the saline lock (see the Nursing Care Guideline: Converting an Intravenous Line box).
  - Tubing is discarded per facility policy and procedures.
  - New tubing is used for each transfusion.
  - Restart the primary infusion if ordered.

Documentation Concerns

- Document the reason for the transfusion.
- Document vital signs before, during, and after the transfusion.
- Record follow-up specifics regarding the transfusion's effectiveness as a treatment for the patient's condition.
- Include the date, starting and ending times for the transfusion, blood type, and the component and amount infused.
- Record the blood product and patient identification information and the blood product expiration date.
- Note any observations made during the required monitoring period during and after the transfusion.
- Document patient intake and output.
- Evaluate pertinent laboratory results before and after the procedure.
- If the patient has an adverse event, document the event in detail, and follow facility policy and procedures.

Evidence-Based Practice

- It is imperative to follow facility policy and procedures for the identification of the patient and the blood product before beginning the transfusion, including use of two nurses during the verification process. The most common reason for a transfusion reaction is inappropriate identification of the patient and matching the blood product to the patient. Technology, such as plastic identification locks, bar code medication verification, and transfusion reading devices, is implemented to reduce errors (Vamvakas and Blajchman, 2010).
- Most reactions to a transfusion occur within the first 15 minutes of initiation. Monitor the patient during this time for signs of a reaction.
- "If policies, procedures, and guidelines are not followed correctly, the patient's safety may be compromised, and this may result in a fatality. Not all transfusion adverse events can be avoided, but early detection and management is essential. Staff should receive appropriate training and have their competency assessed. Nurses should ensure that they are aware of the risks involved and the role and responsibilities throughout the transfusion process" (Watson and Hearnshaw, 2010, pp. 47-48).

clotting, to maintain oncotic pressure, and to protect from infection. When replacing the lost blood components becomes necessary, a blood transfusion is ordered (Nursing Care Guideline: Administering Blood Products box).

QSEN FOCUS!

The use of technology and standardized practices supports safety and quality. The value of standardization for safety is exhibited through the use of bar code scanning before blood product administration.

Complications

The three main types of adverse reactions to blood products are hemolytic, allergic, and febrile. Hemolytic reactions (i.e., destruction of red blood cells) occur because of ABO or Rh incompatibilities between the patient and donor blood. This life-threatening reaction can occur with administration of 10 to 15 mL of incompatible blood. Multiple checks of the patient and donor information are essential.

Allergic reactions are much more common and can range from mild to severe. Allergic reactions occur when a patient has a hypersensitivity response to plasma proteins in the donor's blood.

Febrile nonhemolytic reactions occur when the patient reacts to the white blood cells, platelets, or plasma proteins. It causes a rise of 2°F in the patient's temperature and can occur during or after the transfusion. If patient is febrile at initiation of blood product, verify administration of the infusion with health care provider.

For any adverse reaction, the nurse's first action is to stop the transfusion. The nurse then begins an IV infusion of 0.9% normal saline with new tubing at a keep-vein-open rate, notifies the ordering physician, and closely monitors the patient.

Other complications include fluid overload and bacterial contamination. Table 39-17 lists complications of blood transfusions, symptoms, and nursing care.

TABLE 39-17 Complications of Blood Transfusion

OCCURRENCE	SYMPTOMS	NURSING IMPLICATIONS
Allergic Response		
Fairy common, based on a hypersensitivity response to the foreign plasma proteins	*Mild:* local erythema, hives, itching, asthmatic wheezing *Severe:* laryngeal swelling, dyspnea, tachypnea, chest pain, cardiac arrest	Stop transfusion. Notify ordering physician immediately. Administer antihistamines; in mild cases, may be able to continue transfusion after antihistamine has taken effect. Continue to assess patient and monitor vital signs. Document the reaction, subsequent treatment, and patient response.
Acute Hemolytic Reaction		
Occurs with antigen-antibody reaction due to ABO or Rh incompatibilities Can result from errors in mislabeling crossmatch sample sent to laboratory, improper crossmatching, or errors in patient and blood verification at bedside	Chills, fever, facial flushing, burning along the vein, lumbar or flank pain, chest pain, shock	Stop transfusion immediately. Remove tubing and replace with new IV tubing and normal saline solution at keep-vein-open (KVO) rate. Notify ordering physician immediately. Notify the blood bank. Monitor vital signs. Have emergency equipment available. Send remaining blood, blood tubing and filter, and a sample of patient's blood and urine to the laboratory. Document the reaction, subsequent treatment, and patient response.
Febrile Nonhemolytic Reaction		
Occurs when the patient reacts to the white blood cells in donor blood Occurs in up to 6% of all transfusions	Defined as a 2° F rise in body temperature compared with pretransfusion reading Chills and malaise common	Stop the infusion. Notify ordering physician immediately. Notify the blood bank. Administer antipyretics and/or antihistamines as ordered. Document the reaction, subsequent treatment, and patient response. Can be avoided by using leukocyte-reduced components or washed red blood cells.
Bacterial Contamination		
Occurs when during the donation or preparation of blood, usually by organisms capable of surviving cold temperatures, such as *Pseudomonas* or *Staphylococcus*	Abdominal cramping, chills, diarrhea, fever, shock, onset of renal failure, vomiting	Infuse blood in less than 4 hr; stop infusion after 4 hr. Change administration sets q 4 hr or after each unit. Stop the infusion immediately if symptoms occur. Notify the ordering physician. Administer antibiotics, corticosteroids, and epinephrine as ordered. Have emergency equipment available. If the patient is discharged shortly after transfusion, explain the symptoms of infection, such as fever, chills, diarrhea, and abdominal cramping. Instruct the patient to contact the ordering physician immediately if symptoms occur.
Circulatory Overload		
Usually occurs when whole blood is transfused too quickly or packed red blood cells (PRBCs) lead to a fluid shift from the interstitial to vascular space	Signs of fluid volume excess, including dyspnea, headache, tachycardia, hypertension, and distended jugular veins	Slow or stop infusion. Use packed RBCs instead of whole blood. Notify the ordering physician immediately. Administer oxygen as needed. Administer diuretics as ordered. If the patient is discharged shortly after transfusion, explain the symptoms of fluid overload, such as difficulty breathing, edema, headache, or increased heart rate. Instruct the patient to contact the physician immediately if symptoms occur.

From Weinstein SM, Hagle, ME: *Plumer's principles & practice of infusion therapy,* ed. 9, Philadelphia, 2014, Lippincott Williams & Wilkins.

TOTAL PARENTERAL NUTRITION

Total parenteral nutrition (TPN) is a hypertonic IV solution designed to meet a patient's total nutritional needs. It contains amino acids, glucose, lipids, vitamins, minerals, electrolytes, and trace elements. TPN provides the calories, protein building blocks, and fluid needed to promote wound healing and meet metabolic requirements. It is used when the patient is unable to meet nutritional and metabolic demands through oral intake or when disease (e.g., pancreatitis, ulcerative colitis, bowel obstruction) or surgery requires complete bowel rest. Indications for TPN include debilitating illnesses lasting longer than 2 weeks, loss of more than 10% of pre-illness weight, serum albumin levels less than 3.5 g/dL, or nitrogen loss due to extensive burns or draining wounds.

Infusion

Because of the increased tonicity of TPN, it is infused through central venous access with a PICC, CVC, or implanted port. Often, a multilumen CVC is used, with one lumen dedicated to TPN only. If a patient requires other IV medications or therapy, the other lumens can be used, or a peripheral IV site can be used.

> **! SAFE PRACTICE ALERT**
>
> Never piggyback or administer other medications or blood products into the same line as total parenteral nutrition.

When beginning TPN, the infusion should begin slowly, allowing the pancreas to adjust to the increased glucose levels. The normal amount of TPN is 2.5 to 3 liters infused over 24 hours. A continuous infusion allows for more stable blood glucose control (Nursing Care Guideline: Administering Total Parenteral Nutrition and Lipids box).

Complications

The complications associated with TPN are similar to those for any CVC use: infection, air embolism, or fluid overload. Because of the contents in TPN, the patient is at a higher risk for infection. Strict sterile technique is used during IV care, especially during dressing, bag, and tubing changes. With the high levels of dextrose in TPN, patients, especially those with a history of diabetes, can develop hyperglycemia. Blood sugar levels are checked on a routine basis. Insulin is often ordered by the PCP and added by the pharmacy to the TPN solution to help offset this effect. Rebound hypoglycemia can occur

NURSING CARE GUIDELINE

Administering Total Parenteral Nutrition and Lipids

Background

- Nutritional fluids are administered intravenously when enteral feedings are contraindicated or insufficient.
- Total parenteral nutrition (TPN) is ordered specifically for a patient's needs and is based on laboratory results for the patient.

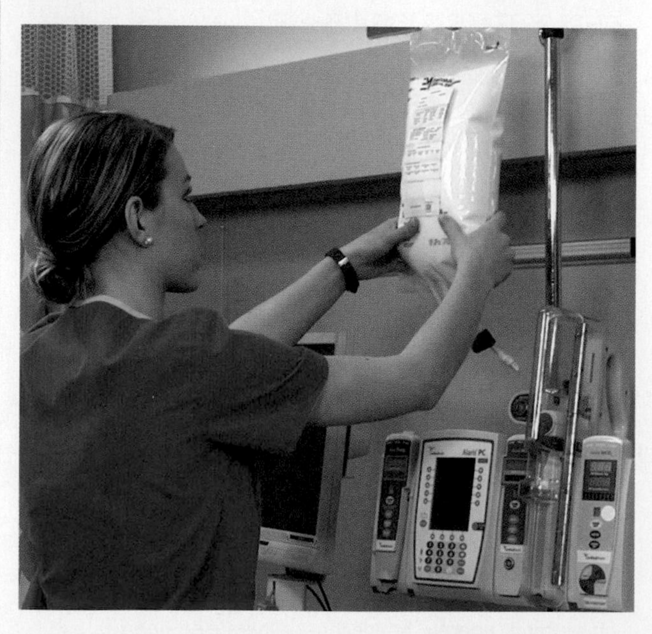

- The primary ingredients are proteins, carbohydrates, and fats (i.e., lipids).

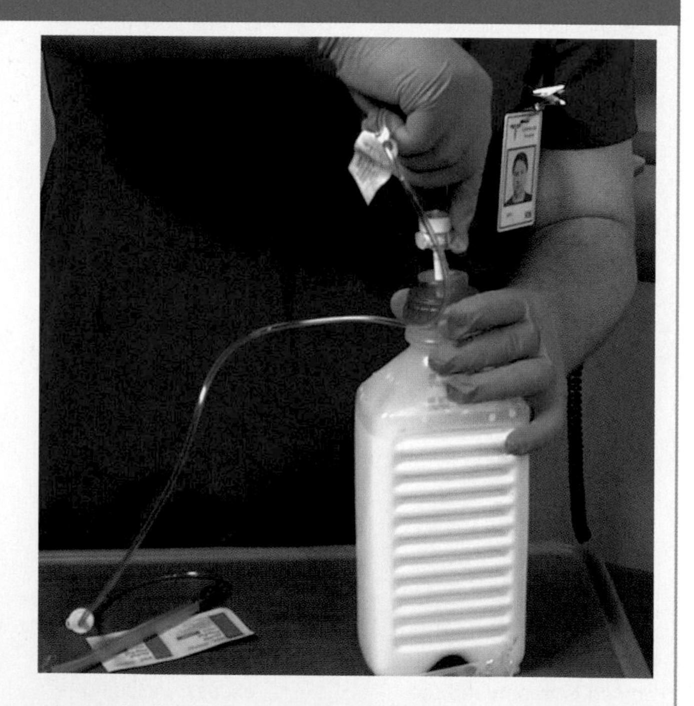

- It also includes electrolytes and vitamins.
- If needed, TPN may include medications.
- Lipids are fatty substances that provide calories and are given as emulsions or in conjunction with TPN.
- TPN is a hypertonic solution (highly concentrated) that easily flows into body fluids.
- Collaboration with the dietician and pharmacist is necessary when caring for a patient receiving TPN.

NURSING CARE GUIDELINE—cont'd

Procedural Concerns

- Ensure sufficient training, education, and competency before performing this skill.
- A central line is used to administer TPN:
  - Designate a separate lumen for TPN.

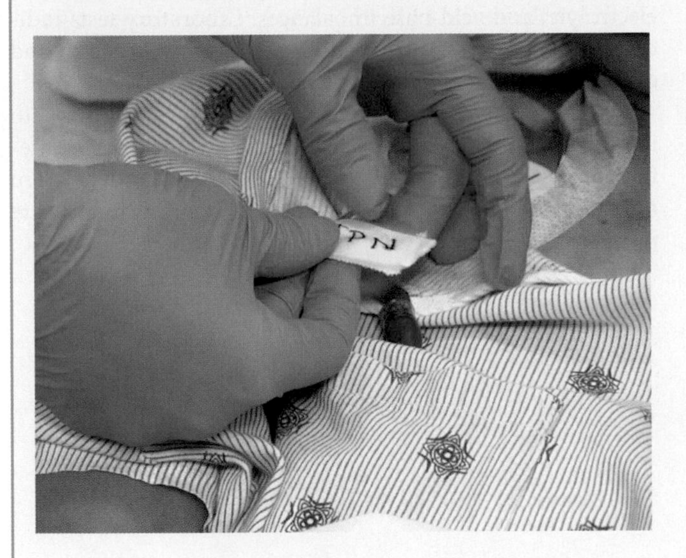

    - Do not infuse any other substances into this line.
    - Keeping TPN separate prevents incompatibility issues with other solutions.
  - TPN is infused using a pump.
- Assess and monitor the patient for the following:
  - Allergies
  - Laboratory results:
    - Electrolytes
    - Blood urea nitrogen (BUN)
    - Clotting factors
    - Glucose (tested every 6 to 24 hours, as ordered)
    - Serum protein
    - Central line patency and insertion site
- Perform the following working with another nurse:
  - Identify the patient.
  - Verify the TPN components against the primary care provider order.
  - Check the expiration date.
  - Ensure vitamin K has been ordered, because vitamin K is produced largely by intestinal bacteria that currently may be absent, but it is needed to produce clotting factors in the gut.
  - Because TPN is considered a medication, ensure compliance with the Six Rights of Medication Administration (see Chapter 35, Nursing Care Guideline: Six Rights of Medication Administration box).
- Maintain sterile technique.
- Prime the infusion set:
  - Use a new infusion set with each infusion.
  - Use an in-line filter with TPN.
  - Do not use a filter with lipids.
- Do not use TPN after it has been hanging for 24 hours; discard any unused solution.
- Assess the following:
  - Patient vital signs at least every 4 hours
  - Daily weight
  - Intake and output
- The administration rate of TPN is increased slowly at the beginning of the infusion and weaned off gradually at the end.
  - Do not suddenly stop a TPN transfusion.
  - The gradual increase and decrease in infusion rate prevents hypoglycemic shock.
- Nurses should never mix medications into TPN.

Documentation Concerns

- Document the reason for administering TPN and lipids.
- Include assessments and monitoring as described in the Procedural Concerns section.
- Note the date, starting and ending times for the infusion, and the second nurse's verification.
- Document the TPN and lipid product information and the patient identification information.
- Describe the observations made during the required monitoring period throughout the infusion.
- Record intake and output.
- If the patient has an adverse event, document the event in detail, and follow facility policy and procedures.

Evidence-Based Practice

- TPN has been determined to be a high risk factor for catheter-related bloodstream infections (CRBSIs) due to the invasive line and the hyperosmolar solution.
- TPN should be used only when absolutely necessary because CRBSIs can cause fatalities (Fraher, Collins, Bourke, et al, 2009, p. 129).

when the TPN solution is abruptly discontinued. TPN infusion rates should be decreased incrementally before completely discontinuing the solution. The nurse must continually monitor the rate to ensure the TPN is infusing at the ordered rate and that new bags are hung promptly to prevent interruptions in the infusion.

With the increased use of long-term CVCs and decreased length of hospital stays, many patients find it necessary to continue IV therapy at home (Home Care Considerations box). This can take the form of continuous IV infusions, such as TPN, or intermittent medication administration, such as long-term antibiotics. The nurse works closely with the patient and family members to ensure correct administration of the therapy and diligent monitoring for signs of complications.

When oral intake is limited, peripheral parenteral nutrition (PPN) can be used to supplement a patient's nutritional status. PPN contains the same ingredients as TPN but at much lower concentrations. It can be infused through a peripheral line, eliminating the need for and avoiding the risks of a CVC.

HOME CARE CONSIDERATIONS

Intravenous Therapy at Home

- Key aspects include the purpose of the IV therapy, initiating the infusion, monitoring the infusion, and assessing for complications.
- Maintaining sterile technique is critical during preparation of the IV, while accessing the site, and during tubing and dressing changes.
- The patient should understand the signs and symptoms of complications and know when to notify the home health nurse or the primary care provider.
- The home health nurse plans frequent visits during the IV infusion, especially when the caregiver is accessing the site and during tubing and dressing changes to assess the family's understanding of the process and their ability to safely administer IV therapy.
- The home health nurse assesses the patient frequently to evaluate the effectiveness of the therapy and signs of complications, especially catheter-related infections.

EVALUATION

To determine the effectiveness of the interventions, the nurse evaluates achievement of the patient goals and outcomes designed to establish and maintain normal fluid, electrolyte, and acid-base balance. Continuous evaluation of goals and revision of the care plan are necessary for patients with fluid, electrolyte, and acid-base imbalances. Laboratory tests indicate the patient's response to fluid and electrolyte therapy and determine whether changes are needed.

Assessing measures of fluid balance allows the nurse to identify problems and intervene early to avoid severe or life-threatening complications. Significant deviations from normal patient responses are reported to the primary care provider.

SKILL 39-1 Starting a Peripheral Intravenous Infusion

PURPOSE

- To provide fluids
- To administer medications
- To replace electrolytes
- To promote comfort
- To provide nutrition
- To maintain emergency access for medications

RESOURCES

- IV Angiocath (16 to 24 gauge, depending on the size of the vein and type of infusion)
- ChloraPrep swab
- 2 × 2 gauze pads
- Tourniquet
- Saline lock extension tubing
- 3- to 10-mL prefilled saline flush
- Dressing supplies (per facility policy and procedures)
- Clean gloves
- Personal protective equipment (PPE) as required

COLLABORATION AND DELEGATION

- Starting a peripheral IV line may not be delegated to unlicensed assistive personnel (UAP).
- UAP may observe a peripheral IV line during care and should report the following to the nurse.
  - Burning, redness, pain, coolness, leaking, bleeding, or swelling at the peripheral IV insertion site
  - Patient concerns or complaints
  - Low volume in an IV bag
  - Alarms sounding on the IV pump
- Many facilities have an IV therapy team that maintains the IV sites. For the comfort and safety of the patient, nurses coordinate with these teams per facility policy and procedures and their own skill level.

EVIDENCE-BASED PRACTICE

- Chlorhexidine antiseptic is used to clean the peripheral IV insertion site for 30 seconds to reduce infections (Moureau, 2009).
- Devices in development are all-in-one IV access devices (including Angiocath, needle, and extension tubing) which are entirely closed insertion devices. More research is needed, but these devices may decrease complications and the need to replace the IV line frequently.

SPECIAL CIRCUMSTANCES

1. **Assess:** Is the nurse unable to obtain IV placement after two attempts?
   Intervention: Seek assistance; do *not* continue attempts.

PREPROCEDURE

I. Check PCP orders and the patient care plan.
Knowledge of patient-specific orders is critical for safe patient care.

II. Gather supplies and equipment.
Preparing for the patient encounter saves time and promotes patient trust.

III. Perform hand hygiene.
Frequent hand hygiene prevents the spread of microorganisms.

IV. Maintain standard precautions.
Use of the correct personal protective equipment (PPE) is required whenever contact with bodily fluids is possible, to reduce the transfer of pathogens.

V. Introduce yourself.
Initial communication establishes the role of the nurse and begins a professional relationship.

VI. Provide for patient privacy.
It is important to maintain patient dignity.

VII. Identify the patient, using two identifiers.
Identifying a patient involves scanning barcodes or comparing the patient's stated name and birthdate to information on the patient's wristband or health record. The correct person must receive the correct treatment.

VIII. Explain the procedure to the patient.
The nurse has a responsibility to inform a patient before initiating care. Information may ease patient anxiety and facilitate cooperation.

PROCEDURE

Starting a Peripheral IV

Follow preprocedure steps I through VIII.

1. Preparing the infusion site: Prepare the necessary supplies on the bedside table.
   a. Obtain an appropriate-size catheter, and have an extra one available.
   b. Connect a 3- to 10-mL, sterile syringe prefilled with normal saline solution (NSS) to the saline lock extension tubing. Inject the saline to prime the tubing, and keep the syringe connected.
   c. Set out gauze, dressing supplies, and tape.
   Preparing items in advance provides organization to facilitate the performance of the procedure by avoiding interruptions. Using a prefilled syringe promotes accuracy. Priming reduces the risk of an air embolus.
2. Raise the bed to working height, and lower a side rail as needed.
   Setting the bed at the correct working height for the provider prevents provider discomfort and possible injury.

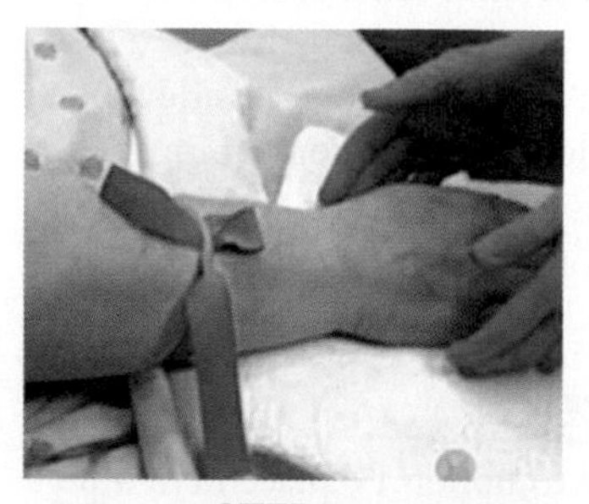

STEP 3a

3. Identify an appropriate site on the most distal area of the patient's nondominant arm, unless contraindicated, and prepare the site:
   a. Apply a tourniquet 4 to 6 inches above the site using a quick-release knot.
   b. Ensure there is a distal pulse.
   c. Move the extremity to a dependent position.
   Using a distal site allows other sites to remain available for subsequent use. Using the patient's nondominant arm if possible promotes patient comfort and allows the patient to perform activities of daily living (ADLs). The tourniquet restricts blood flow and makes the veins more visible and palpable. The quick-release knot allows one-handed release.

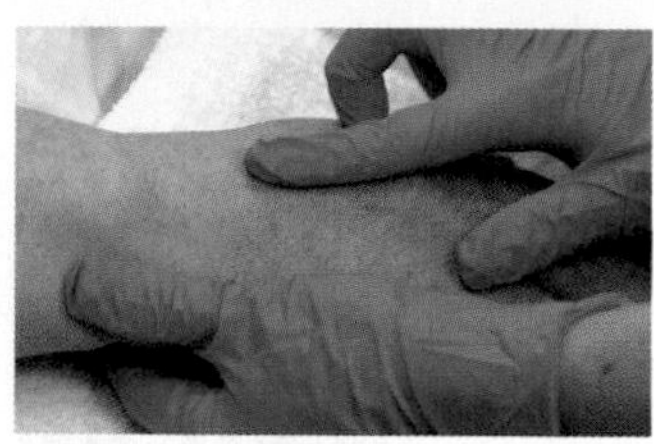

STEP 4

4. Select an appropriate vein:
   a. Preferred veins are the cephalic, basilica, median, radial, and the dorsal veins of the hand.
   b. Use the index finger to trace and palpate the selected vein; it should be bouncy and well dilated.
   The listed veins are preferred due to strength, resilience, and size. Using larger veins reduces the risk of hematoma. Palpation determines the size, depth, and direction of the vein and facilitates accuracy during the procedure.
5. Leave the tourniquet in place for a maximum of 2 minutes and then release.
   Releasing the tourniquet restores blood flow, prevents tissue damage, and promotes patient comfort.
6. After 2 minutes, repeat procedure steps 3 through 5 until an appropriate vein is located. Release the tourniquet.
   Releasing the tourniquet restores blood flow, prevents tissue damage, and promotes patient comfort.
7. Apply clean gloves.
   Using gloves reduces the spread of microorganisms.
8. Repalpate the selected vein.
   Ensure accuracy of the original assessment.
9. Apply the tourniquet, using a quick-release knot.
   The tourniquet restricts blood flow and makes the veins more visible and palpable. The quick-release knot allows one-handed release.
10. Cleanse the site using a 2% chlorhexidine swab and using a brisk motion until all of the solution is used. Allow the site to air-dry.
    Proper antiseptic procedure is used to prevent the spread of microorganisms. There is no specific direction or technique to be used when preparing a site with 2% chlorhexidine. Air-drying prevents contamination.

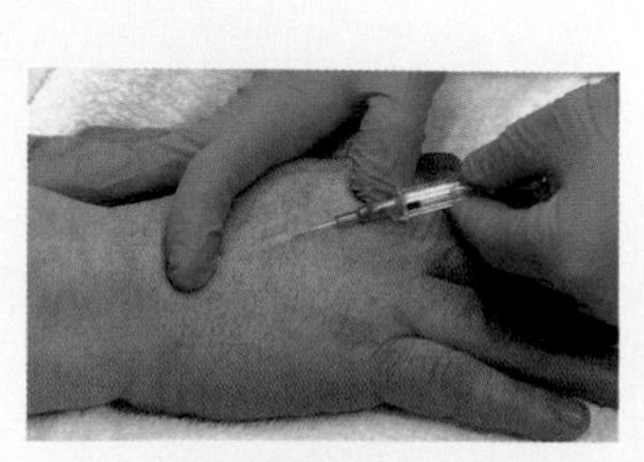

STEP 11

11. Insert the IV Angiocath.
    a. Uncap the needle.
    b. Place the thumb of the nondominant hand below the site.
    c. Use the thumb to apply slight pressure, and pull down toward the wrist.

d. Hold the bevel at a 10- to 30-degree angle below the insertion site.
e. Insert the needle stylet. The initial resistance indicates entry into the vein; advance ¼ inch. If blood returns, stop inserting the needle.
f. Advance the catheter off of the needle stylet.
g. Slide the needle out of the catheter, stabilize the vein and device using gentle pressure 1 to 2 inches above (proximal to) the site to hold the catheter in place, and activate the safety device on the needle stylet.

Proper caregiver hand position stabilizes the patient's arm and vein, which prevents vein rolling or movement, reduces the risk of puncturing a vein, and promotes accuracy and stability during insertion. Using the proper bevel angle prevents accidental needlestick and provider injury. Applying pressure decreases bleeding.

12. Remove the tourniquet with one hand.
Releasing the tourniquet restores blood flow, prevents tissue damage, and promotes patient comfort. Use the gentle pressure to assure the catheter is still secure.
13. Connect the catheter hub to the saline lock extension tubing:
a. Secure the catheter using gentle pressure above the site.
b. Carefully twist the tubing onto the hub.
c. Flush the IV line with NSS (see the Nursing Care Guideline: Flushing an Intravenous Line box).
d. Connect to the IV solution if ordered.
Adding the hub completes the device and closes it from the external environment. Applying pressure assists in securing the device and reduces bleeding. Flushing blood from the line with NSS reduces risk of infection and ensures patency.
14. Secure the device with a dressing per facility policy and procedures.
Dressings decrease bleeding and risk of infection.
15. Label the dressing with initials, date and time of day when it was applied, and the gauge of the catheter.
Proper labeling prevents adverse events and medical errors.
16. Discard the needle that has the safety device engaged into a sharps container.
Proper disposal of the needle reduces the spread of microorganisms and prevents accidental needlestick.

Follow postprocedure steps I through VI.

POSTPROCEDURE

I. Return the bed to its lowest position, raise the top side rails, and verify that the call light is within reach of the patient.
Precautions are taken to maintain patient safety. Top side rails aid in positioning and turning. Raising four side rails is considered a restraint.
II. Assess for additional patient needs and state the time of your expected return.
Meeting patient needs and offering self promote patient satisfaction and build trust.
III. Properly dispose of PPE.
Gloves, gowns, and masks must be appropriately discarded to prevent the spread of microorganisms.
IV. Clean equipment if it was in contact with the patient; see specific manufacturer instructions.
Disinfection eliminates most microorganisms from inanimate objects.
V. Perform hand hygiene.
Frequent hand hygiene prevents the spread of infection.
VI. Document the date, time, assessment, procedure, and patient's response to the procedure.
Accurate documentation is essential to communicate patient care and to provide legal evidence of care.

SKILL 39-2 Maintaining a Peripheral Intravenous Infusion

PURPOSE

- To prevent infections
- To provide fluids
- To administer medications
- To replace electrolytes
- To promote comfort
- To provide nutrition
- To maintain emergency access for medications

RESOURCES

- A 3- to 10-mL prefilled saline flush
- Antiseptic or alcohol wipes
- IV solution per PCP order
- Appropriate infusion set tubing (primary or secondary, appropriate for pump)
- Clean gloves
- IV pole and pump
- Personal protective equipment (PPE) as required

COLLABORATION AND DELEGATION

- Maintaining a peripheral IV line, including changing tubing or solutions, may not be delegated to unlicensed assistive personnel (UAP).
- UAP may observe a peripheral IV line and running infusions during care and should report the following to the nurse:
  - Burning, redness, pain, coolness, leaking, bleeding, or swelling at the site of a peripheral IV line
  - Patient concerns or complaints
  - Low volume in an IV bag
  - Alarms sounding on the IV pump
- Many facilities have an IV therapy team that maintains the IV sites. For the comfort and safety of the patient, nurses coordinate with these teams per facility policy and procedures and their own skill level.

EVIDENCE-BASED PRACTICE

- Peripheral IV sites are changed at least every 72 hours to ensure patency, decrease infection rates, and lower complication risks (Moureau, 2009).

SPECIAL CIRCUMSTANCES

1. **Assess:** Is the IV solution discolored, leaking, or expired?
   Intervention: Discard the IV solution, and obtain a new solution; document per facility policy and procedures.
2. **Assess:** Is the IV solution in a bottle instead of a bag?
   Intervention: Clean the port on the bottle with an antiseptic wipe, and insert a spike into the port on the bottle.
3. **Assess:** Was the tubing spike touched by anything other than the sterile port of an IV bottle?
   Intervention: Discard the spike, and restart with a new one.
4. **Assess:** What should be done if an IV solution does not infuse?
   Intervention: Check the tubing, and assess the IV site.

PREPROCEDURE

I. Check PCP orders and the patient care plan.
Knowledge of patient-specific orders is critical for safe patient care.

II. Gather supplies and equipment.
Preparing for the patient encounter saves time and promotes patient trust.

III. Perform hand hygiene.
Frequent hand hygiene prevents the spread of microorganisms.

IV. Maintain standard precautions.
Use of the correct personal protective equipment (PPE) is required whenever contact with bodily fluids is possible, to reduce the transfer of pathogens.

V. Introduce yourself.
Initial communication establishes the role of the nurse and begins a professional relationship.

VI. Provide for patient privacy.
It is important to maintain patient dignity.

VII. Identify the patient, using two identifiers.
Identifying a patient involves scanning barcodes or comparing the patient's stated name and birthdate to information on the patient's wristband or health record. The correct person must receive the correct treatment.

VIII. Explain the procedure to the patient.
The nurse has a responsibility to inform a patient before initiating care. Information may ease patient anxiety and facilitate cooperation.

PROCEDURE

Maintaining a Peripheral IV Line

Follow preprocedure steps I through VIII.

1. Adhere to the Rights of Medication Administration (see Chapter 35, Nursing Care Guideline: Six Rights of Medication Administration box).
   Avoid possible medication errors by adhering to the Rights of medication administration.
2. Be familiar with and use techniques to reduce medication errors.
   It is critical to reduce medication errors and promote patient safety.
3. Obtain all medications for the assigned time before entering the patient's room.
   Promote patient comfort through minimal interruptions.
4. Ensure medication and solution compatibility.
   Verification of compatibility is critical to reduce medication errors and promote patient safety.
5. Administering IV fluid therapy: Connect the tubing to the IV solution.
   a. Open the tubing package, slide a roller clamp 2 inches below the drip chamber, and roll the clamp closed.
   b. To remove sterile protections, pull or snap off the cover from the port on the bag, and slide off the cover from the spike on the tubing.
   c. Use aseptic technique to insert the spike into the port using a twisting motion. Ensure that it is fully inserted.
   Using a roller clamp ensures the accuracy of drip regulation and prevents wasting of solution during preparation. Maintain sterility while preparing the port and spike to prevent the spread of microorganisms.

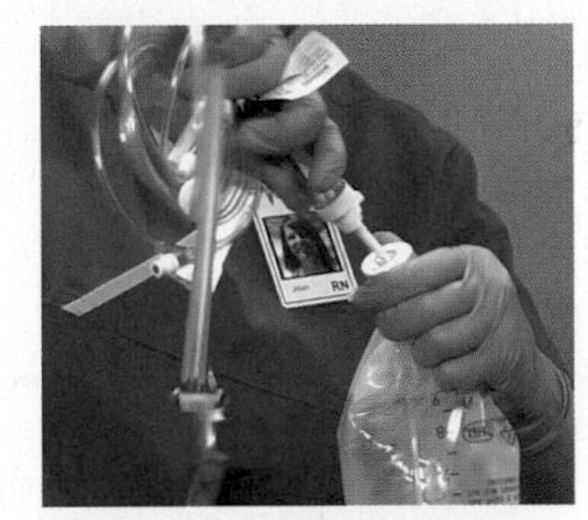

STEP 5

6. Squeeze the drip chamber, and then fill it one-half to one-third full with the IV solution.
   Squeezing removes air from the tubing and creates suction.

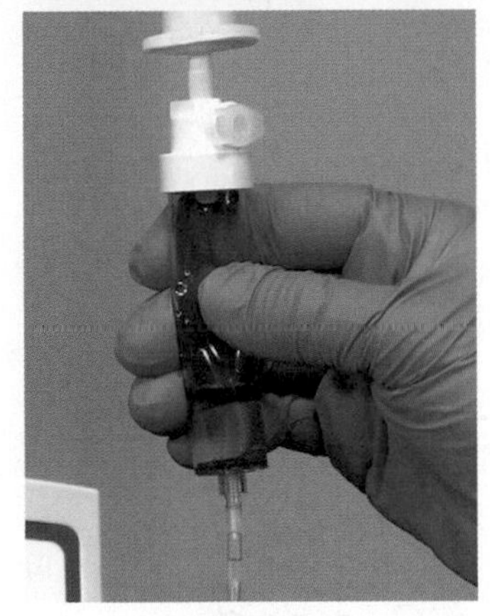

STEP 6

7. Fill the tubing with solution:
   a. Remove the cap on the end of the tubing; do *not* discard it, and keep the cap sterile. Place the end of the tubing over the sink; do *not* touch the sink.
   b. Slowly open the clamp.
   c. Allow the solution to run through the tubing. Hold tubing upside-down, and tap the ports to release the air and fill the ports.
   d. Close the clamp when the tubing is full.
   e. Replace the cap on the tubing.
   Maintain sterility and prevent contamination. Proper preparation of the tubing and ports prevents air from entering the tubing and prevents loss of solution.
8. Inspect the tubing for air; if air is present, tap the tubing to move the air up.
   Remove air from the tubing to prevent adverse events and complications.
9. Connect the tubing to the peripheral IV catheter (see the Nursing Care Guideline: Converting an Intravenous Line box).
10. Program the IV pump for infusion; see manufacturer instructions.
    Use the correct infusion rate to prevent adverse events and medical errors.
11. Ensure the tubing and solution are labeled per facility policy and procedures.
    Proper labeling of solutions prevents adverse events and medical errors.
12. Disconnect the tubing after the infusion is complete (see the Nursing Care Guideline: Converting an Intravenous Line box).

Follow postprocedure steps I through VI.

POSTPROCEDURE

I. Return the bed to its lowest position, raise the top side rails, and verify that the call light is within reach of the patient.
Precautions are taken to maintain patient safety. Top side rails aid in positioning and turning. Raising four side rails is considered a restraint.

II. Assess for additional patient needs and state the time of your expected return.
Meeting patient needs and offering self promote patient satisfaction and build trust.

III. Properly dispose of PPE.
Gloves, gowns, and masks must be appropriately discarded to prevent the spread of microorganisms.

IV. Clean equipment if it was in contact with the patient; see specific manufacturer instructions.
Disinfection eliminates most microorganisms from inanimate objects.

V. Perform hand hygiene.
Frequent hand hygiene prevents the spread of infection.

VI. Document the date, time, assessment, procedure, and patient's response to the procedure.
Accurate documentation is essential to communicate patient care and to provide legal evidence of care.

SKILL 39-3 Central Line Dressing Change and Care

PURPOSE

- To prevent infection
- To provide long-term intravenous (IV) fluids
- To administer long-term IV medications
- To administer rapid infusions
- To administer irritating medications such as hypertonic solutions or total parenteral nutrition (TPN)
- To maintain emergency access for medications

RESOURCES

- Central line dressing kit including two pairs of sterile gloves, two masks, antiseptic scrub, and transparent dressing
- Sterile gloves, if not included in the central venous line dressing kit
- Clean gloves
- Two face masks or shields if not included in kit
- ChloraPrep swab (if required by facility and different from that included in the kit)
- Chlorhexidine gluconate patch (if required by facility)
- Steri-Strips if indicated
- Personal protective equipment (PPE), if appropriate

COLLABORATION AND DELEGATION

- Dressing change and care of the central line may not be delegated to unlicensed assistive personnel (UAP).
- UAP may observe a central line during care and should report the following to a nurse:
  - Burning, redness, pain, coolness, leaking, bleeding, or swelling at the site of the central line
  - Patient concerns or complaints regarding the central line
  - Low solution volume in an IV bag
  - Alarms sounding on the IV pump
  - Changes in vital signs

EVIDENCE-BASED PRACTICE

- Using chlorhexidine as the antiseptic agent for cleaning the central venous catheter site and applying a chlorhexidine gluconate patch are recommended for cleaning and dressing a central venous catheter site.
- Ensuring dressing changes occur every 3 days has been shown to significantly reduce catheter-related infections (*Drug News*, 2009; Ellison, 2009; Suffredini, Masur, Lynch, 2010; Timsit, Schwebel, Bouadma et al, 2009).

SPECIAL CIRCUMSTANCES

1. **Assess:** Has the CVP kit been opened, torn, or contaminated during opening, or has it expired?
   Intervention: Stop the procedure, and obtain a new kit.
2. **Assess:** Has the site or caregiver's dominant hand been contaminated during the procedure?
   Intervention: Stop the procedure, and start over.
3. **Assess:** Is the insertion site red or swollen, or have other signs or symptoms of infection been observed?
   Intervention: Document the observations appropriately, and notify the primary care provider.

PREPROCEDURE

I. Check PCP orders and the patient care plan.
Knowledge of patient-specific orders is critical for safe patient care.

II. Gather supplies and equipment.
Preparing for the patient encounter saves time and promotes patient trust.

III. Perform hand hygiene.
Frequent hand hygiene prevents the spread of microorganisms.

IV. Maintain standard precautions.
Use of the correct personal protective equipment (PPE) is required whenever contact with bodily fluids is possible, to reduce the transfer of pathogens.

V. Introduce yourself.
Initial communication establishes the role of the nurse and begins a professional relationship.

VI. Provide for patient privacy.
It is important to maintain patient dignity.

VII. Identify the patient, using two identifiers.
Identifying a patient involves scanning barcodes or comparing the patient's stated name and birthdate to information on the patient's wristband or health record. The correct person must receive the correct treatment.

VIII. Explain the procedure to the patient.
The nurse has a responsibility to inform a patient before initiating care. Information may ease patient anxiety and facilitate cooperation.

PROCEDURE

Central Line Dressing Change and Care

Follow preprocedure steps I through VIII.

1. Prepare the supplies on a bedside table:
   a. Place the CVC dressing kit on a bedside table.
   b. Place a small bag (to be used for waste disposal) on the bed, making sure that it is lower than the sterile field (ideally, place it at the foot of the bed). Alternatively, use a trash can at the side of the bed.
   Preparing supplies in advance avoids interruption during the procedure and provides organization that facilitates performance of the procedure. Provide a waste receptacle at a location that will not contaminate the sterile field.
2. Raise the bed to working height, and lower the head of the bed.
   Setting the bed at the correct working height for the provider prevents provider discomfort and possible injury. A flat bed provides the optimal position for the procedure.
3. Open the CVC line dressing kit and place a mask on the patient if indicated by facility or manufacturer policy. Have the patient turn his or her face away from the catheter site.
   Having the patient avoid breathing on the site while it is unprotected prevents spread of microorganisms and infection.
4. Put on a face mask or shield and the first pair of gloves from the kit.
   Use of the correct PPE is required whenever contact with bodily fluids is possible to reduce the spread of microorganisms and prevent infection among patients and providers.
5. Remove the dressing and Steri-Strip that is stabilizing the catheter:
   a. Remove the dressing in the direction of catheter insertion. Hold the skin taut and gently pull the dressing away from the taut skin.
   b. Dispose of the dressing into the waste receptacle.
   c. Inspect the insertion site.
   d. Remove the gloves, and dispose them in the waste receptacle.
   e. Perform hand hygiene.
   The dressing is removed to allow assessment of the site and to facilitate the remainder of the procedure. Proper disposal of waste prevents contamination of the sterile field with microorganisms. Hand hygiene reduces the spread of microorganisms and reduces infections.
6. Add Steri-Strips to the sterile field if required by facility policy. Put on sterile gloves (see Chapter 26, Skill 26-2), and prepare items from the kit on the sterile field (see Chapter 26, Skill 26-4).
   Maintain sterile procedure to reduce the spread of microorganisms and prevent infection. Preparing supplies in advance maintains organization and avoids interruption during the procedure.
7. Cleanse the central line site:
   a. Use the nondominant hand to hold the catheter vertically in the air (i.e., off the skin).
   b. With the dominant hand, use a ChloraPrep swab with a vertical and horizontal motion around the site for at least 30 seconds. Cleanse the tubing with the swab. Discard the swab in the waste receptacle. If a ChloraPrep swab is not available, refer to facility policy and procedures for an appropriate antiseptic solution or swab.
   Proper cleansing technique is used to prevent the spread of microorganisms and avoid infection.

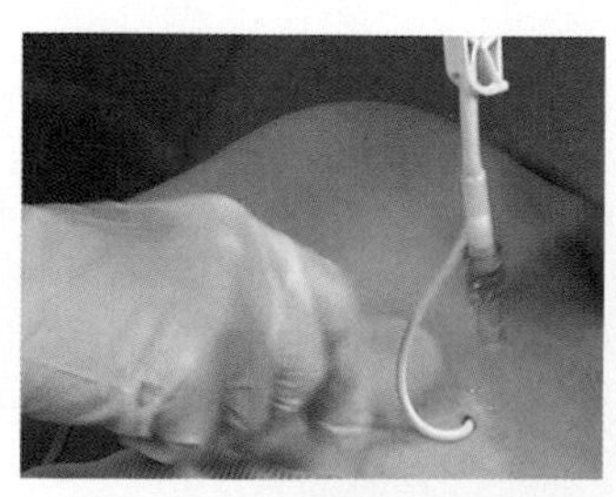

STEP 7

8. Allow the site to air-dry for 30 seconds. Apply skin protectant to the site and allow it to dry.
   Air-drying prevents contamination and reduces infection and the spread of microorganisms. Skin protectant helps the adhesive stick to the skin and protects skin from tearing.

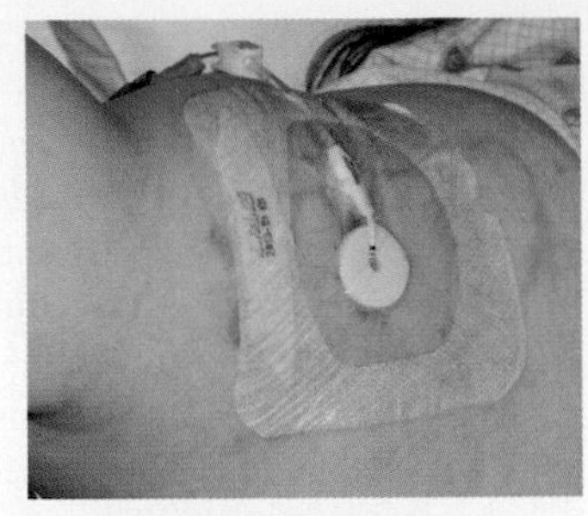
STEPS 9 and 11

9. Apply a chlorhexidine gluconate patch around the catheter and over the site, with the slit positioned over the central line. If a chlorhexidine gluconate patch is not available, refer to facility policy and procedures for an appropriate dressing.
Proper antiseptic equipment and procedures are used to prevent the spread of microorganisms and infection.

10. Apply Steri-Strip to stabilize the catheter if required by facility policy.
Secures the catheter to the skin.

11. Apply a transparent dressing over the site.
Transparency allows for site assessment without removing the dressing.

12. Write initials, date, and time of day on the dressing label; apply the label over the dressing, but do *not* occlude the site.
Proper labeling of the dressing prevents adverse events and medical errors by communicating essential information. Avoid placing labels over the site to prevent infection.

13. Remove gloves, and discard used supplies in a waste receptacle.
Proper disposal of waste prevents the spread of microorganisms.

Follow postprocedure steps I through VI.

POSTPROCEDURE

I. Return the bed to its lowest position, raise the top side rails, and verify that the call light is within reach of the patient.
Precautions are taken to maintain patient safety. Top side rails aid in positioning and turning. Raising four side rails is considered a restraint.

II. Assess for additional patient needs and state the time of your expected return.
Meeting patient needs and offering self promote patient satisfaction and build trust.

III. Properly dispose of PPE.
Gloves, gowns, and masks must be appropriately discarded to prevent the spread of microorganisms.

IV. Clean equipment if it was in contact with the patient; see specific manufacturer instructions.
Disinfection eliminates most microorganisms from inanimate objects.

V. Perform hand hygiene.
Frequent hand hygiene prevents the spread of infection.

VI. Document the date, time, assessment, procedure, and patient's response to the procedure.
Accurate documentation is essential to communicate patient care and to provide legal evidence of care.

SUMMARY OF LEARNING OUTCOMES

LO 39.1 *Discuss the normal structure and function of fluids, electrolytes, acids, and bases in the body:* Fluids can be found in two areas in the body: intracellular and extracellular; extracellular sites include the interstitial, intravascular, and transcellular spaces. Fluid moves by osmosis from areas of lower concentration of solutes to areas of higher concentration. The major electrolytes in the body are sodium, potassium, calcium, magnesium, chloride, and phosphate ions. Movement of electrolytes occurs through diffusion, filtration, and active transport. The body must maintain a normal pH (7.35 to 7.45) to function efficiently. Three mechanisms maintain normal pH levels: buffering systems, respiratory control of carbon dioxide (CO_2), and renal control of bicarbonate (HCO_3^-).

LO 39.2 *Differentiate among common fluid, electrolyte, and acid-base imbalances and their underlying causes:* Common fluid and electrolyte imbalances include fluid volume deficit, fluid volume excess, hyponatremia, hypernatremia, hypokalemia, hyperkalemia, hypocalcemia, hypercalcemia, hypomagnesemia, hypermagnesemia, hypophosphatemia, and hyperphosphatemia. The numerous causes of fluid and electrolyte imbalances include intake and output, medications and IV therapy, and a variety of illnesses. Four acid-base imbalances can occur: respiratory acidosis, respiratory alkalosis, metabolic acidosis, and metabolic alkalosis.

LO39.3 *Outline assessment priorities for patients with fluid, electrolyte, and acid-base imbalances:* Assessment parameters for fluid, electrolyte, and acid-base imbalances include the health history, especially recent changes in fluid intake, diet, and weight; edema and altered skin turgor; and diagnostic test results.

LO39.4 *Identify the most common nursing diagnoses related to fluid, electrolyte, and acid-base imbalances:* Nursing diagnoses related to fluid and electrolyte imbalances include *Readiness for Enhanced Fluid Balance, Risk for Imbalanced Fluid Volume, Deficient Fluid Volume, Excess Fluid Volume,* and *Decreased Cardiac Output.*

LO39.5 *Integrate nursing goals and outcomes into the plan of care for patients with fluid, electrolyte, and acid-base imbalances:* Nursing goals reflect attainment of balanced intake and output, a stable daily weight, normal urine specific gravity, vital signs within the patient's normal limits, and normal serum levels of electrolytes and arterial blood gases.

LO39.6 *Carry out nursing interventions to maintain normal fluid, electrolyte, and acid-base balance or to correct imbalances:* Interventions for fluid imbalances include ongoing focused assessment, restricting or encouraging fluids, restricting or providing supplemental sources of electrolytes, and IV therapy. Blood infusions and total parenteral nutrition may be needed by selected patients.

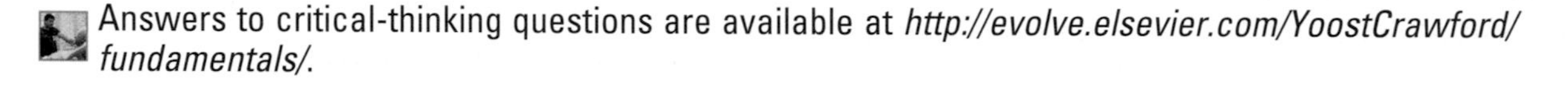
Answers to critical-thinking questions are available at *http://evolve.elsevier.com/YoostCrawford/fundamentals/.*

REVIEW QUESTIONS

1. A patient has reported a 2-kg (4.4-lb) weight gain over the past 3 days. Which factor should the nurse question?
   - **a.** Protein intake
   - **b.** Potassium intake
   - **c.** Calorie intake
   - **d.** Sodium intake
2. A nurse caring for a hospitalized patient is told in the shift change report that the patient's laboratory results are sodium = 140 mEq/L; potassium = 4.1 mEq/L; calcium = 9.5 mg/dL; and magnesium = 3.4 mEq/L. Which abnormal level will the nurse report to the primary care provider?
   - **a.** High sodium level
   - **b.** Low potassium
   - **c.** Low calcium level
   - **d.** High magnesium level
3. For a patient with a nursing diagnosis of *Fluid Volume Deficit,* the nurse is alert to which signs and symptoms? *(Select all that apply.)*
   - **a.** Hypertension
   - **b.** Flushed skin
   - **c.** Dry mucous membranes
   - **d.** Weak, thready pulse
   - **e.** Pale yellow urine
4. The nurse is caring for a patient who needs to increase calcium in her diet but does not like milk. Which food should the nurse encourage the patient to consume?
   - **a.** Cod
   - **b.** Eggs
   - **c.** Spinach
   - **d.** Tomatoes

5. A nurse in the emergency department is caring for an adult patient with numerous draining wounds from gunshots. The patient's pulse rate has increased from 100 to 130 beats/min over the past hour. For which imbalance should the nurse assess symptoms?
   a. Respiratory acidosis
   b. Extracellular fluid volume deficit
   c. Metabolic alkalosis
   d. Intracellular fluid volume excess
6. A 65-year-old female patient is a two pack a day cigarette smoker with a history of chronic obstructive pulmonary disease (COPD). What is the interpretation of her arterial blood gas values (pH 7.34, PCO_2 55 mm Hg, PO_2 82 mm Hg, HCO_3^- 32 mEq/L)?
   a. Partially compensated respiratory alkalosis
   b. Uncompensated metabolic acidosis
   c. Uncompensated respiratory alkalosis
   d. Partially compensated respiratory acidosis
7. A patient with an excessive alcohol intake has a reduced amount of antidiuretic hormone (ADH). Which symptom is the patient likely to exhibit?
   a. Dysuria
   b. Polyuria
   c. Oliguria
   d. Hematuria
8. The nurse is assessing the intravenous (IV) site in the right forearm and notices the area around it is cool, swollen, firm, and tender to touch. Which complication is most likely occurring?
   a. Infection
   b. Speed shock
   c. Infiltration
   d. Phlebitis
9. Which activity is important to include in the plan of care for a client with a peripherally inserted central catheter (PICC)?
   a. Use sterile technique when changing the PICC dressing.
   b. Change the IV tubing every 72 hours.
   c. Take blood pressure in the arm with the PICC line.
   d. Use only macrodrip tubing with IV infusions through the PICC line.
10. The nurse has begun an infusion of fresh frozen plasma (FFP). Which symptom indicates an allergic reaction to the FFP?
   a. Respirations: 30/min
   b. Urine output: 50 mL/hr
   c. Heart Rate: 62 beats/min
   d. Temperature: 39° C (102.2° F)

Answers and rationales to review questions are available at *http://evolve.elsevier.com/YoostCrawford/fundamentals/*.

REFERENCES

American College of Sports Medicine, American Dietetic Association, Dietitians of Canada: Nutrition and athletic performance: A joint position statement. *Med Sci Sports Exerc,* 41(3):709-731, 2009.

Bishop L, Dougherty L, Bodenham A, et al. Guidelines on the insertion and management of central venous access devices in adults. *Int J Lab Hematol,* 29:261-278, 2007.

Centers for Disease Control and Prevention (CDC): Guidelines for the prevention of intravascular catheter-related infections, 2011. Retrieved from *http://stacks.cdc.gov/view/cdc/5916.*

Cronenwett L, Sherwood G, Barnsteiner J, et al: Quality and safety education for nurses. *Nurs Outlook,* 55(3), 122-131, 2007.

Drug News: Catheter-related infection: Antibacterial sponge soaks up risk. *Nursing,* 39(6):53, 2009.

Ellison RT: Benefit found for chlorhexidine dressings. *J Watch Infect Dis,* 2009.

Food and Drug Administration (FDA): Bar code label requirements for blood and blood products, 2011. Retrieved from *www.fda.gov/biologicsbloodvaccines/developmentapprovalprocess/advertisinglabelingpromotionalmaterials/barcodelabelrequirements/ucm133136.htm.*

Fraher MH, Collins CJ, Bourke J, et al.: Cost-effectiveness of employing a total parenteral nutrition surveillance nurse for the prevention of catheter-related bloodstream infections. *J Hosp Infect,* 73(2):129-134, 2009.

Infusion Nurses Society (INS): *Policies and procedures for infusion nursing,* ed. 4, Norwood, Mass., 2011, Infusion Nurses Society.

The Joint Commission: Hospital: 2014 National patient safety goals. Retrieved from *www.jointcommission.org/assets/1/6/HAP_NPSG_Chapter_2014.pdf.*

Lim C: Fluid requirements during physical exercise. *Nutr Today,* 44(1):10-13, 2009.

Macklin D: Catheter management. *Semin Oncol Nurs,* 26(2): 113-120, 2010.

Moureau N: Preventing peripheral intravenous line infections: Recommendations for healthcare facilities. *J Assoc Vasc Access,* 14(4):187-190, 2009.

National Institutes of Health, Office of Dietary Supplements: Vitamin D, 2011. Retrieved from *http://ods.od.nih.gov/factsheets/VitaminD-HealthProfessional/.*

Oh H, Seo W: Alterations in fluid, electrolytes and other serum chemistry values and their relations with enteral tube feeding in acute brain infarction patients. *J Clin Nurs,* 16:298-307, 2007.

Pagana KD, Pagana TJ: *Mosby's manual of diagnostic and laboratory tests,* ed. 5, St. Louis, 2014, Mosby.

Saladin K: *Anatomy & physiology: The unity of form and function,* ed. 6, Boston, 2012, McGraw-Hill Medical.

Suffredini AF, Masur H, Lynch JP III: Determining which component of a "bundle" improves outcomes: Benefit of chlorhexidine-impregnated sponge dressings for venous catheter sites. *Ann Intern Med,* 152(9), 608, 2010.

Timsit JF, Schwebel C, Bouadma L, et al, Dressing Study Group: Chlorhexidine-impregnated sponges and less frequent dressing changes for prevention of catheter-related infections in critically ill adults: a randomized controlled trial. *JAMA*, 301, 1231-1241, 2009.

Vamvakas EC, Blajchman MA: Blood still kills: Six strategies to further reduce allogeneic blood transfusion-related mortality. *Transfus Med Rev*, 24(2), 77-124, 2010.

Watson D, Hearnshaw K: Understanding blood groups and transfusion in nursing practice. *Nurs Stand*, 24(30), 41-48, 2010.

Webster J, Osborne S, Rickard C, Hall J: Clinically indicated replacement versus routine replacement of peripheral venous catheters. *Cochrane Database Syst Rev*, 17(3), CD007798, 2010.

Weinstein SM, Hagle ME: *Plumer's principles & practice of infusion therapy,* ed. 9, Philadelphia, 2014, Lippincott Williams & Wilkins.

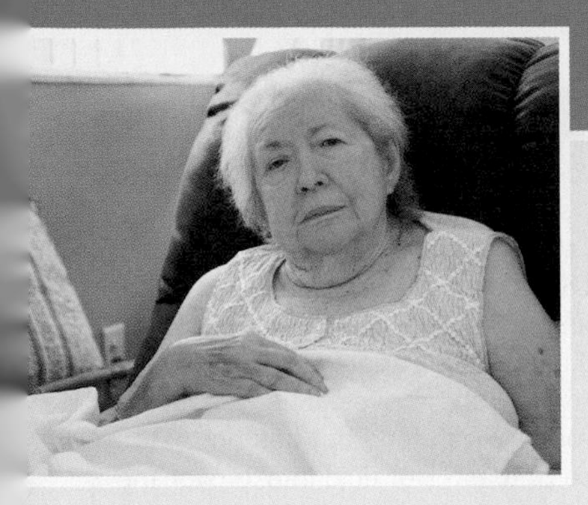

CHAPTER 40

Bowel Elimination

EVOLVE WEBSITE

http://evolve.elsevier.com/YoostCrawford/fundamentals/

- Additional Evolve-Only Review Questions With Answers
- Answers and Rationales for Text Review Questions
- Answers to Critical-Thinking Exercises
- Case Study With Questions
- Video Skills Clips
- Conceptual Care Map Creator
- Animations
- Skill Checklists
- Glossary

LEARNING OUTCOMES

Comprehension of this chapter's content will provide students with the ability to:

LO 40.1 Describe the anatomy and physiology of the gastrointestinal tract and the processes involved in formation, storage, and elimination of waste products.

LO 40.2 Identify common alterations in bowel elimination.

LO 40.3 Integrate components of a comprehensive assessment of the patient to identify issues with bowel elimination.

LO 40.4 Identify nursing diagnoses related to bowel elimination.

LO 40.5 Outline goals for patients experiencing alterations in bowel elimination.

LO 40.6 Implement interventions to maintain normal bowel elimination.

KEY TERMS

cathartic, p. 1052
chyme, p. 1044
colonoscopy, p. 1055
colostomy, p. 1048
***Clostridium difficile*, p. 1046**
constipation, p. 1047
defecation, p. 1046
diarrhea, p. 1046
enema, p. 1059
fecal occult blood test, p. 1054
flatulence, p. 1047
hemorrhoids, p. 1046
ileostomy, p. 1048
impaction, p. 1047
incontinence, p. 1047
lavage, p. 1059
laxatives, p. 1051
ostomy, p. 1048
paralytic ileus, p. 1051
peristalsis, p. 1045
polyps, p. 1054
stoma, p. 1048
suppository, p. 1059
Valsalva maneuver, p. 1047

CASE STUDY

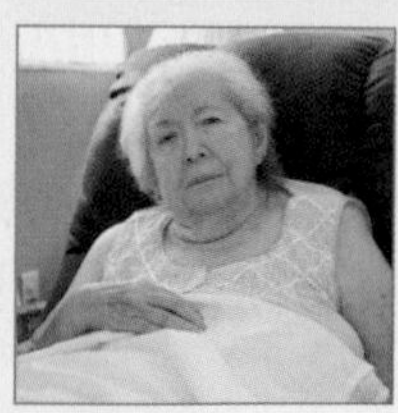

Mrs. Schaffer is an 82-year-old obese female admitted to the rehabilitation center after undergoing surgery for repair of a right hip fracture from a fall at home. At 72 hours postsurgery, she is receiving morphine patient-controlled anesthesia (PCA) for moderate postoperative pain, with results of reduction in reported pain. She has no significant past medical history and no known drug allergies (NKDA). Her DNR document specifies a full code.

Mrs. Schaffer's vital signs are T 37.1° C (98.9° F), P 70 and regular, R 12 and unlabored, and BP 110/76, with a pulse oximetry reading of 97% on room air. She rates her pain as 5 of 10 and refuses additional medication. Mrs. Schaffer is reluctant to move around, stating that the pain is worse when she moves. She needs the assistance of one person to move from bed to chair. She has been ordering her own meals from the cafeteria but has not eaten more than half of the meal that is sent. Her morning tray included eggs with sausage and a slice of toast. Her fluid intake over the past shift was 200 mL in 8 hours and her output was 180 mL. On auscultation, she has hypoactive bowel sounds, and her abdomen is slightly firm and tender to deep palpation. During the evening assessment, the patient informs the nurse that she "feels constipated" and that she has not moved her bowels in a few days.

Treatment orders are as follows:

- Physical therapy for ambulation
- Vital signs q shift
- Regular diet as tolerated
- Intake and output q shift
- Incentive spirometer q 1 hr while awake
- Complete blood count and serum chemistry panel daily

Medication orders are as follows:

- Morphine (MS Contin) PCA 1 mg/hour basal with 0.4 mg q 10 min, with 4 mg/hr lockout
- Enoxaparin (Lovenox) 60 mg subcutaneously daily
- Docusate (Colace) 1 capsule daily

Refer back to this case study to answer the critical-thinking questions throughout the chapter.

In most American households without very young children, bowel elimination is considered a private matter, one that generally is not talked about with others. Within the health care environment, however, the patient's bowel elimination function, or dysfunction, is evaluated, analyzed, and discussed frankly and openly. The nurse must be aware of the patient's discomfort and embarrassment that potentially accompany discussion of bowel elimination, understand the associated issues of self-esteem, and be sensitive to what the patient may regard as a personal matter.

Elimination of solid waste products is a normal function of the body and critical to maintaining nutritional status, hydration, and fluid and electrolyte balance. Regular bowel elimination may be disrupted by various factors, including food and fluid intake, various illnesses and diseases, trauma and surgery, medications, immobility, and psychological issues. The nurse must understand the physiology of elimination, factors that alter elimination, and measures that assist the patient in maintaining bowel function. Alteration in bowel elimination can become a life-threatening medical emergency. Consistent monitoring of bowel patterns is an essential nursing assessment.

NORMAL STRUCTURE AND FUNCTION OF THE GASTROINTESTINAL TRACT LO 40.1

The gastrointestinal (GI) tract is the body system responsible for the digestion of food and absorption of nutrients and fluids. Because this chapter addresses bowel elimination, it focuses on the essential role of the GI system in the formation, storage, and elimination of waste products. The GI system is a series of muscular organs extending from the mouth to the anus (Figure 40-1).

ESOPHAGUS

The esophagus is a collapsible tube, connecting the pharynx to the stomach. From the pharynx, the esophagus passes through the mediastinum and diaphragm and meets the stomach at the location of the lower esophageal sphincter. The primary function of the esophagus is to transport solids and liquids from the mouth, where digestion begins, into the stomach (VanPutte, Regan, Russo, et al, 2014).

STOMACH

The stomach begins at the cardiac sphincter and extends into the duodenum through the pyloric sphincter. Anatomically it is located in the left upper quadrant of the abdomen, slightly inferior to the diaphragm. Food mixes in the stomach with digestive juices, causing the chemical and mechanical breakdown of food into **chyme** before entering the small intestine. Chyme is a thick fluid mass of partially digested food and gastric secretions that is passed from the stomach to the small intestine.

The stomach produces and secretes hydrochloric acid, pepsin, intrinsic factor, and mucus. The hydrochloric acid

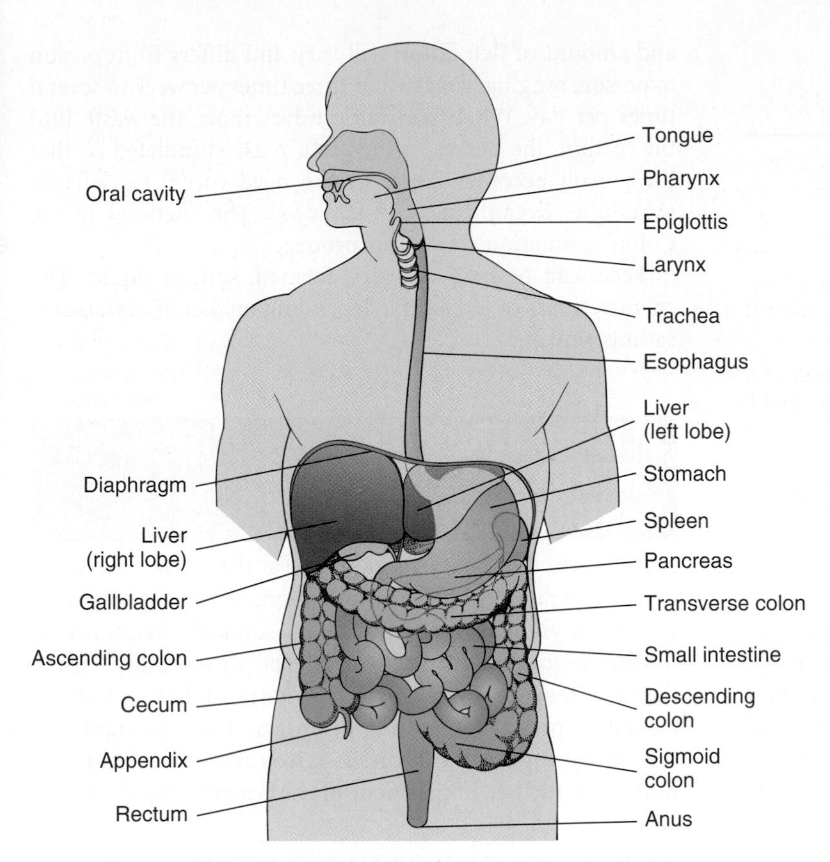

FIGURE 40-1 The gastrointestinal system: Mouth through anus. (From Monahan FD, Sands JK, Neighbors M, et al: *Phipps' medical-surgical nursing: Health and illness perspectives,* ed. 8, St. Louis, 2007, Mosby.)

combines with the digestive enzymes to cause a breakdown of the food structures and helps to kill off harmful bacteria ingested with the foods. Pepsin is an enzyme produced in the mucosal lining of the stomach that acts to degrade protein. Intrinsic factor is a protein produced by cells in the stomach lining. It is needed for the intestines to efficiently absorb vitamin B_{12}, which is needed to produce red blood cells. Mucus protects the stomach mucosa from damage by the gastric acid and enzyme activity (VanPutte, Regan, Russo, et al, 2014).

ⓔ The animations "Hormones and Gastric Secretion," "Hydrochloric Acid Production by Parietal Cells in the Gastric Glands of the Stomach," and "Three Phases of Gastric Secretion" provide further details about production and secretion of enzymes and acids in the stomach.

SMALL INTESTINE

The small intestine is digestive and absorptive in function. Intestinal juices and bile from the liver, gallbladder, and pancreas mix with the chyme for digestion and absorption of nutrients. The small intestine is a hollow cylindrical organ, approximately 6 meters (18 to 21 feet) in length; it contains three segments.

The first section of the small intestine, the *duodenum,* begins at the pyloric sphincter. The duodenum has two secretory functions: In one, hormones are secreted that trigger the pancreas to release pancreatic juice and bile. In the other, the duodenum protects the intestine by secreting chemicals that neutralize the acidity of the chyme from the stomach before it reaches the jejunum.

The midregion of the small intestine, the *jejunum,* controls carbohydrate and protein absorption. The third section, the *ileum,* extends from the jejunum to the ileocecal valve at the cecum of the large intestine. The ileum is responsible for the absorption of fats, bile salts, and water. Contents that remain undigested after passing through the small intestine, such as fiber, the indigestible portion of plant foods, empty into the cecum in the lower right quadrant of the abdomen (VanPutte, Regan, Russo, et al, 2014).

LARGE INTESTINE

The large intestine is shorter in length, 1.5 meters, or 5.5 feet, but wider in diameter than the small intestine; it extends from the ileocecal valve to the anus. The large intestine is composed of the cecum, ascending colon, transverse colon, descending colon, sigmoid colon, rectum, and anus. Anatomically, the large intestine is located on the periphery of the abdominal compartment and surrounds the small intestine and other structures. It is the primary organ of bowel elimination. **Peristalsis**, the mechanism of progressive contraction and relaxation of the walls of the intestine, forces chyme into the large intestine through the ileocecal valve, which prevents

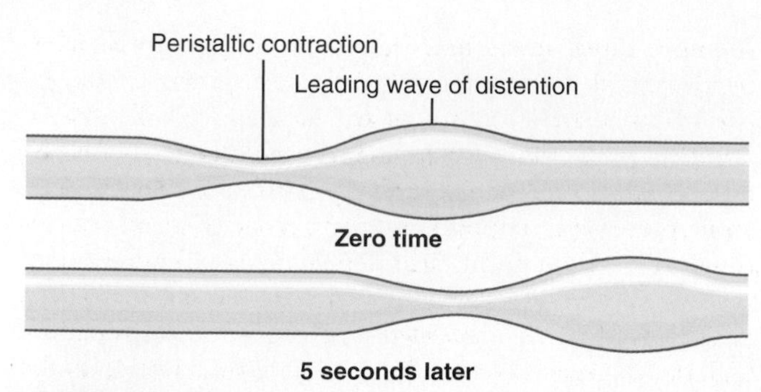

FIGURE 40-2 Peristalsis. (From Hall JE: *Guyton and Hall textbook of medical physiology,* ed. 12, St. Louis, 2011, Saunders.)

regurgitation (backflow) of chyme (VanPutte, Regan, Russo, et al, 2014) (Figure 40-2).

The colon is made up of muscular tissue that is able to expand and contract to accommodate and eliminate varying amounts of waste and gas (flatus). The functions of the colon are absorption, secretion, and elimination. Water is absorbed from indigestible food residue. Nutrients and electrolytes, especially sodium and chloride, are absorbed from digested food that has passed from the small intestine. Bicarbonate is secreted in exchange for chloride. The colon excretes 4 to 9 mEq of potassium daily. Serious electrolyte imbalances may occur with alterations in colonic function. A mucous layer is in place to help to protect the intestinal wall. Waste from the body is eliminated through the formation of feces and expelled from the body by way of the rectum and anus (VanPutte, Regan, Russo, et al, 2014).

RECTUM AND ANUS

The rectum is the final portion of the large intestine; it is approximately 10 to 15 cm (4 to 6 inches) in length. At the distal portion lies the anus, which is 2.5 to 5 cm, or 1 to 2 inches. The rectum has folds of tissue that temporarily hold fecal contents. Each fold contains an artery and a vein that can become distended from pressure during straining. This distention may result in the formation of hemorrhoids. **Hemorrhoids** are swollen and inflamed veins in the anus or lower rectum.

The anal canal contains an internal and an external sphincter, each controlled by the sympathetic and parasympathetic nervous system. The sensory nerves in the anal canal help to control bowel continence (VanPutte, Regan, Russo, et al, 2014). The animation "Organs of Digestion" shows the sequence of the entire digestive system.

DEFECATION

The final act of digestion by which the solid, semisolid, or liquid waste is expelled by the body is the process of **defecation,** or bowel movement. Feces and flatus are expelled from the GI tract through the anal canal and anus. Frequency and amount of defecation will vary and differs from person to person, ranging from two or three times per week to several times per day. When peristaltic waves move the waste into the rectum, the nerves in the rectum are stimulated so that the person becomes aware of the need (urge) to defecate (VanPutte, Regan, Russo, et al, 2014). The "Reflexes in the Colon" animation shows this process.

Feces can be hard and dry, formed, soft, or liquid. The characteristics of feces vary, depending on diet, illness, medications, and age.

ALTERED STRUCTURE AND FUNCTION OF THE GASTROINTESTINAL TRACT

LO 40.2

Many hospitalized patients either are at risk for or have some type of alteration in bowel elimination. The changes may be due to physiologic issues, such as surgical alterations or disease processes, medication effects, or mobility issues. Changes may by psychological in nature related to stress, anxiety, depression, or eating disorders. It is important that the nurse recognize the disorders as well as the associated risks to prevent further impairment of the patient's health status.

ABNORMAL DEFECATION PATTERNS

Because the organs of the GI system process food and fluids for use within the body systems, any alteration may lead to serious issues for the patient. Impaired elimination has serious implications for patient well-being and treatment outcomes.

Diarrhea

Diarrhea is an intestinal disorder that is characterized by an abnormal frequency and fluidity of fecal evacuations. Hyperactive bowel sounds, urgency, abdominal pain, and cramping are all characteristics. Diarrhea is associated with disorders which affect digestion, absorption, and secretion in the GI tract. Ingested materials pass too quickly through the intestine, resulting in a decrease in the amount of time for absorption of fluids and nutrients. Many pathologic conditions and other factors may cause diarrhea, including allergies or intolerance to food, fluids, or drugs; antibiotic use; cathartic or laxative use; communicable foodborne pathogens; diseases of the colon; diagnostic testing of the lower GI tract; enteral nutrition usage; medications; psychological stress; surgery of the GI tract; and ***Clostridium difficile.***

C. difficile is a bacterium that causes diarrhea. It can lead to life-threatening inflammation of the colon. *C. difficile* infection with associated diarrhea, often called simply "C-diff," most commonly affects older adults in hospitals and long-term care facilities and typically occurs after use of antibiotic medications (Simor, 2010). C-diff is easily transmitted, and in recent years, these infections have become more difficult to treat. The most common clinical picture in mild to moderate C-diff consists of occurrence of foul smelling, watery diarrhea three or more times a day for 2 or more days, accompanied by mild abdominal cramping and tenderness (Simor, 2010).

The patient with diarrhea produces an increased number of stools, with passage of liquid or unformed feces, and finds it difficult to control the urge to defecate. In addition to frequent liquid stools, the patient often experiences spasmodic cramps and increased bowel sounds.

Prolonged diarrhea may lead to nutritional and metabolic disturbances, with resultant fatigue, weakness, malaise, and loss of a substantial amount of fat and muscle tissue, making the patient look extremely thin or emaciated. Serious fluid and electrolyte losses can develop within a short time, particularly in infants, small children, and elderly people, causing symptoms of nausea, vomiting, headache, confusion, fatigue, restlessness, and muscle weakness and spasms. With persistent diarrhea, the patient may experience irritation of the anal region, increasing the risk for skin breakdown.

Incontinence

Incontinence refers to the loss of voluntary control of fecal and gaseous discharges through the anus. Incontinence can have a profound impact on the affected person's body image. In many cases, the patient is alert but unable to control defecation. The patient is at risk for skin breakdown and may suffer from social isolation related to embarrassment from the soiling of clothing or use of incontinence products.

Constipation

Constipation is a common problem, affecting the quality of life for many. It is estimated that more than 4 million Americans complain of frequent constipation. Women report constipation more often than men, and adults older than 65 years of age are more likely to have constipation. Constipation is a complication of pregnancy and after surgery (National Institutes of Health [NIH], 2014).

Constipation is defined as having infrequent or difficult bowel movements, as well as having fewer than three bowel movements per week. Slowed intestinal peristalsis and infrequent bowel movements result in increased water absorption in the colon, leading to difficulty passing stool, excessive straining at defecation, the inability to defecate at will, hard feces, and rectal pain. In addition, the patient may experience abdominal cramping, pain, pressure, distention, anorexia, and headache.

Causes of constipation extend across the clinical spectrum. Irregular bowel habits, ignoring the urge to defecate, a diet low in fiber or high in animal fats, hemorrhoids, and low fluid intake are causative factors. Patients with conditions that block nerve impulses to the colon, including spinal cord injury and tumor may have changes in bowel patterns. Metabolic conditions such as hypothyroidism, hypercalcemia, or hypokalemia slow GI motility or increase water absorption. Psychiatric issues, including anxiety, depression, and cognitive impairment, may lead to changes in bowel habits or decreased recognition of defecation urge. Prolonged periods of bed rest or lack of regular exercise will slow GI motility. Medications, including anticholinergics, antispasmodics, anticonvulsants, antidepressants, antihistamines, antihypertensives, antiparkinsonian agents, bile acid sequestrants, diuretics, antacids, iron supplements, calcium supplements, and opioids, have been shown to slow colonic action. Laxative misuse is associated with rebound constipation. Older adults may experience slowed peristalsis related to the loss of muscle elasticity, reduced intestinal mucous secretion, or a low-fiber diet. The patient with hemorrhoids may experience pain and have difficulty passing stool, which can lead to retention of fecal material and contribute to constipation.

Constipation presents a significant health risk to the patient. Straining during defecation can induce elevations in intraocular pressure, increased intracranial pressure, changes in the cardiac rhythms, and hemorrhoids. The **Valsalva maneuver** consists of "bearing down" while holding the breath. The person thus is exerting force against a closed windpipe, creating increased intrathoracic pressure. This maneuver causes an extremely rapid rise in blood pressure, which is followed by a fall in arterial blood pressure. Dizziness, blurred vision, and fainting can result.

Impaction

Impaction refers to the presence of a hard fecal mass in the rectum or colon that the patient is incapable of expelling. Impaction is the result of unresolved constipation. Over time, a mass of stool becomes wedged in the bowel and cannot be moved along for defecation. Impaction is seen most often in debilitated, confused, or unconscious patients.

The patient may report the inability to pass a stool for several days or longer, despite repeated urges to defecate. The cardinal sign of impaction is continuous oozing of liquid stool, with no normal stool. Oozing occurs as the liquid portion of feces higher in the intestines seeps around the mass. Loss of appetite, nausea, vomiting, distention, cramping, and rectal pain accompany the condition. Barium used in radiologic examinations contributes to the risk of impaction. The at-risk patient receiving barium for diagnosis or treatment is encouraged to increase fluids or is given laxatives or enemas to ensure removal of the barium.

Diagnosis of impaction is by digital examination and palpation of the fecal mass. Digital examination, manipulation, and removal of a fecal impaction are within the scope of practice for nurses, although some agencies require an order from a primary care provider (PCP).

FLATULENCE

Flatulence is the production of a mixture of gases in the intestine, by-products of the digestive process. The mixture, known as flatus, is expelled from the mouth (belching) or the anus (passing of flatus). The noises commonly associated with flatulence are caused by air escaping. Discomfort may develop from the buildup of gas pressure. Severe flatulence often is associated with abdominal distention and severe sharp pain.

Flatulence is a normal body function and an important signal of normal activity. It is documented by nursing staff after surgical procedures or other treatments to indicate the return of normal bowel function.

Flatulence results from a variety of sources. Action of bacteria in chyme passing through the large intestine, swallowed air and gases that diffuse between the bloodstream and the intestine, foods such as cabbage and onions, abdominal surgery, and narcotics can lead to changes in the motility of the bowel and may increase flatulence. Movement such as walking and rocking may help relieve pain and promote movement of the gases through the intestines. It may be necessary to insert a rectal tube if excessive gas cannot be expelled through the anus.

BOWEL DIVERSIONS

The terms *ostomy* and *stoma* often are used interchangeably, although they have different meanings. An **ostomy** is a surgically created opening in a GI, urinary, or respiratory organ that is exited onto the skin. A **stoma** ("mouth" in Greek) is any body opening but usually refers to the actual exit point for a GI surgical ostomy, which forms a slight protuberance of mucosa (gut lining tissue) through the skin.

Bowel diversion ostomies are created to divert and drain fecal material. Bowel ostomies are classified as either temporary or permanent and by their anatomic location and technique of stoma construction. Bowel diversions are created for patients with conditions that prevent normal passage of feces from the rectum. The location of the ostomy determines the consistency of the stool. Water reabsorption varies for specific areas of the bowel, leading to differences in the consistency of the stool (for example, very liquid stool with an ileostomy and very formed stool with a descending colostomy).

Colostomy

A **colostomy** is surgically created when a portion of the colon (large intestine) or the rectum is removed and the remaining colon is brought through the abdominal wall. A temporary colostomy is used to allow the lower portion of the colon to rest or heal. Usually created in emergency situations, temporary colostomies are designed to be closed at a later time. The colostomy may have one or two openings (with two, one of them will discharge only mucus).

Permanent colostomies are placed when surgical resection of diseased tissue leads to loss of part of the colon. They are created as a treatment for colorectal cancer, or after the lower digestive tract is removed due to illness or disease. Single stomas are created when one end of the bowel is brought out through an opening onto the anterior abdominal wall. The distal portion of the GI tract usually is removed or sewn closed. This type is referred to as an end, or terminal, colostomy and is permanent.

Sigmoid and descending colostomies are the most common type of ostomy surgeries. The end of the descending or sigmoid colon is brought to the surface of the abdomen, usually on the lower left quadrant (Figure 40-3). The descending colostomy is located higher than the sigmoid colostomy. Both produce solid fecal material. The frequency of discharge with both types can be regulated. Patients with descending or sigmoid colostomies may not need to wear an appliance at all times, and odors usually can be controlled (Deitz and Gates, 2010b).

A transverse colostomy is created in the transverse colon, resulting in one or two openings. It is located in the upper abdomen, in the middle or on the right side (see Figure 40-3). Transverse colostomies produce semiformed liquid drainage, because some liquid has been reabsorbed. The drainage from a transverse colostomy is malodorous and needs to be managed. The patient usually has no control over the frequency of discharge, so appliances are in place at all times (Deitz and Gates, 2010b).

Ascending colostomies are similar to ileostomies. Drainage is liquid and cannot be regulated. Digestive enzymes are present and cause an odor. Ascending colostomies are relatively rare. The opening is in the ascending portion of the colon and is located on the right side of the abdomen (see Figure 40-3) (Deitz and Gates, 2010b).

The loop colostomy is a temporary colostomy created in a surgical emergency; it is on the right abdomen. The loop colostomy consists of one stoma with two openings (Figure 40-4). The proximal end of the stoma is active and discharges stool. The distal end is inactive and may discharge mucus. The loop colostomy is created when a loop of bowel is brought out onto the abdominal wall and supported by a bridge. The loop colostomy procedure results in a large stoma that may be difficult to manage because of its size and inability to be covered with available ostomy products (Deitz and Gates, 2010b).

With the double-barrel colostomy, two ends of bowel are brought out onto the abdominal wall, resulting in two distinct stomas (see Figure 40-3). The proximal end is the functional stoma, and the distal end is the nonfunctional stoma. The bowel between the double-barrel colostomy stomas is surgically severed.

Ileostomy

An **ileostomy** is a surgically created opening in the small intestine, usually at the end of the ileum (Figure 40-5). The intestine is brought through the abdominal wall to form a stoma. Ileostomies may be temporary or permanent and may involve removal of all or part of the colon. An ileostomy bypasses the large intestine. Stools from an ileostomy are frequent and liquid, and drainage cannot be regulated. Drainage contains digestive enzymes, which can be damaging to the skin; therefore patients with ileostomies wear an appliance

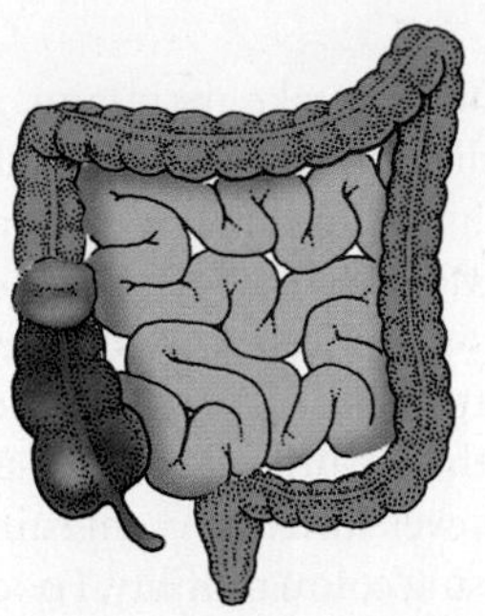

The **ascending colostomy** is used for right-sided tumors.

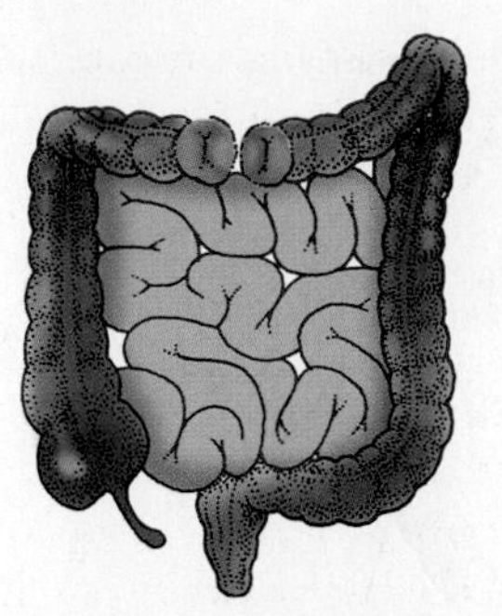

The **transverse (double-barrel) colostomy** is often used in such emergencies as intestinal obstruction or perforation because it can be created quickly. There are two stomas. The proximal one, closest to the small intestine, drains feces. The distal stoma drains mucus.

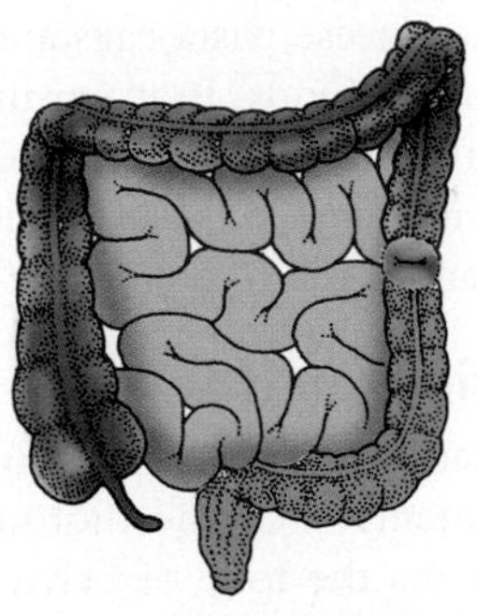

The **descending colostomy** is used for left-sided tumors.

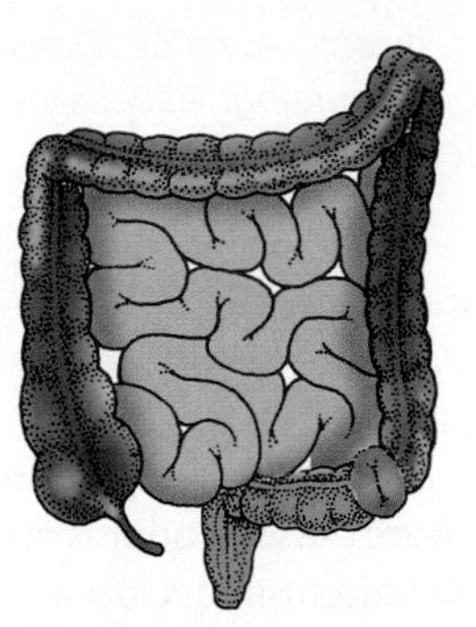

The **sigmoid colostomy** is used for rectal tumors.

FIGURE 40-3 Location of colostomies. (From Ignatavicius DD, Workman ML: *Medical-surgical nursing: Patient-centered collaborative care,* ed. 7, St. Louis, 2013, Saunders.)

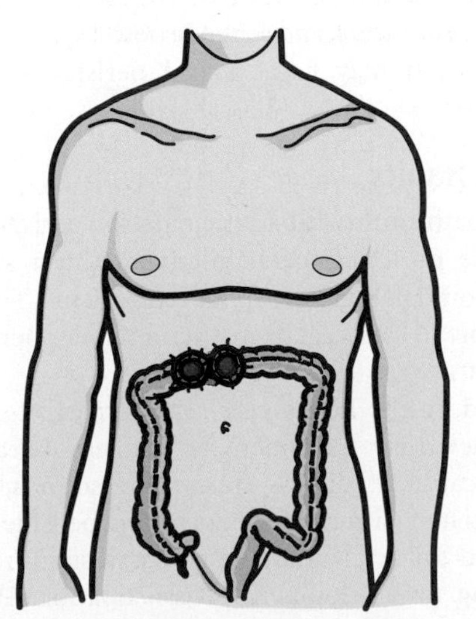

FIGURE 40-4 Loop colostomy. (From Phillips N: *Berry & Kohn's operating room technique,* ed. 12, St. Louis, 2013, Mosby.)

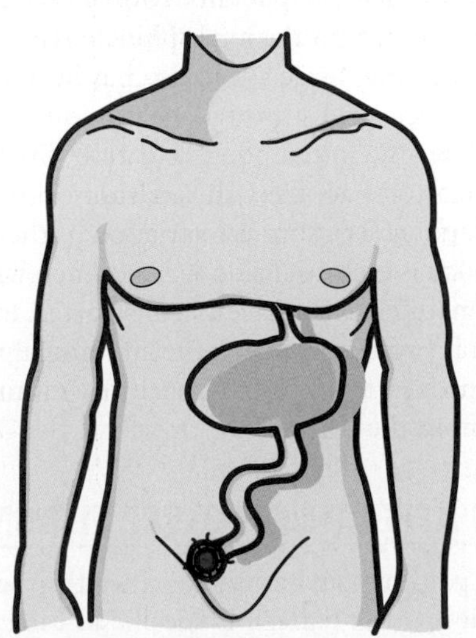

FIGURE 40-5 Ileostomy. (From Phillips N: *Berry & Kohn's operating room technique,* ed. 12, St. Louis, 2013, Mosby.)

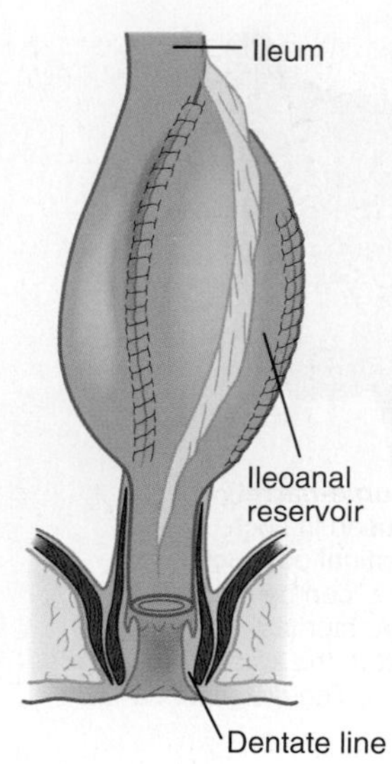

FIGURE 40-6 Ileoanal reservoir. (From Lewis SL, Dirksen SR, Heitkemper MM: *Medical-surgical nursing: Assessment and management of clinical problems,* ed. 9, St. Louis, 2014, Mosby.)

continuously and take special precautions to prevent skin breakdown. Because few bacteria are present, odor is minimal. Fluid and electrolyte balance is monitored closely for the patient who has an ileostomy in place.

The ileoanal pouch is now the most common ileostomy. Technically, it is not an ostomy because there is no stoma. In this procedure, the colon and most of the rectum are surgically removed, and an internal pouch is formed out of the terminal portion of the ileum. An opening at the bottom of this pouch is attached to the anus so that the existing anal sphincter can be used for continence (Figure 40-6). This procedure is performed on patients with ulcerative colitis or familial polyps in whom the anal sphincter is still intact (not removed in previous surgery). It also has been called a pull-through, endorectal pull-through, pelvic pouch, and J-pouch procedure. After the initial pouch creation, the patient has a temporary ileostomy to allow the anastomosis to heal.

The Kock pouch is a surgical variation of the ileostomy. A reservoir pouch is created inside the abdomen with a portion of the terminal ileum. A valve is constructed in the pouch, and a stoma is brought through the abdominal wall. A catheter or tube is inserted into the pouch several times a day to drain feces from the reservoir.

FACTORS AFFECTING BOWEL ELIMINATION

Elimination patterns can be altered in health as well as illness. A regular elimination pattern is specific to each patient, and influenced by age, environment, and culture (Diversity Considerations box). Diet, physical activity, emotional health, and surroundings may affect elimination in either a positive or a negative way.

Diet

Daily food intake maintains peristalsis. Ingestion of a high-fiber diet improves the likelihood of a normal elimination pattern. Fiber in whole grains, fresh fruits, and vegetables flushes fats and waste products more efficiently and helps keep stool soft. It is recommended that adults include 20 to 35 grams of fiber in the diet each day to promote bowel health.

With consumption of gas-producing foods such as onions, cauliflower, and beans, intestinal walls can become distended, increasing colon motility. Food intolerance (e.g., lactose intolerance) results in digestive upset and, in some instances, the passage of watery stools, diarrhea, cramps, or flatulence. Fluid intake or loss affects characteristics of feces. Increased water intake eases the passage of stools. Poor fluid intake increases the risk of constipation because passage of stool is slower, promoting additional water reabsorption with resultant harder stools. Spicy foods produce diarrhea and flatus in some people. Cheese, pasta, eggs, and lean meats can be constipation-producing foods. Bran, prunes, figs, chocolate, and alcohol have a laxative effect. Many people whose lifestyle includes the same mealtimes daily exhibit a regularly timed response to food and a regular pattern of peristaltic activity in the colon.

Physical Activity

Regular physical activity promotes peristalsis and facilitates movement of chyme thorough the colon. Regular activity maintains the tone of pelvic and abdominal floor muscles. Weakened abdominal and pelvic floor muscles resulting from lack of exercise, immobility, or altered neurologic function are often ineffective in increasing the intra-abdominal pressure during defecation, leading to constipation.

Psychological Factors

Emotional stress accelerates the digestive process, and peristalsis is increased. Diarrhea, nausea, and gaseous distention often occur. Diseases associated with stress include colitis, Crohn's disease, ulcers, and irritable bowel syndrome. Patients with depression may have slowed peristalsis, resulting in constipation.

Personal Habits

Sharing a bathroom with another person, privacy concerns, convenience of toileting facilities, and busy schedules all influence bowel habits in hospitalized patients. These patients need support to establish or maintain regular personal elimination habits.

As noted, in the health care setting, patients share bathrooms. They may have activity intolerance and limited balance because of disease states. The sounds, sights, and odors associated with use of bedpans and bedside commodes, or of shared toilet facilities, are embarrassing to the patient, contributing to development of constipation. Patients may ignore the urge to defecate, allowing for increased water absorption in the colon, in turn making feces hard and difficult to expel. When habitually suppressed, the urge to defecate may be lost, and constipation and impaction occur.

DIVERSITY CONSIDERATIONS

Life Span

- Meconium is the first fecal material passed by the newborn. It is black, tarry in consistency, odorless, and sticky.
- Infants have a small stomach, less secretion of enzymes, and a fast transit of food through the GI tract. As a result, they pass stool frequently, often after each feeding. Because the intestine is immature, and water is not well absorbed, infants who are breast-fed have light yellow to golden feces that are soft and liquid. Infants who are fed formula have stool that is dark yellow in color and well formed.
- Control of defecation typically is achieved at the age of approximately 2 years.
- School-age children and adolescents have bowel habits similar to those of adults.
- Constipation may be an issue with school-age children related to lack of privacy, risk of bullying, limited access, and dirty bathrooms. These factors can cause a child to delay defecation during school (Kistner, 2009).
- Older adults may have poor fluid intake, be unable to eat fiber, or have swallowing and chewing difficulties, which may lead to constipation.
- Constipation is the most common bowel management problem in the elderly population.
- Bowel elimination problems are especially prevalent in long-term care facilities.

Culture, Ethnicity, and Religion

- African Americans have the highest incidence of colon cancer in the United States.
- Jews of Eastern European descent have a high risk for colorectal cancer.
- African Americans have a high incidence of lactose intolerance; it is important to check for family history.
- Cultural factors, such as the gender of the caregiver, may affect bowel elimination and nursing care.

Disability

- Patients with physical limitations and mobility problems may have difficulty with constipation and incontinence.
- Patients with impaired mobility may have difficulty getting to the bathroom and may need assistive devices such as bars or raised toilet seats or elevated commodes
- Cognitive impairment such as Alzheimer disease may decrease the ability to respond to urge, contributing to constipation or incontinence.
- Patients with mental limitations may have difficulty recognizing or responding to urge.
- A slowing of nerve impulses to the anal region in some neurologic diseases may make the patient become less aware of the need to defecate, leading to development of irregular bowel movements.
- A reduction in activity levels and muscle weakness decreases peristalsis, and esophageal emptying slows.

Morphology

- Up to 66% of obese people suffer from osteoarthritis, which causes functional impairment and interferes with activities of daily living.
- Obesity can lead to gastroesophageal reflux disease (GERD), stress incontinence, hemorrhoid formation, and abdominal hernias.
- Morbidly obese patients have an increased risk for incontinence related to several factors, among which is the difficulty sitting on a standard size bedpan, bedside commode, or toilet.
- The additional time it takes for the obese patient to get to the toilet, or to move the patient to the toilet, may be responsible for incontinence episodes.
- Pressure of an enlarged abdomen on the bowel in turn places pressure on the sphincter, resulting in stool leakage (Harris, 2008).

Posture

The normal posture during defecation is squatting, which most modern toilets facilitate. The immobilized patient is not able to effectively contract abdominal muscles, making defecation difficult. If permitted, the head of the patient's bed is elevated to allow for a position more likely to facilitate defecation.

Pain

Hemorrhoids, rectal surgery, fistulas, and abdominal surgery will cause patients to suppress the urge to defecate, to avoid pain. With repeated failure to defecate, constipation may result or become worse. Narcotic pain medications also contribute to development of constipation. Stool softeners may be prescribed.

Pregnancy

As the fetus grows, pressure is exerted on the rectum, impairing passage of feces. Straining during defecation or the delivery process can result in hemorrhoid formation. Prenatal vitamins high in iron increase the risk of constipation.

Surgery and Anesthesia

Anesthesia blocks parasympathetic stimulation to the muscles of the colon and cause peristalsis to slow or cease. Surgery that requires manipulation of the intestines causes temporary cessation of intestinal movement. The stoppage of peristalsis is called **paralytic ileus**, which lasts 24 to 48 hours. For patients who remain inactive or are unable to eat after surgery, return of bowel function may be further delayed. Patients whose surgery was conducted with use of spinal or local anesthesia are less likely to experience this problem. Early activity and frequent assessment of bowel sounds are important during this period.

Medications

Some medications interfere directly or indirectly with bowel elimination. **Laxatives** ease defecation, often by stimulating bowel activity. Types of laxatives include bulk-forming agents, osmotics, salines, stimulants, and stool softeners. Cathartics are strong laxatives that stimulate evacuation of the bowel by causing a change in GI transit time. Other medications soften stool, promoting defecation. Some suppress peristaltic activity and are used to control diarrhea and decrease gastric emptying.

Certain medications cause diarrhea or constipation as a side effect. Antibiotics contribute to diarrhea by interfering with the normal bacterial flora in the GI tract. Anticholinergic drugs inhibit gastric acid secretion and depress GI motility. Opioid analgesics also depress GI motility. Histamine antagonists suppress secretion of hydrochloric acid and interfere with digestion of some foods. Calcium supplements and opioids slow colonic action.

Some medications affect the appearance of the feces. Drugs that can cause GI bleeding when taken for extended periods of time, such as nonsteroidal antiinflammatory drugs (NSAIDs), may cause red or black stools, depending on where the bleeding is occurring. Iron salts, which cause constipation, can cause stool to be black. Antacids cause whitish discoloration or white specks.

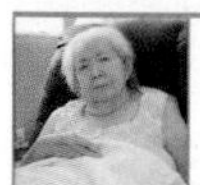

1. Explain the pathophysiology related to Mrs. Schafer's elimination problem.

Diagnostic Tests

Before diagnostic procedures of the bowel, the patient may be placed on a restricted diet or given cleansing enemas. Prescribed bowel preparations to ensure emptying of the bowel are given to facilitate visualization at endoscopic, radiographic, or other examinations. After the procedure, changes in elimination, such as increased gas and loose stools, may persist until the patient returns to a normal eating pattern.

ASSESSMENT LO 40.3

Gathering subjective and objective data for assessment of bowel elimination allows the nurse to identify patterns and abnormalities. The assessment of the GI system includes a focused interview, including past and present health history (Health Assessment Questions box); physical inspection of the abdomen; inspection of the feces; and a focused diet history including chewing difficulties, medications, illnesses, and food intolerance.

While performing the bowel elimination assessment, the nurse considers the patient's physical, mental, and functional abilities, as well as the home environment and family and social support. Attention focuses on identification and prioritization of immediate problems and relief of symptoms, before a full assessment is undertaken.

HEALTH HISTORY

A comprehensive history identifying normal and abnormal patterns of bowel elimination and comparing them to the patient's perception of normal is a crucial step in identifying elimination issues. Include any history of surgeries or illness affecting the GI tract. Family history is evaluated for GI cancer, Crohn's disease, and other GI disturbances with familial links.

ABDOMINAL ASSESSMENT

Before inspecting the abdomen, inspect the patient's mouth, teeth, tongue, and gums for sores, dentition, and moisture. Poor dentition, mucosal dryness, and mouth sores can cause pain or make swallowing difficult. An abdominal assessment should always begin with inspection and auscultation, because palpation and percussion alter peristaltic activity. Percussion is an advanced skill and usually is performed by nurses with special training.

Inspection

The abdominal assessment is performed while the patient is in the supine position with a pillow behind the head and knees. Determine the contour of the abdomen by viewing at eye level. Abdominal contour may appear flat, round, scaphoid, or protuberant in pregnancy, obesity, or ascites. Abdominal distention may appear as a protuberant abdomen with taut skin. Observe the symmetry of the abdomen, noting bulging or masses. Observe the position of umbilicus; if it is protruding or displaced, a mass or hernia may be present. Observe the abdominal wall for movement. Increased peristaltic activity could indicate an obstructive process. The nurse notes scars, stomas, and lesions during inspection.

Auscultation

With the patient in the supine position, auscultation begins in the right lower quadrant and proceeds through each of the remaining quadrants. Assure that the stethoscope is in contact with the patient's skin. Normal bowel sounds are irregular, high-pitched, and gurgling and occur every 5 to 15 seconds. Hyperactive bowel sounds tend to be loud, high-pitched, and rushing; they are commonly heard with diarrhea or inflammatory disorders. Hypoactive bowel sounds are slow and sluggish, with occurrence of less than five sounds per minute. Decreased bowel sounds are common after surgery. Absence of sounds may be a sign of obstruction or paralytic ileus. Patients with ileus or intestinal obstruction require immediate medical attention. The nurse listens for 5 full minutes before documenting the absence of sounds.

Palpation

Palpation determines organ size, organ placement, masses, pain, and presence of fluid. Painful areas are palpated last. Light touch is used over all four quadrants. The abdomen

HEALTH ASSESSMENT QUESTIONS

History

- Have you been diagnosed with an abdominal disease such as cholecystitis, ulcers, diverticulitis, cholelithiasis, or cirrhosis?
- Have you had abdominal surgery or trauma?
- Have you ever been diagnosed with an infection in the abdomen?
- Do you have abdominal changes, or physical problems that affect appetite, bowel function? If so, for how long?
- Do you have a family history of gastrointestinal disturbances?

General Questions

- Have you experienced changes in diet or appetite recently?
- Describe your daily diet and fluid intake.
- What is your current weight? Have you had recent weight changes (planned or unplanned)? What is your height?
- Describe your bowel habits.
- Are you experiencing changes in your bowel habits, including diarrhea or constipation?
- When did the changes start?
- Describe the type of change you have been experiencing?
- Describe the color and consistency of your stool.
- Have you been taking any medication that would cause changes in the consistency of the stool, such as laxatives or cathartics, or antibiotics?
- What do you think may be the cause of the changes?
- What have you done to correct the situation? Have these measures helped?
- Do you experience rectal pain or itching?
- Have you experienced feelings of bloating or gas? What do you do to relieve feelings or symptoms of bloating or gas?
- Are the symptoms related to specific meals, types or quantity of food, or time of day or night?
- Do you have other symptoms that accompany the bloating or gas such as vomiting, headaches, belching, flatulence, heartburn, or pain? If pain is experienced does it radiate to the shoulders or arms?
- Do you use antacid medications? If so how often? Do you notice a positive response to the medication?
- Do you have nausea or vomiting? If so, what is the onset of the nausea or vomiting? Is it related to particular stimuli?
  - Describe the emesis. Are there any associated symptoms?
- Are you using any types of home remedy?
- Are you experiencing any abdominal pain? If so, rate the pain on a 1 to 10 pain scale.
- Describe the onset, location, duration, and characteristics of the pain.
- Does the pain radiate?
- What makes the pain better? What makes it worse?
- Are you taking any medication for the pain?
- Describe your current stress level.
- How do you think you cope with stress? Describe some of your coping skills.
- Do you work with any chemical irritants?
- Have you traveled recently? Where have you traveled?

Pregnant Patient

- Do you suffer from constipation, heartburn, or flatulence?
- Are you experiencing nausea and vomiting? If so, does it occur at certain times of the day or with specific foods?

Older Adult

- Do you experience constipation? If so how often?
- Are you ever incontinent of feces?
- Do you take laxatives? Which one? How often?
- What type of fiber-containing food do you eat during a typical day?
- What types of fluids do you drink? How much fluid do you drink in a day?
- Are you able to get to the store for your groceries?
- Do you eat alone or with someone?
- Do you wear dentures?

should be soft, smooth in contour, and pain-free. The patient should be relaxed during palpation, because tense muscles will interfere with palpating underlying organs or masses. In obese patients, bimanual or deep palpation is required to detect underlying organs.

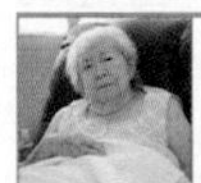

2. Identify the focused assessments that must be completed for Mrs. Schaffer related to her current elimination problem.

LABORATORY TESTS

Laboratory tests are necessary to obtain information on elimination problems. Laboratory testing can help determine the presence of bleeding, inflammation, or infection. Some tests that are performed are stool cultures and stools for occult blood.

Stool Cultures and Occult Blood

A stool culture is used along with other tests to detect parasites in the stool and to help determine the cause of diarrhea. Stool cultures are ordered if the patient complains of diarrhea for several days or when blood or mucus is noted in loose stools. They may be ordered if the history suggests that the patient may have consumed food contaminated with bacteria associated with undercooked meat or raw eggs, or the same food that has made others ill. Recent travel outside the United States may suggest possible food contamination. If the patient has had a previous pathogenic bacterial infection of the GI tract that has been treated or resolved, additional stool cultures may be performed to verify that the pathogenic bacteria are no longer detectable.

Negative results usually reflect the fact that the stool culture was checked for pathogens at several intervals and none were isolated. If the culture is negative for the major pathogens, it is likely that the diarrhea is due to another cause. If the stool culture is positive for pathogenic bacteria, infection is the most likely cause of prolonged diarrhea. The stool sensitivity testing report may identify the causative agent, with appropriate treatment suggestions.

Testing for the presence of blood in the feces is performed using a **fecal occult blood test** (see Skill 34-3). Fecal occult blood tests measure for microscopic amounts of blood in the feces, which can be a sign of a growth in the colon or rectum. Blood may be present in the stool in association with benign (noncancerous) or malignant (cancerous) growths or **polyps** in the colon, hemorrhoids, anal fissures, intestinal infections, ulcerative colitis, Crohn's disease, diverticular disease, and abnormalities of the blood vessels in the large intestine. GI bleeding may be microscopic (occult blood) or may be easily seen as red blood, or black, tar-like stools called melena. A positive fecal occult blood test indicates that blood has been found in the stool. A negative test result indicates that no blood was found in the stool sample. The fecal occult blood test requires the collection of three small stool samples taken 1 day apart. The consecutive specimens are collected separately because colon cancers may bleed intermittently. Fecal occult blood test results are affected by ingestion of certain foods. A special diet is prescribed 48 to 72 hours before the test. Foods that affect the test results and therefore should be avoided are beets, broccoli, cantaloupe, carrots, cauliflower, cucumbers, fish, grapefruit, horseradish, mushrooms, poultry, radishes, red meat, turnips, and vitamin C–enriched foods and beverages.

DIAGNOSTIC EXAMINATIONS

Diagnostic tests provide information about alterations in clinical status that may not be evident from laboratory test results. Many of the diagnostic tests used for patients with alterations in GI function allow for visualization of the organ systems and function. Tissue samples can be obtained during some of the tests. The nurse must be familiar with diagnostic tests and implications of the results, both to prepare the patient for a specific test and to provide care that may be required at completion of the procedure.

Upper GI Series

An upper GI series (barium swallow) is a radiologic study that defines the anatomy of the upper digestive tract to visualize the esophagus, stomach, and duodenum. This series of images assists in the diagnosis of upper GI diseases and conditions such as ulcers, tumors, hiatal hernias, scarring, blockages, and abnormalities of the GI tissues. An upper GI study involves some risk from radiation exposure. Patients who are or may become pregnant should notify the radiology department staff, because such studies carry some risk of harm to the fetus from radiation exposure.

Before the procedure, the patient should not eat or drink anything for 4 to 8 hours. The procedure involves swallowing a liquid that contains barium, which fills and coats the intestinal lining, making the anatomic structures visible. X-ray images are taken at different angles through the chest and abdomen.

A major side effect of the upper GI series is constipation. Patients who undergo an upper GI study are encouraged to drink extra fluids after the test. A laxative may be recommended to promote evacuation of the bowels if the barium is not eliminated completely within 1 or 2 days. Barium has a whitish appearance that may be apparent in the stool for several days after the test.

Lower GI Series

The lower GI series, also known as a barium enema, consists of x-ray imaging of the rectum, colon, and the lower portion of the small intestine to assist in diagnosis of abnormal growths, ulcers, polyps, diverticula, and colon cancer. Barium is inserted into the colon, and then x-ray pictures of the colon and rectum are taken. The barium aids in visualizing the size and shape of the colon and rectum.

The patient undergoing a lower GI series is informed that the barium will cause fullness and pressure in the abdomen and there will likely be the urge to have a bowel movement. The patient is asked to change positions while x-ray pictures are taken, to obtain different views of the colon.

To prepare for the procedure, the patient will have a restricted diet for a few days beforehand, generally a liquid diet for the 2 prior days, clear liquids only for 24 hours, and then a laxative or enema just before the procedure. As in the upper GI series, the barium may cause constipation and cause the stool to turn gray or white for a few days after the procedure.

Endoscopy

An esophagoscopy is an endoscopic procedure to view the inside of the esophagus. A gastroscopy is a procedure to view the inside of the stomach. A duodenoscopy is a procedure to view the inside of the duodenum, the first part of the small intestine. These examinations are performed as a single procedure and are collectively referred to as an upper endoscopy, or esophagogastroduodenoscopy (EGD).

In this procedure, a fiber-optic endoscope, a flexible instrument with a small camera on the end, is passed through the mouth, down the throat, and into the stomach. This examination assists in the diagnosis or clarification of any abnormalities that may have been seen on an x-ray image. Upper endoscopies are prescribed for patients with swallowing difficulties, vomiting, bleeding, gastric reflux, abdominal pain, or chest pain.

Because direct visualization of the structures is necessary, the stomach must be empty; therefore the patient should not have anything to eat or drink for at least 8 hours before the examination. The patient receives medication that causes drowsiness, relaxation, amnesia, and possibly lightheadedness. The throat is sprayed with a numbing medicine that helps prevent discomfort and gagging. The numbness lasts about 30 to 45 minutes. The patient is asked to swallow once or twice during the initial period of insertion to facilitate movement of the endoscope. The tube does not interfere with the patient's ability to breathe and is only mildly uncomfortable after the initial insertion. The examination takes approximately 10 to 20 minutes. During the study and afterward, the patient may have a feeling of fullness, because it requires injection of a moderate amount of air to expand the abdomen, allowing for better visualization.

A biopsy specimen may be obtained for examination, or electrosurgical instruments may be used to treat some medical conditions. Photographs or videos may be taken to document abnormalities. Driving is not permitted for 12 hours after the procedure to allow the sedative time to wear off. The nurse is responsible for checking for return of the gag reflex before allowing the client to eat or drink after the procedure.

Colonoscopy

Colonoscopy is a procedure performed to visualize inflamed tissue, ulcers, and abnormal growths in the anus, rectum, and colon. The procedure is used to look for early signs of colorectal cancer and to diagnose unexplained changes in bowel habits, abdominal pain, bleeding from the anus, and weight loss.

Before the procedure, the patient performs bowel preparation to empty solids from the GI tract by following a clear liquid diet for 1 to 3 days. The patient should not drink beverages containing red or purple dye. A laxative or an enema may be required the night before the colonoscopy. Patients should inform the PCP of all medical conditions and any medications, vitamins, or supplements taken regularly, including aspirin, arthritis medications, anticoagulants, diabetes medications, and vitamins that contain iron. Patients usually are on NPO status for several hours before the procedure.

For colonoscopy, the patient lies on the left side on an examination table. A light sedative, and possibly pain medication, are given to promote relaxation. A long, flexible, lighted tube called a colonoscope, or scope, is inserted into the anus and slowly guided through the rectum and into the colon. A small camera transmits a video image to a computer screen, allowing careful examination of the intestinal lining. Bleeding and puncture of the large intestine are possible but uncommon complications of colonoscopy. During the procedure, growths (polyps) or abnormal tissues may be removed (biopsy) and tested for cancer. Tissue removal and the treatments to stop any bleeding usually are painless. Cramping or bloating may occur during the first hour after the procedure. Driving is not permitted for 12 hours after colonoscopy, to allow time for the sedative effects to wear off.

◆ NURSING DIAGNOSIS LO 40.4

On completion of the nursing assessment of the patient's bowel function, data obtained may reveal the risk for or an actual elimination problem. Accurate assessment is crucial to identify defining characteristics of impaired elimination. To determine the appropriate nursing diagnoses for the patient, the nurse clusters the data.

- *Constipation* related to pain medication use, decreased fluid intake, and decreased mobility as evidenced by no stools for a few days, hypoactive bowel sounds, and a firm, tender abdomen
- *Diarrhea* related to malabsorption as evidenced by bloating, cramping, and loose liquid stools
- *Bowel Incontinence* related to sphincter dysfunction as evidenced by constant dribbling of soft and liquid feces, inability to recognize the urge to defecate, and fecal staining of underclothing
- *Self-Care Deficit: Toileting* related to impaired mobility as evidenced by need for assist of one for toileting and restriction of bedrest
- *Disturbed Body Image* related to bowel diversion as evidenced by refusal to discuss descending colostomy and disinterest in learning about care of ostomy

In addition to the nursing diagnoses for issues related to bowel elimination that are listed, the patient may exhibit *Risk for Constipation* or *Perceived Constipation*. The patient with bowel elimination issues also may have associated nursing diagnoses not directly related to elimination, such as *Risk for Impaired Skin Integrity, Fluid Volume Deficit,* and *Pain.*

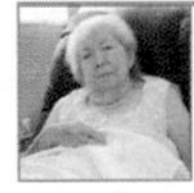

3. Based on the information in the case study, identify three nursing diagnoses with related factors for Mrs. Schaffer, along with patient teaching interventions that may be necessary for each.

◆ PLANNING LO 40.5

The goals for patients with elimination problems are structured around maintaining normal elimination patterns, returning to previous levels of function, and preventing associated risks (Table 40-1). Goals related to reestablishing normal bowel function and prevention of further complications include:

- Patient will pass soft stools daily during hospitalization.
- Patient will defecate formed stools within 24 hours.
- Patient's episodes of bowel incontinence will decrease within 48 hours after starting a toileting program.
- Patient will perform self-care after toileting within 2 days.
- Patient will participate in personal colostomy care during hospitalization.

TABLE 40-1 Care Planning

NANDA-I NURSING DIAGNOSIS LABEL WITH NURSING DIAGNOSIS STATEMENT	NURSING OUTCOME CLASSIFICATION (NOC)	NURSING INTERVENTION CLASSIFICATION (NIC)
Constipation related to pain medication use, decreased fluid intake and decreased mobility, as evidenced by no stools for a few days, hypoactive bowel sounds, and a firm, tender abdomen	*Bowel elimination* (0501) Stool soft and formed (050104)	*Constipation/impaction management* (0450) Encourage increased fluid intake unless contraindicated.

From Bulechek G, Butcher H, Dochterman J, et al (Eds): *Nursing interventions classification (NIC)*, ed. 6, St. Louis, 2013, Mosby; Moorhead S, Johnson M, Maas M, et al (Eds): *Nursing outcomes classification (NOC)*, ed. 5, St. Louis, 2013, Mosby; NANDA International: *Nursing diagnoses: Definitions and classification, 2012–2014*, West Sussex, England, 2012, Wiley-Blackwell. Reprinted with permission from NANDA International, Inc.

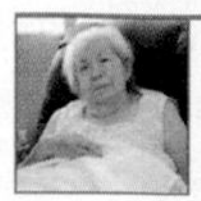

The conceptual care map for Mrs. Schaffer can be found at *http://evolve.elsevier.com/YoostCrawford/fundamentals/*. It is partially completed to indicate how to use the map as a learning tool. Complete the nursing diagnoses using the example conceptual care maps shown in Chapters 8 and 25 to 33.

IMPLEMENTATION AND EVALUATION LO 40.6

The nurse can help patients achieve regular bowel elimination by performing or assisting the client with techniques and habits that promote regular elimination. Nursing measures to aid in bowel elimination include interventions for diarrhea, constipation, impaction, and incontinence, as well as those for patients with bowel diversions.

INTERVENTIONS

After assessing the pattern of the patient's elimination and determining the patient's perception of normal bowel elimination, encourage the establishment of a regular elimination pattern. Variations in diet and personal habits lead to misconceptions regarding the frequency of bowel movements and can lead to overuse of laxatives. In such cases, the patient is warned that ongoing use of laxatives is associated with harmful side effects, such as an increase in constipation and impaction, predisposition to colorectal cancer, dependency, and electrolyte imbalance.

Suggest warm liquids, which stimulate peristalsis and aid in defecation. Emphasize the necessary ingredients for a normal bowel regimen (fluid, fiber, activity, and a regular schedule for defecation). Laxatives may be needed to establish a regular pattern; however, provide laxatives, suppositories, and enemas as needed and as ordered only. Laxative use varies the patient's regular pattern, so the nurse and the patient together establish a goal of eliminating their use. Instruct the patient to avoid straining to defecate. Straining is a form of the Valsalva maneuver and can cause bradycardia and possibly death, especially in patients with cardiac disease.

Every patient with elimination problems is weighed daily, because weight is an important indicator of fluid balance in the body. Dementia, acute confusion, and mental retardation are risk factors for fecal incontinence; therefore, mental status is monitored closely. Patients are monitored closely for impaction, which is more common in elderly than in younger people. The patient is checked for impaction before administration of antidiarrheal medications. Teach appropriate methods of taking these medications and instruct the patient on their side effects. Immobile patients who are incontinent with liquid stool may have a fecal management system inserted to drain the stool. This device is similar to a urinary drainage system and is used to protect the surrounding skin.

The nurse helps to control or prevent diarrhea in patients by following some simple guidelines. Hand washing between caring for patients, after using the bathroom, and before and after preparation of foods will greatly reduce the risk of diarrhea from a foodborne or communicable illness.

Meticulous skin care and containment of fecal drainage are necessary to prevent skin breakdown; a fecal collector can be used if necessary. The skin is protected with barrier creams containing zinc oxide or lanolin or with a petroleum-based product. Barrier creams are wiped off if soiling occurs (Beldon, 2008).

Elderly patients are evaluated for fecal incontinence on entrance to the acute or long-term care facility. The rate of incontinence in the acute care setting is 3%; in long-term care facilities, incontinence rates can be as high as 50%.

Preventive Screening

Patients are encouraged to follow recommended colorectal screening guidelines. The fecal occult blood test is recommended yearly for everyone 50 years of age and older. Sigmoidoscopy and colonoscopy, which are screening tests for colorectal polyps and early signs of cancer, should begin at age 50 for most people—earlier in those with a family history of colorectal cancer, a personal history of inflammatory bowel disease, or other risk factors. The tests are performed every 5 to 10 years, depending on the individual's history and the type of test performed (American Cancer Society, 2014).

Diet

Patients with elimination problems may need to make changes in their diet to promote regular elimination patterns. In general, a diet of high-fiber foods, with adequate fluid intake, is encouraged, although this diet may not be sufficient for the patient with alterations to normal elimination patterns. For more information on a high-fiber diet, see Chapter 30. Daily intake of fiber helps prevent constipation by giving stool bulk (Evidence-Based Practice and Informatics box). Food such as fresh fruits, beans, vegetables, and bran cereals are incorporated into the patient's diet. Fluid intake up to 6 to 8 glasses of liquids per day should be consumed to help prevent hard, dry stools.

EVIDENCE-BASED PRACTICE AND INFORMATICS

Fiber and Bowel Health

Fiber in the diet has many benefits, including:

- Normalization of bowel movements
- Maintenance of bowel integrity and health
- Lowering blood cholesterol levels
- Helping control blood sugar levels
- Aiding weight loss
- Potentially helping to prevent colorectal cancer

The Mayo Clinic website, *www.mayoclinic.com/health/fiber/NU00033,* among others, can guide patients in increasing the amount of fiber in their diet.

The patient with diarrhea benefits from bland, small meals, which may be more easily tolerated. Milk products, spices, food that irritates or stimulates the GI tract, gas-producing foods, and caffeine are avoided. Hot and cold liquids also are avoided because they stimulate peristalsis; liquids of tepid temperatures are preferred. Oral or intravenous intake of fluids to prevent dehydration is necessary for the patient with diarrhea.

The healthy patient should drink at least 6 to 8 glasses of fluid daily. Hot liquids and fruit juices, such as prune juice and apple juice, are encouraged because they stimulate peristalsis, although they are to be avoided by the patient with diarrhea. For the patient with flatulence, gas-forming foods such as cabbage, beans, onions, and cauliflower are avoided.

The patient receiving tube feedings is taught principles of safe food handling, including rinsing feeding containers every 8 hours and replacing the containers every 24 hours to prevent bacterial growth. Rapid administration of tube feeding has been associated with diarrhea; therefore the rate of infusion may need to be adjusted. Bulking agents, including soluble fiber such as psyllium, may be used in tube feedings to prevent diarrhea. The nurse should consult a dietitian when diarrhea occurs, to identify food allergies and intolerance but still maintain the patient's dietary requirements. Close monitoring of the patient's fluid and electrolyte balance will help prevent life-threatening fluid deficiency and electrolyte or acid-base imbalance.

Exercise

Encourage the patient to be out of bed as soon as possible after surgery or illnesses. Exercises such as turning and changing positions in bed and passive or active range-of-motion exercises increase peristalsis and help prevent constipation. Aerobic exercise raises respiratory and heart rates, which stimulates contraction of intestinal muscles.

After eating, blood flow is increased to the stomach and intestines to promote digestion. However, strenuous exercise causes blood to be diverted to the heart and brain. Waiting approximately an hour after a meal to exercise is advised. Walking 10 to 15 minutes per day has been shown to increase digestive function.

Promoting Normal Bowel Patterns in Health Care Facilities

The nurse assists patients in health care facilities achieve regular defecation by providing privacy and assisting in establishing a regular pattern of elimination. The patient is offered toileting opportunities often, because soiling may occur if the patient is forced to wait. The nurse encourages independence with toileting activities when possible, although the need to toilet increases the risk of falls or accidents. Assisting the patient to a commode or to a sitting position facilitates bowel elimination, and the nurse or unlicensed assistive personnel (UAP) may need to stay with a patient who is too weak to be left alone.

Bedpan

Patients who are unable to walk to the bathroom or who are restricted to bed secondary to procedures, illness, injury, or surgery require the use of the bedpan for elimination (Nursing Care Guideline: Assisting the Patient Using a Bedpan box). The caregiver must be quick to respond to the toileting needs of the patient restricted to bed, because frequently there is little time between urge and elimination.

Preserving skin integrity and preventing pain with required positioning are important. Sitting on a bedpan is uncomfortable because the pressure points rest on the hard surface. Time on the bedpan is limited, to prevent skin breakdown and decreased sphincter control. Leaving the patient on the bedpan longer than 10 minutes can result in pressure ulcer formation (Ethical, Legal, and Professional Practice box).

Maintain the patient's privacy during bowel elimination. Pull the curtain closed around the patient. Close bathroom doors. Make certain that treatment routines do not interfere with the patient's routine. Cover the patient with bed linens to maintain comfort and dignity. Allow the patient access to the call light and toilet paper.

Bedpans are assigned for use by a single patient but are washed and disinfected after each use. Always perform hand hygiene and use gloves when handling a bedpan.

NURSING CARE GUIDELINE

Assisting the Patient Using a Bedpan

Background

- When the patient cannot be out of bed, use of a bedpan may be required.
- The two types of bedpans are:
  - A fracture pan is a shallow bedpan that is used for patients with hip or back fractures or to promote comfort in patients who may have to lie flat or are unable to raise their buttocks off the bed. Fracture bedpans are placed with the handle towards the patient's feet.
  - A regular bedpan has higher sides and is more uniquely shaped, similar to a standard toilet seat; it allows the patient to be raised to a more normal position for elimination.

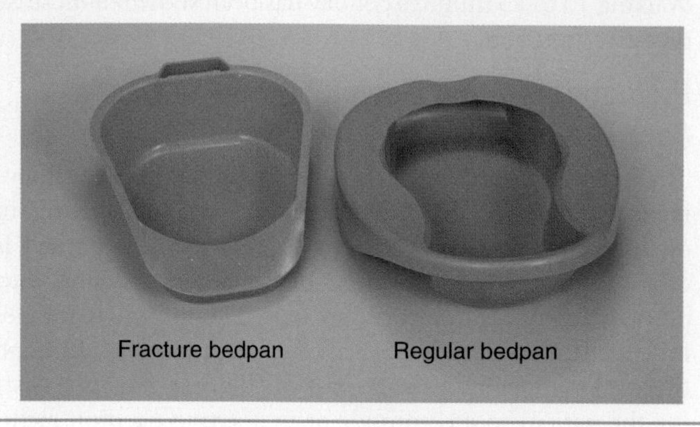

Procedural Concerns

- Always wear gloves when assisting a patient with elimination.
- Place a waterproof pad on the bed.
- The patient must be properly positioned, with buttocks centered on the bedpan.
- If the patient is unable to assist with lifting/movement, roll the patient to one side and place the bedpan on the bed, then roll the patient onto the bedpan.
- Elevate the head of the bed, using Fowler position if it can be tolerated by the patient.
- Do not leave the bedpan in place for longer than 10 minutes; doing so will promote or exacerbate pressure ulcers and/or skin breakdown.
- After bedpan removal, provide perineal care.
- Remove gloves and perform hand hygiene.

Documentation Concerns

- Document patient intake and output.
- Note the patient's tolerance of the procedure.
- Record skin assessment details.

ETHICAL, LEGAL, AND PROFESSIONAL PRACTICE

Care of the Patient With Altered Elimination

The nurse is responsible for providing competent care to the patient to reduce risk of infection and to maintain skin integrity.

- Length of time a patient is left on the bedpan can contribute to pressure ulcer formation. Answer the call bell promptly for the patient with issues in bowel elimination.
- After elimination, wash the area with soap and water and thoroughly dry to help prevent skin breakdown. Apply barrier cream to the skin if there is a risk of breakdown.
- The patient who is incontinent is exposed to moisture and bacteria and requires frequent assessment of skin integrity.
- The nurse is responsible for monitoring and identifying an alteration in elimination. Failure to identify alterations may hold the nurse liable for negligent nursing practice.

SAFE PRACTICE ALERT

Wear appropriate personal protective equipment (PPE) when cleaning a bedpan. There is a possibility of splashing during the cleaning procedure, so PPE should include gloves, a gown, and a mask with an eye shield.

Bedside Commode

The bedside commode is a portable chair with a toilet seat and a receptacle beneath that can be emptied (Figure 40-7). It is used most often with adult patients who can get out of bed but have difficulty with ambulation. Safety is a consideration in moving the patient to the commode.

Early Ambulation

Exercise is important in maintaining GI function. Early ambulation after surgery or an illness stimulates peristalsis and helps maintain function. Therefore the patient is encouraged to be out of bed as soon as possible.

Bowel Patterns

For the patient experiencing bowel elimination problems, a return to previous level of function is the optimal goal. To achieve that goal, additional assistance may be needed in the form of bowel training programs, elimination schedules, and medications.

Antidiarrheal Medications

Antidiarrheal medications are used to slow the motility of the intestine or promote the absorption of excess fluid in the intestine. Antidiarrheal medications are available as over-the-counter products. The most effective agents, however,

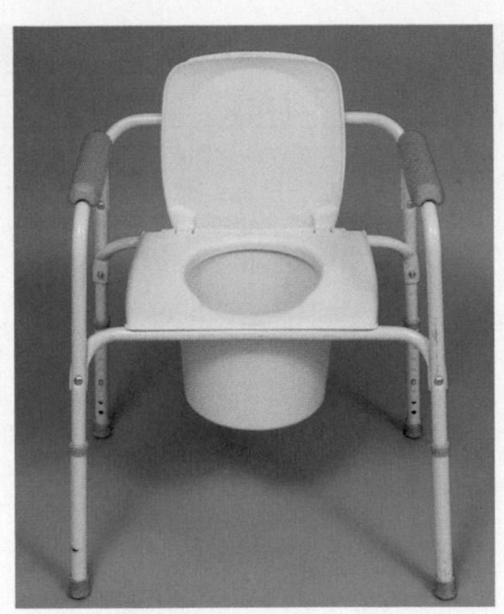

FIGURE 40-7 Bedside commode. (From Sorrentino SA, Remmert L: *Mosby's textbook for nursing assistants*, ed. 8, St. Louis, 2012, Mosby.)

are prescription opiate agents such as loperamide (Imodium), diphenoxylate-atropine (Lomotil), and codeine, which decrease intestinal muscle tone to slow the passage of feces. These drugs are given for 48 to 72 hours. Caution is used with opiates that are habit-forming, such as diphenoxylate-atropine, and codeine. The cause of the diarrhea must be determined.

Laxatives and Stool Softeners

Cathartics and laxatives may be prescribed for a patient who is unable to empty the bowel normally. Although the two terms often are used interchangeably, *cathartics* induce defecation with a stronger effect on the intestines. Laxatives have a milder action, producing soft or liquid stools. Any laxative or cathartic is contraindicated in patients with nausea, vomiting, or undiagnosed abdominal pain. The chronic use of laxatives can weaken the natural response of the bowels, resulting in rebound constipation.

Laxative suppositories are more effective than their oral counterparts because of their stimulant effect on the rectal mucosa. A rectal **suppository** is a drug delivery system that is inserted into the rectum, where it dissolves for medication absorption through the rectal mucosa. The nurse ensures that the suppository is placed in contact with the mucosa and not in stool that is in the rectum. Laxative suppositories work to soften the stool and distend the rectum. These suppositories take approximately 30 minutes to work; therefore the patient should plan accordingly (see Chapter 35, Nursing Care Guideline: Rectal Medication Administration for more information on rectal suppository administration).

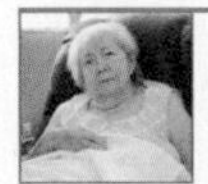

4. Identify three interventions that the nurse should expect to implement for Mrs. Schaeffer, and give the rationale for each.

Enemas

An **enema** is the introduction of solutions into the rectum and sigmoid colon via the anus (Skill 40-1). The increase in the volume of fluid rapidly distends the colon and irritates the intestinal mucosa lining, stimulating complete evacuation of the lower intestinal tract.

Common uses of enemas include relief of constipation, removal of impacted feces, emptying of the bowel before diagnostic tests or surgery, and beginning a program of bowel training. Enemas can be used to instill medications. Several types of enema solutions are used today (Table 40-2).

Nasogastric Intubation

Nasogastric (NG) intubation is necessary when the patient needs decompression of the GI tract, administration of medication or enteral feedings, compression of internal hemorrhage, or gastric lavage. An NG tube is a pliable tube that is inserted through the nasopharynx into the stomach (see Chapter 30, Skill 30-1). The several types of NG tubes available can be broadly categorized as small-bore tubes or large-bore tubes.

Large-bore tubes, size 12 Fr. and larger, are used for decompression, removal of gastric secretions, and lavage. They are used in conditions in which peristalsis is absent, such as surgery, trauma, infections, or obstruction. The common types of large-bore tubes are the Salem sump and Levin tubes (Figure 40-8). The Salem sump tube is preferred for gastric decompression because it has two lumens, one of which serves as an air vent that connects with the second lumen, which is used for suction of gastric contents. When the main lumen is connected to suction, the other provides a continuous air vent.

Irrigation (**lavage**) of the stomach is performed in cases of active bleeding, poisoning, and gastric dilation. Large-bore tubes including the Salem sump, Levin, and Ewald tubes are used for this purpose. For more information on insertion and use of NG tubes (see chapter 30).

Ostomy Care

Ostomy appliances are used to protect skin, collect drainage, and control odor. Pouching systems may include a one-piece or two-piece appliance consisting of a skin barrier or wafer and a collection pouch (Figure 40-9). The pouch attaches to the abdomen by the wafer and collects the stool output. The barrier or wafer protects the skin from the fecal output. Drainable pouches are used when the pouch needs to be emptied frequently (Skill 40-2).

A patient with an ostomy in place will need to learn self-care, and it is crucial that this is begun in the acute care setting (Collaboration and Delegation box). A wound ostomy continence nurse (WOCN) is consulted early to promote self-care and to teach the meticulous regimen necessary to prevent skin damage and infection (Figure 40-10). The WOCN is certified in the management of patients who have had some type of bowel or bladder diversion. This nurse specialist's

TABLE 40-2 Types of Enemas

TYPE OF ENEMA	DESCRIPTION	VOLUME	USES
Cleansing enemas		120-1000 mL	Empty the bowel and remove feces through instillation of fluid Primary action: peristalsis stimulation
Hypertonic	Work by osmotic pressure, drawing fluid out of interstitial spaces into the colon, which then fills with fluids and distends		
Isotonic	Work by expanding the colon, thus promoting peristalsis		
Oil retention enemas	The feces absorb the oil and become softer and easier to pass The patient must retain the enema for 1-3 hr for the best possible results	120-150 mL	Lubricate the rectum and colon
Medication enemas	The patient must retain the enema so that the medication has time to work		Antibiotic or anthelmintic enemas used to treat local infections such as bacteria, worms, and parasites are types of retention enemas
Carminative enemas		60-80 mL	Provide relief from gastric distention by stimulating peristalsis to improve passage of flatus
Return-flow enemas		100-200 mL of solution, administered and then drained from the rectum (often repeated until drainage is clear)	Provide relief from gastric distention by stimulating peristalsis to improve passage of flatus

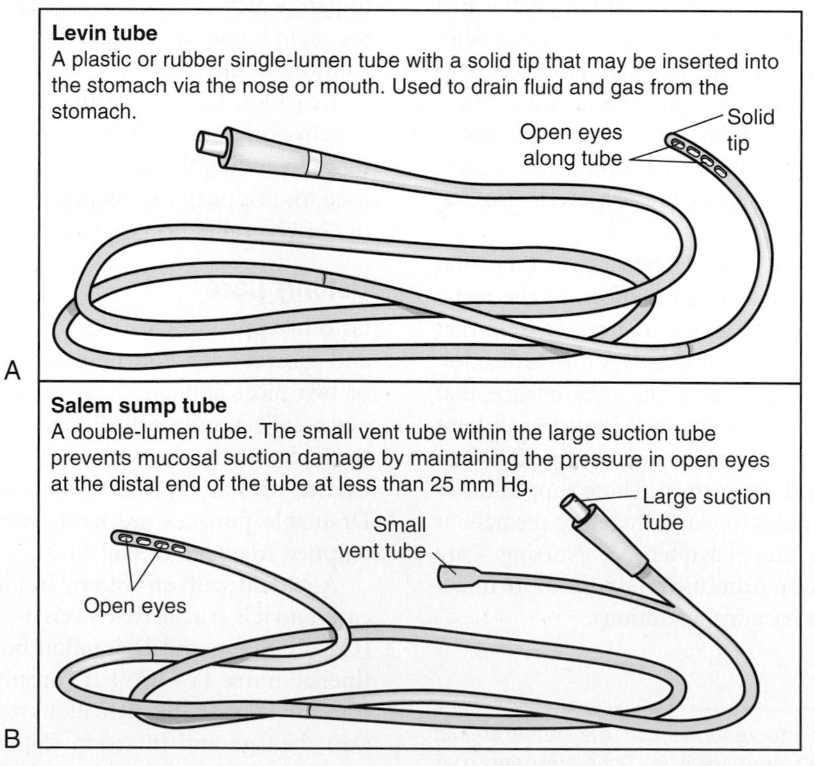

Levin tube
A plastic or rubber single-lumen tube with a solid tip that may be inserted into the stomach via the nose or mouth. Used to drain fluid and gas from the stomach.
Open eyes along tube
Solid tip
A
Salem sump tube
A double-lumen tube. The small vent tube within the large suction tube prevents mucosal suction damage by maintaining the pressure in open eyes at the distal end of the tube at less than 25 mm Hg.
Large suction tube
Small vent tube
Open eyes
B

FIGURE 40-8 Large-bore nasogastric tubes. **A,** Levin tube. **B,** Salem sump tube. (From Silvestri LA: *Saunders comprehensive review for the NCLEX-RN™ examination,* ed. 6, St. Louis, 2014, Saunders.)

COLLABORATION AND DELEGATION

Multidisciplinary Care for Patients With Bowel Elimination Problems

- Patients who are about to undergo ostomy surgery and patients with new ostomy placement should have a consultation with a WOCN. This nurse specialist is certified as an expert in the care of patients with wounds, ostomies, and incontinence.
- Nutrition counseling helps in planning a diet to manage elimination issues.
- Mental health professionals are consulted if issues such as anxiety and depression are affecting the patient's elimination patterns.
- The PCP is consulted for prescriptions and diagnostic evaluation.

areas of expertise include bowel and bladder control and associated skin care issues.

Self-esteem and a positive body image are important to promote in a patient with an ostomy, and emotional support is needed pre- and postoperatively. To address body image and self-esteem concerns, the nurse must recognize the extent of the impact of the ostomy surgery on the patient. The situation in which the ostomy is placed may affect how the patient perceives it. Patients are given the opportunity to express their feelings about their surgery, the changes in their body, and their self-image.

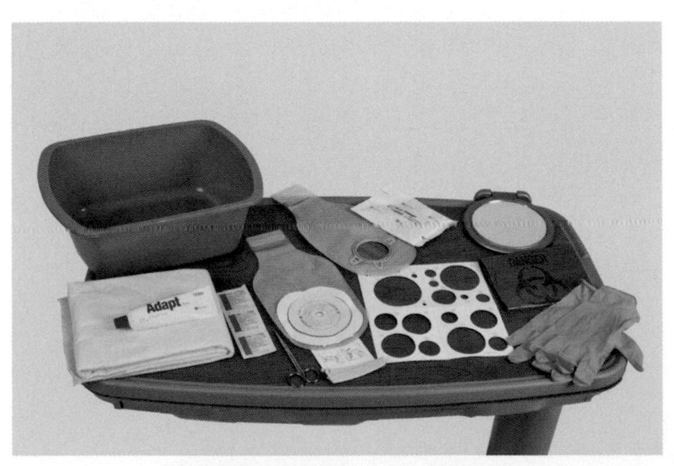

FIGURE 40-9 Ostomy supplies.

QSEN FOCUS!

Patient-centered care empowers the nurse to examine barriers to active involvement of patients in their own ostomy self-care, and to value an active partnership with patients and their families in planning, implementation, and evaluation of care.

Presence of an ostomy may cause disturbed body image, especially if it is permanent. Patients may perceive the ostomy as invasive and disfiguring. A well-placed stoma, however, does not usually interfere with the patient's activity and can be concealed with clothing. Foul odors, spillage or leakage of liquid stools, and inability to regulate bowel movements increase the loss of self-esteem. Patients may have difficulty maintaining or initiating normal sexual relations. Odor control is essential to maintenance of self-esteem, and many ostomy appliances are available that assist with odor control (Home Care Considerations box). Patients should begin to assist the WOCN in caring for the ostomy as soon as possible. Involvement in this process helps the patient build confidence and regain control. Refer patients to colostomy support groups such as the United Ostomy Association or the National Foundation for Ileitis and Colitis.

EVALUATION

Evaluation of the goals and outcomes for the patient with bowel elimination problems is important to achieve the desired outcomes. Whether the goals include a return to normal bowel function or maintaining existing function within the parameters of the patient's condition, it is

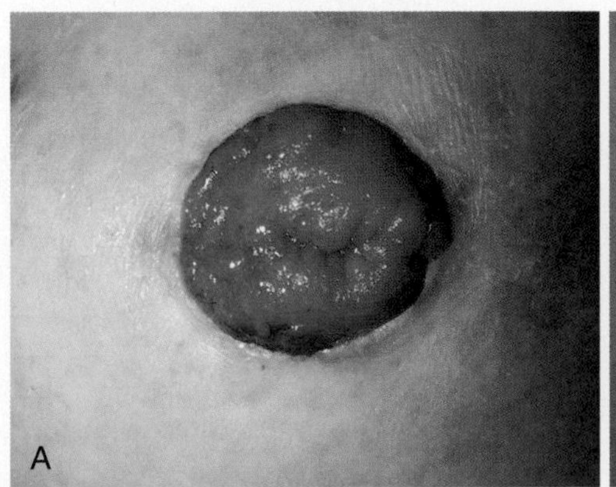

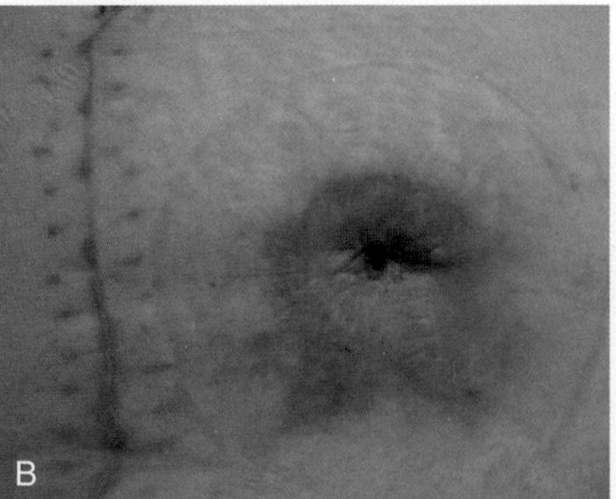

FIGURE 40-10 A, Stoma with intact skin. **B,** Stoma with excoriated skin. (From Evans SRT: *Surgical pitfalls*, Philadelphia, 2009, Saunders.)

HOME CARE CONSIDERATIONS

Patient Education in Colostomy and Ileostomy Care

- Family and significant others are included in ostomy teaching, because this may facilitate the patient's readiness to learn.
- If the patient is apprehensive about touching or looking at the stoma, start slowly and encourage active participation in ostomy care.
- Patients are given a teaching manual with step–by-step instructions, complete with illustrations, and supplemented with DVDs and access to websites.
- Evaluate the patient's home toileting facilities; note the location and availability.
- If the patient consumes gas-producing foods, it may be necessary to manually expel ("burp") trapped air from the bag.
  - In a private setting, the patient can undo the clasp on the flap of the bag and allow the air to be released from the bag.
  - Foods that tend to form gas, such as most beans, broccoli, Brussels sprouts, cabbage, carbonated beverages such as soda and beer, eggs, fish, garlic, onions, some spices, and deep-fried or fatty foods, may be limited or avoided to help control gas and odors.
- Many products are created with an odor barrier film so that odor is contained within the pouch. Commercial deodorizing disks are available.
- Limiting odor-producing foods and emptying the pouch regularly can help reduce odor.
- Some ostomy products have a filter to allow air but not odors to escape from the pouch.

important for the nurse to determine whether they have been met, and if not, why.

If goals have not been met, the nurse reviews the plan of care and considers revising interventions related to bowel elimination. The patient's current food and fluid intake, medication use, activity level, and knowledge are reviewed to determine the effects on GI function. It is important to include the patient during changes in the plan of care. The interim steps may need to be reevaluated and readjusted continuously.

SKILL 40-1 Administering an Enema

PURPOSE

Enemas are used to:
- Promote bowel cleansing
- Relieve constipation
- Empty the bowel for diagnostic testing or surgery
- Begin a bowel training program

RESOURCES

- Noncommercial preparation:
  - Enema bag
  - Tubing
  - Clamp
  - Rectal tube (usually 22 to 30 Fr.)
  - 750 to 1000 mL of appropriate warmed solution (slightly warmer than body temperature or 100° to 105° F)
- *or* commercial prepackaged enema
- Water-soluble lubricant
- Waterproof, absorbent pads
- Toilet tissue
- Basin
- Washcloths, towels
- Clean gloves
- Bedpan, commode, or toilet
- Container for disposal of equipment
- Nonskid footwear

COLLABORATION AND DELEGATION

- Administration of an enema may be delegated to unlicensed assistive personnel (UAP) without a nurse's assistance in some agencies after assessment of the patient has been completed by the nurse. Check with state licensing regulations and facility policies and procedures.
- UAP should report any of the following to the nurse:
  - Changes in vital signs
  - Abdominal pain, cramping, or distention
  - Rectal bleeding
  - Difficulties in performing the procedure or other concerns verbalized by the patient
- UAP also should be instructed in:
  - Appropriate positioning
  - Appropriate equipment usage
  - Appropriate documentation

EVIDENCE-BASED PRACTICE

- Pegram, Bloomfield, and Jones (2008) reiterate that documentation and evaluation of enema effectiveness are imperative, because findings usually affect further treatments or diagnostic tests. The amount and characteristics of stool are documented after an enema.

SPECIAL CIRCUMSTANCES

1. **Assess:** Does the patient demonstrate any contraindications for enema use, such as increased intracranial pressure, glaucoma, or recent rectal or prostate surgery?
   Intervention: Do not perform the procedure; notify the PCP.
2. **Assess:** Has an assessment been made of the patient's abdomen and of external sphincter control, hemorrhoids, and mobility?
   Intervention: The assessment serves two functions:
   - It allows the caregiver to verify that an appropriate enema solution will be used, provides information needed to prepare for the procedure, and confirms the need for the procedure.
   - It establishes a baseline against which findings on subsequent assessments may be compared to determine the effectiveness of the treatment.
3. **Assess:** What position may be used if the patient is unable to be placed in the left side-lying (Sims) position or has poor sphincter control?
   Intervention: Position patient in the dorsal recumbent position on a bedpan.
4. **Assess:** What should be done if the patient's abdomen becomes distended or rigid, if changes in vital signs occur, or if bleeding is noted?
   Intervention: Stop the procedure immediately.
   - Reassess the patient.
   - Notify the PCP of the findings.
5. **Assess:** What should the caregiver do if the patient complains of abdominal pain or cramping during instillation?
   Intervention: Slow the rate of instillation, and reassess the patient.

PREPROCEDURE

I. Check PCP orders and the patient care plan.
Knowledge of patient-specific orders is critical for safe patient care.

II. Gather supplies and equipment.
Preparing for the patient encounter saves time and promotes patient trust.

III. Perform hand hygiene.
Frequent hand hygiene prevents the spread of microorganisms.

IV. Maintain standard precautions.
Use of the correct personal protective equipment (PPE) is required whenever contact with bodily fluids is possible, to reduce the transfer of pathogens.

V. Introduce yourself.
Initial communication establishes the role of the nurse and begins a professional relationship.

VI. Provide for patient privacy.
It is important to maintain patient dignity.

VII. Identify the patient, using two identifiers.
Identifying a patient involves scanning barcodes or comparing the patient's stated name and birthdate to information on the patient's wristband or health record. The correct person must receive the correct treatment.

VIII. Explain the procedure to the patient.
The nurse has a responsibility to inform a patient before initiating care. Information may ease patient anxiety and facilitate cooperation.

PROCEDURE

Administering an Enema

Follow preprocedure steps I through VIII.

1. If the procedure will be performed while the patient is in bed, raise the bed to working height, and lower the side rails on the right side of the bed only, keeping the left top siderail elevated.
   Setting the bed at the correct working height prevents provider discomfort and possible injury.
2. Adhere to the Rights of Medication Administration (see Chapter 35, Nursing Care Guideline: Six Rights of Medication Administration).
   Avoid possible medication errors and promote patient safety by adhering to the Rights of Medication Administration.
3. Follow the principles described in Chapter 35, Nursing Care Guideline: Rectal Medication Administration throughout this skill.
4. Place the patient in the left side-lying (Sims) position with right knee flexed, with waterproof padding under the patient.
   Lying on the left side promotes the flow of solution to the colon by gravity, is the optimal positioning for the procedure, reduces strain on the caregiver, and promotes patient comfort. The waterproof padding protects linens.
5. Make sure a bedpan, commode or toilet are accessible before beginning. Prepare the enema:
   a. If it is a noncommercial preparation, warm the solution from the hospital pharmacy by placing the bag in a basin of warm water. (If it was not provided in a bag, use warm tap water to directly fill the enema bag.) Prime the tubing to remove air, and clamp the tubing.
   b. If it is a commercial preparation, verify the order and inspect the container for the expiration date and any noticeable holes and or damage. Expel any air from the container.
   c. Apply clean gloves.

   Using warm solution prevents abdominal cramping (as would be caused by cold solution) or burning (if hot solution is used). Prime the tube to avoid air infusion, which would cause abdominal distention. Verifying the accuracy of the dose avoids possible medication errors by adhering to the Rights of Medication Administration.

6. Lubricate 6 to 8 cm (3 to 4 inches) of the tip of the rectal tubing or commercial applicator.
   Using lubricant prevents trauma to mucosal tissues and aids insertion.
7. Help the patient to relax by breathing slowly in and out through the mouth. Insert the tip of the tubing or applicator:
   a. Separate buttocks, and locate the anus.
   b. Insert the tip of the tubing/applicator slowly and smoothly 6 to 8 cm (3 to 4 inches) toward the umbilicus.
   c. Hold the tubing/applicator in place.
   Using a slow and smooth motion prevents trauma to the mucosal tissues and prevents perforation of the bowel. Holding the tip in place prevents expulsion of the tubing/applicator via normal contraction of the bowel.
8. Administer the enema:
   a. For a noncommercial preparation, begin by holding the solution at the level of the patient's hip, unclamp the tubing, and raise the enema bag approximately 12 to 18 inches to adjust the flow by gravity so that it flows slowly for 5 to 10 minutes, holding the tubing in place until the enema is complete.
   b. For a commercial preparation, squeeze the tube/bottle slowly and evenly to expel the contents.
   Hold the tubing in place prevents expulsion of solution via stimulation of the bowel and peristalsis from rapid instillation. The enema is administered slowly to prevent distention.
9. Remove the tubing/applicator, covering it with a paper towel as it is being removed.
   Using the paper towel protects the linens from soiling and reduces the spread of microorganisms.
10. Provide the following instructions to the patient:
   a. Retain the solution as long as possible until patient has the urge to defecate (generally 5 to 15 minutes, but the actual time varies, depending on the solution ordered and the patient's reaction).
   b. Do not flush the toilet if the patient is using it to expel the solution.
   Retaining the solution for at least the minimal time allows optimal results. Not flushing the toilet will allow the nurse to assess the outcome of the procedure.
11. Apply nonskid footwear and assist the patient to the bathroom or onto a bedpan.
   Nonskid footwear prevents slipping.
12. Provide perineal care if needed.
   Keeping the perineal area clean and dry prevents skin breakdown.

Follow postprocedure steps I though VI.

POSTPROCEDURE

I. Return the bed to its lowest position, raise the top side rails, and verify that the call light is within reach for the patient.
   Precautions are taken to maintain patient safety. Top side rails aid in positioning and turning. Raising four side rails is considered a restraint.

II. Assess for additional patient needs and state the time of your expected return.
   Meeting patient needs and offering self promote patient satisfaction and build trust.

III. Properly dispose of PPE.
   Gloves, gowns, and masks must be appropriately discarded to prevent the spread of microorganisms.

IV. Clean equipment if it was in contact with the patient; see specific manufacturer instructions.
   Disinfection eliminates most microorganisms from inanimate objects.

V. Perform hand hygiene.
   Frequent hand hygiene prevents the spread of infection.

VI. Document the date, time, assessment, procedure, and patient's response to the procedure.
   Accurate documentation is essential to communicate patient care and to provide legal evidence of care.

SKILL 40-2 Ostomy Care

PURPOSE

- An ostomy pouch effectively collects fecal material (effluent).
- Changing the ostomy pouch is critical to:
  - Maintain skin integrity.
  - Assess stoma healing and integrity.
  - Prevent odors.
  - Promote comfort.
  - Maintain or increase self-esteem and dignity.

RESOURCES

- Pouch:
  - One-piece with attached skin barrier *or*
  - Two-piece ostomy pouch system with separate pouch and skin barrier in the correct size
- Clamp (for drainable pouch; with use of a disposable, closed-end pouch, no clamp is needed)
- Ostomy measurement tool (included in box with ostomy system)
- Ostomy deodorant
- Stoma paste/stomadhesive/barrier paste
- Tape
- Gauze pads
- Washcloths
- Towels
- Waterproof pads
- Basin
- Bedpan
- Graduated container
- Scissors
- Pen
- Clean gloves

COLLABORATION AND DELEGATION

- Changing the pouch of a new ostomy, or care of an ostomy with complications, may not be delegated to unlicensed assistive personnel (UAP).
- Changing the pouch of an established ostomy may be delegated to UAP without a nurse's assistance, after initial assessment of the patient has been completed. Check with state licensing and facility policy and procedure.
- UAP should report any of the following to the nurse:
  - Pain before, during, or after the procedure, either verbalized by the patient or manifested as grimacing or other physical responses
  - Sores, wounds, irritations, or lesions noted
  - Output volume and consistency
  - Difficulties in performing the procedure
- UAP should be instructed in the:
  - Appropriate pouch
  - Appropriate skin barriers
  - Appropriate procedural implementations
  - Appropriate documentation
- Collaborate with wound ostomy continence nurse (WOCN) if available within the facility.
- Collaborate and coordinate the procedure with the PCP or surgeon rounds if dressings or other surgical implementations need to be examined and/or changed.

EVIDENCE-BASED PRACTICE

- WOCNs and teams are specialists with in-depth training in wound and ostomy care, along with knowledge of the specialized products available to treat and prevent complications. The evidence in the United States and Canada has shown that employing and collaborating with WOCNs for care of this specialized population not only are beneficial for patient outcomes but also improve staff education and treatment practices, as well as return on investment in the form of an economical advantage in terms of insurance reimbursement for facilities. It is imperative that the nurse work closely with the WOCN, if available, to promote optimal safe, high-quality patient care (Harris and Shannon, 2008; Jankowski, 2010).
- Soap is not needed in cleaning the stoma or peristomal area, and it can dry the skin and cause complications. Warm water only should be used, along with an adhesive remover if obvious residue remains (Deitz and Gates, 2010a).
- Evidence-based studies on optimal pouch wear time are lacking. It is imperative to be vigilant with assessment of the pouch fitting, stoma, and peristomal skin area. Changing the pouch when not necessary can contribute to the risk of associated skin damage. Reported wear times range from 1 to 7 days, with a "mean ostomy pouch wear time in the United States [of] 4.8 days" (Richbourg, Fellows, and Arroyave, 2008, p. 508).
- It is imperative to take into account the psychological and coping factors of the patient with an ostomy in providing care related to the ostomy appliances. The nurse should assess and incorporate self-image education and promotion during such care. With a more positive body image, the patient is more likely to engage in self-care and health promotion techniques, ultimately leading to better health outcomes (Thorpe, McArthur, and Richardson, 2009; Barnabé and Dell'Acqua, 2008; Simmons et al, 2007).
- Page (2009) described two tools that ostomy care nurses can use to promote optimal care and education for this patient population. Both tools have been shown to be reliable and valid but should be used by specialists. The first is called the *ostomy skin tool* and measures the skin assessment in quantitative terms and then assists in

determining the root cause in order to effect change by altering treatment regimens and products. The second tool is called the *ostomy quality of life tool* (Stoma QoL) and measures four major categories of functioning in the ostomy patient: "sleep, sexual activity, relations to family and close friends, and social relations with people other than family and close friends" (Page, 2009, p. 11). Use of these tools assists all nurses in promoting self-esteem and body image issues in this population.

SPECIAL CIRCUMSTANCES

1. **Assess:** What are the findings on assessment of the stoma?
   Intervention: Check for color, moisture, trauma, healing, and swelling.
   - A normal stoma should be moist, reddish pink, and "budding" slightly above skin level.
     - Dry and purple-black tissue without bleeding indicates necrosis.
       - Assess for circulation and edema.
       - Notify the PCP.
     - Whitish areas indicate fungal infection. Notify the PCP.
     - Open areas, rash, and bleeding may indicate an allergy or a chemical or mechanical reaction. Notify the PCP.
     - If the edges of the stoma are more than "budding" (i.e., are protruding into the pouch):
       - Place the patient supine for 30 minutes.
       - If the site does not return to normal, notify the WOCN and/or the PCP.
   - For a new stoma, the following must be checked:
     - If no flatulence or fecal drainage has occurred by the third day, notify the PCP.
     - Measure the stoma with each assessment to ensure proper equipment sizing secondary to swelling. It takes 6 to 8 weeks for swelling to decrease completely.
     - The opening around the appliance should be less than ⅛ inch in order to:
       - Ensure proper fitting of the equipment
       - Prevent trauma and skin breakdown
       - Facilitate drainage into pouch
2. **Assess:** Does the patient have an established ostomy with the current pouch intact?
   Intervention: Assess the stoma.
   - If there are no complications:
     - The pouching system may stay in place for 3 to 7 days.
     - UAP may be delegated to perform care, in accordance with state and facility guidelines.
   - If there are complications, a pouch change may be required.
     - Make more frequent assessments, and change the pouch as soon as it is not adhering correctly.
     - Leakage is caustic to the skin and stoma; it indicates a need for a different type of pouch or sealant and may require the application of a skin barrier.
     - Consult a WOCN.
     - Care may not be delegated to UAP if there are complications.
3. **Assess:** Is the ostomy new?
   Intervention: Assess the incision, and ensure that placement of the equipment/pouch around the incision will prevent trauma.
   - Ensure accurate measurements are taken. The stoma takes 6 to 8 weeks to shrink to normal size.
   - Notify the PCP or the WOCN of any complications or signs or symptoms of infection.
4. **Assess:** After removal of a used pouch, do some skin barrier fragments remain on the patient's skin?
   Intervention: Use adhesive remover.
   - If the skin barrier is not removed, it can cause skin breakdown and trauma.
   - Do not routinely use adhesive remover.
   - Rinse the site with warm water and pat the site dry with a towel.
   - Do not use alcohol-based products, towelettes, or premoistened products; all of these interfere with skin barrier adhesive.
5. **Assess:** Is odor or excessive gas a problem?
   Intervention: Apply ostomy deodorant, or consider switching appliances.
   - Use only a small amount of deodorant, and do not use homemade mixtures.
   - Appliances with a vent or filter may be a better choice. Consult a WOCN.
6. **Assess:** Does the patient have excessive output?
   Intervention: Empty the ostomy bag when it is one-third to one-half full.
   - Consider switching to a specialty high-output pouch.
   - Consult a WOCN.

PREPROCEDURE

I. Check PCP orders and the patient care plan.
Knowledge of patient-specific orders is critical for safe patient care.

II. Gather supplies and equipment.
Preparing for the patient encounter saves time and promotes patient trust.

III. Perform hand hygiene.
Frequent hand hygiene prevents the spread of microorganisms.

IV. Maintain standard precautions.
Use of the correct personal protective equipment (PPE) is required whenever contact with bodily fluids is possible, to reduce the transfer of pathogens.

V. Introduce yourself.
Initial communication establishes the role of the nurse and begins a professional relationship.

VI. Provide for patient privacy.
It is important to maintain patient dignity.

VII. Identify the patient, using two identifiers.
Identifying a patient involves scanning barcodes or comparing the patient's stated name and birthdate to information on the patient's wristband or health record. The correct person must receive the correct treatment.

VIII. Explain the procedure to the patient.
The nurse has a responsibility to inform a patient before initiating care. Information may ease patient anxiety and facilitate cooperation.

PROCEDURE

Changing a Pouch

Follow preprocedure steps I through VIII.

1. Raise the bed to working height, and lower the side rails as appropriate and safe.
Setting the bed at the correct working height prevents provider discomfort and possible injury.
2. The best timing for changing an ostomy pouch is before a meal but not immediately before it.
Changing the pouch is best performed when the abdomen is comfortable and nondistended, and peristalsis is normal rather than hyperactive. Avoid changing immediately before meals to avoid decreasing the patient's appetite with residual odors from the pouch change.
3. Have the patient in the supine or semi-Fowler position, if possible, with a towel or waterproof pad around area. Alternatively, the patient may stand or sit over the toilet.
The supine or semi-Fowler position facilitates application; the skin should be taut. Using a towel or pad protects the skin and linens.
4. Apply clean gloves. Perform an assessment of the stoma, skin, and fit of the pouch.
Using gloves reduces the spread of microorganisms. The assessment may indicate a need for different appliances or products. Intact drainable pouches may remain in place for up to 7 days.
5. If the patient is using a closed-end pouch, go to Step 6.
If the patient is using a drainable pouch, empty the pouch.
   a. Position the patient over a toilet, bedpan, or graduated container.
   b. Open the clamp, but save it for reuse.
   c. Empty the entire contents of the pouch, and measure the volume, if required. Observe the stool characteristics.
   d. Clean the end of the pouch if needed and reclamp it (see Step 14, below).

e. Determine if the pouch needs to be changed. If so, continue to Step 6. If not, go to Step 11.
f. Remove and dispose of gloves, perform hand hygiene, and apply a new clean pair of gloves.
Positioning over a toilet or bedpan helps to prevent effluent from spilling on the patient during the procedure; effluent is caustic and can break down the skin. Proper disposal of waste prevents the spread of microorganisms and reduces the risk of infection and contamination.

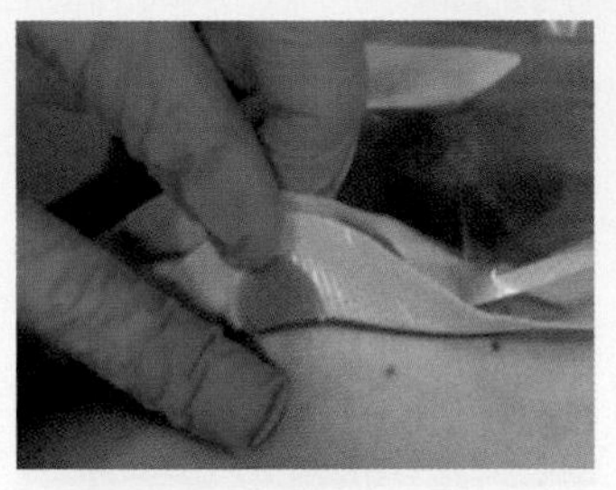

STEP 6

6. Remove the used pouch:
a. Apply clean gloves
b. Gently and smoothly push the skin away from the pouch, keeping the skin taut.
c. Dispose of the pouch per facility policies and procedures.
d. Remove and dispose of gloves, perform hand hygiene, and apply a new clean pair of gloves.
Careful removal of the pouch prevents skin breakdown and trauma, keeps the caustic effluent away from the skin, and prevents patient discomfort. Proper disposal of waste prevents the spread of microorganisms, reduces the risk of infection, and prevents contamination.

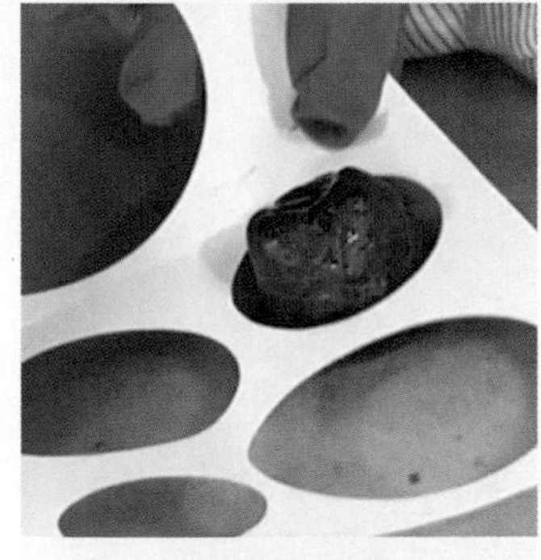

STEP 9

7. Cleanse the area around the stoma:
a. Apply clean gloves. Use warm water and a washcloth to gently clean the area. Do not use premoistened cloths or towelettes.
b. Pat the skin dry with a towel.
c. Place gauze over the stoma if the effluent is liquid or drains continuously.
Proper cleansing prevents skin breakdown and promotes adherence of the appliance to the skin. Because the stoma is vascular in nature, gentle cleansing prevents bleeding. The stoma contains few nerves, so the patient may not feel trauma. Patting the area dry prevents abrasion. Gauze prevents effluent from leaking onto the skin during the procedure.

8. If skin protectant has been ordered or is needed, apply a 2-inch area around the stoma and allow it to completely dry.
Only use skin protectant if needed. It helps to prevent skin breakdown and trauma. The skin protectant must be dry for the pouch to adhere properly to the skin and to avoid leaks.

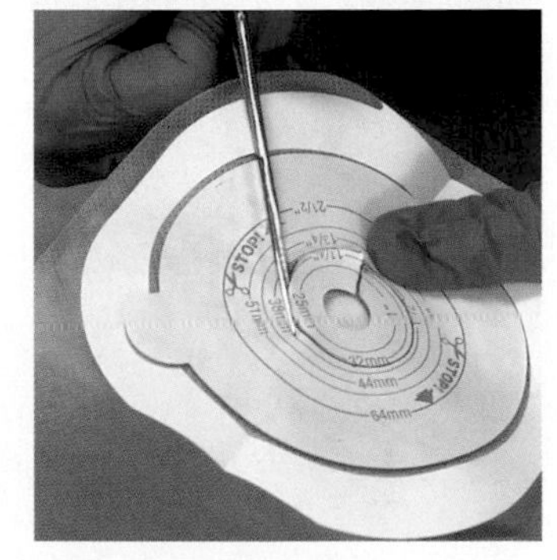

STEP 10c

9. Measure the stoma to verify the correct size appliance will be used.
a. Check the manufacturer directions.
b. Use the measuring guide that is included in the box.
c. Remove and dispose of gloves, perform hand hygiene, and apply a new clean pair of gloves.
Take careful measurements to ensure accuracy and prevents leakage. (Leakage may cause skin breakdown and trauma.) Manufacturers produce various appliances to meet individual needs for optimal outcomes, so it is essential to follow the directions for the specific appliance.

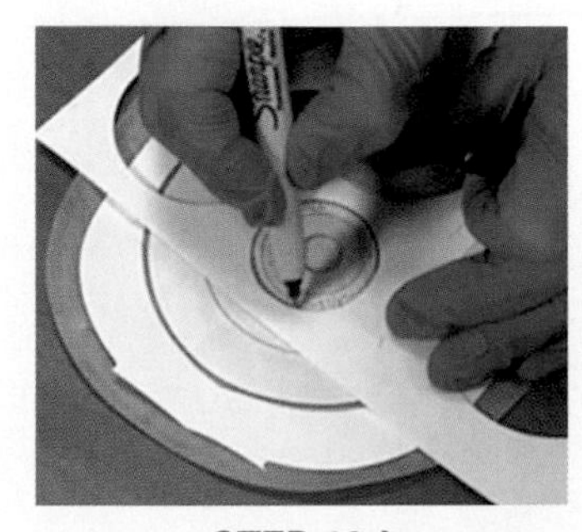

STEP 10d

10. Prepare the pouch by cutting a stoma opening in the back of the wafer/flange:
a. The cut should be $\frac{1}{16}$ to $\frac{1}{8}$ inch larger than the stoma.
b. Use the ostomy measurement guide.
c. If measurements are printed on the back of the pouch or wafer/flange, cut the opening to the appropriate size.
d. If measurements are not provided, center the template over the wafer and trace the correct size; then cut the pouch.
Too large of an opening permits leakage, while too small of an opening irritates the stoma. Use the correct size to prevent leakage and skin breakdown.

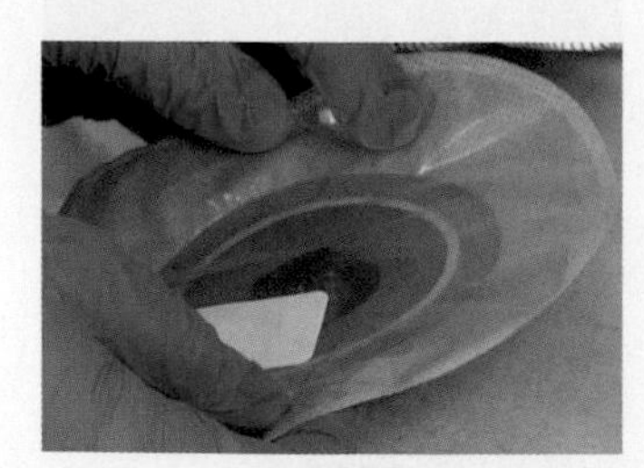

STEP 11a

11. Apply the pouch.
    a. For a one-piece system: remove the backing or apply stomadhesive and allow it to dry. Remove the gauze from the stoma. Center the stoma opening over the stoma, and secure it in place, smoothing the appliance from the stoma outward and ensuring that the seal is complete all around the stoma.
    b. For a two-piece system, apply the wafer/flange first, ensure it is properly adhered to the skin, and snap on the pouch.
    c. Hold a gloved hand over the wafer or have the patient hold a hand over the wafer.

    Secure the pouch in place to prevent leakage and skin breakdown. The back of the pouch or wafer flange acts as a protective skin barrier. A stomadhesive or barrier paste assists as a skin barrier. The skin barrier must dry completely for it to be effective (incomplete drying interferes with the adherence of the appliance to the skin). The body heat from a hand will help the wafer seal to the skin.
12. Assess the seal:
    a. Fill in any leaks with barrier paste.
    b. Maintain pressure to gently hold the pouch in place while the paste dries.
    c. Allow the paste to dry completely.

    Complete the seal to prevent leakage and skin breakdown from caustic effluents. The barrier paste must dry completely for it to be effective.
13. Gently tug on the pouch to ensure that it is securely attached.

    Verify the seal adhered to prevent leakage and skin breakdown from caustic effluents.

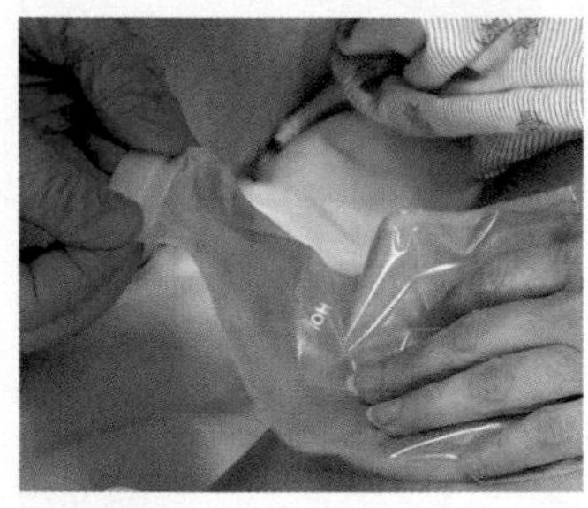

STEP 14

14. If it is a drainable pouch, close the bottom of the pouch by folding it up once and applying the clamp; verify the clamp has snapped shut. Alternatively, follow the manufacturer directions.

    Seal the bottom of the pouch securely to prevent leakage and skin breakdown.
15. Remove and dispose of gloves, perform hand hygiene.

Follow postprocedure steps I though VI.

POSTPROCEDURE

I. Return the bed to its lowest position, raise the top side rails, and verify that the call light is within reach for the patient.
Precautions are taken to maintain patient safety. Top side rails aid in positioning and turning. Raising four side rails is considered a restraint.

II. Assess for additional patient needs and state the time of your expected return.
Meeting patient needs and offering self promote patient satisfaction and build trust.

III. Properly dispose of PPE.
Gloves, gowns, and masks must be appropriately discarded to prevent the spread of microorganisms.

IV. Clean equipment if it was in contact with the patient; see specific manufacturer instructions.
Disinfection eliminates most microorganisms from inanimate objects.

V. Perform hand hygiene.
Frequent hand hygiene prevents the spread of infection.

VI. Document the date, time, assessment, procedure, and patient's response to the procedure.
Accurate documentation is essential to communicate patient care and to provide legal evidence of care.

SUMMARY OF LEARNING OUTCOMES

LO 40.1 *Describe the anatomy and physiology of the gastrointestinal tract and the processes involved in formation, storage, and elimination of waste products:* The GI tract runs from the mouth to the anus. A bolus of food moves from the mouth through the esophagus to the stomach. It then travels through the small intestine into the large intestine, where nutrients and electrolytes, especially sodium and chloride, are absorbed from digested food. Water is absorbed from indigestible food residue. Waste from the body is eliminated through the formation of feces and expelled from the body by way of the rectum and anus.

LO 40.2 *Identify common alterations in bowel elimination:* Diarrhea, constipation, and bowel diversions are the most common alterations in bowel elimination.

LO 40.3 *Integrate components of a comprehensive assessment of the patient to identify issues with bowel elimination:* By understanding normal elimination physiology, the nurse can conduct an in-depth focused assessment of elimination and a physical examination to evaluate alterations in elimination patterns, recent changes, and factors that influence defecation. The nurse understands that the complications of altered elimination include fluid and electrolyte imbalances, body image issues, alterations in skin integrity, imbalanced nutrition, activity intolerance, and pain.

LO 40.4 *Identify nursing diagnoses related to bowel elimination:* Nursing diagnoses related to bowel elimination include *Bowel Incontinence, Constipation, Risk for Constipation, Perceived Constipation, Diarrhea,* and *Toileting Self-Care Deficit.*

LO 40.5 *Outline goals for patients experiencing alterations in bowel elimination:* Patient goals are focused on maintaining current level of function or returning the patient to optimal bowel function.

LO 40.6 *Implement interventions to maintain normal bowel elimination:* By prioritizing the nursing diagnoses related to elimination, the nurse collaborates on a plan of care for the patient and provides interventions based on short-term and long-term goals, with the ultimate aim of returning the patient to an optimal state of health. Ostomy care and teaching of self-care for new ostomy patients constitute a priority nursing intervention. Evaluation and modification of the plan of care are ongoing.

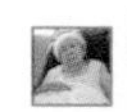

Responses to the critical-thinking questions are available at *http://evolve.elsevier.com/YoostCrawford/fundamentals/.*

REVIEW QUESTIONSBS_SECANCHOR

1. A patient is being discharged from the hospital with a new ileostomy. The patient expresses concern about caring for the ostomy. Before discharge, it is most important for the nurse to coordinate with which member of the health care team?
   a. Home care nurse
   b. Wound ostomy continence nurse
   c. Registered dietitian
   d. Primary care provider
2. The nurse is assigned the care of a patient for whom a cleansing enema has been ordered. What information is most important for the nurse to know before administration of the enema?
   a. The proper way to position the patient
   b. Signs and symptoms of intolerance to the procedure
   c. Vital signs before the procedure
   d. Any past medical or surgical history related to the anus or rectum
3. To prevent constipation in an inactive patient, which early interventions should the nurse implement? *(Select all that apply.)*
   a. Stool softener administration
   b. Enema administration
   c. Increasing fiber in the diet
   d. Increasing physical activity
   e. Increasing fluid intake
4. While performing an abdominal assessment on an unconscious patient, the nurse notes presence of an ostomy. The fecal output is liquid in consistency, with a pungent odor, and the stoma is located in the upper right quadrant of the abdomen. What type of ostomy does the patient have?
   a. Descending colostomy
   b. Ureterostomy
   c. Ileostomy
   d. Ascending colostomy

5. The teaching plan for a patient with diarrhea should include which intervention?
   a. Drinking at least eight glasses of fluid each day
   b. Eating foods low in sodium and potassium
   c. Limiting the amount of soluble fiber in the diet
   d. Eliminating whole-wheat and whole-grain breads and cereal
6. The nurse knows that the teaching for a patient who was recently diagnosed with constipation has been effective if the patient's meal request specifies which food choice?
   a. Hot dog on a bun
   b. Grilled chicken
   c. Tuna sandwich on white bread
   d. Spinach salad with dressing
7. A 40-year-old patient complains of 4 days of frequent loose stools with abdominal cramping. What is the priority nursing diagnosis for this patient?
   a. *Altered Skin Integrity*
   b. *Risk for Imbalanced Fluid Volume*
   c. *Acute Pain*
   d. *Self Care Deficit: Toileting*
8. A patient is scheduled for a colonoscopy. After preprocedure teaching by the nurse, the patient demonstrates understanding when he makes which statement?
   a. "I can have coffee the morning of the procedure."
   b. "I should drink a red sports drink the day before to stay hydrated."
   c. "I should drink clear liquids for 2 days before the procedure."
   d. "I will be able to drive home immediately after the procedure."
9. Which nursing intervention is included for a patient experiencing diarrhea?
   a. Limiting fluid intake to 1000 mL/day
   b. Administering a cathartic suppository
   c. Increasing fiber in the diet
   d. Limiting exercise
10. When administering a cleansing enema, which techniques should the nurse use? *(Select all that apply.)*
   a. Assist the patient to left side-lying (Sims) position.
   b. Perform hand hygiene and apply sterile gloves.
   c. Add room-temperature solution to enema bag.
   d. Lubricate 2 to 4 cm (1 to 2 inches) of tip of rectal tube with lubricating jelly.
   e. Raise container, release clamps, and allow solution to flow to fill tubing.
   f. Hang solution 45 to 60 cm (18 to 21 inches) above anus and instill rapidly.
   g. Clamp tubing after solution is instilled.

Answers and rationales to the review questions are available at *http://evolve.elsevier.com/YoostCrawford/fundamentals/.*

REFERENCES

American Cancer Society: American Cancer Society recommendations for colorectal cancer early detection, 2014. Retrieved from *www.cancer.org/cancer/colonandrectumcancer/moreinformation/colonandrectumcancerearlydetection/colorectal-cancer-early-detection-acs-recommendations.*

Barnabé NC, Dell'Acqua MC: Coping strategies of ostomized individuals, *Rev Lat Am Enfermagem* 16(4):712-719, 2008.

Beldon P: Problems encountered managing pressure ulceration of the sacrum, *Br J Community Nurs* 13:S6-S12, 2008.

Cronenwett L, Sherwood G, Barnsteiner J, et al: Quality and safety education for nurses, *Nurs Outlook* 55(3):122-131, 2007.

Deitz D, Gates J: Basic ostomy management, part 1, *Nursing* 40(2):61-62, 2010a.

Deitz D, Gates J: Basic ostomy management, part 2, *Nursing* 40(5):62-63, 2010b.

Harris C, Shannon R: An innovative enterostomal therapy nurse model of community wound care delivery: A retrospective cost-effectiveness analysis, *J Wound Ostomy Continence Nurs* 35(2):169-183, 2008.

Harris H: Nursing care of the morbidly obese patient, *Nurs Care Made Incredibly Easy!* 6(3):34-43, 2008.

Jankowski IM: Matching patient safety goals to the nursing specialty: Using wound, ostomy, continence nursing services, *J Nurs Admin* 40(1):26-31, 2010.

Kistner M: Dysfunctional elimination behaviors and associated complications in school-age children, *J Sch Nurs* 25(2):108-116, 2009.

National Institutes of Health: Constipation, 2014. Retrieved from *www.nlm.nih.gov/medlineplus/constipation.html.*

Page AC: The ostomy files. Two new tools for your ostomy practice, *Ostomy Wound Manage* 55(12):10-12, 2009.

Pegram A, Bloomfield J, Jones A: Safe use of rectal suppositories and enemas with adult patients, *Nurs Stand* 22(38):39-41, 2008.

Richbourg L, Fellows J, Arroyave WD: Ostomy pouch wear time in the United States, *J Wound Ostomy Continence Nurs* 35(5):504-508, 2008.

Simmons KL, Smith JA, Bobb KA, Liles LL: Adjustment to colostomy: Stoma acceptance, stoma care self-efficacy and interpersonal relationships, *J Adv Nurs* 60(6):627-635, 2007.

Simor A: Diagnosis, management, and prevention of *Clostridium difficile* infection in long-term care facilities: A review, *J Am Geriatr Soc* 58(8):1556-1564, 2010.

Thorpe G, McArthur M, Richardson B: Bodily change following faecal stoma formation: Qualitative interpretive synthesis, *J Adv Nurs* 65(9):1778-1789, 2009.

VanPutte C, Regan J, Russo A, et al: *Seeley's anatomy and physiology*, ed. 10, Boston, 2014, McGraw-Hill.

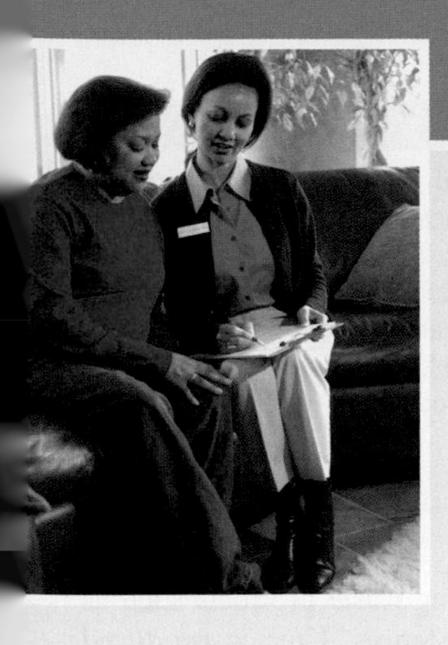

CHAPTER 41

Urinary Elimination

EVOLVE WEBSITE

http://evolve.elsevier.com/YoostCrawford/fundamentals/

- Additional Evolve-Only Review Questions With Answers
- Answers and Rationales for Text Review Questions
- Answers to Critical-Thinking Exercises
- Case Study with Questions
- Video Skills Clips
- Conceptual Care Map Creator
- Animations
- Skills Checklists
- Glossary

LEARNING OUTCOMES

Comprehension of this chapter's content will provide students with the ability to:

LO 41.1 Explain the complexities of the anatomic and physiologic processes of the urinary system.

LO 41.2 Describe abnormal patterns of urinary elimination, including causative factors.

LO 41.3 Carry out a comprehensive assessment of the patient with urinary elimination problems.

LO 41.4 Identify nursing diagnoses related to urinary elimination.

LO 41.5 Create collaborative patient-centered care plans for patients experiencing alterations in urinary elimination.

LO 41.6 Implement interventions to address altered elimination concerns and then evaluate their effectiveness.

KEY TERMS

anuria, p. 1077
dialysis, p. 1077
dysuria, p. 1077
enuresis, p. 1079
functional incontinence, p. 1079
hematuria, p. 1077
hemodialysis, p. 1077
incontinence, p. 1077
irrigation, p. 1087
Kegel exercises, p. 1087
micturition, p. 1077
mixed incontinence, p. 1079
nephrons, p. 1076
nocturia, p. 1077
oliguria, p. 1077
overflow incontinence, p. 1079
peritoneal dialysis, p. 1077
polyuria, p. 1077
stress incontinence, p. 1079
temporary incontinence, p. 1079
urea, p. 1076
urge/urgency, p. 1077
urge incontinence, p. 1079
urinary diversion, p. 1081
urinary incontinence, p. 1078
urinary retention, p. 1079
urinary tract infection, p. 1080

CASE STUDY

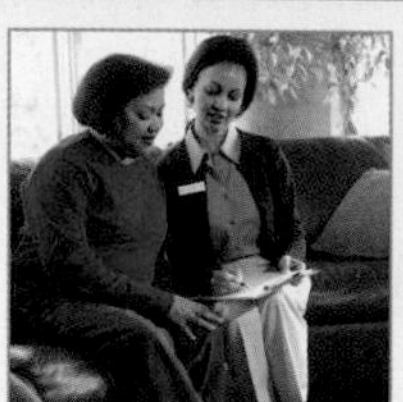

Ms. James is an obese 31-year-old female who comes into the primary care center with complaints of frequency, urgency, burning on urination, and lower abdominal pain rated as 7 on a 0-to-10 scale. Her vital signs are T 38.8° C (101.9° F), P 106 and regular, R18 and unlabored, and BP 110/70.

Significant assessment findings include a history of multiple and frequent bladder infections, occasional vaginal bleeding, right ovarian cyst removal 2 years ago, multiple sexual encounters with her partner in the past 3 weeks, and suprapubic tenderness on palpation. On the basis of diagnostic test results, Ms. James is prescribed an antibiotic, nitrofurantoin (100 mg PO q 6 hr), and the urinary tract analgesic phenazopyridine (2 tablets PO tid PRN) for a bladder infection and told to return to the clinic in a month for a follow-up appointment.

Refer back to this case study to answer the critical-thinking exercises throughout the chapter.

Regular elimination of liquid waste products is an essential body function and is critical to healthy living. Social, cultural, and physical requirements factor into personal urinary elimination habits; therefore privacy and emotional needs, in addition to physical needs, must be addressed to ensure proper care of patients with urinary elimination concerns.

Urine elimination is dependent on factors such as food consumption, fluid intake, medications, and fluid loss through breathing and perspiration. Healthy adults eliminate approximately a quart and a half of urine (1440 mL) each day. Effective elimination of liquid waste material requires proper functioning of the organs of the urinary tract, including the kidneys, ureters, urinary bladder, and urethra, as well as the muscles of the pelvic floor (Figure 41-1). Understanding normal anatomy and physiology related to the urinary system is essential for the nurse to provide optimal care.

NORMAL STRUCTURE AND FUNCTION OF THE URINARY SYSTEM LO 41.1

Nutrients from food are used by the body to maintain all of its functions. The kidneys excrete and reabsorb water and electrolytes from the body. The urinary system controls the composition of blood by removing waste products such as **urea** and conserving useful substances. Urea is produced when protein-rich foods are digested. The urinary system helps to control blood pressure and plays a crucial role in acid-base balance.

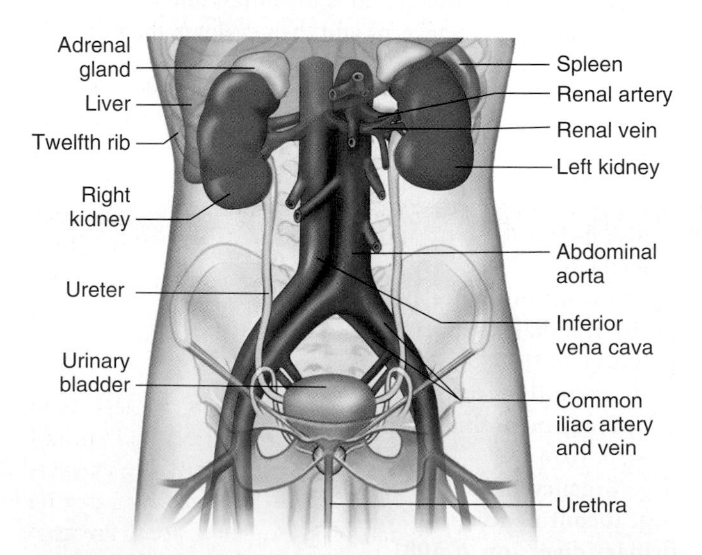

FIGURE 41-1 Organs of the urinary system. (From Patton KT, Thibodeau GA: *Anatomy and physiology*, ed. 8, St. Louis, 2013, Mosby.)

KIDNEYS

The kidneys are the major excretory organs of the body. The two kidneys are located bilaterally below the ribs toward the middle of the back. They filter liquid waste from the blood, balance electrolytes in the blood, regulate blood volume and pressure, produce erythropoietin for red blood cell formation, synthesize vitamin D to help control calcium levels, and maintain the acid-base balance of the extracellular fluid (Shier, Butler, and Lewis, 2012).

Urine is formed by tiny filtering units called **nephrons**, which are the functional units of the kidney. Studies have indicated that the average number of nephrons per kidney is 900,000 to 1 million, with individual kidneys containing between 200,000 to more than 2.5 million nephrons (Bertram, Douglas-Denton, Diouf, et al, 2011). Each nephron consists of the renal corpuscle and a small tube called the renal tubule. The renal corpuscle is made up of a network of blood capillaries called the glomerulus, which is surrounded by Bowman's capsule. The renal tubule is composed of the proximal tubule, the loop of Henle, and the distal convoluted tubule (Shier, Butler, and Lewis, 2012).

Urine formation is a result of three processes. *Filtration* initially occurs in the glomerulus as fluid moves across a membrane as the result of a pressure difference. *Reabsorption* occurs in the renal tubule as most of the filtrate moves back into the blood. At this point waste products, excess solutes, and small amounts of water are not reabsorbed but are secreted. As *secretion* takes place, urine is produced. Urea, water, and other waste substances form urine as they pass through the nephrons down the renal tubules (Shier, Butler, and Lewis, 2012). The online animation demonstrates how the renal system functions. 

URETERS

After exiting the kidneys, urine is carried to the bladder by narrow tubes called the ureters. The ureter wall muscles continually tighten and relax, forcing urine downward. If urine is retained in the kidney or backflows from the bladder toward the kidneys, the patient becomes susceptible to kidney infections.

BLADDER AND URETHRA

From the ureters the urine flows slowly into the bladder, located below the umbilicus and above the symphysis pubis in the lower abdomen, for storage. The bladder walls relax and expand to store urine, and contract and flatten to empty urine through the urethra. Sphincter muscles at the base of the bladder help keep urine from leaking by closing tightly like a rubber band around the opening of the bladder. The urethra transports urine from the bladder to outside the body for elimination and bladder emptying.

The innervation of the bladder signals when it is time to urinate and empty the bladder. This impulse is referred to as **urge** or **urgency**. The brain signals the bladder muscles to tighten and the sphincter muscles to relax, which squeezes urine out of the bladder through the urethra. When all of the signals occur in the correct order, normal **micturition**, or urination, occurs.

NORMAL URINE CHARACTERISTICS

Urine can be produced in small or large amounts. It can be dilute or very concentrated. Normal urine is sterile. It contains fluids, salts, and waste products, but it is free of bacteria, viruses, and fungi. The average adult passes one to two quarts (960 to 1920 mL) of urine per day, depending on the amount of fluids consumed, medications, medical conditions, and dietary intake (such as salt). During the night, urine formation decreases to approximately half of what is produced in the daytime.

ALTERED STRUCTURE AND FUNCTION OF THE URINARY SYSTEM LO 41.2

With the exception of developmental factors associated with age and pregnancy, altered urinary elimination generally is due to some degree of urinary retention or loss of voluntary control of voiding (ability to empty the bladder). Psychosocial factors, food and fluid intake, surgical and diagnostic procedures, pathologic conditions such as hypertension and arteriosclerosis, and urinary tract infections (UTIs) all can affect the structure or function of the urinary system. These factors may alter the volume or characteristics of the urine produced or the effectiveness of excretion.

ABNORMAL URINATION PATTERNS

Abnormal patterns of urination fall into several categories related to failure of the kidneys to produce or excrete more than 50 to 100 mL of urine in 24 hours (**anuria**), a reduced volume of urine typically greater than 100 and less than 500 mL in 24 hours (**oliguria**), excessive production and excretion of urine (**polyuria**), excessive urination at night (**nocturia**), painful urination (**dysuria**), and blood in the urine (**hematuria**). Urinary **incontinence**, the inability to control urination, is prevalent, particularly in women, and can greatly impact quality of life. Urinary retention is the inability to empty the bladder fully and generally is caused by an obstruction or neurologic disorder, enlarged prostate gland, or infection, among other factors.

Anuria

Anuria is the failure of the kidneys to excrete urine. Anuria occurs as a result of any process that limits effective blood flow through the kidneys. Diagnosis of anuria is made when a catheter is passed into the bladder and no urine is present. Inadequate flow or complete obstruction by anything (such as stones or tumors) that blocks both ureters and the bladder, or obstructs the urethra, can lead to an anuric state, resulting in acute or chronic renal failure. Acute anuria is life-threatening and requires emergent investigation to determine the cause. As waste accumulates, the patient becomes at risk for coma or death.

Depending on the severity of anuria and the alterations in the patient's fluid and electrolyte levels, artificial filtering of waste products using renal dialysis may be necessary. **Dialysis** is a technique by which fluids and molecules pass through an artificial semipermeable membrane and are filtered by means of osmosis.

During **hemodialysis**, the patient's blood flows continually from the body through vascular catheters to the dialysis machine. It then goes through the machine's filters, and ultrafiltrate (a liquid from which the blood cells and the blood proteins have been filtered out) is created. The frequency of hemodialysis is dependent on patient status. Once patients with chronic renal failure begin hemodialysis, they typically are required to undergo treatments three times per week or more often. Hemodialysis treatments most often are performed on an outpatient basis (Figure 41-2).

Peritoneal dialysis is performed by instilling dialysis solution into the patient's abdominal cavity through an external catheter. After the solution rests within the peritoneal cavity for a prescribed period of time, it is removed from the body through the catheter. In peritoneal dialysis, the abdominal cavity functions as the dialyzing membrane through which fluid and molecules are exchanged and toxic substances are removed from the body.

Oliguria

Oliguria is defined as reduced urine volume less than 1 mL/kg/h in an infant, less than 0.5 mL/kg/h in children, and less than 400 mL/day in adults (Devarajan, 2012). Oliguria is a symptom of acute or chronic renal failure, which can be classified as prerenal, renal, or postrenal failure. Prerenal failure occurs as a result of reduction in blood flow to the kidneys. Causes of prerenal failure include dehydration, vascular collapse, and low cardiac output. Renal failure is seen

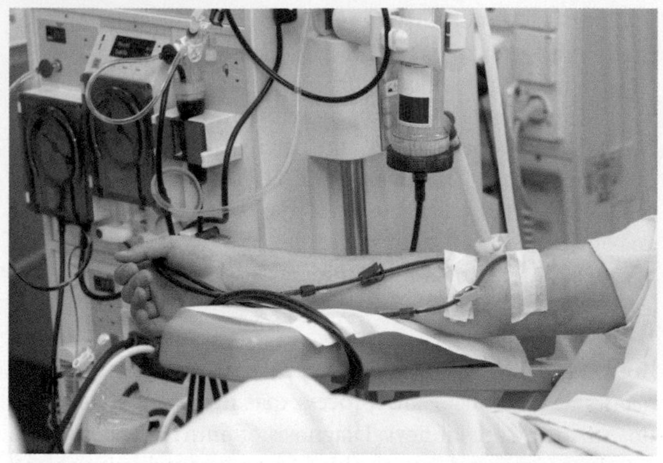

FIGURE 41-2 Patient with chronic renal failure undergoing hemodialysis at an outpatient clinic.

in patients with actual kidney damage. Structural issues with the kidneys, from primary glomerular diseases or vascular lesions, result in renal failure. Postrenal failure is related to a mechanical or functional obstruction of the flow of urine. Oliguria is most easily observed by the nurse through frequent monitoring of the patient's urinary output. Signs and symptoms of oliguria vary according to the underlying cause. The patient may be breathless, with pale, clammy, and cool skin, and have a low blood pressure; there may be signs of edema or anemia; and changes in the heart rhythm, hepatomegaly, and hypertension may be present (Murphy and Byrne, 2010).

The management of oliguria includes treatment for any reversible causes. If the intravascular volume is low, fluids should be administered for restoration. Fluid balance should be monitored and maintained with electrolyte monitoring and correction. Input and output should be recorded, along with daily weights. Potassium retention is common in renal failure. Potassium levels need to be monitored, and dialysis should start when serum potassium exceeds 6.5 mEq/L. Potassium intake should be limited until urine flow is reestablished. Dialysis may be required until the kidneys recover. The overall goal of dialysis is to remove toxins and to maintain fluid, electrolyte, and acid-base balance (Weisberg and Dellinger, 2008).

! SAFE PRACTICE ALERT

Measuring and recording intake and output ("I&O") constitute an essential part of care for a majority of hospitalized patients, especially those experiencing fluid retention or excretion problems. Patients with acute or chronic renal failure may be placed on stringent fluid intake restriction, with orders for the nurse to maintain meticulous intake and output records.

Polyuria

Polyuria is an excessive volume of urine formed and excreted each day. For an adult, this would be 2500 mL or more of urine per day. Polyuria may be caused by consumption of a large amount of fluids, especially fluids that contain caffeine or alcohol, which have a natural diuretic effect; ingestion of too much salt or glucose; use of diuretic medications; diabetes; imaging tests that involve contrast media or dye; or other disease processes.

Nocturia

Nocturia is excessive urination at night. The affected person may awaken several times during the night to urinate, which can disrupt the sleep cycle. Normally, urine decreases in amount and becomes more concentrated at night. Most people can sleep 6 to 8 hours without having to urinate. Nocturia commonly is seen in men with benign prostatic hyperplasia (BPH) and in postmenopausal women as a consequence of decreased bladder tone. It also may be associated with the use of medications such as diuretics, as well as with UTIs, congestive heart failure, cystitis (inflammation of the bladder), and diabetes. Drinking too much fluid before bedtime and sleep disorders also may have an effect. The patient with nocturia should be encouraged to maintain a diary of fluid intake, frequency of urination, urine output, and daily weights, taken at the same time on the same scale, to help determine an appropriate treatment regimen.

Dysuria

Painful urination, known as *dysuria,* may result from a number of factors, including bladder or UTI, cystitis, sexually transmitted disease, yeast infection, kidney or bladder stones, prostatic enlargement, malignancy, and allergic or irritant reaction to soaps, vaginal lubricants, spermicides, contraceptive foams and sponges, tampons, and toilet paper. Patients with dysuria often complain of burning that follows urination. Often a delay in initiating voiding or hesitancy is associated with dysuria (Watring and Mason, 2008).

Hematuria

Hematuria is the abnormal presence of red blood cells in the urine. The bleeding can originate at any point along the urinary tract. Both gross, or visible, and microscopic hematuria may represent serious underlying disease. The color of the urine does not reflect the degree of blood loss. Causes of hematuria include irritation or inflammation of the mucosa and invasion by bacteria. Malignancy, renal stones, trauma, infection, medications, tumors of the kidney, renal cysts, infarction, and arteriovenous malformations (AVM, abnormal connections between arteries and veins) may contribute to hematuria.

Urinary Incontinence

Urinary incontinence is the inability to control the passage of urine. It is prevalent in the United States, affecting up to

51% of adult women and 14% of men, with risk factors including diabetes and obesity (Buckley and Lapitan, 2010; Markland, Richter, Fwu, et al, 2011). Affected individuals may have intermittent or complete inability to hold urine.

Urinary incontinence can be divided into several types. **Stress incontinence** is loss of urine control during activities that increase intraabdominal pressure, such as coughing, sneezing, laughing, or exercise. **Urge incontinence** involves a sudden strong urge to void, followed by rapid bladder contraction. The affected person does not have enough time for toileting between recognition of the urge to urinate and the onset of voiding. **Mixed incontinence** is a combination of both stress and urge incontinence. **Functional incontinence** refers to lack of urine control in the absence of any abnormalities of the urinary tract; it occurs when some physical limitation in functioning, such as difficulty with clothing fasteners or impaired mobility, hinders reaching the toilet before voiding occurs. **Overflow incontinence** is seen in patients who are unable to empty the bladder completely, resulting in a constant dribbling of urine or increased frequency of urination. Overflow incontinence results from weakened muscles of the bladder, which may be a consequence of certain pathologic conditions. **Temporary incontinence** can occur in association with factors such as severe constipation, infections in the urinary tract or vagina, or medication usage.

Urinary incontinence most frequently is seen in elderly people, although not all elderly people become incontinent. Women are more likely than men to suffer from it. Infants and children are not considered incontinent until after toilet training is well established. It is considered normal for children to have occasional accidents (unintentional instances of incontinence) until about age 5 years. Causes of acute urinary incontinence include extended bed rest, medications, increased amount of urine, mental confusion, pregnancy, prostate infection or inflammation, stool impaction, and urinary tract infections. Chronic urinary incontinence issues may be related to bladder cancer, bladder spasms, depression, enlarged prostate, neurologic conditions, pelvic prolapse in woman, pelvic floor muscle damage that may occur with a hysterectomy, spinal injuries, or weakness of the bladder sphincter.

Urinary Retention

Urinary retention is the inability of the bladder to empty. It is caused by an obstruction in the urinary tract or by a neurological disorder. The patient with chronic urinary retention has difficulty starting a stream of urine or emptying the bladder. Once started, the urine flow is weak. Chronic urinary retention causes mild but constant discomfort. During episodes of acute urinary retention, the patient is unable to urinate despite a full bladder. In another presentation, the patient may express the need to urinate frequently and when finished still feel urge. Dribbling may occur between trips to bathroom because the bladder is constantly full. Acute urinary retention is a medical emergency necessitating prompt medical intervention.

Conditions that contribute to urinary retention include vaginal childbirth, infections of the brain or spinal cord, diabetes, stroke, neurologic disorders, heavy metal poisoning, pelvic injury or trauma, prostate enlargement, infection, surgery, bladder stones, rectocele, cystocele, constipation, urethral stricture, and medications such as antihistamines, anticholinergics, antispasmodics, and tricyclic antidepressants.

FACTORS AFFECTING URINARY ELIMINATION

The ability to urinate is influenced by a variety of factors (Diversity Considerations box). These include privacy issues and embarrassment, the effect of specific medications and foods, fluid intake, ambulatory ability, muscle tone that influences the frequency of voiding, the amount of urine produced, the color and other characteristics of the urine, the time of voiding, and voluntary control over actual urination. The cause of **enuresis**, the involuntary passing of urine, may be structural or pathologic, although it may be related to non-urinary problems such as constipation, stress, and illness. Pathologic and surgical conditions may affect the process of urination temporarily or permanently.

Developmental Factors

Individual control of urination changes with age. The infant has no urinary control, and the young child will not gain control until between the ages of 2 and 5 years (Tennant, 2010). Preschoolers may have acquired the ability of independent toileting; however, accidents may occur, and enuresis may be an issue until the age of approximately 5 years. By school age, the child's elimination patterns should be well established. Nocturnal enuresis (bedwetting) is commonly seen in children until full bladder control is established and should not be considered a problem until after age 6 years.

Elderly people are at risk for elimination problems secondary to age-related decreased function of the kidneys. Urgency and frequency often are reported as the muscles supporting the bladder weaken. Retention of urine may lead to nocturia. Prostate enlargement that causes narrowing of the urethra may impair the ability of male patients to completely empty the bladder. Residual urine may predispose the elderly patient to bladder infections.

Psychosocial Factors

Many people consider urination to be a private matter and have established behaviors or habits that are associated with voiding. Alterations in the patient's elimination patterns produce anxiety and contribute to an inability to relax the muscles necessary to initiate voiding. Patients may voluntarily suppress the urge to void secondary to other circumstances, such as unavailability of toileting facilities. These behaviors have been shown to increase the risk of incontinence and UTI.

DIVERSITY CONSIDERATIONS

Life Span

Urinary patterns change over the course of a lifetime.

Age

- Full bladder control is attained between the ages of 3 and 5 years, although nighttime control may not occur until the age of 4 to 5 years.
- Loss of muscle tone in the bladder in older adults contributes to incontinence and frequency. Nocturia is common as well. The bladder does not empty as efficiently in older people.
- Childbirth and gravity tend to weaken the pelvic floor, potentially leading to stress incontinence in older adult women.

Pregnancy

- During pregnancy, the growing fetus compromises bladder space and compresses the bladder, resulting in urinary frequency. Poor abdominal muscle tone also contributes to frequency.
- A 30% to 50% increase in circulatory volume occurs during pregnancy, which increases renal workload and output.
- The hormone relaxin, produced during pregnancy, causes relaxation of the bladder sphincter (Allsworth, Omicioli, Cunkelman, and Homco, 2008).

Gender

- Enlargement of the prostate in men 40 years of age and older may lead to urinary frequency, hesitancy, and retention.
- UTIs are more prevalent in females because of their shorter urethra and because women experience a decrease in pelvic area muscle tone with age and childbirth.

Culture

- Cultural influences may cause patients not to seek treatment for urinary elimination–related difficulties.
- Culture may have an effect on the caregiver's ability to meet the patient's needs. In some cultures it is inappropriate for a member of the opposite sex to care for a patient. Nurses should adjust care plans to reflect cultural sensitivity to the needs of patients and their families.
- Privacy concerns vary culturally. Americans generally regard urination as a private matter (Williams and Hamilton, 2009).

Disability

- Total or partial disability may lead to urinary incontinence or retention.
- Paraplegics can be taught to empty the bladder using straight catheterization, to avoid urinary retention, which may lead to UTIs.
- Lack of privacy in hospitals and assisted care facilities can contribute to incontinence or retention.
- Insufficient time taken to void can lead to changes in urinary elimination patterns.

Morphology

- Pressure of the abdomen lying on the bladder in the obese person can lead to inadequate bladder emptying and incontinence.

Food and Fluid Intake

Changes in the patient's eating or drinking pattern can disrupt normal urination. Dehydration may lead to diminished urinary output. Excessive fluid intake may change the color, odor, or quantity of urine produced. Dietary changes, such as the intake of different food, can cause changes in the color or odor of the urine.

Medication

Certain drugs may alter the production, formation, concentration, clarity, and color of urine. Medications that affect the autonomic nervous system may interfere with the urination process, causing urinary retention. Blood pressure medications, specifically diuretics, change the ratio of water and electrolyte reabsorption within the kidneys, which will alter the concentration of urine.

Muscle Tone

Muscle tone plays a direct role in filling and emptying of the bladder. Poor muscle tone affects the ability of the bladder to contract and expand completely. Changes in the muscle tone of the pelvic floor can alter sphincter control, causing urine leakage.

Surgical and Diagnostic Procedures

Surgical and diagnostic procedures may alter the formation, concentration, color, and passage of urine. Ability to pass urine is affected by swelling. Postoperative bleeding can transform the color and quantity of the urine. Anesthesia contributes to urine retention by decreasing awareness of the need to void.

Pathologic Conditions

Diseases of the kidneys may reduce the production of urine. Heart and circulatory disorders can lead to diminished blood flow to the kidneys, affecting urine production. Calculi may obstruct the ureter, blocking the flow of urine. Dehydration causes water retention, resulting in decreased urinary output. Some pathologic conditions can result in bladder removal. In such instances, urine will need to be diverted from the urinary tract to exit the body.

Urinary Tract Infections

Urinary tract infections (UTIs) are the result of bacteria in the urine. Infection occurs when bacteria from the digestive tract, usually *Escherichia coli,* invade the urethra and multiply. UTI is the single most common hospital-acquired infection

(Centers for Disease Control and Prevention, 2012). It results in more than 1 million hospital admissions each year in the United States alone (Masson, Matheson, Webster, and Craig, 2009). UTI can occur in anyone. Females are more vulnerable than males, with the rate of occurrence gradually increasing with age. Up to 30% of women experience a symptomatic UTI in their lifetime (Masson, Matheson, Webster, and Craig, 2009). The rate for women is believed to be elevated because the female urethra is significantly shorter than that of the male and is located near sources of bacteria (the anus and vagina). The shorter urethra also contributes to the risk of infection associated with sexual intercourse.

People with an elevated risk for infection include those with any abnormality of the urinary tract that obstructs the flow of urine, those with catheters in place, those who have difficulty voiding, and elderly people with bladder control loss. Diabetes or other diseases that suppress the immune system increase the risk of UTI.

Urinary Diversion

A **urinary diversion** is a surgical procedure performed when bladder function is impaired owing to trauma or disease involving the bladder, the distal ureters, or, rarely, the urethra. The diversion may be temporary or permanent and can be classified as continent or incontinent. With cutaneous urinary diversion, urine exits the body through a stoma created on the abdomen (Figure 41-3). With incontinent diversions (ileal conduits, ureterostomies, and other urostomies), an appliance, or bag, must be worn to collect urine as it is excreted from the body. For cutaneous continent diversions (Kock pouch, Mainz pouch, Indiana pouch), a collection reservoir is surgically created using a segment of the intestine; the patient then needs to catheterize the reservoir through a cutaneous stoma every 4 to 6 hours to drain stored urine. The orthotopic bladder substitute (i.e., ileal neobladder) is the most common continent diversion performed today because it most closely resembles the original bladder in both location and function. With this type of urinary diversion, a segment of the intestine is used as a urinary reservoir and is anastomosed (connected) to the patient's native urethra. An orthotopic neobladder eliminates the need for a cutaneous urinary collection device and, in some cases, the need for intermittent catheterization. The type of urinary diversion performed depends on a combination of clinical factors and the patient's preference.

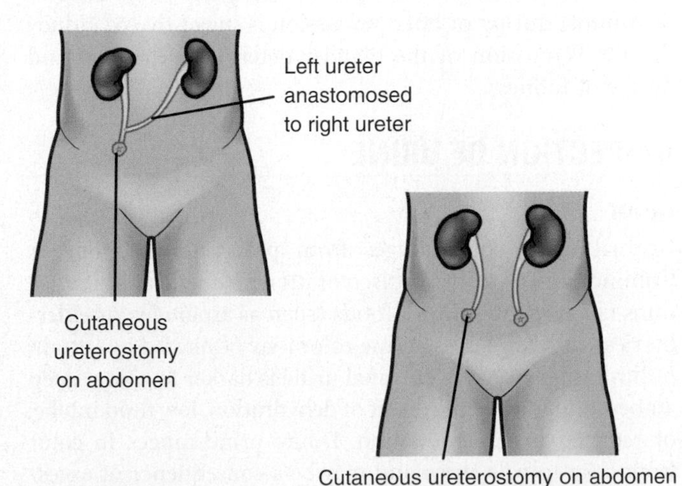

FIGURE 41-3 Cutaneous urinary diversion. (From Lewis SL, Dirksen SR, Heitkemper MM, et al: *Medical-surgical nursing: assessment and management of clinical problems*, ed. 9, St. Louis, 2014, Mosby.)

◆ ASSESSMENT LO 41.3

Open-ended as well as focused questions can be useful in obtaining essential information about the patient's urinary concerns and function. The Health Assessment Questions box contains a variety of questions to guide the interview aspect of the assessment phase.

HEALTH ASSESSMENT QUESTIONS

- Have you ever been diagnosed with kidney or bladder disease?
- Have you ever had surgery or experienced trauma to the urinary system?
- Have you ever had a urinary tract or kidney infection?
- Do you have a family history of kidney disease or urinary problems?
- Do you have any physical problems that may affect the urinary tract, such as high blood pressure, diabetes, kidney stones, multiple sclerosis, Parkinson disease, spinal cord injury, or stroke? If so, have you noticed or experienced any problems with urinary retention?
- Have you experienced changes in your normal urination pattern? If so, have they caused you embarrassment or anxiety, for how long?
- Are you able to control the flow of urine when you urinate?
- Do you ever have to get up at night to urinate?
- Do you have difficulty starting or stopping your flow of urine?
- Have you noticed difficulty initiating the stream of urine? Voiding in small amounts?
- Do you feel the need to void more frequently than in the past?
- Have you noticed any changes in the quality, quantity, color, or odor of the urine? If so, for how long?
- Do you take any vitamins or medications such as antibiotics or diuretics or eat any particular foods that might cause changes in the characteristics of your urine?
- Do you work in an environment or industry that exposes you to harsh chemicals?
- Do you experience pain, burning, itching, or other discomfort associated with urination or pain in the sides of your back or abdomen? If so, describe and rate the pain on a scale of 0 to 10.
- For female patients: How do you cleanse after urination, bowel movements, or intercourse?

During the initial assessment, directed at gathering basic subjective and objective data, the patient's physical and mental abilities must be considered, prioritization of immediate problems identified, and relief of symptoms must be addressed before a full evaluation is undertaken. Signs of distress and the patient's orientation to his or her circumstances should be noted. Changes in mental status may be a symptom of elevated nitrogenous wastes in the blood secondary to kidney dysfunction. Frequent urination and burning during micturition are classic symptoms of UTI. Fatigue is a frequent complaint of patients with kidney disorders.

After completion of a focused interview, including past and present health history, the nurse needs to conduct a physical inspection of the abdomen. Inspection of the urine also is done to evaluate the patient's hydration status and to identify changes related to the use and effects of medications and illnesses. A discussion with the patient focusing on urinary elimination patterns and abnormalities may be difficult, because elimination often is regarded as a private matter; however, it must be done. Refer to the Health Assessment Questions box for health assessment questions to include in the patient's health history interview.

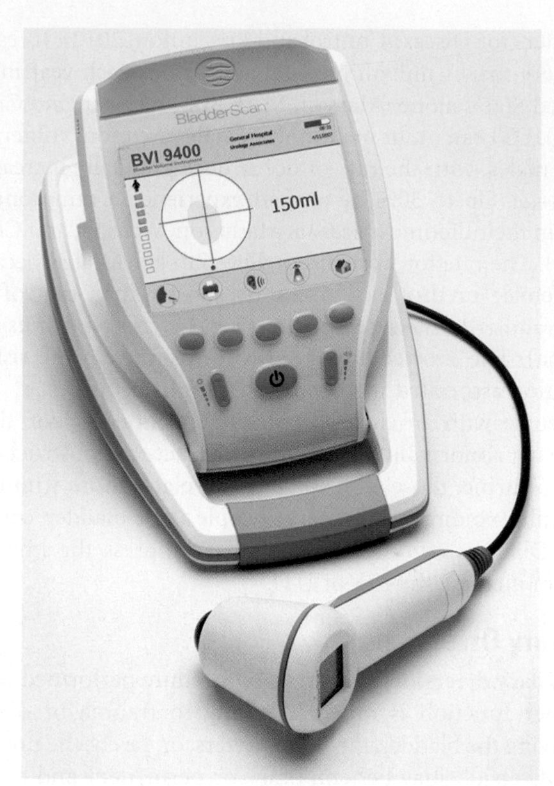

FIGURE 41-4 Determining the level of urinary retention by ultrasound scanning of the bladder can prevent unnecessary catheterization. (Copyright Verathon Inc. Used with permission.)

ABDOMINAL ASSESSMENT

After explaining to the patient what to expect during the abdominal assessment, the nurse should assess the general appearance of the abdomen for dry skin to help determine hydration status and to identify masses, indentations, and scars.

Inspection and Auscultation

The abdomen is inspected for skin color, contour, symmetry, and distention while the patient is in a supine position. Normally, the abdomen is not distended and is symmetric and free of bruises, masses, and swelling. A distended bladder may be visible in the suprapubic area. A bladder scan can be conducted by the nurse with handheld ultrasound equipment to quickly determine the extent of urinary retention (Figure 41-4). Abdominal distention may be seen in conditions such as polycystic kidney disease, pyelonephritis, ascites, and pregnancy. In addition, auscultation of the left and right renal arteries is performed to assess circulation sounds. Normally, no sounds are heard.

Palpation and Percussion

Palpation of the bladder is conducted to determine symmetry, location, size, and sensation. Light palpation should be performed over the lower abdomen. The abdomen should be soft and nondistended. Deep palpation, which can be done to outline the shape of the bladder, usually is performed by the patient's primary care provider (PCP). Using a bimanual technique, the PCP will attempt to palpate the kidneys, which rarely are palpable unless they are enlarged from tumors, cysts, or hydronephrosis. Palpation of an enlarged kidney may be painful for the patient.

Assessment by a PCP may include blunt or indirect percussion to further assess the kidneys. The patient should feel no pain or tenderness with pressure or percussion. Pain or discomfort during or after percussion is suggestive of kidney disease. Percussion of the bladder determines location and degree of fullness.

INSPECTION OF URINE

Color

Normal urine color ranges from pale yellow to amber. Common causes of urine discoloration are medications, vitamins (such as vitamin B), foods (such as asparagus or elderberries), and food dyes. Urine color may be altered by certain health problems. Concentrated urine is darker in color (deep amber) and may be the result of dehydration, low fluid intake, or reduced urine production. Dilute urine ranges in color from clear to pale straw and may be a consequence of excessive fluid intake or the inability of the kidneys to concentrate urine. Red or pink urine may be associated with bleeding, strenuous exercise, UTI, enlarged prostate, kidney or bladder stones, kidney disease, or cancer.

Food

Foods such as beets, blackberries, and rhubarb may discolor the urine pink or red; carrots and carrot juice may turn it orange. Brown or tea-colored urine is associated with consumption of fava beans and aloe. Asparagus consumption may result in blue-green urine (Harvard Health Publications, 2010).

Medication

Certain medications can affect the color of urine. Antimalarial drugs, laxatives, and metronidazole may cause the urine to turn brown or tea-colored. Rifampin, warfarin, and phenazopyridine may turn the urine orange. Blue-green urine can be seen in patients receiving medications such as cimetidine, indomethacin, or promethazine (Harvard Health Publications, 2010).

Pathologic Conditions

Patients with hypercalcemia may have blue-green urine. Those with liver failure from hepatitis and cirrhosis may have brown to tea-colored urine. Severe dehydration can cause urine to range anywhere between dark yellow-orange and tea color.

Clarity

Urine normally is clear. Cloudy urine may indicate the presence of bacteria, blood, sperm, crystals, or mucus. After bladder or kidney surgery, patients may excrete bloody urine containing clots. These patients typically require irrigation of the bladder using a three-way catheter to prevent potential blockage.

Odor

Normal urine usually does not smell very strong. Dehydration may increase the odor of urine as more waste is excreted in smaller volume. Foods (most notably, asparagus) and some diseases are associated with a change in the odor of urine. In uncontrolled diabetes, the urine can have a sweet fruity odor, whereas in infections, a strong, unpleasant odor may be evident.

Amount

The amount of urine that a patient eliminates can vary, depending on factors such as fluid intake, dehydration, and retention. The normal urinary output is approximately equal to fluid intake. Adult urinary output of approximately 60 mL/hour is considered normal.

! SAFE PRACTICE ALERT

Output of less than 30 mL/hour may indicate decreased renal perfusion and should be reported to the patient's PCP immediately.

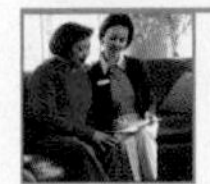

1. Identify three assessment questions that the nurse should ask Ms. James to further investigate her chief complaint.

LABORATORY TESTS

Common tests to evaluate urinary function include measurement of blood urea nitrogen (BUN) and serum creatinine levels to determine kidney function, urinalysis, urine culture to determine the cause of a UTI, and 24-hour urine collection to measure creatinine clearance.

Blood Urea Nitrogen and Creatinine

Blood levels of urea and creatinine are used to evaluate renal function. Urea is the end product of protein metabolism and is measured as BUN. Creatinine is a waste product that is produced in the blood as a by-product of muscle metabolism.

BUN concentration is a measure of the urea level in the blood. Urea is cleared by the kidney, and levels may be increased in the patient who is dehydrated or who has a disease that compromises the function of the kidney. Normal values for BUN in the blood are 7 to 20 mg/dL. Elevated levels may indicate kidney injury or disease as well as conditions such as diabetes, high blood pressure, blockage of the urinary tract, a high-protein diet, severe burns, gastrointestinal bleeding, or problems such as dehydration or heart failure, which affect blood flow. Medications also may elevate BUN levels. Low BUN values may be caused by a low protein diet, malnutrition, liver damage, or drinking excessive amounts of liquids. No pretest preparation is required; however, medications, such as certain antibiotics, corticosteroids, and diuretics, may affect test results.

Creatinine is filtered along with other waste products from the blood by the kidney and eliminated in the urine. It is made at a steady rate, and levels are not affected by diet or by normal physical activities. The patient with kidney damage has decreased urinary creatinine but increased serum levels. The amount of creatinine in the blood is directly related to muscle mass; generally, creatinine levels are higher in men than in women. Normal values of serum creatinine are 0.6 to 1.2 mg/dL for women and 0.8 to 1.4 mg/dL for men.

BUN and serum creatinine are viewed in relationship to each other. Sudden rises in BUN-to-creatinine ratios occur in acute kidney failure associated with shock, dehydration, or severe gastrointestinal bleeding. Low BUN-to-creatinine ratios are seen in patients on low-protein diets or those with severe muscle injury, cirrhosis of the liver, or syndrome of inappropriate antidiuretic hormone (SIADH).

Urinalysis

Urinalysis is an assessment of the urine at a single point in time. Urinalysis is a screening tool for UTI, kidney disease, and other conditions. Single samples can be used for detection or measurement of bacteria, glucose, white blood cells, red blood cells, proteins, and other substances. Urinalysis samples are collected by having the patient void in a specimen cup, or samples may be taken using catheterization. Only small samples of urine (10 to 15 mL) are required for urinalysis testing.

Specific Gravity

Urinalysis for specific gravity monitors the balance of water and solutes (solid matter) in urine. Normal specific gravity in an adult is 1.005 to 1.030. The higher the level of specific gravity, the more solid material is contained in the urine. Fluid intake has a direct relationship to specific gravity. If large volumes of water are consumed, dilute urine is produced, which has a low specific gravity. Specific gravity is high in conditions of dehydration.

pH

The acid-base balance in the body is determined by pH, which reflects the acidity or alkalinity of the urine. Urine normally is slightly acidic, with an average pH of 6. Urine with a pH of 4 is very acidic. A pH of 7 is neutral, and a pH of 9 is very alkaline. The pH is useful in determining the kidneys' response to acid-base imbalances. In metabolic acidosis, the urine pH decreases as the kidneys excrete hydrogen ions; in metabolic alkalosis, pH of the urine increases. Maintaining a healthy pH helps prevent formation of kidney stones.

Urine for Protein

Normally, urine does not contain protein. Protein modules generally are too large to escape from the glomerulus capillaries into filtrate. Protein in the urine may be associated with fever, vigorous exercise, pregnancy, and some diseases, such as kidney disease. In conditions such as glomerulonephritis (inflammation of the glomeruli of the kidney), the cell membrane can become permeable and allow proteins to cross.

Glucose

Normal urine contains very little to no glucose. The urine glucose concentration is used to screen for diabetes and to assess glucose tolerance. Glucose in the urine may be a sign of kidney damage or disease. Urine glucose levels are not an adequate measure of blood glucose levels. In the uncontrolled diabetic patient, glucose may appear in the urine.

Ketones

The presence of ketones in the urine (ketonuria) indicates that fat has broken down for energy. Ketones are normally not passed in the urine. Large amounts of ketones in the urine may indicate diabetic ketoacidosis. A diet low in sugars and carbohydrates, prolonged fasting or starvation, and vomiting also may be associated with ketonuria.

Microscopic Analysis

For microscopic analysis, urine is spun in a centrifuge and sediment settles at the bottom. The sediment is then spread on a slide and checked for red or white blood cells, casts, plugs, or crystals. The presence of crystals in the urine may indicate that stones are present. Bacteria, yeast, and parasites are not normally present in urine and, when present, usually indicate infection.

Suspected Urinary Tract Infection

If a UTI is suspected, urine may be checked for nitrates. Nitrate levels increase when bacteria are present. A leukocyte esterase test determines the level of white blood cells in the urine; elevated levels indicate presence of a UTI.

Culture and Sensitivity Testing

Urine culture and sensitivity testing are performed for diagnosis of a UTI. Urine in the bladder normally is sterile; it does not contain bacteria or organisms. If organisms grow in the culture, sensitivity testing is performed to determine the appropriate antibiotic for treatment.

24-Hour Urine Collection

A 24-hour urine collection usually is performed to determine the amount of creatinine cleared through the kidneys (see Chapter 34, Skill 34-2: Urine Specimen Collection). This timed specimen also is used to measure levels of protein, hormones, minerals, and other chemical compounds in the urine. Creatinine clearance, which measures how well creatinine is removed from the blood by the kidneys, provides information about kidney function. Factors or conditions that may interfere with the accuracy of a 24-hour urine collection include failure to include some portion of the output, continuing the collection beyond 24 hours, spilling the specimen, inability to keep the specimen cool, and previous ingestion of certain foods or medications.

Preparation is not required before initiation of a 24-hour urine collection. The time of the patient's first morning void is the best start time for the 24-hour specimen collection. The first voided specimen is not saved; all urine produced after the first (discarded) specimen is collected in a special opaque container and kept cool. At the completion of the 24 hours, the first voided specimen of the second day (if the collection was started in the morning) is included in the specimen, and the container is transported to the laboratory for analysis. Twenty-four-hour collections may be performed on an outpatient or inpatient basis.

DIAGNOSTIC EXAMINATIONS

In more complicated situations, additional tests may be needed to obtain a more thorough assessment of the urinary system. Diagnostic procedures may be invasive or noninvasive. These tests may require some preparation on the part of the patient before testing. An adequate understanding of each procedure is necessary for the nurse providing care for patients with urologic difficulties to assist them through the diagnostic process.

Ultrasound Assessment of the Bladder or Kidneys

An ultrasound scan may be performed to assess the size, shape, and location of the kidneys; with use of specialized ultrasound technology, blood flow can be monitored during the procedure. Ultrasound studies may be safely conducted in pregnant women and in patients who have allergies to contrast media, because no radiation or contrast dyes are used. Factors or conditions that interfere with ultrasound results include severe obesity, recent barium studies, and excessive flatus or intestinal gas. Generally, no patient preparation such as fasting or sedation is required. If the bladder is to be studied, the patient will be required to drink fluid and refrain from voiding before the procedure. The ultrasound examination itself causes no pain; however, the patient may complain of discomfort from lying still with a full bladder for the duration of the procedure.

Kidney, Ureter, and Bladder X-ray Study

A kidney, ureter, and bladder (KUB) study is a diagnostic x-ray image centered on the iliac crest, typically used to investigate gastrointestinal conditions such as a bowel obstruction or gallstones; it also can detect the presence of kidney stones. In addition, KUB studies are used to assess positioning of indwelling devices such as ureteral stents. A ureteral stent is an indwelling tube placed in the ureter, at a point between the kidney and the bladder. Stents are placed to prevent or treat obstruction of the urine flow through the ureter.

Intravenous Pyelography

An intravenous pyelogram (IVP) is an x-ray study of the kidneys, the bladder, the ureters, and the urethra. The images show the size, shape, and position of the urinary tract. The procedure for IVP involves the injection of contrast material into a vein. X-ray images are then taken at timed intervals. An IVP commonly is performed to identify kidney stones, tumors, or infection; to measure the size of a tumor of the urinary tract; and to look for urinary tract damage after injury. Contraindications for IVP include pregnancy, severe kidney disease, and an allergy to iodine. The patient should not eat or drink for 8 to 12 hours before the test and may need a laxative or enema to ensure that the bowels are empty. Risks involved with IVP are allergic reactions to the contrast material and sudden kidney failure associated with conditions such as diabetes, kidney disease, sickle cell disease, and pheochromocytoma (a rare adrenal gland tumor), as well as medications that affect the kidney (Mayo Clinic Staff, 2014).

Computed Tomography

Computed tomography (CT) of the kidneys, ureters, and bladder is used to diagnose kidney stones, bladder stones, or blockage of the urinary tract. Contrast media may be used during the procedure to help identify blockages, growths, infections, or other diseases. The patient may be required to have nothing by mouth for 8 to 12 hours before the test and may be prescribed a laxative or enema. A sedative may be given to help the patient relax before the procedure. The scan usually takes 30 to 60 minutes but may take up to 2 hours, during which time the patient must lie still. After the procedure, the patient should be encouraged to drink liquids to flush out any contrast material that was given.

Cystoscopy

Cystoscopy is examination of the bladder and urethra through a cystoscope, which is inserted into the urethra and advanced into the bladder. The procedure permits visualization of areas that do not show up well on x-ray images. Cystoscopy is performed to determine the cause of hematuria, dysuria, incontinence, frequency, urgency, or retention. Cystoscopy is used additionally in the diagnosis of conditions that cause blockage of the urethra, as well as for treatment of urinary tract problems. Biopsy of tissues and removal of small stones or growths also can be performed using cystoscopy. Local, spinal, or general anesthesia may be used for the procedure. The patient should take nothing by mouth 8 to 12 hours before the test in case general anesthesia needs to be administered. The entire examination may take up to 45 minutes. The patient may experience a burning sensation and the urge to urinate during the procedure, and lying on the table can become uncomfortable. Risks associated with the test include those associated with anesthesia, temporary swelling of the urethra, difficulty urinating, and mild infection. Puncture of the urethra or bladder is a rare complication. After the procedure, the patient should be encouraged to increase fluid intake, to minimize burning and prevent UTI. Pink-tinged urine commonly is seen for several days after cystoscopy, particularly if a biopsy is performed.

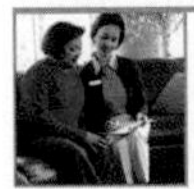

2. What diagnostic studies are most likely to be performed in evaluating Ms. James? Give the rationale for each study.

◆ NURSING DIAGNOSIS LO 41.4

Data obtained during assessment of the patient's urinary elimination function and patterns may reveal existing and potential problems. Accurate assessment and clustering of the data are crucial to identifying the defining characteristics of impaired elimination and to determine the appropriate nursing diagnoses for the patient.

Impaired Urinary Elimination is the nursing diagnosis that addresses several types of urinary dysfunction, including dysuria, frequency, retention, and urgency due to obstructions, infection, sensory impairment, and a variety of other underlying etiologic disorders. *Stress Urinary Incontinence, Functional Urinary Incontinence, Urge Urinary Incontinence,* and *Reflex Urinary Incontinence* are each separate nursing diagnoses. Each of the incontinence diagnoses addresses the unique patient needs associated with that specific type of incontinence. The defining characteristics for each diagnosis are type-specific and allow for selection of individualized nursing interventions.

Although not directly related to urinary elimination, associated nursing diagnoses such as *Risk for Impaired Skin Integrity, Risk for Infection, Disturbed Body Image, Ineffective Coping,* and *Pain* may be appropriately assigned to patients experiencing urinary elimination concerns. Nursing diagnoses specifically related to urinary elimination include the following:

- *Impaired Urinary Elimination* related to microorganisms in the urinary tract as evidenced by urgency, frequency, and reports of burning with urination
- *Urinary Retention* related to post anesthetic state as evidenced by absent urinary output, lower abdominal distension, and residual urine evident on bladder scan
- *Toileting Self-Care Deficit* related to neuromuscular impairment as evidenced by right-sided paralysis, inability to perform proper toileting hygiene, and inability to manipulate clothing during toileting

◆ PLANNING LO 41.5

Goals for the resolution of elimination problems are structured around maintaining normal elimination patterns, returning to previous levels of function, preventing associated risks, or coping with an altered pattern (Table 41-1). The nurse and the patient should work collaboratively to create individualized goals specific for the diagnosis and prioritized according to the patient's need, which may initially have a psychosocial focus (Collaboration and Delegation box). Expected outcomes are related to satisfactory management of incontinence, complete emptying of the bladder, and independent management of toileting tasks. Short-term goals may include:

- Patient will report resolution of UTI symptoms within 5 days of taking prescribed antibiotic treatment.
- Patient will spontaneously empty bladder completely without assistance within 12 hours after surgery.
- Patient will effectively wipe self with left hand after urination within 5 days.

Long-term goals associated with urinary elimination concerns may include:

- Patient will perform self-catheterization without developing a UTI for 6 months after urinary diversion surgery.
- Patient will demonstrate care of urinary diversion before discharge from the hospital.
- Patient will demonstrate ability to safely perform toileting tasks without assistance within 9 months of developing left-sided weakness secondary to a severe cerebrovascular accident.

COLLABORATION AND DELEGATION

Team Approach to Meeting Patient Elimination Needs

- Unlicensed assistive personnel (UAP) often aid patients in toileting. The nurse must communicate necessary actions, such as measuring the amount of urine, noting its color, and determining the frequency of urination. The nurse must stress to the UAP the necessity of documenting voiding patterns.
- Nurse continence specialists may need to be consulted to teach pelvic floor exercises.
- Physical therapists can design a plan to increase overall muscle strength.
- The family may need to alter the home environment to accommodate the patient's elimination needs, depending on physical limitations.
- In some settings, UAP may be permitted to insert a urinary catheter, but it is not routine practice. The UAP may assist with positioning the patient, focusing lighting, maintaining patient position, and providing comfort measures.

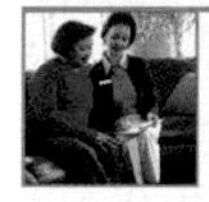

The conceptual care map for Ms. James can be found at *http://evolve.elsevier.com/YoostCrawford/fundamentals/.* It is partially completed to indicate how to use the map as a learning tool. Complete the nursing diagnoses using the example conceptual care maps shown in Chapters 8 and 25 to 33.

TABLE 41-1 Care Planning

NANDA-I NURSING DIAGNOSIS LABEL WITH NURSING DIAGNOSIS STATEMENT	NURSING OUTCOME CLASSIFICATION (NOC)	NURSING INTERVENTION CLASSIFICATION (NIC)
Impaired Urinary Elimination related to microorganisms in the urinary tract as evidenced by urgency, frequency, and reports of burning with urination	*Urinary elimination* (0503) Absence of urinary frequency (050331)	*Urinary elimination management* (0590) Instruct patient to monitor for signs and symptoms of urinary tract infection.

From Bulechek G, Butcher H, Dochterman J, et al (Eds): *Nursing interventions classification (NIC),* ed. 6, St. Louis, 2013, Mosby; Moorhead S, Johnson M, Maas M, et al (Eds): *Nursing outcomes classification (NOC),* ed. 5, St. Louis, 2013, Mosby; NANDA International: *Nursing diagnoses: Definitions and classification, 2012–2014,* West Sussex, England, 2012, Wiley-Blackwell. Reprinted with permission from NANDA International, Inc.

◆ IMPLEMENTATION AND EVALUATION LO 41.6

The implementation phase of the nursing process involves interventions that assist the patient in achieving the goals, including, but not limited to, continence, complete emptying of the bladder, and self-care in toileting. The focus of each goal is directly related to the identified nursing diagnosis, which in turn determines what interventions are most appropriate for each patient. The nurse must focus on activities that will help the patient with compromised urinary elimination return to the normal state of function or adapt to changes in the state of function. Nursing interventions to help patients achieve urinary continence and complete emptying of the bladder and independent toileting include promoting adequate fluid intake, teaching self-care activities, and assisting with voiding. Collaborative interventions require the assistance of the PCP or other professionals, such as a physical therapist or nutritionist.

QSEN FOCUS!

Discussing reliable resources for patient and family referrals will promote informed decision making and support for caregivers after discharge.

Ongoing assessment and follow-up are needed to ensure quality in the care provided and to determine need for further nursing interventions. Patient education is crucial for maintaining urinary tract health (Patient Education and Health Literacy box). Before leaving the acute care facility, the patient needs to demonstrate understanding and competency in assessment of the qualities and characteristics of urine, home catheterization, toileting, fluid intake, and preventing UTIs. An additional important topic for patient education is the relationship between poor hygiene and occurrence of UTIs. Proper hand hygiene can prevent the spread of infection; proper perineal care techniques can prevent cross contamination with bacteria from the anal region. Teaching the female patient pelvic muscle exercises (**Kegel exercises**) helps to strengthen and maintain pelvic floor muscles, thus aiding in the prevention of some types of incontinence.

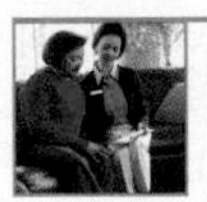

3. List a minimum of three topics that the nurse should discuss with Ms. James before discharging her from the clinic. Include content that the nurse should cover under each topic.

It is necessary to ensure that preparations for the patient's return home have been made before discharge (Home Care Considerations box). The home should be assessed for accessibility of toileting facilities and associated safety issues. The nurse should facilitate the acquisition of needed supplies and equipment and expedite necessary referrals.

PATIENT EDUCATION AND HEALTH LITERACY

Adapting Teaching to Patient Needs

- Instruct patients and families on safe transfer techniques for people with limited mobility needing voiding assistance.
- Instruct patients to respond promptly to urge, to avoid urinary retention and reduce infection risk.
- Emphasize the importance of maintaining fluid intake to help flush the urinary system.
- Instruct patients to promptly report pain or burning on urination; changes in urine color, odor, or clarity; or changes in voiding patterns.
- Reinforce with female patients proper aseptic technique, including washing front to back to maintain perineal cleanliness and voiding after intercourse. Remind male patients to retract foreskin, if present, to thoroughly wash the urinary meatus. Be sure to stress the importance of drying the area thoroughly to prevent skin breakdown or irritation.
- Teach proper care of indwelling catheters and the perineal area, including emptying and cleaning the device, maintaining a closed system, and bladder **irrigation**, or flushing, if necessary.
- Arrange for a wound ostomy continence nurse (WOCN) to teach patients with a urinary diversion appropriate care for the stoma, drainage devices, and skin.
- Teach patients the importance of taking medications as prescribed. Instruct patients and families in desired or adverse drug effects that may influence the urinary elimination pattern. Stress the importance of maintaining fluid intake or restrictions based on medication requirements.

HOME CARE CONSIDERATIONS

Necessary Elimination Resources

- Assessing the home for safety issues related to urinary elimination is important. The patient must have ready access to toilet facilities. Adequate lighting should be ensured.
- Necessary assistive and safety equipment, such as grab bars and raised toilet seats, should be in place in the home before discharge, as needed. Bedpans and a bedside commode, if warranted, should be in the home ahead of time.
- Supplies necessary for catheterization and catheter care, for urinary diversions, and for incontinence care should be purchased.
- Appropriate referrals to home health or social services should be made before discharge. Services such as those of home health aides for assistance with activities of daily living (ADLs) should be confirmed.
- Community resources such as the United Ostomy Association and the National Association for Continence should be identified for patients and their families.

! SAFE PRACTICE ALERT

The home environment should be assessed for factors that may interfere with toileting. Impractical distance to the toilet, inefficient physical layout of the toileting facilities, clutter, stairways, rugs, and inadequate lighting may put ambulatory patients at safety risk.

PROMOTING NORMAL URINARY PATTERNS IN A HEALTH CARE FACILITY

Generally, every patient in a health care facility experiences an alteration in the pattern of elimination. Many people follow routines to promote voiding, but in the health care facility, conflicts with a person's normal routine are common. For example, bed rest, medication use, prescribed medical therapies, and privacy issues can alter the patient's pattern. Proper integration of the patient's habits into daily care will aid in preventing problems with elimination.

! SAFE PRACTICE ALERT

Medications such as diuretics may cause frequency or urgency, potentially compromising patient safety. Instruct patients who are on falls precautions to ask for assistance before ambulation.

Bedpan and Urinal

The patient who is unable to ambulate to the bathroom may require the use of a bedpan or urinal. For many patients, this can be an uncomfortable and embarrassing procedure. Many patients require privacy and an unhurried time to void. Pulling the bedside curtain closed, allowing for adequate time for the patient to void, and encouraging the patient to be in the most normal position possible on the bedpan will help promote elimination.

The bedpan may be warmed before use, because a cold bedpan can cause contraction of the perineal muscles with consequent inhibition of voiding. A high Fowler position increases the intraabdominal pressure and helps stimulate voiding, and flexion of the hip and knees simulates the normal position for a woman. A small pillow or rolled towel placed behind the patient's back will increase comfort. Use of a fracture bedpan is recommended for patients who must remain positioned at an angle less than 30 degrees from horizontal.

Urinals generally are for male use. Urinals for women are available as well, but these rarely are used in the hospital setting (Figure 41-5). The urinal can be used while the patient is standing, sitting, or lying down. The Nursing Care Guideline: Assisting a Patient With a Urinal box outlines the procedure.

To maintain asepsis, hospitalized patients are provided with a bedpan, urinal, or both for personal use that is marked with their name or room number. The bedpan typically is stored in the bathroom. A urinal should be stored out of sight but within reach. It should be kept separate from other equipment used for hygienic care, and aseptic practices prohibit its being kept on the floor, under the bed, or on the over-bed table. Bedpans and urinals should be rinsed thoroughly after each use.

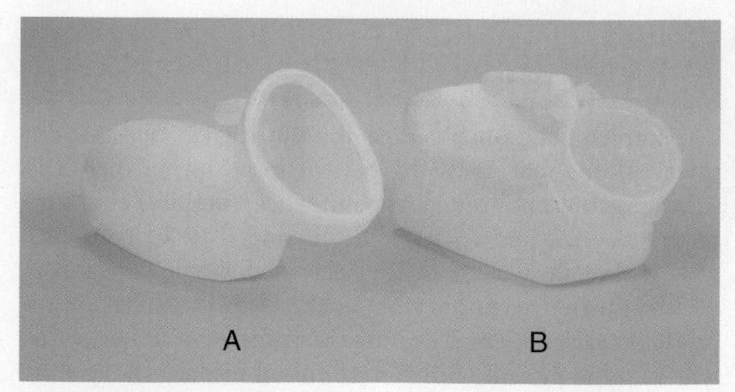

FIGURE 41-5 Male urinals are more commonly used in the acute care setting, although urinals for both females **(A)** and males **(B)** are available.

Bedside Commode

A bedside commode is a chair with a toilet seat top that has a container underneath to collect urine or stool for the patient who is unable to ambulate to the bathroom. The container is removed for emptying and cleaning. A bedside commode is more conducive to elimination than a bedpan. Use of a bedside commode may be appropriate if the patient is weak or unsteady, is at risk for falling, or becomes short of breath when ambulating. It should not be used for the patient who is unable to stand, who is maintained on strict bed rest, or who is at safety risk in an upright position.

Although a bedside commode is not disposable, each hospitalized patient is provided with one for individual use to maintain asepsis; it is cleaned and sanitized between users. The bedside commode container should be emptied and rinsed between each use. Privacy can be an issue with the bedside commode; pulling the privacy curtain and avoiding disruptions are essential.

Privacy

If possible, the patient should be given time and privacy to void. Many patients have difficulty voiding in the presence of others. As noted, pulling the bedside curtain and avoiding disruptions will help to promote elimination. Visitors should be asked to leave the area. If possible, the patient should be provided the use of a private room. If the patient needs to be monitored more closely for safety reasons while using a bedpan or urinal, the nurse should remain at the bedside facing slightly away from the patient and use a cover sheet to allow for privacy.

It may be helpful to provide sensory stimuli that will assist the patient to relax, such as applying warm compresses or blankets to the lower abdomen. Turning on running water

NURSING CARE GUIDELINE

Assisting a Patient With a Urinal

Background

- Routine urination and complete emptying of the bladder will prevent many complications.
- Encourage routine use of the urinal for male patients who are unable to ambulate to the bathroom.

Procedural Concerns

- Patient positioning for using a urinal may be:
  - In bed, where the patient may be:
    - Side-lying or
    - Supine or
    - Supine with the head of the bed elevated
  - Sitting on the side of the bed or
  - Standing
- Apply clean gloves before placing the urinal.
- Place the urinal between the patient's legs, with the penis completely in the urinal.
- Provide privacy, with the call light within reach of the patient.
- Remove the urinal after 10 minutes (whether or not urination has occurred) to prevent skin breakdown.

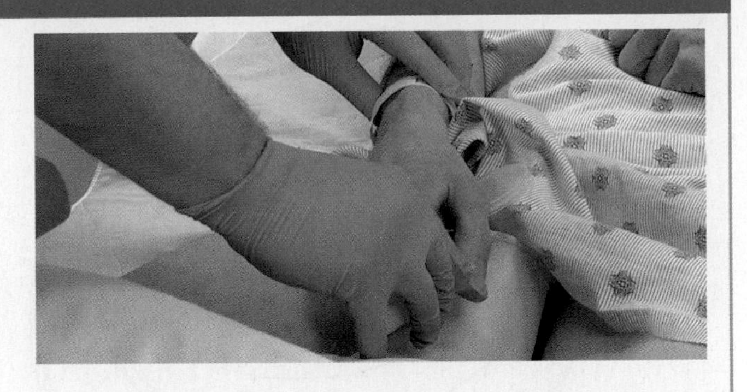

- Provide for patient hand hygiene.
- Assist the patient with cleansing, as needed.
- Implement personal hand hygiene before and after helping the patient with the urinal.

Documentation Concerns

- Document the quantity, color, quality and odor of the urine.
- Note the stream characteristics.
- Monitor frequency of urination.

within hearing distance of the patient may stimulate urge and mask the sound of voiding. These types of interventions help to relieve physical and emotional discomfort.

Toileting Schedule

Determining the patient's toileting pattern may assist the person with urinary elimination. The patient should be encouraged to void at regular intervals whether urge is felt or not. The patient with functional incontinence benefits most from a toileting schedule, which helps improve general control over urination (Morgan, Endozoa, Paradiso, et al, 2008). Create a specific routine based on the patient's normal toileting pattern, then monitor and document episodes of incontinence, looking for patterns. First, establish voiding opportunities on a regular schedule: on awakening, every 1 to 2 hours during the day, before bedtime, and every 4 hours at night; and then gradually increase the time intervals between. Variations to this schedule can be made for bladder retraining to slowly increase the amount of fluid retained and for habit training. Prompted voiding also may be encouraged as the patient develops control.

Fluid Intake

Increasing fluid intake will promote urine production in the patient without renal or cardiac dysfunction. A normal daily intake of 1500 to 2000 mL of fluids usually is adequate to maintain normal micturition. The patient with a history of UTI or urinary calculi should increase that intake to 2000 to 2500 mL for flushing of the urinary tract and prevention of stone formation (Nazarko, 2009b). Although it is important to increase fluid intake, to minimize nocturia, encourage the patient to stop drinking fluids at least 2 hours before bedtime.

! SAFE PRACTICE ALERT

Dehydration can pose a risk for patients trying to control incontinence problems by avoiding adequate fluid consumption. Dehydration may affect the patient's mental status, further contributing to risk.

MONITORING INTAKE AND OUTPUT

For a majority of hospitalized patients, not just those with urinary concerns, it is necessary to monitor and record patient intake and output. Recording of fluid intake and output can be delegated to a qualified UAP, if the nurse takes ultimate responsibility to make sure the intervention is completed satisfactorily. While evaluating intake and output, the nurse should always take into consideration whether the patient has recently undergone surgery, is receiving medications that influence fluid intake and output, or has a medical condition such as kidney or heart failure that affects fluid balance.

Intake includes all food and oral fluids as well as tube feedings and intravenous fluids. In most facilities, solid food intake is documented as an estimated percentage of a meal consumed (e.g., 85% of lunch). Oral fluids are recorded in milliliter (mL) amounts for the size of the container from which they are consumed. A list of volumes for various containers used in a facility, such as coffee cup = 240 mL, juice glass = 120 mL, and water pitcher = 900 mL, should be available for reference before documentation of oral intake. Ice chips are documented as approximately one half of their volume. The volume of tube feedings and intravenous therapies (both maintenance and piggyback) are noted on the can or bag in which they are supplied. Regardless of how liquid intake is "consumed," it is recorded in mL.

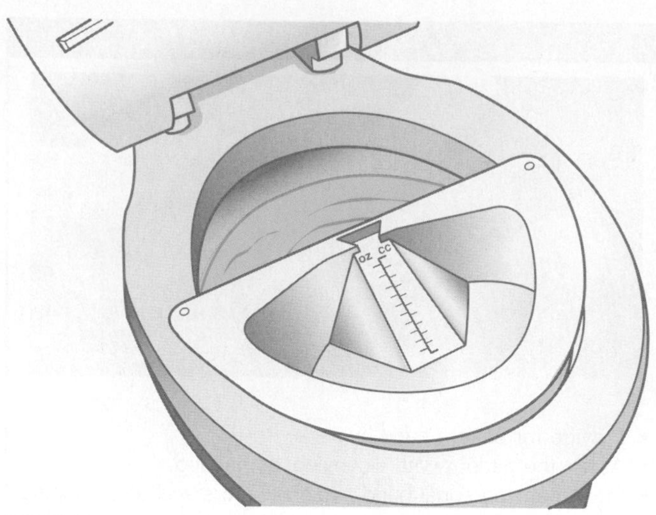

FIGURE 41-6 Urine hats are used to monitor urinary output in ambulatory patients. All liquid output is measured in a disposable graduated container to ensure accuracy of output records. (From Birchenall JM, Streight E: *Mosby's textbook for home care aide,* ed. 3, St. Louis, 2013, Mosby.)

Output is measured by collecting fluid and drainage from bedpans, urinals, urinary catheters, drains, ostomy bags, nasogastric tubes, or collection devices commonly referred to as urine "hats" placed in the front of a toilet or bedside commode (Figure 41-6). All liquid secretions are measured in mL using a disposable, graduated container, which is washed after each use. Each time output receptacles are emptied, the volume is carefully documented. Liquids that are measured and recorded as output include urine, liquid feces, vomitus, blood, and nasogastric and drainage excretions (including those from chest tubes). Irrigation fluid introduced through nasogastric or gastric tubes and catheters should be measured during instillation and subtracted from output before documentation. If a patient is extremely diaphoretic, that is noted, despite its being immeasurable.

! SAFE PRACTICE ALERT

Urine color, clarity, and odor should be assessed before disposal. Urine quantity must be measured before it is discarded to ensure accurate intake and output records.

Once intake and output are recorded, the balance is calculated and documented for assessment. This allows all members of the health care team to determine if a patient has a positive or negative intake-output balance. If the patient has consumed more fluid than has been excreted, the balance is positive. When the patient excretes or loses more fluid than what is consumed, the balance is considered negative (Table 41-2).

TABLE 41-2 Sample Intake and Output (I&O) Calculation

POSITIVE BALANCE	NEGATIVE BALANCE
Intake:	Intake:
Oral fluid = 700 mL	Oral fluid = 100 mL
IV fluid = 1250 mL	Tube feeding = 480 mL
8-hr intake total = 1950 mL	*8-hr intake total* = 580 mL
Output:	Output:
Urine = 940 mL	Urine = 640 mL
Vomitus = 50 mL	Hemovac drainage = 400 mL
8-hr output total = 990 mL	*8-hr output total* = 1040 mL
I&O balance: +960	I&O balance: –460

KEGEL EXERCISES

Kegel exercises are recognized to help keep the female pelvic floor toned, which reduces the risk of incontinence. If performed correctly and regularly, Kegel exercises have been shown to strengthen the pelvic floor muscles that support the uterus, bladder, and bowel (Nursing Care Guideline: Kegel Exercise Techniques box). If the patient has difficulty performing Kegel exercises, biofeedback training may be used. A small monitoring probe is inserted into the patient's vagina or rectum, or small electrodes are placed outside the area, and when the patient contracts the pelvic floor muscles successfully, a measurement will show on the monitor. When Kegel exercises are performed regularly, improvement normally is seen in approximately 8 to 10 weeks.

PREVENTION OF UTIs

Prevention is key to controlling UTIs, especially in women prone to infection. Nurses need to be proactive in instructing all patients, especially those who have experienced UTIs in the past, about ways to prevent infection or recurrence. Patients should be encouraged to avoid wearing tight-fitting clothing, which can irritate the urethra and prevent ventilation of the perineal area. The patient should drink at least eight 8-ounce glasses of water per day to flush the urinary tract. It is important that the patient urinate when the urge is felt; in people who frequently hold urine, a higher incidence of infection has been reported (Nazarko, 2009b). Women and girls should wipe front to back in the perineal area after urination or defecation, to prevent possible entry of bacteria from the gastrointestinal tract into the urethra. Urination right after sexual intercourse may help prevent UTIs as well. Showers are the preferred method of bathing for the patient prone to development of UTI, because bacteria in bathwater can readily enter the urethra. Likewise, it is important that the patient avoid the use of bubble baths, soaps, powders, and sprays in the perineal area, because they may cause inflammation and encourage bacterial growth. Good perineal hygiene, which includes cleansing the urethral meatus after each voiding or bowel movement, is essential. The genital area also should be cleansed before sexual intercourse.

NURSING CARE GUIDELINE

Kegel Exercise Techniques

Background

- Kegel exercises also are known as pelvic floor exercises.
- They improve muscle tone in the pelvic floor, which helps to prevent stress incontinence.
- Exercises can be done while the person is sitting or standing.

Procedural Concerns

Instruct the patient to:

- Tighten the circumvaginal muscles, anal sphincter, and urinary sphincter together for 3 or 4 seconds without tightening the leg muscles or buttocks.
  - When the exercises are practiced during urination, the patient should be able to completely stop the flow of urine if they are being performed properly.
- Relax the muscles for 30 seconds, and immediately retighten the muscle group.
- Repeat the sequence of 10 times for each set, and do five sets per day.
- Increase gradually to three sets of 5 contractions, each held for 10 seconds with a 10-second rest. Rest for 30 seconds between each set.
- Perform one or two sets per week.

Documentation Concerns

- Document that patient education was provided.

Treatment for a UTI requires antibiotics, and the patient often will achieve symptom relief within 1 or 2 days of treatment. However, patients should be instructed to finish their antibiotics even after they are feeling better. Prophylactic (preventative) or short-term suppressive antibiotic therapy is sometimes prescribed for patients with recurrent UTIs. Long term suppressive therapy is not recommended due to potential development of antibiotic resistance. Kidney infections may require several weeks of antibiotic treatment to resolve. Severely ill patients may require hospitalization with intravenous antibiotics. The use of a heating pad, drinking plenty of water, urinary tract analgesic medication, and avoidance of caffeine, alcohol, and spicy foods will help promote symptom relief.

Approximately 80% of UTIs are the result of catheterization (Conway and Larson, 2011). This clear-cut connection makes avoiding the use of indwelling catheters a primary consideration in UTI prevention. Nurses should be aware of and follow care guidelines if catheterization is required.

URINARY CATHETERIZATION

Urinary catheterization most often is performed by introducing a catheter into the patient's urethra to reach the bladder. For urethral catheterization, any of four different kinds of catheters—straight, Foley, triple-lumen, and coudé—may be used (Figure 41-7). *Straight catheters* are single-lumen devices, designed for one-time or short-term catheterization: The catheter is left in place only long enough to drain the patient's bladder. The procedure may be performed to (1) obtain samples of urine for analysis, (2) diagnose infection or kidney dysfunction, (3) drain residual urine found during a bladder scan, (4) empty a continent urinary diversion, or (5) drain the bladder of a paraplegic or quadriplegic who has lost the ability to urinate naturally.

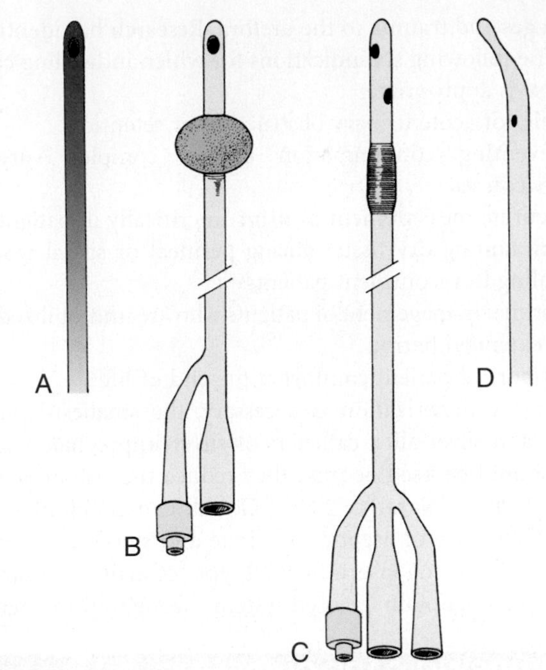

FIGURE 41-7 Urinary catheters. **A,** Straight. **B,** Foley. **C,** Triple lumen. **D,** Coudé. (Modified from Wein AJ: *Campbell-Walsh urology,* ed. 9, Philadelphia, 2007, Saunders.)

Foley and coudé catheters are two lumen *indwelling catheters*. One lumen is for filling a balloon at the tip of the catheter to "anchor" it in place and the other is for draining urine. Coudé catheters are a special type of double-lumen, indwelling catheter that are slightly stiff and bent at the end, allowing the catheter to pass more easily through a partially constricted urethra. They are used mostly in men experiencing prostate enlargement or BPH. Coudé catheters may need to be placed using a metal wire introducer. Placement using an introducer typically is performed by a physician or the patient's urologist, to avoid damaging urethral tissue. Both Foley and coudé catheters are designed to be left in place, draining the bladder continuously or intermittently for an extended period of hours, days, or weeks. Skill 41-1 reviews the procedure for insertion and care of a urinary catheter.

Triple-lumen catheters are used for bladder irrigation. The triple-lumen design allows sterile irrigation fluid to be introduced into the bladder to provide localized antibiotic treatment or to drain blood and blood clots after surgical or diagnostic procedures (Skill 41-2).

Despite its multiple applications, in addition to being the primary cause of UTIs, urinary catheterization may lead to blockages and trauma to the urethra. Research has identified only the following six indications for which indwelling catheter use is appropriate:

1. Relief of acute urinary obstruction or retention
2. Preventing contamination during complex surgical procedures
3. Accurate measurement of urine in critically ill patients
4. Maintaining dry tissue during perineal or sacral wound healing in incontinent patients
5. Optimal management of patients who are immobilized for an extended period
6. Support of patient comfort at the end of life

When catheterization is necessary, the smallest-suitable device and silver alloy catheters or silver-impregnated catheters should be used because they reduce the risk of associated infection (Nazarko, 2009a; Gould, Umscheid, Agarwal, et al, 2009). Use of aseptic technique and sterile equipment is necessary during insertion of all types of urinary catheters. It is best to maintain a closed system throughout the period in which the indwelling catheter is in place, to prevent the introduction of microorganisms into the bladder. Indwelling urinary catheters should be placed only when indicated and should be removed as soon as medically possible (Nursing Care Guideline: Discontinuing an Indwelling Catheter box).

Routine Catheter Care

Catheters should be inserted using aseptic technique and sterile equipment, as recommended by the Centers for Disease Control and Prevention (CDC) (Gould, Umscheid, Agarwal, et al, 2009). Once the catheter is placed, the urethral meatus should be cleansed with soap and water once or twice daily. The routine use of povidone-iodine or neomycin-bacitracin solutions, ointments, or creams with the cleansing routine is not recommended and shows no advantage in infection prevention (Nazarko, 2009a). Catheter bags should be consistently kept below the level of the bladder, to prevent backflow leading to catheter-acquired UTI (CAUTI) (Evidence-Based Practice box).

NURSING CARE GUIDELINE

Discontinuing an Indwelling Catheter

Background

- Indwelling catheters are a primary source of urinary tract infections (UTIs) and should be removed as soon as medically possible.
- The Centers for Disease Control and Prevention (CDC) has issued guidelines for insertion, use, and removal to aid in decreasing catheter-associated UTIs.
- The patient may experience burning and difficulty voiding, as well as frequency or retention, after removal.

Procedural Concerns

- Identify the patient.
- Explain the procedure to the patient.
- Perform hand hygiene and don clean gloves.
- Empty the urinary collection drainage bag.
- Measure urinary output for documentation.
- Obtain urine specimen, if ordered.
- Remove the catheter from the anchoring device.
- Place a disposable waterproof pad under the area from which the catheter is being removed.
- Check the balloon volume.
- Withdraw fluid from the balloon:
  - Connect a sterile syringe to the balloon port.
  - Allow fluid to flow into the syringe.
  - If needed, pull back on the plunger of the syringe to ensure the balloon is fully deflated.
  - Remove the syringe.
- Remove the catheter slowly and smoothly as the patient exhales, placing it lightly on the disposable waterproof pad.
- Ensure that the catheter and the balloon are both intact.
- Dispose of the catheter and waterproof pad.
- Clean the perineal area.
- Remove gloves.
- Perform hand hygiene.
- Monitor the patient's output closely.
  - If the patient is urinating only small quantities, assess for bladder distention.
  - If the patient has not urinated during the 6 to 8 hours after removal of the catheter:
    - Assess for urinary retention via bladder scan.
    - Notify the primary care provider (PCP).
    - Intermittent catheterization with a straight catheter or reinsertion of an indwelling catheter may be necessary.

Documentation Concerns

- Record urinary output.
- Document any difficulties with performing the procedure, as well as the patient's response to the procedure.
- Note any patient education that was done.
- Record the findings of the urinary assessment after catheter removal, including:
  - The quantity of urine, and frequency of urination
  - The color, odor, consistency, and amount (COCA) of the urine
- Include any difficulty encountered by the patient with urinary retention and/or bladder distention.

Evidence-Based Practice

- Postoperative patients should have an indwelling catheter removed within 24 hours of surgery unless there are other appropriate reasons for the catheter to remain in place (Gould, Umscheid, Agarwal, et al, 2009).
- Some studies have been done to address whether or not to clamp the catheter before removing it. The evidence leans slightly in the direction that it is better to leave the catheter unclamped so the urine is flowing freely as the catheter is removed. Additional studies have documented fewer cases of bacteriuria when this practice is applied (Gould, Umscheid, Agarwal, et al, 2009).

EVIDENCE-BASED PRACTICE

Urinary Catheter Infection Prevention

It is imperative that catheter bags be kept below the level of the bladder at all times to prevent reflux of urine into the bladder, which may lead to infection (Gould, Umscheid, Agarwal, et al, 2009).

- When transferring patients with indwelling catheters horizontally from bed to cart, keep the catheter bag below the level of the patient's legs to prevent urine backflow. Do not place the catheter bag on the patient's abdomen or legs during transfer.
- When positioning the catheter bag for a patient lying or sitting in bed, make sure that the bag is hung on the bed frame and not the side rail, even if the rail is in low position. The side rail may be inadvertently raised at any time with the catheter bag attached, causing a reflux of urine.

Preconnected closed-drainage urinary catheterization systems should be used to reduce risk of interruption of the system by staff or the patient's family. Routine irrigation of the indwelling catheter is not recommended for UTI prevention. Arbitrary and routine intervals for changing catheters are not recommended. Catheters should be changed if debris or encrustation of the catheter is noted. Catheter bags should be emptied when two-thirds full.

Suprapubic Catheters

Surgical placement of a suprapubic catheter may be undertaken if urethral catheterization is either contraindicated or unsuccessful. Men and women with urethral obstructions or injuries and men with prostate cancer and BPH are most often candidates for this type of catheter. Suprapubic catheters are placed with use of local or general anesthesia through the abdominal wall approximately 4 to 5 cm above the symphysis pubis and secured with sutures. Urine drains through the suprapubic catheter into an attached bag secured to the patient's leg or abdomen.

Patients with suprapubic catheters are encouraged to drink plenty of fluid, to maintain hydration and to promote urinary excretion. Care should include daily cleansing around the catheter site with soap and water. Patients should be instructed to avoid the use of creams or lotions around the site. The nurse should assess for any seepage around the site and for signs of infection such as redness or discharge. Documentation should include site appearance; the color, volume, and characteristics of excreted urine; and patient tolerance of the catheter if it is newly placed.

Condom Catheters

Condom catheter use is less likely to lead to bacteriuria, UTI, and death than use of indwelling catheters in patients who retain urine (Saint, Kaufman, Rogers, et al, 2006). Use of condom catheters, however, is not without risk: Skin necrosis, penile strangulation, urethrocutaneous fistulas, dermatitis, skin erosion, pain, and localized infection have been reported. Male patients report that condom catheters are more comfortable and less painful than indwelling urethral catheters (Saint, Kaufman, Rogers, et al, 2006).

Hand hygiene should be performed before and after catheter care. A new condom catheter should be placed daily, along with assessment for potential complications. Perform perineal care while the condom catheter is off. Use a clean washcloth with soap and water, and pull back the foreskin if the patient is uncircumcised. Rinse and dry the penis, and pull the foreskin down over the head of the uncircumcised penis to prevent swelling before placing a new catheter. The Nursing Care Guideline: Applying a Condom Catheter box reviews the procedure.

PERINEAL CARE

Skin care is important in patients with urinary elimination issues, including those with indwelling catheters, to help prevent infection. Urine is very irritating to the skin. When urine accumulates on the skin, it is converted to ammonia, which causes the skin to remain moist and possibly become macerated (softened and broken down). The patient is at risk for skin breakdown, ulceration, and infection. Frequent perineal care is necessary, although use of harsh soaps, bubble baths, powder, or sprays, which can irritate the urethra, leading to inflammation and infection, should be avoided. The perineal area should be cleansed frequently with soap and water or no-rinse cleansers and dried thoroughly. In female patients, cleansing is done from front to back, especially after defecation. Skin should be check regularly for redness or signs of breakdown. Skin protectants, such as Baza Protect Moisture Barrier Cream, may be used to help prevent breakdown or heal affected areas. Specialty incontinence pads that draw moisture away from the surface of the skin may be used for the incontinent patient.

URINARY DIVERSION CARE

Special procedures are required for the care of a patient with a urinary diversion to maintain skin integrity and prevent infection (Nursing Care Guideline: Urinary Diversion Care box). Patients should be encouraged to provide their own urinary diversion care, as much as possible. However, in some cases, the nurse will need to assist those requiring help due to physical limitations or self-image issues. Patients who have recently undergone diversion surgery will require a demonstration and patient education on how best to manage and care for their particular type of urinary diversion. In some health care facilities, a WOCN will be assigned to help with patient education. Sensitivity to patient concerns related to self-image is imperative. Participation in a support group of other people with urinary diversions may be helpful in addressing individual patients' concerns.

NURSING CARE GUIDELINE

Applying a Condom Catheter

Background

- A condom catheter (also known as an external catheter or a Texas catheter) may be used as an incontinence solution for the male patient.
- It consists of a condom device with a drainage collection tube that connects to a urinary collection drainage bag.

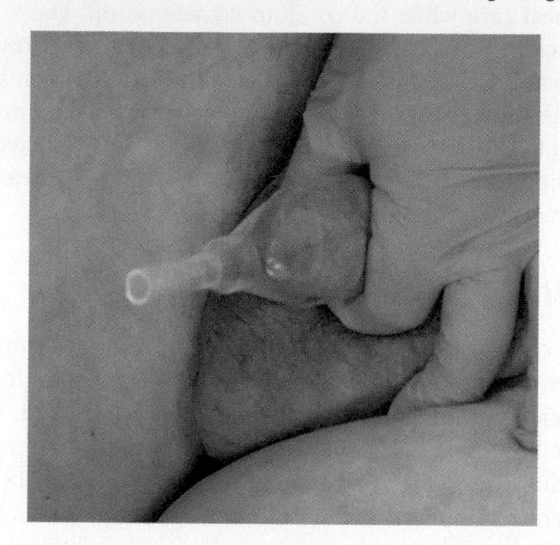

- The catheter is sealed with an adhesive at the base of the penis. It is imperative to monitor the penis for circulatory and integumentary problems while the device is in place.

Procedural Concerns

- Identify the patient.
- Assess skin integrity before applying the device. Do not apply the device if skin changes are noted.
- Perform hand hygiene.
- Don clean gloves.
- Trim the pubic hair as needed to aid in proper placement and prevent complications.
- Clean the perineal area.
- Apply a skin barrier and allow it to dry.
- Apply the catheter: Roll it down over the penis, leaving 1 to 2 inches at the tip of the penis to:
  - Prevent irritation
  - Allow for urine flow
- Hold the bottom of the catheter on the shaft of the penis for 10 to 15 seconds to:
  - Allow the adhesive to bind
  - Prevent skin breakdown and other complications during use
- Connect the drainage tubing to the urinary collection drainage bag.

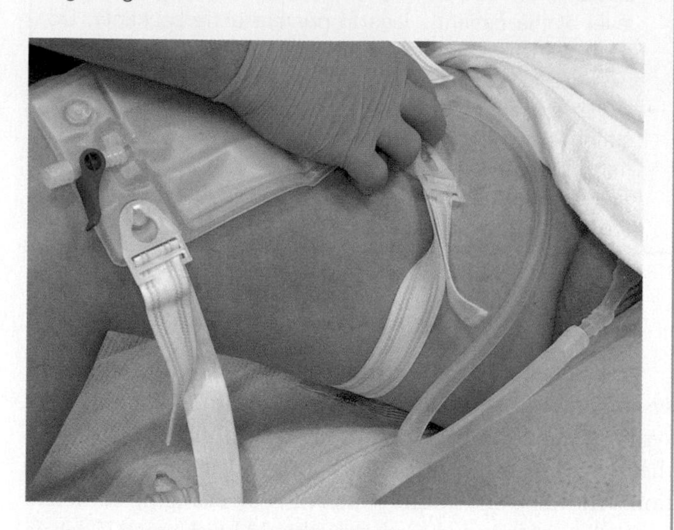

- Dispose of gloves and equipment and perform hand hygiene.

Documentation Concerns

- Record any difficulties encountered with placing the catheter.
- Document urine output and the quantity, color, and odor of the urine.
- Document neurovascular monitoring of the penis.

Evidence-Based Practice

- Saint and colleagues (2006) found that "the use of condom catheters is less likely to lead to bacteriuria, symptomatic UTI, or death than the use of indwelling catheters" (p. 1060).
- It is important to recognize that, without proper care and routine assessment, condom catheters can cause skin breakdown and other complications that can lead to external infections. Use of silicone condom catheters is recommended to facilitate visualization and assessment of the penile shaft on a routine basis, to prevent complications. Using a skin barrier product before application of a condom catheter also is recommended (Newman, 2008).

OBTAINING URINE SPECIMENS

The nurse is responsible for collecting urine specimens. Specimens may be collected for routine urinalysis by having the patient void into a specimen cup or into a clean urinal or bedpan. For culture and sensitivity testing, urine is collected by the clean-catch, or midstream, method, using a sterile specimen cup. Specimens also can be obtained by performing straight catheterization using sterile technique or by removal of a specimen from the tubing of an indwelling catheter or urinary diversion collection bag. Care needs to be taken to ensure that the specimen is not contaminated. See Chapter 34, Skill 34-2: Urine Specimen Collection for additional information and the procedures related to specimen collection.

NURSING CARE GUIDELINE

Urinary Diversion Care

Background

- Various disease processes or disorders, such as cancers, spinal cord injury, or renal calculi, may necessitate the ureters to be diverted externally from the meatus of the bladder to the abdominal wall.
- Types:
  - An ileal conduit is the most common incontinent urinary diversion.
    - A section of small bowel is resected.
    - The ureters are connected to the resected small bowel.
    - The small bowel resection is brought to the abdominal wall.
    - A stoma is created in the abdominal wall.
    - Urine drains through the stoma into a collection bag/device.
  - A ileal neobladder is the most common continent urinary diversion.
    - A section of intestine is used to create a pouch to hold urine.
    - A stoma is created in the abdominal wall.
    - The patient catheterizes the stoma to drain the urine, if necessary.
- Referral to or consultation with a wound/ostomy care nurse may be necessary.

Procedural Concerns

- With the urinary diversion conduit:
  - The collection device usually has a face plate that ensures a good fit around the stoma so that it does not leak.
  - Some patients use a belt with the device/bag.
- With catheterization and a stoma:
  - Assess the normal frequency of catheterization and catheter size.
  - Assess stoma condition (for color, moisture, and skin condition).
  - Check for mucus in the urine (mucus may be normal).
- To reduce odor, empty the collection device at least every 4 to 6 hours.
- The peristomal area can be washed with mild soap and water during the patient's bath.
- Inspect devices and equipment for patency.
- Monitor the stoma for any changes.
  - Potential complications include skin breakdown, ulcerations, and even necrosis.
  - Routine assessment, together with consultation with a wound/ostomy care specialist, is an essential component of stoma care, with implementation of appropriate interventions to prevent infection.

Documentation Concerns

- Document patient urinary intake and output.
- Note stoma condition and skin appearance.
- Record color, odor, consistency, and amount (COCA) of urine.

EVALUATION

Patient goals or outcomes are evaluated to determine their achievement and documented as met, partially met, or unmet. Interventions are evaluated to determine their effectiveness. Care plans are continued, modified, or discontinued, depending on the patient's achievement of the established goal or outcome. The overall aim is to return patients to their previous state of health or to assist patients and families to adapt to functional changes. Sharing evaluation findings with patients helps them recognize goal achievement and move closer to healthy urinary elimination patterns regardless of previous challenges. Prevention of kidney disease, UTIs, and secondary complications such as skin breakdown related to incontinence is a primary concern, whether the patient is in a health care facility or at home. Paying careful attention to detail related to the urinary elimination patterns of patients and providing preventive patient education will help promote positive outcomes. Although the subject often is considered personal in nature, discussions regarding urinary elimination should be encouraged by nurses, to help identify potential problems early and to prevent deterioration of kidney function requiring ongoing lifestyle changes.

SKILL 41-1 Urinary Catheterization: Insertion and Care

PURPOSE

Urinary catheters are used to:
- Accurately monitor urinary output
- Assess bladder function
- Obtain urine specimens
- Relieve bladder distention and discomfort
- Allow for healing after surgical procedures
- Irrigate the bladder
- Instill medications into the bladder
- Manage urinary incontinence
- Manage urinary retention

RESOURCES

- Foley catheter insertion kit (verify that all listed items are available):
  - Sterile fenestrated drape
  - Sterile field square drape
  - Sterile gloves
  - Lubricant
  - Antiseptic cleansing solution (povidone-iodine [Betadine] wipes, or swabs)
  - Cotton balls (if antiseptic solution is provided)
  - Forceps (if antiseptic solution is provided)
  - Prefilled sterile syringe with sterile water
  - Catheter (of the correct size)
  - Tubing and collection drainage bag
  - Leg securing device
- Straight catheter insertion kit:
  - All of the above except: the tubing and collection drainage bag and the leg securing device
  - Drainage collection container (tray from kit)
- Extra sterile gloves (if desired)
- Extra sterile catheter (correct size and type, if desired)
- Clean gloves
- Bath blanket (privacy draping)
- Washcloth, towel, and/or perineal wipes
- Specimen cup, if needed

COLLABORATION AND DELEGATION

- Inserting a straight catheter may be delegated to unlicensed assistive personnel (UAP) without a nurse's assistance following assessment of the patient, depending on the state and the institution's policies and procedures and provided that the UAP has received the appropriate specialized training.
- UAP should report any of the following to the nurse:
  - Patient reports of pain before, during, or after the procedure
  - Sores, wounds, irritations, or lesions noted
  - Difficulties encountered while performing the procedure
- UAP should be instructed in:
  - Sterile technique
  - Appropriate procedure and timing
  - Required documentation

EVIDENCE-BASED PRACTICE

- To prevent catheter-associated urinary tract infections (CAUTIs), "insert catheters only for appropriate indications, and leave in place only as long as needed. For operative patients who have an indication for an indwelling catheter, remove the catheter as soon as possible postoperatively, preferably within 24 hours, unless there are appropriate indications for continued use" (Gould, Umscheid, Agarwal, et al, 2009, p. 45).
- Anchoring of the catheter is imperative, to prevent inadvertent dislodgement and pressure ulcers (Gray, 2008; Siegel, 2008).
- Intermittent catheterization has been shown to carry a lower incidence of urinary tract infections than that for placement of indwelling catheters in acute care facilities, even when accounting for the same time frame of catheter necessity (Niël-Weise and Van den Broek, 2005).

SPECIAL CIRCUMSTANCES

1. **Assess:** Is resistance being encountered with insertion of the catheter?
   Intervention:
   - Pull back the catheter, and attempt a gentle reinsertion/ repositioning.
   - Ensure proper lubrication has been applied to the catheter.
   - Ensure insertion is into the urinary meatus if the patient is female.
   - With gentle pressure, grasp and straighten the male penis, holding it at approximately a 45-degree angle from the abdomen, if resistance is met.
   - Check that the smallest appropriate catheter size is being used.
   - It may be necessary to contact the patient's physician or urologist, per facility policy, to insert a coudé catheter if resistance is persistent.
2. **Assess:** What should be checked if no urinary drainage is seen on insertion of the catheter?
   Interventions: Assess the catheter, its placement, and the urinary system.
   - Verify correct placement:
     - For a female patient, if the catheter has been placed erroneously into the vagina, keeping the catheter there while inserting another sterile catheter into the urinary meatus may avoid inadvertent reinsertion into the vagina.

- For a male patient, the catheter may not move past the prostate. A special coudé catheter with a stiffer, bent tip may be required.
- Check the quantity and time of the last void or catheterization, and check the volume of intake.
- Ask the patient to cough; this increases pressure, which may promote urine flow.
- Ask the patient to take a deep breath in and out to relax the abdominal muscles.
- Check the catheter itself for kinks or other possible obstruction.
- Assess the bladder for distention; perform a bladder scan if necessary and equipment is available.
- Push the catheter in slightly and rotate it; the catheter may not quite be fully inside the bladder, or the opening may be up against the bladder wall.
- Pull the catheter out slightly and rotate it; the catheter may be above the level of urine, or the opening may be blocked.
- Initially drainage may have occurred, but sediment may have been present.
  - Assess the appearance of the urine.
  - Send a specimen to the laboratory for analysis if warranted.
  - Notify the primary care provider (PCP), and obtain orders as needed.
  - Irrigation may be needed.

3. **Assess:** Has urethral discharge been noted when caring for the catheter?
   Intervention: Urethral discharge may be indicative of infection.
   - Ensure catheter care with soap and warm water is performed routinely.
   - Observe the urinary output, and document. Obtain a urine specimen if needed.
   - Communicate the urethral discharge during report, notify the PCP, and document the findings.
   - Continue monitoring and documentation; the possibility of a CAUTI must be kept in mind.
4. **Assess:** Has the catheter been dislodged?
   Intervention: Notify the PCP to determine the need for reinsertion of the catheter.
   - Assess the patient for trauma, and treat if necessary.
   - Inspect catheter to determine whether it is intact.
   - Monitor urinary output.
5. **Assess:** Does your facility allow lidocaine 2% gel (a local anesthetic) to be used as a lubricant?
   Intervention: Check for patient allergy to lidocaine. If none, obtain and substitute lidocaine 2% gel in place of the lubricant in the kit for male catheter insertion.
6. **Assess:** Was sterile equipment contaminated?
   - Continuing with the procedure would increase the risk of the patient contracting a CAUTI.
   - Educate the patient regarding the procedure.
7. **Assess:** Does the patient perform home catheterization utilizing clean technique?
   Intervention: Per the recommendations to prevent CAUTIs, aseptic technique with sterile equipment should be used in the acute care setting.
   - The clean technique is used for chronic, intermittent catheterizations in the home setting:
     - Catheters are washed and reused.
     - The caregiver washes his/her hands with soap and water, and then dons clean gloves.
     - Daily and as needed cleaning of the perineal area is performed.

PREPROCEDURE

I. Check PCP orders and the patient care plan.
Knowledge of patient-specific orders is critical for safe patient care.

II. Gather supplies and equipment.
Preparing for the patient encounter saves time and promotes patient trust.

III. Perform hand hygiene.
Frequent hand hygiene prevents the spread of microorganisms.

IV. Maintain standard precautions.
Use of the correct personal protective equipment (PPE) is required whenever contact with bodily fluids is possible, to reduce the transfer of pathogens.

V. Introduce yourself.
Initial communication establishes the role of the nurse and begins a professional relationship.

VI. Provide for patient privacy.
It is important to maintain patient dignity.

VII. Identify the patient, using two identifiers.
Identifying a patient involves scanning barcodes or comparing the patient's stated name and birthdate to information on the patient's wristband or health record. The correct person must receive the correct treatment.

VIII. Explain the procedure to the patient.
The nurse has a responsibility to inform a patient before initiating care. Information may ease patient anxiety and facilitate cooperation.

PROCEDURE

Insertion: Female

Follow preprocedure steps I through VIII.

1. If you are right-handed, work from the side of the bed closer to the patient's right side; if you are left-handed, work from the side of the bed closer to the patient's left side.
   Using the appropriate hand promotes optimal placement of the catheter and decreases the likelihood of breaking sterile technique.
2. Place the patient in the dorsal recumbent position. Alternatively, use the Sims (or side-lying) position, with the patient's upper leg flexed at the hip.
   This position provides for maximum patient comfort while facilitating insertion of the catheter and minimizing the risk of trauma with insertion.
3. Place a waterproof pad under the patient's buttocks and drape the patient with a bath blanket for privacy, exposing only the perineum.
   A waterproof pad protects bed linens from becoming soiled and draping helps to maintain patient dignity and ease anxiety.
4. Clean the perineal area and dry it thoroughly with a towel.
   Proper cleaning should be used to prevent the spread of microorganisms into the urinary tract, where they may cause infection.
5. After removing your gloves, wash hands before proceeding.
   Hand hygiene is essential before initiating a sterile procedure.
6. Prepare a sterile field and organize supplies.
   a. Use the outer plastic wrapping/container from the kit as a waste disposal receptacle; place it on the bed in a location away from the sterile field (ideally, to the side of the sterile field). Alternatively, use a small bag or trash can at the side of the bed.
   b. Apply sterile gloves.
   c. Place the sterile drape under the buttocks and the fenestrated drape over the perineum.
   d. If using cotton balls in a kit with antiseptic solution, open the solution and pour it over the cotton balls. Place the forceps nearby.
   e. Lubricate 1 to 2 inches of the catheter tip.
   f. If a specimen is needed, open a new sterile specimen container; if it is not needed, remove the specimen container from the sterile field.

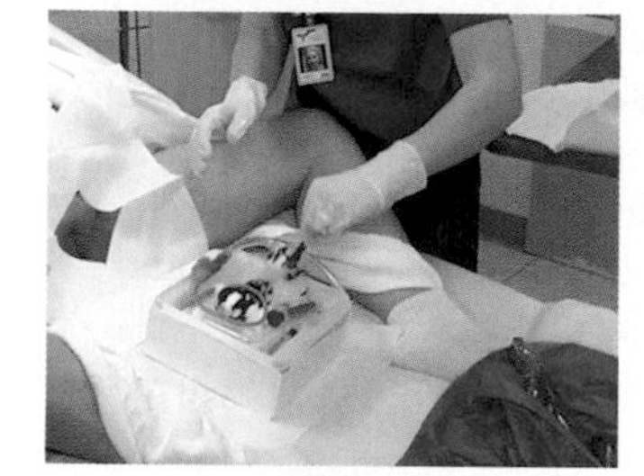

STEP 6f

   Use a sterile field to maintain sterile procedure. Prepare and organize supplies to facilitate the procedure. Place the waste receptacle (for disposing of items during the procedure) at a location that will not contaminate the sterile field. Lubrication prevents trauma by facilitating insertion of the catheter.
7. If the patient is to have an indwelling catheter:
   a. Remove the cap from the prefilled syringe.
   b. Attach the syringe to the injection port.
   c. If the manufacturer instructions do *not* require a testing balloon, go to step 7d. If testing the balloon *is* required, inject the fluid amount indicated on the injection port or in the manufacturer instructions, and observe the balloon for inflation and leaks. Withdraw the fluid and, observe the balloon for complete deflation.
   Prepare and test equipment (if required) to facilitate the procedure; many silicone catheters are pretested during manufacturing, and testing them a second time may result in stretching or damaging the balloon. Balloons without manufacturer pretesting may have faults or be damaged, so testing before insertion of the catheter prevents unnecessarily repeated procedures. Damaged balloons may cause trauma to the tissues in the bladder or urinary tract.
   d. Leave the syringe attached.

8. Designate your nondominant hand as the clean hand: If you are right-handed, use your left hand to hold the labia open. If you are left-handed, use your right hand to hold the labia open and expose the urethral meatus. Do not release the labia. Keep the clean, nondominant hand in place throughout the remainder of the procedure.
   Using the appropriately designated hand maintains sterile procedure and reduces microorganism transmission. Holding the labia open facilitates placement of the catheter; releasing the labia prematurely causes contamination of the urinary meatus and the catheter before insertion.
9. Designate the dominant hand as the sterile hand. Use this hand to pick up antiseptic cleaning swab or the forceps; the forceps will be used to pick up cotton balls soaked in antiseptic solution.
10. Cleanse the urinary/vaginal area:
    a. Use one cotton ball or swab per wipe.
    b. Wipe from front to back (i.e., from anterior end of the labia toward the rectum), using a new cotton ball or swab for each wipe in the following sequence: right labial fold, left labial fold, then directly over the urinary meatus.
    c. Discard each cotton ball or swab in the waste receptacle immediately after use.
    Cleansing from the least-contaminated to the most-contaminated areas while using a fresh cotton ball or swab for each pass maintains sterile procedure, reduces the number of microorganisms in the area where the procedure will take place, avoids introducing microorganisms from the more contaminated area to the cleaner area, and prevents infection.
11. Using your sterile hand, pick up the catheter, ensure that the tip is sufficiently covered in lubricant, and coil the distal end of the catheter in your hand.
    Using the sterile hand maintains sterile procedure. Lubrication prevents trauma by facilitating insertion. Coiling the catheter in your sterile hand reduces risk of contamination.
12. Insert the catheter:
    a. Have the patient bear down.
    b. Insert the tip of the catheter into the urethral meatus; insertion should be for 2 to 3 inches or until urine appears.
    c. Insert the catheter an additional 1 to 2 inches after urine appears.
    d. Release the labia.
    Bearing down relaxes the external sphincter, which assists with insertion and reduces discomfort. Initial insertion length approximates the female urethral length (which usually is 1.5 to 2 inches). The additional 1 to 2 inches of insertion ensures the catheter is firmly placed in the bladder.
13. If a urine specimen is needed, allow urine to flow into the sterile specimen container. If an indwelling catheter is being placed and the collection bag is already attached, wait to obtain a sterile specimen from the collection port on the side of the drainage tubing until after completing the catheterization procedure.
    Once an indwelling catheter is attached to the collection bag, it should not be detached. Maintaining a closed system is recommended to prevent CAUTIs.

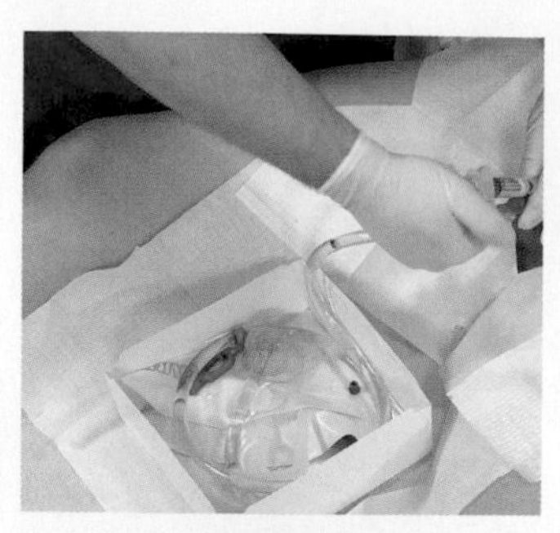

STEP 14a

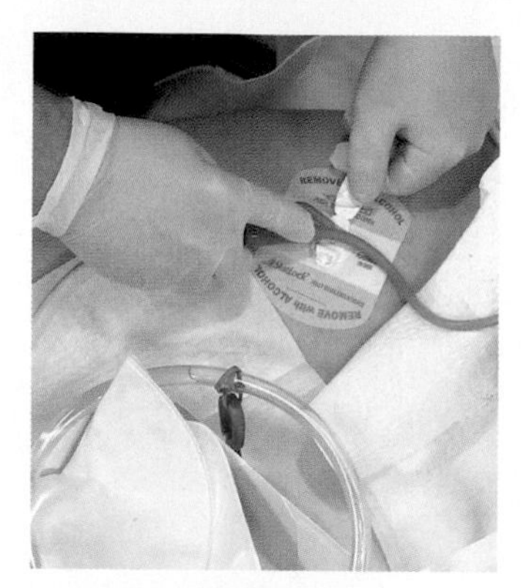

STEP 14b

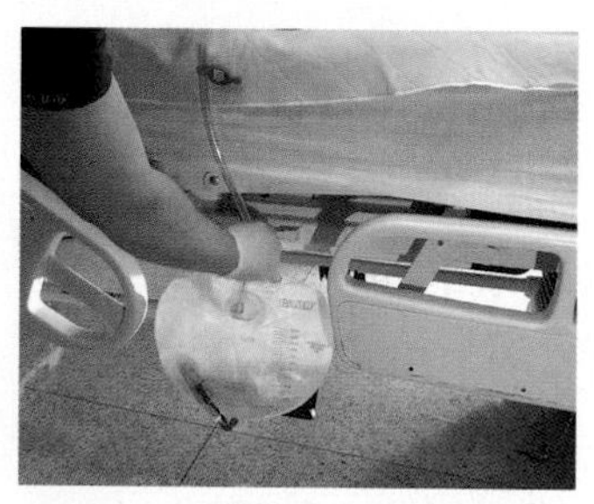

STEP 14c

14. If an indwelling catheter was inserted, inflate the balloon (or attach the sterile water syringe to the injection port and inflate the balloon, if not already in place); gently tug on the catheter; connect the tubing, and secure the catheter with nonallergenic tape or leg securing device. Hang the collection drainage bag from the bed frame.
    Balloons are meant to be inflated with the amount of sterile water marked on the side of the injection port. Tugging gently on the catheter ensures that the balloon rests at the bladder opening. Securing the catheter reduces risk of damage to urinary tissues and inadvertent removal. The collection drainage bag should be consistently maintained below the level of the bladder to prevent backflow of urine and the potential introduction of bacteria into the bladder. Hanging the bag from the bed frame and not the side rail will help to keep the catheter stable and the bag consistently below the bladder.
15. If a straight catheter was inserted, allow complete drainage or drain 1000 mL, clamp the tubing, and wait slightly before additional urine is allowed to drain. Remove the catheter after the bladder is emptied.
    Draining an overdistended bladder too quickly may induce spasms, preventing complete emptying of urine. In patients with spinal cord injuries, rapid decompression of urine may cause hypotension.
16. Reposition the patient for comfort. Dispose of catheterization equipment.

Follow postprocedure steps I through VII.

Insertion: Male

Follow preprocedure steps I through VIII.

1. If you are right-handed, work from the side of the bed closer to the patient's right side; if you are left-handed, work from the side of the bed closer to the patient's left side.
   Using the appropriate hand promotes optimal placement of the catheter and decreases the likelihood of breaking sterile technique.
2. Position the patient in the supine position, with his thighs slightly apart.
   Patient position provides for maximal patient comfort while facilitating insertion of the catheter and minimizing the risk of trauma with insertion.
3. Place a waterproof pad under the patient's buttocks and drape the patient with a bath blanket for privacy, exposing only the penis:
   A waterproof pad protects bed linens from becoming soiled and draping helps to maintain patient dignity and ease anxiety.
4. Provide perineal care.
   Proper cleaning should be used to prevent the spread of microorganisms into the urinary tract, where they may cause infection.
5. After removing your gloves, wash hands before proceeding.
   Hand hygiene is essential before initiating a sterile procedure.
6. If your facility does not allow lidocaine gel injections, proceed to step 7 (below). If it is allowed, inject the lidocaine in accordance with the PCP order and facility policies and procedures:
   a. Usually 10 to 15 mL of gel is used.
   b. Inject approximately 10 mL of the gel directly into the urethra.
   c. Wipe the shaft from the glans toward the testicles.
   d. Wait 2 minutes before insertion of the catheter.
   Lidocaine provides for greater patient comfort during the procedure. Wiping the shaft of penis in downward direction helps to spread medication throughout the urinary tract. The peak analgesia effect of lidocaine gel is obtained at 2 to 5 minutes.

7. Follow steps 6 and 7 for "Insertion: Female, placing the fenestrated drape over the penis."
8. Position the penis upright with your nondominant hand, which is designated as your clean hand. (If you are right-handed, your left hand will be your clean hand; if you are left-handed, the right hand will be your clean hand.)
   a. If the patient is uncircumcised, use your clean hand to retract the foreskin and hold it in the retracted position.
   b. If the patient is circumcised, use the thumb and index finger of your clean hand to hold the penis below the glans.
   c. Do *not* release the positioning or the foreskin until after the catheter is inserted.
   Uncircumcised males have extra skin covering the urethral meatus and glans; this foreskin must be retracted for cleansing to reduce the number of microorganisms and prevent them from entering the urinary tract. The upright penis position straightens the urethra and facilitates insertion. Releasing the position and foreskin will cause contamination of the urethral meatus and the catheter before insertion.
9. Wipe from the urethral meatus outward to the base of glans:
   a. Use a new swab or cotton ball for each wipe.
   b. Discard cotton balls or swabs, as used, in the appropriate waste receptacle.
   c. Repeat the process for a total of three times.
   Cleansing from the least-contaminated to the most-contaminated areas while using a fresh cotton ball or swab for each pass maintains sterile procedure, reduces the number of microorganisms in the area where the procedure will take place, and prevents infection.

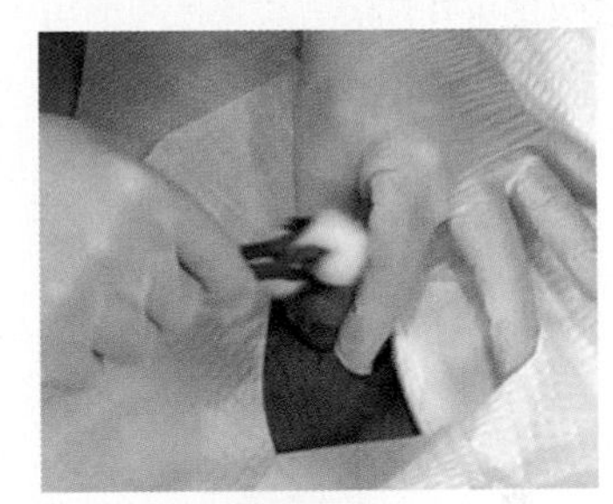
STEP 9

10. Use your dominant hand, designated as your sterile hand, to pick up the catheter, ensure that 5 to 8 inches of the tip are sufficiently covered with lubricant, and coil the distal end of the catheter in your hand.
    Use the dominant hand to prevent unintentional contamination. Lubrication prevents trauma by facilitating insertion. Coiling the catheter in your sterile hand reduces risk of infection.
11. Insert the catheter:
    a. Have the patient bear down.
    b. Insert the tip of the catheter into the urethral meatus while gently rotating the catheter; insertion should be for 7 to 9 inches or until urine appears.
    c. Insert the catheter to the bifurcation ports after urine appears.
    d. Lower the penis, but keep the catheter secure with your clean hand.
    Bearing down relaxes the external sphincter, which assists with insertion and reduces discomfort. Initial insertion length is approximately the male urethral length (which varies). Gentle rotation of the catheter may cause less discomfort for the patient. Inserting the additional length ensures that the catheter is firmly placed in the bladder. Lowering the penis assists the flow of urine via gravity.

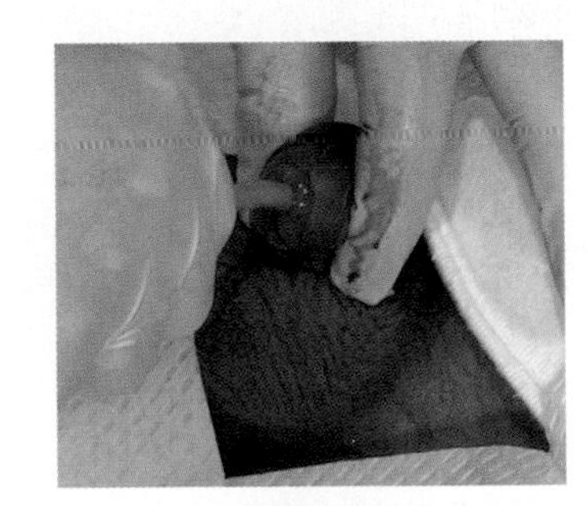
STEP 11

12. Replace foreskin for the uncircumcised male.
13. Follow steps 13 to 16 for Insertion: Female.

Follow postprocedure steps I through VI.

Catheter Care: Indwelling

Follow preprocedure steps I through VIII.

1. Follow steps 1 to 3 for Insertion: Female or Insertion: Male.
2. Clean the perineal area.
   Using the appropriate cleansing technique reduces the number of microorganisms, prevents microorganisms from entering the urinary tract, and prevents infection.
3. For female patients, hold the labia open, and hold the catheter. For male patients, retract the foreskin if needed; hold the penis and catheter.
   Hold the catheter in place to avoid unintentionally dislodging it.

4. Clean the catheter from the urethral meatus downward at least 4 inches with soap and water daily.
   Washing should proceed from the least-contaminated to the most-contaminated area, to prevent the spread of microorganisms and avoid infection.

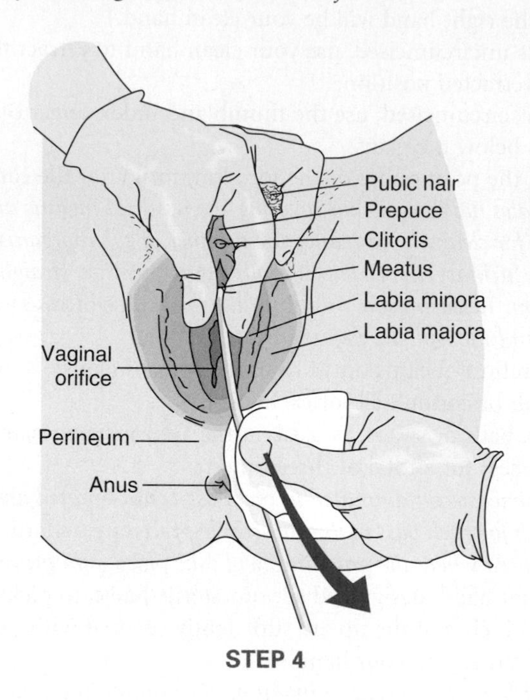

STEP 4

Follow postprocedure steps I through VI.

POSTPROCEDURE

I. Return the bed to its lowest position, raise the top side rails, and verify that the call light is within reach of the patient.
   Precautions are taken to maintain patient safety. Top side rails aid in positioning and turning. Raising four side rails is considered a restraint.

II. Assess for additional patient needs and state the time of your expected return.
   Meeting patient needs and offering self promote patient satisfaction and build trust.

III. Properly dispose of PPE.
   Gloves, gowns, and masks must be appropriately discarded to prevent the spread of microorganisms.

IV. Clean equipment if it was in contact with the patient; see specific manufacturer instructions.
   Disinfection eliminates most microorganisms from inanimate objects.

V. Perform hand hygiene.
   Frequent hand hygiene prevents the spread of infection.

VI. Document the date, time, assessment, procedure, and patient's response to the procedure.
   Accurate documentation is essential to communicate patient care and to provide legal evidence of care.

Step 4 figure from Sorrentino SA, Remmert L: *Mosby's essentials for nursing assistants*, ed. 5, St. Louis, 2014, Mosby.

SKILL 41-2 Closed Bladder Irrigation

PURPOSE

Bladder irrigation is performed to:
- Maintain patency of catheters
- As a postoperative procedure for genitourinary surgeries
- Decrease genitourinary complications (such as infections)

RESOURCES

- Intermittent and continuous irrigation methods:
  - Sterile irrigation solution, per order (room temperature)
  - Antiseptic wipes
  - Catheter clamp for catheter/tubing
  - Clean gloves
  - Waterproof pad
- Intermittent method:
  - Clean gloves
  - Sterile irrigation kit containing the following items (or assemble separately):
    - Graduated container (sterile)
    - Sterile irrigation syringe (60 mL)
- Continuous method:
  - Irrigation tubing (optional Y connector)
  - IV pole
  - Label for irrigation solution bag

COLLABORATION AND DELEGATION

- Bladder irrigation may not be delegated to unlicensed assistive personnel (UAP) without a nurse's assistance. UAP helping to care for the patient should report any of the following to the nurse:
  - Patient complaints of pain before or after the procedure
  - Clots noted in output
  - Change in color, odor, consistency, or amount (COCA) of output
  - Sores, wounds, irritations, or lesions noted
  - Fever or other changes in vital signs

EVIDENCE-BASED PRACTICE

- "Unless obstruction is anticipated (e.g., as might occur with bleeding after prostate or bladder surgery), bladder irrigation is not recommended. Routine irrigation of the bladder with antimicrobials is not recommended" (Gould, Umscheid, Agarwal, et al, 2009, p. 44).

SPECIAL CIRCUMSTANCES

1. **Assess:** Is the wrong catheter currently in use for a patient needing a bladder irrigation procedure?
   Intervention: Change the catheter to the correct type.
   - A single-lumen catheter or straight catheter without a balloon can be used for intermittent bladder irrigation.
   - A double-lumen catheter may be used for:
     - Intermittent irrigation or
     - Continuous irrigation with a sterile Y-connector
   - A triple-lumen catheter is the best choice for closed continuous irrigation.
2. **Assess:** Have you observed bladder distention or the presence of clots, sediment, or mucus in the tubing?
   Intervention: Any of these factors may indicate clogged tubing, bleeding, or tissue sloughing.
   - Check whether output is greater than intake.
   - Check the tubing for patency.
   - Verify that the tubing is placed below the level of the bladder.
   - Milk the tubing, if doing so will not further irritate or damage fragile tissue:
     - Starting at the point at which the tubing exits the patient, squeeze the tubing and release it.
     - Repeat the process while moving along the tube, progressing downward from the patient toward the collection device.
       - Be careful not to tug on the catheter or dislodge it.
       - Milking may release a clot or blockage in the tubing.
     - An alcohol wipe on the outside of the tubing may augment this technique.
3. **Assess:** Is the patient experiencing bladder spasms or discomfort?
   Intervention: Check the temperature of the irrigation solution; cold solutions may cause spasms.
4. **Assess:** What should be done if the irrigation solution does not flow easily with gentle pressure during intermittent irrigation?
   Intervention: Reposition the syringe and check the catheter placement in the bladder.

PREPROCEDURE

I. Check PCP orders and the patient care plan.
Knowledge of patient-specific orders is critical for safe patient care.

II. Gather supplies and equipment.
Preparing for the patient encounter saves time and promotes patient trust.

III. Perform hand hygiene.
Frequent hand hygiene prevents the spread of microorganisms.

IV. Maintain standard precautions.
Use of the correct personal protective equipment (PPE) is required whenever contact with bodily fluids is possible, to reduce the transfer of pathogens.

V. Introduce yourself.
Initial communication establishes the role of the nurse and begins a professional relationship.

VI. Provide for patient privacy.
It is important to maintain patient dignity.

VII. Identify the patient, using two identifiers.
Identifying a patient involves scanning barcodes or comparing the patient's stated name and birthdate to information on the patient's wristband or health record. The correct person must receive the correct treatment.

VIII. Explain the procedure to the patient.
The nurse has a responsibility to inform a patient before initiating care. Information may ease patient anxiety and facilitate cooperation.

PROCEDURE

Intermittent Method

Follow preprocedure steps I through VIII.

1. Empty the drainage bag; accurately measure the amount of urine, noting characteristics of the urine; and document.
Obtaining a volume measurement before performing the procedure provides a baseline assessment. Emptying the drainage bag allows space for the solution drainage and permits accurate assessment of volume and characteristics of output.
2. Verify whether sufficient length of catheter is available to work with, from the anchoring device to the injection port:
   a. If sufficient length is available, leave the catheter anchored.
   b. If there is insufficient length, remove the catheter from the anchoring device and be cautious when working with the catheter.
Sufficient length guards against inadvertently dislodging the catheter.
3. Place a waterproof pad under the catheter at the injection port and point at which the catheter and tubing join.
The pad protects the linens and helps maintain skin integrity by keeping the patient as dry as possible.
4. Put on clean gloves and pour sterile solution into the sterile container.
Use appropriate sterile procedures to maintain sterility within the bladder, thereby avoiding infection.
5. Draw solution into the irrigation syringe from the sterile container using aseptic technique:
   a. Place the tip of the syringe into the sterile solution.
   b. Pull back on the plunger of the syringe to withdraw the prescribed volume of sterile solution.
   c. Cap the syringe tip or place a blunt-tip needle on the syringe.
Using aseptic technique reduces the transmission of microorganisms.
6. Clamp the catheter tubing below the specimen port.
Clamping in this manner allows the solution to flow into the bladder and prevents the solution from draining into the bag.

7. Clean the specimen or injection port with an antiseptic wipe, in accordance with facility policies and procedures.
   Cleaning with antiseptic reduces the spread of microorganisms and the risk of infections.
8. Connect the syringe to the specimen port:
   a. For a needle-less catheter system (Luer-Lok), twist the syringe onto the port.
   b. For a needle system, insert the needle (or blunt-tipped cannula) at a 30-degree angle, with the bevel in the direction of the bladder.
   Using the appropriate method to attach the syringe prevents possible provider injury. The angle of the needle avoids damage to the catheter/specimen port system and allows the solution to flow toward the bladder.

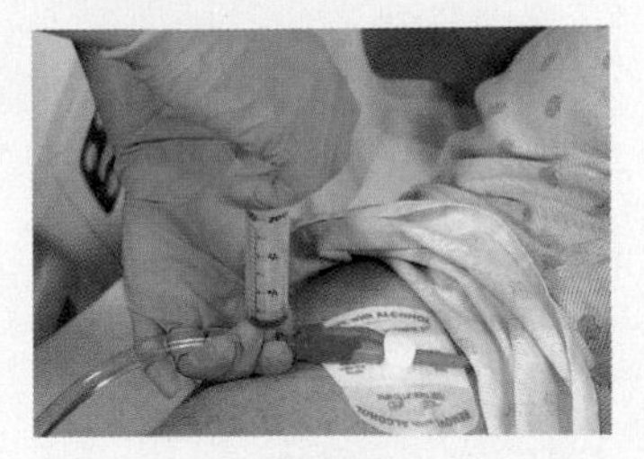
STEP 8

9. Inject the solution slowly, smoothly, and steadily.
   This injection technique decreases the risk of trauma and dislodges clots and sediment.
10. Verify whether the instilled solution is to remain in the bladder for a set amount of time:
   a. If not, withdraw the syringe, insert a new catheter plug, if needed, and remove the clamp to allow the irrigation solution to flow into the collection bag.
   b. If a solution dwell time has been prescribed, withdraw the syringe and keep the clamp on the catheter tubing until the end of the designated time period before releasing the clamp and emptying the bladder.
   c. Secure the catheter again before leaving the patient's bedside.
   Removing the clamp allows drainage by gravity. Securing the catheter reduces the risk of damage to urinary tissues and inadvertent removal of the catheter.

Follow postprocedure steps I through VI.

Continuous Method

Follow preprocedure steps I through VIII.

1. Follow steps 1 to 3 for Intermittent Method.
2. Insert the spike on the irrigation tubing into the port on the irrigation solution bag using an aseptic technique.
   a. Hang the solution bag on the IV pole.
   b. Prime the tubing.
   c. Clamp the tubing.
   Use aseptic technique to prevent the spread of microorganisms.
3. Ensure the solution bag is properly labeled as bladder irrigation solution.
   Proper labeling prevents adverse events and medical errors.
4. Securely attach tubing:
   a. If attaching to a triple-lumen catheter, clean the irrigation port with an antiseptic wipe.
   b. If attaching to a double-lumen catheter, add a sterile Y connector, and clean the connector with an antiseptic wipe.
   Cleaning with antiseptic reduces the spread of microorganisms and the risk of infections, while maintaining sterile procedure.
5. Calculate the drip rate.
   Ensure accuracy and compliance with the PCP order.
6. Open the clamps, and ensure that the fluid is instilling properly.
   Proper instilling decreases the risk of trauma, bladder distention, injury, and discomfort.
7. Note the volume of irrigation solution, determine the appropriate rate for instillation, and pay attention to the period of time the solution is to remain in the bladder, if at all.
   Irrigation fluid may be ordered to run into the bladder and right back out, or it may be ordered to remain for a matter of minutes before draining.
8. Observe color and quality of output from irrigation. Record presence of clots, sediment, or blood.
   Assessment of output is required to determine the effectiveness of the irrigation.
9. Document output and patient tolerance of the procedure.
   Documentation ensures accurate intake and output totals. Records should include patient response to care.

Follow postprocedure steps I through VI.

POST-PROCEDURE

I. Return the bed to its lowest position, raise the top side rails, and verify that the call light is within reach of the patient.
Precautions are taken to maintain patient safety. Top side rails aid in positioning and turning. Raising four side rails is considered a restraint.

II. Assess for additional patient needs and state the time of your expected return.
Meeting patient needs and offering self promote patient satisfaction and build trust.

III. Properly dispose of PPE.
Gloves, gowns, and masks must be appropriately discarded to prevent the spread of microorganisms.

IV. Clean equipment if it was in contact with the patient; see specific manufacturer instructions.
Disinfection eliminates most microorganisms from inanimate objects.

V. Perform hand hygiene.
Frequent hand hygiene prevents the spread of infection.

VI. Document the date, time, assessment, procedure, and patient's response to the procedure.
Accurate documentation is essential to communicate patient care and to provide legal evidence of care.

SUMMARY OF LEARNING OUTCOMES

LO 41.1 *Explain the complexities of the anatomic and physiologic processes of the urinary system:* The kidneys, located bilaterally below the ribs toward the middle of the back, filter liquid waste from the blood, help to control acid-base balance, regulate blood volume and pressure, and contribute to other critical functions of the body. The ureters, bladder, and urethra, located below the kidneys down to the urethral sphincter, work together with the kidneys to eliminate liquid waste from the body.

LO 41.2 *Describe abnormal patterns of urinary elimination, including causative factors:* Changes in body pH, the use of medications, contrast media used in diagnostic procedures, and surgical alterations may have a significant impact on functioning of the urinary system. Alterations in urinary elimination may have a profound psychological effect on the patient.

LO 41.3 *Carry out a comprehensive assessment of the patient with urinary elimination problems:* Accurate assessment and evaluation of urinary system health is necessary for maintenance of urinary health and early identification of alterations. A thorough patient interview, physical exam, and diagnostic testing are often required to determine the underlying etiology of urologic concerns.

LO 41.4 *Identify nursing diagnoses related to urinary elimination:* Nursing diagnoses related directly to urinary elimination are *Impaired Urinary Elimination, Urinary Retention,* and *Self-Care Deficit: Toileting.*

LO 41.5 *Create collaborative patient-centered care plans for patients experiencing alterations in urinary elimination:* Patient goals, established collaboratively with the patient and with other health care professionals during the planning stage of nursing process, should address the degree of dysfunction, establish priority for care measures related to elimination, and focus on the return or adaptation of urinary function to as close to normal as possible.

LO 41.6 *Implement interventions to address altered elimination concerns and then evaluate their effectiveness:* Specific nursing interventions, such as increased patient fluid intake, proper perineal care, and toileting schedules, may help to prevent kidney stone formation, urinary tract infection, urinary incontinence, and urinary retention. Urinary catheterization may be required when elimination patterns and function are altered, but should only be performed when less invasive methods fail. Urinary diversions are surgically performed to drain urine when the bladder is removed. The effectiveness of interventions can be determined on the basis of whether or not patients return to their previous state of health or adapt successfully to functional changes.

Responses to the critical-thinking exercises are available at *http://evolve.elsevier.com/YoostCrawford/fundamentals/.*

REVIEW QUESTIONS

1. A patient with an indwelling catheter reports a need to void. What is the priority intervention for the nurse to perform?
   - **a.** Check to see if the catheter is patent.
   - **b.** Reassure the patient that it is not possible to void while catheterized.
   - **c.** Catheterize the patient again with a larger-gauge catheter.
   - **d.** Notify the primary care provider (PCP).

2. Which nursing instruction is correct when a urine specimen is collected for culture and sensitivity testing from a patient without a urinary catheter?
   - **a.** Tell the patient to void and pour the urine into a labeled specimen container.
   - **b.** Ask the patient to void first into the toilet, stop midstream, and finish voiding into the sterile specimen container.
   - **c.** Instruct the patient to discard the first void and collect the next void for the specimen.
   - **d.** Have the patient keep all voided urine for 24 hours in a chilled, opaque collection container.

3. A female patient has had frequent urinary tract infections. Which statement by the patient indicates that the nurse's teaching on prevention has been effective?
   a. "I will limit my fluid intake to 40 ounces per day."
   b. "I will use bubble bath when bathing."
   c. "I will wait to wear my tight jeans until after my urine is clear."
   d. "I will wipe from the front to back after voiding."
4. A patient is scheduled for an intravenous pyelogram. Which piece of data would be most important to know before the procedure is carried out?
   a. Urinalysis showing negative results on testing for sugar and acetone
   b. History of allergies
   c. History of a recent thyroid scan
   d. Frequency of urination
5. When emptying a patient's catheter drainage bag, the nurse notes that the urine appears to be discolored. The nurse understands that what factors may change the color of urine? *(Select all that apply.)*
   a. Taking the urinary tract analgesic phenazopyridine (Pyridium)
   b. A diet that includes a large amount of beets or blackberries
   c. An enlarged prostate or kidney stones
   d. High concentrations of bilirubin secondary to liver disease
   e. Increased carbohydrate intake
6. What self-care measure is most important for the nurse to include in the teaching plan for a patient who will be discharged with a urostomy?
   a. Change the appliance before going to bed.
   b. Cut the wafer 1 inch larger than the stoma.
   c. Cleanse the peristomal skin with mild soap and water.
   d. Use firm pressure to attach the wafer to the skin.
7. An indwelling catheter is ordered for a postoperative patient who is unable to void. What is the primary concern of the nurse performing the procedure?
   a. Teaching deep-breathing techniques
   b. Maintaining strict aseptic technique
   c. Medicating the patient for pain before the procedure
   d. Positioning the patient for comfort during the procedure
8. The nurse is assessing a patient with an indwelling catheter and finds that the catheter is not draining and the patient's bladder is distended. What action should the nurse take next?
   a. Notify the PCP.
   b. Assess the tubing for kinks and ensure downward flow.
   c. Change the catheter as soon as possible.
   d. Aspirate the stagnant urine in the catheter for culture.
9. The nurse is placing an indwelling catheter in a female patient. She inserts the catheter into the vagina. What is the next action for the nurse to implement?
   a. Collect a urine specimen and notify the PCP.
   b. Leave the catheter in place and insert a new catheter into the urethra.
   c. Remove the catheter from the vagina and place it into the urethra.
   d. Ask another nurse to attempt the catheterization of the patient.
10. What symptom is most likely to be exhibited by the patient who complains of voiding small amounts of urine in relation to his fluid intake?
   a. Nocturia
   b. Polyuria
   c. Anuria
   d. Oliguria

Answers and rationales to review questions are available at *http://evolve.elsevier.com/YoostCrawford/fundamentals/.*

REFERENCES

Allsworth J, Omicioli V, Cunkelman J, Homco J: Discussion: "Reproductive factors associated with nocturia and urgency" by Tikkinen et al, *Am J Obstet Gynecol* 199(2):e1-e3, 2008.

Bertram J, Douglas-Denton, R, Diouf B, et al: Human nephron number: Implications for health and disease, *Pediatr Nephrol* 26(9) 1529-1533, 2011.

Buckley B, Lapitan M: Prevalence of urinary incontinence in men, women, and children—current evidence: Findings of the Fourth International Consultation on incontinence. Epidemiology Committee of the Fourth International Consultation on Incontinence, Paris, 2008, *Urology* 76(2):265, 2010.

Centers for Disease Control and Prevention: Catheter-associated urinary tract infections (CAUTI), Healthcare-associated infections (HAIs), 2012. Retrieved from *www.cdc.gov/HAI/ca_uti/uti.html.*

Conway L, Larson E: Guidelines to prevent catheter-associated urinary tract infection: 1980 to 2010, *Heart Lung* 41:271-283, 2011.

Cronenwett L, Sherwood G, Barnsteiner J, et al: Quality and safety education for nurses, *Nurs Outlook* 55(3):122-131, 2007.

Devarajan P: Oliguria, Medscape Reference: Drugs, Diseases & Procedures, 2012. Retrieved from *http://emedicine.medscape.com/article/983156-overview.*

Gould C, Umscheid C, Agarwal R, et al: Guideline for prevention of catheter-associated urinary tract infections 2009, Atlanta, 2009, Centers for Disease Control and Prevention. Retrieved from *www.cdc.gov/hicpac/pdf/CAUTI/CAUTIguideline2009final.pdf.*

Gray ML: Securing the indwelling catheter, *Am J Nurs* 108(12):44–50, 2008.
Harvard Health Publications: Urine color and odor changes, *Harvard Women's Health Watch* 17(10):7, 2010.
Markland D, Richter E, Fwu C, et al: Prevalence and trends of urinary incontinence in adults in the United States, 2001 to 2008, *J Urol* 186(2):589, 2011.
Masson P, Matheson S, Webster AC, Craig JC: Meta-analyses in prevention and treatment of urinary tract infections, *Infect Dis Clin* 23(2):355-385, 2009.
Mayo Clinic Staff: Tests and procedures: Intravenous pyelogram, 2014. Retrieved from *www.mayoclinic.org/tests-procedures/intravenous-pyelogram/basics/risks/prc-20018949.*
Morgan C, Endozoa N, Paradiso C, et al: Enhanced toileting program decreases incontinence in long term care, *Jt Comm J Qual Patient Saf* 34(4):206-208, 2008.
Murphy F, Byrne G: The role of the nurse in the management of acute kidney injury, *Br J Nurs* 19(3):146, 2010. Retrieved from ProQuest Nursing & Allied Health Source. (Document ID: 2033451171.)
Nazarko L: Providing effective evidence-based catheter management, *Br J Nurs* 18(7):S4-S12, 2009a.
Nazarko L: Urinary tract infection: Diagnosis, treatment and prevention, *Br J Nurs* 18(19):1170-1174, 2009b.
Newman D: Internal and external urinary catheters: A primer for clinical practice, *Ostomy Wound Manage* 54(12):18-35, 2008.
Niël-Weise BS, Van den Broek PJ: Urinary catheter policies for short-term bladder drainage in adults, *Cochrane Database Syst Rev* (3): CD004203, 2005.
Saint S, Kaufman S, Rogers M, et al: Condom versus indwelling urinary catheters: A randomized trial, *J Am Geriatr Soc* 54(7):1055-1061, 2006.
Shier D, Butler J, Lewis R: *Hole's human anatomy and physiology,* ed. 13, New York, 2012, McGraw-Hill.
Siegel TJ: The ins and outs of urinary catheters: Evidence-based management, *Adv Nurse Pract* 16(8):57-60, 2008.
Tennant S: Toilet training more beneficial when started early: Incontinence rates increase in children who begin training later, data show, *Urol Times* 38(4):22, 2010.
Watring NJ, Mason JD: Deciphering dysuria, *Emerg Med* 40(10):29-34, 2008.
Weisberg L, Dellinger R: Management of severe hyperkalemia, *Crit Care Med* 36(12):3246-3251, 2008.
Williams K, Hamilton K: Culturally competent assessment and care of self-mutilation in urological nursing, *Urol Nurs* 29(3):191-194, 2009. Retrieved from CINAHL database.

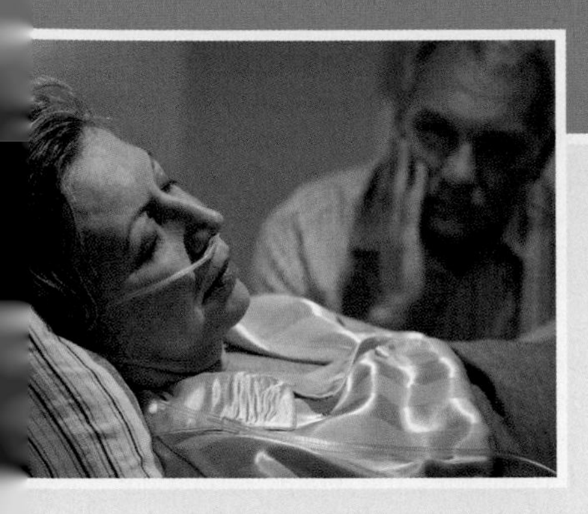

CHAPTER 42

Death and Loss

EVOLVE WEBSITE

http://evolve.elsevier.com/YoostCrawford/fundamentals/

- Additional Evolve-Only Review Questions With Answers
- Answers and Rationales for Text Review Questions
- Answers to Critical-Thinking Questions
- Case Study With Questions
- Glossary

LEARNING OUTCOMES

Comprehension of this chapter's content will provide students with the ability to:

LO 42.1 Describe the process of grief, loss, and bereavement.
LO 42.2 Discuss dysfunctional loss and grieving.
LO 42.3 Identify factors affecting the grief and bereavement process.
LO 42.4 Perform a nursing assessment of patients and their families who are experiencing loss, death, grief, and bereavement.
LO 42.5 Select nursing diagnoses appropriate for people experiencing death and the grieving process.
LO 42.6 Plan appropriate goals and outcomes for dying patients and their families.
LO 42.7 Implement nursing care plans with nursing interventions appropriate for patients and families experiencing death and grief.
LO 42.8 Examine the effects death and loss may have on nurses with appropriate coping strategies.

KEY TERMS

advance directives, p. 1123
algor mortis, p. 1121
anticipatory grief, p. 1113
bereavement, p. 1116
chronic grief, p. 1117
complicated grief, p. 1117
complicated loss, p. 1120
delayed grief, p. 1117
disenfranchised grief, p. 1118
exaggerated grief, p. 1117
grief, p. 1112
hospice, p. 1123
livor mortis, p. 1121
loss, p. 1112
masked grief, p. 1118
mourning, p. 1114
palliative care, p. 1123
rigor mortis, p. 1121
shroud, p. 1128

CASE STUDY

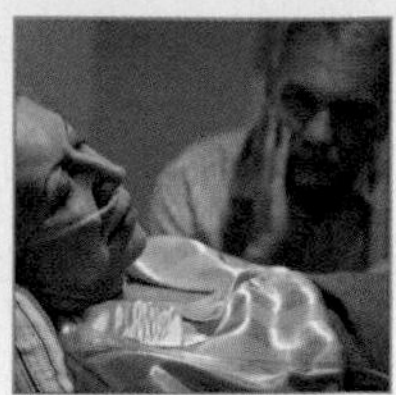

Mrs. Richardson is a 64-year-old hospice patient being cared for at home with the support of the hospice agency staff. She has a 4-year history of colon cancer with metastasis. She underwent surgery, radiation therapy, and various chemotherapy regimens over the last 4 years, until tumor growth continued despite the treatments. Chemotherapy was discontinued 2 months ago, and the metastasis accelerated.

Mrs. Richardson's pain is being controlled by morphine sublingual drops. She is weak but able to use the bedside commode with assistance of one person. She requires assistance with ADLs. Her husband of 41 years helps her during most of the day, but a hospice aide comes in daily for bathing. The hospice nurse visits three times per week. The family has declined hospice spiritual care because they are active with a church. The couple's grown son lives within 30 minutes and visits at least weekly but is busy with his own family and work. Their daughter lives 6 hours away and has been in touch only a couple of times during her mother's illness. When Mrs. Richardson is awake, the couple often reminisce, look at old photos of their family, and talk about funeral plans.

As Mrs. Richardson's condition begins to deteriorate rapidly, the hospice nurse assesses her and tells Mr. Richardson that he should let the children know that their mother will probably live only a few more days. Mr. Richardson agrees to call his children and is openly crying while the nurse comforts him and sits quietly with him. They begin to plan Mrs. Richardson's care for her final days.

Refer back to this case study to answer the critical-thinking questions throughout the chapter.

Death, loss, grief, and bereavement are a part of life for all people. To experience life itself, we must experience loss and grief. This chapter describes various types of loss, the stages of grief and bereavement, and nursing care of the patient and family experiencing loss, grief, and death. Death is a universal aspect of the human experience. Nurses in any setting must be prepared to care for patients who are dying and their families, and for others who are experiencing loss and grief. Through compassionate care, knowledge of the dying process, and excellent skills of communication, quality care can be achieved for patients and families at the time of death or loss.

NORMAL LOSS AND GRIEF LO 42.1

Loss and grief are a normal part of human existence. Everyone, at various stages in life, will experience loss with the accompanying grief response. The terminology describing loss and grief is defined in this section, in which theories or stages of the grieving process also are explored. People cope with various types of loss and experience grief in a very individualized manner. Nurses are instrumental in assisting this coping process as they provide comfort and support to patients and families experiencing loss and grief.

LOSS

Many definitions of *loss* can be found in the nursing literature. **Loss** often is defined as the absence of something to which the affected person has formed an attachment and can involve people, places, or things. Examples are loss of a family member to death, loss of a body part to disease or accident, loss of health or independence to illness or old age, loss of financial stability to catastrophe, and even loss of choice to dementia or other illness that affects cognition. Loss is a separation from someone or something that is of personal importance. The meaning of loss is determined by the person affected by it; thus loss is a subjective experience.

Loss and the resulting grieving process are experienced by everyone over the course of a lifetime. Developmental life changes may be associated with significant losses, which can include moving out of a parental home, changing jobs, loss of a job, retirement, change in friendships, loss of a pet, or loss of a dream for self or family. The nature of loss varies widely: Death, the effects of acute or chronic illness, changes in physical or mental health status, a decrease in self-esteem, loss of hopes, and loss of personal possessions all may precipitate a grief response, discussed next.

GRIEF

Loss elicits a grief response that often is determined by the value placed on the person, place, or thing that is lost. **Grief** is described as the emotional response to a loss. It is the set of individualized and deeply personal feelings and responses experienced with real, perceived, or anticipated loss (Kissane, 2011). Grief produces feelings including anger, frustration, loneliness, sadness, guilt, regret, a sense of resolution, and peace. As noted, specific feelings attached to the grief response are extremely subjective and vary in nature and intensity over time and from person to person. As the significance of the loss increases, a deeper level of grief along with more acute feelings of loss can be expected.

Feelings of loss and grief after a death are experienced over the affected person's lifetime. People who have suffered loss related to a death are faced with a reemergence of the sensations of grief for years after the initial loss. These feelings often return on the anniversary of the loss or death, and at other special times such as birthdays, holidays, family celebrations, graduations, and other developmental milestones in the lives of families. Reminders of the loss, even years later, can elicit the grief response. The reminders include people, places, sights, and sounds such as hearing a favorite song or visiting a vacation destination. The strength and intensity of the emotions experienced during the grieving process will diminish over time, but the feelings never completely go away. It is important for the grieving person to understand that these feelings are a normal part of the grieving process and that measures can be taken to promote coping during these times. Reminiscing about the loved one and talking about the loss to family and friends can provide a positive focus during the grieving process. Rituals and development of new traditions help keep the memory of the deceased alive in a positive manner.

THEORIES AND STAGES OF GRIEF

Grief is described according to its characteristics, signs and symptoms, and responses to the loss that the person is experiencing. Normal grief is described as feelings, behaviors, and reactions to loss; it can be physical, emotional, cognitive, and behavioral in nature (Table 42-1). An important nursing consideration is that active grieving can take months to years, with significant variability in how it progresses.

Certain patterns or similarities in the grieving process have been identified over time. Such work has led to the perspective that grief is a process with a probable course toward resolution of the identified loss. Several theorists, including Kübler-Ross, Bowlby, and Sheldon, have identified stages and tasks of grief and grieving, which are outlined in Table 42-2. Kübler-Ross (2003) first identified five stages of grief while working with patients who were diagnosed with a serious or terminal illness and who were dying. These stages were later adapted to apply to people who have experienced other types of loss. The stages Kübler-Ross described are still considered today by both researchers and clinicians attempting to gain a full appreciation of the experience and emotions of people who are dying and of those suffering grief and loss. Stages identified by Bowlby (1982) begin with numbness as an initial reaction to loss and proceed to reorganization and then recovery. Sheldon's stages (1998) include initial shock, grief, despair, and adjustment. Each of these theories specifies stages and goals for achievement at each stage as people move successfully through the process of grieving.

Research continues related to theories of grief and their application to various patient populations and different types of loss. In addition, none of these theorists would suggest a stepwise progression through the stages of loss and grief as they are outlined. These stages are to be regarded simply as a guide to understanding the process of grief, with no specific timeline detailing when people "should be" in a certain stage or "should" move from one stage to the next. Nurses need to understand these stages, and the feelings and emotions that are common in each stage, so that nursing interventions can be focused on the stage that a patient is experiencing, or the task that the person is attempting to complete related to the process of grief.

TABLE 42-1 Reactions to Loss

AFFECTED DOMAIN	SIGNS AND SYMPTOMS
Physical	• Tightness in the chest and throat • Oversensitivity to noise • Breathlessness • Muscular weakness • Lack of energy • Fatigue • Sleep disturbances • Changes in appetite
Emotional	• Numbness • Loneliness • Sadness • Sorrow • Guilt • Shock • Anxiety • Depression • Anger • Agitation • Lack of interest or motivation • Lower level of patience or tolerance
Cognitive	• Preoccupation with the deceased • Forgetfulness • Preoccupation with the loss • Inability to concentrate • Inability to retain information • Disorganization • Feeling confused
Behavioral	• Crying • Insomnia • Restlessness • Withdrawal • Irritability • Apathy • Impaired work performance

ANTICIPATORY GRIEF

Lindemann (1944) coined the term *anticipatory grief.* This term is used in nursing in the context of caring for dying patients and their families. **Anticipatory grief** is defined as the cognitive, affective, cultural, and social reactions to an *expected death,* felt by the patient as well as family members and friends. This type of grief is experienced before an actual loss occurs and can arise when a person is initially diagnosed with an acute illness, chronic disease, or terminal disease.

Nursing interventions for anticipatory grieving include provision of emotional support with a positive presence,

TABLE 42-2 Theories and Stages of Grief and Loss

THEORY	STAGE	CHARACTERISTICS
Kübler-Ross's five stages of grief	Denial	• A temporary defense to assist in the coping process • The dying person: *"No, it can't be me!"* • The person experiencing loss: *"He did not die in an accident!"*
	Anger	• Occurs after denial when true realization of the circumstances of the loss begin to emerge • The dying person: *"Why me? This is not fair."* • The person experiencing loss: *"Whose fault is it? I am going after them!"*
	Bargaining	• Beginning understanding of the loss with the hope that negotiation can change the circumstances • The dying person: *"I will change my ways and behave if I can live longer—I just want to live!"* • The person experiencing loss: *"I will do anything to have him back."*
	Depression	• Understanding of the certainty of impending death or loss occurs, and the process of grieving, which includes crying and sadness, is able to begin • The dying person: *"It doesn't matter anymore—I am going to die anyway."* • The person experiencing loss: *"It doesn't matter anymore—he is gone and not going to return—why live?"*
	Acceptance	• Coming to terms with the reality of the loss • The dying person: *"Somehow this is going to be okay."* • The person experiencing loss: *"Life will go on somehow!"*
Bowlby's model of grief (1982)	Shock and numbness	• Describes the time immediately after the loss, when the bereaved person feels numb; this is thought to be a natural defense mechanism that allows the person to survive the emotional response to the loss
	Searching and yearning	• Time when the grieving person longs for the deceased and emotions such as anger, fear, anxiety, and confusion may occur
	Disorganization and despair	• Yearning for the deceased decreases while apathy, withdrawal, and anguish begin to surface
	Reorganization	• A new state of normal begins with a decreased intensity of the negative emotions related to the loss, and a sense of enjoyment of life begins to return
Sheldon's stages of grief (1998)	Initial shock	• *Common emotions and experiences:* Numbness, disbelief, relief • *Task:* Accept the reality of the loss
	Pangs of grief	• *Common emotions and experiences:* Sadness, anger, guilt, feelings of vulnerability and anxiety, regret, insomnia, social withdrawal, transient auditory and visual hallucinations of the dead person, restlessness, searching behavior • *Task:* Experience the pain of grief
	Despair	• *Common emotions and experiences:* Loss of meaning and direction in life • *Task:* Adjust to an environment in which the deceased is missing
	Adjustment	• *Common emotions and experiences:* Develop new relationships or interests • *Task:* Emotionally relocate the deceased to an important but not central place in bereaved person's life and move on

active listening, and reassurance while encouraging verbalization of the anticipated loss. Reminiscence and life review (Butler, 1963) are used to assist those experiencing anticipatory grief with the realization that death is approaching. During the dying process, many people develop a sense of their own mortality and impending death and they often contemplate their life. This sense of mortality allows the dying person and significant others to look back and reassess their lives in view of imminent death. Butler views life review as a process essential to resolve potential conflicts, which may assist in the process of accepting death.

MOURNING

Mourning is the outward, social expression of loss. It is demonstrated on an individual basis related to the person's cultural norms, customs, rituals, traditions, and religious or spiritual beliefs. Life experiences and personality traits influence the outward expression of loss.

Nurses working with patients experiencing grief and loss should be aware of cultural characteristics of grief, mourning, death, and loss. Assessment of a person's cultural beliefs related to death rituals, common responses to death and grief, meaning of the afterlife, disposition of the body after death, and any other practices specific to the culture or religion is the responsibility of the nurse. Individualized assessment of each family's beliefs of death and the dying process are necessary to consider while developing nursing interventions and communication strategies (Figure 42-1).

An overview of the beliefs of several cultural and religious groups regarding death and dying as well as grief and bereavement is shown in the Diversity Considerations box. Assessment of personal knowledge, as well as a willingness to learn about various religious and cultural responses to death, loss, grief, and bereavement allows the practicing nurse to provide care that is culturally competent and sensitive to the needs of the patient and their families. For more information about the health beliefs of common world religions, see Chapter 22.

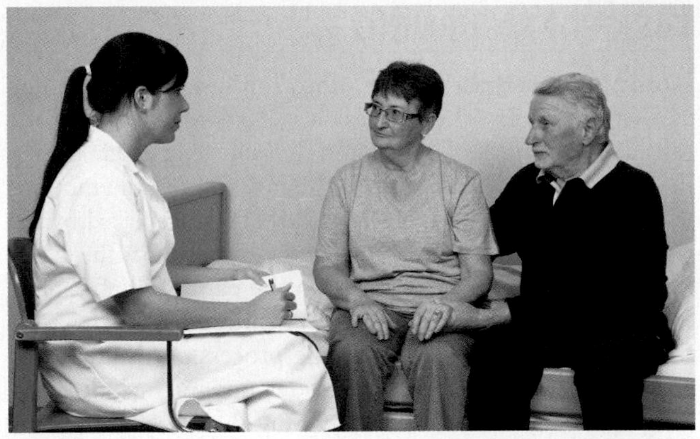

FIGURE 42-1 The nurse assesses the family's beliefs about death.

DIVERSITY CONSIDERATIONS

Culture, Ethnicity, and Religion

African American

- Friends and family often gather at the home of the deceased to offer support and share in the grief process.
- Wakes with music and singing are common.
- A meal is often shared after the wake and funeral.

Asian American

- Consider practices of the various cultural backgrounds: Chinese, Korean, Japanese, Vietnamese, and Laotian.
- Dying at home may be considered bad luck.
- Respect is shown for the body by providing warm clothes for the burial.
- A shrine to the deceased may be displayed in the home.

European American

- Friends and family often gather at the home of the deceased following the death to offer support and share in the grief process.
- Funeral director and clergy assist in planning the funeral and burial.
- Visitation at a funeral home followed by a religious service in a place of worship as well as the gravesite is common.

Hispanic/Latino American

- Diverse cultural backgrounds in this population.
- The rosary is said, often at the home of the deceased.
- Many Hispanic survivors commemorate the loss of a loved one with a promise or commitment that is taken very seriously.

Native American

- Different tribes have different belief systems.
- The Medicine Man or spiritual leader usually moderates the funeral service.
- Some tribes call on their ancestors to come to join the deceased to help with the transition.

Buddhism

- Family may bring religious implements: incense, flowers, fruit, prayer beads, or images of Buddha; and may request a teacher or monk.
- Incense is lit in the room.
- Family may wash the body. Cremation is preferred.

Christianity

- Family may request a visit from a minister or priest for prayers.
- Sacrament of the Sick may be administered by a Catholic priest.
- Cremation and burial both are acceptable.
- Organ donation and autopsy are permissible.

Hinduism

- Priest, family, and friends visit.
- Grief is visually displayed.
- Family may wash the body.
- Cremation is preferred, with ashes scattered in sacred rivers.

Islam

- Family and friends visit to provide emotional support.
- Body is treated with respect. After death, body is moved to face Mecca.
- Autopsy is conducted only for medical or legal reasons.
- Ritualistic washing of the body is performed by a person of the same gender.
- Burial takes place as soon as possible.

Judaism

- Visitors include family, friends, the rabbi, and possibly 10 men from the synagogue; prayers for the sick.
- Body is treated with respect. Autopsy is discouraged.
- Burial takes place as quickly as possible. Embalming is discouraged. Cremation is not appropriate.

Adapted from End of Life Nursing Education Consortium (ELNEC): *Graduate training program,* 2005, 2011. Retrieved from *www.aacn.nche.edu/ELNEC.*

TASKS OF MOURNING

Worden (2008) describes the process of grief and mourning as a series of tasks. The first task is to accept the reality of the loss, as the feelings of shock and disbelief that occur during the initial stage of grieving are the most common emotions felt by those experiencing a loss. Disbelief is replaced by the reality of the actual loss. The second task occurs as the grieving person begins to work through the pain of grief, experiencing the physical, emotional, cognitive, and behavioral responses common to the grieving process. Adjusting to an environment in which the deceased is missing includes rearranging, restructuring, and redefining the roles that person had in the life of the person experiencing the loss. This process of adjustment relates to the emotional, physical, financial, and other existing roles that the dying person once had in the life of the survivor who is grieving. Making life adjustments is necessary as implications of the loss are recognized and dealt with over a period of time. The final task is to emotionally relocate the deceased and move on with life. This task begins the resolution stage of the initial loss. At this time, people who are grieving accept that the deceased person is really gone and become less conscious of the loss and less preoccupied with the deceased. This final task allows survivors to reinvest energy in other relationships and move on with life while still maintaining the deceased person's presence in memories and through religious faith.

BEREAVEMENT

The term **bereavement** includes both grief and mourning, and can be described as the inner feelings and outward expressions that people experiencing loss are demonstrating. Bereavement has been described as a "period of time" that the person experiencing the loss feels the pain of the loss, experiences the grieving process, and begins to adjust to life without the person, place, or thing that has been lost.

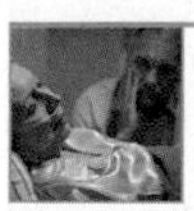

1. Which type of grief is Mr. Richardson experiencing right now? What type of grief reaction would the nurse expect from Mr. Richardson after his wife's death?

NURSING KNOWLEDGE NECESSARY FOR CARE OF THE DYING PATIENT AND THE PATIENT'S FAMILY

Field and Cassel (1997), through the Committee on Care at the End-of-Life of the Institute of Medicine, identified four areas of knowledge and skill that health care professionals need to provide high-quality end-of-life care. These areas are scientific and clinical knowledge, interpersonal skills, sound ethical and professional principles, and skills of organization. All members of the health care team must have the necessary knowledge and skills to promote high-quality care for dying patients in a safe and effective manner at the end of life.

Scientific and Clinical Knowledge

Scientific and clinical knowledge that relates to the underlying disease process and the biologic basis of dying related to specific illness and injury is an essential component of nursing care at the end of life. Assessment of symptoms at the end of life that occur with individual disease processes will allow the nurse to rapidly respond to potentially difficult and distressing problems. Valid and reliable assessment tools are available for health care providers and allow efficient evaluation of a patient's condition. Understanding the pathophysiology, physiologic, and emotional aspects of pain is essential, because pain is the most common symptom in the dying process. Understanding of the treatment of pain and other symptoms requires knowledge of pharmacology for effective treatment to promote high-quality care at the end of life. In addition, understanding the effects as well as limits of life-prolonging interventions is necessary while educating patients and families about options for care.

Interpersonal Skills

Interpersonal skills include the ability to listen to patients and families, as well as other members of the health care team. Empathy and sensitivity to religious, ethnic, and individual differences in care and treatment will enhance effective communication. Being able to convey difficult or bad news and providing information related to prognosis and options for treatment allow the patient and family the ability to make informed decisions. Effective communication is important in understanding and managing the response of patients and families to loss and the dying process.

Ethical and Professional Principles

Ethical principles include doing good and avoiding harm. Determining and respecting patient and family preferences are essential at the end of life. Professional activities include acting as a role model while demonstrating clinical proficiency, integrity, and compassion. Other concerns related to end-of-life care are delineated in the Ethical, Legal, and Professional Practice box.

Patients or families may insist on futile medical care. Futile care is described as treatment that will not change the course of the disease process and offers no hope of survival. If futile efforts at sustaining life put the patient in jeopardy of further harm, nursing communication with the patient, family, and other members of the health care team can enhance the decision-making process and allow for a dignified death (Collaboration and Delegation box).

ETHICAL, LEGAL, AND PROFESSIONAL PRACTICE

Decisions at End-of-Life

- All patients need to consider whether potential burdens of treatment outweigh the benefits. Nurses assist patients and their families in the decision to continue or forego treatment by providing factual information. Quality of life issues are evaluated and determined.
- Patient self-determination and informed decision making are key aspects of end-of-life care. Nurses can advocate for patients to ensure that they are aware of their options for care that include interventions, treatments, anticipated outcomes, as well as risk and benefits of any decision made related to medical care.
- Decision-making capacity is determined on an individual basis. Each person who is making a decision related to end-of-life care must be declared able to make an informed decision based on rational thought and decision-making abilities.
- The decision to withhold or withdraw treatment is a difficult decision that many patients as well as families make as they consider treatment options. Quality of life considerations are taken into account during these potentially difficult times.
- Assisted suicide and euthanasia are not legal (except in a few states where assisted suicide is viewed as medical treatment if provided by a physician for a terminally ill patient) or accepted practice by health care organizations in the United States. If patients or families request assisted suicide in an effort to hasten death, the patient and family needs a comprehensive assessment to determine their mental status, level of comfort, and goals for end-of-life care.
- The American Nurses Association position statement on Euthanasia, Assisted Suicide, and Aid in Dying (2013) prohibits nurses' participation in assisted suicide and euthanasia. Such activities would be a violation of the ethics of the profession.

COLLABORATION AND DELEGATION

End-of-Life Care

- Nurses can facilitate shared decision making related to end-of-life care as patients and families interact with various members of the health care team in either acute care or long-term care settings, or when receiving hospice care. Collaboration during the decision-making process is essential for high-quality end-of-life care.
- Patients and families need consistent information and communication about options for care, treatment measures, and prognosis. Nurses are in the most advantageous position to enhance communication through collaborative efforts with the primary care provider (PCP) and other members of the health care team.
- Nurses are integral members of the health care team. Interdisciplinary care requires the nurse to act independently and also to delegate tasks as appropriate so that high-quality care measures are met for the dying patient as well as the family.
- Unlicensed assistive personnel (UAP) provide assistance with ADLs.
- Social workers provide assistance with referrals to agencies, especially if the dying patient is being discharged to home or a care facility.
- Patients seek control of symptoms in all domains of quality of life. The nurse's role is to meet the needs of the patient in a safe and timely manner.

DYSFUNCTIONAL LOSS AND GRIEF LO 42.2

There are several circumstances during which loss or grief is dealt with in a dysfunctional manner. When the bereaved person is unable to progress through the stages of grief, complicated grief occurs. Another type of dysfunctional grief is disenfranchised grief.

COMPLICATED GRIEF

Complicated grief, called unresolved grief, occurs when the affected person is not able to progress through the normal stages of grieving. It is characterized by distressing symptoms lasting at least 6 months after the death of a significant person. This type of grief is described in the *Diagnostic and Statistical Manual of Mental Disorders* (DSM-5) (American Psychiatric Association, 2013). Risk for complicated grief increases when death is related to trauma, suicide, homicide, or any other sudden and unexpected death. The pain and sadness after a loss are never completely resolved, and the grieving process is so severe that it does not allow a person to continue normal life processes. Symptoms of complicated grief include intense longing for the deceased, denial of the death or sense of disbelief, imagining that the loss has not occurred, searching for the person in familiar places, extreme anger or bitterness over the loss, and avoiding things that are reminders of the loss. Daily life routines are not maintained, and the person's emotional as well as physical health becomes threatened.

Four types of complicated grief have been identified:

1. **Chronic grief** is characterized by grief reactions that do not diminish over time and continue for an indefinite period or very long period of time.
2. **Delayed grief** is characterized by suppression of the grief reaction while the grieving person consciously or unconsciously avoids the pain that has occurred with the loss.
3. **Exaggerated grief** occurs when the survivor is overwhelmed by grief and cannot function in daily life. In such instances, the affected person may use self-destructive behaviors, such as drugs or alcohol, as a coping mechanism. The potential for suicide with exaggerated grief cannot be overlooked by the health care team.

4. The final type of complicated grief is described as **masked grief** and occurs when the behaviors of the survivor interfere with normal functioning, but that person is not aware that these behaviors are concealing the actual grieving process.

Complicated grief reactions are uncharacteristic of the normal grief process and may include a greater intensity of denial, anger, or shock; verbalization of helplessness or hopelessness; panic attacks; substance abuse; or chronic depression. Complicated grief can lead to long-lasting physical problems and serious mental health issues.

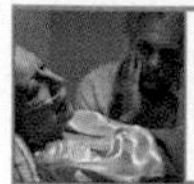

2. What type of grief reaction would the nurse expect from the Richardsons' two children?

DISENFRANCHISED GRIEF

Disenfranchised grief was defined by Doka (2002) as any loss that is not validated or recognized. This type of grief is encountered when a loss happens that cannot be openly acknowledged or publicly shared by the grieving person. It occurs when society does not want to acknowledge the grief, or does not know how to deal with the loss or with the response of the grieving person. Persons at risk for this type of grief include ex-spouses, ex-partners, friends, lovers, mistresses, co-workers, mothers of stillborn babies, and even those who have terminated a pregnancy. Disenfranchised grief can complicate grieving and stress because the loss is not grieved in a manner that is beneficial or advantageous to the afflicted person.

FACTORS AFFECTING THE PROCESS OF GRIEF AND BEREAVEMENT LO 42.3

Various identified factors have an effect on each person's grieving process. The intensity of the emotional and physical responses to loss varies according to the factors described. It is essential to recognize that people experience grief and loss in their own way, with their own set of coping skills, which include life experiences, cultural norms, religious beliefs and spiritual practices. Factors related to grief and bereavement include the importance that was attributed to the loss, the circumstances of the death, and the nature of the relationship to the deceased.

AGE OF THE BEREAVED AND AGE OF THE DECEASED

Chronologic age has an impact on the process of grief and bereavement as well as the age of a person at the time of their death. As people age and gain valuable life experiences, their ability to adapt to loss and grief evolves. Life events that occur over time can promote the person's ability to cope with loss. Coping strategies are adapted over a lifetime as knowledge and experience expand. With age come wisdom and experience, which help the person through the process of grief and bereavement.

Losses are experienced by people across the lifespan. Each stage of life brings specific developmental tasks and different challenges related to loss, grief, and bereavement. Coping strategies and the process of grief and bereavement differ for each age group and developmental level or stage of life. Children experience the grieving process in ways that vary according to their age and developmental stage of life. The End-of-Life Nursing Education Consortium (ELNEC) Project (2005) Module 7: Loss, Grief, and Bereavement outlines age-appropriate views of death and presents suggestions for how nurses can facilitate the grieving process for children up to the age of 18 years.

Adults work through the process of grieving as outlined by the theorists identified in this chapter. They often feel intense emotions while working toward resolution of the loss. Coping styles vary considerably in the adult population. Loss and grief in the older adult population need to be examined, particularly in view of the continued growth of this population. Older adults experience a myriad of losses throughout a lifetime. Many such losses occur during the process of growing older, such as the potential loss of function or of the ability to perform activities of daily living (ADLs).

Gender and gender role differences related to loss, grief, and bereavement have been hypothesized in various types of research during the past 50 years. No definitive findings have been established through research to date. It is thought that gender does have an impact on grief and bereavement, because men and women experience grief differently in relation to how they experience, express, and manage or adapt to loss and grief. Some societies teach that it is not acceptable for males to express emotions; it is more acceptable for women to demonstrate strong emotions when grieving.

Loss of a child often produces an intense grieving process for parents. Many people in Western societies have a greater sense of acceptance and understanding of death when the deceased is an older adult who has "lived a long and good life." The death of someone who is close in age to the survivor may affect the grieving process because it is a reminder of personal mortality.

HEALTH STATUS OF THE SURVIVOR

Physical and emotional health influence the grieving process. Optimal physical and psychological health results in a greater capacity to cope with loss. When the survivor has acted as the caregiver for any length of time, the person's own needs for health care often have been neglected. Once the grieving process begins, undiagnosed and untreated health problems can become a major concern.

COGNITIVE STATUS OF THE SURVIVOR

People with diminished cognitive function have different needs during the time of bereavement and are considered a vulnerable population in the context of loss and grief. Older adults with cognitive impairment, such as dementia, will have difficulty processing their loss and may even forget that they have lost a loved one to death. In addition, families may have difficulty grieving when they are asked on a regular basis about the deceased and why the deceased is not available.

RELATIONSHIP TO THE DECEASED

The relationship of the survivor to the deceased, and the type and quality of their relationship, will affect the grieving process. Examples of difficult losses with the potential for complicated grief are miscarriage, loss of a child, and loss of a first-degree relative or spouse.

For other people experiencing loss, the nature of the relationship may be more distant, so that the sensations associated with grief and bereavement are minimized. Examples are minor grief reactions to the loss of an ex-spouse or an abusive spouse and to the loss of a family member or friend who has been absent from the life of the survivor. The quality or value of the relationship has an impact on the grief felt by the bereaved.

COPING STYLES AND CONCURRENT STRESSORS

Coping skills have an impact on the process of grief and bereavement. These include both past and present coping skills as well as healthy versus unhealthy patterns of coping. People who have lived through previous loss will have used various coping skills and thus have an array of strategies available for dealing with a current loss. Accepting support and expressing emotions are healthy coping strategies. Coping styles that include suppressing feelings or avoidance of difficult situations by running away may ultimately result in a prolonged and more painful experience of loss.

Loss is a stressor, and concurrent stressors have an impact on the grieving process. The process of bereavement is multiplied with an increased number of stressors and may be extended or interrupted. Stressors in daily life are numerous and can include family issues, caregiving concerns, financial problems, workplace demands, and lack of a support system. Multiple stressors can complicate the grieving process, resulting in a crisis situation.

AVAILABLE SUPPORT SYSTEMS

Social support is essential during the process of grieving. Sources of support include family members and friends, fellow members of a religious or spiritual community, and support groups for people who have experienced a similar loss. Professional counseling with a grief counselor is an option to recommend for people experiencing intense emotions that have not abated despite use of other sources of support.

SOCIOECONOMIC STATUS

The implications of financial circumstances cannot be overlooked when working with the grieving person and the family. Availability of funds has an effect on the grieving process related to affordability of necessary services. Funerals are expensive, and many families do not have the resources necessary to provide the proper or desired burial for their loved one. In addition, the death of a loved one may mean loss of income for surviving family members. People with higher levels of education and higher incomes have demonstrated a greater ability to obtain necessary support throughout the process of grieving.

RELIGION AND SPIRITUALITY

Religious or spiritual beliefs have an impact on ability to cope with death and loss. Many people derive strength from their religious or spiritual beliefs, customs, and rituals. They find comfort and support in counsel from their religious and spiritual leaders. The grieving process is made less painful as meaning is found in the midst of loss. Others feel that God is punishing them when something bad happens in their lives. Anger toward God may lead to feelings of guilt and even greater anguish over the loss.

TYPE OF LOSS

Loss related to a suicide often leads bereaved family and friends to feel shame, fear, guilt, rejection, and anger. Shame is a common feeling for these suicide survivors related to the societal stigma of suicide. Nurses can review the events leading up to the death, to help the survivor understand that the suicide was actually a long-term process and not just a singular event. Families are encouraged to talk about the death together. When survivors feel that anxiety, depression, and a suicidal tendency are familial traits, fear of another family member's having such traits may intensify the loss. Denial includes the potential need to disguise the real cause of the death, which complicates the grieving process. Guilt may include the potential for self-blame or a feeling of moral failure. Anger arising as an emotional response to this type of loss frequently is misdirected at the deceased, evoking a further sense of guilt.

When a loss is related to a murder or other wrongful death, the survivor's personal sense of security is threatened and a sense of control is lost. Grief reactions usually are severe, intense, exaggerated, and complicated. It is difficult to comprehend the loss after a murder has occurred, which complicates the grieving process. Survivors may experience a sense of vulnerability or fear of being murdered. Revengeful thoughts can bring normal anger to a point of rage. Interaction with law enforcement officials the court system, and news media may complicate the grieving process while the survivor becomes a victim to the intrusion of outside forces.

COMPLICATED LOSS

Many conditions or situations are recognized to complicate the grief process. **Complicated loss** occurs with a sudden death, a violent or traumatic death, multiple deaths, loss that is related to a social stigma, and with the death of a young person. Sudden death does not allow the survivor time to prepare for the impending loss, and this type of event can leave the survivor with a sense of feeling out of control and wondering about the meaning of the death and even of life itself. Any violent or traumatic death such as a suicide, homicide, or accident can lead to a sense of shock and disbelief that is a normal part of the grieving process but is much stronger with a violent type of loss. When people experience a series of losses, the ability to grieve becomes difficult, because the emotions may leave a person feeling numb. This type of loss may include multiple losses over time or the loss that occurs when several people are killed in one accident. The age of the deceased can result in complicated loss, especially with the death of a child or of someone close to the survivor's own age.

Complicated loss can occur with a catastrophic event such as a natural disaster, loss of the home and its contents, or violent acts such as murder, rape, war, bombings, or other events such as the September 11, 2001 attack on New York's World Trade Center towers. These losses may involve violation of basic human rights and can affect an individual person, a family unit, or an entire nation. During this time of loss, symbolic losses can include a loss of security, trust, liberty, and pursuit of happiness.

Loss of a house to a fire involves loss of the home and its contents, loss of personal control of security, and loss of past lifestyle. Emotional stresses of this type of loss include a sense of powerlessness, the horror at witnessing suffering, and possibly the difficulty of identifying victims. Complicated loss associated with catastrophe typically leaves a visual as well as a cognitive imprint, with reminders often encountered on a daily basis.

The experience of miscarriage or stillbirth affects not only the mother but also other members of the grieving family. Parents and other relatives are asked to say good-bye before they have said hello (Humphrey and Zimpfer, 2007), and hopes and plans for a new family member cannot be realized. This type of loss is considered a complicated loss in that the bereaved are grieving a dream. Often, however, the mother is left to grieve this loss essentially alone, because she, unlike the father or any other member of the family, started the attachment process to the baby during the pregnancy, with development of a unique physical bond. Her feelings and experiences during the period of loss and bereavement will therefore differ (O'Leary, 2004). For the mother, grief may be experienced physically as a sense of acute emptiness, aching arms, and a potential sense of unreality. Emotional symptoms may include sadness, anger, guilt, depression, a sense of "what might have been," and a potential sense of failure. For effective grieving to occur, parents need to be allowed to see and hold the infant if possible. This may include dressing and rocking the baby and selecting clothes for the funeral (Humphrey and Zimpfer, 2007).

◆ ASSESSMENT LO 42.4

Assessment of grieving is customized for each circumstance. Asking both focused and open-ended questions will give the nurse information on how to best support and care for dying persons and their loved ones (Health Assessment Questions box).

HEALTH ASSESSMENT QUESTIONS

Assessment of the Grieving Individual and Family
- What are you feeling right now? Are there other feelings that you have been experiencing?
- How are you coping with these feelings?
- Do you have other stressors or concerns in addition to this loss?
- Have you coped with a loss in the past?
- Who is able to support you during this very difficult time?
- Is this loss affecting your physical health? Do you have concerns related to your physical health?
- What are your needs from the healthcare team?

Assessment of Anticipatory Grief
- Will your loved one's death result in loss of financial support?
- Are you and your family having difficulty making decisions?
- Are there other losses that you are still dealing with?
- Has your loved one's diagnosis or determined prognosis been recent (less than 6 months)?
- Has the illness been of long duration (greater than 12 months)?
- Have you had suicidal thoughts or do you feel unable to cope with this crisis?

Assessment of Potential Dysfunctional Grieving
- Do you feel that your support system is inadequate?
- Are you using more alcohol, tobacco, drugs, or prescribed medications?
- Do you have more difficulty sleeping than usual?
- Have you lost or gained weight?
- Has your grief subsided or intensified in the last few weeks?
- Are you able to carry out your day-to-day activities including work, social commitments, and household responsibilities?
- Do you have new health concerns?

GENERAL ASSESSMENT

Grief assessment should include the patient, family members, and significant others. Assessment of grief within a family system includes understanding relationships within the family and where support can be obtained for the individual members. A functional family (one that is characterized by love, mutual respect, and support among its individual members) is better prepared to deal with the feelings, stresses, and changes that occur during the time of loss.

ASSESSMENT OF THE CAREGIVER

Persons providing care for those at the end of life experience stressors related to the role of provider of care. Many caregivers do not care for themselves while they are caring for a loved one who is dying. Assessment of the needs of the caregiver is an essential component of the nursing care that is provided to patients. Caregivers need to take steps to preserve their own health and well-being (Mayo Clinic, 2012). The caregiver assessment includes:

- General health checkup
- Focused assessment of physical, mental, or emotional symptoms
- Assessment of nutritional status
- Sleep evaluation
- Examination of the caregiver's ability to maintain work and family roles
- Maintenance of dental and visual health
- Assessment of social network
- Evaluation of support systems

Signs and symptoms of caregiver stress include feeling tired and overwhelmed, getting too much or not enough sleep, and significant weight gain or loss. Caregivers may lose interest in activities they formerly enjoyed (Mayo Clinic, 2012).

ASSESSMENT TOOLS

Specific tools for assessment of grief are available from the Toolkit of Instruments to Measure End of Life Care: Grief and Bereavement, developed as a project funded by the Robert Wood Johnson Foundation *(www.chcr.brown.edu/pcoc/griefa.htm)*. Common assessment parameters pertinent to nursing included in these tools are consideration of the relationship to the deceased (and the quality of that relationship), type of loss (sudden or expected, traumatic or disease based), current coping strategies, available support systems, health status (physical as well as emotional), religious or spiritual beliefs, any concurrent stressors, financial or socioeconomic status, history of previous loss, family assessment, and satisfaction with current relationships.

PHYSICAL ASSESSMENT OF THE DYING PATIENT

Caring for patients who are dying requires excellent skills of physical assessment. Many families of patients who are dying ask the nurse, "When is death going to occur?" Although nurses are not in a position to predict the time of death, knowledge of the physical signs and symptoms of death will allow the nurse to support families when death appears imminent. Physical symptoms at the end of life include weakness and fatigue, increased drowsiness, and sleeping more and responding less. A decrease in oral intake and a decrease in the swallow reflex may occur. Surges of energy may occur as the dying person begins to make the transition to death. Changes in bowel and bladder elimination are common and include constipation, diarrhea, and potential incontinence. Patients and families need to know that these are normal changes, and education about these changes will enhance coping abilities during the time of anticipatory grief.

Signs and Symptoms of Impending Death

Universal manifestations of imminent death include a decrease in urine output, cold and mottled extremities, and changes in vital signs, in that the blood pressure decreases and heart rate often increases but can decrease. Changes in breathing patterns, with the occurrence of periods of apnea that increase as the body shuts down, and apparent respiratory congestion or the "death rattle" from the inability to swallow secretions also are common manifestations of impending death.

Signs and Symptoms of Death

Signs and symptoms of actual death include absence of heartbeat and respirations, an involuntary release of stool and or urine, lack of any response to verbal or tactile stimuli, and a drop in body temperature as the body begins to cool. This cooling is called **algor mortis**, or cooling after death. The eyes may remain open, the jaw will drop as the mouth appears to be open, and the color of the skin becomes pale and then bluish (**livor mortis**) as blood settles. After a period of time, **rigor mortis**, or stiffening of the joints of the body, will set in.

◆ NURSING DIAGNOSIS LO 42.5

NANDA-I defines grieving as a "normal, complex process that includes emotional, physical, spiritual, social, and intellectual responses and behaviors by which individuals, families, and communities incorporate an actual, anticipated, or perceived loss into their daily lives." Common NANDA-I nursing diagnoses that grieving persons may experience are *Compromised Family Coping, Ineffective Coping, Interrupted Family Processes, Ineffective Health Maintenance, Insomnia, Powerlessness, Spiritual Distress,* and *Risk for Spiritual Distress.*

Sample nursing diagnostic statements related to grieving and death are:

- *Grieving* related to the anticipated death of spouse as evidenced by crying when told that wife will live only a few more days.
- *Complicated Grieving* related to an unexpected loss of a family member as evidenced by extreme fatigue, feelings of disbelief and lack of acceptance of the death, inability to participate in family functions, and verbalization of blame for the death—"I should have been there."
- *Risk for Complicated Grieving* with risk factors of lack of social support during the grieving process, statements of loneliness, isolation, and lack of interest in verbalizing feelings.
- *Chronic Sorrow* related to continued sadness and depression after amputation of left leg as a result of a motorcycle accident as evidenced by statements of fear, helplessness, hopelessness, low self-esteem, and continued self-blame and sadness.
- *Death Anxiety* related to beginning understanding of terminal diagnosis and prognosis of less than 6 months to live as evidenced by statement of fear of dying, fear of suffering while dying, fear of leaving family members at the time of death, and a feeling of powerlessness over the dying process.

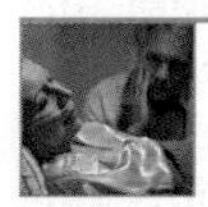

3. Identify an appropriate nursing diagnosis for Mr. Richardson, and give reasons why it is appropriate.

PLANNING LO 42.6

Examples of goals or outcome statements related to the sample NANDA-I nursing diagnoses listed in the Nursing Diagnosis section include (Table 42-3):

- Husband will express his feelings toward the anticipated loss of his wife during her last few days.
- Family members will be able to talk about the loss and the meaning the loss has for the family during therapy session.
- Patient/family will identify any factors that may affect the grieving process during visit to PCP.
- Patient will identify personal strengths within 1 month of amputation.
- Patient will accept assistance from friends, family, and significant others during the process of grief within 2 weeks of diagnosis.

IMPLEMENTATION AND EVALUATION LO 42.7

Providing nursing care to dying patients and their families can be a challenging as well as a rewarding responsibility. It is important for the nurse to develop trust and rapport while using skills of therapeutic communication to acknowledge their experience of loss.

CARE OF THE DYING PATIENT AND THE PATIENT'S FAMILY

People who are grieving need to know that they are heard and understood as they are trying to make sense of the loss and the emotions of grief. Providing education about the stages of grief will assist in the provision of appropriate nursing interventions as communication techniques vary according to the stage of grief. Simply understanding that what they are feeling is normal can assist in the grieving process. Encouraging healthy behaviors, such as exercise, rest and sleep, adequate diet, journaling, stress-relieving techniques, and other healthy coping mechanisms identified by the affected person, will facilitate movement toward resolution of the loss.

An important nursing intervention is listening while patients or their families tell the story of their loss, because verbalization of the loss allows the process of bereavement to begin. Including the entire family or significant others in the assessment and planning of nursing interventions for grief and bereavement also is essential, both because grief work involves the entire family and because family dynamics affect each person's grieving process (Becvar, 2003). Using community resources and making appropriate referrals may help enhance coping while providing the grieving person with additional and ongoing sources of support.

TABLE 42-3 Care Planning

NANDA-I NURSING DIAGNOSIS LABEL WITH NURSING DIAGNOSIS STATEMENT	NURSING OUTCOME CLASSIFICATION (NOC)	NURSING INTERVENTION CLASSIFICATION (NIC)
Grieving related to the anticipated death of spouse, as evidenced by crying when told that wife will live only a few more days.	Coping (1302) Uses effective coping strategies (130212)	Grief Work Facilitation (5290) Support progression through personal grieving stages

From Bulechek G, Butcher H, Dochterman J, et al (Eds): *Nursing interventions classification (NIC)*, ed. 6, St. Louis, 2013, Mosby; Moorhead S, Johnson M, Maas M, et al (Eds): *Nursing outcomes classification (NOC)*, ed. 5, St. Louis, 2013, Mosby; NANDA International: *Nursing diagnoses: Definitions and classification, 2012–2014,* West Sussex, England, 2012, Wiley-Blackwell. Reprinted with permission from NANDA International, Inc.

ADVANCE DIRECTIVES FOR END OF LIFE

Advance directives are legal documents that allow people to communicate their wishes about what type of medical care they would like to receive at the end of life. It is a nursing responsibility to be aware of types of advance directives available and to discuss the options with patients and families. A copy of the patient's advance directives should be part of the medical records. Advance directives are discussed in greater detail in Chapter 11.

HOSPICE AND PALLIATIVE CARE

Some confusion has arisen among the general public as well as health care providers about the difference between hospice and palliative care. *Palliative care* includes hospice care, but not all palliative care is considered hospice care. *Hospice care* is provided to patients with a life expectancy of 6 months or less who decide to forego curative treatment. Palliative care begins at the time of a diagnosis and includes curative measures.

Hospice

Hospice is defined by the National Hospice and Palliative Care Organization (NHPCO) as a program that provides comfort and supportive care for terminally ill patients and their families, either directly or on a consulting basis with the patient's physician or another community agency. The whole family is considered the unit of care, and care extends through their period of mourning (NHPCO, 2014). When the patient or a surrogate decision maker accepts or chooses the hospice benefit, curative treatments are no longer a focus of care. The goal becomes symptom control and quality-of-life measures. It is important for nurses to understand that patients who choose the hospice benefit can live longer than 6 months and remain on the hospice program. Medicare benefits include an initial 90-day benefit period, a second 90-day benefit period, and then unlimited 60-day benefit periods so long as progression of the terminal illness is documented. Patients who enter a hospice program and later decide that they want to pursue treatment for a cure can revoke the hospice benefit and seek curative treatment.

The care provided by hospice occurs in various settings with a focus on symptom control and with the understanding that dying is a part of the normal life cycle. Care is provided to patients and families in the home, residential or long-term care facilities, dedicated inpatient settings, designated hospital beds, and prisons, and even to homeless populations (Home Care Considerations box). Several tools are used to assist members of the health care team determine prognosis. General tools include the Karnosfsky Performance Scale, the Palliative Performance Scale, and the Functional Assessment Staging Tool (FAST). These guidelines assess functional status such as ambulation and self-care, nutritional intake, evidence of disease, cognitive function, and level of consciousness.

> **HOME CARE CONSIDERATIONS**
>
> **Hospice Care in the Home**
>
> Patients receiving hospice in the home require skilled, knowledgeable nurses to provide a high level of care because many needs are specific for the dying patient and the family of that patient. Care includes:
>
> - Assessment of safety in the home related to the physical as well as social environment
> - Physical as well as psychosocial assessment conducted in an independent and thorough manner
> - Coordination with all members of the health care team
> - Assurances that family care providers are knowledgeable and able to provide the necessary physical care
> - Safe use of equipment that is being used in the home and provision of necessary services

Hospice care is provided by an interdisciplinary team that includes nurses, physicians, pharmacists, social workers, spiritual care providers, massage therapists, art therapists, and music therapists. Physical therapy or occupational therapy may be included in the individualized plan of care if the patient's goal is to regain strength to improve quality of life. Care includes durable medical equipment, medications related to the terminal illness, respite care, homemaker services, home health services, and volunteer services (Figure 42-2). Grief and bereavement services are recognized as a core component of any hospice or palliative care program, according to the National Consensus Project for Quality Palliative Care (2013). These services are available for at least 13 months after the death of the patient, and risk assessments are routinely conducted.

Palliative Care

Palliative care emerged in response to the needs of patients who were not terminally ill but needed high-quality symptom control for a serious or life-threatening illness. This type of care is appropriate for anyone who has a chronic, debilitating condition.

The World Health Organization (WHO, 2014) states that **palliative care** "improves the quality of life of patients and families who face life-threatening illness, by providing pain

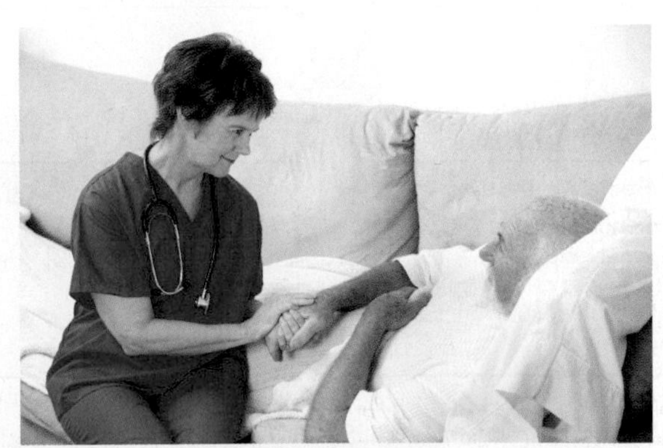

FIGURE 42-2 A hospice patient is cared for at home.

and symptom relief, spiritual and psychosocial support from diagnosis to the end of life and bereavement." Palliative care provides relief from pain and other distressing symptoms, affirms life and regards dying as a normal process, intends to neither hasten nor postpone death, integrates the psychological and spiritual aspects of patient care, and offers a support system to help patients live as actively as possible until death. Palliative care includes hospice care along with curative measures. Palliative care is appropriate early in the course of illness. It is used in conjunction with other therapies that are intended to prolong life, such as chemotherapy or radiation therapy, and includes those interventions needed to manage distressing clinical complications.

The WHO defines palliative care for children as follows: "The principles apply to other pediatric chronic disorders and include the active total care of the child's body, mind and spirit, and involves giving support to the family" (2014). Pediatric palliative care begins when an illness is diagnosed, and continues regardless of whether or not a child receives treatment for the identified disease.

INTERVENTIONS FOR SYMPTOM MANAGEMENT AT THE END OF LIFE

Effective symptom management at the end of life is essential to meet the care needs of patients and families specific to this period. The City of Hope Pain and Palliative Care Resource Center (2014) has identified four domains of quality of life that are significant to people facing the end of life (Figure 42-3). Attention to management of the physical symptoms common at the end of life will improve quality of life for the patient, who can then expect to maintain an optimal level of psychological, social, and spiritual well-being.

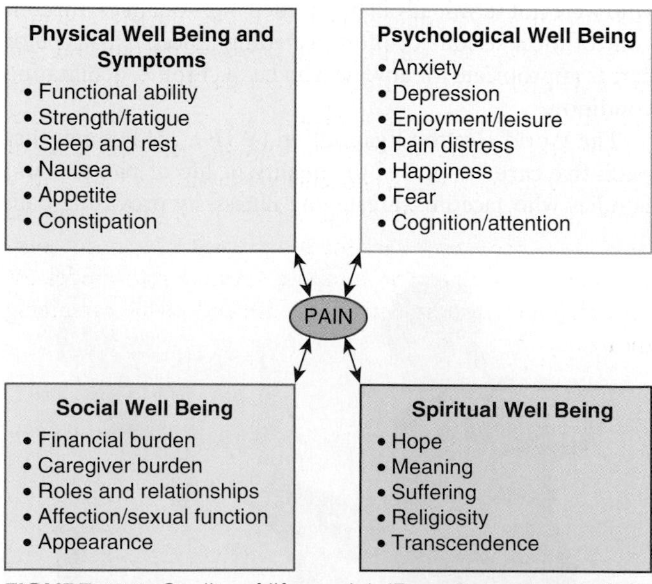

FIGURE 42-3 Quality-of-life model. (From Betty Ferrell, PhD, FAAN, and Marcia Grant, DNSc, FAAN, City of Hope Medical Center, Duarte, California.)

Adequate control of symptoms at the end of life requires ongoing assessment and evaluation of interventions. Common physical and psychological symptoms at the end of life include pain, dyspnea, anorexia and cachexia, constipation, diarrhea, nausea and vomiting, fatigue, anxiety, and depression. Nurses need to be knowledgeable in the management of these symptoms. Aggressive management of symptoms will promote a peaceful death for the patient and facilitates the grieving process for the surviving family members.

> **! SAFE PRACTICE ALERT**
>
> Families need a great deal of education and support if distressing symptoms are present. Education and support to the patient as well as the family are essential as nurses work promptly to control patient symptoms with pharmacologic and nonpharmacologic measures.

CARE OF THE DYING PATIENT

Dying has been described as a physical, psychological, social, and spiritual event (End-of-Life Nursing Education Consortium [ELNEC], 2010). In delivery of care for a dying person, the patient and family are considered the unit of care. The provision of nursing care to the dying patient may occur in any setting, including acute care, long-term care, and home care.

The Care Environment

The provision of a supportive environment is essential in caring for the dying patient. Patients are encouraged to bring some of their favorite belongings with them if they are not at home. These may include a pillow, blanket, stuffed animal, photographs, or other treasured mementos. Photographs provide comfort to the dying person as well as the family, allow life review to occur, help families reminisce, and facilitate nurses' knowledge of the family dynamics. A major benefit of having photos of the dying person is that nurses can see that person as once-healthy with a lifetime of experiences that does not include only illness and approaching death.

Allowing pets to visit brings comfort and companionship. Families are allowed unrestricted visiting hours, time for privacy, and space necessary for closeness and intimacy. Interventions to provide a supportive environment for the dying patient and family require the nurse to be creative while advocating for patient and family needs and choices.

For the person who is "actively dying," a change of setting, such as transfer from a nursing home to a hospital, or from a hospital to a hospice facility, can be disruptive and distressing. The setting is changed only if the patient or family requests a change. If the person prefers to die at home, for example, that request would be honored. Patients and families are given options for where they want the death to occur, and the nurse provides support while advocating for the wishes of the patient and family.

Each member of the health care team ensures that diagnostic tests and procedures are conducted only if treatment measures will be implemented. Vital signs may not be necessary unless they are being obtained to update a family member about a dying patient's status.

Communication With Dying Patients and Their Families

Open and honest communication is essential as death is approaching. Informed decision making is a necessary requirement in an effort to gain trust of the patient and family. It is only through honest communication that is sensitive, caring, and compassionate that trust is facilitated and high-quality care is provided (Evidence-Based Practice and Informatics box). Information at the end of life is given in simple, uncomplicated terms, while avoiding overloading or overwhelming the patient or family members. The provision of simple answers to questions that consider the patient's and family members' understanding and readiness for information is essential. Family members often are tired, have difficulty concentrating, and cannot focus on information that is provided to them. The nurse may need to answer the same questions while providing information repeatedly so that the family can integrate what they are learning as the patient's condition changes. Patients may be aware that they are dying and ask the nurse about the dying process. Nurses need to be honest while exploring any potential concerns or fears that the patient may be having.

QSEN FOCUS!

Through patient-centered care of dying patients and their families, the nurse demonstrates understanding of pain and suffering; assesses the extent of the pain and suffering as well as the levels of physical and emotional comfort; and recognizes the specific beliefs of patients and families.

EVIDENCE-BASED PRACTICE AND INFORMATICS

Recommendations for Patients in End-of-Life Intensive Care Unit

- Recommendations for end-of-life care in the intensive care unit have been published by the Agency for Healthcare Research and Quality that relate to not only physical care of the dying patient but also the need for improved communication.
- Consideration of the value of family conferences as a tool for communication, interdisciplinary team rounds, and development of an environment that supports open communication are described.
- More information is provided in a published consensus statement by the American College of Critical Care Medicine, available at *www.ncbi.nlm.nih.gov/pubmed/18431285.*

Providing education and accurate information as death approaches is an essential component of nursing care at the end of life. Honest and factual information can empower patients and families. Educational needs of patients and families are noted in the Patient Education and Health Literacy box.

PATIENT EDUCATION AND HEALTH LITERACY

End-of-Life Care

- Teach patients and families the signs and symptoms of the dying process in terms they can understand. Knowing what to expect can empower family caregivers during this very difficult time.
- Explain measures used to control symptoms and to maintain quality of life for the patient. Knowing that efforts are being made to keep their loved one comfortable can decrease the stress family members may feel while caring for the dying person.
- Provide assurance that members of the health care team are available and ready to provide assistance and support.
- Educate caregivers about how to provide physical care measures to allow the family to provide safe care in a manner that will allow comfort for the patient as well as the family.

When a person is imminently dying, the family may want to be at the bedside constantly. This period often is termed the *death vigil.* Other families may be uncomfortable being with the dying person for very personal reasons. Fear often is a common feeling for families who have not faced death or who have experienced death in a detrimental manner. Common fears include fear of being alone with the patient, fear of their loved one having a painful or otherwise symptomatic death, fear that they will witness suffering, and fear of not knowing if the patient has actually died. Families who are fearful need an increased level of support by various members of the interdisciplinary team. Increased presence of family members, friends, and spiritual support will help allay some of these fears. It is the responsibility of the nurse to reassure the family that the patient will be kept as comfortable as possible. The nurse serves as a role model for how and when to implement effective end-of-life caregiving measures.

! SAFE PRACTICE ALERT

Be aware that families may react with anger and fear as their loved one is dying. Nurses should ensure their own safety in any environment in which they practice. Always be aware of the potential for aggressive behaviors, and bring a calm and reassuring manner to interactions with patients as well as their families.

It can be a very difficult but necessary task for the nurse to communicate to families that their loved one has died. Telling the family that the patient has died is done in an open and honest manner with compassion and support. Providing information in small amounts, repeatedly if necessary, allows the family to process that information. Many families are shocked and overwhelmed at the time of death and will need time to process that death has just occurred. If the family is expecting the death, they may have been prepared in advance through the process of anticipatory grieving. Family members may feel numb and lost at this time; the nurse assists them in understanding what they need to do after the death. It is helpful for the nurses to ask what family members are capable of doing at that point—for example, making telephone calls to other family members.

CARE OF THE PATIENT WHO IS IMMINENTLY DYING

Care of the patient who is imminently, or actively, dying demands the most basic nursing care measures provided with a high level of caring and compassion. Gentle bathing is necessary, with peri-care performed on a regular basis unless symptoms such as pain or shortness of breath are intolerable. Oral care is essential because many dying patients breathe through the mouth. Use of a moistening agent and care of the lips to prevent dryness will promote comfort. Turning and repositioning are necessary to prevent skin breakdown, which could result in pain and discomfort. If the patient is agitated or restless, decreasing environmental stimuli while playing soothing music may promote a sense of peace and comfort. The most important intervention is to ensure that symptoms are controlled. Frequent and attentive assessment to ongoing or new symptoms with prompt intervention will promote comfort and prevent any undue distress or suffering.

Symptom management and keeping a dying patient comfortable are priority nursing goals. Pain medication is given as needed, often in the form of sublingual drops or suppositories. Supplemental oxygen may help a patient who is struggling to maintain oxygenation. Patients who experience nausea or vomiting are treated with medication in suppository form. Use of alternative therapies such as guided imagery, massage, distraction techniques, and herbal therapies may be helpful.

Patients who are actively dying may lose the ability to swallow, so that secretions may build up, causing congestion and difficulty breathing. Secretions can be controlled through medications to decrease oral and respiratory secretions, and suctioning if it does not cause the patient undue distress.

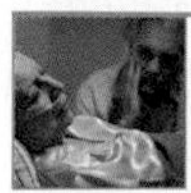

4. What nursing interventions are appropriate for the Richardsons during Mrs. Richardson's last few days?

Nearing Death Awareness

Nearing death awareness has been described as a special communication of the dying, which occurs when patients are approaching death or imminently dying. Not all people will have this experience, but the nurse must be aware of the signs that nearing death awareness is occurring. People who are experiencing nearing death awareness may appear confused and report speaking to or seeing already deceased persons, such as a parent or spouse. Many people in this state describe spiritual beings and bright lights, together with a sense of peace and beauty. Making hand gestures, such as reaching or picking, or holding unseen objects is common. Nurses caring for patients exhibiting these signs should not assume that they are confused or hallucinating or having a reaction to medications. Many professionals experienced in the field of end-of-life care have witnessed these signs and believe that the dying person is undergoing a transition from this life to the next. The person may actually be trying to communicate his or her experience to the family or health care providers. This conveyed experience often is viewed as a type of symbolic communication, perhaps trying to ask for permission to die or resolving previous conflicts. *Final Gifts: Understanding the Special Awareness, Needs, and Communications of the Dying,* by Maggie Callanan and Patricia Kelley (1992) describes this process.

It is important to recognize that these experiences can be comforting to the dying patient, and nurses should not contradict or argue with the person. It is imperative to simply be present with the person, listen, and be open to any attempts to communicate. It is acceptable to ask gentle questions such as "What are you seeing?" or "How does that make you feel?" Having an open discussion with the family while describing what is occurring may provide further insight to the nurse as the health care provider, as well as promoting a sense of understanding and acceptance for the family.

If a death is expected, such as with a terminal illness, the final days or hours before a person dies may be one of the most significant events that the dying person and loved ones experience. It is a time to say good-bye and complete end-of-life or life-closure tasks. Nurses facilitate this process as they provide care, education, support, and advocacy during this time. The goal is to provide dignified end-of-life care to patients and their families in any practice setting.

POSTMORTEM CARE: CARE OF THE PATIENT AT THE TIME OF DEATH

The procedure to pronounce death begins with identifying the patient. The nurse notes the general appearance of the body, lack of reaction to verbal or tactile stimuli, lack of response of the pupils to light, absence of a pulse on palpation or a heartbeat on auscultation, no blood pressure, and no audible respirations on auscultation of the lungs. If family members are present, they may be reassured to watch the nurse assess for signs of death as a sense of reality of the actual death is determined. Once death has been confirmed, the nurse, in any setting, determines that the death occurred without "unusual circumstances." Any signs of foul play or of suicide or missing medications are reported to the appropriate authorities, which may include the police and the coroner. Documentation of the time of death includes the patient's name, the time the call was made to the appropriate health care provider related to notification of the death, and actual findings on the physical examination. The physician caring for the patient and other health care providers involved in the patient's care are notified as well.

Nurses need to be aware of the policies and procedures at their individual places of employment related to pronouncement of death and the actions that need to be taken at the time of death. Each state has practice guidelines that determine who can pronounce death. If the patient is an organ donor, it is necessary to follow policies and procedures appropriate to the organ(s) donated. In addition, if an autopsy is going to be performed as required by law or family request, any invasive tubes or lines must remain in the body. Such devices include IV lines, nasogastric tubes, tracheostomy appliances, endotracheal tubes, Foley catheters, drainage tubes, and any other invasive device that was used before death.

After death in any setting, any medical equipment or tubes in the body are removed from the room unless an autopsy is to be performed. Any unnecessary items related to prior care of the patient are removed from the room, and the room is cleaned. Bathing and dressing the body demonstrate respect and dignity for the deceased and help the family in the grieving process. Proper positioning of the body and covering the body appropriately after death demonstrate respect, because a peaceful last impression of the deceased is important for the family. At this time it is necessary to ask the family if any special religious or cultural practices need to be followed. Physical care of the body may be dictated by cultural practices. The Nursing Care Guideline box details preparing a body for the morgue.

CARE OF THE FAMILY AT THE TIME OF DEATH

Skills of interpersonal communication, which include empathy, unconditional positive regard, genuineness, attention, and listening skills are essential at this time. Nurses must be comfortable "being with" the dying patient and family. Being present, by being in the room or close to the area and through active listening, is an essential part of caring for those at the end of life.

Collaborative care is necessary because care for the dying is an interdisciplinary activity. Identifying which members of the health care team have developed relationships with the family during the illness and supporting their continued involvement with the family after the death of the patient can allow for enhanced grieving, both for the family and for the health care provider. Continued therapeutic communication by physicians, nurses, social workers, chaplains, and even dietary and housekeeping staff can assist the family in the grieving process.

Another important nursing intervention is to provide the family time with the deceased so they can say goodbye and begin to let go. Nurses can offer to call for spiritual support in accordance with the wishes of the family. Pastoral care assists in the decision-making process about funeral arrangements as necessary. If the death is expected, funeral arrangements may have already been made, and the funeral home may be contacted by telephone or other means by the nurse or the family.

Bereavement Support

After a death, bereavement support begins immediately. The nurse begins by providing support and compassion, while being present with active listening. Assessment of grief reactions and risk factors for complicated grief is completed at this time. Follow-up bereavement support is provided by phone calls, cards, and possible attendance at funeral services, depending on the care setting. If the bereaved are in need of further support, referral to community bereavement resources such as hospice or other support groups is necessary.

Death of an infant or child is an extremely difficult experience for many parents and families. At the time of death, babies are wrapped snugly in a blanket, and parents are encouraged to hold their child. Siblings are allowed to participate in this process as well.

When children are close to the deceased, caregivers are encouraged to openly and honestly answer any questions they may have. The child's responses to the loss are evaluated while determining if the child should attend the funeral. If young children are going to attend the funeral, they need to be prepared for what they will see, who will be there, what they may feel, how they may see other people grieving, and what they will be doing during the time that they are at the funeral. It is essential to explain to the child what the body will look like, and the fact that the deceased will not talk, move, or breathe.

Health care providers often fear expressing emotions in front of their patients and families. This fear causes many to avoid discussing potentially difficult topics that are essential to end-of-life care. Nurses and others who work with dying patients need an outlet to express their emotions. For more information, see section later in this chapter: The Nurse: Experiences of Caring for the Dying. Some health care providers experience a sense of guilt or failure when they cannot cure their patients, which may lead to lack of communication related to needs at the end of life. Other common fears are

NURSING CARE GUIDELINE

Preparing a Body for the Morgue

Background

- Policy regarding postmortem care differs among states and between facilities. Be sure to be familiar with your institution's policy and procedures before care of the body after death.
- It is imperative that the body be treated with the same respect and dignity given during life.
- Care of the body postmortem can be delegated to UAP with appropriate education regarding institution procedures.
- Dependent upon culture, family may wish to take part in final care. Assist the family in appropriate postmortem care as necessary.

Procedural Concerns

- *Positioning*: The body is placed in a supine position (on the back) in normal anatomic position, to prevent abnormal pooling of the blood.
  - Arms at side (palms down) or across the abdomen
  - Head/shoulders elevated on one pillow (to prevent discoloration of the face secondary to blood pooling)
  - Dentures and or other prosthetics are inserted if available to maintain normal anatomic appearance.
  - Close the eyes and hold them closed for several seconds so that they remain shut.
  - Jewelry is removed (with the exception of a wedding ring, which often is taped in place); check institution policy for specific details.
- *Medical tubes/paraphernalia:* Policies regarding medical equipment (such as IV lines, nasogastric tubes, chest tubes, or endotracheal tubes) vary among institutions/states.
  - Some require they remain in/attached to the body exactly as they were at the time of death
  - Some states/institutions allow the paraphernalia to be cut to a specified length but require that the tubes still remain in place.
  - Still other facilities/states may allow them to be removed completely.
  - Remove any extraneous movable equipment from the room out of respect for the family viewing the body.
- *Washing the body:* The family may wish to participate in this procedure or may complete this procedure in private. Health care personnel should abide by their wishes as much as possible.
  - Clean any soiled areas on the body (a full bath is not necessary).
  - Place absorbent pads under the buttocks (when the muscles relax, urine and feces will be expelled).
  - Apply a clean gown.
  - Brush the patient's hair.
  - Replace and straighten top sheets.
  - Remove any soiled linens from the room.
- *Religious concerns*: Certain religions may require a specialized person to perform this portion of the procedure, whereas other religions might forbid washing of the body. Accommodation of the family's religious wishes should be made if possible. Regardless, the mortician will ultimately wash the body before final discharge.
- After the family has left the hospital or health care facility, the body may be wrapped in a **shroud**, a cloth, sheet, or bag, for transportation to the morgue or funeral home.

Documentation Concerns

- Ensure that the death certificate has been signed.
- Follow through with any organ donation arrangements. Ensure adherence to institutional and state policy and procedures.
- *Identification*: The hospital ID band is left in place. Many facilities require additional identification—check with institution procedure/policy for specific information, but common locations for ID tags or labels are the ankle/foot and the outer shroud in which the body is wrapped for transport. Personal items not taken by the family are identified and documented.
- Appropriately document all of the procedural applications in a final note on the patient's chart. In addition, be sure to include to whom any personal items were dispersed, the time of body transfer, and any other special circumstances.

related to the uncertainty of making a prognosis and determining appropriate treatment measures for individual patients.

Effective communication includes the need for the powerful skill of listening. Sensitive listening requires energy and involvement and being present physically, mentally, and emotionally.

EVALUATION

Evaluation of the nursing care provided to the grieving patient and family, or to the dying patient and family, focuses on the consideration of the goals of that person and the family unit. Careful attention to the specific loss, related factors, and risk factors for potential decreased quality of life are important considerations. People who are grieving need to demonstrate that they can talk about the meaning of their loss, use available support systems, and deal with the loss as they move through the stages of grief. Identification of feelings, any change in health, and effective coping strategies are essential to the grieving process. A return to life and a level of functioning, physically, socially, emotionally, and spiritually, that existed before the loss is evaluated.

For those who are experiencing death anxiety, an ability to discuss their concerns about their death and feelings associated with dying are findings that demonstrate effective nursing interventions and individual coping. Goal setting and gaining a realistic perspective related to the disease process and prognosis are indicators of development toward meeting the goals of nursing care and quality end of life care.

THE NURSE: EXPERIENCES OF CARING FOR THE DYING LO 42.8

In a majority of health care settings, nurses will experience death and loss. Many nurses experience a multitude of losses in their clinical practice, and possibly in their personal lives. Cumulative loss is a succession of loss experienced by nurses who work with those who are dying. When the nurse is exposed to frequent loss and death, available time may be inadequate to resolve grief issues of one patient before another patient dies. Accumulation of loss can result in unresolved grief and potential chronic grief and bereavement (Vachon and Huggard, 2010).

Working with dying patients can create a personal sense of loss and fear about the nurse's own mortality. Some nurses develop defense mechanisms to cope with loss and grief in the practice setting. These defenses allow the nurse to temporarily alleviate the discomfort related to death and dying. Focusing only on physical care needs while overlooking the emotional or psychosocial nature of nursing care allows a nurse to avoid uncomfortable feelings and fears related to death and loss. These behaviors result in emotional distancing, avoidance, and potential withdrawal from dying patients and their families when supportive care from the nurse is most needed.

A nurse's comfort level with dying patients and families is affected by personality, past experience with loss and grief, and cultural, social, and spiritual belief systems. To effectively care for the dying, nurses need to explore their personal feelings regarding death. Self-exploration and reflection through personal death awareness exercises, and discussion of beliefs concerning life and death with friends, peers, coworkers, and pastoral care workers will promote an understanding and acceptance of death as a part of life. Nurses should be aware of their own fears, feelings, responses, and reactions to death and dying so that they have the ability to communicate effectively and to convey caring, acceptance, and respect for patients and families who are experiencing death, loss, and grief. Verbalization of feelings to others and expression of emotions help nurses process their own reactions to the grieving process.

Nurses who experience cumulative losses need to have support systems in place and be able to explore and express their feelings associated with anxiety, loss, and grief. These support systems may be formal, informal, or spiritual, or may be in the form of continuing education in end-of-life care (Vachon and Huggard, 2010). Self-care is an important aspect of the nurse's overall health and ability to handle the stressors of working with the dying patient. Proper diet, exercise, sleep, time for relaxation, and vacations all are aspects of self-care that will strengthen the nurse's ability to continue providing effective care.

SUMMARY OF LEARNING OUTCOMES

LO 42.1 *Describe the process of grief, loss, and bereavement:* Loss is determined by the affected person and is a subjective experience that elicits a grief response. Grief is the emotional response to loss while mourning is considered the outward signs of grief demonstrated by the person based on his or her personal, cultural, and religious or spiritual beliefs. Bereavement is the feelings and expressions that people experiencing loss demonstrate.

LO 42.2 *Discuss dysfunctional loss and grieving:* Dysfunctional loss and grieving include complicated grief, which occurs when a person does not progress through the normal stages of grief, and disenfranchised grief when a person cannot openly grieve a loss.

LO 42.3 *Identify factors affecting the grief and bereavement process:* Various factors including developmental level, gender, socioeconomic status, religion and spirituality, health status of the survivor, the relationship to the deceased and the strength of that relationship, coping styles, concurrent stressors, available support systems, and the type of loss experienced affect the grief and bereavement process.

LO 42.4 *Perform a nursing assessment of patients and their families who are experiencing loss, death, grief, and bereavement:* Nurses must assess individual patients as well as families during the grieving process. Valid and reliable tools have been developed that will allow a complete and thorough assessment.

LO 42.5 *Select nursing diagnoses appropriate for people experiencing death and the grieving process:* Nursing diagnoses for grief and death include *Grieving, Complicated Grieving, Chronic Sorrow,* and *Death Anxiety.*

LO 42.6 *Plan appropriate goals and outcomes for dying patients and their families:* Goals for dying patients and their families relate to the specific nursing diagnosis and to the stage of grieving.

LO 42.7 *Implement nursing care plans with nursing interventions appropriate for patients and families experiencing death and grief:* Nursing care for patients and families experiencing death and loss is individualized. Therapeutic communication, being present for the patient and family, treating symptoms that cause discomfort, and educating the patient and family are all part of nursing care. Evaluation of the care plan is ongoing because changes may occur rapidly when a patient is near death.

LO 42.8 *Examine the effects death and loss may have on nurses with appropriate coping strategies:* Nurses experience death and loss on a recurring basis while providing care in most any health care setting. Working with dying patients requires nurses to develop their own awareness and understanding of death and dying as well as loss and grief.

Answers to the critical-thinking questions are available at *http://evolve.elsevier.com/YoostCrawford/fundamentals/.*

REVIEW QUESTIONS

1. While caring for a female patient with advanced multiple sclerosis, the nurse is discussing the difference between hospice and palliative care. Which statement by the patient indicates understanding of the difference between hospice and palliative care?
   - **a.** "I will need to get hospice care if I want my symptoms controlled."
   - **b.** "I can get palliative care right now— even though I am not going to die anytime soon."
   - **c.** "My doctor has to make the decision if I have hospice care."
   - **d.** "I can't get any other treatments, even if they are experimental, if I choose palliative care."
2. The nurse is orienting new staff to a clinical unit that provides palliative care. A new employee asks what "grief" is exactly. Which statement indicates that the nurse has correctly defined grief?
   - **a.** The emotional response to a loss
   - **b.** The outward, social expression of a loss
   - **c.** The depression felt after a loss
   - **d.** The loss of a possession or loved one
3. The nurse has been caring for a 65-year-old male patient who has just died. In planning for follow-up bereavement care, the nurse knows that which person is at risk for disenfranchised grief?
   - **a.** A daughter who lives in a different state
   - **b.** The son who was with the client when he died
   - **c.** An estranged ex-wife of the patient who lives nearby
   - **d.** The 16-year-old grandchild of the patient
4. The mother of two children, 8 and 10 years of age, has just experienced the death of her mother, the children's grandmother. The mother is concerned about the emotional impact attending the funeral may have on her children. She asks the nurse what she should do in relation to her children attending the funeral. What is the nurse's best response?
   - **a.** "Take them to the funeral—they need closure, and seeing their grandma in the casket will assist them in knowing that she has died and will not return. Many children attend funerals in today's society."
   - **b.** "Do not take them to the funeral—they are too young to be exposed to the emotions that are demonstrated at funerals. Many children who attend funerals have adverse psychological reactions."
   - **c.** "Talk to your children about how they feel about attending the funeral and encourage them to ask questions and talk about their concerns. If they want to go, they will need to be prepared for what will happen at the funeral."
   - **d.** "Talk to your children about what your mother meant to you and how much she cared for them as her grandchildren and then see if they really want to attend the funeral. If they want to go it is okay to take them."
5. The nurse has been caring for a patient who has just died. What is the preferred outcome in caring for the body after death?
   - **a.** Make sure the body is sent to the morgue within an hour after death.
   - **b.** Have the family members participate in the bathing and dressing of the deceased.
   - **c.** Notify in person or by phone all family and team members immediately after the patient's death.
   - **d.** Demonstrate respect for the body and provide a clean, peaceful impression of the deceased for the family.

6. Several theorists have identified stages of the grieving process. The nurse understands these stages and knows that people progress through them in an individualized manner. Which statement is true regarding the steps of the grieving process?
   a. There is a definite "timetable" or period of time specific to each stage of the grieving process.
   b. Nursing interventions are generalized across all stages of the grieving process.
   c. Tasks to be achieved at each stage have been identified by each theorist.
   d. There is a common stepwise progression through each stage of the grieving process.
7. Which statement is true regarding advance directives?
   a. Advance directives apply only when the person has a chronic illness.
   b. Advance directives should be drawn up by family members of people who are incompetent.
   c. Discussion of advance directives is a nursing responsibility.
   d. Advance directives should be kept in a safety deposit box until the person dies.
8. In which scenario is hospice care provided?
   a. Only in the homes of the terminally ill
   b. For any terminal illness that requires symptom control
   c. For cancer patients only in their last weeks of life
   d. In hospital settings based on the seriousness of the illness
9. In caring for a dying patient, what is an appropriate nursing action to increase family involvement?
   a. Insisting that all bedside care be performed by the family
   b. Asking family members what they would like to do for their loved one and allowing them to participate
   c. Expecting the family to be able to perform the patient's daily needs and to meet them consistently
   d. Refusing all assistance from the family, to decrease family stress
10. The nurse caring for a dying patient understands that "nearing death awareness" is occurring when the patient asks which question?
    a. "Where are my shoes? I need to get ready for the trip."
    b. "Is my daughter from California going to come and visit before I die?"
    c. "When do you think that I am going to die?"
    d. "How much longer can I live without food or water?"

Answers and rationales for the review questions are available at *http://evolve.elsevier.com/YoostCrawford/fundamentals/.*

REFERENCES

American Nurses Association: Euthanasia, assisted suicide and aid in dying, 2013. Retrieved from *www.nursingworld.org/euthanasiaanddying.*

American Psychiatric Association: *Diagnostic and statistical manual of mental disorders*, ed. 5, Washington, D.C., 2013, Author.

Becvar DS: *In the presence of grief: Helping family members resolve death, dying, and bereavement issues*, New York, 2003, Guilford Press.

Bowlby J: *Attachment and loss*, ed. 2, New York, 1982, Basic Books.

Butler RN: The life review: An interpretation of reminiscence in the aged, *Psychiatry* 26:65-76, 1963.

Callanan M, Kelley P: *Final gifts: Understanding the special awareness, needs, and communications of the dying*, New York, 1992, Poseidon Press.

City of Hope Pain and Palliative Care Resource Center: Quality of life pain impact model, 2014. Retrieved from: *http://prc.coh.org/pdf/pain_QOL_model.pdf.*

Cronenwett L, Sherwood G, Barnsteiner J, et al: Quality and safety education for nurses, *Nurs Outlook* 55(3):122-131, 2007.

Doka K: *Disenfranchised grief: New directions, challenges, and strategies for practice*, Champaign, Ill., 2002, Research Press.

End-of-Life Nursing Education Consortium: *Graduate training program*, Washington, DC, 2005, City of Hope and the American Association of Colleges of Nursing.

End-of-Life Nursing Education Consortium: *Core curriculum*, Washington, D.C., 2011, City of Hope and the American Association of Colleges of Nursing.

Field M, Cassel C (eds): *Approaching death: Improving care at the end of life*, Committee on Care at the End of Life, Division of Health Care Services, Institute of Medicine, Washington, D.C., 1997, National Academy Press.

Humphrey GM, Zimpfer DG: *Counseling for grief and bereavement*, Thousand Oaks, Calif., 2007, Sage Publications.

Kissane DW: Bereavement. In G Hanks, NI Cherney, NA Christakis, et al (eds), *Oxford textbook of palliative medicine*, ed. 4, Oxford, UK, 2011, Oxford University Press.

Kübler-Ross E: *On death and dying*, New York, 2003, Macmillan.

Lindemann E: Symptomatology and management of acute grief, *Am J Psychiatry* 101:141-148,1944.

Mayo Clinic: Caregiver stress: Tips for taking care of yourself, 2012. Retrieved from *www.mayoclinic.org/healthy-living/stress-management/in-depth/caregiver-stress/art-20044784.*

National Consensus Project for Quality Palliative Care: Clinical practice guidelines for quality palliative care, ed. 3, 2013. Retrieved from *www.nationalconsensusproject.org*.

National Hospice and Palliative Care Organization: Hospice and palliative care, 2014. Retrieved from *www.nhpco.org/about/hospice-care*.

O'Leary J: Grief and its impact on prenatal attachment in the subsequent pregnancy, *Arch Womens Ment Health* 7(1):7-18, 2004.

Sheldon F: ABC of palliative care: Bereavement, *Br Med J* 316(7129):456-458, 1998.

Vachon ML, Huggard J: The experience of the nurse in end-of-life care in the 21st century: Mentoring the next generation. In BR Ferrell, N Coyle (eds), *Oxford textbook of palliative nursing*, New York, 2010 Oxford University Press.

Worden JW: *Grief counseling and grief therapy: A handbook for the mental health practitioner*, ed. 4, London, 2008, Springer.

World Health Organization: Palliative care is an essential part of cancer control, 2014. Retrieved from *www.who.int/en*.

APPENDIX A

Abbreviations, Roots, Prefixes, and Suffixes

COMMONLY USED ABBREVIATIONS

NOTE: Abbreviations in common use can vary widely from place to place. Each institution's list of acceptable abbreviations is the best authority for its records.

Abbreviation	Definition
ac	before meals
ACLS	advanced cardiac life support
ad lib	as desired
ADA	American Diabetes Association
ADD	attention deficit disorder
ADLs	activities of daily living
AIDS	acquired immunodeficiency syndrome
ALS	advanced life support; amyotrophic lateral sclerosis
AM, am	morning
AMI	acute myocardial infarction
ASD	atrial septal defect
AST	aspartate aminotransferase (formerly SGOT)
A-V, AV, A/V	arteriovenous; atrioventricular
BCLS	basic cardiac life support
BE	barium enema
bid, b.i.d.	twice a day (bis in die)
BM	bowel movement
BMR	basal metabolic rate
BP	blood pressure
BPH	benign prostatic hypertrophy
bpm	beats per minute
BR	bedrest
BRP	bathroom priviledges
BSA	body surface area
BSC	bedside commode
BSE	breast self-examination
BUN	blood urea nitrogen
Bx	biopsy
c̄	with
CABG	coronary artery bypass graft
CAD	coronary artery disease
CAT	computerized (axial) tomography scan
CBC, cbc	complete blood count
CCU	coronary care unit; critical care unit
CF	cystic fibrosis
CHD	congenital heart disease; coronary heart disease
CHF	congestive heart failure
CK	creatinine kinase
CMV	cytomegalovirus
CNS	central nervous system
c/o	complaint of
CO	carbon monoxide; cardiac output
CO_2	carbon dioxide
COPD	chronic obstructive pulmonary disease
COX	cyclooxygenase
CP	cerebral palsy; cleft palate
CPAP	continuous positive airway pressure
CPK	creatine phosphokinase
CPR	cardiopulmonary resuscitation
CSF	cerebrospinal fluid
CT	computed tomography
CVA	cerebrovascular accident; costovertebral angle
CVP	central venous pressure
D&C	dilation (dilatation) and curettage
dc, DC, D/C	discontinue
DIC	disseminated intravascular coagulation
diff	differential blood count
DKA	diabetic ketoacidosis
DM	diabetes mellitus; diastolic murmur
DNA	deoxyribonucleic acid
DNR	do not resuscitate
DOA	dead on arrival
DOB	date of birth
DOE	dyspnea on exertion
DPT	diphtheria-pertussis-tetanus
DRG	diagnosis-related group
DSM	*Diagnostic and Statistical Manual of Mental Disorders*
DT	delirium tremens
DVT	deep vein thrombosis
D_5W	dextrose 5% in water
Dx	diagnosis
EBV	Epstein-Barr virus
ECG, EKG	electrocardiogram; electrocardiograph

Continued

Abbreviation	Definition
ECHO	echocardiography
ECT	electroconvulsive therapy
ED	emergency department
EDD	estimated date of delivery
EEG	electroencephalogram; electroencephalograph
EENT	eye, ear, nose, and throat
ELISA	enzyme-linked immunosorbent assay
EMG	electromyogram
EMS	emergency medical service
EMT	emergency medical technician
ENT	ear, nose, and throat
ER	emergency room (hospital)
ERV	expiratory reserve volume
ESR	erythrocyte sedimentation rate
ESRD	end-stage renal disease
ET	endotracheal tube
ETOH	ethyl alcohol
FBS	fasting blood sugar
FEV	forced expiratory volume
FH, Fhx	family history
FHR	fetal heart rate
FOB	foot of bed
FTT	failure to thrive
fx	fracture
GB	gallbladder
GC	gonococcus; gonorrheal
GI	gastrointestinal
Grav I, II, etc.	pregnancy one, two, three, etc. (gravida)
GSW	gunshot wound
gtt	drops (guttae)
GU	genitourinary
Gyn	gynecology
H&P	history and physical
HA	headache
HAV	hepatitis A virus
Hb, HGB	hemoglobin
HBV	hepatitis B virus
HCG	human chorionic gonadotropin
HCT	hematocrit
HDL	high-density lipoprotein
HEENT	head, eye, ear, nose, and throat
HIV	human immunodeficiency virus
HOB, hob	head of bed
h/o	history of
HOH	hard of hearing
H_2O_2	hydrogen peroxide
HR, hr	heart rate; hour
hs	bedtime
HSV	herpes simplex virus
HT, HTN, ht	hypertension; height
hx, Hx	history
I&O	intake and output
IBW	ideal body weight
ICP	intracranial pressure
ICU	intensive care unit
Ig	immunoglobulin
IM	intramuscular
INR	international normalized ratio
IUD	intrauterine device
IV	intravenous
IVP	intravenous pyelogram; intravenous push
IVPB	intravenous piggyback
KCl	potassium chloride
KUB	kidney, ureter, and bladder
KVO	keep vein open
L	liter
lab	laboratory
lb	pound
L&D	labor and delivery
LDL	low-density lipoprotein
LE	lower extremity; lupus erythematosus
LMP	last menstrual period
LOC	level of consciousness
LP	lumbar puncture
LR	lactated Ringer's
LVH	left ventricular hypertrophy
MAP	mean arterial pressure
mcg	microgram
MD	muscular dystrophy
MDI	medium dose inhalant; metered dose inhaler
mEq	milliequivalent
mg	milligram
MI	myocardial infarction
mL, ml	milliliter
mm Hg	millimeters of mercury
MMR	maternal mortality rate; measles-mumps-rubella
MRI	magnetic resonance imaging
MVA	motor vehicle accident
N/A	not applicable
NaCl	sodium chloride
NANDA-I	North American Nursing Diagnosis Association–International
NAS	no added salt
N&V, N/V	nausea and vomiting
NG, ng	nasogastric
NICU	neonatal intensive care unit
NKA	no known allergies
NKDA	no known drug allergies
NPO, n.p.o.	nothing by mouth (non per os)
NSAID	nonsteroidal antiinflammatory drug
NSR	normal sinus rhythm
O_2	oxygen
OB	obstetrics
OBS	organic brain syndrome
OOB	out of bed

Abbreviation	Definition
OR	operating room
OTC	over-the-counter
oz	ounce
$\bar{p}$	after
PACU	postanesthesia care unit
PALS	pediatric advanced life support
pc	after meals
PCA	patient-controlled analgesia
PE	physical examination
PEEP	positive end-expiratory pressure
PERRLA	pupils equal, regular, react to light and accommodation
PET	positron emission tomography
PICC	percutaneously inserted central catheter
PID	pelvic inflammatory disease
PKU	phenylketonuria
PM, pm	evening
PMH	past medical history
PMI	point of maximal impulse
PMN	polymorphonuclear neutrophil leukocytes (polys)
PMS	premenstrual syndrome
PO, p.o.	orally (per os); by mouth
POD	postoperative day
PRN, p.r.n.	as required (pro re nata); as needed
pro time	prothrombin time
pt	pint
PT	prothrombin time; physical therapy
PTT	partial thromboplastin time
PVC	premature ventricular contraction
q	every
qh	every hour
qid	four times a day
qt	quart
R	respiration; right; Rickettsia; roentgen
RBC, rbc	red blood cell; red blood count
RDA	recommended daily/dietary allowance
RDS	respiratory distress syndrome
Rh	rhesus factor in blood
RNA	ribonucleic acid
R/O	rule out
ROM	range of motion
ROS	review of systems
RR	recovery room; respiratory rate
R/T	related to
RX, Rx	prescription
$\bar{s}$	without
SCD	sequential compression device
SGOT	serum glutamic oxaloacetic transaminase
SGPT	serum glutamic pyruvic transaminase
SIDS	sudden infant death syndrome
SLE	systemic lupus erythematosus
SOB	shortness of breath
S/P, s/p	status post
s/s	signs and symptoms
Staph	staphylococcus
stat	immediately (statim)
STD	sexually transmitted disease
STI	sexually transmitted infection
Strep	streptococcus
Sx	symptoms
T	temperature; thoracic
T&A	tonsillectomy and adenoidectomy
TB	tuberculosis
TBL, tbsp, T	tablespoon
TENS	transcutaneous electrical nerve stimulation
TIA	transient ischemic attack
tid	three times a day
TMJ	temporomandibular joint
TPN	total parenteral nutrition
TPR	temperature, pulse, and respiration
TSE	testicular self-examination
TSH	thyroid-stimulating hormone
TSP, tsp, t	teaspoon
Tx	treatment
UA	urinalysis
URI	upper respiratory infection
UTI	urinary tract infection
VC	vital capacity
vol	volume
VS, v.s.	vital signs
VSD	ventricular septal defect
WBC, wbc	white blood cell; white blood count
WNL	within normal limits
WT, wt, wgt	weight

From *Mosby's dictionary of medicine, nursing, and health professions,* ed. 8, St. Louis, 2009, Mosby.

ROOTS

Root	Definition
aden/o	gland
adip/o, lip/o, steat/o	fat
albin/o, leuk/o, leuc/o	white
angi/o, vas/o	vessel
anter/o	front, before
arteri/o	artery
arthr/o	joint
audi/o	hearing

Continued

Root	Definition
blast/o	embryonic
brachi/o	arm
bronch/o	airway
carcin/o	cancer
cardi/o	heart
cephal/o	head
cerebr/o, encephal/o	brain
cervic/o	neck
chol/e	bile, gall
cholecyct/o	gallbladder
chondr/o	cartilage
cirrh/o, jaund/o, xanth/o	yellow
cleid/o	clavicle
col/o	colon
colp/o	vagina
cost/o	rib
crani/o	skull
crypt/o	hidden
cutane/o, dermat/o, derm/o	skin
cyan/o	blue
cyst/o	urinary bladder, cyst
cyt/o	cell
dactyl/o	finger or toe
elast/o	elastic
enter/o	intestines
erythem/o, erythr/o, rube/o	red
gastr/o	stomach or ventral
glomerul/o	glomerulus
gloss/o	tongue
gon/o	genitals
gynec/o, gyn/o	female
hem/o, hemat/o	blood
hepat/o	liver
hist/o	tissue
hol/o	entire, complete
home/o	like, similar
hydr/o	water, liquid, hydrogen
hypn/o	sleep
hyster/o, metr/o	uterus
idi/o	distinct, unknown
ile/o	ileum
ili/o	ilium, flank
irid/o	iris of the eye
kerat/o	horny substance, cornea
labi/o	lip, labial
lact/o	milk, lactic acid
laryng/o	larynx
later/o	side or lateral
lith/o	stone
lymph/o	lymph
mamm/o, mast/o	breast
medi/o	middle
medull/o	medulla
melan/o	black, darkness
men/o	menses
menig/o	meninges
my/o	muscle
myel/o	spinal cord, marrow
myring/o	eardrum
nas/o, rhin/o	nose
necr/o	death
nephr/o	kidney
neur/o	nerve, nervous tissue
nucle/o	nucleus
ocul/o, ophthalm/o	eye
odont/o	teeth
onc/o	tumor, mass
onych/o	nail
oophor/o, ovari/o	ovary
orchid/o	testicle
oste/o	bone
ot/o	ear
path/o	disease
ped/o	foot, children
phag/o	ingestion, eating
phleb/o	vein
pneum/o	air, breath
poster/o	behind, posterior
proct/o	anus, rectum
proxim/o	near
psych/o	mind, mental
py/o	pus
pyel/o	pelvis
pylor/o	pylorus
rachi/o	spine
radi/o	radioactive
ren/o	kidney
salping/o	tube
scler/o	hard
splen/o	spleen
squam/o	scale
thorac/o	chest, chest wall
thromb/o	blood clot
tox/o	poison
trache/o	trachea, windpipe
trich/o	hair
ur/o	urine
ureter/o	ureter
urethr/o	urethra
ventr/o	abdomen, ventral
vesic/o	bladder, vesicle
viscer/o	body organs

PREFIXES

Prefix	Definition
a-	before, without
ab-	away from
acu-	clarity, sharpness
ad-	toward
all-, allo-	divergence
ambi-	both
an-	not, without
ante-	before
anti-	against
arch-, arche-, archi-	first, beginning
aur-, auro-	ear
auto-	self
bar-, baro-	weight, pressure
bi-, di-, diplo-	two, double
bili-	bile
bio-	life
brady-	slow
bucco-	cheek
caud-	tail
chemo-	chemical
circum-	around
co-	together
contra-, counter-	against
cryo-	cold
de-	from, removal
demi- hemi-, semi-	half
dia-	through
dis-	removal, separation
duct-	carry
dys-	abnormal, difficult, painful
ecto-	outside
endo-, ento-, im-, in-, intra-	within
epi-	upon, over
episio-	perineum
esthesi-	sensation, feeling
etio-	causation
eu-	normal, good, true
ex-	out
exo-	outside of
extra-	outside, in addition to
fasci-, fascio	fibrous membrane, band
fibro-	fibrous tissue
hetero-	other, different
homo-, homeo-	same
hyper-	high, increased, above
hypo-, sub-	under, decreased
iatro-	medicine, healing
immuno-	free from, immune
in-, im-	not
infra-, sub-	below, under
inter-	between
intra-	within
intro-	on the inside
iso-	equal, same
juxta-	near
macro-	large
mal-	bad, poor
megalo-	abnormally large
meso-	middle
meta-	beyond, over
micro-	abnormally small
mono-, uni-	one
multi-	many
neo-	new
nocto-	night
non-	not
oligo-	little
oo-	egg
ortho-	straight, correct
pan-	all
para-	beside, near
per-	by, through
peri-	around
poly-	many
post-	after, behind
pre-, pro-	before, in front of
prim-	first
pseudo-	false
quad-	four
re-	back, again
retro-	backward, behind
super-	above, excessive
supra-	above
syn-, sym-	together
tachy-	fast
trans-	through, across
tri-	three
ultra-	beyond
un-	not

SUFFIXES

Suffix	Definition
-ac, -al, -ary, -eal, -ic, -ory, -ous	pertaining to
-acro	extremity, extreme point
-agogue	producer, secretor
-agra	sudden, severe pain
-algia, dynia	pain
-ase	enzyme
-asis, -ia, -ism, -osis	condition
-asthenia	weakness
-ather, -athero	fatty plaque
-cardia	action of the heart
-cardio	heart
-cele	swelling, hernia
-centesis	puncture of a cavity
-cide	destroying, killing
-clysis	washing, flushing
-crine	secrete
-crit	separate
-cyte	cell
-desis	binding, fixation
-ectasis	expansion, dilation
-ectomy	cutting out
-emia	blood condition
-form	in the shape of
-gen, -genic	produce, production
-gram	writing, record
-graph	instrument used to write or record
-graphy	process of writing or recording
-iatric	medicine
-ics	body of knowledge
-itis	inflammation
-lith	stone
-logy	study of
-lysis	dissolving, separating
-malacia	softening
-megaly	abnormal enlargement
-meter	measuring instrument
-metry	to measure
-odynia	pain
-oid	resembling
-ole, -ule	small
-oma	tumor
-para	to bear, give birth
-pathy	disease, feeling
-penia	deficiency
-pexy	surgical fixation
-phagia	eating, ingestion
-phasia	speech
-philia, -phile, -philic	affinity for
-plasia	formation, molding
-plasty	plastic repair
-plegia	paralysis
-pnea	breathing
-poiesis	growth, formation
-rrhage, -rrhagia, -rrhagy	burst forth
-rrhaphy	surgical repair
-rrhea	flow, discharge
-rrhexis	rupture
-scope	instrument for viewing
-scopy	visual examination
-stasis	stoppage of flow
-stenosis	narrowing
-stomy	surgical opening
-tome, -tomy	cutting
-tripsy	crushing
-trophy	nutrition, growth
-tropia, -tropic	deviation from normal, have influence on
-uria	presence of a substance in urine

APPENDIX B

NANDA-I Diagnostic Labels

2012–2014 NANDA-I APPROVED NURSING DIAGNOSES

Activity Intolerance
Risk for **Activity Intolerance**
Ineffective **Activity Planning**
Risk for Ineffective **Activity Planning**
Risk for **Adverse Reaction to Iodinated Contrast Media**
Ineffective **Airway Clearance**
Risk for **Allergy Response**
Anxiety
Risk for **Aspiration**
Risk for Impaired **Attachment**
Autonomic Dysreflexia
Risk for **Autonomic Dysreflexia**
Disorganized Infant **Behavior**
Readiness for Enhanced Organized Infant **Behavior**
Risk for Disorganized Infant **Behavior**
Risk for **Bleeding**
Risk for Unstable **Blood Glucose Level**
Disturbed **Body Image**
Risk for Imbalanced **Body Temperature**
Insufficient **Breast Milk**
Ineffective **Breastfeeding**
Interrupted **Breastfeeding**
Readiness for Enhanced **Breastfeeding**
Ineffective **Breathing Pattern**
Decreased **Cardiac Output**
Caregiver Role Strain
Risk for **Caregiver Role Strain**
Ineffective **Childbearing Process**
Readiness for Enhanced **Childbearing Process**
Risk for Ineffective **Childbearing Process**
Impaired **Comfort**
Readiness for Enhanced **Comfort**
Readiness for Enhanced **Communication**
Acute **Confusion**
Chronic **Confusion**
Risk for Acute **Confusion**
Constipation
Perceived **Constipation**
Risk for **Constipation**
Contamination
Risk for **Contamination**
Readiness for Enhanced Community **Coping**
Defensive **Coping**
Ineffective **Coping**
Readiness for Enhanced **Coping**
Ineffective Community **Coping**
Compromised Family **Coping**
Disabled Family **Coping**
Readiness for Enhanced Family **Coping**
Death Anxiety
Decisional Conflict
Readiness for Enhanced **Decision-Making**
Ineffective **Denial**
Impaired **Dentition**
Risk for Delayed **Development**
Diarrhea
Risk for **Disuse Syndrome**
Deficient **Diversional Activity**
Risk for **Dry Eye**
Risk for **Electrolyte Imbalance**
Disturbed **Energy Field**
Impaired **Environmental Interpretation Syndrome**
Adult **Failure to Thrive**
Risk for **Falls**
Dysfunctional **Family Processes**
Interrupted **Family Processes**
Readiness for Enhanced **Family Processes**
Fatigue
Fear
Ineffective Infant **Feeding Pattern**
Readiness for Enhanced **Fluid Balance**
Risk for Imbalanced **Fluid Volume**
Deficient **Fluid Volume**
Excess **Fluid Volume**
Risk for Deficient **Fluid Volume**
Impaired **Gas Exchange**
Risk for Dysfunctional **Gastrointestinal Motility**
Dysfunctional **Gastrointestinal Motility**
Risk for Ineffective **Gastrointestinal Perfusion**
Grieving

NANDA International: *Nursing diagnoses: Definitions and classification, 2012–2014,* West Sussex, England, 2012, Wiley-Blackwell. Reprinted with permission from NANDA International, Inc.

Complicated **Grieving**
Risk for Complicated **Grieving**
Risk for Disproportionate **Growth**
Delayed **Growth and Development**
Deficient Community **Health**
Risk-Prone **Health Behavior**
Ineffective **Health Maintenance**
Impaired **Home Maintenance**
Readiness for Enhanced **Hope**
Hopelessness
Risk for Compromised **Human Dignity**
Hyperthermia
Hypothermia
Readiness for Enhanced **Immunization Status**
Ineffective **Impulse Control**
Functional Urinary **Incontinence**
Overflow Urinary **Incontinence**
Reflex Urinary **Incontinence**
Stress Urinary **Incontinence**
Urge Urinary **Incontinence**
Risk for Urge Urinary **Incontinence**
Bowel **Incontinence**
Risk for **Infection**
Risk for **Injury**
Insomnia
Decreased **Intracranial Adaptive Capacity**
Neonatal **Jaundice**
Risk for Neonatal **Jaundice**
Deficient **Knowledge**
Readiness for Enhanced **Knowledge**
Latex Allergy Response
Risk for **Latex Allergy Response**
Sedentary **Lifestyle**
Risk for Impaired **Liver Function**
Risk for **Loneliness**
Risk for Disturbed **Maternal–Fetal Dyad**
Impaired **Memory**
Impaired Bed **Mobility**
Impaired Physical **Mobility**
Impaired Wheelchair **Mobility**
Moral Distress
Nausea
Noncompliance
Readiness for Enhanced **Nutrition**
Imbalanced **Nutrition:** Less Than Body Requirements
Risk for Imbalanced **Nutrition:** More Than Body Requirements
Imbalanced **Nutrition:** More Than Body Requirements
Impaired **Oral Mucous Membrane**
Risk for **Other-Directed Violence**
Acute **Pain**
Chronic **Pain**
Impaired **Parenting**
Readiness for Enhanced **Parenting**
Risk for Impaired **Parenting**
Risk for **Perioperative Positioning Injury**
Risk for **Peripheral Neurovascular Dysfunction**
Disturbed **Personal Identity**
Risk for Disturbed **Personal Identity**
Risk for **Poisoning**
Post-Trauma Syndrome
Risk for **Post-Trauma Syndrome**
Readiness for Enhanced **Power**
Powerlessness
Risk for **Powerlessness**
Ineffective **Protection**
Rape-Trauma Syndrome
Ineffective **Relationship**
Readiness for Enhanced **Relationship**
Risk for Ineffective **Relationship**
Impaired **Religiosity**
Readiness for Enhanced **Religiosity**
Risk for Impaired **Religiosity**
Relocation Stress Syndrome
Risk for **Relocation Stress Syndrome**
Risk for Ineffective **Renal Perfusion**
Impaired Individual **Resilience**
Readiness for Enhanced **Resilience**
Risk for Compromised **Resilience**
Parental **Role Conflict**
Ineffective **Role Performance**
Readiness for Enhanced **Self-Care**
Bathing **Self-Care** Deficit
Dressing **Self-Care** Deficit
Feeding **Self-Care** Deficit
Toileting **Self-Care** Deficit
Readiness for Enhanced **Self-Concept**
Risk for **Self-Directed Violence**
Chronic Low **Self-Esteem**
Situational Low **Self-Esteem**
Risk for Chronic Low **Self-Esteem**
Risk for Situational Low **Self-Esteem**
Ineffective **Self-Health Management**
Readiness for Enhanced **Self-Health Management**
Risk for **Self-Mutilation**
Self-Mutilation
Self-Neglect
Sexual Dysfunction
Ineffective **Sexuality Pattern**
Risk for **Shock**
Impaired **Skin Integrity**
Risk for Impaired **Skin Integrity**
Sleep Deprivation
Readiness for Enhanced **Sleep**
Disturbed **Sleep Pattern**
Impaired **Social Interaction**
Social Isolation
Chronic **Sorrow**
Spiritual Distress
Risk for **Spiritual Distress**

Readiness for Enhanced **Spiritual Well-Being**
Impaired **Spontaneous Ventilation**
Stress Overload
Risk for **Sudden Infant Death Syndrome**
Risk for **Suffocation**
Risk for **Suicide**
Delayed **Surgical Recovery**
Impaired **Swallowing**
Ineffective Family **Therapeutic Regimen Management**
Risk for **Thermal Injury**
Ineffective **Thermoregulation**
Impaired **Tissue Integrity**
Ineffective Peripheral **Tissue Perfusion**
Risk for Decreased Cardiac **Tissue Perfusion**
Risk for Ineffective Cerebral **Tissue Perfusion**
Risk for Ineffective Peripheral **Tissue Perfusion**
Impaired **Transfer Ability**
Risk for **Trauma**
Unilateral Neglect
Impaired **Urinary Elimination**
Readiness for Enhanced **Urinary Elimination**
Urinary Retention
Risk for **Vascular Trauma**
Dysfunctional **Ventilatory Weaning Response**
Impaired **Verbal Communication**
Impaired **Walking**
Wandering

Helpful Hints for Answering NCLEX-Style Questions

Mastering the ability to analyze NCLEX-style questions is one of the greatest challenges new nursing students face as they begin their professional education. It requires strong foundational knowledge in the physical and social sciences and nursing, as well as advanced critical thinking skills and sound clinical judgment. Most nursing students enter college highly qualified with a history of excellent grades, so they initially focus more on grades than the much more important issues of learning and patient safety. Ultimately, nursing students must overcome the tendency to focus on their GPA and instead concentrate more on understanding, applying, and synthesizing nursing content to provide safe, patient-centered care.

NCLEX questions focus primarily on the responsibilities of the nurse and how those relate to providing comprehensive, informed care. There are a variety of item formats that appear on the NCLEX licensing exam. Types of NCLEX exam questions (National Council of State Boards of Nursing, 2014) include the following:

- Multiple-choice with only one correct answer out of four possible options
- Multiple-response that require students to choose all of the correct options from a list of five
- Ranked, priority-based that ask students to put a list in order of importance in a given situation
- Fill-in-the blank or "hot spot" that require calculation of a dosage or identification on an illustration
- Medical record review that present a patient problem to solve
- Audio and graphics that ask for an aural or visual review of content

This material seeks to provide fundamentals nursing students with strategies for answering multiple-choice questions correctly.

Most faculty-developed NCLEX-style exam questions focus on some aspect of the nursing process. They expect the student to know what data are significant in a given situation or what additional information is needed. Some questions ask the student to prioritize care. Others ask about what can be delegated, or what interventions should be implemented. Still others require students to identify how best to evaluate changes in a patient's condition or situation. NCLEX-style questions contain a stem (the actual question), the correct response (answer), and various numbers of distractors (incorrect responses) if they are multiple-choice or multiple-response test items.

Some general guidelines for answering NCLEX-style multiple-choice questions include the following:

- Read the stem and the response options of the question through once, without answering the question. Read the stem again and underline or circle key words that provide a context in which the item is to be answered. Read the possible responses and cross out any that are obviously not correct. Then re-read the stem a third time to determine which of the responses is **best in the identified situation** before choosing an answer.
- Eliminate all responses that contain information you recognize as incorrect before selecting an answer.
- Avoid reading into the stem of the question by assuming additional information that is not in the test item.
- Look for similarity in the response options provided for multiple-choice questions. When only one response is to be chosen, selecting an answer that is the same as another option, worded differently, is obviously going to be wrong.
- Note qualities of the patient or subject of the question such as patient age, disease process, diagnostic test, or specific circumstance (i.e., preoperative status).
- Answer questions according to book, class, or laboratory instructional materials rather than by referencing experiences with relatives, friends, or from observing nurses or aides in the clinical setting.
- Focus on key words or phrases in the stem that indicate timing or importance. These may include first, immediately, urgent, most critical, best, next, of greatest concern, or highest priority.
    - If there is an indication of priority, use Maslow's hierarchy of needs theory or the ABCs of health care facility CPR to decide on the correct response.
    - Remember that physiological needs are the first priority according to Maslow, followed by safety, love and belonging, esteem, and self-actualization. See Figure

Compiled from National Council of State Boards of Nursing: Alternate item formats FAQs, 2014. Retrieved from *https://www.ncsbn.org/2334.htm*.

1-6 and Table 8-1 in the text for further information on Maslow's theory as it relates to nursing.

Examples

1. Which action would the nurse undertake **first** when beginning to **formulate a patient's plan of care**?
   a. List possible treatment options
   b. Identify realistic outcome indicators
   c. Consult with health care team members
   d. Rank patient concerns from assessment data
   *In this question, the key word is **first** indicating a need to pay attention to timing and the focus is **formulating a patient's care plan**. All of the responses are actions that the nurse will undertake; however, the question is asking which action comes **first**.*
   The correct response is **d**. Prioritizing or ranking patient needs precedes the identification of outcome indicators, consulting with team members, or consulting with interdisciplinary team members.
2. A patient is being discharged from the hospital with a new ileostomy. The patient expresses **concern about caring for the ostomy**. Before hospital discharge, it is **most important** for the nurse to coordinate with which member of the health care team?
   a. Home care nurse
   b. Wound ostomy continence nurse
   c. Registered dietitian
   d. Primary care provider
   *Key phrases in this stem are **most important** and **concern about caring for the ostomy**. These indicate a need to address priority and focus on a specific patient circumstance.*
   The correct answer is **b**. The wound ostomy continence nurse (WOCN) is the most important person to contact to schedule teaching sessions and follow-up care. This nurse specialist is certified in the treatment of patients who have a bowel or bladder diversion. Although team input is important, the contribution of the WOCN is paramount to help the patient achieve competence and comfort with self-care before discharge.

- In most cases, avoid responses that include the words "always" or "never" or those that imply limits with words such as "all" or "only." Each patient situation is unique and requires the nurse to determine what is most appropriate in that specific context.
  - Exceptions to this may be safety-related circumstances such as the following:
    - "Always" is appropriate in a situation such as checking patient identity before administering medications.
    - "Never" is applicable if a student is asked about giving a medication by a route that is not recommended or safe.

  Other than in these types of safety situations, options with the words "always" or "never" are rarely correct.

Examples

1. What would be the **best** therapeutic response to a patient who expresses **indecision** about recommended chemotherapy treatments?
   a. "Can you tell me why you are undecided?"
   b. "It is **always** a good idea to have chemotherapy."
   c. "What are you thinking about the treatments at this point?"
   d. "You should follow whatever your health care provider recommends."
   *The key words in this question stem are **best** and **indecision**. Response b can immediately be omitted as a response option since it contains the word **always** in what is not specifically a safety-related circumstance.*
   The correct response is **c**. Asking open-ended questions allows patients to share freely on a subject. "Why" questions, using closed-ended questions, and giving advice such as, "It is always a good idea to have chemotherapy" are all examples of nontherapeutic communication that limit patient reflection and sharing on topics of concern.
2. In which scenario is **hospice care** provided?
   a. **Only** in the homes of the terminally ill
   b. For any terminal illness that requires symptom control
   c. For cancer patients **only** in their last weeks of life
   d. In hospital settings based on the seriousness of the illness
   *This question focuses on a specific context (**hospice care**) and two of the distractors contain the word **only**, which is restrictive and not applicable. Those two possible responses can be omitted immediately.*
   The correct answer is **b**. Hospice care is provided in a variety of settings, including home care, freestanding inpatient units, hospitals, long-term care facilities, and prisons, as well as to the homeless, for patients with any disease or illness that has been determined to be life-limiting (prognosis of 6-month survival). Any patient who is experiencing symptoms—physical, psychological, or spiritual—can benefit from hospice support and symptom control at the end of life.

- If there is a response that refers to assessment, that most often will be the correct answer. Assessment is the first step of the nursing process that guides the actions of the health care team. The item response may not use the word "assess" specifically, but may use words or phrases such as: look for, observe, listen, check, verify, identify, recognize, determine, note, gather, or collect.
- Before selecting a response that is similar to "Notify the patient's primary care provider," consider if any of the other options indicates a nursing action that would provide pertinent patient data that should be collected or addressed before calling the physician or nurse practitioner.

Examples

1. While auscultating a patient's lungs the nurse notes diminished breath sounds at the base of the right lung. What action should the nurse take next?
   a. Refer the patient for a chest x-ray.
   b. **Listen** to the base of the patient's left lung.
   c. **Notify the patient's primary care provider** (PCP).
   d. Palpate the patient's lung fields bilaterally.

   This question illustrates the concepts of recognizing alternative words for assessment (in this case, ***listen****) and* ***an action that should be carried out before notifying the patient's PCP****.*

   The correct response is **b**. When auscultating a patient's lungs, the nurse should follow a pattern that compares lung fields side to side in each area, making listening to the base of the patient's left lung the next step for this nurse to take. Referring the patient for an x-ray, palpating the patient's lung fields, and notifying the patient's physician might be indicated later, depending on the outcome of the full respiratory assessment.
2. The nurse is caring for a 6-year-old patient in the emergency department who just had a full left leg cast placed for a fracture. As the nurse is reviewing the discharge instructions with the patient's mother, she states, "You don't have to go over those—I'll read them at home." What should the nurse do?
   a. **Contact the physician** immediately.
   b. Consider the possibility of health literacy limitations and **assess** further.
   c. Stop the teaching, because the mother obviously has taken care of casts before.
   d. Explain to the mother that reading the instructions with her is required.

   This question illustrates an ***alternative wording for PCP*** *and actually uses the word* ***"assess,"*** *even though it is not the first word in the answer.*

   The correct response is **b**. The patient's mother may have limited reading skills or health literacy and should be further assessed. Contacting the physician in this situation would not be appropriate because ensuring that the patient and family understand discharge instructions is the responsibility of the nurse. Assuming that the mother has taken care of casts in the past may be inaccurate. Stating that reading the instructions with the nurse is a requirement does not ensure that the patient or mother comprehend the instructions.

Ultimately the keys to analyzing and answering NCLEX-style multiple choice questions are as follows:

1. Knowing foundational information
2. Determining the subject, focus, and/or circumstance of the stem, and
3. Recognizing the priority, context, and nuances of each possible response.

Practice taking as many NCLEX-style questions as possible. Mastering the art of applying nursing knowledge to patient care situations enhances your clinical decision-making skills and enables you to provide safe patient care now and for the rest of your nursing career!

GLOSSARY

abnormal reactive hyperemia The persistent redness that occurs during a stage I pressure ulcer due to excessive vasodilation caused by pressure.

absorption Movement of smaller elements through the walls of the digestive tract and into the blood. The passage of a drug from the administration site into the bloodstream.

abstinence Voluntarily avoidance of sexual intercourse.

abuse Anything offensive, harmful, or injurious to an individual, that can pose a direct safety threat. The four major types of abuse are physical, psychological/emotional, sexual, and financial.

accidents Incidents that occur at random and may be unavoidable.

accommodation Changing the pattern of behavior when encountering new similar objects. The ability of the eyes to focus on near objects.

accountability The concept of being answerable for one's actions.

acculturation Cultural change achieved through the exchange of cultural features resulting from firsthand contact between groups.

accuracy To represent something in a true and correct way.

acid A chemical that releases hydrogen ions.

activated partial thromboplastin time Coagulation blood test used to detect bleeding disorders caused by abnormalities of the intrinsic clotting system and to monitor the effectiveness of heparin therapy.

active range of motion Demonstration of full, independent movement of each joint.

active transport The movement of a solute from areas of lower to higher concentration which requires energy.

activities of daily living (ADLs) Activities that include bathing, mouth care, grooming, toileting, dressing, and eating.

actual nursing diagnoses NANDA-I diagnostic labels for existing problems or concerns of a patient.

acute illness An illness typically characterized by an abrupt onset and short duration (less than 6 months).

acute pain Pain that lasts for less than 6 months.

acute wound A wound that progresses through the phases of wound healing in a rapid, uncomplicated manner.

adaptation The process of adjusting schemes in response to stimuli within the environment.

adaptive cognition The idea that thought is more responsive to context and less constrained by the need to find only one answer to a question.

a-delta fibers Large-diameter, myelinated fibers with rapid conduction that cause sharp, acute pain.

advance directives Consists of three documents: (1) living will, (2) durable power of attorney, and (3) health care proxy, commonly referred to as a *durable power of attorney for health care.*

Advanced Practice Registered Nurse (APRN) A registered nurse who has met advanced educational and clinical practice requirements at a minimum of a master's level and provides at least some level of direct care to patient populations.

adventitious breath sounds Abnormal sounds that originate in the lungs and airways.

adverse effects Severe, unintended, unwanted, and often unpredictable drug reactions.

advocacy Supporting or promoting the interests of others or of a cause greater than oneself.

advocate Someone who supports and promotes the interests of others.

aerobic exercise Physical activity that requires increased work by the heart and lungs for oxygen metabolism to produce energy.

afebrile Maintaining normal body temperature between 36.5° to 37.5° C; (97.6° to 99.6° F).

affective domain A form of learning that recognizes the emotional component of integrating new knowledge.

agents of disease Causes of a disease.

agnostic A person who believes that the nature or existence of God is unknowable.

airborne transmission Microorganisms are dispersed by air currents and inhaled or deposited on the skin of a susceptible host.

airway obstruction A potentially life-threatening emergency caused by blockage of the pharynx either by the tongue or another object.

alanine aminotransferase (ALT) An enzyme found primarily in the liver and also found in the kidneys, heart, and skeletal muscle.

albinism A congenital loss of pigmentation characterized by a generalized lack of melanin pigment in the eyes, skin, and hair or, in rare instances, in the eyes alone.

albumin The major plasma protein, primarily responsible for maintaining fluid balance by providing colloidal osmotic pressure in the blood.

aldosterone A hormone that acts on the distal convoluted tubule of the kidney to increase the reabsorption of water and sodium back into the bloodstream.

algor mortis A drop in body temperature as the body begins to cool after death.

alkaline phosphatase (ALP) An enzyme found primarily in the liver levels, which is a useful indicator of liver and bone disease.

allergic reactions Unpredictable immune responses to medications.

allostasis The means by which homeostasis is reestablished. Its purpose is to assist the body in maintaining stability .

alopecia Permanent or temporary hair loss.

Alzheimer's disease The most common type of dementia in which protein fragments called amyloid plaques build up between the nerve cells of the brain, blocking electrical and chemical connections between neurons.

ambulatory care Care that takes place in a physician's office or outpatient clinic.

amino acids The "building blocks" of proteins that must be consumed in food every day.

amyloid plaques Protein fragments.

anabolism The use of energy to change simple materials into complex body substances and tissue.

anaerobic exercise Physical activity that does not require oxygen metabolism.

analgesic Pain-reducing medication.

analytic epidemiology Generates a hypothesis of why the disease might be occurring in the community and then tests the hypothesis.

anaphylactic reaction A severe allergic reaction.

anesthesia An inhaled or injected pharmacologic agent that makes the patient insensitive to pain and sensation during a procedure or surgery.

anger An emotion that involves antagonism toward another person or situation. It is evoked when an individual feels wronged.

angina pectoris The crushing chest pain that is the first indication of an oxygen-deprived heart.

angioplasty The balloon surgery that flattens fatty deposits to open blood flow in blocked arteries.

anonymity A person's identity or personal information is not known.

anorexia nervosa A very serious disorder in which the person exhibits life-threatening practices as a result of an altered mental state. There is a distortion of body image with the intense fear of gaining weight or being viewed as "fat," despite the fact that the individual's weight is less than healthy or normal.

anorexia A loss of appetite by patients experiencing illness or side effects from allergies, medications, or treatments, such as chemotherapy, that suppress the desire to eat.

anorgasmia Inability to achieve orgasm.

anosmia The complete loss of the sense of smell.

antagonism A drug's effect is decreased by taking it with another substance.
anthropometry The study of measurements of the human body.
antibodies Immunoglobulin molecules that recognize foreign invaders.
ANTICipate model A handoff mechanism endorsed by the Agency for Healthcare Research and Quality in which administrative data (A) must be accurate; new clinical information (N) must be updated; tasks (T) performed by the provider must be clearly explained; illness (I) severity must be communicated; and contingency plans (C) for changes in clinical status must be outlined to assist cross-coverage of the patient.
anticipatory grief The cognitive, affective, cultural, and social reactions to an expected death, felt by the patient as well as family members and friends.
antidiuretic hormone A hormone secreted by the pituitary gland that maintains serum osmolality by controlling the amount of water excreted in the urine.
antiembolism hose Tightly fitting elastic stockings that are used to promote blood flow of venous return and prevent edema in the lower extremities, deep vein thrombosis, venous stasis, and pulmonary emboli.
antigen Protein molecules on the surface of foreign invaders or nonliving substances such as toxins, chemicals, drugs, or particles that trigger the immune response.
anuria The failure of the kidneys to excrete urine.
anxiety A response to stress that causes apprehension or uncertainty. there are various levels and types of anxiety.
aphasia Speech or language impairment.
apical pulse A central pulse that can be auscultated over the apex of the heart at the point of maximal impulse.
APIE note Adds *A*, assessment, combining subjective and objective data to the PIE format.
apnea An absence of breathing; brain damage occurs after 4 to 6 minutes of apnea.
applied research Testing the application of theories in different situations with different populations.
approximated Brought together.
arrhythmia An irregular heartbeat that can prevent the heart from pumping adequate blood.
arterial blood gas (ABG) A diagnostic test that examines arterial blood to assess a patient's oxygenation status and acid-base balance.
ascites An abnormal collection of fluid in the peritoneal cavity.
asepsis Freedom from and prevention of disease-causing contamination.
aspartate aminotransferase (AST) An enzyme found primarily in the heart, liver, and muscle which is released after cell death or injury.
aspiration Inhalation of fluid or foreign matter into the lungs and bronchi.
assault A threat of bodily harm or violence caused by a demonstration of force by the potential perpetrator. A feeling of imminent harm or feeling of immediate danger must exist for assault to be claimed.
assertiveness The ability to express ideas and concerns clearly while respecting the thoughts of others.
assessment The organized and ongoing appraisal of a patient's well-being.
assimilation Attempting to use a new object in the same way that more familiar objects are used. The process by which individuals from one cultural group merge with, or blend into, a second group.
assisted suicide A person causes his or her own death with the assistance of oral medication or an intravenous injection supplied by a physician or health care provider.
asthma A chronic respiratory disorder characterized by airway spasms, bronchial narrowing or obstruction, mucus accumulation and airway inflammation.
atelectasis The collapse of all or part of the lung.
atheist A person who believes that a god or higher powers do not exist.
atherosclerosis The buildup of plaque in coronary arteries around the heart.
atrial natriuretic peptide A hormone secreted by cells in the atrium of the heart in response to an increase in blood pressure causing an increase in glomerular filtration rate, which leads to increased excretion of water in urine.
atrophy Wasting away of muscles; a decrease in size.
auricle The outer ear.
auscultation Listening, with the assistance of a stethoscope, to sounds within the body.
auscultatory gap During blood pressure measurement, absence of Korotkoff sounds noted in some patients after the initial systolic pressure.
autocratic leader A leader who exercises strong control over subordinates. This type of leader assumes that followers are motivated by external forces such as the need for approval by the supervisor and the need to avoid punishment.
autonomy The freedom to make decisions supported by knowledge and self-confidence.
axilla Armpit.

bacteria Single-cell organisms that are capable of causing disease, but that also live on and in the skin, eyes, nose, mouth, upper throat, lower urethra, lower intestine, and large intestine as normal flora.
bag-valve-mask (BVM) device Also known as an Ambu bag; a resuscitator bag used to assist ventilation.
bar-code medication administration (BCMA) After using a portable scanner to sign into the electronic medication administration record (eMAR) by scanning his or her id badge, the nurse then electronically scans the bar codes on the patient's wristband and the drug to determine that the right patient is getting the right drug and dose at the right time. An alert on the eMAR signals a potential error, and it is the nurse's responsibility to verify all information before administering the medication to the patient.
basal metabolic rate (BMR) The minimum amount of energy required to maintain body functions at rest while awake.
bases Substances that accept hydrogen ions.
basic research Research conducted to generate theories.
basophils A type of white blood cell that is involved in the inflammatory response to injury.
battery Actual physical harm caused to another person.
Behavioral Risk Factor Surveillance System (BRFSS) An ongoing, state-based, random-digit-dialed telephone survey of the noninstitutionalized U.S. population over 18 years old. BRFSS collects data on health risk behaviors and preventive health services related to leading causes of death.
behavioral theories Theories that assume that leaders learn certain behaviors. These theories focus on what leaders do, rather than on what characteristics they innately possess.
beliefs A mental representation of reality or a person's perceptions about what is right, true, or real, or what the person expects to happen in a given situation.
beneficence Doing good; nurses demonstrate beneficence by acting on behalf of others and placing priority on the needs of others rather than on personal thoughts and feelings.
bereavement The inner feelings and outward expressions that people experiencing loss demonstrate.
bias An inclination or tendency toward favoritism or partiality.
bier block A regional anesthetic involving injection of an agents into the venous circulation of an extremity.
bilirubin A components of bile that is synthesized in the liver, spleen, and bone marrow.
bingeing The intake of excessive amounts of food, as many as 2000 to 3000 calories at one time.
bioburden Bacterial load.
bioethics The study of ethical and philosophical issues in biology and medicine.
biopsy Removal of a sample of cells to detect cancer.
bioterrorism The deliberate release of biological agents such as bacteria, viruses, and other germs to cause illness or death in people, animals, or plants.
bisexual An individual who is emotionally or sexually attracted to people of either sex.

blog A type of social media that is usually maintained by an individual and has regular entries of commentary, descriptions of events, or other material such as graphics or videos.

blood pressure The measurable pressure of blood within the systemic arteries.

blood urea nitrogen A kidney function test that measures urea in the blood.

body mass index (BMI) A helpful tool for determining the extent of obesity and its potential health complications.

borborygmi Hyperactive bowel sounds audible without a stethoscope.

bradycardia A slow heart rate of less than 60 beats per minute in the adult.

bradypnea A decrease in respiratory rate to less than 10 breaths per minute in the adult.

brain natriuretic peptide (BNP) A hormone produced by myocardial cells and released from the ventricle during times of increased pressure or overload.

breadth To consider a topic, problem, issue, etc., from every relevant viewpoint.

bronchodilators Oral or inhaled medications that increase the diameter of the bronchioles, which decreases wheezing and improves oxygenation.

bruit An abnormal swooshing sound audible on auscultation over an aneurysm, the carotid artery, or an arteriovenous (AV) fistula.

bruxism The clenching of teeth or the grinding of teeth from side to side that occurs during sleep.

buccal Medication administered against the mucous membrane of the cheek.

bulimia nervosa An eating disorder that involves an obsession with bingeing followed by purging. In an effort not to gain weight from the excessive amount of food eaten; the person may use self-induced vomiting or excessive exercise.

bureaucratic leader A leader that assumes that followers are motivated by external forces. This type of leader relies on policies and procedures to direct goals and work processes.

burnout Mental or physical exhaustion due to constant stress or activity.

C fibers Smaller, unmyelinated fibers with slow conduction that cause a diffuse, dull, and longer-lasting pain.

cachexia Physical wasting.

capillary closing pressure The minimum pressure required to collapse a capillary.

capillary refill An indication of peripheral blood perfusion, measured in seconds.

carbohydrates Chemical substances compiled from carbon, hydrogen, and oxygen molecules.

carbon monoxide A colorless, odorless gas that can cause sudden illness and even death.

cardiac murmurs Blowing or swishing sounds heard on systole or diastole, caused by increased or abnormal blood flow through the valves of the heart.

caring Having concern or regard for that which affects the welfare of another.

case law Judicial decisions from individual court cases. It was historically referred to as "common law."

case manager Coordinator of care.

catabolism The breaking down of substances from complex to simple, resulting in a release of energy.

cataplexy The sudden loss of voluntary muscle tone.

cataracts A condition that causes the lens of the eye to become cloudy and impair vision.

cellular immunity A defense by the white blood cells—lymphocytes—in response to foreign microorganisms.

Centers for Medicare and Medicaid Services (CMS) The federal organization that certifies all Medicare- and Medicaid-participating hospitals.

central venous catheter A central venous access device that is inserted into a major vein in the arm or chest with the tip of the catheter lying in the superior vena cava, just outside the right atrium.

centration Focusing on only one aspect of an object.

cerebrovascular accident (CVA) Injury to the brain that occurs when an area of the brain is deprived of blood flow; also called a stroke.

cerumen Earwax.

chafing Inflammation of the skin due to friction.

channel The method of communication. Any of the five senses may be used as channels.

charting by exception (CBE) Documentation that records only abnormal or significant data. It reduces charting time by assuming certain norms. In this type of charting each facility must define what is normal. Any assessment finding outside normal is charted as an exception.

cheilitis Dry, cracked lips.

chemical restraint A medication that is administered to a patient to control behavior.

chemoreceptors Sensory nerve endings that react to chemicals.

chief complaint The patient's presenting problem, reason for seeking care.

cholesterol A waxy, fatlike substance that is found in all cells of the body.

chronic bronchitis A disorder associated with chronic obstructive pulmonary disease that is characterized by inflammation of the larger airways, increased production of mucus, and chronic cough.

chronic grief A type of complicated grief characterized by grief reactions that do not diminish over time and continue for a long period of time.

chronic illness Any condition characterized by a loss or abnormality of body function that lasts longer than 6 months and requires ongoing long-term care.

chronic obstructive pulmonary disease (COPD) A general term used for a group of disorders characterized by impaired airflow in the lungs.

chronic pain Pain that lasts for longer than 6 months.

chronic wound A wound that fails to progress to healing in a timely manner, often remaining open for an extended period of time.

chyme Semiliquid product of digestion that travels from the stomach through the intestines.

cilia Tiny hairs lining the nasal passages.

circadian rhythms Day-night, 24-hour biological cycle.

circulating nurse A registered nurse who is the patient's advocate in the operating room, and a liaison between scrubbed personnel and the surgical team.

circumcision Surgical removal of the foreskin of the penis that is considered a religious rite for those of the Jewish and Muslim faiths.

civility Acting politely, showing respect.

clarity To be easily understood, clear in thought or style.

clean contaminated wound A wound that is similar to a clean wound, but because the surgery involves organ systems that are likely to contain bacteria, the risk for infection is greater.

clean wound A wound in which there is no infection and the risk for development of an infection is low.

clinical manifestations Signs and symptoms.

clinical reasoning Using critical thinking, knowledge, and experience to develop solutions to problems and make decisions in a clinical setting.

clinical research Research that is used when testing theories about the effectiveness of interventions.

clonus A repetitive vibratory contraction of the muscle that occurs in response to muscle and tendon stretch.

closed wound A wound in which the skin is still intact.

Clostridium difficile A bacterium that causes diarrhea and inflammation of the colon; often called "C. diff."

clustering Organizing patient assessment data into groupings with similar etiologies (underlying causes).

coanalgesic medications Medication that works synergistically with standard pain medications to enhance pain relief and to treat side effects of the medication.

code of ethics A formalized statement that defines the values, morals, and standards guiding practice within a specific discipline or profession.

codependency A dysfunctional relationship in which the person who wants to help acts in a manner that enables harmful behavior by another person.

cognition Knowing influenced by awareness and judgment; it comprises skills that include language, calculation, memory, attention, reasoning, learning, problem solving, and decision making.

cognitive domain A form of learning based on knowledge and material that is remembered.

collaboration Two or more people work together towards a common goal. In nursing, collaboration occurs when RNs, UAP, LPN/LVNs, primary care providers, social workers, clergy, and therapists all interact productively to provide quality patient care.

colloids Substances that do not dissolve easily.

colonized wound A wound in which one or more organisms are present on the surface of the wound when a swab culture is obtained but there is no overt sign of an infection in the tissue below the surface.

colonoscopy A procedure performed through a scope to visualize inflamed tissue, ulcers, and abnormal growths in the anus, rectum, and colon.

colostomy Surgically created bowel diversion when a portion of the colon is brought through an opening created in the abdominal wall.

community-based nursing Care for individuals within specific areas such as schools, prisons, or businesses.

comorbid Two or more medical conditions existing simultaneously.

complicated grief A grieving person is not able to progress through the normal stages of grief.

complicated loss Loss that occurs with a sudden death, a violent or traumatic death, multiple deaths, loss that is related to a social stigma, and with the death of a young person.

computed tomography (CT) A radiological procedure in which the use of a special scanner allows cross-sectional images of an organ to be visualized.

computer literacy Knowledge of computers and the ability to use them efficiently.

computerized provider order entry (CPOE) Orders are entered into a computer by clinicians and sent directly to the appropriate department.

conception The process of a sperm and an ovum uniting.

conceptual framework or model A collection of interrelated concepts that provides direction for nursing practice, research, and education. A conceptual model addresses the four concepts of the nursing metaparadigm: optimal functioning of the person or patient, how people interact with the environment, illness and health promotion, and nursing's role.

condom A thin rubber sheath that covers the penis to prevent sperm from entering the vagina.

cones A type of photoreceptors present in the retina that detect sharp, color images.

confidentiality The ethical principle that a health professional will hold secure all information relating to a patient unless the patient gives consent for disclosure.

conservation The ability to recognize that objects remain the same even if they change in appearance.

consistency The measurement of organ location and size against the expected anatomic norm, any distention or masses, and vibration or pulsation associated with movement.

constipation Infrequent or difficult bowel movements, or having fewer than three bowel movements per week.

constitutional law Laws derived from a formal written constitution that defines the powers of government and the responsibilities of its elected or appointed officials.

contact One person's body surface touching the surface of another's body or object.

contaminated wound A wound with bacteria present resulting from trauma, a break in sterile technique during surgery or spillage of bowel contents or other bacteria-laden material during surgery.

continuous theories A theory of development that subscribes to the belief that development occurs in a smooth and gradual process from infancy to adulthood.

contraception Techniques used for birth control, to prevent pregnancy.

contracture Permanent fixation of a joint.

control group The group in an experiment that does not receive the treatment.

controlled substance Drugs with regulated manufacturing, prescribing, and dispensing requirements.

coping The dynamic cognitive and behavioral efforts to manage demands (internal or external) that are appraised as exceeding immediately available resources.

core temperature The temperature of deep tissues.

correlational research Research used to explore a relationship between two variables.

C-reactive protein A protein produced by the liver in response to inflammation, tissue damage, and infection.

creatine kinase An enzyme found primarily in skeletal muscle, cardiac muscle, and brain tissue.

creatinine A waste product of skeletal muscle metabolism that is excreted via the kidneys.

creativity The ability to think differently.

crepitation (crepitus) Crackling or rubbing felt as a result of air in superficial tissues.

criminal law The body of state and federal laws written to prevent harm to the country, state, and individual citizens.

crisis intervention Short-term assistance provided to an individual with the goal of regaining equilibrium in a time of physical or emotional upheaval.

critical appraisal A balanced evaluation of the strengths and benefits as well as the weaknesses and flaws of the research.

critical closing pressure The minimum pressure required to collapse a capillary.

critical thinking A complex process that involves reflection while thinking to provide for a more clear, precise, accurate, relevant, consistent, and fair thought process.

Cross-Linking Theory of Aging The theory that suggests that, over time, protein fibers that make up the body's connective tissue form bonds, or crosslinks, with one another causing tissue becomes less elastic and leading to negative outcomes such as loss of flexibility, clouding of the lens of the eye, clogged arteries, and damaged kidneys.

crystallized intelligence Skills that depend on accumulated knowledge, experience, good judgment, and mastery of social conventions.

crystalloids Solutes that dissolve easily in water.

cue A hint or an indication of a potential disease process or disorder.

cultural competence The complex integration of an individual's knowledge, attitudes, beliefs, skills, and encounters with those of persons from different cultures.

cultural openness A lifelong stance that promotes cultural self-awareness and continuing development of transcultural skills.

cultural sensitivity The recognition that there are differences among cultures.

culturally congruent care The use of culturally based knowledge in sensitive, creative, safe, and meaningful ways to promote the health and well-being of individuals or groups.

culture The learned, shared, and transmitted knowledge of values, beliefs, and ways of life of a particular group that are generally transmitted from one generation to another and influence the individual's thinking, decisions, and actions in patterned or certain ways. May change over time.

cyanosis Bluish discoloration of the skin and mucous membranes, caused by decreased oxygen levels in arterial blood.

dandruff Scaling and flaking of the skin of the scalp.

dangling Sitting up on the side of the bed prior to standing.

DAR note A charting format that is based on Data collected about the patient problems, the Action initiated, and the patient's Response to the actions.

data Information collected by the researcher from the participants in the research and is expressed either as numbers or words.

data analysis Specific procedures used to summarize the words or numbers and create a meaningful result for interpretation.

debridement The removal of necrotic tissue.

decision making Choosing a solution or answer from among different options; often considered a step in the problem-solving process.

decision support system (DSS) A computerized system that supports decision making activities such as choosing appropriate diagnoses or medications, and improving the quality of care through reminders and safe-practice alerts.

decode The receiver's interpretation of the message. Numerous factors may affect the ability of the receiver to accurately decode a message. The message may be misinterpreted if clarity is not sought and achieved by the receiver.

decussate To cross over.

dedication The ability to spend the time necessary to accomplish a task.

deductive reasoning Generating facts or details from a major theory, generalization, or premise (i.e., from general to specific).

defamation of character Public statements made by an individual that are false and injurious to another person.

defecation The final act of digestion by which the solid, semisolid, or liquid waste is expelled by the body through the anus.

defense mechanisms Unconscious strategies that allow an individual to decrease or avoid unpleasant circumstances.

defining characteristics Cues or clusters of related assessment data that are signs, symptoms, or indications of an actual or health-promotion nursing diagnosis.

dehiscence The partial or complete separation of the tissue layers during the healing process; usually occurs in connection with surgical incisions.

dehydration A hypertonic form of fluid volume deficit, which occurs with excessive loss of water or inadequate intake of fluid.

delayed grief A type of complicated grief characterized by suppression of the grief reaction while the grieving individual consciously or unconsciously avoids the pain that has occurred with the loss.

delegation A transfer of responsibility that gives a competent individual the authority to perform a selected nursing task in a specific situation.

delirium A reversible state of acute confusion characterized by a disturbance in consciousness or a change in cognition that develops over 1 to 2 days and is caused by a medical condition.

dementia A permanent decline in mental function over a period of time that is characterized by the decline in many cognitive abilities, including reasoning, use of language, memory, computation, judgment, and learning.

democratic leader A leader that believes that employees are motivated by internal means and want to participate in decision making. Views self as equal to followers.

dentures Artificial teeth.

deontology An ethical theory that stresses the rightness or wrongness of individual behaviors, duties, and obligations without concern for the consequences of specific actions.

dependent nursing interventions Tasks the nurse undertakes that are within the nursing scope of practice but require the order of a physician or PCP to be implemented.

dependent variable The outcome that is affected by the independent variable.

depression A mood disorder characterized by a sense of hopelessness and persistent unhappiness.

depth Exploring a topic or problem below the surface to identify and manage related complexities.

dermis Thick, middle layer of skin between the epidermis and the deeper subcutaneous layer.

descriptive epidemiology Studies that are conducted once a disease is evident.

descriptive research Identifies data and characteristics about a population or phenomenon.

detumescence Loss of blood from erectile tissue.

development The increasing maturation of physical ability, thought processes, and behaviors over time.

diabetic retinopathy A complication of diabetes mellitus in which the blood vessels of the retina become damaged.

diagnosis label A concise term or phrase that represents a pattern of related clustered data.

dialysis A technique by which fluids and molecules pass through an artificial semipermeable membrane and are filtered via osmosis.

diaphragm A flexible, round rubber dome placed in the vagina for contraception.

diarrhea An intestinal disorder characterized by an abnormally high frequency and increased fluidity of fecal evacuations.

diastolic pressure The lowest pressure on arterial walls, which occurs when the heart rests.

diffusion The movement of solutes across a selectively permeable membrane from areas of higher concentration to areas of lower concentration until equilibrium has been reached.

digestion The breaking down of food into smaller particles of nutrients.

diplopia Double vision.

direct care Interventions that are carried out by having personal contact with patients.

discipline A specific field of study or branch of instruction or learning.

discontinuous theories A theory that describe development as progressing through a series of distinct and predictable stages triggered by inborn factors.

discrimination Policies and practices that harm a group and its members.

disenfranchised grief Any loss that is not validated or recognized, occurring when the loss cannot be openly acknowledged or publicly shared by the grieving individual.

disinfection The removal of pathogenic microorganisms.

dissemination The communication and distribution of research information and findings.

distress Stress that is beyond the ability of an individual to cope with or adapt to effectively.

distribution The process of delivering a medication to tissues, organs, and, ultimately, the specific site of action.

disuse osteoporosis Loss of bone mass due to lack of activity.

do-not-resuscitate (DNR) order Directions given by patients who are faced with life-threatening illness, or their designated family members acting as health care proxies, to refuse or limit extraordinary measures that may prolong the patient from experiencing natural death.

droplet transmission The mucous membranes of the respiratory tract (nose, mouth, or conjunctiva) are exposed to the secretions of an infected individual.

drug Any substance that either positively or negatively alters physiologic function.

drug incompatibility Mixing medications in a solution that causes precipitation, or combining a drug with another drug that causes an adverse chemical reaction.

drug tolerance An adaptation to medication, which eventually leads to less effective pain relief.

dualistic thinking Dividing information, values, and authority into right and wrong, good and bad, we and they.

durable power of attorney A legal document that allows a designated person to make legal decisions on behalf of an individual who is unable or not permitted to make legal decisions independently.

dyspareunia Painful intercourse.

dysphagia Difficulty swallowing.

dyspnea Difficult, labored breathing, usually with a rapid, shallow pattern and sometimes painful.

dysrhythmia An irregular rhythm in the pulse, caused by an early, late, or missed heartbeat.

dyssomnias Disorders associated with getting to sleep, staying asleep, or being excessively sleepy.

dysuria Painful urination.

early intervention Strategies introduced at the first detection of a possible health problem.

ecchymosis Bruising.

edema Swelling.

effleurage A massage technique that employs long hand movements along the length of the back muscles.

ego The part of the mind that functions in reality and allows people to seek out pleasure within the norms of society.

egocentric A stage of development in which children believe that everyone else sees the world exactly as they see it.

elective surgery A surgical procedure that is planned in advance and performed to improve the patient's quality of life.
electrical shock The energy flows through the body, or a portion of the body, to the ground when a person comes in contact with an energy source .
electrocardiogram (ECG) A recording of the electrical current generated by the heart during depolarization and repolarization of the cardiac muscle.
electrolytes Positively or negatively charged ions that conduct electrical impulses across cells.
electronic health record (EHR) A longitudinal record of health that includes the information from both inpatient and outpatient episodes of health care from one or more care settings.
electronic infusion device Intravenous infusion pump used for a more precise delivery of intravenous fluids.
electronic medical record (EMR) A record of one episode of care, either an inpatient stay or an outpatient appointment.
embryo A developing zygote after 3 weeks up until 2 months after conception.
emergency surgery A surgical procedure that is unanticipated and is performed immediately to preserve the life of the patient, a body part, or body function.
emerging adulthood Prolonged transition phase between adolescence into adulthood.
emic A perspective that focuses on the local, indigenous, and insider's culture.
emphysema A disorder associated with chronic obstructive pulmonary disease that is characterized by inflamed and damaged alveolar walls in the lungs.
encode The translation of the sender's thoughts and feelings into communication with a receiver.
enculturation The process whereby a culture is passed from generation to generation.
endoscopy An examination of the interior of an organ or cavity by means of a fiberoptic scope.
endotracheal tube Semirigid, curved airway tube with a cuff at the distal end that seals to prevent aspiration of gastric contents into the lung, allows positive pressure for ventilation, and keeps air from leaking out of the airway.
enema The introduction of solutions into the rectum and sigmoid colon via the anus.
enteral feeding Tube feeding.
enuresis The involuntary passing of urine.
environmental (extrinsic) factors Environmental variables such as food sources, vectors of disease or socioeconomic influences.
enzymes Proteins responsible for catalyzing most chemical reactions in the body, such as digesting food and synthesizing new compounds.
eosinophils A type of white blood cell that destroys parasites and is involved in allergic reactions.
epidemiology The study of disease incidence and prevalence.
epidermis The outermost layer of the skin and the thinnest of the layers, which regenerates every 4 to 6 weeks.
epidural anesthesia A regional anesthesia in which an agent is injected into the epidural space through the lumbar or thoracic region.
epistaxis Nosebleed.
epithelial tissue Tissue that lines tubes, cavities, and the surface of the skin.
equilibration The process by which a balance between present understanding and new experiences is restored.
equilibrium Balance.
erectile dysfunction (ED) The inability to achieve or maintain a penile erection for sexual intercourse.
erythema Redness of the skin caused by congestion or dilation of the superficial blood vessels in the skin, signaling circulatory changes to an area.
erythrocytes Red blood cells.
eschar Necrotic tissue.
ethics The standards of moral conduct within a society. The main concepts in nursing ethics are accountability, advocacy, autonomy, beneficence, confidentiality, fidelity, justice, nonmaleficence, responsibility, and veracity.
ethnicity An individual's identification with or membership in a particular racial, national, or cultural group and observation of the group's customs, beliefs, and language.
ethnocentrism The belief that one's own culture is superior to that of another while using one's own cultural values as the criteria by which to judge other cultures.
ethnography A focus on the sociology of meaning through close field observation of a sociocultural phenomenon.
etic A perspective that focuses on the outsider's world and especially on professional views.
etiologic factors Causes of a disease.
eupnea Normal respiration with a normal rate and depth for the patient's age.
eustress Motivational stress that is associated with effective coping and adaptation.
euthanasia The act of painlessly ending the life of another.
evaluation Examination of goal or outcome attainment by focusing on the patient and the patient's response to nursing interventions.
evidence-based practice (EBP) The integration of best research evidence with clinical expertise, patient values and needs, and the delivery of quality, cost-effective health care.
evisceration The total separation of the tissue layers, allowing the protrusion of visceral organs through the incision.
exacerbation Worsening of clinical manifestations.
exaggerated grief A type of complicated grief where the survivor is overwhelmed by grief and cannot function in daily life.
excoriation An abrasion due to rubbing or scratching.
excretion A process that removes the less active drug or its metabolites.
experimental research Research that explores the causal relationships between variables.
extracellular fluid Body fluid that is outside the cells.
fairness Avoiding bias or prejudice and dealing with a situation in a just manner.
faith A belief beyond oneself that is based on trust and life experience rather than scientific data.
falls An events in which an individual unintentionally and through the force of gravity drops to the ground, floor, or some other lower level.
false imprisonment The unauthorized restraint or detention of a person.
fat-soluble vitamins Vitamins A, D, E, and K are fat-soluble vitamins that are stored in the liver and fat tissue. Toxicity may result if excessive amounts are taken.
febrile Elevated body temperature.
fecal occult blood test A test that measures microscopic amounts of blood in the feces.
feedback The response of the receiver to avoid misinterpretation of a message.
felony A serious crime that results in the perpetrator's being imprisoned in a state or federal facility for more than 1 year.
fetus The term for an embryo beyond 2 months after conception.
fever A rise in body temperature above normal, caused by trauma or illness.
fiber A complex carbohydrate classified as either soluble or insoluble.
fiberoptics A system in which flexible glass or plastic fibers are used to transmit light around curves and corners which allows direct visualization of the area of interest.
fibrinogen An essential component of blood clotting that converts into fibrin threads in the presence of ionized calcium.
fidelity Keeping promises or fulfilling agreements made with others.
fight-or-flight response A physiologic response to stress, whether physical or psychological, that activates the autonomic nervous system, resulting in an increase in heart rate, blood pressure, and respirations along with pupil dilation and a decrease in gastric motility and blood flow to the skin.
filtration The process by which fluid and solutes move together from an area of higher pressure to one of lower pressure.
first-order beliefs The foundation or the basis of an individual's belief system.
fistula Abnormal connections between two internal organs or between an internal organ and, through the skin to the outside of the body.
flaccidity Lack of muscle tone.

flatulence The production of a mixture of gases in the intestine as a byproducts of the digestive process.
fluid intelligence The ability to detect relationships among stimuli, the speed with which information is analyzed, and the capacity of working memory.
fluid volume excess A fluid imbalance that occurs when fluid intake exceeds output.
focused assessment An examination in which only specific, relevant areas are examined.
footdrop One of the more common joint contractures that results in permanent plantar flexion.
forced expiratory flow The maximal flow rate that is attained during the middle of the forced vital capacity maneuver.
forced expiratory volume in 1 second (FEV_1) The volume of air expelled in 1 second from the beginning of the forced vital capacity.
forced vital capacity (FVC) Part of pulmonary function tests that measures the volume of air the patient can forcefully expel after the maximum amount of air is breathed in.
formal leadership Leadership that is part of an official position, which may or may not be a management position.
fraction of inspired oxygen (FIO_2) The percentage of oxygen in inspired air.
free radicals Naturally occurring, highly reactive chemicals that form in the presence of oxygen and can cause harmful alterations in cellular function similar to those seen in aging.
friction Rubbing.
frostbite Ice crystals form inside the cells due to exposure to subnormal temperatures, which may cause permanent circulatory and tissue damage.
full-thickness wound A wound that extends through the dermis to the subcutaneous layer and may extend farther, to the muscle, bone, or other underlying structures.
functional incontinence Lack of urine control in the absence of any abnormalities of the urinary tract.
functional residual capacity The volume of air that remains in the patient's lung after normal expiration.
fungi Single-cell organisms, such as yeast and mold, that are capable of causing infection.
futile care Care that is perceived as useless and that prolongs the time until death rather than restoring life.

gait The patient's manner of walking.
gamma-glutamyltransferase (GGT) An enzyme found primarily in the liver and biliary tract that assists in transporting amino acids across cell membranes.
gay A term most often associated with male homosexuality.
gender identity An individual's self-concept with respect to being a male or female.
gender role The outward behavior of a person as a male or female and the perception of what constitutes gender-appropriate actions.
general adaptation syndrome (GAS) The physical response to stress.
general anesthesia A combination of inhaled or intravenous anesthetic agent is used to cause central nervous system depression and put the patient in a drug-induced coma.
generalization Broad statements or ideas about people or things.
generalized anxiety disorder Unrealistic levels of worry and tension with or without an identifiable cause.
generativity Reaching out to others in ways that guide and give to the next generation.
generic name The official drug name assigned by the U.S. Adopted Names Council, which is simpler than the chemical name.
genetic vulnerability The risk of disease expression based on genotype.
gingivae Gums.
gingivitis Inflammation of the gums.
glaucoma A serious medical condition of the eye that causes increased intraocular pressure, which puts pressure on the optic nerve, leading to loss of peripheral visual fields and possibly blindness.
globulins Plasma proteins classified as alpha, beta, and gamma globulins; some function as antibodies, while others are responsible for enzymatic functions and the transport of lipids, iron, and copper in the blood.
grand theory A global conceptual framework that defines broad perspectives for nursing practice and provides ways of looking at nursing phenomena from a distinct nursing perspective.
granulation tissue The new tissue created to fill the wound that is beefy red in appearance.
grief The emotional response to loss.
grounded theory research Research that attempt to derive a theory from the data collected in the research.
growth Increase in height and weight.
guarding Positioning to prevent movement of a painful body part.
gustation The sense of taste.

half-life The time it takes for the blood concentration of a drug to measure half of the original dose due to drug elimination.
halitosis Unpleasant breath odor.
handoff The real-time process of passing patient-specific information from one caregiver to another or among interdisciplinary team members to ensure continuity of care and patient safety. A handoff can be oral or written.
healing ridge A 1-cm-wide ridge, or area of induration along an incision that indicates that collagen synthesis has taken place in a wound.
health belief model (HBM) Developed by psychologists Hochbaum, Rosenstock, and Kegels. It explores the relationship between patient attitudes and beliefs and how those factors predict health behavior.
health care proxy The specific durable power of attorney for medical care.
health care–associated infections (HAIs) Infections acquired while the patient is receiving treatment in a health care facility such as a hospital, long-term care facility, clinic, or primary care office.
health history Includes all pertinent information collected during initial or early contact with a patient that can guide the development of a patient-centered plan of care.
Health Insurance Portability and Accountability Act (HIPAA) Act passed in 1996 that created federal standards for the protection of personal health information, whether conveyed orally or recorded in any form or medium. the act clearly mandates that protected health information may be used only for treatment, payment, or health care operations. Nurses share the responsibility of preventing a breach of confidentiality.
health literacy The unique ability of the patient to understand and integrate health-related knowledge.
health promotion model (HPM) A health model by Pender that relies on the premise that a multidimensional interaction exists between an individual and the environment in which health promotion consists of a collection of behaviors directed at improving the individual's well-being.
health promotion Behavior motivated by the desire to increase well-being and optimize health status.
health protection Includes intentional behaviors aimed at circumventing illness, detecting it early, and maintaining the best possible level of mental and physiologic function within the boundaries of illness.
health A state of complete physical, mental and social well-being and not merely the absence of disease or infirmity.
health-promotion nursing diagnoses NANDA-I diagnostic labels used in situations in which patients express interest in improving their health status through a positive change in behavior.
Healthy People 2020 An initiative designed to track, over 10-year increments, risk factors and personal behaviors related to physical activity, access to health services, tobacco use, substance use, responsible sexual behavior, mental health, immunizations, injury and violence prevention.
heat exhaustion Profound sweating resulting in excessive water and electrolyte loss following environmental heat exposure.
heatstroke Prolonged exposure to the sun or high environmental temperatures overwhelm the body's heat-loss mechanisms. This health emergency has a high mortality rate.
hematuria Blood in the urine.
hemiparesis Weakness on one side of the body.

hemiplegia Paralysis of one side of the body.
Hemoccult A test for hidden blood in the stool.
hemodialysis Mechanical filtration of impurities and waste products from the blood of patients who have acute or chronic renal failure.
hemoglobin (Hgb) A protein primarily responsible for oxygen transport to and carbon dioxide transport from the erythrocytes.
hemolysis Red blood cell destruction.
hemolytic reactions The life-threatening destruction of red blood cells.
hemoptysis The presence of blood in the sputum.
hemorrhage A large amount of bleeding.
hemorrhoids Swollen and inflamed veins in the anus or lower rectum.
Hemovac drain A closed drainage system in which a soft drain is attached to a springlike suction device.
heterosexual A person who has sexual interest in or sexual intercourse exclusively with partners of the opposite sex.
high-density lipoprotein cholesterol A lipoprotein that transports excess cholesterol from the tissues back to the liver, where it is broken down and excreted in bile.
higher-order beliefs Ideas derived from a person's first-order beliefs using inductive or deductive reasoning.
hirsutism A condition affecting both men and women in which hair growth on the upper lip, chin, and cheeks becomes excessive and vellus body hair becomes thicker and coarser.
historical research Research that studies historic documents to determine an accurate picture of a historical event or time period.
holistic health models Models based on the philosophy that a synergistic relationship exists between the body and the environment.
holistic Treating the patient's physical, mental, emotional, spiritual, and social self; address the many dimensions necessary to fully care for a patient.
home health care nursing Care for a patient that takes place in a residential, home setting.
homeostasis The body's regulation of systems to maintain a steady state of equilibrium.
homocysteine An amino acid formed in the conversion of methionine to cysteine.
homosexual A person who has sexual interest in or sexual intercourse exclusively with members of his or her own sex.
hope A confident expectation.
hospice care End-of-life care for the terminally ill.
host (intrinsic) factors Individual variables such as genetics, age, or gender.
host (reservoir) The source of infection; can be inanimate objects, human beings, and animals.
human subject An individual about whom an investigator conducting research obtains (1) data through intervention or interaction with the individual; or (2) identifiable private information.
humanistic The promotion of human welfare.
humility The ability to recognize that no one is superior to another.
humoral immunity A defense system that involves antibodies and white blood cells that are produced to fight antigens which allows the body to produce substances such as interferon and interleukin-1, which cause fever.
hydrocephalus An accumulation of cerebrospinal fluid in the ventricles of the brain.
hydrostatic pressure The force of the fluid pressing against the blood vessel which is controlled by the force of myocardial contraction, rate of contraction, and blood flow.
hygiene Practices such as cleanliness that promote and preserve health.
hypercalcemia Increased serum calcium level greater than 10.5 mg/dL.
hypercapnia High levels of carbon dioxide.
hyperglycemia Increased blood glucose levels.
hyperkalemia Increased serum potassium level greater than 5.0 mEq/L.
hyperlipidemia Elevation of plasma cholesterol, triglycerides, or both.
hypermagnesemia increased serum magnesium level greater than 2.1 mEq/L.
hypernatremia Serum sodium levels greater than 145 mEq/L. This imbalance is due to either a greater loss of water compared to sodium or a greater intake of sodium.
hyperphosphatemia Increased serum phosphorus levels greater than 2.6 mEq/L.
hypersomnia Excessive daytime sleepiness lasting at least 1 month, causing impairment in occupational or other areas of a person's life.
hypertension Elevated blood pressure; it is the leading cause of cardiovascular disorders and the most important risk factor for stroke.
hyperthermia High body temperature.
hypertonic A solution with higher osmolarity than body fluids that pulls water from the cell to the extracellular fluid compartment, leading to cell shrinkage.
hypertonicity An increase in muscle tone.
hyperventilation Exhibited by deep, rapid respirations; it is often caused by stress or anxiety.
hypnotics Medications that induce unnatural sleep that disturbs REM and NREM sleep.
hypocalcemia Decreased serum calcium levels less than 8.5 mg/dL.
hypokalemia Decreased serum potassium level less than 3.5 mEq/L.
hypomagnesemia Decreased serum magnesium levels less than 1.3 mEq/L.
hypophosphatemia Decreased serum phosphorus levels less than 1.7 mEq/L.
hypotension A systolic blood pressure of less than 90 mm Hg (or 20 to 30 mm Hg below the patient's normal blood pressure) or diastolic blood pressure of 60 mm Hg or less.
hypothermia Low body temperature.
hypothesis A statement about two or more variables and their relationship to each other.
hypotonic A solution with a lower osmolarity than body fluids that causes excess water to move into cells.
hypotonicity A decrease in muscle tone.
hypoventilation Slow, shallow respirations; it is associated with drug overdose and obesity, as well as COPD and cervical spine injury.
hypovolemia A decrease in fluid volume.
hypoxemia Low oxygen levels in the blood.

id The part of personality consisting of instincts, operating on an unconscious level not based in reality.
idiosyncratic reaction An unpredictable patient response to medication.
ileostomy A surgically created opening in the small intestine, usually at the end of the ileum.
illness A state of health characterized by a decrease or impairment in an individual's abilities to engage in physical or mental functioning that was previously experienced.
immune response The body's attempt to recognize and protect itself from substances that are foreign and harmful, triggered by an antigen.
immunization The process by which an individual develops immunity against a specific agent.
impaction The presence of a hard fecal mass in the rectum or colon that the patient is unable to expel.
implementation Initiation of appropriate interventions designed to meet the unique needs of each patient.
incidence Occurrence.
incontinence The loss of ability to voluntarily control urine or feces.
independent nursing interventions Tasks within the nursing scope of practice that the nurse may undertake without a physician or PCP order.
independent variable A concept that is thought to have an effect on another concept.
indirect care Nursing interventions that are performed to benefit patients but do not involve face-to-face nurse-patient contact.
inductive reasoning Using specific facts or details to make conclusions and generalizations; proceeding from specific to general.
infected wound A wound that shows clinical signs of infection, including redness, warmth, and increased drainage that may or may not be purulent (contain pus), and has a bacterial count in the tissue of at least 10^5 per gram of tissue sampled when cultured.
infection A disease state caused by an infectious agent that occurs when a pathogen multiplies in a susceptible host.
inferences Conclusions.
infertility When a couple has not conceived after 12 months of contraceptive-free intercourse if the female is under the age of 34, or

after 6 months of contraceptive-free intercourse if the female is over the age of 35.

inflammatory phase The body's initial response to wounding of the skin that lasts about 3 days.

inflammatory response A local response to cellular injury or infection that causes capillary dilation and leukocyte infiltration.

informatics A broad academic field encompassing artificial intelligence, cognitive science, computer science, information science, and social science.

information literacy The ability to recognize when information is needed and to locate, evaluate, and effectively use the needed information.

informed consent Permission granted by a patient after discussing each of the following topics with the physician, surgeon, or advanced practice nurse who will perform the surgery or procedure: (1) exact details of the treatment, (2) necessity of the treatment, (3) all known benefits and risks involved, (4) available alternatives, and (5) risks of treatment refusal.

infrastructure Provides the basic necessities of life.

inhalation Medications taken into the body through the respiratory tract.

insomnia The most common dyssomnia; characterized by difficulty in falling asleep or staying asleep, sleep that is too light, or early morning awakenings.

inspection The use of vision, hearing, and smell to closely scrutinize physical characteristics of a whole person and individual body systems.

institutional review board A review committee established to help protect the rights and welfare of human research subjects.

instruments The data collection tools used to collect information.

integrity Aligning one's actions with their stated values.

integumentary system The body system comprised of skin, nails, hair, sweat glands, and sebaceous glands.

intentional injuries Injuries that result from deliberate acts of violence or abuse and often involve fatal consequences such as suicide and homicide.

intentional torts Wrongs committed by individuals who deliberately seek to injure or hurt another person.

intermittent infusion device A saline lock or prn adapter that allows periodic or emergency venous access.

International Classification for Nursing Practice (ICNP) Provides an international standard that facilitates the description and comparison of nursing practice locally, regionally, nationally, and internationally.

international normalized ratio A coagulation blood test that is a standardized ratio to monitor the effect of anticoagulant therapy.

internet The shared global computing network.

interpersonal communication Takes place between a minimum of two people; it may be formal or informal and conversational, and it may or may not have a stated goal or purpose.

interstitial fluid Fluid between the cells of an organ or tissue.

intracellular Body fluid that is within the cell.

intradermal (ID) A shallow injection into the dermis skin layer, just under the epidermis.

intramuscular (IM) An injection into a muscle of adequate size to accommodate the amount and type of medication.

intraoperative The second phase of surgery that begins when the patient enters the operating room and ends when the patient is transferred to the post anesthesia care unit.

intrapersonal communication Occurs within oneself and focuses on personal needs and has the potential of having an impact on a person's well-being.

intrauterine device (IUD) A contraceptive device placed through the cervix into the uterus that may contain progesterone or copper, which changes the uterine lining, thus reducing the chance of implantation.

intravascular Blood plasma.

intravenous (IV) An injection into a vein.

invasion of privacy Public disclosure of private information, use of a person's name or likeness without permission, intrusion into a person's place of solitude, and meddling into another's personal affairs.

irrigation Flushing of the bladder.

ischemia Reduced blood flow.

Isometric exercise Physical activity that requires tension and relaxation of muscles without joint movement.

isotonic exercise Active movement with constant muscle contraction.

isotonic A solution that has the same osmolarity as blood plasma.

Jackson-Pratt drain A closed drainage system in which a soft drain is attached to a bulblike suction device.

jaundice A yellow hue to the skin, mucous membranes, or eyes of both light- and dark-skinned individuals.

judgment The result or decision related to the processes of thinking and reasoning.

justice Acting fairly and equitably.

Kegel exercises An exercise that helps to keep the female pelvic floor toned, which reduces the risk of incontinence.

ketones Organic chemical compounds that result from incomplete fat oxidation when carbohydrates are not available.

kilocalorie The amount of heat energy it takes to raise the temperature of 1000 g of water 1° C.

Korotkoff sounds The sounds for which the nurse listens when assessing blood pressure.

kwashiorkor A lack of protein accompanied by fluid retention.

kyphosis An outward curvature of the thoracic spine.

labyrinths The intricate communicating passageways that make up the inner ear.

lactation The production and release of milk by the breasts (mammary glands).

laissez-faire leader A leader who provides little or no direction to followers. The followers develop their own goals and make their own decisions. Few policies and procedures are in place.

laryngospasm Causes the laryngeal muscle to briefly spasm causing the patient to have trouble speaking and difficulty breathing.

lavage Irrigation of the stomach.

laxatives Medications that ease defecation by stimulating bowel activity.

lead poisoning A public health issue that occurs when lead builds up in the blood over a period of months or years; it can affect all of the body systems.

leadership The ability to influence, guide, or direct others. Leadership focuses on relationships, using interpersonal skills to persuade others to work toward a common goal.

learning Acquiring knowledge or skills through instruction or experience.

lesbian A term most often associated with female homosexuality.

leukocytes White blood cells.

libel Written forms of defamation of character.

licensure The granting of a license, which provides legal permission to practice.

life expectancy The average number of years of life remaining at a given age.

lipids Fat found within the body, including true fats and oils such as fatty acids, cholesterol, and phospholipids.

listserv A computer program that automatically sends messages to multiple e-mail addresses on a mailing list.

literature review A critical analysis of current information on a specific subject that will be studied or discussed in a research project or scholarly article.

living will A document that specifies the treatment a person wants to receive in circumstances in which that person is unconscious or no longer capable of making decisions independently.

livor mortis The color of the skin becomes pale, then bluish after death.

local adaptation syndrome (LAS) Inflammation, reflexive response to pain, or hypoxia secondary to catecholamine release that results from the direct affect of stress on body tissues.

local anesthesia The regional application or injection of anesthetic drugs subcutaneously to a specific area of the body.

logic To have a mutually supporting and sensible combination of combined thoughts, whereby the conclusion follows from presented facts.

logrolling Moving the whole body as a unit in straight alignment.
long-term goals Goals that take weeks, months, or longer to achieve.
lordosis An inward lumbar curvature just above the buttocks area.
loss The absence of something or someone to which a person has formed an attachment.
low-density lipoprotein A lipoprotein that transports cholesterol from the liver to various parts of the body.
lymphocytes A type of white blood cell that recognizes foreign antigens, produces antibodies, and creates memory cells.

maceration Breakdown of the skin caused by fluid.
macronutrients Nutrients that are needed in large amounts.
macular degeneration Damage to the area of the retina that provides central vision leading to loss of vision in the central visual fields.
magnanimity Giving credit where credit is due.
magnetic resonance imaging (MRI) A superconducting magnet and radio frequency waves cause hydrogen nuclei to emit signals that are translated by a computer into a well-defined image of the structure.
major surgery A surgery in which there is a higher risk to the life of the patient and the surgery involves reconstruction or alteration of a body part.
malabsorption Problematic or inadequate absorption of nutrients in the intestinal tract.
malignant hyperthermia A rare, hereditary, and potentially life-threatening condition that can occur in susceptible individuals when inhaled general anesthesia is administered.
malnutrition An imbalance in the amount of nutrient intake and the body's needs.
malpractice Negligence committed by a person functioning within a professional role.
mammogram Soft tissue x-rays that allow visualization of the underlying breast tissue.
management The process of coordinating others and directing them toward a common goal. Management is focused on the task at hand.
marasmus A protein and caloric deficiency.
masked grief A type of complicated grief where the behaviors of the survivor interfere with normal functioning, but the person is not aware that these behaviors are concealing the actual grieving process.
Maslow's hierarchy of needs A model used to understand the interrelationship between the elements of basic requirements for survival and the desires that drive personal growth and development.
mastication Chewing.
maturation phase The last phase of wound healing which lasts for up to a year.
medical asepsis Clean technique used to prevent infection and break the chain of infection.
medication A drug specifically administered for its therapeutic effect on physiologic function.
medication administration record (MAR) A list of ordered medications, along with dosages and times of administration, on which the nurse initials medications given or not given. A paper MAR includes a signature section in which the nurse is identified by linking the initials used with a full signature.
medication error Any preventable event that may cause or lead to inappropriate medication use or patient harm while the medication is in the control of the health care professional, patient, or consumer.
medication interaction A drug's action is modified by the presence of a certain food, herb, or another medication.
meditation Mindful reflection or contemplation; another form of intrapersonal communication. Some people use it regularly as a means of self-encouragement and reassurance.
menopause The permanent cessation of menstrual activity.
menstruation The female's cyclic periodic discharge of body fluid from the uterus during the reproductive years, from approximately 12 to 50 years of age.
message The content transmitted during communication.
meta-analysis An analysis that merges statistical results from related studies for the purpose of discovering similarities and differences between the studies.
metabolic acidosis High acid content in the blood, with a pH less than 7.35, and a bicarbonate level less than 22 mEq/L.
metabolic alkalosis An excess of bicarbonate ions, which raises the pH above 7.45 and bicarbonate levels greater than 26 mEq/L.
metabolism The process of chemically changing nutrients, such as fats and proteins, into end products that are used to meet the energy needs of the body or stored for future use, thereby helping to maintain homeostasis in the body. The process by which a drug is altered to a less active form to prepare for excretion.
metaparadigm A global set of concepts that identify and describe the central phenomena of the discipline and explain the relationship between those concepts.
micronutrients Nutrients needed by the body in limited amounts.
micturition Urination.
middle-range theory A moderately abstract theory that has a limited number of variables. Middle-range theories are more concrete and narrowly focused on a specific condition or population than are grand theories.
milliequivalent The ability of cations to bond with anions to form molecules.
minerals Chemicals needed for energy, muscle building, nerve conduction, blood clotting, and immunity to diseases.
minor surgery Surgical alteration that is minimal with low risk to the life of the patient.
misdemeanor A crime of lesser consequence that is punishable by a fine or incarceration in a local or county jail for up to 1 year.
mixed incontinence A combination of both stress and urge incontinence.
mode of transmission The microorganism's form of transportation to travel from the source to the susceptible host.
moderate sedation Conscious sedation or an altered state of consciousness providing a moderate to deep level of sedation, amnesia, and analgesia that minimizes pain and discomfort achieved by use of pain medications and sedatives.
monocytes A type of white blood cell involved in phagocytosis; they become macrophages.
monounsaturated fatty acids Have only one double bond between per molecule and are components of triglycerides.
mourning The outward, social expression of loss.
mucous membranes Lining of the passages and cavities of the body, such as nasal, oral, vaginal, urethral, and anal areas.
mucus Fluid secreted by mucous membranes.
multimodal analgesia The use of more than one means for controlling pain.
multimodal learner A person who does best when more than one teaching strategy is used or who is able to adapt to a variety of teaching strategies.
myocardial infarction (MI) The blockage of blood flow to the coronary arteries of the heart.
myoglobin An oxygen-transporting and storage protein found in cardiac and skeletal muscle.
myopia Nearsightedness that causes a person to be able to see clearly only a short distance.

NANDA-I NANDA International, Inc., formerly North American Nursing Diagnosis Association.
narcolepsy A chronic neurologic disorder caused by the brain's inability to regulate the sleep-wake cycle normally, resulting in an uncontrollable desire to sleep.
nasopharyngeal airway An airway placed through the nostril into the pharynx.
nature versus nurture The debate over whether development is predetermined at birth (nature) or whether the child's environment (nurture) controls how development progresses.
necrosis Death of cells, tissues, or organs.
negative reinforcement A form of learning that occurs when behavior results in the removal of an unpleasant stimulus, increasing the chance that the behavior will be repeated.

negative self-talk Internal conversation that is potentially harmful or destructive and may damage the ability of an individual to achieve his or her greatest potential or to overcome adversity.
negligence Creating a risk of harm to others by failing to do something that a "reasonable person" would ordinarily do or doing something that a "reasonable person" would ordinarily not do.
nephron The tiny filtering units in the kidneys that form urine.
nerve block Regional anesthetic that is injected into a particular nerve, group of nerves, or surrounding tissue.
neurofibrillary tangles Twisted fragments of protein that clog the nerve cells which interrupts nutrient delivery to brain cells.
neuropathic pain Pain that results from nerve injury; the pain continues even after the painful stimuli are gone.
neurotransmitters Inflammatory substances that are released into the extracellular space as a result of tissue damage.
neutrophils A type of white blood cell that act as first defenders against bacterial and fungal infections, foreign antigens, and cell debris.
nits Lice eggs.
nociceptive pain The most common type of pain; occurs when nociceptors are stimulated in response to an injury or tissue damage from surgery or trauma or to inflammation.
nociceptors The free endings of afferent nerve fibers, which are sensitive to thermal, mechanical, or chemical stimuli.
nocturia Excessive urination at night.
nocturnal enuresis Bedwetting at night.
nonmaleficence "First, do no harm;" the avoidance of harm.
non-opioid analgesics Drugs that do not contain narcotics that are used in the treatment of many types of mild to moderate pain.
non–rapid eye movement (NREM) sleep The phases of sleep in which REM sleep does not occur, growth hormone is released to repair epithelial and brain cells, cell division for skin and bone marrow renewal occurs, and energy is conserved.
nonsteroidal anti-inflammatory drugs (NSAIDs) Nonnarcotic drugs that do not contain steroids that are used in the treatment of many types of mild to moderate pain.
nontherapeutic communication Can be hurtful and potentially damaging to interaction. Changing the subject or sharing personal opinions, serves to limit conversation between the nurse and the patient and discourages open conversation on sensitive topics.
nonverbal communication Wordless transmission of ideas in the form of body language, gestures, touch, attire, facial expressions, and eye contact.
normal flora Non-disease-causing microorganisms, such as bacteria, fungi, and protozoa that live within or on the body.
nurse practice acts Laws that provide the scope of practice defined by each state or jurisdiction and are the legal limits of nursing practice. These acts are laws that the nurse must be familiar with to function in practice.
nursing diagnosis Identification of an actual or potential problem or response to a problem.
nursing informatics A specialty area of informatics that addresses the use of health information systems to support nursing practice.
nursing interventions classification (NIC) A comprehensive, research-based, standardized classification of multidisciplinary interventions and associated activities.
nursing minimum data set (NMDS) Standardized collection of essential nursing data used on a regular basis by the majority of nurses in the delivery of care across settings.
nursing outcomes classification (NOC) Standardized vocabulary used for describing patient, family, or community responses to nursing interventions.
nursing process The systematic method of critical thinking used by professional nurses to develop individualized plans of care and provide care for patients.
nursing theory A group of concepts that can be tested in practice and can be derived from a conceptual model.
nursing The protection, promotion, and optimization of health and abilities, prevention of illness and injury, alleviation of suffering through the diagnosis and treatment of human response, and advocacy in the care of individuals, families, communities, and populations.
nutrients The necessary substances obtained from ingested food that supply the body with energy; build and maintain bones, muscles, and skin; and aid in the normal growth and function of each body system.
nutrition The body's intake and use of adequate amounts of necessary nutrients for tissue growth and energy production.
nystagmus Rapid, shaking, involuntary movement of the eyes.

obesity The result of a person's energy intake consistently exceeding energy use.
object permanence An object still exists even when it is out of sight.
objective data Data that can be measured or observed. The nurse's senses of sight, hearing, touch, and smell are used to collect objective data. Also called signs.
obstructive sleep apnea (OSA) Absence of breathing during sleep caused by collapse of the upper airway despite respiratory effort.
olfaction The sense of smell.
oliguria A reduced urine volume less than 1mL/kg/hr in an infant; less than 0.5 mL/kg/hr in children; and less than 400 mL/day in adults.
oncotic pressure The presence of plasma proteins, specifically albumin. because these plasma proteins are too large to pass through the capillary membrane, they hold the fluid in the intravascular space.
onset of action The time the body takes to respond to a drug after administration.
open wound A wound characterized by an actual break in the skin's surface.
openness A leader's ability to listen to other points of view without prejudging them or shutting them down.
operant conditioning A form of learning based on reinforcement or punishment.
opioid analgesics The most effective agents for relief of moderate to severe pain. These narcotic drugs work by binding to the opioid receptors in the nervous system, which are sites of endorphin action.
opportunistic infections Harmless organisms that become pathogenic.
oral By mouth.
orthopnea Difficulty in breathing when in positions other than upright.
orthostatic hypotension A sudden drop of 20 mm Hg in systolic pressure and 10 mm Hg in diastolic pressure when the patient moves from a lying to sitting to standing position.
osmolality Ionic concentration.
osmolarity The number of osmols per liter of solvent.
osmoreceptor Located in the hypothalamus, monitor the osmolarity of blood plasma.
osmosis The movement of water across cell membranes.
osmotic pressure The force created when two solutions of different concentrations are separated by a selectively permeable membrane.
ossicles The three small bones in the middle ear.
ostomy A surgically created opening in the gastrointestinal, urinary, or respiratory organs, which is exited onto the skin.
outcome identification Observable behaviors or actions that indicate attainment of a goal.
outcome indicators Criteria on which goal attainment is observed or measured.
overflow incontinence A condition in which a person is unable to empty the bladder completely, resulting in a constant dribbling of urine or frequency in urination.
oxygen saturation Amount of oxygen in the arterial blood.

pain threshold The point at which the brain recognizes the stimulus as pain.
pain tolerance The intensity or duration of pain that a patient is able or willing to endure.
pain Physical suffering or discomfort caused by illness or injury.
palliative care Comfort care offered to patients at any stage of a serious illness.
pallor Pale skin tone, that is usually uniformly disseminated throughout the skin surface. Pallor can be caused by illness, emotional shock or stress, decreased exposure to sunlight, anemia, or genetics.

palpation Physical examination using touch to assess body organs and skin texture, temperature, moisture, turgor, tenderness, and thickness.

papillary dermis Projections that provide the "stick" that anchors layers of the skin together, preventing them from sliding back and forth.

paracentesis A needle aspiration that involves removing fluid from the peritoneal cavity.

paradigm A person's worldview.

paralytic ileus The stoppage of peristalsis.

paraplegia Lower-body paralysis.

parasite Organisms that live on or in other organisms and are capable of causing disease.

parasomnias Abnormal sleep behaviors.

parenteral Medication administration by injection or infusion.

paresthesia Numbness or tingling.

parish nursing A specialty within nursing in which specially educated registered nurses provide counseling, referrals, and spiritual care.

partial-thickness wound A wound that involves the epidermis and the dermis but does not extend through the dermis to the subcutaneous layer.

passive range of motion Passive movement of each joint of the body of another person to the point of resistance while evaluating the person's comfort level.

pathogen Any infectious, disease-causing agent; can include bacteria, viruses, fungi, and parasites.

pathologic bone fractures Spontaneous bone breaks without trauma.

patient interview A formal, structured discussion in which the nurse questions the patient to obtain demographic information, as well as data about current health concerns and past medical and surgical history.

patient-controlled analgesia (PCA) A system in which an electronically controlled infusion pump immediately delivers a prescribed amount of analgesic to the patient when he or she activates a button, without the need for a nurse to administer it.

peak plasma level The highest serum (blood) concentration of a drug.

pediculosis A contagious scalp infection most commonly known as head lice.

Penrose drain An open drain that is a flexible piece of tubing; is usually not sutured into place.

perception The way the brain perceives information.

percussion Tapping the patient's skin with short, sharp strokes that cause a vibration to travel through the skin and to the upper layers of the underlying structures.

perimenopause The phase prior to the onset of menopause and the first year after menopause.

perineal care Cleansing of the genital area, urinary meatus, and anus.

perioperative nursing The nursing specialty that provides for patients before, during, and after surgery.

perioperative period The three phases of surgery.

peripheral neuropathy Nerve damage away from the center of the body.

peripheral pulse Pulses that can be palpated over arteries located away from the heart.

peripherally inserted central catheter (PICC) A catheter inserted by a physician or specially trained nurse into the cephalic or basilic veins or antecubital space and threaded up until it rests in the superior vena cava right outside the right atrium. It can remain in place for weeks to months and does not have the risk of pneumothorax associated with its use; and it is associated with fewer catheter-related infections.

peristalsis Progressive wave action causing movement of contents through the gastrointestinal system.

peritoneal dialysis A procedure to remove waste products from the body of a patient in chronic renal failure that is performed by instilling dialysis solution into the patient's abdominal cavity through an external catheter.

personal protective equipment (PPE) The equipment that health care personnel use to protect against the spread of infection. Gloves, masks, goggles, face shields, gowns, caps, and shoe coverings are all examples.

petechiae Tiny, dark red spots that indicate hemorrhage under the skin.

pétrissage A massage technique performed by using a kneading motion with the fingers and thumb along the patient's back and shoulders.

phantom pain Occurs after an amputation when the brain continues to receive messages from the area of the amputation.

pharmacodynamics The process in which a medication interacts with the body's cells to produce a biologic response.

pharmacokinetics The study of how a medication enters the body, moves through the body, and is excreted.

phenomenological research Research that explores the lived experiences of a specific group of people experiencing a similar event in their lives.

phenomenon An aspect of reality that can be observed or experienced.

philosophy A statement about the beliefs and values of nursing in relation to a specific phenomenon such as health.

phlebitis Inflammation of a vein.

physical assessment A comprehensive data collection followed by an extensive physical examination of every body system.

physical restraint A device, such as material or equipment attached or adjacent to the patient's body, used to restrict movement.

PICO An acronym used to formulate a research question that stands for: P: patient, population, or problem; I: intervention; C: comparison intervention; O: outcomes.

PIE A format for problem oriented documentation that stands for Problem, Intervention, Evaluation.

planning Phase of the nursing process during which the nurse prioritizes a patient's nursing diagnoses, establishes short- and long-term goals, chooses outcome indicators, and identifies interventions to address patient goals.

pleural effusion Fluid accumulation in the pleura of the lungs.

pneumonia Inflammation of the lungs usually caused by an infection or foreign material.

poisoning The intentional or unintentional ingestion, inhalation, injection, or absorption through the skin of any substance that is harmful to the body.

polyps Benign or malignant tissue growth in the colon.

polysomnography The recording of brain waves and other physiologic variables, such as muscle activity and eye movements, during sleep.

polyunsaturated fatty acids Fatty acids with multiple pairs of double carbon bonds.

polyuria An excessive volume of urine formed and excreted each day.

portal of entry The means by which the microorganism enters the susceptible host.

portal of exit The means by which the pathogen escapes from the reservoir, or source of infection.

positive self-talk Internal conversation that provides motivation and encouragement; it may be used to build self-esteem and self-confidence.

postformal thought Cognitive development past Piaget's formal operational stage consisting of gradual change in thinking in the face of reality and adult responsibility.

postoperative The third phase of surgery that begins when the patient is admitted to the postanesthesia care unit and ends when the patient has completely recovered from the surgical procedure, which in some cases is several months.

post-traumatic stress disorder (PTSD) A very serious mental health condition characterized by flashbacks and erratic behaviors that results from exposure to a horrifying experience. PTSD may develop when an individual's ability to cope is exceeded by the trauma that was experienced.

postural drainage A therapeutic way to position a patient to use gravity to help mobilize respiratory tract secretions.

prayer A form of meditation traditionally directed to a deity.

prealbumin A plasma protein synthesized by the liver and considered a precise measure of nutritional status.

precision To provide sufficient detail, resulting in the understanding of exactly what was meant.

preemptive analgesia The administration of medications prior to a painful event to minimize pain.
prejudice A preformed opinion, usually an unfavorable one, about an entire group of people that is based on insufficient knowledge, irrational feelings, or inaccurate stereotypes.
preoperative The first phase of surgery that begins when the patient decides to have surgery and ends when the patient is taken to the operating room.
presbycusis Age-related hearing loss.
presbyopia Farsightedness, or an age-related decrease in the ability to focus on near objects.
prescription Medications dispensed by a pharmacist on receipt of written directions from a medical provider legally permitted to prescribe drugs.
pressure ulcer Pressure sores, bedsores, or decubitus ulcers that may develop on areas damaged due to tissue ischemia secondary to compression and inactivity.
prevalence Pervasiveness or extent of a disease.
preventive action A lifestyle change along with information gathering about a health topic that leads to actual change in behavior.
primary data Data that comes directly from the patient.
primary intention Wounds that tend to heal quickly and result in minimal scar formation because the edges of the skin can be brought together.
primary prevention The stage of an individual's health when it is possible to keep disease from becoming established, either by removing the potential causes or by increasing resistance.
privacy The right to be free from intrusion or disturbance in a person's private life or affairs.
problem solving A systematic, analytic approach to finding a solution.
problem-oriented medical record (POMR) Integrates charting from the entire care team in the same section of the record. The POMR is usually structured to provide a focus for the documentation.
profession An occupation that requires at a minimum specialized training and a specialized body of knowledge.
proliferative phase A phase in wound healing that repairs the defect; fills the wound bed with new tissue, called granulation tissue; and resurfaces the wound with skin.
proprioception An awareness of posture and movement.
positive reinforcement A form of learning that occurs when a behavior is met with a positive consequence increasing the likelihood of repeating the behavior.
prosthetic Artificial.
prothrombin time A coagulation blood test that detects bleeding disorders caused by abnormalities of the extrinsic clotting system, and used to monitor the effectiveness of warfarin sodium (coumadin) therapy.
proxemics The study of the spatial requirements of humans and animals.
pruritus Itching.
psychogenic pain Pain that is perceived by an individual but has no physical cause.
psychomotor domain A form of learning that incorporates physical movement and the use of motor skills into learning.
ptosis Abnormal drooping of the eyelid.
puberty A time of great change as a child matures into an adult, both physically and socially; also referred to as adolescence.
public health nursing Examines the greater community as a whole—the city, county, state, nation, continent, world—and designs collaborative and interdisciplinary strategies to keep the population healthy by preventing or controlling disease and threats to human health.
pulmonary embolism A blood clot that detaches and lodges in the pulmonary artery.
pulse deficit Occurs when the apical pulse rate exceeds the radial pulse rate.
pulse oximetry Measures the amount of oxygen available to tissues, is typically assessed with respirations.
pulse The palpable, bounding blood flow created by the contraction of the left ventricle of the heart.
purging Intentional vomiting.
purpura Bleeding underneath the skin.
purulent Containing pus.

quadriplegia Inability to move all four extremities.
qualitative research Research that focuses on personal beliefs, thoughts, and feelings that produces data in the form of comments or observations.
quantitative research Research that focuses on measurable, objective data that usually produces information in the form of numbers.
quasi-experimental research Research that examines a causal relationship between variables, but it may not meet the strict guidelines of experimental research.
questioning Someone who is unsure or exploring his or her sexual orientation or gender identity.

RACE A fire emergency response acronym. R: rescue all patients in immediate danger and move them to safe areas. A: activate the manual-pull station and/or fire alarm and have someone call 911. C: contain the fire by closing doors, confining the fire and preventing the spread of smoke. E: extinguish the fire if possible after all patients are removed from the area.
race A socially constructed concept that tends to group people by common descent, heredity, or physical characteristics.
racism A belief that race is the primary determinant of human traits and capacities and that racial differences produce an inherent superiority of a particular race.
radial pulse Palpated by placing the first two or three middle fingers of one hand over the radial artery at the groove along the radial, or thumb side, of the patient's inner wrist.
radiating pain Pain that extends to another area of the body.
radiography The use of x-rays to visualize bones, organs, and soft tissues for abnormalities.
range of motion Degrees of movement.
rapid eye movement (REM) sleep Quick scanning movements of the eyes that occur during sleep, associated with dreaming.
reasoning Logical thinking that links thoughts, ideas, and facts together in a meaningful way; used in scientific inquiry and problem solving.
rebound tenderness Discomfort experienced after stimulation is discontinued.
receiver The person who receives and decodes, or interprets, the communication.
referent The initiating event or thought that leads one person to interact with another, may be anything, including something related to one of the senses.
referred pain Pain that occurs in one area but hurts in another area, such as pain from a myocardial infarction or heart attack.
reflection The process of contemplating experiences, sometimes even life-changing experiences, and searching for meaning in those events.
regional anesthesia Anesthesia that disrupts the transmission of nerve impulses to a specific area of the body.
regulatory law Laws, established by administrative bodies, such as state boards of nursing, that outline how the requirements of statutory law will be met.
related factors The underlying cause or etiology of a patient problem.
relativist thinking The ability to recognize multiple, conflicting versions of "truth" representing legitimate alternatives occurring as adolescents become aware of the diversity of opinions on any topic.
relevance To focus on facts and ideas directly related and pertinent to the subject at hand.
religion Provides a structure for understanding spirituality and involves rites and rituals within a faith community.
remission A period of relief from symptoms during chronic illness.
renin–angiotensin system Regulates blood pressure and fluid balance through vasoconstriction and excretion or reabsorption of sodium.
replication Reproduction or duplication.
research use The application of research findings to clinical practice.
reservoir masks Masks that have a bag that inflates with oxygen and deliver higher levels of oxygen to a patient.

residual volume The amount of air remaining in the lungs after maximum expiration. The expected finding is 1.2 liters.

respiration The frequency of breaths per minute (bpm). One inhalation and one exhalation is one breath.

respiratory acidosis High acid content in the blood, with a pH less than 7.35, and the partial arterial pressure of carbon dioxide ($Paco_2$) is increased to greater than 45 mm Hg.

respiratory alkalosis pH is increased to greater than 7.45 and the partial arterial pressure of carbon dioxide ($Paco_2$) is decreased to less than 35 mm Hg.

responsibility The concept of being dependable and reliable.

restless legs syndrome A familial sleep disorder characterized by disagreeable-feeling leg movements resulting from intense, abnormal, lower-extremity sensations of crawling or tingling.

rete ridges Projections that provide the "stick" that anchors layers of the skin together, preventing them from sliding back and forth.

retina Innermost layer of the eye that contains photoreceptors (rods and cones).

reversibility An important development in thinking patterns that enables older children and adults to change direction in their thinking to return to the starting point.

rigor mortis The stiffening of the joints of the body after death.

risk factor reduction The step-by-step improvement of individual health factors that, when combined, lower the likelihood of developing a certain disease.

risk factors Environmental, physical, psychological, or situational concerns that increase a patient's vulnerability to a potential problem or concern.

risk nursing diagnoses NANDA-I diagnostic labels used when there is an increased potential or vulnerability for a patient to develop a problem or complication.

rituals Formal, stylized, repetitive, and stereotyped actions performed in special places at special times.

rods Types of photoreceptors present in the retina that are sensitive to light and therefore provide vision in dim light.

role boundaries The limits and responsibilities of individuals within a given setting.

rule of descent The arbitrary assignment of a race to a person on the basis of a societal dictate that associates social identity with ancestry.

safety The condition of being free from physical or psychological harm and injury.

salivary glands Glands in the mouth secrete mucus, enzymes, and a watery fluid, which mix to form saliva.

sample The actual individuals in the population from whom the data will be collected.

sandwich generation Refers to middle-aged adults who are the caretakers of more than one generation of their families.

sanguinous Drainage that usually indicates bleeding and is bright red.

sarcopenia Loss of flesh; the process of decreasing muscle tissue (muscle mass) and muscle strength that begins in the 30s.

saturated fatty acids Contain as many hydrogen atoms as the carbon atoms can bond with and no double carbon bonds.

SBAR A communication format specifically suggested for use in nurse-physician interactions and as a handoff tool. Stands for Situation, Background, Assessment, Recommendation.

scar tissue An avascular mass of collagen that gives strength to the repaired wound.

scoliosis Sideways or S-shaped curvature of the spine that is always abnormal.

scrub nurse Specially trained nurse who prepares the surgical set-up, handles instruments, maintains surgical asepsis while draping, and assists the surgeon by passing instruments, sutures, and supplies.

sebaceous glands Glands in the dermis that secrete an oily substance that keeps the hair and skin soft.

secondary data Information shared by family members, friends, or other members of the health care team.

secondary intention New tissue fills in from the bottom and sides of the wound until the wound bed is filled.

secondary prevention The stage of an individual's health when a disease process has evolved far enough that it is detectable by medical tests but the patient may still be asymptomatic.

secondary sleep disorders Sleep problems caused by underlying medical or psychiatric disorders.

sedation A state of calm or reduced anxiety.

selectively permeable membrane The cell membrane that allows water to move across but not the solutes.

self-actualization The highest level of optimal functioning that involves the integration of cognition, consciousness, and physiologic utility into a single entity.

self-concept The way in which individuals perceive unchanging aspects of themselves, such as social character or abilities, physical appearance, body image, and ways of thinking.

self-efficacy The belief in one's own ability to perform a task.

semicircular canal A second set of labyrinths in the inner ear with receptors that interpret the head's position.

sender The person who initiates and encodes the communication. Senders may be individuals or groups who have a message to share.

senescence Biological aging.

sensation A feeling, within or outside the body, of conditions resulting from stimulation of sensory receptors.

sense of coherence (SOC) A characteristic of personality that references one's perception of the world as comprehensible, meaningful, and manageable.

sensory adaptation Process by which some impulses are ignored by the brain during times of alertness because they are not prioritized as important.

sensory deprivation Decreased stimulation from the environment.

sensory overload An overabundance of stimuli from the environment and from internal sources such as pain.

sentinel event An unexpected occurrence involving death or serious physical or psychological injury, or the risk of injury. Such events are called "sentinel" because they signal the need for immediate investigation and response.

sequential compression devices (SCDS) Inflatable sleeves that wrap around the legs of patients and are attached to an air source which inflates and deflates creating a massaging action for the lower extremities.

seriation The ability to arrange things in a logical order.

serosanguineous Drainage that is pink to pale red and contains a mix of serous fluid and blood.

serous Drainage that contains clear, watery fluid from plasma.

sex Classification of male or female determined by the internal and external genitalia. The term often used to express "sexual intercourse."

sexual orientation A person's attraction to his or her own sex, the opposite sex, or both sexes when choosing a sexual partner.

sexuality The collective characteristics that mark the differences between male and female.

sexually transmitted disease (STD) A disease acquired as a result of sexual intercourse or other intimate contact with an infected individual.

sexually transmitted infection (STI) An infection acquired as a result of sexual intercourse or other intimate contact with an infected individual without actual signs of disease.

shear The result of the relationship between friction and gravity; causes a hyperangulation and stretching of the blood vessels, damaging them and their ability to transport blood.

shock A life-threatening condition in which the circulatory system fails to maintain adequate perfusion to the vital organs.

short-term goals Goals that are achievable within less than a week.

shroud A cloth, sheet, or bag, for transportation of the body to the morgue or funeral home.

side effects Predictable but unwanted and sometimes unavoidable reactions to medications.

significance To concentrate on the most important information in one's reasoning and take into consideration the most important concepts, facts, or ideas.

signs Data that can be measured or observed. the nurse's senses of sight, hearing, touch, and smell are used to observe signs. also called objective data.

sinus tract A tunnel or narrow passageway extending outward from the edge of the wound.

situational theories The theory that leaders change their approach depending on the situation. The situation includes a number of factors, such as characteristics of the group, the type of business, and the economic climate.

sitz baths Baths for soaking a patient's perineal area.

skipped generation The parents of the approximately 4% to 5% of the child population in the United States who lives with grandparents and apart from parents.

slander Oral defamation of character.

sleep A naturally occurring altered state of consciousness regulated by the central nervous system.

sleep apnea Absence of breathing (apnea) or diminished breathing during sleep.

sleep deprivation A prolonged, inadequate quality and quantity of sleep.

smegma A whitish substance under the foreskin.

SOAP note A format for documentation. Stands for Subjective data, Objective data, Assessment, Plan.

SOAPIE note A format for documentation. Stands for Subjective data, Objective data, Assessment, Plan, Intervention, Evaluation.

SOAPIER note A format for documentation. Stands for Subjective data, Objective data, Assessment, Plan, Intervention, Evaluation, Revisions to plan.

social determinants of health Identifiable variables that affect health and wellness that are key components in guiding health promotion activities and preventive behaviors.

social media Include various online technologies such as Facebook, Twitter, and LinkedIn that allow people to communicate easily via the internet to share information and resources.

social structure Influences how people interact with one another.

socialization The process of being reared and nurtured within a culture and acquiring its characteristics.

solute Substances that dissolve in a liquid.

solvent The liquid a solute dissolves in.

somatic pain Pain that occurs with injury to skin, muscles, bones, and joints.

somnambulism Sleepwalking.

spasticity Increased muscle tone.

spinal anesthesia An anesthetic agent injected into the subarachnoid space.

spirit The expression of spirituality through a person's capability for thought, contemplation, and exploration of meaning and purpose in life.

spiritual care A mutual, purposeful, interactive process between a nurse and other members of the health care team, and a patient, which may include family, to promote the patient's spiritual health.

spiritual distress A disruption in a belief or value system.

spirituality The expression of meaning and purpose in life.

stage I pressure ulcer A wound resulting from pressure on tissue characterized by intact, nonblistered skin with nonblanchable erythema, or persistent redness, in the area that has been exposed to pressure.

stage II pressure ulcer A partial-thickness wound resulting from pressure on tissue that involves the epidermis and/or dermis but does not extend below the level of the dermis. it can present as a blister or open wound.

stage III pressure ulcer Full-thickness wound resulting from pressure on tissue that extend into the subcutaneous tissue but do not extend through the fascia to muscle, bone, or connective tissue.

stage IV pressure ulcer Full-thickness wound resulting from pressure on tissue that is deeper than a stage iii pressure ulcer and involves exposure of muscle, bone, or connective tissue such as tendons or cartilage.

stages of illness model A model that best describes illness behavior and how individuals arrive at the coping mechanisms necessary for the management of disease conditions.

stagnation Self-centered and narcissistic.

stakeholder Someone who is an integral part of the process, either the end user of the process or anyone who may be affected by the process.

standardized nursing terminology A structured vocabulary that provides a common means of communication among nurses.

standards of care The minimum requirements for providing safe nursing care. federal and state laws, rules and regulations, accreditation standards, and institutional policies and procedures are used to formulate nursing standards of care.

standards The minimum set of criteria of practice.

statutory law Laws created by legislative bodies such as the U.S. congress and state legislatures. state statutes must be consistent with all federal laws.

steatorrhea Fecal fat.

stenosis Narrowing.

stereotype An idea about a person, a group, or an event that is thought to be typical of all others in that category.

sterilization A process used to destroy all microorganisms, including their spores.

stimulus A change in the environment sufficient to evoke a response.

stoma The protuberance of the gastrointestinal, urinary, or respiratory organs through the skin.

strabismus Crossed eyes.

stratum corneum The outermost of the epidermal layers.

stratum germinativum The innermost of the epidermal layers.

stress appraisal The process by which a person interprets a stressor as either a threat or a challenge.

stress incontinence A loss of urine control during activities that increase intra-abdominal pressure, such as coughing, sneezing, laughing, or exercise.

stress A demand from the internal or external environment that exceeds the person's immediately available resources or ability to respond.

stressor An event or stimulus that disrupts a person's sense of equilibrium.

striae Stretch marks resulting from pregnancy and weight loss or gain.

subcutaneous layer A layer of adipose tissue, or fat, that attaches the dermis to the underlying muscles and bone, delivers the blood supply to the dermis, provides insulation, and has a cushioning effect.

subcutaneous An injection into the subcutaneous tissue just below the skin.

subjective data Spoken information that cannot be authenticated. generally, subjective data are gathered during the interview process if patients are well enough to describe their symptoms.

sublingual Medication administration under the tongue.

suffocation A state in which air no longer reaches the lungs because of smothering, drowning, or choking, resulting in a loss of respiration.

sundowning A worsening of agitation and confusion in the evening.

superego The moral branch of personality, referred to as the conscience.

superficial wound A wound that involves only the epidermis.

superstructure Provides a belief system that helps people identify themselves, their society, and the world around them.

supervision Monitoring an activity being carried out by someone else and making sure that it is performed correctly.

suppositories A drug delivery system that is inserted into the rectum, where it dissolves for medication absorption by coming into contact with the rectal mucosa.

surgical asepsis Sterile technique used to prevent the introduction of microorganisms from the environment to the patient.

susceptible host Someone exposed to an infectious disease who is likely to contract the disease. Increased susceptibility is associated with people at the extremes of age, those who are nutritionally compromised, and those who have experienced recent trauma or surgery.

suspected deep tissue injury An area of intact skin that is purple or maroon or a blood-filled blister indicating damage under the skin.

sutures Threads or metal staples used to bring the edges of a wound together to speed wound healing and reduce scar formation.

symbols Signs, sounds, clothing, tools, customs, beliefs, rituals, and other items that represent meaningful concepts.

symptoms Subjective description of a disease process or problem by a patient.

synergistic effect The combined effect of substances is greater than the effect of either substance if taken alone.

systematic review Provides a comprehensive, unbiased analysis through the use of a strict scientific design to select and assess various related research studies.

systolic pressure The peak of the pressure wave on the arterial wall.

tachycardia An excessively fast heart rate (>100 bpm in the adult).

tachypnea An increase in respiratory rate to more than 24 bpm in the adult.

tactile fremitus A palpable vibration transmitted through the chest wall that occurs with the movement of the vocal cords during speech.

tactile Touch.

tapotement A massage technique that involves a tapping or percussion motion with the side of the palm or ulnar side of the hand.

target population (population of interest) Groups of individuals who are of concern or at risk for injury, disease, or disability, including those most vulnerable.

taxonomy A unified language classification system.

teaching Imparting knowledge or giving instruction.

telecommunications device for the deaf (TDD) An electronic device that sends text communications through a telephone line.

telehealth/telemedicine The use of the internet to link medical experts with other clinicians, patients, or patient information, allowing for remote consultations with clear video images and high-fidelity links.

temperature The sensible heat of the human body.

temporary incontinence Urinary leakage that results from issues such as severe constipation, infections in the urinary tract or vagina, or medication usage.

tertiary intention A delay in wound healing between injury and closure.

tertiary prevention Occurs when a condition or illness is permanent and irreversible. The aim of care is to reduce the number and impact of complications and disabilities the individual experiences as a result of the disease process or medical condition.

The Joint Commission An independent, not-for-profit group in the United States that accredits hospitals and other health care-related agencies and focuses on the goal of patient safety.

therapeutic communication A beneficial, positive interaction that focuses on the patient in a nurse-patient interaction.

therapeutic effect The intended effect; the desired result or action of a medication.

thoracentesis A needle aspiration that removes fluid from the pleural space.

thrill Abnormal vibration felt on palpation over an aneurysm, the carotid artery, or an arteriovenous (AV) fistula.

thrombophlebitis Inflammation of the vein with the formation of a blood clot.

tinnitus Ringing in the ears.

tonicity The level of osmotic pressure of a solution.

toothette A disposable foam swab used for oral care.

topical Medication administration on the skin or mucous membranes.

topical anesthesia A type of local anesthesia applied to surface areas of the skin and mucous membranes, used to decrease discomfort.

torts Wrongs committed against another person that do not involve a contract.

tortuosity Bending and twisting.

total parenteral nutrition (TPN) Intravenous nutrition given through a peripherally inserted central catheter line or central venous catheter by means of an infusion pump. TPN may be the only feasible option for patients who do not have a functioning GI tract, or it may be given when patients are unable to ingest, digest, or absorb essential nutrients.

toxic effects The buildup of medication in the blood due to impaired metabolism and excretion, or an overdose.

toxins A wide variety of substances that can poison or harm a living organism or individual through mechanisms such as ingestion, inhalation, and environmental exposure.

tracheostomy tube A tube placed directly in the trachea through the neck to control the airway.

trade name A registered name assigned by the drug manufacturer; brand name.

trait theories Theory that assumes that leaders are born with the personality traits necessary for leadership, which few people were thought to possess.

transformational leaders Leaders who employ methods that inspire people to follow their lead. Transformational leaders work toward transforming an organization with the help of others.

transactional leaders Leaders who use reward and punishment to gain the cooperation of followers.

transcellular Extracellular fluid that is in cerebrospinal, synovial, peritoneal, pleura, and pericardial fluids.

transcendence The process of moving beyond who one is in the moment and toward who one will become in the future.

transcultural nursing The comparative human-caring differences and similarities among the beliefs, values, and patterned life ways of cultures to provide culturally congruent, meaningful, and beneficial health care.

transdermal patch A topical preparation designed to deliver medication slowly for long-term systemic effects.

***trans*-fatty acids** Composed of partially hydrogenated fatty acids, and saturated fats; are known to raise the body's total cholesterol.

transgendered A person who has a gender identity or gender perception different from the phenotypic gender.

transsexual A person who self-identifies as a member of the opposite sex. The sexual anatomy is not consistent with the gender identity.

transvestite A person who has the desire to dress in the clothes of and be accepted as a member of the opposite sex.

trapeze A triangular device suspended above the bed to assist with movement and transfers.

triglycerides The most abundant lipids in food. Although the intake of a limited amount of triglycerides is important, an excess can be unhealthy.

troponin I and troponin T Proteins found exclusively in cardiac muscle and released during myocardial damage.

trough The lowest serum level of the medication.

tubal ligation Female sterilization; the ligation of the fallopian tubes; the tubes are tied off or severed.

tunnel A narrow passageway extending outward from the edge of the wound.

turgor Tension due to fluid content.

ultrasound A procedure that provides visualization of soft tissue organs by recording and measuring the reflection of ultrasonic waves.

undermining An area of tissue loss present under intact skin, usually along the edges of the wound, forming a "lip" around the wound.

unintentional injuries Unplanned incidents causing injury such as falls, motor vehicle crashes, poisonings, drownings, fire-associated injuries, suffocation by ingested objects, and firearms.

unintentional poisoning Unplanned ingestion, inhalation, injection, or absorption through the skin of any substance harmful to the body.

unintentional torts Omissions or acts by individuals that cause unintended harm.

unstageable pressure ulcer A full-thickness wound in which the amount of necrotic or slough tissue in the wound bed makes it impossible to assess the depth of the wound or the involvement of underlying structures.

urea Waste products in the blood that are removed by the urinary system.
urge incontinence A sudden strong urge to void, followed by rapid bladder contraction.
urge/urgency Innervation of the bladder that signals a person when it is time to urinate and empty the bladder.
urgent surgery Surgery that needs to be performed within the next 24 hours.
urinary diversion A surgical procedure performed when bladder function is impaired due to trauma or disease involving the bladder, distal ureters, and, rarely, urethra.
urinary incontinence Inability to control the passage of urine.
urinary retention Inability of the bladder to empty.
urinary tract infection The result of bacteria in the urine. Infection occurs when bacteria, usually *Escherichia coli,* from the digestive tract invade the urethra and multiply.
urobilinogen Substance produced by the breakdown of bilirubin in the intestines.
utilitarianism An ethical theory in which behaviors are determined to be either right or wrong based on how they benefit the greater good.

vaginismus Contraction of the vaginal muscles to the degree that the penis cannot be inserted.
validation The process of gathering information to determine whether the information or data collected are factual and true.
validity The strength or the degree to which a concept, conclusion, or measurement is justifiable and corresponds accurately to the real world.
Valsalva maneuver Bearing down while holding the breath; usually done while defecating.
values clarification A process used to help individuals reflect on, clarify, and prioritize personal values to increase self-awareness or to make decisions.
values conflict When a person's values are inconsistent with his or her behaviors or when the person's values are not consistent with the choices that are available.
values system A set of somewhat consistent values and measures that are organized hierarchically into a belief system on the basis of a continuum of relative importance.
values Enduring ideas about what a person considers is good, best, and the right thing to do—and the bad, worst, and wrong thing to do—and about what is desirable or has worth in life.
variable A concept with different values that can be measured, manipulated, or controlled in the study.
vasectomy Male sterilization; the severing of the vas deferens, which carry sperm out of the testes.
vasoconstriction Narrowing of blood vessels throughout the body that increases arterial blood pressure.
vectors Insects or animals that carry pathogens from one host to another.
venipuncture Insertion of a needle directly into a vein.
veracity Truthfulness.
verbal communication may be spoken, written, or electronic.
vertigo Disequilibrium, spinning sensation.
vibration External manipulation of the thorax by gently shaking a flat hand against the chest; used during postural drainage therapy.
virus The smallest microorganisms; they reproduce inside living cells and are responsible for causing many different types of disease.
visceral pain Pain that arises from the organs of the body and occurs in such conditions as appendicitis, pancreatitis, inflammatory bowel disease, bladder distention, and cancer.
vital signs (VS) A basic but very important component of the physiologic assessment of a patient; used to monitor the functioning of body systems. VS consist of body temperature (T), pulse (P), respirations (R), blood pressure (BP), and pain assessment.
vitamins Organic compounds that contribute to important metabolic and physiologic functions within the body.
vitiligo A loss of skin pigment.
vulnerable populations Those at high risk for a disease or problem.

water-soluble vitamins Vitamins that dissolve in the body and are excreted in the urine. They are easily destroyed by air, light, and cooking. Water-soluble vitamins must be ingested daily through dietary sources or supplements because they are not stored in the body. Examples are C and B complex vitamins.
wear-and-tear theory of aging A theory first introduced in 1882 by Dr. August Weismann, a German biologist, that the body wears out from hard use.
wellness The active process of self-care through being aware of and making choices toward a healthy life.
windshield survey An initial needs assessment that involves collecting data through observation of the community's geography, population, environment, industry, education, recreation, communication, transportation, and public services.
wound Disruptions in the skin's integrity that lead to a loss of the skin's normal functioning.

zygote A fertilized ovum; begins as a single cell.

GLOSSARY

urge incontinence [illegible]

urinary retention [illegible]

validation [illegible]

values [illegible]

values clarification [illegible] When a person's values are in conflict with those [illegible] the person [illegible] the [illegible]

value system [illegible] that a person [illegible]

values [illegible]

variable A factor that can [illegible]

vasoconstriction Narrowing of blood vessels [illegible] blood pressure.

venipuncture [illegible]

verbal communication [illegible]

vertigo [illegible]

vibration [illegible]

virus [illegible]

vitamin [illegible]

vulnerable populations [illegible]

water-soluble vitamins [illegible]

wellness [illegible]

wound [illegible]

INDEX

A

Page numbers followed by "f" indicate figures, "t" indicate tables, and "b" indicate boxes.

B

H

J

X

Y

Z